Laboratory medicine
HEMATOLOGY

Laboratory medicine
HEMATOLOGY

JOHN B. MIALE, M.D.

Professor Emeritus of Pathology,
University of Miami School of Medicine,
Miami, Florida

SIXTH EDITION

With **1173** illustrations and **64** color plates

The C. V. Mosby Company

ST. LOUIS • TORONTO • LONDON   1982

A TRADITION OF PUBLISHING EXCELLENCE

Editor: Don E. Ladig
Manuscript editor: Karen Edwards
Design: Susan Trail
Production: Debbie Wedemeier

SIXTH EDITION

The C.V. Mosby Company
11830 Westline Industrial Drive, St. Louis, Missouri 63141

Library of Congress Cataloging in Publication Data

Miale, John B.
  Laboratory medicine.

  Bibliography: p.
  Includes index.
  1. Hematology. 2. Blood—Diseases. I. Title.
[DNLM: 1. Hematologic diseases. WH 100 M618L]
RB145.M47 1982   616.1′5   81-14153
ISBN 0-8016-3422-9   AACR2

TS/VH/VH 9 8 7 6 5 4   02/A/223

To my wife
Emily

Preface

Every author appreciates that the preface to a book is in fact an epilogue. Yet there are great differences between the two. If it were feasible, or even advisable, to write a preface before undertaking the writing or the revision, it would be done with the optimism and enthusiasm that accompany the undertaking of a new project. An epilogue, on the other hand, is after the fact, and although a certain degree of optimism persists that the work will be well received, much of the enthusiasm has been consumed during the many preceding months. Thus this new edition is presented with the hope only that it will be received at least as well as the previous one.

The deletion of old material and the addition of new information have been unavoidably arbitrary. The volume of new literature since the previous edition is not only larger than ever, but also reveals greater sophistication in the study of hematologic disorders. The pertinence of research data to clinical application is not always obvious; I hope to be forgiven if I have omitted studies that later will prove to be clinically significant. Nevertheless, almost every chapter contains revisions, with some minor and some major updating and rewriting. As in previous editions, the emphasis is on the pathogenesis of hematologic abnormalities as they relate to the clinical picture and laboratory diagnosis.

Once again I want to acknowledge my gratitude for the editorial assistance of my associate, Jessie W. Kent. Her meticulous attention to detail in the text, tables, figures, and references has been invaluable. My secretary, Rita Sliauzis, has responded nobly to the challenge of deciphering my handwriting and is due special thanks.

John B. Miale

And ever, as the story drained
   The wells of fancy dry,
And faintly strove that weary one
   To put the subject by,
"The rest next time—" "It is the next time!"
   The happy voices cry.

Thus grew the tale of Wonderland
   Thus slowly, one by one,
Its quaint events were hammered out—
   And now the tale is done,
And home we steer, a merry crew,
   Beneath the setting sun.

Lewis Carroll
Alice's Adventures In Wonderland

Contents

1   The reticuloendothelial system. I. Hemopoiesis, 1

2   The reticuloendothelial system. II. Phagocytosis, pinocytosis, lysosomal storage diseases, and the spleen, 35

3   The reticuloendothelial system. III. Lymphocytes and the immunocyte complex, 73

4   Morphology of blood and bone marrow cells, 116

5   The bone marrow, 211

6   The blood, 350

7   Application of statistics and quality assurance in hematology, 367

8   Oxygen transport and delivery: iron-deficiency anemia, 388

9   Folic acid, vitamin B_{12}, and macrocytic anemia, 416

10   The erythrocyte: porphyrin and hemoglobin metabolism, 445

11   The erythrocyte: abnormal forms and immunology, 475

12   Transfusion of blood, blood products, and blood substitutes, 524

13   Anemia due to decreased erythrocyte survival—congenital and acquired hemolytic anemias, 550

14   Anemia due to decreased erythrocyte survival—the hemoglobinopathies, 602

15   Leukocytes: leukocytosis, leukopenia, and functional abnormalities, 658

16   Aplastic anemia, myeloproliferative disorders, leukemia, and lymphoma, 689

17   Hemostasis and blood coagulation, 772

Appendix   Methods, 859

References, 939

Laboratory medicine
HEMATOLOGY

COLOR PLATES

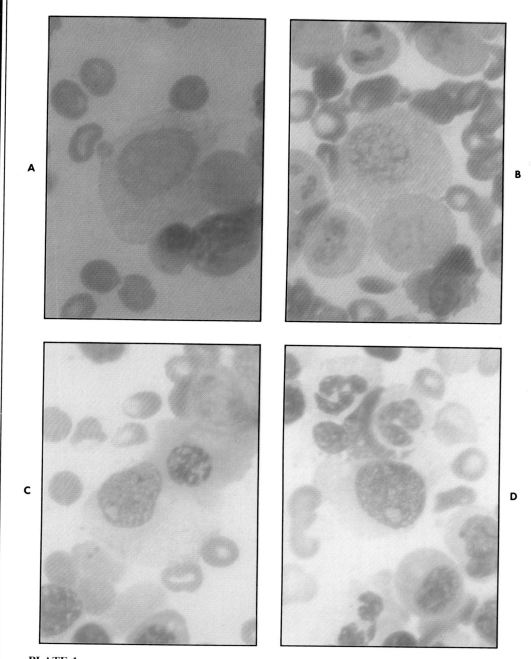

PLATE 1

The reticulum cell. Traditionally, the term "reticulum cell" is not applied to the cell in the stem cell compartment but rather to a cell that has differentiated into a phagocyte. The cytoplasm is abundant and often contains iron pigments and cellular debris. The nucleus is characteristically large and vesicular and contains a large blue nucleolus. As defined here, this cell is found in small numbers in normal bone marrow. It may be encountered more frequently in proliferating bone marrow. The cells of some very primitive types of leukemia have many of the features of the reticulum cell.

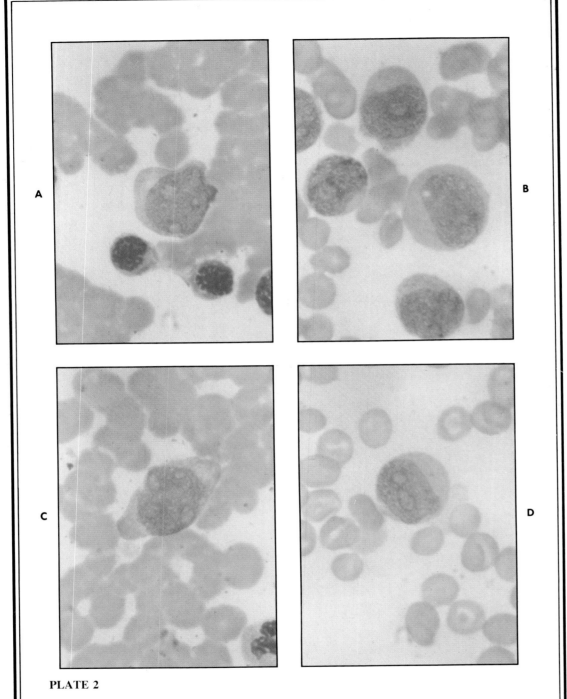

PLATE 2

The myeloblast. The cell is usually about 3 times the diameter of a red blood cell but may be only 2 times the diameter in some acute leukemias of the micromyeloblastic type. The high nucleus/ cytoplasm ratio, the leptochromatic and delicately structured nucleus, and the nucleoli indicate the blast nature of these cells. As shown, the nucleoli may be multiple or single and are usually more numerous than in the lymphoblast, but this is not a reliable differential feature.

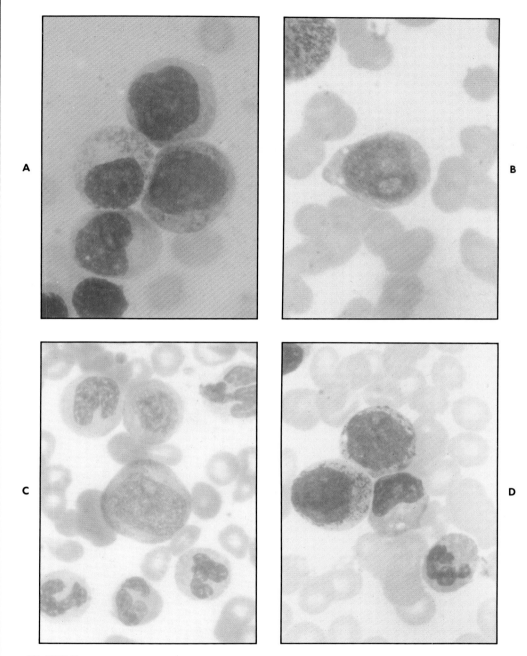

PLATE 3

The progranulocyte. **A,** The two cells on the right have immature nuclei with faintly visible nucleoli and a few cytoplasmic granules, the cell on the left above is a late myelocyte, the cell below a metamyelocyte. **B,** An early progranulocyte with an unusually large nucleolus. **C,** A classic progranulocyte, with four band neutrophils and one metamyelocyte in the field. **D,** Progranulocyte (top cell) with heavy, nonspecific granulation and an immature nucleus. There is not enough nuclear maturation to classify this cell as a myelocyte. The cell on the left is an early myelocyte.

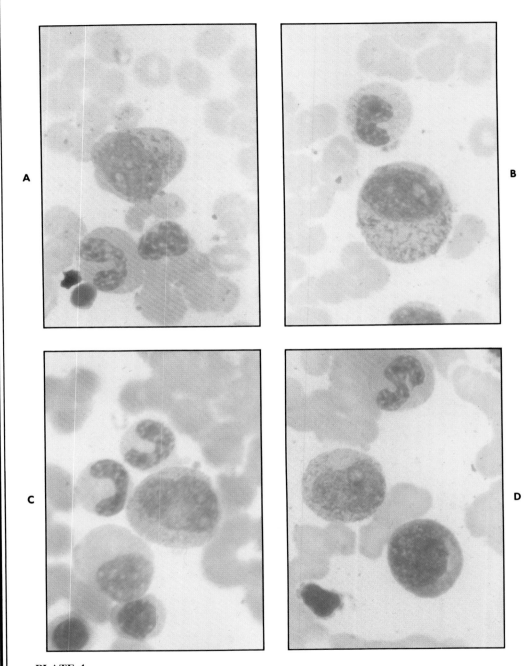

PLATE 4

The myelocyte. **A,** Shows a still immature nucleus with several nucleoli and prominent, nonspecific, coarse granulation of the cytoplasm (center). The typical myelocyte seldom shows more than one nucleolus, and this is usually obscured by overlying granules. Two band neutrophils are also shown: **B,** a myelocyte somewhat older than **A,** as judged by the nucleus/cytoplasm ratio and **C,** an atypical myelocyte in chronic myelocytic leukemia. The nucleus is immature and contains two nucleoli, but the granulation in the cytoplasm is not as coarse as in the typical cells shown in **A** and **B.** Also shown in **C** are two band neutrophils (above and left), a poorly granulated neutrophil metamyelocyte (below and left), and two orthochromic normoblasts; **D** shows a myelocyte similar to **C** (center), a basophilic normoblast (lower right), and a band neutrophil (above).

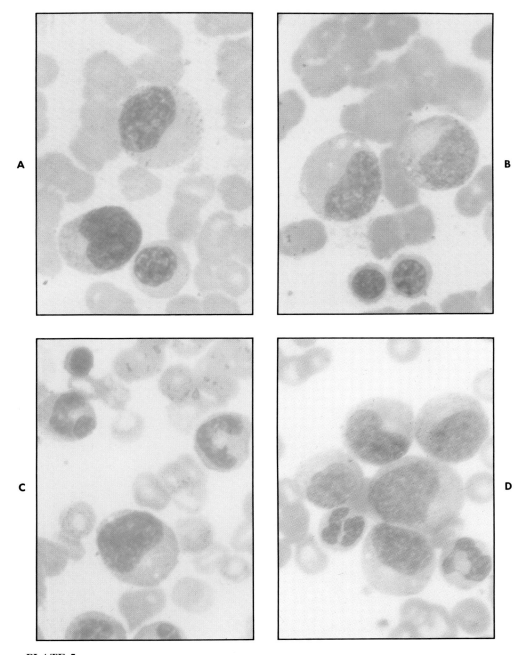

PLATE 5

The metamyelocyte. **A,** The cell at top center is a neutrophilic metamyelocyte that has remnants of nonspecific granules. Note the myeloid spot. The cell at 7 o'clock is a more mature metamyelocyte. The cell at 6 o'clock is an atypical, unusually small metamyelocyte. **B,** Two metamyelocytes, the one on the right less mature than the one on the left, both with toxic vacuoles. The two small cells are normoblasts. **C,** A normal mature neutrophilic metamyelocyte and two stab neutrophils. **D,** Five neutrophilic metamyelocytes and two segmented neutrophils.

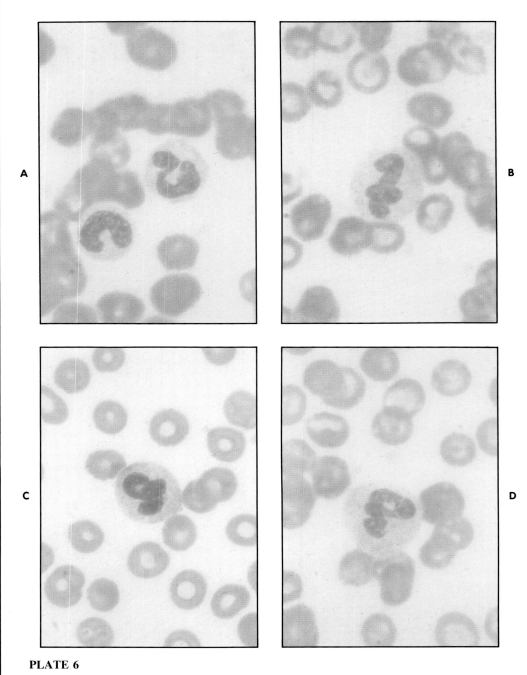

PLATE 6

The band neutrophil. **A,** The cell below is a young band form, more mature than the metamyelocyte but with a thick nucleus; the cell above is older, with beginning constriction of the nucleus. **B-D,** Bands in which the nucleus is folded on itself. Note that a filament is not seen in any of these cells.

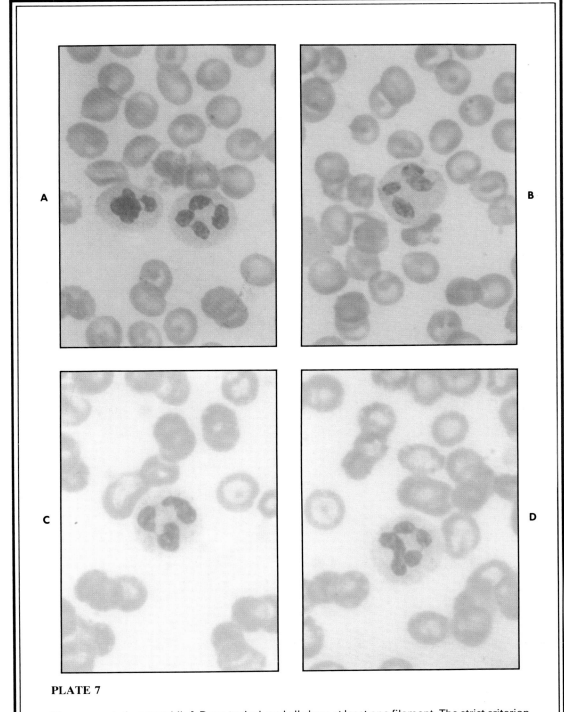

PLATE 7

The segmented neutrophil. **A-D** are typical, and all show at least one filament. The strict criterion for a filament is that it represents a bilayer of nuclear membrane with no chromatin in between. The cell to the left in **A** shows a little thicker filament than this but still acceptable.

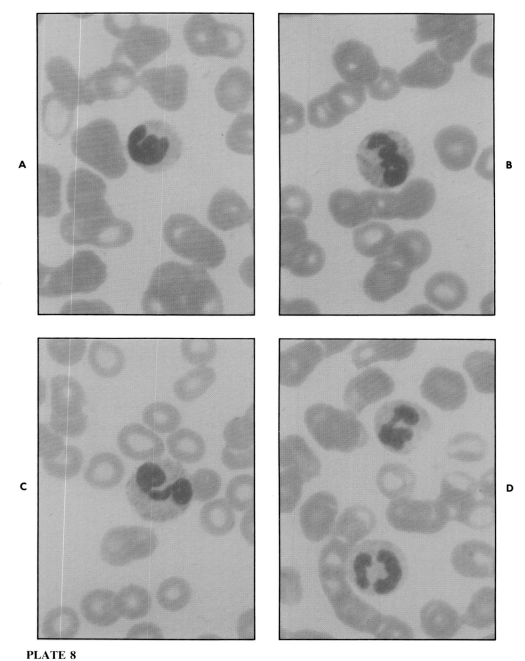

PLATE 8

Segmented and band neutrophils. The morphology of an old controversy or, what is a segmented cell? A segmented cell is one in which a *filament* connects two or more lobes. The filament must be visible, not assumed to be there but lying under a lobe. **A,** A band neutrophil that would be called, erroneously, a segmented cell by the criterion ''when in doubt call it a segmented cell.'' **B,** Also a band neutrophil. **C,** A band neutrophil because the constriction is too thick to qualify as a filament. In **D** the cell on the top is a band neutrophil, the one on the bottom a segmented neutrophil. Sometimes the filament connecting two lobes of a segmented cell is broken, or at least not visible, and this cell is of course a segmented cell and not a band.

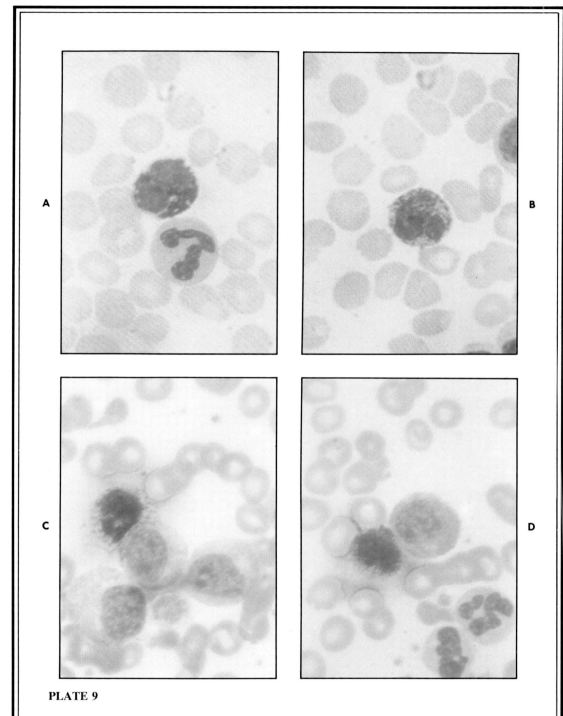

PLATE 9

The basophil and eosinophil leukocytes. **A,** A typical basophil (above) and a band neutrophil. **B,** A typical basophil. **C,** A basophil (above) and three neutrophilic metamyelocytes. **D,** A basophil (left center), an eosinophil (right center), a segmented neutrophil (4 o'clock), and a band neutrophil (5 o'clock). The typical basophil in normal blood, **A** and **B,** is characterized by an abundance of blue-black granules that vary in size and usually obscure the nucleus. Basophils in chronic myelocytic leukemia or myeloproliferative syndromes often seem fragile, with loss of cellular membrane and leaching out of granule material, **C** and **D. D** shows the difference between a basophil and an eosinophil. Note that although the eosinophil granules are not a pure orange-red color, they are uniform in size and have pale centers.

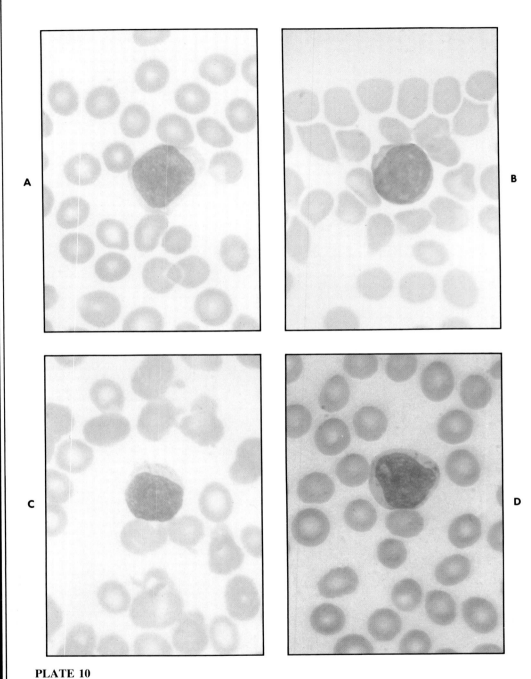

PLATE 10

The lymphoblast. Lymphoblasts are not found in normal blood, and those illustrated are from a patient with acute lymphocytic leukemia. As shown in **A,** the lymphoblast usually has fewer nucleoli and a more irregular nuclear outline, sometimes even indented, than the myeloblast. The nucleus/cytoplasm ratio is usually very high, **B.** In some cases the cytoplasm contains fine to coarse inclusions, **C** and **D,** which should not be mistaken for the granules of granulocytes. Vacuolization of the cytoplasm is common. The characteristic PAS reaction is shown in Plate 50.

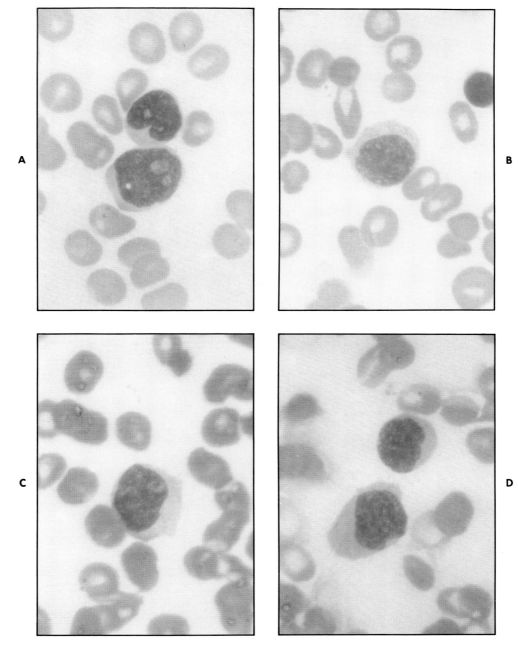

PLATE 11

The prolymphocyte. Prolymphocytes are not present in normal blood, and those illustrated are from cases of acute lymphocytic leukemia where they are found in variable number. Lying between the lymphoblast and the lymphocyte in the maturation sequence, prolymphocytes exhibit a wide variation in morphology. It is in fact simpler to define the prolymphocyte as a cell that is more mature than a lymphoblast and not as mature as the lymphocyte. **A** shows a prolymphocyte (above) and a lymphoblast (below). **B** and **C** are classified as prolymphocytes. **D** shows a prolymphocyte (above) and a monocyte (below). In general the prolymphocyte has a coarser nuclear pattern and more abundant cytoplasm than the lymphoblast. One nucleolus may be visible. Prolymphocytes are considerably larger than lymphocytes and the nuclear pattern is not heavily pachychromatic.

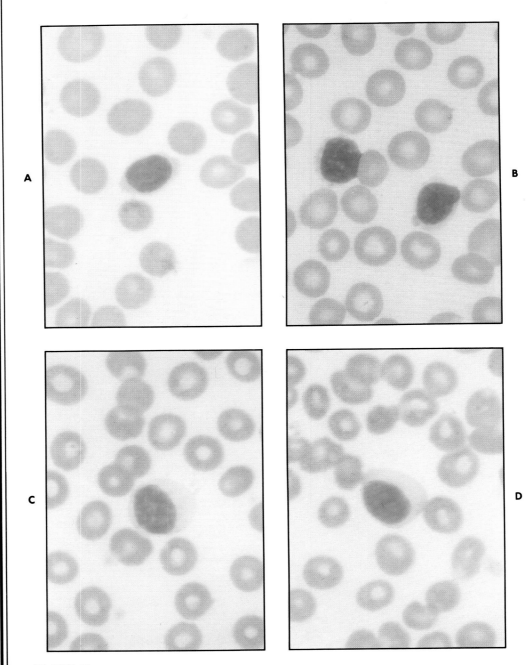

PLATE 12

The lymphocyte. The cell in **A** is the typical small lymphocyte found in normal blood. Note the dense, pachychromatic nucleus and the smudged chromatin-parachromatin junction. The cytoplasm is clear, but normal lymphocytes may have small cytoplasmic granules. These are, however, peroxidase negative. The cells in **B** are also from normal blood, and the slight fraying of the cellular membrane should not be mistaken for that of "hairy cell" leukemia (Plate 55). The cells in **C** and **D** are large lymphocytes, but, although more common in infants, have no significance.

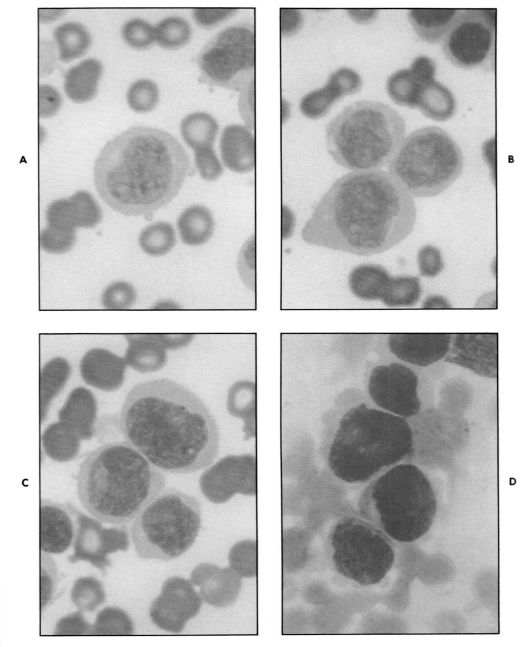

PLATE 13

The monoblast. The monoblast is not found in normal blood and although there may be a rare monoblast in normal bone marrow it is not possible to identify it with certainty. The cells illustrated here are from a patient with acute monocytic (histiocytic) leukemia. There are no reliable morphologic criteria for distinguishing these from other blasts. Cytochemical reactions are also of little value, since the cytochemical reactions of normal monocytes (Table 4-8) may not help to identify monoblasts. Perhaps the most helpful hint, other than the presence of pro-monocytes in the same smear, is the irregularity and delicate structure of the nucleus, but even this is not diagnostic. Neither is the cytoplasmic budding seen in **D**.

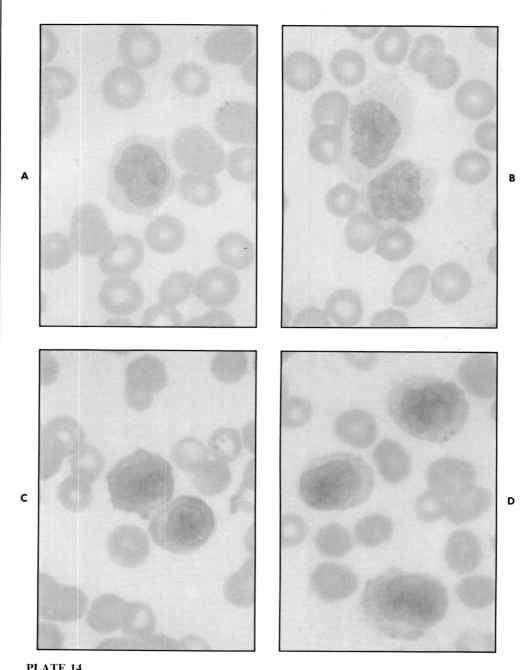

PLATE 14

The promonocyte. The cells illustrated are from a case of acute monocytic (histiocytic) leukemia. Note the typical delicate and folded "monocytoid" nucleus. The cytoplasm contains very small pink granules, and, by definition, a cell containing granules is more mature than a blast. Whether the morphology of monocytic cells in monocytic leukemia can be used to define the morphology of the normal series remains to be established.

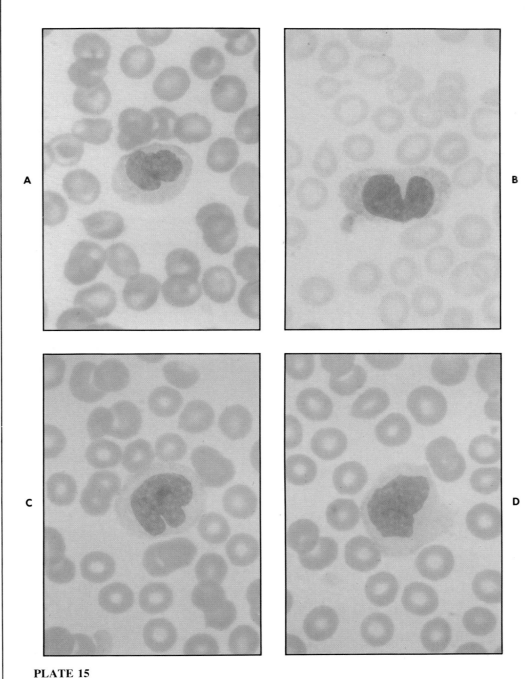

PLATE 15

The monocyte. All these cells are from normal blood and are considered typical. Note the monocytoid nucleus and the very fine, dust-like, pink, cytoplasmic granules. These characteristics can be obscured by overstaining or if the stain is not good. The most common error is to call a poorly stained monocyte a neutrophilic metamyelocyte.

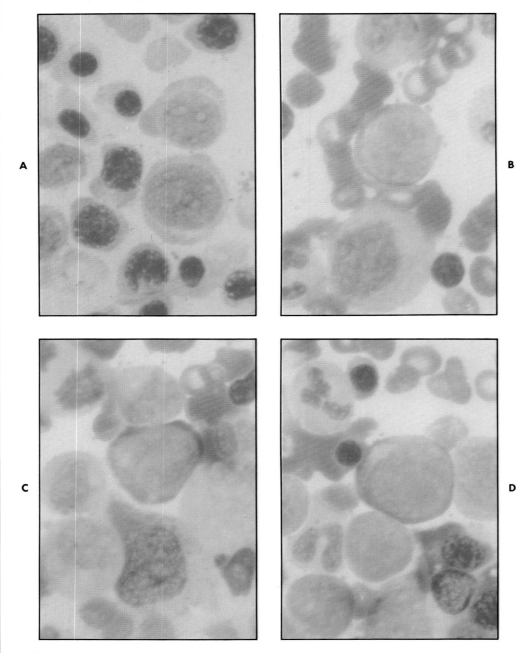

PLATE 16

The pronormoblast. The pronormoblast is sometimes difficult to distinguish from other blasts, but characteristically the nucleus tends to be round rather than oval and the cytoplasm more abundant than in the myeloblast. Some of its features, especially the blue nucleoli, which are sometimes very prominent, **A,** are similar to what is assumed to characterize hemopoietic stem cells. When immature cells such as those illustrated here are found in a bone marrow showing severe erythroid hyperplasia, as in **A,** it is safe to assume that they are pronormoblasts. The cells in **C** and **D** are classified as pronormoblasts because, in spite of the cytoplasmic basophilia, the nucleus is still immature and very delicate in structure. **A** also shows many polychromatophilic and orthochromic normoblasts. The large cell below the pronormoblast in **C** is a phagocytic reticulum cell.

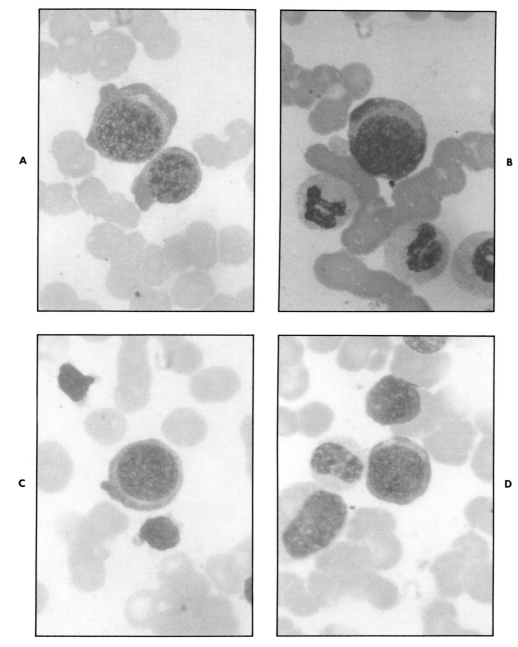

PLATE 17

The basophilic normoblast. The basophilic normoblast is distinguished from the pronormoblast by the coarser nuclear structure and the intense basophilia of the cytoplasm. The intense basophilia reflects the greater content of RNA preceding the synthesis of hemoglobin. At this stage of erythroid maturation, we see the roundness of the nucleus, which is characteristic of this and more mature erythroid cells. **A** shows two basophilic normoblasts, the one on the bottom being unusually small. The cell in **D** is the most mature.

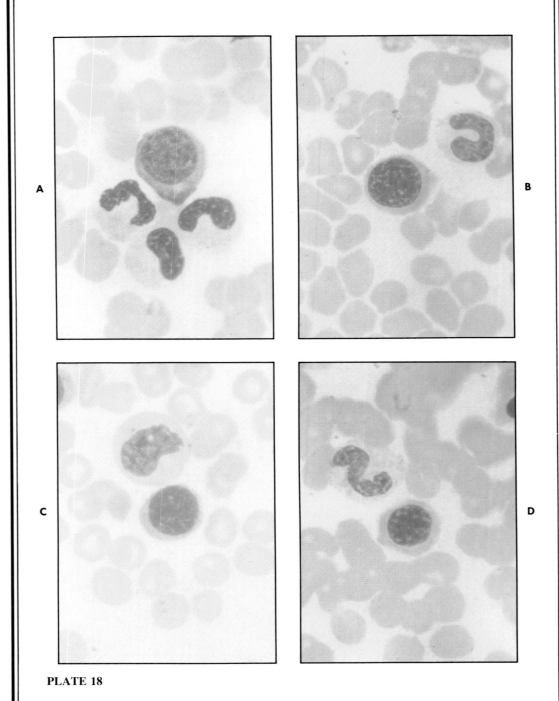

PLATE 18

The polychromatophilic normoblast. This cell is characterized by progressive nuclear maturation and by the appearance of hemoglobin in the cytoplasm. In an early cell, **A,** only a few very faint areas of orange tint are seen and much basophilia remains in the cytoplasm. **B** shows a typical polychromatophilic normoblast. In a late cell, **C** and **D,** there is more hemoglobin and less basophilia in the cytoplasm, and the nucleus is dense with a coarse structure and sharp chromatin-parachromatin distinction.

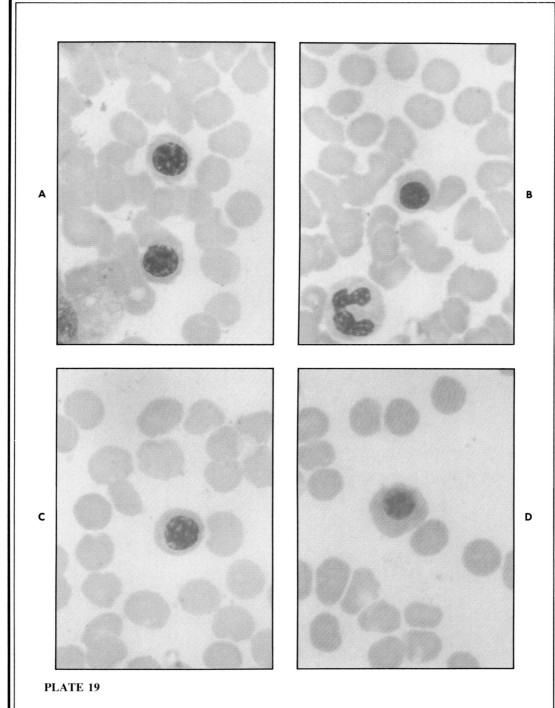

PLATE 19

The orthochromic normoblast. The nucleus is now round, dense, and small. The cytoplasm is fully hemoglobinated, and, typically, the color of the cytoplasm is orange-pink with little or no basophilia, **A** to **D**. In bone marrow smears, however, it is not uncommon to find that cells having all the other features of orthochromic normoblasts do not have a pure orthochromic cytoplasm, **D**.

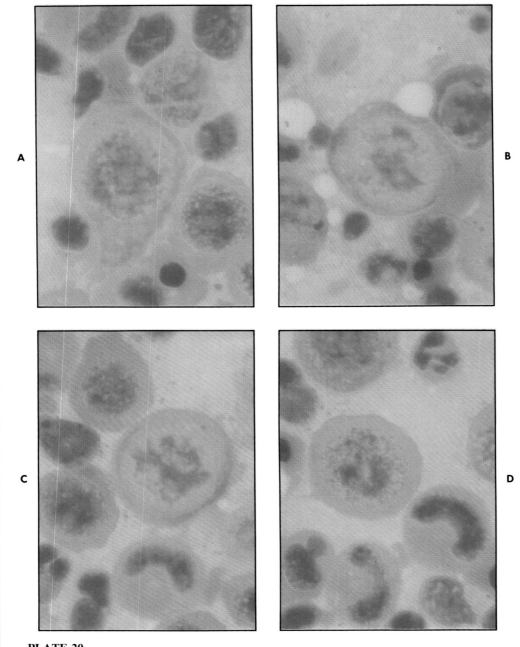

PLATE 20

The promegaloblast. Megaloblastic dyspoiesis is characterized by gigantism of the cells as well as by asynchronism of nuclear and cytoplasmic maturation. The asynchronism and nuclear atypism make it difficult to categorize the megaloblastic cells with confidence. The least mature cell, the promegaloblast, is a very large cell with many of the features of a reticulum cell. It may show the typical net-like structure of the megaloblastic nucleus, as in **D**, or present irregular condensations of chromatin and nucleolar material, **A-C**. In **A**, the cell to the right of the large promegaloblast is probably a polychromatophilic megaloblast. In **C**, note the giant stab neutrophil below the promegaloblast; two polychromatophilic megaloblasts are above and left. Two giant stabs are seen in **D**.

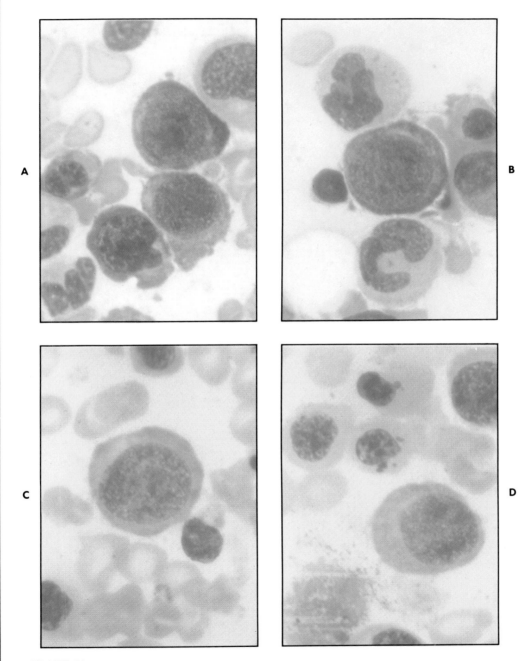

PLATE 21

The basophilic megaloblast. This cell is characterized by a nucleus that is more mature than that of the promegaloblast, with the appearance of the net-like pattern of nuclear chromatin that is characteristic of the megaloblastic series. The basophilia of the cytoplasm varies from intense, **A** and **B,** to moderate, **C** and **D,** and, because of atypical development, the basophilia tends to disappear later than in the normoblastic series. In my experience the classification of the cells of the megaloblastic series on the basis of cytoplasmic maturation is usually equivocal and I base the degree of maturation mostly on the nuclear structure. Note the two giant stab neutrophils in **B,** a very helpful sign of folate or vitamin B_{12} deficiency. **D** also shows three orthochromic megaloblasts (upper left).

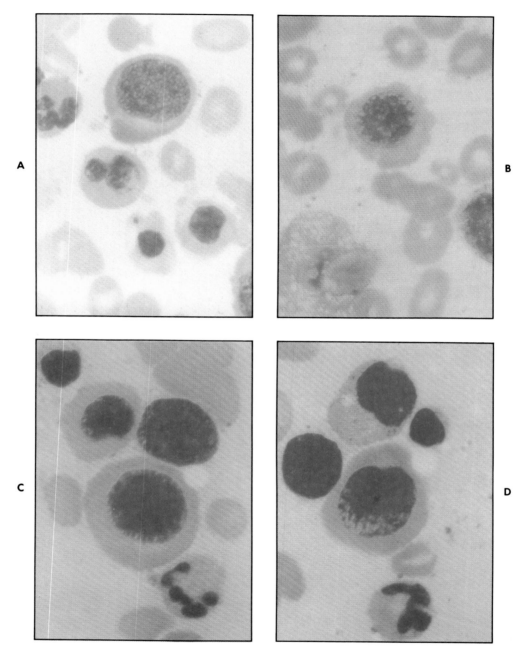

PLATE 22

The polychromatophilic megaloblast. The maturation of the megaloblastic series is characterized by occasional extreme asynchronism of nuclear and cytoplasmic maturation. The cell illustrated in **A** can be considered a typical, very early polychromatophilic megaloblast, that in **B** a more fully developed cell. The cells in **C** and **D** show atypism of the nucleus, gigantism, and well established hemoglobination of the cytoplasm. In **C** there is an orthochromic megaloblast (above) and a hypersegmented neutrophil (below). Three orthochromic normoblasts are also shown in **A**.

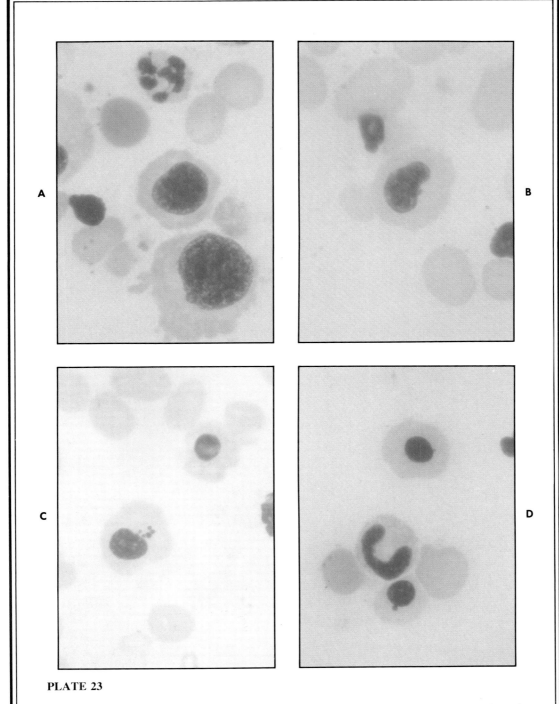

PLATE 23

The orthochromic megaloblast. In spite of a sometimes bizarre nuclear shape, orthochromic megaloblasts are easily identified by their large size and abundant cytoplasm. The cytoplasm contains hemoglobin and basophilia may persist, as in **A,** or is no longer present, **B-D.** Note the hypersegmented neutrophil in **A** and the nuclear fragments in **C.** In **A,** the cell below the orthochromic megaloblast is probably a polychromatophilic megaloblast.

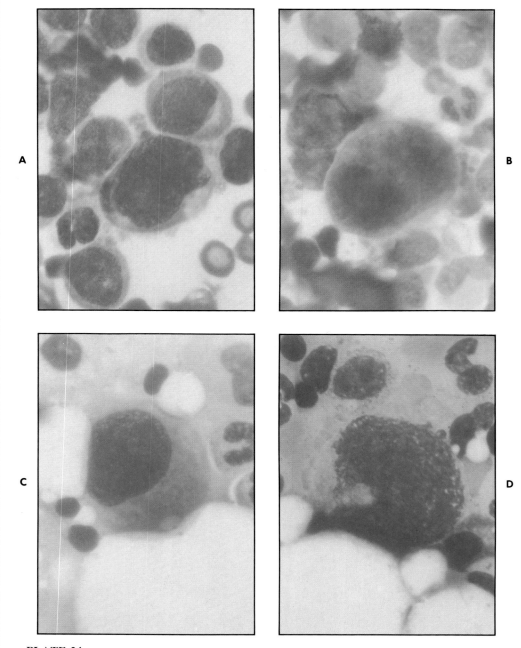

PLATE 24

The megakaryoblast. The cells illustrated are all early forms in the megakaryocytic series and the distinction between the megakaryoblast and the promegakaryocyte is based on the presence of platelet formation in the latter. This is sometimes difficult to determine with certainty. I would classify **A-C** as megakaryoblasts, while **D** might easily be considered more mature. If in doubt, PAS positivity of the cytoplasm would indicate platelet formation (Plate 26).

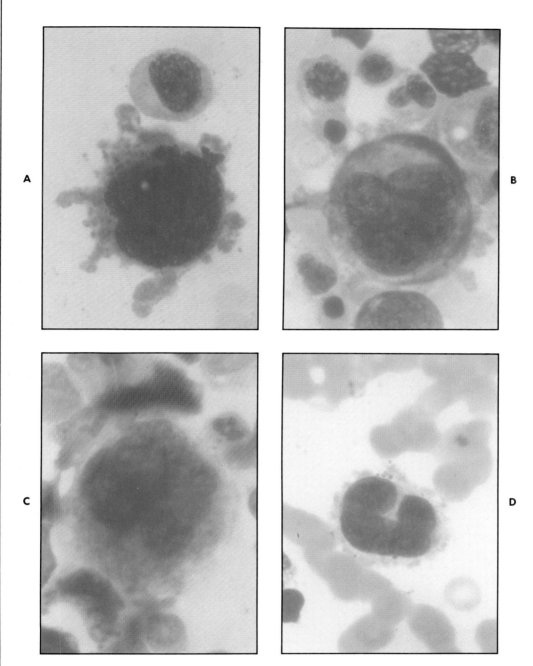

PLATE 25

The promegakaryocyte. At this stage of megakaryocytic maturation there is unmistakable plate-let formation in the cytoplasm, but the cytoplasm is still scanty. The cell illustrated in **D** is an atypical "dwarf" promegakaryocyte.

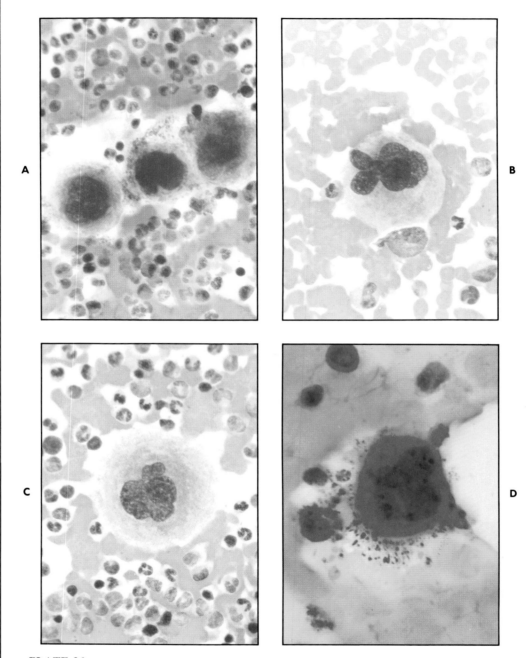

PLATE 26

The megakaryocyte. This is a very large cell and these photomicrographs are taken at a lower magnification than the others. In **A,** there is good platelet formation. The cells in **B** and **C** are from a case of idiopathic thrombocytopenic purpura; there is poor platelet formation, seen frequently in this disease but not diagnostic. **D** is a PAS stain showing the very strong PAS positivity of platelets.

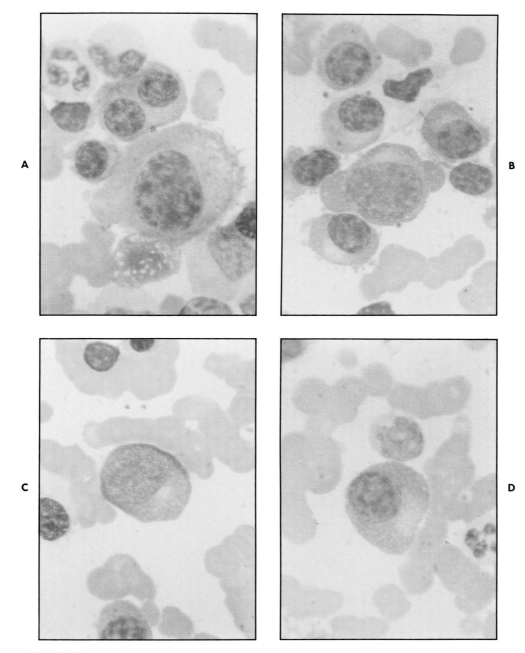

PLATE 27

The plasmablast. All examples are from multiple myelomas. There is one feature of the plasmablast, the relatively abundant cytoplasm, that helps to distinguish it from other blasts, but usually one depends on the many other cells of the series, as in myeloma, in determining that an immature cell is a plasmablast. Note the other plasma cells in **A** and **B,** and the rouleau formation in all four examples.

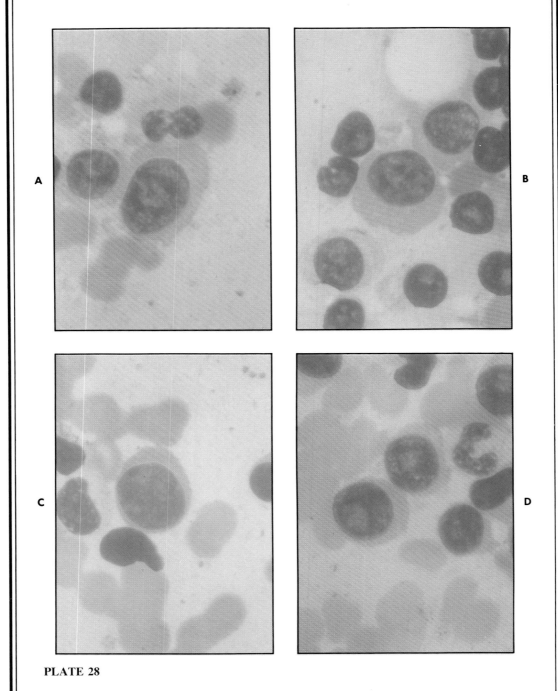

PLATE 28

The proplasmacyte. The cells illustrated are from cases of multiple myeloma. The proplasmacyte has a more mature nucleus than the plasmablast and the cytoplasm is scantier than in the normal adult plasma cell.

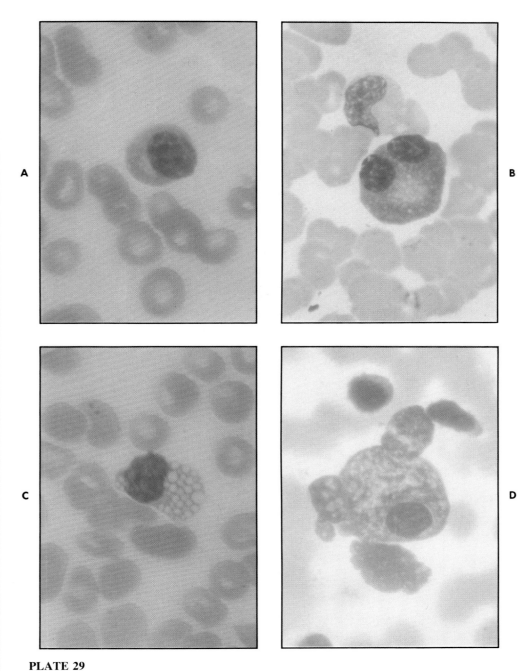

PLATE 29

The plasmacyte. Multinucleated plasma cells such as **B** are often seen in multiple myeloma but may be found in nonmyelomatous bone marrows; the one illustrated here was encountered in a normal bone marrow. The cell in **C** is of the "grape-cell" type. **D** shows a plasma cell with a "flaming" red cytoplasm in a bone marrow that was invaded by metastatic carcinoma.

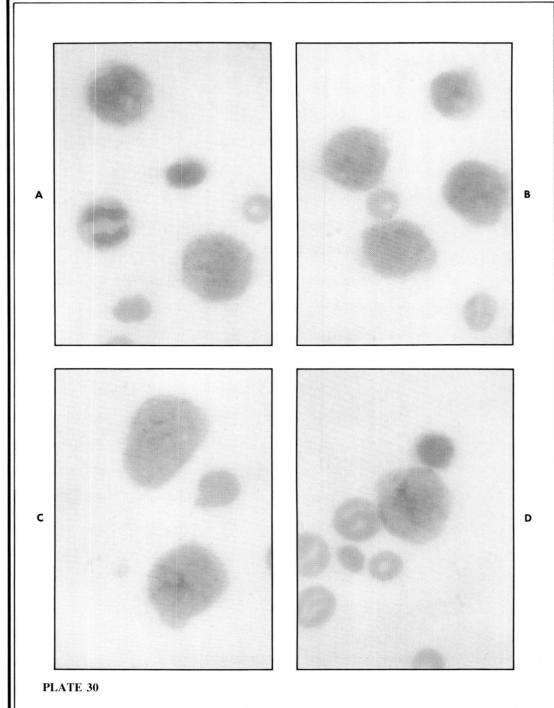

PLATE 30

Cytochemistry of blood cells: naphthol ASD chloroacetate esterase. **A-D,** Acute progranulocytic leukemia. **A** shows two progranulocytes, a segmented neutrophil, and a lymphocyte. The cells in **B** and **C** are progranulocytes. **D** shows one progranulocyte and one lymphocyte. (Smear courtesy Dr. T. Dutcher.)

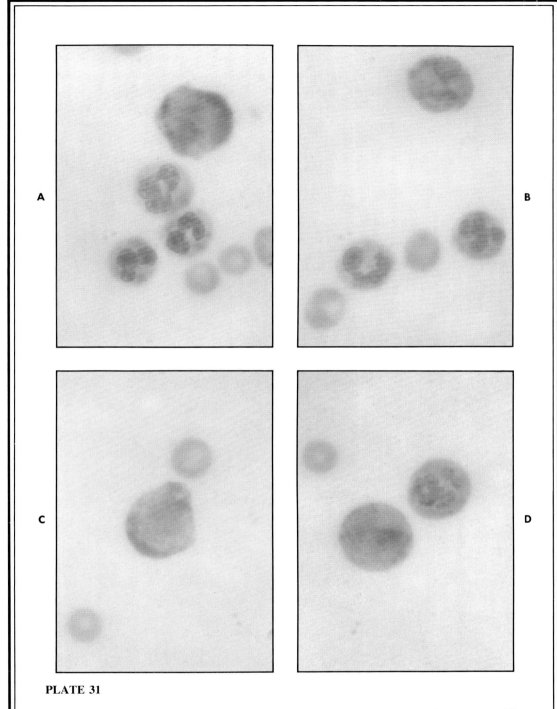

PLATE 31

Cytochemistry of blood cells: peroxidase. **A,** One segmented neutrophil, two band neutrophils, and one myelocyte. **B,** One band neutrophil, one segmented neutrophil, and one eosinophil. **C,** One progranulocyte. **D,** One segmented neutrophil and one progranulocyte. Acute progranulocytic leukemia. (Smear courtesy Dr. T. Dutcher.)

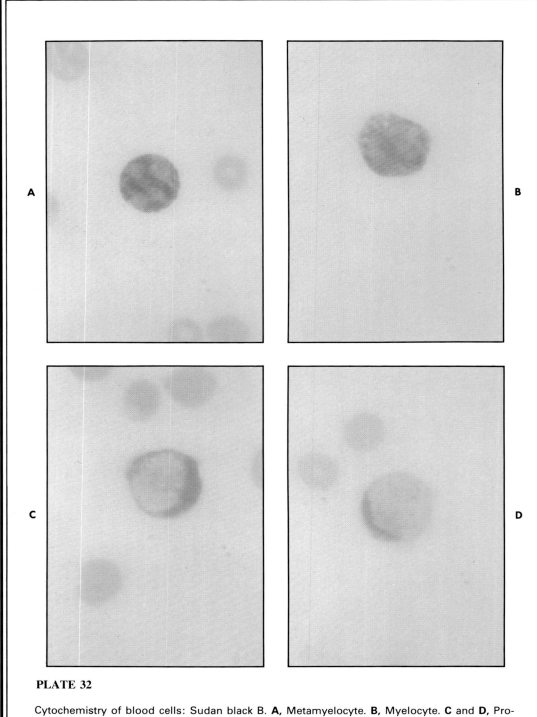

PLATE 32

Cytochemistry of blood cells: Sudan black B. **A,** Metamyelocyte. **B,** Myelocyte. **C** and **D,** Progranulocytes. Acute progranulocytic leukemia. (Smear courtesy Dr. T. Dutcher.)

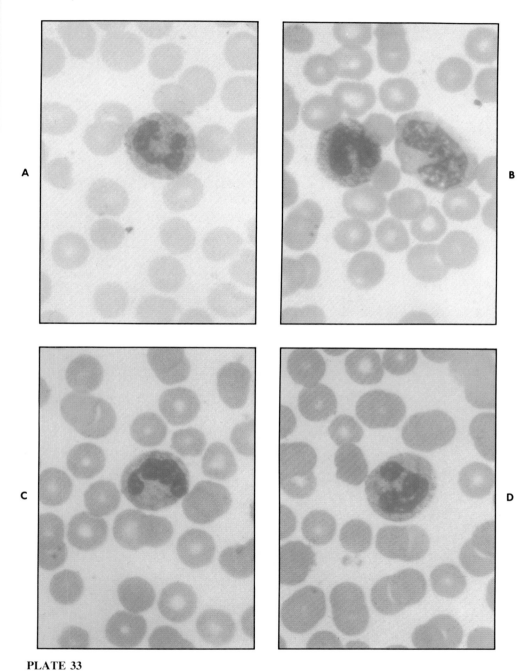

PLATE 33

Toxic granulation of neutrophils. The cytoplasm contains granules that are very prominent and slightly larger than the normal neutrophilic granules. Toxic granulation is never as intense as the abnormal granulation seen in the Alder-Reilly (Plate 34) or Chediak-Higashi (Plates 35 and 36) anomalies.

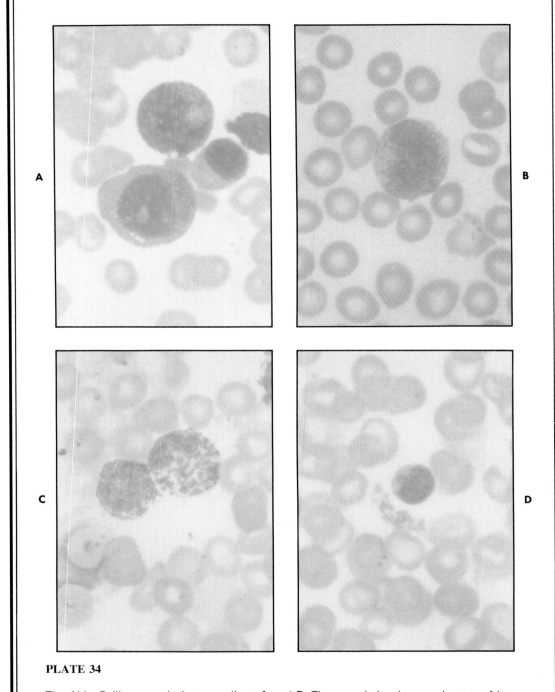

PLATE 34

The Alder-Reilly anomaly in gargoylism. **A** and **B,** The granulation in granulocytes of intermediate maturity is abundant and coarse. **C** shows a second type of anomalous granule, rod- or comma-shaped. **D** shows an inclusion in a lymphocyte (Mittwoch cell).

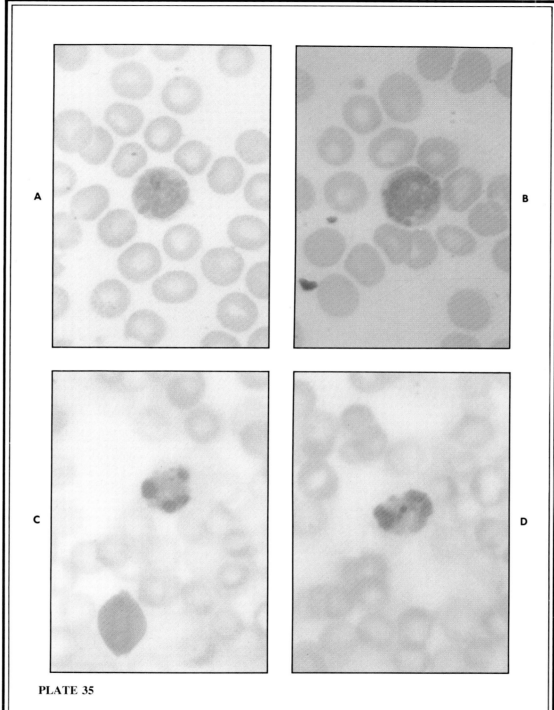

PLATE 35

The Chediak-Higashi anomaly. Peripheral blood. **A** and **B**, Wright's stain. **C** and **D**, Peroxidase stain. Note that the abnormal inclusions are strongly peroxidase positive. **C** also shows a peroxidase negative cell (below).

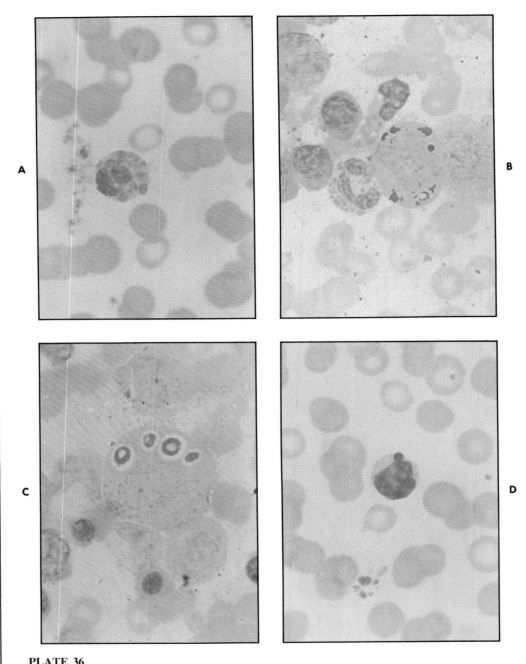

PLATE 36

The Chediak-Higashi anomaly. Bone marrow. **A,** A neutrophil with small inclusions, similar to the neutrophil abnormality usually seen in the peripheral blood (Plate 35). **B** and **C,** Extreme gigantism of the lysosomal inclusions. **D,** An inclusion in a lymphocyte, indistinguishable by itself from the lymphocytic inclusions in the Alder-Reilly anomaly (Plate 34).

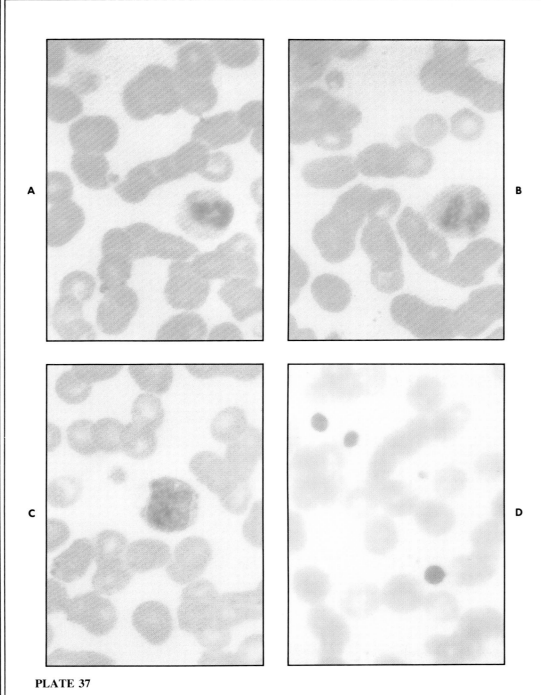

PLATE 37

The May-Hegglin anomaly. Peripheral blood. **A** and **B,** Döhle bodies in band neutrophils with sparse giant platelets. **C,** Döhle body in a metamyelocyte and giant platelet. **D,** Giant platelets.

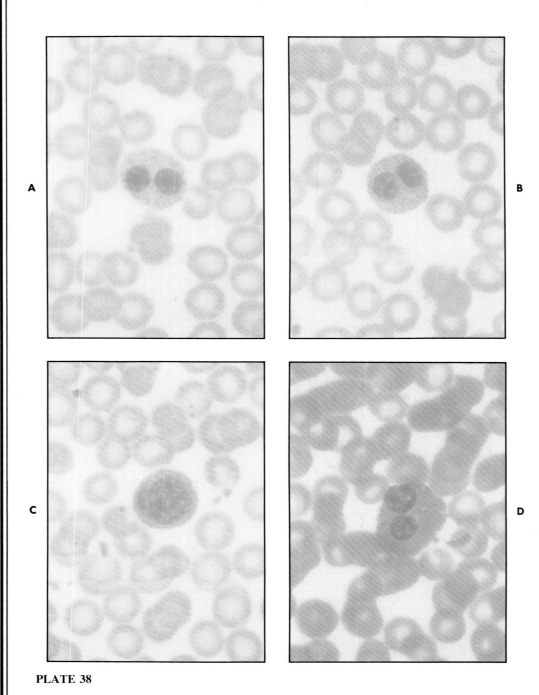

PLATE 38

Congenital Pelger-Huët anomaly. Peripheral blood. **A** and **B**, Typical bilobed pince-nez forms of adult neutrophils. **C**, A metamyelocyte with a round nucleus. **D**, A bilobed eosinophil.

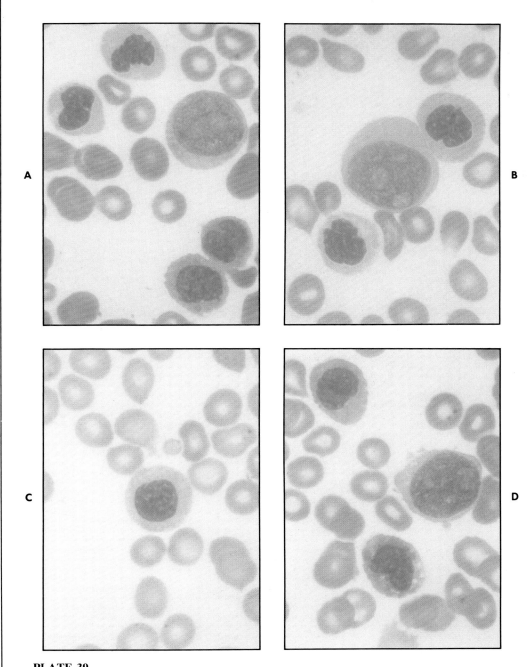

PLATE 39

Acquired Pelger-Huët anomaly. Chronic granulocytic leukemia, peripheral blood. **A,** A myeloblast, three neutrophils, and an eosinophil that show nuclear hyposegmentation. **B,** A myeloblast and two hyposegmented neutrophils. **C,** A neutrophil with a round nucleus. **D,** A myeloblast and two hyposegmented eosinophils.

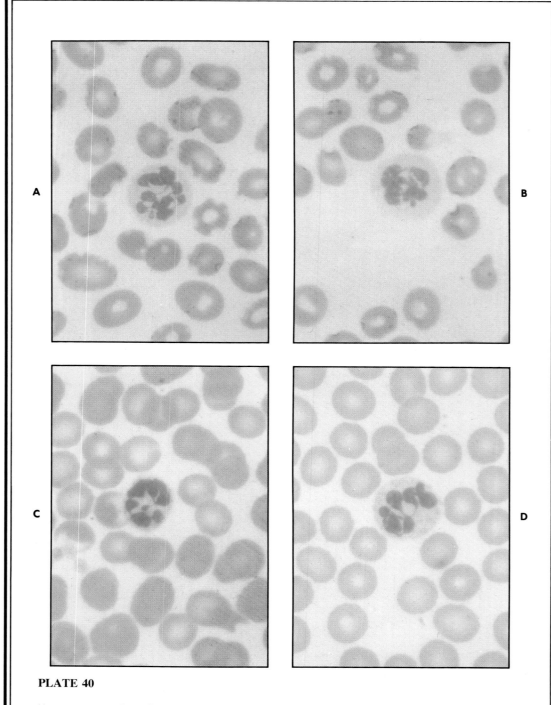

PLATE 40

Hypersegmentation of neutrophils. **A** and **B,** In pernicious anemia, peripheral blood. **C** and **D,** Familial hypersegmentation. Note that in familial hypersegmentation there is no macrocytosis or anisocytosis of the red blood cells. (Courtesy Dr. U. Undritz.)

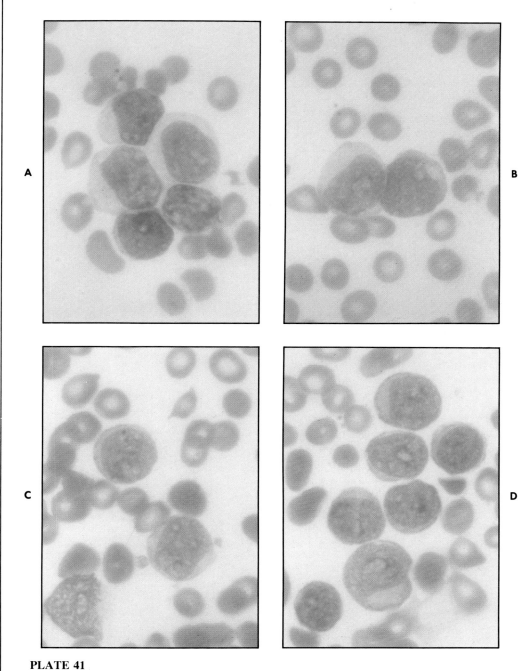

PLATE 41

Acute granulocytic leukemia. All the cells illustrated are myeloblasts. Note the variability in size and number of the nucleoli. Some irregularly contracted red blood cells give evidence of red cell fragmentation.

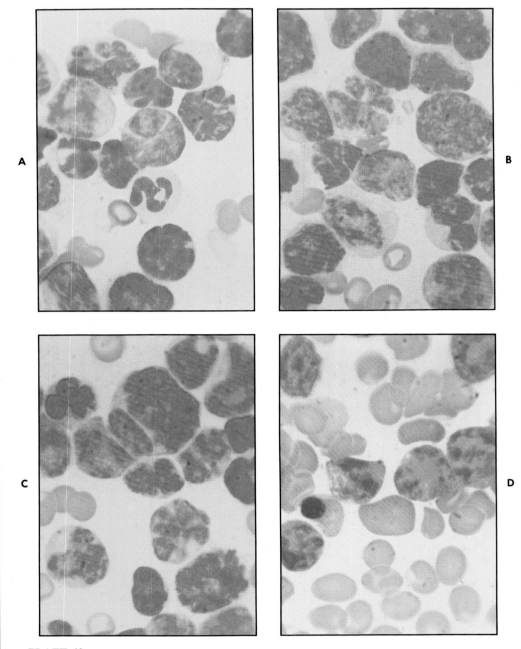

PLATE 42

The Rieder nuclear malformation. Bone marrow, acute granulocytic leukemia. The "Rieder cell" is characterized by an irregularly bizarre or cloverleaf-like malformation of leukemic blasts, usually induced when the cells are exposed to an anticoagulant.

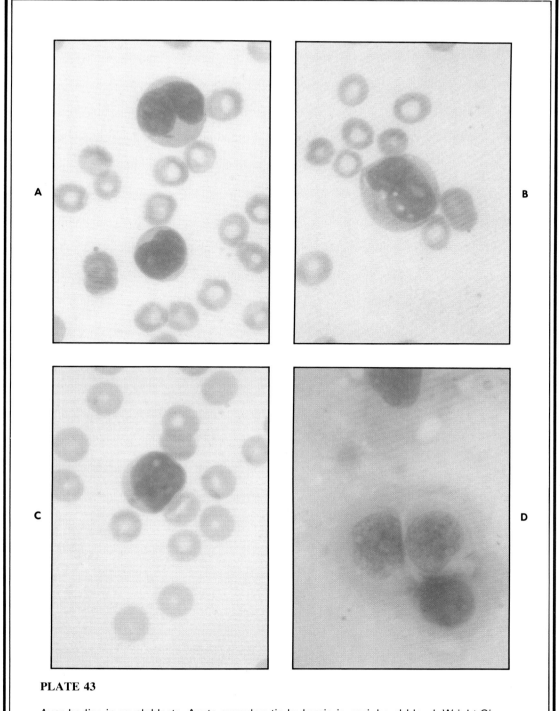

PLATE 43

Auer bodies in myeloblasts. Acute granulocytic leukemia in peripheral blood, Wright-Giemsa stain. **A-C,** Note that the shape varies from rods to ovoid forms. **D,** Auer body in myeloblasts, acute granulocytic leukemia with meningeal involvement, and touch preparation from surgically excised tumor mass causing pressure symptoms.

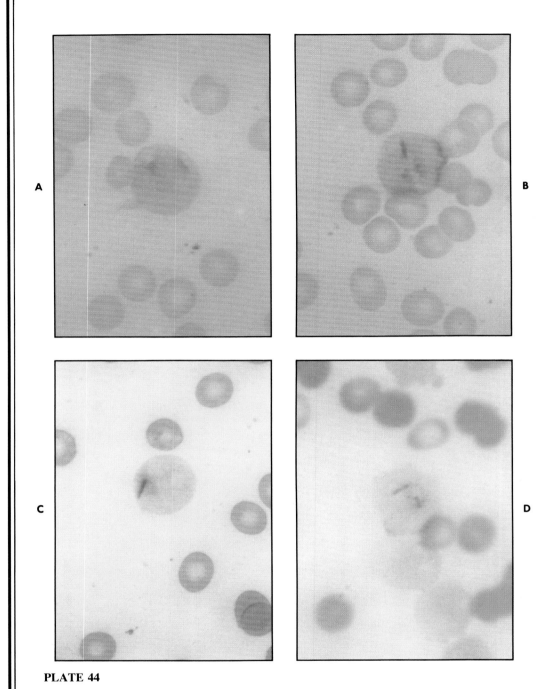

PLATE 44

Auer bodies in myeloblasts: cytochemical reactions. **A** and **B,** Peroxidase. **C,** Sudan black B. **D,** Naphthol ASD chloroacetate. (Courtesy Dr. T. Dutcher.)

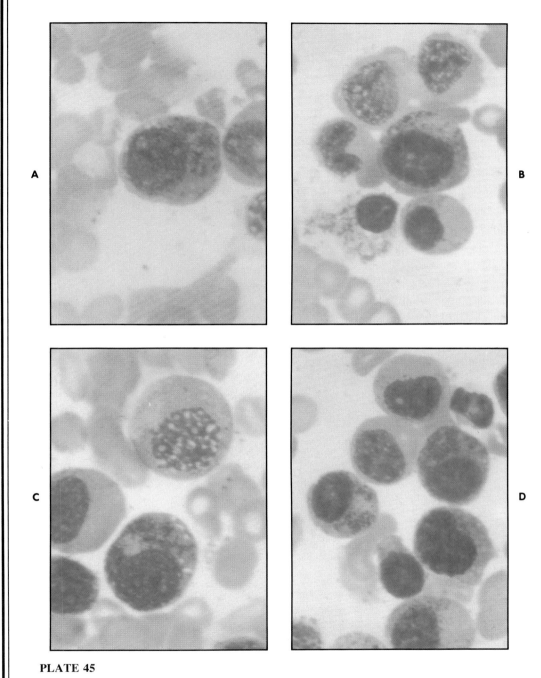

PLATE 45

Acute progranulocytic leukemia. Bone marrow. The immature granulocytes, the progranulo-cytes in **A-C,** and the myelocytes in **D** contain large, coarse, sometimes rod-shaped granules that make this a characteristic morphologic variant.

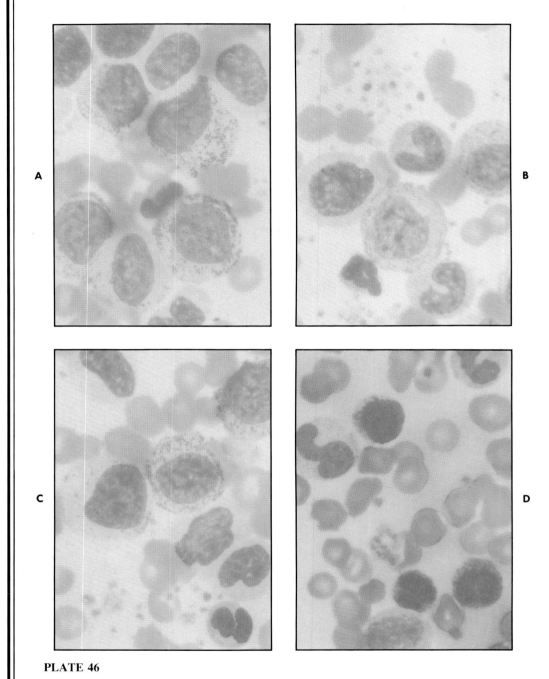

PLATE 46

Chronic granulocytic leukemia. Peripheral blood. The cell population is entirely granulocytic, and progranulocytes and myelocytes are predominant. Note the striking increase in platelets in **B** and **C**. **D,** Three basophils, another characteristic finding in chronic myelocytic leukemia.

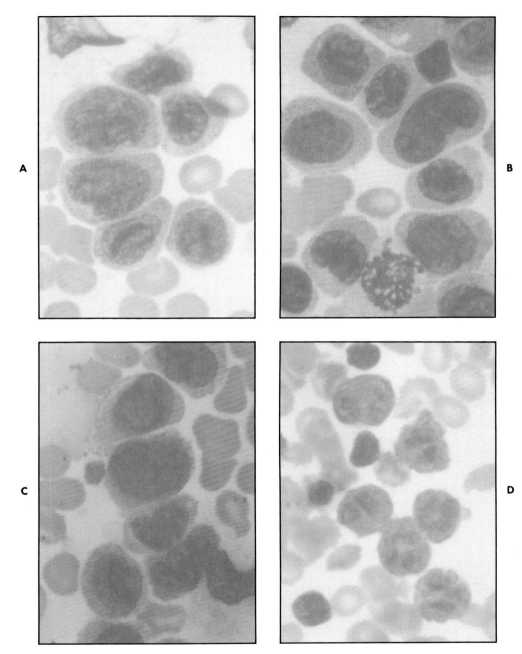

PLATE 47

Acute myelomonocytic leukemia. Peripheral blood. The cells in **A** show a delicate monocytoid nucleus and only faint granulation of the cytoplasm, but in **B** and **C** the granulocytic nature of the cytoplasm is more conspicuous. Represented is a mixture of myelomonoblasts and more mature cells (progranulocytes, myelomonocytic). **D** is a buffy coat preparation, from a different case, prepared from citrated blood, showing the Rieder cell malformation in acute myelomonocytic leukemia.

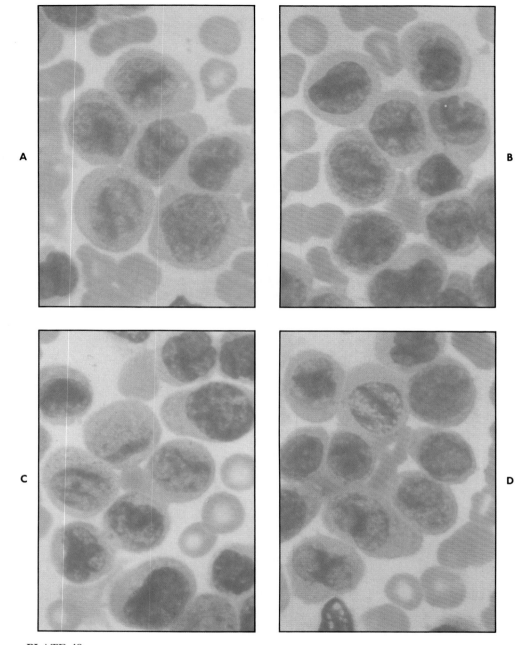

PLATE 48

Acute myelomonocytic leukemia. The combination of monocytoid nucleus with some of the cells having cytoplasmic granules of the myeloid type. This patient had a very short survival with clinically acute leukemia. The atypicality of this cell type makes it difficult to classify the cells into traditional categories.

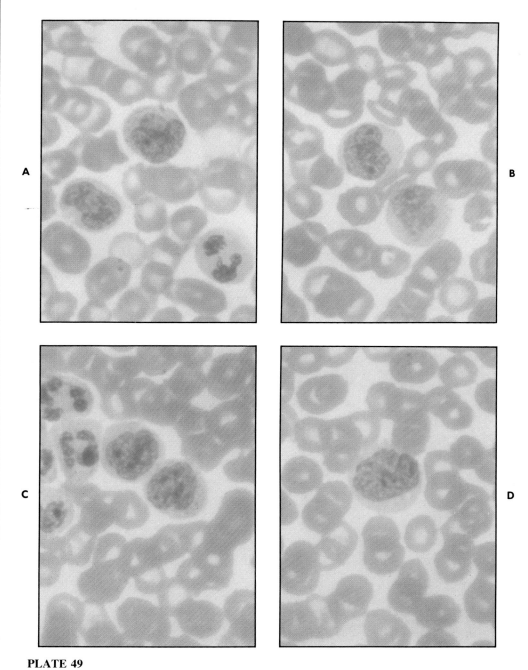

PLATE 49

Chronic myelomonocytic leukemia. The cells are more mature than those seen in the clinically acute cases; this patient's clinical course was not acute. Although the nucleus is typically mono-cytoid, the cytoplasmic granules are not prominent in this example.

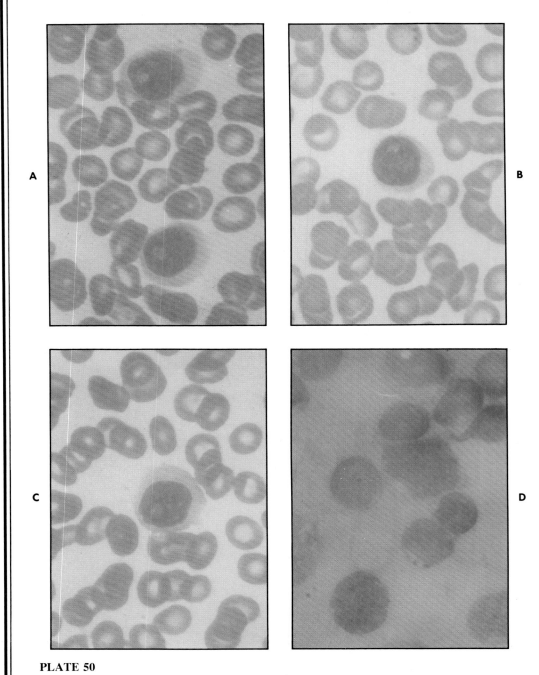

PLATE 50

Acute lymphocytic leukemia. **A-C** show lymphoblasts, Wright-Giemsa stain. **D** is a PAS stain showing the PAS-positive cytoplasmic inclusions.

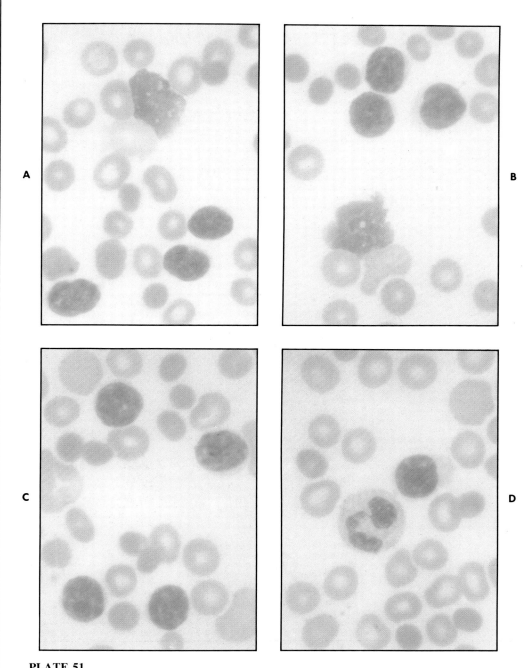

PLATE 51

Chronic lymphocytic leukemia. Peripheral blood. The cells illustrated are all small lymphocytes, not unusual in morphology except for the indentation and folding of the nucleus in **A** and **B**. Microspherocytosis is striking, a feature of the autoimmune hemolytic anemia that sometimes complicates an otherwise rather benign course. Degenerated lymphocytes (smudge forms) are usually more numerous than in this example. **D** shows a segmented neutrophil below the lymphocyte.

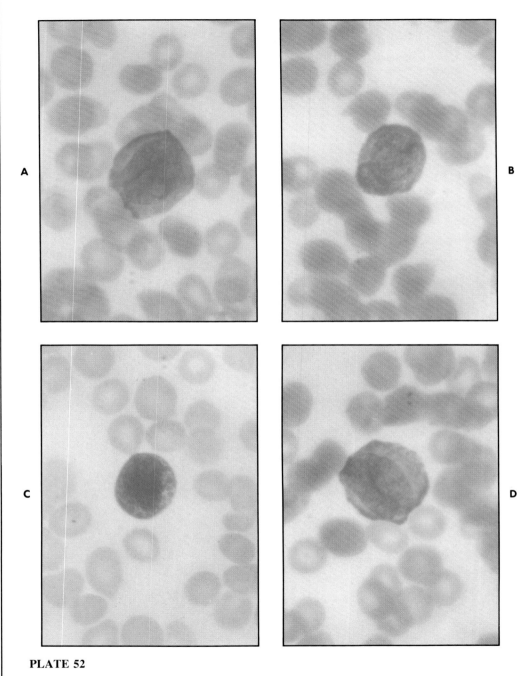

PLATE 52

Mast cell leukemia. Peripheral blood smear. The cells are bizarre, and the nucleus is obscured by blue-black granules. Toluidine blue positivity is characteristic of these granules. (Courtesy Dr. J. W. Rebuck.)

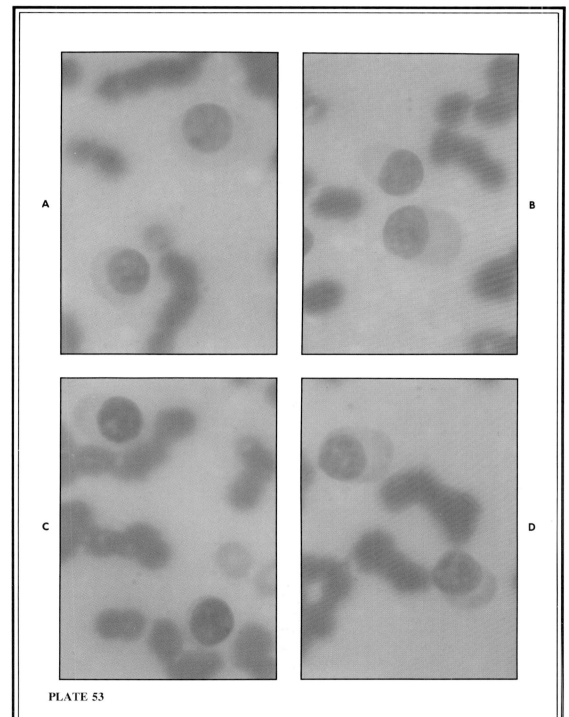

PLATE 53

Plasma cell leukemia. Peripheral blood from a patient with multiple myeloma, leukemic phase. The leukocyte count was 76,000/mm³ (76 × 10⁹/l) with 84% plasma cells as shown. Note the rouleau formation of the red cells.

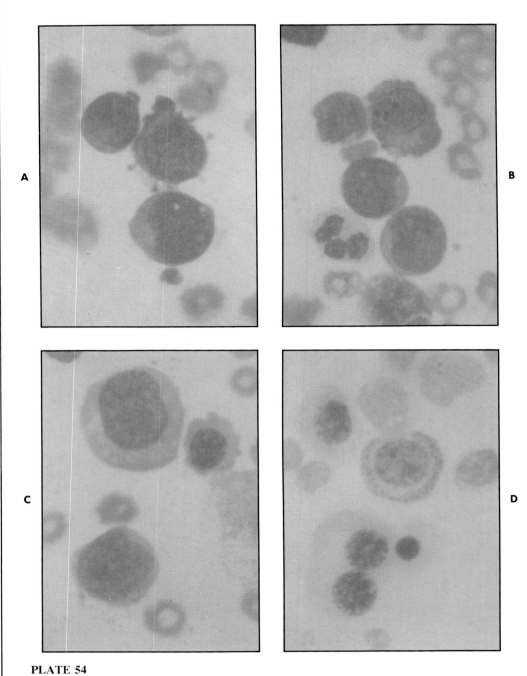

PLATE 54

Acute erythremic myelosis. Bone marrow. **A-C,** Wright-Giemsa stain. **D,** PAS stain. **A-C** show a mixture of myeloblasts and megaloblastic cells. The characteristic PAS positivity of the red cell series is shown in **D,** which also shows large orthochromic megaloblasts.

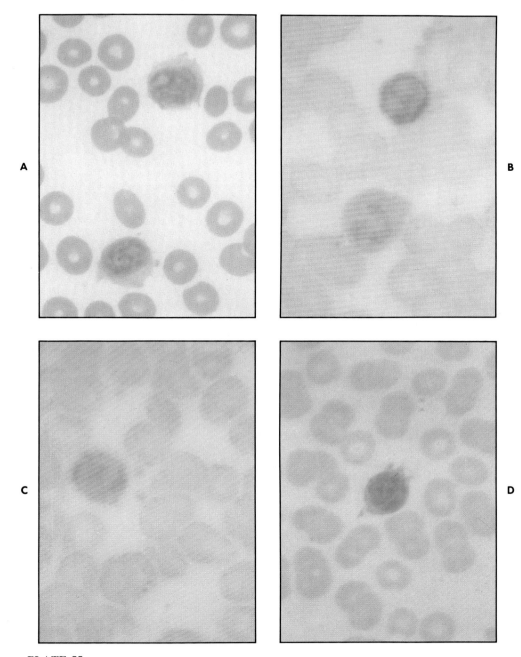

PLATE 55

Leukemic reticuloendotheliosis ("hairy cell leukemia"). **A,** A blood smear, showing the typical frayed edge of the cell outline. **B,** Acid phosphatase stain showing the strongly acid phosphatase–positive leukemic cell and a very slightly positive segmented neutrophil. **C,** Acid phosphatase reaction with tartrate added, showing no inhibition by tartrate. **D,** A "hairy cell" from a case of proved infectious mononucleosis, to show that not all "hairy" cells are leukemic. Note that this cell appears otherwise normal and that a nucleolus is not visible.

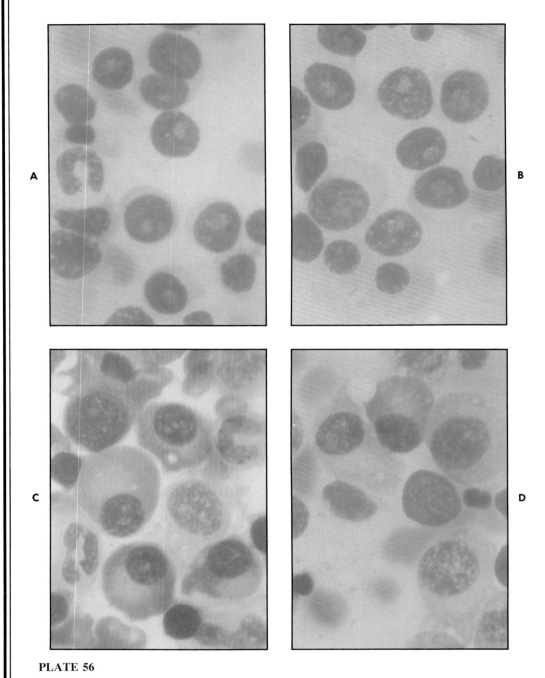

PLATE 56

Multiple myeloma. Bone marrow aspirations from four different patients showing different degrees of plasma cell immaturity.

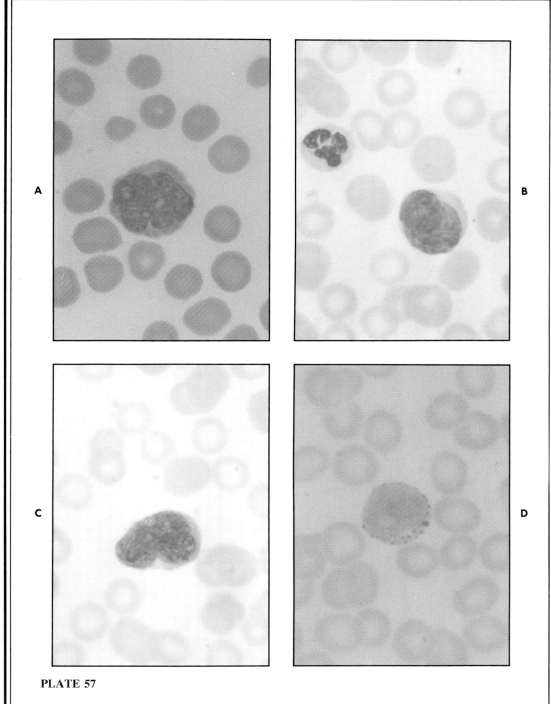

PLATE 57

The Sézary cell. **A-C,** Wright-Giemsa stain. **D,** PAS stain. Note that the typical cell is large and has a bizarre nucleus. **D** shows numerous PAS-positive granules.

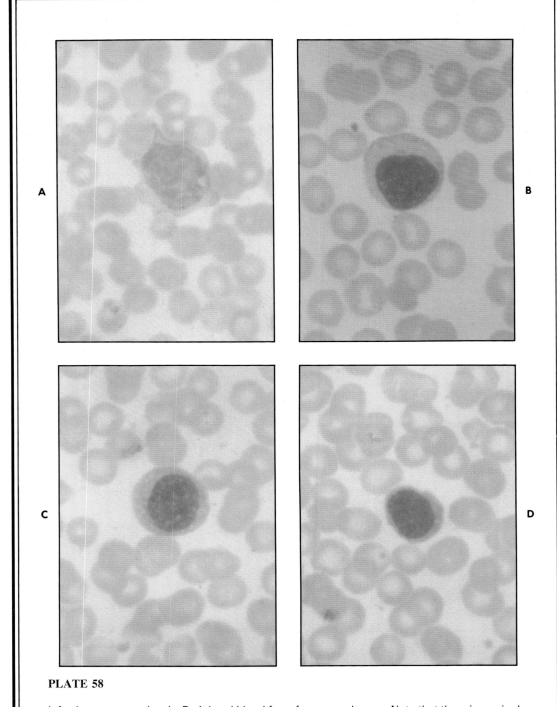

PLATE 58

Infectious mononucleosis. Peripheral blood from four proved cases. Note that there is no single morphologic type of reactive lymphocyte in infectious mononucleosis. The cell in **A** is probably the most characteristic of this disease, whereas the other three resemble the reactive lymphocytes seen in other diseases or reactions.

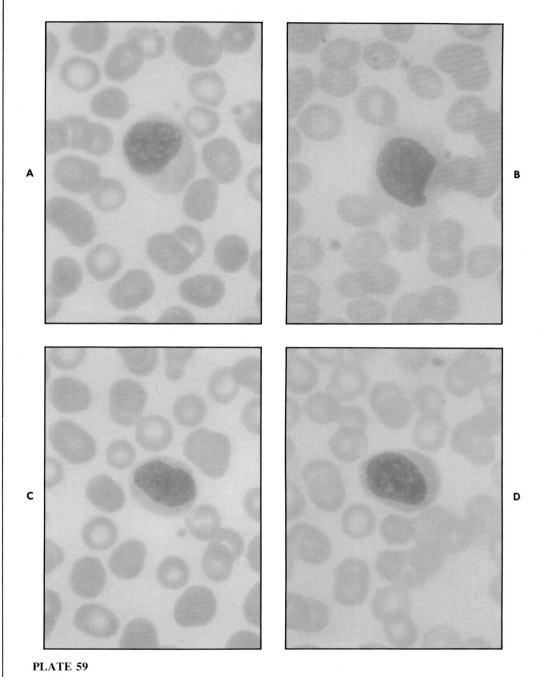

PLATE 59

Reactive lymphocytes. Viral infections, not infectious mononucleosis.

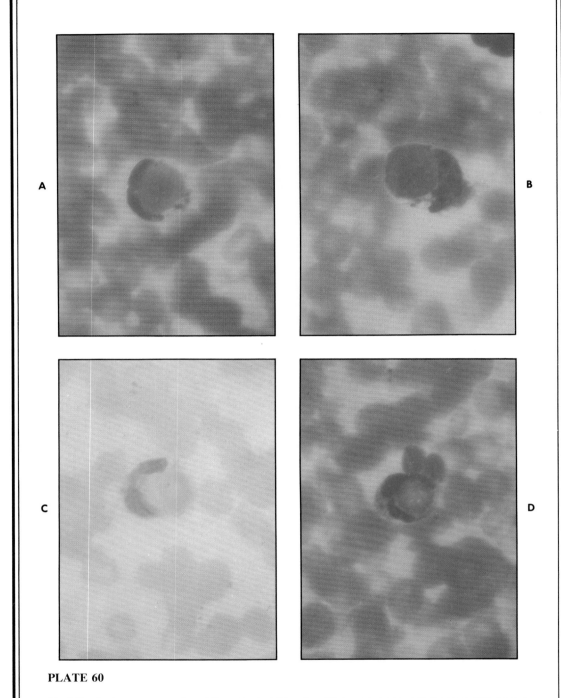

PLATE 60

The LE cell phenomenon. **A** and **B** are typical LE cells with homogeneous inclusions. **C** is from a positive LE preparation and shows ingestion of homogeneous material by an eosinophil. **D** is a "tart" cell, the ingested material retaining some evidence of nuclear structure and not sufficiently homogeneous to qualify as an LE cell.

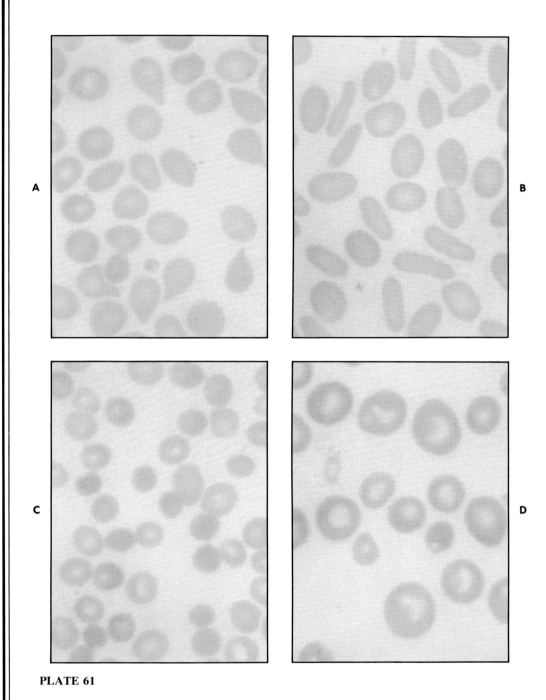

PLATE 61

Abnormal forms of the red blood cell. **A,** Teardrop red blood cells in blood, myeloproliferative syndrome (myelofibrosis with splenomegaly). **B,** Blood, congenital elliptocytosis. **C,** Blood, hereditary spherocytic hemolytic anemia. **D,** Blood, pernicious anemia, showing macrocytosis and 4+ anisocytosis.

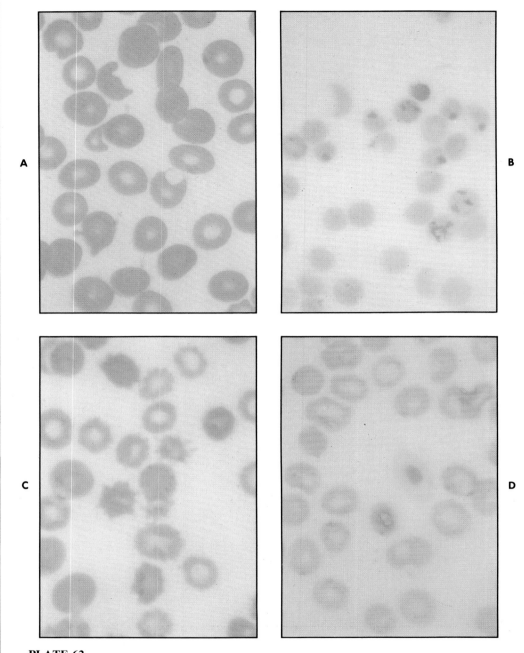

PLATE 62

Abnormal forms of the red blood cell. **A,** A "blister" red blood cell, hemolytic anemia. **B,** Reticulocytes and Heinz bodies, hemolytic anemia caused by enzymatic deficiency. **C,** Acanthocyte formation in acute liver disease. **D,** Artifact, a nucleated avian red blood cell found in blood contaminated with Dade Reagents hematology control material. (Smear courtesy Dr. F. Lynn Leverett.)

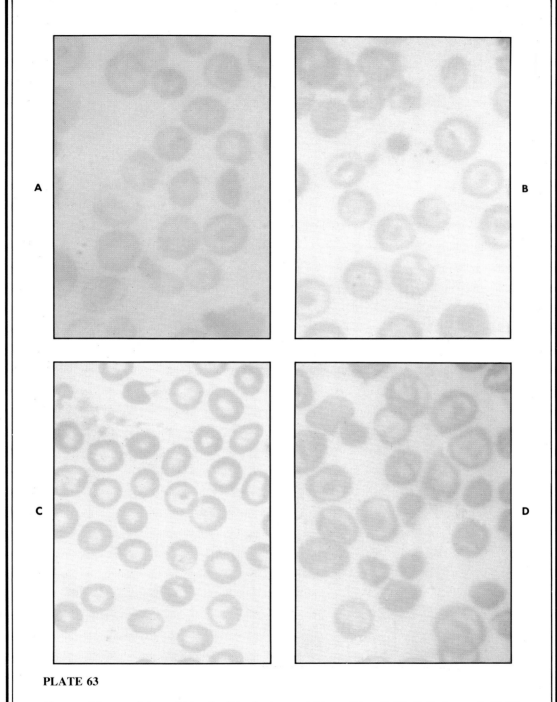

PLATE 63

Abnormal forms of the red blood cell in the hemoglobinopathies. **A,** Hb S–thalassemia. **B,** Hb S–C hemoglobinopathy. **C,** Thalassemia minor. **D,** Homozygous Hb C disease. Note the intraerythrocytic crystals in **B** and **D.**

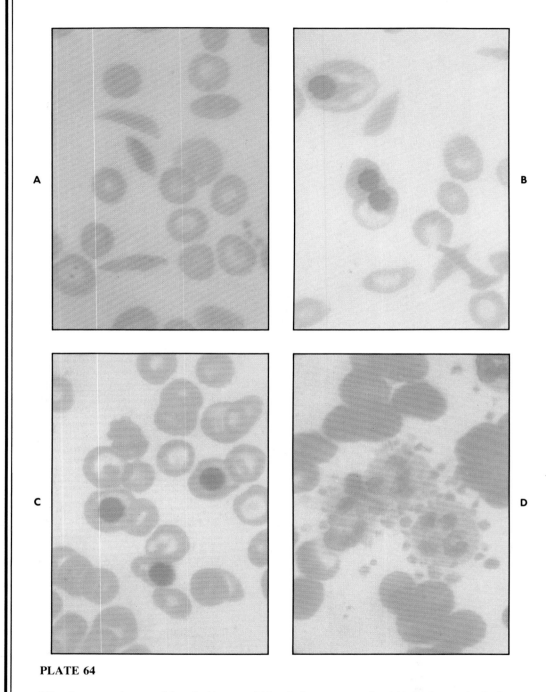

PLATE 64

Miscellaneous abnormalities. **A,** Untreated blood, drepanocytes in sickle cell anemia. **B,** Drepanocytes and normoblasts in blood, sickle cell anemia, and hemolytic crisis. **C,** Normoblastosis, blood, myeloproliferative syndrome (metastatic breast carcinoma to bone marrow). **D,** Platelet satellism.

1

"Nous savons depuis longtemps que les globules blancs du sang et les anticorps participent à la défense de l'organisme. Un troisième élément entre en jeu, dont l'étude est en plein dévelopment: le système réticuloendothélial."

Pasteur Vallery-Radot

The reticuloendothelial system
I. Hemopoiesis

INTRODUCTION
THE RETICULOENDOTHELIAL SYSTEM
PATHOPHYSIOLOGY OF THE RES
  Cellular composition
  Functions and reactions
HEMOPOIESIS
  Derivation of blood cells
  The stem cell
  Hemopoiesis in the embryo
    Mesoblastic period
    Primitive erythroblasts versus definitive normoblasts
    Control of erythropoiesis in the fetus and newborn
    Hepatic hemopoiesis
    Medullary hemopoiesis
  Kinetics of hemopoietic proliferation
    Quantitative aspects
    "Feedback" rate-regulating systems
  Nucleic acids in hemopoiesis
  Endocrines in hemopoiesis
    Pituitary
    Adrenals
    Sex hormones
    Thyroid
  Neurogenic control of hemopoiesis
  Erythropoiesis
    Erythropoietin
      Assay and normal values
      Chemistry of erythropoietin
      Immunology of erythropoietin
      Formation and metabolism
      Physiologic and pathologic significance
    Quantitative aspects of erythropoiesis
      The erythron
      Normal erythropoiesis
      Effective versus total erythropoiesis
  Leukopoiesis
    Kinetics of granulocytopoiesis
      Stem cell compartments
      Progranulocyte compartment
      Myelocyte compartment
      Metamyelocyte, band, and segmented compartments
    Granulocytopoiesis and leukocytosis
    Inhibitors of granulocytopoiesis
    Lymphocytes
      Definition
      Origin
      Life span
      Fate of blood lymphocytes
      Adrenocortical influence on lymphocytes and lymphoid tissue
      Lymphocytes and the immune system
  Thrombocytopoiesis
  Extramedullary hemopoiesis
    Ectopic versus extramedullary hemopoiesis
    Bone marrow embolism distinguished from ectopic hemopoiesis
    Relation between fetal and extramedullary hemopoiesis
    Possible mechanisms of extramedullary activity
    Extramedullary hemopoiesis in normal infants
    Hemopoietic potential of mesenchymal cells
    Extramedullary hemopoiesis in liver and spleen
    Extramedullary hemopoiesis simulating tumor
    Relation of medullary to extramedullary hemopoiesis
    Sites of extramedullary hemopoiesis
  Release of blood cells

INTRODUCTION

The quantitative and qualitative abnormalities found in the peripheral blood are the result of imbalances between *cell production, cell release,* and *cell survival* or *cell loss.* Under normal conditions the cells made in hemopoietic tissues are morphologically normal; also, the rates of cell production, cell release, and cell destruction are so well regulated that the peripheral blood counts are not only normal, but remarkably constant. If, however, one of the three basic mechanisms becomes abnormal, upsetting the equilibrium, deviations from the norm will soon be found in the peripheral blood. For example, anemia may result from a combination of (1) reduced erythrocyte production, normal release, and normal survival; (2) normal erythrocyte production, normal release, and reduced survival; or (3) increased erythrocyte production, normal release, and severely shortened survival or excessive cell loss. Simple and obvious as this concept may seem, it is the basis of hematologic diagnosis. Our understanding of these basic processes grows year by year but is as yet incomplete. Cell production (hemopoiesis) and cell survival are now measurable with a high degree of confidence; the process of cell release is still poorly understood. Still, the application of what is known makes possible increasingly accurate and specific diagnosis based on pathogenesis. From this follows rational and effective therapy.

In recent years the hematologist has learned that, although classic morphology remains an important facet of hematologic diagnosis, it is the normal and abnormal biochemical function at the cellular level that tells him what is normal and what has gone wrong. Function can be examined in the laboratory, and when correlated with clinical findings yields the most complete picture obtainable.

The concept of the *reticuloendothelial system* (RES) is one unifying concept at the cellular level, for in one way or another it is involved in all normal and pathologic hematologic processes.

THE RETICULOENDOTHELIAL SYSTEM

The term "reticuloendothelial system," or RES, was coined by Aschoff and Kiyono (1913) to define, by an inclusive term, a system of cells found both inside and outside of organs and characterized by (1) phagocytic activity and (2) staining by vital dyes. They thus recognized the common biologic and functional nature of cells seemingly of diverse nature, such as the clasmatocytes of Ranvier, the adventitial cells of Marchand, the fixed histiocytes of Maximow, the endothelial sinusoidal cells in lymph nodes, bone marrow, adrenal cortex, hypophysis, and spleen, and the Kupffer cells in the liver. The presence of argentophilic fibrils (reticulum) in association with the supravitally stainable stellate cells and with endothelial cells lining vascular channels suggested a morphologic unit consisting of "reticulum cells," endothelial cells, and reticulum—the RES.

Metchnikoff (1905), years before Aschoff, became convinced that the body had an active cellular defense mechanism. This romantic with a flair for the spectacular wrote:

One day, when the family had gone to the circus to see some extraordinary trained monkeys, I remained alone at my microscope looking at the motile cells of a transparent starfish larva, when a new idea came to me all of a sudden. I had the idea that similar cells must serve as a defense mechanism against harmful invaders. I said to myself that, if my supposition were correct, a splinter introduced into a starfish larva having neither blood vessels nor nervous system should be quickly engulfed by the motile cells, such as is found in a person who has a splinter in a finger. No sooner said than done . . . this experiment served as the basis for the theory of phagocytosis, to the development of which I devoted the next twenty-five years of my life.

He also observed that in another species of aquatic animal, fungus spores were engulfed and digested by leukocytes and, after noting the same phenomenon with bacteria, postulated a close relationship between immunity and phagocytosis. He referred to the neutrophilic leukocytes of the blood as *microphages* and to the fixed tissue histiocytes as *macrophages*. One who knew this remarkable man described him as "naïf et idéaliste, aux yeux gris-bleu pleins de bonté, aux cheveux ébouriffés qui cachaient un cerveau dans la matière duquel il y avait du génie. Coeur sans défense devant l'existence, en lui vivaient à la fois Tourguenieff et Tolstoï. Et sur son âme lyrique semblait avoir passé le souffle de Moussorgsky" (Vallery-Radot, 1957).

At about the same time other investigators (Behring, Kitasato, Pasteur, Roux, Bordet) were studying the role of immunologic defenses against infection. For a time it seemed that the cellular and the immunologic mechanisms were complementary but unrelated. In fact, when Aschoff and Kiyono (1913) proposed the concept of the RES (As-

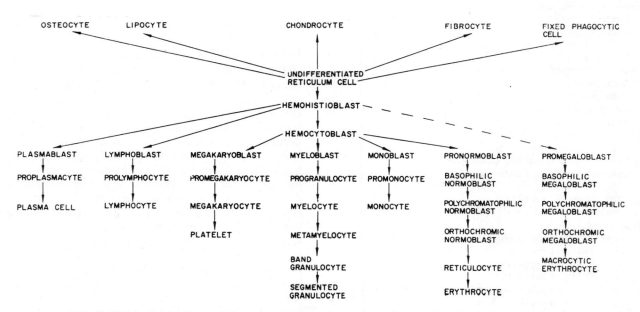

Fig. 1-1. RES from the standpoint of its multipotentiality and derivation of blood cells. This scheme is intended also to establish a standard nomenclature for blood cells. The current scheme of cell derivation is given in Fig. 1-5 (p. 6).

choff, 1925) the concept was primarily cellular and included only the physiologic function of phagocytosis. Morphologically, so long as it was assumed that reticulum cells are phagocytic, stain with vital dyes, and form the argentophilic reticulum, it seemed possible for all to agree on what was meant by the term "reticulum cell." However, it then became apparent, chiefly because of the histochemical studies of Hortega, that the glial cells in the brain and similar cells at extracerebral sites have argentophilic cytoplasm and cytoplasmic processes but are neither phagocytic nor stainable with vital dyes until altered by an inflammatory reaction. This gave rise to polemics over nomenclature, and criticism of the term "reticulum cell" has extended into recent years. Most recently, Gall (1958) has emphasized the difficulties of defining this cell exactly; he prefers to use "histiocyte" instead. Note, however, that the validity of this and other arguments is diminished when based on purely morphologic criteria, for what a cell is and is capable of becoming cannot be determined accurately by its morphology alone. In fact, the importance of the concept of the RES is not in the definition of its cellular components but in its central role in the protective functions to be discussed in later pages.

We now look at the RES in a broader sense, including two important concepts. The first is that the reticuloendothelial cells and their derivatives make up a cellular and immunologic defense system. The second is that the undifferentiated and still primitive cells of the RES are multipotential, one of the lines of differentiation being in the hemopoietic direction, other differentiations being into phagocytic and non-phagocytic histiocytes and into fibroblasts and other connective tissue cells (Fig. 1-1).

Beginning with those who scoffed at Metchnikoff, many have been reluctant to accept such a diffuse federation of cells as a system or have become lost in the minutiae of cell nomenclature. Inevitably, other terms have been proposed, such as *reticulohistiocytic system, mononuclear phagocyte system,* or *reticular system.* None of these terms are better than the original; in fact, some define a totally different concept. For example, the recommended nomenclature of "mononuclear phagocytic system" (Langevoort et al, 1970) specifically excludes cells that are not highly phagocytic, such as endothelial cells. Others (Diebold, 1973) include fibroblasts in the RES, claiming an interchangeable transformation of fibroblasts and monocytes. In my opinion, there is little to criticize of the classic concept of the RES, and these attempts to modify it beyond recognition can only lead to confusion.

PATHOPHYSIOLOGY OF THE RES
Cellular composition

The cells of the RES lie either within the vascular system or extravascularly. Those within the vascular system are the *blood monocytes,* able to migrate into extravascular spaces and to transform into tissue or fixed macrophages, and the *endothelial cells* in special situations (capillaries of the liver, lymph nodes, adrenals, and hypophysis and of splenic sinuses). The cells of the RES that lie outside the vascular system are the *reticulum cells* and *lymphoid cells* in the spleen, lymph nodes, bone marrow, and thymus, and the *fixed phagocytic cells* or *fixed macrophages* (the macro-

phages of Metchnikoff, clasmatocytes of Ranvier). The term "histiocyte," introduced by Aschoff on the basis of his opinion that the phagocytic cell in tissues is of tissue origin, is obviously inappropriate.

Functions and reactions

The functions and reactions of the RES (in the broad sense, the undifferentiated reticular cell and its derivatives; in the anatomic sense, the organs and specialized tissues containing these cells—the spleen, liver, lymph nodes, thymus, and bone marrow) can be classified as follows:

1. *Hemopoiesis,* the production and maintenance at physiologic levels of the blood and bone marrow cells
2. *Immunologic reactions,* humoral and cellular (Wissler et al, 1960)
3. *Storage* or *accumulation* of metabolites and *phagocytosis* of senescent or abnormal blood cells, of cellular breakdown products, and of other particulate matter, bacteria, fungi, and parasites (Cotran, 1965; Saba, 1970; Van Furth, 1970)
4. *Metabolic activity,* biotransformation and excretion of cholesterol, conservation and utilization of hemoglobin iron, drug detoxification, clearance and detoxification of endotoxin, clearance of intravascular fibrin aggregates and other macromolecular substances in disseminated intravascular coagulation, and clearance and biotransformation of steroids (Hyman and Paldino, 1960; Trubowitz and Masek, 1968)
5. *Benign and malignant proliferation* (hyperplasia and neoplasia)

In this chapter we will consider the first of these functions, hemopoiesis. Immunologic reactions of the RES are discussed in Chapter 3, storage and phagocytic functions in Chapter 2, conservation and utilization of hemoglobin iron in Chapters 8 and 10, clearance of macromolecular substances in Chapter 17, and benign and malignant proliferation in Chapter 16.

HEMOPOIESIS
Derivation of blood cells

The derivation and sequences of maturation shown in Fig. 1-1 are intended primarily to define a standard nomenclature for the blood cells we see in blood and bone marrow smears. It is now apparent, however, that regardless of how modified, such a scheme does not reflect all of the events that take place in the differentiation of stem cells or in the interaction between differentiating cell lines.

In the 1960s the study of hemopoiesis was taken away from the speculative morphologist when it was shown that bone marrow cells could form hemopoietic colonies when cultured in soft agar (Plunznik and Sachs, 1965; Bradley and Metcalf, 1966). Another valuable technic was to inject bone marrow cells into heavily irradiated mice. Within a few days colonies of blood cells developed in the spleen (Till and McCulloch, 1961; Becker et al, 1963; Curry and Trentin, 1967; Curry et al, 1967; Wu et al, 1968).

Data from these and more recent publications (Cairnie et al, 1976; Metcalf, 1978; Trentin, 1978; Cline and Golde, 1979a; Cline and Golde, 1979b) show that: (1) there is indeed a multipotential stem cell, (2) pluripotential stem

Table 1-1. Terms used in current investigations of hemopoiesis.*

Term	Definition
CFU-S	Stem cell–forming hemopoietic colonies in the spleen of irradiated mice
CFU-C	Stem cell–forming hemopoietic colonies in tissue culture; require CSF
BFU-E	Burst-forming erythroidal unit; primitive RBC precursor
CFU-E	Colony-forming unit for erythroid cells; the erythropoietin-responsive cell (ERC)
CFU-Eo	Colony-forming unit for eosinophil line
CFU-M	Colony-forming unit for megakaryocytic line
CFU-G,M (CFU-D)	Granulocyte-monocyte precursor
CFU-L	Stem cell committed to lymphocytic line
CFU-TL	Colony-forming unit for T-lymphocytic line
CFU-BL	Colony-forming unit for B-lymphocytic line
CSF	General term for a colony-stimulating factor, also called colony-stimulating activity (CSA)
GM-CSF	General terms for colony-stimulating factors for granulocytes and monocytes

*Lamerton (1976) calls this "alphabetic hematology."

cells replenish themselves to maintain the population of the stem cell compartment, (3) pluripotential stem cells are influenced to become unipotential and then give rise to the various cell types, and (4) proliferation and differentiation of hemopoietic stem cells depend not only on glycoproteins having specific stimulatory properties but also on interactions between cell lines. The nomenclature used in discussing these effects is given in Table 1-1.

The stem cell

The hemopoietic stem cell is the most primitive cell type. It is in a sense uncommitted regarding what cell type it will produce, yet committed as a hemopoietic precursor. It is capable of division, thus maintaining a compartment in a functional but not anatomic sense of like cells. Some stem cells remaining unmodified in the stem cell compartment are truly pluripotential, whereas some are influenced to become unipotential and give rise to various blood cell types.

The evidence favoring the existence of pluripotential stem cells is convincing: (1) irradiated mice given infusions of cells bearing marker chromosomes generate blood cells that have the marker chromosome (Trentin et al, 1967; Wu et al, 1968), i.e., the derivative cells are clonal; (2) a characteristic marker, the Philadelphia chromosome, is found not only in leukemic granulocytes but also in megakaryocytes, normoblasts, and monocytes (Trujillo and Ohno, 1963; Stryckmans, 1974; Golde et al, 1977a); (3) the proliferating cells in polycythemia vera as determined by common G-6-PD–marker isoenzymes (Adamson et al, 1976) are clonal; and (4) hemopoietic colonies in the spleen are established from a single precursor cell (Till and McCulloch, 1961). It is found in lymphocytic-rich cell fractions of blood and bone marrow and looks like a small lymphocyte (Dicke et al, 1973; Rubinstein and Trobaugh, 1973) (Fig. 1-2).

Stem cells are designated as CFU-S or CFU-C depending on whether spleen or agar colonies are produced. The multipotential stem cell is the CFU-S, while CFU-C cells are committed to the formation of blood cells and require CSF for proliferation (Hays and Craddock, 1978). The distinction between CFU-S and CFU-C is more than conceptual, for CFU-S cells share an antigen found in mouse brain that differs from the theta (Θ) antigen and is not found on CFU-C cells (Van Den Engh and Golub, 1974). Also, CFU-c cells are more dense (Worton et al, 1969), and more are in the S phase of the cell cycle (Iscove et al, 1970).

Normally, only a small fraction of the cells in the stem cell compartment are in mitosis, a fraction sufficient to maintain a steady state in the population of blood cells (Fig. 1-3). When the demand for blood cells increases, the fraction of dividing stem cells, uncommitted and committed, increases (Fig. 1-4). The stem cell compartment must be considered a functional rather than anatomic entity, because multipotential stem cells are found not only in the bone marrow but also in blood (Loutit, 1968; Nowell and Wilson, 1971). In lethally irradiated dogs with complete destruction of the bone marrow, the bone marrow can be repopulated by injecting autologous leukocytes (Cavins et al, 1964) as well as by injecting autologous bone marrow. The stem cells responsible for recovery are present in the blood in small numbers, about 1/100,000 leukocytes. More are present in bone marrow: 10/10,000 cells (Cronkite and Feinendegen, 1976). Suspensions of autologous thymic, lymph node, or thoracic duct lymphocytes do not effect repopulation of the bone marrow (Storb et al, 1968).

If isologous bone marrow cells are transferred into severely irradiated mice, hemopoietic colonies will develop in the spleen 5 to 10 days later (Becker et al, 1963). Some of the colonies are made up of erythroid cells, others of granulocytic, megakaryocytic, or mixed population (Curry and Trentin, 1967). Transplantation of cells from splenic colonies of a single cell type yields colonies that are of either pure or mixed cell types, indicating that the original colony also contained uncommitted and still multipotential stem cells. Furthermore, Trentin et al (1967) and Nowell et al (1970) showed that it is also possible to repopulate depleted lymphoid organs with cells from hemopoietic splenic colonies and that the new lymphocytes are capable of producing immunoglobulins and can be either T or B cells (Trentin, 1971). Thus the conclusion is made that the CFU-S stem cell is truly multipotential (Lala and Johnson, 1978). Fig. 1-5 outlines the current views of the derivation of various cell types.

Although it is accepted that the stimulus to differentiate and proliferate in each cell line is mediated by glycoprotein inducers (hemopoietins) such as erythropoietin (p. 17), thrombopoietin (p. 24), and various leukopoietins (p. 27), the proliferation of uncommitted stem cells is probably not dependent on these glycoprotein inducers. For example, in the erythroid series erythropoietin does not act on uncommitted stem cells but on a committed erythropoietin-sensitive stem cell one step removed from the pluripotential stem cell. Also, the development of hemopoietic colonies in the spleen and bone marrow of irradiated animals shows that various types of colonies have a predilection for a characteristic geographic distribution in the host organ.

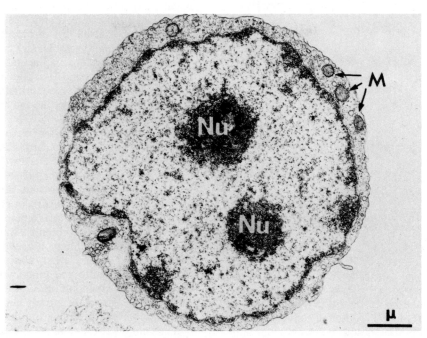

Fig. 1-2. Electron microphotograph of the candidate stem cell, human bone marrow. **Nu,** nucleoli; **M,** mitochondria. (From Dicke, K.A., et al: Identification of cells in primate bone marrow resembling the hemopoietic stem cell in the mouse, Blood **42:**195-208, 1973, by permission.)

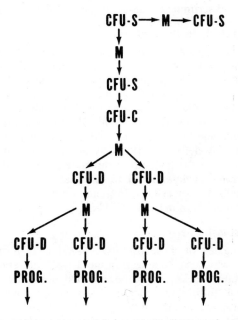

Fig. 1-3. Homoplastic (normal) hemopoiesis using granulopoiesis as a model. Symbols as in Fig. 1-5: *M,* mitosis; *PROG.,* progranulocyte. The uncommitted stem cell compartment is maintained by mitosis of CFU-S cells.

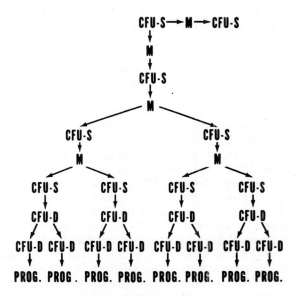

Fig. 1-4. Heteroplastic (stimulated) hemopoiesis. Labels as in Fig. 1-3.

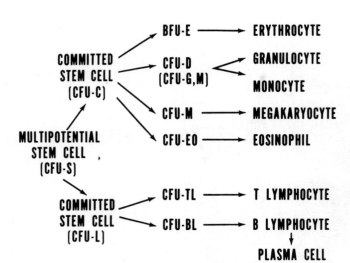

Fig. 1-5. Current views of the derivation of various cell types. See Table 1-1 for nomenclature.

In the spleen of such a host the subcapsular area favors the formation of erythroid colonies, whereas the deeper parenchyma and the bone marrow favor differentiation toward granulocytes (Curry et al, 1967). Although some investigators believe that the location of various colony types is simply a random seeding (Till et al, 1964), it is likely that the line of differentiation is influenced by the nature of the environment in which an uncommitted stem cell finds itself. Trentin (1978) uses the term "hemopoietic inducive microenvironment" (HIM) and suggests that induction is the result of interaction between the stem cells and the stromal and other cells in a given location. The characteristics of the membrane of the colony-forming cells may also be important (Tonelli and Meints, 1978).

Cline and Golde (1979b) discuss granulopoiesis as a model to study these cellular interactions. They point out that three major categories of interaction can be defined: (1) the interaction between mononuclear phagocytes and other blood cells; (2) the interaction of T-lymphocytes with precursors of granulocytes, mononuclear phagocytes, eosinophils, and erythroid cells; and (3) the cellular interactions of the stromal cells of the host organ. The interaction probably depends on the production of colony-stimulating activity (CSA or CSF) by monocytes, macrophages, and antigen-stimulated T-lymphocytes. CSA may be related to the production of glycoproteins having specific stimulatory activities (Metcalf, 1977), but other substances, such as prostaglandins (Kurland and Moore, 1977), act as modulating factors. Those of the F series stimulate while those of the E series inhibit colony formation (Miller et al, 1978). Other inhibitors have been described (Herman et al, 1978).

The uncommitted stem cell compartment is affected in the cyclic pancytopenia in gray collie dogs; this condition is called "canine cyclic hematopoiesis" (CH). Dunn et al (1977; 1978) have shown that the cyclic fluctuation in peripheral blood neutrophils, monocytes, platelets, and reticulocytes parallels fluctuations in CSA and CFU-C as measured by the diffusion chamber technic. Patt et al (1973)

proposed that the fluctuation of the number of blood cells in this canine disorder is caused by cyclic feedback stimulation of the stem cell compartment. Moore et al (1974) believe that CSF is produced by monocytes, with a negative or neutral influence exerted by mature granulocytes. It is not unlikely that hematologic diseases considered to be clonal in nature (polycythemia vera, acute leukemia, and aplastic anemia of the Diamond-Blackfan type) can be restudied from the standpoint of an abnormality either in the uncommitted stem cell pool or of the interaction of stem cells in a given environment.

Most investigations of stem cell compartments and colony-forming cells have been carried out in animals, but Cline et al (1977) studied bone marrow recolonization in four patients who had aplastic anemia and received transplants of bone marrow. By the fourteenth day discrete hemopoietic colonies had formed, consisting of clusters of 8 to more than 200 cells. The majority of colonies were of a single cell type; about 2% of the colonies were classified as mixed, almost always containing only two cell types. The mean distribution of colony types was: 26.8% erythroid, 31% myeloid (neutrophilic and monocytic), 33.7% undifferentiated, 14.2% eosinophilic, 2.4% megakaryocytic, and 1.8% mixed. These data from humans suggest that there may be important differences in the pattern of repopulation in man from those found in the spleen of the mouse; at about the same stage of development in man, mixed colonies are rare (1.8% versus 23% to 47% in mouse spleens) while eosinophil colonies occur more frequently. Admittedly, these differences could be caused by some alteration of the microenvironment in aplastic anemia, but they also warn against indiscriminate transfer of animal data to humans.

Hemopoiesis in the embryo

In the embryo the mesenchymal stem cells of the yolk sac differentiate into groups of cells characterized by a large nucleus containing spongy chromatin, one or two nucleolar chromatin condensations, and a deeply basophilic cytoplasm (Fig. 1-6). These are the primitive blood cells called *hemocytoblasts* by Maximow and Bloom, *hemohistioblasts* by Ferrata and Di Guglielmo, and *lymphoidocytes* by Pappenheim. By definition, if not by unmistakable morphology, this cell is the transition from an undifferentiated reticulum or mesenchymal cell to one that can produce only blood cells Yoffey (1971). In modern terminology this cell is the colony-forming unit (CFU-S), p. 24.

Mesoblastic period

Aggregates of these primitive blood cells form *blood islands*, which are first seen in the 2-week-old embryo. In the next few weeks, during the so-called mesoblastic period, these cells fulfill their function of fetal erythropoiesis. Later they disappear as the liver gradually becomes the chief hemopoietic organ. During the mesoblastic period the blood islands become connected by primitive endothelial tubes formed by the transformation of peripherally located mesenchymal cells into endothelial cells. Thus the primitive blood cells come to be enclosed in endothelium-lined spaces (Fig. 1-7). Upon further differentiation into cells recognizable as

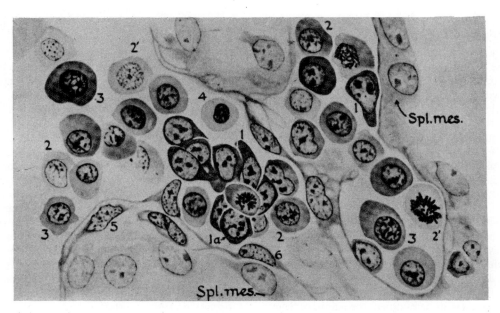

Fig. 1-6. Hemopoiesis in an 18-somite human fetus (about 4 weeks old). **1,** Primitive reticuloendothelial cells (called hemocytoblasts in the original article, now CFU-S); **2-4,** primitive erythroblasts; **6,** endothelial cell. **Spl. mes.,** Splanchnic mesothelium. (From Bloom and Bartelmez, 1940; original Plate 1, p. 47.)

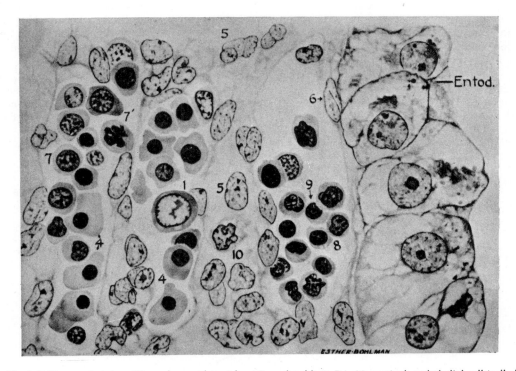

Fig. 1-7. Hemopoiesis in a 20-mm human fetus (about 8 weeks old). **1,** Primitive reticuloendothelial cell (called hemocytoblast in the original article, now CFU-S); **4,** primitive erythroblasts; **9,** definitive orthochromic normoblasts; **10,** histoid wandering cell. **Entod.,** Entoderm. (From Bloom and Bartelmez, 1940; original Plate 1, p. 47.)

erythroblasts, and with the secretion of plasma, *blood* is established as a definitive somatic component.

Primitive erythroblasts versus definitive normoblasts

Leukocytes and megakaryocytes are seldom found during the earliest phase of mesoblastic hemopoiesis. The predominant cell is the primitive erythroblast, a large cell, 15 to 25 μ in diameter, with coarse clumped chromatin in the nucleus, several nucleoli, and homogeneous basophilic cytoplasm. Since these primitive erythroblasts differentiate by elaborating a primitive hemoglobin, they probably serve the oxygen needs of the embryo for some time before being replaced by definitive normoblastic cells. In the yolk sac of the 9-week-old embryo about one half of the cells are primitive erythroblasts, and the rest are definitive normoblasts (Fig. 1-8).

The natural history of primitive erythroblasts is particularly interesting because they apparently do not develop into mature erythrocytes. They appear very early, elaborate some hemoglobin, and then die, being replaced by normoblastic cells that do differentiate into adult erythrocytes. The primitive erythroblasts have a striking resemblance to the megaloblastic cells seen in hemopoietic principle deficiencies (Wintrobe and Shumacker, 1935, 1936). Since fetal liver contains very little of this substance, it is possible that the primitive erythroblast is a reflection of a deficiency state in the fetus, which has its counterpart in the megaloblastic dyspoiesis of postnatal hemopoietic principle deficiencies.

Rosenberg (1969) studied an 11-week-old fetus (4.7 cm) and found that the hemoglobin in liver homogenates consisted of 37% Hb A and 63% Hb F; the peripheral blood of the same fetus contained about 4% Hb A and 96% Hb F. It would seem that the definitive normoblasts are active in the synthesis of Hb A even though relatively few of the derivative erythrocytes are released into the peripheral blood at that time. The fetal liver also contains a distinctive fetal form of G-6-PD and the fetal type of hexokinase.

Control of erythropoiesis in the fetus and newborn

Most of the studies on erythropoietin (p. 17) have dealt with its role in regulating erythropoiesis in the adult. The fetus and newborn are, however, perhaps in even greater need for control of erythropoiesis. There is first the need to build the red cell mass from zero to neonatal levels, then to adjust the polycythemic state at birth to normal levels, and then to adjust to the switch from fetal to adult hemoglobin (Chapter 17). Only then can erythropoiesis be said to have reached the adult system.

In utero, in the normal fetus, there is a gradual increase in plasma erythropoietin with increasing gestational age (Finne and Halvorsen, 1972). At term the erythropoietin level in cord blood is very high, and it must be assumed that relative hypoxia in utero culminates in excess production of erythropoietin and secondary polycythemia at birth. Amniotic fluid concentration parallels the plasma concentration. Fetal anemia, as in isoimmune hemolytic disease of the newborn (Chapter 13) is accompanied by high levels of erythropoietin in the amniotic fluid. Since the kidney is thought to be the chief organ involved in the synthesis or activation of erythropoietin (p. 20) and since the earliest development of primitive erythroblasts, in the yolk sac stage, precedes the development of the kidneys, it is not unreasonable to suggest that primitive erythroblast formation is either not erythropoietin-dependent or is regulated by extrarenal erythropoietin (i.e., liver, p. 20) while the definitive red cell is regulated by renal erythropoietin.

Immediately after birth, with improved oxygenation, the erythropoietin level drops to undetectable levels and, with red cell breakdown exceeding production, the red cell mass decreases and the concentration of serum bilirubin increases (physiologic hyperbilirubinemia of the newborn). The red cell mass begins to increase again after the second or third month. At that time, the switching mechanism from fetal to adult hemoglobin is fully operative. Since adult hemoglobin is a more efficient deliverer of oxygen, there may be no

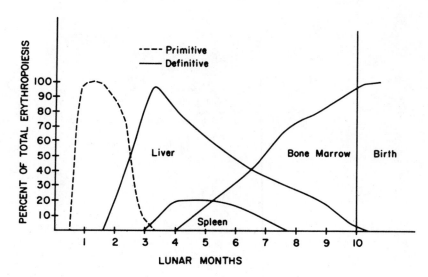

Fig. 1-8. Erythropoiesis in the fetus. Comparison of primitive and definitive erythroid precursors and estimate of relative contribution of liver, spleen, and bone marrow to the total of normoblastic cells.

hypoxia, and in fact it has been suggested that the activity of 2,3-DPG (p. 390) is more important than the ratio of Hb A to Hb F (Oski and Delivoria-Papadopoulos, 1970).

Hepatic hemopoiesis

By the third month (Rosenberg, 1969) mesoblastic hemopoiesis is no longer an important factor, and the liver has become the chief site of blood cell formation (Fig. 1-9). It is not known whether hemopoietic cells arise from mesenchymal cells in the liver or by colonization from stem cells circulating in the blood (Yoffey, 1971). This second phase is referred to as the period of hepatic hemopoiesis (Fig. 1-10, *A*). It reaches peak activity during the third or fourth month and remains active until a few weeks before birth. Only a few hemopoietic foci are normally present in the liver and spleen of infants born after a normal period of gestation. There is evidence that the incident of birth, as an independent factor, accelerates the loss of hemopoietic

activity from the liver, for the high degree of hepatic hemopoiesis found in the premature infant disappears long before an age equivalent to maturity is reached.

Although hepatic hemopoiesis is the chief mechanism for production of blood cells during the middle third of fetal development, there are significant contributions by the spleen (Fig. 1-10, *B*), thymus, and lymph nodes (Fig. 1-11, *A*). The spleen is at first active in erythropoiesis, myelopoiesis, and lymphopoiesis, but by the fifth month, myelopoiesis has become minimal. Splenic erythropoiesis continues until the end of normal gestation, and lymphopoiesis continues throughout life. The lymph nodes first show lymphopoiesis between the fourth and fifth fetal months and then continue to be active throughout life.

The second or hepatic phase in the fetus has an important counterpart in the adult. Normal hemopoiesis in the adult is almost entirely a function of the bone marrow, *medullary hemopoiesis*, but under the stimulus of abnormal require-

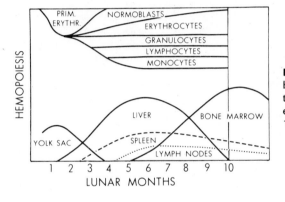

Fig. 1-9. Hemopoietic sequences in the fetus and the time of release of blood cells into the circulation. There is evidence (Rosenberg, 1969) that leukopoiesis may begin in the shafts of the femur and humerus as early as the eleventh week of fetal life. (Modified from Wintrobe, 1974.)

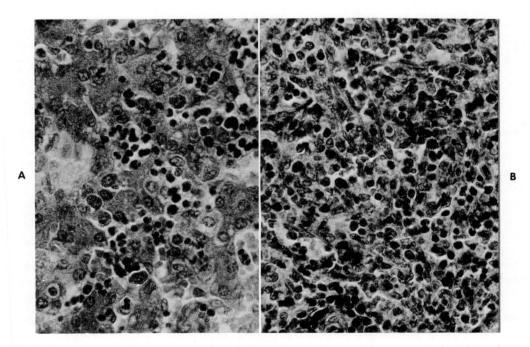

Fig. 1-10. A, Hemopoiesis in the liver of a 7-month-old human fetus. **B,** Hemopoiesis in the spleen of a 7-month-old human fetus. (Hematoxylin-eosin stain; ×450.)

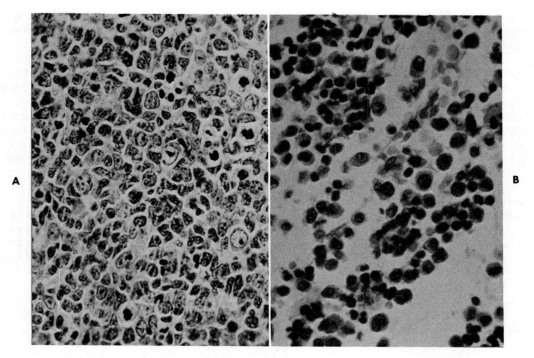

Fig. 1-11. Lymphopoiesis in the lymph node of a 7-month-old human fetus. **B,** Normal hemopoiesis in the bone marrow at birth. (Hematoxylin-eosin stain; ×450.)

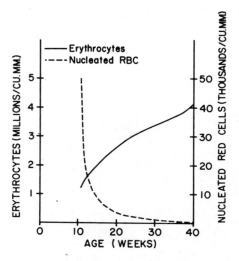

Fig. 1-12. Average erythrocyte and nucleated RBC counts during fetal life. (Data from Thomas and Yoffey, 1962.)

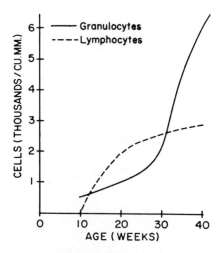

Fig. 1-13. Average granulocyte and lymphocyte count during fetal life. (Data from Thomas and Yoffey, 1962.)

ments the organs active during fetal life again develop hemopoietic activity so that striking blood cell formation may be seen in the liver, spleen, and other organs. This *extramedullary hemopoiesis* in postnatal life reflects the potential of resting hemopoietic cells to again become functional if the need arises.

Medullary hemopoiesis

The final phase is that in which the bone marrow assumes the chief role in hemopoiesis, the *medullary period*. This begins at about the fifth month when islands of mesenchymal cells in the bone marrow, remaining after resorption of cartilage, differentiate into blood cells of all types. The activity increases during the last trimester, and at term the marrow is, and then remains, the chief site of normal hemopoiesis. At birth, if there are no abnormal demands, the bone marrow is very active (Fig. 1-11, *B*) and extramedullary hemopoiesis is negligible except for lymphopoiesis in the spleen, lymph nodes, and thymus.

The first appearance of each cell type in the peripheral

blood corresponds roughly to maximal hemopoietic activity in the parent tissue. Early in fetal life many nucleated red blood cells are present (Fig. 1-12), but their number gradually diminishes, until at birth a normal infant almost never shows more than 10/100 leukocytes. Nonnucleated erythrocytes gradually increase, and first granulocytes, then lymphocytes (Fig. 1-13), and finally monocytes and platelets can be recognized in the peripheral blood.

In the normal infant and adult the marrow is the only site of erythropoiesis, granulocytopoiesis, and thrombocytopoiesis. The marrow at birth is extremely cellular, and the marrow cavities of the shafts of the long bones are filled with active red marrow. In the digits, replacement of red by fatty marrow begins before birth and the marrow is completely fatty by the age of 1 year (Emery and Follett, 1964). The marrow volume in the digits is, however, small, and in general the newborn infant has little marrow reserve. Increased cell production, if needed, must take place at extramedullary sites. As the body grows and the marrow cavities enlarge, not all of the potential hemopoietic tissue is needed, so that fatty marrow is found in gradually increasing amounts. In the adult, red marrow is normally seen only in the sternum, vertebrae, pelvis, ribs, skull, and proximal portions of the long bones. During periods of increased need, fatty marrow can be rapidly transformed to active red marrow by proliferation and differentiation of young and stem cells, a reserve that can be mobilized in a relatively short time.

Kinetics of hemopoietic proliferation

Under normal conditions cell replication involves an orderly series of cellular changes: the "cell cycle." The cycle is described in terms of phases G1, S, G2, and M (Studzinski, 1974).

A newly replicated but resting cell destined for another mitotic episode begins to prepare for DNA replication and is designated as being in the G1 phase. Here it receives a stimulus, largely unknown but possibly involving cyclic AMP (Willingham et al, 1972), polyamines (Russell and Snyder, 1968), poly (ADP-ribose) (Shall, 1972), or nonhistone chromosomal proteins (Wang, 1968). One or several of them act to trigger replication of chromosomal DNA. A cell in the G1 phase may not be destined for another mitosis but for maturation and functional expression; it is then said to be in the G0 phase. In response to a specific stimulus a cell in the G0 phase can enter the G1 compartment and become part of the mitotic cycle. Examples of this are the regeneration of somatic cells following injury to that organ and probably proliferation of normal functional cells responding to a neoplastic stimulus.

When replication of chromosomal DNA is initiated, the cell is in the S phase. Over a period of about 8 hours there is a continuum of DNA synthesis, and the regions of the chromosome that replicate as a unit have been called "replicons." A model for replication of the double helix has been proposed by Sugino and Okazaki (1973).

When replication of chromosomal DNA in the S phase is complete, the cell enters a relatively short premitotic period, the G2 phase. Characteristic of this phase are accelerated metabolic reactions, including synthesis of cytoplasmic lipids, membrane phospholipids, proteins, and RNA. The successive characteristics of maturing blood cells are developed during this phase. The G2 phase is followed by mitosis, the M phase, normally resulting in the formation of two like cells each having the normal complement of chromosomes. The M phase is the shortest of the phases of cell proliferation, requiring about 30 minutes in normal mammalian cells. "Spindle poisons" such as colchicine can prolong the M phase or even arrest the dividing cell in metaphase, leading to degeneration of the cell or recovery to form a multinucleated cell.

Quantitative aspects

The derivation of quantitative data on hemopoiesis depends on several assumptions: (1) the hemopoietic sequence can be considered as series of compartments and subcompartments representing definite stages in the maturation sequence; (2) since it is extremely difficult to measure how many cells may reenter a compartment once they have left it (Warner and Athens, 1964), it is generally assumed that reentry of cells does not significantly affect the population of a compartment; (3) in some compartments, representing those of younger cells, there is active mitosis, while in the later postmitotic compartments, mitosis is negligible; (4) in mitotic compartments the generative cycle consists of four successive stages; a postmitotic rest, a stage of DNA synthesis identifiable by labeling with tritiated thymidine or other DNA labels, a premitotic rest stage, and the final mitotic stage; and (5) the total time required for the progression through the four phases is called the generation time for a given stage of the development of a given cell line and it is generally assumed that the generation time is about equal in successive compartments.

Various investigators, accepting some or all of these assumptions and utilizing such technics as DNA-labeling and the mitotic index, have derived quantitative estimates of the hemopoietic sequence for various cell types. In spite of the many assumptions and the technical problems involved, the various estimates agree remarkably well.

One of the earliest estimates of the number and distribution in compartments of the various cell lines was calculated by Osgood (1954). His estimates are presented in Figs. 1-14 to 1-16 and in Table 1-2. Cronkite et al (1959) have made calculations from the *mitotic index* (ratio of the number of dividing cells to total cells) of human bone marrow. They assumed that the time span in each multiplication and division compartment was the same. The mitotic index for the red cell series was 44.8/1,000 cells capable of division, and for the granulocytic series it was 20.2/1,000. By counting mitotic figures containing labeled RNA in serial aspirations of bone marrow, some other approximations can be made; e.g., using the formula $t_G = t_M/M$ (t_G = generation time; t_M = mitotic time; M = mitotic index), it can be calculated that the average generation time of the myeloid precursors is between 0.5 and 1.5 hours, and the same figures are derived for the erythroid precursors. The size of the polychromatophilic normoblast compartment can be estimated on the basis of there being twice as many orthochromic as poly-

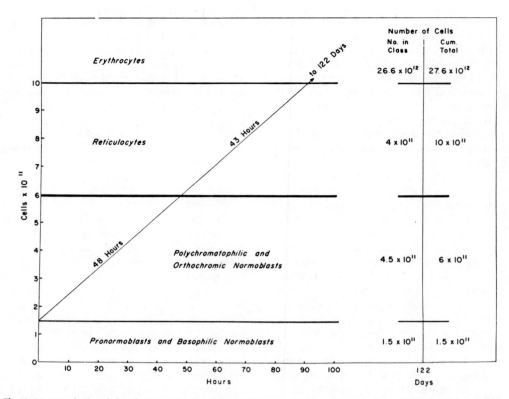

Fig. 1-14. Number and distribution of cells of the erythrocytic series. Lowest horizontal line is drawn at 1.5 × 10^{11}, representing total number of dividing cells. Intermitotic interval is about 16 hours. Slope of diagonal line defines the time course of a single cell that underwent mitosis at time 0. (Redrawn from Osgood, 1954.)

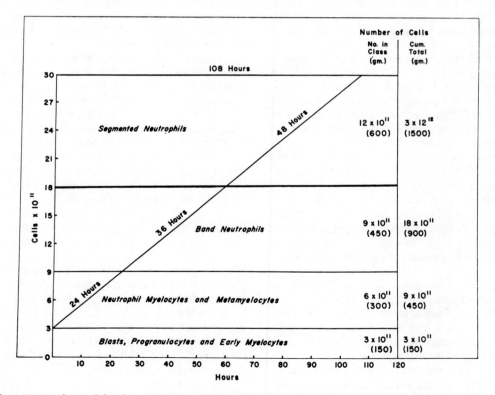

Fig. 1-15. Number and distribution of neutrophilic leukocytes; see legend for Fig. 1-14. Intermitotic interval is 12 hours. (Redrawn from Osgood, 1954.)

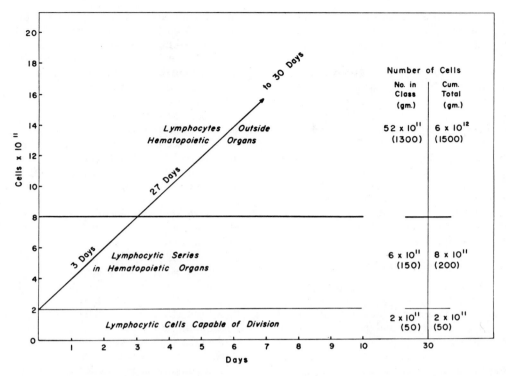

Fig. 1-16. Number and distribution of lymphocytic cells; see legend for Fig. 1-14. Intermitotic interval is 24 hours. (Redrawn from Osgood, 1954.)

Table 1-2. Number and distribution of blood cells in normal person weighing 70 kg*

| Cell type | In hemopoietic organs | | Outside hemopoietic organs | | | Total blood cells in body (grams) |
	Bone marrow (grams)	Lymphoid tissue and spleen (grams)	In peripheral blood and hemopoietic organs (grams)	Outside peripheral blood and hemopoietic organs (grams)	Ratio of cells within blood to cells outside blood	
Erythrocytic	100	0	2,500	0		2,600
Granulocytic	900	0	10	600	1:60	1,500
Lymphocytic	100	100	3	1,300	1:433	1,500
Monocytic, plasmocytic, thrombocytic, and disintegrated cells	200	200	1	400	1:400	800

*After Osgood, 1954.

chromatophilic normoblasts—polychromatophilic normoblasts label immediately and are capable of division, and orthochromic normoblasts are labeled only by division of the precursor cell. Therefore:

(1) $$\text{No. formed per day} = \frac{2N_p}{t_G}$$

(2) $$\text{No. dying per day} = \frac{N_{RBC}}{t_{RBC}}$$

since

(3) $$\frac{2N_p}{t_G} = \frac{N_{RBC}}{t_{RBC}}$$

then

(4) $$N_p = \frac{N_{RBC}}{t_{RBC}} \times \frac{t_G}{2}$$

where:

N_p = No. of polychromatophilic normoblasts
$2N_p$ = No. of orthochromic normoblasts
t_G = Generation time (0.94 day, average)
N_{RBC} = Total RBC in 60-kg man (2.07×10^{13})
t_{RBC} = Life span of erythrocyte (120 days)

and

(5) $$N_p = \frac{2.07 \times 10^{13}}{120} \times \frac{0.94}{2} = 8.1 \times 10^{10}$$

If we assume the compartment ratio of $1:2: \ldots 2^n$, the total number of erythroid precursors is 3.14×10^{11}, or 5.23×10^9/kg of body weight. Most investigators' results are roughly the same as these.

Similar calculations can be made for neutrophils, but so many assumptions must be made and so many contradictions ignored (i.e., time spent in blood, number in the blood versus number in extravascular or noncirculating compartments, life span after extrusion from blood, the possibility of recycling between blood and sequestration sites, etc.) that the derived numbers are only approximations. It is estimated that the mitotic phases take 5 to 7 days and the postmitotic phases 5 to 6 days (Bainton et al, 1971).

The advanced student may want to consider the mathematics of hemopoietic kinetics as presented by Harris (1959), Von Foerster (1959), Rigas (1959), Quastler (1959), and Killmann et al (1964).

"Feedback" rate-regulating systems

The number of blood cells of all types in the peripheral blood shows only minor fluctuations and is in fact remarkably constant. This steady state (homeostasis) implies a balance between the rate of production and the rate of destruction (Boggs, 1966; Erslev, 1971a). Since an increased rate of production does not by itself initiate accelerated destruction it follows that the steady state must be maintained by signals, originating peripherally, that somehow regulate the rate of blood cell proliferation centrally.

Various hypotheses can be postulated as to the source of the signals and the cells they stimulate. In physiologic situations, it is probable that cytopenia, the reduction in circulating blood cells, is the major activator of the proliferating stimulus. It is unlikely that the products of cellular disintegration serve as major rate-regulating stimuli, for the intensity of the proliferative response is not significantly greater when the cytopenia is the result of extensive cellular disintegration than when it is the result of simple cellular removal. And yet, it may not be justified to generalize, for there is some evidence that products of erythrocyte lysis or hemoglobin breakdown exert some influence on erythropoiesis

and hemoglobin synthesis (Waksman and Rabinovitz, 1966; Sanchez-Medal et al, 1969) even though the principal erythropoietic stimulus is erythropoietin (p. 18).

As for the cells stimulated by the signal, the possible receptors are three: (1) uncommitted stem cells, (2) committed stem cells, and (3) immature cells in compartments where mitosis is still possible.

When there is a deficiency of only one cell type, compensatory proliferation of only that type occurs. If uncommitted stem cells were affected there should be simultaneous proliferation of several cell types unless one assumes that the same stimulus directs the proliferating uncommitted stem cells to become committed to one cell lineage. In pathologic states, such as the myeloproliferative syndromes (Chapter 16), we do see simultaneous proliferation of several types of blood cells and infer from this that the stimulus acts primarily on uncommitted stem cells.

The second possibility, that the signal acts specifically on committed stem cells, is undoubtedly operative in erythrocyte mass homeostasis (Lajtha, 1964). It is proposed that erythropoietin stimulates blast cells committed to the erythroid line (BFU-E) to accelerated mitosis as well as to differentiation into the next stages of maturation, so as not to deplete the stem cell pool while providing the more mature cells. We can suppose that this mechanism applies to systems regulating the production of other types of blood cells, but as we will see the nature of the controlling systems for these is poorly understood.

The third possibility, that the signal acts through intermediate compartments, cannot be excluded and may in fact merely modify the second concept. If, for example, the signal causes proliferation and accelerated maturation and release from a mitotic compartment, then depletion of that compartment could act as a signal for more intense activity of the preceding compartment until there would be ultimately an effect on the stem cell compartment (Fig. 1-17). It may be that this sequence is more important in leukopoiesis, where release phenomena play such a striking role, than in erythropoiesis and thrombopoiesis where release reactions are less intense.

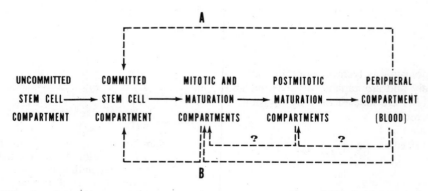

Fig. 1-17. General model of the two most likely feedback and rate-regulating mechanisms in normal homeostasis of blood cells. In **A,** a deficiency in the peripheral compartment acts as a signal for directly stimulating the stem cell compartment. In **B,** the stem cell compartment is also stimulated, but by intermediate stimuli derived from intermediate compartments.

Nucleic acids in hemopoiesis

In common with all nucleated cells, blood cells contain nucleic acids that are involved in the synthesis of cytoplasmic components. The nuclear chromatin in the resting cell and the chromosomes of a dividing cell are composed of deoxyribonucleic acid (DNA), with a small amount of ribonucleic acid (RNA) in the parachromatin (nucleoplasmic RNA or heterogeneously sedimenting RNA or Hn RNA) while the nucleolus contains ribosomal precursor RNA (r-pre-RNA). The cytoplasm contains only RNA, and this is heterogeneous, there being at least four fractions differing in sedimentation coefficients and function: transfer RNA (tRNA), messenger RNA (mRNA), ribosomal and polyribosomal RNA (rRNA), and mitochondrial associated RNA (m^t-RNA). The amount of DNA is approximately the same in all blood cells, but RNA is directly proportional to the volume of cytoplasm (Henry et al, 1967) and to the rate of metabolic activity.

For directed and specific synthesis of proteins to take place, the directive from a given locus on a strand of DNA is transcribed into RNA, which in turn determines the sequence of the amino acid subunits. Synthesis takes place in ribosomes and the various RNAs contribute to directing and effecting the synthetic process in these organelles. Transfer RNA (tRNA) (Madison, 1968) is responsible for recognizing amino acids and sequences and for their proper alignment. Accordingly, there are many variants of tRNA having some general features in common but also many structural differences to allow interaction with specific amino acids. It is thought that tRNA is active, or "charged," in the aminoacyl-tRNA form. Messenger RNA (mRNA) was first postulated by Jacob and Monod (1961) for an *E. coli* system, and its role in mammalian protein synthesis has been confirmed (Lockhard and Lingrel, 1969; Gross and Goldwasser, 1971). Messenger RNA directs the synthesis of polypeptide chains by the ribosomes (Perry, 1966), with tRNA acting as the dispatcher. Ribosomes are the actual site of protein synthesis and contain a variety of RNAs (structural) known collectively as ribosomal RNA (rRNA). The information from mRNA is imparted to groups of ribosomes, several of which make up the polysomes (Gierer, 1963).

Although this concept is somewhat mechanistic, I like to think of a long strand of programmed mRNA in opposition to a polysome, the beginning of the mRNA strand dictating that the polypeptide chain to be assembled should begin with an N-terminal, and to other polysomes fitting the conformation of the mRNA so as to build sequentially a polypeptide chain. As an extrapolation from studies with bacteria (Capecchi and Klein, 1969) we can assume that in the synthesis of mammalian proteins the end of the mRNA strand is so coded as to signal the termination of the polypeptide chain. As a final event, polypeptide chains having an affinity for each other (light and heavy chains of immunoglobulins, alpha and beta chains of normal hemoglobin, etc.) combine to form complex molecules.

It can be predicted that the synthetic sequence can go wrong at several points, and in fact it is surprising that it does so only seldomly. Perhaps there is a "self-destruct"

system that eliminates perpetuation of errors of synthesis. In some cases there is an additional interaction between the completed polypeptide chains and a nonprotein, as between the polypeptide chains of hemoglobin and the heme moiety, a deficiency of one or the other affecting the amount of the final product. Finally, there are ratelimiting reactions that must be regulated by either the amount of mRNA or its reactivity; also "switching mechanisms" that initiate changes in the information system (Chapter 14).

Endocrines in hemopoiesis

The evidence that hormones play a part in hemopoiesis is both clinical and experimental. As discussed in the following sections, hormonal imbalances may be accompanied by significant hematologic changes, and deficiencies respond to hormonal therapy. Experimentally, the technic of tissue culture has been used to define the effect of various hormones on erythroid and granulocyte-monocyte colony formation (Table 1-3). It is almost certain that those hormones that stimulate erythropoiesis do so by potentiating the effect of erythropoietin. According to Gorshein et al (1974), androgenic steroids increase the size of the stem cell pool responsive to erythropoietin, the BFU-E. The potentiation is probably the result of increased intracellular cyclic AMP, since other agents that increase cAMP (theophylline, epinephrine) potentiate the response to erythropoietin. Stimulation and inhibition of granulocyte-monocyte proliferation is effected by potentiating or inhibiting CSF. Thus none of the hormones can substitute for erythropoietin or CSF factors. The observed in vitro effects do not always parallel the clinical situation; i.e., estrogens have demonstrable hemopoietic effect in vivo but are not active in vitro.

Pituitary

In its role as the governor of the function of all other endocrine organs, the effects of pituitary dysfunction are

Table 1-3. Effect of hormones on erythroid (CFU-E) and granulocyte-monocyte (CFU-C) colony formation in tissue culture[a]

Hormone	CFU-E	CFU-C
Androgens[b]	↑[c]	↑
Adrenergic antagonists	↑	—
Dexamethasone[d]	↑	↓
Estrogen	—	—
Growth hormone[e]	↑	—
Prolactin	—	—
Progesterone	—	—
Prostaglandin E$_2$[f]	↑	↓
Thyroxin[g]	↑	—

[a]Modified from Golde and Cline (1978).
[b]See above.
[c]↑, stimulation; ↓, inhibition; —, no effect.
[d]Stimulation of CFU-E and inhibition of CFU-C blocked by progesterone or deoxycortisol.
[e]Stimulation of CFU-E is direct (not involving eyrthropoietin); characteristic species specificity (Golde et al, 1977b)
[f]Prostaglandins of A and F series have no effect.
[g]Blocked by β-adrenergic antagonists (Popovic et al, 1976).

mediated almost exclusively through other than pituitary hormones. Hypophysectomy produces a significant anemia in experimental animals (Crafts and Meineke, 1959). Hypopituitarism in the human is also usually accompanied by anemia. Pituitary extracts used in replacement therapy tend to correct the anemia, but no better than treatment with nonpituitary hormones such as thyroxin or the sex hormones (Fisher and Crook, 1962). In fact, the most effective treatment for the anemia of hypopituitarism has been testosterone proprionate (Shirakura, 1968). Some patients respond to combinations of "end organ" hormones such as thyroid, adrenal, and sex hormones. Hyperactivity of the pituitary gland such as occurs in pituitary Cushing's syndrome may be accompanied by elevation of the red blood cell count above normal (Thompson and Eisenhardt, 1943). The effect on erythropoiesis of pituitary hormones and of other hormones under pituitary control is produced by stimulation or suppression of release of erythropoietin (Meineke and Crafts, 1968).

Adrenals

The adrenal glands are probably responsible for mediating the hematologic changes that accompany hypopituitarism or hyperpituitarism. ACTH from the pituitary gland stimulates the adrenal cortex to liberate a large number of adrenocortical hormones having various effects on hemopoietic tissues (Yoffey et al, 1954). As a result of adrenocortical hyperactivity, there is an increase in circulating erythrocytes, neutrophils, and platelets, and a reduction in lymphocytes. Characteristically, the number of circulating eosinophils is reduced, possibly because their release from the bone marrow is inhibited (Hudson, 1964). The inhibition of lymphoid tissue has an important effect on antibody formation (Dougherty et al, 1964). The beneficial effects of corticosteroid administration in autoimmune diseases is a result of suppression of immunologic responsiveness; the anti-inflammatory activity is caused by interference with the mobilization and function of neutrophils and by the diminished phagocytic activity of macrophages (Greendyke et al, 1965). Hypoadrenalism, as in Addison's disease, is often accompanied by anemia, granulocytopenia, and lymphocytosis (Saphir, 1967).

Sex hormones

While proper balance between sex hormones is necessary for normal hemopoiesis, an imbalance of these hormones seldom produces severe hematologic disturbances. Castration of the adult male, animal or human, produces a mild anemia that usually responds to androgen therapy (Crafts, 1946). Ovariectomy in female animals has been reported to produce a rise in the erythrocyte count (Steinglass et al, 1941), which returned to normal when estradiol was given. It is tempting to ascribe the lower normal erythrocyte and hemoglobin values in women to an estrogen preponderance, but it is more likely that it is the male who has higher values because of androgen stimulation of erythropoiesis.

In the experimental animal, androgens stimulate and estrogens inhibit erythropoiesis (Dukes and Goldwasser, 1961). In the polycythemic mouse, testosterone propionate stimulates erythropoiesis as measured by the uptake of iso-

topically labeled iron (Fried and Gurney, 1968). It has been suggested that the inhibitory effect of estrogens is related to an inhibition of erythropoietin action either by neutralizing erythropoietin (Piliero et al, 1968) or by inhibiting the proliferation of stem cells (Jepson and Lowenstein, 1966, 1967). Androgens, on the other hand, enhance erythropoiesis (Shahidi, 1973) either by increasing the production of erythropoietin (Rishpon-Meyerstein et al, 1968) or by enhancing the effect of erythropoietin on the stem cell compartment (Naets and Wittek, 1968). Using the isolated perfused dog kidney as the model for erythropoietic production, Paulo et al (1974) found that the androgens that stimulate erythropoietin production are characterized by a double bond at the 4 to 5 position in the androstan nucleus, a methyl group at the 19 position, and an α-configuration of the hydrogen at position 5. The erythropoietic effect of androgens may be potentiated by an increase in erythrocyte 2,3-DPG (Parker et al, 1972). I have studied two elderly men with erythrocytosis (secondary polycythemia) caused by high-dose therapy with testosterone given to increase sexual potency.

The erythropoiesis-stimulating action of androgens has been documented in women receiving androgen therapy for advanced carcinoma of the breast (Fig. 1-18). There is also evidence for stimulation of erythropoiesis by androgens in anemia associated with myeloproliferative disorders (Gardner and Nathan, 1966), in aplastic anemia (Allen et al, 1968; Sanchez-Medal et al, 1969), and in idiopathic refractory sideroblastic anemia (Kushner et al, 1971).

Thyroid

Anemia is found in about one half of the cases of hypothyroidism, and thyroidectomy usually produces anemia in both humans and animals (Tudhope and Wilson, 1960). In intact experimental animals, thyroid hormone stimulates erythropoiesis (Shalet et al, 1966). This effect is abolished when the kidneys are removed or by the administration of antierythropoietin antiserum, and it must be concluded that the effect of thyroid hormone is mediated by erythropoietin (Lucarelli et al, 1967).

In hypothyroidism there are also many metabolic effects, including intestinal malabsorption of iron and folate. Although the anemia is usually hypochromic and microcytic (Larsson, 1957), it may be macrocytic as a result of a deficiency of folate (Hines et al, 1968). The anemia may be masked by the reduced plasma volume (Muldowney et al, 1957); when thyroid hormone is given, the plasma volume increases earlier than does the erythrocyte count, so that early in the course of therapy the anemia may seem to become more severe.

In hyperthyroidism the blood picture is usually normal (Rivlin and Wagner, 1969). Many years ago Kocher (1883) described a pattern in hyperthyroidism consisting of mild leukopenia with relative neutropenia, lymphocytosis, and eosinophilia. This "Kocher blood picture" has not withstood the test of a number of subsequent studies, but we have found that hyperthyroid patients often show a relative and absolute lymphocytosis. This lymphocytosis is probably the result of the generalized hyperplasia of lymphoid tissue seen in hyperthyroidism (Ernström, 1965).

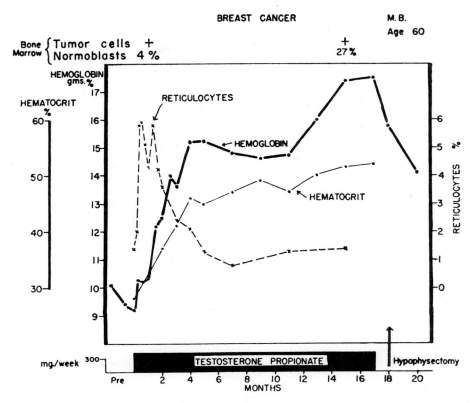

Fig. 1-18. Increase in reticulocytes, hemoglobin, and hematocrit during androgenic hormone therapy for advanced cancer of breast. (From Kennedy, 1962.)

Neurogenic control of hemopoiesis

The evidence for neurogenic control of hemopoiesis is reviewed by Moeschlin (1954). Although the neurogenic regulation is related in part to endocrine activity, it may also act independently (Halvorsen, 1966). Stimulation of the hypothalamus (Paulo et al, 1973a) effects an increase in reticulocytes released from the bone marrow, probably the result of vasoconstriction. Experimental irritation of the diencephalon by needle puncture or by parenteral administration of foreign proteins or inflammatory exudates produces a leukocytosis that is independent of the pyrogenic effect. The leukocytosis is thought to be produced, first, through direct parasympathetic stimulation of the bone marrow and, second, through sympathetic stimulation of the liver via the anterior roots of the sympathetic ganglia and the splanchnic nerves. The liver reacts to this stimulus by elaborating a leukocytosis-stimulating substance called leukopoietin that stimulates leukopoiesis in the marrow. This type of leukocytosis occurs in hypophysectomized and adrenalectomized animals and is therefore independent of pituitary or adrenal activity. It should be added that hypophysectomized animals eventually lose their reactivity to the leukocytosis stimulus, a reactivity that can be restored by giving ACTH.

Erythropoiesis

The maintenance in a normal individual of a remarkably constant erythrocyte count and erythrocyte mass in the peripheral blood implies the existence of an erythropoietic stimulus that under physiologic conditions so regulates the rate of production of new erythrocytes as to balance the rate of normal destruction. Under some unphysiologic conditions such as acute blood loss, sufficient stimulation of erythropoiesis occurs to restore the peripheral blood values to normal. After this, there is a return to the physiologic rate. Under other conditions such as hypoxia or residence at high altitude, erythropoiesis is stimulated beyond that at sea level, and an increase in the erythrocyte count and circulating erythrocyte mass results (secondary polycythemia).

Various mechanisms have been postulated to explain physiologic and pathologic erythropoiesis: endocrine, nervous and splenic mechanisms, local hypoxia in the bone marrow, and a humoral erythropoietic factor. Some of these, lacking experimental confirmation, have not progressed beyond the original speculations. One, the concept of a humoral erythropoietic factor, is substantiated by a considerable body of experimental data. This humoral factor is called erythropoietin. Comprehensive reviews are presented by Krantz and Jacobson (1970) and by Fisher (1972).

Erythropoietin

What has been called the erythropoietin era actually began in 1906. In that year Carnot and Deflandre (1906) injected serum from an anemic rabbit into a normal rabbit and noted that after a single injection of 9 ml of serum the erythrocyte count of the recipient rose from 5.5 million to 8 million/mm³ (5.5 to 8.0 × 10^{12}/1). The serum of the anemic animal was presumed to contain a substance, *hemopoietin*,

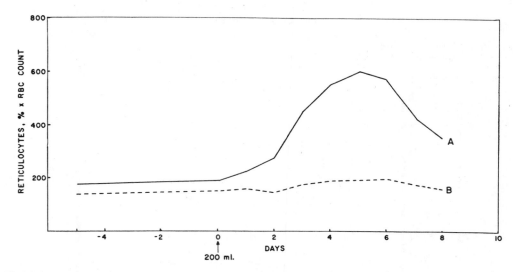

Fig. 1-19. A, Reticulocyte response in rabbits receiving "anemic" plasma compared to, **B,** control animal receiving normal plasma. Two hundred milliliters of plasma given on day 0. (Modified from Erslev, 1953.)

that stimulated erythropoiesis. Bonsdorff and Jalavisto (1948) focused attention on the erythropoiesis-stimulating activity of the humoral factor by calling it *erythropoietin*. With some exceptions, the same phenomenon has been observed by most of those who have tried the experiment; e.g., Erslev (1953) produced significant reticulocytosis in rabbits by giving 200 ml of plasma from anemic donors (Fig. 1-19).

Other even more imaginative experiments have provided stronger evidence for a humoral factor. Reissmann (1950) made rats parabiotic by inducing capillary anastomoses between each pair. In parabiotic pairs the elaboration in one of a substance with a measurable effect will produce the same effect in the parabiotic twin. By subjecting one of the parabiotic rats to hypoxia while the other breathed normal air, Reissmann found that both animals developed erythroid hyperplasia of the bone marrow. He concluded that hypoxia in one rat had caused the elaboration of a substance that stimulated the bone marrow of both. Furthermore, stimulation of erythropoiesis in the rat exposed to normal oxygen tension had occurred in the presence of a normal arterial oxygen saturation, eliminating hypoxia per se as the erythropoietic stimulant.

Stohlman et al (1954) took brilliant advantage of the opportunity to study the humoral erythropoietic factor in a patient having polycythemia secondary to a patent ductus arteriosus. In this patient, the oxygen saturation and tension were normal in brachial artery blood and low in femoral artery blood. This circumstance represents, in effect, a parabiotic system in a single individual, one region of the body being normally oxygenated while another is hypoxic. The bone marrow supplied by normally oxygenated blood was hyperplastic, indicating that hyperplasia occurred in response to a humoral substance produced at another site rather than to local hypoxia. Note that oxygenation of the brain centers in this case was normal, tending to exclude a central neurogenic effect.

Evidence for the humoral nature of the stimulus is also provided by experiments with hypoxic lactating rats. Grant (1956) has shown that newborn rats nursed by hypoxic mothers have a larger total red blood cell mass than litter mates nursed by normal mothers. It is supposed that the erythropoiesis-stimulating factor is therefore present in the milk of hypoxic mothers. As will be discussed later, it is possible to demonstrate that the urine of anemic animals also has erythropoiesis-stimulating activity.

These classic experiments, admirable for their directness and simplicity, established erythropoietin as the humoral erythropoietic factor and initiated extensive investigations into its origin and function.

ASSAY AND NORMAL VALUES. Although the development of in vitro assay technics would be very useful and practical, none so far devised has been judged adequate. Dunn and Napier (1978) emphasize that bioassays cannot be considered to be quantitative unless three doses of both the test and reference materials are used and the data analyzed by acceptable methods. Unfortunately, many of the data on erythropoietic levels in health and disease have been derived from one-dose studies. The chief drawback is the problem of obtaining a sufficiently concentrated and pure antigen for immunologic technics (Krugers Dagneaux et al, 1968; Lange et al, 1969); except with erythropoietin of highest purity, most of the immunologic reactions are probably caused by contaminants. Using as the antigen an erythropoietin preparation having about 8,000 units/mg of protein, Fisher et al (1971) describe a radioimmunoassay sensitive to 0.045 microunits of erythropoietin.

Acceptable in vivo assay methods have been devised, based on direct and indirect evidence of stimulated erythropoiesis in experimental animals. Jacobson et al (1959) define erythropoietin as the factor that, when given to a test animal, will (1) stimulate incorporation of ^{59}Fe into red cells, (2) stimulate a reticulocyte response, or (3) increase the total red cell mass. Borsook (1964) proposed more rigid criteria. He suggested that response to increasing amounts of erythropoietin appears in the following order: reticulocy-

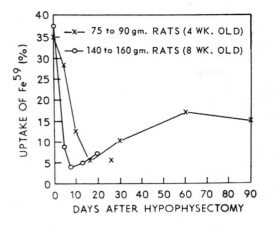

Fig. 1-20. Percentage incorporation of ^{59}Fe into red blood cells of rats hypophysectomized at 4 and 8 weeks of age. (From Jacobson et al, 1959.)

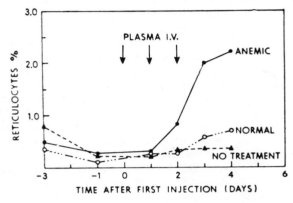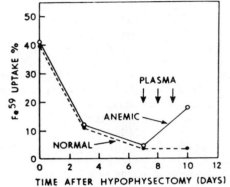

Fig. 1-21. Effect of "anemic" plasma on reticulocyte values and on incorporation of ^{59}Fe of hypophysectomized rats. (From Jacobson et al, 1959.)

tosis, increased red cell mass, increased hematocrit, increased red cell count, and increased hemoglobin concentration. Not all workers have used all these criteria, most having concentrated on single effects such as reticulocytosis, increased red cell mass, or, most commonly, increased uptake of ^{59}Fe. Often, preparations of erythropoietin are found capable of producing only one or two of the several erythropoietic responses. Lange et al (1971) describe a hemagglutination-inhibition assay for erythropoietin, but Kolk-Vegeter et al (1975) found a commercial kit based on this technic to be unreliable.

Great difficulty is encountered in in vivo assays when the erythropoietin activity is low in the material assayed. While some investigators believe that an agent that is the physiologic governor of erythropoiesis should be able to produce a statistically significant response in a normal animal, this is not the case, and most investigators use animals "conditioned" to be very sensitive to the effect of erythropoietin. Many investigators (Fried et al, 1956; Jacobson et al, 1959) have shown that when young rats are hypophysectomized the red cell mass falls (Fig. 1-20) and the animals become very sensitive to erythropoietic substances (Fig. 1-21). Animals can be conditioned also by irradiation (Stohlman and Brecher, 1956), fasting (Fried et al, 1957), dehydration

(Rambach et al, 1961), polycythemia (DeGowin et al, 1962), or by treatment with nitrogen mustard (Korst et al, 1958). The polycythemic mouse is the favorite assay animal. It is small, requires small amounts of assay material, and it is easily made polycythemic, with complete suppression of erythropoiesis, by intraperitoneal injections of mouse erythrocytes. It is also the most sensitive assay system (DeGowin et al, 1962). Polycythemia in mice can also be produced by exposure to a hypoxic atmosphere of 90% nitrogen and 10% oxygen (Boivin and Eoche-Duval, 1965) or by using enclosures covered with a dimethyl silicone membrane more permeable to carbon dioxide than to oxygen (Lange et al, 1968a).

Whatever the assay method, an erythropoietin reference or standard is needed. Based on the observation that cobalt stimulates erythropoietin production in some species, the *cobalt unit* was proposed (White et al, 1960). This is defined as the response of the Sprague-Dawley strain of rat to 5 micromoles of cobalt. Miller et al (1974) have shown that the production of erythropoietin after administration of cobaltous chloride to normal animals can be related to the development of respiratory alkalosis, the increased affinity for oxygen by hemoglobin, and to the resulting hypoxia at the cellular level. Schooley and Mahlmann (1975) have shown that acidosis inhibits the initiation of erythropoietin production by hypoxia. Other investigators relate the cobalt effect to release of lysosomal enzymes by a direct toxic effect (Smith et al, 1974). Rodgers et al (1972) implicate a cAMP-dependent mechanism involving a renal protein kinase. The first crude erythropoietin standard was designated *Standard A* (Cotes and Bangham, 1966), and was prepared from sheep plasma. Arbitrarily, 0.05 mg of Standard A was designated as one unit, equivalent to one cobalt unit. Erythropoietin *Standard B* has now been designated as the *International Reference Preparation for Erythropoietin* and the international unit defined as the activity in 1.48 mg of the International Reference Preparation. Even this is not as pure or concentrated as needed. In fact, Dukes et al (1969) report that the log dose-response slopes of several erythropoietin preparations, including the International Reference Preparation, are not identical.

Assay of urinary erythropoietin using the concentration method least likely to result in loss of activity shows that men excrete more erythropoietin than women and prepubertal boys: normal men, 2.8 ± 1.3 units/24 hr; normal women, 0.9 ± 0.4 units/24 hr; prepubertal boys, 1.0 units/24 hr (Alexanian, 1966; Adamson et al, 1966). Using a radioimmunoassay method, Fisher et al (1971) found urinary erythropoietin in three normal subjects to be 4.93 to 30 mg/24 hr while in four anemic patients (type of anemia not given) it was 72.5 to 303 mg/24 hr.

CHEMISTRY OF ERYTHROPOIETIN. Erythropoietin is a glycoprotein. Sheep erythropoietin contains 24% carbohydrate; the human hormone contains 34% carbohydrate (Espada et al, 1972). It requires the terminal sialic acid for activity in vivo but not in vitro (Goldwasser et al, 1974). Reported molecular weights vary widely, from 27,000 (Ruhenstroth-Bauer, 1950) to 61,000 (Lukowski and Painter, 1968), but the best data favor 20,000 to 30,000 (O'Sullivan et al, 1970; Dorado et al, 1974; Lewis et al, 1975). Erythropoietin has been purified to an activity of 9,000 units/mg of protein (Goldwasser and Kung, 1968).

IMMUNOLOGY OF ERYTHROPOIETIN. Antisera to human urinary erythropoietin show highly specific *biologic* activity (Schooley et al, 1968), neutralizing human, sheep, mouse, rat, and rabbit plasma erythropoietin as well as erythropoietin in cyst fluids and tumors (Rosse and Waldmann, 1964). Antihuman erythropoietin antiserum does not neutralize avian erythropoietin (Rosse and Waldmann, 1966). It should be noted that although antierythropoietin antisera can neutralize erythropoietin, impurities in the antigen void any claim that a pure immunologic system is operative. In fact, Lange et al (1968b, 1969) showed that one antierythropoietin antiserum contained two different types of antibody, one neutralizes erythropoietin while the other caused hemagglutination.

FORMATION AND METABOLISM. Jacobson et al (1959) showed that although extirpation of various organs does not impair the ability of the animal to produce erythropoietin, neither the rat nor the rabbit can respond after bilateral nephrectomy. These classic studies established the kidney as the chief organ involved in the production of erythropoietin, but there followed other investigations showing that the situation is not so simple.

For one thing, there are reports that erythropoietin is present in a few instances of the renoprival state (absence of kidneys) in humans (Naets and Wittek, 1968; Nathan et al, 1968a). This has not been found to be the case in animals. In humans, severe bilateral renal disease is usually accompanied by anemia, erythroid hypoplasia of the bone marrow, and decreased or absent plasma erythropoietin. Following successful renal transplantation, erythropoietin is again detectable (Abbrecht and Greene, 1966) and there is a simultaneous reticulocytosis and improvement of the anemia (Hoffman, 1968). The observation (Mirand and Prentice, 1957) that hypophysectomized and nephrectomized rats do produce erythropoietin in response to hypoxia also suggests that erythropoietin can be produced elsewhere than in the kidney (Mirand et al, 1968). The source of extrarenal erythropoietin is not known, nor is it clear how it relates to the major portion of erythropoietin from the kidney.

Instances of secondary polycythemia presumably caused by extrarenal sources of erythropoietin are well documented in pathologic states: hypernephroma (Shalet et al, 1967; Waldmann et al, 1968), Wilms' tumor (Thurman et al, 1966), solitary renal cysts and polycystic kidney disease (Rosse et al, 1963a; Mirand et al, 1968), hydronephrosis (Mirand et al, 1968), nephrocalcinosis (Cöster, 1961), renal adenomas (Waldmann et al, 1968), cerebellar hemangioblastomas (Hennessy et al, 1967), Lindau's disease (Sweeney, 1965), hepatoma (Scott and Theologides, 1974), hamartoma of the liver (Josephs et al, 1962), and uterine fibromyomata (Ossias et al, 1973). In most instances, it has been shown that plasma or urine erythropoietin is increased, that cyst fluid or tumor tissue contain erythropoietin, and this erythropoietin can be neutralized by antierythropoietin antiserum. In some instances it has been postulated that compression of normal kidney tissue by the cyst or tumor causes ischemia of renal tissue and production of erythropoietin (Mitus et al, 1964).

At the molecular level, Schooley and Mahlmann (1971) report that prostaglandins PGE_1 and PGE_2 stimulate erythropoiesis in polycythemic mice and that the stimulation is erythropoietin dependent. Prostaglandins also have a direct erythropoiesis-stimulating effect (Dukes et al, 1973). The prostaglandin effect is accompanied by an increase in kidney cyclic AMP (cAMP) (Paulo et al, 1973b), just as cobalt-induced erythropoiesis is accompanied by increased cAMP (Rodgers et al, 1972). One can speculate that renal hypoxia, cAMP activity, and release or accelerated synthesis of erythropoietin are interrelated.

The actual site in the kidney where erythropoietin is formed is still debated. Fisher et al (1965) and Busuttil et al (1971) have shown that erythropoietin is found in the glomeruli but not in the tubules, but since erythropoietin is found in urine it may be present in the glomeruli in the course of clearance from the blood stream rather than because it is produced there. Gruber et al (1977) have shown by immunofluorescence that in the rat the Kupffer cells in the liver are the primary site of erythropoietin production during the first 2 weeks of life, whereas erythropoietin is formed both in the Kupffer cells and the glomeruli of the kidney in older animals. Zanjani et al (1977) also believe that the liver is the primary site of erythropoietin formation in the mammalian fetus (sheep). There are some claims that the juxtaglomerular apparatus is involved in the synthesis of erythropoietin (Mitus et al, 1968) but others do not agree (Fisher and Balcerzak, 1969). There are interesting reports (Jepson and McGarry, 1968; Erkelens and Statius van Eps, 1973) of patients with histologically proved hypertrophy of the juxtaglomerular apparatus (Bartter's syndrome) who also had polycythemia and increased concentration of erythropoietin in both plasma and urine. Prostaglandins of renal origin may be involved in erythropoietin production, notably PGE$_2$ (Gross et al, 1976), and it is of interest that Bartter's syndrome is characterized by high levels of urinary prostaglandins (Gill et al, 1976).

The role of the kidney may be, in fact, to provide either a system for activating plasma erythropoietin made elsewhere or by providing an inhibitor that is blocked by hypoxia. There is better evidence for the first possibility. It has been shown that when a subcellular fraction of kidney tissue is incubated with normal serum, the erythropoietin titer of the serum is increased (Contrera et al, 1966; Zanjani et al, 1967). The kidney activity has been named the *renal erythropoietic factor* (REF) and the inactive erythropoietin precursor the *erythropoietinogen* or *erythrogenin* (Fig. 1-22) (Gordon et al, 1967). Erythropoietinogen (erythrogenin) has a molecular weight between 30,000 and 50,000 and can be found in the urine of anemic patients (Lewis et al, 1975).

The activation is thought to be an enzymatic first order reaction (DuBose et al, 1977). Erythropoietin is inactivated not only by homogenates of kidney tissue, but also of liver and spleen (Erslev and Kazal, 1968) and by hepatic lysosomes (Briggs et al, 1973). There is good evidence that the liver in vivo inactivates erythropoietin, but the significance of this is not obvious. Some investigators (Fletcher et al, 1973; Halvorsen, 1974) favor the hypothesis that erythropoietic stimulation represents a balance between erythropoietin and an erythropoietic inhibitor. In fact, the failure to extract erythropoietin from kidney tissue is related to the presence of a lipid inhibitor in the kidney (Abaidoo, 1974). A potent inhibitor is also present in lipid extracts of rabbit stomach. The presence of inhibitors in plasma has been detected in newborn infants (Skjaelaaen et al, 1971), in hypertransfused animals (Whitcomb and Moore, 1964), and in subjects returning to sea level from a high altitude (Reynafarje, 1968).

PHYSIOLOGIC AND PATHOLOGIC SIGNIFICANCE. Erythropoietin provides the mechanism whereby the bone marrow produces more erythrocytes when there is an acute need, such as in anemia, or when there is a need for increased oxygen-carrying capacity, as in hypoxia. The small amount of erythropoietin present in the plasma of normal individuals may be part of the mechanism for maintaining the erythrocyte mass at a remarkably constant level. Erythropoietin in excess, as when it is produced by cysts or tumors, produces secondary polycythemia, for apparently the bone marrow cannot distinguish between a physiologic and pathologic stimulus.

It is not difficult to envision how erythropoietin acts when there is an acute need, as in anemias of various types, or when the situation mimics anemia, as in hypoxia. One cannot be satisfied with all aspects of the mechanisms proposed

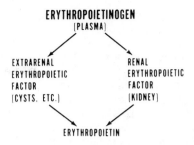

Fig. 1-22. The formation of erythropoietin. This scheme assumes that the precursor in plasma (erythropoietinogen or erythrogenin) is converted to erythropoietin either by renal erythropoietic factor (**REF**) or by extrarenal erythropoietic factor or factors.

both for the stimulation of erythropoietin production and for its action, but the general outline is acceptable. The case for hypoxia as a stimulant for erythropoietin production is clear (Gurney et al, 1965; Carmena et al, 1967), and some would go so far as to say that hypoxia is the final pathway for increasing erythropoietin. When, as in anemia, the red cell mass is reduced, it would follow that the decreased oxygen-carrying capacity would produce hypoxia, which then would stimulate production of erythropoietin. However, in some anemias erythropoietin is increased, as expected, but in others it is normal or decreased. Erythropoietin is increased in thalassemia (Gordon et al, 1964a), in sickle cell anemia (Hammond et al, 1968), in iron deficiency anemia (Movassaghi et al, 1967), in aplastic anemia (van Dyke et al, 1966; Rishpon-Meyerstein et al, 1968) and in red cell aplasia (River, 1966). Since in aplastic anemia and red cell aplasia there is little or no production of erythrocytes it has been suggested variously that (1) there is an inhibitor of erythropoietin or (2) the marrow is unresponsive to erythropoietin. Both explanations are logical and equally likely or unlikely. Erythropoietin is either normal or decreased in the anemia of chronic renal insufficiency (Adamson, 1968).

Erythropoietin acts on the stem cell compartment—not on the portion of uncommitted stem cells but on stem cells committed to erythropoietic differentiation (Bruce and McCulloch, 1964; Schooley et al, 1968). Functionally, the stem cell responding to erythropoietin has been called the *erythropoietin-responsive cell* (ERC or BFU-E). There is evidence that the action of erythropoietin is not limited to the stem cell compartment, but that it also influences maturation rates in later compartments (Necheles et al, 1968; Eaves and Eaves, 1978; Adamson et al, 1978) and release of reticulocytes from the bone marrow (Gordon et al, 1962). Chamberlain et al (1975) suggest that erythropoietin also acts on the wall of bone marrow sinuses, enhancing release of erythroid cells from the bone marrow.

Van Vliet and Huisman (1964) have shown that sheep having only hemoglobin A respond to erythropoietin by producing a population of red cells containing a new hemoglobin, hemoglobin C. This reaction is blocked by antierythropoietin antiserum (Lewis et al, 1970). This is compatible with the suggestion that erythropoietin acts on erythropoietin-responsive cells by inducing a new kind of mRNA. Once stimulated, BFU-E can continue to proliferate for a time in the absence of erythropoietin (O'Grady and Lewis, 1970). It is difficult to relate this to the observation (Schooley and Mahlmann, 1972) that synthesis of erythropoietin, once triggered, continues for some time after the hypoxia is terminated.

The distinction between CFU-S and BFU-E is also compatible with our concept of the genesis of the myeloproliferative disorders (Fig. 16-1). In one of the myeloproliferative disorders, polycythemia vera, there is no increase in erythropoietin in spite of the fact that the erythrocyte count and mass are abnormally high (Adamson and Finch, 1970; Spivak and Cooke, 1976). We postulate that proliferation of several cell lines at the same time is caused by the stimulation of the uncommitted stem cell compartment, equivalent to CFU-S. Erythropoietin is not responsible for multilinear differentiation; in fact, secondary polycythemia such as secondary to cysts and tumors is characterized by both high erythropoietin levels, important in differentiating polycythemia vera from secondary polycythemia, and unilinear (erythrocytic) proliferation only. Furthermore, if erythropoietin is added to marrow cells from polycythemia vera patients it does not stimulate incorporation of ^{59}Fe (Zucker et al, 1972).

The role of erythropoietin in physiologic homeostasis of red cell mass is not clear. The presence of small amounts in normal plasma suggests that it should be implicated, and yet the fluctuations found normally in the red cell count and mass are so small that it is difficult to conceive that any organ can be so sensitive to such minute changes in oxygen as to turn the erythropoietin mechanism on and off. Erslev (1971b) suggests that erythropoietic cells may be sensitive to hemoglobin or hemoglobin degradation products.

Quantitative aspects of erythropoiesis

THE ERYTHRON. The concept of the erythron as all the erythroid tissue of the body is a useful symbol of the physiologic unity of that tissue. It encourages the approach to diagnosis in terms of erythropoiesis, cell release, and cell destruction and provides a convenient term to remind us that the study of only one component may yield data that are inconclusive or misleading.

The cells of the erythron for which quantitative data are available are the nucleated red blood cells in the marrow, the reticulocytes in the marrow, the reticulocytes in the peripheral blood, and the adult red blood cells.

NORMAL ERYTHROPOIESIS. Several methods have been employed to estimate the total number of cells in the erythron. One method is to count the erythroid cells in a marrow aliquot and to calculate cellularity from the ratio of aliquot to total marrow as determined by tagging with ^{59}Fe. Using this method, Finch (1959) calculates the composition of the erythron in normal humans to be as follows: nucleated red cells, 5.0×10^9/kg; marrow reticulocytes, 4.7×10^9/kg; circulating reticulocytes, 3.1×10^9/kg; and mature red blood cells, 308×10^9/kg.

Osgood's (1954) calculations (Fig. 1-14) are based on the assumption that one-fourth of the nucleated red cells are capable of division, and the maturation time of the other three fourths is 48 hours. He estimates the total cells in each category (not related to body weight) as pronormoblasts plus

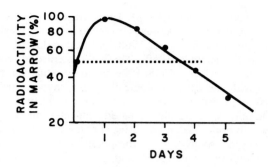

Fig. 1-23. Marrow turnover of ^{59}Fe. (Adapted from Finch, 1959.)

basophilic normoblasts, 1.5×10^{11}; polychromatophilic plus orthochromic normoblasts, 4.5×10^{11}; reticulocytes, 4×10^{11}; and mature red blood cells, 26.6×10^{12}. Expressed as cells per kilogram of body weight (70 kg), Osgood's calculated number of nucleated red cells in the marrow is 8.6×10^9/kg. The agreement obtained by different methods of calculation is remarkably good.

An estimate of the time that nucleated red blood cells and reticulocytes spend in the marrow can be made by measuring the marrow transit time of ^{59}Fe (Fig. 1-23). Radioiron injected intravenously disappears rapidly from the plasma and soon can be detected in circulating erythrocytes. The amount incorporated into erythrocytes is assumed to represent that taken up by normoblasts and reticulocytes in the bone marrow. Thus the time interval between 50% disappearance from the blood to 50% release by the marrow (82 hours) represents the transit time of ^{59}Fe in the marrow and is assumed to also represent the amount of time normoblasts and reticulocytes spend in the marrow.

EFFECTIVE VERSUS TOTAL ERYTHROPOIESIS. We are indebted to Finch (1959) for emphasizing the physiologic importance of *effective* in contrast to *total* erythropoiesis. Effective erythropoiesis represents the number of viable and functional erythrocytes available for physiologic needs, reflecting a balance between number of cells produced and their life span. Total erythropoiesis, on the other hand, merely records the total number of cells, with no indication as to whether an adequate number of erythrocytes is being made available.

Not all methods used to study erythrokinetics measure effective erythropoiesis. The erythroid-myeloid ratio determined from smears, plus the estimate of bone marrow cellularity from paraffin sections, the measurement of plasma iron turnover, and the measurement of fecal urobilinogen excretion are parameters of total erythropoiesis, the first two measuring total erythrocyte production and the third measuring total hemoglobin catabolism. Effective erythropoiesis is measured by the number of reticulocytes entering the peripheral blood, the erythrocyte count, and the red cell uptake of iron on the one hand and by red blood cell survival or life span on the other.

The reticulocyte count, particularly when expressed as the absolute count (percent reticulocytes times erythrocyte count), is of practical importance, for it reflects effective erythropoiesis. To evaluate an anemia without this simple

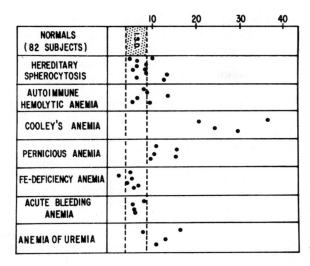

Fig. 1-24. In vitro maturation (hours, T½) of reticulocytes in normal persons and in various types of anemia. (From Baldini and Pannacciulli, 1960.)

Table 1-4. Effective and total erythropoiesis in anemias*

Erythrokinetic classification	Effective erythropoiesis†		Total erythropoiesis†	
	Reticulocyte count	RBC ^{59}Fe uptake	Erythroid tissue in bone marrow	Plasma iron turnover
Hyperfunction				
Hereditary spherocytosis (Case 1)	6.8	3.6	6.4	5.3
Hereditary spherocytosis (Case 2)	8.8	4.2	4.7	5.3
Relative hypofunction				
Myelofibrosis	0.8	1.3	—	1.9
Cirrhosis	0.9	1.3	2.0	1.1
Hypofunction				
Uremia	0.2	0.3	0.2	0.6
Erythroid hyperplasia of marrow	0.2	0.1	0.1	0.5
Dysfunction				
Thalassemia	0.7	0.6	11.0	6.5
Pernicious anemia	—	1.2	—	2.8

*Finch, 1959.
†Multiples of the normal value taken as 1.0.

but necessary determination is like undertaking a trip without knowing the starting point or the destination, an apt simile for the "iron—plus B$_{12}$—plus intrinsic factor—plus multivitamins—let's see what happens" therapists.

Baldini and Pannacciulli (1960) have studied the in vitro maturation rate of reticulocytes and shown the average half-life of normal reticulocytes to be 4.8 hours (SD ± 1.9). This value is less than estimates of reticulocyte half-life in vivo, but since in vitro and in vivo estimates were found to be proportional, in vitro studies were used to determine reticulocyte maturation rates in various anemias. The maturation time was found to be prolonged in thalassemia, in pernicious anemia in relapse, and in anemia of chronic uremia (Fig. 1-24). This increase was attributable not only to the presence of young reticulocytes but also to the relatively longer time necessary for complete loss of reticulum. These investigators concluded that the reticulocyte count in peripheral blood is the result of three variables: (1) the rate of release of reticulocytes from the bone marrow, (2) the degree of immaturity of the freshly released reticulocytes, and (3) the rate of

disappearance of reticulum. The last introduces a variable not usually taken into account.

Nevertheless, under normal and most abnormal conditions the relationship between absolute reticulocyte count and number of erythrocytes produced in the bone marrow is linear. This relationship becomes less regular when the duration of the reticulocyte stage is altered, usually by premature release of marrow reticulocytes into the peripheral blood. This shortens the time spent in the marrow and increases the number of heavily reticulated "young" reticulocytes in the peripheral blood. Thus the number of reticulocytes in the peripheral blood may be doubled, without any corresponding increase in erythropoietic activity in the marrow. This situation can be recognized if sufficient attention is paid to the degree of maturity of the reticulocytes. It is also helpful to remember that an increased rate of release of reticulocytes is often accompanied by the release of normoblasts, easily identified in a blood smear. In some anemias, notably pernicious anemia, the marrow is hyperplastic but few reticulocytes will be found in the peripheral blood.

In the megaloblastic anemias the reticulocyte stage in the bone marrow is of longer duration than normal, and maturation of the reticulocytes in the bone marrow often progresses to complete loss of reticulum before the cells are released. In other anemias the combination of hyperplastic marrow and reticulocytopenia of the peripheral blood has led to the concept of maturation arrest, attractive but difficult to prove. Whatever the mechanism involved, it is important to appreciate that marrow erythropoiesis may be intense yet ineffective.

A comparison between effective erythropoiesis and total erythropoiesis in the anemias is given in Table 1-4.

Leukopoiesis
Kinetics of granulocytopoiesis

The preceding material on erythropoiesis will seem more complete and definitive than the following discussion of leukopoiesis for two reasons: (1) there is more information available concerning erythropoiesis and (2) some of the fundamental difficulties encountered in dealing with leukopoiesis do not apply to erythropoiesis. On one hand, the only blood cells that can be completely accounted for in the bone marrow and peripheral blood are those of the erythrocytic series. These cells remain in the peripheral blood from the time they enter the vascular system until they die, about 120 days later. Leukocytes, on the other hand, enter and leave the blood several times between birth and death, a nomadic restlessness that makes census taking difficult. Those counted in the peripheral blood represent cells in temporary residence and a small fraction of the total population. To carry the simile further, this transient population includes members of various independent tribes, each governed by its own laws, each independent of the other, and each genetically conditioned to a different life cycle. When erythrocytes die, the remains are disposed of in a predictable way that yields known catabolic products from which the number of original cells can be determined with accuracy. Leukocytes, on the other hand, do not contain so convenient and characteristic a substance as hemoglobin. It has taken considerable ingenuity to learn what we do know about the processes of leukopoiesis. Even so, what is known about leukopoiesis is far from being complete. By analogy with erythropoiesis it must be assumed that one or more stimulatory substances exist that deserve to be called leukopoietins. Assuming that such leukopoiesis-stimulating activity or activities exist, we must deal with striking differences between erythropoiesis and leukopoiesis, namely, that leukopoiesis produces a variety of cell types and that the study of leukopoiesis involves not only proliferative phenomena but also the release of leukocytes from the bone marrow. Leukocytosis produced by injecting a substance into an experimental animal may therefore be either a stimulus for proliferation of precursor cells or a stimulus for release of maturing or mature cells from the bone marrow or even a stimulus for altering the ratio of sequestered to circulating cells. Erythropoietin, on the other hand, acts primarily on erythropoietin-sensitive stem cells, and to a minor degree on the maturation sequelae, but it has only a slight effect on the release of reticulocytes and no known effect on the redistribution of red cells in the blood.

STEM CELL COMPARTMENTS. The stem cell compartment consists of two subcompartments—the *uncommitted stem cell compartment* and the *committed stem cell compartment* (p. 4). The uncommitted (multipotential) stem cell compartment contains CFU-S. The stem cell committed to granulopoiesis, CFU-C (Fig. 1-5), is the myeloblast, and it is probable that there is no morphologic distinction between CFU-C and the further committed stem cells BFU-E, CFU-D, etc. Thus it is possible to consider the derivation of bone marrow cells as being monophyletic, if one goes entirely by morphologic criteria, or polyphyletic, if one considers functional categories.

PROGRANULOCYTE COMPARTMENT. Progranulocytes are clearly granulocyte precursors. They are capable of mitosis and differentiate into myelocytes. Generation time, from progranulocyte to myelocyte, is estimated at 24 hours. There are roughly about three times as many progranulocytes in this compartment as there are myeloblasts in the preceding compartment.

MYELOCYTE COMPARTMENT. Myelocytes are also capable of mitosis. They differentiate into metamyelocytes, with a generation time from myelocyte to metamyeloctye of about 100 hours. There are roughly 16 times as many myeloctyes in this compartment as there are progranulocytes in the preceding compartment.

METAMYELOCYTE, BAND, AND SEGMENTED COMPARTMENTS. From the kinetic standpoint, these compartments are similar in that the metamyelocyte, band, and segmented granulocyte are postmitotic cells, i.e., incapable of undergoing mitosis and synthesizing DNA. Since they undergo only successive maturation, the size of the three compartments is approximately equal, roughly the same as the myelocyte compartment. The maturation time for each stage is about 40 to 50 hours.

The mature granulocyte, the segmented cell, deserves special consideration, for it represents the functional end product of the maturation sequence. The total granulocyte compartment can be broken down into two major subcompartments, one portion in circulating blood, the *circulating granulocyte pool,* the other in the vascular system but not circulating because it is temporarily immobilized by marginating in the blood flow and adhering to the walls of capillaries and venules, the *marginated granulocyte pool.* Osgood (1954) calculated that out of the total population of granulocytes (in bone marrow, in circulation, and not in circulation) only a small fraction is present in circulating blood, about $\frac{1}{60}$ of the total (Table 1-2). Most are in the bone marrow, about 60%, and in the marginated compartment, about 40%. These estimates are remarkably close to later estimates (Cartwright et al, 1964; Alexanian and Donohue, 1965), that about half of the neutrophils are in the marginated pool. This marginated pool, distributed anatomically among large organs with rich vasculature (lungs, liver, and spleen), represents a huge reserve quickly available for mobilization into flowing blood, to be increased, if the need is sufficiently great, by accelerated maturation and release from the bone marrow.

There is strong evidence that the high granulocyte count in the peripheral blood in chronic myelocytic leukemia is attributable only in part to increased production in and release from the granulocyte compartments. The life span of leukemic granulocytes is significantly longer than that of normal cells, so that the leukemic leukocytosis in the peripheral blood is caused in part by the accumulation of longer-lived cells (Bierman, 1967). The lymphocyte in chronic lymphocytic leukemia is also long-lived, and the high lymphocyte count in the peripheral blood in this disease is also related to the longer life span.

Granulocytopoiesis and leukocytosis

The precursor that proliferates to form granulocytes and monocytes (CFU-D or CFU-G,M) requires the action of a class of substances, colony-stimulating factor (CSF) or colony-stimulating activity (CSA), in order to proliferate in tissue culture. There is good evidence that in man CSF is produced by monocytes and macrophages (Chervenick and LoBuglio, 1972; Golde and Cline, 1972; Golde and Cline, 1974a; Moore et al 1974; Boggs, 1975). CSF production is stimulated by bacterial endotoxin (Ruscetti and Chervenick, 1974), which also stimulates the release of neutrophils, indicating that the monocyte-macrophage complex serves a double role in bacterial infection, stimulating both the production and the release of neutrophils. CSF is also produced by stimulated lymphocytes (Cline and Golde, 1974). The chemical nature of colony-stimulating factor or factors is not known. One CSF isolated from human urine is a glycoprotein with a molecular weight of about 45,000 (Metcalf, 1972).

The second feature of granulocytopoiesis involves leukocytosis-inducing and leukocyte-releasing reactions. There is considerable literature on substances, occurring naturally or evoked by various stimulants, that cause the mobilization of leukocytes (Gordon et al 1964b; Golde and Cline, 1974b). These substances modify the distribution of granulocytes in the three compartments (bone marrow, marginated pool next to the wall of blood vessels, and the circulating pool) and so are responsible for regulating the level of circulating cells. They do not act on the stem cell pool. Leukocytosis-inducing substances have various degrees of specificity for individual leukocyte types (Miller and McGarry, 1976).

Inhibitors of granulocytopoiesis

A number of inhibitors of granulocytopoiesis have been described: chalones, lipoprotein inhibitors, and prostaglandins (Vogler and Winton, 1975; Broxmeyer et al, 1977; Cline et al, 1978). These are products of neutrophils, macrophages, and lymphocytes. Inhibitors may provide the feedback mechanism for slowing stimulated leukopoiesis. Those derived from lymphocytes may play a part in lymphocyte-mediated suppression of hemopoiesis in some cases of aplastic anemia (Hoffman et al, 1977) and red cell aplasia (Hoffman et al, 1976; Litwin and Zanjani, 1977). Inhibitors, especially the chalones, are thought to act by inhibiting CSF, but the suggestion that they are specific inhibitors of the action of CSF on granulocytic precursors cannot be confirmed.

Lymphocytes

In the last few years the lymphocyte and the lymphoid systems have been shown to occupy a major position in the scheme of the body's defense mechanism. The immunobiology of this system deserves a complete discussion, and this is given in Chapter 3. In this section we will deal only with some basic considerations of lymphocytopoiesis.

DEFINITION. One by-product of the new appreciation of the central role of the lymphocytic system in immune reactions is the disturbing feeling that we are no longer certain what a lymphocyte is. A purely morphologic description, such as is given in Chapter 4, is not sufficient once we realize that the lymphocytes make up a mixed population, some short-lived and some long-lived, some dealing with cellular and others with humoral immunity, some with one repopulation capacity and others with a different capacity. These problems will be considered in Chapter 3. What is considered in this section is, in the classic sense, a purely morphologic approach to lymphocytopoiesis.

ORIGIN. Organs concerned exclusively with the formation of lymphocytes (lymph nodes and lymphoid nodules) are found only in mammals and some birds. In species lower than birds, lymphatic tissue is not discrete, and lymphocytes, along with granulocytes and other blood cells, are formed throughout hemopoietic tissues. Just as the purely lymphocyte-forming organs and tissues appear late in phylogenetic progression, so do they appear late in human embryonic development. Likewise, the appearance of human lymphocytes precedes the full development of lymph nodes. Lymph nodes can be found first in the third month and are well developed by the fifth month of gestation.

The development of lymph nodes in the human embryo is first seen in embryos of 30 mm in size, occurring first in the walls of the cervical lymph sacs. Later, node formations can be found in other lymph sacs and still later along peripheral lymphatics. These early foci are first composed of proliferating stem cells that, as Bloom (1960) points out, *look* like lymphocytes. If they are lymphocytes then, as in the scheme of cell derivation of Maximow and Bloom, the lymphocyte is the stem cell from which other blood cells are derived, for the early primordia soon contain myelocytes and often a few erythroblasts and megakaryocytes. As the embryo grows, these hemopoietic primordia cease making cells other than lymphocytes and normally continue as pure lymphocytic nodules.

LIFE SPAN. In addition to the lymph nodes, the bone marrow, the spleen, the thymus, and the lymphoid tissue in the gastrointestinal tract contribute to the number of lymphocytes in the blood. As we will see later, at least two populations of lymphocytes are derived from these various tissues. Those in the bone marrow and thymus have a short life span (3 to 5 days). Those in the spleen and lymph nodes have life spans of months or even years. The long-lived lymphocytes pass in and out of the blood, tissue spaces, and lymphoid tissue. They are capable of mitotic division, as shown by two examples. First, lymphocytes from donors irradiated for ankylosing spondylitis some years earlier showed chromosomal abnormalities attributable to the radiation when stimulated to undergo mitosis in tissue culture. Second, DNA-labeled lymphocytes from male donors injected into newborn female mice formed clones of lymphocytes having both the male Y chromosome and the labeled DNA.

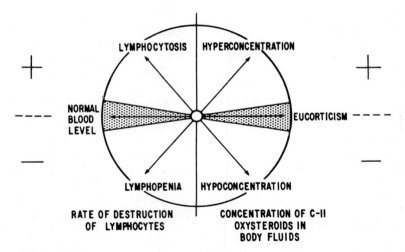

Fig. 1-25. Relationship between blood concentration of adrenocortical hormones and number of lymphocytes in blood. (From Dougherty, 1959.)

FATE OF BLOOD LYMPHOCYTES. The thesis of recirculation of lymphocytes presented by Mann and Higgins (1950), by Gowans (1957), and by Everett et al (1964) seems to be based on good evidence. When the thoracic duct of a rat is cannulated, the lymph collected the first day contains many lymphocytes. After this the lymphocyte count falls considerably. This fall can be prevented if the collected lymph is reinfused into the animal. Further, if lymph collected from another animal is, at the same time, given intravenously to the rat with the thoracic duct fistula, the lymph collected from the cannula remains high in lymphocytes. It can also be shown by isotopic labeling that these lymphocytes come from the transfused lymph and not from the animal's own lymphoid tissue. If this recirculation hypothesis is correct, then it is likely that lymphocytes migrate from the blood to the lymph nodes and thence back into the blood. This recirculation is postulated for the small lymphocytes only, cells constituting 90% of thoracic lymph lymphocytes. Medium and large lymphocytes probably have a life history that is quite different since in vivo they are labeled quite promptly and uniformly. Large lymphocytes also label promptly in vitro with ^{3}H-thymidine, whereas small lymphocytes do not. Since labeling with ^{3}H-thymidine is dependent on active DNA synthesis, it must be concluded that medium and large lymphocytes are actively synthesizing DNA, whereas small lymphocytes are not. The output of thoracic duct lymphocytes varies markedly in different species, being highest in the rat (about 115×10^6 cells/kg/hr) and lowest in man (about 4×10^6/kg/hr).

ADRENOCORTICAL INFLUENCE ON LYMPHOCYTES AND LYMPHOID TISSUE. No discussion of the life cycle of lymphocytes would be complete without some mention of the effect of adrenocortical steroids on lymphoid tissue. Although the effect is predominantly that of producing lymphopenia, it bears on the question of lymphopoiesis and lymphocyte survival.

Dougherty and White (1944) reported that administration of ACTH produced a rapid loss of lymphocytes from the blood, followed within 24 hours by a return to the normal level. This two-phased reaction is called the *lymphopenic response*. The response is not produced by ACTH if the animal is adrenalectomized, but can be produced by the adrenocortical hormones cortisol (compound F) and cortisone (compound E). Cortisol is the major lymphopenia-producing steroid in humans. It is rapidly metabolized, the half-life of free cortisol being about 40 to 50 minutes. Prolonged lymphopenia is thus dependent on a continuous supply of excess cortisol or on interference with its degradation, as in liver disease. Conversely, when there is an inadequate supply of cortisol, there is a tendency toward lymphocytosis (Fig. 1-25). The stress reaction (emotional stimuli, starvation, exposure to cold, etc.) also causes lymphopenia but differs from the lymphopenia produced by cortisol administration in that the lymphopenia is three-phased, there being a first brief period of lymphocytosis (Fig. 1-26). Occasionally a fourth phase, called the "lymphocytotic overshoot" by Dougherty (1959) is seen in which lymphocytosis follows the recovery to normal levels. He suggests that this lymphocytotic response is caused by a relative adrenocortical insufficiency, corresponding to the first phase of the stress reaction in the intact animal.

Many investigators have shown that following adrenocortical stimulation or corticosteroid administration, lymphatic tissue changes follow the same pattern as the changes in blood lymphocytes; e.g., short-term administration of cortisol produces acute involution of the thymus, lymph nodes, and other lymphoid aggregates, followed by restitution to normal. If cortisol administration is prolonged, there is a prolonged suppression of lymphoid tissue, but restitution does occur when hormone administration is stopped. Conversely, there is an increase in lymphatic tissue mass following adrenalectomy. The loss of lymphatic tissue mass following corticosteroid administration has been attributed to three effects: (1) shedding of lymphocyte cytoplasm, (2) pyknosis and, with larger doses of corticosteroids, karyorrhexis, and (3) inhibition of lymphocytopoiesis. It is note-

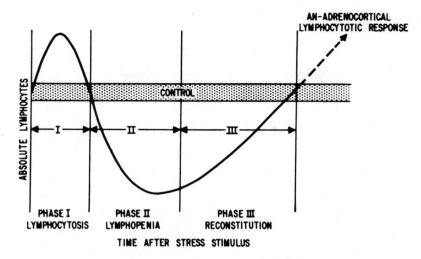

Fig. 1-26. Lymphocytic responses to stress. (From Dougherty, 1959.)

worthy that the small lymphocytes are more susceptible to these hormone effects than are the immature (reticular) lymphocytes.

LYMPHOCYTES AND THE IMMUNE SYSTEM. This subject is discussed in detail in Chapter 3.

Thrombocytopoiesis

Platelets are cytoplasmic fragments of a specialized cell called the megakaryocyte. Three stages of megakaryocyte maturation can be described (Bessis, 1977): the basophilic megakaryocyte (MK1), the granular megakaryocyte (MK2), and the platelet-forming megakaryocyte (MK3). The MK1 cell has a basophilic cytoplasm and a diploid nucleus (p. 148) and normally is classified as a megakaryoblast. The nucleus becomes increasingly polyploid as the cell becomes older, and MK3 cells may have as much as 64 times the normal number of chromosomes. Fragmentation of the cytoplasm of an MK3 cell liberates platelets.

In embryonic life, megakaryocytes are found in most hemopoietic tissues, but in the normal adult it is thought that platelet production occurs principally in the bone marrow. In hemopoietic disorders characterized by abnormal and extramedullary hemopoiesis, megakaryocytes may again be seen in fetal locations, but it is not certain that these function normally in platelet production. Megakaryocytes may be normal, increased, or decreased in thrombocytopenic states (Chapter 17).

Matter et al (1960) have produced thrombocytopenia in rats by exchange transfusions of platelet-poor blood and found that the platelet count began to rise on the second day, rose to higher than normal on the fourth to sixth day, and returned to normal by the seventh day. The new platelets were larger than normal, an interesting observation since large platelets are often seen in human thrombocytopenic purpura. The megakaryocytes in the bone marrow showed no marked increase in number, but by electron microscopy, profound morphologic changes could be seen, consisting of a reduction in cytoplasmic mass and a loss of platelet demar-

cation membranes. The data suggest that the platelet number was restored not by proliferation of precursors but rather by stimulating existing megakaryocytes to make more platelets. This is true, at least, for a situation in which an acute reduction in the number of circulating platelets is produced. The increased number of megakaryocytes, many immature, in the bone marrow in chronic thrombocytopenias indicates that proliferation of megakaryocytes does occur in chronic states.

The observation that plasma from patients with idiopathic thrombocytopenic purpura is able to stimulate thrombocytosis has led to the suggestion that thrombocytosis is stimulated by a humoral facor called *thrombopoietin* or *thrombopoietic stimulating factor,* TSF. Thrombopoietin can be congenitally deficient (Lewis, 1974; McDonald and Green, 1977). A sensitive method for demonstrating the activity of the plasma factor is to inject the plasma into rats in a transient state of thrombocytopenia. De Gabriele and Penington (1967) have shown that the factor is inactivated or removed by platelets and suggest that this may represent a thrombopoietic "feedback" mechanism. Shreiner and Levin (1973) state that the production of platelets by megakaryocytes is controlled by the number of circulating platelets. Krizsa et al (1977) have shown that platelet homogenates inhibit thrombocytopoiesis, inducing a dose-dependent thrombocytopenia and a reduction in the number of megakaryocytes in the bone marrow. Intact platelets are not very inhibitory. McDonald (1973, 1974a, 1974b) has partially purified TSF from sheep blood, produced a rabbit anti-TSF serum, and used this to devise a hemagglutination-inhibition assay of thrombopoietin. Antithrombopoietin antiserum depresses thrombocytopoiesis while having no direct effect on circulating platelets (McDonald, 1978). The immediate effect of antithrombopoietin is to produce a severe thrombocytopenia followed by thrombocytosis. The rebound thrombocytosis is accompanied by proliferation of megakaryocytes in the bone marrow, supposedly because of compensatory increase in TSF (McDonald and Clift, 1979). Newly generated platelets

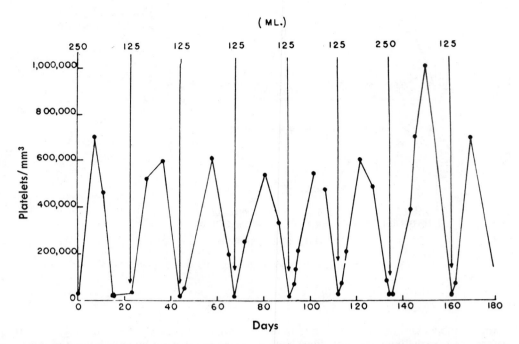

Fig. 1-27. Thrombocyte responses to transfusions of fresh frozen plasma to a patient with thrombocytopenia and after splenectomy. (From Schulman et al, 1960.)

are larger than old ones (Karpatkin and Garg, 1974). In rats, bilateral nephrectomy abolishes their ability to have the rebound thrombocytosis; one possible reason is that the kidneys play a role in the synthesis of TSF (McDonald, 1976). Fetal mouse cells in culture produce both TSF and erythropoietin (Ogle et al, 1978), but not always of equal activity, supporting the suggestion that the two hemopoietins are separate entities (Evatt et al, 1976).

Schulman et al (1960, 1965) first presented evidence that chronic thrombocytopenia may be caused by the deficiency of a factor present in normal plasma and necessary for megakaryocyte maturation and platelet production. Transfusion of normal whole blood, plasma, or fresh frozen plasma was followed by a significant increase in the platelet count, this increase being remarkably constant both in degree and in duration (Fig. 1-27). Of particular interest is the observation that this transfusion effect was more noticeable after splenectomy. It has been observed repeatedly that the platelet count rises sharply after splenectomy, particularly in thrombocytopenic states, indicating that the spleen normally serves as a regulating mechanism, if not in thrombocytopoiesis, then in platelet sequestration and release.

The same investigators have shown that normal plasma is capable of stimulating thrombopoiesis in rats and in humans suffering from idiopathic thrombocytopenic purpura. The activity of normal plasma is reduced by storage at 4° and −20° C. There is some evidence that the thrombopoietin activity is higher than normal in plasma from animals with induced thrombocytopenia. Thrombopoietin activity is demonstrable also in normal plasma (Linman and Pierre, 1962) and in plasma from thrombocythemic patients (Linman and Pierre, 1963). The effectiveness of transfusion of fresh blood in thrombocytopenic states has long been appre-

ciated. While fresh blood is used to supply platelets, these studies make us wonder how much of its beneficial effect may be a result of its thrombocytopoiesis-stimulating activity.

It can be calculated that about 20,000 to 40,000 new platelets per mm³ (0.02 to 0.04 × 10^{12}/1) of blood are produced each day (Mustard et al, 1966) if, as seems evident from various data, the life span (or, better, survival) is 8 to 9 days. Platelets are concerned with hemostasis (see Chapter 17 for the role of platelets in hemostasis and for a discussion of their reactions and function); therefore two types of death can be postulated, one caused by senescence and the other incidental to fulfilling hemostatic functions.

Extramedullary hemopoiesis

The development of extramedullary hemopoietic foci is not infrequent in hematologic disorders. It may be minimal or extreme in degree, the latter accounting for some syndromes characterized by splenomegaly or hepatomegaly. There has been a tendency to separate these syndromes and the phenomenon of extramedullary hemopoiesis into a group of somewhat exotic, poorly understood diseases. Actually an understanding of the basic processes of extramedullary hemopoiesis is more important than the system of classification. In this section the process is discussed in general as well as in specific terms, and it is correlated with problems of cell derivation on the one hand and with hematologic disorders on the other. (See Chapter 16 for complete discussion of myeloproliferative disorders.)

Ectopic versus extramedullary hemopoiesis

Ectopic hemopoiesis may be defined as the process of blood cell formation in sites other than those that are nor-

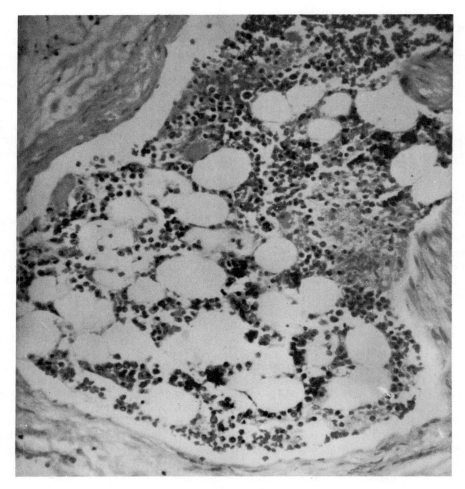

Fig. 1-28. Embolism of bone marrow to lung. The blood vessel is occluded by a fragment of bone marrow composed of a mixture of hemopoietic cells and fat. (Hematoxylin-eosin stain; ×350.)

mally active. The term "extramedullary hemopoiesis," i.e., outside of the bone marrow, is sometimes used synonymously with "ectopic hemopoiesis," but these terms are synonymous only when, as in the normal adult, the chief hemopoietic organ is the bone marrow. The term "ectopic" is also applicable when there is an ectopic formation of blood cells that are normally formed in the bone marrow, such as the granulocytes. In the case of lymphocytes, which are produced chiefly in lymph nodes, spleen, and other lymphoid tissue, extramedullary lymphopoiesis may be considered normal, whereas ectopic lymphopoiesis would refer to production of lymphocytes in organs other than those just mentioned.

Bone marrow embolism distinguished from ectopic hemopoiesis

Embolism of bone marrow and fat to the lungs is a common complication of fractured bones (Fig. 1-28). Embolism also occurs in the absence of fracture, having been reported as a complication of eclampsia and other convulsive states as well as after closed-chest cardiac massage (Carstens, 1969). Whatever the cause, marrow emboli are distinguished from ectopic hemopoiesis in that they represent embolism of foreign tissue without implantation and continuing activity.

Relation between fetal and extramedullary hemopoiesis

As stated in the discussion of hemopoiesis (p. 6), extramedullary hemopoiesis is a normal process in the young fetus—the liver and spleen being responsible for hemopoiesis until the bone marrow takes over this function. After birth, in a normal situation, marrow hemopoiesis is sufficient to take care of the normal requirements for new granulocytes, erythrocytes, and platelets. The liver and spleen are inactive at this time, although their hemopoietic potential is preserved throughout life. If, for any reason, there is an intense hemopoietic stimulus that cannot be satisfied adequately by increased marrow activity, these organs are capable of reverting to the fetal hemopoietic phase. When this happens various degrees of extramedullary blood cell formation occur in these organs.

Possible mechanisms of extramedullary activity

There has been much speculation as to the mechanism by which this dormant potential is activated. Some have suggested that in case of extreme hemopoietic stimulation, immature cells are swept out of the bone marrow to lodge in other organs, where they proliferate and give rise to an extramedullary focus. This has been referred to as the "colonization" theory. It is doubtful that this process operates in a nonneoplastic situation, particularly when immature cells cannot be found in the peripheral blood. In some leukemias, on the other hand, it is likely that at least part of the tissue "infiltration" by leukemic cells represents a sequestration of cells that may be present in the peripheral blood in large numbers.

Most of the evidence favors the concept that extramedullary foci arise from a local transformation of cells that have hemopoietic potentials. Regardless of which theory of blood cell formation one favors, it is apparent that mesenchymal cells with hemopoietic potentials capable of differentiating in various directions, depending on the need, are to be found at numerous sites throughout the body. It is not correct to speak of this process as metaplasia since it involves only the differentiation of primitive cells in a hemopoietic direction.

Extramedullary hemopoiesis in normal infants

Careful histologic studies in infants and children have revealed that small foci of extramedullary hemopoiesis occasionally persist for 1 or 2 months after birth. In the newborn infant, extramedullary foci have been found in the prostate, adrenals, kidneys, renal pelvis, mammary glands, and the corium of the skin of the sole of the foot. It has been suggested that these foci in the skin occur in relation to sweat glands or sweat gland derivatives; e.g., in the sole of the foot, extramedullary foci are usually found in the neighborhood of sweat glands. Extramedullary foci are more common in the mammary gland of the newborn female than in that of the male, and the interesting suggestion is made that there may be a connection between the location of the hemopoietic foci in the breast and prostate and the tendency of carcinomas arising at these points to metastasize to bone. In normal infants, extramedullary foci are almost never found after the second month of life.

Hemopoietic potential of mesenchymal cells

It seems reasonable to suppose that, although the hemopoietic activity in the spleen, liver, and other extramedullary sites normally disappears after birth, primitive cells remain at these sites that can be called upon to differentiate in the hemopoietic direction by either physiologic or pathologic stimuli. In addition, these "resting" cells are probably capable of differentiating along alternate lines into granulocytes, erythrocytes, megakaryocytes, and possibly lymphocytes. Under the influence of various stimuli the population of an extramedullary focus may consist principally of any one cell type; e.g., in response to an intense need for erythrocytes the foci may consist principally of normoblasts, whereas in other cases the extramedullary foci consist principally of granulocytes.

Extramedullary hemopoiesis in liver and spleen

The spleen is particularly susceptible to hemopoietic stimuli, as evidenced by the frequency of splenomegaly in hemopoietic disorders. This suggests that organs such as the spleen and liver, which are of major importance in fetal hemopoiesis, are more readily stimulated than tissues of minor importance. This may be merely an expression of the larger amount of potential hemopoietic tissue in these organs. In either case the ready detection on physical examination of an enlarged spleen or liver has tended to focus attention on these organs. One unfortunate result has been that the underlying relationship between medullary and extramedullary hemopoiesis has been obscured by the number and variety of "splenic" syndromes, so arbitrarily classified that interrelations and basic mechanisms are not appreciated.

Extramedullary hemopoiesis simulating tumor

Extramedullary hemopoiesis is found not only in organs such as the liver and spleen. Occasionally a mass of extramedullary hemopoietic tissue arises in a location in which a primary neoplasm might be suspected. The underlying hematologic disorder most commonly found is a hemolytic anemia (Coventry and LaBree, 1960). Intrathoracic and paravertebral masses of hemopoietic tissue make up one characteristic group; i.e., Hanford et al (1960) described two instances of massive thoracic extramedullary hemopoiesis in patients having hemolytic anemia (hereditary spherocytosis). One patient also had gout, which is not infrequent in chronic hemolytic anemia. Splenectomy was performed in both; in neither case did the thoracic mass decrease in size. Knoblich (1960) described a patient with thalassemia minor whose hemolytic anemia was diagnosed only after the intrathoracic tumors were found to consist of hemopoietic tissue. Fig. 1-29 illustrates one instance of extramedullary hemopoiesis in a lymph node.

One special type of extramedullary hemopoietic mass has been called *myelolipoma*. It applies to a fairly distinct mass usually found in or adjacent to the adrenal gland and composed of a mixture of fat and hemopoietic tissue. Myelolipomas are usually small and asymptomatic, but Parsons and Thompson (1959) reported the surgical removal of one such mass weighing 1,250 Gm. It is questionable whether this particular location of extramedullary hemopoiesis should be glorified by a special name. Certainly the adrenal gland is not an uncommon site of diffuse foci of extramedullary hemopoiesis. Perhaps the chief difference between myelolipomas and other hemopoietic nodules is that the myelolipomas reported have been a more or less incidental finding at necropsy or surgery; there is apparently no concomitant hematologic disease. Corwin and Nettleship (1959) reported finding in the liver a tumor 15 cm in diameter consisting principally of erythroid cells, which they called *solitary erythroblastoma*.

Relation of medullary to extramedullary hemopoiesis

The relationship between medullary and extramedullary hemopoiesis is shown in Fig. 1-30. In the normal adult the blood cell precursors in the bone marrow produce adult cells under the influence of a maturation stimulus, the intensity of which is in delicate balance with the normal rate of cell survival. Adult or nearly adult cells are then liberated into the peripheral blood to fulfill their physiologic function and

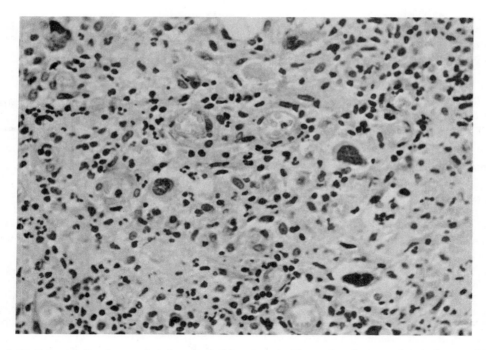

Fig. 1-29. Extramedullary hemopoiesis in a cervical lymph node. The section shows a mixture of neutrophils, mononuclear cells, and the large megakaryocytes. (Hematoxylin-eosin stain; ×250.)

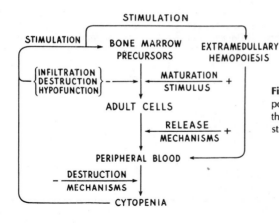

Fig. 1-30. Interrelationships of medullary and extramedullary hemopoiesis in the adult. There is evidence that, in the case of granulocytes, there are inhibitory mechanisms that are operative at the proliferative stages (p. 25).

eventually die. It may be supposed that the rate of cell survival or destruction is the principal regulator of the intensity of the hemopoietic stimulus to the marrow. If one accepts that the life span of a normal blood cell is constant, then it is the marrow that must compensate for increased or decreased needs. The hemopoietic stimulus is intensified if cell survival is shortened, producing peripheral cytopenia. As a result, the hemopoietic activity of the marrow increases. Depending on the intensity of the stimulus, there may be at first increased proliferation of precursors, followed by replacement of fatty tissue by active hemopoietic tissue and in children by an increase in total marrow mass by resorption of cortical bone and enlargement of the marrow cavities. At any stage the marrow response may be sufficient to satisfy the need, in which case either the peripheral blood picture returns to normal or a state of balance is produced

between increased rate of destruction and increased hemopoietic activity, thus maintaining the peripheral blood values at a constant, though lower than normal, level.

Let us suppose that marrow compensation has been maximal, but the need for more blood cells remains unsatisfied. Hemopoietic reserves are then called in, and extramedullary hemopoiesis takes place wherever cells exist having this special potential. It is assumed that blood cells formed outside the marrow also find their way into the peripheral blood. It is possible, however, that some extramedullary foci merely reflect the response to the stimulus and are not physiologically important.

Finally, there are situations in which the bone marrow is functionally abnormal because of infiltration with foreign tissue, destruction by toxic agents, or metabolic suppression. In these cases the marrow cannot respond to the hemopoietic stimulus, which may then be directed to extramedullary sites. If there is no demonstrable marrow activity, hemopoiesis will be dependent on the degree of extramedullary response.

This schematic, partially hypothetical outline may be helpful in understanding the pathologic physiology of the myeloproliferative disorders and some of the otherwise puzzling findings in the aplastic or aregenerative anemias (Chapter 16).

Sites of extramedullary hemopoiesis

Extramedullary hemopoiesis has been reported in a variety of clinical and experimental conditions (Jordan, 1942) (Table 1-5) and ectopic hemopoiesis has been found in many sites (Table 1-6). Fig. 1-31, *A*, illustrates extramedullary hemopoiesis in the spleen of an infant with hemolytic anemia caused by Rh incompatibility. Hemopoiesis in this case is almost entirely restricted to erythropoiesis since it is the erythrocytes that are destroyed at an excessive rate. In the same case there was striking extramedullary hemopoiesis in other tissues such as the liver (Fig. 1-31, *B*) and the subepicardial fat (Fig. 1-31, *C*). Fig. 1-31, *D*, illustrates extramedullary hemopoiesis in an adult with agnogenic myeloid metaplasia. Extramedullary hemopoiesis (erythropoiesis) may be found in renal vessels in instances of shock (Fig. 1-32) and has been described in the skin in neonatal infants suffering from cytomegalovirus or rubella virus infection (Brough et al, 1967).

Extramedullary hemopoiesis, whether compensatory or neoplastic, may be suspected when physical examination reveals enlargement of the spleen, liver, or lymph nodes. It may be confirmed by aspiration biopsy of these organs.

Release of blood cells

It can be calculated that, in a steady state situation in man, 2×10^{11} erythrocytes, 1×10^{10} granulocytes, and 4×10^{11} platelets leave the extravascular spaces in the bone marrow and enter the vascular sinuses and then the peripheral blood. Since the number of blood cells released from the marrow can be increased on demand, the release mechanism is somehow controlled and is not random. There is a difference of opinion as to whether cells are released by an active transport through the endothelial cells (emperipolesis) (Farr and DeBruyn, 1975; DeBruyn et al, 1977) or through endothelial cell junctions (Chamberlain and Lichtman, 1978; Tavassoli and Shaklai, 1979). What is true for one cell type is not necessarily true for all others. In fact, although emperipolesis may be involved in the release of lymphocytes from lymph nodes, most of the other blood cells are released from the bone marrow by squeezing through gaps between endothelial cells.

Electron microscopy has shown that the gaps are much smaller than the blood cells so that a great deal of deformability is required for egress of the cell. Normoblasts passing through such gaps lose their nucleus so that normally very few nucleated erythrocytes are found in the blood. When erythropoiesis is intravascular instead of extravascular, as seen normally in birds and partially in some myeloproliferative syndromes in man (Tavassoli and Weiss, 1973), nucle-

Table 1-5. Conditions in which extramedullary hemopoiesis has been described

A. Clinical
1. Hemolytic anemias
2. Pernicious anemia
3. Anemia associated with liver disease
4. Myelofibrosis
5. Myelosclerosis
6. Hodgkin's disease
7. Leukemia
8. Erythremia
9. Anemia associated with sepsis
10. Myeloproliferative syndromes (aplastic anemia, etc., see Chapter 16)
11. Neoplasms metastatic to bone marrow
12. Severe infectious diseases (congenital syphilis, scarlet fever, diphtheria, septicemia, tuberculosis, pneumonia, kala-azar)
13. Hemochromatosis

B. Experimental
1. Anemia produced by experimental bleeding
2. Injection of hemolysins and other cytotoxins
3. Splenectomy followed by bleeding or ionizing radiation
4. Ionizing radiation
5. Experimental leukemia or transplantable tumors
6. Injection of viable or killed bacteria
7. Injection of cell emulsions or cell breakdown products

Table 1-6. Sites at which ectopic hemopoiesis has been reported

1. Spleen	15. Lungs
2. Liver	16. Pleura
3. Lymph nodes	17. Thyroid gland
4. Adrenal glands	18. Skeletal muscle
5. Renal parenchyma	19. Choroid of eye
6. Renal pelvis	20. Arterial walls in tuberculous areas
7. Ureter	
8. Sole of foot	21. Pancreas
9. Breast	22. Epicardium
10. Subcutaneous tissues	23. Nasal polyps
11. Calcified arterial plaques	24. Endometrial polyps
12. Wall of vena cava	25. Various malignant tumors
13. Cardiac valves	26. Subserosal fat of intestine
14. Tonsils	27. Prostate

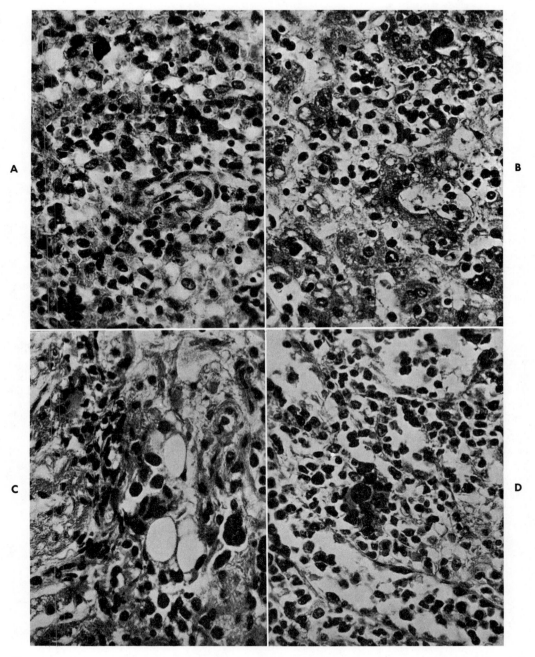

Fig. 1-31. A-C, Extramedullary hemopoiesis at various sites in an infant with hemolytic anemia. **A,** Spleen (most of the cells are normoblasts). **B,** Liver (most of the cells are normoblasts). **C,** Subepicardial fat (most of the cells are normoblasts, but some myeloid cells and one megakaryocyte are also present). **D,** Extramedullary hemopoiesis in the spleen of an adult with agnogenic myeloid metaplasia.

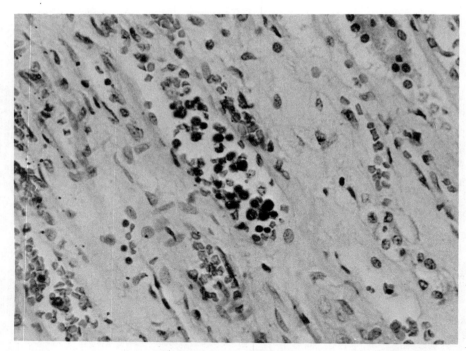

Fig. 1-32. Extramedullary hemopoiesis (erythropoiesis) in the kidney in shock. Note the normoblasts. (Hematoxylin-eosin stain; ×250.)

ated erythrocytes are present in blood. In the granulocytic series it is probable that adult cells are more easily deformed than immature cells (Lichtman, 1970). Megakaryocytes are located very near the walls of bone marrow sinuses (Lichtman et al, 1978). Platelets are released by penetration of a bud of platelet-rich cytoplasm through the sinus wall, the nucleus remaining in the original extravascular location. The cytoplasmic fragment undergoes further fragmentation in the circulation to liberate the platelets. Only rarely, and then in myeloproliferative diseases, do entire cells or nuclear fragments penetrate the sinus wall and enter the circulation.

2

"She snatched at those berries
that grew on that vine.
She gobbled down four, five, six,
seven, eight, nine!
And she didn't stop eating,
young Gertrude McFuzz,
Till she'd eaten three dozen!
That's all that there was."

Dr. Seuss: *Gertrude McFuzz*

The reticuloendothelial system

II. Phagocytosis, pinocytosis, lysosomal storage diseases, and the spleen

INTRODUCTION
INGESTIVE AND DIGESTIVE FUNCTIONS
  Endoplasmic reticulum and lysosomes
  Digestive capacity of lysosomes
LYSOSOMES AND STORAGE DISEASES
  Gaucher's disease (glucosyl ceramide lipidosis)
    The sphingolipids
    The metabolic defect
    Clinical features
    Diagnosis
  Niemann-Pick disease (sphingomyelin lipidosis)
    The metabolic defect
    Clinical features
    Diagnosis
  The sea-blue histiocyte syndrome
  The Chediak-Higashi syndrome
  Lysosomal storage of lipomucopolysaccharides
  RES proliferation: idiopathic histiocytosis
THE SPLEEN AS AN ORGAN OF THE RES
  Structure of the spleen
  Functions of the spleen
    A hemopoietic and immunologic organ
    Storage of iron and other normal metabolites
    Phagocytosis of foreign particles and microorganisms
    Sequestration and destruction of blood cells
  Congenital anomalies
  Atrophy
  In systemic infections
  In hemolytic anemia
  In other diseases of blood and blood-forming organs
  In autoimmune diseases
  Biopsy of the spleen
    Indications and contraindications
    Site of puncture
    Puncture technic
    Normal and abnormal splenograms**

INTRODUCTION

In Chapter 1 we described the role of the RES in hemopoiesis. In this chapter we turn our attention to a second major function, that of disposing of blood cells and metabolites that, for one reason or another, are no longer useful and must be disposed of lest the body be glutted with garbage. At the same time, the RE cells are endowed with exquisite discrimination, for under normal conditions only damaged or senescent blood cells are attacked. Furthermore, some by-products are eliminated while others are conscientiously returned to metabolic pools, e.g., hemoglobin iron and globin.

When the RE cells are normal we see them performing these functions neatly and efficiently. In some instances the amount of metabolite is so large that the cells' storage ability is taxed to the limit and they gorge themselves to death, so to speak. As an example, this is the case when for one reason or another the intake of iron is so great that the phagocytes become engorged with iron-containing pigments. In other situations the phagocytic RE cell is gentically defective and its lysosomal digestive processes deficient in the necessary enzymes to degrade metabolic products taken into the cell. In these important abnormalities the unaltered metabolite is retained by the RE cell and its cytoplasm becomes engorged with accumulated metabolite. This unfortunate situation gives rise to a group of *RE storage diseases* or, more accurately, to *lysosomal storage diseases* that are classified on the basis of the genetically deficient lysosomal enzyme and the metabolite stored in excess.

We will have to deal with this subject at both the cellular and organ level. At the cellular level we have the physical and biochemical processes by which substances to be destroyed or metabolized enter the phagocytic cell, what

35

they encounter when they get there, and what happens to them under normal or abnormal conditions. At the organ level we have the spleen, liver, and bone marrow as major and identifiable organs of the RES, rich in phagocytic cells so that they become involved, and enlarged in the case of the spleen (splenomegaly) and the liver (hepatomegaly), whenever large numbers of RE cells are involved. Thus splenomegaly and hepatomegaly are common indicators of RE reaction or malfunction. Furthermore, there are some special functions of the spleen, which, so far as is known, are not shared by other collections of RE cells, and this is still another reason for not limiting the discussion to what happens at the cellular level. Finally, it is impossible to cover some subjects, however interesting, in great detail in a text devoted to hematology, so that in general we will emphasize those disorders of the RES that have hematologic expression.

The events at the cellular and biochemical levels will occupy our attention first. The interested reader will find complete reviews of the lysosomal storage diseases in Hers and Van Hoof (1973), Van Furth (1975), Unanue (1976), and Stanbury et al (1978).

INGESTIVE AND DIGESTIVE FUNCTIONS

All normal and abnormal metabolic and storage functions of macrophages depend on the ability of the cell to take in metabolites and foreign material. Early classic studies showed that colloidal dyes or particulate substances injected intravenously are cleared from the blood and found in the cytoplasm of the phagocytic cells of the RES, the macrophages or phagocytic histiocytes. At first the ingestion of these substances was referred to as phagocytosis (from the Greek *phagein,* to eat). As noted in the preceding chapter, it was this cellular function that fascinated Metchnikoff and which led to the concept of "cellular immunity." At about the same time Von Behring and others were studying the role of the blood in the immune response, so that for a time cellular immunity and "humoral immunity" seemed to be parallel but unrelated defense mechanisms. Some years later Wright and Douglas (1903) showed that serum contains a substance that stimulates phagocytosis of bacteria by leukocytes. They named the serum factor *opsonin,* from the Greek *opsonein,* to buy or prepare food. Differing from previous investigators, they suggested that opsonins acted not on the cell but on the bacteria, conditioning them for phagocytosis. However, in spite of the conciliation of the two classic defense mechanisms, the investigative tools then available were not adequate to explain the basic mechanisms involved.

Developments in enzyme chemistry, cytochemistry, and electron microscopy have provided the means to uncover the intricacies of phagocytic function, and have revealed a number of cytoplasmic organelles and their function.

Endoplasmic reticulum and lysosomes

Lysosomes are cytoplasmic granules or vesicles that are involved with the catabolism or destruction of substances or organisms ingested by phagocytic cells. The general term used for ingestion by whatever process is *endocytosis.* As shown in Fig. 2-1, ingestion of metabolites by macrophages is accomplished by the process called *pinocytosis.* This function is peculiar to the macrophage and is not shared by neutrophilic leukocytes. Microorganisms, cellular debris, and other large particulate matter are ingested by *phagocytosis.* In primitive animal species, ingestion of bacteria and other foreign cells involves nonspecific interactions between glycoproteins in the cell membrane of macrophages and carbohydrates in the foreign cell wall (Weir and Ögmundsdóttir, 1977). In vertebrates there is an additional mechanism involving opsonins in general and, specifically, receptors at the macrophage surface for the Fc component of immunoglobulins and the C3 component of the complement system. The macrophage membrane also binds fibrinogen, probably at sites distinct from those for immunoglobulins and complement (Colvin and Dvorak, 1975). In either case, there is an invagination of the cell membrane, forming the *pinocytic vacuole* or *phagocytic vacuole,* respectively, that in turn comes to lie entirely within the cell in the form of a free digestive vacuole (*endocytic vacuole* or *phagosome*). Once this is accomplished, lysosomes come into play.

Primary lysosomes, derived from endoplasmic reticulum and from the Golgi apparatus, normally fuse with the endocytic vacuole and supply it with lysosomal enzymes (hydrolases) active against all classes of molecules—lipids, polysaccharides, and proteins. After fusion with the endocytic vacuole, a *secondary lysosome* is formed. It is here that enzymatic degradation of the contents of the vacuole takes place. The hydrolases are active at an acid pH, and acid phosphatase is a key marker for lysosomal hydrolases. The "storage diseases" to be discussed later are caused by the lack of a specific lysosomal enzyme resulting in a given metabolite not being degraded and accumulating to excess. The primary (nonspecific) azurophilic granules of granulocytes and monocytes are primary lysosomes stained by the complex dyes in Wright's stain. The basophilic granules of basophil leukocytes must also be presumed to be lysosomes since these cells undergo degranulation under certain conditions. In the case of neutrophil leukocytes, a phagocytosed bacterium is first found in the endocytic vacuole. This is followed by fusion of the endocytic vacuole with lysosomes so that these lose their identity, and "degranulation" is said to take place (Egeberg et al, 1969). The primary lysosomes bring to the endocytic vacuole a bactericidal substance or substances, probably of a basic protein nature distinct from acid phosphatase, alkaline phosphatase, or lysozyme (Zeya and Spitznagel, 1969). When the primary lysosomes are deficient in the bactericidal component, bacteria are ingested but not killed; this is the pathogenesis of "chronic granulomatous disease of childhood" (Holmes and Good, 1972) (p. 664), characterized by recurrent multiorgan infections. Deficiency of primary lysosomal myeloperoxidase of neutrophil leukocytes has been described (Lehrer and Cline, 1969). Myeloperoxidase is one of the few lysosomal enzymes that is not an acid hydrolase, and according to Klebanoff (1970) it is part of the bactericidal system of neutrophils. A myeloperoxidase is also present in the granules of eosinophils and monocytes (Bainton and Farquhar, 1970). An asymptomatic deficiency of myeloperoxidase has been reported (Joshua et al, 1970). The most spectacular lysosomal abnormality of leukocytes is the Chediak-Higashi syndrome. This is discussed on p. 45.

As shown in Fig. 2-1, primary lysosomes are derived from both the endoplasmic reticulum and the Golgi apparatus, but it must be noted that the endoplasmic reticulum is the source not only of lysosomal enzymes but also of non-lysosomal enzymes, proteins, and lipids that are found in the cytoplasm *(cytosol)* of the cell. One special class of enzymes is found in the *peroxisomes* and *microperoxisomes,* characterized by having catalase and peroxide producing and destroying activity. The endoplasmic reticulum also initiates the process of *autophagy* whereby metabolites are segregated in endoplasmic dilations that are then incorporated into lysosomes. This process is responsible for forming inclusions, *residual bodies* or *dense bodies,* of metabolites not subject to enzymatic action, such as the accumulation of iron-containing pigments, the accumulation of α-chains in β-thalassemia (Chapter 14) and of lipofuscin pigment. Residual bodies are also the end product of enzymatic action in secondary lysosomes formed by pinocytosis or phagocytosis. The term *crinophagy* has been used to describe the process of intracellular regulation of endogenous secretory products. In this process, secretory granules fuse directly with primary lysosomes so that the material secreted in excess is immediately sequestered.

The process of *exocytosis* is the reverse of pinocytosis and phagocytosis and accounts for the extrusion of metabolites from the cell. It is debatable whether residual bodies are spit out of the cell by this method, but exocytosis is one of the mechanisms for the liberation of cellular enzymes into the extracellular fluid, the other mechanism being death of the cell and total disruption of the cell membrane. Cell death can, of course, result from a variety of cytotoxic effects, but in the context of this section we should mention the "suicide bag hypothesis," which supposes that self-digestion of lysosomes leads to the release into the cell of lysosomal enzymes, which then cause cell death. The importance or frequency of this sequence is still being debated, but seems to be well documented in the case of gout. Shirahama and Cohen (1974) believe that urate crystals taken up by leukocytic lysosomes damage the lysosomal membrane, causing death of the leukocytes and liberation of hydrolytic enzymes into the joint fluid. The same type of lysosomal damage is produced by phagocytized silica particles in pneumoconiosis.

Digestive capacity of lysosomes

There are many lysosomal enzymes, each with varying degrees of substrate specificity, as will be discussed later,

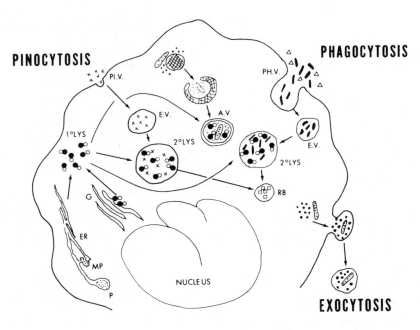

A.V.= AUTOPHAGIC VACUOLE
PI.V.= PINOCYTIC VACUOLE
PH.V.= PHAGOCYTIC VACUOLE
E.V.= ENDOCYTIC VACUOLE
RB= RESIDUAL BODY
ER= ENDOPLASMIC RETICULUM
P= PEROXISOME
MP= MICROPEROXISOME

x= MOLECULAR MATERIAL
I= MICROORGANISM
•= PRIMARY LYSOSOMES
○= HYDROLASE AND OTHER ENZYMES
⋮= CYTOPLASMIC MATERIAL
⬚= MITOCHONDRION
□= DIGESTIVE REMNANTS
△= OPSONINS
G= GOLGI APPARATUS

Fig. 2-1. Schema of the subcellular ingestive and digestive processes taking place in cells capable of endocytosis.

Table 2-1. Some lysosomal enzymes active in intracellular catabolic processes

Enzymes active against proteins
Cathepsin A
Cathepsin B
Cathepsin C
Cathepsin D
Neutral proteinase
Cathepsin IV
Dipeptidylaminopeptidase II
Thyroid acetylphenylalaninetyrosine hydrolase
Collagenases

Enzymes active against carbohydrates
Glucosidases
Xylosidase
Galactosidases
Fucosidases
Mannosidase
Glucuronidase
Hexoseaminidase
Glucoraminidase
Galactoseaminidase
Neuraminidase
Hyaluronidase
Lysozyme

Enzymes active against lipids
Acid lipase
Phosphatidate phosphatase
Phospholipases
Acid sphyngomyelinase
Ceramidase
Galactocerebrosidase
Glucocerebrosidase
Arylsulfatases

but in general lysosomal enzymatic activity attacks most classes of substances that are constituents of cells and tissues (Table 2-1). Except for simple molecules, breakdown of large or complex molecules involves several enzymes acting sequentially (Vaes, 1973) or at specific parts of the molecule. The end products of digestion are either sufficiently small molecules that pass through the lysosomal membrane into the cytoplasmic matrix or, if too large, remain in lysosomes as residual bodies.

LYSOSOMES AND STORAGE DISEASES

The term "storage disease" is much older than the current knowledge of lysosomal pathology. In general, lysosomes become overloaded by one of three mechanisms: (1) lysosomal enzymatic activity is normal but the metabolite is either inert or is resistant to lysosomal digestion (accumulation of lipofuscin pigment in the course of normal cell aging, accumulation of iron-containing pigments when there is excessive breakdown of hemoglobin, accumulation of mycobacteria species whose lipid capsule is resistant to lysosomal digestion), (2) lysosomal enzymatic activity is normal but the rate of pinocytosis exceeds lysosomal catabolic activity (protein accumulation in the tubular cells in nephrosis), or (3) an inborn error of metabolism is present in which a lysosomal enzyme is deficient, the ingested metab-

olite cannot be degraded, and the lysosomes become engorged with that metabolite.

The storage diseases considered here have the third pathogenesis. It must be assumed that some genetic mutation is responsible for the suppression of synthesis of a given enzyme (protein) molecule or, more likely, for the modification of the molecule so that it no longer functions normally. A second mechanism may be involved—the lack of cofactors called *corrective factors,* elaborated by normal cells and capable of correcting the enzymatic defect. When a given enzymatic activity is demonstrably absent, plus the demonstration of reduced enzymatic activity in heterozygous relatives, this is sufficient for concluding that the defect is genetically derived. Identification of heterozygotes is important also from the standpoint of genetic counseling. In most human storage diseases, there is often an increased activity of related enzymes along with a deficiency of the specific enzyme. Van Hoof and Hers (1972) suggest that the storage material has a high affinity for hydrolases that protects them against denaturation or digestion.

Since the bone marrow, spleen, and liver have the greatest concentration of the phagocytes involved in abnormalities of lysosomal storage it is not unexpected to find these organs to be greatly altered, both microscopically and grossly, in the storage diseases. Hematologic expression of the cellular abnormality is not uncommon, at least when the bone marrow and spleen are involved. While there are storage diseases that primarily affect nerve tissue, and these are also lysosomal abnormalities, we must limit our discussion to those that do present problems in the differential diagnosis of hematologic abnormalities or show unusual morphologic changes in blood cells.

Traditionally, the storage diseases have been classified as lipidoses, mucopolysaccharidoses, and so on, depending on whether the accumulated material was thought to be a lipid or mucopolysaccharide. As better definitions of the storage material have become available, it seems obvious that the traditional classification is inexact. A better understanding of the abnormalities at the cellular level makes it obvious that the basic defect is of lysosomal enzymes, and that the nature of the storage material, whether it be lipid, carbohydrate, or both, is determined by the enzymatic defect. While the sequential degradation of lipid or carbohydrate molecules gives some unity to storage diseases where the material is primarily of one class of substance, this is no longer an important aspect of classification.

Gaucher's disease (glucosyl ceramide lipidosis)

There are good reasons for placing Gaucher's disease at the top of the list of lysosomal storage diseases. It is not only the most common, but it is the first storage disease in which the composition of the accumulated material was established and the first in which the enzymatic deficiency was related to the storage abnormality. The elucidation of the basic defect in this disease naturally led to biochemical and enzymatic studies in other storage abnormalities. An interesting historical aside is that when Phillipe Gaucher reported the first case in 1882 he believed it to be a case of "epithelioma" of the spleen. It was Marchand (1907) who recognized that the abnormal cells are engorged with a "foreign" sub-

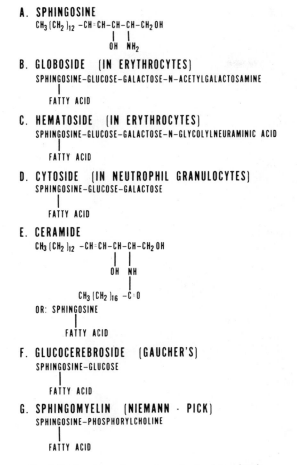

A. SPHINGOSINE

$CH_3(CH_2)_{12} -CH=CH-CH-CH-CH_2OH$
                         OH NH₂

B. GLOBOSIDE (IN ERYTHROCYTES)

SPHINGOSINE-GLUCOSE-GALACTOSE-N-ACETYLGALACTOSAMINE
      |
    FATTY ACID

C. HEMATOSIDE (IN ERYTHROCYTES)

SPHINGOSINE-GLUCOSE-GALACTOSE-N-GLYCOLYLNEURAMINIC ACID
      |
    FATTY ACID

D. CYTOSIDE (IN NEUTROPHIL GRANULOCYTES)

SPHINGOSINE-GLUCOSE-GALACTOSE
      |
    FATTY ACID

E. CERAMIDE

$CH_3(CH_2)_{12} -CH=CH-CH-CH-CH_2OH$
                        OH NH
                            |
          $CH_3(CH_2)_{16} -C=0$

OR: SPHINGOSINE
      |
    FATTY ACID

F. GLUCOCEREBROSIDE (GAUCHER'S)

SPHINGOSINE-GLUCOSE
      |
    FATTY ACID

G. SPHINGOMYELIN (NIEMANN · PICK)

SPHINGOSINE-PHOSPHORYLCHOLINE
      |
    FATTY ACID

Fig. 2-2. Structure of some important sphingolipids.

stance and Lieb and Mladenović (1929) who later showed that the substance was a cerebroside. This is another example of what is undesirable about eponyms.

The sphingolipids

Since Gaucher's disease and some other lysosomal storage diseases are characterized by the accumulation of lipid substances, it is desirable to review briefly some basic aspects of lipid metabolism as they relate to the subject.

Sphingolipids are so named because they are lipid complexes identified originally in brain tissue. The chief sphingolipid is sphingosine (Fig. 2-2, A), which occurs as a number of amino alcohol congeners depending on substitutions at carbon-1. Various classes of sphingolipids are determined by the nature of the substitution at carbon-1 or carbon-2. In sphingomyelin the hydroxyl group is esterified with phosphorylcholine while in cerebrosides, gangliosides, and other glycolipids, molecules of glucose or galactose are glycosidically linked to carbon-2. The basic unit of sphingolipids is *ceramide* (Fig. 2-2, E), the N-acyl derivative with a long-chain fatty acid attached to the amino group on carbon-2 through an amid linkage. Ceramide by itself is not a storage material except in Farber's disease (Van Hoof and Hers, 1973), but when complexed with one or more molecules of hexose (glucose or galactose) it accumulates in various storage diseases. When any of the ceramide trisaccharides are substituted with one or more N-acetylneuraminic acid radicals, the compounds are called *gangliosides*. Storage of various gangliosides is found in some lysosomal storage diseases which are outside the scope of this book.

The metabolic defect

The enzymatic defect is a deficiency of lysosomal glucocerebrosidase resulting in accumulation of glucocerebroside (ceramide glucose or ceramide glucosyl) (Brady, 1978a). Jervis et al (1962) report one case in which the stored material was cytoside rather than glucocerebroside. The chief source of glucocerebroside is ceramide lactoside (cytoside) (Fig. 2-2, D), the major neutral glycolipid of neutrophil leukocytes. Other glycolipids are derived from the stroma of red cells, the major component being globoside and a minor component of hematoside. Under normal conditions these glycolipid wastes of leukocyte and erythrocyte breakdown are degraded to ceramide and the carbohydrate component. Even when there is no enzymatic defect there may be accumulation of glycolipids when more are available than normal lysosomal function can accommodate. Thus in chronic myelocytic leukemia, the breakdown of large numbers of granulocytes accounts for the finding of Gaucher-like foamy cells in the bone marrow and spleen, probably reflecting the accumulation of ceramide lactoside (Kattlove et al, 1969; Brady, 1978a). However, Kirchen and Marshall (1976) could not demonstrate glucocerebroside in non-Gaucher's storage cells. They also noted differences at the ultrastructural level.

Clinical features

Some authors (Hsia et al, 1962) have estimated that more than 300 cases of Gaucher's disease have been reported, but it is likely that the actual number is several times greater since it is probable that only cases of unusual interest become a matter of record. Gaucher's disease has been reported in all age groups, from the newborn to an 86-year-old person (Brinn and Glabman, 1962). Because of the wide age distribution and the varied symptoms, the disease is classified as either type 1 (adult form), type 2 (infantile form), and type 3 (juvenile form). The most common is type 1 (Brady, 1978a). The earlier the onset, the more severe the disease and the shorter the life expectancy. The following features are common to all forms: splenomegaly, hepatomegaly, destruction of bone, hypochromic anemia, leukopenia, thrombocytopenia, and pigmentation of the skin in exposed areas. Pingueculae (triangular yellowish spots on the conjunctiva, usually on the nasal side) are common but not diagnostic. Lymphadenopathy may be present but is uncommon. The disease (other than the cerebral form) has a higher frequency among Ashkenazic Jews than in Oriental Jews and other ethnic groups. The inheritance pattern is autosomal recessive.

In type 2, the infantile form (onset—birth to 1 year of age), the disease is rapidly progressive and death usually occurs before 2 years of age. Characteristically, neurologic signs overshadow all others, with hyperextension of the head, internal strabismus, other motor disturbances, and

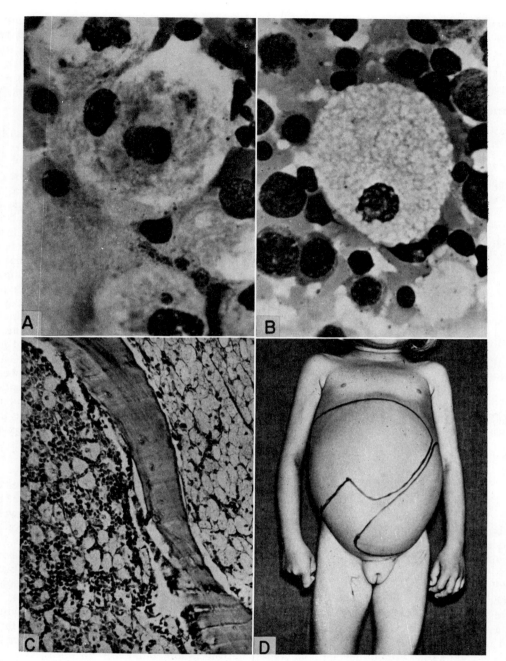

Fig. 2-3. Gaucher's disease. **A** and **B,** Bone marrow smears. (Wright's stain; ×950.) **C,** Necropsy section of the bone marrow. (Hematoxylin-eosin stain; ×100.) **D,** Photograph of the patient during life. The liver and spleen are outlined.

History and physical examination: This 7-year-old girl was apparently well until she was 3 years of age. At that time her mother noticed that she was becoming pale. There was progressive enlargement of the abdomen, accompanied by vomiting and diarrhea for 3 months before admission to the hospital. During the preceding few years the mother had also noticed a brownish pigmentation to the skin. Physical examination revealed a child who appeared chronically ill. The body temperature was 37.7° C. There were generalized lymphadenopathy, splenomegaly, and hepatomegaly, **D.**

Laboratory data: Hb 9.7 Gm/dl of blood, RBC 2.98 million/mm³ (2.98 × 10¹²/l), WBC 43,000/mm³ (43 × 10⁹/l); leukocyte differential count normal; platelet count 11,600/mm³ (0.012 × 10¹²/l). Many Gaucher's cells were found in the bone marrow aspiration.

Discussion: The terminal illness was characterized by cardiac decompensation, hypoproteinemia, and ascites. At necropsy the liver weighed 1,150 Gm and the spleen 1,340 Gm.

mental retardation. The cerebral type of Gaucher's disease is rare among Jews. If a sibling of an infant with cerebral Gaucher's develops the disease, it is likely to be of the same type. The spleen, liver, bone marrow, and other tissues show infiltration with Gaucher cells, but the nervous system does not. In fact, no characteristic changes have been described in the nervous system, and the question of the reason for the severe nervous dysfunction remains unanswered. There is normally a rapid turnover of gangliosides (ceramide-glucose-galactose-*N*-acetylgalactosamine-galactose plus *N*-acetylneuraminic acid linked to the middle and terminal molecules of galactose) in the brain during neonatal life. The turnover involves degradation of glucocerebroside, and it is suggested that if there is sufficient glucocerebrosidase in the neuronal cells, the infants and children will escape damage to the central nervous system.

In type 3, the juvenile form (onset—1 to 8 years of age), there is only occasional involvement of the nervous system. There is rapidly progressive splenomegaly and hepatomegaly (Fig. 2-3). Thrombocytopenia and easy bruising are common. Episodes of unexplained abdominal pain and fever are also common. Destruction of bone, with rarefaction of the distal shafts and erosion of the cortex, is often accompanied by pain.

In type 1, the adult form of Gaucher's disease, the course is usually chronic and splenomegaly may not be detected until the patient is in the teenage years or much older. Diagnosis usually follows the discovery of splenomegaly, thrombocytopenia, leukopenia, or anemia. In some cases the thrombocytopenia may be responsible for abnormal bleeding as the first symptom.

Diagnosis

Anemia is usual and is more intense in the acute infant and juvenile forms than in the chronic adult variant. There is no evidence of decreased red cell survival, and the anemia is normocytic and hypochromic. *Leukopenia* in the range of 2,000 to 3,000 leukocytes/mm^3 (2 to 3 $\times$ 10^9/1) is the rule, with relative lymphocytosis and, at times, monocytosis. *Thrombocytopenia* is usually moderate, 50,000 to 100,000/mm^3 (0.05 to 0.10 $\times$ 10^{12}/1), but may be so severe as to be accompanied by purpura and abnormal bleeding. Characteristically, the *serum acid phosphatase* activity is markedly elevated. Mercer et al (1977) have found the increase to be in acid phosphatase isoenzyme 5, in contrast to elevated isoenzyme 2, which is more prominent when acid phosphatase activity is increased in carcinoma of the prostate. It should be noted that there is no increase in serum acid phosphatase activity in Niemann-Pick disease.

There are reports of Gaucher cells being found in the peripheral blood (Gött and Pexa, 1964), but they are found in abundance in bone marrow and the spleen (Figs. 2-3 and 2-4). They are also found in the liver and in the sinuses of lymph nodes, and at necropsy, in kidney, adrenal, thyroid, and alveolar capillaries. Frederickson (1966a) reports a case in which obstruction of lung capillaries by Gaucher cells led to the development of pulmonary hypertension.

The Gaucher cell is large, 20 to 80 μ, and has a relatively small eccentric nucleus with a coarsely clumped cytoplasm that is filled with a fibrillar pale-staining lipid giving it a "crumpled tissue-paper" appearance (Fig. 2-5). The cytoplasmic arrangement of the lipid is seen beautifully by electron microscopy (Fig. 2-6). The glucocerebroside forms

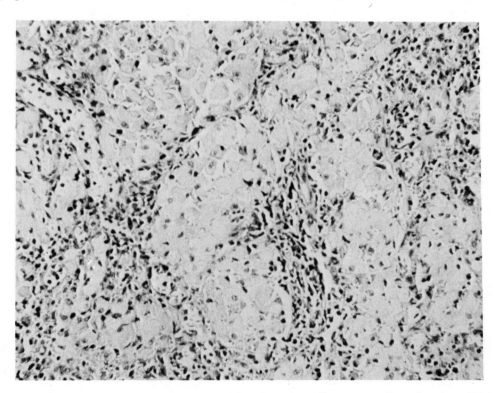

Fig. 2-4. Spleen, Gaucher's disease. Note the nodules of Gaucher cells. (Hematoxylin-eosin stain; ×250.)

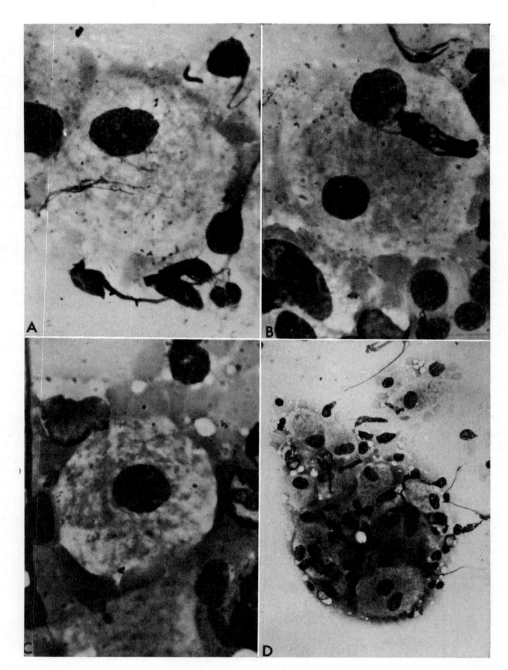

Fig. 2-5. Gaucher's disease, spleen imprints. A 2½-year-old white girl previously diagnosed as suffering from Gaucher's disease, subjected to splenectomy because the spleen had become so enlarged as to produce respiratory distress. Excised spleen weighed 2,100 Gm. Touch preparation was made from the freshly cut surface. (Leishman's stain; **A-C,** ×900; **D,** ×250.) (Courtesy Dr. John W. Rebuck.)

inclusions bounded by a single membrane and obscuring normal intracellular organelles. It is generally agreed that the cytoplasm is PAS-positive, acid-phosphatase-positive, Oil-red-O-negative, faintly positive in frozen sections, negative in paraffin embedded sections (Fig. 2-7), and Sudan-black-B-negative. However, Brady (1972) states that Gaucher cells are Oil-red-O-positive.

Since Gaucher's disease is an expression of a genetically determined deficiency of a lysosomal enzyme, the defect is also present in other than RE cells. The level of activity of glucocerebrosidase in leukocytes from the peripheral blood parallels that in phagocytes, and this provides an additional diagnostic tool (Peters et al, 1975). This technic has been found reliable in identifying heterozygotes. Brady (1978a) and Guibaud et al, (1978) report the use of fetal cells, taken from amniotic fluid obtained by amniocentesis and grown in tissue culture, to monitor pregnancies thought to have a high risk of Gaucher's disease. Cultured skin fibroblasts can also

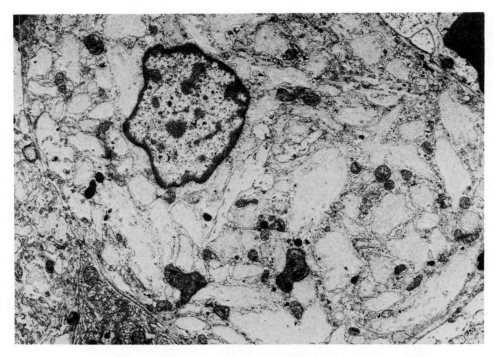

Fig. 2-6. Gaucher cell. (Electron photomicrograph.) (Courtesy Dr. James A. Freeman.)

be used to identify homozygotes and heterozygotes (Guibaud et al, 1978). These technics can be applied to other storage diseases (Kolodny, 1972).

Various approaches to therapy, notably enzyme replacement, are discussed by Peters et al (1977). Dale and Beutler (1976) report on a high-yield method for purifying glucocerebrosidase from human placental tissue. Pentchev et al (1978) compared the properties of glucocerebrosidase obtained from normal spleen and that obtained from Gaucher's spleen and concluded that the enzyme from Gaucher's spleen is structurally altered and catalytically deficient.

Niemann-Pick disease (sphingomyelin lipidosis)

This disease was first reported by Niemann (1914) in a patient with a Gaucher-like syndrome. In 1927, Pick reviewed a number of cases and identified them as a separate entity that he called "lipoid cell splenomegaly." It is the second most common lipid storage disease, with something under 200 cases reported (Fredrickson, 1966b). It is also the second of three inherited metabolic diseases having a predilection for Jewish children (the third is Tay-Sachs disease). There is evidence that this disease is more heretogeneous than Gaucher's.

The metabolic defect

Most authors (Brady, 1972; Brady and King, 1973b) feel that the storage material is *sphingomyelin* (Fig. 2-2, *G*) and that the metabolic defect is a deficiency of sphingomyelinase (Brady et al, 1966b). However, Fredrickson (1966b) points out that in a high percentage of cases the involved spleen and other organs also contain large amounts of cholesterol, in some cases exceeding the amount of sphingo-

myelin on a molar basis. Since the two lipids are derived from different biochemical pathways, it has been suggested that the accumulation of cholesterol is secondary to the storage of sphingomyelin. The accumulation of cholesterol may, however, indicate a poorly understood heterogeneity of Niemann-Pick cases, for in the Nova Scotia variant (p. 44) there is normal sphingomyelinase activity in cultured skin fibroblasts (Sloan et al, 1969) and the primary underlying defect may be of cholesterol metabolism (Brady and King, 1973b). Another lipid found frequently in the foamy cells is *ceroid* (? lipofuscin). Its presence varies from cell to cell. The accumulation of ceroid in Niemann-Pick cells bears on the problem of the ceroid storage diseases (p. 45).

Clinical features

The general features of Niemann-Pick disease are splenomegaly, hepatomegaly, and severely impaired mental development. About 30% of cases have a characteristic cherry-red spot in the macula of the retina caused by degeneration of retinal neurons. The liver involvement may result in mild jaundice. It affects infants primarily, though there are reports of an occasional patient who has been diagnosed in adult life (Pfändler, 1946). Rarely, the disease may develop in utero (Burne, 1953). Death usually occurs between the second and third year. It affects girls more often than boys and about 40% are Jewish.

As noted, the disease is probably heterogeneous, and the patients have been divided into five groups (Brady, 1978b). Group A consists of the classic type, with onset in early infancy, death within a year or two, massive hepatosplenomegaly, and severe brain damage. Group B consists of those with massive hepatosplenomegaly but no brain dam-

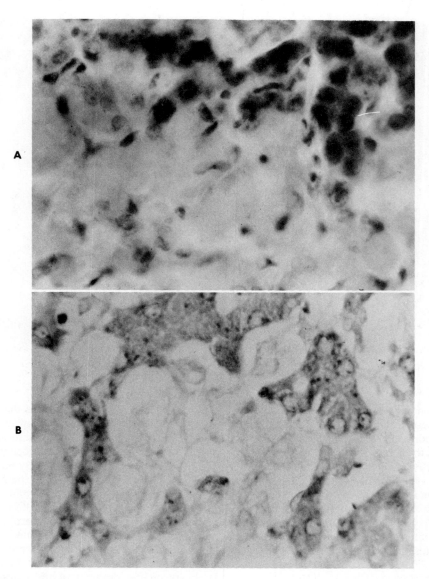

Fig. 2-7. Cytochemical reactions of Gaucher cells. (**A,** Oil red O stain; ×450. **B,** Acid-fast stain; frozen sections, ×450.) Note that Gaucher cell is oil red O negative or faintly positive and acid-fast negative. Compare with Fig. 2-8.

age. Group C consists of patients with less striking enlargement of the spleen and liver, a more chronic course, and late onset of brain damage. Group D consists of a variant known as the Nova Scotian, after patients clustered in that geographic region, and characterized by normal sphingomyelinase activity and a relatively large storage of cholesterol. Group E consists of a small number of adults with moderate hepatosplenomegaly and foam cells in the liver and spleen but no neurologic involvement. Sphingolipid storage is most marked in groups A and B.

Diagnosis

The clinical picture of hepatosplenomegaly and neurologic damage strongly suggests one of the lysosomal storage diseases, and the diagnosis depends on finding Niemann-Pick cells in the bone marrow and other tissues. There are no significant abnormalities in routine laboratory tests. Anemia and thrombocytopenia are uncommon and are mild if present. Occasionally, lymphocytes with cytoplasmic vacuoles are found in the peripheral blood (Crocker and Farber, 1958), but these are not diagnostic as they are also found in Tay-Sachs disease, in neuronal ceroid lipofuscinosis, and other storage diseases (Table 2-4, p. 52). In contrast to Gaucher's disease, the serum acid phosphatase level is usually normal.

The Niemann-Pick cell is found in the bone marrow, spleen, liver, lungs, and lymph nodes. It is as large as the Gaucher cell, 20 to 80 μ. The cytoplasm is engorged with droplets of sphingomyelin so that it appears filled with globular rather than wrinkled material as in the Gaucher cell. The cytochemical reactions depend on varying amounts of sphingomyelin, ceroid, and cholesterol, each of which has

Table 2-2. Cytochemical reactions of some storage cells in fresh smears or frozen sections*

Stain	Gaucher's	Niemann-Pick	Ceroid storage†
Hematoxylin-eosin	Colorless	Greenish-yellow	Brownish-yellow
Wright-Giemsa	Colorless	Blue-green‡	Blue-green
PAS	Positive	Variable	Positive
Oil red O	Negative to slight	Positive‡	Positive
Sudan black B	Slight	Positive‡	Positive
Baker's acid hematin	Negative	Positive	Positive
Luxol fast blue	Negative	Positive	Doubtful
Acid-fast	Negative	Positive	Positive
Autofluorescence	Positive (diffuse)	Positive (nodular)	Positive (nodular)
Acid phosphatase	Positive	Negative	Negative

*Formalin fixation and paraffin embedding removes phospholipid from Niemann-Pick cells, voiding the positive reaction for phospholipid with Baker's acid hematin and Luxol fast blue.
†Primarily the sea-blue histiocyte syndrome, but applies to other accumulations of ceroid-like material.
‡Varies from cell to cell.

individual reactions (Table 2-2). The cytochemical reactions are best studied as smears and imprints, since formalin fixation of tissues removes an unpredictable amount of lipids from the Niemann-Pick cell.

The sea-blue histiocyte syndrome

Since we have noted the blue-green staining of the cytoplasm of Niemann-Pick cells when stained with Wright-Giemsa stain, it is appropriate to discuss conditions in which similar cells may be found in the bone marrow, spleen, liver, and lymph nodes, as well as the significance of otherwise unspecified "foam cells."

If we accept the assumption that the blue-staining material is ceroid (Rywlin et al, 1971a; Reidbord et al, 1972), the term coined by Lillie et al (1942) for an autofluorescent insoluble lipid pigment in the livers of rats with nutritional cirrhosis, we can generalize that this pigment is stored in the lysosomes of phagocytes in a wide variety of conditions. Ceroid is the result of oxidation and polymerization of unsaturated lipids (Hartroft and Porta, 1965).

In the "sea-blue histiocyte syndrome" (Silverstein et al, 1970), splenomegaly and hepatomegaly are present in most cases, purpura and thrombocytopenia in about half of the cases, and occasional neurological damage. The bone marrow and spleen contain many histiocytes with blue or blue-green-staining cytoplasm (Fig. 2-8). The cytochemical reactions are given in Table 2-2. There is evidence that the syndrome is hereditary and probably has an autosomal recessive inheritance (Jones et al, 1970; Blankenship et al, 1973). There are some who have not accepted this condition as a specific syndrome (Kattlove et al, 1970) on the basis that blue-staining histiocytes are seen in many diseases. To further complicate matters, Sawitsky et al (1972) find that the sea-blue granules contain glycolipid, phospholipid, and sphingolipid. The nature of both the stored lipid and the enzymatic defect, if one is present, needs further clarification.

In contrast with the syndrome of sea-blue histiocytosis, similar cells are found in association with a variety of conditions (Table 2-3). In the syndrome, sea-blue histiocytes are numerous, whereas in the secondary conditions, there are usually only a few, usually in the bone marrow,

sometimes in the spleen, and almost never in the liver, and there are often foamy Gaucher-like cells that do not stain blue. Kirchen and Marshall (1976) have observed significant ultrastructural differences between Gaucher and other storage cells. Although it would be comforting to know the exact nature of the stored lipids in such a wide variety of diseases, we can assume that lipids derived from excessive breakdown of leukocytes, erythrocytes and platelets (Kattlove et al, 1970) accumulate in lysosomes of phagocytic cells and that the cytochemical characteristics vary with the lipid that is stored.

The case illustrated in Fig. 2-9 is interesting in that the foam cells were Gaucher-like, but proved to be histiocytes engorged with atypical mycobacteria.

The Chediak-Higashi syndrome

This syndrome may be the most spectacular of the lysosomal diseases, at least to hematologists. Originally an unexplained anomaly of leukocytes, it has now assumed its proper place among the lysosomal disorders (Davis and Douglas, 1972; Van Hoof and Hers, 1973).

The first known instance of the disease came to the attention of Dr. Béguez César and Dr. Montero who, in 1940, referred a 4-year-old Cuban girl to Dr. M. Chediak. Abnormalities in the leukocytes were recognized as unusual and not previously described. In 1952, Chediak reported a full account of the hematologic findings in four members of the original family. In 1954, Higashi reported the same anomaly in an 11-month-old Japanese infant, stressing the strongly peroxidase-positive reaction of the cytoplasmic granules. In 1955, Sato called attention to the similarity of the two reports and suggested the name Chediak-Higashi syndrome. The first report was in fact that of Steinbrinck (1948), and in the European literature his name is often associated with the syndrome.

The disease is inherited as an autosomal recessive characteristic. It affects infants and children, and death usually occurs before the early teens from recurrent infection; but sometimes the necropsy findings are puzzling and have been interpreted as lymphosarcoma (Giloon et al, 1960), lymphoma and leukemia (Efrati and Jonas, 1958), or lymphoma (Padgett et al, 1967). The disease is often associated with

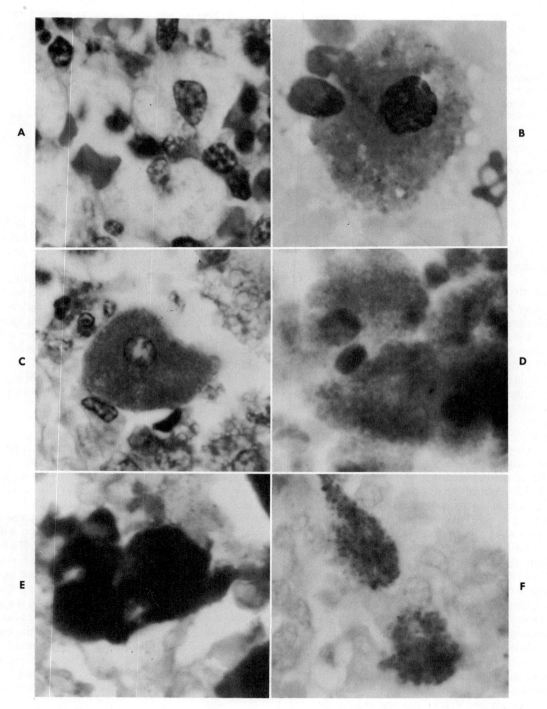

Fig. 2-8. Syndrome of sea-blue histiocytosis. **A,** Spleen. (Hematoxylin-eosin stain; ×450.) **B,** Spleen imprint. (Wright's stain; ×950.) **C,** Spleen, paraffin section. (Sudan black; ×950.) **D,** Spleen, frozen section. (Oil red O; ×950.) **E,** Spleen, paraffin section. (PAS stain; ×950.) **F,** Spleen, paraffin section. (Acid-fast stain; ×950.)

Table 2-3. Conditions in which Gaucher-like foam cells or sea-blue-staining phagocytes have been found

Condition	Reference
Atheromatous plaques	Györkey et al, 1967
Ceroid granuloma of gallbladder	Amazon and Rywlin, 1980
Ceroid histiocytosis in ITP	Rywlin et al, 1971a
Ceroid histiocytosis in a vegetarian	Winkler et al, 1969
Ceroid pigmentophagia in albinos	Bednar et al, 1964
Ceroid storage disease in childhood	Oppenheimer and Andrews, 1959
Chronic granulocytic leukemia	Kattlove et al, 1969; Dosik et al, 1972
Chronic granulomatous disease of childhood	Bartman et al, 1967
Drug-treated hypertension	Imoto et al, 1971
Erythremic myelosis	Karayalcin et al, 1971
Familial lecithin-cholesterol acyl-transferase deficiency	Jacobsen et al, 1972
Familial lipochrome histiocytosis	Ford et al, 1962
Hermansky-Pudlak syndrome	White et al, 1973
Hyperlipoproteinemia	Yamamoto et al, 1970; Rywlin et al, 1971b
Idiopathic thrombocytopenic purpura	Rywlin et al, 1971a
Lymphoma	Mason et al, 1978
Mycosis fungoides	Robinowitz et al, 1975
Nueronal ceroid lipofuscinoses	Zeman and Siakotos, 1973
Niemann-Pick disease	Crocker, 1969
Polycythemia vera	Sundberg et al, 1964
Porphyria and infectious mononucleosis	Ghosh, 1972
Sea-blue histiocyte syndrome	Silverstein et al, 1970
Sea-blue histiocytosis with acid phosphatemia	Blankenship et al, 1973
Sickle cell anemia	Kattlove et al, 1969
Tay-Sachs disease	Kristensson and Sourander, 1966
Thalassemia	Zaino et al, 1971
Wolman's disease	Lowden et al, 1970
Congenital dyserythropoietic anemia	Van Dorpe et al, 1973

partial albinism of the skin and hair and decreased pigment in the retina. The most prominent abnormalities are splenomegaly, hepatomegaly, and abnormal granulation of both granulocytic and lymphocytic cells. Leukopenia and thrombocytopenia are common. An acquired form, the pseudo-Chediak-Higashi anomaly, has been reported in acute leukemia (Van Slyck and Rebuck, 1974; Tulliez et al, 1979), in chronic granulocytic leukemia with myelofibrosis (Tsai et al, 1977), and in progranulocytic leukemia (Toolis et al, 1978). While the blood cell abnormalities are striking (Figs. 2-10 and 2-11), it has been found that abnormal cytoplasmic inclusions are present in many other tissues including skin and hair (Windhorst et al, 1968) and the peripheral (Lockman et al, 1967) and central (Sung et al, 1969) nervous system. Abnormal granules have been seen in all types of blood cells, including megakaryocytes and platelets (Parmley et al, 1979), and surprisingly even in erythroid cells

(Efrati and Danon, 1968). Deprez et al (1978) describe the giant melanosomes in epidermal melanocytes. However, the clinical symptomatology of lack of resistance to infection has focused attention on the granules in neutrophil cells and macrophages.

The abnormal inclusions in neutrophil cells vary on Wright's staining from moderately coarse azurophilic granules in immature cells to large red-purple inclusions in more mature cells. Cytochemical studies show that the giant granules in neutrophils, eosinophils, monocytes, and phagocytic reticulum cells are strongly peroxidase positive. The inclusions in lymphocytes are peroxidase negative. There is some disagreement in the interpretation of stains for lipids, but in general the anomalous granules in the granulocytes and phagocytes are moderately sudanophilic and give a positive lipid reaction by Baker's method. The inclusions in lymphocytes are reported as either sudanophilic or nonsudanophilic by various authors. There is also some disagreement as to the results of the PAS reaction. Some report all anomalous granules to be PAS positive, while others report that only the inclusions in lymphocytes are PAS positive. Mauri and Silingardi (1964) report that the anomalous granules can be either PAS positive or PAS negative, but more often PAS negative or weakly positive, that the inclusions in lymphocytes and phagocytes are PAS positive, and that the reaction is negative after digestion with saliva or diastase.

In addition to humans, the syndrome has been reported in mink (Leader et al, 1963), cattle (Padgett et al, 1964), the beige mouse (Bennett et al, 1969), cats (Kramer et al, 1977), and a killer whale (Taylor and Farrell, 1973). This unusual occurrence has enabled investigators to study an abundance of material (Prieur and Collier, 1978). Ultrastructural studies have shown that early granulocytes lack the primary azurophilic granules and instead form pleomorphic abnormal granules from precursor vacuoles derived from the Golgi apparatus. These undergo fusion to form the striking inclusions in mature granulocytes. The same sequence, with some differences in the structure of the large inclusions, occurs in all species. There is no abnormality of formation of secondary definitive (neutrophilic) granules (not to be confused with secondary lysosomes), which are present in addition to the abnormal granules. The abnormal granules are acid-phosphatase positive, possibly abnormally permeable lysosomes (White, 1966). The only enzymatic abnormality, an increased serum lysozyme activity, may reflect the abnormal permeability of the lysosomal membranes for this lysosomal enzyme.

There is no satisfactory explanation of the severe susceptibility to infection. Defective mononuclear leukocyte chemotaxis has been demonstrated (Gallin et al, 1975) and abnormal neutrophils behave normally during phagocytosis, but have a moderately reduced capacity to kill some bacteria in vitro (Root et al, 1972). According to Boxer et al (1979), microtubule assembly is defective in the neutrophils; this can be corrected by ascorbic acid. This is in contrast to chronic granulomatous disease of childhood in which defective bactericidal activity is accompanied by impaired biochemical activity (oxidation of glucose through the hexose monophosphate shunt) (Nathan and Baehner, 1971).

Text continued on p. 53

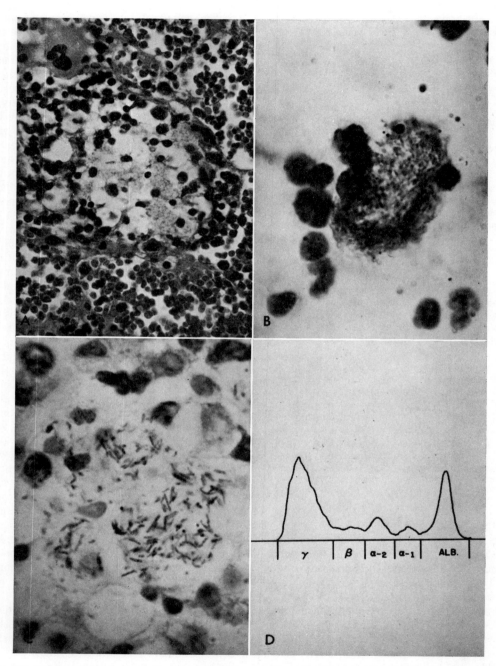

Fig. 2-9. Disseminated infection with atypical mycobacteria (scotochromogen, Group II) mimicking Gaucher's disease and presenting as thrombocytopenic purpura. **A,** Paraffin section of bone marrow. (Hematoxylin-eosin stain; ×400.) **B,** Bone marrow smear, (Acid-fast stain; ×950.) **C,** Paraffin section of bone marrow. (Acid-fast stain; ×950.) **D,** Serum electrophoretic pattern, tracing from filter paper. (Case used by courtesy of Dr. D. Traggis.)

Bone marrow differential count

Cell		Percent	Cell	Percent
Myeloblasts		2.0	Lymphocytes	27.0
Progranulocytes		0.5	Monocytes	1.5
Myelocytes		3.0	Plasmacytes	0.5
Neutrophilic	2.5		Pronormoblasts	2.0
Eosinophilic	0.5		Basophilic normoblasts	6.0
Metamyelocytes		14.0	Polychromatophilic normoblasts	20.0
Neutrophilic	12.0		Orthochromic normoblasts	6.0
Eosinophilic	2.0		Reticulum cells	2.0
Bands		13.5	Atypical histiocytes	4.0
Segmented		2.0		

Discussion: This interesting and unusual case history covers a period of almost 3 years of intensive investigation into this child's problem and is best presented by deviating from the form usually adopted. This white girl died at the age of 3 years. She had been ill intermittently since birth, first with skin rashes that were thought to have an allergic etiology, then with repeated upper respiratory infections that on three occasions were accompanied by high fever and convulsions. At the age of 2 she was admitted to another medical center for a complete evaluation of her various supposed allergies, and at that time was found to have a low platelet count, slight splenomegaly, and minimal lymphadenopathy. An axillary node was excised, but the histopathologic findings indicated only nonspecific hyperplasia. Aspiration biopsy of the bone marrow revealed nothing of note. The diagnosis of idiopathic thrombocytopenic purpura was made, and she was given prednisone, 15 mg/day.

She was seen by our staff shortly after that, and because her platelet count was still low (50,000/mm^3, 0.05×10^{12}/l), prednisone was increased to 30 mg/day. In 2 weeks the platelet count returned to normal (250,000, 0.25×10^{12}/l), and steroid therapy was stopped. However, 1 week later she developed severe purpura, ecchymoses, and pulmonary hemorrhage. The platelet count was markedly decreased (2,000/mm^3, 0.002×10^{12}/l). She again responded to prednisone, 30 mg/day, and blood and platelet transfusions, and within 2 weeks was hematologically normal.

Four weeks later she was again admitted to the hospital, this time because of fever (40° C), nasopharyngitis, and otitis media. She had been on a maintenance dose of 10 mg prednisone per day, and the platelet count had remained normal; during her stay in the hospital the platelet count dropped to 24,000/mm^3 (0.024×10^{12}/l), and prednisone was again increased to 30 mg/day. Bone marrow was obtained by aspiration and cultured for mycobacteria and fungi. Some weeks later, after she improved and was discharged, the bone marrow culture revealed growth of an atypical mycobacterium classified as a scotochromogen Group II. Serum protein electrophoresis at this time was normal; total serum protein was 5.9 Gm/dl, with 2.60 Gm of albumin and 1.25 Gm of γ-globulin.

She was admitted to the hospital for the last time 6 months later, and at that time had splenomegaly, hepatomegaly, and fever. She had prominent Cushing-like features by then, having been on prednisone for about 1 year. Another aspiration biopsy of the bone marrow revealed what seemed at first to be lipid-filled histiocytes of the Gaucher type, but acid-fast stains showed the histiocytes to be engorged with acid-fast bacilli rather than lipid. Culture again yielded growth of atypical mycobacteria, scotochromogen Group II. Atypical mycobacteria were also recovered from tracheal washings and urine. At this time the serum electrophoretic pattern was abnormal with total serum protein of 6 Gm/dl, albumin 1.5 Gm, and gamma globulin 3.16 Gm.

In spite of treatment with kanamycin, ETA, and prednisone, she died at the age of 3 years, 2 months, about 9 months after the first positive culture for atypical mycobacteria. Necropsy established the immediate cause of death to be aspiration pneumonitis; there was disseminated involvement of lungs, spleen, liver, lymph nodes, and bone marrow. There was some tubercle formation in the liver and spleen, but the inflammatory reaction was generally diffuse, and histiocytes that appeared foamy on routine staining were actually filled with acid-fast organisms.

Several interesting questions were raised: (1) Was the overwhelming infection with atypical mycobacteria opportunistic and made possible by long-term prednisone treatment? or (2) Was the thrombocytopenia secondary to the infection rather than idiopathic? In favor of the first possibility, that the thrombocytopenia was of the idiopathic type, is the finding of several normal bone marrow biopsies prior to the one that yielded the positive culture. Histiocytes filled with mycobacteria were not found until late in the disease. Their superficial resemblance to Gaucher cells makes one wonder how often the two diseases have been confused.

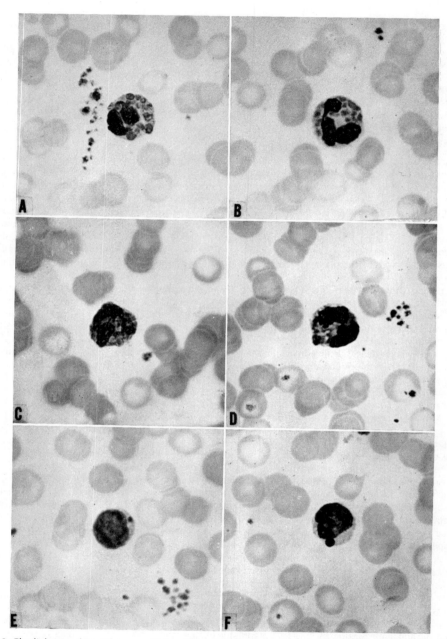

Fig. 2-10. Chediak-Higashi syndrome, peripheral blood. **A-D,** Neutrophils. **E** and **F,** Lymphocytes. (See also Plates 35 and 36.) (Wright's stain; ×750.) (Courtesy Dr. W.L. Donohue.)

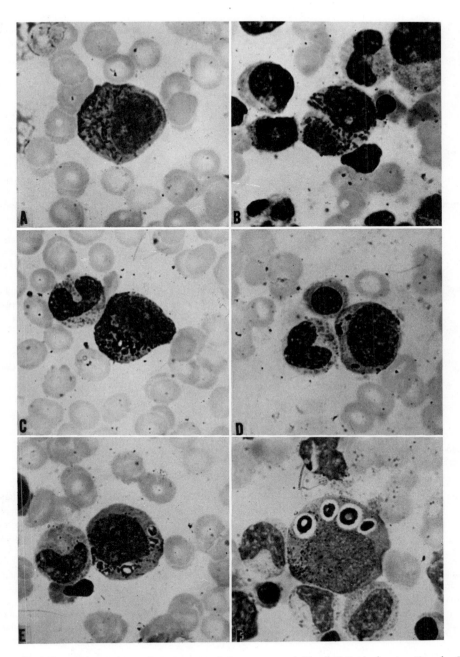

Fig. 2-11. Chediak-Higashi syndrome, bone marrow. **A,** Immature myeloid cell. **B-F,** Myelocytes. (See also Plates 35 and 36.) (Wright's stain; ×750.) (Courtesy Dr. W.L. Donohue.)

Table 2-4. Features of the storage diseases involving mucopolysaccharides*

Number	Eponym	Clinical manifestations	Genetics	Urinary MPS	Enzyme-deficient	Blood cell abnormalities†
MPS I H	Hurler	Clouding of cornea; grave manifestations; Death usually before age 10	Homozygous for MPS IH gene	Dermatan sulfate; heparan sulfate	α-L-Iduronidase	AG;V
MPS I S	Scheie	Stiff joints; cloudy cornea; aortic valve disease; normal intelligence and (?) life span	Homozygosity for MPS I S gene	Dermatan sulfate; heparan sulfate	α-L-Iduronidase	AG;V
MPS I H/S	Hurler-Scheie	Intermediate phenotype	Genetic compound of MPS I H and MPS I S genes	Dermatan sulfate; heparan sulfate	α-L-Iduronidase	AG;V
MPS II-XR severe	Hunter, severe	No corneal clouding; Milder course than in MPS IH; death before 15 years	Hemizygous for X-linked gene	Dermatan sulfate; heparan sulfate	Iduronate sulfatase	AG;V
MPS II-XR, mild	Hunter, mild	Survival to 30s to 60s; fair intelligence	Hemizygous for X-linked allele	Dermatan sulfate; heparan sulfate	Iduronate sulfatase	AG;V
?MPS II-AR	?Autosomal Hunter	Same as mild or severe MPS II-XR	Homozygous for autosomal gene	Dermatan sulfate; heparan sulfate	Iduronate sulfatase	AG;V
MPS III A	Sanfilippo A	Indistinguishable phenotype: mild somatic; severe central nervous system effects	Homozygous for Sanfilippo A gene	Heparan sulfate	Heparan N-sulfatase (sulfamidase)	AG(rare); V
MPS III B	Sanfilippo B		Homozygous for Sanfilippo B gene	Heparan sulfate	N-acetyl-α-D-glucosaminidase	?
MPS III C	Sanfilippo C		Homozygous for Sanfilippo C gene	Heparan sulfate	Acetyl-CoA: α-glucosaminide N-acetyltransferase	?
MPS IV A	Morquio A	Severe, distinctive bone changes; cloudy cornea; aortic regurgitation; thin enamel	Homozygous for Morquio A genes	Keratan sulfate	Galactosamine-6-sulfate sulfatase	AG
MPS IV B	Morquio B (O'Brien-Arbisser)	Mild bone changes; Cloudy cornea; hypoplastic odontoid; normal enamel	Homozygous for Morquio B gene	Keratan sulfate	β-galactosidase	AG
MPS VI, severe	Maroteaux-Lamy, classic severe	Severe osseous and corneal change; valvular heart disease; Striking WBC inclusions; normal intellect; survival to 20s	Homozygous for Maroteaux-Lamy (M-L) gene	Dermatan sulfate	Arylsulfatase B (N-acetylgalactosamine 4-sulfatase)	AG;V
MPS VI, intermediate	Maroteaux-Lamy, intermediate	Moderately severe changes	Homozygous for allele at M-L locus or genetic compound	Dermatan sulfate	Arylsulfatase B (N-acetylgalactosamine 4-sulfatase)	AG;V
MPS VI, mild	Maroteaux-Lamy, mild	Mild osseous and corneal change; normal intellect; aortic stenosis	Homozygous for allele at M-L locus	Dermatan sulfate	Arylsulfatase B (N-acetylgalactosamine 4-sulfatase)	AG;V
MPS VII	Sly	Hepatosplenomegaly dysostosis multiplex; Mental retardation; WBC inclusions	Homozygous for mutant gene at β-glucuronidase locus	Dermatan sulfate; heparan sulfate	β-Glucuronidase	AG;V
MPS VIII	DiFerrante	Short stature; mild dysostosis multiplex; Ring-shaped metachromasia of lymphocytes	Homozygous for MPS VIII gene	Keratan sulfate; heparan sulfate	Glucosamine-6-sulfate sulfatase	?

*Modified from McKusick, 1978.
†AG, abnormal cytoplasmic granulation; V, vacuolated lymphocytes and other blood cells.

Lysosomal storage of lipomucopolysaccharides

Following the description by Hunter (1917) of two brothers having a syndrome of coarse features, hepatosplenomegaly, and chondrodystrophy, and of two similar unrelated patients by Hurler (1919), a general classification of similar cases as *Hunter-Hurler syndrome* became common usage. As variants were described, new eponyms were added, not easily distinguished on clinical findings, with a proliferation of descriptive terms such as gargoylism (for the facial appearance) and dysostosis multiplex (for the skeletal changes). The demonstration of a lipid component in the stored material gave rise to the term lipochondrodystrophy, but it was Brante (1952) who showed that the stored material in the liver cells is acid mucopolysaccharide (modern terminology: glycosaminoglycuronoglycan), while that in neurons is ganglioside. Later studies confirmed that both mucopolysaccharides and mucolipids are involved in the storage defect, and the term lipomucopolysaccharidosis may more accurately describe the biochemical storage. Groover et al (1972), Van Hoof (1973), Kolodny (1976), and McKusick et al, 1978) review in detail the clinical and biochemical findings.

The term "gargoylism" obviously includes several variants of mucopolysaccharide storage abnormality. McKusick (1969) distinguished six phenotypic variants in the group, but the original McKusick classification has since been modified (McKusick, 1978; McKusick et al, 1978) (Table 2-4). Hurler's syndrome (mucopolysaccharidosis I) is the most frequent and shows all of the signs of classic gargoylism: moderate dwarfism, enlarged skull, flat nose, thick lips, deformed thorax, hepatomegaly, splenomegaly, flexion deformities of the joints of arms, legs, and hands, severe mental and motor retardation, and marked opacity of the cornea. The neurologic lesions are characteristic (Fig. 2-12). A vivid but somewhat cruel description of children afflicted with gargoylism is that of Jackson et al (1954): "ugly, blind, weak, pasty, hoarse, big-eared, bushy-eyebrowed, snub-nosed, open-mouthed, hairy, claw-fingered, pot-bellied, knock-kneed, knobby-jointed, dwarfed idiots." Most patients die before 10 years of age, usually of cardiopulmonary disease. Renteria et al (1976) describe the nature of the myocardial damage, which includes infiltration with deposits of mucopolysaccharides and deposition of collagen.

Studies with cultured fibroblasts have been responsible for a potentially important therapeutic approach, the discovery of "corrective factors" (Brady, 1975). These are specific proteins elaborated by fibroblasts and other cells that are capable of correcting the metabolic defect. For example, not only do normal fibroblasts elaborate corrective factors for various mucopolysaccharidoses, but fibroblasts from patients with different syndromes are capable of mutual correction of the storage defect.

Lysosomal storage of mucopolysaccharides is reflected in cytoplasmic vacuolization and enlarged secondary lysosomes in the cells of many organs. Our special interest here is in changes found in blood cells.

Alder (1939) described an anomaly of leukocytes characterized by prominent azurophilic granulation in neutrophils, eosinophils, basophils, and some of the monocytes and lymphocytes. While this was originally thought to be a leukocytic anomaly unrelated to any metabolic defect, the two siblings described by Alder developed skeletal deformities at puberty. In the light of later definitions of metabolic disorders, it must be assumed that Alder's cases suffered from a generalized metabolic disease, a skeletal dystrophy similar to or identical with gargoylism or one of the related mucopolysaccharide storage diseases.

A more specific association of abnormal granulation and gargoylism was reported by Reilly (1941). Like Alder, who did not relate his findings to gargoylism, Reilly did not relate his to Alder's. However, it was subsequently assumed that the leukocytic anomaly described by Alder and that described by Reilly are identical and that they both are stigmata of gargoylism or, in modern terms, of abnormal mucopolysaccharide storage. Accordingly, the literature abounds with references to the Alder anomaly and of Reilly cells in gargoylism.

I must confess that eponymic fuzziness is disturbing in general and in this case in particular. There is no argument with the many well-documented observations that abnormal lysosomal storage of mucopolysaccharides and other metabolites is responsible for the abnormal vacuolization and granulation seen in blood and other cells in the diseases listed in Table 2-4. However, some years ago I had occasion to study peripheral blood and bone marrow smears from two elderly (67 and 72 years old), clinically healthy and normal men (Fig. 2-13). The changes in the granulocytes are indistinguishable from those in Alder's anomaly and in Reilly cells. Yet there was no evidence of generalized metabolic disease of any of the recognized types. The generally accepted association of Alder and Reilly cells with various syndromes does not fit these cases, even though there is little doubt that some lysosomal abnormality is present. My original designation of these cells as Alder's is as unsatisfactory as any other.

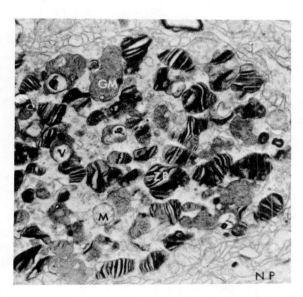

Fig. 2-12. Gargoylism (mucopolysaccharidosis I), brain. The granulomembranous bodies, **GM,** and "zebra bodies," **ZB,** are characteristic. (Electron photomicrograph.) (Courtesy Dr. Fernando P. Aleu.)

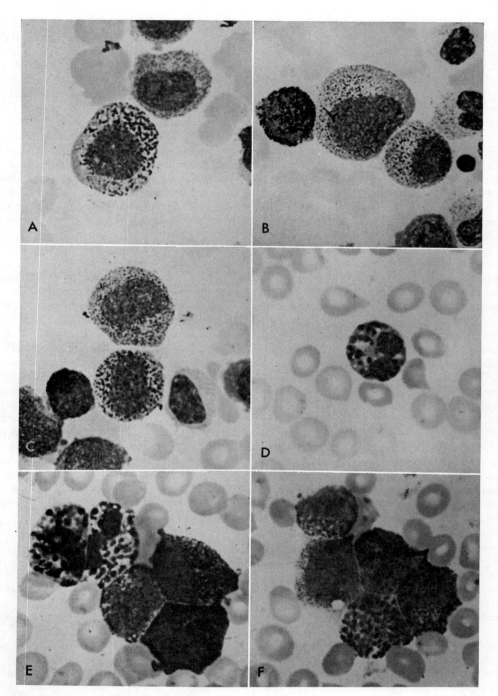

Fig. 2-13. Alder-like or Reilly-like abnormal granulation in blood cells from two healthy and clinically normal, elderly men, 67 years old (case 1, **A-C**) and 72 years old (case 2, **D-F**).

There are other problems of nomenclature and the specificity of eponyms. As noted, "gargoylism" was at one time applied to various syndromes in the group of mucopolysaccharidoses, or at least to the two now thought to be different, Hurler's syndrome and Hunter's syndrome. Groover et al (1972) and Van Hoof (1973) both mention many as yet incompletely defined and unnamed variants. Eponyms have been attached to some of the cellular abnormalities and, although descriptive, should not be accepted as being highly diagnostic. For example, vacuolated lymphocytes are sometimes called *Mittwoch cells* (Mittwoch, 1961, 1963) and are thought to be characteristic of "gargoylism" in the absence of abnormal granulation in granulocytes, but they are found in many other storage diseases (Table 2-4 and Fig. 2-14). These lymphocytes in smears stained routinely show either clear vacuoles caused by leaching out of the mucopolysac-

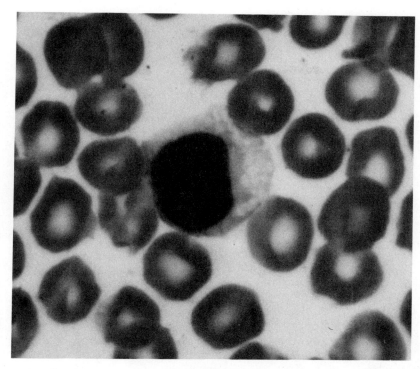

Fig. 2-14. Vacuolated lymphocyte in peripheral blood in familial amaurotic idiocy (neuronal ceroid lipofuscinosis, juvenile type of Spielmeyer-Vogt). Strouth et al (1966) reported that in 12 of 16 children having familial amaurotic idiocy there was abnormal cytoplasmic granulation in granulocytes, the appearance being that of Alder cells.

charide or some residual material that stains dark red-purple with Wright-Giemsa stain and metachromatically with toluidine blue. Lymphocytes showing stainable inclusions are also known as *Gasser cells*. Large histiocytes in the bone marrow containing large red-purple inclusions on staining with Wright-Giemsa and that stain metachromatically with toluidine blue are known as *Buhot's cells*. In one series of cases (Pearson and Lorincz, 1964) these abnormally granulated histiocytes were found in the bone marrow in the absence of abnormal granulocytes in the peripheral blood.

The cytochemistry and ultrastructure of the abnormal lymphocytes in the genetic mucopolysaccharidoses is described by Belcher (1972). In three cases of Hurler's syndrome, one case of Hunter's syndrome, and one case of Sanfilippo's syndrome, 18% to 39% of the lymphocytes in peripheral blood contained 5 to 10 cytoplasmic granules that stained metachromatically with acidic toluidine blue. The lymphocytes tended to be more strongly acid phosphatase positive than normal cells. Electron microscopy revealed cytoplasmic vacuoles, sometimes containing some electron-dense material, enclosed by a unit membrane and sometimes appearing to arise from the Golgi zone.

Rampini and Adank (1964) have emphasized the variability of the presence of the various abnormal cells in the peripheral blood and bone marrow and it is important that both are studied. They reported the hematologic findings in 16 cases of gargoylism. They found the granulocytic anomaly to be present in all 16; 2 were classified as the *complete* anomaly, 14 as the *incomplete*. Of the 14 in the incomplete

group, 12 were classified as the lymphocytic type, showing the anomalous granulation in both the peripheral blood and the bone marrow; 1 was classified as the lymphocytic type, but the anomaly was found only in bone marrow cells.

The *complete* form involves cells in both the peripheral blood and the bone marrow, all of the granulocytes, some of the lymphocytes, and occasional monocytes (Figs. 2-15 and 2-16). After May-Grünwald-Giemsa staining, the neutrophils contain large and coarse, dark purple to black granules. The basophils contain even larger black-purple or grayish granules and contain the same type of granule as the eosinophil, making a distinction between these two cell types difficult. In the lymphocytes the granules are round, dark blue, and usually surrounded by a clear halo. The same type of granulation, but sparser, is found in some of the monocytes.

After Wright's staining the granulation is still obviously abnormally coarse, but not as striking as in May-Grünwald-Giemsa staining. Instead of the normal small neutrophilic granules, neutrophilic leukocytes contain numerous, fairly coarse azurophilic granules. Sometimes the granules obscure the nucleus, which characteristically stains lighter than in normal cells. Eosinophilic leukocytes are even more bizarre, the granules being deeply azurophilic, sometimes greenish gray rather than brick red. The anomalous eosinophilic and neutrophilic granules are strongly peroxidase positive. In contrast with toxic granulation (p. 157) the granules are not strongly alkaline-phosphatase-positive. The basophils are also abnormal, containing prominent azuro-

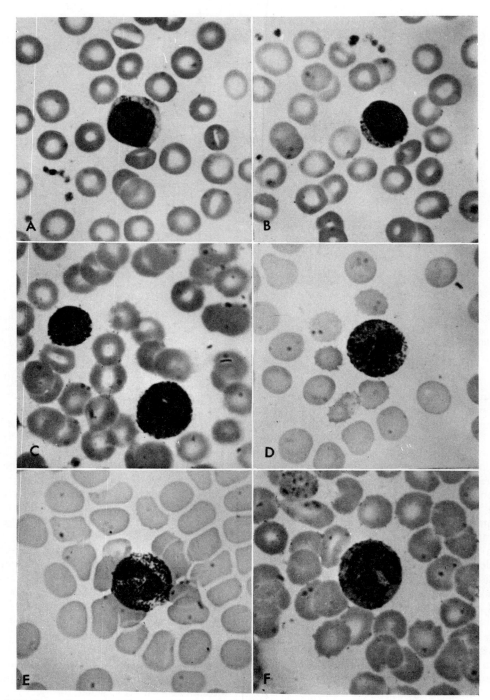

Fig. 2-15. Gargoylism (mucopolysaccharidosis I), peripheral blood. **A** and **B,** Lymphocytes with abnormal granulation. **C,** A lymphocyte (left) and a neutrophil. **D-F,** Neutrophils. (May-Grünwald-Giemsa stain; ×950.) (Case 6 from Rampini and Adank, 1964.)

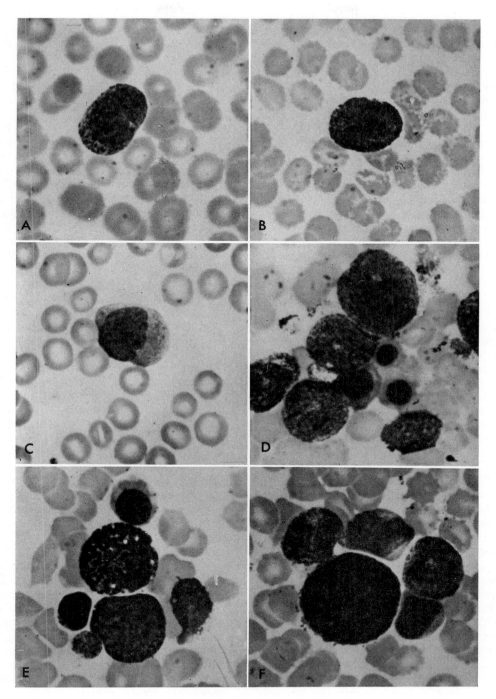

Fig. 2-16. Gargoylism (mucopolysaccharidosis I), peripheral blood and bone marrow. **A** and **B,** Neutrophils, peripheral blood. **C,** Monocyte, peripheral blood. **D-F,** Neutrophils and myelocytes, bone marrow. (May-Grünwald-Giemsa stain; ×950.) (Case 6 from Rampini and Adank, 1964.)

philic granules similar to those in eosinophils. They can be distinguished from eosinophils only by the peroxidase reaction, which remains negative in basophils, and by positive toluidine blue staining. Monocytes also have abundant azurophilic granules, that vary in the intensity of staining; the monocytoid nucleus is preserved. The affected lymphocytes contain few or many coarse azurophilic granules.

The bone marrow cells in the complete form are severely affected. All the myeloid stages except the myeloblast show the same type of abnormal granulation seen in the granulocytes in the peripheral blood. Some of the lymphocytes and occasionally osteoblasts, mast cells, and endothelial cells are also affected.

In the *incomplete* form (lymphocytic type) a few to as many as half of the lymphocytes in the peripheral blood are abnormal, containing large round darkly basophilic granules frequently surrounded by a clear halo (Fig. 2-17). Monocytes are rarely affected, neutrophils never. In the bone marrow, Rampini and Adank (1964) reported abnormalities in most cases, but not so obvious as to be found on casual search. The most frequent finding is abnormal granulation in large cells thought to be phagocytic reticulum cells. Abnormal lymphocytes are present in small number. They describe abnormal granulation also in occasional plasma cells and osteoblasts.

In summary, it seems likely that abnormal granulation is to be found in all cases of classic gargoylism; the anomalous granulation is quite obvious in the complete form of the anomaly, but in the incomplete form it must be searched for diligently. Whereas the complete form affects the granulocytic series in both the peripheral blood and marrow and some of the lymphocytes as well, in the incomplete form the most commonly affected cells are the lymphocytes in the peripheral blood and the phagocytic reticulum cells in the bone marrow, and only in rare cases are neutrophils in the peripheral blood affected.

RES proliferation: idiopathic histiocytosis

The proliferation capacity of the RES at its most malignant—the leukemias and lymphomas—will be discussed in subsequent chapters. Idiopathic histiocytosis is discussed here because it lies somewhere between the storage diseases and the malignant proliferations.

The three diseases falling into this category are *eosinophilic granuloma of bone, Hand-Schüller-Christian syndrome,* and *Letterer-Siwe disease.* In many ways they are quite different, localized eosinophilic granuloma being usually benign, but Letterer-Siwe disease has a serious prognosis. In other aspects, they are often not easily distinguished by pathologic criteria alone, and have at times been thought, without much justification, to transform from one entity to the other. Because of these difficulties and the still unsupported suspicion that three diseases, presenting proliferation of histiocytes as a common feature, might be caused by the same agent, infectious or another type, it was suggested (Lichtenstein, 1953) that they represented variants of a single entity with the suggested name of *histiocytosis-X.* This concept has not been accepted universally (Otani, 1957). Vogel and Vogel (1972) review this subject critically and make yet another suggestion that there are two, not three, entities,

eosinophilic granuloma and Hand-Schüller-Christian disease being one and Letterer-Siwe disease the other.

It is not surprising that basically little progress has been made in resolving these problems of classification and diagnosis, for so far the approach has been necessarily unsophisticated and limited to clinical acumen and pure morphology. Without the basic understanding of the stimulus and response that lead to malignant transformation, or even the more elementary control of normal proliferation of cells, it is not likely that understanding can come by restructuring the available evidence.

In any case, there are two important points to be made:
1. Foam cells, in this case histiocytes containing cholesterol (sudanophilic), are present in tissue from all three cases, many in Hand-Schüller-Christian disease and usually sparse in the other two. Since cholesterol storage is characteristic of the rare Wolman's disease (Patrick and Lake, 1973) and of Tangier disease (Fredrickson, 1966c), and is one of the elements of the storage material in Niemann-Pick disease, these now considered lysosomal storage disorders, it must be assumed that the element of cholesterol storage in idiopathic histiocytosis probably is also a lysosomal defect.
2. While localized eosinophilic granuloma produces no hematologic changes, and in Hand-Schüller-Christian there may be only mild anemia, there is usually hepatosplenomegaly, anemia, thrombocytopenia, and leukopenia in Letterer-Siwe disease.

In Letterer-Siwe disease there is proliferation of histiocytes in all tissues, but particularly the spleen, lymph nodes, and bone marrow. There may be diffuse or nodular infiltration with large mononuclear cells and occasional multinucleated giant cells (Fig. 2-18). Foamy histiocytes are usually present but in small number and are smaller than the foam cells in other diseases. They contain cholesterol an are sudanophilic. Usually the spleen is only moderately enlarged, but it may be very large in affected older infants. Thrombocytopenia and purpura are common. A characteristic rash, papular and sometimes hemorrhagic, may be the first sign of the disease. Infants and children less than 2 years of age are affected and death usually occurs within weeks or a few months after the onset.

Hand-Schüller-Christian disease, on the other hand, is benign and chronic. It affects older children. The most severely affected tissue is bone, and radiologic evidence of multifocal bone destruction usually overshadows the relatively moderate lymphadenopathy and splenomegaly. The osteolytic lesions occur most commonly in the skull, and involvement of the sella turcica and sphenoid bone leads to diabetes insipidus and sometimes exophthalmos. The bone marrow is normal. The histologic picture varies with the stage of the disease, the earliest lesions showing only histiocytic proliferation and eosinophilia while in the late stages there are many foamy histiocytes (Fig. 2-19) that contain cholesterol and are sudanophilic.

Eosinophilic granuloma of bone is confined to bone and is usually limited to a single locus. In order of decreasing frequency, the bones involved are the skull, the femur, the ribs, the mandible, the vertebrae, and the pelvis. The dis-

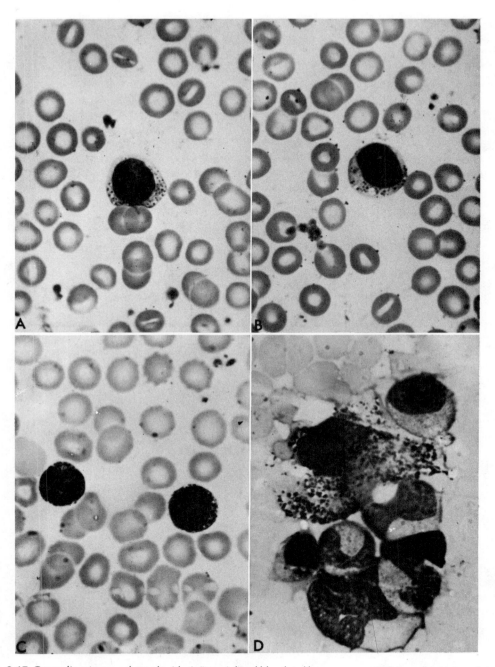

Fig. 2-17. Gargoylism (mucopolysaccharidosis I), peripheral blood and bone marrow. **A-C,** Lymphocytes, peripheral blood. **D,** Histiocyte with abnormal inclusions, bone marrow. (May-Grünwald-Giemsa stain; ×950.) (**A-C,** Case 3; **D,** Case 1 from Rampini and Adank, 1964.)

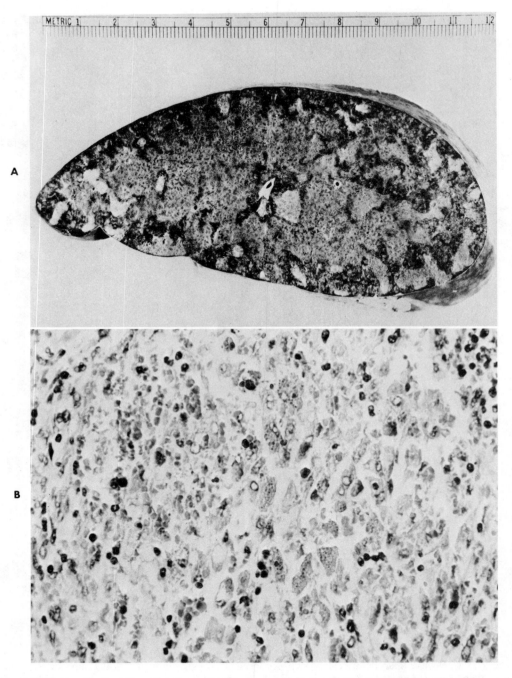

Fig. 2-18. Spleen, Letterer-Siwe disease. **A,** Gross appearance. **B,** Paraffin section. (Hematoxylin-eosin stain; ×250.)

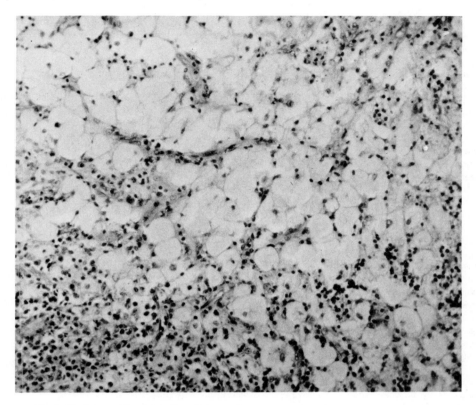

Fig. 2-19. Spleen, Hand-Schüller-Christian disease. (Hematoxylin-eosin stain; ×250.)

ease affects adolescents and young adults, and the prognosis following curettage and radiation therapy is excellent. There are no changes in the bone marrow or peripheral blood, and there is no lymphadenopathy or splenomegaly. Biopsy shows histiocytic proliferation, many eosinophils, and a few cholesterol-containing foam cells.

THE SPLEEN AS AN ORGAN OF THE RES

The entire RES is involved in cytolytic, phagocytic, and storage functions, but some may find it difficult to ascribe such important activities to a diffuse, anatomically indistinct tissue. Since the spleen represents a major portion of the RES, its participation in cell survival and destruction can be taken as a model for these processes in other locations. In addition, the anatomic structure of the spleen is such that there is a sluggish flow of blood through the complex of sinuses. Because of these anatomic characteristics, blood cells, erythrocytes particularly, are exposed in a semistagnant situation to the lytic and phagocytic functions of the RES.

Enlargement of the spleen (splenomegaly) is a feature of many hematologic disorders (Table 2-5) and is sometimes the first sign of hematologic disease. Silverstein and Maldonado (1970) report that asymptomatic splenomegaly is most often caused by portal hypertension, myeloproliferative disorders, Gaucher's disease, or splenic cyst. At one time or another, physicians may detect an enlarged spleen for which there is no explanation.

Structure of the spleen

The spleen comprises the largest single collection of lymphocytes and reticuloendothelial cells in the body. The capsule consists of a thin band of connective tissue with elastic fibers, covered by serous endothelium. In humans, there is no smooth muscle in the capsule and thus, unlike in some animal species, it has no contractile capability. The parenchyma consists of a lymphoid component, the white pulp, seen as tiny gray-white lymphoid nodules, and the red pulp (the "cords of Billroth"), containing erythrocytes in the sinuses and phagocytic reticulum cells, some granulocytes, and occasional plasma cells adjacent to the vascular channels.

The vascular system of the spleen (Fig. 2-20) is not like that in any other organ. The splenic artery usually divides into several branches. These enter the organ at different points along the hilus and travel centrally in the large trabeculae of the capsule. When one of these arterioles leaves the trabecula, it becomes ensheathed with lymphocytes and becomes the *follicular artery* of the white pulp. Distally, the follicular arteries leave the white pulp and enter the red pulp as straight *penicillar arterioles*. These then empty into the venous sinusoids.

There are several opinions as to the nature of the transition between the arterial and the venous vessels. One opinion is that the penicillar arteries open directly into the sinusoids (the "closed" theory); others think that the artery opens first into the cords of the red pulp, from which blood enters

Table 2-5. Classification of causes of splenomegaly according to various splenic functions

I. Splenomegaly primarily due to hemopoietic activity
  A. Granulopoiesis
    1. Reactive hyperplasia to acute and chronic infections
      a. "Acute splenic tumor" of various acute infections
      b. Tuberculosis
      c. Congenital syphilis
      d. Malaria
      e. Trypanosomiasis
      f. Histoplasmosis
      g. Schistosomiasis
      h. Leishmaniasis
      i. Echinococcosis
    2. Myeloproliferative syndromes
    3. Granulocytic leukemia
  B. Lymphopoiesis
    1. Generalized lymphocytic reactions
      a. Infectious mononucleosis
      b. Other viral infections
      c. Hyperthyroidism
    2. Lymphocytic leukemia
    3. Lymphomas
  C. Erythropoiesis
    1. Hemolytic anemias
    2. Chronic anemias
    3. Myeloproliferative syndromes, including polycythemia vera
    4. Erythroleukemia
  D. Other cell types
    1. Plasmacytosis
    2. Multiple myeloma
    3. Monocytic leukemia

II. Splenomegaly primarily due to destructive activity
  A. Hemolytic anemias
  B. Thrombocytopenic purpura
  C. Splenic neutropenia
III. Splenomegaly due to reticuloendothelial hyperactivity
  A. Reticuloendothelial hyperplasia in acute and chronic infections
  B. Disseminated lupus erythematosus
  C. Rheumatoid arthritis
  D. Felty's syndrome
  E. Hemochromatosis and hemosiderosis
  F. Lysosomal storage disease
  G. Amyloidosis
  H. Diabetes mellitus
  I. Lymphomas
IV. Splenomegaly due to vascular factors (congestive splenomegaly)
  A. Cirrhosis of liver
  B. Portal vein blockage
  C. Splenic vein thrombosis and other obstructions
  D. Cardiac failure
  E. Infarction
V. Splenomegaly due to other causes
  A. Primary neoplasms and cysts
  B. Metastatic neoplasms
  C. Macrosomia

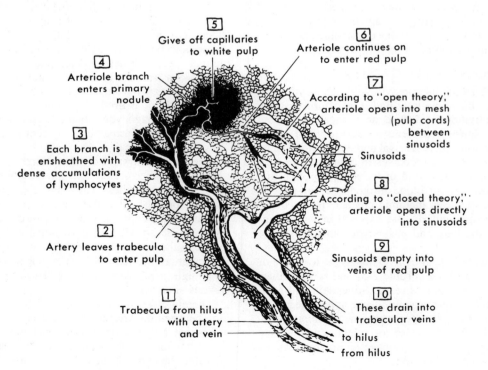

Fig. 2-20. Vascular system of the spleen. (From Blaustein, 1963.)

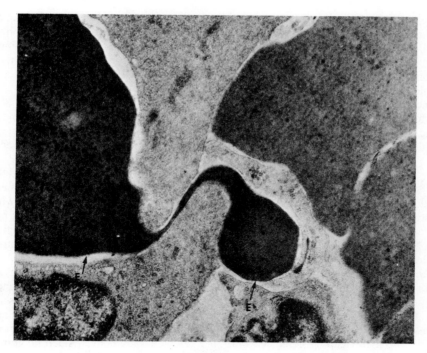

Fig. 2-21. Erythrocyte, **E,** lying partially inside (smaller portion) and partially outside a sinusoid. Spleen, Hb H disease. (Electron photomicrograph.) (From Wennberg and Weiss, 1968.)

the sinusoids through a discontinuous endothelial lining (the "open" theory). Knisley (1936) described yet another system (in the nonhuman spleen), one portion being open and another a closed capillary shunt connecting arterioles and venules (Weiss, 1974).

In any case, it is agreed that blood flow through the sinusoids and red pulp is sluggish. The discontinuous nature of the sinusoidal wall has been confirmed by electron microscopy (Fig. 2-21).

Functions of the spleen
A hemopoietic and immunologic organ

The functions of the spleen can be classified under two general headings (Table 2-6): functions that reflect the function of the RES and special functions characteristic of the organ (Crosby, 1959).

The production of cells capable of making antibodies (lymphocytes and plasma cells) and the role of the spleen as an immunologic organ go hand in hand. The immunocyte system is discussed in Chapter 3. As a discrete and surgically accessible portion of the system, the spleen is sometimes excised when it is suspected to be hyperactive in the production of antibodies. From the diffuseness and complexity of the immunologic system, one can predict that excision of a portion of it would not be expected to achieve much. Indeed, splenectomy has little or no effect on antibody production. For example, if an adult person who has had a splenectomy for nonhematologic reasons (i.e., traumatic rupture) is challenged with certain antigens, that person will form antibodies in no less titer than a normal person with an intact spleen. Supposedly, the antibody-producing role is assumed by other immunologically competent tis-

Table 2-6. Functions of spleen

I. Functions related to spleen as organ of RES
  A. Production of lymphocytes and plasma cells
  B. Production of antibodies
  C. Storage of iron and other normal metabolites
  D. Storage of abnormal metabolites
  E. Phagocytosis of foreign particles and microorganisms
  F. Destruction of blood cells
II. Functions characteristic of organ
  A. Related to erythrocytes
    1. Maturation of surface membrane
    2. Reservoir function
    3. "Culling" function
    4. "Pitting" function
    5. Disposal of senescent or abnormal erythrocytes
  B. Related to platelet life span
  C. Related to leukocyte life span

---

sues. However, there is delayed production of antibodies against capsular antigens of bacteria that the host has not encountered previously (Kitchens, 1977). It has also been found that in the challenged postsplenectomy patient there is production of IgM but poor production of IgG (Sullivan et al, 1978).

Bisno (1971) and Torres and Bisno (1973) reviewed the incidence of infection in splenectomized adults and concluded that postsplenectomy pneumococcal infection is not uncommon. It may occur many years after splenectomy (Haque et al, 1980). Smith et al (1957) presented 19 cases of severe and often fulminating infection in children who had been subjected to splenectomy. In two children, the splenectomy was performed for traumatic rupture and in the others for various hematologic disorders. The different susceptibility to infection in infants and children has been ascribed to "serologic immaturity" of the entire immunologic system. Most authors also agree that the hematologic disorders that are often indications for splenectomy are also accompanied by an immunologic deficiency or abnormality. In this group the incidence of postsplenectomy infection is high. Splenectomy performed to stage Hodgkin's disease is a prime example (Trigg, 1979). Of the 403 children in this group, 7.9% developed serious infections and 16 of those (50%) died.

Storage of iron and other normal metabolites

Phagocytosis of erythrocytes and breakdown of the hemoglobin occur in the entire RES, but normally about half of this catabolic activity takes place in the spleen. In splenomegaly, most hemoglobin breakdown occurs in the spleen. Hemoglobin-derived iron is stored in phagocytic histiocytes. These can be seen to be engorged with hemosiderin (Fig. 2-22) when there is accelerated erythrocyte destruction, as in the hemolytic anemias. When there is a marked increase in stored iron, the spleen is said to be "siderotic." In iron overload, from whatever cause, not only the spleen but other tissues, notably the liver (Kupffer cells), become siderotic.

Phagocytosis of foreign particles and microorganisms

Exogenous substances (such as carbon particles, macromolecular carbohydrate aggregates, and colloid particles) and endogenous pigments (such as hematin and melanin) are cleared from the blood by the phagocytic histiocytes in the spleen and other organs. Phagocytosis of microorganisms contributes to the defense mechanism. As an example, it was noted some years ago that splenectomized dogs succumb to an overwhelming infection with *Bartonella* (Knutti and Hawkins, 1935). This infection, common in dogs, is kept under control as long as the spleen removes and destroys the infected erythrocytes.

Sequestration and destruction of blood cells

In a normal person the spleen contains only about 20 to 30 ml of erythrocytes, but in splenomegaly the reservoir function is increased markedly and the abnormal enlarged spleen contains many times this volume of red blood cells. The transit time is then lengthened, and the erythrocytes are subject to lytic effects for a long time. In part, stasis causes consumption of glucose, upon which the erythrocyte is dependent for the maintenance of normal metabolism, and the erythrocyte is destroyed. Selective destruction of abnormal erythrocytes is also accelerated by the splenic pooling.

As erythrocytes pass through the spleen, the organ inspects them for imperfections and destroys those that it recognizes as abnormal or senescent. This is called the "culling" function. Even more remarkable is the "pitting" function, by which the spleen removes granular inclusions (Howell-Jolly bodies, siderotic granules, etc.) and parasites (Schnitzer et al, 1972) without destroying the erythrocyte. This normal function of the spleen keeps the number of circulating erythrocytes with inclusions to a minimum; by the same token after splenectomy the peripheral blood reflects the loss of the pitting effect. Thus the *postsplenectomy peripheral blood film* (Lipson et al, 1959) (Fig. 2-23) shows Howell-Jolly bodies, siderotic granules, and flat target cells, the latter a consequence of the loss of normal maturation of the surface membrane. The "postsplenectomy blood pic-

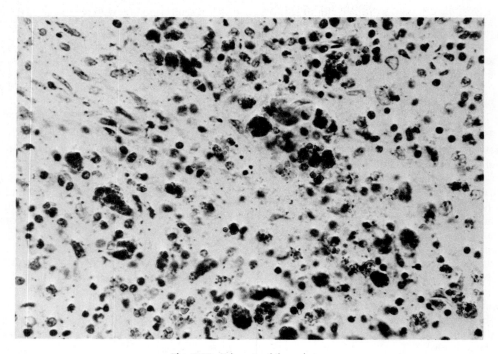

Fig. 2-22. Siderosis of the spleen.

ture" may be useful in detecting torsion of the spleen (De-Bartolo et al, 1973), a nonfunctioning spleen, asplenia, or splenic infarction (Larrimer et al, 1975).

The spleen also pools platelets in large numbers, and the entry of platelets into the splenic pool and their return to the circulation is extensive. In splenomegaly the splenic pool may be so large as to produce thrombocytopenia (Chapter 17). This lowering of the platelet count in splenomegaly has sometimes been erroneously interpreted as increased destruction of platelets in the spleen. Sequestration of leukocytes in the enlarged spleen may, in similar fashion, produce leukopenia.

The concept of "hypersplenism," then, is that in some cases the splenic sequestering effect on one or more of the three types of circulating blood cells (erythrocytes, granulocytes, and platelets) is so striking as to reduce the content of these cells in the peripheral blood (Jandl and Aster, 1967; Jacobs, 1974). This sequestering effect can be demonstrated by the finding that isotope-labeled erythrocytes and platelets accumulate in the enlarged spleen, as evidenced by increased radioactivity of the organ. Hereditary splenomegaly with hypersplenism is reported in several members of three related families by Rao et al (1974).

Congenital anomalies

Congenital absence of the spleen (asplenia or agenesis of the spleen) is rare and by itself causes no difficulties. Quite often asplenia is associated with congenital heart disease (defects or absence of the atrial or ventricular septum, persistent common atrioventricular canal, pulmonary stenosis or atresia, transposition of the great vessels, anomalous con-

nections of the pulmonary veins, and presence of both superior venae cavae with absent coronary sinus) (Aguilar et al, 1956). These abnormalities usually produce cyanotic disease in the young infant but are seldom amenable to surgical correction, in contradistinction to other types of congenital heart disease in which the spleen is normally present. The combination of cyanotic heart disease and a peripheral blood picture characteristic of lost splenic function (Howell-Jolly bodies, target cells and siderocytes) makes this an easily detected syndrome. Extracardiac anomalies are also common in asplenia (Freedom, 1972; Majeski and Upshur, 1978).

A more common congenital anomaly is the occurrence of accessory spleens. This should be distinguished from splenosis, the implantation of splenic tissue on peritoneal surfaces following splenic rupture (Brewster, 1973). In one series of necropsies, accessory spleens were found in about 10% of the cases. One out of every six accessory spleens is located in the tail of the pancreas. Lesions affecting the main spleen usually affect the accessory spleen. It is difficult to distinguish between "congenital polysplenia" (multiple spleens) and the not uncommon finding of "accessory spleens." Rodin et al (1972), among others, have pointed out the frequent occurrence of severe congenital heart disease in polysplenia, but it is not logical to differentiate between polysplenia and accessory spleens by the presence or absence of congenital heart disease.

The least common congenital anomaly is fusion of the spleen and gonads.

Atrophy

Atrophy of the spleen is not uncommon in elderly individuals. It may also occur in wasting diseases. In chronic hemolytic anemias, particularly sickle cell anemia, there is progressive loss of pulp, increasing fibrosis, scarring from multiple infarcts, and incrustation with iron and calcium deposits. The fibrosis and deposition of iron and calcium salts sometimes forms siderotic nodules or Gamna-Gandy bodies (Fig. 2-24). In the final stage of atrophy the spleen may be so small as to be hardly recognizable (Fig. 2-25). Advanced atrophy is sometimes referred to as "autosplenectomy." The peripheral blood then shows all the features of the "postsplenectomy" blood picture (Fig. 2-23).

In systemic infections

Enlargement of the spleen is common in acute systemic infections. The enlarged, soft cellular organ is then said to show "acute reactive hyperplasia." Other terms used are "acute inflammatory splenomegaly," "septic splenitis," or "acute splenic tumor."

The splenomegaly is caused in part by a true reactive hyperplasia of the granulocytic and lymphocytic cells of the pulp and in part by a congestion with erythrocytes. In reacting to the systemic infection, the spleen acts as a concentrated RES defense. The reaction may be to pathogenic organisms, but most often it is to the products of inflammation, substances responsible for the mobilization of neutrophils, lymphocytes, and eosinophils. The spleen can also react to foreign substances not the product of inflammation, such as foreign protein.

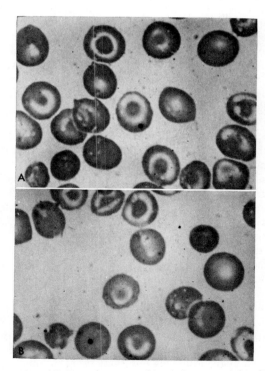

Fig. 2-23. A and **B,** Postsplenectomy blood picture, peripheral blood. Note target cells and Howell-Jolly bodies. (Wright's stain; ×1,100.)

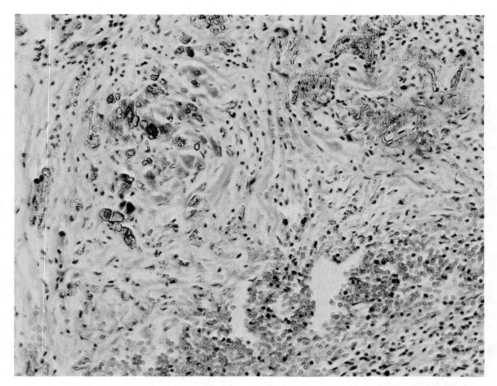

Fig. 2-24. Siderotic nodule (Gamna-Gandy body), spleen, sickle cell anemia. (Hematoxylin-eosin stain; ×125.)

Acute reactive hyperplasia is characterized by an increase in the cells of the red pulp. Neutrophils are numerous, and some may be of intermediate maturity. There is also an increase in phagocytic cells, both of the mononuclear type and of the fixed histiocyte type. These contain ingested debris from dead leukocytes and erythrocytes, and sometimes bacteria and other organisms. A number of plasma cells can also be found. The lymphoid follicles are usually hyperplastic, although the lymphoid hyperplasia may be obscured by the marked congestion of the red pulp. Sometimes the follicles have large reactive centers showing much phagocytic activity.

The large soft spleen in infectious mononucleosis is easily subject to rupture. This complication, necessitating splenectomy, has provided most of the histologic material for study. The spleen is enlarged to three or four times the normal size. Characteristic changes are as follows: (1) large number of reactive lymphocytes (virocytes) (Chapter 3, Plate 59) such as those found in the peripheral blood, bone marrow, and lymph nodes are seen in the red pulp and in the sinusoids, (2) the follicles are usually not hyperplastic, and (3) the virocytes usually infiltrate the capsule, the trabeculae, the adventitia of the arteries, and the subintima of the veins and sinusoids. It is thought that the cellular infiltration and edema of the capsule accounts for the high incidence of rupture.

In hemolytic anemia

Hemolytic anemia is the general term applied to diseases in which anemia is referrable to a decreased life span of the erythrocytes (Chapters 13 and 14). When the rate of destruction is greater than can be compensated for by the bone marrow, anemia results. When there is accelerated destruction of erythrocytes, the spleen's normal role in disposing of damaged erythrocytes is exaggerated and so, in that sense, the spleen plays an important role in hemolytic disease. However, study of the pathologic anatomy of the spleen in these conditions contributes relatively little to an understanding of their pathogenesis, just as a study of the city's garbage disposal plant provides only a superficial impression of contemporary society.

Decreased erythrocyte survival is the result of one of the two abnormal situations: (1) the erythrocyte is itself abnormal, an *intrinsic* defect, and therefore not able to survive normally, or (2) there is an *extrinsic* influence that damages an otherwise normal erythrocyte and shortens its life span. In either case, the spleen seems to dispose of the defective erythrocytes, but especially when the erythrocytes are intrinsically abnormal.

In *congenital spherocytic hemolytic anemia* (hereditary spherocytosis) (Chapter 13) the intrinsic abnormality of the erythrocytic membrane gives rise to erythrocytes that are small and spheroid, rather than the normal flattened biconcave disks with a decreased life span. The two components of the disease are production by the bone marrow of spherocytic erythrocytes and increased destruction of these cells in the spleen. The spleen destroys spherocytes selectively, as shown by the following observations: (1) normal erythrocytes transfused into a person having hereditary spherocytosis survive for a normal time, (2) erythrocytes from a person

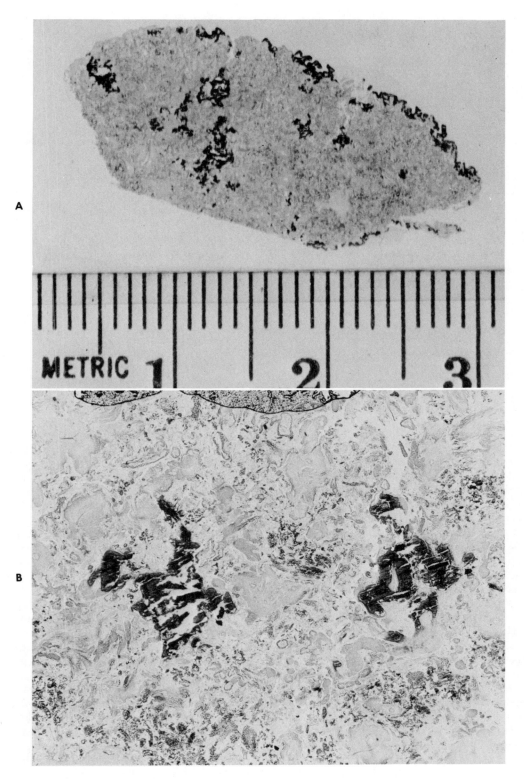

Fig. 2-25. Atrophy of spleen in long-standing sickle cell anemia. **A,** Gross appearance of bisected organ. Photograph shows actual size of spleen bisected along its greatest dimension. **B,** Paraffin section. (Hematoxylin-eosin stain; ×25.) Note complete loss of normal architecture and replacement by fibrous tissue, pigment, and calcium deposits.

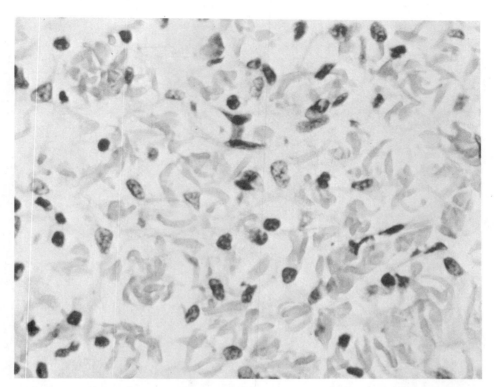

Fig. 2-26. Sickled erythrocytes, spleen, sickle cell anemia. (Hematoxylin-eosin stain; ×450.)

with hereditary spherocytosis transfused into a normal recipient are rapidly destroyed, (3) erythrocytes from a person with hereditary spherocytosis transfused into a recipient previously subjected to splenectomy survive for a normal time, and (4) in hereditary spherocytosis, splenectomy completely cures the hemolytic disease even though the bone marrow continues to make spherocytes and the appearance of the peripheral blood smear is unchanged (Jacobs, 1969).

The spleen is always enlarged and weights of 500 to 1,000 Gm are not uncommon. The cut surface is deep red and hemorrhagic. The characteristic microscopic features are: (1) marked congestion of the red pulp, possibly because the spheroid erythrocytes do not pass readily through the sinusoidal walls, (2) hyperplasia of the endothelial cells lining the sinusoids, (3) relatively empty sinusoids, and (4) little or no hemosiderin, in contrast to many other hemolytic anemias. If accessory spleens are present, they not only exhibit the same morphology but, if not excised along with the principal spleen, will take over the destructive function and the original splenectomy will be ineffective.

In *sickle cell disease* as well as in some severe variants such as Hb S—Hb C or Hb S—thalassemia combinations (Chapter 14), the spleen is severely involved. The changes are progressive and are most severe in cases of long standing. As in hereditary spherocytosis, the defect in the erythrocytes is intrinsic, the content of Hb S causing them to assume rigid, bizarre, sickle-like shapes under hypoxic conditions. Their rigidity and peculiar shape cause them to plug up small blood vessels, and most of the clinical findings can be explained on the basis of microthrombi. In the spleen they do not pass out of the red pulp, so that it is markedly congested and contains many sickled erythrocytes (Fig. 2-26). Later the spleen shows the effect of repeated hemorrhages and infarcts, the hemorrhages leading to diffuse fibrosis with scattered siderotic nodules, while repeated infarction produces many large depressed scars. The most severe degree of fibrosis and atrophy has already been discussed and illustrated (p. 65 and Fig. 2-25). The microscopic features that distinguish the spleen in sickle cell disease are: (1) the sickled erythrocytes, always prominent in formalin-fixed tissue, (2) the large amount of hemosiderin (as opposed to the spleen in congenital spherocytosis), (3) progressive fibrosis, and (4) numerous infarcts. It should be noted that some sickled erythrocytes are seen in any hemoglobinopathy where Hb S is one of the hemoglobins; thus they may be seen in sickle cell trait (Hb S plus Hb A). Here, however, the spleen is relatively normal.

The spleen is also severely involved in thalassemia (Cooley's anemia or Mediterranean anemia). This hemoglobinopathy differs from the others in that an abnormal molecular form of hemoglobin is not present (Chapter 14). Rather there is suppression of synthesis of beta polypeptide chains (β-thalassemia) or alpha polypeptide chains (α-thalassemia), resulting in deficient synthesis of otherwise normal hemoglobin. Suppression of normal hemoglobin synthesis is accompanied by increased amounts of Hb A_2 or Hb F. The erythrocytes are not only deficient in normal hemoglobin (hypochromic) but are also abnormal in shape, many being

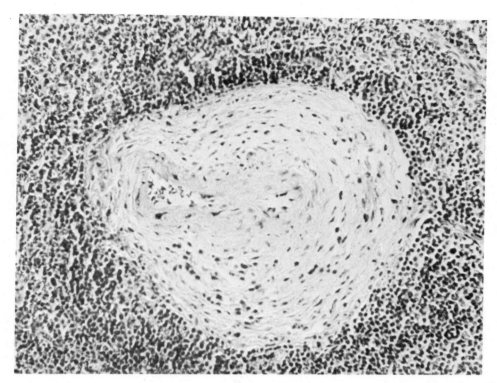

Fig. 2-27. Spleen, disseminated lupus erythematosus, showing typical "onionskin" appearance of arteriolar wall. (Hematoxylin-eosin stain; ×125.)

target cells, while the others vary markedly in size and shape. Their life span is short because they are destroyed in large numbers by the spleen.

The disease ranges in severity from mild to very severe; the changes in the spleen are greatest in the severe form called thalassemia major. The spleen is very large often seeming to fill the abdominal cavity. The organ is firm and the capsule often thickened. The cut surface is dark red. Microscopically, there is marked congestion, fibrosis, and hyperplasia of reticuloendothelial cells. The one feature that is characteristic is the presence of foci of blood cell formation, extramedullary hemopoiesis. Also characteristic, but not as frequent, is the presence of foam cells in the red pulp. These are large and show a foamy cytoplasm that contains PAS-positive mucopolysaccharide. Siderotic nodules are sometimes found, but these are seen also in other hemolytic anemias.

In other diseases of blood and blood-forming organs

The spleen, as one organ of the RES, seldom escapes being involved in proliferative reactions that classically are described as having their genesis in other organs such as lymph nodes or bone marrow. Thus, in addition to the conditions already discussed, which may be considered to primarily involve some special splenic function, splenomegaly is found in hematologic disorders involving granulocytopoiesis, lymphopoiesis, erythropoiesis, and proliferation of other cell types (Table 2-5).

In autoimmune diseases

The concept of "autoimmune disease," a direct and noxious attack by specific immunologic agents against cells and tissues, is based on firm experimental evidence. For example, allergic encephalomyelitis and thyroiditis can be produced by injecting organ extracts into animals, while graft-versus-host reactions may involve such evidence of generalized disease as Coombs'–positive hemolytic anemia, polyarthritis, myocarditis, nephritis, etc. While the experimental autoimmune diseases are usually characterized by the presence of tissue-specific antibodies in the blood, it does not necessarily follow that when they are present, antibodies in the blood in human diseases thought to be of the autoimmune type are in every instance directly toxic to cells and tissues. Nevertheless, it would seem that a fairly common denominator is the reaction of connective tissue in these diseases. Since the spleen is often involved, the pathologic changes in this organ deserve brief mention.

Splenomegaly, with or without characteristic histologic alterations, is common to the entire group. In rheumatoid arthritis, for example, the spleen is usually enlarged but presents no characteristic histologic changes. The spleen in systemic lupus erythematosus usually shows foci of degenerating collagen in the capsule and the characteristic periarterial "onionskin" lesion (Fig. 2-27) that affects the central and penicillary arteries.

There are two types of thrombocytopenic purpura in which the spleen shows recognizable involvement. In idiopathic thrombocytopenic purpura (immunologic thrombocy-

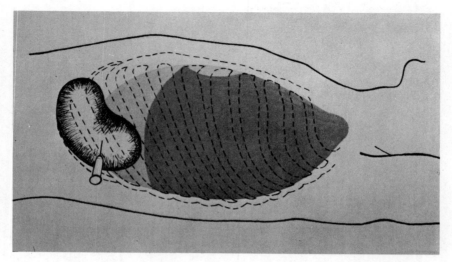

Fig. 2-28. Relationship of spleen to thoracic cage and preferred site for splenic puncture.

Table 2-7. Normal and abnormal splenograms*

	Normal (%)	Myelofibrosis (%)	Sepsis (%)	Chronic myelocytic leukemia (%)	Chronic lymphocytic leukemia (%)	Hemolytic anemia (%)
Reticulum cells†	0.5-1.8	0.3	4.2	—	—	3.1
Normoblasts	0.1-0.2	5.3	0	6.6	—	9.3
Myeloblasts	0	0	0	2.4	—	—
Progranulocytes	0-0.1	0.7	—	11.0	—	—
Myelocytes	0.05-0.2	12.0	1.7	25.6	0.1	0.7
Metamyelocytes	0-0.1	10.3	—	14.6	—	—
Band neutrophils	1.0-7.0	7.3	63.1	22.4	0.2	7.6
Segmented neutrophils	8.0-25.0	3.3	9.2	10.4	0.5	7.5
Eosinophils, mature	0.2-1.5	—	0.2	1.1	—	1.2
Basophils, mature	0.1-1.1	—	—	4.0	—	1.5
Monocytes	1.2-2.4	1.7	1.2	0.5	0.3	3.6
Reticulolymphocytes‡	0-0.1	—	—	—	—	—
Lymphoblasts	0-0.2	—	0.1	—	—	—
Lymphocytes, young	1.0-10.5 ⎫	59.0	1.9 ⎫	1.4	4.4	2.6
Lymphocytes, mature	57.0-84.5 ⎭		17.2 ⎭		94.1	62.8
Plasma cells	0-0.3	—	1.2	—	—	—
Megakaryocytes	0	Present	—	Present	—	—

*Data from Moeschlin, 1951.
†Macrophages, fat cells, plasmacytoid reticulum cells, tissue mast cells, and pulp cells.
‡Correspond to the germinal center cells of lymphoid nodules.

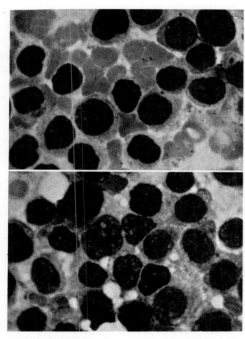

Fig. 2-29. Splenic aspiration, acute myelomonocytic leukemia. (Wright's stain; ×850.)

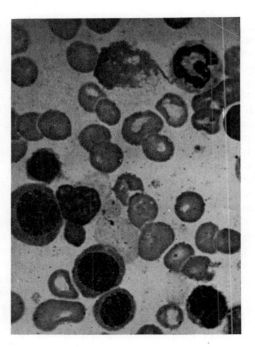

Fig. 2-30. Smear from splenic puncture, hemolytic anemia. Note typical normoblasts.

topenic purpura) the spleen is usually unremarkable; occasionally the lymphoid follicles are hyperplastic, megakaryocytes may be found in the red pulp, and there may also be occasional lipid-filled histiocytes (Table 2-3). In thrombotic thrombocytopenic purpura, characteristic microthrombi can be found (p. 852).

Biopsy of the spleen

Aspiration of splenic tissue for biopsy may yield corroborative or diagnostic information in a large number of conditions (Block and Jacobson, 1950; Chatterjea et al, 1952). Splenic puncture was first performed by Widal, who used it to obtain material for culture in typhoid fever. It was frequently used to diagnose parasitic diseases such as leishmaniasis, malaria, and trypanosomiasis, particularly in geographic areas in which these diseases are common. It remains a potentially dangerous procedure, but as the technic of splenic puncture has been improved and standardized, it has become an important adjunct in hematologic diagnosis. However, the indications and contraindications should be respected. Moeschlin's (1951) monograph is an excellent and comprehensive study of all phases of splenic puncture.

Indications and contraindications

Splenic puncture is primarily an aid to hematologic diagnosis and therefore should be performed only when it is anticipated that information of value will be obtained. Splenic aspiration for the diagnosis of bacterial or protozoan diseases is not widely practiced in this country. Most researchers believe that puncture is inadvisable for children or adults who may be unable or unwilling to cooperate.

However, many successful punctures on infants have been reported. It is generally recommended that soft spleens, as in acute infections and infectious mononucleosis, should not be punctured. Splenic puncture is contraindicated in splenic hypertension, such as in portal hypertension, and splenic vein thrombosis.

Site of puncture

It is generally recommended that the puncture be done at the ninth or tenth left intercostal space, at the midaxillary line or the point of maximal dullness to percussion (Fig. 2-28). However, some feel that splenomegaly must be present before splenic aspiration biopsy is considered, and in such cases the transabdominal route is preferred. It is claimed that, because the needle is more mobile and the diaphragm is not punctured, there is less chance of a major tear in the splenic capsule when the transabdominal route is used.

Puncture technic

With the patient lying flat on his back on a firm bed or treatment table, the splenic area is percussed to determine the limits of resonance on inspiration and expiration. The ninth or tenth interspace is located at the midaxillary line, and this point is marked if it is at least 5 cm below the point of resonance on deep inspiration. The skin is cleansed and painted with an antiseptic, and the area is suitably draped with sterile towels or drapes. Moeschlin (1951) recommends meticulous attention to the sterility of solutions and needles. After cutaneous infiltration a 20-gauge, 10-cm needle attached to a syringe containing procaine (Novocain) solution is inserted perpendicularly to the skin. When a point is reached at which the patient feels a little pain, the peritoneum has been reached. On further careful penetration the tip of the needle can be felt to scratch against the spleen. The depth of penetration at this point is marked on the needle, and the needle is withdrawn. This measurement is transferred to the splenic puncture needle, and the guard is set 1 to 2 cm beyond this point. The special needle used for splenic puncture has a sharp bevel and stylet. Some have used a spinal puncture needle, although it has no guard to mark the depth of penetration. Others have omitted local anesthesia.

After these preliminaries, the puncture needle is pushed through the skin, the stylet is removed, a dry 10-ml syringe is attached, and the patient is instructed to take a deep breath and hold it. The patient is instructed to close his mouth and pinch his nose shut. Puncture is then performed quickly. The needle is thrust into the spleen in the predetermined direction and to the marked depth. Quick forceful suction is then exerted. The suction is released, and the needle is quickly withdrawn. The material obtained, usually very little, is expressed from the needle, and smears are made and stained with Wright's stain. The patient should remain quietly on his back for 1 hour and in bed for 4 to 6 hours after the puncture.

Normal and abnormal splenograms

In most cases it is sufficient to study the cells on the smears microscopically, without performing differential cell counts. With experience one comes to recognize the appearance of normal splenic material, which contains roughly 75% lymphocytes, the remainder of the cells being chiefly band and segmented neutrophils with scattered reticulum cells and macrophages. Normally only a very few normoblasts or myeloblasts will be found. Abnormal cells such as Reed-Sternberg cells, epithelioid cells, giant cells, megakaryocyte, normoblasts, and megaloblasts have the same appearance as on bone marrow smears.

If quantitative data are desired, a differential count of 1,000 cells is done, and the results are compared with the normal splenogram (Table 2-7).

The information obtained is interpreted along with other hematologic and clinical data and often yields a more complete hematologic picture than that obtainable from the peripheral blood and bone marrow alone. Imprints made from a freshly cut surface of spleen removed surgically or obtained at necropsy sometimes help in the interpretation of the tissue sections (Cowling et al, 1978). At times, notably in specimens from Niemann-Pick disease, the cytochemical features are better demonstrated in smears and imprints than in tissue sections. Splenic aspiration is particularly rewarding in the study of multiple myeloma, myeloproliferative syndromes, leukemia (Fig. 2-29), leukemoid reactions, and reactions characterized by normoblastic proliferation (Fig. 2-30).

3

"May I remind you that scientific truth can be defined as that corpus of facts and provisional generalizations which, in the consensus of competent scholars, has not yet been shown to be wrong."

Sir McFarlane Burnet

The reticuloendothelial system
III. Lymphocytes and the immunocyte complex

INTRODUCTION
THE LYMPHOCYTIC SYSTEM
  Introduction
  The lymphocyte
    Morphology
    Lymphocytopoiesis
    Life span
    Sites of formation
  The duality of the lymphocytic system
  Role of the bone marrow
  Role of the thymus
  Lymphocytic migration streams
  Transformation of lymphocytes
    In vitro transformation to blastoid cells
    In vivo transformations
  Lymphocyte function: T-, B-, and null cells
    Introduction
    T-lymphocytes
      Lymphocytotoxin
      Migration inhibition factor (MIF)
      Transfer factor (TF)
      Lymphocyte transforming factor (LTF)
      Lymph node permeability factor
      Eosinophilotropic factor
      Helper and suppressor T-cells
    B-lymphocytes
    Null cells
    Interrelations in the immune response
    Perspective
  The lymphocyte in immunologic reactions
    Cellular immunity
      The delayed hypersensitivity reaction (DHR)
      Antilymphocytic serum (ALS)
      Transplantation reactions
      Cancer immunology
      In pregnancy
    Humoral immunity: the immunoglobulins
      Definition
      Structure
      Function
      Genetics of immunoglobulin synthesis
      Allotypes
      Synthesis

    Normal serum concentrations
    Catabolism
  Immunoglobulinopathies
    Classification
  Primary immunodeficiencies
    X-linked agammaglobulinemia
    Thymic hypoplasia
    Immunodeficiency with thymoma
    Severe combined immunodeficiency
    Immunodeficiency with normal immunoglobulins or
      hyperglobulinemia
    Immunodeficiency with thrombocytopenia and eczema
    Immunodeficiency with ataxia-telangiectasia
    Immunodeficiency with hematopoietic hypoplasia
    Selective immunoglobulin deficiencies
  Hyperimmunoglobulinemia
    Immunoblastic (angioimmunoblastic) lymphadenopathy
    Lymphadenopathy with sinus histiocytosis
    Giant lymph node hyperplasia
    Gamma heavy chain disease
    Chronic lymphocytic leukemia
    Infectious mononucleosis
    Drug-induced lymphadenopathy
  Laboratory diagnosis of immunodeficiency
    In thymus-dependent cellular immunity deficiencies
      Lymph nodes
      Hematologic data
      Skin tests for delayed hypersensitivity reactions
      Evaluation of lymphocyte transformation
      Release of MIF
      Presence or absence of the thymus
      Measurement of complement components
    In humoral (immunoglobulin) deficiencies
      Measurement of serum immunoglobulins
      Presence of natural and acquired antibodies
      Antibody response to immunization
      Presence of plasma cells
      Assessment of lymphoid mass
  Lymph nodes
    Normal structure: histologic
    Normal structure: cytologic
    Function
    Aspiration and imprint preparations

INTRODUCTION

In the preceding chapter we noted that one of the functions of the RES is phagocytosis. Normally this activity is responsible for gobbling up microbial invaders so that the host is not overwhelmed. At about the same time that Metchnikoff was elaborating this concept of immunity as a cellular process, Von Behring and Kitasato showed that the blood of animals given an injection of tetanus toxin contained a substance capable of specifically neutralizing the toxin. The specific substance produced by the body in response to the injection of a foreign material (antigen) was later called an *antibody,* and subsequent investigations showed that antibodies are induced by a wide variety of foreign proteins. In 1937 Tiselius localized the antibody activity in the γ-globulin fraction of serum. At first, "γ-globulin" and "antibody" were synonymous, but then it was found that antibody is not always of the γ type, the nongamma type being of several varieties. The term "immunoglobulin" was suggested by Heremans in 1959 and adopted by the World Health Organization in 1964 to cover the entire spectrum of antibodies, and with the immunoelectrophoresis technic, plus other technics of immunochemistry and protein chemistry, five *classes* of immunoglobulins have been defined: IgA, IgG, IgM, IgD, and IgE.

In contrast to the classic cellular immunity reactions dependent on phagocytic activity, the immunoglobulins are responsible for humoral immunity reactions. However, the discovery that antibody production is dependent on the activity of lymphoid tissues has modified the classic dichotomy of cellular and humoral immunity with the lymphocyte sometimes participating in cellular immune reactions, as in the rejection of a graft, and at other times (or at the same time) contributing to humoral immunity.

Macrophages, plasma cells, and lymphocytes are all involved in the formation of antibodies, and these cells make up a functional, though cellularly heterogeneous, unit of the RES. In searching for a suitably descriptive term for the cells of this functional unit, it was first proposed that they be called *immunologically competent cells.* In 1963 Dameshek proposed the terms "immunoblast" and "immunocyte," the former for the primitive cell and the latter for the plasma cells and lymphocytes derived from it. These terms are now in common use, but it should be remembered that Dameshek's philosophical suggestion was an attempt to express *functional* unity and was not intended to define the immunologically competent cells as morphologic entities. In order to fit the concept of the immunoblast into the modern schemes of cell derivation (Fig. 1-2), it can be assumed that it is equivalent to the CFU-L, the cell committed to the lymphocytic line.

THE LYMPHOCYTIC SYSTEM
Introduction

The lymphocytic system in humans consists of aggregates of lymphocytes and the lymphatic channels in which the lymph flows. The formation, flow, and function of lymph is a subject of great interest and importance but will not concern us here. That subject is thoroughly covered by Yoffey and Courtice (1970). We will turn out attention to the cellular portion of the system, consisting of both diffuse and discrete aggregates of lymphoid cells: the *thymus,* the *lymph nodes,* the *spleen,* the *lymphoid nodules in the intestine (Peyer's patches),* and the *bone marrow.* Yoffey and Courtice (1970) group all these tissues under the term "lymphomyeloid complex." In lower forms the lymphomyeloid complex is primarily responsible for hemopoiesis, but in higher forms, particularly warm-blooded vertebrates, the hemopoietic role is minor while there is found a full expression of the immunologic role of lymphoid cells. This role is the subject of this chapter.

In recent years there has been an explosive growth of interest in the function of the lymphocytic system. Although infections and neoplastic involvement of lymph nodes were recognized for many years, considerations of lymphoid function were few and remarkably unscientific. Two are noteworthy. The concept that the tonsils served as the portal entry for the streptococcus responsible for rheumatic fever and as foci of "hidden infection" was responsible for many thousands of "prophylactic" tonsillectomies in the 1940s. Even earlier was the thesis that the thymus had a direct connection with otherwise unexplained death in children—"status thymicolymphaticus." Hammar (1921) finally disposed of this myth by showing that there is neither gross nor microscopic difference between the thymus glands of children dying from trauma and those previously thought to be diagnostic of status thymicolymphaticus. As a result, investigators showed no interest in the thymus for many years

Good and co-workers (MacLean et al, 1956) studied a man who had a benign thymic tumor (thymoma) and agammaglobulinemia. They thought that the association of two very rare conditions in the same patient might be meaningful rather than coincidental. The assumption that a nonfunctioning thymus causes agammaglobulinemia was tested by injecting an antigen, bovine serum albumin, into thymectomized adult rabbits; the researchers were disappointed to find a normal antibody response. In retrospect, we now know that thymectomy in an adult does not affect any of the immunologic responses.

The explanation of the association between the thymus and immune reactions did not come from such direct attacks on the problem.

There are two gut-associated lymphoid aggregates in the chicken. One is the thymus, analogous in structure and location to that in higher species. The other, the bursa of Fabricius, is found only in birds and is located at the other end of the gut just above the cloaca. Surgical excision of the bursa of Fabricius in the newly hatched chick was found to suppress the ability of the adult chicken to produce immunoglobulin antibodies. The same inability to form antibodies can be produced by injecting testosterone into the egg during the hatching period; this produces chicks without a bursa of Fabricius, "chemical bursectomy." In the absence of the bursa, however achieved, chickens retain those immunologic responses not dependent on immunoglobulin production, i.e., delayed hypersensitivity and homograft rejection, but lose the ability to make immunoglobulins. Thus it was concluded that the bursa of Fabricius is essential to the humoral defense mechanism (immunoglobulin dependent) but not to the cellular defense mechanism (cell dependent).

On the other hand, excision of the thymus in the newborn

results in defective lymphocytopoiesis, abolishment of the delayed hypersensitivity reaction (DHR), and homograft rejection. These can be reversed by transplanting fetal thymic tissue, and it can be shown that the new lymphocytes that are formed come from the thymic graft. DiGeorge's syndrome in human infants is characterized by the absence of thymic tissue, and transplantation of fetal thymic tissue has successfully restored lymphocytopoiesis and immunocompetence (Cleveland et al, 1968).

We are told that B. Glick, in the course of studying the role of the bursa of Fabricius in the sexual development of chicks, learned that bursectomized chickens are poor antibody producers. He published this finding in *Poultry Science* (Glick et al, 1956) after *Science* turned down the manuscript on the grounds that it was not of general interest (in modern terms we would say "not pertinent"). Glick's report went unnoticed until Good became interested in the problem. The dissociation of immunologic responsiveness in fowl was proposed by Warner et al (1962).

These important and fundamental observations stimulated extensive investigations of the role of the lymphocytic system in immune reactions. The duality of the chicken lymphocytic system has been transferred to the human, with the popular concept of two types, at least, of lymphocytes: the T-lymphocytes, which are thymus dependent, and the B-lymphocytes, which are equivalent to bursa-dependent cells. In the following discussion it is well to remember that this duality, quite sharp in many respects, is in another sense somewhat artificial, for not only are all lymphocytes derived from the same hemopoietic stem cell, but they also interact and do not always operate as independent effectors of the immunologic responses.

The lymphocyte
Morphology

As the subject of this chapter is developed, we will often find ourselves confronted with the problem of defining the lymphocyte on the basis of function. A morphologic definition is not so difficult.

The lymphocyte may be small or large. The small lymphocyte is more common and is 6 to 8 μ in diameter. The large lymphocyte may measure up to 18 μ in diameter. The small lymphocyte has a dense *pachychromatic* (coarse chromatin pattern) nucleus, smudged and indistinct parachromatin, and very scanty pale cytoplasm. The large lymphocyte has more abundant cytoplasm and a less dense and slightly larger nucleus that is still pachychromatic. The distinction between small and large lymphocytes is modified by the tendency of small lymphocytes to round up in the thick portion of a smear and to flatten in the thin portion (Fig. 4-13). This is most striking in the lymphocytes of chronic lymphocytic leukemia, as illustrated.

The nucleus is round or ovoid, usually smooth, but sometimes notched. The chromatin pattern, described as pachychromatic, is coarse and irregularly clumped. Characteristically, the chromatin-parachromatin zones are indistinct and smudged, as a pencilled drawing over which a finger has been rubbed. The nucleus usually contains one nucleolus, not usually evident in routine smears because of the density of the nucleus, but obvious on phase or electron microscopy.

The cytoplasm of resting lymphocytes is pale blue on Wright-stained smears and may contain fine azurophilic granules, particularly in large or reactive lymphocytes. Other inclusions may be present and of unknown significance.

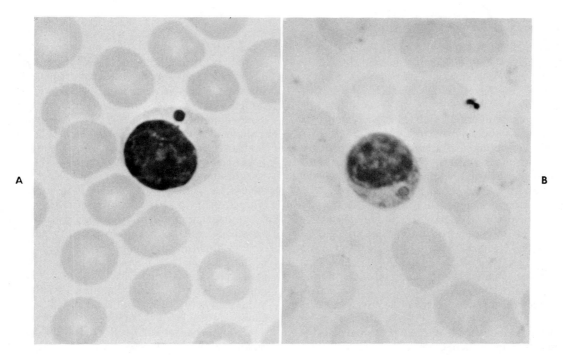

Fig. 3-1. Lymphocyte with single large inclusion, unnamed, from a 73-year-old man in good health. **A,** Peripheral blood. (Wright's stain; ×1,250.) **B,** Peripheral blood. (PAS stain; ×1,250.)

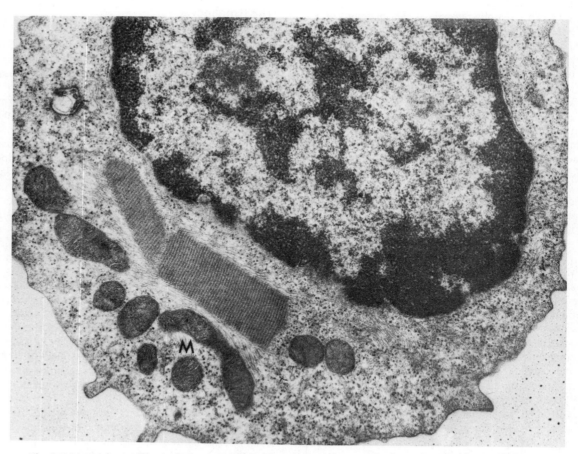

Fig. 3-2. Unusual crystalline inclusion in circulating lymphocyte of a normal subject, lying between the nucleus and mitochondria **(M).** Original magnification ×19,000. (From Zucker-Franklin, D.: The ultrastructure of lymphocytes, Semin. Hematol. **6:**4-27, 1969, by permission.)

One large spherical inclusion is shown in Fig. 3-1. The inclusion described by Gall (1936) is faint and difficult to see with routine stains but is obvious by phase microscopy. Crystalline inclusions have also been described (Zucker-Franklin, 1969) (Fig. 3-2).

By standard electron microscopy the inactive lymphocyte is seen to have scanty round or ovoid mitochondria, little or no endoplasmic reticulum, and a small and unremarkable Golgi apparatus (Figs. 3-3 and 3-4). The ribosomes in the cytoplasm of a nonstimulated lymphocyte are dispersed and do not form clusters.

Cytochemical reactions do not show a highly active cytoplasmic system. Normal and, more commonly, leukemic and lymphomatous cells may contain PAS-positive inclusions (Quaglino and Hayhoe, 1959) usually small and few in normal cells, numerous and coarse in malignant cells. A few small sudanophilic granules may be present in the area of nuclear indentation. Lymphocytes are peroxidase negative, alkaline phosphatase negative, esterase negative, and acid phosphatase positive (Hayhoe et al, 1964). The acid phosphatase positivity is abolished by tartrate in normal cells but is tartrate resistant in leukemic reticuloendotheliosis (p. 725).

Lymphocytes are actively motile, the nucleus usually occupying the forward portion and the cytoplasm streaming behind. In peripheral blood films lymphocytes arrested in this state of locomotion present the "hand-mirror" appearance or the nucleus is sometimes centrally placed and the cytoplasm streams away from it fore and aft. Their active locomotion may contribute to their supposed ability to pass through the cytoplasm of endothelial cells (Marchesi and Gowans, 1964), a process called *emperipolesis* (Ioachim, 1965). However Schoefl (1972) has shown that lymphocytes migrate across vascular endothelium by insinuating themselves between endothelial cells and not by passing through them (p. 105). Nishi et al (1979) have confirmed this by scanning electron microscopy. Schoefl views the endothelial cells as being compressible so that they again close behind the migrating lymphocyte and thus avoid loss of fluid. Specialized interactions are required between the membranes of endothelial cells and that of lymphocytes for migration to take place (Stamper and Woodruff, 1976; Weissman et al, 1978). In the acute inflammatory reaction neutrophil leukocytes also migrate out of the vascular system between endothelial cells, but in that case the inflammatory response has caused the endothelial cells to round up and the open intercellular spaces are exposed to both cells and fluid.

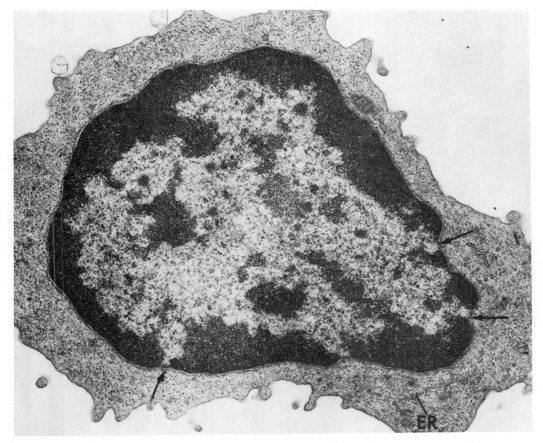

Fig. 3-3. Small "inactive" lymphocyte. Arrows point to nuclear pores. Ribosomes are scattered singly throughout the cytoplasm. There is one small profile of endoplasmic reticulum **(ER).** Original magnification ×1,700. (From Zucker-Franklin, D.: The ultrastructure of lymphocytes, Semin. Hematol. **6:**4-27, 1969, by permission.)

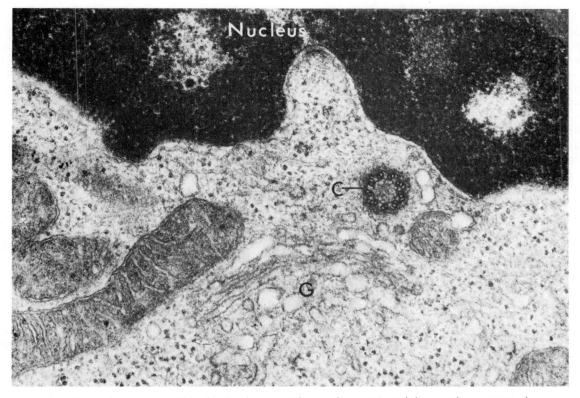

Fig. 3-4. Detail of an "inactive" lymphocyte showing Golgi membranes **(G)** and the complex structure of a centriole **(C)** with its nine triplet rods in perfect cross section. Original magnification ×44,000. (From Zucker-Franklin, D.: The ultrastructure of lymphocytes, Semin. Hematol. **6:**4-27, 1969, by permission.)

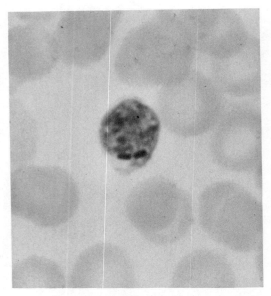

Fig. 3-5. Phagocytic lymphocyte, ingestion of *E. coli* in vitro. (Wright's stain; ×950.) (Courtesy Dr. Stanley B. Smith.)

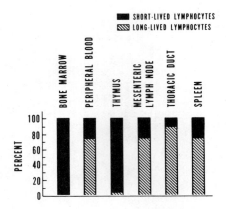

Fig. 3-6. Relative content of short-lived and long-lived lymphocytes in various tissues. (Data for rat from Everett et al, 1964.)

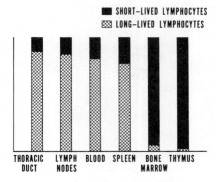

Fig. 3-7. Probable distribution of long-lived and short-lived lymphocytes in human tissues.

There is no longer doubt that some small lymphocytes can be phagocytic (Fig. 3-5). Phagocytosis of mycoplasma (Zucker-Franklin et al, 1966) of *Leishmania* and *Histoplasma* organisms (Rebuck et al, 1958), of erythrocyte fragments (Hughes, 1966), and of streptococci (Hertzog, 1938) has also been reported.

Lymphocytopoiesis

At one time the lymphocyte was a monotonously uninteresting cell. Morphologically, it showed no colorful characteristics on routine staining, and electron microscopy only added to the disappointment; the absence of endoplasmic reticulum, the rudimentary Golgi apparatus, and the sparse mitochondria hardly suggested a metabolically important cell.

Nevertheless, the suspicion persisted that lymphocytes must play an important, albeit obscure role in the body. Surely it would be a cruel joke to be endowed with a variety of cell whose only role was to transform into lethal leukemias and lymphomas!

Until a few years ago one could only list unrelated observations that kept the suspicion alive. For one thing, Maximow (1932) had from the earliest publications considered "lymphocyte" and "hemocytoblast" as synonymous, a concept later rejected but now considered partially valid. Also, lymphocytes appeared "atypical" at times, as for example the Downey cells of infectious mononucleosis and the "virocytes" that appeared often in association with viral infections. Even when not atypical, lymphocytes predominate in the chronic stage of the inflammatory response, while infiltration of lymphocytes around tumor nodules led to speculation that they might be involved in the reaction of the host to the tumor tissue. Also, the total lymphocyte mass in the body, 1,500 Gm according to Osgood (1954) and 1,600 Gm according to Pulvertaft (1959), is equal to the total granulocyte mass, so that lymphoid tissue can hardly

be considered a minor component. Finally, there was speculation that the lymphocyte might undergo some transformation when suitably stimulated, but because it was thought to be incapable of mitosis and was in that sense an "end cell," it did not seem that transformation processes could be quantitatively important. We can appreciate why at one time the lymphocyte was described as a "phlegmatic spectator watching the turbulent activities of the phagocytes" (Arnold Rich).

Life span

Because of the recirculation so characteristic of lymphocytes, life span cannot be measured by transfusing isotopically labeled cells into a recipient animal. In vivo labeling (Ottesen, 1954), on the other hand, has shown that about 15% of the lymphocytes have a life span of about 4 days whereas the others have a life span as long as 170 days. The small lymphocyte in chronic lymphocytic leukemia has an even longer life span—3 months to 3 years. This accounts partially for the extremely high counts in the peripheral blood in this disease (Chapter 16).

There have been few opportunities to study the life span of labeled lymphocytes in humans. Confirmation of the double population has been obtained by another technic, the use of chromosome markers. Ionizing radiation produces unstable chromosome aberrations, unstable in the sense that cells so altered cannot undergo mitotic division, and the chromosome abnormality persists for the duration of the cell's life span. Such chromosomal abnormalities have been produced in persons given therapeutic X-irradiation for ankylosing spondylitis, and a study of the karyotype of the lymphocytes has shown that some have a life span of 10 years or longer (Claman, 1966). Similar data (life span of 3 years) have been derived for lymphocytes of women irradiated for carcinoma of the cervix.

In the rat, different tissues vary in the relative proportion of short-lived and long-lived lymphocytes (Fig. 3-6). These proportions hold for humans (Fig. 3-7), and studies with various mammals show only one species that behaves differently, the pig.

Sites of formation

The lymphocytes found in the peripheral blood are cells in transit from one lymphoid tissue to another or to sites of inflammation. In this sense it can be generalized that the sites of formation of blood lymphocytes are the various lymphoid tissues. However, if one asks which tissue or organ is primarily responsible for lymphocytopoiesis, the question requires a complicated answer.

It was once thought that the centers of lymphoid follicles were the chief source for genesis of new lymphocytes. The evidence seemed good, for the centers showed much mitotic activity as well as a population of apparently younger lymphocytes. Later it became clear that the follicle centers are in fact a site of antibody formation and represent zones of reaction rather than the site of small lymphocyte production.

The search for quantitative data on lymphocyte production was complicated at first by the finding that the lymphocyte population is in a state of constant flux and migration. Since almost all the lymphocytes in peripheral blood come from the major lymphatic ducts emptying into major veins, there should be a direct quantitative relationship between the number of lymphocytes in thoracic duct lymph and the number in the blood. Estimates of the number of thoracic duct lymphocytes entering the blood per unit time revealed that, based on the number of lymphocytes in the thoracic duct and in the blood, enough cells entered the blood to replace those in the blood several times each day. With no evidence for a high rate of destruction, and indeed with the new evidence that the thoracic duct lymphocyte has a very long life span, it was obvious that lymphocytes must somehow leave the bloodstream.

Gowans (1964) investigated this by labeling thoracic duct lymphocytes with a radioactive tag and then returning them to the donor animal or another animal of the same inbred strain. He found that when tagged lymphocytes were given intravenously, they reappeared in the lymph of the thoracic duct. They could also be traced from the blood to the cortex of lymph nodes, to Peyer's patches, and to the white pulp of the spleen. Significantly, they did not enter the thymus. Two important concepts came from thse and other studies: (1) there is a constant recirculation of small lymphocytes through the blood and lymph, and (2) the small lymphocyte that is found in the thoracic duct sooner or later migrates to various lymphoid organs and tissues with the notable exception of the thymus. These various migrations and "homing" effects have given rise to the concept of the duality of the lymphoid system as the *central* lymphoid tissue and the *peripheral* lymphoid tissue.

The duality of the lymphocytic system

It has become fashionable to consider the lymphocytic system as developing along two functionally distinct lines, the *thymus dependent* and the *bursa dependent*. This has been a useful concept, but it must be pointed out that although normally there are two (possibly three) distinct functional types of lymphocytes, they all originate from bone marrow stem cells and only by remote analogy can some of them be considered "bursa dependent." As noted earlier, ablation of the bursa of Fabricius in fowl abolishes the ability to produce immunoglobulins and there is no doubt that in that species the cellular and humoral immune systems are quite separate. However, it is only by analogy that the "gut-associated" lymphoid tissue (Peyer's patches, appendix, tonsils, and diffuse collections of lymphocytes under the epithelium of the intestine) is considered the counterpart of the bursa of Fabricius. Certainly, thymus dependent and bursa dependent do not indicate a separate source of lymphocytes. For example, repopulation of Peyer's patches in neonatally thymectomized mice does not depend on thymic lymphocytogenesis (Evans et al, 1967). Furthermore, the functionally distinct types of lymphocytes are not restricted to one or the other location, for in any sample from blood or thoracic duct there is a mixture of the two, as evidenced by the production of both cellular and humoral responses when given to suitable hosts (Gowans et al, 1962; Porter and Cooper, 1962). In any case, the concept has given rise to the nomenclature of T-lymphocytes (for thymus dependent) and B-lymphocytes (for bursa dependent) (Cooper et al, 1968a).

There is probably more justification for considering the lymphoid system under two categories, the *central* and the *peripheral* (Fig. 3-8). The central system consists of the bone marrow and the thymus. Cells from both the bone marrow and the thymus populate all other lymphoid tissues, the peripheral system. This functional duality is reflected in the structure of the lymphoid nodule (Fig. 3-9): the corona of small lymphocytes is made up of T-lymphocytes and is involved in cellular immunity, whereas the reactive center contains B-lymphocytes and represents a site of antibody synthesis.

Role of the bone marrow

The marrow contains many lymphocytes, about 20% of all cells (Osmond, 1975). Most are scattered among the other cells, but occasionally form nodules (Fig. 5-19) and these occasionally form reactive centers (Fig. 3-10). The bone marrow is involved in three phases of lymphocytopoiesis. First, it is the source of the stem cell compartments. Second, it is the site of primary lymphocytogenesis. Third, it receives lymphocytes from all other lymphoid aggregates with the exception of the thymus.

In primary lymphocytogenesis in the bone marrow the "virgin" lymphocytes have at first neither the characteristics of T- or of B-cells. These characteristics are acquired

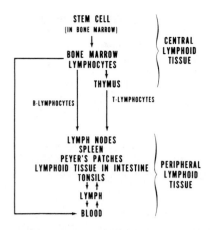

Fig. 3-8. The separation of central and peripheral lymphoid tissue. Not all the migration streams are shown. (See Fig. 3-11.)

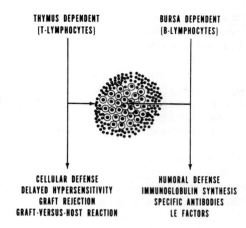

Fig. 3-9. The dual derivation of the cells of a lymphoid nodule.

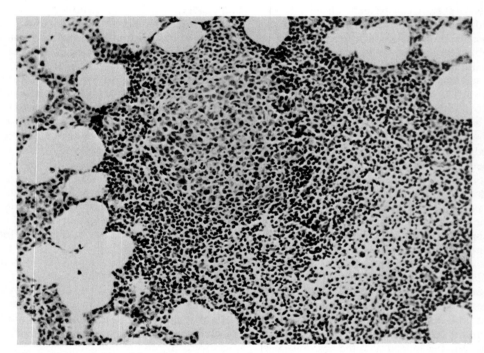

Fig. 3-10. Lymphoid nodule with reactive center, bone marrow. (Hematoxylin-eosin stain; ×125.)

later, after the cells migrate either to the thymus or to peripheral lymphoid tissues (p. 81). Lymphocytes originating in the thymus presumably acquire T characteristics in situ, but this may also occur after recirculation. Lymphocytes originating in peripheral lymphoid tissues are presumably also "virgin" cells until they recirculate to bone marrow or peripheral lymphoid sites (lymph nodes, spleen, gastrointestinal tract). Gupta and Good (1980) refer to these cells as pre-T- and pre-B-cells (p. 87).

Role of the thymus

The thymus is the first portion of the lymphoid system to develop fully in the fetus. It is fully developed in late fetal life, continues to enlarge until late childhood, when slow involution occurs. In mammals it is derived from the endoderm of the third and fourth pharyngeal pouches and from the ectoderm of the brachial cleft. At first it is predominantly an epithelial organ. At about the third month of fetal life the first lymphocytes appear, supposedly derived from cells of epithelial origin with endodermal cells providing the initial stimulus for differentiation. As it develops, it forms a lobulated organ, each lobe divided into a cortex and a medulla. The cortex contains small pachychromatic lymphocytes primarily, called "thymocytes" because of their location. They are morphologically similar to the small lymphocyte in blood and in other lymphoid tissues. The medulla consists of a syncytium of reticular cells and the characteristic Hassall's corpuscles. The reticular cells are normally partially obscured by lymphocytes, but are prominent when lymphocytes are depleted.

Lymphocytopoiesis in the thymus precedes lymphocytopoiesis in the peripheral lymphoid tissues. The priority of thymic lymphocytopoiesis is more striking in rodents than in humans and some other mammals. In humans, structurally and functionally mature peripheral lymphoid tissue is present at birth, provided that the thymus is normal. It appears that thymus-induced maturity of peripheral lymphoid tissues occurs early in fetal life.

The thymus is the site of extremely active lymphocytopoiesis (Andreasen and Christensen, 1949; Metcalf, 1967). In addition, lymphocytes from other sites enter the thymus and large numbers leave it via the lymphatics (Harris and Templeton, 1968) and efferent blood vessels (Ernström et al, 1965). The efferent lymphocytes (thymofugal) go to the peripheral lymphoid tissue, primarily lymph nodes and spleen (Linna, 1968), a process called *peripheralization.* This is essential for the initial population of peripheral lymphoid tissues and also for repopulation when they are depleted of lymphocytes. The lymphocytes entering the thymus (thymopetal) are primarily of bone marrow origin (Barnes et al, 1967) and probably contribute stem cells as well. Various authors have claimed that some lymphocytes from the thoracic duct and the peritoneal cavity migrate to the thymus, but if this occurs at all it is of very minor importance. Efferent thymic lymphocytes are long-lived T-lymphocytes (Parrot and DeSousa, 1971) that, as noted, populate the corona of lymphoid follicles and make up the periarteriolar sheath of lymphocytes in the white pulp of the spleen.

There is much unresolved discussion about whether lymphocytes must actually migrate to the thymus before acquiring T-characteristics, whether those characteristics can be induced by a humoral thymic factor, or whether both mechanisms are operative. The existence of a humoral factor, called lymphocyte stimulating factor (LSF) or more specifically *thymosin* (Goldstein et al, 1966), seems well established. The immunologic deficiency in thymectomized newborn animals can be restored either by implantation of thymic tissue enclosed in a millipore chamber that allows diffusion of fluid but not the escape of cells (Osoba, 1965; Metcalf, 1967); or by administration of thymic extracts (Trainin and Linker-Israeli, 1967), not necessarily from the same species. According to Incefy et al (1975), the differentiation of precursor cells to T-lymphocytes by thymic extracts is the result of changes in cytoplasmic RNA, which in turn dictates the synthesis of T-specific membrane features. The term "thymus-derived lymphocyte" should be used when referring to the efferent cell stream and "thymus-dependent lymphocyte" for the cell that has, under thymic influence, acquired immunologic competence. The thymic factor is essential for the normal function of immunologically competent lymphocytes but not for the initial processing of the antigen by macrophages (Rosenoer et al, 1970).

Lymphocytic migration streams

In the preceding sections we have referred to various migrations of lymphocytes between tissues and fluids.

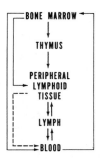

Fig. 3-11. Lymphocytic migration streams. The stream shown by the dotted line is important only when the peripheral lymphoid tissue is reacting strongly to an antigenic stimulus.

These migrations, the chief ones shown in Fig. 3-11, are well established and serve an important function not only in lymphocytopoiesis and lymphocytic function, but also in total hemopoiesis. It must be assumed that some sort of tropism or "homing" mechanism organizes the localization of some lymphocytes in certain tissues, depending on their origin and destiny (Woodruff, 1974). The nature of the regulating mechanisms is not known, but they do remind us of other compulsory migrations, as in birds and aquatic animals, that are also a source of wonder and are no better understood.

It might seem that the very multiplicity of migration streams could be interpreted as nothing more than random recirculation, but the evidence points instead to striking selectivity. Labeled thoracic duct lymphocytes injected intravenously localize in the cortex of lymph nodes, in Peyer's patches, and in the white pulp of the spleen but *not* in the thymus; labeled bone marrow lymphocytes injected intravenously are found in the bone marrow and thymus but *not* in the peripheral lymphoid organs; tagged thymic lymphocytes localize in lymph nodes, Peyer's patches, and spleen but *not* in the bone marrow.

Migration streams are related in part to the distinction between long-lived and short-lived lymphocytes. For example, most of the small lymphocytes in the bone marrow are of the short life span type (Brahim and Osmond, 1970), while a smaller fraction is of the long life span type (Rosse, 1971; Gale et al, 1975). Using normal parabiotic guinea pigs, Rosse (1972) found that the majority of labeled long-lived lymphocytes from one parabiont migrated to the bone marrow of the other, obviously via the blood, and also that there was complete intermixing of long-lived lymphocytes in lymph, lymph nodes, and spleen, but not in the thymus of the parabionts.

Transformation of lymphocytes

Lymphocytes undergo specific and important transformations both in vitro and in vivo. In many ways the study of in vitro transformations has supported many of the concepts of in vivo transformations. The study of these transformations dealt the final blow to the concept that lymphocytes are "end cells" not capable of mitosis or transformation. Transformations are interesting also in explaining some of the "atypical" features of lymphocytes in viral diseases, drug reactions, immune reactions, etc, for there is no doubt that the atypicality of these lymphocytes is nothing more than the expression of their reactivity to various antigens.

In vitro transformation to blastoid cells

Under certain conditions lymphocytes grown in tissue culture undergo a transformation to a large immature cell. This cell has the appearance of a blast cell, hence the term "blastoid," and the transformation is called the *blastoid transformation*. The formation of blastoid cells from lymphocytes is important for many reasons. For one thing, it is another indication that the lymphocyte is not an inert cell; it is capable of dedifferentiation to an immature cell, and this is not seen, as far as we know, in any other blood cell. The transformation to an immature cell may reflect the mechanism by which some small lymphocytes can function as multipotential stem cells in the bone marrow stem cell compartment. As we will see, the transformation to blastoid forms can be used to study cellular function in some immunologic diseases.

The changes that accompany blastoid transformation are striking (Naspitz and Richter, 1968). The earliest changes occur in the nucleus, which enlarges and changes from pachychromatic to leptochromatic, and one or more nucleoli can be seen. Later the cytoplasm becomes more abundant, basophilic, pyroninophilic, and usually contains many small vacuoles. Cytoplasmic budding or pseudopod formation is present. Electron microscopy shows the cytoplasm to be rich in clustered ribosomes, and there is some formation of endoplasmic reticulum. The Golgi apparatus is well developed. Blastoid cells show active synthesis of DNA and RNA (McIntyre and Ebaugh, 1962). Blastoid cells make immunoglobulin (Lerner et al, 1971), complement components (Glade and Chessin, 1968), interferon (Minnefor et al, 1970), mediators of cellular immunity (Granger et al, 1970), and β-2-microglobulin (Bernier and Fanger, 1972). Stimulated lymphocytes also release a macrophage migration inhibition factor (MIF) (Bloom and Bennett, 1968), a cytotoxic factor (Williams and Granger, 1969), a blastogenic factor (Kasakura and Lowenstein, 1965), leukotactic factors (Ward et al, 1969), and a transfer factor (Lawrence, 1969). Hütteroth et al (1972) used the mixed antiglobulin reaction to study surface immunoglobulins of normal lymphocytes and found the surface receptors to have μ heavy chain and κ light chain specificity, with some individual differences among lymphocytes from various sources. Klein et al (1968) found the same specificities for the surface receptors of cultured Burkitt's lymphoma lymphocytes. Production of LATS (long-acting thyroid stimulator), a characteristic γ-globulin in hyperthyroidism, was first described in PHA-stimulated lymphocyte cultures from patients with that disease (Kriss et al, 1964). Blastoid cells are actively mobile and can and do undergo mitosis. Stimulated lymphocytes (by PHA) produce enhanced repopulation of the hemopoietic system in sublethally irradiated recipients (Lopez and Lozzio, 1972). Blastoid transformation is accompanied by increases in the activity of several lysosomal enzymes (acid phosphatases, aryl sulfatase, and α-glucosidase) and of some nonlysosomal enzymes (G-6-PD and LDH) (Rabinowitz and Dietz, 1967; Nadler et al, 1969).

Transformation can be produced by "nonspecific" antigens, by "specific" antigens, and in mixed leukocyte cultures. Nonspecific antigens are phytohemagglutinin (PHA), pokeweed mitogen (PWM), streptolysin S (SLS), staphylococcal endotoxin, and antilymphocyte globulin (ALG). Stimulation by these agents is nonspecific in that there need not be prior sensitization of the lymphocytes to the antigen. Nonspecific stimulation is more powerful than that of specific antigens. The specific antigens are active only when the lymphocytes have been sensitized to the antigen, such as tuberculin, diphtheria toxoid, streptolysin O, filtrate of cultures of staphylococci, smallpox vaccine, polio vaccine, measles vaccine, isoniazid, and penicillin.

PHA is a mucoprotein found in aqueous extracts of the red kidney bean *(Phaseolus vulgaris)*. It is able to agglutinate erythrocytes, hence the term "phytohemagglutinin," and for many years it was used to remove erythrocytes from biologicals or suspensions of mixed cells. It was realized later that it also stimulated mitosis and other changes in lymphocytes, hence the term "mitogen." When added to a culture of small lymphocytes, PHA interacts with the lymphocyte membrane (Kornfeld and Kornfeld, 1969), stimulates synthesis of nucleic acids, first RNA and then DNA (McIntyre and Ebaugh, 1962), and converts the cells to a mitotically active blastoid state. According to Jones and Roitt (1972), responsiveness to PHA is a characteristic of T-lymphocytes, but Lischner et al (1973) have shown that under some conditions B-lymphocytes also respond to PHA. The response to PHA is dose dependent and can also vary with various commercial reagents (Eddie-Quartey and Gross, 1978). Crude PHA can be purified into two mitogenic proteins. One, high titer phytohemagglutinin (H-PHA), binds strongly to red blood cells and causes mixed agglutination of lymphocytes and red blood cells. The other, low titer phytohemagglutinin (L-PHA), binds poorly to red blood cells and has weak red blood cell–lymphocyte agglutinating activity. The addition of autologous red blood cells potentiates the lymphocyte mitogenic activity of H-PHA, and Yachnin et al (1972) propose that the potentiation can be explained by a matrix hypothesis, which supposes that orientation of PHA molecules on the surface of lymphocytes is such as to produce stimulation of PHA levels that would otherwise be ineffective. Another mitogen, concanavalin A, may be a specific activator of T-lymphocytes (Gery et al, 1972).

Pokeweed mitogen (PWM) is an extract of pokeweed *(Phytolacca americana)*. Its action is slightly different from that of PHA in that it induces two types of blastoid cells, one similar to that produced by PHA and another that has the ultrastructural features of a plasma cell (Barker et al, 1965; Douglas and Fudenberg, 1969). Barker et al (1966) have reported plasmacytosis in the peripheral blood of two technicians accidentally inoculated with PWM. One other difference between PHA and PWM is that PWM stimulates B-lymphocytes primarily (Greaves et al, 1972), but PWM can stimulate T-lymphocytes also (Lischner et al, 1973).

The "mixed leukocyte reaction" refers to the formation of blastoid lymphocytes in cultures seeded with an equal number of leukocytes from a different individual (Bain et al,

1964). The thought that the reaction is caused by antigenic differences between the two cell populations is supported by the observation that cells from monozygotic twins do not transform in the mixed leukocyte reaction. Accordingly, the mixed leukocyte reaction has been suggested as an additional test of histocompatibility in graft or transplant situations (Rubin et al, 1964).

Blastoid transformation, induced by various technics and agents, has been used to study the competence of lymphocytes and the immune response in various diseases. Stimulated lymphocytes from persons with macroglobulinemia produce macroglobulin, those from persons with multiple myeloma produce the same globulin found in the serum, while those from agammaglobulinemic subjects fail to synthesize immunoglobulins (Bach et al, 1969). Gotoff (1968) reports normal PHA response in Bruton-type agammaglobulinemia, in the Wiskott-Aldrich syndrome, and in one child thymectomized at birth. PHA response was abnormal in an infant with thymic dysplasia and variable in cases of ataxia-telangiectasia. In many instances the abnormality is manifested by decreased blastoid transformation. This has been noted in lymphocytes from patients with inoperable carcinoma of the lung (Han and Takita, 1972), chronic lymphocytic leukemia (Bernard et al, 1964; Douglas et al, 1973), Hodgkin's disease (Corder et al, 1972), and some types of lymphoma (Papac, 1970; Greally et al, 1973). Depressed transformation in mycosis fungoides is related to the stage of the disease, being most depressed when the disease is in stage IV (DuVivier et al, 1978). Opelz et al (1973) report that aspirin has a marked inhibitory effect on PHA-induced transformation.

Because most of the genetically determined enzyme systems can be found in cultured lymphocytes, cultures of lymphocytes are useful in the detection and study of both heterozygous and homozygous inherited metabolic disorders (Hirschhorn et al, 1969). Lymphocytes grow readily in culture, and a number of lymphoid cell lines have been established, from normals (Gerber and Monroe, 1968), from benign and malignant lymphoproliferative disorders (Clarkson et al, 1967; Glade et al, 1969), and from subhuman primates (London and Ellis, 1969). Lymphocytes in long-term culture produce all the metabolic products produced as a result of mitogen-induced transformation (p. 82). Furthermore, they retain special features of the original cell (Povey et al, 1973), e.g., the giant lysosomes of the Chédiak-Higashi syndrome (Blume et al, 1969), and specific enzyme deficiencies: Lesch-Nyhan syndrome (Choi and Bloom, 1970) and ganglioside storage disease (O'Brien et al, 1971).

Blastoid cells in tissue culture tend to aggregate around macrophages, a phenomenon called *peripolesis*. It has been suggested that macrophages are attracted to the ameboid projections on the surface of blastoid cells (uropodasis). This is in line with the concept that antibody production is a transfer of "processed" antigen from macrophages to lymphocytes. The sensitized lymphocyte (also called "activated," "committed," or "conditioned") then produces specific antibody. In so doing, it develops the characteristics of a plasma cell. By analogy the "virocytes" and "reactive lymphocytes" seen in the peripheral blood in infectious mononucleosis and lymphoproliferative disorders (Chapter 15) represent stimulated and reactive lymphocytes.

In vivo transformations

As already noted, it is almost certain that the in vivo transformation of small lymphocytes to "atypical lymphocytes," "virocytes," or "reactive lymphocytes" is the counterpart of the blastoid transformation in vitro. In addition, various transformations are known to take place in reactive states, whereas others are possible but not confirmed. It is accepted that lymphocytes can transform in vivo into macrophages, which may also be derived from blood monocytes, and that lymphocytes can transform into plasma cells (Roberts et al, 1957; Rebuck and LoGrippo, 1961; Zlotnik, 1967).

Dormant B-lymphocytes have immunoglobulins on the cell membrane, but the secretion of antibody is stimulated by helper T-cells in two ways. T-cells activated by concanavalin A or phytohemagglutinin produce a nonspecific B-cell activator, but in the presence of a specific antigen the antibody produced by the B-cells is specific for that antigen. It is assumed that B-cells stimulated by nonspecific activator plus antigen make up a clone of specific antibody-producing cells. Some of these clonal cells retain their specificity of antibody production after the antigenic stimulus is dissipated, so that at a later time they again react specifically to that antigen. Because of this property, they are called "memory cells."

Lymphocyte function: T-, B-, and null cells
Introduction

In the preceding discussion we have described the derivation of the concept of the duality of the lymphocytic system, expressed as two major classes of lymphocytes, T and B. Most lymphocytes can be classified as one or the other, with subpopulations of each (Cahill et al, 1977), but some, notably in lymphoproliferative disorders, have the characteristics of neither and are called null cells. It has been suggested that all lymphocytes originate as null cells and acquire T or B characteristics during maturation (Davis, 1975).

T- and B-lymphocytes have different primary roles in the immune response, but equally important are cell interactions between T- and B-lymphocytes and macrophages. Some of the interactions are cell-to-cell interactions; some are mediated by soluble factors produced by activated T-cells.

When sensitized T-cells are activated, they produce soluble substances called "lymphokines." Some interactions between T-lymphocytes, B-lymphocytes, and macrophages are mediated by lymphokines, and some may depend on direct contact between T-cells and macrophages. In any case, T-cells may act as *effector T-cells,* which are involved in the delayed hypersensitivity reaction and the graft-versus-host reaction, they may act as *helper T-cells,* which enhance antibody production by B-lymphocytes, or they may act as *suppressor T-cells,* which inhibit antibody production by B-cells. The evidence points to helper and suppressor cells being distinct cell lines (Steinberg and Klassen, 1977); suppressor T-cells bear receptors for the Fc portion of IgG, whereas helper T-cells have receptors for the Fc portion of IgM.

T-lymphocytes

T-lymphocytes in the mouse have a characteristic surface antigen (θ antigen) not present in human cells (Raff, 1971). Human T-lymphocytes also have a characteristic surface marker, uncovered after treatment with neuraminidase, that binds purified A hemagglutinin from the snail *Helix pomatia* (Hammarström et al, 1973). Another marker of T-lymphocytes may be β-2-microglobulin, shown to be a synthetic product of lymphocytes and a constituent of the cell membrane (Bach et al, 1973; Fanger and Bernier, 1973). T-lymphocytes are thought to have a relatively smooth surface

when viewed by scanning electron microscopy (Polliack et al, 1973), in contrast to the complex villous pattern of B-lymphocytes (Fig. 3-12). However, Alexander and Wetzel (1975) believe that the difference is artifactual and that the two types cannot be differentiated by scanning electron microscopy. T-lymphocytes are the predominant lymphocyte in blood and lymph (60% to 80% of the lymphocytes in the peripheral blood) (Nowell et al, 1975). In lymph nodes T-lymphocytes localize in the dense corona of lymphoid follicles and in the interfollicular and subfollicular zones; in the spleen they are found in the outer mantle of the periarteriolar sheath. They have no, or very few, immunoglobulin receptors on the surface membrane (Crone et al, 1972). Most lymphocytes transformed by PHA are T-cells (Jones and

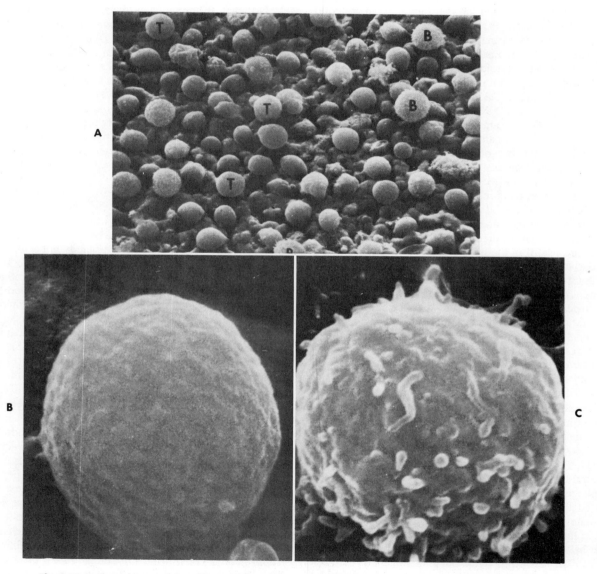

Fig. 3-12. Surface characteristics of T- and B-lympocytes. Scanning electron microscopy. **A,** Smooth T-lymphocytes and villous B-lymphocytes. **B,** Higher magnification of T-lymphocyte. **C,** Higher magnification of B-lymphocyte. Note dissenting opinion of Alexander and Wetzel (1975). (From Polliack, A., et al: Identification of human B and T lymphocytes by scanning electron microscopy, J. Exp. Med. **138:**607-624, 1973.)

Roitt, 1972). T-lymphocytes form rosettes (E rosettes) with sheep red blood cells not coated with human complement (Ross et al, 1973). T-lymphocytes have increased β-glucuronidase activity. By immunofluorescence, T-lymphocytes can be shown to bind antithymocyte antibody at the surface membrane (RC Williams et al, 1973). T-lymphocytes can recognize and respond to antigen, and an immunoglobulin-like T-cell receptor has been postulated (Marchalonis et al, 1978). T-lymphocytes can be identified in smears from blood or tissues by using bacteria coated with anti-T antiserum (Teodorescu et al, 1976). T-lymphocytes can be shown to be positive for esterase activity when a modified procedure is used (Higgy et al, 1977), whereas B-lymphoctyes are esterase negative. Under different conditions Pangalis et al (1978) found T-lymphocytes to be strongly esterase positive.

Matchett et al (1973) present evidence for depletion of T-lymphocytes from the peripheral blood in Hodgkin's disease. This is consistent with the hypothesis (Order and Hellman, 1972) that the lesion of Hodgkin's disease is caused by unaffected T-lymphocytes reacting with stimulated lymphocytes to produce a cell-to-cell chronic host-versus-graft reaction. Concurrently, a depletion of the stimulated cells can be expected.

There is a growing consensus that cellular immunity reactions mediated by T-lymphocytes are important in the biology of various neoplasms (Ritts and Neel, 1974), and developments in this field certainly should be followed closely.

T-lymphocytes are long-lived and are responsible for cellular immune reactions such as graft rejection and delayed hypersensitivity reactions. Sensitized T-lymphocytes interacting with antigen or mitogen liberate a number of products. These are the *lymphokines* (Dumonde, 1970), generally chemical mediators of *cellular* immune responses, the best established being (1) cytotoxic and growth-inhibiting factor (lymphocytotoxin), (2) migration inhibition factors (MIF), (3) transfer factor (TF), (4) mitogenic or blastogenic factor (cell stimulatory or lymphocyte transforming factor [LTF]), (5) lymph node permeability factor, and (6) eosinophilotropic factor. There is no certainty that these are distinct factors, for the possibility exists that a few substances could exhibit different activities depending on concentration of the factor, the target cell on which it acts, and other variables (Lawrence and Valentine, 1970; Kay, 1971).

LYMPHOCYTOTOXIN. Specifically sensitized lymphocytes (lymphocytes stimulated by mitogens and incubated with tissue cells or target cells containing the specific antigen) elaborate lymphocytotoxin (Granger and Kolb, 1968; Kolb and Granger, 1968; Williams and Granger, 1969; Granger et al, 1970). They then become "aggressor lymphocytes" and destroy the target cell. The high concentration of T-cells in and around primary tumors suggests that they play an important part in tumor immunobiology (Husby et al, 1976). It is probable that release of lymphocytotoxin is primarily dependent in the lymphocyte undergoing blast transformation either by specific antigens or by mitogens. Stimulated lymphocytes produce lymphocytotoxin and release it into the surrounding medium, where it disrupts the cell membrane of the target cell either directly or by an effect on the internal metabolic systems. It has been sup-

posed that the aggressor cell and the target cell must be in contact to effect destruction of the target cell, but most hypothetical cell-cell interactions can be explained equally well by the greater concentration of active agent in proximity to the aggressor cell.

Lymphocytes are resistant to lymphocytotoxin (in fact, lymphocytes are generally resistant to their own products) except in the presence of a high concentration of lymphocytotoxin. Epithelial cells are most susceptible to the cytotoxic effect, followed in order of decreasing susceptibility by fibroblasts, renal tubular cells, and hepatocytes. Lymphocytotoxin is obviously important in cellular immunity reactions in which foreign cells are destroyed.

Release of lymphocytotoxin is blocked by inhibitors of protein synthesis such as puromycin and cyclohexamide and by inhibitors of oxidative phosphorylation such as dinitrophenol. Since blocking DNA or RNA synthesis does not block release of lymphocytotoxin, it is assumed that the blockage is at the mRNA level; thus it is postulated that lymphocytotoxin production is controlled by mRNA. Cortisone also inhibits lymphocytotoxin release, but the mechanism is not known.

MIGRATION INHIBITION FACTOR (MIF). A variety of antigens can induce sensitized lymphocytes to secrete a factor that inhibits the migration of macrophages (Bloom and Bennett, 1966, 1970; David, 1966; Mackaness, 1969; Bloom and Jiminez, 1970; Remold et al, 1970). Since sensitized lymphocytes play a key role in the first step of the delayed hypersensitivity reaction (DHR), the secretion of MIF, in in vitro studies seems to be the counterpart of the DHR in vivo. The reaction at an injection site can be produced either by the injection of antigen that reacts with previously sensitized lymphocytes causing the release of MIF, as in the tuberculin reaction, or by injection of cell-free MIF into nonsensitized animals. MIF is responsible for the accumulation of macrophages around bacteria and other antigens and may or may not be identical with a factor called "macrophage chemotactic factor" that is said to be responsible for attracting macrophages to the lesion.

MIF or MIF-like substances are liberated also from lymphocytes infected by viruses (PA Ward et al, 1972), and Cohen et al (1974) report that the serum from most patients with Hodgkin's disease (10 of 13), non-Hodgkin's lymphomas (14 of 16), and chronic lymphocytic leukemia (4 of 5) has MIF activity. Since chronic lymphocytic leukemia is a B-cell disease (p. 87), the elaboration of MIF in this disease may be an example of MIF production by B-cells as a result of "nonspecific" stimulation (Yoshida et al, 1973).

TRANSFER FACTOR (TF). In animals the delayed hypersensitivity reaction can be achieved only by transfer of viable lymphocytes, and it was assumed for some time that the same requirement held for humans. However, passive transfer in humans was found to require many fewer viable lymphocytes and to last much longer. It was then found that cell-free extracts of lymphocytes were equally effective, and the agent responsible for transfer of delayed hypersensitivity was called TF (Lawrence et al, 1960; Jensen et al, 1962; Bloom and Chase, 1967; Adler and Smith, 1969). Unlike MIF, TF is antigen specific in that every antigen stimulates release of a TF specific for that antigen and no other. It can be assumed that an antigen stimulates a clone of T-lymphocytes to produce TF. Once released, TF also confers on noncommitted lymphocytes the capacity to respond to the specific antigen (Rosenfeld and Dressler, 1974), and the recruited noncommitted lymphocytes undergo blast transformation only when exposed to the specific antigen. TF is nonimmunogenic and is produced only by human lymphocytes.

LYMPHOCYTE TRANSFORMING FACTOR (LTF). During incubation of sensitized lymphocytes with antigen a substance or substances (LTF) are formed that induce nonspecific blast transformation of other lymphocytes (Maini et al, 1969; Spitler and Lawrence, 1969; Valentine and Lawrence, 1969; Janis and Bach, 1970). This is also called mitogenic, blastogenic, or cell stimulatory factor. As with many of the other factors, there is no certainty that this is in fact an effect attributable to a specific substance different from other factors inducing blast transformation, such as TF. Unlike TF, however, LTF is produced by both animal and human lymphocytes.

LYMPH NODE PERMEABILITY FACTOR. This factor is said to increase the permeability of vascular endothelium in lymph nodes (Willoughby et al, 1964). Note, however, that some other factors, notably MIF, also provoke hyperplastic reactions in lymph nodes.

EOSINOPHILOTROPIC FACTOR. It has been shown that the induction of eosinophilia in *Trichinella* infection is mediated by lymphocytes. Sensitized lymphocytes supposedly liberate the so-called eosinophilotropic factor (Basten and Beeson, 1970). McGarry et al (1971) demonstrated the dependence of the eosinophilic response to tetanus toxoid on T-lymphocytes without assuming the existence of eosinophilotropic factor. I have seen one case of the Sézary syndrome, a T-lymphocyte proliferation, with striking blood eosinophilia.

HELPER AND SUPPRESSOR T-CELLS. In addition to the various activities of T-cells expressed by the lymphokines, T-cells are involved in helping B-cells to produce antibodies. In addition, T-cells can also suppress antibody production, and it is probable that helper T-cells and suppressor T-cells are distinct cell lines (Steinberg and Klassen, 1977).

B-lymphocytes

B-lymphocytes are short lived, bone marrow derived, and bursa equivalent. They have surface immunoglobulin receptors and contribute to the immune response by participating in the elaboration of immunoglobulins—the humoral defense mechanism. They are in the minority in blood (20% of the lymphocytes) but make up the bulk of peripheral lymphoid tissue. They bear a complement receptor (C3) and form rosettes with sheep erythrocytes coated with human complement, EAC rosettes (Bianco et al, 1970). B-lymphocyte rosettes are characterized by contact through both villous and nonvillous areas by scanning electron microscopy (PS Lin et al, 1973). B-lymphocytes also bear receptors for aggregated γ-globulin, probably by means of surface receptors for the Fc portion of IgG (Dickler and Kunkel, 1972; Huber et al, 1974). B-lymphocytes can also be identified by the use of antibody-coated bacteria (Teodorescu et al,

1976). B-lymphocytes also bind untreated *Brucella malitensis* (Teodorescu and Mayer, 1978).

The specificity of the immune response is dependent on recognition of antigen by specific antigen-recognizing receptors on the surface of lymphocytes (Katz and Benacerraf, 1972). It is now accepted that B-lymphocytes have immunoglobulin receptors on the surface membrane (Pernis et al, 1970) that are distributed at random and average about 10^5/cell (Unanue et al, 1973). The class of immunoglobulin identified on the surface of normal lymphocytes varies greatly in different species and somewhat among reports by various investigators: about half of human lymphocytes have IgM (Pernis et al, 1970), almost all rabbit lymphocytes bear IgM (Perkins et al, 1972), the predominant class in the guinea pig is IgG. Human lymphocytes that do not bear IgM receptors usually bear IgA, IgG, IgD, or IgE receptors. Ross (1977) reviews some of the technical difficulties in identifying surface markers of T- and B-cells. Scanning immunoelectron microscopy has been used to distinguish between the various surface immunoglobulins (Ito et al, 1978).

Null cells

Many investigators have encountered lymphocytes that have *neither* T nor B characteristics (Lay et al, 1971; Mendes et al, 1973; Seligmann et al, 1973). The significance of these "null" cells is not clear at this time. Null cells have been encountered in leukemia and lymphomas (Table 3-1), and it may be assumed that these cells, because of their immaturity, have not yet acquired B or T characteristics. It might be added that a very few lymphocytes having *both* T and B characteristics are found in normal blood and in some leukemias resembling chronic lymphocytic leukemia (Shevach et al, 1974).

Interrelations in the immune response

As shown in Fig. 3-13, the total spectrum of the immune response requires some degree of cellular interdependence. In its simplest terms, antigen is phagocytized by macrophages and is either restricted to lysosomes and destroyed or processed to be passed on to receptor lymphocytes. Soluble antigens are poorly processed, and the availability is increased by adjuvants that help to present the antigen as particulate. Antigen is passed on directly to contiguous lymphocytes as processed antigen consisting of a complex of antigen and macrophage RNA (AA Gottlieb et al, 1967) and accepted by the receptor lymphocytes at their surface immunoglobulin sites (Greaves et al, 1972). The processing role of the macrophage is more than a simple preparation of antigen for the receptor lymphocyte, for macrophage RNA carries the specific code for antibody synthesis (Haurowitz, 1970). An excess of nonprocessed antigen may combine with the receptor sites and block the acceptance of processed antigen. Having recognized and accepted the processed antigen, the lymphocytes become immunologically active either in cellular or immune responses. At the same time, "memory cells" remain in each clone (Burnet, 1969) with the capacity to respond to the same antigen at a future time. There is also evidence that some T-lymphocytes act as "helper cells" to B-lymphocytes (Claman and Chaperon, 1969).

Table 3-1. Types of lymphocytes found in various lymphoproliferative disorders

Disorder	T-lymphocyte	B-lymphocyte	Null lymphocyte[j]
Acute lymphocytic leukemia	25%[d]	2%[h]	Majority[h]
Chronic lymphocytic leukemia	Rare[e]	Majority[i]	Rare
Leukemic reticuloendotheliosis[a]	Rare	Predominant	0
Sézary's syndrome	Predominant[f]	0	0
Hodgkin's disease[b]	Decreased	0	0
Non-Hodgkin's lymphoma[c]	Predominant	Rare	Rare
Infectious mononucleosis	Predominant[g]	0	0

[a]Hairy cell leukemia. HJ Cohen et al (1979).
[b]In blood. In splenic tissue T-lymphocytes are increased (de Sousa et al., 1978).
[c]Varies in different types. B-lymphocytes predominant in nodular lymphomas (Mann et al., 1979) and most diffuse poorly differentiated lymphomas (Brouet et al., 1975c). Some diffuse lymphomas are of T-cell or null cell type (Gajl-Peczalska, 1975; ES Jaffe et al., 1975).
[d]Kersey et al., (1975).
[e]Brouet et al., (1975b); characteristically, patients have splenomegaly without lymphadenopathy.
[f]Broder et al., (1976).
[g]Sheldon et al., (1973).
[h]Brouet et al., (1975a).
[i]Gupta and Good (1980).
[j]Some cells previously classified as null may in fact be pre-B-cells (lack surface IgG but contain intracytoplasmic IgM) (Vogler et al., 1978; Gupta and Good, 1980).

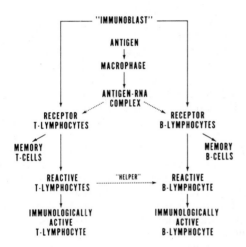

Fig. 3-13. Interrelations in the immune response.

Cyclic AMP compounds inhibit various of the immunologic reactions, and some inflammatory mediators (histamine, prostaglandins) limit the intensity of the inflammatory and immune reaction (Bourne et al, 1974). It is suggested that lymphocytes have or acquire receptors for these substances at the surface and that the immune response is inhibited or modified by (1) inhibition of mitogen- or antigen-induced blast transformation (Smith et al, 1971), (2) inhibition of immune cytolysis (Lichtenstein et al, 1973), (3) inhibition of production or release of lymphocytic factors (interferon, MIF, etc.) (Bourne et al, 1974), and (4) prevention of the antibody response by inhibition of the proliferation of antibody-forming cells (Watson et al, 1973) or by inhibition of the production or release of antibody (Melmon et al, 1974).

Perspective

There is no doubt that one of the greatest advances in our understanding of disease has been the clarification of the role of lymphocytes in cellular and humoral immunity and parallel developments in the field of structure and functions of the immunoglobulins. when it became obvious that lymphocytes are important cells indeed, they became, and continue to be, the object of intensive study from all possible angles, from electron microscopy to the characterization of membrane receptors. The study of normal human lymphocytes soon revealed that T-cells and B-cells can in fact be distinguished on the basis of several individual membrane characteristics.

It was natural that the lymphoproliferative disorders should be studied next, with the hope that application of the methods used to distinguish normal lymphocytes would lead to a better understanding of benign and malignant lymphoproliferations, perhaps even to a sound and stable classification of the lymphomas.

Few of these hopes have been fulfilled (Table 3-1), but I would venture the prediction that an unequivocal classification of lymphocytic leukemias and lymphomas according to cell type should not be expected. It is probable that "virgin" lymphocytes have no characteristics, and that the differentiation into B and T types occurs later as they are exposed to a multiplicity of immunologic environments and cellular interactions. If this is the case, then it can be expected that the cell characteristics of a given lymphocytic leukemia or lymphoma do not prove the origin from a given cell type but rather reflect variable modifications imposed on pre-cells or null cells in the course of the disease.

The lymphocyte in immunologic reactions

When an antigen is injected intradermally into a recipient previously sensitized to that antigen, two types of immune reactions can be observed. The first occurs within minutes or 1 to 2 hours, depends on the reaction between the antigen and the specific immunoglobulin antibody, and cannot be transferred by sensitized lymphocytes. This *immediate hypersensitivity reaction* is, therefore, *humoral*. The second type of reaction is slower in developing, 6 to 24 hours, is not dependent on the presence of a specific immunoglobulin antibody, and can be transferred by suspensions of sensitized lymphocytes. This *delayed hypersensitivity reaction* is, therefore, *cellular*.

Immunologic diseases are the result of one or another of these two reactions, with the exception of immunologic deficiency states where disease is caused by failure of either cellular or humoral defense mechanisms. For a complete discussion of immunologic diseases the reader is referred to Samter (1965). We will limit the discussion here to some of the basic reactions.

Cellular immunity

THE DELAYED HYPERSENSITIVITY REACTION (DHR). The classic DHR (Raffel, 1965) can be induced with tuberculin or PPD, but there are many other agents to which the body reacts in this way. The reaction is not limited to the skin, since bacterial, viral, parasitic, and contact antigens can produce the DHR in internal organs such as the mucosa of the bladder, colon, vagina, and uterus as well as in the joints, liver, and cornea. While the DHR in the skin has been studied intensively, the reaction has a much broader biologic significance, e.g., allograft rejection and allergic encephalomyelitis.

Landsteiner and Chase (1940) showed that the cellular portion of the peritoneal exudate of guinea pigs sensitized to a simple chemical substance (picryl chloride, 2,4,6-trinitrochlorobenzene) could, when injected into a normal guinea pig, produce a delayed inflammatory response. A few years later (1945) Chase showed that sensitivity to tuberculin could be transferred passively by suspensions of cells from lymph nodes and spleen. Other investigators have demonstrated passive transfer of hypersensitivity to various bacteria and bacterial products (tetanus toxoid, streptococci, *Pasteurella tularensis,* and *Brucella*), viruses (cowpox, mumps, and lymphogranuloma venereum), fungi (*Coccidioides, Candida, Trichophyton, Blastomyces,* and *Histoplasma*), parasites (*Trichinella, Ascaris, Schistosoma,* and *Echinococcus*), contact antigens of plant origin (poison ivy and poison oak), and contact-active chemicals (O-chlorobenzoyl chloride, *p*-nitrosodium methylaniline, and beryllium sulfate).

Histologically, the DHR is characterized by infiltration with mononuclear cells, commonly surrounding small vessels to produce the "perivascular island" effect. The infiltrating cells are lymphocytes, some of the blastoid type, and macrophages.

The mediator of the DHR is the small lymphocyte. Most investigators think that a two-stage reaction is involved. First, a relatively small number of lymphocytes are sensitized to the antigen, either through specific receptor sites at the surface or by a transfer of information from macrophages to lymphocytes in the form of a complex of macrophage RNA and ingested antigen. During this first stage the lymphocytes are "conditioned" to the antigen; some call this process "induction," and the lymphocytes can be said to thus acquire "immunologic memory." Conditioned lymphocytes then proliferate and are numerically sufficient to effect the immune response. In the case of immediate hypersensitivity reactions the conditioned lymphocytes transform

to immunoglobulin-synthesizing cells ("plasma cells" and "lymphocytes") that provide circulating antibody. In the delayed reaction the sensitized lymphocytes are responsible for the reaction without the component of circulating antibody. As expected, antilymphocyte antiserum will inhibit the DHR.

Skin allografts can be made to survive if mobilization of sensitized lymphocytes does not occur. This has been accomplished by depleting the lymphoid tissues of lymphocytes by using irradiation, corticosteroids, antimetabolites, or antilymphocyte antiserum. Depletion of circulating lymphocytes by chronic drainage of thoracic duct lymph is also effective. The graft will also survive if lymphocytes have no access to it, as in the case of transplants to avascular tissues, such as the cornea of the eye, or to the brain.

ANTILYMPHOCYTIC SERUM (ALS). The properties and potential of ALS deserve special mention (Russell and Monaco, 1967; Woodruff, 1967; Sell, 1969; Lance, 1970). Because it was shown to prolong the survival of skin allografts in rats at the same time that the work with human organ transplants was being intensified, ALS became an important adjunct to preventing organ rejection. As Medawar (1968) points out, however, it is not a new concept. He cites its use by Metchnikoff in the late 1800s and by other investigators in the early 1900s. Also, I cannot resist reference to my own work with antispleen serum (Miale, 1947) and the lymphocyte changes produced by it.

ALS is produced by injecting lymphocytes into a host animal. The antiserum used in humans is usually produced by injecting human lymphocytes into horses. The antiserum contains a mixture of antilymphocyte antibodies. It acts by blocking surface immunoglobulin (Paraskevas et al, 1972) and by cytolysis of circulating (long-lived, thymus-dependent) lymphocytes (Tyler at al, 1969), which are then removed by reticuloendothelial phagocytes. This destructive effect is complement dependent. ALS does not directly attack the lymphocytes in lymphoid organs; the lymphocytes will be depleted, however, as a consequence of the continued destruction of circulating lymphocytes.

ALS has several important advantages over other immunosuppressive agents (irradiation, alkylating agents, steroids, antifolates, etc.). It does not inhibit or destroy antibody-producing cells, and thus the recipient is able to respond normally to infection by bacteria or viruses. It erases the body's immunologic memory for previous reactions to antigens and may be useful in the treatment of autoimmune syndromes in which the body continues to react against antigens that behave as though they were foreign. Finally, it makes the body less sensitive to antigenic differences between the graft and the host, so that xenografts are within the realm of possibility.

There has been some interest in antithymocyte serum (Nagaya, 1970; Ablin et al, 1972; Aisenberg et al, 1973b) but its potential is still under investigation.

TRANSPLANTATION REACTIONS. The graft-versus-host reaction can be produced by injecting lymphocytes into a host animal that is incapable of rejecting them, i.e., an animal that has been heavily irradiated, a newborn animal that has not yet developed the capacity to reject a graft, or an animal that is·antigenically similar. The classic demonstration of the reaction showed that when two inbred mouse strains (genetic designation *AA* and *BB,* respectively) are crossed, a hybrid (genetic designation *AB*) is produced that possesses the antigens of both parents. If lymphocytes from one parent *(AA)* are injected into the *AB* hybrid, they will not be rejected because *AA* is not foreign to *AB.* However, the *AA* cells will become sensitized to cells carrying the B determinant from the other parent and will eventually attack and destroy them. The damage results in a syndrome characterized by hepatosplenomegaly; lymphocytic depletion and atrophy of lymph nodes, Peyer's patches, and the thymus; alopecia; wasting; and eventual death—the "runt disease" or "wasting syndrome." The injection of a small number of lymphocytes produces a more chronic disease; many of these animals have terminal leukemia.

Understanding and modifying transplantation immunity are basic to success in tissue and organ transplantation. The antigens that impart an acceptable "sameness" or a catastrophic "difference" to a cell are known as histocompatibility, or H, antigens and are related to specific genetic loci called histocompatibility loci making up the HL-A system (Ceppellini and van Rood, 1974; van Rood, 1974) (Chapter 11).

CANCER IMMUNOLOGY. One other area of great interest is the relationship of transplantation immunity reactions to the resistance or susceptibility of the host to invading tumor tissue (Kahan and Reisfeld, 1969; Kissmeyer-Nielsen et al, 1972). A lymphocytic infiltrate of T-cells is commonly seen around tumor nodules in human material as well as animal transplant experiments (Fisher and Fisher, 1972; Husby et al, 1976). This can be interpreted variously, of course, but the possibility exists that this represents a weak and apparently ineffective rejection reaction toward the tumor tissue. We know that tumors have tumor-specific antigens that are not present in the cells of the host. These are weak antigens, and investigators working this field have encountered many difficulties. Nevertheless, it is not outside the realm of possibility, and of hope, that the prevention or treatment of neoplasms may someday be based on a more complete understanding of cellular or humoral immunity reactions (Ritts and Neel, 1974).

IN PREGNANCY. During pregnancy the fetus presents a potential homograft situation. Since the mother in most cases fails to reject the fetus, it has been assumed that the maternal response to fetal histocompatibility antigens is somehow altered. Walknowska et al (1969) and Schröder and de la Chapelle (1972) have shown that fetal lymphocytes enter the maternal circulation and can be found in the mother's blood as early as the fourteenth week of gestation. It is not unlikely that the transplacental passage of lymphocytes contributes to the altered maternal reactivity to fetal antigens (Billingham, 1964; Hellström et al, 1969; Carr et al, 1973).

Humoral immunity: the immunoglobulins

DEFINITION. The term "immunoglobulins" is used to encompass the whole group of antibody proteins as well as related proteins found in pathologic states, such as multiple myeloma, Waldenström's macroglobulinemia, etc., that have little or no antibody function. As is so often the case,

the study of pathologic conditions has been a major factor in clarifying the normal physiologic state. We find, therefore, that while this section deals with the role of immunoglobulins in the immune response, some references to pathologic states cannot be avoided. These pathologic states, the immunoglobulinopathies, are covered in detail in Chapter 16.

Within a relatively few years our knowledge of the structure and function of the immunoglobulins has progressed from the elementary to the complex. The original salting-out technics gave an inexact separation of serum proteins into two fractions, "albumin" and "globulin." More critical separation technics such as the ethanol precipitation schemes of Cohn yielded many fractions and subfractions, particularly of globulin proteins. Moving boundary electrophoresis on various constantly improved media identified five major categories: albumin, α_1-globulins, α_2-globulins, β-globulins, and γ-globulins. Ultracentrifugal separation of serum proteins allows separation according to molecular weight in terms of Svedberg units (S). Three major constituents can be identified: the A or 4S fraction (molecular weight about 70,000 and consisting mostly of albumin), the G or 7S fraction (molecular weight about 160,000 and consisting mostly of γ-globulin), and the M or 19S fraction (molecular weight about 1 million, the macroglobulins). The technic of immunoelectrophoresis yields the most specific and critical separation (20 or more serum proteins are identifiable with polyvalent antisera) (Fig. 3-14), whereas the use of monospecific antisera allows identification and quantification of individual proteins and protein subunits.

STRUCTURE. Five *classes* of immunoglobulins (Ig) have been described: IgG, IgA, IgM, IgD, and IgE. The basic structure of all immunoglobulin molecules consists of two pairs of polypeptide chains, two *heavy chains* (H chains) and two *light chains* (L chains), linked by interchain covalent disulfide bonds (Fig. 3-15). Detailed reviews of the genetics, structure, and function of the immunoglobulins are given by Metzger (1970, Milstein and Pink (1970), Edelman (1971), Gally and Edelman (1972), Solomon and McLaughlin (1973), and Natvig and Kunkel (1973).

The nomenclature follows the recommendations in Bull WHO **41**:975, 1969:

1. It is recommended that the variable and constant regions be termed the "V region" and the "C region," respectively.
2. The symbols "V_L" and "C_L" are used for the variable and constant regions of the L chains.
3. The symbols "V_H" and "C_H" are used for the variable and constant regions of the H chains.
4. If it is desired to specify a particular class or subclass of H chain, the symbol "subscript H" should be replaced by the symbol of the class or subclass. For example, the C_H region of the H chain of a molecule of the γG1 subclass would be designated "$C_{\gamma 1}$ region." Similarly, if it is desired to specify a particular type of L chain, the symbol "subscript L" should be replaced by the symbol for the chain, e.g., "V_κ region," "C_λ region."
5. It is suggested that half-cystinyl residues be designated by Roman numerals, the first residue being that

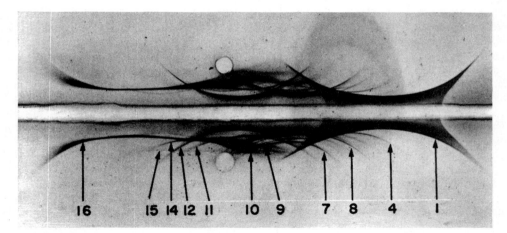

Fig. 3-14. Proteins of normal serum. Immunoelectrophoresis, normal serum against polyvalent antiserum (anti-goat): **1**, albumin; **4**, antitrypsin; **8**, haptoglobin; **7**, ceruloplasmin; **9**, α_2-macroglobulin; **10**, β-lipoprotein; **11**, hemopexin; **12**, transferrin; **14**, IgA globulin; **15**, IgM globulin; **16**, IgG globulin.

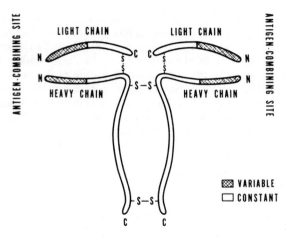

Fig. 3-15. Structure of immunoglobulin molecule. It is, like the hemoglobin molecule, a tetramer of polypeptide chains. Two are L chains and two are H chains. The *N*-terminals are the antigen-combining sites. The diagram shows the disulfide bond connecting the C-terminal portion of each L chain to its neighbor H chain and the disulfide bonds connecting the long portions of the H chains. Not shown are the disulfide bonds within the polypeptide chains, two within each L chain and four within each H chain. The L chains are the same in all classes of immunoglobulins; the specific class of immunoglobulin is determined by the H chains.

closest to the amino terminus. An Arabic number, as a subscript, corresponds to the number of the amino acid residue.

6. All variable regions associated with an L chain of a given type are defined as a "group." Subdivisions are called "subgroups" and are designated by Roman numerals in order of decreasing frequency.

7. These new symbols are used to represent the structure of immunoglobulin molecules:

$$[(V_\kappa I C_\kappa) (V_\gamma C_\gamma I)] = \text{a dimer } _\gamma G1 \text{ molecule}$$
with κ light chains of group I

Each *class* of Ig is characterized by a specific heavy chain: γ in IgG, α in IgA, μ in IgM, δ in IgD, and ε in IgE. Subclasses of heavy chains characterize *subclasses* within some of the classes. There are four γ subclasses, γ^1, γ^2, γ^3, and γ^4, and they characterize IgG subclasses IgG1, IgG2, IgG3, and IgG4, respectively. Likewise, there are two IgA subclasses, IgA1 and IgA2, characterized by α-chain subclasses α^1 and α^2, and two IgM subclasses, IgM1 and IgM2, characterized by μ-chain subclasses μ^1 and μ^2.

IgG subclasses vary in their capacity to bind complement (Augener et al, 1971), the order being IgG3 > IgG1 > IgG2 > IgG4, the last having very little or no affinity. IgA subclasses show striking structural differences, with IgA2 lacking the interchain disulfide bonds that link H and L chains in all other immunoglobulins (Grey et al, 1968; Jerry et al, 1972). Lacking disulfide bonds, IgA2 may be stabilized by secretory IgA. Normal serum contains about 90% IgA1 and 10% IgA2, whereas about 50% of secretory (salivary) IgA consists of IgA2.

IgG subclasses have different metabolic properties (Morell et al, 1970). The average half-life of IgG1, IgG2, and IgG4 is 21 days, but that of IgG3 is only 7 days. In addition, IgG3 has a higher turnover rate and a slower rate of synthesis (3.4 mg/kg/day as compared with 25.4 mg/kg/day for IgG1). The normal relative concentrations of IgG subclasses are 65% IgG1, 23% IgG2, 8% IgG3, and 4% IgG4.

IgG subclasses also show individual immunologic specificities. For example, anti-Rh antibodies consist primarily of IgG1 and IgG3 (Natvig et al, 1967), as do most red blood cell autoantibodies and isoantibodies (Abramson and Schur, 1972). Of the four subclasses, only IgG4 is not involved in complement fixation. All four pass equally through the placenta.

Heavy chains interact with one or the other of two types of L chains, κ or λ, to form the tetramer immunoglobulin molecule. For example, the general molecular formula for IgG is either γ2κ2 or γ2λ2, while for subclass IgG1 the molecular formula is either $\gamma^1 2\kappa 2$ or $\gamma^1 2\lambda 2$ (Table 3-2).

Table 3-2. Complete terminology of the heavy and light chains of human immunoglobulins

H chain

Region:	V Region
Subgroups:	V_{HI}, V_{HII}, H_{HIII}
Region:	C Region ($C_H{}^1$, $C_H{}^2$, $C_H{}^3$)
Class:	C_γ, C_α, C_μ, C_δ, C_ϵ
Subclass:	$C_{\gamma 1}$, $C_{\gamma 2}$, $C_{\gamma 3}$, $C_{\gamma 4}$, $C_{\alpha 1}$, $C_{\alpha 2}$, $C_{\mu 1}$, $C_{\mu 2}$

L chain

Type:	Kappa (κ)
Region:	V Region (V_κ)
Subgroups:	$V_{\kappa I}$, $V_{\kappa II}$, $V_{\kappa III}$
Region:	C Region (C_κ)
Allotypes:	$C_\kappa Leu^{191}$ (In V1, In V2)
	$C_\kappa Val^{191}$ (In V3)
Type:	Lambda (λ)
Region:	V Region (V_λ)
Subgroups:	$V_{\lambda I}$, $V_{\lambda II}$, $V_{\lambda III}$, $V_{\lambda IV}$, $V_{\lambda V}$
Region:	C Region (C_λ)*
Allotypes:	$C_\lambda Ser^{154}Arg^{191}$ (Kern⁻, Oz⁻)
	$C_\lambda Ser^{154}Lys^{191}$ (Kern⁻, Oz⁺)
	$C_\lambda Gly^{154}Arg^{191}$ (Kern⁺, Oz⁻)
	$C_\lambda Gly^{154}Lys^{191}$ (Kern⁺, Oz⁺)

*Also described are Mz⁺, Mz⁻; Mcq⁺, Mcq⁻ (Solomon, 1976).

Immunoglobulins containing κ light chains are sometimes called type K and those containing λ chains are type L.

Each polypeptide chain is composed of two regions designated "constant region" (C region) and "variable region" (V region) (Fig. 3-15). In the L chain both the V region and the C region contain 107 amino acids. In the H chain the V region contains 121 amino acids and the C region contains 325. As is implied, the amino acid composition of the C regions is constant. The C_H region consists of three homologous regions of about equal length designated C_H1, C_H2, and C_H3. In the V regions various substitutions of amino acids are possible, allowing the assembly of immunoglobulin molecules having different immunologic specificities. The V regions are located distally (Fig. 3-15), and it is here that antigen binding takes place.

The distinction of C and V regions and the determination of the amino acid sequences in each have given rise to an additional subclassification of H and L chains based on the structure of the C and V regions (Table 3-2). This takes into account three subgroups of L κ-chains ($V_{\kappa I}$, $V_{\kappa II}$, and $V_{\kappa III}$), five subgroups of L λ-chains ($V_{\lambda I}$, $V_{\lambda II}$, $V_{\lambda III}$, $V_{\lambda IV}$, and $V_{\lambda V}$), and three subgroups of the V region of the H chain (V_{HI}, V_{HII}, and V_{HIII}). The genetic markers InV are identified with the amino acid at position 191 of C_κ (C region of κ light chain). Variations in the amino acids at positions 191 and 154 of C_λ account for the immunochemical designations Kern⁺, Kern⁻ (Hess and Hilschmann, 1971) and Oz⁺, Oz⁻ (Ein and Fahey, 1967). Mz⁺, Mz⁻ represents variations at positions 147/174. Mcq⁺, Mcq⁻ represents variations at positions 116/118/167 (Solomon, 1976).

A third type of polypeptide chain, designated J, has been found in association with polymeric secretory IgA and with IgM polymers (Mestecky et al, 1971, 1972). This is a small chain, molecular weight 23,000 to 26,000, involved in the polymerization of the monomers of IgA or IgM (Parkhouse, 1972). J chains have not been found in association with IgG, IgD, or IgE.

The stereochemical configuration of an immunologic molecule is shown in Fig. 3-16. Proteolytic digestion of the immunoglobulin molecule yields a number of polypeptide subunits (Fig. 3-17). Amino acid analysis of these has not only given the primary structure of the entire polypeptide chains, but also some hypotheses of the genetic control over their synthesis.

The molecule of IgG (molecular weight 160,000) and IgD (molecular weight 180,000) immunoglobulins contains two H chains and two L chains. IgA molecular weights are multiples of 160,000, so that it may be a dimer (Fig. 3-18) or a trimer of the basic molecule.

Immunoglobulins are present in almost every external secretion but not always in the same ratio as in normal blood. In part, the difference is illustrated by the opposite behavior of IgG and IgA regarding transplacental transport (IgG passes from mother to fetus, whereas IgA does not). Only anti-Rh antibodies of the IgG type pass from the mother to the fetus and have the potential of producing isoimmune hemolytic disease. In part, the difference is qualitative. For example, secretory IgA is qualitatively different from serum IgA. The molecule of secretory IgA is larger than the corresponding serum IgA dimer, has a sedimentation coefficient of 11S rather than 7S, and its disulfide bonds are not readily reduced by sulfhydryl reagents. IgA has an additional nonimmunoglobulin "secretory" component with a molecular weight of about 60,000. This secretory piece was once thought to be acquired when the IgA molecule from serum passed through the epithelial cells of the secreting organ. It has been shown that secretory IgA levels are not related to serum IgA levels, and it is more likely that secretory IgA is synthesized within the cells of the salivary glands (Tomasi, 1972; Walker and Hong, 1973). As noted above, the J chain is associated with polymeric secretory IgA.

An excess formation of immunoglobulins is present in multiple myeloma (Chapter 16). In most cases the excess immunoglobulin is of only one class, e.g., IgG, IgA, IgD, or IgE. In Waldenström's macroglobulinemia the immunoglobulin is IgM. Only in rare cases have two distinct electrophoretic peaks been found in one serum. In myeloma there may also be excretion in the urine of protein composed of only L chains, the Bence Jones proteins. In each case the molecular character of the immunoglobulin is homogeneous, and yet it has been found that myeloma proteins from different patients are seldom identical. The same is true of Bence Jones proteins. It would seem that an almost unlimited number of substitutions are possible in the variable portion of the polypeptide chains. The immunoglobulins in myeloma do not have any of the known antibody functions.

Bence Jones proteins are complete immunoglobulin L chains in the form of monomers and dimers (Edelman and

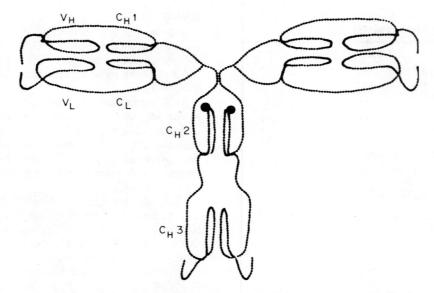

Fig. 3-16. Model of immunoglobulin molecule. (Courtesy Dr. Gerald M. Edelman.)

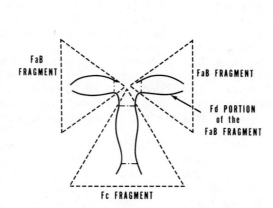

Fig. 3-17. Digestion by papain of a molecule of immunoglobulin yields two FaB and one Fc fragment. Note that cleavage occurs between sites of disulfide bonding. If digestion is by pepsin, the cleavage point is below the upper disulfide bond connecting the H chains.

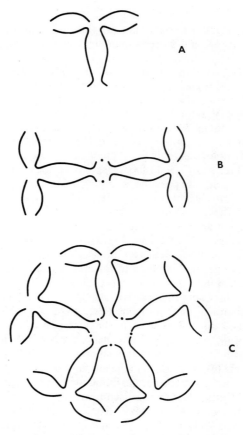

Fig. 3-18. Polymerization of a single immunoglobulin molecule, **A,** to form an IgA dimer, **B,** and an IgM pentamer, **C.**

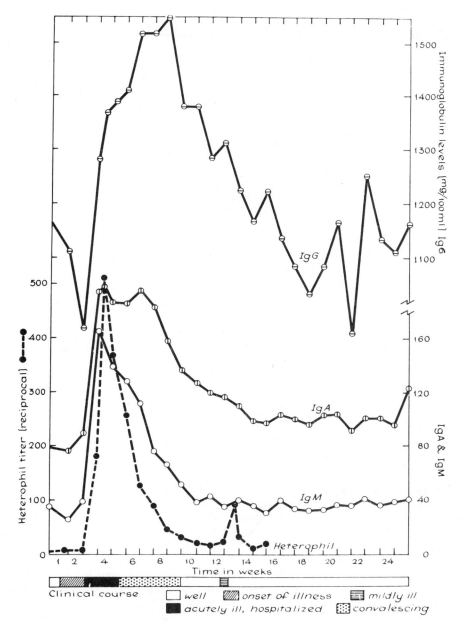

Fig. 3-19. Immunoglobulin and heterophil antibody levels in the course of infectious mononucleosis in a 23-year-old man. (From Allansmith, M., and Bergstresser, P.: Sequence of immunoglobulin changes resulting from an attack of infectious mononucleosis, Am. J. Med. **44:**124, 1968.)

Galley, 1962). They are therefore either type κ or type λ. Fragments of chains can be found in urine from patients with Bence Jones proteinuria (Cioli and Baglioni, 1968). They are precipitated out of urine at between 40° and 60° C at pH 5; they redissolve at 100° C at an acid pH. They are most specifically identified by immunoelectrophoresis using anti-κ or anti-λ antisera. Urine may contain portions of immunoglobulin molecules, as in "H-chain disease" when the F fragment of H chains is excreted. These are not precipitated on heating.

FUNCTION. The immunologic functions of the normal immunoglobulins are summarized in Table 3-3. A striking example of immunoglobulin responses to infection is presented in Fig. 3-19. The subject was a young man whose immunoglobulin levels were being measured weekly when he developed infectious mononucleosis.

The most recently discovered class of immunoglobulin, IgE, deserves special mention (Bennich and Johansson, 1971). As shown in Table 3-3, it is the only immunoglobulin having reaginic activity. Reaginic antibody is responsible for allergic reactions. It was so named by Prausnitz and Küstner when they showed that skin-sensitizing antibody

Table 3-3. Characteristics of human immunoglobulins

Characteristics	IgG	IgA	IgM	IgD	IgE
H chain*	γ	α	μ	δ	ϵ
L chain*	κ or λ	κ or λ	κ or λ	κ or λ	κ or λ
Molecular formula	$\gamma 2\kappa 2$ or $\gamma 2\lambda 2$	$(\alpha 2\kappa 2)n$ or $(\alpha 2\lambda 2)n$	$(\mu 2\kappa 2)5$ or $(\mu 2\lambda 2)5$	$\delta 2\kappa 2$ or $\delta 2\lambda 2$	$\epsilon 2\kappa 2$ or $\epsilon 2\lambda 2$
Subclasses	IgG1, IgG2, IgG3, IgG4	IgA, IgA2	IgM1, IgM2	IgD1, IgD2	—
J chain	0	+†	+‡	0	0
Genetic factors					
Gm	+§	0	0	0	0
InV	+	+	+	+	?
Molecular weight	160,000	(160,000)n	900,000	180,000	200,000
Sedimentation constant	7S	7, 9, 11, 13S	18, 24, 32S	7S	8S
Immunologic function					
First detectable antibody	0	0	+	0	0
In secondary response	+	0	0	0	0
Binds complement	+‖	0	+	0	0
Placental transport	+	0	0	0	+
Guinea pig skin sensitizer	+	0	0	0	+
Reacts with rheumatoid factor	+	0	0	0	0
Reaginic antibody	0	0	0	0	+
Serum concentration (mg/dl) mean ± 1 SD	1,244 ± 220	390 ± 90	120 ± 35	3(range 0-30)	0.01-0.07
Total circulating pool (mg/kg)	494	95	37	1.1	0.02
Half-life (days)	23	6	5	2.8	2.4
Synthetic rate (mg/kg/day)	34	24	6.9	0.4	0.017

*For subgroups see Table 3-2.
†Polymeric secretory IgA only.
‡IgM pentameter only.
§See Kunkel et al, 1970.
‖Capacity varies with subclass.

could be passively transferred by intradermally injecting the serum of an allergic individual (Küstner) into a normal recipient (Prausnitz). Challenge with the specific allergen (fish) by injection into the site previously injected with the serum produced a wheal-and-flare reaction in the normal recipient. The reagin had been passively transferred in what came to be known as the Prausnitz-Küstner test.

When the first four classes of immunoglobulin were identified, it was shown that none of them had reaginic activity. In 1966 Ishizaka and his co-workers showed that the reaginic antibody in the serum of persons sensitive to ragweed was a distinct class of immunoglobulin, which they called IgE (Ishizaka and Ishizaka, 1969). Shortly after, myelomas of the IgE type were found (Ogawa et al, 1969). An apparently new class of immunoglobulin, designated IgND, was found in both a myeloma serum and in normal sera by Johansson and Bennich (1967) and Johansson et al (1968). These authors did not discover its reaginic role, but the other properties of IgND are identical with those of IgE. In 1968 Bennich et al (1968) drafted a WHO report recommending the official designation IgE for this new immunoglobulin.

Human IgE is unique in its action. Its specificity for reaginic antibody is shown by its blocking of passive sensitization of the skin by reaginic antibody, and an intracutaneous injection of anti-IgE induces the typical erythemawheal reaction. The IgE molecule attaches to receptor sites on the cell membrane of basophils (Sullivan et al, 1971) and mast cells, which then release histamine when exposed to antigen (Ishizaka and Ishizaka, 1970; Becker et al, 1973; Metzger, 1978), the cells showing a degranulation reaction as the result. IgE is present in the serum in minute amounts, 10 to 70 µg/dl. Serum IgE levels are elevated in patients having allergic disorders (hay fever, asthma, atopic eczema) (Johansson et al, 1970). Elevated IgE levels are also found in parasitic infections (Hogarth-Scott et al, 1969; Rosenberg et al, 1970). Buckley et al (1972) report the cases of two adolescent boys who had recurrent pyogenic infections, normal serum concentrations of IgG, IgA, IgM, and IgD, extremely elevated IgE, depressed anamnestic antibody responses to diptheria and tetanus antigens, and no response to primary immunization. IgE deficiency, combined with IgA deficiency, is a feature of ataxia-telangiectasia (Ammann et al, 1969) and may be a factor in respiratory diseases (Polmar et al, 1972).

GENETICS OF IMMUNOGLOBULIN SYNTHESIS. Hill et al (1966) postulate that the evolutionary origin of the modern immunoglobulin molecule involves the evolution of subunits beginning with a primitive type of L chain (Fig. 3-20). According to this hypothesis, the first type of polypeptide (preimmunoglobulin) was a short chain (107 amino acids) of the L type, which then duplicated and doubled in length (to 214 amino acids) to form a primitive L chain. It is assumed there was duplication as well of an ancestral gene for the preimmunoglobulin, with further gene duplications to con-

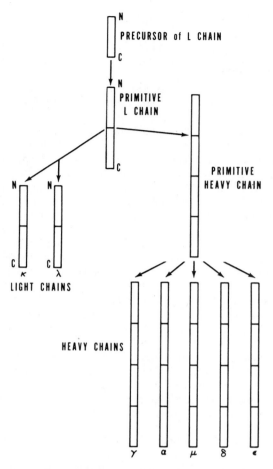

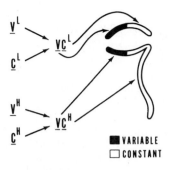

Fig. 3-21. Genetic control of L and H chains of immunoglobulin molecule according to the concept that each chain is coded by a paired gene, one portion of which controls the synthesis of the variable portion while the other controls the synthesis of the constant portion. Some think that the five types of H chains are coded by separate (allelic) genes.

Fig. 3-20. Evolutionary history of polypeptide chains of immunoglobulin molecule. (From Hill et al, 1966.)

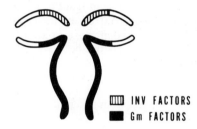

Fig. 3-22. Location of InV and Gm factors on IgG molecule.

trol not only the synthesis of a new type of chain (H) containing 446 amino acids, but ultimately the several types of L and H chains.

The genetic control of the modern immunoglobulin molecule is still obscure, and no one hypothesis accounts satisfactorily for the diversity of the variable portions of the two chains. The simplest concept is that two basic structural genes, *V* and *C,* are involved (Hood, 1972) for each chain, that these fuse to form a *VC* gene, the V portion coding the variable portion of the chain and the C portion coding the constant portion (Fig. 3-21). Problems arise at the next step—how to account for the diversity and control of subgroups (Edelman, 1971). At least ten loci appear to control the classes and subclasses of H chains (Natvig and Kunkel, 1968), two loci are involved in the control of L chain types, and an undetermined, seemingly infinite number of loci are needed to control the variable portions of the chains. It is probable that this genetic system is based on closely linked alleles at each locus, possibly controlled by exclusion or suppression effects and possibly by the receptors on the cell surface (Dubiski, 1972). The study of antigenic determinants on immunoglobulins of nonhuman primates promises to shed some light on these questions (van Loghem and Litwin, 1972).

Only vertebrates can produce immunoglobulins in response to antigenic stimulation. The elasmobranchs (sharks) are phylogenetically the most ancient vertebrates. In one species (lemon shark), Clem et al (1967) have found that only IgM-type immunoglobulin is formed. This finding is consistent with the hypothesis of Marchalonis and Edelman (1965) that, from the standpoint of evolutionary history, the IgM class is younger than the IgG and IgA classes, and therefore μ-chain formation precedes that of γ-chains or α-chains. It is possible, of course, that divergent evolution might have taken place before or after the primitive vertebrates (Gitlin et al, 1973).

ALLOTYPES. If we consider immunoglobulins to be protein antigens, and in fact the preparation of specific antisera is based on their antigenicity, three types of immunoglobulin protein antigens can be distinguished: (1) antigens present in all normal sera are called *isotypes,* the normal immunoglobulin classes, subclasses, and fragments, (2) antigens present in some normal sera, their presence being genetically controlled, are called *allotypes,* and (3) antigenic properties related to one specific antibody population represent individual specificities and are called *idiotypes* (Natvig and Kunkel, 1973). It is probable that the Xh antigen (Dunston and Gershowitz, 1973), identical with Pa_1 antigen, is isotypic. We are concerned here with allotypes in the immunoglobulin system, responsible for *genetic polymorphism* within the system. Since allotypes are genetically controlled, they are also called *genetic markers* or *genetic factors*. In addition to the genetic and anthropologic importance, allotypes can be responsible for transfusion reactions (Ropartz, 1971).

Some allotypes (Gm, Am, and ISF) are related to heavy chains, whereas others (InV) are related to light chains (Fig. 3-22). Gm allotypes are found only in immunoglobulins of the IgG type, and each IgG subclass possesses distinctive Gm factors (Kunkel et al, 1970) (Table 3-4). The factors are inherited according to simple mendelian principles. Allotypic phenotype is expressed in terms of the factors present, e.g., Gm(1,2), whereas genotype designation follows the usual custom, e.g., $Gm^{1,2}/Gm^{1,2}$. The incidence of Gm and other factors varies in different population groups. Among whites 40% to 65% are Gm(1) positive and none are Gm(15) positive; among blacks 100% are Gm(1) positive and 14% to 21% are Gm(15) positive. The most frequent combination in various racial groups is given in Table 3-5.

The second H chain genetic markers, Am1 and Am2, have been found on the C_2 chain of non-disulfide-linked IgA2. IgA1 and disulfide-linked IgA2 lack Am and are designated Am2 negative (Kunkel et al, 1969). Am1 was described by Vyas and Fudenberg (1969). The relationship between Am1 and Am2 has not been worked out. Am1 is found in 98% of whites, 52% of blacks, 76% of Japanese, and 56% of Chinese. About the same frequencies apply for Am2.

The third H chain genetic marker (ISF) is found on the H chain of IgG1 (Ropartz et al, 1967, 1968). It is unrelated to the Gm and Am systems, and the frequency varies with the age of the individuals (Ropartz, 1971)—20% of children, 40% of adults, and 60% over 70 years of age—and with

race—98% of British Nigerian blacks being phenotype ISF(1).

The InV genetic markers (InV1, InV2, and InV3) are found only on L chains of most classes of immunoglobulins. They also have different incidences in various racial groups. Whites are 11% to 20% InV2 positive, whereas 53% to 58% of blacks are InV2 positive. Twenty percent of whites are InV1 positive, whereas 94% of Venezuelan Indians are InV1 positive (Gallango and Arends, 1965). InV3 has a high frequency in all populations, and 95% of whites and 82% of blacks are heterozygous for InV1 and InV3 (Steinberg, 1969). The InV allotypes are transmitted by three alleles, InV^1, InV^2, and InV^3, and the rare phenotype InV1,2,3-negative may be attributable to a fourth gene, InV^- (Steinberg et al, 1962), or to a suppression or deletion phenomenon.

SYNTHESIS. The role of the lymphoid system in the establishment of humoral immunity is reviewed in the early part of this chapter. The cells responsible for the synthesis of immunoglobulins are the plasma cells and lymphocytes.

Usually only one class of immunoglobulin is synthesized in a given immunocyte, and a clone of immunocytes supposedly synthesizes the same immunoglobulin. In rare instances, two or three different immunoglobulins have been demonstrated in a single plasma cell (Levin et al, 1971; Natvig and Kunkel, 1973). The presence of a given immunoglobulin plus Bence Jones protein in single plasma cells in myeloma is considered to represent excess production of L chains rather than the synthesis of two different immunoglobulins.

The synthetic mechanism depends on the phagocytosis of antigen by macrophages, the binding of antigen to low molecular weight RNA, and the transfer of antigen-RNA to the immunocyte. Adjuvants (Freund's adjuvant, aluminum hydroxide, etc.) probably act as does RNA to keep antigen

Table 3-4. Allotypes on H chains in relation to immunoglobulin subclasses*

Gm markers	Immunoglobulin subclass	Gm markers	Immunoglobulin subclass
1	IgG 1	15	IgG 3
2	IgG 1	16	IgG 3
3 (4)	IgG 1	17	IgG 1
4 (3)	IgG 1	18	IgG 1
5 (12)	IgG 3	19	IgG 3
6	IgG 3	20	IgG 1
7	IgG 1	21	IgG 3
8	IgG 1	22	IgG 1
9	IgG 1	23	IgG 2
10 (13)	IgG 3	24	IgG 3
11	IgG 3	25	IgG 3
12 (5)	IgG 3	**Am markers**	
13 (10)	IgG 3	1	IgA 2
14	IgG 3	2	IgA 2

*Modified from Ropartz, 1971; Natvig and Kunkel, 1973.

Table 3-5. Most frequent combinations of Gm allotypes in various racial and population groups*

Population	Gm allotypes
Whites	Gm (1, 17, 21), Gm (1, 2, 17, 21), Gm (3, 5, 14, 17)
Blacks	Gm (1, 5, 13, 14, 17), Gm (1, 5, 14, 17), Gm (1, 5, 6, 14, 17)
Mongoloids	Gm (1, 17, 21), Gm (1, 2, 17, 21), Gm (1, 13, 17), Gm (1, 3, 5, 13, 14)
Bushmen (Africa)	Gm (1, 17, 21), Gm (1, 5, 17), Gm (1, 13, 17), Gm (1, 5, 13, 14, 17)
Pygmies	Gm (1, 5, 6, 7), Gm (1, 5, 13, 14, 17)
Micronesians	Gm (1, 17, 21), Gm (1, 3, 5, 13, 14)
Melanesians (New Guinea)	Gm (1, 17, 21), Gm (1, 2, 17, 21), Gm (1, 3, 5, 13, 14)
Melanesians (Bougainville)	Gm (1, 17, 21), Gm (1, 2, 17, 21), Gm (1, 3, 5, 13, 14)

*Data from Steinberg, 1969.

Table 3-6. Concentrations of immunoglobulins in serum of normal subjects at different ages*

Age	No. of subjects	Level of γG		Level of γM		Level of γA		Level of total γ-globulin	
		mg/dl† (range)	% of adult level	mg/dl† (range)	% of adult level	mg/dl† (range)	% of adult level	mg/dl† (range)	% of adult level
Newborn	22	1,031 ± 200 (645-1,244)	89 ± 17	11 ± 5 (5-30)	11 ± 5	2 ± 3 (0-11)	1 ± 2	1,044 ± 201 (660-1,439)	67 ± 13
1-3 mo	29	430 ± 119 (272-762)	37 ± 10	30 ± 11 (16-67)	30 ± 11	21 ± 13 (6-56)	11 ± 7	481 ± 127 (324-699)	31 ± 9
4-6 mo	33	427 ± 186 (206-1,125)	37 ± 16	43 ± 17 (10-83)	43 ± 17	28 ± 18 (8-93)	14 ± 9	498 ± 204 (228-1,232)	32 ± 13
7-12 mo	56	661 ± 219 (279-1,533)	58 ± 19	54 ± 23 (22-147)	55 ± 23	37 ± 18 (16-98)	19 ± 9	752 ± 242 (327-1,687)	48 ± 15
13-24 mo	59	762 ± 209 (258-1,393)	66 ± 18	58 ± 23 (14-114)	59 ± 23	50 ± 24 (19-119)	25 ± 12	870 ± 258 (398-1,586)	56 ± 16
25-36 mo	33	892 ± 183 (419-1,274)	77 ± 16	61 ± 19 (28-113)	62 ± 19	71 ± 37 (19-235)	36 ± 19	1,024 ± 205 (499-1,418)	65 ± 14
3-5 yr	28	929 ± 228 (569-1,597)	80 ± 20	56 ± 18 (22-100)	57 ± 18	93 ± 27 (55-152)	47 ± 14	1,078 ± 245 (730-1,771)	69 ± 17
6-8 yr	18	923 ± 256 (559-1,492)	80 ± 22	65 ± 25 (27-118)	66 ± 25	124 ± 45 (54-221)	62 ± 23	1,112 ± 293 (640-1,725)	71 ± 20
9-11 yr	9	1,124 ± 235 (779-1,456)	97 ± 20	79 ± 33 (35-132)	80 ± 33	131 ± 60 (12-208)	66 ± 30	1,334 ± 254 (966-1,639)	85 ± 17
12-16 yr	9	946 ± 124 (726-1,085)	82 ± 11	59 ± 20 (35-72)	60 ± 20	148 ± 63 (70-229)	74 ± 32	1,153 ± 169 (833-1,284)	74 ± 12
Adults	30	1,158 ± 305 (569-1,919)	100 ± 26	99 ± 27 (47-147)	100 ± 27	200 ± 61 (61-330)	100 ± 31	1,457 ± 353 (730-2,365)	100 ± 24

*From Stiehm and Fudenberg, 1966a.
†Mean ± 1 SD.

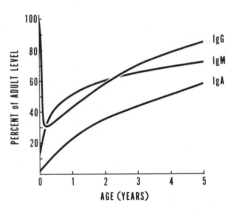

Fig. 3-23. Serum concentrations of IgG, IgA, and IgM from birth to 5 years of age. (Data from Stiehm and Fudenberg, 1966a.)

in a particulate state as well as in the original immunogenic configuration. There is evidence that the level of a given immunoglobulin in the blood is proportional to the number of plasma cells shown to be active in its synthesis. The half-life of IgA is about 6 days, that of IgG about 23 days, and that of IgM about 5 days.

NORMAL SERUM CONCENTRATIONS. IgG is the only immunoglobulin that crosses the placenta from the mother to the fetus; at birth the newborn's serum contains a nearly normal adult concentration of IgG but very little IgA and IgM. There is a sharp reduction of IgG shortly after birth (Fig. 3-23), a reflection of its being consumed in some unknown fashion. The first new immunoglobulin formed is IgM, and the rate of synthesis of IgM and new IgG is somewhat greater than that of IgA. Synthesis of the immunoglobulins is dependent on the infant leaving the germ-free environment of the womb and being exposed to the antigen-polluted world. If an animal is reared in a germ-free environment, the concentration of all the immunoglobulins is about one-fourth that found in conventional animals, and the sharp increase in the concentration of IgM does not occur. By the same token, if a newborn infant's serum contains high levels of IgM and IgA, this can only be the result of perinatal (twenty-eighth week of gestation to seventh day postpartum) infection (Hardy, 1971). An increased level of IgM can be associated with the following infections in infants: *E. coli* diarrhea, urinary tract infection, enteroviral infection, aseptic meningitis, bacteremia, congenital syphilis, rubella, toxoplasmosis, and cytomegalovirus infection (Alford et al, 1967).

Table 3-6 (p. 97) presents data on the concentration of immunoglobulins in serum, according to age. Most other published data are comparable (Buckley et al, 1968). Maddison et al (1975) give normal values, in international units, for healthy adults (1 IU = 80.4 μg of IgG, 14.2 μg of IgA, and 8.47 μg of IgM). The normal values for IgA and IgG do not show a sex difference, but the concentration of IgM from about 5 years of age to adulthood is slightly but significantly higher in females (Butterworth et al, 1967). Low levels of IgG are reported in "small-for-date" babies (Yeung and Hobbs, 1968). American black men and women have slightly but significantly higher levels of serum IgG,

IgA, and IgM (Karayalcin et al, 1973). Data for normal values of 21 serum proteins, including immunoglobulins, are presented by Weeke and Krasilnikoff (1972). Schur et al (1979) have determined the concentration of the four IgG subclasses in children from birth to age 16.

CATABOLISM. It can be assumed that the immunoglobulins are in dynamic equilibrium comparable to other proteins. More is known about rates of synthesis and half-lives than about their degradation and fate. One probable catabolic mechanism is destruction or elimination by the gastrointestinal tract. This has been estimated variously as accounting for 20% to 70% of the antibody loss. A small amount is probably lost in the urine, as fragments rather than whole immunoglobulin molecules. The liver accounts for about 30% of IgG catabolism; its participation in degrading other classes is suspected but not proved.

Immunoglobulinopathies
Classification

In addition to multiple myeloma and Waldenström's macroglobulinemia, there is a large number of disorders characterized by deficient or excess synthesis of immunoglobulins. In most of those accompanied by excess immunoglobulin synthesis the immunoglobulin has the physicochemical characteristics of its class and, in spite of polymorphisms, can be considered normal. In a few the disorder is characterized by an excess of immunoglobulin fragments that are not found in normal serum or urine. Some of the disorders are considered "primary" in the sense that there is no association with neoplasm, infection, etc., whereas others are "secondary" because such an association does exist (Ritzmann et al, 1975). Yet some of the "primary" deficiencies are associated with well-defined anatomic lesions in the thymus and other lymphoid organs, whereas some of the "secondary" disorders are associated with primary lesions of the immunocyte system such as lymphomas. Finally, not all the syndromes are completely clarified with respect to pathogenesis or to the features that distinguish one from the other.

These are some of the reasons why no one classification is completely satisfactory. An additional difficulty is the problem of nomenclature. Early in the game the scanty knowledge was adequately covered by terms such as "hypogammaglobulinemia," "agammaglobulinemia," "hyperproteinemia," "gammopathy," "paraproteinemia," and "dysgammaglobulinemia." Most of these terms can now be reexamined in the light of additional knowledge and found wanting. For example, whereas some are disorders of γ-globulin (IgG) synthesis, others involve the other classes of immunoglobulins; the term "gammopathy" can no longer cover them all. Likewise, the term "dysgammaglobulinemia" is no longer applicable. If the prefixes "dys" and "para" are used at all, they should be restricted to the situation when a truly abnormal protein is found, e.g., "dysimmunoglobulinemia" should be restricted to H chain disease, L chain disease, and possibly also to cryoglobulinemia and pyroglobulinemia.

Three classifications are presented here. The first is a general classification of the immunoglobulin abnormalities, and Table 3-7 adopts two of the terms, "hypoimmunoglobu-

Table 3-7. Classification of immunoglobulinopathies*

I. Hypoimmunoglobulinemia
  A. Primary (see Table 3-8)
  B. Secondary
    1. Associated with leukemia and lymphoma
    2. Associated with autoimmune diseases (unusual)
    3. Associated with chronic infection (bronchiectasis)
    4. Associated with hypoalbuminemia
      a. In nephrotic syndrome
      b. In protein-losing enteropathy
      c. In extreme malnutrition or malabsorption
    5. Associated with pernicious anemia
  C. Physiologic (newborn)
II. Hyperimmunoglobulinemia
  A. Primary
    1. Related to race (African and American blacks)
    2. Familial (in nondiseased relatives of patients with autoimmune disease or Waldenström's macroglobulinemia)
    3. Familial Wiskott-Aldrich syndrome (eczema, thrombocytopenia, and chronic infection)
    4. In myeloma group (Chapter 16)
      a. Multiple myeloma
      b. Waldenström's macroglobulinemia
      c. H chain disease
      d. L chain disease
      e. Para-amyloidosis
    5. Immunoblastic lymphadenopathy
  B. Secondary
    1. Secondary to bacterial infection
    2. In trypanosomiasis
    3. Associated with neoplasm
      a. Leukemia
      b. Lymphoma
      c. Carcinoma
    4. Associated with RE storage diseases (Gaucher's disease)
    5. Idiopathic
      a. Hyperimmunoglobulinemia in apparently healthy individuals (some precede classic myeloma or neoplasm)
      b. Cryoglobulinemia (may be associated with neoplasm or autoimmune disease)
      c. Pyroglobulinemia (may be associated with neoplasm)
    6. In miscellaneous diseases
      a. Liver disease (chronic active hepatitis)
      b. Sarcoidosis
      c. Infectious mononucleosis
      d. Charcot's syndrome (tropical splenomegaly with macroglobulinemia)
      e. Benign hyperglobulinemic purpura
      f. In sulfonamide hypersensitivity (sulfisoxazole)
      g. Equine infectious anemia (horses)
      h. Aleutian disease (mink and ferret)
      i. Myeloproliferative disorders
      j. Associated with amyloidosis

*Modified from Engle and Wallis, 1969.

Table 3-8. Classification of primary immunodeficiencies*

Deficiency	B-lymphocytes (a)†	B-lymphocytes (b)	T-lymphocytes	Inheritance X-linked	Inheritance Autosomal recessive	Other‡
X-linked agammaglobulinemia	X	(X)§		X		
Thymic hypoplasia			X			X
Severe combined immunodeficiency	X	X	X	X	X	X
With dysostosis	X	?	X		X	
With ADA‖ deficiency	X		X		X	
Immunodeficiency with generalized hematopoietic hypoplasia	X		X		X	
Selective Ig deficiency						
IgA	?	X	(X)			X
Others (IgM, IgE)		?				X
X-linked immunodeficiency with increased IgM		X		X		
Immunodeficiency with ataxia-telangiectasia		X	X		X	
Immunodeficiency with thrombocytopenia and eczema (Wiskott-Aldrich syndrome)			X	X		
Immunodeficiency with thymoma		X§	X			X
Immunodeficiency with normal or hypergammaglobulinemia	X	X	(X)			X
Transient hypogammaglobulinemia of infancy		X				X
Variable immunodeficiencies (largely unclassified and very frequent)	X	X	(X)		(X)	X

*From Cooper et al, 1973.
†(a) indicates absent or very low, (b) easily detectable or increased, and (X) less frequent occurrence than X.
‡Other implies multifactorial or unknown genetic basis or no known genetic basis.
§Some cases with circulating B lymphocytes without detectable surface immunoglobulins have been found.
‖Adenosine deaminase.

Table 3-9. Incidence of association of hyperimmunoglobulinemia and lymphadenopathy

Group A. Very high incidence of association
1. Immunoblastic (angioimmunoblastic) lymphadenopathy
2. Lymphadenopathy with sinus histiocytosis
3. Giant lymph node hyperplasia
4. Gamma heavy chain disease
5. Chronic lymphocytic leukemia
6. Infectious mononucleosis
7. Drug-induced lymphadenopathy

Group B. Low to moderately high incidence of association
1. Multiple myeloma (Shustik et al, 1976)
2. Waldenström's macroglobulinemia (Krajny and Pruzanski, 1976)
3. Mu heavy chain disease (Forte et al, 1970)
4. Primary amyloidosis (Ko et al, 1976)
5. Some lymphomas (Palutke and McDonald, 1973)
6. Rheumatoid arthritis (Calabro et al, 1976)
7. Felty's syndrome (Sienknecht et al, 1977)
8. Disseminated lupus erythematosus (Dubois, 1974)
9. Arthralgia-purpura syndrome (Peetoom-Meltzer syndrome) (Meltzer et al, 1966)
10. Cytomegalic inclusion body disease (Turner and Wright, 1973)
11. Toxoplasmosis (Turner and Wright, 1973)
12. Syphilis (Turner and Wright, 1973)
13. Sarcoidosis (Siltzbach et al, 1974)
14. Vaccination and immunization (Hartsock, 1968)
15. Sjögren's syndrome (Anderson and Talal, 1971)
16. Kaposi's sarcoma (Lubin and Rywlin, 1971)

linemia'' and ''hyperimmunoglobulinemia,'' proposed by Engle and Wallis (1969). I have not adopted their third, ''paraimmunoglobulinopathy,'' because, as stated previously, almost all these disorders are accompanied by the presence of an excess of one or another class of *normal* immunoglobulin, and I see no reason to separate them from the other hyperimmunoglobulinemias.

The second (Table 3-8) is a report of a special committee (Cooper et al, 1973) that modifies and updates a previous classification of primary immunoglobulin deficiencies. This second classification takes into account the new information on the role of T- and B-lymphocytes but is no doubt subject to future modification.

The third (Table 3-9) lists the immunglobulinopathies accompanied by lymphadenopathy and may be clinically useful.

In the following section we will outline the chief features of those immunodeficiency states that are most clearly defined and discuss an approach to their diagnosis. The discussion of multiple myeloma, Waldenström's macroglobulinemia, H chain disease, L chain disease, etc. will be found in Chapter 16.

Primary immunodeficiencies
X-linked agammaglobulinemia

This is the Bruton-type agammaglobulinemia (Bruton, 1952; Craig et al, 1954; Janeway et al, 1956; Baron et al, 1962; Cooperband et al, 1968), a B-lymphocyte defect resulting in extreme deficiency of all classes of immunoglobulins. Serum isohemagglutinins are absent or of extremely low titer. Inheritance is X-linked recessive; only males are affected. There is extreme susceptibility to recurrent pyogenic infections, and the disease, because it usually manifests at about 6 to 9 months of age, is sometimes called infantile X-linked agammaglobulinemia. One-third to one-half the affected children develop a rheumatoid arthritis-like syndrome before therapy is begun; others develop signs and symptoms of other collagen diseases. The number of circulating lymphocytes is usually normal, since B-lymphocytes make up only a small proportion of the circulating lymphocytes, and as expected the circulating lymphocytes have T but not B characteristics. Lymphocyte transformation is normal. In the peripheral lymphoid tissues, those areas populated by B-lymphocytes, the germinal centers of lymphoid follicles, are depleted of cells, and the mass of lymphoid tissue is reduced. Following antigenic stimulation, there is no tissue response in the form of germinal centers and no plasma cells are present. The paracortical regions of lymph nodes are normal. Likewise, there is no immunoglobulin response to antigenic stimulation. Cellular immunity responses are normal.

Thymic hypoplasia

This is also known as DiGeorge's syndrome (DiGeorge, 1965; Huber et al, 1967; Lischner et al, 1967). The basic defect is failure of the thymus to develop, so that there is a defect of T-lymphocytes. B-lymphocytes are normal, serum immunoglobulins are normal, and plasma cells are normal, but in spite of this there may be deficient response to some antigens. The number of circulating lymphocytes is usually normal but may be decreased. Because the primary defect is of T-lymphocytes, all cellular immunity responses are deficient. In the peripheral tissues, those areas populated by T-lymphocytes, the paracortical areas of lymph nodes, are depleted by lymphocytes, whereas germinal centers are normal. There may also be an absence of parathyroid glands, causing tetany of the newborn. Cardiovascular abnormalities are frequent. The mode of inheritance is not known.

Immunodeficiency with thymoma

This is also known as Good's syndrome (Good and Zak, 1956; Jeunet and Good, 1968) and is characterized by a deficiency of all classes of immunoglobulins in association with thymoma of the spindle cell type. The peripheral blood shows progressive lymphopenia to very low levels and eosinopenia. In peripheral lymphoid tissues there is a deficiency or absence of germinal centers and of paracortical lymphoid tissue. The bone marrow shows an absence of plasma cells and eosinophils. Humoral antibody responses are deficient, as are cellular immunologic responses.

Severe combined immunodeficiency

This term is the recommended substitute for a complex of terms for the immunodeficiency showing both a humoral and cellular defect associated with poorly developed thymic tissue (thymic dysplasia) (Tobler and Cottier, 1958; Rosen and Janeway, 1966; Miller, 1967; Hitzig et al, 1968; Rosen and Merler, 1972). Perhaps the term most often used in the older literature is "Swiss type of agammaglobulinemia"; others are "alymphocytosis," "thymic alymphoplasia," "thymic dysplasia," "lymphopenic agammaglobulinemia," and "Glanzmann and Riniker's lymphocytophthisis." Part of the nomenclature problem can be attributed to the now accepted fact that inheritance can be either autosomal recessive or X-linked recessive, with no clear distinction between cases of one type or another.

The peripheral blood shows very low concentrations of immunoglobulins, severe lymphopenia, eosinophilia, and absent granulocytosis response in infections. The bone marrow shows a deficiency of lymphocytes and plasma cells. The peripheral lymphoid tissue shows depletion of both B- and T-lymphocyte regions, with only a few scattered lymphocytes and mast cells and an occasional eosinophil. The thymus is extremely small, in the neck rather than in the anterior mediastinum, and histologically shows a few spindle cells but no lymphocytes or Hassall's corpuscles. A deficiency of T-cell maturation secondary to the thymic hypoplasia is postulated (Dosch et al, 1978). Because of combined B- and T-lymphocyte deficit, there is no immunologic response, humoral or cellular, to a variety of challenges. The affected children have no resistance to infection and usually die of bacterial or viral infections before 2 years of age. If vaccination is done, fatal generalized vaccinia is inevitable. The transplantation of bone marrow does not always correct the immunodeficiency (Bortin and Rimm, 1977) but is considered the treatment of choice (O'Reilly et al, 1978).

Immunodeficiency with normal immunoglobulins or hyperglobulinemia

This syndrome, also known as Nezelof's syndrome, is characterized by a hypoplastic thymus, lacking both lymphocytes and Hassall's corpuscles, lymphopenia, deficient lymphocytes in the peripheral lymphoid organs with only a few germinal centers, and deficient cellular immunity responses (Nezelof et al, 1964; Fulginiti et al, 1966; Schaller et al, 1966; Goldman et al, 1967). In contrast, the serum levels of immunoglobulins are normal or elevated and there is no lack of plasma cells. Since the affected child seems very susceptible to a variety of microorganisms, it is probable that anitbody function is deficient is spite of normal immunoglobulins. Indeed, antigenic stimulation results in little or no specific antibody response. On the other hand, there is a high incidence of antiglobulin-positive hemolytic anemia and of other autoimmune phenomena. The case reported by Rothbach et al (1979) is an interesting variant, the features being normal lymph node histology, normal T- and B-lymphocytes in the blood, normal concentrations of immunoglobulins, but no antibody response to diphtheria toxoid, tetanus toxoid, influenza A vaccine, or six pneumococcal polysaccharides.

Immunodeficiency with thrombocytopenia and eczema

This is commonly called the Wiskott-Aldrich syndrome (Krivit and Good, 1959; Blaese et al, 1967; Stiehm and McIntosh, 1967; Cooper et al, 1968b) and is characterized by a normal thymus, thrombocytopenia, abnormal platelet function (Chapter 17), eczema, lymphopenia, normal or decreased germinal centers, normal plasma cell population, decreased lymphoid tissues of thymic origin (paracortical area of lymph nodes), and a high frequency of lymphoreticular malignancy. Immunoglobulins usually show some abnormality, with the class, degree, and direction of change selectively but variably involved. There is markedly decreased resistance to infection and variable antibody response to some antigens. Isohemagglutinins are regularly absent.

Immunodeficiency with ataxia-telangiectasia

Ataxia-telangiectasia is an autosomal recessive disease involving several organ systems (Thieffry et al, 1961; Epstein et al, 1966; Lévêque et al, 1966; Meshaka et al, 1966; Peterson et al, 1966; Stobo and Tomasi, 1967; McFarlin et al, 1972). It derives its name from the combination of cerebellar ataxia with telangiectasia (dilated venules and capillaries) in the sclerae and of exposed or friction areas of the skin. The chief immunologic lesion is a thymus of the embryonic type lacking cortical and medullary organization and Hassall's corpuscles. Kaufman and Miller (1977) propose that ataxia-telangiectasia is an autoimmune disorder associated with a cytotoxic antibody to thymus and brain. The disturbed immunologic responses are of the combined type, with low or absent IgA and secretory IgA in about three-fourths of the cases, deficient antibody response to some antigens, and deficient cellular immunity response to some antigens. In addition to the IgA deficiency, most patients have a deficiency of IgE, and the serum contains IgM of low molecular weight. Mild lymphopenia occurs in about one-third of the patients.

The small proportion of patients with the clinical signs and symptoms of the syndrome but without immunologic deficiency are not subject to infections, but those with combined humoral and cellular defects have severe and usually fatal respiratory and other infections. It is interesting to note that many of the immunodeficiency diseases are associated with neoplasms of either lymphoid or other tissues, and the incidence of neoplasia in ataxia-telangiectasia is among the highest (Waldmann and Blaese, 1972). An elevated α-fetoglobulin level is common (Sugimoto et al, 1978).

Immunodeficiency with hematopoietic hypoplasia

This rare immunodeficiency, originally described as "reticular dysgenesia," is characterized by the usual features of the immunodeficiency states (thymic dysplasia, lymphopenia, lymphoid depletion, and immunoglobulin deficiency) plus severe neutropenia and severely diminished or absent granulocytic precursors in the bone marrow (De Vaal and Seynhaeve, 1959; Gitlin et al, 1964; Alonso et al, 1972). This devastating combination makes survival past the first few weeks of life impossible. The necropsy described by Alonso et al (1972) showed almost complete depletion of peripheral lymphoid tissues and a severely hypoplastic bone marrow lacking granulocytic precursors and containing only a few megakaryocytes and normoblasts. Although the granulocytic defect is most striking, it would seem that the nearly total hemopoietic and lymphocytic aplasia must be caused by failure of the stem cell compartment in early embryonic life.

Selective immunoglobulin deficiencies

This heterogeneous group of not uncommon immunoglobulin deficiencies has, as a common denominator, an anatomically normal thymus and peripheral lymphoid tissue and a deficiency or absence of one or two immonoglobulins (Rosen et al, 1961; Jamieson and Kerr, 1962; Hinz and Boyer, 1963; Rosen and Bougas, 1963; Rockey et al, 1964; Bachman, 1965; Barth et al, 1965; Hermans et al, 1966; Stiehm and Fudenberg, 1966b; Crabbe and Heremans, 1967; Stocker et al, 1968). There may be a selective deficiency of IgA alone, IgA and IgG (usually with elevated IgM), IgM alone, IgG alone, IgA and IgM, or IgE.

The deficiency may be hereditary or acquired, symptomatic or asymptomatic. Some, but not all, in the hereditary group show an autosomal recessive pattern. The acquired group includes loss of immunoglobulins in the urine in the nephrotic syndrome or in the stool in the protein-losing enteropathies (intestinal lymphangiectasia, steatorrheas, sprue), in the lymphomas and leukemias, in some of the autoimmune diseases, or as the result of immunosuppressive therapy. Patients in the symptomatic group have recurrent pyogenic, viral, or mycotic infections.

Primary adult hypoimmunoglobulinemia may or may not be included in this group. Classically, the onset is in adult life and there is a moderate decrease in all classes of immunoglobulins, but at any given time one immunoglobulin may show a disproportionate decrease. Patients in this group have a high incidence of lymphomas, leukemias, and other neoplasms, the hypoimmunoglobulinemia sometimes preceding the onset of the malignancy by many years.

Immunoglobulin deficiency associated with nodular lymphoid hyperplasia of the intestine (Hermans et al, 1966; Kirkpatrick et al, 1968) can also be included in this group, since there is an absence of IgA and IgM with only moderate decrease of IgG. The lymphoid hyperplasia is easily visualized in barium-contrast roentgenograms of the bowel and is caused by massive hyperplasia of the lymphoid follicles. Absence of plasma cells in the lamina propria is characteristic of this syndrome as well as of other gastrointestinal abnormalities accompanied by IgA deficiency.

Patients who lack IgA can become sensitized to transfused IgA and form anti-IgA antibodies (Vyas et al, 1969). These antibodies can cause anaphylactoid and urticarial transfusion reactions (Chapter 12), and patients having anti-IgA should be transfused, if necessary, with thoroughly washed red cells (Vyas et al, 1968). It is possible that in other immunoglobulin deficiency states transfused immunoglobulins may cause the production of anti-immunoglobulin antibodies that could account for transfusion reactions.

Hyperimmunoglobulinemia

A classification of hyperimmunoglobulinemia is given in Table 3-7, p. 99, and Table 3-9, p. 100. The most important, that caused by myelomatous disease, is discussed in Chapter 16. One other, immunoblastic lymphadenopathy, is of particular interest to hematologists.

Immunoblastic (angioimmunoblastic) lymphadenopathy

Immunoblastic lymphadenopathy (angioimmunoblastic lymphadenopathy with dysproteinemia) is a recently described syndrome (Frizzera et al, 1974; Lukes and Tindle, 1975; Schultz and Yunis, 1975; Mathe et al, 1976; Palutke et al, 1976; Pruzanski et al, 1976). The disease resembles lymphoma. The histopathologic features of the lymph nodes are (1) loss of normal architecture, (2) proliferation of large lymphocytes (immunoblasts), plasma cells, "plasmacytoid lymphocytes," and histiocytes, (3) vascular (endothelial) proliferation, and (4) amorphous, PAS-positive, acidophilic material deposited between cells. There is a deficiency of T-lymphocytes and a proliferation of B-lymphocytes. There is hyperimmunoglobulinemia, usually polyclonal but occasionally monoclonal; cold agglutinins of anti-**I** specificity may be present; and IgM-IgG cryocomplexes have been identified in some cases. The urine may contain Bence-Jones λ-chains. Antiglobulin-positive hemolytic anemia is common. The blood shows thrombocytopenia, leukocytosis, and lymphocytoid plasma cells.

Clinically, the onset is acute and the disease usually affects older men and women. There is rapidly progressive lymphadenopathy and hepatosplenomegaly, high fever, and skin rash. The disease is considered benign on the basis of the histologic findings but is clinically malignant with a poor prognosis. A histologically malignant variant, immunoblastic sarcoma, has been described by Lukes and Tindle (1975).

The etiology is unknown, but some speculate that it may represent (1) a graft-versus-host reaction, (2) exaggerated proliferation of B-lymphocytes in an abnormal immune state, or (3) a hyperimmune response to unknown antigens, infectious agents, or drugs. Response to steroids and chemotherapy is variable.

Lymphadenopathy with sinus histiocytosis

The characteristic features of this disease, also called sinus histiocytosis with massive lymphadenopathy (SHML), are massive lymphadenopathy and hypergammaglobulinemia (Dorfman and Warnke, 1974). The histologic appearance of the lymph nodes is described by Rosai and Dorfman (1969). The predominant immunoglobulin is IgG, with minor increases in IgA and IgM.

Giant lymph node hyperplasia

This has also been called angiomatous lymphoid hamartoma. It is characterized by very large lymphoid tumors in the mediastinum, but huge lymph nodes may be found at other sites (Keller et al, 1972). The hypergammaglobulinemia is usually polyclonal with increased IgG and IgA (Kahn et al, 1973; van den Ende et al, 1975).

Gamma heavy chain disease

Lymphadenopathy is very common (Frangione and Franklin, 1973). The hypergammaglobulinemia is usually polyclonal, and there is extensive production of H chains, γ type.

Chronic lymphocytic leukemia

This is the only leukemia in which lymphadenopathy and hypergammaglobulinemia or other immunoglobulin abnormalities are frequently associated (p. 726).

Infectious mononucleosis

The increase in immunoglobulins is usually of the IgG type (Fig. 3-19).

Drug-induced lymphadenopathy

This is usually seen in some individuals receiving anticonvulsant drug therapy (Greene, 1975). A typical case is presented in Fig. 3-31, p. 113. Various patterns of immunoglobulin increases are reported (Holland and Mauer, 1965; Dorfman and Warnke, 1974).

Laboratory diagnosis of immunodeficiency

Before the role of the laboratory in the identification of immunologic disease is discussed, it should be emphasized that, as in all medicine, diagnosis relates to a patient and not to a specimen. Before costly and time-consuming analyses are undertaken, there should be reasonable suspicion that an immunologic disease may be present. This may be suspected by the family history in the case of a newborn. Recurrent severe infectious disease should initiate immunologic investigations, as should hematologic abnormalities such as lymphopenia or agranulocytosis. However, repeated infections such as colds or respiratory disease in the asthmatic child or in the child with cystic fibrosis are not indications to search for a primary immunologic disease. Infections caused by organisms resistant to therapy, or inadequately treated, might seem to indicate a primary immunologic disease when in fact the problem is one of accurate diagnosis and adequate treatment.

In thymus-dependent cellular immunity deficiencies

The assessment of thymus-dependent immunity is based on (1) gross and microscopic examination of lymph nodes, (2) hematologic data, (3) skin tests for delayed hypersensitivity reactions, (4) evaluation of lymphocyte transformation, (5) measurement of release of MIF (migration inhibitory factor), (6) roentgenographic verification of the presence or absence of the thymus, and (7) measurement of complement factors.

LYMPH NODES. Normal infants, even newborn, and children have easily palpable lymph nodes, and the inability to detect lymph nodes suggests lymphocyte depletion. Biopsy of a node usually helps to differentiate cellular from humoral disorders. In thymus-dependent disease the germinal centers are normal or, if reduced, are still of normal cellularity while there is lymphocyte depletion in the deep cortical areas. In antibody-dependent deficiencies, there is a partial or complete loss of germinal centers with no plasma cells and the deep cortical areas are usually normal. Biopsy and microscopic examination of a lymph node 5 to 7 days after regional antigenic stimulation (Good, 1955) will show absence of plasma cells if the disease is humoral or combined cellular-humoral and a normal plasma cell response in pure cellular immunity deficiencies. Lymph node biopsy should not be done if the diagnosis of combined immunodeficiency is obvious or suspected.

HEMATOLOGIC DATA. The peripheral blood examination gives information on the number and morphology of lymphocytes and granulocytes, the number of platelets, and changes in red blood morphology. The total white blood cell count and the differential count are used to calculate the absolute number of circulating lymphocytes (p. 670), and normality is judged on the basis of data for normals for the age group in question (Table 15-4, p. 668). Lymphopenia, when present, usually indicates a T-lymphocyte deficiency. An initial normal lymphocyte count does not exclude the diagnosis (Gitlin and Craig, 1963), and serial counts may be needed to reveal progressive lymphopenia. The morphology of lymphocytes is normally that of the typical small lymphocyte (Heyn et al, 1973). Thrombocytopenia can be estimated from the blood smear or determined by a direct platelet count. In those conditions accompanied by hemolytic anemia the erythrocytes may show spherocytosis or the presence of schizocytes (see Chapter 13).

Examination of the bone marrow is usually of little help with the exception of providing information on the presence or absence of plasma cells (Steiner and Pearson, 1966). Plasma cells can be very sparse in children less than 1 year of age.

SKIN TESTS FOR DELAYED HYPERSENSITIVITY REACTIONS. The delayed hypersensitivity reaction is dependent on a normal cellular immune system and is used as a specific indicator of the integrity of the thymus-dependent lymphocyte function. The newborn is soon exposed to a variety of microbial antigens and, if normal, is sensitized to them, so that subsequent skin testing with the antigens will produce the typical delayed hypersensitivity skin reaction. The older the child, the more likely that sensitization will have occurred. Five antigens are commonly used for intradermal injection (details in Fudenberg et al, 1971, and Moore and Meuwissen, 1973): tuberculin, *Candida* extract, *Trichophyton* extract, streptococcal antigens, and mumps skin testing antigen. Additional antigens can be used if prevalent in a given area, e.g., coccidioidin where coccidiosis is endemic. Most children over 6 years of age will react to at least one of the antigens, but failure to react might be a result of lack of exposure, so that a negative result does not necessarily prove a T-lymphocyte defect.

When the results of intradermal tests are inconclusive, active sensitization can be tried. The agent used, 2:4-dinitrochlorobenzene (Dupuy and Preud'homme, 1968), is applied to the skin and sensitization determined by a second application of the agent to the same site 14 to 21 days later (Fudenberg et al, 1971). If there is a reaction marked by erythema, induration, and vesiculation, it can be concluded that the subject tested has a normal T-dependent system.

EVALUATION OF LYMPHOCYTE TRANSFORMATION. In vitro blastoid transformation of lymphocytes stimulated by specific or nonspecific stimuli is a function primarily of

T-lymphocytes (p. 81) and can be used to evaluate T-lymphocyte depletion (Douglas et al, 1969).

RELEASE OF MIF. When sensitized T-lymphocytes are challenged with the specific antigen, they release a number of factors, one of which is the migration inhibitory factor (MIF) (p. 85). Release of MIF, as measured by the inhibition of migration of guinea pig macrophages, is a good indication of normal T-lymphocyte function (Thor et al, 1968; Rocklin et al, 1970).

PRESENCE OR ABSENCE OF THE THYMUS. A normally developed thymus lies in the upper anterior mediastinum and usually can be identified on a lateral roentgenogram of the newborn. Absence of a thymic shadow is compatible with a deficient cellular immune system.

MEASUREMENT OF COMPLEMENT COMPONENTS. Complement is a complex of components (p. 556) present in fresh normal serum and capable of entering into many antigen-antibody reactions (Lepow, 1965). Since complement is a mediator of cellular injury, it plays a role in cellular immune reactions, particularly cytolysis and phagocytosis. Measurement of complement components C_2, C_3, and C_5 may be indicated, the latter particularly if there is a phagocytic defect. However, there is no obvious value in measuring complement components in other types of immunodeficiencies.

In humoral (immunoglobulin) deficiencies

Assessment of the humoral immunity system is based on the following: (1) measurement of serum immunoglobulins, (2) presence of natural antibodies, (3) antibody response to immunization, (4) presence of plasma cells in lymphoid tissue, bone marrow, and intestine, and (5) assessment of lymphoid mass.

MEASUREMENT OF SERUM IMMUNOGLOBULINS. The quantification of immunoglobulins in serum is based on the combination of the immunoglobulin to be measured with its specific antiserum. The *single radial diffusion* method of Mancini et al (1965), modified by Fahey and McKelvey (1965) and others, is accurate to a coefficient of variation of about 10% and requires at least 24 hours of diffusion. A method based on *immunoelectrodiffusion* (Freeman and Smith, 1970) gives greater precision and sensitivity than single radial diffusion. A single radial diffusion method using *isotopically tagged antisera* (Rowe, 1969) is still more sensitive, capable of detecting protein at a concentration of about 100 μg/ml. *Radioimmunoassay methods* (Wide and Porath, 1966) have the highest sensitivity. Immunoglobulin levels may show a week-to-week variance of as much as 20% in some individuals (Veys et al, 1977). Variations because of age, race, and sex must be taken into account (Maddison et al, 1975).

Variation in the standards used, regardless of the method, introduces a greater variation than the methodologic error, as evidenced by the report (Rowe et al, 1970) that reasonable interlaboratory agreement in the measurement of immunoglobulin concentration was achieved when all used the same WHO reference preparation. It is recommended that the WHO reference preparations be used. These are available for the five classes of immunoglobulins and can be obtained from the WHO Regional Reference Center for Immunoglobulins, National Cancer Institute, Bethesda, Maryland 20014. These reference materials are standardized in terms of international units (IU). The conversion of international units to the more familiar mg/dl or mg/l is based on the following equivalents: 1 IU is equivalent to 80.4 μg of IgG, 14.2 μg of IgA, and 8.47 μg of IgM (Humphrey and Batty, 1974). Some antisera and standards available from commercial sources are sometimes unsatisfactory (Fudenberg et al, 1971). Reliability can be achieved only by strict quality control measures. The sensitivity of the method should also be matched to the purpose; e.g., immunoglobulins present in low concentrations, such as IgD and IgE, require methodology of the highest degree of sensitivity.

Subclasses can be determined by using specific subclass antisera, either in the standard technics or by hemagglutination inhibition (Yount et al, 1970).

PRESENCE OF NATURAL AND ACQUIRED ANTIBODIES. Immunologically normal persons have natural antibodies (agglutinins) of the A-B-O system in their serum. The serum of a group O child normally contains anti-**A** and anti-**B,** that of a group A child contains anti-**B,** and that of a group B child contains anti-**A.** The predicted agglutinin may be absent and is then an indication of the inability to form specific antibodies, even when the concentration of immunoglobulins in serum is not abnormally low.

ANTIBODY RESPONSE TO IMMUNIZATION. Antibodies acquired following immunization indicate a normal humoral response. A child immunized against diphtheria will show no local reaction when tested with diphtheria toxin (Schick test) if antibodies to diphtheria are present. The presence or absence of antibodies to other immunizations such as against tetanus, typhoid, and paratyphoid also assesses the competence of the humoral response.

In the absence of prior immunization, active immunization with any of several microbial vaccines can be carried out and the antibody response measured (Fudenberg et al, 1971). Failure to form specific antibody is evidence of deficient humoral immunity. Live vaccines of any type must not be used for this purpose, for if the child is not immunocompetent, fatal overwhelming infection can result.

PRESENCE OF PLASMA CELLS. Plasma cells are the effectors of humoral responses. Their presence usually indicates a normal humoral system; their absence, an abnormal one. Plasma cells should be searched for in the germinal centers of lymph nodes, after regional antigenic stimulation if possible, in the bone marrow, and in the lamina propria of rectal mucosa obtained by rectal biopsy (Crabbe and Heremans, 1967). Absence of plasma cells in the gastrointestinal tract usually indicates an IgA defect.

ASSESSMENT OF LYMPHOID MASS. Palpable lymphoid tissue and identifiable tonsillar and adenoidal tissue are reduced in classic X-linked agammaglobulinemia. In most other primary humoral immunodeficiencies there is no significant reduction in lymphoid mass.

Lymph nodes
Normal structure: histologic

Lymph nodes are discrete nodules of lymphoid tissue located at anatomically constant points along the course of lymphatic vessels. Lymphoid tissue is not found exclusively in lymph nodes; lymphoid aggregates are present in the submucosa of the intestinal tract and bronchi, in normal bone marrow, in the spleen, and diffusely in the thymus. However, as in the case of the spleen, lymph nodes represent circumscribed and identifiable structures whose enlargement is easily discovered by palpation. As discrete structures, they can be excised and subjected to detailed bacteriologic, cytologic, and histologic study.

Lymph nodes have a fibrous capsule from which connective tissue trabeculae extend into the node in a roughly radial arrangement. The connective tissue framework between the trabeculae consists of a network of reticulum fibers, and this stroma supports primitive reticuloendothelial cells, scattered phagocytic histiocytes, and the predominant lymphocytes. In the *medullary* or *paracortical* (central) portion of the lymph node the small lymphocytes are packed tightly in sheets and cords. In the peripheral or cortical portion the lymphocytes are condensed into roughly spherical *lymphoid nodules*. These may consist entirely of small lymphocytes when the lymph node is in a completely resting or nonreactive state. When stimulated, the primary lymphoid nodules develop *germinal* or *reactive centers* that consist of medium and large lymphocytes (some in mitosis), scattered reticulum cells that may or may not be phagocytic, and some plasma cells. The proliferating germinal center is usually pale staining and sharply circumscribed by the crowded dark-staining small lymphocytes at the periphery that form a *corona* around the reactive center. The corona and the deeper paracortical areas of the node are populated by T-lymphocytes, whereas the germinal centers are composed of B-lymphocytes and their progeny is active in the sythesis of immunoglobulin.

Lymph enters the node through afferent vessels and empties into a distinct subcapsular sinus that is continuous with sinuses running along the trabeculae. These ultimately form efferent lymphatics that leave the node at the hilus. The sinuses are lined by flat *littoral* or *lining* cells, sometimes called endothelial, which are quite different when studied by electron microscopy. The chief difference is that littoral cells are phagocytic, and as such they are active in performing a house-cleaning function on the lymph. Under pathologic conditions these cells hypertrophy, multiply, become detached, and become free phagocytes in the lymph sinus, the ''Sinuskatarr'' of German authors.

Normal structure: cytologic

Study of the morphology of individual cells, as seen in imprints from the freshly cut surface of a lymph node or from smears of aspirated material (Hajdu and Melamed, 1973), is a useful adjunct to the histopathologic appearance. Histologic sections are essential for determining the relationship of cells to each other and to the architecture of the tissue, but cellular details are partially obscured by fixation and by the thickness of the section. On the other hand, imprints make possible a study of individual cells, as in a blood smear, and often reveal details or morphology that, in combination with the histologic appearance, are extremely useful in arriving at the correct diagnosis.

Imprints of a normal node show a predominance of small lymphocytes, a few less mature lymphoid cells, and scat-

Table 3-10. Differential counts from normal lymph node imprints*

Cell	Percent
Reticulum cells	0- 0.1
Mast cells	0- 0.5
Lymphoblasts	0.1- 0.9
Prolymphocytes	5.3-16.4
Lymphocytes	67.8-90.0
Monoblasts	0- 0.5
Promonocytes	0- 0.5
Monocytes	0.2- 7.4
Plasmablasts	0- 0.1
Proplasmacytes	0- 0.5
Plasma cells	0- 4.7
Neutrophils	0- 2.2
Eosinophils	0- 0.3
Basophils	0- 0.2

*Modified from Lucas, 1955.

tered cells of other types (Table 3-10). When the node is abnormal, quantitative and qualitative abnormalities will be found.

Function

The functions of the lymph nodes are three: formation of lymphocytes, production of antibodies, and filtration of the lymph.

The lymph nodes are responsible for a portion of the total lymphocyte-producing capacity of lymphoid tissue. There is as yet no information on how many lymphocytes enter the total lymphocyte pool from lymph nodes and how many are produced elsewhere. On the basis of weight, lymph nodes contain about 100 Gm of lymphoid tissue as compared to 70 Gm in the bone marrow and 1,300 Gm scattered throughout other tissues. Lymphocytes originating in lymph nodes enter the lymph channels on the efferent side. Some enter the bloodstream directly by passing through the walls of capillary vessels. The lymph nodes not only generate new lymphocytes but are also populated by lymphocytes originating in the central tissues.

The role of the lymphocyte in the production of antibodies has already been mentioned (p. 89). With reference to lymph nodes, immunologic activity is a property of the lymphoid nodules: the small lymphocytes in the corona are responsible for cellular immunity (homograft rejection, delayed hypersensitivity, and graft-versus-host reactivity), whereas the plasma and other cells in the reactive center are responsible for humoral immunity (production of immunoglobulins and specific antibodies).

Lymph nodes play an obvious but relatively unimportant role as filters of particulate matter (anthracotic pigment, cellular debris, and bacteria). Tumor cells carried by the lymph from the primary site to regional lymph nodes may implant and grow to form metastases.

Aspiration and imprint preparations

Excision of superficial lymph nodes is usually a minor surgical procedure recommended over biopsy by aspiration. However, the histopathologic diagnosis of lymph node

Text continued on p. 115.

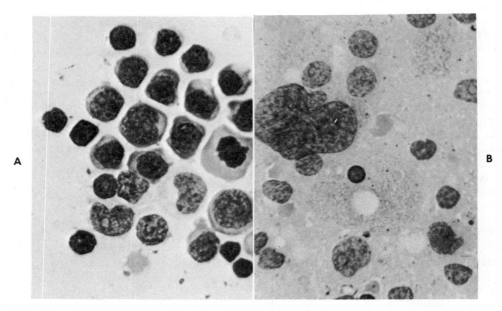

Fig. 3-24. Lymph node imprint, extramedullary hemopoiesis. **A,** Lymphocytes and normoblasts. **B,** Megakaryocyte. (Wright's stain; ×450.) (Courtesy Dr. J. C. Sieracki.)

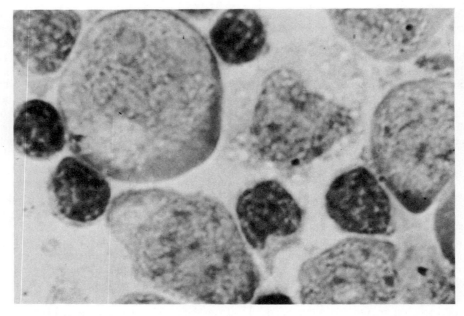

Fig. 3-25. Lymph node imprint, infectious mononucleosis. (Wright's stain; ×1,200.) (Courtesy Dr. J. C. Sieracki.)

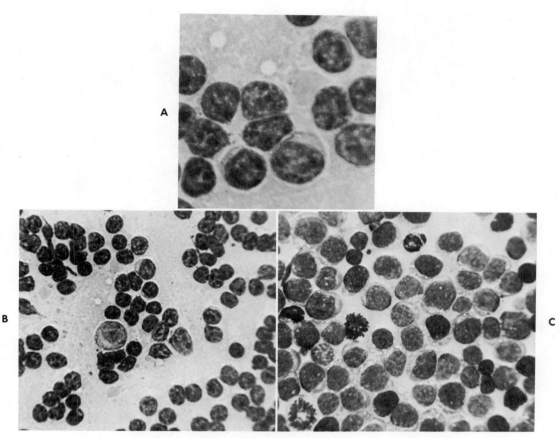

Fig. 3-26. Lymph node imprints, lymphocytic lymphoma. **A,** Well differentiated. (Wright's stain; ×1,200.) **B,** Well differentiated. (Wright's stain; ×450.) **C,** Poorly differentiated. (Wright's stain; ×450.) (Courtesy Dr. J. C. Sieracki.)

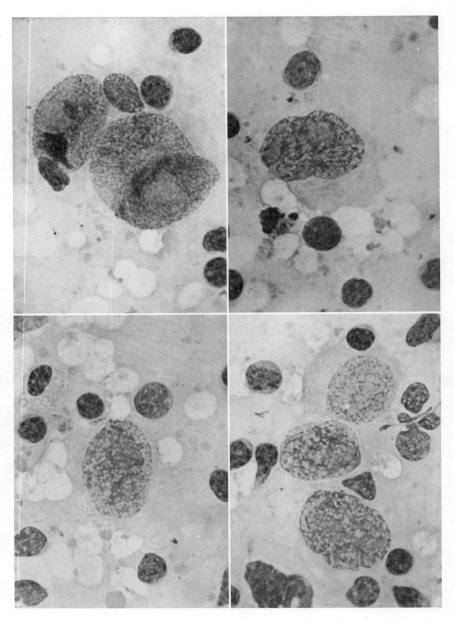

Fig. 3-27. Hodgkin's disease, cervical lymph node imprints. A 22-year-old white man with fever and lymphadenopathy. Posterior cervical lymph node excised and imprints made from freshly cut surface. The large nucleoli are pale blue. (Hematoxylin-eosin stain; ×1,000.)

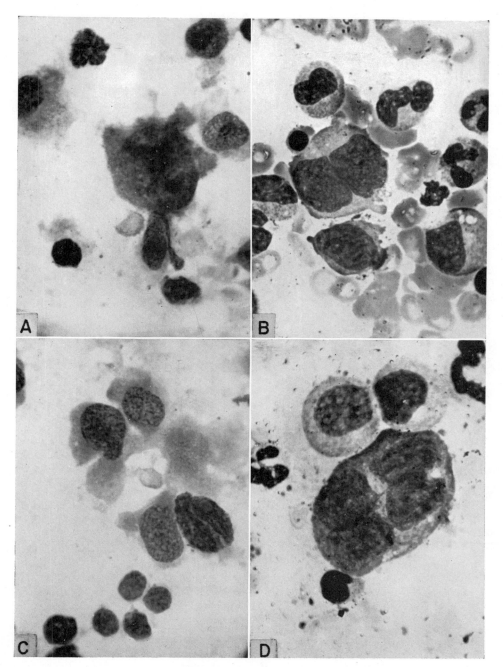

Fig. 3-28. Hodgkin's disease, lymph node aspiration. Smears made from lymph node aspiration. (Wright's stain; ×950.)

History and physical examination: This 56-year-old man had complained of abdominal pain and intermittent fever for 3 months. The pain was usually felt in the right lower quadrant. He was thought to have appendicitis and was operated on. The findings were a normal appendix and a large retroperitoneal mass, which after biopsy was diagnosed as Hodgkin's granuloma. After surgery, large matted right inguinal lymph nodes soon appeared as well as splenomegaly and hepatomegaly.

Laboratory data: Hb 8.7 Gm/dl of blood; RBC 3.15 million/mm³ (3.15 × 10¹²/l). Other findings, except for this moderate anemia, are not pertinent.

Discussion: Bone marrow smears in this case did not reveal abnormal cells, but paraffin sections showed granulomatous areas compatible with the diagnosis of Hodgkin's disease. Aspiration of an inguinal lymph node was carried out, and the smears revealed atypical reticulum cells of the Reed-Sternberg type, **A-D.**

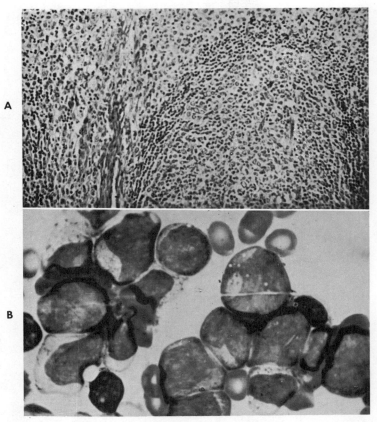

Fig. 3-29. Lymphoma, non-Hodgkin's, posterior cervical lymph node. A 4-year-old boy with generalized lymph-adenopathy, minimal splenomegaly, fever, and thrombocytopenia. Histopathologic findings are not clearly indicative of lymphoma, but imprints show atypical lymphoblasts. **A,** Paraffin section. (Hematoxylin-eosin stain; ×120.) **B,** Imprint. (Wright's stain; ×950.)

Fig. 3-30. Non-Hodgkin's lymphoma, nodular, moderately differentiated, posterior cervical lymph node. **A,** Paraffin section. (Hematoxylin-eosin stain; ×120.) **B** and **C,** Imprints. (Wright's stain; ×950.) **D,** Lymphangio-gram showing involvement of para-aortic nodes.

History and physical examination: This patient is a 20-year-old white man. He was referred for diagnosis 1 year ago, with complaints of low-grade fever, malaise, and lymphadenopathy. He had firm, discrete, nontender posterior cervical lymph nodes, 1 to 2 cm in diameter, and similar but larger bilateral inguinal nodes. Peripheral blood picture was normal, and there was no elevation of heterophil titer. Aspiration biopsy of sternal marrow was carried out, and smears and sections were interpreted as normal. A posterior cervical lymph node was excised; sections showed only nonspecific hyperplasia.

During the next year he was never entirely well subjectively, but he seemed to feel worse periodically, with fever and malaise. During these episodes the adenopathy seemed more marked. One year after onset he reported a weight loss of 15 pounds and vague abdominal distress. Peripheral blood picture remained normal with the exception of an occasional immature lymphocyte in blood smears. Bone marrow biopsy was repeated and was again normal. Cervical node excision was done, and the findings on this examination are illustrated.

Discussion: Paraffin sections of lymph node were submitted to a number of capable pathologists, and the opinions varied from benign hyperplasia to frank lymphoma. Having the advantage of close clinical contact with the patient and the cytology of the imprints, which I believed indicated a lymphoma, I thought that the correct diagnosis was nodular non-Hodgkin's lymphoma, albeit in an early stage of development. Lymphangiograms supported this opinion. Once again, lymph node imprints can be most helpful in problem cases.

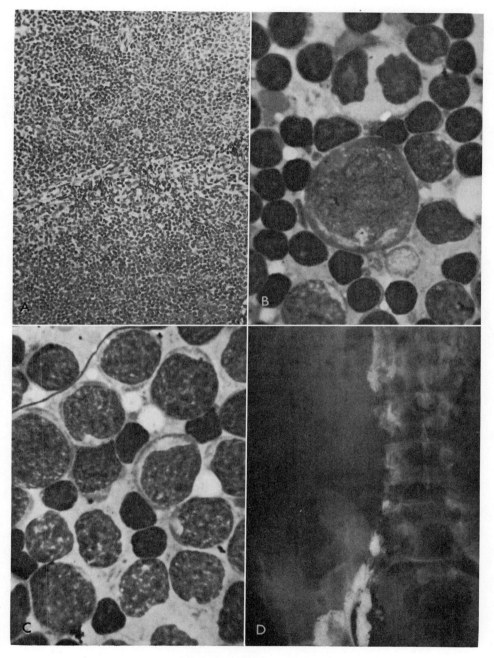

Fig. 3-30. For legend see opposite page.

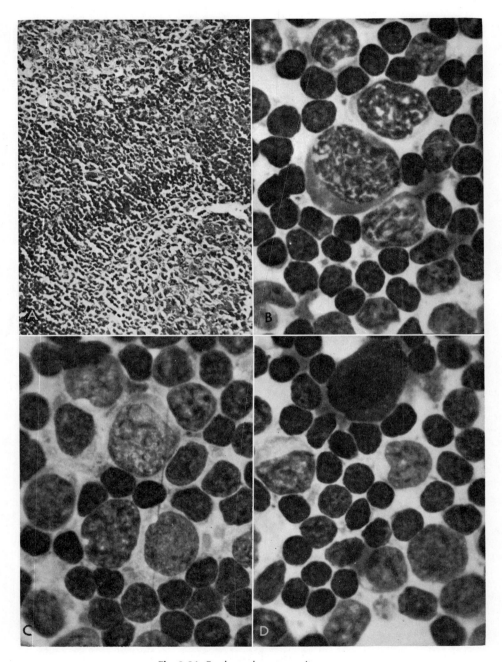

Fig. 3-31. For legend see opposite page.

Fig. 3-31. Lymphadenopathy and splenomegaly, lymphoid hyperplasia probably due to anticonvulsant drug (Celontin). **A,** Paraffin section. (×120.) **B-D,** Lymph node imprints. (Wright's stain; ×950.) (Patient of Dr. S. Rosen.)

Differential count from node imprint

Cell	Percent
Reticulum cells	0.2
Mast cells	0.1
Lymphoblasts	7.0
Prolymphocytes	9.0
Lymphocytes	80.0
Neutrophils	1.0
Eosinophils	0.2
Atypical lymphocytes	2.5

History and physical examination: This patient was a 13-year-old white girl. She was an epileptic, having suffered grand mal seizures since the age of 4. Epileptic state had been fairly well controlled by Dilantin, but 6 weeks before admission Celontin was substituted for Dilantin. Her first unusual episode, however, occurred 1 month before this change in therapy. At that time there was an acute onset of purpura and ecchymoses. The platelet count was very low, and the diagnosis of idiopathic thrombocytopenic purpura was made. Prednisone was given, and the platelet count promptly returned to normal, but when the medication was reduced, there was recurrence of thrombocytopenia with severe vaginal bleeding. She was admitted to the hospital for complete evaluation of the thrombocytopenic state.

On physical examination the only positive findings were the following: (1) moderate purpura of extremities with a few ecchymoses, (2) enlarged spleen, 2 fingerbreadths below the costal margin, and (3) moderate cervical lymphadenopathy, more marked on right.

Laboratory data: Blood Hb 11.2 Gm/dl, WBC 7,700 (7.7×10^9/l); leukocyte differential count: segmented neutrophils 21%, stab neutrophils 6%, lymphocytes 67%, monocytes 1%, eosinophils 5%. Many of the lymphocytes appeared somewhat atypical. Platelet count on admission was 20,000/mm³ (0.02×10^{12}/l), which stayed within the range of 15,000 to 20,000 (0.015 to 0.02×10^{12}/l). Urinalysis was normal. Direct antiglobulin test, LE preparations, and heterophil antibody studies were negative.

Discussion: Because of the lymphadenopathy and the atypical lymphocytes in the peripheral blood smear, it was thought that additional information should be obtained before the thrombocytopenic purpura was labeled idiopathic. There was also the question of the anticonvulsant drugs being the culprits. Accordingly, a 2 × 2.5 cm lymph node was excised from the right subdigastric chain, and bone marrow was obtained by aspiration biopsy.

As recommended, the lymph node was bisected immediately after surgery, and imprints were made from the fresh cut surface. The tissue was then processed for routine paraffin sections. The differential count from the imprints is given above. It was thought that the cytology from the imprints was compatible with the type of reaction caused by the anticonvulsant drugs (Saltzstein and Ackerman, 1959; Bajoghli, 1961; Rosenfeld et al, 1961). Paraffin sections showed only hyperplastic changes. Therapy was changed from Celontin to Mysoline, and the adenopathy disappeared and has not returned.

As for the thrombocytopenia, it recurred whenever corticosteroid therapy was reduced, and eventually a splenectomy was done. Following splenectomy the platelet count rose to a high of 660,000/mm³ (0.66×10^{12}/l) and then returned and has remained at a normal level. Since the thrombocytopenia preceded the lymphadenopathy, it is probably unrelated to anticonvulsive therapy and has been classified as idiopathic. One cannot be sure that this is justified.

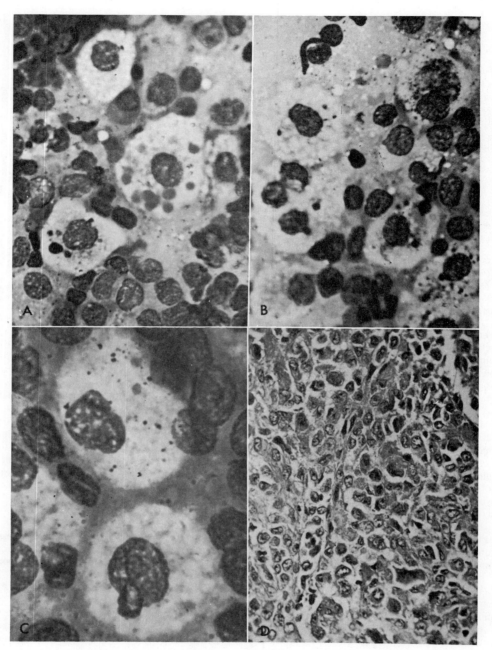

Fig. 3-32. Letterer-Siwe disease. **A-C,** Smear of lymph node aspiration. (Wright's stain; **A** and **B,** ×400; **C,** ×950.) **D,** Paraffin section, lymph node. (Hematoxylin-eosin stain; ×400.)

History and physical examination: This child was noted to have petechiae, ecchymoses, lymphadenopathy, and slight splenomegaly at birth. He was in the hospital for 6 months, and there is a great deal of clinical and laboratory data that is not pertinent to this presentation. The diagnosis was made at the age of 1 month by aspiration biopsy of a large cervical node and by histopatholgic examination after excision. Bone marrow aspiration biopsy was also performed.

Laboratory data: At birth and for some time thereafter the hematologic and other laboratory data were normal. Later there were anemia, leukopenia, and thrombocytopenia, which followed treatment with methotrexate and x-irradiation. He also received large doses of corticosteroids.

Discussion: The reticuloendotheliosis is quite striking in the lymph node aspirate and in the paraffin section of the lymph node. Note the foam cells, which resemble Gaucher cells but do not have the reticular cytoplasm. The distinction among the various dyslipidoses is not always easy to make with confidence on cytologic or histopathologic criteria alone.

lesions is difficult and calls for experience as well as clinicopathologic correlation. Sometimes any additional cytologic evidence available is of great value. I have found this true of imprints made from the freshly excised node. Imprints are made by gently touching (not smearing) the freshly cut surface of the node to a glass slide. The imprints are then stained with Wright's stain. Feinberg et al (1980) stain imprint preparations with a modified Papanicolaou technic and also use special cytochemical stains (oil red O, α-naphthyl acetate esterase, acid phosphatase, tartrate-resistant acid phosphatase, and methyl green–pyronine). It is occasionally desirable to obtain material from a lymph node by means of needle aspiration. The procedure is simple and safe. After the overlying skin is infiltrated with an anesthetic agent, the node is fixed between the thumb and index finger of one hand while aspiration is performed with the other, using a 20-gauge needle, as for splenic puncture. Smears are made from the material obtained and stained with Wright's stain.

Examples of lymph node cytology are shown in Figs. 3-24 to 3-32.

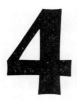

"The shape of things,
their colours, lights
and shades, changes,
surprises. . . ."
R. Browning: *Fra Lippo Lippi*

Morphology of blood and bone marrow cells

PRINCIPLES OF NORMAL CELL MATURATION
  Cytoplasmic differentiation
    Loss of basophilia
    Cytoplasmic granules
    Elaboration of hemoglobin
  Nuclear maturation
    Structure and cytochemistry
    Changes in shape
  Reduction in cell size
PRINCIPLES OF ABNORMAL CELL MATURATION
  Abnormal cytoplasmic maturation
  Abnormal nuclear maturation
  Abnormal size
  Multinuclearity
  Hiatus leukemicus
NOMENCLATURE
DESCRIPTION OF WRIGHT-STAINED BLOOD AND BONE
  MARROW CELLS
  Reticulum cell
  Myeloblast
  Progranulocyte
  Myelocyte
  Metamyelocyte and juvenile
  Band granulocyte
  Segmented granulocyte
  Lymphoblast
  Prolymphocyte
  Lymphocyte
  Monoblast
  Promonocyte
  Monocyte
  Pronormoblast
  Basophilic normoblast
  Polychromatophilic normoblast
  Orthochromic normoblast
  Promegaloblast
  Basophilic megaloblast
  Polychromatophilic megaloblast
  Orthochromic megaloblast
  Megakaryoblast
  Promegakaryocyte
  Megakaryocyte
  Plasmablast
  Proplasmacyte
  Plasmacyte
ABNORMAL FORMS IN BLOOD AND BONE MARROW
  Toxic granulation

  Auer bodies
  Pelger-Huët anomaly
  May-Hegglin anomaly and Döhle bodies
  Sézary's syndrome
  Virocytes and reactive lymphocytes
  Jordans' anomaly in progressive muscular dystrophy
  Cytochemically abnormal neutrophils and eosinophils (Alius-Grignaschi anomaly)
  Cystine crystals in cystinosis
  Miscellaneous leukocytic inclusions
  Constitutional hypersegmentation of neutrophilic leukocytes
  Endothelial cells in peripheral blood
  Tumor cells in peripheral blood
  Phagocytic cells in peripheral blood
  Phagocytosis in bone marrow
SEXUAL DIMORPHISM OF LEUKOCYTES
  Human chromosomes
  Chromosomal content of blood cells
  Nuclear sex and sex chromatin
  The drumstick as a sex characteristic
MORPHOLOGY OF BLOOD AND BONE MARROW CELLS WITH
  SPECIAL TECHNICS
  Supravital methods
    General considerations
      Advantages of method
      Technical considerations
      Vital staining plus phase contrast
  Phase contrast microscopy
    General considerations
    Time-lapse photography
  Electron microscopy
    General considerations
    Ultrastructure of a blood cell
    Normal blood cells
      Granulocytes
      Monocytes
      Lymphocytes
      Plasma cells
      Megakaryocytes and platelets
      Normoblasts
    Ultrastructure of abnormal blood cells
      Leukemic cells
      Plasma cells in myeloma
      Phagocytic histiocytes
      Gaucher cells
      Pelger-Huët anomaly
      May-Hegglin anomaly

Cytochemistry of blood cells
 Peroxidase (myeloperoxidase)
 Lipids
 Glycogen
 Alkaline phosphatase
 Acid phosphatase
 Esterases
 Application of cytochemistry to the study of leukemia

PRINCIPLES OF NORMAL CELL MATURATION

Before outlining the characteristics of individual cells it is advisable to discuss the general features of cell maturation. It is important for the student to understand these principles. Simply memorizing the features of each cell type does not enable the student to analyze the appearance of abnormal cells such as those found in the leukemias and other examples of abnormal hemopoiesis. Experience in teaching morphology has repeatedly confirmed the importance of analyzing the appearance of a cell according to the basic principles of normal and abnormal cell maturation. These principles are quite simple.

In any cell series an almost infinite gradation of cells exists between the most immature "blast" form and the mature definitive cell. The mature cell is described and identified by certain specific features that develop in the course of maturation. These features gradually appear as the cell matures, so that each cell must evolve gradually and appear at some stage of maturation. Since this is normally an orderly process, blood cells exhibit recurring features that have led to the description of typical stages. It cannot be emphasized too strongly, however, that cell development does not occur in instantaneous steplike transformations but by gradual transition, and the stages described for convenience are merely typical frames from a continuous strip. It cannot be expected, therefore, that all the cells present in a blood or bone marrow smear will conform exactly to the description of the "typical" cell. Failure to appreciate this may result in frustration and failure to become adept at cell identification. One other basic consideration is that since a cell is composed of several component parts, each must undergo transformation. Normally the changes are simultaneous and parallel, a developmental *synchronism* that simplifies description and analysis. However, abnormal hemopoiesis may be characterized by different rates of maturation for the nucleus and cytoplasm called *asynchronism,* producing cells often called atypical or bizarre but whose structure is just as easily analyzed as that of normal cells.

The transformation from an immature to a mature cell always involves changes in the cytoplasm and nucleus and is generally accompanied by reduction in cell size. It is only for convenience that each is described and diagrammed separately (Fig. 4-1).

The following discussion of normal and abnormal maturation serves also as an index to the three features that must be considered, first separately and then together, when identifying a blood cell. Each is important, but one, cell size, is worthy of special emphasis. I have found that students beginning the study of blood cell morphology usually learn quickly to view objectively the nuclear and cytoplasmic features of cells but are often misled by neglecting to consider whether the cell being studied is large or small. I like to use as reference the red blood cell—one is usually present in the field, its size normally varying but little from a mean diameter of about 7.2 μ, and deviations from this size are usually easier to detect than in other cells. In addition, the students who train themselves to use such a ready-made reference for size will not find it difficult to change to a microscope of different magnification.

Cytoplasmic differentiation
Loss of basophilia

Cytoplasmic differentiation is accompanied by profound changes in the cytochemistry of cytoplasm, including elaboration of enzymes and changes in nucleic acid content. The cytoplasm of immature cells is generally deeply basophilic, basophilia referring to the affinity for a basic dye such as the methylene blue present in Wright's and other polychrome

Cytoplasmic differentiation

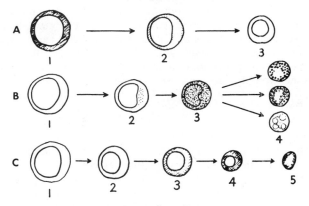

Nuclear maturation

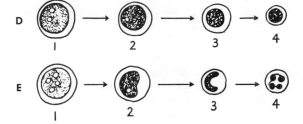

Reduction in cell size

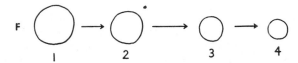

Fig. 4-1. Principles of normal cell maturation. **A,** Loss of cytoplasmic basophilia. **B,** Elaboration and differentiation of cytoplasmic granules. **C,** Elaboration of specific cytoplasmic constituent (hemoglobin). **D,** Reduction in nuclear size, condensation of chromatin, and reduction of nucleoli. **E,** Alteration of nuclear shape. **F,** Reduction in cell size.

stains. Basophilia is proportional to the cytoplasmic content of ribonucleic acid (RNA). As the cell matures, there is a gradual loss of cytoplasmic RNA and cytoplasmic basophilia. In general, therefore, the more basophilic the cytoplasm, the less mature the cell.

Cytoplasmic granules

In myeloid cells cytoplasmic differentiation is characterized by the appearance of granules. These are probably concerned with enzyme systems, but they also differ chemically. Three types are commonly distinguished on the basis of individual staining properties. Some common properties such as lipid content or the presence of peroxidase and other enzymes exist and may be useful in distinguishing myeloid granules from all others.

When cytoplasmic granules first appear, they are few, coarse, and wine red, the "nonspecific" granules. As the granulocyte matures, three types of "specific" granules appear. (See p. 206 for a discussion of the cytochemistry of nonspecific and specific granules.) The number gradually increases, and the granules differentiate into three types. In a mature cell one of these types will predominate. Each type has an affinity either for acid or for basic dyes. Those that are *acidophilic* or *eosinophilic* stain orange-red and are characteristic of the eosinophil leukocyte. The *basophilic* granules are blue-black and identify the basophil leukocyte, whereas those that stain with both the basic and the acid dyes of a compound stain, called *neutrophilic,* characterize the neutrophilic leukocyte and are purplish.

Elaboration of hemoglobin

A different type of cytoplasmic differentiation is seen in the synthesis of a characteristic cytoplasmic constituent such as hemoglobin. This is a special feature of the maturation of erythroid cells. At first the immature cell contains no visible hemoglobin, though Turpin (1970) finds that the greatest rate of hemoglobin synthesis occurs in the pronormoblast and basophilic normoblast. However, this is obscured by the basophilia of cytoplasmic RNA in stained smears, and it is only when the RNA content is reduced that hemoglobin becomes visible. It appears, then, that as the normoblast matures it elaborates more and more hemoglobin until, at the orthochromic stage, it contains a great deal of orange-staining hemoglobin and no basophilic RNA. Gradually a little appears and then a great deal, the most mature normal cell containing a standard and maximal amount of this respiratory pigment. At this stage of development the nucleus is apparently no longer necessary and is eliminated by extrusion.

Nuclear maturation

Nuclear maturation is concerned with changes in the structure and chemical composition of the nuclear chromatin and nuclei, reduction in size of the nucleus with condensation of chromatin, and in some cases with striking changes in nuclear shape.

Structure and cytochemistry

The immature nucleus is round or oval. The nucleus-to-cytoplasm (N/C) ratio is high, and the netlike or spongelike nuclear chromatin is very delicate. As the cell matures, the chromatin strands become increasingly coarse and clumped, while their staining properties change from purplish to blue. Simultaneously a reduction in the number of nucleoli is noted. These are usually invisible in a mature cell. At the same time there are striking changes in the distribution of nucleic acids. The nucleus of the young cell is characterized by nuclear chromatin that is rich in deoxyribonucleic acid (DNA). The nucleoli contain RNA and are therefore Feulgen negative (Bernhard, 1966). As the cell matures, the RNA-positive nucleoli disappear, and in their place is found DNA-positive, nucleolus-associated heterochromatin.

Changes in shape

Nuclear maturation of some cell types produces striking changes in shape. This is particularly true of the granulocytes in which the end result is a nucleus containing two or more lobulations connected by filaments of nuclear membrane. The more mature the cell, the more polymorphous the nuclear structure. Of two young cells, the older is the one showing the more striking deviation from the primitive round or oval nuclear shape.

Reduction in cell size

Reduction in cell size is a feature of maturity in all cells except those of the megakaryocytic series, in which the youngest cell (diploid) is smaller than the fully developed megakaryocyte (polyploid). In general, however, a mature cell is smaller than an immature one. In most cells nuclear condensation is greater than the reduction in total cell volume. The nucleus-to-cytoplasm ratio is therefore *high* in the young cells and *low* in mature cells.

PRINCIPLES OF ABNORMAL CELL MATURATION

In pathologic hemopoiesis, striking deviations in one or more of these orderly sequences can be seen. They result in atypical cells abnormal with respect to nuclear maturation, cytoplasmic differentiation, or size. In addition, the normal synchronous maturation of nucleus and cytoplasm and synchronous reduction in size may instead be asynchronous, producing cells showing greater or less maturity of one with respect to the other. To classify such cells is sometimes difficult; e.g., one may encounter a cell having a well-differentiated segmented nucleus, thus presumably an adult neutrophil, but whose cytoplasm is immature, the granules being primitive, atypical, or absent. It may be assumed then that nuclear maturation is normal but cytoplasmic maturation is retarded. In such instances it is often necessary to classify age and degree of differentiation according to nuclear features, assuming the abnormal features to be inaccurate indices of maturity. In other instances hereditary anomalies of nuclear or cytoplasmic development can be recognized as specific cases of anomalous maturation.

Abnormal cytoplasmic maturation

Abnormal cytoplasmic maturation is most commonly seen in the granulocytes. Accelerated proliferation, whether leukemic or benign, often leads to asynchronism in the maturation of nucleus and cytoplasm, the latter often so much retarded that a poorly granular or even agranular cytoplasm may be found in cells otherwise qualifying as myelocytes, metamyelocytes, or even adult neutrophils. Bessis (1973c) refers to this developmental asynchronism as "maturation anarchy." At times granules are present but remain primitive and azurophilic. In granulocytic leukemia Ullyot and Bainton (1974) and Bainton et al (1977) describe several interesting abnormalities of cytoplasmic maturation: mature neutrophils containing both nonspecific and specific granules but lacking peroxidase, mature neutrophils lacking specific granules, mature neutrophils lacking nonspecific granules, and the packaging of peroxidase into Auer rods surrounded by single-unit membranes (p. 157). In the erythrocytic series, stimulated proliferation sometimes leads to retarded cytoplasmic maturation, with persistent cytoplasmic basophilia and late hemoglobination. The megaloblastic family of cells must be considered totally atypical and will be discussed later. It should be mentioned here, however, that one often encounters megaloblastic cells with abundant cytoplasm exhibiting basophilia late in the series. Abnormal cytoplasmic inclusions such as Döhle bodies (infectious diseases), Auer bodies (leukemia), and toxic granulation (infection and poisons affecting the marrow) are evidence of abnormal cytoplasmic maturation.

Abnormal nuclear maturation

As discussed later in this chapter, abnormally large nuclei may be a manifestation of polyploidy. Sometimes two or more nuclei are present, usually in severe disturbances such as leukemia; one nucleus may be diploid and the other polyploid. Individual nuclei may show either accelerated or retarded reduction in nucleoli. Hypersegmented nuclei in neutrophils are seen in reaction to sepsis and in megaloblastic dyspoiesis due to deficiency of hemopoietic principle. In leukemic proliferation there is often a tendency toward irregularity in the nuclear outline in cells such as lymphocytes, which normally have a round or oval nucleus. The nucleus then shows indentation. Leukemic lymphocytes with such indented (buttock) nuclei are sometimes called *Rieder cells*. In acute myelocytic leukemia the myeloblasts sometimes show bizarre nuclear shapes (see Plate 42). These also are called Rieder cells.

Abnormal size

Recognition of abnormal size is of more practical importance. Cells that are either larger or smaller than normal often supply important diagnostic information; e.g., giant myelocytes, metamyelocytes, and stab forms are not uncommon in myelocytic leukemia and in reactive leukocytic proliferation. Giant myeloblasts are sometimes seen in leukemia, often exhibiting polyploidy in the nucleus as well. In the erythroid series the megaloblastic cells are examples of larger than normal size and are apparent at even the adult nonnucleated macrocytic erythrocyte stage. Granulocytes are also abnormally large in megaloblastic dyspoiesis, the giant metamyelocytes and stab forms being highly characteristic of folic acid and vitamin B_{12} deficiency.

The one important example of the abnormally small cell is the micromyeloblast, an abnormally small myeloblast sometimes encountered in acute myelocytic leukemia. These small blast cells may be as small as lymphocytes and may be mistaken for them by inexperienced observers. The small size is due to a reduction in the amount of cytoplasm, which is sometimes so scanty that the cell resembles a naked nucleus. The nucleus, however, usually shows one or more nucleoli.

Multinuclearity

Cells containing more than one nucleus (polykaryons) are common in pathologic material. Chambers (1978) discusses the mechanisms of cell fusion and the condition accompanied by polykaryon formation. The most common pathologic polykaryons are seen in inflammatory reactions (granulomas of various types and some neoplasms). The osteoclast is considered a normal polykaryon, although it may represent a reaction to bone as a foreign body. Binucleated or multinucleated plasma cells are sometimes found in an otherwise normal bone marrow.

Hiatus leukemicus

In leukemia, particularly granulocytic, the bone marrow often shows blasts (myeloblasts) and mature cells (mature granulocytes) without any intermediate forms. Bessis (1973b) believes that this maturation abnormality, so named by Naegeli, represents immature leukemic cells that fail to mature and normal granulocytes derived from the maturation of the few remaining normal precursors.

NOMENCLATURE

Differences in terminology, although fewer than in former years, are always a problem. Such variations reflect different opinions regarding the origin of blood cells as well as the impulse to improve on familiar names. A revision and clarification of existing hematologic nomenclature was undertaken in 1949 by a special committee of the American Society of Clinical Pathologists. A real contribution was made in proposing a standard and acceptable nomenclature for most cell types. The nomenclature proposed for cells of the erythrocytic series, however, seems awkward and artificial. We use instead the terminology outlined in Table 4-1, which, for comparison, also lists the recommendations of the Committee.

DESCRIPTION OF WRIGHT-STAINED BLOOD AND BONE MARROW CELLS

See Summary in Table 4-2.

Reticulum cell (Fig. 4-2)

The use of the term "reticulum cell" is not easy to defend. As discussed in Chapter 1, the primitive reticuloendothelial or mesenchymal cell differentiates in various directions. One of these is a transformation to hemopoietically oriented primitive cells, now called colony-forming units (CFU) (Table 1-1, p. 4). CFUs are stem cells, and, although they can be defined on the basis of colony formation in tissue culture, there are no morphologic criteria by which they can be distinguished from other primitive blasts. In a differential count on bone marrow the name "reticulum cell" can be used for two cells, one having a rather abundant frayed cytoplasm, immature nucleus, and large blue nucleolus, the other being obviously phagocytic.

Table 4-1. Nomenclature used in this text compared with that proposed by American Society of Clinical Pathologists, Committee for Clarification of the Nomenclature of Cells and Diseases of the Blood and Blood-Forming Organs

Nomenclature used in this text	Nomenclature proposed by A.S.C.P.
Myeloblast	Myeloblast
Progranulocyte	Progranulocyte
Myelocyte	Myelocyte
Metamyelocyte	Metamyelocyte
Band granulocyte	Band granulocyte
Segmented granulocyte	Segmented granulocyte
Lymphoblast	Lymphoblast
Prolymphocyte	Prolymphocyte
Lymphocyte	Lymphocyte
Monoblast	Monoblast
Promonocyte	Promonocyte
Monocyte	Monocyte
Plasmablast	Plasmoblast
Proplasmacyte	Proplasmocyte
Plasmacyte	Plasmocyte
Megakaryoblast	Megakaryoblast
Promegakaryocyte	Promegakaryocyte
Megakaryocyte	Megakaryocyte
Platelet	Thrombocyte
Pronormoblast	Rubriblast
Basophilic normoblast	Prorubricyte
Polychromatophilic normoblast	Rubricyte
Orthochromic normoblast	Metarubricyte
Promegaloblast	Rubriblast, pernicious anemia type
Basophilic megaloblast	Prorubricyte, pernicious anemia type
Polychromatophilic megaloblast	Rubricyte, pernicious anemia type
Orthochromic megaloblast	Metarubricyte, pernicious anemia type

Table 4-2. Summary of characteristics of blood and bone marrow cells (Wright's stain)

Cell	Size (μ)	Nucleus	Nucleoli	Cytoplasm	N/C ratio	Comments
1. Reticulum cell	15-25	Irregularly oval; delicate membrane; delicate chromatin; sharply demarcated parachromatin	1-3, irregular and faint	Abundant, pale blue, mottled, usually no granules but may have a few azurophilic granules	1:1	In marrow smears, cell outlines usually indistinct; cytoplasm usually mottled and may appear vacuolated; nucleus often shows thickenings at intersections of chromatin strands
2. Myeloblast	10-20	Large, oval or round; thin membrane; stippled or finely reticulated chromatin; sparse, sharply demarcated parachromatin	2-5, distinct	Sparse, no granules, deeply basophilic	5:1-7:1	Usually does not show clear perinuclear halo as in lymphoblast, nor is chromatin as coarse as in lymphoblast nucleus; in pathologic proliferation these cells may be very large (macromyeloblasts) or about the size of young lymphocytes (micromyeloblasts); latter easily mistaken for lymphocytes, but micromyeloblast contains finer chromatin
3. Progranulocyte	14-20	Large, round or oval; thin membrane; chromatin netlike with some clumping next to nucleoli; parachromatin sparse	1-3, not as prominent	Sparse, basophilic but not as intense as in myeloblast	5:1	Distinguished from myeloblast chiefly by presence of granules and from later cells by small number of granules; at times granules large and round, but usually fine and irregular
4. Myelocyte a. Neutrophilic b. Eosinophilic c. Basophilic	10-18	Indistinct when cell heavily granulated; chromatin fairly coarse; parachromatin sparse	0-1, indistinct	Moderate, heavily granulated (granules may obscure nucleus)	2:1	Most heavily granulated of blood cells; granules may be purplish at early stage of development, later differentiate into basophilic, eosinophilic, or neutrophilic
5. Metamyelocyte a. Neutrophilic b. Eosinophilic c. Basophilic	10-18	Kidney shaped; heavy nuclear membrane; chromatin coarse; parachromatin sparse	0	Fairly abundant, pinkish, contains specific granules smaller and more variable in size than in myelocyte	1.5:1	Indentation of nucleus indicates greater maturity; granules of neutrophilic metamyelocytes vary in size; in eosinophilic or basophilic cells, granules remain large and usually obscure nuclear outline
6. Band granulocyte a. Neutrophilic b. Eosinophilic c. Basophilic	10-15	Sausage or band shaped; coarse, deeply staining purple chromatin; parachromatin very scanty	0	Abundant, pinkish, contains specific granules (fine when neutrophilic)	1:2	Nucleus may be constricted at one or more points, but as long as there is visible chromatin between nuclear membranes, cell called band form; when nucleus folded but constriction not visible, should be classified as a band form; nuclear outline in basophilic and eosinophilic cells usually obscured by granules
7. Segmented granulocyte a. Neutrophilic b. Eosinophilic c. Basophilic	10-15	Lobules of dense chromatin connected by one or more thin filaments	0	Abundant, pinkish, contains specific granules	1:3	Presence of one or more thin filaments identifies cell as segmented granulocyte; neutrophilic granules very fine; eosinophilic and basophilic granules large and round, obscuring the nucleus
8. Lymphoblast	10-18	Round or oval; definite nuclear membrane; chromatin in thin strands or stippled, light red-purple	1-2	Homogeneous and moderately basophilic, often shows lighter perinuclear zone	7:1-5:1	Not easily distinguished from other blast cells; lighter perinuclear zone may be helpful; also relatively few nucleoli
9. Prolymphocyte	10-18	Oval or slightly indented; chromatin varies from fine to slightly coarse; parachromatin indistinct	1	Sparse, moderately basophilic, homogeneous	5:1	At times difficult to distinguish prolymphocytes from lymphoblasts, particularly in lymphocytic leukemia; may contain a very few azurophilic granules

Continued.

Table 4-2. Summary of characteristics of blood and bone marrow cells (Wright's stain)—cont'd

Cell	Size (μ)	Nucleus	Nucleoi	Cytoplasm	N/C ratio	Comments
10. Lymphocyte	6-18	Round or oval, slightly or deeply indented; chromatin in coarse clumps; indistinct sparse parachromatin	0	Sky blue or medium blue, clear and glassy	5:1-2:1	Vary in size, chiefly because of variation in amount of cytoplasm; may contain number of large azurophilic granules; sky blue, clear cytoplasm characteristic
11. Monoblast	14-18	Round or oval; thin membrane; chromatin fine and delicate; parachromatin abundant	1-2	Basophilic, homogeneous, nongranulated	6:1	Differentiated with difficulty from other blast cells; is said to have more basophilic cytoplasm than myeloblast and less basophilic cytoplasm than lymphoblast; actually all gradations seen in monocytic leukemias
12. Promonocyte	14-18	Moderately indented; thin membrane; chromatin in coarse clumps; indistinct sparse parachromatin	0-1	Moderately abundant, gray-blue and opaque, few extremely fine pink granules	5:1	Characterized by presence of very fine pink granules, "azurophilic dust"; however, demonstration of such granules requires most critical staining technic
13. Monocyte	12-18	Indented or folded, delicate, pale staining; fine chromatin with much parachromatin	0	Gray or gray-blue, opaque, very fine pink granules	4:1	Adult monocyte easily identified in thin well-stained smear, but in thick or overstained smears characteristics lost; one helpful feature is that monocytic nucleus stains much lighter than similar cells
14. Pronormoblast	14-19	Round or very slightly oval, central or slightly eccentric; fine reticular chromatin; sparse indistinct parachromatin	1-2, very faint	Scanty, deeply basophilic, homogeneous, opaque	8:1	Superficially similar to other blast cells, but characterically has rounder, more centrally placed nucleus
15. Basophilic normoblast	10-15	Round, slightly eccentric; chromatin coarse and dark staining; parachromatin sparse but distinct	0-1	More abundant, intensely to moderately basophilic, opaque, royal blue	6:1	Distinguished from pronormoblast by coarse chromatin of nucleus, from lymphocytes by opaque basophilic cytoplasm; cytoplasmic basophilia characteristically vivid royal blue
16. Polychromatophilic normoblast	8-12	Round, eccentric; chromatin coarse and dark staining; parachromatin distinct	0	More abundant, pink to orange hemoglobin localized in patches or diffused throughout orange-tinged cytoplasm	4:1	Distinguished from earlier cell of erythrocytic series by appearance of hemoglobin, from lymphocytes by distinct parachromatin and opaqueness of cytoplasm
17. Orthochromic normoblast	7-10	Small and shrunken, dense; may be round or bizarre; no parachromatin visible	0	Orange-red as in adult cell	1:2	Gradations between polychromatophilic normoblasts and orthochromic normoblasts commonly seen
18. Promegaloblast	19-27	Round or slightly oval; chromatin in strands or fine punctate masses; abundant pink or blue parachromatin, sharply demarcated	1-2, pale and indistinct	Relatively abundant, lightly basophilic, may be mottled	6:1	Distinguished from normoblastic cells by typical nuclear structure; is usually larger than pronormoblast; cytoplasm in larger cells relatively more abundant

	Size (μm)	Nucleus	Nucleoli	Cytoplasm	N:C ratio	Remarks
19. Basophilic megaloblast	15-22	Round; chromatin and parachromatin as in promegaloblast	0	Relatively abundant, more basophilic than promegaloblast, royal blue or deep purple	4:1	Nuclear structure characteristic; generally larger than corresponding normoblast
20. Polychromatophilic megaloblast	10-18	Round; chromatin coarser but parachromatin still sharp and abundant	0	Varying amounts of orange hemoglobin in basophilic cytoplasm	2:1	Characteristically sharp and abundant parachromatin remains even with moderate coarseness of chromatin; generally larger than corresponding normoblast
21. Orthochromic megaloblast	8-15	May or may not show parachromatin	0	Pink to orange, moderately abundant	1:1	May or may not have typical megaloblastic nuclear pattern; tends to be larger than corresponding normoblast, with more abundant cytoplasm
22. Megakaryoblast	25-35	Oval, indented, sometimes indistinctly bisected; chromatin fine and delicate; parachromatin sparse and pink	2-6	Very scanty, irregularly basophilic	10:1	Usually so much larger than other blast cells that it is easily identified; when small, identification may be difficult
23. Promegakaryocyte	25-50	Irregular and polylobulated, quite large; darker staining than younger cell	0-2	Moderately to faintly basophilic, few to many fine azurophilic granules near nucleus	6:1	Nucleus usually more irregular than megakaryoblast, larger and more delicate than megakaryocyte
24. Megakaryocyte	40-100	Multilobular and bizarre; chromatin irregularly clumped	0-many	Abundant, pale, with granular pink aggregates	1:1-1:2	Cell appearance so varied that typical cell is not easily described; may seem to be multinucleated, but must be distinguished from osteoclasts, which are truly multinucleated and in which each nucleus contains a sharply defined nucleolus
25. Plasmablast	15-25	Round or oval, eccentric; chromatin reticulated; parachromatin distinct	2-4	Moderately to deeply basophilic; granules absent	1:1-2:1	Cell has same nuclear structure as reticulum cell except for less parachromatin and somewhat coarser chromatin strands
26. Proplasmacyte	15-25	Oval or round, eccentric; chromatin moderately coarse	1-2	Azure blue, with lighter perinuclear zone	1:1-2:1	Characteristic brilliant basophilia of plasmacyte appears in this precursor and is usually typical; may resemble basophilic normoblast (and vice versa) but in normoblast blue is darker
27. Plasmacyte	10-20	Round or oval, eccentric; very coarse clumped chromatin; sharp but sparse parachromatin	0	Azure blue, with lighter perinuclear zone	1:2	Nucleus quite eccentrically located; color of cytoplasm typical

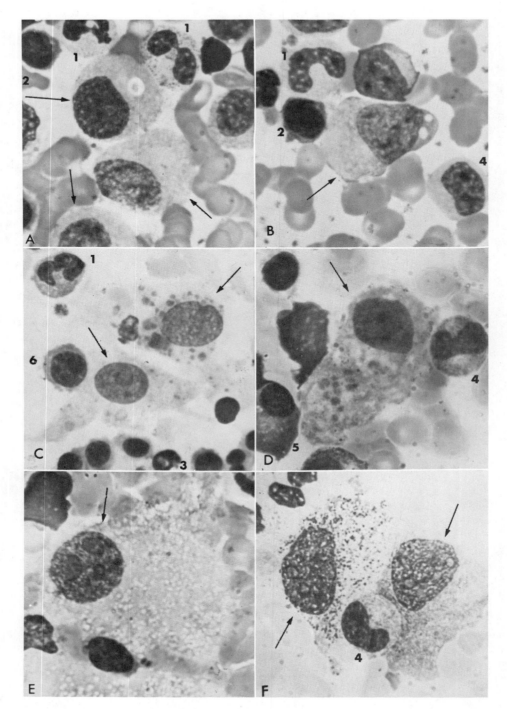

Fig. 4-2. Reticulum cell (arrows). **A,** Bone marrow, brucellosis. One of the reticulum cells contains a vacuole. **B,** Bone marrow, infection. **C** and **D,** Bone marrow, chronic hemolytic anemia. Reticulum cells contain iron and other particulate matter. **E,** Bone marrow, atypical reticulum cell in Hodgkin's disease. **F,** Normal bone marrow. Reticulum cells of Ferrata type. Other cells in fields: **1,** stab neutrophil; **2,** lymphocyte; **3,** group of orthochromic normoblasts; **4,** neutrophilic metamyelocyte; **5,** plasma cell; **6,** polychromatophilic normoblast. (Wright's stain; ×950.)

Size: 15 to 25 μ; usually irregular in outline.

Nucleus: Usually oval; delicate nuclear membrane. Nuclear chromatin forms an irregular network of light violet strands and small irregular clumps. The parachromatin is light blue or pink and sharply demarcated from the chromatin. Nodular thickenings are common where chromatin strands cross.

Nucleoli: 1-3; irregular in shape, somewhat hazy in outline, and usually light blue.

Cytoplasm: Abundant; nucleus-to-cytoplasm ratio 1:1 or less; pale blue and mottled. It usually is not granular but may contain a few large azurophilic granules or a large number of red granules or strands (Ferrata reticulum cell). The cytoplasm of the phagocytic reticulum cell contains cellular debris, iron granules, and sometimes parasites.

Myeloblast (Fig. 4-3)

Size: 10 to 20 μ; round.

Nucleus: Round or oval; thin nuclear membrane. The chromatin is abundant, stippled, finely reticulated, and light purple. The parachromatin is sparse, pale blue or pink, and sharply demarcated.

Nucleoli: 2 to 5; rather well outlined; round or oval; pale blue. The chromatin tends to be clearer next to the nucleoli.

Cytoplasm: Sparse to moderately abundant; nucleus-to-cytoplasm ratio 5:1 to 7:1; variously basophilic and usually not lighter in the perinuclear zone. It contains no granules, but the phagocytic cell contains cellular debris, iron, and sometimes parasites.

Progranulocyte (Fig. 4-4)

The chief identifying feature of this cell is that it contains a few azurophilic granules. Some differences in terminology exist. Sabin classified all immature cells with granules as myelocytes, calling those cells with fewer than 10 granules myelocytes A, those with a moderate number of granules myelocytes B, and those with a maximum number of granules myelocytes C. I prefer to call cells with a few granules progranulocytes and cells with either a moderate or a maximum number of granules myelocytes. Note that progranulocytes are sometimes slightly larger than myeloblasts or myelocytes.

The cytoplasm of granulocytes contains two types of granules. The large, coarse azurophilic *nonspecific* granules appear first in the progranulocytes and are very numerous in the myelocytes. *Specific* granules (neutrophilic, eosinophilic, or basophilic) appear first in late myelocytes and characterize the later metamyelocytes, bands, and segmented forms. On Wright-stained smears the numerous nonspecific granules in myelocytes disappear as the specific granules develop, and this was once thought to represent either a loss of nonspecific granules or a conversion of nonspecific to specific granules as the cells matured. However, electron microscopy combined with cytochemical reactions shows that (1) nonspecific granules are peroxidase positive, (2) nonspecific granules having peroxidase activity persist even in the most mature granulocytes, and (3) specific granules are peroxidase negative and alkaline phosphatase positive

(Bainton et al, 1971; Spitznagel et al, 1974; Bainton, 1975a), although West et al (1974) find that alkaline phosphatase activity is not granule-related. Since electron microscopy proves the persistence of nonspecific granules, the failure to see them in mature cells stained with Romanowsky-type stains must be a result of altered staining characteristics. The nonspecific granules are classified as primary lysosomes (Chapter 2), whereas the specific are thought to be nonlysosomal.

Size: 14 to 20 μ; round or oval.

Nucleus: Large, round, or oval; thin nuclear membrane. The chromatin is in the form of a network, slightly coarse and with some slight clumping, especially near the nucleoli.

Nucleoli: 1 to 3; less prominent than in the myeloblast; pale blue; round or oval.

Cytoplasm: Sparse; nucleus-to-cytoplasm ratio about 5:1; basophilic but lighter than myeloblast. It contains a few purplish granules that may be either large and round or fine and irregular.

Myelocyte (Fig. 4-5)

No distinction is made between the early and the late myelocyte.

Size: 10 to 18 μ; round or oval.

Nucleus: Indistinct; thin nuclear membrane, particularly if the cell is heavily granulated. The chromatin network is coarse with irregular patches of blue- or pink-staining parachromatin.

Nucleoli: Usually absent or invisible; rarely more than one.

Cytoplasm: Moderate in amount; nucleus-to-cytoplasm ratio about 2:1. The granules are large and in the early stage of development are azure (purplish blue). As the cell differentiates, the nonspecific granules decrease, while more and more specific granules appear. Thus myelocytes in the bone marrow normally tend to show varying proportions of granules of each type. In more mature cells the specific granules appear as definitely *eosinophilic* (brick red), *basophilic* (deep blue), or *neutrophilic* (lilac). When present in large numbers, the cytoplasmic granules usually obscure the nuclear outline.

Metamyelocyte and juvenile (Fig. 4-6)

In common usage most hematologists consider the terms "metamyelocyte" and "juvenile" synonymous. However, the two are not so considered in Europe, where they are classified as one or the other depending on the degree of nuclear maturity. Accordingly, the juvenile is considered the more mature by a few hours. The distinction has been emphasized by the different pattern noted when these cells are labeled with tritiated thymidine. Nevertheless, there seems to be no practical value in distinguishing between the metamyelocyte and the juvenile, and we will continue to use the two terms synonymously.

At this stage the nucleus first shows a definite alteration from a round to a kidney shape. Nuclear condensation coarsens the chromatin, and the nucleolus is not visible. As in the myelocyte, different types of granules will be found in the

Text continued on p. 131.

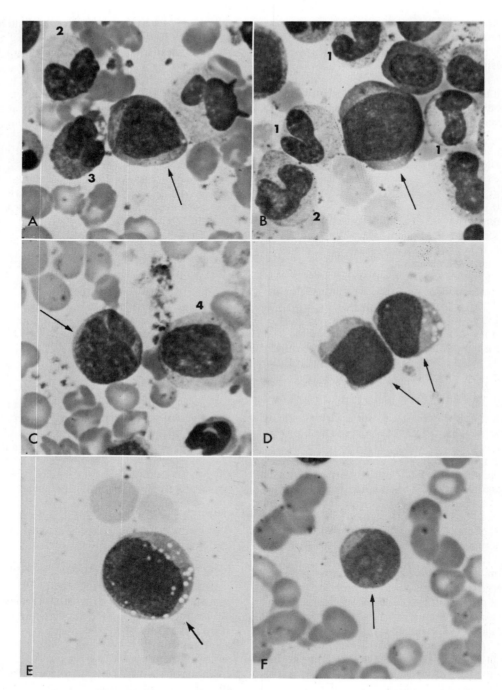

Fig. 4-3. Myeloblast (arrows). **A,** Normal bone marrow. **B,** Bone marrow, chronic myelocytic leukemia. **C,** Bone marrow, acute myelocytic leukemia. **D** and **E,** Peripheral blood, acute myelocytic leukemia. **F,** Micromyeloblast, peripheral blood, acute myelocytic leukemia. Other cells in fields: **1,** stab neutrophil; **2,** neutrophilic metamyelocyte; **3,** eosinophil; **4,** progranulocyte. (Wright's stain; ×950.)

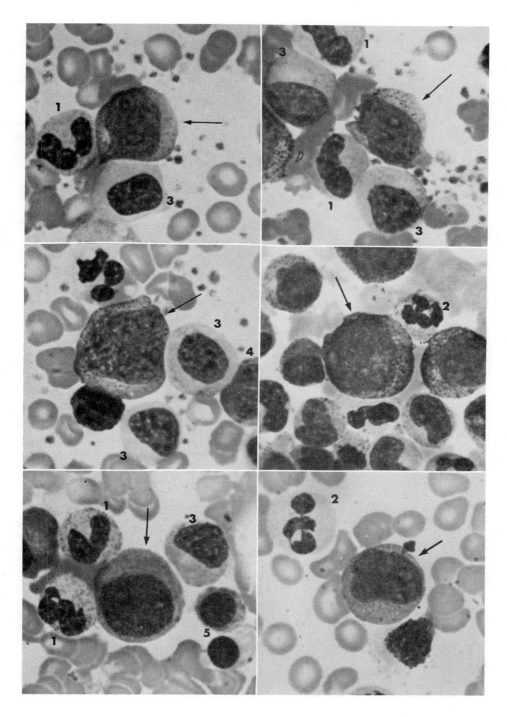

Fig. 4-4. Progranulocyte (arrows). Bone marrow, chronic myelocytic leukemia. Other cells in fields: **1,** band neutrophil; **2,** segmented neutrophil; **3,** neutrophilic metamyelocytes; **4,** eosinophil; **5,** polychromatophilic normoblast. (Wright's stain; ×950.)

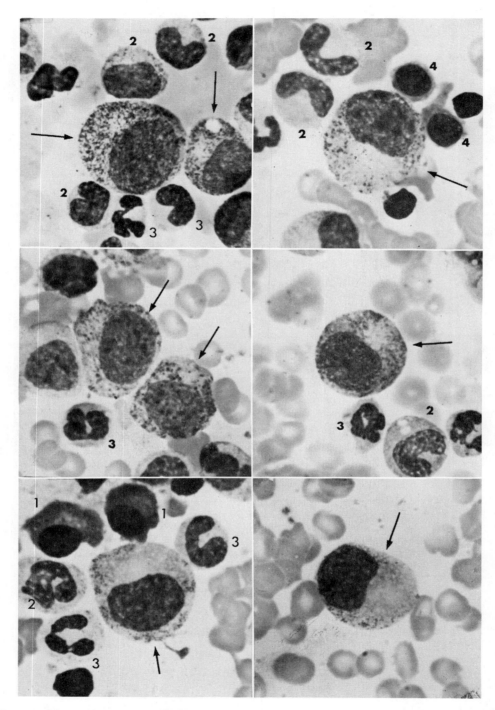

Fig. 4-5. Myelocyte (arrows). Bone marrow, arranged roughly in order of maturity, from the least mature, **A,** to the most mature, **F.** Other cells in fields: **1,** plasma cells; **2,** metamyelocytes; **3,** band neutrophils; **4,** polychromatophilic normoblasts. (Wright's stain; ×950.)

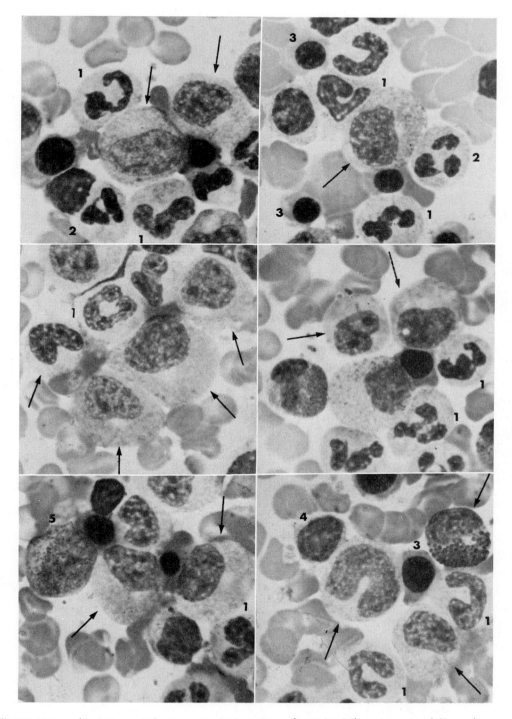

Fig. 4-6. Metamyelocyte (arrows). Bone marrow, various stages of maturity. **F** shows an eosinophilic myelocyte. Other cells in fields: **1,** stab neutrophils; **2,** segmented neutrophil; **3,** orthochromic normoblast; **4,** lymphocyte; **5,** myelocyte. (Wright's stain; ×950.)

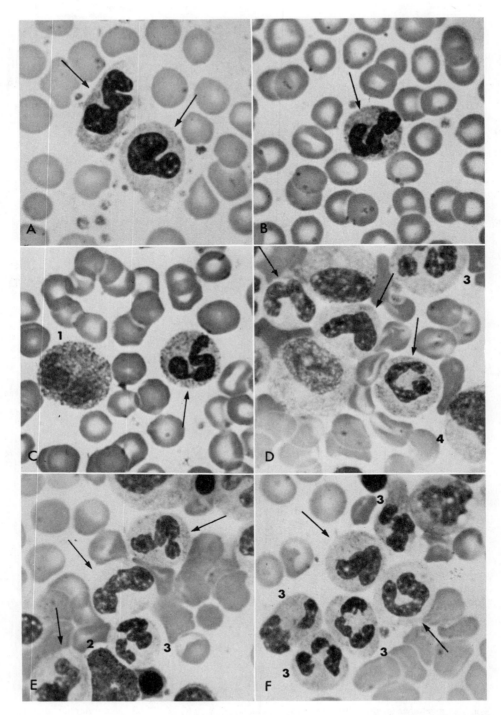

Fig. 4-7. Band granulocyte (arrows). **A** and **B,** Peripheral blood. **C-F,** Bone marrow. Other cells in fields: **1,** segmented eosinophil; **2,** band eosinophil; **3,** segmented neutrophil; **4,** metamyelocyte. (Wright's stain; ×950.)

neutrophilic metamyelocyte, the *eosinophilic* metamyelocyte, and the *basophilic* metamyelocyte.

Size: 10 to 18 μ.

Nucleus: Kidney shaped; nuclear membrane heavy. The chromatin is coarse or in thick strands, staining deep purple, and much darker than in younger cells. The parachromatin is scanty but distinct. The nucleolus is not usually visible.

Cytoplasm: Fairly abundant; nucleus-to-cytoplasm ratio about 1.5:1. The cytoplasm is pink. The specific granules are either eosinophilic, basophilic, or neutrophilic and are smaller than in the myelocyte and less uniform in size.

Band granulocyte (Fig. 4-7)

Here the nucleus undergoes further condensation, forming a sausage-shaped band or stab form (*stabkernige*). The shape of the nucleus in eosinophils and basophils becomes increasingly difficult to see because of the large obscuring granules.

Size: 10 to 15 μ.

Nucleus: Sausage or band shaped. It may be constricted at one or more points, but a significant amount of chromatin is seen in the constriction. The chromatin is coarse and deep purple-blue. The parachromatin is scanty; the nucleolus is not visible.

Cytoplasm: Abundant; pale blue or pink; nucleus-to-cytoplasm ratio about 1:2. It contains fine lilac granules (neutrophil), large blue-black granules (basophil), or brick red granules (eosinophil) that have the appearance of small hollow spheres.

Segmented granulocyte (Figs. 4-8 and 4-9)

Adult granulocytes are characterized by segmentation of the nucleus into lobes connected by fine filaments of nuclear membrane within which no chromatin can be seen. The dividing line between band and filament form is not always clear. In some laboratories, if a nucleus appears to be lobulated but is without a visible filament, the cell is classified as a segmented cell on the assumption that a filament must be present. I think, however, that such an assumption cannot be made and that cells should be classified as segmented forms *only when a filament is visible* (Plate 8).

In 1904 Arneth concluded that the older the nucleus, the greater the degree of segmentation and number of segments. He proposed a classification of neutrophilic granulocytes based on the shape of the nucleus and the number of lobes. This, with subclassifications, resulted in a rather complex system that is now thought to have little practical value. However, two concepts have persisted: (1) that maturation of the nucleus is characterized by increasing lobulation and (2) his concept of the shift to the left. Since his method of tabulation placed young cells in the left-hand columns, an increase in the number of immature cells gave greater weight to the left side. Hence any condition that caused an increase in young forms produced a shift to the left in the differential count.

In 1911 Schilling proposed that granulocytes be classified into four types: (1) myelocytes, (2) juveniles (metamyelocytes), (3) *stabkernige* cells (band forms), and (4) seg-

mented neutrophils. He did not further subdivide the segmented cells. According to Schilling, two types of shift to the left occur. One is a regenerative shift, indicating the increased liberation of young cells in response to marrow stimulation. The other is a degenerative shift in which a depression of bone marrow function interferes with normal maturation and results in the liberation of immature cells.

Other systems such as those proposed by Cooke and Ponder (five classes corresponding to the number of lobes in the nucleus) or by Haden (filamented and nonfilamented forms) have joined the original Arneth and Schilling classifications in the limbo of medical history. None of those systems offers anything more than the standard differential count now in common use, which is a simplification of the original schemes.

Size: 10 to 15 μ.

Nucleus: Chromatin coarse and dense; staining deep purple-blue, with scant parachromatin. Two or more lobes of nuclear chromatin are connected by thin filaments.

Cytoplasm: Abundant; nucleus-to-cytoplasm ratio about 1:3; light pink or blue. Specific granules are fine and pink or lilac (neutrophilic), large and brick red (eosinophilic), or large and blue-black (basophilic) (Plate 9).

Lymphoblast (Fig. 4-10)

This cell is either absent in normal bone marrow or present in extremely small numbers. The features described are those observed in cases of lymphocytic leukemia. The origin of lymphocytes is the lymphoid tissue of the body and the marrow to a significant degree.

Size: 10 to 18 μ.

Nucleus: Fairly centrally located; definite nuclear membrane. The chromatin is in thin strands or stippled light red-purple. The parachromatin is moderately abundant, sharply demarcated, and light blue. The nucleus is generally round or oval, with no indentation.

Nucleoli: 1 to 2; small; pale blue.

Cytoplasm: Homogeneous and moderately to heavily basophilic; sparse, with nucleus-to-cytoplasm ratio 5:1 to 7:1. Often, but not always, it shows a lighter perinuclear zone. There are no granules.

Prolymphocyte (Fig. 4-11)

Whereas the lymphoblast and the adult lymphocyte vary but little from their fellows, the prolymphocyte includes cells that morphologically are judged to be too old to be lymphoblasts and cells that are almost, but not quite, adult. Thus this classification includes a large spectrum of intermediates.

Size: 10 to 18 μ; average smaller than lymphoblast.

Nucleus: Round or oval; may be slightly indented. The chromatin is more clumped than in the lymphoblast but is still relatively fine and dark red-purple. The parachromatin is generally not as well defined as in the lymphoblast or as smudged as in the adult lymphocyte.

Nucleoli: Usually one; round, blue, and sharply outlined.

Text continued on p. 137.

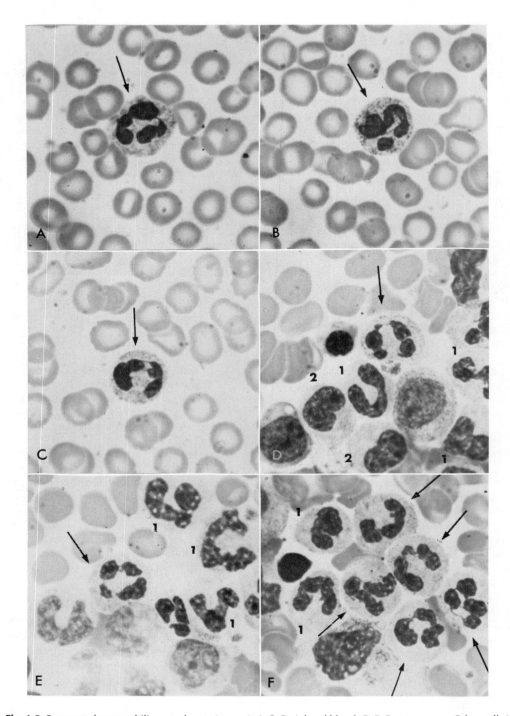

Fig. 4-8. Segmented neutrophilic granulocyte (arrows). **A-C,** Peripheral blood. **D-F,** Bone marrow. Other cells in fields: **1,** stab neutrophil; **2,** neutrophilic metamyelocyte. (Wright's stain; ×950.)

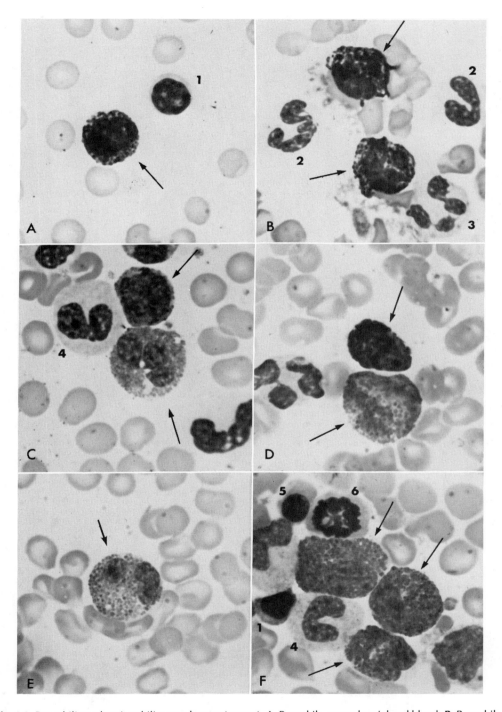

Fig. 4-9. Basophilic and eosinophilic granulocytes (arrows). **A,** Basophils, normal peripheral blood. **B,** Basophils, peripheral blood, chronic myelocytic leukemia. **C** and **D,** Basophil (above) and eosinophil (below), peripheral blood, chronic myelocytic leukemia. **E,** Eosinophil, normal bone marrow. **F,** Eosinophilic myelocyte and meta-myelocyte, bone marrow, eosinophilic leukemia. Other cells in fields: **1,** lymphocyte; **2,** stab neutrophil; **3,** segmented neutrophil; **4,** neutrophilic metamyelocyte; **5,** orthochromic normoblast; **6,** cell in mitosis. (Wright's stain; ×950.)

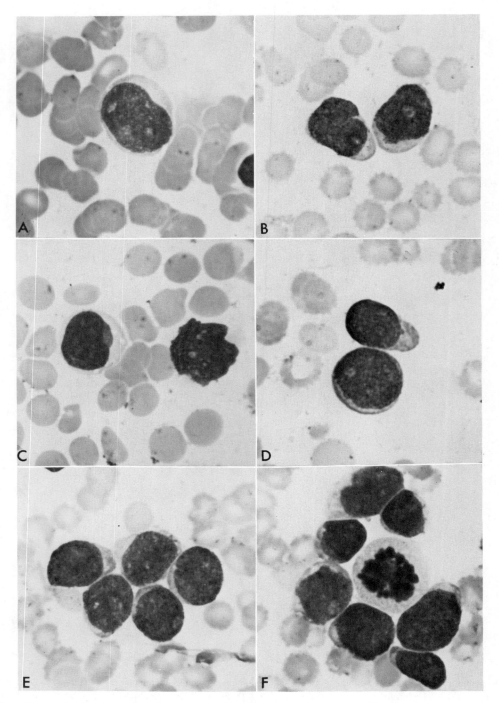

Fig. 4-10. Lymphoblast. Acute lymphocytic leukemia. **A-D,** Peripheral blood. **E** and **F,** Bone marow. All the cells are lymphoblasts except for a smudge form in **C** and a cell in mitosis in **F.** (Wright's stain; ×950.)

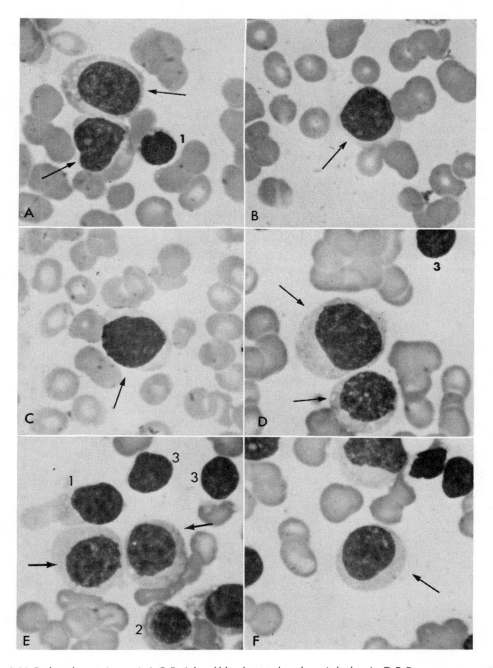

Fig. 4-11. Prolymphocyte (arrows). **A-C,** Peripheral blood, acute lymphocytic leukemia. **D-F,** Bone marrow, acute lymphocytic leukemia. Other cells in fields: **1,** mature lymphocyte; **2,** polychromatophilic normoblast; **3,** naked lymphocytic nuclei. (Wright's stain; ×950.)

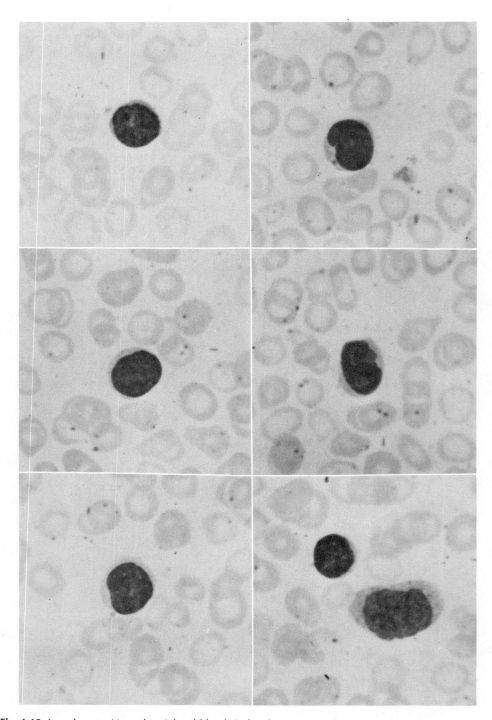

Fig. 4-12. Lymphocyte. Normal peripheral blood. **F** also shows a normal monocyte. (Wright's stain; ×950.)

Cytoplasm: Tends to be more abundant than in the lymphoblast; nucleus-to-cytoplasm ratio closer to 5:1; light blue to medium dark blue. Occasionally it has azurophilic granules.

Lymphocyte (Fig. 4-12)

The presence of small, medium, and large lymphocytes in the blood of the adult and the predominance of medium and large lymphocytes in the blood of infants are common observations. Whether or not this implies that the large cell is younger than the small is a moot point (Chapter 1). The size can be so easily changed by the thickness of the smear (Fig. 4-13) that the classification of lymphocytes into large, medium, and small is technically untrustworthy and of doubtful significance.

Size: Small, 6 to 8 μ; medium, 8 to 14 μ; large, 8 to 18 μ.

Nucleus: Round or oval; may be slightly or deeply indented; usually somewhat eccentric. The nuclear membrane is heavy. The chromatin is in the form of large coarse clumps blending into sparse pale blue to pink parachromatin, so that the differentiation between chromatin and parachromatin is not sharp, i.e., the parachromatin is usually described as "smudged."

Nucleoli: One may occasionally be seen in the larger cells; generally none. Nucleoli can be demonstrated by special staining (Ridway and Garrett, 1974).

Cytoplasm: Typically sky blue, but may be medium blue; clear and homogeneous. There are occasional azuro-

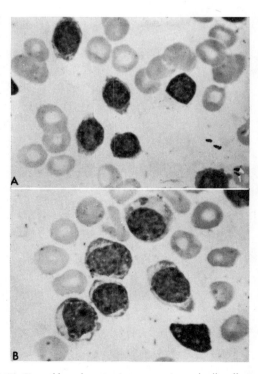

Fig. 4-13. Size of lymphocytes in a smear is markedly affected by the thinness of the smear. These cells are the same but have been photographed from thick, **A,** and thin, **B,** portions of the same peripheral blood smear (chronic lymphocytic leukemia). (Wright's stain; ×750.)

philic granules. The large and medium lymphocytes occasionally contain a moderate number of azurophilic granules. These are normal cells, and the significance of the azurophilic granules is not known.

Monoblast (Fig. 4-14)

The monocytic cell was originally described by Ehrlich as a transitional cell between the lymphocyte and the granulocyte. This concept has been generally abandoned. The origin of the monocyte is described differently by different authors. According to modern thinking, monocyte cells, whether purely histiocytic or myelomonocytic, are derived from CFU-G,M.

Size: 14 to 18 μ.

Nucleus: Round or oval; thin nuclear membrane. The chromatin structure is similar to the reticulum cell or myeloblast, but appears to stain lighter. The parachromatin is abundant, sharply demarcated, and pale pink or blue.

Nucleoli: 1 to 2.

Cytoplasm: Moderate; basophilic; no granulation in the blast stage. The presence of fine lilac granules indicates maturation to the promonocyte or monocyte stage.

Promonocyte (Fig. 4-15)

Size: 14 to 18 μ.

Nucleus: Moderately indented; thin nuclear membrane. The chromatin is fine and threadlike, giving the nucleus a pale appearance by comparison with other cells. The parachromatin is abundant.

Nucleoli: 0 to 1.

Cytoplasm: Gray-blue; opaque, with very fine lilac granules, smaller than in any of the other cells, sometimes referred to as azurophilic dust.

Monocyte (Fig. 4-16)

This cell is easily identified in a well-prepared and well-stained smear, but if it is badly stained, the typical features are lost and the characteristic very fine lilac granules are not seen. Overstaining often produces large scattered purplish granulation, which leads to mistaking this cell for a metamyelocyte. It should be remembered that the nucleus in the monocyte is definitely lighter staining than in other cells. This is a very helpful criterion.

Size: 12 to 18 μ.

Nucleus: Indented or folded over; delicate; pale staining. The chromatin is in fine strands; the parachromatin is abundant and distinct.

Nucleoli: Usually none; occasionally one.

Cytoplasm: Light gray or gray-blue; opaque; characteristic numerous, fine, dustlike lilac granules.

Pronormoblast (Fig. 4-17)

This, the most immature cell in the normoblast series, is not far removed from the BFU-E (Fig. 1-5, p. 6). Its nucleus is very similar to that of the reticulum cell, with its delicate chromatin and somewhat indistinct blue nucleoli. As the primitive mesenchymal cell differentiates into the normoblastic series, its cytoplasm becomes more abundant

Text continued on p. 142.

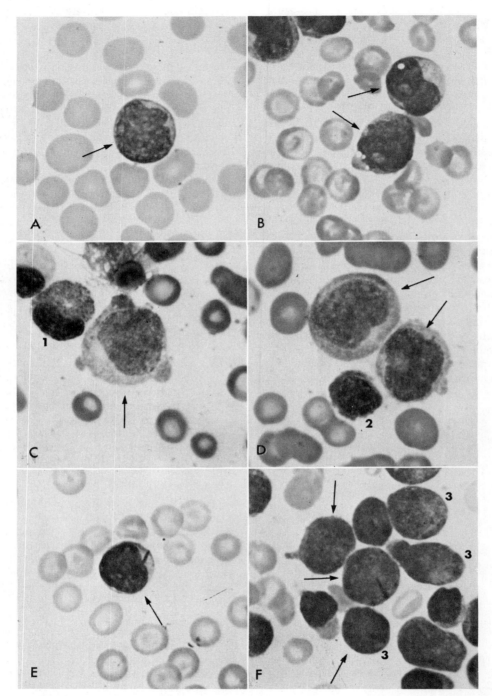

Fig. 4-14. Monoblast (arrows). **A** and **B,** Peripheral blood, acute leukemia, myelomonocytic. **C** and **D,** Bone marrow, acute monocytic (histiocytic, Schilling-type) leukemia. **E** and **F,** Peripheral blood and bone marrow, acute leukemia, myelomonocytic. Note the Auer bodies in **E** and **F.** It is not always possible to judge a cell as being a monoblast on the basis of the morphology of that one cell alone. The cells illustrated here are blast cells found in patients diagnosed as having acute leukemia, myelomonocytic or histiocytic. Note that the morphology is quite variable. Other cells in fields: **1,** eosinophil; **2,** normoblast (? polychromatophilic); **3,** promonocytes in myelomonocytic leukemia. (Wright's stain; ×950.)

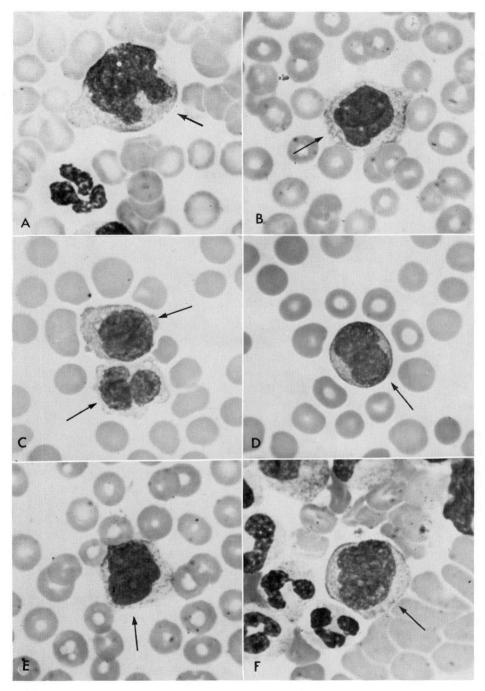

Fig. 4-15. Promonocyte (arrows). **A-E,** Peripheral blood, monocytic leukemia. **F,** Normal bone marrow. (Wright's stain; ×950.)

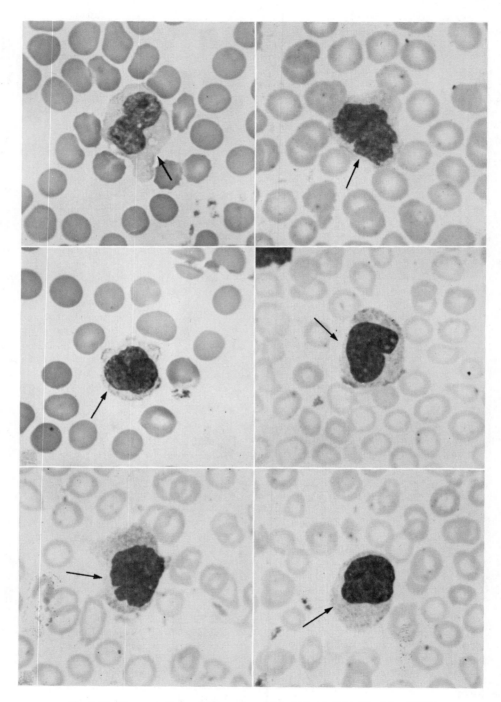

Fig. 4-16. Monocyte (arrows). Normal peripheral blood. (Wright's stain; ×950.)

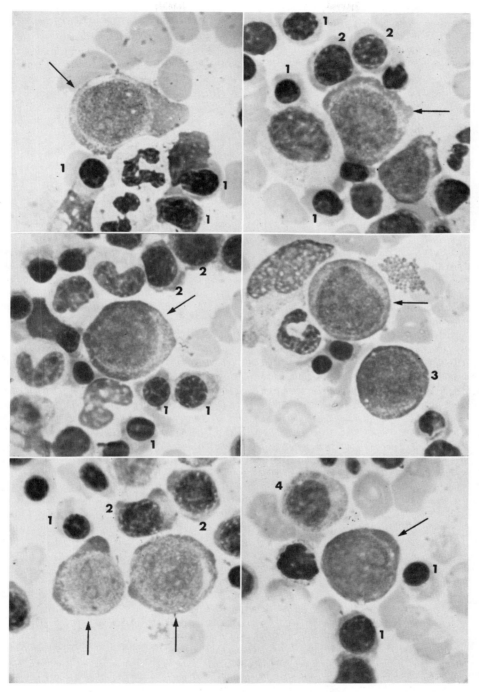

Fig. 4-17. Pronormoblast (arrows). Bone marrow, erythroid hyperplasia. Other cells in fields: **1,** orthochromic normoblast; **2,** polychromatophilic normoblast; **3,** basophilic normoblast; **4,** metamyelocyte. (Wright's stain; ×950.)

and more basophilic. These are probably the two characteristics of the pronormoblast as compared to the primitive mesenchymal cell. Also, a more abundant cytoplasm distinguishes the pronormoblast (and the basophilic normoblast to follow) from the myeloblast and other blast cells.

In the transition from pronormoblast to basophilic normoblast, the cytoplasmic basophilia becomes intense, the nuclear chromatin coarsens, and the nucleoli are lost or become invisible.

Size: 14 to 19 μ.

Nucleus: Round or slightly oval; thin nuclear membrane; may be central or slightly eccentric. The chromatin varies from finely reticular, as in the myeloblast, to coarsely reticular with a tendency to clumping. The parachromatin is indistinct and scant.

Nucleoli: 1 to 2; usually very faint and pale blue.

Cytoplasm: Small in amount; nucleus-to-cytoplasm ratio usually greater than in myeloblast but smaller than in the promegaloblast; moderately basophilic, homogeneous, and opaque.

Basophilic normoblast (Fig. 4-18)

This cell is similar to the pronormoblast but obviously more adult, since nucleoli are generally absent and the nuclear chromatin is coarser. The degree of basophilia varies from intense to moderate and is greater than in the pronormoblast.

Basophilic normoblast can usually be distinguished from other blast cells because (1) the nucleus is generally rounder, (2) the cytoplasm is more abundant and is clearly visible all around the somewhat eccentrically placed nucleus, (3) the nuclear chromatin is coarse and thus the nucleus stains darker and is more bluish, and (4) the nucleoli are generally not visible.

Size: 10 to 15 μ.

Nucleus: Smaller than in the pronormoblast; generally round and slightly eccentric; nuclear membrane thin. The chromatin is coarse and irregular, so that the nucleus stains dark. The parachromatin is sparse but distinct.

Nucleoli: 0 to 1.

Cytoplasm: Appears more abundant than in the pronormoblast because of the smaller nucleus. It varies from intense to moderately basophilic and is royal blue and opaque.

Polychromatophilic normoblast (Fig. 4-19)

This cell is characterized by the first appearance of visible hemoglobin, usually perinuclear, so that the cytoplasm stains pink to basophilic, either irregularly if the hemoglobin is localized or diffusely blue-orange where the hemoglobin is distributed throughout the cytoplasm.

Size: 8 to 12 μ.

Nucleus: Round and smaller than in precursors; usually eccentric; thick nuclear membrane. The chromatin is very coarse and clumped, so that the nucleus stains very dark. The parachromatin is distinct in contrast to the lymphocyte, with which it may be confused if the hemoglobin content is not recognized.

Nucleoli: None.

Cytoplasm: Relatively more abundant than in precursors; varies from basophilic, with perinuclear areas of pink-staining or orange/staining hemoglobin, to diffusely lilac (polychrome).

Orthochromic normoblast (Fig. 4-20)

This classification applies to the fully hemoglobinated form of the normoblast. When found in the peripheral blood (hemolytic disease, etc.), the cytoplasm is truly orthochromic, i.e., the normal color of the adult nonnucleated erythrocyte. There is usually no trace of basophilia. In bone marrow smears, however, it is unusual to find orthochromic normoblasts with a pure orange cytoplasm, most showing various degrees of basophilia.

This cell is not capable of undergoing mitosis, and the bizarre shape sometimes seen in the nucleus is pyknosis preceding extrusion of the nucleus to form the adult nonnucleated erythrocyte.

Size: 7 to 10 μ.

Nucleus: Small and shrunken; dense and dark staining because of marked condensation of chromatin. Little structure is recognizable, with the parachromatin no longer distinguishable. It may be round, oval, or have various bizarre forms and is usually eccentric.

Nucleoli: None.

Cytoplasm: Orange-red, as in adult erythrocyte.

Promegaloblast (Fig. 4-21)

Size: 19 to 27 μ.

Nucleus: Round or oval; slightly eccentric; thin nuclear membrane. The chromatin is fine and delicate, as thin chromatin strands or fine punctate masses sharply demarcated from abundant pink parachromatin. The general effect is that of a lighter staining, stippled nucleus, more finely reticulated than in the pronormoblast. Occasionally nuclear parachromatin is so abundant that it suggests the structure of the reticulum cell nucleus.

Nucleoli: 1 or 2; pale, large, irregular, and indistinct.

Cytoplasm: Abundant, in absolute amount as well as relative to nuclear size, with much lower nucleus-to-cytoplasm ratio than in pronormoblast. It is lightly basophilic and mottled, with irregular patches of colorless hyaloplasm. According to Kass (1974a), the cytoplasm of early megaloblasts in pernicious anemia, but not in folate deficiency, stains pink with alizarin red S. Normoblasts do not stain pink.

Basophilic megaloblast (Fig. 4-22)

This cell corresponds to the basophilic normoblast stage but shows the special nuclear features of the megaloblast nucleus as well as being larger than the basophilic normoblast.

Size: 15 to 22 μ.

Nucleus: Round or oval and usually eccentric; thin nuclear membrane. The chromatin, as in the promegaloblast, is occasionally slightly coarse but definitely finer than in the basophilic normoblast. The parachromatin is abundant and sharply demarcated.

Nucleoli: Usually none, or one is seen with difficulty.

Text continued on p. 148.

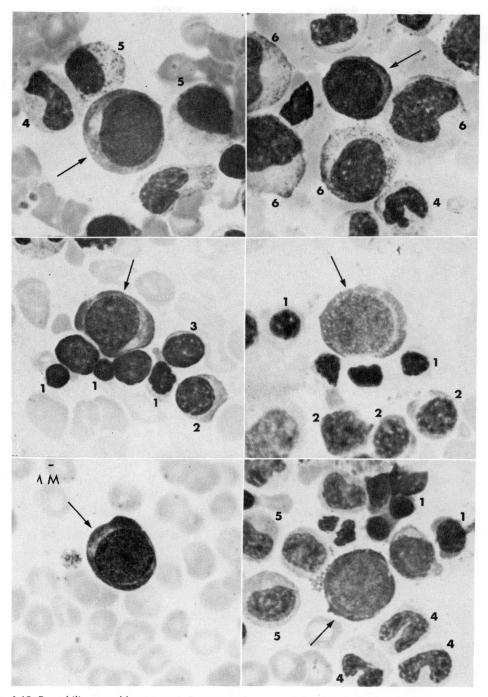

Fig. 4-18. Basophilic normoblast (arrows). Bone marrow smears. Other cells in fields: **1,** orthochromic normoblast; **2,** polychromatophilic normoblast; **3,** lymphocyte; **4,** band neutrophil; **5,** neutrophilic metamyelocyte; **6,** myelocyte. (Wright's stain; ×950.)

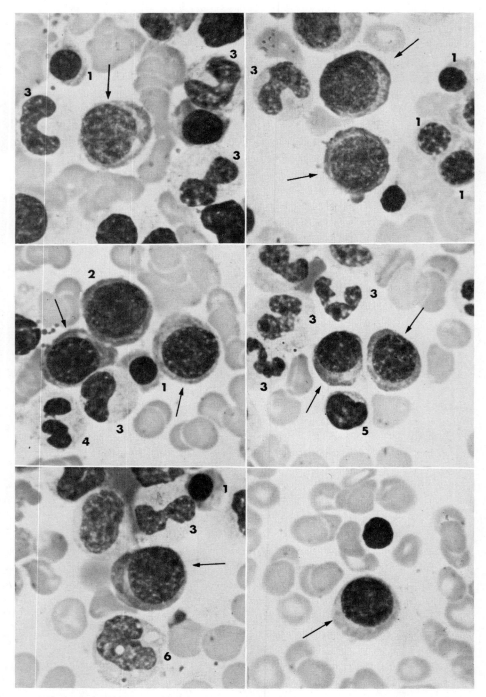

Fig. 4-19. Polychromatophilic normoblast (arrows). Bone marrow. Other cells in fields: **1,** orthochromic normoblast; **2,** basophilic normoblast; **3,** stab neutrophil; **4,** segmented neutrophil; **5,** lymphocyte; **6,** monocyte. (Wright's stain; ×950.)

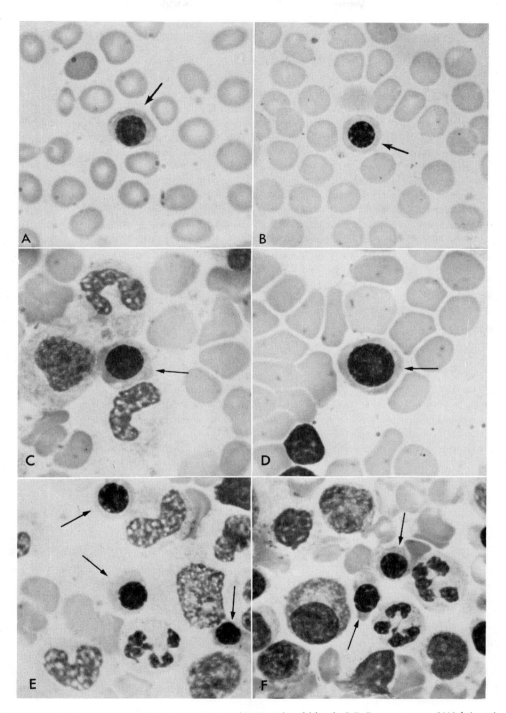

Fig. 4-20. Orthochromic normoblast (arrows). **A** and **B,** Peripheral blood. **C-F,** Bone marrow. (Wright's stain; ×950.)

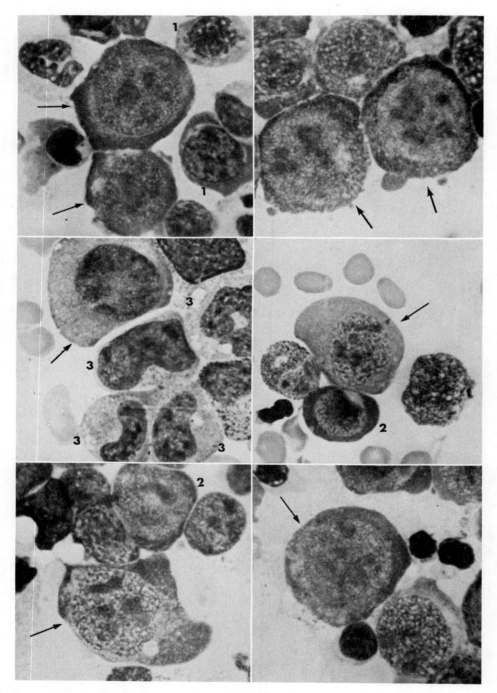

Fig. 4-21. Promegaloblast (arrows). Bone marrow, pernicious anemia. Other cells in fields: **1,** orthochromic megaloblast; **2,** basophilic megaloblast; **3,** giant neutrophilic metamyelocytes and stabs. (Wright's stain; ×950.)

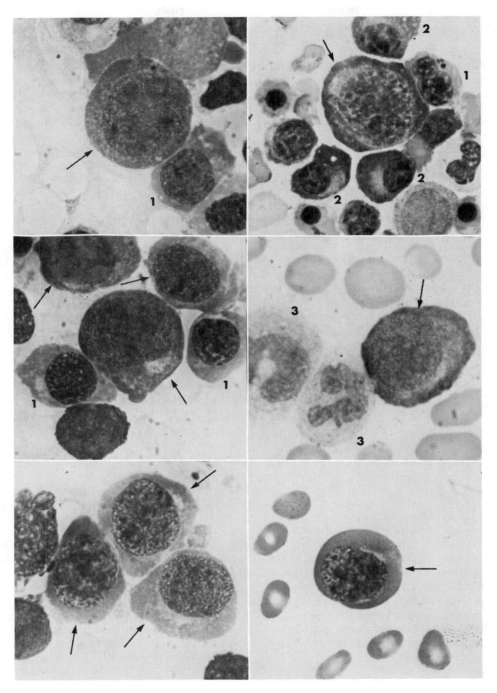

Fig. 4-22. Basophilic megaloblast (arrows). Bone marrow, pernicious anemia. Other cells in fields; **1,** polychromatophilic megaloblast; **2,** plasma cell; **3,** giant metamyelocyte. (Wright's stain; ×950.)

Cytoplasm: Abundant; more than in basophilic normoblast, but less than in the promegaloblast. It usually shows slight mottling. Characteristically, it is more basophilic than in promegaloblastic cells, staining a vivid royal blue.

Polychromatophilic megaloblast (Fig. 4-23)

This cell corresponds to the polychromatophilic normoblast but is larger, with more cytoplasm, and still shows the characteristic megaloblastic nuclear structure.

Size: 10 to 18 μ.

Nucleus: Round and eccentric; nuclear membrane moderately thick. The chromatin is slightly coarser but not as coarse as in the polychromatic normoblast. The parachromatin is still abundant.

Nucleoli: None.

Cytoplasm: As in the polychromatophilic normoblast, but more abundant. It varies, from patchy areas of pink and orange in a basophilic field to a uniform violet color. In pernicious anemia in relapse the cytoplasm may be opaque and hyalin-like with vaguely concentric mottling.

Orthochromic megaloblast (Fig. 4-24)

The completely hemoglobinated form is similar to an orthochromic normoblast but larger. The nuclear characteristics of the series remain, and differentiation from normoblasts is also based on cell size. It occasionally contains two or three abnormal nuclei and may be three or four times the size of an orthochromic normoblast.

Size: 8 to 15 μ.

Nucleus: Varies from a somewhat coarse network to a dense chromatin mass. The parachromatin is abundant, but the looser structure is not visible when the nucleus is dense.

Nucleoli: None.

Cytoplasm: Completely hemoglobinated; pink to orange; more abundant than the corresponding normoblast.

Megakaryoblast (Fig. 4-25)

The megakaryocytic series is characterized by several unusual features: (1) the youngest cell type is generally much smaller than the adult; (2) repeated nuclear division without cellular division takes place, so that instead of the usual diploid nucleus present in other cells the megakaryocytic nucleus is polyploid; (3) the functional end product, the blood platelet, is a cytoplasmic fragment.

Bessis (1977) divides the maturation of the cells in this series into three stages: MK1 (the basophilic megakaryocyte), MK2 (the granular megakaryocyte), and MK3 (the platelet-forming megakaryocyte).

Size: 25 to 35 μ.

Nucleus: Round or oval; large; with delicate purple-staining chromatin and sparse parachromatin.

Nucleoli: 2 to 6; small and indistinct.

Cytoplasm: Scanty; nucleus-to-cytoplasm ratio about 10:1; irregularly basophilic; occasionally shows blunt extrusions.

Promegakaryocyte (Fig. 4-26)

Size: 25 to 50 μ.

Nucleus: Irregular and large; coarser than in the megakaryoblast. It may appear to be lobulated, and sometimes two or more distinct nuclei are seen.

Nucleoli: 0 to 2; difficult to see.

Cytoplasm: Moderately basophilic with some polychromasia. It contains a few fine azurophilic granules in the perinuclear area. Sometimes there is early platelet formation at the periphery.

Megakaryocyte (Fig. 4-27)

This is the largest of the blood cells and varies so much in appearance that it is difficult to describe a single typical form. It usually has a single nucleus showing extreme pleomorphism. Occasionally in pathologic conditions the nucleus will be segmented or polynuclear. Such a cell must be differentiated from an osteoclast.

Size: 40 to 100 μ.

Nucleus: Multiform; usually resembles a staghorn calculus. The chromatin is coarse and irregularly clumped.

Nucleoli: None to many; usually not visible, but in a thinned-out cell many small nucleoli may be seen, reflecting polyploid endomitotic divisions of the nucleus.

Cytoplasm: Abundant, pale, with azurophilic granules either evenly dispersed or clumped. It may show pseudopod-like projections and shedding of the cytoplasm to form platelets.

Plasmablast (Fig. 4-28)

The assumption that plasma cells are derived from lymphoid cells accounts for the similarity in descriptions of plasmablasts and lymphoblasts. In plasmacytomas, however, the youngest cells seen in tissues and bone marrow resemble reticulum cells more than the lymphocytes. The following description of plasmablasts is from pathologic material. This may or may not be justified. I do not believe that a distinction should be made between plasma cells and myeloma cells.

Size: 15 to 25 μ.

Nucleus: Round or oval; eccentric. The chromatin is reticulated and slightly coarse, and the parachromatin is distinct and moderate in amount.

Nucleoli: 2 to 4.

Cytoplasm: Moderately to deeply basophilic; fairly abundant; nucleus-to-cytoplasm ratio about 1:1 or 2:1. It may be mottled; granules are absent.

Proplasmacyte (Fig. 4-29)

Size: 15 to 25 μ.

Nucleus: Oval or round; eccentric; moderately coarse. It may be as large as that of the plasmablast.

Nucleoli: 1 to 2; may be very large in abnormal forms.

Cytoplasm: Brilliant blue or azure, with lighter perinuclear zone common; appears opaque; nucleus-to-cytoplasm ratio 1:1 or 2:1.

Text continued on p. 157.

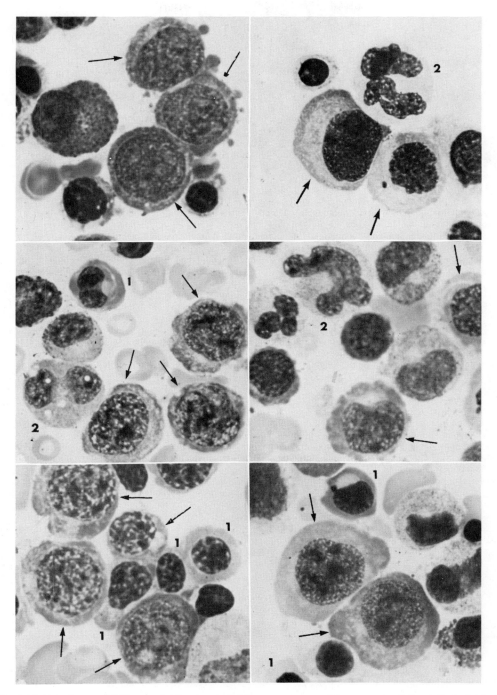

Fig. 4-23. Polychromatophilic megaloblast (arrows). Bone marrow, pernicious anemia. Other cells in fields: **1,** orthochromic megaloblast; **2,** giant metamyelocyte. (Wright's stain; ×950.)

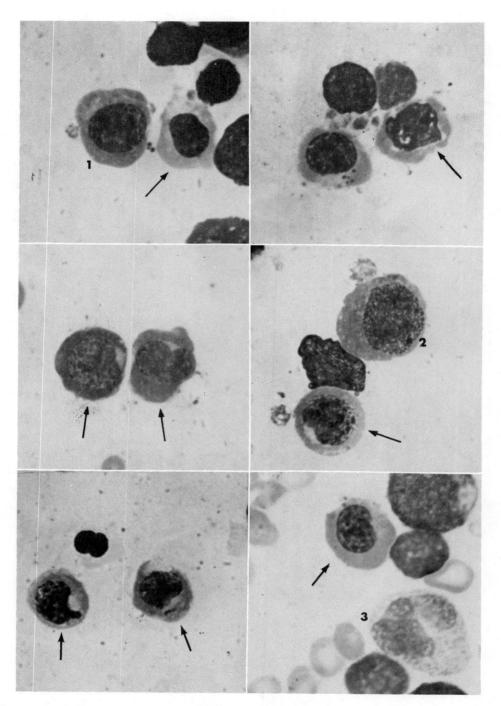

Fig. 4-24. Orthochromic megaloblast. Bone marrow, pernicious anemia (arrows). Other cells in fields: **1,** polychromatophilic megaloblast; **2,** basophilic megaloblast; **3,** giant metamyelocyte. (Wright's stain; ×950.)

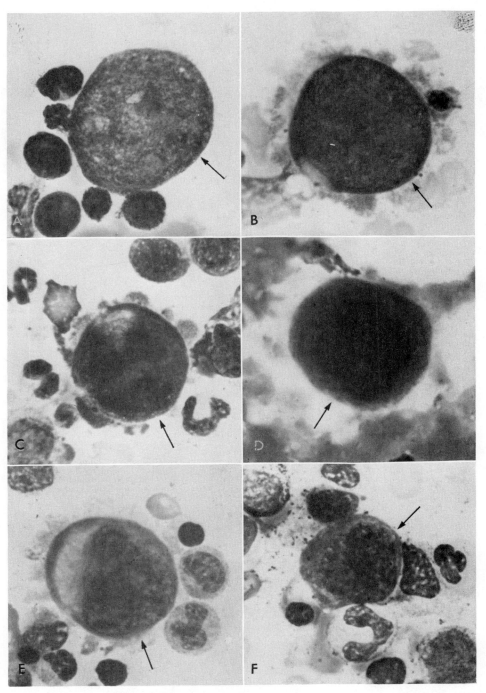

Fig. 4-25. Megakaryoblast (arrows). Bone marrow. Cell pictured in **A** is from a myeloproliferative disorder, and the cell is atypical. Cells in **B-F** show some evidence of being more mature than the true blast stage, but some degree of differentiation helps to identify the cell as an immature megakaryocyte. Strictly speaking, nuclear division and evidence of platelet formation would place the cell in the next stage, the promegakaryocyte. (Wright's stain; ×950.)

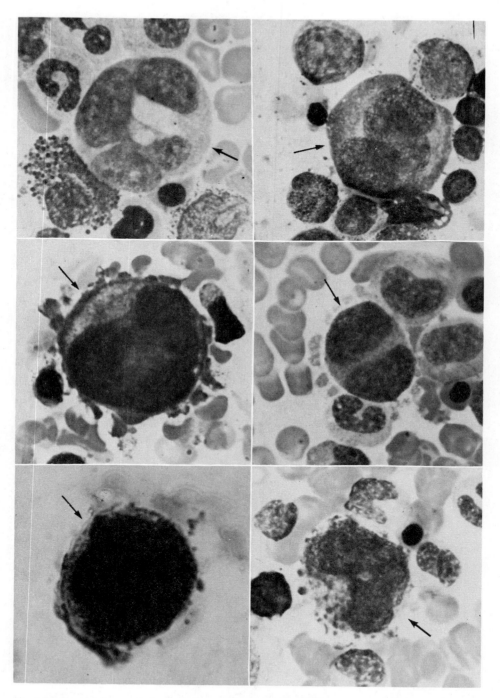

Fig. 4-26. Promegakaryocyte (arrows). Bone marrow. See legend for Fig. 4-25. (Wright's stain; ×950.)

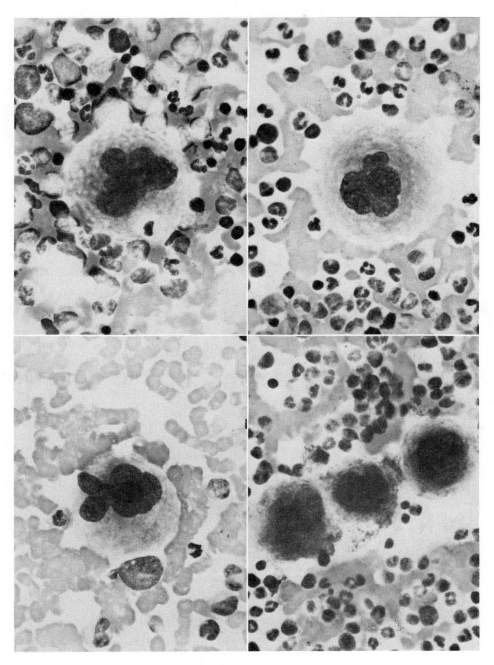

Fig. 4-27. Megakaryocyte. Bone marrow. (Wright's stain; ×400.)

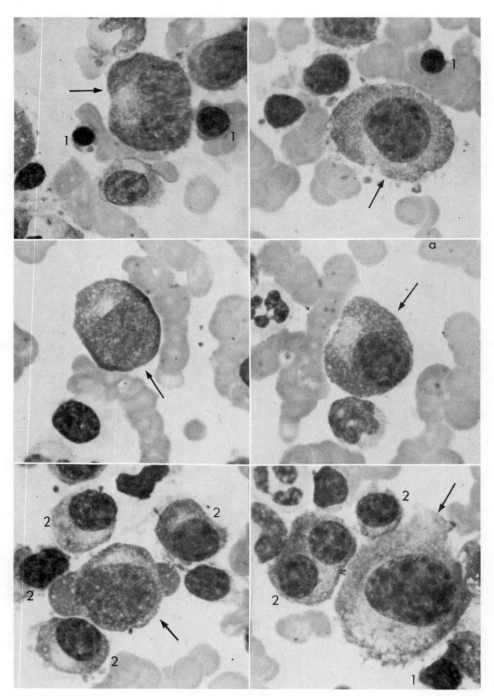

Fig. 4-28. Plasmablast (arrows). Bone marrow, multiple myeloma. Other cells in fields: **1,** orthochromic normoblast; **2,** plasmacytes. (Wright's stain; ×950.)

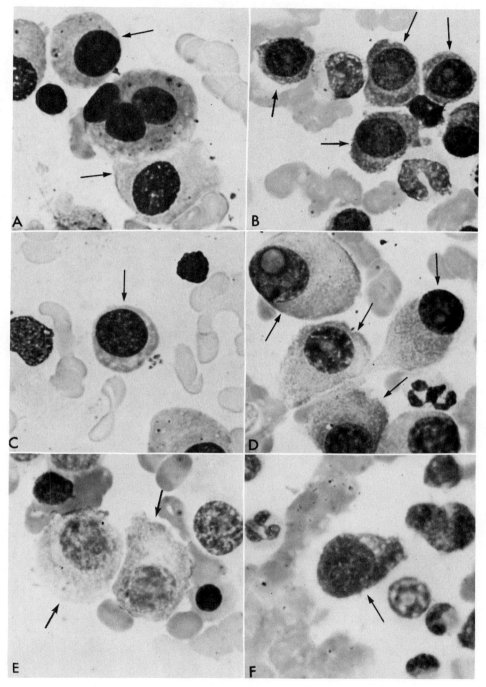

Fig. 4-29. Proplasmacyte (arrows). Bone marrow, multiple myeloma. Note the prominent nucleoli in **A, B,** and **D.** (Wright's stain; ×950.)

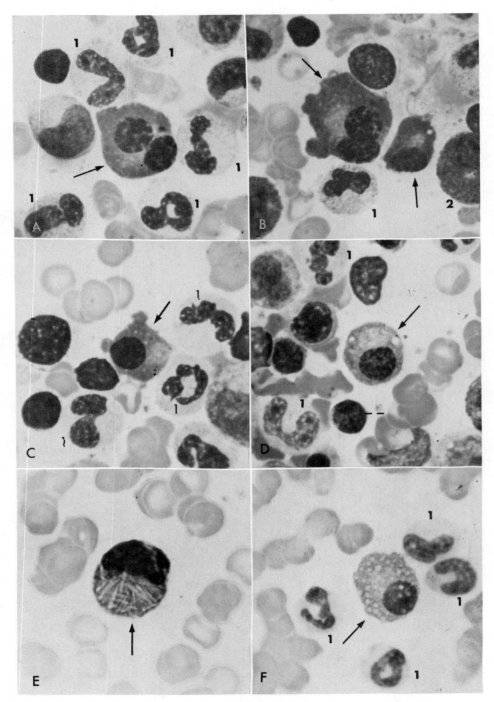

Fig. 4-30. Plasmacyte (arrows). **A-D,** Bone marrow. **E** shows a plasmacyte with crystalline inclusions. **F** shows a plasmacyte with globular inclusions (Russell bodies). Other cells in fields: **1,** stab neutrophils; **2,** eosinophils. (Wright's stain; ×950.)

Plasmacyte (Fig. 4-30)

Size: 10 to 20 μ.

Nucleus: Round or oval; eccentrically placed. It has coarse, clumped chromatin, with sparse but sharp parachromatin. The "wheelspoke" pattern is seldom seen in bone marrow smears, since this appearance in tissue sections is probably due to fixation.

Nucleoli: None in normal cells. One giant nucleolus is usually present in abnormal forms.

Cytoplasm: Brilliant azure, with pale perinuclear zone in normal cell; may contain clear distinct vacuoles; nucleus-to-cytoplasm ratio 1:2.

ABNORMAL FORMS IN BLOOD AND BONE MARROW

We are concerned here with a number of characteristic morphologic abnormalities of leukocytes resulting from abnormal maturation of the nucleus, cytoplasm, or both. Many of the cytoplasmic abnormalities reflect an abnormality of lysosomes and situations in which this is clearly the case, as in the Chédiak-Higashi syndrome, are discussed in Chapter 2. Others are probably also lysosomal abnormalities but are discussed in this chapter, which also deals with nuclear abnormalities. Abnormal forms of red blood cells are discussed in Chapter 11.

Toxic granulation

The specific granules in stab and segmented neutrophils are fine and lilac, whereas the nonspecific granules in young granulocytes are coarse and dark purple. In severe infections or other toxic states the neutrophilic metamyelocytes, stabs, and segmented forms may contain coarse, dark purple granules resembling the nonspecific azurophilic granules (Fig. 4-31). As noted (p. 206), adult neutrophils do contain nonspecific granules whose characteristics are changed, so that normally they do not stain with Romanowsky-type stains. In toxic granulation the cytoplasmic environment is altered, so that there is a persistence of the primitive staining characteristics of the primary lysosomes, which may in fact reflect the need for increased lysosomal activity.

Toxic granulation is seen so frequently on peripheral blood smears from hospitalized patients that it has little diagnostic significance. When found in a supposedly healthy person, it may indicate unsuspected disease or infection. Toxic granulation is sometimes accompanied by vacuolization of the cytoplasm, but this is not indicative of bacteremia or viremia as claimed (Malcolm et al, 1979).

It is important to distinguish this acquired abnormality from the abnormal granulation of severe congenital abnormalities such as in the storage diseases or the Chédiak-Higashi syndrome. Large intracytoplasmic, nonlysosomal inclusions in neutrophils have been observed in colchicine intoxication (Powell and Wolf, 1976).

Auer bodies

In 1906 Auer described what have come to be known as Auer bodies in an article entitled *Some Hitherto Undescribed Structures Found in Large Lymphocytes of an Acute Leukemia*. In spite of apparent confirmation of these unusual bodies in lymphoblasts by such illustrious names as Pap-penheim, Ottenberg, and Naegeli, subsequent investigators established that they do not occur in lymphoblasts—Auer had confused lymphoblasts and myeloblasts—and they are found only in myelocytic leukemia, in monocytic and myelomonocytic leukemia, and occasionally in plasma cells of multiple myeloma. It must be noted that plasma cells sometimes contain crystalline inclusions composed of immunoglobulin. These may have the appearance of Auer bodies on Wright-stained smears, but may not show all the cytochemical reactions of true Auer bodies (see below). One investigator, Inoue (1924), recorded their presence even in mature neutrophils in chronic myelocytic leukemia.

Auer bodies, sometimes called Auer rods, are usually found in the region of the centrosome and indentation of the nucleus. Although they are usually rodlike or spindle shaped, they are sometimes oval or even round. On Wright-stained smears they are red-purple (Fig. 4-32) rods, 1 to 6 μ long, and usually less than 1.5 μ thick. Cytochemically, they are peroxidase positive, sudanophilic, RNA positive, acid phosphatase positive, and ASD chloroacetate positive (Plate 44). They show negative reactions for DNA, alkaline phosphatase, and glycogen. They contain mucopolysaccharides, RNA, lecithin, and acetyl lipid. They are not digested by pepsin or trypsin and are insoluble in all of the common solvents. Arbitrarily, a crystalline inclusion must show the indicated cytochemical reactions, characteristic of the inclusions found in acute granulocytic leukemia, to be called an Auer body. Dutcher (1974) discusses a case of chronic lymphocytic leukemia with inclusions resembling Auer rods in the lymphocytes that were, however, Sudan black B negative, peroxidase negative, and naphthol ASD chloracetate negative, so that they could not be called Auer bodies.

Of the various mechanisms proposed for the genesis of Auer bodies, the one recently substantiated by electron microscopy indicates that they are formed by coalescence of azurophilic granules within the matrix of endoplasmic reticulum (Freeman, 1966; Fukushi et al, 1972).

Pelger-Huët anomaly

This anomaly of leukocytic maturation was first described by Pelger in 1928 in two patients suffering from tuberculosis. He believed it to indicate a poor prognosis. Huët, in 1931, established that the anomaly was hereditary. It is characterized by (1) decreased segmentation of the nucleus of granulocytes, (2) marked condensation of nuclear chromatin in granulocytes, lymphocytes and normoblasts, and (3) normal cytoplasmic maturation. In human beings, cases fall into two categories: (1) the familial and congenital anomaly (true Pelger-Huët) and (2) the acquired pseudo-Pelger-Huët anomaly. Genetically, the defect is usually heterozygous and benign, but an instance of the homozygous defect in humans is reported by Begemann and Campagne (1952). The mother and father of the homozygous patient were, as expected, each heterozygous with respect to the Pelger-Huët anomaly. Another homozygous human case was reported by Bernard et al (1965). In rabbits, selective breeding of Pelger-Huët heterozygous animals produces a lethal homozygous form.

The incidence of the anomaly is different in various geographic regions: in the United States the overall incidence is

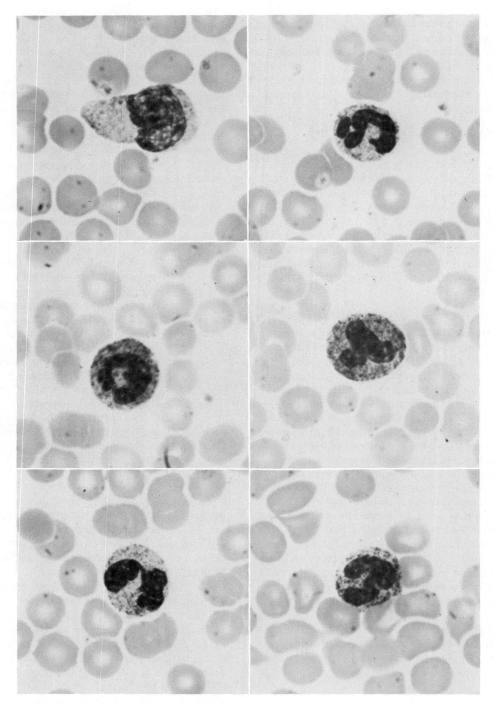

Fig. 4-31. Toxic granulation of neutrophilic leukocytes. Peripheral blood. (Wright's stain; ×950.)

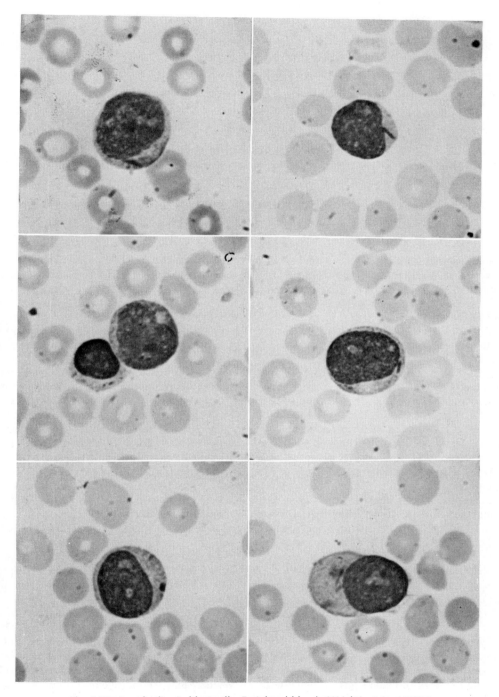

Fig. 4-32. Auer bodies in blast cells. Peripheral blood. (Wright's stain; ×950.)

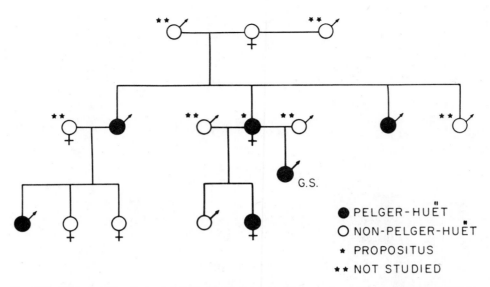

Fig. 4-33. Pedigree of family having Pelger-Huët anomaly. (Redrawn from Rosse and Gurney, 1959.)

1:5,000 to 1:10,000 (Skendzell and Hoffman, 1962), but in one area (Spokane, Washington) the incidence is 1:43,000 (Ludden and Harvey, 1962); in Germany the incidence is 1:1,000 (Nachtsheim, 1950); in India it is 1:320 (Gehlot and Monga, 1973). The anomaly has been found in America, Europe, Asia, Australia, and in one African black family (Lanzkowsky et al, 1965).

The dominant and non-sex-linked features of the inheritance pattern are shown in Fig. 4-33. G.S. is a 2-day-old child, illustrating that the anomaly is both familial and congenital. Other congenital or familial anomalies accompany the Pelger-Huët defect at times. The propositus and some other members of the family shown in Fig. 4-33 also had various degrees of elliptocytosis. Most investigators interested in this anomaly have followed the classification of neutrophilic cells into type A, B, or C cells as suggested by Harm (1955). Type A neutrophils are normal. Type B cells are intermediate in nuclear abnormality. Type C neutrophils are those showing the most striking abnormalities. The usual heterozygous human case shows a preponderance of type B and C neutrophils, whereas in the homozygous smear about 95% of the neutrophils are type C, 5% or less showing any segmentation. Undritz (1937, 1954) described a third variant, the so-called partial carrier, in which cell types A, B, and C are present simultaneously. The inheritance pattern of partial carriers is the same as for the classic form, but an affected family apparently has either the partial-carrier form or the classic form, never both.

The morphology of Pelger-Huët cells is shown in Plate 38. Most striking are the neutrophils that have two lobes or none; three lobes are seldom encountered. When two lobes are present, they often present the characteristic pince-nez form, two symmetric lobes connected by a filament. Sometimes the lobes are asymmetric. When there is no segmentation, the nucleus may be round or oval or may resemble the stab form. The nuclear chromatin is very coarse and dense and stains deeply. The cytoplasmic granulation remains normal even when the nuclear abnormality is most marked, Pelger cells showing the usual cytochemical reactions. Superficially, then, the cells might be thought to be normal stab neutrophils or metamyelocytes, but the coarseness of the nuclear chromatin, the pince-nez appearance, and the absence or scarcity of segmented forms should alert the observer to the possibility of a nuclear anomaly. Rosse and Gurney (1959) discuss one patient admitted to the hospital because of abdominal pain in the right lower quadrant; appendicitis was suspected. The leukocyte count was 6,200/ mm^3 (6.2 × 10^9/1); the differential count revealed 24% segmented neutrophils, 35% stabs and metamyelocytes, 34% lymphocytes, 4% monocytes, 2% eosinophils, and 1% basophils. The leukocytes were recognized as being Pelger-Huët cells, the apparent shift to the left was correctly interpreted as a failure of segmentation, and surgery was avoided. Anomalous nuclear structure in eosinophils, monocytes, and lymphocytes may also aid recognition of this defect. However, whereas these cells are markedly affected in the homozygous anomaly, in the usual heterozygous form the nuclear abnormality is variable and sometimes slight. When megaloblastic anemia occurs in a person with this anomaly, the neutrophils have three or four lobes and might be considered normal if they were not originally Pelger-Huët cells. After adequate treatment with vitamin B$_{12}$ or folic acid, the neutrophils again show the typical Pelger-Huët morphology.

The pseudo-Pelger-Huët anomaly is seen most often in chronic myelocytic leukemia (Thiele, 1953; Darte et al, 1954), but it has been described in acute leukemia and myeloid metaplasia (Dorr and Moloney, 1952), enteritis (Heckner, 1948), Fanconi's panmyelopathy (Ulrich and Wiedemann, 1953), myeloproliferative disorders (Rado and Hammer, 1959), exanthem subitum (Degenhardt and Wiedemann, 1953), malaria (Undritz, 1954), mongolism (Davidson et al, 1954), agranulocytosis (Heilmeyer, 1942), severe myxedema (Shanbrom and Tanaka, 1962), multiple myeloma (Böttner and Reinecke, 1955), various myeloproliferative syndromes (Muratore et al, 1973), and megaloblastic

(Taylor, 1973) and sideroblastic anemia (Lejeune et al, 1974). The anomaly may affect only eosinophils (Chilosi et al, 1979). Plum et al (1978) describe one patient with multiple congenital defects and Pelger-Huët cells. The acquired anomaly and the familial form are morphologically identical, though some of the leukocytes in the acquired type associated with myelocytic leukemia resemble the severely affected cells of the homozygous form. The distinction, then, between the acquired pseudo-Pelger-Huët and the true familial Pelger-Huët anomaly rests on (1) the absence of the anomaly in the parents and other members of the family and (2) the presence of disease states known to produce the acquired anomaly. The case reported by Darte et al (1954) is particularly interesting in this regard. As the chronic myelocytic leukemia in their patient progressed to a fatal end, the absolute number of atypical Pelger-Huët leukocytes increased in proportion to the rising total leukocyte count. The acquired anomaly has also been described in rats having chronic myelocytic leukemia (Hlavay and Svec, 1958). Very occasionally myelocytic leukemia or some other leukocytic disorder has occurred in persons having the heterozygous Pelger-Huët anomaly. Thiele (1953) reported one such combination in a patient having aleukemic myelosis, Alder and Schaub (1952) reported one in a patient with chronic myelocytic leukemia, Huber (1939) reported one in a patient with myelocytic leukemia, and Ardeman et al (1963) reported one in a patient with pernicious anemia. The anomaly has been found in foxhounds (Bowles et al, 1979).

Nothing is known about the basic abnormality in nucleic acid metabolism presumed to be responsible for the abnormal nuclear maturation. It is known that the administration of colchicine to rabbits heterozygous for Pelger-Huët anomaly results in more striking nuclear changes, the leukocytes then resembling those in the homozygous state (Harm, 1953). It may be assumed that the acquired form in chronic myelocytic leukemia also reflects abnormal nucleic acid metabolism.

Aside from the theoretical interest stimulated by this anomaly, three practical points can be made: (1) recognition of the Pelger-Huët anomaly and its distinction from a reactive shift to the left are of obvious importance when the patient is suspected of having an infectious disease, particularly if there is a possibility of surgical intervention; (2) there is agreement that the anomaly is transmitted as a dominant non-sex-linked characteristic (Schneiderman et al, 1969) and, although I know of no instance of its being so applied, this could conceivably be helpful in a case of disputed parentage; and (3) the blood of a patient with this anomaly contains cells that are sufficiently different from normal to make them useful in studying leukocytic survival, life span, and intravascular residence time. This technic was used by Rosse and Gurney (1959) in determining that most transfused leukocytes are removed from the circulating blood within 24 hours.

May-Hegglin anomaly and Döhle bodies

In toxic conditions such as scarlet fever, septicemia, pneumonia, burns, or measles, the cytoplasm of neutrophilic leukocytes contains oval or spindle-shaped inclusions, light blue or blue-gray in color (Plate 37). These were described by Döhle in 1912 in blood smears from persons ill with scarlet fever and were thought by him to be a characteristic and possibly a diagnostic finding in this disease. Amato, in 1923, described similar inclusions, believing them to be viral structures; they are sometimes called Amato bodies. We know now that Döhle bodies can be found in a variety of toxic states. They have been found most commonly in the infectious diseases mentioned previously, but can be found in small numbers in pernicious anemia, chronic myelocytic leukemia, myeloproliferative syndromes, and hemolytic anemia. Itoga and Laszlo (1962) found Döhle bodies in as many as 6% of the neutrophilic granulocytes in patients receiving cyclophosphamide (Cytoxan) for various neoplastic diseases. They have also been found in women with uncomplicated pregnancies (Abernathy, 1966). Döhle bodies are not true inclusions but rather areas free of specific granules and rich in RNA. They are more distinct in smears made from fresh capillary blood than in those from blood that contains an anticoagulant. They stain red with methyl green–pyronine.

Inclusions similar to Döhle bodies are also found in a syndrome described by May in 1909 and by Hegglin (1945). In addition to the basophilic cytoplasmic inclusions, May-Hegglin anomaly is characterized by thrombocytopenia and the presence of giant platelets (Plate 37). Furthermore, whereas Döhle bodies accompany a toxic condition and disappear when the patient recovers, Hegglin's inclusions persist throughout life. The cytoplasmic inclusions in May-Hegglin syndrome are usually larger and have a structure that is different from Döhle bodies (Cawley and Hayhoe, 1972) and are spindle or crescent shaped and light blue; they can be found in adult neutrophilic leukocytes, eosinophils, basophils, monocytes, and occasionally even in lymphocytes. The inclusions are pyroninophilic and peroxidase, Sudan black B, alkaline phosphatase, acid phosphatase, and PAS negative. Their appearance by electron microscopy is shown in Fig. 4-34. Basophilic spindle-shaped inclusions may be found in metamyelocytes, band neutrophils, and even myelocytes when the bone marrow is studied in this syndrome.

The second feature of the syndrome, giant platelets often accompanied by thrombocytopenia, has been studied by Rebuck et al (1961). When observed under the electron microscope, these abnormal platelets fail to show the usual striking extension of pseudopods. The mean platelet volume was found to be 37 to 50 μ^3, as compared with the normal of 10 to 20 μ^3.

The abnormality is familial and shows an autosomal dominant inheritance (Najean et al, 1966; Vargas, 1970). Roughly one-third of the more than 80 cases reported have mild to severe hemorrhagic disease (Godwin and Ginsburg, 1974) manifested by easy bruising, recurrent epistaxis, gingival bleeding, profuse menstrual periods, or abnormal bleeding following dental extractions or surgery. In great part, the clinical and laboratory findings are related to the thrombocytopenia, most platelet counts being in the range of 40,000 to 80,000/mm^3 (0.04 to 0.08 × 10^{12}/l). A few extremely low platelet counts and a very occasional normal count are recorded. The pathogenesis of the thrombocytope-

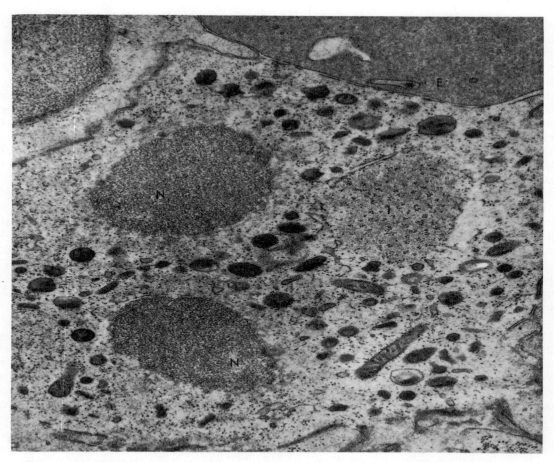

Fig. 4-34. May-Hegglin anomaly. The illustration shows a portion of an anomalous leukocyte containing two nuclear masses, **N,** and an atypical Döhle body—like inclusion. **I.** A portion of an adjacent erythrocyte is labeled **E.** (Electron microscopy.) (From Jordan and Larsen, 1965.)

nia is not clear, platelet survival being either normal (Godwin and Ginsburg, 1974) or moderately decreased (Najean et al, 1966). The number of megakaryocytes in the bone marrow is normal, but some show large hypergranular platelets in the cytoplasm (Rebuck et al, 1971; Kass, 1974b), suggesting an intrinsic fault in cytoplasmic maturation.

There may be an element of abnormal platelet function, but many of the reports are contradictory. Rebuck et al (1961) report abnormal pseudopod formation, but Volpe et al (1974) found platelet morphology to be normal by electron microscopy. Tests of platelet function usually show no abnormality, and the decreased platelet adhesiveness reported by Godwin and Ginsburg (1974) and deficient platelet factor 3 release reported by Lusher et al (1968a) were not found by other investigators (Goudemand et al, 1970). The prolonged bleeding time and deficient clot retraction seem to be proportional to the thrombocytopenia. Platelet aggregation by collagen, epinephrine, and ADP is normal (Godwin and Ginsburg, 1974).

Sézary's syndrome

Sézary's syndrome consists of chronic erythrodermia and "abnormal" mononuclear cells in the peripheral blood, lymph nodes, and skin infiltrate. The abnormal cell is called the Sézary cell, and, because it has been found in the blood of patients with mycosis fungoides (Clendenning et al, 1964), some have defined the Sézary syndrome as the combination of mycosis fungoides and Sézary cells in the blood. In fact, Sézary cells are found also in patients having various inflammatory dermatoses (Duncan and Winkelmann, 1978) and in only a small percentage of the cases of mycosis fungoides (Winkelman and Hoagland, 1980). Meyer et al (1977) found that normal blood may contain 6% to 8% Sézary cells, as judged by the presence of a cerebriform nucleus by electron microscopy. It must be assumed that the morphologic features reflect the nuclear changes in a lymphocyte undergoing either benign or malignant transformation.

During the years between 1938 and 1959 Sézary (1959) wrote a number of articles describing the combination of erythrodermia and large mononuclear cells (*cellules monstrueuses*) in the peripheral blood and tissue infiltrates. His findings seemed to separate out of the general group of erythrodermia one particular variety, that in which large monocytoid or reticulum-like cells are found in the peripheral blood. The cell is large and has a monocytoid nucleus (Plate 57). Other European writers (Wilson and Fielding, 1953; Bureau et al, 1959; Main et al, 1959) adhered to the

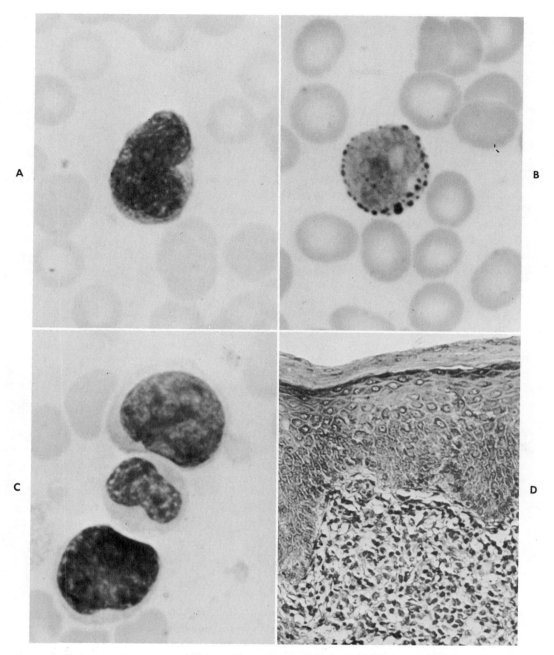

Fig. 4-35. Sézary's syndrome, typical "large cell" variant. **A,** Peripheral blood. (Wright's stain; ×1,250.) **B,** Peripheral blood. (PAS stain; ×1,250.) **C,** Bone marrow. (Wright's stain; ×1,250.) **D,** Skin. (Hematoxylin-eosin stain; ×250.)

original description of the Sézary cell in their reports, all appearing in either French or British journals.

Then, in 1961, there appeared the first article in an American journal (Taswell and Winkelmann, 1961). The authors described seven cases of chronic erythrodermia that they diagnosed as being instances of the Sézary syndrome. The Sézary cell described by them is, however, totally unlike that described by Sézary. Whereas Sézary describes and illustrates the cell as a large monocytoid mononuclear cell with abundant clear cytoplasm (PAS stain not done), Tas-

well and Winkelmann's cells are obviously small lymphocytes showing a vacuolated cytoplasm and PAS-positive granules. Brody et al (1962) adopted the American version of the Sézary cell. Olansky and McCormick (1963) adopted uncritically the features of the Sézary cell proposed by Taswell and Winkelmann and added still another case of the Sézary syndrome to the American literature.

Within recent years the controversy has been mitigated somewhat by the opinion of several investigators (Lutzner et al, 1973; Flandrin and Brouet, 1974) that there exists a

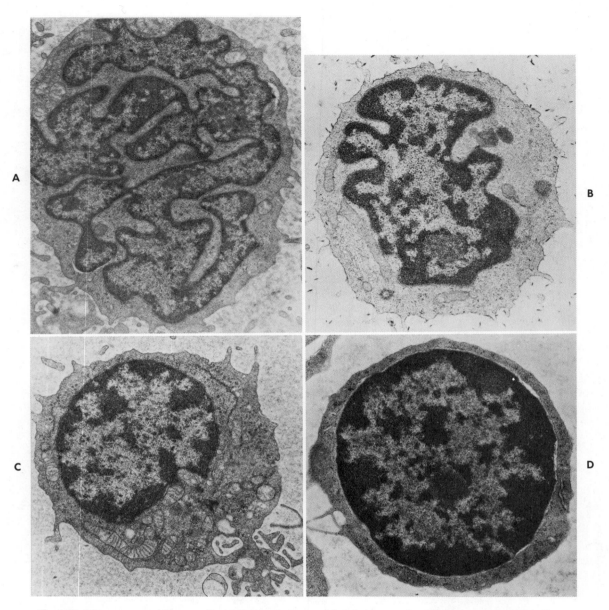

Fig. 4-36. Ultrastructure of Sézary cells. **A,** The classic Sézary cell with the typical cerebriform nucleus. **B,** Small cell variant. **C,** "Atypical" Sézary cell lacking the cerebriform nucleus but not having the features of a normal lymphocyte. **D,** Small lymphocyte from a patient with chronic lymphocytic leukemia. (Fron Edelson, R. L., et al: Morphologic and functional properties of the atypical leukocytes of the Sézary syndrome, Mayo Clin. Proc. **49:**558, 1974.)

"small cell variant" of the typical Sézary cell. This was the predominant cell in the peripheral blood in 16 of 25 cases studied by Flandrin and Brouet (1974). The large Sézary cell was predominant in 8 cases. In 6 of the cases there was a mixture of large and small cells, and in 1 of the cases there was a significant percentage of cells intermediate in size between the large and the small.

Only within recent years have there been cytochemical, immunologic, and ultrastructural data that are basic in answering the question, "What is the Sézary cell?"

On routinely stained peripheral blood smears, that large cell variant is a large cell, 12 to 20 μ in diameter, with a convoluted monocytoid nucleus and a cytoplasm devoid of granules but sometimes vacuolated (Fig. 4-35). The small cell variant looks like a fairly normal lymphocyte except for the presence of nuclear grooves that are usually difficult to see because the nuclear chromatin is highly condensed and the nucleus stains very dark.

One of the important features of the Sézary cell is the appearance of its nucleus by electron microscopy (Lutzner and Jordan, 1968; Edelson et al, 1974; Zucker-Franklin, 1974). As shown in Fig. 4-36, the classic large Sézary cell shows a convoluted, serpentine, cerebriform nucleus. This nuclear feature is also characteristic of the small cell variant.

Table 4-3. Cytochemical reactions of Sézary and related cells*

Reaction	Normal lymphocytes	Sézary cells	Hairy cells†	Monocytes	Macrophages
PAS	Neg.	Pos.‡	Neg.	Neg.	Neg.
β-Glucuronidase	Pos.‡	Pos.‡	Neg.	Pos.‡	Pos.
Acid phosphatase	Pos.‡	Pos.‡	Pos.§	Pos.‡	Pos.‡
Peroxidase	Neg.	Neg.	Neg.	Pos.‡	Neg.
Alkaline phosphatase	Neg.	Neg.	Neg.	Neg.	Neg.
Naphthol ASD esterase	Neg.	Neg.	Pos.	Pos.	Pos.

*Data from Flandrin and Brouet, 1974.   ‡Most but not all.
†Leukemic reticuloendotheliosis, "hairy cell" leukemia, p. 725.   §Not inhibited by tartrate.

According to Edelson et al (1974), the cells of chronic lymphocytic leukemia do not show the cerebriform nuclear structure, but Flandrin and Brouet (1974) state that in one case of chronic lymphocytic leukemia some leukemic cells were typically cerebriform.

The cytochemical reactions of Sézary and related cells are shown in Table 4-3. Perhaps the most characteristic reaction is the periodic acid–Schiff (PAS) for glycogen (Fig. 4-35, Plate 57). The reaction is usually abolished by diastase digestion; but if the inclusions are of the fetal type of glycogen, they are diastase resistant (Menefee et al, 1978). Many, but not all, large Sézary cells are PAS positive, and a higher percentage of small cells are PAS positive. However, PAS positivity per se does not make a Sézary cell, for lymphocytes in lymphocytic leukemia (Plate 50) and lymphosarcoma infrequently contain PAS-positive granules (Hayhoe et al, 1964). Sézary cells are strongly positive for β-glucuronidase activity, granular pattern as in normal lymphocytes, whereas hairy cells are negative. Sézary cells are acid phosphatase positive (reaction inhibited by tartrate) (Faramarz Naeim et al, 1979), peroxidase negative. In general the cytochemical reactions are more like those of lymphoid cells than of the cells of the macrophage system.

Immunologic studies usually show that Sézary cells are related to T-lymphocytes (Brouet et al, 1973; Winkelmann, 1973), since they have no receptors for antibody or complement and do form rosettes with uncoated sheep erythrocytes. Occasionally, Sézary cells fail to react as T-lymphocytes (Braylan et al, 1975) and behave as null cells.

The question of defining a Sézary cell remains in spite of all this information (Flandrin and Brouet, 1974). Unresolved questions are: (1) Do the variants, according to cell size, represent hypodiploidy and hyperdiploidy (Prunieras, 1974)? (2) What accounts for the cerebriform transformation of the nucleus? (3) Granted that the Sézary cell has a characteristic cerebriform nuclear structure, what similar cells are found in classic chronic lymphocytic leukemia and other lymphocytic disorders? and (4) Is there any significance, related to diagnosis, therapy, and prognosis, to the two or three size variants?

Virocytes and reactive lymphocytes

A common morphologic variant of lymphocytes is frequently seen in the peripheral blood. This refers to mononuclear cells, almost certainly of lymphocytic origin, which are neither normal nor leukemic. For want of a better term, these have sometimes been referred to as atypical lymphocytes. Attention was drawn to these cells by Türk (1907), who found them in the peripheral blood of a patient who later recovered from what was thought to be acute leukemia. This is probably one of the earliest recorded cases of the disease we now call infectious mononucleosis. Türk's description of an atypical cell having a somewhat immature nucleus and a basophilic cytoplasm similar to that of a plasma cell established in medical literature the term "Türk cell." To this day there is no general agreement as to what a Türk cell is or was. Türk's own description was not definitive. We are fairly certain, however, that cells so described are reactive lymphocytes (Plate 59) falling within the virocyte group.

The atypical lymphocytes for which Litwins and Leibowitz (1951) proposed the term "virocytes" are usually indistinguishable from the lymphocytes found in the peripheral blood of persons having infectious mononucleosis. Atypical lymphocytes of the virocyte type are sometimes found in the peripheral blood of clinically well children. Fichtelius and Vahlquist (1955) found such lymphocytes in many children up to 3 years of age. It may be assumed that these children are "well" insofar as they have no clinically obvious respiratory infection. There is another clinical syndrome that I accept, called pseudomononucleosis by Vahlquist et al (1958). In this syndrome the patient presents signs and symptoms compatible with infectious mononucleosis, plus the usual virocytes in the peripheral blood, but has negative serologic findings. These cases are due to infection with other viruses. I believe that the characteristic serologic reaction is indispensable to a diagnosis of infectious mononucleosis (p. 676). In the other diseases listed, fewer virocytes are seen than is usual in infectious mononucleosis and pseudomononucleosis; in fact, it is seldom that more than 15% of the leukocytes are virocytes.

Virocytes (Plate 59) are usually large, up to 20 μ in diameter, though they can be smaller. The cytoplasm is moderately to deeply basophilic and foamy or patchy, occasionally with a few small vacuoles. The nucleus shows a coarse chromatin pattern, not usually as lumpy as that of a normal lymphocyte and with a sharper chromatin-parachromatin distinction. It is usually possible to recognize one or another feature of type I, II, and III cells, as described by Downey et al (1923), in infectious mononucleosis, but virocytes usually resemble type III cells.

Atypical lymphocytes are cells that are reacting to an abnormal stimulus. In the case of known viral infection the term "virocyte" is a good one. There are, however, other

Table 4-4. Conditions in which virocytes or other reactive lymphocytes are found in peripheral blood

I. Reaction to viral infection (virocytes)
  A. Infectious mononucleosis
  B. Pseudomononucleosis
  C. Acute viral hepatitis
  D. Herpes zoster
  E. Herpes simplex
  F. Roseola infantum
  G. Viral pneumonitis
  H. Upper respiratory infection (viral)
  I. Mumps
  J. Rubeola
  K. Rubella
  L. Hemorrhagic fever (Argentina)
II. Reaction to nonviral infection (reactive lymphocytes)
  A. Tuberculosis
  B. Rickettsialpox
  C. Syphilis (congenital, secondary, and tertiary)
  D. Diphtheria
  E. Malaria
  F. Scarlet fever
  G. Typhus

III. Reaction to drugs (reactive lymphocytes)
  A. PAS hypersensitivity
  B. Dilantin and Mesantoin hypersensitivity
  C. Lead intoxication (early stage only)
  D. Barbiturate poisoning
  E. Butazolidine hypersensitivity
  F. Tetrachlorethane toxicity
  G. Trinitrotuluene toxicity
IV. Reaction in miscellaneous conditions (reactive lymphocytes)
  A. After open-heart surgery
  B. After massive blood transfusion
  C. After lung resection
  D. Overexposure to ionizing radiation
  E. Agranulocytosis
  F. Dermatitis herpetiformis (arsenical)
  G. Serum sickness
  H. Pemphigus vulgaris
  I. Ulcerative colitis
  J. Acute myocardial infarction
  K. Addison's disease

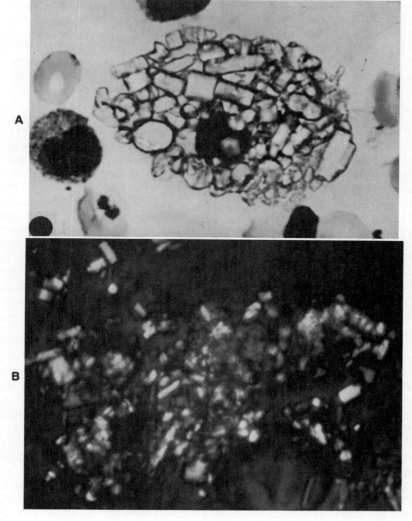

Fig. 4-37. Cystinosis, crystals in bone marrow. **A,** Phagocyte containing cystine crystals. (Standard illumination; ×950.) **B,** Cystine crystals by polarized light. (**A** courtesy Dr. C. L. Conley; **B** from Frazier, 1965.)

reactive states in which the stimulus is nonviral (Table 4-4). In these states the cells should be called reactive lymphocytes, since they have been shown to have an accelerated DNA synthesis and are analogous to the "transformed" lymphocyte in tissue culture under the influence of phytohemagglutinin or specific antigen.

Jordans' anomaly in progressive muscular dystrophy

Jordans (1953) has described the presence of sudanophilic inclusions in the cytoplasm of granulocytes in two brothers suffering from progressive muscular dystrophy. Rozenszajn et al (1966) have found the same anomaly in two sisters who had ichthyosis. The sudanophilic inclusions are also found in some monocytes and lymphocytes in the peripheral blood and in progranulocytes, myelocytes, metamyelocytes, and an occasional plasma cell in the bone marrow. Routine Wright-stained smears show only vacuolization of the involved cells, and lipid staining should be done to identify the abnormality. The vacuoles do not give any other cytochemical reactions.

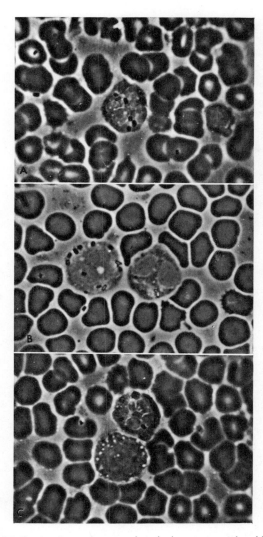

Fig. 4-38. Cystinosis, cystine crystals in leukocytes, peripheral blood. (Phase contrast microscopy.) (Courtesy Dr. D. Korn.)

Cytochemically abnormal neutrophils and eosinophils (Alius-Grignaschi anomaly)

Grignaschi et al (1963) described two siblings whose neutrophils and monocytes were peroxidase negative and Sudan negative. Presentey (1968) has reported an anomaly of eosinophils characterized by hyperlobulation, hypogranulation, and negative peroxidase and lipid staining of the eosinophilic granules. Bozdech et al (1980) have described a partial peroxidase deficiency in neutrophils and eosinophils in a patient with ceroid lipofuscinosis (Kufs' disease). The abnormality was not demonstrable with the benzidine peroxidase reaction but was detectable with the reagent 4-chloro-1-naphthol (Elias, 1980), the reagent used in the Technicon Hemalog D.

Cystine crystals in cystinosis

Cystinosis (cystine storage disease, Lignac-Fanconi disease) is an inherited (recessive or incompletely recessive) disease characterized by aminoaciduria—specifically, excessive amounts of cystine, lysine, arginine, and ornithine in the urine. Cystine crystals in the urine are usually found in homozygotes, who are also prone to form cystine calculi in the urinary tract. Crystals of cystine are also deposited in the reticuloendothelial cells in the liver, spleen, lymph nodes, and bone marrow; they are easily seen with the slit lamp in the cornea and conjunctiva. The crystals are strongly birefringent and have been found not only in bone marrow (Fig. 4-37), but also in neutrophilic leukocytes (Fig. 4-38) and monocytes in the peripheral blood. Although only hexagonal plate crystals form spontaneously in urine, the crystals in the bone marrow and peripheral blood cells are described as rectangular or square. They must, therefore, be distinguished from oxalate crystals, which are sometimes found in neutrophilic leukocytes in oxalated blood (Fig. 4-39).

Miscellaneous leukocytic inclusions

Isolated reports of unusual inclusions are difficult to evaluate. Powell and Wolf (1976) describe cytoplasmic inclusions in neutrophils in a case of suicidal ingestion of colchicine. Smith (1967) describes similar inclusions in a 16-week-old infant having congenital atresia of the bile ducts and livedo reticularis. Tracey and Smith (1978) studied a family, several members of which had inclusions in both eosinophils and basophils. Valenzuela et al (1976) found unusual fibrillary inclusions in neutrophils of human renal allografts.

Constitutional hypersegmentation of neutrophilic leukocytes

In the peripheral blood of a normal person the segmented neutrophils seldom have more than five lobes, with an average of three. Undritz and Schäli (1964) described a family showing a hereditary constitutional hypersegmentation of the neutrophils in which the neutrophils had an average of four lobes, with some having six or seven (Plate 40). The condition is benign but must be distinguished from the hypersegmented macropolycyte in megaloblastic dyspoiesis. Davidson et al (1960) described another instance of what is probably the same benign anomaly, but they have stressed the large size of the neutrophilic leukocytes.

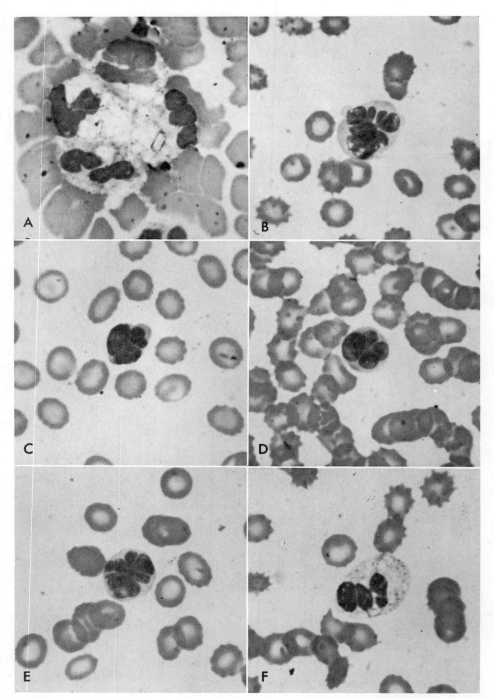

Fig. 4-39. Oxalate crystals and cellular artifacts due to oxalate anticoagulant. **A,** Oxalate crystals. **B-E,** Cloverleaf artifact in nucleus of lymphocytes. **F,** Segmented neutrophil containing oxalate crystals. Note also the crenated erythrocytes in **B, C, D,** and **F.**

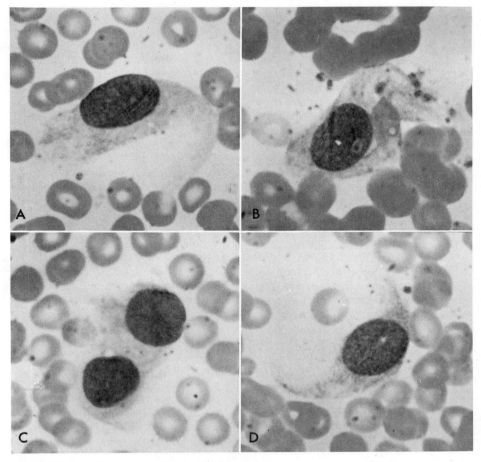

Fig. 4-40. Endothelial cells, peripheral blood smear. These cells may be encountered when blood is drawn by venipuncture. They originate from the endothelial lining of the vein.

Endothelial cells in peripheral blood

When blood smears are made from venous blood, they will occasionally contain endothelial cells derived from the vein lining (Fig. 4-40). These have no significance but must be distinguished from tumor and other pathologic cells.

Tumor cells in peripheral blood

It is now well established that tumor cells can be found in the peripheral blood of persons having malignant tumors. Observations dating back many years show that tumor cells are sometimes found by chance in routine peripheral blood smears. Ashworth (1869) found tumor cells in the blood of a patient with multiple malignant skin tumors. Schleip (1906) described tumor cells in the blood of a patient with carcinoma of the stomach. Ludman and Spear (1957) reported finding Reed-Sternberg cells in the peripheral blood of a patient with Hodgkin's disease. Except for the unusual patient in whom there is massive terminal dissemination through the bloodstream (Myerowitz et al, 1977), finding tumor cells in simple smears of the peripheral blood is a matter of chance. The incidence increases strikingly if concentration methods are used. Engell (1955) destroyed the erythrocytes in venous blood with saponin and examined paraffin sections of the sediment for tumor cells. He found tumor cells in venous blood draining from the tumor area in a surprisingly large percentage of the patients: 59% of 107 patients with carcinoma of the colon or rectum, 75% of 8 patients with carcinoma of the stomach, 3 out of 4 patients with carcinoma of the lung, and 3 out of 4 patients with carcinoma of the breast. In 7 out of 14 patients with advanced carcinoma, tumor cells were found in preparations made from blood drawn from the antecubital vein.

Moore et al (1957) reported their experience with a concentration technic in which the sedimentation of erythrocytes was accelerated by adding fibrinogen and smears made from the sediment of the centrifuged supernate. They reported positive smears from the peripheral blood in 93 out of 179 patients with malignant tumor. The incidence when blood was obtained from the regional vein was 60 out of 109. Rarely, tumor cells may be so numerous in the blood as to suggest leukemia (Carey et al, 1976).

The method described by Malmgren et al (1958) has been adopted by many workers. It consists of destroying the erythrocytes and leukocytes with streptolysin, filtering through a Millipore filter, and then staining the cells directly on the filter. When this technic has been used, the yield of positive preparations has ranged from 17% to 39%. Difficulties in identification should not be underestimated. In a significant article, Raker et al (1960) pointed out that many large and apparently atypical cells in concentrated blood specimens may instead be normal megakaryocytes. In examining blood from 144 patients with malignant tumors, they found only 2 with unequivocal tumor cells. In 60 patients (42%), the tumor cells at first reported were, on reappraisal, thought to be megakaryocytes instead. Jackson (1962) found megakaryocyte fragments in 26 of 26 blood samples from subjects with cancer and no cells that would be identified as cancer cells.

The import of tumor cells in peripheral or regional blood is not clear. The data available generally show a significant increase in positive preparations as the result of surgical manipulation (Long et al, 1960; Roberts et al, 1960). The fate of these cells is not known, however. No one has yet convincingly shown that the prognosis of patients having tumor cells in the peripheral blood is worse than that of patients who do not. Nor is there any apparent relationship between the number of cells and the patient's survival, although it is true that numerous tumor cells are found in patients with far-advanced tumors and usually few or none in those with early tumors. As far as we know, cancer cells, or tumor emboli, in the blood do not necessarily give rise to distant metastases (Wood, 1958; Zeidman, 1965).

Phagocytic cells in peripheral blood

The presence of phagocytic cells in the peripheral blood has been commented on by a number of authors. Some have called them histiocytes or atypical phagocytic cells. In the German literature these cells, when seen in the blood in subacute bacterial endocarditis, are called endocarditis lenta cells.

Phagocytic cells are found in the peripheral blood in a variety of conditions (Table 4-5). The list is so long as to have limited practical importance. Indeed, except in one disease, subacute bacterial endocarditis, phagocytic cells may or may not be present, and when present, the number is usually small. In subacute bacterial endocarditis, however, phagocytic cells are seen frequently, and often in large numbers. The series of 273 patients having subacute bacterial endocarditis reported by Hill and Bayrd (1960) showed phagocytic cells in 8% of the 228 patients with positive blood cultures and in 26.6% of the 45 patients with negative blood cultures. Their report of an additional 23% of non-phagocytic cells in the positive blood culture group and 33.3% in the negative blood culture is difficult to interpret. They stated that transitional forms between these and typical monocytes were numerous. Whether one report may be compared with another, therefore, depends on the method of classification. Joseph (1925), for example, reported that 80% of the leukocytes in his patient's blood were monocytes. The frequency with which monocytosis accompanies many of the diseases listed should be emphasized. In subacute bacterial endocarditis the presence of cells showing phagocytosis is of greater significance than is the presence of nonphagocytic forms.

Both types are shown in Figs. 4-41 and 4-42. Some technical points need emphasis. The number of phagocytic cells varies markedly from hour to hour. In addition, since both phagocytic and nonphagocytic cells tend to marginate when the blood is smeared, the result of the differential count depends on whether special emphasis is placed on marginal areas. An intriguing finding, substantiated by many authors, is that a large number of phagocytic cells may be found in blood obtained from the earlobe, whereas they are usually scarce or absent in venous blood or blood from a finger puncture. The total leukocyte count also may differ greatly, that in blood from the earlobe frequently being much higher. Daland et al (1956) also stated that the first drop of blood contains many more phagocytic cells than the second and subsequent drops.

The cytoplasm of phagocytic cells usually contains cellular debris and other unidentifiable material. On occasion there may be phagocytosis of recognizable microorganisms, as in the unusual example shown in Fig. 4-43.

Phagocytosis in bone marrow

Evidence of phagocytic activity is usually seen in marrow smears from normal subjects. This is a normal function of the reticuloendothelial cells, seen as ingestion of cell nuclei, nuclear fragments, and debris. A special but still essentially normal type of phagocytosis is seen in the ingestion of extruded normoblastic nuclei by phagocytic reticuloendothelial cells (*Rundkern-macrophagen*). Usually one sees phagocytosis of one or two normoblastic nuclei. When this type of phagocytosis is striking, the marrow often shows an increase in erythropoietic activity.

Phagocytosis of lymphocytes and platelets is not seen in smears of normal marrow. This and other types of phago-

Table 4-5. Diseases in which phagocytic cells may be found in peripheral blood*

1. Subacute bacterial endocarditis
2. Septicemia
3. Rheumatic fever with active myocarditis
4. Tuberculosis
5. Perinephric abscess
6. Hepatic abscess
7. Infectious mononucleosis
8. Mastoiditis
9. Ulcerative colitis
10. Chronic sinusitis
11. Subsiding hepatitis
12. Subsiding acute appendicitis
13. Trichinosis
14. Trypanosomiasis
15. Malaria
16. Typhoid fever
17. Typhus
18. Smallpox
19. Cholera
20. Hemolytic anemia
21. Thrombocytopenic purpura
22. Disseminated lupus erythematosus
23. Carcinoma
24. Lymphoma
25. Leukemia
26. Agranulocytosis

*Collected from Connal, 1911; Dameshek, 1931; Cole et al, 1958; Engle and Koprowska, 1959; and Hill and Bayrd, 1960.

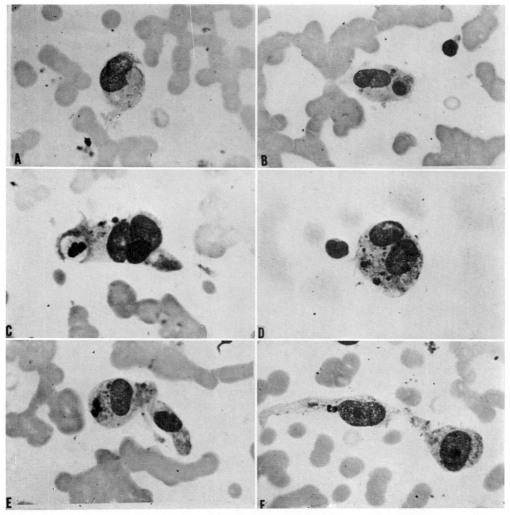

Fig. 4-41. Phagocytic cells, peripheral blood, subacute bacterial endocarditis. **A,** Histiocyte with ingested red blood cell. **B,** Histiocyte with ingested lymphocyte. **C,** Giant multinucleated histiocyte with ingested leukocytes. **D,** Multinucleated histiocyte with pigment granules in cytoplasm. **E,** Histiocytes, one with ingested degenerating neutrophil. **F,** Large histiocytes having drawnout cytoplasmic streamers. (From Engle and Koprowska, 1959.)

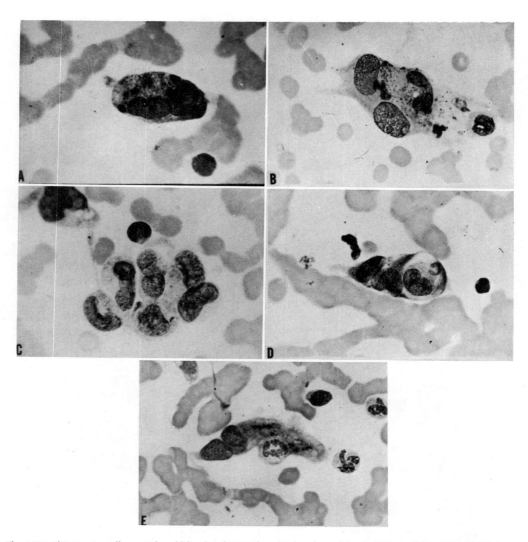

Fig. 4-42. Phagocytic cells, peripheral blood, subacute bacterial endocarditis. **A,** Giant multinucleated histiocyte with prominent nucleolus. **B,** Giant multinucleated histiocyte with neutrophilic leukocyte and debris in cytoplasm. **C,** Clump of histiocytes having elongated vesicular nuclei. **D** and **E,** Giant multinucleated histiocytes with ingested leukocytes. (From Engle and Koprowska, 1959.)

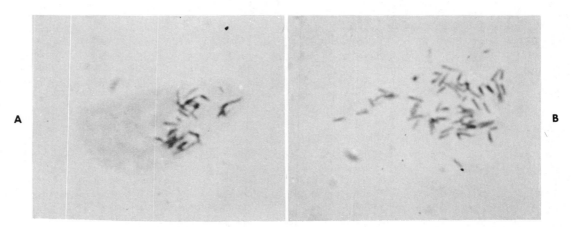

Fig. 4-43. *Mycobacteria leprae,* peripheral blood, acute lepromatous crisis. **A,** In a mononuclear cell, probably a monocyte. **B,** Lying free. (Acid-fast stain; ×1,400.) (Courtesy Dr. J. F. Lopez.)

Table 4-6. Frequency of pathologic phagocytosis in bone marrow in various diseases*

Disease	Percent phagocytes
Hemolytic anemia	1.7
Chronic infectious diseases (except tuberculosis)	1.68
Hodgkin's disease	1.14
Cavitary pulmonary tuberculosis	0.92
Other tuberculosis	0.85
Pernicious anemia	0.7
Acute pneumonia	0.6
Neoplasms	0.54
Iron deficiency anemia	0.35
Boeck's sarcoid	0.32
Hepatitis and cirrhosis	0.30
Chronic rheumatoid arthritis	0.17
Leukemia	0.02

*From Horster, 1957.

cytosis by reticuloendothelial cells, monocytes, eosinophils, and neutrophils is pathologic; e.g., phagocytosis of altered nuclear material is now recognized as characteristic of disseminated lupus erythematosus. Horster (1957) has written authoritatively on pathologic phagocytosis. A summary of the incidence and extent of pathologic phagocytosis derived from a study of 155 abnormal marrows is given in Table 4-6. Marked histiocytic proliferation and phagocytosis are reported in the bone marrow of infants having hemolytic anemia (Zinkham and Diamond, 1952).

SEXUAL DIMORPHISM OF LEUKOCYTES

Prior to 1949 maleness and femaleness were considered rather obvious traits in spite of occasional puzzling deviations from the norm. Barr and Bertram (1949) initiated a new age of scientific sexology by reporting that the nerve cells of female cats contain a distinct nuclear structure that in male cats was either extremely small or not visible. They first called this structure a nucleolar satellite because of its juxtaposition to the nucleolus. It has also been called the heterochromatin mass. Later, when it became apparent that this structure reliably distinguished female cats from male cats, it was called the sex chromatin. The latter term expressed a belief held by Barr and Bertram from the first that the heterochromatin mass was indeed an expression of the chromosome content of the nucleus, i.e., presence of the larger XX mass in the female versus the smaller XY mass in the male. Indeed, Graham and Barr (1952) showed that all the body cells of the cat could be sexed by the presence or absence of the heterochromatin mass. Moore and Barr (1954) showed that the same applies to the somatic cells of humans. It has now been established that this criterion also applies to other mammals, including the dog, mink, marten, ferret, raccoon, skunk, goat, and deer.

Two interesting sidelights are worth mentioning; they teach important lessons. First, after Barr and Bertram's report most of us wondered how such a structure, so obvious once it was pointed out, could have been looked at for many years without being seen. Surely this is a lesson in objective observation! The second sidelight is the report of Coidan

(1951) denying the validity of Barr and Bertram's observations. Unfortunately he investigated rats and mice, which have no heterochromatin mass in the nerve cells. This is also true of the hamster, ground hog, rabbit, and pigeon. In cattle the nerve cells are sexable, but other cells are not.

Davidson and Smith (1954) described a morphologic sex difference in the polymorphonuclear leukocytes, the characteristic drumstick. For a time it was thought the drumstick was also an expression of chromosomal sex. We now think this is not so. It is necessary to provide some background to bring this characteristic of blood cells into proper relationship with other aspects of nuclear sexing.

In perspective, investigation of nuclear sexing has followed three paths: (1) the geneticists' studies on chromosomes, (2) the studies on nuclear sexing according to nuclear heterochromatin, and (3) observations on the satellite body or drumstick of leukocytes.

Human chromosomes

The geneticists' attempts to count and identify chromosomes were originally limited to nonvertebrate cells and those having fewer chromosomes than mammalian cells. The only mammalian cell that offered any hope was the tubular cell of the testis, which in meiosis exhibits fairly distinct chromosomes. In this cell, Painter (1923) counted 48 as the normal number of chromosomes. He also established the XY male configuration. Hsu (1952) introduced a tissue culture method that caused the chromosomes to swell and disperse, making it possible for the first time to see and chart accurately the chromosomal content of mammalian cells. There followed many refinements of this technic. The result was that Tjio and Levan (1956) established the normal human diploid chromosome number to be 46, not 48. These can be arranged into 22 pairs (Fig. 4-44), the remaining 2 being the sex chromosomes XY (in the male) or XX (in the female). Such an arrangement is called a *karyotype* (Fig. 4-45). In accordance with the recommendations of the Human Chromosomes Study Group, the term "idiogram," though used interchangeably by many to refer to such an arrangement of chromosomes, is best reserved for the diagrammatic representation of karyotype.

Many syndromes with chromosomal abnormalities have been studied, revealing chromosomal trisomy, monosomy, triploidy, mosaicism, translocations, abnormal satellites, and abnormal size of chromosomes. Meanwhile, normal chromosome patterns have been found in a dozen or more other diseases. For further details, Eggen's book (1965) on cytogenetics is highly recommended.

Chromosomal content of blood cells

In spite of recent interest in the chromosomal content of blood and somatic cells in persons having syndromes such as Turner's, Klinefelter's, etc., little can be found in the literature about the chromosomal content of blood cells in hematologic disorders. The work of Rothlin and Undritz (1946) and of Undritz (1951) suggests that even under normal conditions some blood cells undergo polyploid development and that polyploidy is frequently characteristic of neoplastic proliferation.

All normal human cells with the exception of male and female germ cells contain 46 chromosomes. A primitive

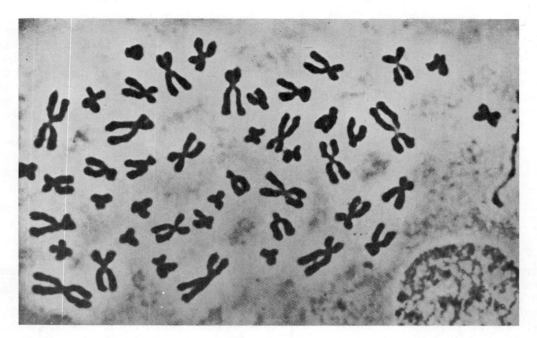

Fig. 4-44. Chromosomes of a normal male, peripheral blood cell culture. (×2,000.) (From Human Chromosomes Study Group, 1960.)

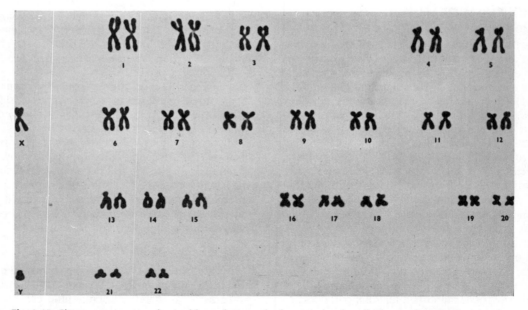

Fig. 4-45. Chromosomes cut and paired from photograph of a normal male cell. The numbering is in accordance with the recommendation of the Human Chromosomes Study Group, University of Colorado Medical Center. (From Human Chromosomes Study Group, 1960.)

germ cell in the process of maturation undergoes meiotic division, in the course of which two germ cells (spermatozoa or unfertilized ova) are formed, each having half the full complement of chromosomes. In humans, therefore, normal *germ cells* are *haploid* and contain 23 chromosomes. Most other normal cells contain 46 chromosomes and are called *diploid*. Some cells, notably normal adult megakaryocytes and some abnormal somatic and hemic blood cells, contain more than 2 sets of chromosomes (23 per set) and are therefore called *polyploid*. Polyploidy may be tetraploid (4 sets of chromosomes), hexaploid (6 sets), octaploid (8 sets), etc. A polyploid cell may owe its increased chromosomal content to nuclear mitosis without cytoplasmic cleavage, thus forming a multinucleated cell (normal osteoclasts, some multinucleated plasma cells in myeloma, Reed-Sternberg cells in Hodgkin's granuloma, and some neoplastic cells). The individual nuclei are diploid, however. Other cells are polyploid as a result of repeated incomplete mitoses without either nuclear or cytoplasmic cleavage and form a single large polyploid nucleus (megakaryocytes and some neoplastic cells). Still others (some megakaryocytes and neoplastic cells) contain several nuclei, some polyploid and some diploid.

Prior to the development of technics for counting chromosomes the diploidy or polyploidy of blood cells could be determined only roughly from mitoses encountered by chance in blood and bone marrow smears. Thus cells showing an unusually large number of chromosomes would be considered polyploid; those showing other than the usual bipolar spindle would certainly be polyploid. The presence of abnormally large chromosomes speaks for pathologic mitosis, the chromosomes doubling in size but failing to separate. Such cells usually have giant nucleoli. Probable polyploidy can be ascribed to multinucleated cells or to cells having abnormally large nuclei. According to these criteria, the following blood cells are normally diploid: normoblasts, megaloblasts, basophilic granulocytes, monocytes, lymphocytes, and plasma cells. Polyploidy is common in neoplastic cells, but may be seen in the apparently benign proliferation of normoblasts, megaloblasts, granulocytes, monocytes, lymphocytes, and plasma cells. Polyploidy, by itself, is therefore not a reliable criterion of neoplasia.

In 1960 Nowell and Hungerford described a minute chromosome in cultured blood cells of patients having chronic myelocytic leukemia. This chromosome has been called the Philadelphia chromosome, or Ph^1 chromosome (see p. 727 and Fig. 16-20). There are many reports of other chromosomal abnormalities in leukemia: endoreduplication in acute leukemia (Bottura and Ferrari, 1963); 45 chromosomes, including an abnormally large acrocentric chromosome (acute leukemia) (Hungerford and Nowell, 1962); 47 chromosomes, the extra one in the number 7 to 12 group (acute leukemia) (Hungerford and Nowell, 1962); and the presence of the Ph^1 chromosome in erythroid cells in the acute terminal phase of chronic myelocytic leukemia (Trujillo and Ohno, 1963).

Nuclear sex and sex chromatin

The determination of nuclear sex has become a standard laboratory procedure and, although not entirely within the province of hematology, bears on the significance of the sexual dimorphism of leukocytes.

We have already referred to the pioneer work of Barr and several of his associates in describing the presence in females of a chromatin body first called the nucleolar satellite and later the sex chromatin body or Barr body. The sex chromatin usually lies against the nuclear membrane and is about 1 μ in maximum dimension (Figs. 4-46 and 4-47). The outer aspect conforms to the outline of the nuclear membrane; the inner aspect may be round, oval, or pointed. In some cells, notably the nonepithelial cells, the body may lie away from the membrane; it is then round or oval. It is composed of DNA, as evidenced by its staining reaction with the Feulgen, methyl green–pyronine, and ribonuclease-gallocyanin stains. No stain or technic has yet shown any difference between sex chromatin and the other chromatin of the nucleus. The nucleolar chromatin is, of course, different, containing RNA rather than DNA.

In technically good preparations, whether paraffin sections or smears, the number of nuclei containing the sex chromatin in material from a normal female varies from 25% to 50% of the nuclei suitable for counting. The percent of cells showing chromatin bodies may be decreased (1) postpartum, where the incidence of positive cells may be less than 10% during the first 3 days postpartum, (2) in newborn females, also during the first 3 days, and (3) with corticosteroid or estrogen administration. It is accepted that even in the best preparations up to 10% of the nuclei in tissue or cells from a normal female show no visible chromatin body. Sex chromatin is absent from normal male cells, though here again it is accepted that a few cells may contain a typical body.

Chromosomal sex, as determined by the presence of the sex chromatin, is established early in embryonic life, even preceding gonadal differentiation, and remains a stable component of the nucleus. It cannot be changed by castration, administration of hormones, or any other means. Even when, as in the adrenogenital syndrome in females, the body habitus becomes markedly masculine, the nuclear sex chromatin remains unaffected. If the placenta is studied, it is found that the cells on the maternal side are sex chromatin positive, those on the fetal side being chromatin positive or negative, depending on the sex of the fetus. The studies on freemartins are also interesting. Twin births in cattle sometimes result in one normal male, whereas the other is intersexual and sterile and hence useless as a sire. The useless twin is called a freemartin. Although scientifically interesting, to the farmer he is an economic liability. It has long been thought that the freemartin is really a female that, under the influence of male hormones in utero, assumes the male configuration. Moore et al (1955) have indeed shown this assumption to be correct. They were able to demonstrate that cells from the freemartin contain sex chromatin and hence the freemartin is a genetic female. A human parallel to this is the production of pseudohermaphroditism in the female fetus having congenital adrenal hyperplasia or, less commonly, when the mother receives progestinic steroids during pregnancy.

It was originally thought that the chromatin body was derived in equal parts from two X chromosomes. It is now

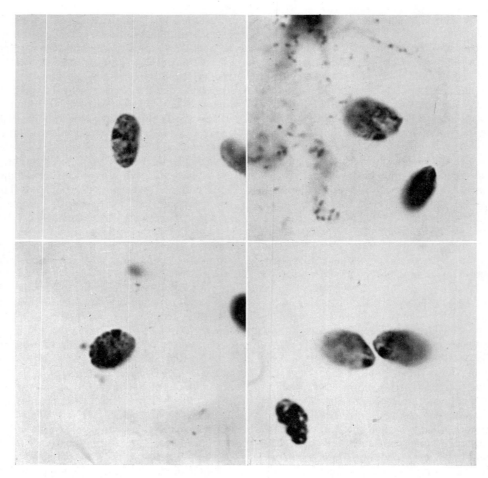

Fig. 4-46. Nuclear sex chromatin, buccal smear. (Hematoxylin-eosin stain.)

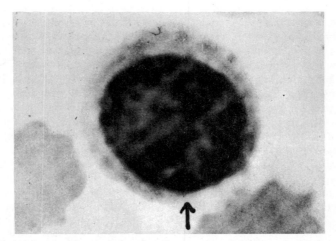

Fig. 4-47. Nuclear sex chromatin in a lymphocyte. (From Murthy and von Haam, 1958.)

Table 4-7. Nuclear, chromosomal, and leukocytic sex patterns in normal and some abnormal states

	Sex chromatin	Chromosomes	Drumsticks
Normal male	Negative	46 (XY)	Absent*
Normal female†	Positive	46 (XX)	Present*
Female pseudohermaphroditism‡	Positive	46 (XX)	Present
Male pseudohermaphroditism§	Negative	46 (XY)	Absent
Gonadal dysgenesis‖	Positive	45XO/46XX	Present
	Negative	45XO/46XY	Absent
	Positive	45XO/47XXX	Present
	Positive	45XO/46XX/ 47XXX	Present
Seminiferous tubule dysgenesis¶	Positive	46XX/47XXY	Present
	Positive	46XY/47XXY	Present
	Positive	48XXXY/49XXXXY	Present
	Negative	46XY/47XXY	Absent
True hermaphroditism#	Negative	45XO/46XY	Absent
	Positive	46XX/47XXX	Present

*See text.

†Two instances of "superfemales" with XXX configuration (and others with XXXX) have been described. Neither was, as a female, the superbly endowed epitome of womanhood of poets and dreamers (male). Rather, one had amenorrhea, underdeveloped breasts, and infantile genitalia. The other was, in addition, mentally defective.

‡Congenital hyperadrenalism, adrenal hyperplasia, or adrenogenital syndrome; maternal virilization during gestation from tumor (arrhenoblastoma) or androgenic therapy.

§Hereditary; thought to be due to a deficiency of male hormone during fetal life; appearance of internal and external sex organs extremely variable. Sex chromatin negative in persons externally female suggests the syndrome of testicular feminization.

‖Gonadal agenesis, ovarian agenesis, Turner's syndrome, or Bonnevie-Ullrich syndrome; confirmed by finding chromatin-negative cells. The presence of chromatin-positive cells does not exclude the diagnosis.

¶Klinefelter's syndrome and variants. Usually chromatin positive.

#Both ovarian and testicular tissue present; more often chromatin positive than negative.

thought that the chromatin body is derived from one entire X chromosome. The number of chromatin bodies is related to the number of X chromosomes (n) by the expression n − 1. Thus, if the patient has a complement of two X chromosomes, one chromatin body is formed. If there are three X chromosomes, two chromatin bodies are formed.

The chromatin body therefore does not truly express genetic sex. Genetic sex is determined by the presence in males and the absence in females of the Y chromosome. In a normal XY male there will be no chromatin body, but in the (abnormal) XXY male there will be a chromatin body. By the same token, a phenotypic female showing no chromatin bodies probably has an XO chromosome pattern. Chromatin body counts should be followed by karyotyping when a complete study is indicated.

By definition, then, we can determine the *nuclear sex* of an individual by the presence or absence of the sex chromatin body. This technic determines only one facet of the sex status of the person being studied, for at least seven variables of sex have been listed (Hampson et al, 1955): (1) chromosomal (nuclear) sex, (2) gonadal sex, (3) hormonal sex, (4) sex according to internal genital organs, (5) sex according to external genital organs, (6) sex of assignment and rearing, and (7) psychosexual sex according to gender and orientation. Gender is used in the sense of "all those things that a person says or does to disclose himself or herself as having the status of a boy or man, girl or woman." A single test, such as would determine whether a person's

nuclei are sex chromatin positive or sex chromatin negative, does not therefore determine in the medicolegal sense whether that person is male or female.

Nuclear sex in normal and abnormal states is shown in Table 4-7, which also summarizes the chromosomal content and leukocytic sex.

The drumstick as a sex characteristic

This finding has been amply confirmed. Artifacts with which the drumstick might be confused have been fully described. The drumstick, characteristically found in 1% to 7% of the polymorphonuclear leukocytes in females, must be distinguished from small clumps and racquets, which are found in both sexes (Fig. 4-48). The sessile nodules are also considered by some investigators to be characteristic of female cells.

Most have agreed with Davidson and Smith (1954) that the drumstick in a leukocyte represents the equivalent of the nuclear sex chromatin in somatic cells. Thus each would be equivalent to an XX chromosome pair. Some sloppiness of terminology is found in the literature because of this assumption; the phrase "sex chromatin in the leukocytes" is commonly used or even "sex chromatin" alone, the text explaining whether this is in the blood or in the somatic cells. It seems to me that Ashley (1957) clearly showed the drumstick to be a structure unrelated to either the nuclear sex chromatin of somatic cells or the XX chromosome pair in every female cell. His opinion was based on the finding of

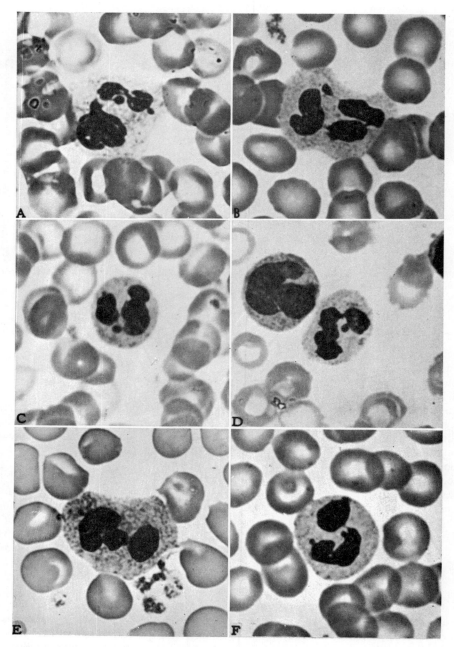

Fig. 4-48. Sexual dimorphism of leukocytes, peripheral blood. **A-C,** Drumsticks. **D-F,** Artifacts. (Wright's stain; ×1,450.)

typical sessile drumsticks in cells that also showed nuclear sex chromatin. If one accepts this, it follows that an additional sexual dimorphism, characteristic of neutrophilic leukocytes, is indicated. To avoid confusion in terminology, this should not be referred to as the sex chromatin in leukocytes. As a matter of fact, a nuclear sex chromatin body can be readily found in blood cells of females. Sex chromatin is usually difficult to distinguish from other aggregates in the dense nucleus of neutrophilic leukocytes, but occasionally is quite obvious. It can be seen in some lymphocytes and more easily in the monocytes (Fig. 4-47). It is remarkable to note the complete agreement between nuclear and leukocytic sexing in both normal and abnormal states. It appears that this dimorphic feature of neutrophilic leukocytes is just as reliable as the nuclear sexing of somatic cells. Furthermore, the pitfalls in distinguishing true drumsticks from artifacts are more easily avoided than those encountered in nuclear sexing, and the preparations are easier to make. A dimorphism independent of chromosomal makeup remains an empiric criterion of sex until an adequate explanation for this nuclear feature can be made.

Our laboratory uses good thin blood smears made by the slide method and stained by the routine Wright method. Fresh capillary blood is used. Oxalated blood may be used, but the number of artifacts increases, and it becomes somewhat difficult to distinguish true drumsticks. Special stains such as Wright-Giemsa, May-Grünwald-Giemsa, or Feulgen have been used but offer no advantages. When stained by the Feulgen technic, both drumsticks and artifacts are Feulgen positive, though artifacts stain less intensely. As is true of nuclear sex chromatin, no known histochemical reaction distinguishes between other nuclear chromatin and the characteristic drumstick.

Given a well-stained thin smear, the criteria for leukocytic sex are sharp and reliable. True drumsticks are always about 1.5 μ in diameter and are easily visible at a magnification of ×90. The dense bulbous end is joined to the nucleus by a very thin filament, presumably composed only of nuclear membrane. No more than one drumstick to a cell has ever been found. Drumsticks occur only in neutrophilic and eosinophilic leukocytes, not only adult polymorphonuclears but also stab forms and metamyelocytes.

According to the criteria of Davidson and Smith (1954), drumsticks are found in 1% to 7% of the segmented neutrophils in females and in less than 1% of the neutrophils in males. Accumulated data show a wider normal range for normal females, from 0.2% (1 in 500 leukocytes, polymorphonuclears, stabs, and metamyelocytes) to 8%. In one instance as many as 17.8% of neutrophils contained drumsticks. Quite positive but contradictory opinions are recorded about the frequency of true drumsticks in leukocytes of the normal male. Some authors say they are never found, and others say that they do occur in small number. I have seen structures I thought to be typical drumsticks in smears from men, but since data on their reproductive history and nuclear sex are lacking, this observation does not necessarily cast doubt on the reliability of this feature. Since this is a rare finding (no drumsticks were seen in hundreds of others smears from men), it is also possible that it represents an undiscovered problem of intersex. This has not, to my

knowledge, been investigated. Another interesting possibility is suggested by Davidson et al (1958), who found that in dissimilar twins there may be drumstick-positive leukocytes in the blood of the male twin. They explain this chimera, also occurring as serologically dissimilar erythrocytes, as an exchange of hemopoietic elements between the twins, possibly in both directions.

The artifacts to be distinguished from drumsticks present no great problem after some experience has been gained. Nuclear tags, small clumps, or small clubs may also be joined to the nucleus by a thin filament but are much smaller than the drumsticks. The racquet artifact is as large as a drumstick but instead of being solid shows a hollow or pale-staining center. In hypersegmented neutrophils one sometimes sees accessory lobes of nuclear material. These are usually larger and more irregular than drumsticks but are not infrequently joined to other nuclear material by two filaments. I agree with several authors who state that the sessile nodule (a nuclear appendage the same size as a drumstick but attached to the nucleus by a broad base rather than a filament) should be considered an artifact but that it does not occur in blood cells from males. This is of some practical importance, the finding of one or more sessile nodules suggesting that the search for typical drumsticks should be continued beyond the usual limit of counting 500 leukocytes.

MORPHOLOGY OF BLOOD AND BONE MARROW CELLS WITH SPECIAL TECHNICS

Although diagnosis in hematology has been and will continue to be based primarily on the standard technics of Romanowsky staining of films and hematoxylin-eosin staining of paraffin-embedded tissue, the special technics of supravital staining, phase contrast microscopy, electron microscopy, and cytochemistry have each contributed to the understanding of the structure and function of blood cells.

The technics of cytochemistry are currently the most useful, although studies on the ultrastructure of blood cells by electron microscopy are equally exciting. In both areas interesting developments are to be expected. Supravital staining and phase microscopy have been thoroughly explored and fall into the category of near-standard technics.

Supravital methods
General considerations

The historical observations made by Sabin et al (1925) on the supravital characteristics of blood cells demonstrated the usefulness of this technic and, in fact, led these authors to draw certain conclusions as to the derivation of blood cells. The resulting theory of blood cell derivation has not received uniform acceptance. The supravital method, however, has survived as an important tool in hematology. Its chief virtue is the study of blood cells in a living state, in some cases providing differential features not apparent in fixed and stained smears.

Many advances were made possible by this method, particularly in the study of monocytic and phagocytic cells. Because it did not allow a clear differentiation between normoblasts and megaloblasts, some concluded that these cells were identical, thus supporting an erroneous concept. Such a shortcoming should not entirely condemn the method. Adverse criticism carried too far has at times overshadowed the many advantages of the supravital method.

ADVANTAGES OF METHOD. I do not urge the use of the supravital method as a routine procedure for the study of blood and bone marrow cells. I do believe that it is a helpful method in studying cells of doubtful morphology on stained smears. In my experience it has been most useful in the identification of monocytes, in the diagnosis of monocytic leukemia, and in the differentiation of lymphocytes from micromyeloblasts. I agree that the method is not suitable for the routine study of normal and abnormal erythropoiesis and that stained dried smears are superior for this purpose. It is recommended for studying imprints from lymph nodes and other tissues. Finally, it is often applicable to special hematologic problems. I used this method to study the mononuclear response following the administration of antispleen serum to dogs. In these studies the cells found in the peripheral blood were extremely difficult to identify in Wright-stained smears, but by the supravital method were found to have features common to both lymphocytes and monocytes.

TECHNICAL CONSIDERATIONS. The care taken in making a preparation and the quality and adjustment of the optical system have a great deal to do with obtaining satisfactory results. It is essential that the microscope be adjusted so that Köhler illumination is achieved. This depends on the use of a field diaphragm as well as of an adjustable condenser. In microscopes equipped with substage mirrors it is preferable to use the flat side of a surface-coated mirror. It is also best to work in a darkened room. Above all, the preparations must be thin, and the cells must be well separated. As just mentioned, it is not necessary to use a warm stage. As a matter of fact, the preparations are useful for a longer time at room temperature, since the cells remain well preserved for 1 to 2 hours. Extra preparations may be kept at refrigerator temperature to retard cellular degeneration for an even longer period.

VITAL STAINING PLUS PHASE CONTRAST. In 1955 Ackerman and Bellios published two articles on the morphology of blood and bone marrow cells in vital films when viewed with the phase microscope. This combination of vital staining and phase microscopy is superior.

Phase contrast microscopy
General considerations

The development of good and relatively inexpensive phase equipment has provided the hematologist with yet another means of studying blood cells. Prior to this development, two types of illumination were used. In the first, the light was simply reduced by shutting down the substage diaphragm or lowering the condenser; in the second, illumination was by dark field. Both of these revealed somewhat more of the structure of the cell than standard bright-field illumination. However, the loss in resolving power of the objective results in an image that is not sharp and is further obscured by diffraction. Dark-field illumination provides a sharper image. One sees clearly the tiny platelets, the ameboid movement of cells, and intercellular reactions such as phagocytosis and agglutination. However, little more than the specific granules of the cells can be distinguished.

Phase microscopy, on the other hand, intensifies relatively minute differences in optical density and allows one to see the intimate details of cells and cytoplasmic structures. The chromatin of the nucleus, the mitochondria, the centrosome, and specific granules of the cytoplasm are all clearly visible in the living unstained and undamaged cell. Platelets are seen so distinctly with this illumination that they can be counted directly in a special counting chamber.

Phase contrast microscopy depends on two optical principles: (1) light waves out of phase cancel each other entirely or partially, depending on whether they are of the same or different amplitudes, and (2) the speed of light passing through a substance varies with the refractive index of the substance. The chief features of a phase microscope (Fig. 4-49) are the following. Instead of the usual Abbe condenser used in standard microscopes there is a special phase condenser containing an annular diaphragm below the lowermost lens, which transmits light only around the annulus at the circumference, the center being blacked out. Phase objectives are also different; a ring of fine film is applied at

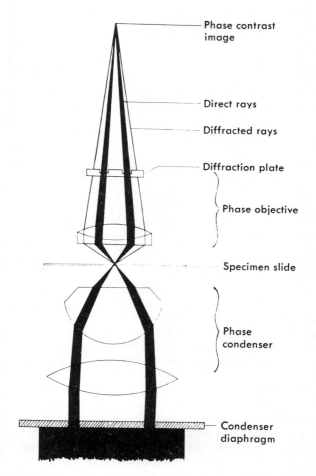

Fig. 4-49. Optics of phase microscopy (schematic). The phase contrast image is produced by two superimposed light wave systems, not in phase with each other, so that minute differences in optical density are intensified. The objective in a phase system acts essentially as a diffraction grating, whereas the position of the phase condenser determines the degree of phase contrast.

the rear focal plane, either on a separate disk or directly on the surface of the rear lens. This film acts as diffraction grating, the light passing through it being thrown out of phase. When the phase optical system is viewed through the special centering eyepiece, the phase-shifting annular film of the objective appears black, whereas the image of the condenser annulus is bright. When the two rings are exactly concentric and superimposed, the optical system is such that light rays, diffracted but little while passing through a specimen, are out of phase by one-fourth of a wavelength with rays that are diffracted more and that pass chiefly through the center of the objective. That portion of the specimen that is a greater impediment to light waves because of greater thickness or diffraction is seen as a dark structure against the lighter background made by areas that diffract light waves less. Differences are thus markedly accentuated. Structures invisible by standard microscopy because they differ little from adjacent areas in refraction thus become clearly delineated. In standard microscopy, differential staining is used to bring out such structures, but at the expense of killing the cell and subjecting its components to harsh chemical insults. With phase microscopy, on the other hand, the living and undistorted cell can be examined. The experience of looking at living cells and distinguishing minute structural details is an exciting one.

Time-lapse photography

It might be interesting to mention some of the observations made by Bessis and Bricka (1952), who have studied cells with cinematography, or time-lapse photography. Living neutrophils so studied have revealed some features not apparent with other technics. One of these is the hyaloplasmic veil at the periphery of the cell, which is clearly visible during the process of locomotion and ingestion of foreign particles. Bessis recorded erythrophagocytosis in a film in which one remarkable sequence shows an erythrocyte partially ingested by a neutrophil, one portion being taken into the cell while the other is discarded. Three other phenomena are quite easily studied by this method. One is the spreading phenomenon, in which granulocytes and monocytes spread on surfaces and become greatly flattened. The cell then becomes immobile, and the fine internal structure can be seen very clearly. Another is that of the movements of intracytoplasmic structures, the most remarkable being that of the centrosome. This structure moves rather rapidly around the circumference of the nucleus, which appears to be indented by its adjacent centrosome. The specific granules seem to follow the centrosome, so that there is always a concentration of granules around it regardless of its position. Bessis estimated the amplitude of the movement to be from 5 to 10 μ and its occurrence to be approximately every 30 seconds. The type of movement that the entire cell exhibits can also be recorded. Each type of blood cell has a characteristic movement and assumes a characteristic shape. Myeloblasts have a wormlike movement; lymphoblasts and lymphocytes take on a hand-mirror form; monocytes show broad pseudopods, with a terminal, irregular cauliflower-like fringe. Finally, as the preparations age, all the stages of cellular degeneration can be studied, such as frangmentation, karyolysis, pyknosis, the formation of bullae, and vacuolization.

Electron microscopy
General considerations

Whereas images obtained by phase contrast microscopy are due to different optical densities of the cell structures with respect to the passage of light out of phase, those obtained with the electron microscope are caused by differences in density to the passage of electrons. When ultrathin (0.02 to 0.03 μ) sections are studied by electron microscopy, a very high degree of resolution is made possible—2 to 3 mμ as compared to the optimum resolving power of the standard microscope, 0.2 μ. Thus the resolving power of the electron microscope approaches that needed to visualize monolayers of macromolecules.

In revealing the ultrastructure of cells, the electron microscope has provided an unprecedented look at the fine anatomy of cell structure as well as a better understanding of the relationship between structure and function; e.g., Braunsteiner and Pakesch (1955) investigated the changes occurring in thyroid cells stimulated by thyrotropic hormone and found that the appearance of fine, tortuous filaments (*secretory lamellae*) parallels the increase in secretory activity of the cell. They also found that, of all the blood cells, the plasma cell is the only one that shows a similar lamellar structure. The lamellae are composed of two layers, approximately 200 Å thick, separated by a clear space of 200 to 300 Å. If, as it seems, the lamellae reflect secretory activity, this ultrastructural feature of plasma cells is consistent with the view that plasma cells elaborate globulin proteins. Another example of the relationship between ultrastructure and cell physiology is provided by studies of the erythrocyte membrane. By electron microscopy this has been shown to have evenly spaced depressions that may correspond to immunologically specific loci and to the sites at which antigen-antibody reactions take place.

Perhaps the greatest disappointment so far has been the inability of the electron microscope to reveal the etiologic agent of human leukemia. To those who are convinced of the viral etiology of human leukemia this is an almost personal affront. The failure to identify an intracellular virus does not, of course, settle anything, for it is possible for such viral particles to have the same density to the searching electron stream as other protein particles normally present in cells. Nor can it be assumed that every leukemic cell would be uniformly infected with the virus, since even the known virus sarcoma may have the infective agent present in only 1% of the cells. Also, the virus particles are not necessarily found within leukemic cells. Some investigators have even suggested that submicroscopic particles found free in the plasma of persons having leukemia may represent the infectious agent in this disease.

Ultrastructure of a blood cell

The ultrastructural composite features of blood cells are shown in Fig. 4-50 and in the illustrations that follow. For more detailed descriptions refer to Low and Freeman (1958) and Bessis (1973b).

The nucleus appears very much the same as in phase contrast images. It is denser and darker than the remainder of the cell, the density increasing in older cells as the chromatin condenses. The internal structure is a confused network of chromatin strands with no obvious organization. The

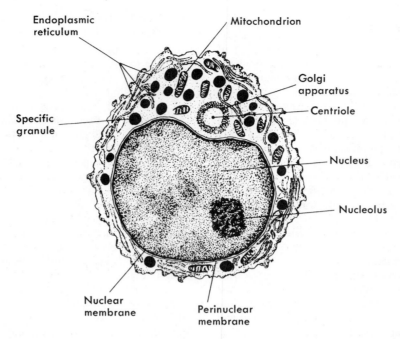

Fig. 4-50. Diagram of the ultrastructure of a blood cell, in this case a neutrophilic myelocyte.

nucleus is surrounded by a dense *nuclear membrane,* enveloped in turn by an extremely delicate *external membrane.* The space between the two membranes, the *perinuclear space,* connects with the cytoplasmic matrix and contains cytoplasmic rather than nuclear material. The nucleolus presents as a dark granular or netlike structure.

The matrix of the cytoplasm is a reticular network of flattened bags or canals, and this network is called the *endoplasmic reticulum* (Fig. 4-51). This structure is found in all cells except the mature erythrocyte. It is abundant in young cells, where it takes the form of flattened parallel lamellae. In older cells it is sparse and presents as isolated bags. The endoplasmic reticulum has been likened to a network of canals, defined at one end by the cytoplasmic membrane and at the other end by the perinuclear space. The *granules of Palade* are minute (100 to 200 Å, 10 to 20 nm) granules adhering to the external surface between the canals. They are electron dense and therefore dark in photographs and may represent units of riboprotein.

On electron microscopy the mitochondria are seen to have a complex structure. They are rounded, oval, or elongated, depending on the type of cell (Figs. 4-52 to 4-55, 4-60, 4-61, 4-65 and 4-67). Each mitochondrion is limited by a membrane, 10 to 25 mμ thick, which then extends toward the interior in the form of *cristae* appearing sometimes villous, sometimes lamellar. When greatly magnified, the outer membrane and the cristae are seen to consist of two layers each about 8 mμ thick and separated by a space about 5 mμ wide. In the matrix of the mitochondrion one sees small (2 to 3 mμ) granules.

The granules of leukocytes are striking and characteristic for each type of granulocyte. The nonspecific (undifferentiated) granules of early myeloid cells, staining deeply azurophilic with Romanowsky stains, are round, rather homo-geneous, and usually larger and paler than the specific granules (Fig. 4-55). Neutrophilic granules are smaller, denser, and slightly elongated (Figs. 4-52, 4-56 and 4-57). Basophilic granules are large, very dense, and homogeneous (Figs. 4-53 and 4-59). Eosinophilic granules differ from the others in that they contain dense crystalloid inclusions (Figs. 4-52 and 4-58). They vary in size and shape but are generally rectangular or trapezoidal.

Normal blood cells

GRANULOCYTES. The ultrastructure of granulocytes has been extensively investigated and the maturation sequence well established.

The *myeloblast* (Fig. 4-54) is characterized by prominent masses of nucleolar material, a finely granular cytoplasm with minimally developed endoplasmic reticulum, and small swollen mitochondria. There are no cytoplasmic granules.

In the *progranulocyte* the cytoplasm contains nonspecific granules that are round, of medium density, homogeneous, and surrounded by a thin membrane. The nucleus is slightly denser than that of the myeloblast, with some coarsening of chromatin around the periphery.

The *myelocyte* (Fig. 4-55) shows further condensation of nuclear material. Depending on the degree of maturation, there are many or few nonspecific granules, fewer as the number of differentiated granules in the cytoplasm increases. The endoplasmic reticulum is abundant, but mitochondria are few and filamentous.

Metamyelocytes (Fig. 4-56) show the predicted changes in nuclear shape and chromatin clumping. The granules, almost all of the specific type, fill the cytoplasm. Mitochondria are sparse.

Band and *segmented forms* (Fig. 4-57) show the granules

Text continued on p. 192.

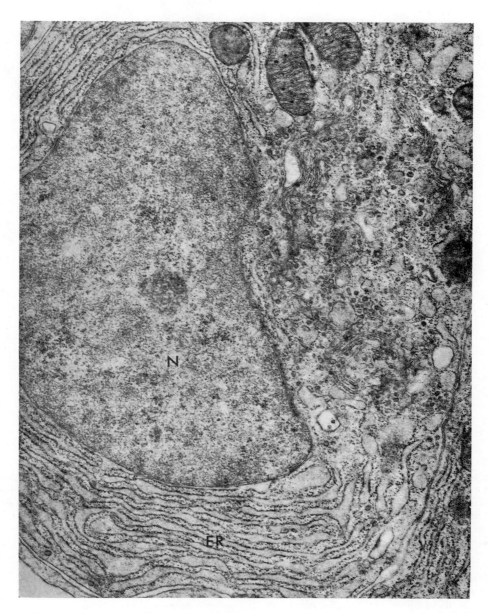

Fig. 4-51. Endoplasmic reticulum. The granules of Palade are seen as granular condensations on the endoplasmic reticulum. The cell illustrated here is a normal plasma cell. **N,** Nucleus; **ER,** endoplasmic reticulum. (Electron photomicrograph.) (Courtesy Dr. George D. Sorenson.)

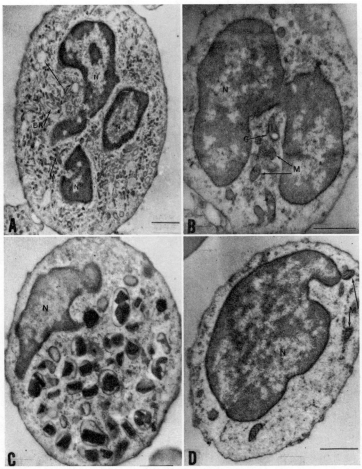

Fig. 4-52. Electron photomicrographs of blood cells. Length of black line = 1 μ. **A,** This normal neutrophil shows three lobes of the nucleus, **N,** and many cytoplasmic granules. A long rodlike mitochondrion at **M** has indistinct cristae. Light granules with a denser periphery are the endoplasmic reticulum of Palade, **ER.** The larger pale areas are more truly vesicular in nature, **V.** There are also many smaller granules of varying density. The whole is embedded in a matrix of very fine grained cytoplasmic protein. A portion of a platelet is in the lower left corner. **B,** This is a normal monocyte. The nuclear cytoplasmic ratio is lower than in the lymphocytes. There is also a distinct Golgi structure, **G,** in the hof of the nucleus, **N;** the double membrane of the nucleus is quite evident. **C,** This is a normal eosinophil, with its nucleus, **N,** in the upper left portion. The many cytoplasmic granules with the dense inclusions are the eosinophilic structures that characterize this cell type. Some granules have multiple inclusions and show greater variety of form than in rat and guinea pig eosinophils. No mitochondria are present in this cut; however, they have been seen in other human cells and resemble those seen in the neutrophil. **D,** This normal lymphocyte has a large nucleus, **N,** and a few large conspicuous mitochondria, **M,** with well-defined cristae. Frequently lymphocytes show even less cytoplasm. The cytoplasm has very few granules other than mitochondria. The nuclear wall is a double membrane like those of the granulocytic series. (From Goodman et al, 1957.)

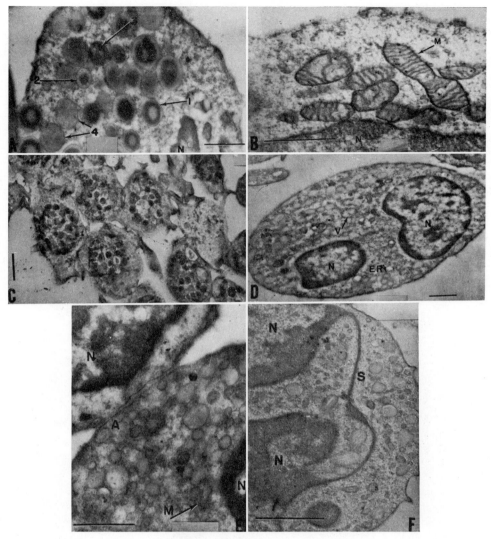

Fig. 4-53. Electron photomicrographs of blood cells. Length of black line = 1 μ. **A,** This is a portion of a basophil's cytoplasm from a patient with myelocytic leukemia (13% basophils in peripheral blood). The tip of a nuclear lobe is seen at **N.** All large basophil granules are round or slightly ovoid. There are at least two and perhaps three types of these large granules. Those with the ring of dense material and a light central core are shown at arrow **1.** The arrangement at arrow **2** is a cut through one end of the hollow-ball type. The mottled core type as shown at arrow **3** may be another version of the dense inclusion-type granule. There is a group of granules that are more vesicular (arrow **4**). These are apparently completely lacking in the denser material and in general appear structureless. All these large granules have a double-walled peripheral membrane. **B,** This portion of a lymphocyte shows the large mitochondria, **M,** and the well-developed cristae system. The cell nucleus, **N,** is at the bottom. **C,** These are a group of platelets showing fairly uniform dense granules. A few vesicles and spicules are also present. **D,** This is another normal neutrophil with two nuclear lobes, **N,** and a fairly extensive distribution of endoplasmic reticulum, **ER,** with a few vesicles and smaller granules, but apparently no mitochondria. The double wall of the nucleus is apparent in the larger lobe in the original print. **E,** Portion of a normal neutrophil on the right is in close apposition to a lymphocyte in the upper left. This shows clearly the sharpening of the outer cell wall at point of contact with another cell. The thickness of the membrane at **A** was measured with an ocular micrometer and found to be 80 Å. A portion of the nucleus, **N,** of each cell is present. A portion of a mitochondrion, **M,** is present in the neutrophil. **F,** This is a portion of the strand, **S,** connecting two lobes of the nucleus, **N.** The double-walled nature of the nuclear membrane can be seen, and at higher magnifications it becomes apparent that the dense nuclear material is continuous the full length of the strand. The scalloped nature of the cell surface is also evident. (From Goodman et al, 1957.)

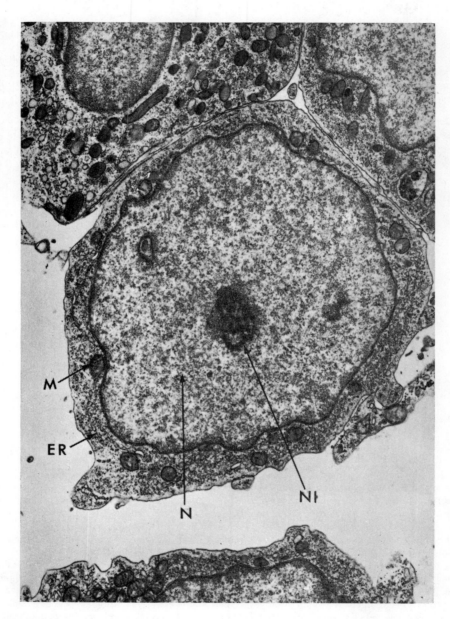

Fig. 4-54. Myeloblast. **NI,** Nucleolus; **N,** nucleus; **ER,** endoplasmic reticulum; **M,** mitochondrion. (Electron photomicrograph.) (Courtesy Dr. James A. Freeman.)

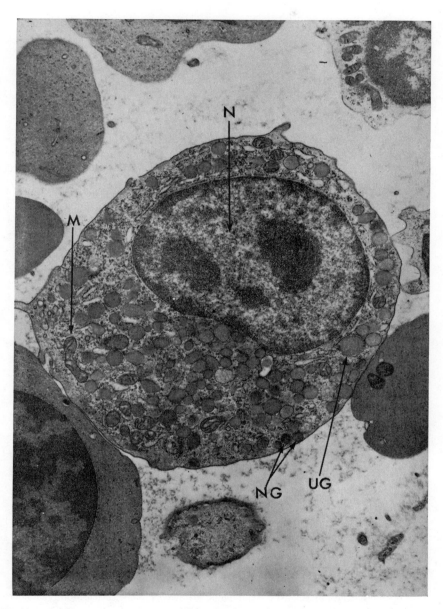

Fig. 4-55. Neutrophilic myelocyte. **UG,** Undifferentiated granule; **NG,** neutrophilic granule; **N,** nucleus; **M,** mitochondrion. (Electron photomicrograph.) (Courtesy Dr. James A. Freeman.)

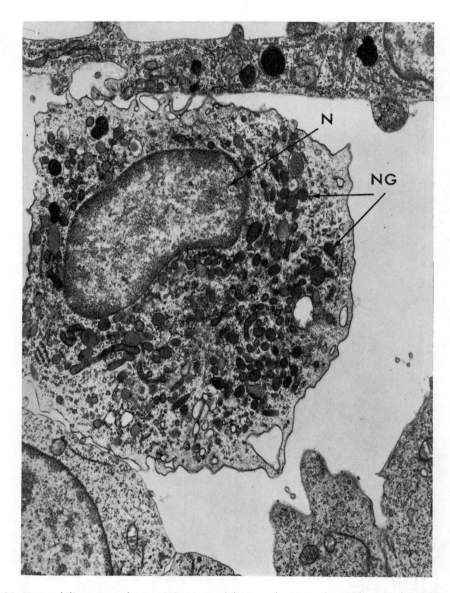

Fig. 4-56. Neutrophilic metamyelocyte. **NG,** Neutrophilic granule; **N,** nucleus. (Electron photomicrograph.) (Courtesy Dr. James A. Freeman.)

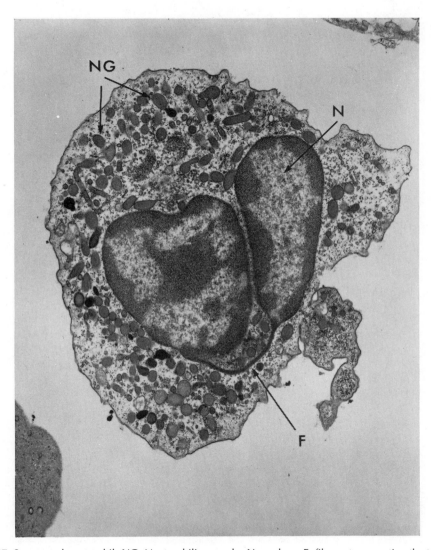

Fig. 4-57. Segmented neutrophil. **NG,** Neutrophilic granule; **N,** nucleus; **F,** filament connecting the two lobes. (Electron photomicrograph.) (Courtesy Dr. James A. Freeman.)

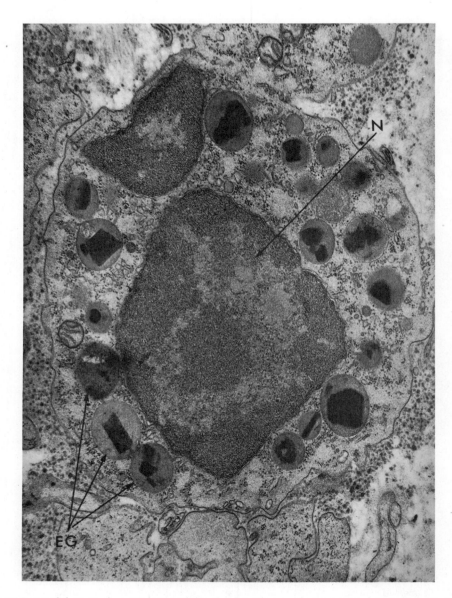

Fig. 4-58. Eosinophil. **N,** Nucleus; **EG,** eosinophilic granules. (Electron photomicrograph.) (Courtesy Dr. James A. Freeman.)

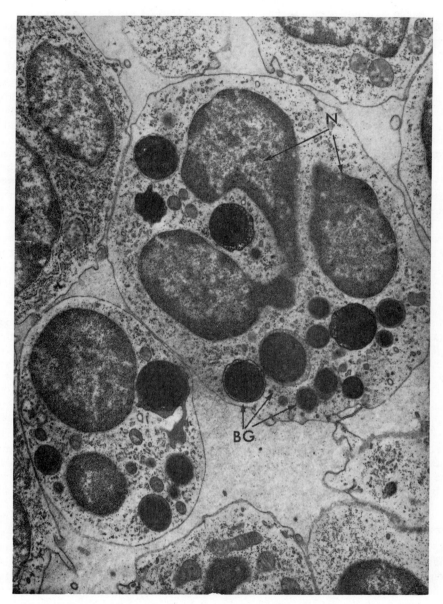

Fig. 4-59. Basophils (from dog thoracic duct). **BG,** Basophilic granules; **N,** nucleus. (Electron photomicrograph.) (Courtesy Dr. James A. Freeman.)

characteristic for each cell type. In the illustrated segmented neutrophil the filament is clearly seen to be made up of nuclear membrane only. An eosinophil is illustrated in Fig. 4-58, and a basophil in Fig. 4-59.

MONOCYTES. The ultrastructure of the cells of this series has been described by several authors. The pale vesicular nucleus seen in ordinary smears has its counterpart in the pale and delicate indented structure seen by electron microscopy (Figs. 4-52, 4-62, and 4-63). The cytoplasm contains small granules that are fewer and smaller than those of granulocytes. Mitochondria are numerous and smaller than in granulocytes.

LYMPHOCYTES. The nucleus is round, seldom indented, and has fine reticular chromatin. The cytoplasm is usually less dense than in other leukocytes. A few small electron-dense granules are sometimes present. The mitochondria are round or oval, smaller, and paler than those of granulocytes. In general the cytoplasm contains fewer structures than that of other cell types (Figs. 4-52 and 4-65).

PLASMA CELLS. The cytoplasm is characterized by a very abundant endoplasmic reticulum that assumes the configuration of parallel lamellae (Figs. 4-63 and 4-66 to 4-69). The mitochondria are large, with prominent cristae. The nucleus shows coarse chromatin clumping.

MEGAKARYOCYTES AND PLATELETS. The cytoplasm of the megakaryocyte has, in addition to endoplasmic reticulum and small mitochondria, many homogeneous granules that, when particles of cytoplasm are shed, become the circulating blood platelet. Characteristically, the surface of the cell often shows blebs that do not contain cytoplasmic organelles. From various descriptions of megakaryocytes it seems obvious that the different appearances recorded reflect different degrees of cellular activity. The intact circulating platelet shows distinct zones (Fig. 4-53); when altered by adhesion to a foreign surface or after treatment with thrombin, platelets assume bizarre stellate shapes.

NORMOBLASTS. The chief feature distinguishing normoblasts from other cells is the greater electron density of the cytoplasm that accompanies the elaboration of hemoglobin in the cell (Fig. 4-60). The nucleus is generally coarse, resembling that of the lymphocyte. Fortuitous sectioning sometimes reveals the process of nuclear extrusion to form a nonnucleated erythrocyte (Fig. 4-61).

Ultrastructure of abnormal blood cells

LEUKEMIC CELLS. In blast forms and progranulocytes several investigators have found a characteristic perinuclear structure that has been called the *crescentic zone* or the fibrillar formation. When fully developed, it consists of a barrel-shaped fibrillar formation enclosing electron-dense granular material. No other ultramicroscopic feature has so far been reported that might be said to differentiate leukemic from normal cells. Leukemic cells show variable swelling of the endoplasmic reticulum. The mitochondria of leukemic cells often appear swollen and larger than in the corresponding normal cell.

In myelocytic, monocytic, and myelomonocytic leukemia and in multiple myeloma, Auer bodies (p. 157) are sometimes encountered. By electron microscopy (Fig. 4-62) these have been shown to be made up of laminated, homogeneous, crystalline plaques parallel to the long axis of the Auer body. A monoblast from acute monocytic leukemia is shown in Fig. 4-63. Myelomonocytic cells are shown in Fig. 4-64, and here the mixture of monocytoid nuclear structure and myelocytic cytoplasm is well shown. Small lymphocytes in chronic lymphocytic leukemia are illustrated in Fig. 4-65.

PLASMA CELLS IN MYELOMA. The ultrastructure of myeloma cells clearly shows these to be plasma cells having exaggerated features, and thus there is additional evidence for not considering the myeloma cell a separate cell type. In any given case myeloma cells are similar, but they can differ appreciably from case to case; this has long been recognized to be true on the basis of routine stains. The nucleolar formation is generally very prominent; the endoplasmic reticulum is very striking, pleomorphic, and has prominent granules of Palade (Figs. 4-66 and 4-67). The mitochondria are normal or increased in number; sometimes they are quite elongated and bizarre. Occasionally the ergastoplasmic sacs are distended, presumably by abnormal globulin synthesis and accumulation (Fig. 4-68). When condensed in certain areas, homogeneous *Russell bodies* are formed (Fig. 4-69).

PHAGOCYTIC HISTIOCYTES. Phagocytic histiocytes (Fig. 4-70) show the typical vesicular nucleus of the reticulum cell. The cytoplasm contains a variety of debris and sometimes erythrocytes and nuclear fragments.

GAUCHER CELLS. Gaucher cells are quite spectacular by ordinary microscopy, but are even more so by electron microscopy. The cell, a histiocyte, becomes engorged with cerebroside. It is this ingested lipid that gives the Gaucher cell the foamy appearance seen in Wright-stained smears. As shown by electron microscopy, the cytoplasm contains numerous irregular, spindle-shaped structures varying greatly in size but generally 700 to 800 mμ in length (Fig. 4-71). Inside the spindles there are small branching tubular structures that average 32 mμ in diameter. It is assumed that this peculiar formation is that assumed by cerebroside after it enters the histiocyte. It is of interest, also, that this structural feature of the Gaucher cell is said to be different from the ultrastructure of xanthoma cells and the histiocytes in Tay-Sachs disease, adult hereditary cerebromacular degeneration, and Niemann-Pick disease.

PELGER-HUËT ANOMALY. The cells shown in Fig. 4-72 are from a patient with the homozygous anomaly. Electron microscopy shows that the nuclear abnormality is not limited to neutrophils and other leukocytes but is found in all hemopoietic cells, including megakaryocytes, plasma cells, and normoblasts. The abnormality of the nucleus lies in evaginations of both the nuclear and perinuclear membrane to form club-shaped extrusions into which nuclear "sap" but no chromatin extends. There is no demonstrable abnormality of cytoplasmic structure.

MAY-HEGGLIN ANOMALY. Neutrophils showing the May-Hegglin anomaly have been studied by electron microscopy (Fig. 4-34). The Döhle bodies seem to be composed of patches of fibrils, presumably RNA fibrils. Platelets have been shown to have a normal ultrastructure when in a fresh and unmodified state. When the release reaction begins, the ultrastructure becomes abnormal.

Text continued on p. 206.

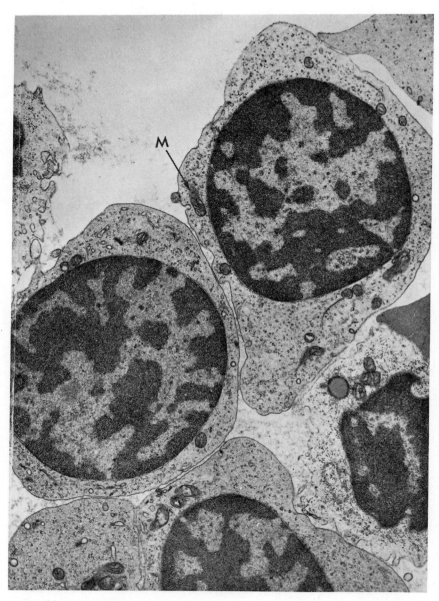

Fig. 4-60. Normoblasts, intermediate in development, probably polychromatophilic. **M,** mitochondrion. (Electron photomicrograph.) (Courtesy Dr. James A. Freeman.)

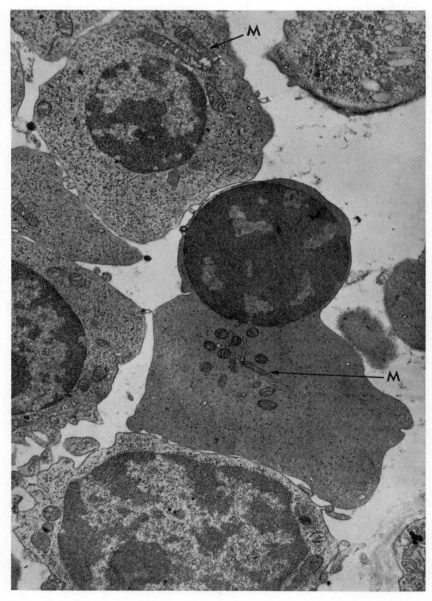

Fig. 4-61. Orthochromic normoblast extruding its nucleus. **M,** Mitrochondrion. (Electron photomicrograph.) (Courtesy Dr. James A. Freeman.)

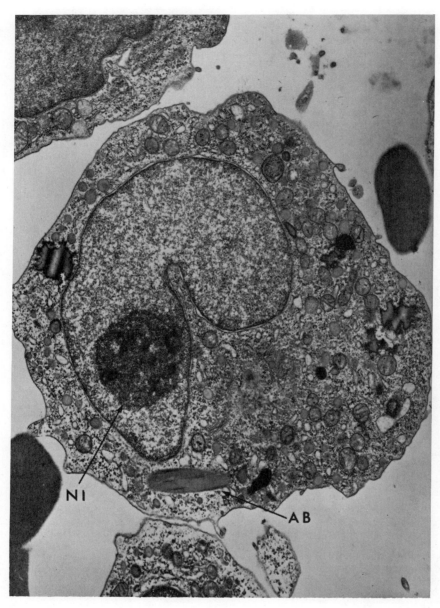

Fig. 4-62. Monoblast with Auer body. **AB,** Auer body; **NI,** nucleolus. (Electron photomicrograph.) (Courtesy Dr. James A. Freeman.)

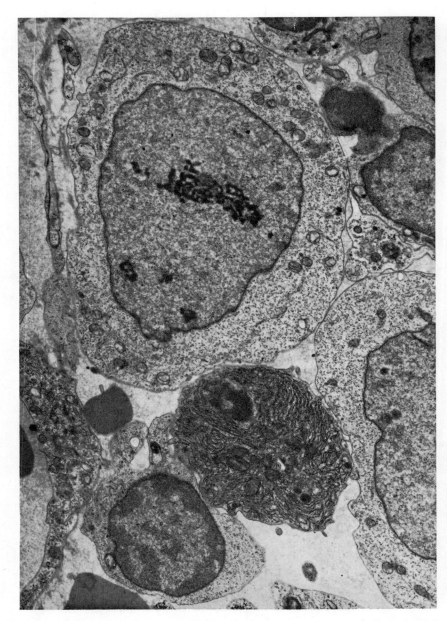

Fig. 4-63. Monoblast (above) and plasma cell (below). (Electron photomicrograph.) (Courtesy Dr. James A. Freeman.)

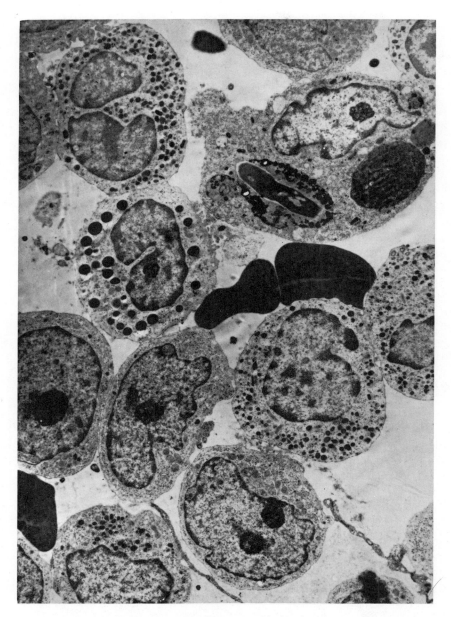

Fig. 4-64. Chronic myelomonocytic leukemia. Cell at upper right-hand corner is a phagocytic histiocyte containing an ingested erythrocyte. (Electron photomicrograph.) (Courtesy Dr. James A. Freeman.)

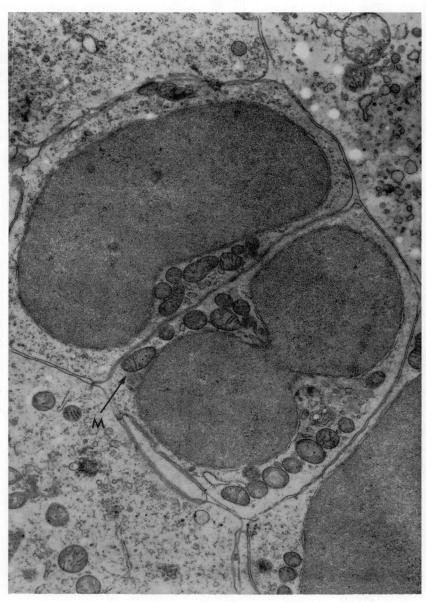

Fig. 4-65. Lymphocytes, chronic lymphocytic leukemia. **M,** Mitochondrion. (Electron photomicrograph.) (Courtesy Dr. James A. Freeman.)

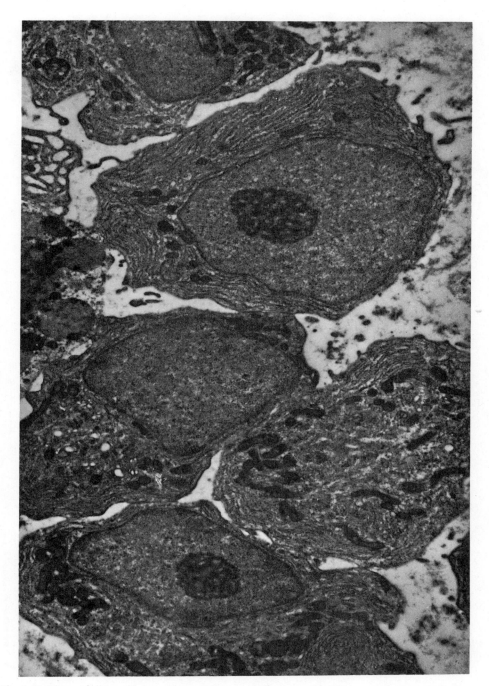

Fig. 4-66. Plasma cells, multiple myeloma. (Electron photomicrograph.) (Courtesy Dr. George D. Sorenson.)

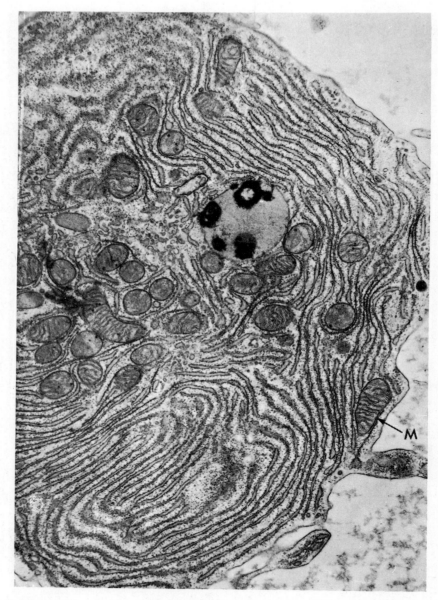

Fig. 4-67. Plasma cell, multiple myeloma. **M,** Mitochondrion. The prominent endoplasmic reticulum is shown beautifully. (Electron photomicrograph.) (Courtesy Dr. James A. Freeman.)

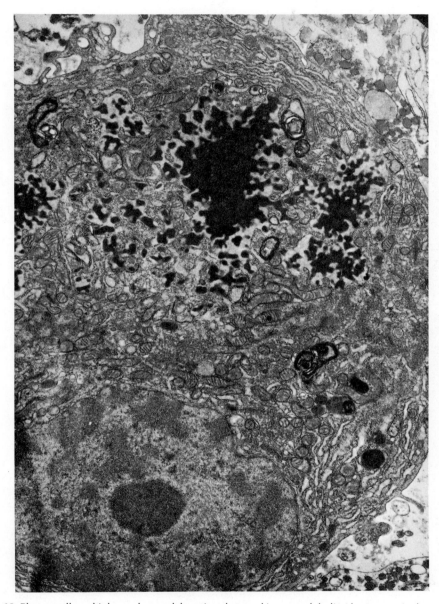

Fig. 4-68. Plasma cell, multiple myeloma, elaborating abnormal immunoglobulin (dense areas in the cytoplasm). (Electron photomicrograph.) (Courtesy Dr. James A. Freeman.)

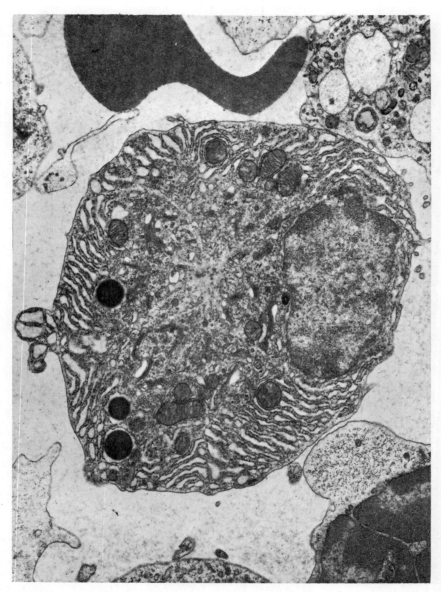

Fig. 4-69. Plasma cell, multiple myeloma, containing Russell bodies. (Electron photomicrograph.) (Courtesy Dr. James A. Freeman.)

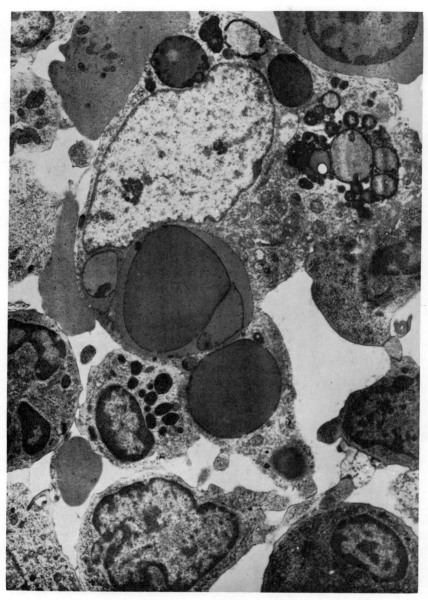

Fig. 4-70. Phagocytic histiocyte, bone marrow, containing ingested erythrocytes. (Electron photomicrograph.) (Courtesy Dr. James A. Freeman.)

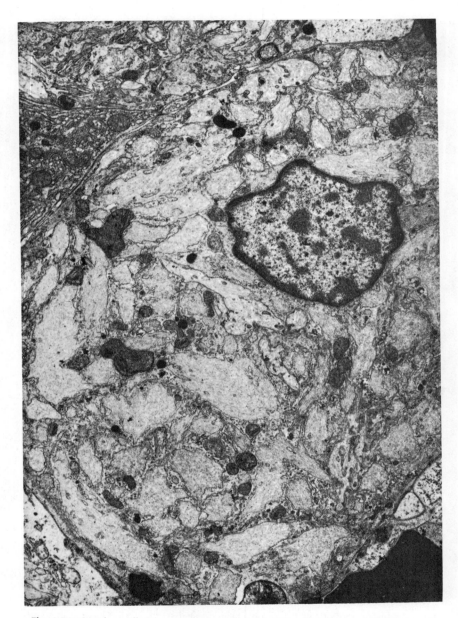

Fig. 4-71. Gaucher cell. (Electron photomicrograph.) (Courtesy Dr. James A. Freeman.)

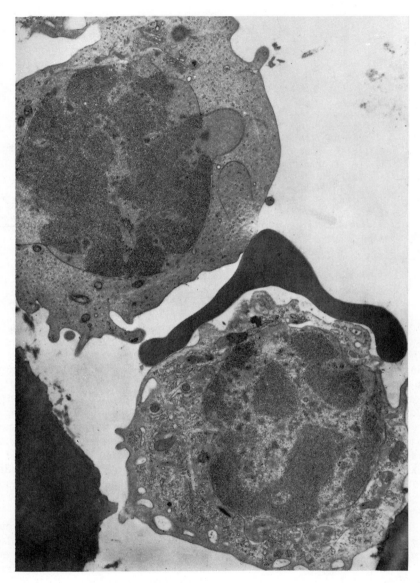

Fig. 4-72. Pelger-Huët anomaly (homozygous), bone marrow. Normoblast (above) and granulocyte (below). (Electron photomicrograph.) (Courtesy Dr. James A. Freeman.)

Table 4-8. Cytochemical reactions in normal and abnormal blood cells

Cell	Peroxidase	Sudan	PAS	Alkaline phosphatase
Normal				
Myeloblast	Neg.	Neg.	Neg.	Neg.
Progranulocyte	++++	++++	++	±
Myelocyte	++++	++++	++++	±
Metamyelocyte	++++	++++	++++	+
Adult neutrophil	++++	++++	++++	+ to ++++
Eosinophil	++++	++++	Neg. to +	Neg.
Basophil	Neg.	++++	Neg. to +	Neg.
Lymphocyte	Neg.	Neg.	Neg.[a]	Neg.
Monocyte	± to ++	± to +	± to +	Neg.
Megakaryocyte	Neg.	±	++++	Neg.
Platelet	Neg.	±	++++	Neg.
Normoblast	Neg.	Neg.	Neg.	Neg.
Abnormal				
Leukemic lymphoblast	Neg.	Neg.	+ to +++[b]	Neg.
Myelomonocytic cell	Neg. to +++[c]	Neg. to +++[c]	Neg. to +++[c]	Neg.
Monocytic (histiocytic) leukemic cell	Neg. to ±	Neg. to ±[c]	Neg. to +	Neg.
Leukemic myeloblast	Neg.	Neg.[d]	±	Neg.
Erythroleukemic cell	Neg.	Neg.	+++	Neg.
Lymphocyte in chronic lymphocytic leukemia	Neg.	Neg.	+ to ++	Neg.
Auer bodies	++++	++++	Neg.	Neg.

[a]A few normal lymphocytes may show fine to medium-sized PAS-positive inclusions.
[b]PAS-positive inclusions are coarse.
[c]Varies with maturity; blasts are negative, whereas more mature cells are positive.
[d]Mitochondria may stain faintly.

Cytochemistry of blood cells

Cytochemical reactions should be used as an adjunct to standard morphology. When used properly, cytochemical reactions may be helpful in the identification of the cell line of leukemias of uncertain type, but too much reliance on these reactions can confuse rather than help. Cytochemical reactions in leukemia are discussed by Hayhoe et al (1964) and Scott (1978).

Cytochemical reactions are most useful in (1) distinguishing among some of the leukemias, (2) distinguishing between granulocytic leukemia and a granulocytic leukemoid reaction, (3) distinguishing between classic Auer rods and other crystalline inclusions, (4) identifying the lymphocyte of leukemic reticuloendotheliosis, and (5) identifying the ringed sideroblasts in the sideroblastic anemias. Tables 4-8 and 4-10 summarize the major cytochemical reactions.

Peroxidase (myeloperoxidase) (Plate 31)

The peroxidase reaction has been used for many years as a specific marker for the granules of cells of the myeloid series. The peroxidase in granules is called myeloperoxidase to distinguish it from other, nonspecific peroxidases (Yam et al, 1971).

Myeloperoxidase is present exclusively in azurophilic (nonspecific) granules. Synthesis of myeloperoxidase begins at the progranulocyte stage (Bainton, 1975b), so that progranulocytes, myelocytes, metamyelocytes, and band and segmented neutrophils are strongly peroxidase positive. Since the more mature cells are peroxidase positive but no azurophilic granules are seen in Wright-stained smears, it must be assumed that the tinctorial properties of azurophilic granules change as the cell matures. Eosinophils are strongly peroxidase positive; the peroxidase is located within the matrix of specific granules (Cotran and Litt, 1969) and may be different from the myeloperoxidase of neutrophils (Yam et al, 1971). Lymphocytes are peroxidase negative. Basophils are peroxidase negative by the usual benzidine technique, but when 3,3'-diaminobenzidine tetrahydrochloride is used, the granules are peroxidase positive (Ackerman and Clark, 1971). Monocytes show only a few peroxidase-positive granules.

By definition the myeloblast contains no azurophilic granules; however, some peroxidase activity may be present, associated with the rough endoplasmic reticulum and Golgi apparatus from which the azurophilic granules are derived (Bessis and Maigné, 1970). The cells of myelomonocytic leukemia usually are strongly peroxidase positive, whereas those of pure monocytic (histiocytic) leukemia are peroxidase negative or very weakly positive. Turpin et al (1978) found an absence of neutrophilic peroxidase in a case of diffuse mastocytosis. Cech et al (1979) report finding myeloperoxidase-deficient neutrophils, supposedly as a hereditary deficiency, in a diabetic patient.

The peroxidase reaction depends on the oxidation by hydrogen peroxide of a suitable substrate to form a chromogenic oxidized product. The substrate may be benzidine (Graham, 1918), benzidine dihydrochloride (Kaplow, 1965), diaminobenzidine (Graham and Karnovsky, 1966), 3,3′,5,5′-tetramethylbenzidine dihydrochloride (Liem et al, 1979), ortho-tolidine (Hayhoe and Flemans, 1970), or 4-chloro-1-naphthol (Elias, 1980). In my opinion the carcinogenicity of benzidine and benzidine derivatives as laboratory reagents has been exaggerated.

Peroxidase is unstable, and the reaction must be performed on freshly made smears. If the smears are not fresh, the lipid and esterase reactions can be used to identify granulocytes.

Lipids (Plate 32)

Most studies on cellular lipids have been carried out with Sudan black B, which reacts with a variety of lipids, including neutral fats, phospholipids, and steroids. With this stain the granules of neutrophils and basophils stain intensely, black or gray. In contrast, the granules of eosinophils stain only on the surface, giving the impression that they have an external lipid envelope. Myeloblasts contain minute sudanophilic mitochondria, which are obscured in more mature cells by the intensely sudanophilic granules. Lymphocytes usually show only a few variably sudanophilic mitochondria. Monocytes have a few very small sudanophilic granules that are usually concentrated near the hof of the nucleus. Megakaryocytes show fine punctate staining of the cytoplasm, and platelets are faintly sudanophilic. The cerebroside in Gaucher cells is not sudanophilic.

All structures that are peroxidase positive are also sudanophilic, except that peroxidase is unstable, demonstrable only in fresh smears, whereas sudanophilia is not affected by storage of smears.

Identification of lipids has been refined by the use of Baker's method. This is based on the acid hematin reaction for phospholipids, pyridine extraction serving as the control. Acid hematin is specific for phospholipids or phospholipid-protein complexes removed by pyridine extraction. By Baker's method the granules of the leukocytes stain various shades of gray to black, and mitochondria are more easily visualized than with Sudan black B. The mitochondria seen with Baker's method correspond in size, shape, and distribution to those seen in supravital preparations. In granulocytes the mitochondria are obscured by the heavily stained granules. The mitochondria of lymphocytes are easily identified. Cells of the erythrocytic series do not stain with this method but do show mitochondria.

Glycogen

Glycogen is stained by the periodic acid–Schiff (PAS) reaction. Periodic acid splits C—C bonds of glycogen at CHOH—CHOH groups, producing aldehydes (CHO). The Schiff reagent then reacts with the aldehydes to form a colored product, magenta when basic fuchsin is used. The reaction must be timed carefully because prolonged exposure to periodic acid can oxidize the aldehydes and cause a false-negative reaction. Glycogen is the only diastase-sensitive PAS-positive substance, so that saliva or malt diastase is used to check the specificity of the reaction. Cytochemical studies using this reaction have yielded the following interesting data:

1. Normal lymphocytes occasionally show PAS-positive granules but generally are PAS negative.

2. Normal lymphoblasts are PAS negative, but leukemic lymphoblasts and the small lymphocytes of chronic lymphocytic leukemia have numerous fine to coarse PAS-positive granules.

3. In the granulocytic series, PAS positivity increases in the maturation sequence: the myeloblasts are PAS negative, the adult polymorphonuclear cells are strongly PAS positive, and cells of intermediate maturity show intermediate PAS positivity. The granules of eosinophils are PAS negative, but the cytoplasm shows diffuse staining. The same is true of basophils.

4. Monocytes often show fine or moderately coarse PAS-positive granules.

5. Megakaryocytes and platelets are strongly PAS positive. Megakaryoblasts are PAS negative, and promegakaryocytes are intermediate.

6. Normal normoblasts are PAS negative, but the abnormal normoblasts or megaloblasts in erythroleukemia show strong PAS positivity. A small proportion of weakly positive normoblasts is found in acquired hemolytic disease. Many normoblasts in severe iron-deficiency anemia and in thalassemia major are strongly PAS positive. Megaloblasts in pernicious anemia are PAS negative.

7. Lymphosarcoma cells in the peripheral blood and bone marrow contain increased amounts of glycogen and are moderately to strongly PAS positive.

8. In many benign lymphoproliferative diseases (infectious mononucleosis and other viral diseases) the lymphocytes show PAS positivity. It is thought, then, that the presence of glycogen is not by itself an index of malignant transformation in lymphoid tissue, but rather accompanies proliferative activity.

9. Some believe that B-cell lymphoproliferative diseases are more likely to show PAS positive cells than T-cell diseases (Catovsky et al, 1974a), but other investigators have found no significant difference (Brouet et al, 1976). The cells of Sézary's syndrome, of T-cell origin, contain many coarse PAS-positive inclusions (Fig. 4-35).

10. Plasma cells and Russell bodies are PAS negative on smears but PAS positive in tissue sections (Goldberg and Deane, 1960).

Alkaline phosphatase

The determination of the alkaline phosphatase activity in leukocytes has very practical applications. Phosphatases, more specifically phosphomonoesterases, are enzymes that liberate orthophosphoric acid from alcohol or phenolic monoesters. There is probably a wide spectrum of phosphomonoesterases in body cells and fluids, but, based on pH requirements, two types are commonly distinguished, acid phosphatase and alkaline phosphatase. There are differences other than in optimum pH; e.g., magnesium ions are strong activators of alkaline phosphatases but not of acid. Manganese, zinc, and cobalt ions are weaker activators of alkaline phosphatase than are magnesium ions. Fluorides inhibit the acid but not the alkaline enzyme. By analogy with alkaline phosphatase in the kidney, it has been suggested that there are at least two alkaline phosphatases, one activated by zinc ions and glycine and inhibited by iodoacetate and the other inhibited by the same concentration of zinc ions and glycine. More specifically with respect to leukocytes, Trubowitz et al (1957) proposed that at least two alkaline phosphatases are present in leukocytes, one being activated by magnesium ions and the other by zinc ions. They also suggested that the zinc-activated enzyme is involved in the elevated phosphatase activity seen in infection and leukemoid reactions. Indeed, zinc is known to be an important constituent of leukocytes. In leukemic leukocytes, zinc is low, particularly when the count is high and the disease in relapse. This may explain why the cells in chronic granulocytic leukemia seem to have little alkaline phosphatase. In contrast to peroxidase activity, alkaline phosphatase activity is a property of specific granules. Young neutrophils have a lower alkaline phosphatase activity than the older neutrophils (Bondue et al, 1980).

Except in one special situation (hypophosphatasia), there is little or no correlation between serum and leukocyte alkaline phosphatase. The enzyme in the leukocyte is not absorbed from the serum, for it cannot be increased by incubating leukocytes in serum having a high alkaline phosphatase activity. In hypophosphatasia the leukocytes have no alkaline phosphate activity and neither does the serum, but here there is an inborn error of metabolism affecting all tissues.

In common with other enzymes, leukocyte alkaline phosphatase activity reflects intracellular metabolic activity. It has been suggested that this enzymatic activity is controlled by a gene on chromosome 21. This suggestion is based on the association between abnormalities in this chromosome and low leukocyte alkaline phosphatase activity; e.g., high activity is found in mongolism, in which gene 21 is trisomic, and low in chronic myelocytic leukemia, in which there is a partial deletion of this gene. In "classic" chronic myelocytic leukemia this gene forms the characteristic Ph^1 chromosome. However, some patients with chronic granulocytic leukemia lack the Ph^1 chromosome and are called "atypical." In general, alkaline phosphatase activity is low in both Ph^1-positive and Ph^1-negative cases. In a study of chronic granulocytic leukemia in childhood, Rosen and Nishiyama (1968) found the leukocyte alkaline phosphatase scores to be significantly higher in the Ph^1-negative children than in the Ph^1-positive children. Also, the phosphatase score increased more in intercurrent infection in the Ph^1-positive children than in the atypical ones. In adults, both Ph^1-positive and Ph^1-negative cases of chronic granulocytic leukemia show low phosphatase scores.

Biochemical methods for measuring alkaline phosphatase activity in leukocyte suspensions are cumbersome and impractical. In addition, it has been noted that in some situations (multiple myeloma and chronic lymphocytic leuke-

Table 4-9. Alkaline phosphatase reaction in neutrophils in various disorders scored according to method of Kaplow (1963)

Disease	No. of cases	Score	
Normal*	100	15- 70; average, 30	
Leukocytosis†	80	105-265; average, 136	High
Leukemoid reaction‡	33	150-365; average, 280	
Acute lymphocytic leukemia	24	93-213; average, 130	
Polycythemia vera	17	87-314; average, 209	
Myeloproliferative disorders, various§	7	4-280; average, 186	
Hodgkin's disease (active)	8	90-294; average, 238	
Chronic lymphocytic leukemia	29	11-149; average, 64	Normal
Secondary polycythemia‖	31	10- 61; average, 35	
Lymphosarcoma	9	15- 85; average, 44	
Multiple myeloma	18	21- 95; average, 52	
Chronic myelomonocytic leukemia	21	12- 50; average, 23	
Chronic myelocytic leukemia	37	0- 24; average, 11	Low
Acute myelocytic leukemia	11	0- 11; average, 4	
Acute monocytic leukemia	14	7- 48; average, 21	
Infectious mononucleosis¶	47	4- 31; average, 16	
Paroxysmal nocturnal hemoglobinuria	1	11; —	
Congenital hypophosphatasia#	1	0; —	

*Alkaline phosphatase scores in the high range (100 to 150) may be found in women taking oral contraceptives. The score is also high in the normal newborn infant (200 to 250), decreasing to the normal adult value by 6 months of age.

†Score depends on degree of leukocytosis, being highest when the leukocyte count is very high. Range represented here is 15,000 to 50,000 leukocytes/mm³ of blood (15 to 50 × 10⁹/1). Normal values are reported in sickle cell anemia with leukocytosis (Wajima and Kraus, 1968).

‡All myelocytic. Range is 50,000 to 170,000 leukocytes/mm³ of blood (50 to 170 × 10⁹/1).

§Other than polycythemia vera. This is the only low value in our series, in a patient with terminal (nonleukemic) leukopenia and anemia.

‖Includes stress erythrocytosis (3 cases), polycythemia associated with tumor (1 renal and 1 uterine), congenital heart disease (19 cases), and pulmonary fibrosis syndromes (7 cases).

¶During acute phase. Values rise gradually to normal during recovery.

#Reported by Beisel et al, 1959.

mia) the cytochemical score is in the high normal range, whereas the biochemical measurement shows low activity.

The *cytochemical* demonstration of alkaline phosphatase depends on the formation of a colored precipitate at the site of hydrolysis of substrate. The method of Gomori, modified slightly by several investigators, depends on incubating smears with glycerophosphate at pH 9 in the presence of calcium and magnesium ions. Insoluble calcium phosphate is formed at the site of reaction and is then visualized by being converted to black cobalt sulfide. Kaplow's modification (1955) of earlier technics uses fixation in 10% formalin in absolute methanol at 0° C, sodium α-naphthyl phosphate in the substrate, and fast blue RR as the diazonium salt. This method gives results that are clear-cut and reproducible.

In 1963 Kaplow (1963) described a modification of the original method that gives very good results. The new method uses naphthol AS-BI phosphate and fast red violet LB buffered with propanediol at pH 9.7. The final coupled product is brilliant ruby red, and the smears are somewhat easier to "score" as to degree of alkaline phosphatase activity.

Kaplow (1963, 1968) proposed rating the degree of positivity of phosphatase staining in each neutrophil on the basis of a 0 to 4 scale, the score for a given smear being the sum of ratings for 100 neutrophilic leukocytes. The criteria for rating a given cell are as follows:

0 Colorless
1 Diffuse but slight positivity, with occasional granules
2 Diffusely positive, with moderate number of granules
3 Strongly positive, with numerous granules
4 Very strongly positive, with very dark confluent granules

When these criteria are used, a semiquantitative expression of leukocytic alkaline phosphatase is possible. In actual practice it is usually possible to distinguish a normal smear from an abnormal smear by simple inspection, scoring being done in the less obvious case.

The result of alkaline phosphatase studies in various disease states is given in Table 4-9. Different observers may vary in the interpretation of the intensity of staining, the variation between trained observers being about 10%. In general only myeloid cells show alkaline phosphatase, and these but weakly when normal. Increased phosphatase activity is noted in the leukocytosis caused by various infections. Very striking increases are noted in leukemoid reactions and most myeloproliferative disorders but not in chronic myelocytic leukemia. Thus the alkaline phosphatase reaction is often useful in differentiating both leukemoid states from leukemia and polycythemia vera from erythrocytosis (Mitus et al, 1959). It must be noted that this generalization is modified by the clinical stage of the disease or by response to treatment (Kelemen, 1973). It has been noted, for example, that the usually elevated alkaline phosphatase score in a myeloproliferative disorder will drop when the disease is in transformation to the leukemic state. On the other hand, leukocyte alkaline phosphatase values will often rise when chronic myelocytic leukemia responds to chemotherapy (Myleran) (Xefteris et al, 1961). Low alkaline phosphatase

activity has been reported in sideroblastic anemia (Lehrer et al, 1972).

Leukocyte alkaline phosphatase is high in the newborn and in a variety of stress situations. Administration of ACTH produces high values; cortisone does not. Elevated values are often encountered in normal pregnancy, as early as the fifth week after the last menstrual period (Beal et al, 1967). Activity is high in Down's syndrome (Alter et al, 1962). Low values have been reported in idiopathic thrombocytopenic purpura, in paroxysmal nocturnal hemoglobinuria, and in collagen diseases.

Acid phosphatase

Acid phosphatase is found in almost all cells (Rozenszajn et al, 1963) and therefore has little application in the identification of blood cells. An important exception is in leukemic reticuloendotheliosis (p. 725). Whereas the acid phosphatase reaction in most blood cells is inhibited by tartrate, it is not inhibited in the "hairy cells" of this disease (Plate 55). Tartrate resistance (no inhibition by tartrate) is a feature also of Sézary cells and prolymphocytic leukemia (Katayama and Yang, 1979).

Esterases (Plate 30)

Leukocytes contain esterases, a group of lysosomal enzymes that hydrolyze both aliphatic and aromatic esters. Esterases are associated with the azurophilic (nonspecific) granules (Rindler et al, 1971). Li et al (1973) separated nine esterase isoenzymes having different cell distribution and substrate specificity: isoenzymes 2, 7, and 9 in neutrophils, isoenzyme 6 in plasma cells, and isoenzymes 4 and 5 in monocytes.

The substrates commonly employed for the demonstration of esterases are naphthol ASD chloroacetate, naphthol ASD acetate, α-naphthyl acetate and α-naphthyl butyrate. The latter is considered more specific for monocytic esterase than is α-naphthyl acetate (Ansley et al, 1971). As shown in Table 4-10, the reactions with naphthol ASD chloroacetate are seen chiefly in granulocytes. Monocytes react more strongly with naphthol ASD acetate, and this reaction, as well as a similar one in the cells of pure monocytic leukemia, is inhibited by fluoride. Positivity in granulocytes is not inhibited by fluoride. Naphthol ASD acetate also shows strong reactions with megakaryocytes, whereas α-naphthyl acetate reacts strongly only with monocytes and plasma cells.

Data on esterase reactions in various leukemias are contradictory (Leder, 1970; Bennett and Reed, 1975; Castoldi et al, 1975). It is agreed that the cells of acute lymphocytic leukemia are esterase negative. In myelomonocytic leukemia the blasts are usually negative or weakly positive, whereas the more mature cells with cytoplasmic granulation are esterase positive with no inhibition by fluoride. In pure monocytic (histiocytic) leukemia the cells are variably esterase positive, and when positive the reaction is inhibited by fluoride. Auer rods are esterase positive. The abnormal erythroid cells in erythroleukemia are strongly positive (Kass, 1975b). According to Tavassoli et al (1979), naphthol ASD chloroacetate is considered to be a specific substrate for

Table 4-10. Cytochemical reactions: esterase

Cell	NAS-DC*	NAS-DA†	NAS-DAF‡	α-NB§
Myeloblast, (normal)	Neg.	Neg.	Neg.	+
Myeloblast, leukemic	++++	++++	++	Neg.
Auer bodies	++++	++++	++	+
Progranulocyte	++++	++++	++++	+
Neutrophil, adult	+++	+++	+++	+
Basophil	+	+	+	Neg.
Eosinophil	Neg.	+	+	+
Monocyte	+	+++	0 to +	+++
Lymphocyte	Neg.	Neg.	Neg.	Neg.
Plasma cell	Neg.	+	Neg.	++
Myelomonocytic leukemia	+ to ++	+ to ++	+ to ++	+
Monocytic leukemia	+ to +++	+ to +++	Neg.	+++
Erythroleukemia	+++	+++	+++	++
Acute lymphocytic leukemia	Neg.	Neg.	Neg.	Neg.

*NAS-DC = Naphthol ASD chloroacetate.
†NAS-DA = Naphthol ASD acetate.
‡NAS-DAF = NAS-DA reaction after inhibition by fluoride.
§α-NB = α-naphthyl butyrate.

granulocytic esterase, whereas α-naphthyl butyrate is monocyte specific. They found that by consecutive staining of the same preparation with the two substrates (Yam et al, 1971), the cells of granulocytic leukemia are positive with naphthol ASD chloroacetate, those of monocytic leukemia are positive with α-naphthyl butyrate, and those of myelomonocytic leukemia react with both substrates. Knowles and Holck (1978) have shown that the esterase for α-naphthyl acetate is specific for T-lymphocytes, producing a single nodule of reaction product, whereas monocytes stain diffusely, and B-lymphocytes are negative.

In summary, the esterase reactions seem to be most useful in (1) differentiating esterase-negative lymphoid cells from other cell types, (2) characterizing the cells of acute monocytic leukemia by the inhibition of the esterase reaction by fluoride, and (3) studying cells in tissue embedded in paraffin and in old smears (because of the great stability of esterases).

Application of cytochemistry to the study of leukemias

An accurate classification of leukemias is based on all the available evidence, clinical and morphologic. Cytochemistry is merely an adjunct to standard morphology. The skilled morphologist can correctly classify most of the leukemias using standard Wright-stained or Wright-Giemsa–stained smears of blood and bone marrow. In a very few instances cytochemistry is helpful in resolving a specific problem. In rare instances one must deal with an "unclassifiable leukemia" or one so primitive that the stem cells have no morphologic or cytochemical features that identify the cell line.

Depending on the enthusiasm of the investigator for cytochemical studies, one can find numerous reports indicating either limited or promising results when cytochemistry is applied to a variety of leukemias. The report of Bennett and Reed (1975) is acceptably objective. They found that the diagnosis according to cytochemical findings in 32 cases of acute nonlymphocytic leukemia showed poor correlation with the morphologic diagnosis, only 40% of the cases showing agreement between the two.

Nevertheless, cytochemistry is useful if applied to specific problems (1) esterase reactions are useful in differentiating acute monocytic leukemia from myelomonocytic leukemia (Flandrin and Daniel, 1973; Shaw and Nordquist, 1975; Sultan, 1977), although it should be noted that in most cases the differentiation is made easily without cytochemistry; (2) the PAS reaction is helpful in differentiating benign from malignant lymphoproliferative disorders; (3) the alkaline phosphatase score is helpful in differentiating between granulocytic leukemoid reactions and granulocytic leukemia; (4) cytochemical reactions are useful in differentiating between Auer bodies and other crystalline inclusions (p. 209); (5) the acid phosphatase reactions are useful as markers for the hairy cells of leukemic reticuloendotheliosis; (6) the PAS reaction is useful in identifying the abnormal erythroid cells in erythroleukemia (Kass, 1977c); (7) the PAS reaction is useful in identifying the Sézary cell; (8) the PAS reaction is useful for distinguishing between PAS-positive megakaryocytes and polymorphic giant tumor cells; (9) the PAS reaction reveals intranuclear PAS positivity in Waldenström's macroglobulinemia; and (10) staining for intracellular iron identifies the ringed sideroblast of sideroblastic anemia.

5

"View them in composition with other things."
I. Watts

The bone marrow

OBTAINING MARROW TISSUE BY BIOPSY
TECHNICS FOR OBTAINING MARROW TISSUE
OBTAINING MARROW BY ASPIRATION
  Local analgesia
  Sites for aspiration
    Sternal marrow aspiration technic
    Iliac marrow aspiration technic
    Vertebral marrow aspiration technic
    Posterior ilium aspiration technic
    Tibial marrow aspiration technic
    Rib marrow aspiration technic
    Preparation of marrow tissue for study
OBTAINING MARROW BY TREPHINE BIOPSY
POSTMORTEM MARROW
NORMAL MARROW AND THE SIGNIFICANCE OF DEVIATIONS
  FROM NORMAL
  Normal marrow
  Qualitative abnormalities
  Quantitative abnormalities
  Illustrative cases

Examination of the peripheral blood reveals its cellular content at the time of sampling and yields data necessary for qualitative and quantitative classification of abnormalities, but it gives limited information about the pathogenesis of an abnormal state. If treatment is guided by trial and error rather than by an appreciation of the pathogenesis of disease, it cannot fail to have disappointing, confusing, or even harmful results.

Hematologic diagnosis depends on knowing as much as possible about three processes: cell production, cell release, and cell survival. Since the mechanisms of cell release are least understood, diagnosis is usually based on a determination of the balance between rate and quality of hemopoietic activity on the one hand and rate of cell survival on the other. Qualitative and quantitative data on *medullary hemopoiesis* are obtained by examination of marrow tissue. Significant hemopoiesis at other sites is called *extramedullary hemopoiesis*. When it occurs, tissue from both the bone marrow and these other sites must be obtained for study.

Under normal conditions almost all hemopoiesis takes place in the bone marrow. Hematologic disorders caused by abnormal cell production are usually induced by abnormal medullary hemopoiesis. For this reason study of the bone marrow is the most frequently used adjunct to the diagnosis of blood disorders. The book by Schleicher (1973) on bone marrow biopsy and the monograph by Rywlin (1976) on the histopathology of the bone marrow are highly recommended.

OBTAINING MARROW TISSUE BY BIOPSY

Obtaining marrow tissue by aspiration or trephine biopsy is no longer a dramatic procedure and need not be a traumatic one. In skilled hands, morbidity and mortality are negligible. In some patients, diagnosis can be made from microscopic examination of the marrow alone; in others the information obtained will confirm other findings or exclude some diseases that might be considered in the differential diagnosis. However, as with other laboratory examinations, marrow should be examined only when specifically indicated, i.e., when the physician is seeking a specific answer to a specific question. Indications and contraindications for examining the marrow are given in Table 5-1.

Properly handled marrow tissue can give a wealth of information. Wright-stained or Wright-Giemsa–stained smears give excellent cytologic details, and duplicate smears may be stained for peroxidase or other cytochemical reactions (Rywlin, 1976). A differential count can give the relative proportion of different cell types but is not a measure of the number of cells present in the marrow. This information is best obtained from paraffin sections of isolated marrow particles. Sections not only give an accurate measure of the relative cellular and fat content but also are essential for diagnosis in the granulomatous diseases such as tuberculosis in which the histologic pattern is more reliable than the morphology of individual cells. The use of direct marrow cell counts and hematocrit readings to obtain quantitative data is advocated by some, but we feel that paraffin sections are more reliable for this purpose. Marrow tissue may also be cultured to isolate and identify bacteria and other pathogenic agents or may well be used for animal inoculation studies. It is well, therefore, to plan the handling of the tissue specimen in advance to include technics that might give useful information. Our routine practice is to prepare both thin smears and paraffin sections of marrow particles. In special cases, marrow tissue is cultured and used for animal inoculation.

211

Table 5-1. Indications and contraindications for bone marrow studies

I. Marrow examination indicated
  A. Macrocytic anemias
  B. Clinical evidence for blood dyscrasia (otherwise unexplained lymphadenopathy, splenomegaly, hepatomegaly, etc.)
  C. Peripheral blood findings suggestive of leukemia
  D. Unexplained anemia, thrombocytopenia, or leukopenia
  E. Roentgenologic evidence of bone lesions possibly caused by a blood dyscrasia
  F. Cases of carcinoma, with or without roentgenologic evidence of metastases
  G. Identification of parasites sometimes found in the bone marrow (leishmania, histoplasma, plasmodium, trypanosomes)
  H. For bacteriologic and histologic investigations of granulomas
  I. Disseminated lupus erythematosus (peripheral blood studies preferred)
  J. Prior to splenectomy to determine functional state of bone marrow
  K. Diagnosis of lipid storage diseases
  L. Following progress of therapy in anemais, leukemias, etc.
  M. Iron-deficiency anemia (estimation of iron content of marrow)
II. Marrow examination usually not helpful
  A. Hemolytic anemias (not associated with leukemia or lymphoma)
  B. Chronic lymphocytic leukemia (histologic examination of lymph node tissue more reliable)
III. Marrow examination contraindicated
  A. Hemophilia and related congenital hemorrhagic disorders

TECHNICS FOR OBTAINING MARROW TISSUE

The technics for obtaining marrow consist of *aspiration, trephination,* and *surgical excision.*

Aspiration is the most common technic and will usually yield an adequate specimen. Occasionally a "dry tap" occurs when aspiration fails to yield marrow tissue. Sometimes aspiration at another site will be successful, and it is not always possible to explain why the first failed. Dry taps sometimes occur when the marrow is involved with metastatic tumors, lymphomas, sarcoidosis, histoplasmosis, or miliary tuberculosis. Occasionally they will be experienced in pernicious anemia of leukemia because of the difficulty of aspirating a thick, hypercellular or gelatinous marrow. In other cases, failure to obtain a specimen by aspiration is later explained when acellular, fibrous, or sclerotic marrow is demonstrated by different technics.

In no case should a diagnosis of aplastic or fibrous marrow be based only on a failure to obtain marrow by aspiration. If repeated aspirations fail, trephination or surgical excision must be performed.

OBTAINING MARROW BY ASPIRATION

Needles of various designs are available. All are satisfactory, the use of one or the other usually being a matter of personal preference. I prefer the University of Illinois sternal puncture needle* (Fig. 5-1). This is an excellent needle, large and heavy enough to allow a firm grip and absolute control at all times. The "guard" added to prevent too deep a penetration is, in practice, superfluous. The need for a guard would indicate a poor puncture technic. It can be used, however, to secure a good grip. The fingertips are pressed against the guard, and the body of the needle is grasped frimly in the palm of the hand. Entrance into the marrow cavity is effected by firm but controlled pressure while the needle is rotated alternately clockwise and counterclockwise. In this manner the dense cortex can be penetrated gradually and without loss of control over the depth of penetration.

---

*V. Mueller & Co., Chicago, Ill.

Local analgesia

Local analgesia is achieved by infiltrating the area with a 1% solution of procaine hydrochloride or other local anesthetic. The patient should always be asked if he or she is allergic to local anesthetics. A small amount is first injected intradermally at the site chosen for puncture. The fine hypodermic needle is then thrust through the bleb, perpendicular to the skin surface, until the bone is encountered. Some anesthetic may be injected as the needle traverses the subcutaneous tissues, but this is probably of little value. If too much is injected, it may actually obscure valuable landmarks. Two potentially painful areas must be carefully infiltrated. They are the skin and the periosteum. Effective subperiosteal infiltration is accomplished by firmly fixing the point of the hypodermic needle in the bone and injecting the analgesic agent under pressure. Adequate periosteal analgesia will eliminate much of the patient's pain and discomfort.

Recently Dyment et al (1978) have reported their experience with jet anesthesia using an instrument (Syriijet II) that delivers 0.35 ml of 2% lidocaine with a force of 2,600 psi. This method was found to be safe and effective and deserves serious consideration.

Sites for aspiration

The sternum, ilium, vertebral spinous processes, and other sites usually yield comparable samples, but at times aspiration will be unsuccessful at one site and successful at another. There seems to be no statistically significant quantitative difference between samples from different sites. At any site a single specimen is hardly representative of the entire marrow, which, particularly when abnormal, may be totally different in adjacent areas (Fig. 5-2). In early acute leukemia it is possible to have the aspirate from one site show leukemic infiltrations while that from another site is normal or shows only erythroid hyperplasia. The choice of site for aspiration is usually a matter of personal preference but may be based on specific indications; e.g., the very thin cartilaginous sternum of infants makes sternal puncture difficult and dangerous. A site other than the sternum is also

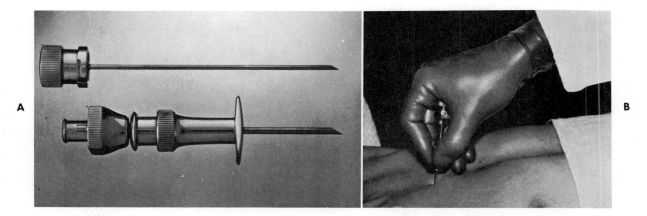

Fig. 5-1. University of Illinois marrow aspiration needle. **A,** Natural size. Although originally designed as a sternal marrow needle, it is suitable for puncture at any other site. A smaller model is available for use in infants and children. **B** illustrates proper method of holding needle.

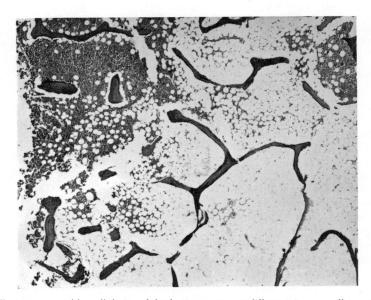

Fig. 5-2. Illustrating variable cellularity of the bone marrow at different sites, paraffin section. Diagnosis was aplastic anemia, etiology undetermined. Aspiration biopsy revealed an acellular marrow. (Hematoxylin-eosin stain; ×22.)

indicated in the presence of congenital anomalies of the sternum and in the case of an apprehensive adult. In special cases the best site for puncture is at a point of bone tenderness or destruction. Not uncommonly aspiration of marrow at a point showing an abnormality in roentgenograms will yield diagnostic tissue, whereas aspiration at another site chosen at random may yield only normal marrow. Likewise, marrow from the ilium of a patient with carcinoma of the prostate may reveal more than would sternal marrow. The skilled hematologist should be ready to perform marrow aspiration at whichever site circumstances dictate.

STERNAL MARROW ASPIRATION TECHNIC. (Fig. 5-3). The preferred point of aspiration is the body of the sternum opposite the second interspace. Here the sternum is firmly fixed and congenital anomalies are infrequent. At this level

in the adult the outer lamina averages 1.35 mm and the inner lamina 1.42 mm, with an average marrow cavity depth of 7.5 mm (Fig. 5-4). These measurements are only a rough guide, for in any given patient they may differ both as to thickness of the cortex and depth of the marrow cavity.

The skin is carefully cleansed, using green soap followed by Merthiolate or a similar disinfectant. In males it is best to shave the area at the site of puncture. Thorough washing of the operator's hands is sufficient; sterile surgical gloves are unnecessary. After adequate analgesia is achieved, the second interspace is located, the index finger and thumb of the left hand outlining the lateral borders of the sternum. The needle point is then centered exactly midway between the borders of the sternum. Held as previously described and perpendicular to the skin, the needle is inserted with a bor-

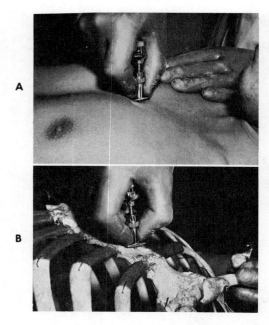

Fig. 5-3. Aspiration of sternal marrow. **A,** Photograph of actual aspiration. **B,** Anatomic relationships.

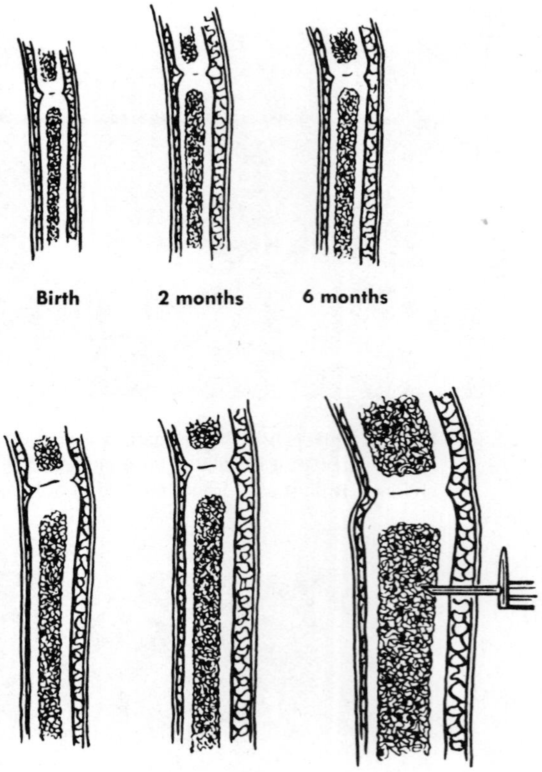

ing motion and steady but not excessive pressure. There is usually no need to incise the skin if the needle is sharp and smooth. The boring pressure is continued until skin, subcutaneous tissue, and outer lamina are penetrated. The classic desciption of a ''give'' when the marrow cavity is entered is not only unreliable but also actually indicates loss of control. The pressure should be so gauged as to avoid any sudden penetration when resistance is lessened. A more reliable test for penetration of the outer lamina is made by gently tilting the needle. When the outer cortex has been penetrated, the needle will be fixed at one point but can be tilted. If the needle point is touching the posterior lamina, however, it will be fixed at two points and cannot be tilted. When it is determined that the needle is in the marrow cavity, the stylet in unlocked and removed, a tightly fitting 10 ml syringe is inserted in its place, and forceful aspiration is effected. *No more than 0.2 ml of marrow should be aspirated,* thus minimizing dilution of the marrow with sinusoidal blood. This first material obtained is used to prepare thin smears. A second syringe is then applied and about 1 ml of marrow is aspirated, from which additional marrow particles for particle smears and permanent paraffin sections can be obtained. When aspiration has been completed, the needle is withdrawn and a dry sterile dressing is applied to the site of puncture.

In infants and young children, aspiration from the iliac crest or spinous process is easier than from the sternal site, but sternal aspiration is possible. There are a few special considerations. The miniature Klima-Rosseger needle* or any other small needle should be used for infants and children under 3 years of age. Since the sternal lamina in infants is largely cartilaginous, resistance to penetration is less, and

*V. Mueller & Co., Chicago, Ill.

Birth **2 months** **6 months**

1 year **10 years** **Adult**

0 .1 2
cm.

Fig. 5-4. Midsagittal sections through sternum showing in actual size the average thickness of the laminae and the depth of the marrow cavity at different ages.

pressure must be applied with extreme caution. When the anterior lamina is traversed, cancellous bone of a somewhat different consistency is encountered in the marrow cavity. Only a few drops of marrow can be expected. Indeed, continued suction in an attempt to obtain more marrow only results in dilution of the specimen with sinusoidal blood. Since 0.1 mm³ of marrow contains on the average 10,000 cells, one or two well-made smears should be sufficient for routine studies.

ILIAC MARROW ASPIRATION TECHNIC. (Figs. 5-5 to 5-7). The ilium can be penetrated in one of several places. Usually the patient lies flat on his back, and a point 1 inch below and 1 inch behind the superior iliac spine is located. The needle is then inserted as described for sternal aspiration, but in a horizontal direction. There is a geater likelihood of marrow dilution with sinusoidal blood in iliac puncture than in sternal puncture.

The iliac crest proper in adults is usually too dense to be penetrated easily, but it is easily pierced in infants and children. At a point halfway between the anterior and posterior spines, the crest can be outlined between the thumb and

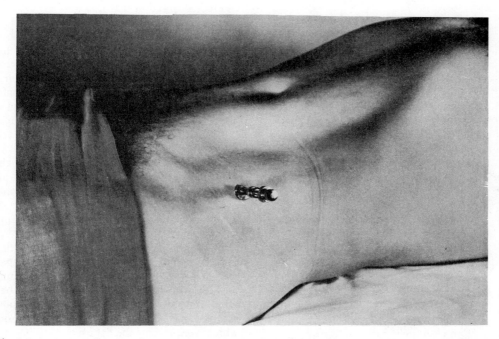

Fig. 5-5. Aspiration of anterior iliac crest marrow. Needle is fixed at a point 1 to 2 inches below and behind the anterosuperior spine.

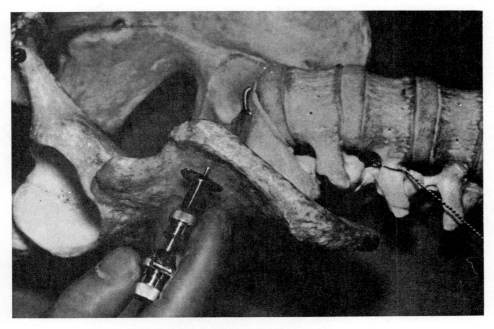

Fig. 5-6. Anatomic relationships, anterior iliac crest.

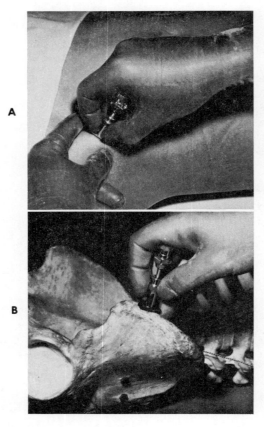

Fig. 5-7. A, Marrow aspiration at iliac crest. B, Anatomic relationships.

forefinger of the left hand. The needle is inserted in a vertical direction, oriented so that it moves downward parallel to the inner and outer cortex, until the marrow cavity is entered. Aspiration performed in the usual way.

Leffler (1957) advocates using the anterosuperior iliac spine rather than the crest of the ilium. The spine is easily outlined, and the cortex is less dense here than at the crest. With the subject lying on his back, the needle is directed downward and slightly cephalad. Aspiration is carried out as usual. When the marrow cavity has been entered in the center of the highest part, there is a good deal of leeway as to direction of the needle and depth of penetration.

VERTEBRAL MARROW ASPIRATION TECHNIC. (Figs. 5-8 and 5-9). Spinous process puncture is another reliable technic for obtaining marrow tissue. Its chief advantages are: (1) the aspiration is performed out of sight of the patient, (2) the spinous process is a firmer structure on which to apply pressure than the sternum, and (3) when a series of aspirations is required, several spinous processes are available (from D_{10} to L_4).

The aspiration is usually performed with the patient sitting up and leaning forward while braced against the back of a chair or the edge of the bed. The recumbent facedown position is sometimes advocated and may be better for children. With the patient sitting up and leaning forward, the spinous processes of L_2, L_3, and L_4 are quite prominent, whichever presents the flattest surface being the one usually chosen. Analgesia and method of aspiration are the same as for other sites. It is claimed that marrow tissue from the spinous process gives a hemogram similar to sternal marrow. It is also claimed that the spinous process contains

Fig. 5-8. Aspiration of bone marrow from a spinous process. The patient is in a sitting position.

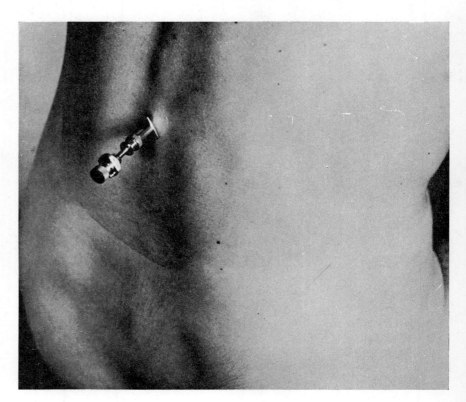

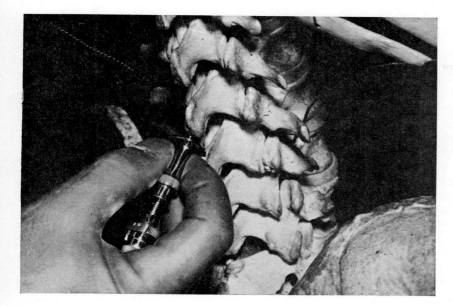

Fig. 5-9. Anatomic relationships, spinous process puncture.

Fig. 5-10. A, Aspiration of bone marrow from posterior ilium. **B,** Anatomic relationships.

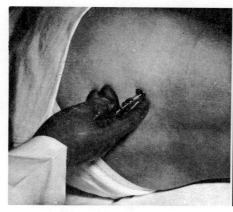

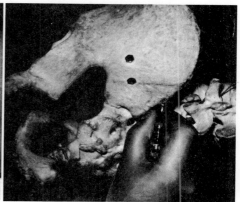

Fig. 5-11. Bone marrow preparations. **A,** Thin smear. **B,** Particle smear. **C,** Paraffin section.

A   B   C

active red marrow later in life than the sternal marrow (Loge, 1948).

POSTERIOR ILIUM ASPIRATION TECHNIC. (Fig. 5-10). The posterior ilium is in many ways an ideal site for bone marrow puncture. Bierman and Kelly (1956) pointed out that the marrow cavity here is quite large. Furthermore, the direction of the aspirating needle can be parallel to the inner and outer cortex, thus avoiding the risk of perforating the deep bony table. One can take advantage of this to obtain marrow tissue by biopsy at this site by using a Vim-Silverman or other biopsy needle (p. 220). Another advantage of this method is that the patient cannot see the instrument and is usually less apprehensive. One minor disadvantage is that in persons who are obese it is more difficult to palpate the landmarks of the posterior ilium.

Aspiration is carried out with the subject positioned as for a lumbar puncture, lying on his side with his knees drawn up and his back comfortably flexed. It is more comfortable for the operator if the subject is at the near edge of the bed. After the usual infiltration of skin and periosteum with procaine (Novocain), puncture is done at a point 1 cm cephalad to the posterosuperior iliac spine. The posterior iliac crest is penetrated with the usual clockwise and counterclockwise boring motion, the needle being directed toward the anterosuperior iliac spine. After the marrow cavity has been entered, aspiration is carried out in the usual manner.

TIBIAL MARROW ASPIRATION TECHNIC. Tibial marrow aspiration is sometimes performed in infants but is not recommended for older children. Since the cortex becomes increasingly dense with age, penetration becomes more difficult. I know no special indication for choosing the tibia over a site such as the ilium, but occasionally an alternate site is useful. The puncture is done at the medial aspect of the head of the tibia, below the medial condyle and the tibial

BONE MARROW STUDY

Name_____ Age_____ Date_____

Doctor_____ Ward_____ Chart No._____

			Normal	Range	Observed
		Blasts, unclassified			
70%	57.4%	Myeloblasts	1.2	0.3- 5.0	
		Progranulocytes	3.0	1.0- 8.0	
		Myelocytes	8.7	0.9-20.3	
		Neutrophilic	7.0	5.0-19.0	
		Eosinophilic	1.4	0.5- 3.0	
		Basophilic	0.3	0 - 0.5	
		Metamyelocytes	11.0	13.0-32.0	
		Neutrophilic	9.0	5.6-22.0	
		Eosinophilic	1.5	0.3- 3.7	
		Basophilic	0.3	0 - 0.3	
		Band cells	17.9	6.1-36.0	
		Neutrophilic	16.0	15.0-30.0	
		Eosinophilic	1.6	0.2- 2.0	
		Basophilic	0.2	0 - 0.3	
		Segmented	15.6	8.7-27.0	
		Neutrophils	13.4	7.0-30.0	
		Eosinophils	2.0	0.5- 4.0	
		Basophils	0.2	0 - 0.7	
	12.6%	Lymphoblasts			
		Prolymphocytes	9.8	2.7-24.0	
		Lymphocytes			
		Monoblasts			
		Promonocytes	1.4	0.7- 2.8	
		Monocytes			
		Plasmoblasts			
		Proplasmocytes	0.6	0.1- 1.5	
		Plasmocytes			
		Megakaryoblasts			
		Promegakaryocytes	0.2	0.03-0.4	
		Megakaryocytes			
19.1%	19.1%	Promegaloblasts			
		Basophilic megaloblasts	0	0	
		Polychromatophilic megaloblasts			
		Orthochromic megaloblasts			
		Pronormoblasts	0.5	0.2- 4.0	
		Basophilic normoblasts	2.4	1.5- 5.8	
		Polychromatophilic normoblasts	11.7	5.0-26.4	
		Orthochromic normoblasts	4.5	1.6-21.0	
10.9%	10.9%	Unidentified	1.7	0.02-3.3	
		Disintegrated cells	9.2	1.1-20.8	
		Reticulum cells	0.2	0.2- 2.0	

Fig. 5-12. Useful form for reporting results of bone marrow examination. Fig. 5-13 shows reverse side of this form.

tuberosity (Pochedly, 1969). The technic is the same as for other sites.

RIB MARROW ASPIRATION TECHNIC. The ribs may be used for marrow aspiration, but the puncture is technically difficult because of the narrow and flexible surface presented by the rib. This site should be reserved for instances in which there is roentgenographic evidence of a lesion in the rib. Care should be taken to avoid the intracostal vessels and nerves.

PREPARATION OF MARROW TISSUE FOR STUDY. The first material aspirated, *about 0.2 ml of marrow,* is used for the preparation of several thin smears. A 24-gauge needle is attached to the syringe, and small drops are individually placed on clean glass slides or coverslips. These are smeared out as for a peripheral blood smear. By delivering a very small drop of marrow through the small-gauge needle, good thin smears can be prepared (Fig. 5-11). If particle smears are desired as well, the remaining material from the first aspiration is expressed on a slide, and the small particles are identified, transferred to another slide, crushed gently, and then smeared.

Material from the second aspiration is expressed into a small test tube containing 1 drop of standard full-strength heparin solution, then mixed thoroughly with the anticoagulant, and used to make paraffin sections of marrow particles. There are various ways of collecting these particles,

one of the simplest being that of straining material through lens paper or some similar type of fine hard filter paper (Rywlin, 1976). After straining, the particles remaining on the paper are pushed together with an applicator stick and immediately fixed in Bouin's or other fixing fluid. Handling from this point on is the same as for any tissue specimen. The Giemsa stain recommended by Cramer et al (1973) gives excellent results.

I have been impressed by the magnificent sections prepared by fixing marrow particles in glutaraldehyde, embedding in methacrylate, and staining ultrathin sections with the Giemsa stain. These ultrathin sections provide not only the usual information obtainable from sections but also excellent cytologic detail. The ultrathin sections can also be used for iron stains and other special stains (Oberling et al, 1973).

If marrow aspiration is carried out chiefly for bacteriologic diagnosis, the second aspiration is expressed into a sterile tube containing 1 ml of 1% sodium citrate and mixed thoroughly. From this, routine and special bacteriologic studies can be made. Routine bacteriologic examination includes inoculation of thioglycollate broth, blood agar plates, and poured blood agar plates. Identification of *Mycobacterium tuberculosis* is best accomplished by culturing fresh marrow tissue or by guinea pig inoculation of the sediment or buffy coat after centrifugation.

Description:

Diagnosis:

NORMAL VALUES FOR CHILDREN	Control Figures for Various Age Groups									
	1-2 Mo.	3-12 Mo.	1-2 Yr.	3-4 Yr.	5-6 Yr.	7-8 Yr.	9-10 Yr.	11-12 Yr.	13-14 Yr.	15-16 Yr.
Myeloblasts	1.6	1.9	0.7	1.4	1.8	1.0	1.4	1.1	1.2	1.3
Progranulocytes	5.6	1.8	3.4	3.2	3.2	1.8	2.0	1.7	1.1	1.9
Myelocytes	18.1	16.7	13.3	15.9	17.2	17.4	16.5	15.31	16.4	16.8
Metamyelocytes	25.6	23.9	21.8	22.0	22.9	23.4	26.1	22.2	21.6	23.2
Bands and segs	9.3	7.2	14.1	16.4	12.6	12.3	10.9	12.2	12.2	13.3
Pronormoblasts	0.8	0.6	0.8	0.4	0.5	0.4	0.3	0.2	0.4	0.5
Basophilic normoblasts	1.9	2.1	1.2	1.0	1.2	1.7	1.6	1.8	1.3	2.2
Polychromatophilic normoblasts	12.6	14.5	19.5	16.4	17.3	19.4	19.1	21.8	18.3	15.1
Orthochromic normoblasts	1.6	2.5	2.1	1.2	3.6	3.4	2.4	2.7	3.1	2.5
Lymphocytes	19.7	25.4	19.3	18.6	17.5	13.6	13.6	16.0	18.0	17.4
Myeloid: erythroid ratio	5.5	3.5	2.5	3.4	2.8	2.6	2.9	2.3	2.7	3.3

Fig. 5-13. Reverse side of form shown in Fig. 5-12. These normal values were obtained years ago in our laboratory. Rosse et al (1977) have tabulated the normal values for 88 infants and children as they matured from birth to 18 months of age. Forty-five children were followed up for the entire 18 months. Their values differ significantly from the above, primarily showing a change in the percentage of lymphocytes after the first month from 14.42% ± 5.54% to values of more than 40%.

Maximum information will be obtained only when the method of handling the aspirated material is guided by a specific purpose. It is seldom desirable to perform a bone marrow aspiration in the hope that out of a mass of cytologic and bacteriologic data the diagnosis will manifest itself. The pathologist should decide on the procedure after seeing the patient and evaluating the circumstances.

Smears are stained with Wright's stain for routine studies, and a minimum of 500 nucleated cells is enumerated for a differential count. A form such as that shown in Figs. 5-12 and 5-13 is useful for reporting the results. Interpretation is made, of course, in conjunction with a study of the peripheral blood and other laboratory investigations after a visit to the bedside and a thorough study of the patient's clinical picture. Special cytologic studies such as supravital preparations, phase microscopy, electron microscopy, and cytochemical investigations are sometimes required.

OBTAINING MARROW BY TREPHINE BIOPSY

The technic of McFarland and Dameshek (1958), which uses the Vim-Silverman needle to perform a biopsy of bone marrow from the posterior iliac crest, is highly recommend-

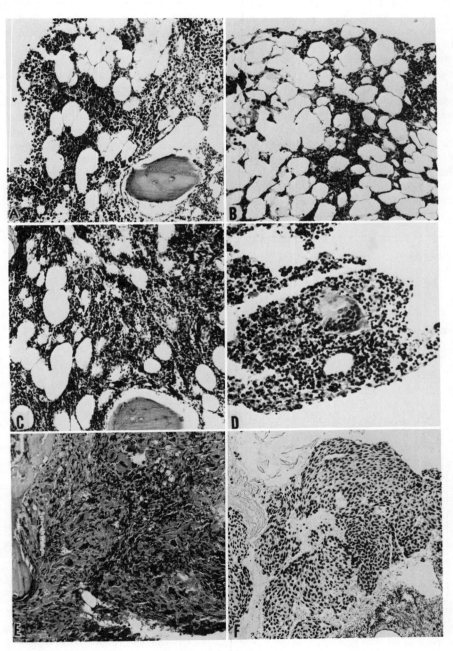

Fig. 5-14. Paraffin sections of bone marrow tissue obtained with Vim-Silverman needle. **A,** Normal marrow. **B,** Hypoplastic marrow. **C,** Chromic lymphocytic leukemia. **D,** Granuloma. **E,** Myeloproliferative syndrome with myelofibrosis. **F,** Metastatic carcinoma. (Hematoxylin-eosin stain; ×100.)

ed. It yields adequate specimens and is easily mastered. The technic is basically the same as that used for an aspiration biopsy at the posterior iliac crest. A 2⅜-inch Vim-Silverman needle with obturator in place is inserted through the posterior crest and inclined toward the iliac crest in a slightly cephalad direction. When the point of the needle has just entered the marrow cavity, the obturator is removed and the biopsy blades are inserted. The biopsy blades are then advanced their full length by steady forward pressure without rotation. The outer portion of the needle is then advanced over the biopsy needle by a gentle clockwise and counterclockwise rotation. When it can be advanced no farther, the units are withdrawn together. The plug of marrow tissue is then gently expressed. One or more particles can be teased out and used for smears. The greater portion of tissue is used to prepare histologic sections (Fig. 5-14). Dancey et al (1976) recommend fixation in acrolein, embedding in methyl methacrylate, and sectioning at 2 mm thickness. This technic gives even fixation and avoids distortion and shrinkage of the cells. However, they found these sections do not stain well with Wright's or Giemsa's stain and recommend staining with eosin Y and azure II and staining for esterase activity for better visualization of neutrophil granules.

Ellis et al (1964) reported their experience with a modified Vim-Silverman needle (Fig. 5-15), which is an improvement over the standard needle. The modified needle yields large specimens and is more durable. In 1,455 needle biopsies they had only a 5% failure rate. In 157 cases the biopsy specimen obtained by this technic enabled them to make a diagnosis not apparent by the aspiration specimen (Table 5-2). In 96 other cases the tissue section confirmed

the diagnosis made from the aspiration specimen (polycythemia vera, acute leukemia, chronic myelocytic leukemia, chronic lymphocytic leukemia, multiple myeloma, and Gaucher's disease). The value of bone marrow biopsy using the Jamshidi-Swaim biopsy needle (Jamshidi and Swaim, 1971) in the diagnosis of bone marrow lesions and in the staging of Hodgkin's and non-Hodgkin's lymphomas is substantiated by Bearden et al (1974) and Dick et al (1974). Similar results have been obtained using other types of trephine needles (Brunning et al, 1975). Surely the hematologist who "doesn't believe" in tissue sections of bone marrow will be limited not only in diagnostic success but also in chances of going to heaven.

Table 5-2. Diagnoses made from paraffin sections, not apparent in aspiration biopsy material (total of 1,445 needle biopsies)*

Miliary tuberculosis	6
Sarcoidosis	2
Histoplasmosis	1
Granuloma, ? type	1
Myelofibrosis	36
Aplastic marrow	39
Metastatic tumor	25
Osteitis fibrosa cystica	9
Paget's disease	2
Hodgkin's disease	7
Lymphosarcoma	23
Reticulum cell sarcoma	5
Thrombotic thrombocytopenic purpura	1
TOTAL	157

*From Ellis et al, 1964.

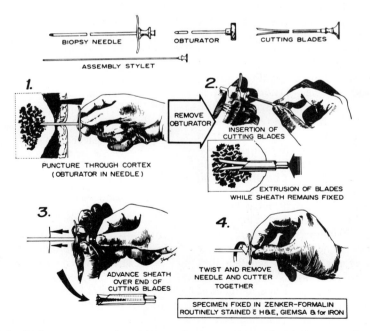

Fig. 5-15. Obtaining bone marrow tissue from posterior iliac crest with modified Vim-Silverman needle. (Courtesy Dr. M. P. Westerman; from Ellis et al, 1964.)

POSTMORTEM MARROW

Marrow obtained during necropsy and processed routinely yields paraffin sections that are generally adequate with regard to cellular detail. In fact, Krumbhaar (1936) studied an archaeologic skeleton estimated to be 600 to 1,000 years old and found the marrow sections to have surprisingly good cellular detail. If, however, one obtains postmortem marrow by aspiration and prepares smears in the usual manner, it will be found that within a very few hours after death there is considerable autolysis and that even those cells not showing degenerative changes stain poorly. Adult granulocytes, particularly, autolyze rapidly; lymphocytes are the best preserved. In general, aspiration biopsy of bone marrow yields acceptable smear specimens up to 3 hours after death, but in some cases autolysis will be well advanced by this time. Refrigeration does not seem to alter significantly the quality of specimens obtained during the first 3-hour period.

The addition of bovine albumin to marrow prior to preparing smears restores cytologic detail and yields good preparations for as long as 23 hours postmortem (Rickert and Vidone, 1968). The albumin technic was originally advocated by Berenbaum (1956), who suggested that the rapid postmortem change is not the result of the autolysis but rather increased susceptibility of the cells to shearing when smeared. Albumin may protect the cells from this damage because of its high viscosity.

NORMAL MARROW AND THE SIGNIFICANCE OF DEVIATIONS FROM NORMAL

There is general agreement that at birth all marrow spaces are filled with active red marrow and that in the normal adult some of the marrow space is occupied by fatty tissue. By 20 years of age, the shafts of the long bones normally contain only fatty (yellow) marrow, red marrow being found only in the proximal epiphyseal end. The marrow-containing bones in the adult are skull, clavicles, scapulae, sternum, ribs, vertbrae, pelvis, and proximal end of the long bones. With advancing age, even the marrow in these bones changes in the amount of fatty tissue it contains; whereas the bone marrow in a normal young adult is half fatty and half red, that of men and women of advanced age (late sixties, seventies, and eighties) is normally two-thirds fatty and one-third red.

The mean weight of all marrow, fatty and red, in a normal person weighing 70 kg has been estimated to be about 3,600 Gm. The mass of marrow in all bones normally containing some red marrow is likewise estimated to be about 2,100 Gm. The normal weight of red marrow only is calculated by Ellis (1961) to be 1,459 Gm for a 70 kg man. It can be seen, therefore, that the mass of functioning marrow in the adult is about that of the liver. Table 5-3 summarizes the distribution of functioning marrow in a normal adult; Table 5-4 gives the distribution of marrow spaces regardless of whether they contain fatty marrow, red marrow, or both. Values for bone marrow volume in the fetus and newborn are comparable with the exception of a relatively greater volume in the newborn skull (Hudson, 1965). When there is stimulation of hemopoiesis, for whatever reason, fatty marrow is replaced by red marrow to various degrees. When hemopoiesis is very active, as in pernicious anemia or leukemia, not only is

Table 5-3. Distribution of red marrow by weight in bones of normal 40-year-old man*

Site	Weight of red marrow (grams)	Percent of total red marrow
Cranium and mandible	136.6	13.1
Humeri, scapulae, and clavicles	86.7	8.3
Sternum	23.4	2.3
Ribs	82.6	7.9
Vertebrae	297.8	28.4
Pelvis	418.6	40.0

*From Ellis, 1961.

Table 5-4. Distribution of marrow spaces in adult human skeleton*

Bone	Percent of total marrow space
Humeri	5.98
Ulnae	1.38
Radii	1.34
Hands and wrists	2.74
TOTAL, UPPER LIMBS	11.44
Femora	17.06
Tibiae	10.92
Fibulae	1.54
Patellae	0.82
Ankles and feet	8.42
TOTAL, LOWER LIMBS	38.76
Ribs, 1-4	2.08
Ribs, 5-8	3.36
Ribs, 9-12	1.90
TOTAL, RIBS	7.34
Cranium	6.33
Mandible	0.60
TOTAL, HEAD	6.93
Scapulae	2.38
Clavicles	0.76
Sternum	1.38
Pelvis	16.28
TOTAL	20.80
Cervical vertebrae	1.78
Dorsal vertebrae	7.29
Lumbar vertebrae	5.61
TOTAL, SPINE	14.68

*From Woodard and Holodny, 1960.

all marrow red but, even within this, very little fatty tissue can be seen. In infants and children, the marrow spaces being already filled with red marrow, increased hemopoietic activity, as in hemolytic anemia, is accommodated by an enlargement of the marrow space that produces typical roentgenographic findings (Fig. 5-16).

The use of isotopes to estimate marrow mass and to locate areas of increased activity has fired the enthusiasm of some investigators but seems to have little practical value and possibly some danger. Isotopes, especially the colloidal ones,

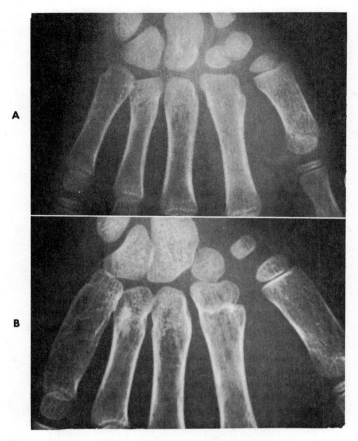

Fig. 5-16. Typical roentgenographic findings in severe erythroid hyperplasia. Enlargement of marrow space due to increased hemopoietic activity. **A,** Hand of normal 9-year-old child. **B,** Hand of 9-year-old child having marked erythroid hyperplasia (sickle cell anemia). (Courtesy Dr. Catherine Poole.)

are removed from the bloodstream by reticuloendothelial cells, and the uptake in the marrow is said to correlate close-ly with hemopoietic activity. Edwards et al (1964) used [198]Au and obtained some interesting graphic representation of the mass of marrow in various bones. It is extremely doubtful, however, whether the use of such an isotope hav-ing a long half-life is justified merely to obtain pretty pic-tures.

The values for a normal differential count shown in Fig. 5-12 are derived from counts on marrows from 500 suppos-edly normal adults. The results are similar to other published normal values. In some categories the range is wide as may be expected when one realizes that aspiration samples a very small volume of marrow tissue. Further, the usual differen-tial count done on 500 cells is not based on a sufficiently large number of cells to provide a critically narrow range of normal values. Since it is customary in our laboratory to count 500 marrow cells, the control values are based on 500-cell differential counts of normal marrows. Fig. 5-13 shows control values for children (see legend).

Normal marrow

We consider a marrow specimen normal if the differential count falls within the normal range, if it is normally cellular as determined by a paraffin section, and if no foreign or abnormal cells are present.

Normal constituents such as osteoclasts and osteoblasts (Fig. 5-17) should not be confused with metastatic tumor cells or atypical megakaryocytes. They are found most fre-quently in specimens from infants and children but may also be seen in adult specimens. *Osteoblasts* have a deeply baso-philic cytoplasm and an eccentric nucleus. These two fea-tures give the osteoblast an appearance superficially similar to a plasma cell. Differential features are as follows: (1) an osteoblast is about twice the size of a plasma cell, (2) an osteoblast almost always shows an irregularly round area of pale-staining cytoplasm not related to the nucleus, whereas the lighter staining area of the plasma cell surrounds the nucleus, and (3) the nucleus of the osteoblast usually shows one or more distinct nucleoli. *Osteoclasts* may be confused with megakaryocytes since both are large, but they can usu-ally be distinguished from these by the presence of an even number of distinct round or oval nuclei, all of which are identical in appearance. Fat cells and mast cells (Fig. 5-18) should not be mistaken for pathologic cells.

Another normal finding is illustrated in Fig. 5-19, which shows a lymphoid nodule. These areas are usually sharply defined and consist of small lymphocytes. Rywlin et al (1974) and Rywlin (1976) have made a detailed study of normal and abnormal lymphoid nodules in the bone mar-row. They found them to be more common in normal mar-row than recorded in previous reports. It is probable that

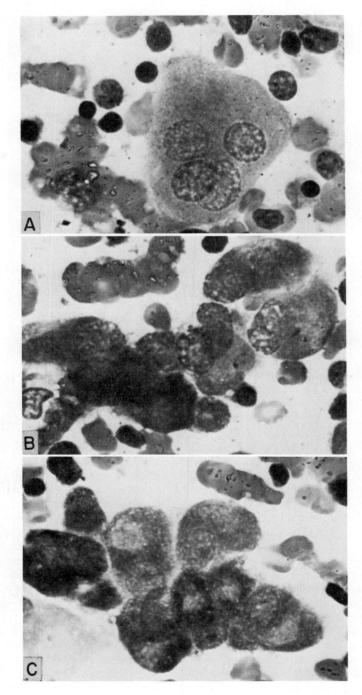

Fig. 5-17. Osteoclasts and osteoblasts found in normal marrow. **A,** Osteoclast. **B** and **C,** Osteoblasts. (Wright's stain; ×950.)

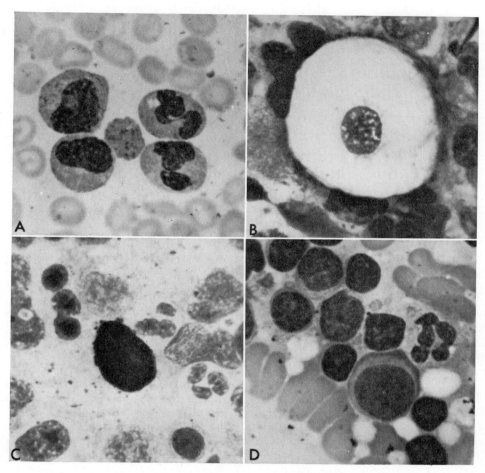

Fig. 5-18. Miscellaneous cells. **A,** Fragment of cytoplasm of a granulocyte surrounded by four intact cells, bone marrow. **B,** Fat cell, bone marrow. **C,** Mast cell, bone marrow. **D,** Very primitive cell, lymph node imprint. (Wright's stain; ×950.)

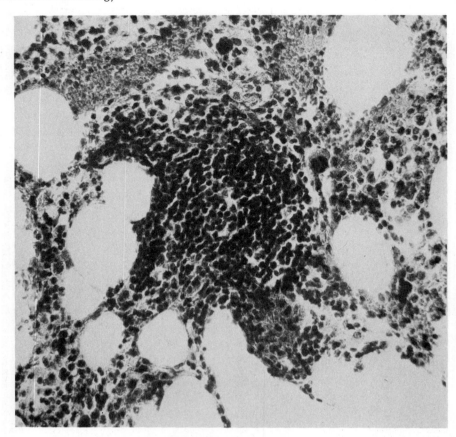

Fig. 5-19. Lymphoid nodule found in normal marrow, paraffin section. (Hematoxylin-eosin stain; ×450.)

they contribute to the lymphocytic population of the normal marrow. It is important to recognize them as normal marrow structures.

Deviations from the normal may be qualitative or quantitative. These are summarized in Table 5-5.

Qualitative abnormalities

Qualitative abnormalities may be caused by cells having an abnormal morphology, such as immature or atypical cells, or by the presence of cells foreign to the marrow, such as metastatic tumor cells (Lake-Lewin et al, 1975; Rosenberg, 1975; Garrett et al, 1976; Anner and Drewinko, 1977; Pasmantier et al, 1977; Singh et al, 1977; Savage et al, 1978). In some cases there are quantitative changes as well as qualitative abnormalities; e.g., infiltration of the marrow with tumor cells is often accompanied by a reduction in the number of normal marrow cells. This is not due to "crowding out" of normal cells by the abnormal ones but rather to poorly understood metabolic effects. In other cases of metastatic invasion there may be increased proliferation of normal marrow cells, with increased cellularity and decreased fat content.

Qualitative abnormalities are identified by a careful microscopic study of the smears and sections. It is strongly recommended that these be studied first under low magnification to avoid overlooking clumps of abnormal cells. In *multiple myeloma* the characteristic cells are often present in large numbers and may be identified easily under low mag-

nification. Nonmyelomatous (reactive) *plasmacytosis* (greater than 4% plasma cells) is seen in cirrhosis of the liver, in infectious diseases, and in immunologic reactions (Hyun et al, 1976). An increase in *mast cells* may be found in chronic lymphocytic leukemia, macroglobulinemia, miliary tuberculosis, carcinoma metastatic to the bone marrow, and various lymphoproliferative diseases (Nixon, 1966; Yoo et al, 1978). *Megaloblastic cells* may also be easily identified under low power, but other features of megaloblastic dyspoiesis require oil-immersion magnification and attention to minute details. *Tumor cells* are usually present in clumps (Fig. 5-20) that are visible under low magnification. These clumps may be numerous, particularly if aspiration has been carried out at a site of bone destruction. A number of slides may have to be searched before they are found. The *lipid storage diseases* such as Gaucher's, Niemann-Pick, and Hand-Schüller-Christian disease usually show such a strikingly abnormal picture that the diagnosis is obvious at first glance. These and other lipid-containing macrophages are discussed in Chapter 2. Conn and Sundberg (1961) reported three cases of primary amyloidosis with involvement of the bone marrow; in one case the diagnosis of amyloidosis was first made from the sternal marrow biopsy. Necrotic tumor tissue or necrotic bone marrow tissue caused by ischemia should not be confused with artifactual changes (Brown, 1972). Drug sensitivity reactions may account for the eosinophilic fibrohistiocytic lesions described by Rywlin et al (1972). Rywlin and Ortega (1972)

Table 5-5. Classification of abnormalities that may be present in bone marrow

I. Qualitative abnormalities
  A. "Myeloma" cells
  B. Megaloblastic dysplasia
  C. Tumor cells
  D. "Storage cells"—Gaucher's, Niemann-Pick, Hand-Schüller-Christian, etc.
  E. LE cells
  F. Lymphoma cells
  G. Porphyria erythropoietica
  H. Granulomas (tuberculosis, brucellosis, infectious mononucleosis)
  I. Parasites (plasmodia, leishmania, trichinae)
  J. Bacteria and fungi
  K. Vacuolization of normoblasts in chloramphenicol toxicity
  L. Vacuolization of normoblasts in phenylketonuria
  M. Vacuolization of normoblasts in acute alcoholism
  N. Amyloidosis
  O. Necrotic tissue (tumor or ischemic infarct)
II. Quantitative abnormalities
  A. Hyperplasia
    1. Generalized
      a. Myeloproliferative syndromes
      b. Reaction to pancytopenia
    2. Selective
      a. Lymphocytic
        (1) Lymphocytic leukemia
        (2) Infectious mononucleosis
        (3) Infectious lymphocytosis
        (4) Various viral infections
        (5) Lymphocytic leukemoid reaction
        (6) Relative because of decrease in other cell types
        (7) Lymphomas
      b. Granulocytic
        (1) Infection
        (2) Myelocytic leukemia
        (3) Myelocytic leukemoid reaction (myeloproliferative syndrome, myelocytic type)
        (4) Relative because of decrease in other cell types
      c. Monocytic
        (1) Monocytic leukemia
        (2) Relative because of decrease in other cell types
      d. Plasmacytic
        (1) Multiple myeloma
        (2) Rheumatoid arthritis
        (3) Hypersensitivity states
        (4) Syphilis
        (5) Hepatic cirrhosis
        (6) Hodgkin's disease

        (7) Waldenström's macroglobulinemia
        (8) Amyloidosis
        (9) Malignant tumors
        (10) Weber-Christian disease
        (11) Ulcerative colitis
      e. Normoblastic
        (1) Chronic blood loss
        (2) Hemolytic anemias
        (3) Iron-deficiency anemias
        (4) Erythremia
        (5) Treated megaloblastic anemia
        (6) Myeloproliferative syndrome, erythroid type
        (7) Relative because of decrease in other cell types
      f. Megakaryocytic
        (1) Thrombocytopenias
        (2) Myeloproliferative syndrome, megakaryocytic type
      g. Histiocytic
        (1) Congenital rubella
        (2) Bacterial infection
        (3) Parasitic infection
        (4) Kyasanur Forest disease
        (5) Lymphomas
      h. Mast cells
        (1) Mast cell disease
        (2) Osteoporosis of aging
  B. Hypoplasia
    1. Generalized
      a. Myelofibrosis
      b. Myelosclerosis
      c. Osteopetrosis
      d. Caused by myelotoxic agents (chemicals, ionizing radiation, etc.)
      e. Caused by tumor or other infiltrations
      f. Virus infection (Venezuelan equine encephalitis, dengue fever, rubella)
      g. "Burned-out" erythremia
      h. Physiologic in old age
      i. "Idiopathic"
    2. Selective
      a. Granulocytic
        (1) Agranulocytosis
        (2) Ionizing radiation (early effect)
        (3) Relative
      b. Normoblastic
      c. Megakaryocytic
        (1) Thrombocytopenic purpura (some types)
        (2) Benzol poisoning
      d. Plasmacytic in agammaglobulinemia

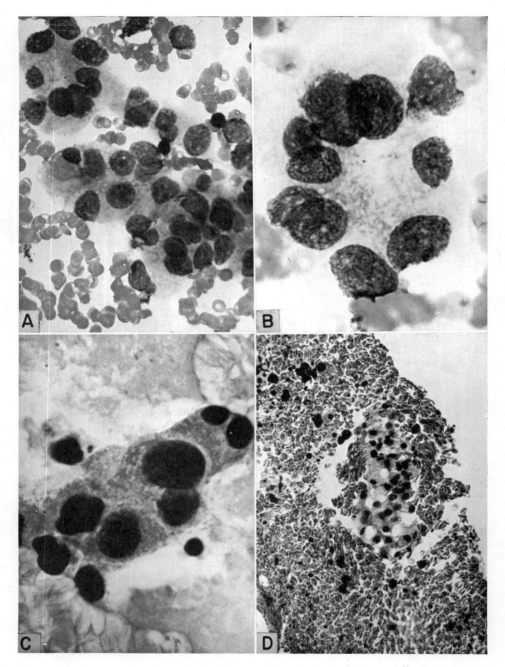

Fig. 5-20. Metastatic tumor cells in marrow aspirates. **A,** Metastatic adenocarcinoma of prostate. (Wright's stain; ×450.) **B,** The same. (×950.) **C,** Carcinoma of prostate, undifferentiated. (Wright's stain; ×950.) **D,** Carcinoma of breast, paraffin section. (Hematoxylin-eosin stain; ×450.)

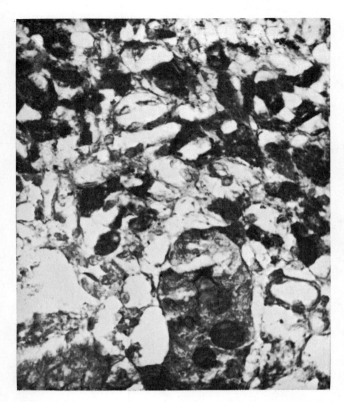

Fig. 5-21. Bone marrow, Whipple's disease, paraffin section. (PAS stain; ×1,600.)

describe lipid granulomas. Granulomas are also found in Q fever (Okun et al, 1979). I encountered a case of Whipple's disease in which the aspirated marrow showed the diagnostic PAS-positive intracellular material (Fig. 5-21). An interesting case of anthracosis of the bone marrow has been described by Miller (Fig. 5-22).

Peripheral blood preparations and antinuclear antibody identification have largely replaced marrow studies in the search for the *LE phenomenon* in disseminated lupus erythematosus. Nevertheless, excellent preparations may be produced if the marrow is handled as recommended. Schmid et al (1955) have called attention to a qualitative abnormality of the normoblasts in *porphyria erythropoietica*. As shown in Fig. 5-23, some of the normoblasts show a characteristic nuclear inclusion of hemoglobin that is usually apparent in routine preparations. Diagnosis of the *lymphomas* rests largely on the presence of morphologically abnormal cells, but usually these cases are accompanied by striking quantitative abnormalities.

Parasites (malaria, trypanosomiasis) may be seen easily in Wright-stained smears, although some advocate the Giemsa stain for this purpose. *Histoplasma* is seen easily with either Wright's stain or a silver stain (Fig. 5-24). Tuberculosis of the bone marrow shows typical tubercles (Fig. 5-25). Acid-fast organisms of various kinds can be demonstrated by the acid-fast stain (Fig. 5-26). Special cultures should supplement morphologic identification of microorganisms.

Finally, some qualitative abnormalities are best revealed

by paraffin sections of marrow particles. In diseases characterized by a granulomatous tissue reaction the characteristic conformation may be clearly revealed in a paraffin section but may be destroyed or obscured in a smear.

Necrosis of bone marrow tissue may be found in a variety of diseases: neoplastic, infectious, or nutritional (Kiraly and Wheby, 1976; Norgard et al, 1979). There is no common etiology, with the possible exception of vascular occlusion caused by sickle cell disease or Hb S/C hemoglobinopathy (Charache and Page, 1967), or disseminated intravascular coagulation (Harigaya et al, 1977). Necrosis of bone marrow tissue may produce bone pain (Kinney et al, 1977).

Quantitative abnormalities

Quantitative abnormalities may be relative or absolute. Aplasia, hypoplasia, or hyperplasia may affect the marrow as a whole or may be selective for only one cell type. If all cell types are affected, the differential count may be normal, and the quantitative abnormality becomes apparent only on study of the paraffin sections. If one cell type is predominantly affected, the differential count will reveal the relative disproportion among cell types, and the paraffin section determines whether the increase or decrease is relative or absolute.

Fong et al (1979) compared three types of bone marrow preparations for the estimation of cellularity: (1) needle biopsy sections, (2) smears of aspirated marrow particles, and (3) aspirated clot sections. Cellularity was estimated by both the usual survey method and by the point-counting method of Hartsock et al (1965). The point-counting method, although the more accurate, is time consuming—requiring about 1 hour per specimen—and is poorly reproducible by different observers. I still feel that an estimation made from a paraffin section of particles or from a core biopsy is sufficient, remembering that there may be a great deal of variation in the cellularity from one biopsy site to another. Smears and sections should be prepared from every biopsy specimen.

One of the common indications for a biopsy of the bone marrow is to estimate storage iron, which is reported as decreased, normal, or increased. Note that the estimation of storage iron should be done on smears rather than from histologic sections of tissue obtained by core biopsy (Fong et al, 1977). It is probable that the loss of stainable iron is caused by decalcification procedures, because histologic sections prepared from formalin-fixed particles compare favorably with the smear preparations.

Normal bone marrow has a supporting lattice of lacy connective tissue, referred to generally as reticulin. It consists of two types of fibers, those staining by silver impregnation but not with the trichrome stain (true reticulin) and those staining with the trichrome stain (collagenous reticulin). Reticulin is increased in most pathologic marrow (Rywlin, 1976), such as is present in agnogenic myeloid metaplasia, lipid granulomas, chronic lymphocytic leukemia, monoclonal macroglobulinemia, myeloma, polycythemia vera, and myelofibrosis. Manoharan et al (1979) found increased reticulin in acute leukemia and reported that effective antileukemic therapy resulted in resolution of some or all of the increased reticulin.

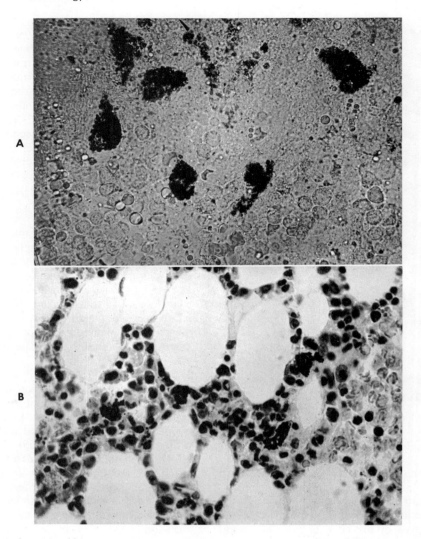

Fig. 5-22. Anthracosis of bone marrow. **A,** Unstained marrow tissue. **B,** Paraffin section. (Hematoxylin-eosin stain.) (From Miller, 1959.)

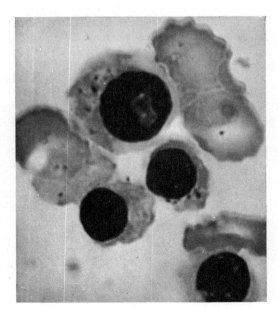

Fig. 5-23. Normoblasts, porphyria erythropoietica. (Courtesy Dr. R. Schmid.)

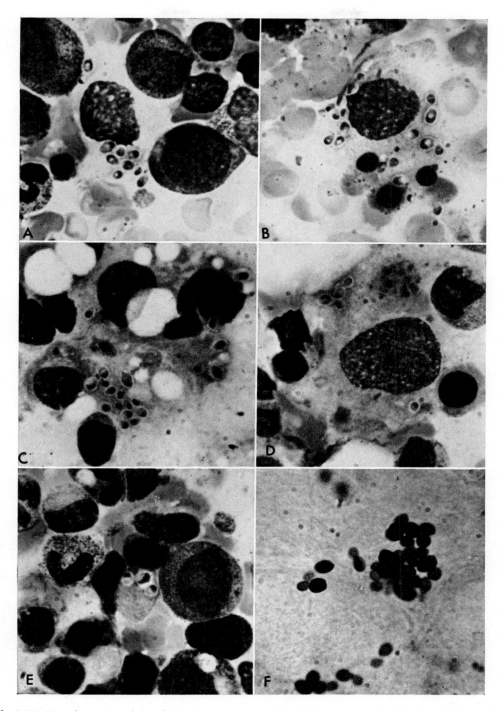

Fig. 5-24. *Histoplasma capsulatum,* bone marrow smears. (**A-E,** Wright's stain; ×950. **F,** Gomori silver stain.) (Courtesy Dr. A. A. Cooperburg.)

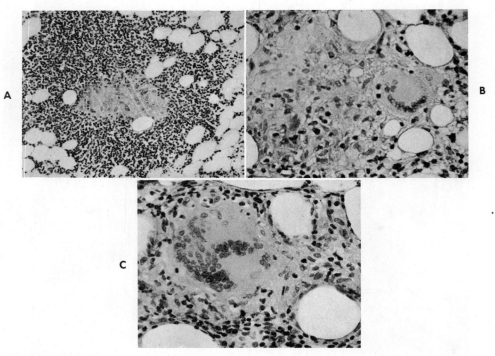

Fig. 5-25. Tubercle (*Mycobacterium tuberculosis* infection), bone marrow. (Hematoxylin-eosin stain; **A,** ×120; **B** and **C,** ×400.)

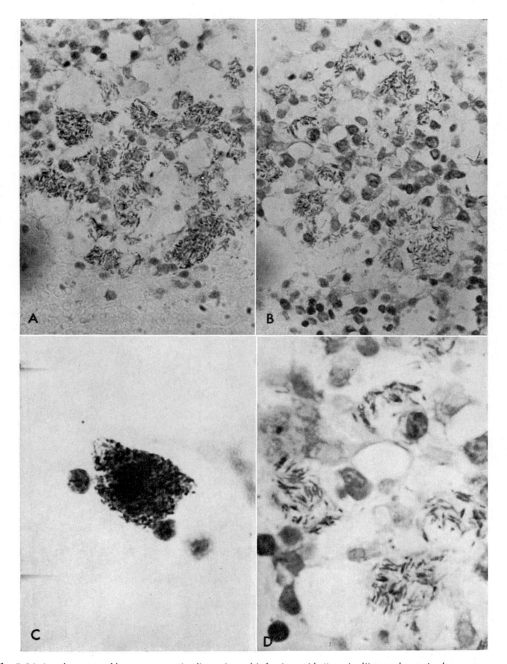

Fig. 5-26. Involvement of bone marrow in disseminated infection with "atypical" mycobacteria, bone marrow smears. **C** shows a histiocyte engorged with acid-fast bacilli. (**A** and **B,** Acid-fast stain; ×400. **C** and **D,** Acid-fast stain; ×950.)

Illustrative cases

Cases from our files are presented and illustrated in Figs. 5-27 to 5-83. It cannot be emphasized too strongly that hematologic diagnosis begins at the bedside. Laboratory studies may be all important in establishing the diagnosis but can seldom be divorced from the history and physical examination. Many pitfalls await the physician who attempts to make a diagnosis solely on the basis of marrow morphology. The stethoscope and examining finger are as necessary to the pathologist as the microscope.

Fig. 5-27. Case 1. Normal bone marrow. **A-C,** Marrow smears. (Wright's stain; ×950.) **D,** Paraffin section of marrow. (Hematoxylin-eosin stain; ×450.)

Bone marrow differential count

Cell	Percent		Cell	Percent	
Myeloblasts		0.8	Segmented (total)		10.2
Progranulocytes		2.8	Neutrophils	9.6	
Myelocytes (total)		7.4	Eosinophils	0.4	
Neutrophilic	6.7		Basophils	0.2	
Eosinophilic	0.6		Prolymphocytes		0.4
Basophilic	0.1		Lymphocytes		6.2
Myelocytes (total)		16.0	Monocytes		1.2
Neutrophilic	15.6		Plasmacytes		1.8
Eosinophilic	0.3		Megakaryocytes		0.6
Basophilic	0.1		Normoblasts (total)		24.2
Band cells (total)		28.0	Pronormoblasts	0.6	
Neutrophilic	26.6		Basophilic normoblasts	4.2	
Eosinophilic	1.4		Polychromatophilic normoblasts	16.6	
			Orthochromic normoblasts	2.8	
			Reticulum cells		0.4

History and physical examination: Normal 23-year-old medical student in apparent good health. Physical examination was normal.

Laboratory data: Peripheral blood studies revealed Hb 14.6 Gm/dl, RBC 4.87 million/mm^3 (4.87 × 10^{12}/l), WBC 10,700/mm^3 (10.7 × 10^9/l); leukocyte differential count: 5% stab neutrophils, 49% segmented neutrophils, 37% lymphocytes, 4% monocytes, 4% eosinophils, and 1% basophils; erythrocyte morphology, normal; platelet count 247,000/mm^3 (0.247 × 10^{12}/l) (phase microscopy).

Discussion: Marrow differential count shows a normal distribution of cell types. Values fall within limits of control values. Note the normal cellularity in **D.**

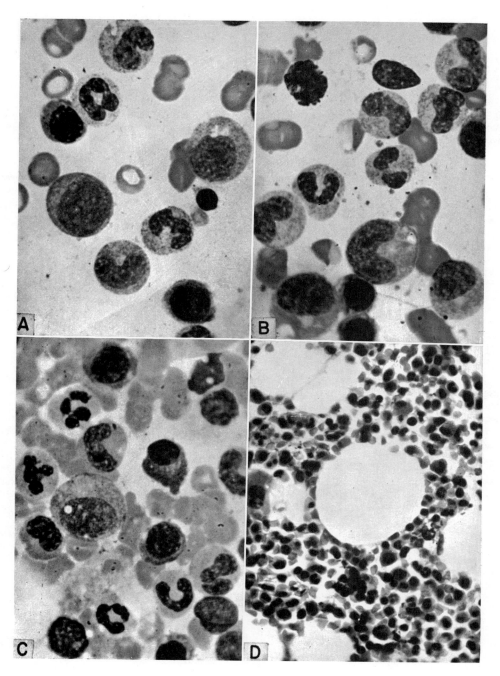

Fig. 5-27

Fig. 5-28. Case 2. Hyperplasia of the myeloid series secondary to infection (pneumonia). **A,** Marrow smear. (Wright's stain; ×450.) **B** and **C,** Marrow smear. (Wright's stain; ×950.) **D,** Paraffin section of marrow. (Hematoxylin-eosin stain; ×450.)

Bone marrow differential count

Cell	Percent		Cell	Percent
Progranulocytes		1.0	Prolymphocytes	1.0
Myelocytes (total)		10.0	Lymphocytes	5.6
Neutrophilic	7.6		Monocytes	2.4
Eosinophilic	2.2		Proplasmacytes	0.2
Basophilic	0.2		Plasmacytes	3.8
Metamyelocytes (total)		13.0	Megakaryocytes	0.4
Neutrophilic	12.4		Polychromatophilic normoblasts	1.8
Eosinophilic	0.6		Orthochromic normoblasts	8.4
Band cells (total)		36.2	Reticulum cells	0.2
Neutrophilic	36.0			
Eosinophilic	0.2			
Segmented (total)		16.0		
Neutrophils	15.0			
Eosinophils	1.0			

History and physical examination: Two days before admission the patient, a 40-year-old man, had an acute onset of fever and chills. One day before admission there was a cough productive of rusty sputum and sharp pleural pain on the right side. Examination revealed dullness and decreased breath sounds over the right posterior thorax. Roentgenogram showed a moderate amount of fluid at the base of the right lung and patchy opacities in the right lower lobe. There was moderate generalized lymphadenopathy. The spleen was firm and easily palpable 3 cm below the costal margin.

Laboratory data: Hb 12.5 Gm/dl of blood, RBC 4.5 million/mm^3 (4.5×10^{12}/l), WBC 18,700/mm^3 (18.7×10^9/l); leukocyte differential count: 47% segmented neutrophils, 28% stab neutrophils, 17% lymphocytes, 7% monocytes, and 1% eosinophils; total protein 6.26 Gm/dl of serum (albumin 3.71 Gm and globulin 2.55 Gm/dl of serum). Culture of sputum revealed an almost pure culture of *Diplococcus pneumoniae.* Urinalysis showed mild proteinuria, 35 mg/dl, and on microscopic examination, occasional leukocytes and erythrocytes were found in the sediment.

Discussion: Bone marrow aspiration was performed because of the lymphadenopathy and splenomegaly. The marrow was much more cellular than normal, **D,** with only occasional noncellular fat spaces. Bone marrow differential count showed a relative increase of myeloid cells, mostly in the band forms, suggesting that the stimulus was relatively mild. In severe infections there may be striking proliferation with metamyelocytes as well, so that both the marrow and the peripheral blood may contain immature myeloid cells. These "leukemoid" reactions must be differentiated from myelocytic leukemia.

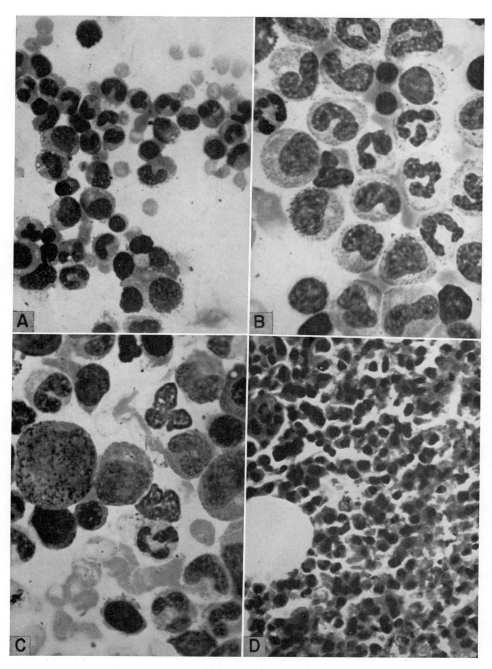

Fig. 5-28

Fig. 5-29. Case 3. Generalized hyperplasia of the bone marrow with toxic changes due to sepsis, bone marrow smears. (Wright's stain; ×950.) Toxic changes illustrated consist chiefly of cytoplasmic vacuoles with moderate toxic granulation of the neutrophilic cells.

Bone marrow differential count

Cell	Percent		Cell	Percent
Myeloblasts		1.0	Segmented (total)		12.6
Progranulocytes		2.0	Neutrophils	11.8	
Myelocytes (total)		21.6	Eosinophils	0.8	
Neutrophilic	21.6		Lymphocytes		9.0
Metamyelocytes (total)		24.0	Monocytes		0.2
Neutrophilic	24.0		Plasmacytes		0.4
Band cells (total)		22.4	Pronormoblasts		0.2
Neutrophilic	22.0		Basophilic normoblasts		0.2
Eosinophilic	0.4		Polychromatophilic normoblasts		6.0
			Reticulum cells		0.4

History and physical examination: This 69-year-old woman had been ill at home for about 2 weeks. During this time she had a spiking fever (as high as 105° F, 40° C), progressive weakness, anorexia, and considerable weight loss. For some years she had dysuria and frequency of urination, complaints that became more severe about a month before admission. She was found to be acutely ill, dehydrated, and emaciated. Her temperature was 105° F (40° C). There was marked bilateral costovertebral angle tenderness. The spleen was tender and palpable 4 cm below the costal margin.

Laboratory data: Peripheral blood Hb 8.2 Gm/dl, RBC 2.86 million/mm³ (2.86×10^{12}/l), WBC 44,950/mm³ (44.95×10^9/l); leukocyte differential count: 12% neutrophilic myelocytes, 33% stab neutrophils, 39% segmented neutropolis, 7% lymphocytes, 8% monocytes, and 1% basophils; erythrocyte and platelet morphology normal. Urine contained 115 mg protein/dl, acetone, and clumps of leukocytes. Many gram-negative bacilli were found in a gram-stained smear of the urine sediment. Blood and urine cultures were positive for *Escherichia coli.*

Discussion: The marrow was extremely cellular and the differential count showed a marked preponderance of neutrophilic cells. Toxic changes were striking, with vacuolization of the cells and heavy coarse granulation. Similar changes were seen in the neutrophils of the peripheral blood. It is interesting to note that the myeloid hyperplasia in the marrow does not involve the eosinophils. This patient apparently had been suffering from chronic, and later acute, pyelonephritis complicated by bacteremia. The myeloid hyperplasia of the bone marrow and the peripheral blood leukocytosis speak not only for the severity of the septic state but also for a considerable degree of hemopoietic reactivity in spite of the patient's advanced age. In view of the hematologic response, the prognosis was good, and, indeed, prompt and effective antibiotic therapy resulted in complete recovery from the acute episode.

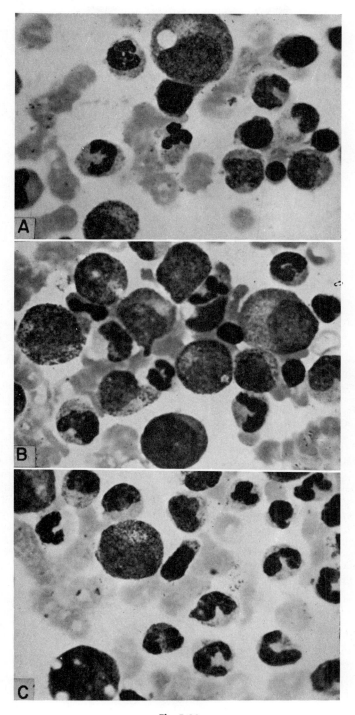

Fig. 5-29

Fig. 5-30. Case 4. Normoblastic hyperplasia due to chronic hemorrhage; bone marrow smears showing a preponderance of normoblastic cells. (Wright's stain; ×950.)

Bone marrow differential count

Cell	Percent		Cell		Percent
Myeloblasts		1.5	Segmented (total)		18.5
Progranulocytes		0.5	Neutrophils	15.0	
Myelocytes (total)		8.0	Eosinophils	3.5	
Neutrophilic	7.0		Lymphocytes		2.0
Eosinophilic	1.0		Monocytes		0.5
Metamyelocytes (total)		3.0	Plasmacytes		8.0
Neutrophilic	3.0		Megakaryocytes		2.0
Band cells (total)		7.0	Pronormoblasts		0.5
Neutrophilic	7.0		Basophilic normoblasts		8.0
			Polychromatophilic normoblasts		10.0
			Orthochromic normoblasts		30.5

History and physical examination: This 77-year-old man had been suffering from complications of benign prostatic hypertrophy. This had required his regular attendance at the urology outpatient clinic for about 2 years. On one occasion a blood count showed that he had severe anemia. When questioned, he admitted noticing tarry stools for 1 year. Since, in his mind, this had nothing to do with his difficulty in urination, he had not called anyone's attention to it. Subsequent laboratory tests showed a persistently and strongly positive reaction for occult blood in the stool. Gastrointestinal roentgenograms showed extensive diverticulosis.

Laboratory data: Peripheral blood studies revealed Hb 4.8 Gm/dl, RBC 1.83 million/mm^3 (1.83 × 10^{12}/l), WBC 18,850/mm^3 (18.85 × 10^9/l); leukocyte differential count: 41% segmented neutrophils, 4% band neutrophils, 1% neutrophilic metamyelocytes, 51% lymphocytes, and 3% eosinophils; reticulocyte count 4.2%. Urine was cloudy and alkaline, with specific gravity of 1.007, trace of protein, and no sugar. Microscopic examination showed 70 to 80 leukocytes per high-power field and many bacteria in the sediment. Urea nitrogen was 23 mg/dl of serum.

Discussion: Normoblastic hyperplasia of the marrow is typical in chronic blood loss. Chronic hemorrhage eventually produces an iron deficiency that is reflected in hypochromic and usually microcytic anemia. The normoblastic hyperplasia represents an attempt to compensate for the peripheral deficiency of hemoglobin mass and may be expected whenever iron deficiency, in the broad sense, exists. One characteristic feature of this type of anemia is the low serum iron and low iron content of the marrow and other body depots. In anemia due to chronic infection there is usually normoblastic hyperplasia and normal or increased amounts of iron in the marrow.

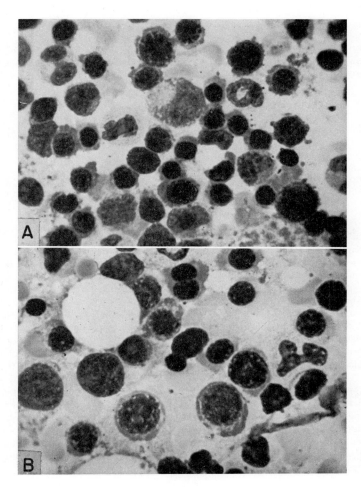

Fig. 5-30

Fig. 5-31. Case 5. Normoblastic hyperplasia associated with iron-deficiency anemia. **A,** Bone marrow smear. (Wright's stain; ×450.) **B** and **C,** Bone marrow smears. (Wright's stain; ×950.) **D,** Peripheral blood smear. (Wright's stain; ×950.) Note the extreme hypochromia, anisocytosis, and poikilocytosis of the erythrocytes illustrated in **D.**

Bone marrow differential count

Cell	Percent		Cell	Percent	
Myeloblasts		0.8	Segmented (total)		2.4
Myelocytes (total)		5.2	Neutrophils	2.4	
Neutrophilic	5.2		Lymphocytes		12.4
Metamyelocytes (total)		6.6	Monocytes		0.4
Neutrophilic	5.8		Pronormoblasts		3.2
Eosinophilic	0.8		Basophilic normoblasts		7.6
Band cells (total)		12.6	Polychromatophilic normoblasts		19.2
Neutrophilic	12.6		Orthochromic normoblasts		29.6

History and physical examination: This 18-month-old black child was brought to the hospital because of an upper respiratory infection, fever, and cough. Delivery at birth had been uneventful, and development was normal except for numerous colds. She appeared well nourished but was acutely ill and listless. On admission her temperature was 100.6° F (38.5° C). There was inflammation of the pharynx and an apical systolic murmur. Roentgenograms showed moderate cardiac enlargement.

Laboratory data: Peripheral blood studies revealed Hb 2.2 Gm/dl, RBC 1.6 million/mm³ (1.6×10^{12}/l), WBC 14,500/mm³ (14.5×10^9/l); leukocyte differential count: 3% neutrophilic metamyelocytes, 8% stab neutrophils, 10% segmented neutrophils, 69% lymphocytes, and 10% monocytes. On the peripheral blood smear, 4 normoblasts/100 leukocytes were found and erythrocytes showed 3+ anisocytosis, 4+ hypochromia, and 2+ poikilocytosis. Reticulocyte count was 4.8% and platelet count 338,000/mm³ (0.338×10^{12}/l). Tests for sickle cells were negative.

Discussion: The pathogenesis of severe anemias of this type is discussed in Chapter 8. This case falls into the category of iron-deficiency anemia of infancy, characterized by a startlingly severe anemia of the hypochromic and microcytic types. Infants so affected are usually well nourished and even obese. White infants do not show the degree of pallor that would be expected in anemias with such low values. Biopsy of the bone marrow is necessary to distinguish anemias of the iron-deficiency type from the true megaloblastic anemia of infancy and childhood. Iron-deficiency anemia shows normoblastic hyperplasia, as in this case, whereas the other type shows megaloblastic dyspoiesis.

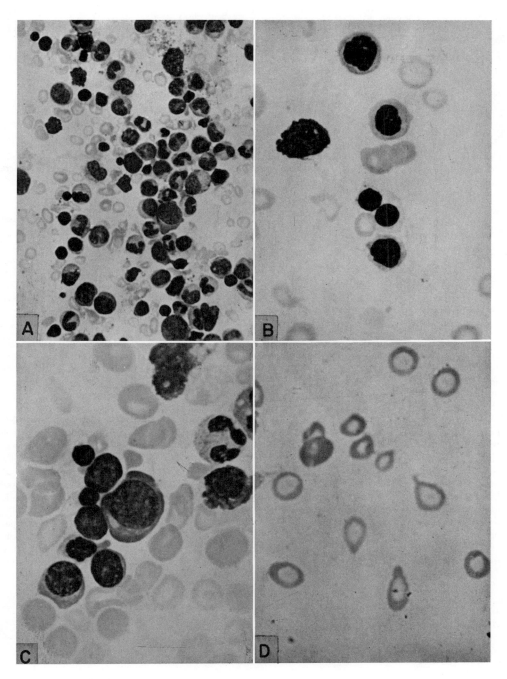

Fig. 5-31

Fig. 5-32. Case 6. Normoblastic hyperplasia of the bone marrow associated with an acute hemolytic crisis of sickle cell anemia. **A,** Peripheral blood smear. (Wright's stain; ×950.) **B** and **C,** Bone marrow smears. (Wright's stain; ×950.) Note the sickle cells and the single normoblast in the peripheral blood smear.

Bone marrow differential count

Cell	Percent		Cell	Percent
Myelocytes (total)		5.7	Lymphocytes	1.8
Neutrophilic	5.7		Plasmacytes	0.3
Metamyelocytes (total)		19.5	Pronormoblasts	0.3
Neutrophilic	19.5		Basophilic normoblasts	3.3
Band cells (total)		10.8	Polychromatophilic normoblasts	16.0
Neutrophilic	10.8		Orthochromic normoblasts	39.0
Segmented (total)		3.3		
Neutrophils	3.3			

History and physical examination: This 24-year-old black woman was admitted to the hospital because of malaise and jaundice. She had been pregnant for 5 months. Five days before admission she had a gradual onset of malaise, fever, chills, generalized aching, and anorexia. Two days later the urine became very dark. When admitted, there was definite icterus of the sclerae, her temperature was 103° F (39.5° C), pulse 112/minute, and BP 140/70. The liver edge was palpable 3 fingerbreadths below the costal margin. The spleen was not palpable. She stated that she had been hospitalized several times "for anemia."

Laboratory data: Peripheral blood studies showed Hb 7.3 Gm/dl, RBC 1.86 million/mm³ (1.86 × 10¹²/l), WBC 23,000/mm³ (23 × 10⁹/l) (corrected for normoblasts to 17,968/mm³, 17.968 × 10⁹/l); leukocyte differential count: 8% stab neutrophils, 62% segmented neutrophils, 25% lymphocytes, 4% monocytes, and 1% eosinophils. There were 28 normoblasts/100 leukocytes. Erythrocytes showed 2+ anisocytosis, and many were sickle cells. Platelet count was 303,800/mm³ (0.3038 × 10¹²/l) (phase microscopy) and reticulocyte count 14.3%. Bisulfite test showed 95% sickling. Total bilirubin was 25.8 mg/dl of serum, with 12.6 mg/dl of serum at 1 minute. Urine test for bile was positive and urine urobilinogen test strongly positive. Fecal urobilinogen output was 544 mg/100 Gm of feces. Electrophoresis revealed a hemoglobin pattern of sickle cell anemia (Hb S—Hb S).

Discussion. Normoblastic hyperplasisa of the bone marrow is usual in all chronic hemolytic anemias but may be striking after a crisis of the hemolytic type, as in this case. There are a few reports of acute clinical exacerbation of sickle cell anemia in which there was no reticulocytosis in the peripheral blood and in which the bone marrow revealed hypoplasia of the erythrocytic precursors. These findings suggest that this type of crisis is "aplastic."

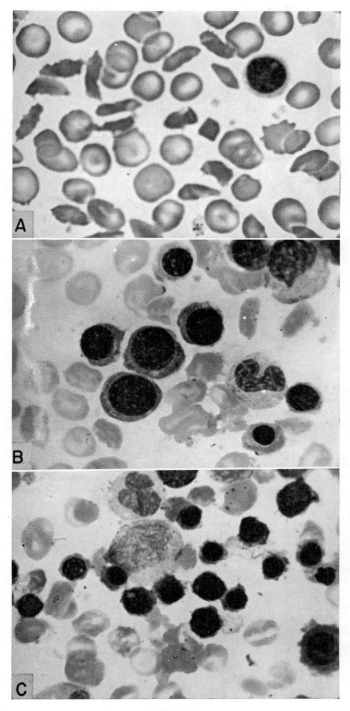

Fig. 5-32

Fig. 5-33. Case 7. Normoblastic hyperplasia of the bone marrow associated with macrocytic anemia of liver disease and hemolytic anemia. **A** and **B,** Bone marrow smears. (Wright's stain; ×950.) **C,** Peripheral blood smear. (Wright's stain; ×950.) **D,** Paraffin section of marrow. (Hematoxylin-eosin stain; ×450.)

Bone marrow differential count

Cell	Percent		Cell	Percent
Myeloblasts		1.6	Lymphocytes	9.0
Progranulocytes		1.0	Monocytes	0.2
Myelocytes (total)		6.4	Plasmablasts	0.2
Neutrophilic	6.2		Proplasmacytes	0.8
Eosinophilic	0.2		Plasmacytes	8.8
Metamyelocytes (total)		6.2	Megakaryocytes	0.4
Neutrophilic	6.2		Pronormoblasts	1.8
Band cells (total)		8.4	Basophilic normoblasts	8.0
Neutrophilic	8.0		Polychromatophilic normoblasts	5.4
Eosinophilic	0.4		Orthrochromic normoblasts	38.0
Segmented (total)		4.0		
Neutrophils	3.4			
Eosinophils	0.6			

History and physical examination: The patient was a 52-year-old woman. For many years her diet had included one bottle of whiskey per day—"sometimes more on rainy days." About 6 weeks before admission she had a severe upper respiratory infection and fever, and 2 weeks later she noted the onset of jaundice that gradually increased in intensity. She said that her urine had been dark for 2 weeks, but her stools were normal in color. The only significant findings on examination were deep jaundice of the skin and sclerae, an enlarged, slightly tender liver 6 fingerbreadths below the costal margin, and moderate splenomegaly. There was ascites but no edema.

Laboratory data: Peripheral blood studies revealed Hb 8.1 Gm/dl of blood, RBC 2.54 million/mm³ (2.54 × 10^{12}/l), WBC 13,850/mm³ (13.85 × 10^9/l); leukocyte differential count: 1% myelocytes, 2% neutrophilic metamyelocytes, 26% stab neutrophils, 48% segmented neutrophils, and 23% lymphocytes. Erythrocytes showed macrocytosis, moderate anisocytosis, and poikilocytosis. MCV was 126 fl. Erythrocyte fragility studies showed decreased osmotic fragility (initial hemolysis at 0.40% salt concentration, complete hemolysis at 0.22%, normal control values 0.46 and 0.32%). Reticulocyte count was 7%. Total bilirubin was 6 mg/dl of serum, 3.8 mg/dl at 1 minute. Results of liver function tests were compatible with moderately severe liver dysfunction. Urine test for bile was positive, and 30.1 mg of urobilinogen was excreted in the urine between 2:00 and 4:00 P.M. Direct antiglobulin (Coombs') test was negative.

Discussion: The anemias associated with liver disease include normochromic normocytic anemia, macrocytic anemia, and hemolytic anemia. About one third of the patients with chronic liver disease have normochromic normocytic anemia, and the marrow is usually normal, occasionally moderately hypoplastic. The macrocytic anemias usually show a normoblastic marrow, but megaloblastic dyspoiesis has been described. Hemolytic anemia with decreased erythrocyte survival may accompany liver disease and may be superimposed on either of the other two types of anemia. In this case the normoblastic hyperplasia and reticulocytosis suggest that a hemolytic component was present. It is impossible to be sure of this in the absence of erythrocyte survival studies, since the antiglobulin test is usually negative, and pigment excretion studies are untrustworthy in the presence of parenchymatous liver involvement.

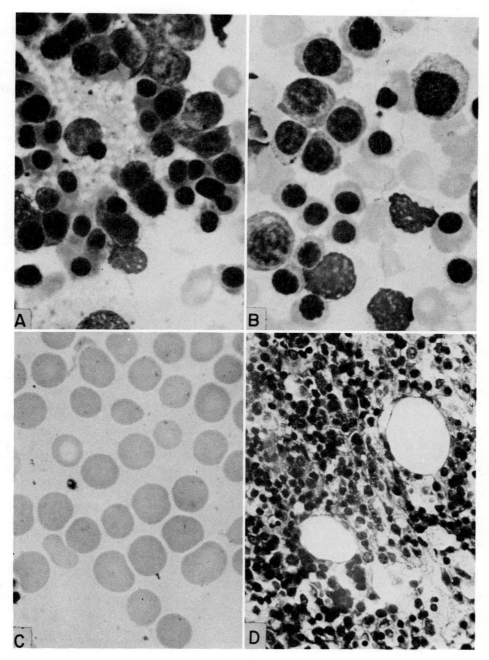

Fig. 5-33

Fig. 5-34. Case 8. Aplastic bone marrow and pancytopenia following therapeutic x-irradiation. **A** and **B,** Bone marrow before therapy. **C** and **D,** Bone marrow after therapy. **A,** Bone marrow smear. (Wright's stain; ×950.) **B,** Paraffin section of marrow. (Hematoxylin-eosin stain; ×450.) **C,** Bone marrow smear. (Wright's stain; ×950.) **D,** Paraffin section of marrow. (Hematoxylin-eosin stain; ×450.)

Bone marrow differential count

Cell	Percent		Cell	Percent
Myeloblasts		0.6	Prolymphocytes	0.6
Progranulocytes		1.4	Lymphocytes	12.0
Myelocytes (total)		7.6	Monocytes	1.8
Neutrophilic	7.0		Plasmacytes	0.4
Eosinophilic	0.6		Megakaryocytes	0.6
Metamyelocytes (total)		10.6	Pronormoblasts	0.2
Neutrophilic	10.4		Basophilic normoblasts	1.0
Eosinophilic	0.2		Polychromatophilic normoblasts	11.0
Band cells (total)		21.2	Orthochromic normoblasts	1.2
Neutrophilic	19.0		Reticulum cells	0.8
Eosinophilic	2.2			
Segmented (total)		29.0		
Neutrophils	25.0			
Eosinophils	4.0			

History and physical examination: Four years before final admission this 54-year-old white woman had noticed a mass in the right side of her neck. A biopsy of this mass was performed and diagnosed as lymphosarcoma (reticulum cell type). The mass disappeared following x-ray therapy, and the patient remained well until about 3 months before her final illness. At that time she was admitted to the hospital complaining of gradual abdominal enlargement and increasingly severe backaches. She was found to have a large, ill-defined midabdominal mass. The liver and spleen were not enlarged. An exploratory laparotomy revealed a huge retroperitoneal mass that proved to be a lymphosarcoma of the same type as the original mass in the neck. Following surgery she was given deep x-irradiation (total dosage of 3,000 R) to the abdomen and mediastinum.

Laboratory data: On admission the peripheral blood findings were not strikingly abnormal—Hb 11.3 Gm/dl, RBC 3.95 million/mm³ (3.95×10^{12}/l), WBC 2,950/mm³ (2.95×10^9/l); leukocyte differential count: 10% stab neutrophils, 82% segmented neutrophils, 5% lymphocytes, 1% monocytes, and 2% eosinophils; platelet count 234,000/mm³ (0.234×10^{12}/l) (phase microscopy). Bone marrow was normally cellular, with a normal differential count as reproduced above.

Following x-ray therapy, however, severe pancytopenia developed. As the patient's general condition deteriorated, the peripheral blood values dropped to very low levels—Hb 5.6 Gm/dl of blood, RBC 2.0 million/mm³ (2.0×10^{12}/l), WBC 1,250/mm³ (1.25×10^9/l); leukocyte differential count: 87% lymphocytes; platelet count 18,000/mm³ (0.018×10^{12}/l). Two biopsies of the marrow showed extreme hypocellularity. Marrow smears contained too few cells to warrant a differential count. Many reticulum cells were present.

Discussion: The lethal effects of ionizing radiation are strikingly demonstrated in this case. Therapy was undertaken with caution, partially because of the leukopenia, and serial marrow examinations during the course of treatment showed little change. It was not until the full course was completed that irreversible pancytopenia developed. The illustrations reveal almost complete fatty replacement of the marrow, with no evidence of regeneration.

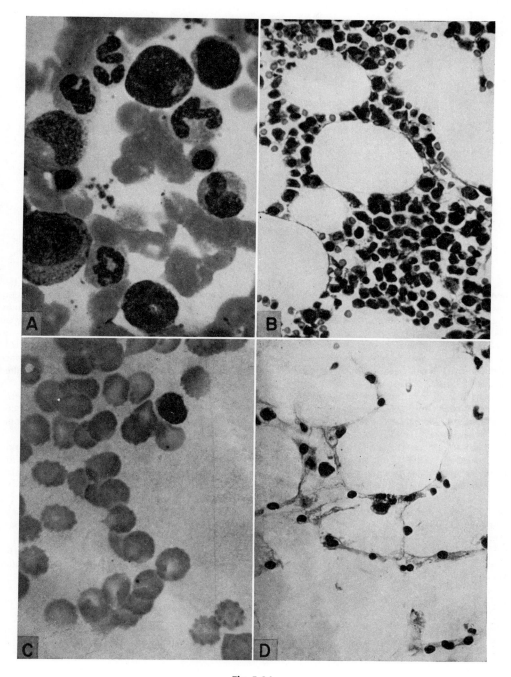

Fig. 5-34

Fig. 5-35. Case 9. Aplastic bone marrow and pancytopenia following the administration of chloramphenicol. **A,** Bone marrow smear. (Wright's stain; ×950.) **B,** Paraffin section of marrow. (Hematoxylin-eosin stain; ×100.) **C,** Paraffin section of marrow. (Hematoxylin-eosin stain; ×450.) (Courtesy Dr. U. Jonsson.)

Bone marrow differential count

Cell	Percent		Cell	Percent
Band cells (total)		8.0	Lymphocytes	69.6
Neutrophilic	8.0		Plasmacytes	0.6
Segmented (total)		21.8		
Neutrophils	21.2			
Eosinophils	0.6			

History and physical examination: Five weeks prior to her admission the patient, a 35-year-old woman, had contracted a severe "cold" while living in a Northern city. Her physician prescribed chloramphenicol. For about 1 week she took four 250 mg capsules each day. Hoping that a mild climate would help overcome her infection, she decided to come to Florida for a short vacation. Upon arrival in Florida, about a week after she had stopped taking the chloramphenicol, she began to feel ill again. She had six capsules of chloramphenicol with her and took them over a period of 1½ days, hoping to stave off a recurrence of her illness. Within 24 hours she noticed severe bruising even after minimal trauma. Soon after, spontaneous hemorrhages appeared over the entire surface of the body. She consulted a physician who, after finding that she had thrombocytopenia and hematuria, admitted her to the hospital.

Examination in the hospital revealed multiple petechiae on both legs. Multiple subcutaneous hemorrhages, 1 cm or more in diameter, were present on the chest, arms, thighs, and buttocks. One small hemorrhage was found in the sclera of the right eye. Petechiae were on the hard palate and nasopharynx. There was no lymphadenopathy, hepatomegaly, or splenomegaly.

Laboratory data: On admission, blood findings were Hb 11.0 Gm/dl of blood, RBC 3.72 million/mm^3 (3.72×10^{12}/l), WBC 1,150/mm^3 (1.15×10^9/l); leukocyte differential count: 100% small normal lymphocytes; platelet count 1,000/mm^3 (0.001×10^{12}/l) (phase microscopy); reticulocyte count 0.05%. Urine was grossly bloody. Stool was tarry, and the guaiac reaction for occult blood was 4+.

Discussion: She was treated with vitamin B$_{12}$, folic acid, and transfusions of fresh whole blood collected in plastic containers, but no improvement in the thrombocytopenia resulted. On the tenth hospital day she had an acute cerebral hemorrhage. She died on the following day. Necropsy revealed a massive cerebral hemorrhage and hemorrhages in body cavities, viscera, and retroperitoneal tissues.

The figures illustrate the microscopic appearance of the bone marrow aspirated when she was admitted to the hospital. An almost complete marrow depression is apparent. The history strongly suggests that chloramphenicol was the myelotoxic agent.

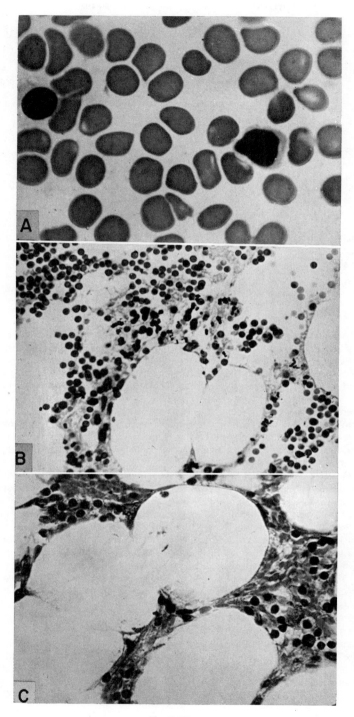

Fig. 5-35

Fig. 5-36. Case 10. Pancytopenia with hyperplastic bone marrow and megaloblastosis. **A-C,** Bone marrow smears. (Wright's stain; ×950.) **D,** Paraffin section of marrow. (Hematoxylin-eosin stain; ×450.)

Bone marrow differential count

Cell	Percent		Cell	Percent
Myeloblasts		0.2	Lymphocytes	7.4
Progranulocytes		0.6	Monoblasts	0.2
Myelocytes (total)		8.8	Promonocytes	0.6
Neutrophilic	8.6		Monocytes	0.2
Eosinphilic	0.2		Proplasmacytes	0.2
Metamyelocytes (total)		6.0	Plasmacytes	2.2
Neutrophilic	5.6		Promegaloblasts	1.2
Eosinophilic	0.4		Basophilic megaloblasts	7.6
Band cells (total)		0.8	Polychromatophilic megaloblasts	6.4
Neutrophilic	0.8		Orthochromic megaloblasts	4.8
Segmented (total)		1.4	Pronormoblasts	2.4
Neutrophils	1.0		Basophilic normoblasts	0.8
Eosinophils	0.4		Polychromatophilic normoblasts	6.2
Lymphoblasts		0.2	Orthochromic normoblasts	40.0
Prolymphocytes		1.4		

History and physical examination: This patient, a 28-year-old mentally retarded black male, complained of weakness and dizziness. He had apparently been in good health until 1 month before admission. At that time he had an acute onset of fever, sore throat, and a painful swelling on the left side of his neck. He was given four injections of penicillin by his physician. The sore throat improved, but otherwise he felt progressively worse, with loss of weight and severe headaches. On the day before admission he had vomited bloody material and passed a bright red stool.

He had suffered very severe headaches and for relief took a patent medicine popular in his neighborhood. It was later found to contain 10 Gm of aminopyrine per fluid ounce. The directions on the bottle recommended a dosage of 1 teaspoonful, "to be repeated every 3 hours if necessary." However, the patient said that he had taken the medicine in doses of one-half bottle at a time since he could not read and in any case did not own a spoon. Physical examination revealed no abnormalities.

Laboratory data: Hb 4.8 Gm/dl of blood, RBC 1.44 million/mm³ (1.44×10^{12}/l), WBC 700/mm³ (0.7×10^9/l); leukocyte differential count: 1% myelocytes, 2% neutrophilic metamyelocytes, 8% stab neutrophils, 6% segmented neutrophils, 81% lymphocytes, and 2% eosinophils; reticulocyte count 0.4%; platelet count 14,000/mm³ (0.014×10^{12}/l) (phase microscopy). Erythrocytes on the peripheral blood smear showed macrocytosis, basophilic stippling, 3+ anisocytosis, and 1+ poikilocytosis. Also on the smear were 5 normoblasts/100 leukocytes. Tests for sickle cells were negative. Direct antiglobulin (Coombs') test was negative. Total bilirubin was 0.6 mg/dl serum. Gastric analysis was normal. Bone marrow was hyperplastic, with a relative increase in erythrocyte precursors, of which 20% were megaloblasts.

Discussion: This case is an excellent example of the difficulties occasionally encountered in hematologic diagnosis. The hyperplastic marrow is not incompatible with the peripheral pancytopenia if it is assumed that the marrow hyperplasia is a "compensatory" process. Megaloblastosis has been described as a feature of rapidly proliferating marrows regardless of the primary stimulus. It is of interest that the administration of folic acid plus vitamin C, vitamin B_{12}, and all three in combination failed to produce any elevation of the low reticulocyte count. Folic acid plus vitamin C did, however, produce a conversion of the bone marrow morphology to a true normoblastic picture. No therapy affected either the leukopenia or the thrombocytopenia, and the patient died 13 months after the onset of the disease. The final peripheral blood counts and bone marrow studies were essentially the same as on admission. It was felt that this case represented pancytopenia due to aminopyrine.

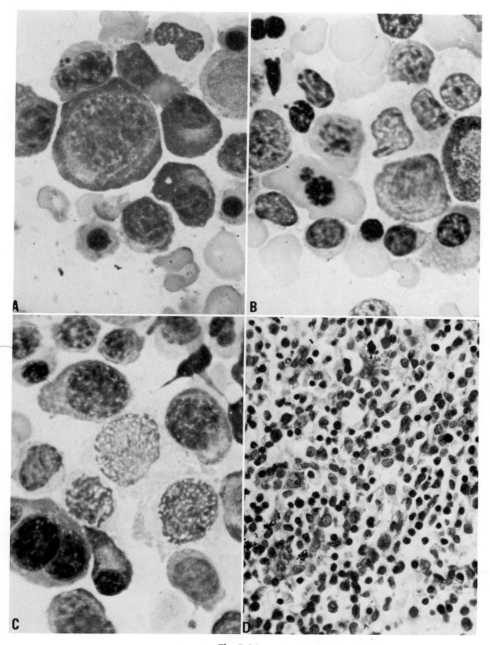

Fig. 5-36

Fig. 5-37. Case 11. Leukemoid reaction of the myelocytic type associated with chronic pyelonephritis, azotemia, and cerebral hemorrhage. **A** and **B,** Bone marrow smears. (Wright's stain; ×950.) **C,** Paraffin section of marrow. (Hematoxylin-eosin stain; ×450.)

Bone marrow differential count

Cell	Percent		Cell	Percent	
Myeloblasts		0.6	Segmented (total)		30.4
Progranulocytes		1.8	Neutrophils	29.4	
Myelocytes (total)		15.8	Eosinophils	1.0	
Neutrophilic	15.2		Lymphocytes		7.0
Eosinophilic	0.6		Proplasmacytes		4.6
Metamyelocytes (total)		12.2	Megakaryocytes		0.4
Neutrophilic	12.2		Orthochromic normoblasts		6.0
Band cells (total)		21.2			
Neutrophilic	20.2				
Eosinophilic	1.0				

History and physical examination: This 62-year-old woman was semicomatose when admitted to the hospital. She had been chronically ill for about 1 year, complaining of severe headaches, abdominal pain, anorexia, and marked loss of weight. Four days before admission she had a sudden onset of very severe headache and vomiting, followed by blurring of vision. Her temperature on admission was 102° F (38.9° C).

Laboratory data: Hb 10.4 Gm/dl of blood, RBC 3.89 million/mm³ (3.89×10^{12}/l), WBC 82,000/mm³ (82×10^9/l); leukocyte differential count: 2% neutrophilic myelocytes, 3% neutrophilic metamyelocytes, 15% stab neutrophils, 71% segmented neutrophils, 6% lymphocytes, 2% monocytes, and 1% eosinophils; platelet count 728,000/mm³ (0.728×10^{12}/l) (phase microscopy); NPN 165 mg/dl of blood. Urinalysis showed 250 mg protein per dl. Urine sediment contained countless pus cells per high-power field. Grossly bloody fluid was obtained by spinal puncture. The bone marrow showed myeloid hyperplasia.

Discussion: The patient died 1 week after admission, and necropsy revealed extensive subdural, subarachnoid, and intracerebral hemorrhages. There was also bilateral chronic pyelonephritis and acute hemorrhagic cystitis.

A high leukocyte count and the presence of immature cells in the peripheral blood suggest a differential diagnosis between leukemia and leukemoid (or leukemia-like) reactions. The distinction is not always easy to make. The diagnosis of a leukemoid reaction is based on (1) a leukocyte count above 50,000/mm³ (50×10^9/l), (2) the presence of immature cells in the pripheral blood, (3) exclusion of leukemia by bone marrow biopsy or splenic aspiration, and (4) the subsequent course of the illness. It has been noted that in myelocytic leukemoid reactions the bone marrow usually shows a larger number of mature cells than it does in myelocytic leukemia. Leukemoid reactions of the lymphocytic and monocytic type have also been described but are not as common.

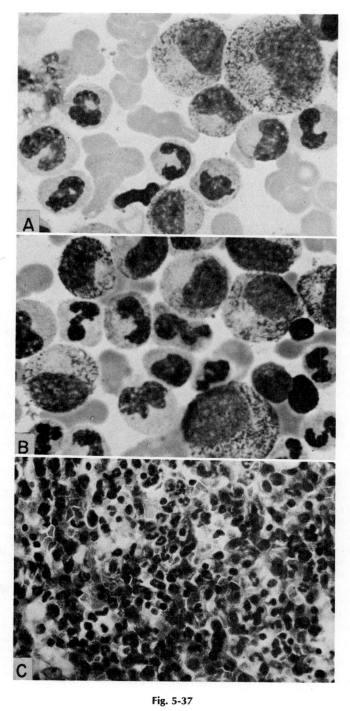

Fig. 5-37

Fig. 5-38. Case 12. Hyperplasia of the eosinophilic series associated with sarcoidosis. **A** and **B,** Bone marrow smears. (Wright's stain; ×950.) **C,** Paraffin section of marrow. (Hematoxylin-eosin stain; ×450.) **D,** Paraffin section of a lymph node. (Hematoxylin-eosin stain; ×70.) **A** and **B** illustrate the large number of eosinophilic cells seen in the smears. **C** shows the hypercellularity of the marrow. **D** is a photomicrograph of the lymph node showing sarcoidosis.

Bone marrow differential count

Cell	Percent		Cell	Percent	
Myeloblasts		0.4	Segmented (total)		20.0
Progranulocytes		0.8	Neutrophils	5.2	
Myelocytes (total)		5.4	Eosinophils	14.8	
Neutrophilic	2.4		Lymphocytes		3.4
Eosinophilic	3.0		Monocytes		0.2
Metamyelocytes (total)		16.4	Plasmacytes		1.8
Neutrophilic	7.8		Pronormoblasts		1.0
Eosinophilic	8.6		Basophilic normoblasts		3.6
Band cells (total)		37.0	Polychromatophilic normoblasts		7.6
Neutrophilic	17.0		Orthochromic normoblasts		2.4
Eosinophilic	20.0				

History and physical examination: This 29-year-old black man was admitted to the hospital because of weakness, abdominal pain, and ulcers of both legs. He described the weakness as having been progressive for months and accompanied by loss of appetite and weight. For about 1 week he had suffered dull, generalized abdominal discomfort and occasionally moderate pain. He appeared to be chronically ill. Physical examination disclosed diffuse lymphadenopathy. The spleen was firm, and the edge was 5 cm below the costal margin. The liver was also firm and nontender, the edge being palpable 3 cm below the costal margin.

Laboratory data: Peripheral blood studies showed Hb 9.7 Gm/dl, RBC 3.4 million/mm³ (3.4 × 10¹²/l), WBC 57,000/mm³ (57 × 10⁹/l); leukocyte differential count: 15% segmented neutrophils, 4% lymphocytes, 80% eosinophils, and 1% monocytes; platelet count 256,000/mm³ (0.256 × 10¹²/l) (phase microscopy); reticulocyte count 0.7%; total protein 5.92/dl of serum (albumin 3.0 Gm and globulin 2.9 Gm/dl of serum); thymol turbidity 3.5 units. Sickle cell test (bisulfite) showed 90% sickling of erythrocytes. Paper electrophoresis of hemoglobin revealed Hb A-Hb S (sickle cell trait). Kahn and VDRL tests on blood were 4+. No ova or parasites were found in the stool. Skin test for trichinosis was negative. A cervical lymph node biopsy showed sarcoidosis, **D.** Roentgenograms of the chest revealed bilateral infiltrations.

Discussion: The eosinophilia of the peripheral blood and bone marrow in this case was extreme. Eosinophilia is not common in sarcoidosis but has been recorded. It is more common in Hodgkin's disease (about 20% of the cases) but is seldom as high as in this case. Marrow eosinophilia of various degrees has been reported in a variety of other conditions (Rohr, 1952): asthma, urticaria, Löffler's syndrome, myositis, intestinal and visceral parasitic infestation, trichinosis, "mycosis fungoides," pernicious anemia after treatment with liver extract, periarteritis nodosa tumors, and myelocytic leukemia. Generally it is accompanied by eosinophilia in the peripheral blood, but following the administration of ACTH there are reports of eosinophilia in the marrow, with eosinopenia in the peripheral blood. It has been suggested that eosinopenia produced by stress or ACTH is caused by inhibited release of eosinophils from the bone marrow.

The provisional diagnosis in this case included most of the conditions listed above. The adenopathy and splenomegaly favored a diagnosis of Hodgkin's disease, but biopsy of a lymph node revealed Boeck's sarcoid. An intensive and successful attempt was made to rule out other conditions that might have accounted for the eosinophilia.

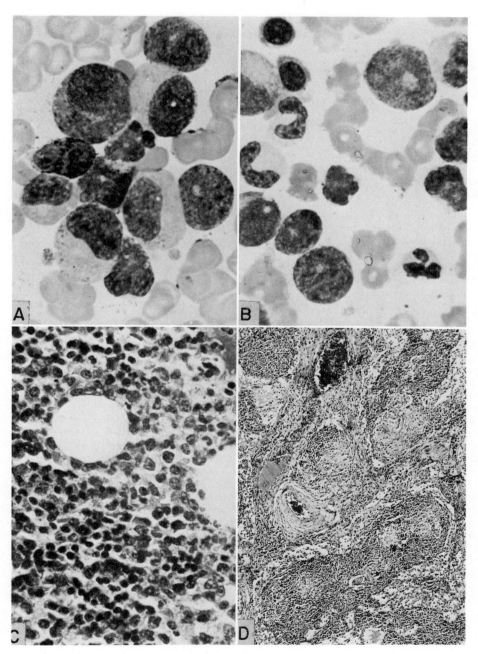

Fig. 5-38

Fig. 5-39. Case 13. Eosinophilic leukemia. **A,** Peripheral blood. **B,** Bone marrow. (Wright's stain; ×950.) **C,** Heart, left ventricle. (Hematoxylin-eosin stain; ×150.) **D,** Spleen. (Hematoxylin-eosin stain; ×400.)

Bone marrow differential count

Cell	Percent		Cell	Percent
Myeloblasts		8.0	Segmented (total)	31.5
Progranulocytes		8.5	Neutrophils	4.0
Myelocytes (total)		5.0	Eosinophils	20.5
Neutrophilic	1.0		Basophils	7.0
Eosinophilic	4.0		Lymphocytes	5.0
Metamyelocytes (total)		8.5	Monocytes	0.5
Neutrophilic	4.5		Pronormoblasts	0.5
Eosinophilic	4.0		Basophilic normoblasts	1.0
Band cells (total)		23.0	Polychromatophilic normoblasts	6.5
Neutrophilic	8.0		Orthochromic normoblasts	2.0
Eosinophilic	15.0			

History and physical examination: This 53-year-old white male was admitted to the hospital in a semicomatose state. He had been well up to 1 week before, at which time there was onset of headache, then generalized aching, then weakness and disorientation. Physical examination showed no abnormalities; temperature and blood pressure were normal. Studies directed toward the neurologic symptoms were not helpful except for a spinal fluid protein of 56 mg%. Blood examination for bromides and barbiturates was negative. However, routine blood counts revealed a peripheral blood leukocyte count of 76,000/mm³ (76 × 10⁹/l) with striking eosinophilia. Aspiration biopsy of the bone marrow was then performed.

Laboratory data: Peripheral blood findings included Hb 14.6 Gm/dl, RBC 5.3 million/mm³ (5.3 × 10¹²/l), WBC 76,000/mm³ (76 × 10⁹/l); leukocyte differential count: 7% segmented neutrophils, 8% stab neutrophils, 5% lymphocytes, 1% monocytes, 71% eosinophils, 2% eosinophilic myelocytes, 5% basophils, and 1% myeloblasts; platelet count 66,000/mm³ (0.066 × 10¹²/l). Alkaline phosphatase stain of peripheral blood smear showed only an occasional weakly phosphatase-positive neutrophil; the eosinophilic cells were uniformly phosphatase negative.

Discussion: The patient deteriorated rapidly in spite of treatment with steroids, nitrogen mustard, and methotrexate, and death occurred 7 days later. The illness was marked by increasing stupor, labored respiration, and fever to 104° F (40° C). Necropsy revealed pulmonary edema, extensive mural thrombi in the right atrium, left ventricle, and right ventricle, accompanying leukemic infiltration of the myocardium, subendocardial necrosis, and organization of mural thrombus. There was eosinophilic infiltration of the liver and spleen. A mesenteric lymph node showed massive infiltration with myelocytes, only a few of which were eosinophilic. The brain was extensively damaged by ischemic infarcts in both cerebral and cerebellar hemispheres. Many blood vessels were found to be occluded by masses of fibrin and entrapped eosinophilic leukocytes.

There is some difference of opinion whether "eosinophilic leukemia" is a clinical and hematologic entity. Eosinophilia sometimes accompanies chronic myelocytic leukemia and in such cases does not seem to deserve separate classification. However, there are reports of cases similar to the one presented here that indicate a typical entity on the basis of (1) an acute course, (2) eosinophilia accompanied by myeloblastic proliferation, (3) frequent involvement of myocardium and endocardium with necrosis and organizing mural thrombi, and (4) frequent involvement of the central nervous system (see Bentley et al, 1961).

Goh et al (1965) studied the cytogenetics of two cases of eosinophilic leukemia. In neither case was the Philadelphia chromosome identified. Since the Philadelphia chromosome has been found in almost all cases of chronic myelocytic leukemia, the implication is that eosinophilic leukemia is not simply a variant of myelocytic leukemia.

The myocardial and endocardial lesion with extensive thrombus formation is very similar to that found in fibroplastic parietal endocarditis with eosinophilia (see Fig. 5-40, Case 14), supposedly not a leukemic process. The endocardial thrombus formation in this case and Case 14 is histologically similar except for the expected greater degree of organization in the more chronic case. The chief differentiation is the immaturity of the bone marrow proliferation in the case called eosinophilic leukemia. Other types of eosinophilia are illustrated and discussed in Figs. 5-38 to 5-42.

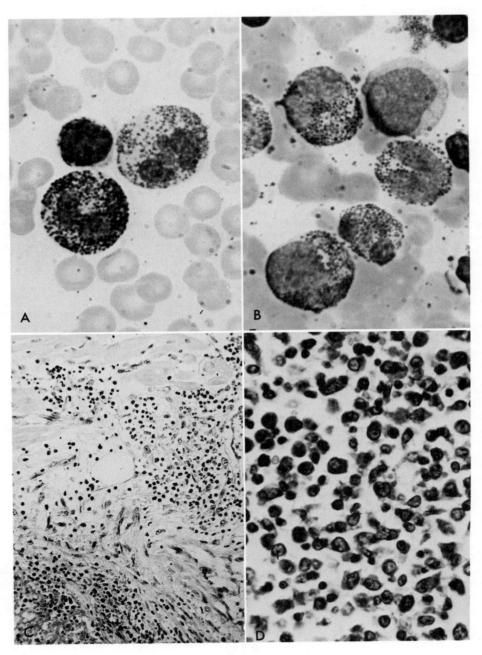

Fig. 5-39

Fig. 5-40. Case 14. Fibroplastic parietal endocarditis with eosinophilic leukocytosis. **A** and **B,** Bone marrow smear. (Wright's stain; ×950.) **C,** Photomicrograph of mural thrombus in left ventricle. (Hematoxylin-eosin stain; ×120.) **D,** Gross appearance of mural thrombus in left ventricle.

Bone marrow differential count

Cell	Percent		Cell	Percent
Myeloblasts		1.2	Segmented (total)		46.7
Progranulocytes		3.8	Neutrophils	18.0	
Myelocytes (total)		5.8	Eosinophils	28.0	
Neutrophilic	1.0		Basophils	0.7	
Eosinophilic	4.8		Lymphocytes		4.8
Metamyelocytes (total)		8.4	Monocytes		0.2
Neutrophilic	2.4		Pronormoblasts		0.6
Eosinophilic	6.0		Basophilic normoblasts		1.1
Band cells (total)		22.1	Polychromatophilic normoblasts		7.5
Neutrophilic	8.0		Orthochromic normoblasts		1.8
Eosinophilic	14.1				

History and physical examination: This 19-year-old white medical student was admitted with signs and symptoms of cardiac failure. Seven months before he developed an upper respiratory infection and was then found to have eosinophilic leukocytosis (WBC 19,000/mm³, 19 × 10⁹/l, 52% eosinophils). He recovered without treatment, and within 9 days the eosinophilia disappeared. Within 2 months, however, he developed fatigability, orthopnea, dyspnea on exertion, and nonproductive cough. There was an accompanying gain of 25 pounds in body weight and evidence of pleural effusion and ascites. He improved when treated with digitalis and diuretics, but 2 months later there was relapse with recurrence of the signs and symptoms of cardiac failure. Past history was otherwise unremarkable.

The pertinent findings on physical examination were the following: BP 160/100; macular rash over the chest, abdomen, and back; distended neck veins; moderate cyanosis; orthopnea; evidence of bilateral hydrothorax; cardiomegaly with a high-pitched, blowing systolic murmur audible over the cardiac apex and along the left sternal border; liver palpable 3 cm below the costal margin. There was no splenomegaly or lymphadenopathy.

Laboratory data: Hb 14.7 Gm/dl, WBC 21,500/mm³ (21.5 × 10⁹/l), leukocyte differential count, segmented neutrophils 24%, stab neutrophils 2%, lymphocytes 18%, and eosinophils 50%; platelet count 45,000/mm³ (0.045 × 10¹²/l). Urinalysis showed 75 mg of protein per dl, sediment unremarkable except for 8 to 14 hyaline casts/hpf; serum protein studies not remarkable; serum urea nitrogen 37 mg/dl; stools repeatedly negative for ova and parasistes; skin tests for trichinosis showed no reaction. Roentgenograms of the chest showed no pulmonary infiltration but confirmed the bilateral hydrothorax and the cardiomegaly. Electrocardiograms showed right axis deviation, probable subendocardial ischemia, and incomplete left bundle branch block. Several blood preparations for the LE factor were negative. Sternal bone marrow obtained by aspiration is reported above. Biopsy of gastrocnemius muscle revealed no abnormality.

Discussion: At first there seemed to be some clinical improvement on a regimen of prednisone, 100 mg/day, and the leukocytosis and eosinophilia also improved (WBC 13,600/mm³, 13.6 × 10⁹/l, 13% eosinophils). However, he developed an atrial tachycardia first and then, on the next day, an episode of acute dyspnea. The following day, while eating, he suddenly gasped for breath and died.

In addition to the expected findings of cardiac failure, necropsy showed multiple bilateral pulmonary emboli, both old and fresh, and recent infarcts. The heart was hypertrophied (540 Gm). The epicardium was normal. There were old organizing and recent mural thrombi in the right and left ventricles, chiefly in inflow tracts, with involvement of papillary muscles and severe reduction in ventricular volumes. There was a fresh hemorrhagic infarct in the right auricular appendage. There was patchy myocardial fibrosis, **C,** and obvious, but not severe, eosinophilic infiltration.

No more than 40 cases of this syndrome have been reported, and they are thoroughly reviewed by Brink and Weber (1963), who also discuss the differential diagnosis of similar endocardial involvement. Two additional points should be made: (1) eosinophilic leukocytosis is reported in 38 of the 40 cases, thus justifying inclusion of this syndrome in the differential diagnosis of eosinophilia and (2) the mural thrombi found here are very similar to those described in the case of eosinophilic leukemia, suggesting the possibility that the endocarditis may have as a common denominator injury by the eosinophilotactic stimulus or possibly by breakdown products of eosinophils.

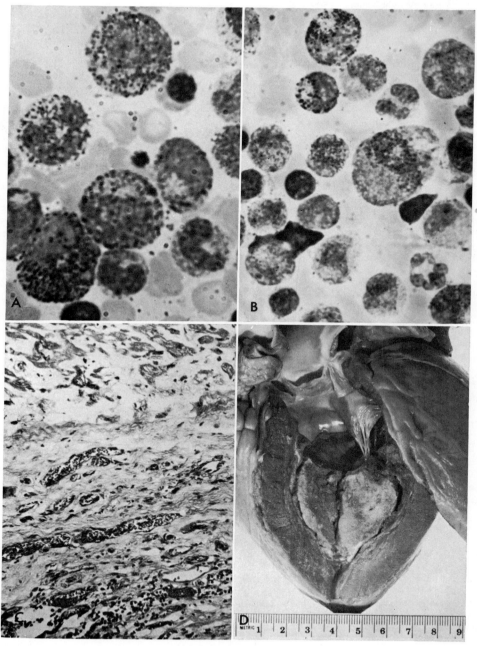

Fig. 5-40

Fig. 5-41. Case 15. Eosinophilic leukocytosis of unknown etiology (? cyclic). **A** and **B,** Peripheral blood. **C** and **D,** Bone marrow. (Wright's stain; ×950.)

Bone marrow differential count

Cell	Percent		Cell	Percent
Myeloblasts		0.3	Segmented (total)		24.0
Progranulocytes		1.1	Neutrophils	5.0	
Myelocytes (total)		6.4	Eosinophils	18.7	
Neutrophilic	2.2		Basophils	0.3	
Eosinophilic	4.2		Lymphocytes		3.4
Metamyelocytes (total)		15.8	Monocytes		2.0
Neutrophilic	3.1		Plasmacytes		1.0
Eosinophilic	12.7		Pronormoblasts		1.0
Band cells (total)		36.0	Basophilic normoblasts		6.0
Neutrophilic	12.0		Polychromatophilic normoblasts		8.0
Eosinophilic	24.0		Orthochromic normoblasts		5.0

History and physical examination: This 22-year-old white male was admitted for investigation of the eosinophilia discovered a few days before by his physician. He had been well until 2 weeks before admission, at which time he visited his doctor with complaints of fever, chills, and nonproductive cough. Roentgenogram of the chest was normal, but the leukocyte count was 72,000/mm³ (72 × 10⁹/l), and the differential count showed 80% eosinophils. About 1½ years before, while serving in the Navy, he had been admitted to a Naval hospital because of weight loss of 20 pounds, dull epigastric pain, and malaise. Leukocytosis and eosinophilia (45,700/mm³, 45.7 × 10⁹/l, with 72% eosinophils) were the only abnormalities found in spite of a very extensive investigation. While hospitalized he showed symptomatic improvement, and the leukocytosis and eosinophilia reverted to normal. No diagnosis was estabished, and he was returned to full active duty.

The experience in our hospital was an almost exact duplicate of the episode 18 months previously. In addition to the above, it was learned that during his tour of duty in the Navy he had visited the Caribbean, Mediterranean, and South American areas. There was a suggestive allergic background, evidenced by nonseasonal rhinorrhea and sneezing. On physical examination the findings were entirely normal.

Laboratory data: On admission the blood Hb was 15.5 Gm/dl, hematocrit 49%, and WBC 51,600/mm³ (51.6 × 10⁹/l). The leukocyte differential count was 8% segmented neutrophils, 7% lymphocytes, 2% monocytes, and 80% eosinophils (half of the eosinophils were stab forms). Urinalysis showed microscopic hematuria (14 to 16 RBC/hpf), but a complete investigation of the urinary tract revealed only mild posterior urethritis. Repeated examination of stools and urine never revealed the presence of parasites. All liver function studies were normal, including liver tissue obtained by biopsy for histologic examination. The patient's blood was group A, and the anti-B titer was not elevated as is sometimes seen in infection with visceral larva migrans. Serum protein electrophoresis showed the α₂-fraction to be moderately elevated (1.04 Gm/dl as compared to our normal range of 0.32 to 0.66 Gm/dl). Roentgenographic studies of chest and gastrointestinal tract showed no abnormalities. Aspiration biopsy of bone marrow showed eosinophilic hyperplasia with preponderance of adult forms. Family studies showed the following:

Father: WBC 7,300, 1% eosinophils
Mother: WBC 7,200, 5% eosinophils
Sister: WBC 7,300, 3% eosinophils
Brother: WBC 10,200, 10% eosinophils

Discussion The patient's eosinophilia spontaneously decreased and within 17 days completely disappeared. On the seventeenth day of his hospital stay the WBC was 8,800/mm³ (8.8 × 10⁹/l), and the differential count showed only 8% eosinophils.

Eosinophilic leukocytosis is defined by an absolute eosinophil count (WBC count times the percent of eosinophils) higher than 400/mm³ of blood. The usual causes of eosinophilia are well documented (Chapter 15), and the other case studies (Figs. 5-38 to 5-42) illustrate some of them. As far as I know, a case similar to this has not been described. The cyclic nature of the disease, as shown by the two like episodes 18 months apart, is striking. There is a suggestion that the disease may be familial in the case of the brother, but familial eosinophilia is not cyclic nor of the degree shown by this patient.

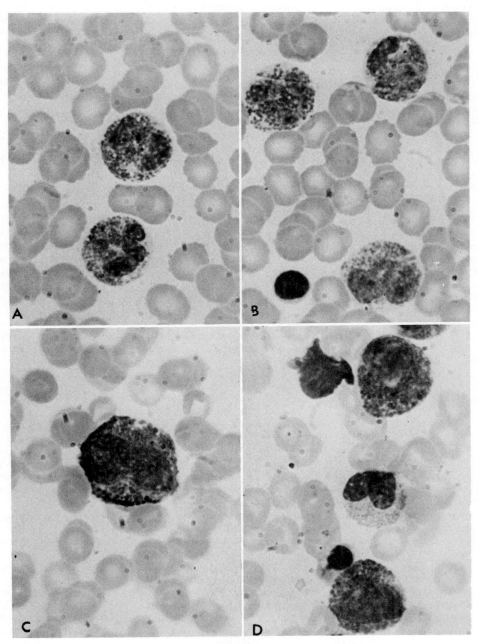

Fig. 5-41

Fig. 5-42. Case 16. Eosinophilic leukemoid reaction, etiology unknown. **A-C,** Bone marrow smear. (Wright's stain; ×950.) **D,** Paraffin section of bone marrow. (Hematoxylin-eosin stain; ×400.) (Referred by Dr. Wm. E. Cowell.)

Bone marrow differential count

Cell	Percent		Cell	Percent
Blasts		3.0	Segmented (total)		35.2
Progranulocytes		3.2	Eosinophils	25.6	
Myelocytes (total)		3.6	Neutrophils	9.6	
Eosinophilic	2.0		Lymphocytes		33.6
Neutrophilic	1.6		Monocytes		0.3
Metamyelocytes (total)		6.9	Pronormoblasts		0
Eosinophilic	3.3		Basophilic normoblasts		0.3
Neutrophilic	3.6		Polychromatophilic normoblasts		3.0
Bands (total)		19.3	Orthochromic normoblasts		4.3
Eosinophilic	11.0				
Neutrophilic	8.3				

History and physical examination: This 5-month-old white girl was admitted to the hospital because she had splenomegaly, hepatomegaly, and a leukocyte count of 106,000/mm³ (106 × 10⁹/l) with 84% eosinophils. Up to that time she had been seen regularly by her pediatrician; growth and development were normal, and she had been well except for mild upper respiratory infections. At the age of 18 weeks she was seen in the pediatrician's office for a routine follow-up visit, and for the first time the spleen was palpable 3 fingerbreadths below the costal margin.

Physical examination in the hospital showed an irritable child with low-grade fever (99.6° F, 37.5° C). Otherwise she was well nourished, alert, and did not appear ill. The spleen was enlarged and firm, the edge smooth and 2½ fingerbreadths below the costal margin, and the notch palpable just below the costal margin. The liver edge was 2 fingerbreadths below the right costal margin. There was no lymphadenopathy or other positive findings.

Laboratory data: The leukocytosis and eosinophilia persisted throughout the 7 days that the child was in the hospital:

> 3/5: WBC 51,018, 64% eosinophils
> 3/6: WBC 60,200, 81% eosinophils
> 3/7: WBC 54,100, 69% eosinophils
> 3/8: WBC 53,700, 68% eosinophils
> 3/9: WBC 64,500, 84% eosinophils

The platelet count was normal (260,000/mm³, 0.26 × 10¹²/l). Stools were negative for ova and parasites. Nasal secretion did not contain eosinophils. The mother's leukocyte count and differential count were normal. Roentgenograms of the chest, long bones, and skull were normal. Aspiration biopsy of tibial bone marrow was performed; the differential count is given above.

Discussion: While in the hospital the course was uneventful, and there was no change in the physical signs. She seemed to be a normal healthy child except for the hepatosplenomegaly and eosinophilia. She was discharged, and no therapy was given. The eosinophilia gradually disappeared, as shown by the following counts:

> 4/8: WBC 26,000, 55% eosinophils
> 4/29: WBC 13,300, 4% eosinophils

Two and one-half years later, the child was entirely normal. There was neither splenomegaly nor hepatomegaly. No further follow-up was possible.

This case illustrates a failure that is not uncommon—that of failing to establish the etiology of the eosinophilia. While this is more common in moderate eosinophilias, we have been frustrated by several cases like this one, in which the eosinophilic leukocytosis is so striking that it seems difficult to accept the conclusion that an etiologic diagnosis is not possible.

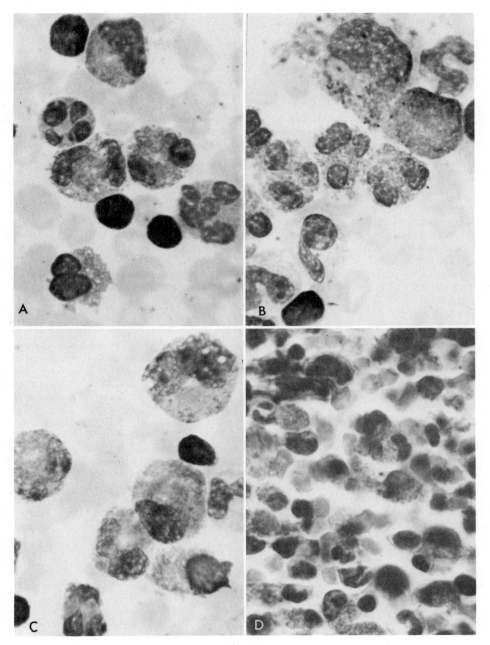

Fig. 5-42

Fig. 5-43. Case 17. Polycythemia vera. **A,** Bone marrow smear. (Wright's stain; ×450.) **B** and **C,** Bone marrow smears. (Wright's stain; ×950.) **D,** Paraffin section of marrow. (Hematoxylin-eosin stain; ×450.) Note the hypercellularity, the large number of megakaryocytes, and the large platelet mass in **C.**

Bone marrow differential count

Cell	Percent		Cell	Percent
Myeloblasts		2.2	Lymphocytes	5.6
Progranulocytes		2.2	Monocytes	0.8
Myelocytes (total)		8.0	Proplasmacytes	0.8
Neutrophilic	8.0		Megakaryocytes	2.0
Metamyelocytes (total)		8.8	Pronormoblasts	1.6
Neutrophilic	8.8		Basophilic normoblasts	4.4
Band cells (total)		26.4	Polychromatophilic normoblasts	6.6
Neutrophilic	26.4		Orthochromic normoblasts	8.4
Segmented (total)		22.2		
Neutrophils	20.2			
Eosinophils	2.0			

History and physical examination: This patient was a 62-year-old woman who had the fortunate combination of polycythemia vera and a gastric ulcer that periodically produced severe bleeding and thus served as an autotherapeutic method for reducing the erythrocyte count and blood volume. After one of these episodes the patient was asked to return to the hospital at a later date for a complete hematologic study. On physical examination the only significant finding was splenomegaly, the edge of the spleen being palpable 4 fingerbreadths below the costal margin.

Laboratory data: Peripheral blood studies showed Hb 16.8 Gm/dl of blood, RBC 7.9 million/mm^3 (7.9 × 10^{12}/l), WBC 57,750/mm^3 (57.75 × 10^9/l), leukocyte differential count: 1% myelocytes, 3% neutrophilic metamyelocytes, 12% stab neutrophils, 69% segmented neutrophils, 6% lymphocytes, 4% monocytes, 2% eosinophils, and 3% basophils; platelet count 3,700,000/mm^3 (3.7 × 10^{12}/l) (phase microscopy); reticulocyte count 2.9%. All bone marrow specimens showed a strikingly hypercellular marrow with numerous megakaryoctes.

Discussion: The hematologic findings clearly illustrate that in polycythemia vera there is diffuse hyperplasia of the marrow involving all cell series. Not only is this apparent in the marrow smears and sections but also the peripheral blood findings of polycythemia, leukocytosis, and thrombocytosis reflect hyperactivity of the marrow. Such findings justify the concept that polycythemia vera properly belongs in the group of myeloproliferative syndromes.

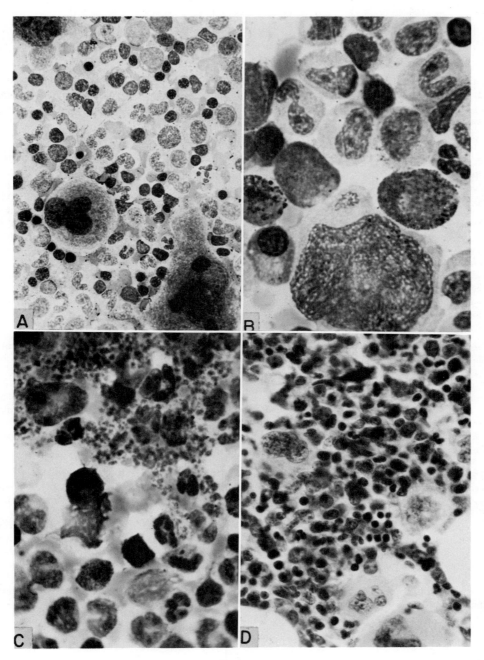

Fig. 5-43

Fig. 5-44. Case 18. Myeloproliferative syndrome (agnogenic myeloid metaplasia of the spleen without myelofibrosis). **A,** Bone marrow smear. (Wright's stain; ×450.) **B,** Paraffin section of marrow. (Hematoxylin-eosin stain; ×450.) **C** and **D,** Necropsy sections of liver and spleen, respectively, illustrating extramedullary hemopoiesis. (Hematoxylin-eosin stain; ×450.) Note the extramedullary megakaryocytosis.

Bone marrow differential count

Cell	Percent		Cell	Percent
Myeloblasts		1.6	Lymphocytes	4.0
Myelocytes (total)		4.2	Plasmacytes	0.2
Neutrophilic	4.0		Pronormoblasts	2.0
Eosinophilic	0.2		Basophilic normoblasts	4.8
Metamyelocytes (total)		3.6	Polychromatophilic normoblasts	22.0
Neutrophilic	3.6		Orthochromic normoblasts	39.0
Band cells (total)		10.4	Reticulum cells	1.2
Neutrophilic	10.0			
Eosinophilic	0.4			
Segmented (total)		7.0		
Neutrophils	6.4			
Eosinophils	0.4			
Basophils	0.2			

History and physical examination: Until 3 months prior to admission this 74-year-old man had been in excellent health. At this time he noticed a gradual enlarging of the abdomen, first on the left side and then on the right. Dyspnea, epigastric discomfort, anorexia, and a 15-pound loss of weight followed.

Examination revealed a few petechiae on both forearms and in the buccal mucosa. The liver was palpable 4 fingerbreadths below the costal margin, and the splenic outline extended to the umbilicus and down to the iliac crest. There was no lymphadenopathy. Other findings were compatible with arteriosclerotic cardiovascular disease.

Laboratory data: Hb 8.2 Gm/dl of blood, RBC 2.89 million/mm^3 (2.89×10^{12}/l), WBC (corrected for normoblasts) 16,500/mm^3 (16.5×10^9/l); leukocyte differential count: 3% myeloblasts, 6% myelocytes, 15% neutrophilic metamyelocytes, 36% stab neutrophils, 27% segmented neutrophils, 8% lymphocytes, 4% eosinophils, and 1% basophils. On the peripheral blood smear there were 49 normoblasts per 100 leukocytes, and erythrocytes showed striking polychromasia and stippling. Reticulocyte count was 6.9%; platelet count 260,000/mm^3 (0.26×10^{12}/l). Direct antiglobulin (Coombs') test was negative. Total bilirubin was 0.8 mg/dl of serum, with 0.1 mg/dl at 1 minute.

Discussion: Bone marrow specimens obtained during life revealed generalized hyperplasia, with a differential count indicating extreme normoblastic hyperplasia. This case is an example of a myeloproliferative syndrome with striking extramedullary splenic hemopoiesis. Exact classification is difficult and perhaps unwarranted. Similar cases have been variously referred to as agnogenic myeloid metaplasia, erythroleukemia, and Di Guglielmo's syndrome.

The patient did not respond to conservative treatment. At necropsy the spleen weighed 1,360 Gm (normal weight about 150 Gm).

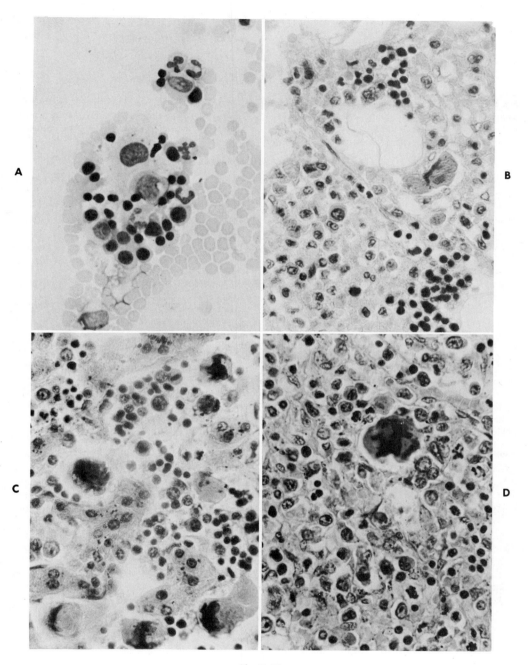

Fig. 5-44

Fig. 5-45. Case 19. Megaloblastic bone marrow (pernicious anemia). **A** and **B,** Bone marrow smears. (Wright's stain; ×950.) **C,** Peripheral blood smear. (Wright's stain; ×950.) **D,** Paraffin section of marrow. (Hematoxylin-eosin stain; ×450.) Note the megaloblasts in **A** and **B** and also the giant metamyelocytes. A hypersegmented neutrophil and macrocytic erythrocytes are shown in **C.**

Bone marrow differential count

Cell	Percent		Cell	Percent
Myelocytes (total)		1.2	Lymphocytes	3.4
Neutrophilic	1.2		Plasmacytes	1.8
Metamyelocytes (total)		15.0	Megakaryocytes	0.2
Neutrophilic	14.8		Promegaloblasts	2.0
Eosinophilic	0.2		Basophilic megaloblasts	12.6
Band cells (total)		20.8	Polychromatophilic megaloblasts	8.0
Neutrophilic	20.8		Orthochromic megaloblasts	2.8
Segmented (total)		9.4	Pronormoblasts	10.0
Neutrophils	7.4		Basophilic normoblasts	6.4
Eosinophils	1.6		Polychromatophilic normoblasts	0.8
Basophils	0.4		Orthochromic normoblasts	5.6

History and physical examination: This patient was a 66-year-old white man. The diagnosis of pernicious anemia had been made 10 years previously. Intramuscular liver extract had proved to be effective therapy. He decided not to continue his liver injections, however, and had been without this therapy for 4 years. His complaints on admission were progressive weakness, loss of appetite, dyspnea, and orthopnea.

When examined, he was pale, with a yellowish tinge. BP was 120/70. The heart was enlarged to the midaxillary line and the sixth interspace. The spleen was not palpable, but the liver edge was 3 cm below the costal margin. The tongue showed atrophy of the papillae. Neurologic examination revealed absent knee and ankle reflexes, with loss of vibratory sense.

Laboratory data: Hb 5.6 Gm/dl of blood, RBC 1.25 million/mm^3 (1.25×10^{12}/l), WBC 4,500/mm^3 (4.5×10^9/l); leukocyte differential count: 3% stab neutrophils, 54% segmented neutrophils, 42% lymphocytes, and 1% eosinophils. On the peripheral blood smear the erythrocytes showed 4+ anisocytosis and poikilocytosis, and there were 3 normoblasts/100 leukocytes. MCV was 152 fl, MCH 44.8 pg, and MCHC 29.4%; hematocrit reading 19% cell volume; platelet count 114,000/mm^3 (0.114×10^{12}/l). Total bilirubin was 2.6 mg/dl of serum, with 0.4 mg/dl at 1 minute. No free hydrochloric acid was found in gastric analysis, even after histamine stimulation.

Discussion: Pernicious anemia is one of the macrocytic anemias characterized by megaloblasts in the bone marrow. As discussed in Chapter 9 and illustrated in the following cases, the presence of megaloblasts in the marrow is not, of itself, diagnostic of pernicious anemia. It does, however, confirm the diagnosis when supported by clinical and other laboratory criteria. It is important to realize that a deficiency of hemopoietic factor will be revealed in the abnormal morphology of leukocytes and megakaryocytes as well as in megaloblastosis. Involvement of all the constituents of the marrow suggests a total hemopoietic defect (dyspoiesis) that produces anemia, leukopenia, and thrombocytopenia in the peripheral blood.

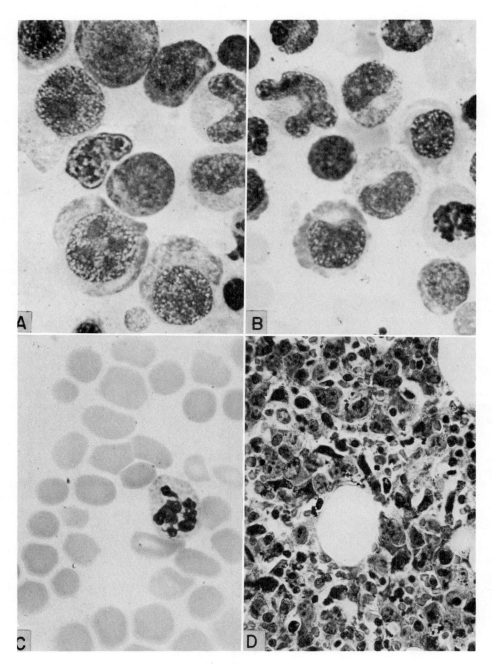

Fig. 5-45

Fig. 5-46. Case 20. Megaloblastic bone marrow (tropical macrocytic anemia). **A-C,** Bone marrow smears. (Wright's stain; ×950.) **D,** Peripheral blood smear. (Wright's stain; ×950.)

Bone marrow differential count

Cell	Percent		Cell	Percent
Myelocytes		7.2	Lymphocytes	9.6
Neutrophilic	7.2		Plasmacytes	0.8
Metamyelocytes (total)		9.0	Megakaryoblasts	0.2
Neutrophilic	8.8		Megakaryocytes	0.2
Eosinophilic	0.2		Basophilic megaloblasts	2.2
Band cells (total)		18.8	Polychromatophilic megaloblasts	6.4
Neutrophilic	18.0		Orthochromic megaloblasts	8.2
Eosinophilic	0.8		Basophilic normoblasts	5.6
Segmented (total)		14.4	Polychromatophilic normoblasts	6.0
Neutrophils	12.0		Orthochromic normoblasts	11.2
Eosinophils	2.4		Reticulum cells	0.2

History and physical examination: This patient was a 37-year-old Puerto Rican who had been in good health. A year prior to admission he started to suffer from nausea after eating, gaseous distention, vague abdominal pain, and diarrhea. These complaints continued until a few weeks before admission, when he began to vomit and have generalized crampy abdominal pain. He felt progressively weaker and lost about 20 pounds in weight. On examination he was found to be pale and emaciated. The liver edge was felt 4 cm below the costal margin, but the spleen was not palpable. The tongue was smooth and red. There were no neurologic abnormalities.

Laboratory data: Hb 8.2 Gm/dl of blood, RBC 2.54 million/mm^3 (2.54 × 10^{12}/l), MCV 105 fl, MCH 30 pg, MCHC 29%, WBC 3,000/mm^3 (3.0 × 10^9/l); leukocyte differential count: 1% stab neutrophils, 35% segmented neutrophils, 50% lymphocytes, 2% monocytes, 11% eosinophils, and 1% basophils; reticulocyte count 1.2%; platelet count 431,800/mm^3 (0.4318 × 10^{12}/l) (phase microscopy); total protein 5.22 Gm/dl of serum (3.55 Gm albumin and 1.67 Gm globulin/dl of serum). A normal amount of fat and hookworm ova were found in the stool. Roentgenograms of the gastrointestinal tract after a barium meal showed a normal bowel pattern. Gastric analysis showed normal free HCl.

Discussion: THe megaloblastic dyspoiesis in the bone marrow is striking, but by itself is not diagnostic. The diagnosis of tropical macrocytic anemia is based partially on other evidence such as the presence of free acid in the gastric juice and absence of neurologic abnormalities as well as on the patient's residence in a subtropical country. After specific therapy this patient had a maximum reticulocytosis of 35.8%.

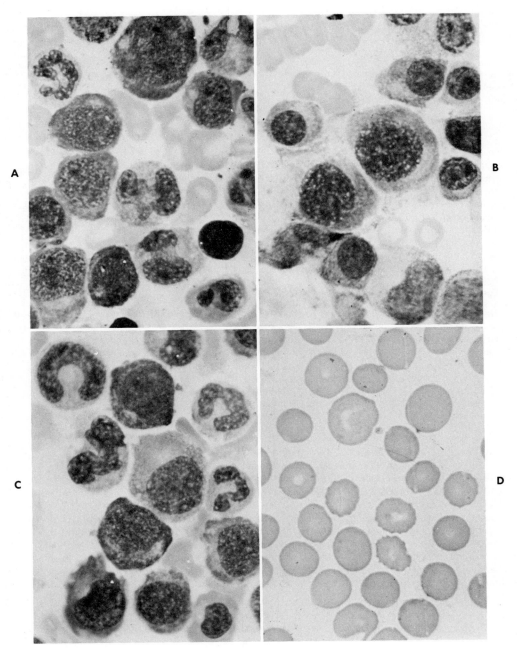

Fig. 5-46

Fig. 5-47. Case 21. Megaloblastic bone marrow (macrocytic anemia of pregnancy in a patient with sickle cell disease). **A,** Bone marrow smear. (Wright's stain; ×950.) **B,** Peripheral blood smear. (Wright's stain; ×950.) **C,** Paraffin section of marrow. (Hematoxylin-eosin stain; ×450.)

Bone marrow differential count

Cell	Percent		Cell	Percent
Myeloblasts		0.2	Lymphocytes	3.0
Progranulocytes		0.6	Plasmacytes	2.0
Myelocytes (total)		1.6	Megakaryocytes	0.6
Neutrophilic	1.6		Promegaloblasts	7.4
Metamyelocytes (total)		4.6	Basophilic megaloblasts	7.0
Neutrophilic	4.6		Polychromatophilic megaloblasts	2.1
Band cells (total)		9.6	Orthochromic megaloblasts	1.9
Neutrophilic	9.0		Basophilic normoblasts	11.6
Eosinophilic	0.6		Polychromatophilic normoblasts	40.8
Segmented (total)		4.2	Orthochromic normoblasts	2.0
Neutrophils	3.6		Reticulum cells	0.8
Eosinophils	0.6			

History and physical examination: This 18-year-old black girl was admitted to the hospital because of bilateral leg ulcers and for study of marked anemia associated with pregnancy. Two years previously she had been treated for leg ulcers due to sickle cell disease. At that time the Hb was 7.3 Gm/dl of blood, and the RBC was 2.8 million/mm³ (2.8×10^{12}/l). The pregnancy was of 8 months' duration, and she had no complaints except for the painful leg ulcers.

Examination revealed that the height of the fundus of the uterus corresponded to the period of gestation, and the fetal heart was heard in the right lower quadrant. Each ankle was swollen, indurated, discolored, and scarred. Open ulcers with surrounding inflammation were present on the lateral aspects.

Laboratory data: Hb 4.8 Gm/dl, RBC 1.85 million/mm³ (1.85×10^{12}/l), WBC (corrected for normoblasts) 17,590/mm³ (17.59×10^9/l); leukocyte differential count: 5% stab neutrophils, 62% segmented neutrophils, 31% lymphocytes, 1% monocytes, and 1% eosinophils. Erythrocytes on peripheral blood smear showed macrocytosis, 4+ anisocytosis, and poikilocytosis. Blood smear also showed 102 normoblasts/100 leukocytes. Reticulocyte count was 21.1%; platelet count 566,000/mm³ (0.566×10^{12}/l) (phase microscopy). Bisulfite test showed 71% sickling of erythrocytes. Electrophoresis of hemoglobin showed Hb S–Hb S pattern (sickle cell disease). Total bilirubin was 2.25 mg/dl of serum, with 1.06 mg/dl at 1 minute. Free hydrochloric acid was found on gastric analysis.

Discussion: The megaloblastic marrow and macrocytic anemia led to a diagnosis of macrocytic anemia of pregnancy superimposed on sickle cell anemia. This unusual combination presented a number of interesting features. Most of the erythrocytes on the peripheral blood smears were frankly macrocytic, but many were microcytic and all were hypochromic. The high reticulocyte count can be attributed to sickle cell anemia. After folic acid therapy there was no additional reticulocytosis, even though the number of normoblasts in the peripheral blood dropped from 112 to 35/100 leukocytes. Also there was a satisfactory rise in hemoglobin and the number of erythrocytes.

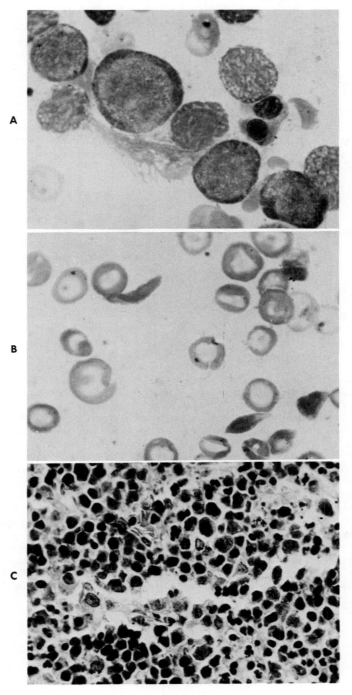

Fig. 5-47

Fig. 5-48. Case 22. Megaloblastic bone marrow associated with primary hemochromatosis. **A-C,** Bone marrow smears. (Wright's stain; ×950.) **D,** Paraffin section of liver. (Hematoxylin-eosin stain; ×450.) Note the typical megaloblastic dyspoiesis in **A-C** and the fibrosis and the iron-containing pigment in **D.**

Bone marrow differential count

Cell	Percent		Cell	Percent
Myeloblasts		0.4	Lymphocytes	9.0
Progranulocytes		0.8	Plasmacytes	1.4
Myelocytes (total)		12.8	Basophilic megaloblasts	1.0
Neutrophilic	12.4		Polychromatophilic megaloblasts	2.0
Eosinophilic	0.4		Orthochromic megaloblasts	5.0
Metamyeloctyes (total)		19.0	Pronormoblasts	6.2
Neutrophilic	18.4		Basophilic normoblasts	2.8
Eosinophilic	0.6		Polychromatophilic normoblasts	2.2
Band cells (total)		25.0	Orthochromic normoblasts	8.0
Neutrophilic	25.0			
Segmented (total)		4.4		
Neutrophils	3.4			
Eosinophils	1.0			

History and physical examination: This patient's illness had been of about 6 years' duration. She was a 40-year-old housewife who was well until she noticed an increasing skin pigmentation, weakness, and easy fatigability. At first the diagnosis was Addison's disease, but later a diagnosis of hemochromatosis was confirmed by a biopsy of the skin. She had never received blood transfusions. Her symptoms gradually became worse, and recently there had been progressive anemia. Physical examination showed the liver to be very firm, and the edge was palpable 3 fingerbreadths below the costal margin. The spleen was just palpable. The skin showed a diffuse gray-bronze color, most noticeable in exposed areas. There were no abnormal neurologic findings.

Laboratory data: Peripheral blood findings were Hb 7.0 Gm/dl, RBC 2.4 million/mm^3 (2.4×10^{12}/l), WBC 4,750/mm^3 (4.75×10^9/l); leukocyte differential count: 40% segmented neutrophils, 57% lymphocytes, and 3% eosinophils. Blood smear showed scattered macrocytosis, 2+ anisocytosis, poikilocytosis, hypochromia of erythrocytes, and a few hypersegmented neutrophils. Platelet count was 274,000/mm^3 (0.274×10^{12}/l) (phase microscopy). Urinalysis was normal. Gastric analysis revealed a normal amount of hydrochloric acid. Blood glucose, NPN, and electrolytes were normal.

Discussion: A biopsy of the marrow was done to determine the degree of erythropoiesis in relation to the anemia. The finding of megaloblasts was not unexpected in view of previous reports of megaloblastic marrows in hemochromatosis. The absence of neurologic dysfunction and the presence of free hydrochloric acid in the gastric juice are typical. A biopsy of the liver showed cirrhosis and large amounts of stainable iron.

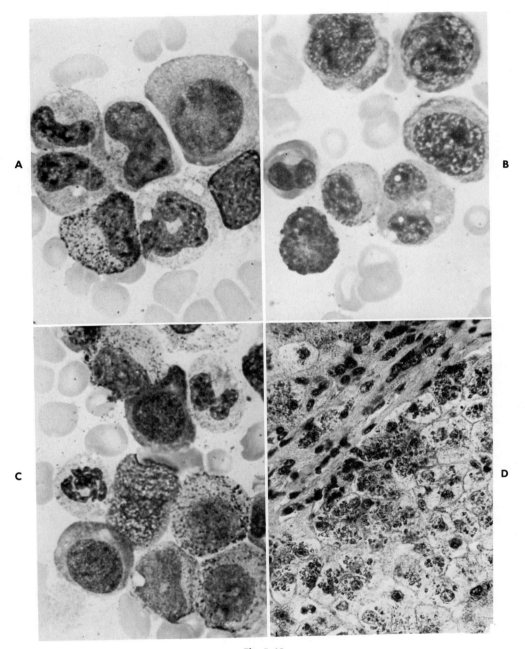

Fig. 5-48

Fig. 5-49. Case 23. Acute monocytic (histiocytic, Schilling type) leukemia. **A** and **B,** Peripheral blood. **C** and **D,** Bone marrow. (Wright's stain; ×950.)

Bone marrow differential count

Cell	Percent	Cell	Percent
Monoblasts	34.2	Segmented neutrophils	1.0
Promonocytes	43.8	Stab neutrophils	1.0
Progranulocytes	3.2	Lymphocytes	1.4
Myelocytes	3.0	Normoblasts	10.4
Metamyelocytes	2.0		

History and physical examination: This patient was a 45-year-old white male admitted to the hospital with severe pseudomembranous tonsillitis of 4 days' duration. There had been frequent attacks of tonsillitis and upper respiratory infection in the past, but this time there was high fever and chills and he had not responded to treatment at home.

Physical examination revealed a temperature of 101° F (38.3° C), palpable cervical, preauricular, and submaxillary lymph nodes, and a diffusely inflamed throat with swollen, bulging tonsils. The spleen was palpable 3 cm below the costal margin.

Laboratory data: On admission the blood Hb was 13.2 Gm/dl, RBC 4.25 million/mm³ (4.25 × 10¹²/l), WBC 39,500/mm³ (39.5 × 10⁹/l); leukocyte differential count: segmented neutrophils 7%, stab neutrophils 5%, lymphocytes 24%, monoblasts 20%, promonocytes 32%, monocytes 8%, and eosinophils 4%; platelet count 53,000/mm³ (0.053 × 10¹²/l). Blood cultures showed no growth, and the heterophil antibody titer was 1:7.

Discussion: Although the infectious disease raised the question of a leukemoid reaction at first, the peripheral blood and bone marrow are typical of monocytic leukemia (pure histiocytic type of Schilling). Antibiotics brought the body temperature to normal within 2 days, but the leukocyte count, differential count, and platelet count did not improve. Death occurred in a few weeks.

The term "monocytic leukemia" should be applied only to cases such as this one, in which the cells show purely monocytic features. The delicate monocytoid nucleus and cytoplasm, the latter containing fine pink granules, is illustrated very nicely in this case. When the nucleus is monocytoid but the cytoplasm contains granules of the myeloid type, the term "myelomonocytic leukemia" should be used (see Figs. 5-50 to 5-53).

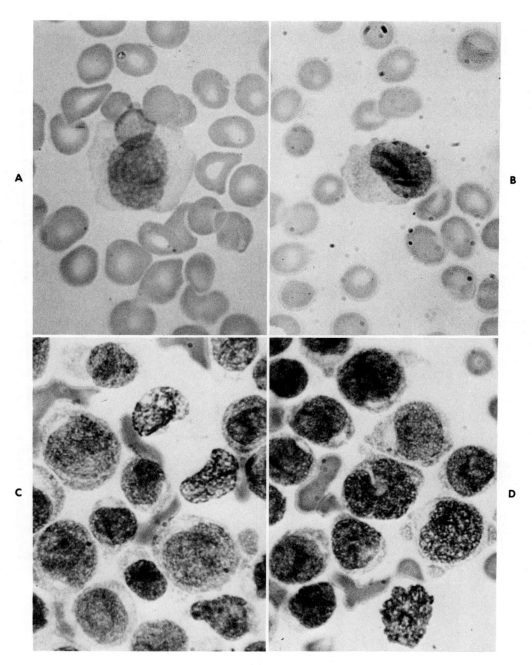

Fig 5-49

Fig. 5-50. Case 24. Acute myelomonocytic leukemia (Naegeli type). **A-C,** Bone marrow smears. (Wright's stain; ×950.) **D,** Peripheral blood smear. (Wright's stain; ×950.) Note the Auer body in a myelomonoblast in **B** and **D.**

Bone marrow differential count

Cell	Percent	Cell	Percent
Monoblasts (myelomonocytic)	82.4	Lymphocytes	1.6
Myelocytes (monocytoid)	11.6	Basophilic normoblasts	0.4
Band neutrophils	0.4	Polychromatophilic normoblasts	0.4
Segmented neutrophils	1.6	Orthochromic normoblasts	1.6

History and physical examination: This patient, a 54-year-old black woman, was in a semicomatose state when admitted to the hospital. Three months before, she began to feel weak and eventually was not able to leave her bed. She was unable to eat and frequently vomited bloody material. When examined, she was acutely ill. The body temperature was 101° F (38.3° C). There were numerous hemorrhages in the skin. There was lymphadenopathy in the cervical, supraclavicular, axillary, and inguinal regions. The liver was slightly enlarged, but the spleen was not palpable.

Laboratory data: On admission the blood findings were Hb 5.5 Gm/dl of blood, RBC 1.78 million/mm³ (1.78 × 10¹²/l), WBC 134,000/mm³ (134 × 10⁹/l); leukocyte differential count: 32% monoblasts, 59% promonocytes, 2% neutrophilic metamyelocytes, 6% stab neutrophils, and 1% segmented neutrophils. There were 3 normoblasts/100 leukocytes on the smear. Platelet count was 20,000/mm³ (0.02 × 10¹²/l) (phase microscopy).

Discussion: As shown in the illustrations, all the abnormal cells found in the peripheral blood and bone marrow show the same morphologic features. These cells are sometimes not easy to classify. At first glance they resemble cells of the myelocytic series, but the convoluted or folded nucleus in some of the cells suggests a monocytoid structure. At times the best that can be done is to classify these cells as myelomonocytic forms. The blast forms are usually characteristic in that, in spite of a very immature nucleus, the cytoplasm contains a few granules that are peroxidase positive. The atypical morphology of these cells may be thought of as an indication of the common derivation of myelomonocytic and myelocytic forms from the myeloblast. In this leukemic variant the cells therefore show features common to both series *(Naegeli type).* Monocytic leukemias of a pure monocytic (histiocytic) type are much rarer. These are referred to as the *Schilling type* (see Fig. 5-49, Case 23).

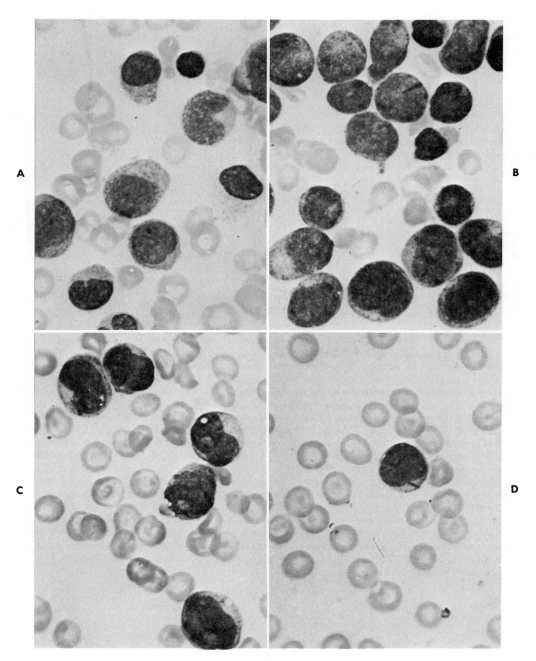

Fig. 5-50

Fig. 5-51. Case 25. Acute myelomonocytic leukemia (Naegeli type). **A,**Bone marrow smear. (Wright's stain; ×950.) **B,**Peripheral blood smear. (Wright's stain; ×950.) **C,** Peripheral blood smear. (Peroxidase stain; ×950.) **D,** Paraffin section of marrow. (Hematoxylin-eosin stain; ×450.) The monocytoid nuclear structure is clearly seen in **A** and **B.** Note the blast cells in **C** that contain a few peroxidase-positive granules.

Bone marrow differential count

Cell	Percent		Cell	Percent
Monoblasts (myelomonocytic)	22.4		Segmented (total)	0.4
Promonocytes (myelomonocytic)	42.8		Basophils	0.4
Monocytes	2.4		Lymphocytes	17.6
Progranulocytes	4.0		Plasmacytes	0.8
Myelocytes (total)	3.6		Basophilic normoblasts	0.4
Neutrophilic	2.0		Polychromatophilic normoblasts	0.4
Basophilic	1.6		Orthochromic normoblasts	2.0
Metamyelocytes (total)	1.6		Disintegrated cells	1.6
Neutrophilic	0.8			
Eosinophilic	0.8			

History and physical examination: The patient, a 29-year-old white man, was well until 1 week before admission to the hospital. At that time he had an acute onset of weakness, malaise, anorexia, and fever. When examined, he was acutely ill and apprehensive. His temperature was 101.2° F (38.5° C). There was hypertrophy of the gums and petechiae on the oral mucosa. Small, discrete posterior cervical lymph nodes were palpable. The edge of the liver was palpable 2 fingerbreadths below the costal margin, and the spleen was easily palpable 4 fingerbreadths below the costal margin. A few petechial hemorrhages were found on the legs.

Laboratory data: On admission the blood studies showed Hb 8.2 Gm/dl of blood, RBC 2.7 million/mm³ (2.7 × 10¹²/l), WBC 31,000/mm³ (31 × 10⁹/l); leukocyte differential count: 87% monoblasts, 12% promonocytes, and 1% segmented neutrophils; platelet count 22,000/mm³ (0.022 × 10¹²/l). The results of numerous other laboratory tests were normal.

Discussion: The diagnosis of acute leukemia was obvious when this patient was first seen. Biopsy of the bone marrow was confirmatory, the predominant cells being myelomonocytic in morphology, the nucleus monocytoid, and the cytoplasm containing coarse granules that were strongly peroxidase positive. Typically, most cells, including the early blast forms, were peroxidase positive. The course of the illness was rapidly progressive in spite of chemotherapy and blood transfusions. Cutaneous and mucosal hemorrhages became numerous, followed by bloody stools, respiratory difficulty, and hemoptysis. The platelet count 1 week after admission was 8,000/mm³ (0.008 × 10¹²/l), and the WBC rose to 179,000/mm³ (179 × 10⁹/l). The patient died 2 weeks after admission. The terminal WBC was 240,000/mm³ (240 × 10⁹/l).

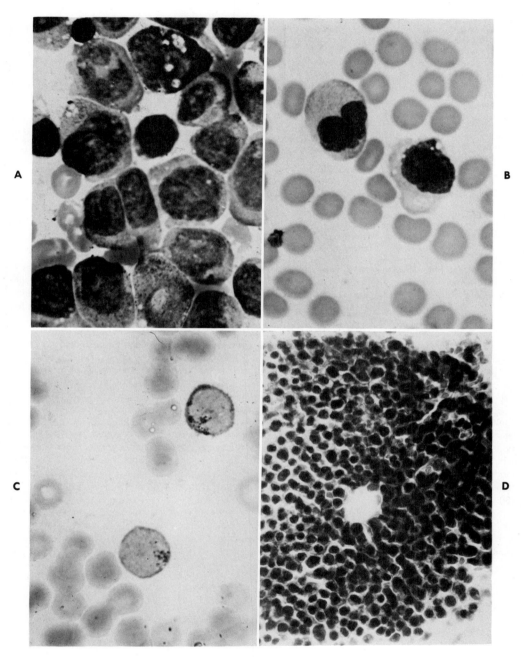

Fig. 5-51

Fig. 5-52. Case 26. Acute myelomonocytic leukemia. **A-C,** Peripheral blood. (Wright's stain; ×950.) **D,** Spleen. (Hematoxylin-eosin stain; ×400.)

Bone marrow differential count

Cell	Percent
Blasts (myelomonoblasts)	72
Promonocytes	10
Myelocytes	10
Metamyelocytes	3
Erythroid cells	5

History and physical examination: This 66-year-old white male was admitted to the hospital with complaints of simultaneous onset of malaise and skin rash 2 weeks previously. He had been in good health before that with no significant history of prior illness. The skin rash began on the legs, spread to the trunk and arms, and varied from flat nodular indurations to papulomacular and hemorrhagic nodules. During this 2-week period he felt increasingly tired and weak.

On physical examination the skin lesions described above were noted to be present over the entire surface but more numerous on the legs. He appeared acutely ill but had no fever. There was hepatomegaly (5 finger-breadths) and splenomegaly (4 fingerbreadths). There was no lymphadenopathy.

Laboratory data: Blood Hb 7.8 Gm/dl, RBC 2.48 million/mm³ (2.48 × 10¹²/l), WBC 273,000/mm³ (273 × 10⁹/l); leukocyte differential count: blasts (myelomonoblasts) 92%, myelomonocytes 5%, and lymphocytes 3%; platelet count 24,000/mm³ (0.024 × 10¹²/l). ECG showed a complete right bundle branch block.

Discussion: Although acutely ill when admitted, his death 40 hours later was impressively rapid. The rapid disintegration of terminal acute leukemia is often startling, something like the awesome rapidity of a prairie fire. I remember a 17-year-old girl whose acute lymphocytic leukemia had undergone complete remission for 14 months who relapsed and died within a 24-hour period. She was seen for a routine periodic check and was found to be anemic for the first time since the onset of the leukemia. Her leukocyte count was 24,000/mm³ (24 × 10⁹/l), and there were 10% lymphoblasts. She was admitted to the hospital; 2 hours later the leukocyte count was 40,000/mm³ (40 × 10⁹/l), 6 hours after that it was 175,000/mm³ (175 × 10⁹/l), and 4 hours after that it was 380,000/mm³ (380 × 10⁹/l). She died 24 hours after admission.

The patient presented here had increasing respiratory difficulty and cyanosis. The blood pressure dropped to 80/75, the pulse gradually faded, and he became comatose and died. At necropsy there was leukemic infiltration of the lungs, epicardium, myocardium, spleen, liver, bone marrow, kidneys, testicles, mucosa of the stomach, small bowel and colon, and the skin.

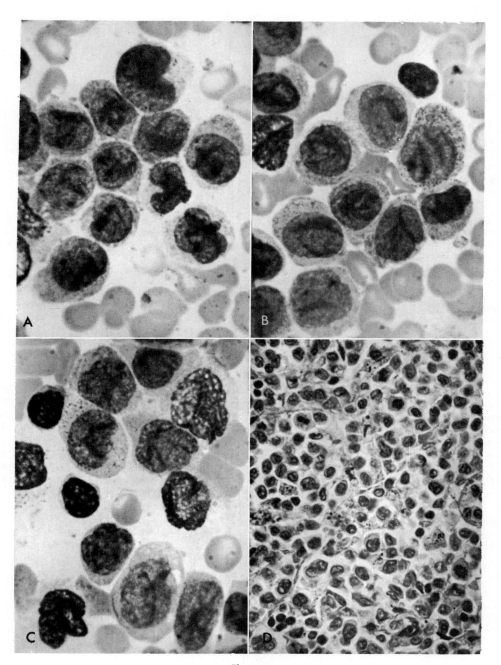

Fig. 5-52

Fig. 5-53. Case 27. Chronic myelomonocytic leukemia. **A** and **B,** Bone marrow smears. (Wright's stain; ×950.) **C,** Paraffin section of a skin nodule. (Hematoxylin-eosin stain; ×450.) **D,** Paraffin section of marrow. (Hematoxylin-eosin stain; ×450.)

Bone marrow differential count

Cell		Percent	Cell	Percent	
Monoblasts (myelomonocytic)		2.4	Segmented (total)		8.4
Promonocytes (myelomonocytic)		21.8	Neutrophils	5.6	
Monocytes		4.8	Eosinophils	2.4	
Myelocytes (total)		7.8	Basophils	0.4	
Neutrophilic	6.6		Prolymphocytes		1.2
Eosinophilic	1.2		Lymphocytes		5.6
Band cells (total)		16.0	Plasmacytes		0.6
Neutrophilic	15.0		Basophilic normoblasts		4.4
Eosinophilic	1.0		Polychromatophilic normoblasts		24.0
			Orthochromic normoblasts		4.4
			Reticulum cells		1.6

History and physical examination: When admitted to the hospital, the patient, a 67-year-old black woman, said she had been "ailing" for some months. She had lost 15 pounds in weight during the previous year, her appetite had been poor, and from time to time she had felt feverish. About a month before admission she first noticed small "lumps" in the skin of her body and arms, followed by large nontender masses in the back of her neck. Examination showed numerous small, slightly raised and indurated nodules in the skin of the abdomen and arms. There were large nontender posterior cervical nodes. The spleen was barely palpable, and the liver edge was felt 3 cm below the costal margin.

Laboratory data: Hb 10.2 Gm/dl of blood, RBC 4.39 million/mm³ (4.39×10^{12}/l), WBC 11,350/mm³ (11.35×10^9/l); leukocyte differential count: 67% promonocytes, 30% segmented neutrophils, 2% stab neutrophils, and 1% eosinophils; platelet count 161,000/mm³ (0.161×10^{12}/l) (phase microscopy).

Discussion: The peripheral blood and marrow contained many promonocytes characterized by irregular and vesicular nuclei. The cytoplasmic granules in these cells were generally very fine, and most gave a positive reaction for peroxidase. Biopsies were taken from a cervical lymph node and from one of the nodules in the skin. Both showed diffuse infiltration with the same type of cell.

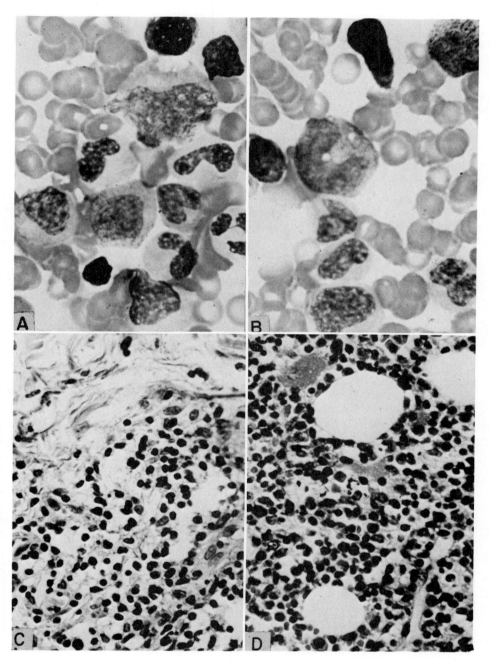

Fig. 5-53

Fig. 5-54. Case 28. Terminal acute relapse of chronic myelomonocytic leukemia. **A** and **B,** Bone marrow smears. (Wright's stain; ×950.) **C,** Paraffin section of marrow. (Hematoxylin-eosin stain; ×450.) Note the mitoses in **B.**

Bone marrow differential count

Cell	Percent		Cell	Percent	
Monoblasts (myelomonocytic)	37.0		Metamyelocytes		1.0
Promonocytes (myelomonocytic)	35.8		Band cells (total)		3.0
Monocytes	12.0		Neutrophilic	1.2	
Progranulocytes	1.3		Eosinophilic	1.8	
Myelocytes (total)	3.9		Segmented		0.6
Neutrophilic	3.6		Lymphocytes		4.6
Eosinophilic	0.3		Proplasmacytes		0.6
			Unidentified		0.2

History and physical examination: This 42-year-old woman had had myelomonocytic leukemia for at least 1 year. She had been treated with cortisone and numerous blood transfusions, but with little benefit. When admitted to the hospital, she complained of severe substernal pain, epigastric pain, nausea, vomiting of coffee-ground—like material, epistaxis, and hemoptysis. Her temperature was 101° F (38.3° C), and she was acutely ill. She had numerous petechiae on her skin and mucous membranes, hepatomegaly, and splenomegaly.

Laboratory data: On admission, blood studies showed Hb 7.9 Gm/dl of blood, RBC 2.7 million/mm³ (2.7 × 10^{12}/l), WBC 14,950/mm³ (14.95 × 10^9/l); leukocyte differential count: 25% monoblasts, 35% promonocytes, 2% stab neutrophils, 6% segmented neutrophils, and 32% lymphocytes; platelet count 9,000/mm³ (0.009 × 10^{12}/l) (phase microscopy).

Discussion: A comparison of the bone marrow smears with those obtained 1 year earlier shows a striking change toward the acute phase. The first marrow contained a preponderance of relatively adult myelomonocytic forms, and the last marrow showed many blast forms. Death occurred 2 weeks after admission, and the necropsy revealed a subarachnoid hemorrhage as well as hemorrhages and leukemic infiltration into other tissues and viscera. It is noteworthy that during the last week of illness there was progressive leukopenia, the last WBC being 2,000/mm³ (2 × 10^9/l).

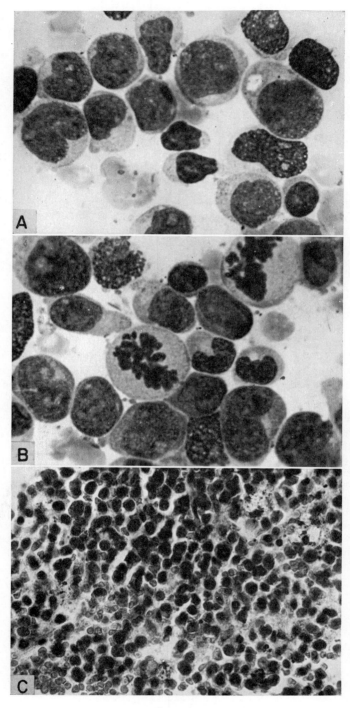

Fig. 5-54

Fig. 5-55. Case 29. Chronic myelocytic leukemia. **A,** Bone marrow smear. (Wright's stain; ×450.) **B** and **C,** Bone marrow smears. (Wright's stain; ×950.) **D,** Paraffin section of marrow. (Hematoxylin-eosin stain; ×450.)

Bone marrow differential count

Cell	Percent		Cell	Percent	
Myeloblasts		1.0	Band cells (total)		15.6
Progranulocytes		10.0	Neutrophilic	12.0	
Myelocytes (total)		41.2	Eosinophilic	3.6	
Neutrophilic	40.0		Segmented (total)		2.2
Eosinophilic	0.2		Neutrophils	2.2	
Basophilic	1.0		Lymphocytes		5.0
Metamyelocytes (total)		23.6	Monocytes		0.2
Neutrophilic	22.0		Plasmacytes		1.2
Eosinophilic	0.6				
Basophilic	1.0				

History and physical examination: This patient was a 70-year-old white man. For the previous 10 days he had complained of increasingly severe dizziness, shortness of breath, and weakness. On admission to the hospital his body temperature was 99.4° F (37.4° C). There were scattered petechiae on the abdomen and right arm. Slightly enlarged nodes were palpable in the left axilla and posterior cervical areas. The edge of the liver was palpable 2 fingerbreadths below the costal margin and the spleen 4 fingerbreadths.

Laboratory data: Hb 4.3 Gm/dl of blood, RBC 1.29 million/mm³ (1.29×10^{12}/l), WBC 56,000/mm³ (56×10^9/l); leukocyte differential count: 2% myeloblasts, 4% progranulocytes, 11% myelocytes, 10% metamyelocytes, 29% stab neutrophils, 17% segmented neutrophils, 22% lymphocytes, 1% monocytes, 3% eosinophils, and 1% basophils. An occasional normoblast was found on the peripheral blood smear. Platelet count was 42,000/mm³ (0.042×10^{12}/l) (phase microscopy). Venous coagulation time was 8 minutes. Capillary bleeding time was 23 minutes. Tourniquet test was strongly positive.

Discussion: Both the peripheral blood and the bone marrow showed a preponderance of myeloid cells with relatively few blast forms. The granulocytes often showed an asynchronism between nuclear and cytoplasmic maturation, which made accurate classification difficult. The low platelet count explains the hemorrhagic manifestations. Occasionally, however, chronic myelocytic leukemia is accompanied by a striking increase in platelets in the peripheral blood.

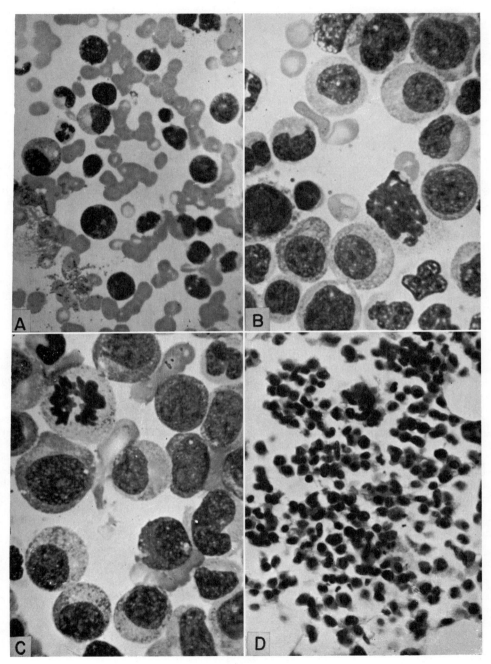

Fig. 5-55

Fig. 5-56. Case 30. Acute myelocytic leukemia. **A** and **B,** Peripheral blood. **C** and **D,** Bone marrow. (Wright's stain; ×950.)

Bone marrow differential count

Cell	Percent		Cell	Percent	
Myeloblasts		52.0	Stab neutrophils		16.0
Progranulocytes		5.0	Segmented (total)		7.0
Myelocytes (total)		12.5	Neutrophils	6.5	
Neutrophilic	8.0		Basophils	0.5	
Eosinophilic	0.5		Lymphocytes		6.0
Basophilic	4.0		Basophilic normoblasts		0.5
Metamyelocytes (total)		9.5	Orthochromic normoblasts		0.5
Neutrophilic	9.0				
Basophilic	0.5				

History and physical examination: This 64-year-old white female had admission complaints of progressive weakness for some weeks, chills, and fever of 2 days' duration. Two months previously she had an episode of "flu," with diarrhea, fatigue, progressive weakness, and dyspnea on exertion, from which she seemed not to recover.

On physical examination the BP was 160/80, pulse 110/minute, respiration 20/minute, and temperature 100.2° F (37.9° C). She was obese, pale, and seemed acutely ill. There were scattered ecchymoses on her thighs and arms, petechiae of her palate, and herpes simplex of her lips. Spleen and liver were not palpable in the obese abdomen.

Laboratory data: Blood Hb 5.5 Gm/dl, hematocrit 15%, WBC 19,500/mm^3 (19.5 × 10^9/l); leukocyte differential count: blasts 37%, progranulocytes 2%, myelocytes 3%, basophils 2%, segmented neutrophils 10%, band neutrophils 24%, metamyelocytes 1%, lymphocytes 15%, and monocytes 6%, platelet count 15,000/mm^3 (0.015 × 10^{12}/l). Sternal marrow aspiration biopsy as above.

Discussion: In spite of transfusions and chemotherapy, she died 16 days after admission. Permission for necropsy was refused.

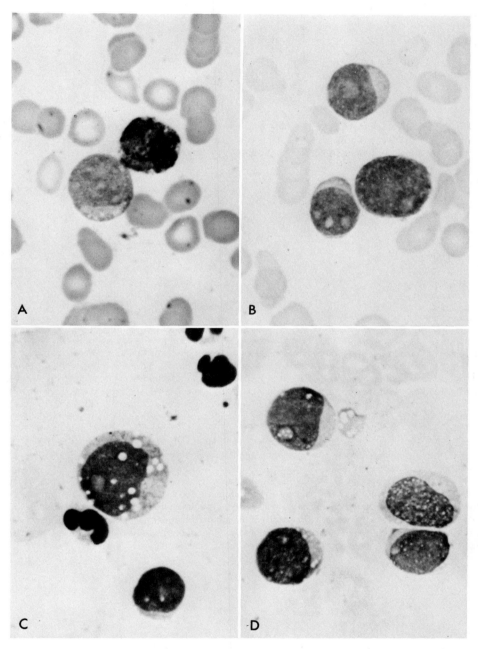

Fig. 5-56

Fig. 5-57. Case 31. Acute myelocytic leukemia with retrobulbar leukemic tumor (chloroma). **A** and **B,** Bone marrow smears. (Wright's stain; ×950.) **C,** Paraffin section of retrobulbar tumor. (Hematoxylin-eosin stain; ×450.) **D,** Paraffin section of marrow particle. (Hematoxylin-eosin stain; ×450.)

Bone marrow differential count

Cell	Percent		Cell	Percent	
Myeloblasts		25.0	Segmented (total)		8.0
Progranulocytes		5.2	Neutrophils	7.0	
Myelocytes (total)		10.2	Eosinophils	1.0	
Neutrophilic	10.0		Lymphocytes		16.0
Eosinophilic	0.2		Monocytes		5.0
Metamyelocytes (total)		10.0	Plasmacytes		0.8
Neutrophilic	10.0		Polychromatophilic normoblasts		2.0
Band cells (total)		14.0	Orthochromic normoblasts		0.2
Neutrophilic	13.6		Unidentified		2.2
Eosinophilic	0.4		Reticulum cells		1.4

History and physical examination: This 2-year-old white boy's illness began with the complaint of being unable to see with his left eye. The ophthalmologist found exophthalmos due to a retrobulbar tumor mass. A frozen section biopsy of the mass was interpreted as a malignant tumor, and the eye was then enucleated. The tumor mass was described as gray-green and soft. Permanent paraffin sections were interpreted by several skilled pathologists who agreed on the diagnosis of reticulum cell sarcoma. For 2 weeks the postoperative course was uneventful; then the boy developed a spiking fever, and there was loss of appetite and weight. The body temperature rose to 102.8° F (39.2° C). The other findings were scattered petechiae and an ecchymosis around the remaining eye.

Laboratory data: Hb 5.5 Gm/dl of blood, RBC 1.78 million/mm³ (1.78×10^{12}/l), WBC 10,650/mm³ (10.65×10^9/l); leukocyte differential count: 7% myeloblasts (micromyeloblasts), 3% progranulocytes, 9% myelocytes, 5% neutrophilic metamyelocytes, 25% stab neutrophils, 18% segmented neutrophils, and 33% lymphocytes; platelet count 11,000/mm³ (0.011×10^{12}/l) (phase microscopy).

Discussion: Bone marrow smears showed 25% myeloblasts and a striking increase in the myeloid-erythroid ratio. Paraffin sections of marrow particles were also strikingly abnormal and showed both abnormal and immature myeloid cells. When compared with sections of the tumor, the abnormal cells were identical. In retrospect we must conclude that the tumor of the eye represented an unusual onset of acute myelocytic leukemia. Because of their greenish color, tumors of this type have been called "chloromas."

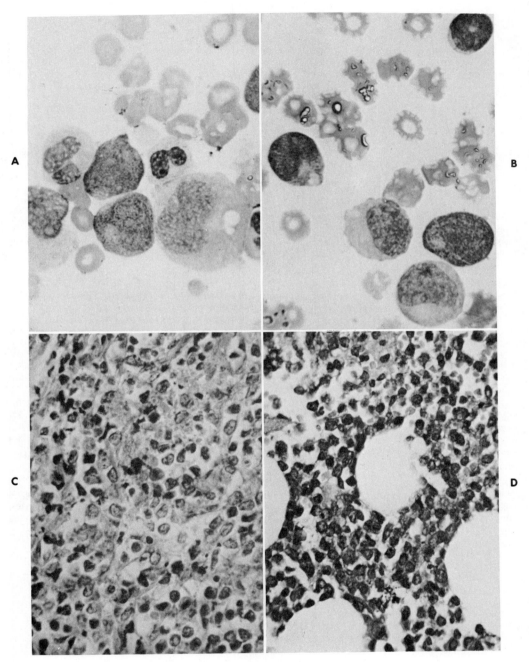

Fig. 5-57

Fig. 5-58. Case 32. Acute myelocytic leukemia (micromyeloblastic). **A-C,** Bone marrow smears. (Wright's stain; ×950.) **D,** Paraffin section of marrow. (Hematoxylin-eosin stain; ×450.)

Bone marrow differential count

Cell	Percent		Cell	Percent	
Myeloblasts		36.0	Band cells (total)		5.8
Progranulocytes		4.2	Neutrophilic	5.8	
Myelocytes (total)		9.0	Segmented (total)		11.0
Neutrophilic	8.2		Neutrophils	10.4	
Eosinophilic	0.6		Eosinophils	0.6	
Basophilic	0.2		Lymphocytes		1.2
Metamyelocytes (total)		3.4	Pronormoblasts		1.8
Neutrophilic	3.2		Basophilic normoblasts		4.2
Eosinophilic	0.2		Polychromatophilic normoblasts		20.8
			Reticulum cells		2.6

History and physical examination: The patient, a 63-year-old white man, complained of increasing weakness. By the time he was admitted he was too weak to walk unassisted. The onset of this illness dated back 1 month when he had a tooth extracted. The extraction was followed by bleeding, which stopped 2 days later. On examination there were no pertinent findings.

Laboratory data: Peripheral blood Hb 8.6 Gm/dl, RBC 3.35 million/mm^3 (3.35 × 10^{12}/l), WBC 234,000/mm^3 (234 × 10^9/l); leukocyte differential count: 27.5% myeloblasts, 9% progranulocytes, 16% myelocytes, 5.5% neutrophilic metamyelocytes, 19.5% stab neutrophils, 19.5% segmented neutrophils, 2.5% lymphocytes, and 0.5% eosinophils. On the smear there were 12 normoblasts/100 leukocytes. Reticulocyte count was 13.9%, and platelet count was 8,000/mm^3 (0.008 × 10^{12}/l) (phase microscopy). Venous coagulation time was 10 minutes. Capillary bleeding time was 1 hour.

Discussion: Many blast cells were present in the peripheral blood and bone marrow. These were smaller than usual and represented a cell type referred to as micromyeloblasts. The variability in size of blast cells is not important except for the difficulty sometimes encountered in distinguishing micromyeloblasts from lymphocytes. The presence of other immature myeloid cells is usually helpful in classifying this type of myeloblast. Note the Auer body in **C.**

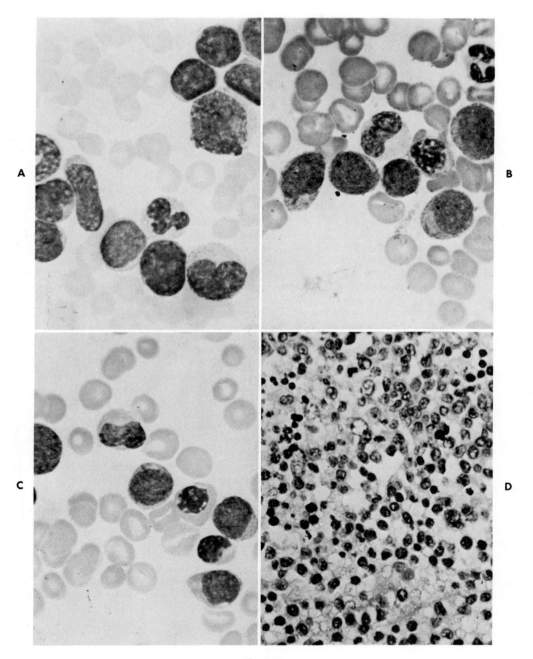

Fig. 5-58

Fig. 5-59. Case 33. Acute myelocytic leukemia (Rieder cells) with hypergammaglobulinemia. **A,** Peripheral blood. **B** and **C,** Bone marrow. (Wright's stain; ×950.) **D,** Scan of serum protein separation on filter paper. Note the abnormal gamma peak. (Referred by Dr. R. Werner Kraatz.)

Bone marrow differential count

Cell	Percent	Cell	Percent
Myeloblasts	51.4	Eosinophils	1.0
Progranulocytes	1.22	Basophils	1.0
Myelocytes	4.6	Lymphocytes	2.0
Metamyelocytes	8.4	Plasma cells	0.5
Stab neutrophils	6.0	Normoblasts	7.5
Segmented neutrophils	7.0		

History and laboratory data: This 50-year-old white male died 4 months after the onset of symptoms; he had been admitted to the hospital several times. The onset was characterized by vertigo, nausea, vomiting, and weakness, and on the first admission the physical examination and the peripheral blood picture were normal. Generalized weakness persisted, and on the second admission 2 weeks later he had moderate leukopenia (3,450/mm^3, 3.45 × 10^{12}/l), a markedly elevated sedimentation rate (92 mm/hour), and moderate anemia (10.9 Gm/dl). Total serum protein concentration was 10.2 Gm/dl, and the electrophoretic pattern was abnormal. On ultracentrifugal separation, the serum protein distribution was as follows: 0.17 Gm/dl S19 macroglobulin, 4.47 Gm/dl S7 globulin, and 0.8 Gm/dl S4 albumin. Sia test was negative. urine was positive for Bence Jones protein. Roentgenograms showed translucent areas in the left and right ischium, left intertrochanteric area, and the head of the left femur. Roentgenograms of the skull were normal.

On his final admission he had extreme weakness and numerous nose bleeds. The blood Hb was 4.5 Gm/dl, WBC 16,500/mm^3 (16.5 × 10^9/l); leukocyte differential count: blasts 77%, adult granulocytes 15%, lymphocytes 7%, and monocytes 1%. There were a few normoblasts. Platelet count was 10,000/mm^3 (0.01 × 10^{12}/l). He was given blood transfusions and corticosteroids but died 5 days later.

Discussion: The unusual feature of this case is the unusual morphology of the myeloblasts. The term "Rieder cells" refers to deep indentation, pseudolobulation, and cloverleaf formation in a nucleus otherwise round or oval. The term has been applied to both the lymphocytes of chronic lymphocytic leukemia and to the myeloblasts of acute myelocytic leukemia.

Bessis (1973b) has shown that leukemic myeloblasts often undergo a nuclear shape change from round to tetrafoliate and quadrifoliate when observed in the living state in a wet coverslipped preparation. He attributes this to interference with the cell's normal metabolic activity. Since the Rieder change occurs within minutes and affects almost all cells in an hour, it is not improbable that it reflects interference with the cell's metabolism through anoxia and other artificial circumstances. It should be noted that nonleukemic cells will undergo the same change after prolonged standing in the wet state, so that the formation of Rieder cells, thought to occur only in leukemia, is probably due to the rapidity with which the change occurs rather than to a primary nuclear abnormality.

Lymphocytes in chronic lymphocytic leukemia are often deeply indented, and these forms are also called Rieder cells. These, however, appear on routine smears and may not have the same pathogenesis as the Rieder myeloblast. It must be noted, also, that when normal oxalated blood stands for many hours before smears are made, normal lymphocytes assume cloverleaf shapes (Fig. 4-9).

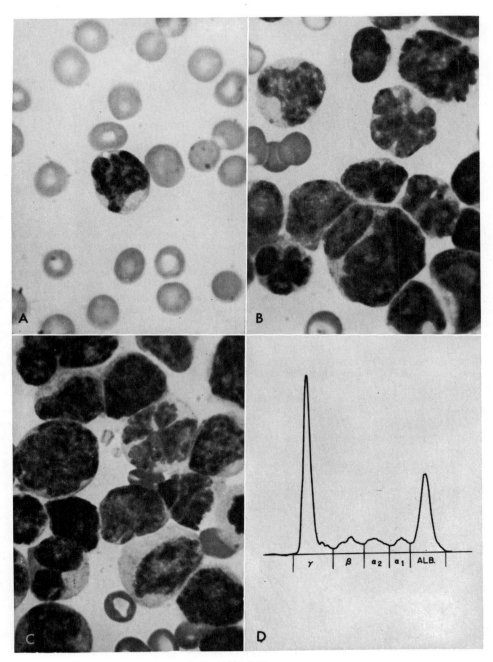

Fig. 5-59

Fig. 5-60. Case 34. Acute promyelocytic leukemia with hemorrhagic diathesis, bone marrow. (Wright's stain; ×1,250.) All the cells illustrated are "atypical" progranulocytes with very large coarse, elongated granules. (Courtesy Dr. G. Pardo.)

History and physical examination: This patient was a 44-year-old female. Two months before admission she noted ecchymoses on her arms and legs. Three days before admission there was an onset of weakness, dizziness, and profuse vaginal bleeding. Two days before admission she developed a high fever and mental confusion. She appeared acutely ill, disoriented, and very pale. There was profuse vaginal bleeding and many ecchymoses.

Laboratory data: Hb 3.2 Gm/dl, hematocrit 12%, WBC 13,600/mm³ (13.6 × 10⁹/l); differential leukocyte count 80% atypical progranulocytes; platelet count 22,000/mm³ (0.022 × 10¹²/l); plasma fibrinogen less than 50 mg/dl. Bone marrow aspiration showed 90% of the cell population to be progranulocytes.

Course: She responded to blood transfusion and heparin, with marked improvement in the bleeding and a rise in the plasma fibrinogen concentration. She was then started on prednisone but had a second episode of bleeding; the laboratory findings were the same as before. Heparin therapy was only partially successful. She died of pneumonia 2 months after she was first seen. Permission for necropsy was refused.

Discussion: There are many reports of hypofibrinogenemia in acute leukemia (Chapter 16). Bleeding is not uncommon, and there is the additional factor of thrombocytopenia. Some feel that there is evidence for a characteristic association of hypofibrinogenemia and acute promyelocytic leukemia. The pathogenesis is probably diffuse intravascular deposition of fibrin (Chapter 17).

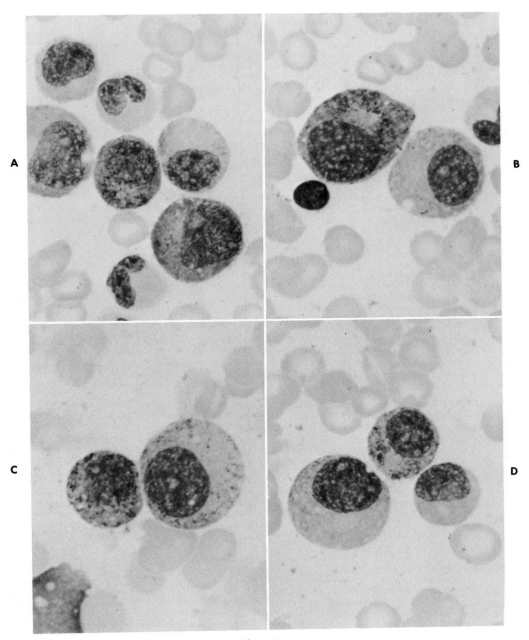

Fig. 5-60

Fig. 5-61. Case 35. Acute "congenital" lymphocytic leukemia. **A** and **B,** Peripheral blood. **C** and **D,** Bone marrow. (Wright's stain; ×950.) (Courtesy Dr. D. Traggis.)

Bone marrow differential count

Cell	Percent
Lymphoblasts	23.0
Prolymphocytes	49.0
Lymphocytes	25.0
Stab neutrophils	2.0
Normoblasts	1.0

History and physical examination: This little girl was first seen at the age of 4 weeks because she had an upper respiratory infection and had passed one blood-streaked stool. She had been previously well except for diminished appetite for 1 week.

On physical examination she did not appear acutely ill and was afebrile. The spleen was enlarged to 7 cm below the costal margin; the liver was also enlarged to 7 cm below the costal margin. Both were firm. There was 1 cm lymphadenopathy in the axillary and inguinal regions, but there was no cervical or epitrochlear lymphadenopathy.

Laboratory data: Blood Hb 9.3 Gm/dl, RBC 2.9 million/mm³ (2.9 × 10¹²/l), hematocrit 26% WBC 458,000/mm³ (458 × 10⁹/l); leukocyte differential count: blasts 55%, prolymphocytes 23%, lymphocytes 18%, stab neutrophils 1%, segmented neutrophils 2%, and eosinophils 1%; platelet count 12,000/mm³ (0.012 × 10¹²/l); reticulocyte count 2.4%. The smear showed an occasional normoblast and many smudged cells. The serum uric acid concentration was 8.6 mg/dl.

Discussion: Acute leukemia can occur at any age, but that seen at birth has been called congenital. Whether an acute leukemia detected first at the age of 4 weeks deserves to be called congenital depends on whether one assumes that it was present at birth. This child had no previous blood counts, and certainly by the age of 4 weeks the disease was well established. It is reported that congenital leukemias are usually of the acute myelocytic variety. This case is lymphocytic, as evidenced by the majority of cells being lymphoblasts, prolymphocytes, and lymphoctyes. Pregnancy and delivery had in this case been uneventful, and the mother had no known leukemogenic exposure.

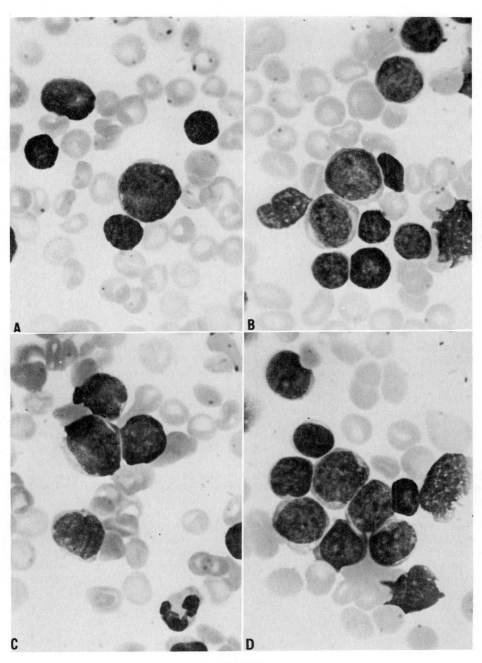

Fig. 5-61

Fig. 5-62. Case 36. Erythremic myelosis (Di Guglielmo) with terminal acute myelocytic leukemia. **A** and **B,** Bone marrow, first admission. (Wright's stain; ×950.) **C** and **D,** Peripheral blood smear, second admission. (Wright's stain; ×950.)

Bone marrow differential count

Cell	Percent		Cell	Percent	
Myeloblasts		24.0	Segmented (total)		7.0
Progranulocytes		8.0	Neutrophils	6.0	
Myelocytes (total)		17.0	Eosinophils	1.0	
Neutrophilic	12.5		Lymphocytes		1.0
Eosinophilic	4.0		Monocytes		1.0
Basophilic	0.5		Plasmacytes		1.0
Band cells (total)		13.0	Normoblasts		8.0
Neutrophilic	11.0		Megaloblasts (total)		20.0
Eosinophilic	1.0		Promegaloblasts	4.0	
Basophilic	1.0		Basophilic	6.0	
			Polychromatophilic	8.0	
			Orthochromic	2.0	

History and physical examination: This 66-year-old retired steel worker was admitted to the hospital because of vomiting and epigastric distress of 3 weeks' duration. On physical examination he appeared chronically ill and pale. He was afebrile, and there were no significant physical findings. There was no enlargement of the liver or spleen.

Laboratory data: Blood Hb 8.6 Gm/dl, hematocrit 21%, WBC 5,150/mm³ (5.15 × 10⁹/l); leukocyte differential count: myeloblasts 3%, myelocytes 4%, metamyelocytes 10%, stab neutrophils 7%, segmented neutrophils 49%, lymphocytes 40%, eosinophils 3%, basophils 3%, and monocytes 1%. The smear showed 3+ anisocytosis and 2+ poikilocytosis. Platelets were decreased in number and large and bizarre in size. Platelet count 80,000/mm³ (0.08 × 10¹²/l); reticulocyte count 0.6%; stools negative for blood.

Discussion: The obvious anemia was at first thought to be due to a bleeding gastric ulcer, but when no evidence for bleeding was found, an aspiration biopsy of the bone marrow was done. The picture of erythremic myelosis was typical, with an increase in blasts and bizarre megaloblastic erythroid forms. A nonleukemic megaloblastic dyspoiesis was ruled out by a normal Schilling test and failure to respond to folic acid. He was given a number of blood transfusions and improved enough to be discharged. However, 3 weeks later he developed a large furuncle on the face and was readmitted. At this time his WBC was 67,000/mm³ (67 × 10⁹/l); leukocyte differential count: blasts 10%, progranulocytes 24%, myelocytes 3%, metamyelocytes 2%, segmented neutrophils 10%, monocytes 38%, lymphocytes 10%, and eosinophils 3%; platelet count 16,000/mm³ (0.016 × 10¹²/l). There were hepatomegaly and splenomegaly. Aspiration biopsy of the bone marrow showed a preponderance of myeloblasts and progranulocytes. In spite of therapy he developed staphylococcal bacteremia and generalized furunculosis. He died 2 weeks after the second admission.

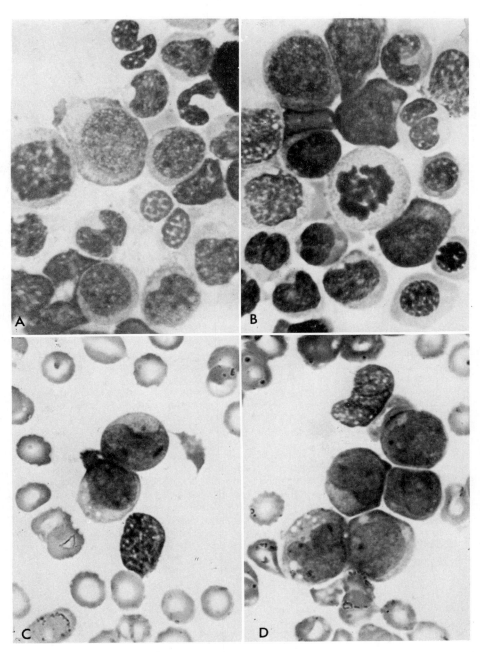

Fig. 5-62

Fig. 5-63. Case 37. Erythroleukemia (Di Guglielmo). **A,** Peripheral blood. **B-D,** Bone marrow. (Wright's stain; ×950.)

Bone marrow differential count

Cell	Percent	Cell	Percent
Myeloblasts	30.0	Plasma cells	1.0
Progranulocytes	4.2	Reticulum cells	6.0
Myelocytes	3.4	Basophilic monoblasts	1.0
Metamyelocytes	7.6	Polychromatophilic normoblasts	2.1
Band neutrophils	2.2	Orthochromic normoblasts	5.6
Segmented neutrophils	7.6	Promegaloblasts	10.2
Lymphocytes	1.0	Basophilic megaloblasts	10.0
Monocytes	2.2	Polychromatophilic megaloblasts	1.1
		Orthochromic megaloblasts	4.8

History and physical examination: The patient was a 26-year-old black female who had been in good health until about 4 weeks previously when she saw her family physician because of lightheadedness. Blood examination revealed a hemoglobin concentration of 6.2 Gm/dl. She was given an oral iron preparation but showed no improvement, the blood hemoglobin concentration a few weeks later being 4.4 Gm/dl. She then complained of recent blurring of vision.

On physical examination, neither splenomegaly nor lymphadenopathy was found. Funduscopic examination showed flame hemorrhages in both fundi.

Laboratory data: On admission to the hospital the peripheral blood showed the following: blood Hb 5.2 Gm/dl, WBC 21,000/mm³ (21 × 10⁹/l); leukocyte differential count: myeloblasts 40.1%, progranulocytes 0.4%, myelocytes 1.4%, metamyelocytes 6.8%, band neutrophils 10.1%, segmented neutrophils 14.1%, lymphocytes 10.0%, monocytes 1.0%, normoblasts 3%, and megaloblasts 14.1%; platelet count 30,000/mm³ (0.03 × 10¹²/l). Direct antiglobulin test was negative.

Discussion: The nomenclature of the variants of Di Guglielmo's syndrome is discussed in Chapter 16. The mixed erythroid and myeloblastic proliferation in this case places it in the erythroleukemia category, at least at this time. It has been pointed out that the myeloproliferative disorders do, if the patient survives for some time, show transformations quite different from the first manifestation. Characteristic of the Di Guglielmo type of erythroleukemia, and distinguishing it from acute myelocytic leukemia, is the megaloblastic proliferation in the bone marrow, the numerous nucleated red cells in the peripheral blood—these are usually megaloblastic—and the PAS positivity of the abnormal erythroid cells. In other megaloblastic proliferations, primary and secondary, the megaloblasts are PAS negative. Also, the megaloblastosis of the Di Guglielmo syndrome does not respond to vitamin B_{12}.

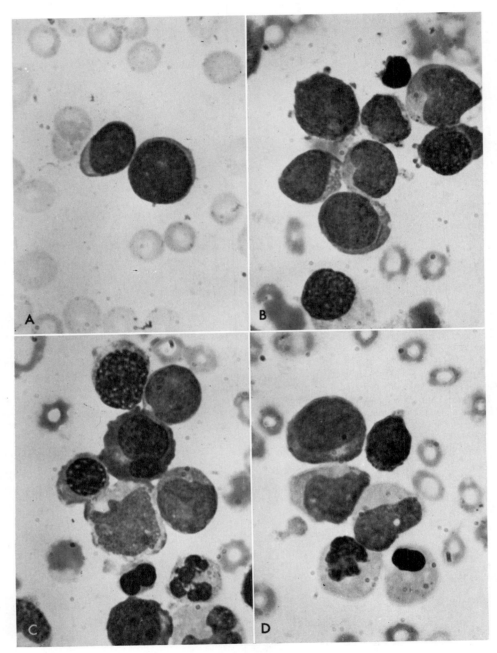

Fig. 5-63

Fig. 5-64. Case 38. Acute lymphocytic leukemia. **A** and **B,** Bone marrow smears. (Wright's stain, ×950.) **C,** Peripheral blood smear. (Wright's stain; ×950.)

Bone marrow differential count

Cell	Percent	Cell	Percent
Lymphoblasts	50.6	Band cells (total)	3.6
Prolymphocytes	28.2	Neutrophilic	3.6
Lymphocytes	14.8	Segmented (total)	2.8
		Neutrophils	2.8

History and physical examination: One month before admission this 17-year-old schoolgirl had an acute onset of fever, chills, and weakness. She became progressively weaker and complained of generalized aching. Her private physician found that she had an abnormally high leukocyte count. When admitted to the hospital, her body temperature was normal. She was pale and apprehensive but did not appear acutely ill. Examination revealed a striking splenomegaly, the edge of the spleen being 2 fingerbreadths above the iliac crest.

Laboratory data: Hb 6.0 Gm/dl of blood, RBC 2.24 million/mm³ (2.24×10^{12}/l), WBC 37,450/mm³ (37.45×10^9/l); leukocyte differential count: 56% lymphoblasts, 22% prolymphocytes, 18% lymphocytes, 2% stab neutrophils, and 2% segmented neutrophils; platelet count 70,000/mm³ (0.07×10^{12}/l).

Discussion: The peripheral blood and bone marrow showed a preponderance of lymphocytic forms, many of which were lymphoblasts and prolymphocytes. The presence of many immature lymphocytes is typical of lymphocytic leukemia.

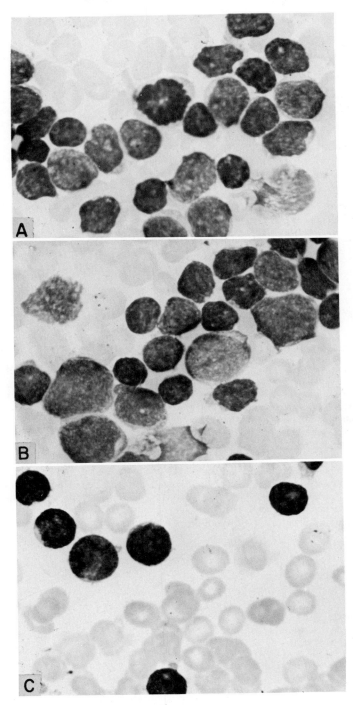

Fig. 5-64

Fig. 5-65. Case 39. Acute lymphocytic leukemia. **A** and **B,** Peripheral blood. **C** and **D,** Bone marrow. (Wright's stain; ×950.)

Bone marrow differential count

Cell	Percent	Cell	Percent
Progranulocytes	1.0	Lymphoblasts	31.2
Myelocytes	2.0	Prolymphocytes	28.8
Metamyelocytes	2.0	Lymphocytes	16.4
Segmented neutrophils	0.6	Pronormoblasts	1.0
Stabs	0.8	Polychromatophilic normoblasts	8.0
Plasma cells	0.2	Orthochromic normoblasts	6.0
Reticulum cells	3.0		

History and physical examination: The onset of this 14-year-old's illness was difficult to determine. For the previous 6 months he had been unusually listless and had done poor work in school. About 6 weeks before he was seen by his physician, he had a flulike episode of generalized aching and fever up to 101° F (38.3° C). The fever had persisted, and when it rose to 103° F (39.44° C), he was seen by the family physician.

Physical examination showed a pale, moderately obese boy. The only positive findings were moderate hepatomegaly and splenomegaly.

Laboratory data: Blood Hb 7.7 Gm/dl, RBC 2.73 million/mm³ (2.73×10^{12}/l), hematocrit 23%, WBC 9,100/mm³ (9.1×10^9/l); leukocyte differential count: lymphoblasts 60%, prolymphocytes 29%, lymphocytes 10%, and neutrophilic metamyelocytes 1%; platelet count 17,000/mm³ (0.017×10^{12}/l).

Discussion: This case presented no problem in diagnosis once peripheral blood studies were carried out. Clinically, however, the onset was insidious. The malaise of leukemia and other serious illnesses, particularly when accompanied by low-grade fever, is often thought to be caused by "flu" unless discovered to be otherwise by laboratory and physical findings.

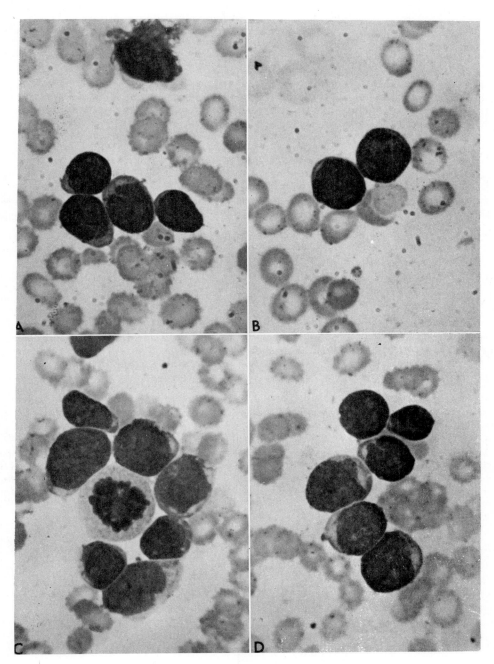

Fig. 5-65

Fig. 5-66. Case 40. Chronic lymphocytic leukemia with terminal acute exacerbation. **A** and **B,** Bone marrow smears. (Wright's stain; ×950.) **C,** Peripheral blood smear. (Wright's stain; ×950.)

Bone marrow differential count

Cell	Percent	Cell	Percent
Lymphoblasts	8.8	Band cells (total)	0.2
Prolymphocytes	33.0	Neutrophilic	0.2
Lymphocytes	56.8	Segmented (total)	1.2
		Neutrophils	0.8
		Eosinophils	0.4

History and physical examination: Seven months before admission to the hospital this 64-year-old white man had a coronary thrombosis. Routine hematologic studies at that time revealed a leukocyte count of 235,000/mm³ (235×10^9/l), with a leukocyte differential count of 99% small lymphocytes. The platelet count was normal. He recovered from the coronary thrombosis, but 1 month before admission began to complain of increasing weakness. On examination he was found to have generalized lymphadenopathy, hepatomegaly, and splenomegaly.

Laboratory data: Hb 8.4 Gm/dl of blood, RBC 2.69 million/mm³ (2.69×10^{12}/l), WBC 290,000/mm³ (290×10^9/l); leukocyte differential count: 8% lymphoblasts, 56% prolymphocytes, 34% lymphocytes, and 2% segmented neutrophils; platelet count 17,000/mm³ (0.017×10^{12}/l) (phase microscopy).

Discussion: The patient's disease was rapidly fatal, death being due to cerebral hemorrhage. It must be supposed that he had had chronic lymphocytic leukemia for at least 7 months and that the terminal episode was an acute exacerbation. Morphologically, this case shows features of both acute lymphocytic leukemia (Fig. 5-64) and chronic lymphocytic leukemia (Fig. 5-67). An acute terminal phase of chronic lymphocytic leukemia is extremely rare.

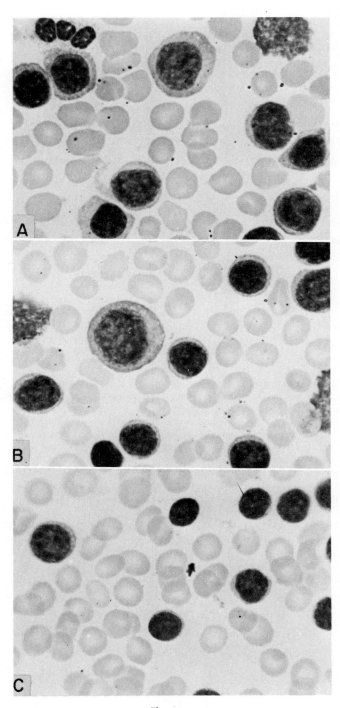

Fig. 5-66

Fig. 5-67. Case 41. Chronic lymphocytic leukemia. **A,** Bone marrow smear. (Wright's stain; ×950.) **B,** Peripheral blood smear. (Wright's stain; ×950.) **C,** Paraffin section of marrow. (Hematoxylin-eosin stain; ×450.)

Bone marrow differential count

Cell	Percent		Cell	Percent	
Progranulocytes		0.2	Segmented (total)		0.2
Myelocytes (total)		0.6	Neutrophils	0.2	
Neutrophilic	0.4		Lymphoblasts		0.2
Eosinophilic	0.2		Prolymphocytes		1.0
Metamyelocytes (total)		0.4	Lymphocytes		94.6
Neutrophilic	0.4		Basophilic normoblasts		0.8
Band cells (total)		0.8	Polychromatophilic normoblasts		1.0
Neutrophilic	0.8		Orthochromic normoblasts		0.2

History and physical examination: Three years prior to admission to the hospital this patient, a 56-year-old man, was found to have chronic lymphocytic leukemia. After receiving a course of x-ray therapy, he felt well. Three days before admission he noted a swelling in the right groin. This soon became exquisitely tender, and he developed fever. When examined, the right inguinal area was tender and contained a raised ecchymosis 4 × 8 cm in dimension. A smaller, but similar, hemorrhage was present on the inner aspect of the thigh. There were generalized lymphadenopathy, hepatomegaly, and splenomegaly.

Laboratory data: Hb 9.2 Gm/dl of blood, RBC 4.0 million/mm³ (4.0 × 10¹²/l), WBC 234,000/mm³ (234 × 10⁹/l); leukocyte differential count: 99% lymphocytes and 1% segmented neutrophils; platelet count 144,000/mm³(0.144 × 10¹²/l). Venous coagulation time was 9 minutes, and capillary bleeding time was 2.5 minutes.

Discussion: The spontaneous hemorrhages subsided after several blood transfusions, and the patient has remained asymptomatic for 7 years. The morphology of chronic lymphocytic leukemia is typical. The peripheral blood usually contains a very high proportion of small mature lymphocytes. Characteristically, there are many disintegrated or smudged cells. The same picture is seen in the bone marrow smears.

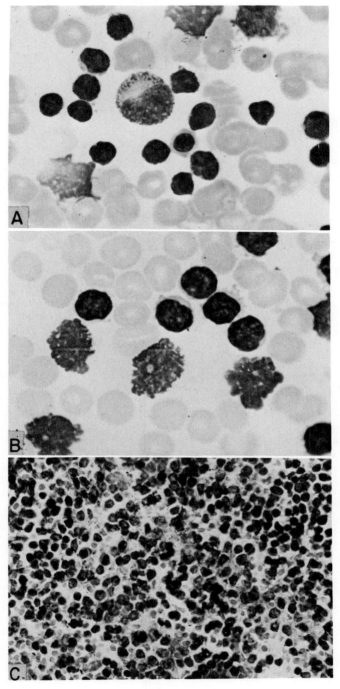

Fig. 5-67

Fig. 5-68. Case 42. Multiple myeloma. **A** and **B,** Bone marrow smears. (Wright's stain; ×950.) **C,** Paraffin section of marrow. (Hematoxylin-eosin stain; ×450.)

Bone marrow differential count

Cell	Percent		Cell	Percent
Myelocytes (total)		5.4	Lymphocytes	12.8
Neutrophilic	5.4		Monocytes	0.2
Metamyelocytes (total)		6.6	Plasmablasts	0.2
Neutrophilic	6.2		Plasmacytes	24.6
Eosinophilic	0.4		Megakaryocytes	0.2
Band cells (total)		16.2	Basophilic normoblasts	2.6
Neutrophilic	15.4		Polychromatophilic normoblasts	19.0
Eosinophilic	0.8		Orthochromic normoblasts	0.8
Segmented (total)		10.6	Reticulum cells	0.8
Neutrophils	9.0			
Eosinophils	1.6			

History and physical examination: This 58-year-old black man was first seen in the outpatient clinic. He complained of backache that had been constant for about 2 years. There was one area of tenderness over the right eighth rib. He had received a number of chiropractic treatments without benefit. When examined, there were pain and swelling in the areas over the right anterior eighth and tenth ribs, spasm of the back muscles, limitation of back motion, and tenderness over the first and second lumbar vertebrae.

Laboratory data: Hb 11.6 Gm/dl of blood, RBC 4.3 million/mm³ (4.3×10^{12}/l), WBC 7,000/mm³ (7.0×10^9/l); leukocyte differential count: 1% stab neutrophils, 55% segmented neutrophils, 37% lymphocytes, 4% eosinophils, and 3% monocytes. Erythrocytes on the peripheral blood smear showed striking rouleau formation. Total protein was 11.71 Gm/dl of serum (albumin 3.65 Gm and globulin 8.06 Gm/dl of serum). Several urine tests for Bence Jones protein were negative. Roentgenograms revealed diffuse skeletal lesions compatible with those found in multiple myeloma.

Discussion: There are several morphologic variants of multiple myeloma. The cells in this case are largely of a mature plasma cell type, with a few larger plasmablasts. In such cases the diagnosis of multiple myeloma must be supported by evidence other than that of plasmacytosis in the marrow.

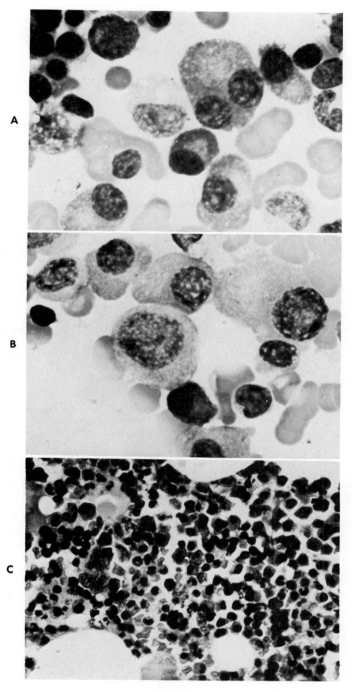

Fig. 5-68

Fig. 5-69. Case 43. Multiple myeloma, bone marrow smears. (Wright's stain; ×950.)

Bone marrow differential count

Cell	Percent		Cell	Percent
Band cells (total)		3.2	Lymphocytes	13.6
Neutrophilic	3.2		Proplasmacytes	3.4
Segmented (total)		4.0	Plasmacytes	75.6
Neutrophils	4.0		Orthochromic normoblasts	0.2

History and physical examination: This 41-year-old black woman had been in good health until 4 weeks before admission to the hospital. At this time there was a sudden onset of pain in the left shoulder and lower back. The pain was at first intermittent, but later became constant and was made worse by motion. Just before admission there were symptoms of cardiac failure. When examined, she was found to have moderate hypertension, distention of the neck veins, cardiac enlargement, and an enlarged tender liver. The spleen was palpable 2 finger-breadths below the costal margin. There was an area of extreme tenderness in the left scapula.

Laboratory data: Hb 4.2 Gm/dl of blood, RBC 1.53 million/mm³ (1.53×10^{12}/l), WBC 4,800/mm³ (4.8×10^9/l); leukocyte differential count normal; platelet count 132,000/mm³ (0.132×10^{12}/l) (phase microscopy); erythrocyte sedimentation rate 71 mm in 1 hour, corrected for the low hematocrit reading to 12 mm in 1 hour; total protein 11.82 Gm/dl of serum (albumin 2.61 Gm and globulin 9.21 Gm/dl of serum). The urine for Bence Jones protein was positive.

Discussion: In this case the laboratory findings are typical of multiple myeloma. The myeloma cells in the bone marrow are much larger than the adult type of plasma cell found in the preceding case (Fig. 5-68). Note also the huge nucleoli characteristic of these cells. The patient was also found to have a bilateral pleural effusion. It is interesting to note that this fluid, when aspirated, contained an abnormally high amount of protein, 8.36 Gm/dl.

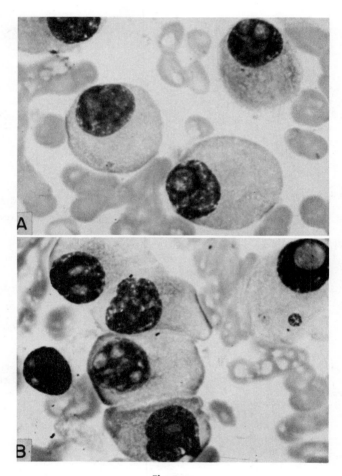

Fig. 5-69

Fig. 5-70. Case 44. Multiple myeloma. **A** and **B,** Bone marrow smears. (Wright's stain; ×950.) **C,** Paraffin section of marrow. (Hematoxylin-eosin stain; ×450.) **D,** Filter paper electrophoretic pattern of serum proteins. Note the striking increase in the β-globulin fraction.

Bone marrow differential count

Cell	Percent		Cell	Percent
Myelocytes (total)		1.2	Lymphocytes	11.6
Neutrophilic	1.2		Plasmablasts	2.0
Metamyelocytes (total)		0.8	Plasmacytes	77.0
Neutrophilic	0.8		Megakaryocytes	0.4
Band cells (total)		2.2	Polychromatophilic normoblasts	4.0
Neutrophilic	2.2			
Segmented (total)		0.8		
Neutrophils	0.4			
Eosinophils	0.4			

History and physical examination: This 79-year-old woman was admitted to the hospital with complaints of progressive weakness, dizziness, and fatigue. Physical examination revealed a pale, tired, elderly person. There were no significant findings except for signs of hypertensive cardiovascular disease.

Laboratory data: Hb 5.5 Gm/dl of blood, RBC 2.7 million/mm^3 (2.7 × 10^{12}/l), WBC 7,000/mm^3 (7.0 × 10^9/l); leukocyte differential count normal; total protein 9.19 Gm/dl of serum (albumin 1.90 Gm and globulin 7.29 Gm/dl of serum). Six different urine specimens gave negative tests for Bence Jones protein.

Discussion: An initial blood count revealed the patient's anemia, and an intensive search was made to find the etiology. A large number of tests were normal as well as roentgenograms of the chest and gastrointestinal tract. Finally, after 2 weeks of futile search, serum protein tests were ordered, and when these showed hyperglobulinemia, the bone marrow aspiration was performed.

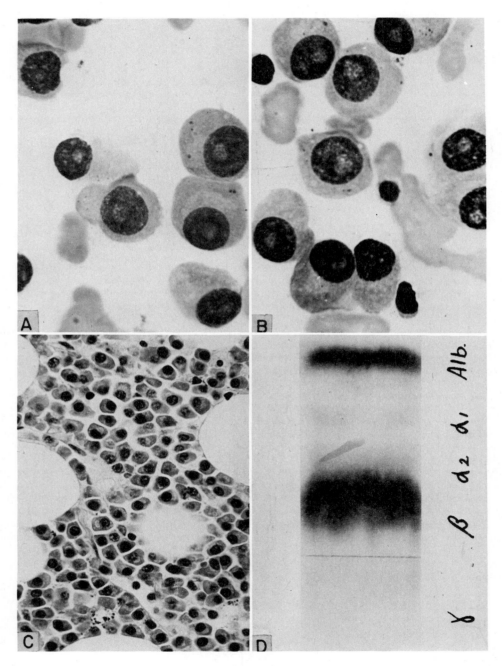

Fig. 5-70

Fig. 5-71. Case 45. Multiple myeloma with no serum protein abnormalities. **A-C,** Bone marrow. (Wright's stain; ×950.) **D,** Serum electrophoretic pattern, tracing from filter paper.

Bone marrow differential count

Cell	Percent	Cell	Percent
Myelocytes	0.5	Plasmablasts	48.0
Metamyelocytes	1.0	Proplasmacytes	12.0
Bands	4.0	Plasmacytes	11.0
Segmented	8.5	Basophilic normoblasts	0.5
Lymphocytes	10.0	Polychromatophilic normoblasts	3.5
Monocytes	2.0		

History and physical examination: On first admission to the hospital this white woman was 45 years old. She had, 5 months before, a sudden onset of back pain as the result of collapse of the eighth dorsal vertebral body. Continued pain and weight loss dictated admission to the hospital for more complete study. Physical examination was unremarkable except for tenderness when pressure was applied over the thoracic vertebrae, ribs, and sternum.

Laboratory data: Peripheral blood studies revealed Hb 12.0 Gm/dl, RBC 4.19 million/mm^3 (4.19 × 10^{12}/l), WBC 7,500/mm^3 (7.5 × 10^9/l); leukocyte differential count unremarkable; platelet count 180,000/mm^3 (0.18 × 10^{12}/l). Serum calcium 11.8 mg/dl, phosphorus 4.2 mg/dl, alkaline phosphatase 3.3 BU. Serum protein fractionation showed a total protein concentration of 6.0 Gm/dl and a normal pattern on paper electrophoresis. Urine was negative for Bence Jones protein. Roentgenographic survey of the skeleton showed compression fractures of the fourth and eighth dorsal vertebrae and radiolucent lesions in the fifth, sixth, and seventh vertebrae, in the right clavicle, posterior ribs, both ischial tuberosities, and in the cranium.

Discussion: She was given chemotherapy, steroids, and deep x-ray therapy to selected areas. At first she showed a striking response, with relief of symptoms and reversion of the bone marrow to an almost normal picture. In spite of this the skeletal disease continued to be progressive, and after the one remission there was progressive anemia, thrombocytopenia, and hypercalcemia (up to 19.0 mg/dl of serum). Repeated blood and urine studies never showed hyperproteinemia, immunoglobulinopathy, or Bence Jones proteinuria. She died about 2 years after the first symptoms.

Necropsy showed diffuse infiltration of skeletal structures with myelomatous tissue. The spleen contained diffuse deposits of eosinophilic, methyl violet–positive amyloid.

This otherwise typical case study is made unusual by the absence of the expected abnormalities in plasma protein. The number of cases is very small in which an acceptably intensive effort to detect serum or urine abnormalities was made and still uncovered no abnormalities, roughly 2% of all cases of multiple myeloma. It is reported that, as in this case, those patients having secondary amyloidosis are the ones who fail to show immunoglobulinopathy.

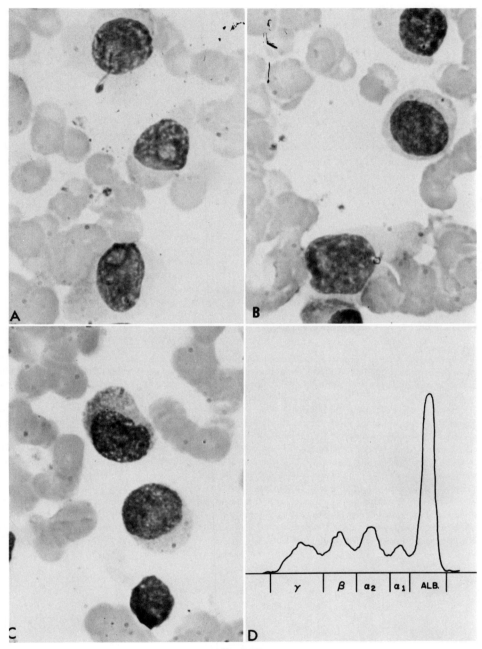

Fig. 5-71

Fig. 5-72. Case 46. Amegakaryocytosis of the bone marrow and thrombocytopenic purpura associated with lymphosarcoma. **A,** Smear from lymph node aspiration. (Wright's stain; ×450.) **B** and **C,** Smears from lymph node aspiration. (Wright's stain; ×950.) **D,** Paraffin section of lymph node. (Hematoxylin-eosin stain; ×450.)

Bone marrow differential count

Cell	Percent		Cell	Percent	
Myeloblasts		0.5	Segmented (total)		18.8
Progranulocytes		0.5	Neutrophils	18.0	
Myelocytes (total)		3.6	Eosinophils	0.8	
Neutrophilic	3.3		Lymphocytes		18.0
Eosinophilic	0.3		Monocytes		0.8
Metamyelocytes (total)		10.5	Plasmacytes		0.5
Neutrophilic	10.0		Pronormoblasts		0.2
Eosinophilic	0.5		Basophilic normoblasts		2.5
Band cells (total)		18.3	Polychromatophilic normoblasts		23.8
Neutrophilic	17.5		Orthochromic normoblasts		1.5
Eosinophilic	0.8		Reticulum cells		0.5
			(No megakaryocytes found)		

History and physical examination: The onset of this 47-year-old man's illness was 6 months prior to admission to the hospital. At that time a tooth extraction was followed by severe bleeding. Three months later bleeding began spontaneously from the same site. An osteopathic physician gave him vitamin K, but this had no effect on the bleeding. There was no previous history of abnormal bleeding, and 1 year before he had undergone cholecystectomy without difficulty. On physical examination his general condition appeared good. There was oozing of blood from the site of the tooth extraction, numerous petechiae of the skin, hemorrhages in the ocular fundi, and generalized lymphadenopathy. The liver and spleen were not enlarged.

Laboratory data: Hb 5.0 Gm/dl of blood, RBC 1.97 million/mm^3 (1.97 × 10^{12}/l), WBC 11,450/mm^3 (11.45 × 10^9/l); leukocyte differential count: 68% segmented neutrophils, 24% lymphocytes, 6% eosinophils, and 2% monocytes; platelet count 6,000/mm^3 (0.006 × 10^{12}/l) (phase microscopy). Venous coagulation time was 8 minutes. Capillary bleeding time was 24 minutes. Clot retraction was very poor.

Discussion: The bone marrow aspiration in this case yielded a normally cellular marrow, which, however, contained no megakaryocytes. The diagnosis of lymphosarcoma was confirmed by aspiration biopsy and surgical biopsy of a cervical lymph node. The patient died 13 days after admission. Necropsy revealed cerebral and other hemorrhages and a spleen weighing 300 Gm.

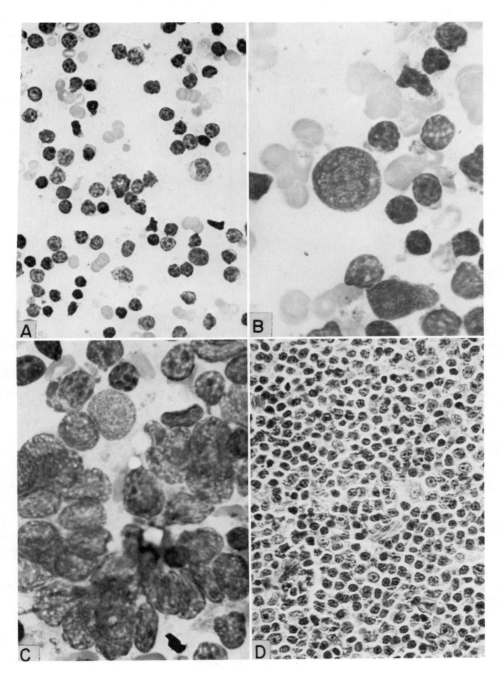

Fig. 5-72

Fig. 5-73. Case 47. Thrombocytopenic purpura associated with a mesenchymal tumor of the stomach (? Hodgkin's, ? megakaryocytoma). **A,** Bone marrow smear. (Wright's stain; ×450.) **B,** Paraffin section of bone marrow particle. (Hematoxylin-eosin stain; ×450.) **C,** Paraffin section of gastric tumor. (Hematoxylin-eosin stain; ×450.) **D,** Megakaryocytes found in bone marrow section. **E,** Giant cells from the tumor. (Hematoxylin-eosin stain; ×950.)

Bone marrow differential count

Cell		Percent	Cell	Percent
Myeloblasts		1.0	Lymphocytes	3.0
Myelocytes (total)		5.4	Plasmacytes	0.4
Neutrophilic	5.0		Megakaryoblasts	0.8
Eosinophilic	0.4		Promegakaryocytes	1.0
Metamyelocytes (total)		14.0	Megakaryocytes	3.0
Neutrophilic	14.0		Pronormoblasts	1.0
Band cells (total)		24.2	Basophilic normoblasts	4.0
Neutrophilic	24.0		Polychromatophilic normoblasts	5.0
Eosinophilic	0.2		Orthrochromic normoblasts	30.8
Segmented (total)		6.4		
Neutrophils	5.0			
Eosinophils	1.4			

History and physical examination: This 75-year-old man had been in good health until he woke one morning to find that he had a great number of skin hemorrhages. As these became more numerous, his stool became black. He was admitted to the hospital 3 days after the onset. On physical examination the skin was pale, and there were numerous petechial hemorrhages on the legs and buttocks, fewer on the trunk and arms, and only an occasional one on the face. The spleen was not palpable, and there was no lymphadenopathy.

Laboratory data: Hb 7.3 Gm/dl of blood, RBC 2.6 million/mm³ (2.6×10^{12}/l), WBC 9,500/mm³ (9.5×10^9/l); leukocyte differential count: 5% band neutrophils, 83% segmented neutrophils, 8% lymphocytes, 3% monocytes, and 1% eosinophils. Peripheral blood smear showed 2+ polychromasia, 2+ anisocytosis, poikilocytosis, hypochromia of the erythrocytes, and 1 normoblast per 100 leukocytes. Reticulocyte count was 8% and platelet count 2,000/mm³ (0.002×10^{12}/l) (phase microscopy). Capillary bleeding time was 30 minutes. Venous coagulation time was 15 minutes. Clot retraction was very poor. Total bilirubin was 1.1 mg/dl of serum.

Discussion: The bone marrow revealed a striking increase in megakaryocytes, both adult and immature, some of which presented degenerative changes. In most there was no evidence of platelet formation. These morphologic features are thought by some to be pathognomonic of immunologic (idiopathic) thrombocytopenia purpura, and the marrow was at first interpreted as compatible with this diagnosis.

In spite of the failure of ACTH and cortisone to improve the thrombocytopenia, his physician recommended that a splenectomy be performed. This was done, but there was no significant postoperative improvement in the platelet count, the highest being 21,920/mm³ (0.0219×10^{12}/l). The spleen weighed 260 Gm and was histologically normal. On the fourth postoperative day the patient bled heavily from the surgical incision, had massive hemoptyses, and died.

Necropsy revealed no accessory spleens. In the stomach, however, there were two nodules of gray tumor tissue; one was 2 cm in diameter and was located in the prepyloric area, while the other was 4 cm in diameter and was in the cardia. The lymph nodes in the gastric mesentery were firm and enlarged, and a 2 cm nodule of tumor tissue was found in the liver. Sections of the tumors, **C,** revealed a pleomorphic neoplasm characterized by giant cells that were indistinguishable from the megakaryocytes in the bone marrow. There has been no agreement on the exact pathologic classification of this tumor. The cells in the bone marrow, if they are megakaryocytes, are indistinguishable from those in the tumor, **D.**

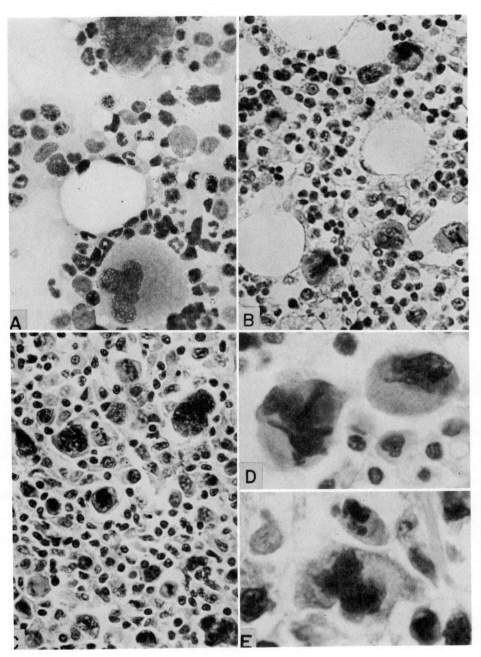

Fig. 5-73

Fig. 5-74. Case 48. Lymphoma, non-Hodgkin's, involving the bone marrow. **A,** Skin. (Hematoxylin-eosin stain; ×100.) **B,** Paraffin section of bone marrow. (Hematoxylin-eosin stain; ×100.) **C** and **D,** Bone marrow smear. (×950.) (Case submitted by Dr. R.I. Sakolsky.)

Bone marrow differential count

Cell	Percent
Lymphoblasts	83
Myelocytes	2
Progranulocytes	5
Metamyelocytes	1
Normoblasts	9

History and physical examination: This was a 22-year-old black female who had been well until 2 months before admission. At that time she noted "lumps" under the skin, first on the knees, then on the arms, and recently on the neck and abdomen. Pain in the knee, wrist, and elbow joints as well as nosebleeds was observed.

On physical examination she did not appear ill but complained of malaise. The temperature was elevated to 101° F (38.3° C). There were enlarged lymph nodes in the neck, axillae, epitrochlear areas, supraclavicular areas, and inguinal region, ranging from 1 to 2 cm in diameter, firm, and nontender. In the subcutaneous tissue of the abdominal wall there were firm nodules varying up to 1 cm in diameter and showing no discoloration of the overlying skin. The spleen was palpable 3 cm below the left costal margin.

Laboratory data: On admission the blood Hb was 12.5 Gm/dl, WBC 3,050/mm^3 (3.05 × 10^9/l); leukocyte differential count: segmented neutrophils 36%, stab neutrophils 8%, metamyelocytes 6%, lymphoblasts 7%, lymphocytes 40%, and monocytes 3%. There were 3 orthochromic normoblasts and 7 polychromatophilic normoblasts per 100 WBC. Platelet count was 120,000/mm^3 (0.12 × 10^{12}/l). Other laboratory data were within normal limits. Aspiration biopsy of the bone marrow and surgical biopsy of one of the skin nodules were interpreted as lymphoma, non-Hodgkin's type.

Discussion: Treatment with steroids, Cytoxan, and 6-MP had no effect, and the patient died about 4 months after the onset of treatment. Terminally, there was severe anemia (blood Hb 3.0 Gm/dl), and although the WBC was not abnormal (5,700/mm^3, 5.7 × 10^9/l), the peripheral blood smear showed that 95% of the leukocytes were bizarre lymphoblasts, similar to those illustrated in the bone marrow smear. When these cells are found in the peripheral blood in the terminal phase of lymphoma, they are often called leukosarcoma or lymphosarcoma cells (see also Fig. 16-19). Permission for necropsy was refused.

The lymphomatous process in this case was very aggressive and within a span of 4 months involved not only the spleen and lymph nodes but also the bone marrow and peripheral blood. Those fond of classifying disease into well-defined categories find little support from cases like this one, for indeed the distinction between the leukemias and the lymphomas often depends on how the disease presents and how carefully it is followed.

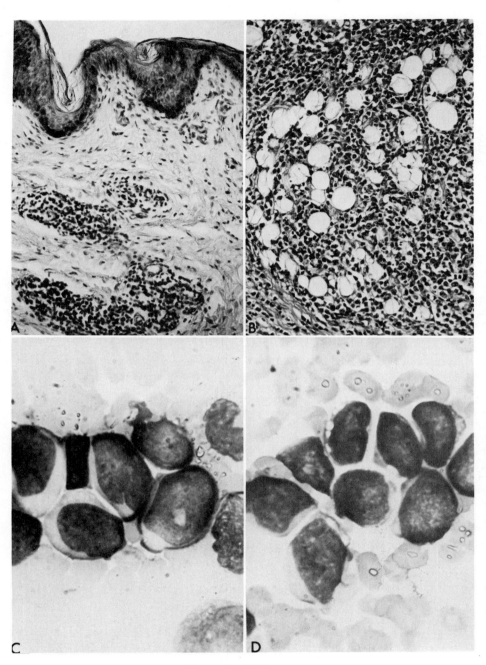

Fig. 5-74

Fig. 5-75. Case 49. Lymphoma, non-Hodgkin's, involving the bone marrow. **A** and **B,** Bone marrow smear. **C,** Peripheral blood. (Wright's stain; ×950.) **D,** Paraffin section, lymph node. (Hematoxylin-eosin stain; ×400.) (Case used by courtesy of Dr. Lowell Stone.)

Bone marrow differential count

Cell	Percent
Atypical lymphosarcoma cells	87
Myeloid cells	10
Erythroid cells	3

History and physical examination: About 10 years before the onset of the present illness, this 56-year-old white male had an episode of massive gastrointestinal bleeding, requiring many blood transfusions and ultimately an exploratory laparotomy. No cause for the bleeding was found, but he continued to have periodic gastrointestinal bleeding requiring hospitalization and blood transfusions. Recently there was a change in his condition, with acute onset of petechiae over the arms, legs, and chest. There was at the same time severe deep pain in the rib cage, sternum, and pelvis. He admitted moderate malaise for the previous year and a weight loss of 15 pounds.

On physical examination he showed generalized petechiae and severe pain on pressure over the ribs and sternum. There was cervical and axillary lymphadenopathy. The liver was down 3 cm below the right costal margin, and the spleen was 10 cm below the left costal margin. Both were firm and nontender.

Laboratory data: Blood Hb 8.1 Gm/dl, WBC 4,500/mm³ (4.5 × 10⁹/l); leukocyte differential count: segmented neutrophils 33%, stab neutrophils 8%, metamyelocytes 1%, lymphocytes 55%, and monocytes 3%. A few of the lymphocytes appeared abnormal, being large with scant cytoplasm and immature lobulated nucleus. There were also occasional normoblasts. Platelet count was 117,000/mm³ (0.117 × 10¹²/l). Roentgenograms showed no bone lesions and after barium enema, isolated diverticula. The illustrations are from marrow obtained by aspiration biopsy from the sternum and from a posterior cervical lymph node.

Discussion: Subjective bone pain is not a common symptom in leukemia or lymphoma, multiple myeloma excepted. Pain on pressure is encountered in one-half to three-fourths of cases of chronic leukemia if the entire sternum is examined. Pain on pressure over the sternum or long bones is sometimes seen in acute leukemia. Bone pain as described in the case presented here is certainly unusual in lymphosarcoma. The patient described was treated with nitrogen mustard and showed a remarkable response; within 4 days the bone pain disappeared and the spleen shrank to 2 cm below the costal margin.

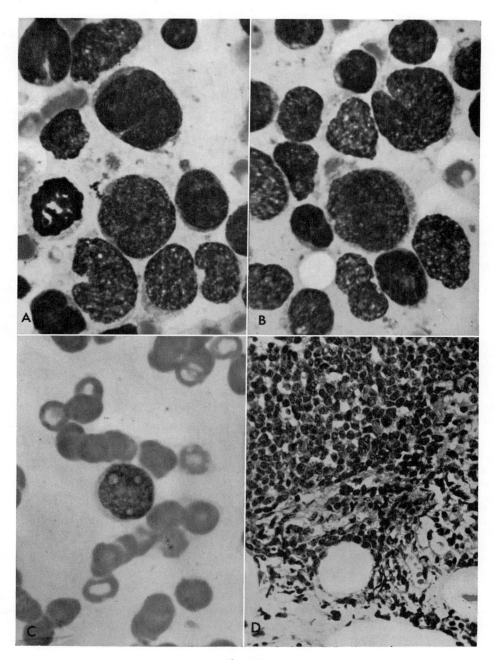

Fig. 5-75

Fig. 5-76. Case 50. Monoclonal immunoglobulinopathy associated with neoplasm (lymphoma of bone marrow). **A,** Bone marrow smear. (Wright's stain ×950.) **B,** Paper and starch gel electrophoresis of serum proteins. **C,** Immunoelectrophoretic patterns, normal control above and patient below. (Case used by courtesy of Dr. Charles Tate.)

Bone marrow differential count

Cell	Percent		Cell	Percent
Myeloblasts		3.0	Lymphocytes	23.0
Progranulocyte		1.0	Monocytes	1.0
Myelocytes (total)		10.0	Plasma cells	3.0
Metamyelocytes (total)		16.0	Pronormoblast	1.0
Neutrophilic	14.0		Basophilic normoblasts	3.0
Eosinophilic	2.0		Polychromatophilic normoblasts	9.0
Band cells (total)		17.0	Orthochromic normoblasts	11.0
Neutrophilic	16.0			
Eosinophilic	1.0			
Segmented		2.0		

History and physical examination: This 46-year-old white female had a 5-year history of recurrent bouts of pneumonitis. She had had one hemoptysis 5 years previously, but bronchoscopy revealed no abnormalities. Since then, she had numerous episodes of cough productive of thick purulent sputum, usually with fever and chest pain. In each instance, roentgenograms of the chest had shown evidence of pneumonitis, but the location varied from time to time. Response to antibiotics was generally good. The most recent admission followed a recurrence of pulmonary symptoms, with chest pain, cough productive of greenish sputum, but without fever. She was a nonsmoker.

Physical examination was not remarkable. Several observers noted the absence of lymphadenopathy and splenomegaly at that time. She was afebrile.

Laboratory data: There was extensive laboratory investigation of the problem presented by this patient, and with the exception of the serum electrophoretic studies and the bone marrow findings, it can be assumed that the results of various cultures, agglutinations, and blood chemical studies were not helpful. Bronchoscopy was done, and the findings, gross, cultural, and cytologic, were normal.

The peripheral blood showed the following: Hb 13.1 Gm/dl, hematocrit 40%, WBC 5,900/mm³ (5.9 × 10⁹/l); leukocyte differential count: segmented neutrophils 42%, stab neutrophils 14%, lymphocytes 40%, and monocytes 4%.

Electrophoresis of serum showed the total protein concentration to be 7.7 Gm/dl. There was a sharp peak in the gamma area, and partition of fractions was as follows: albumin 3.54 Gm, α_1-globulin 0.33 Gm, α_2-globulin 0.66 Gm, β-globulin 0.78 Gm, γ-globulin 2.39 Gm. Starch gel and immunoelectrophoretic findings are given in the discussion. Urine samples were repeatedly negative for protein.

Because of the monoclonal peak, aspiration biopsy of sternal marrow was carried out. There was noted the presence of atypical lymphoid cells, both single and in clumps. The diagnosis was lymphomatous infiltration of the bone marrow. Aspiration biopsy and electrophoretic studies were repeated 3 months later, and the previously noted abnormalities were confirmed. At this time there was splenomegaly, 3 cm below the costal margin for the first time.

Discussion: The abnormal globulin component was found to resolve into several bands on starch gel. By immunoelectrophoresis it was found to be of the γ-G type. This case is a good example of the importance of modern methods for the study of proteins. It emphasizes the point recently made by several authors that immunoglobulinopathy is not as pathognomonic of multiple myeloma as it was once thought. We have encountered it several times in lymphomas particularly. A discussion of the immunoglobulinopathies is presented in Chapter 16.

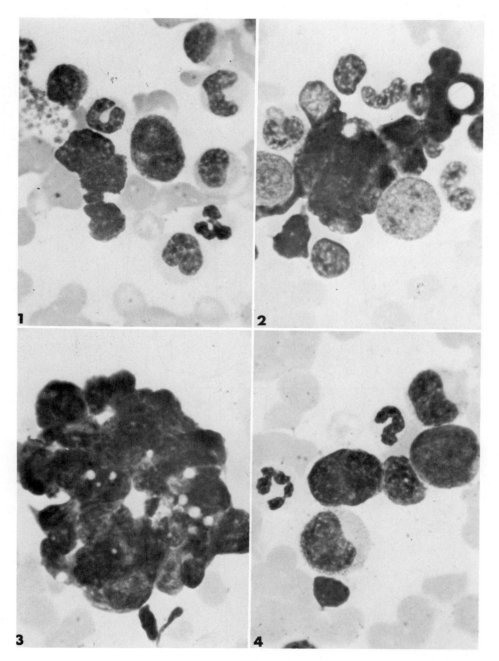

Fig. 5-76   *Continued.*

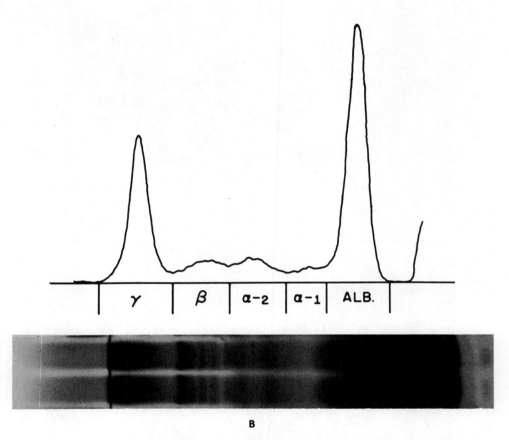

B

Fig. 5-76, cont'd. For legend see p. 332.

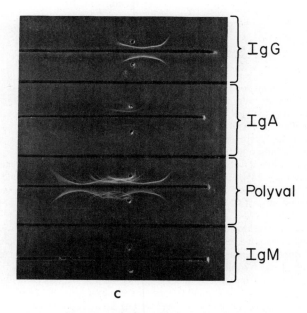

c

Fig. 5-76, cont'd. For legend see p. 332.

Fig. 5-77. Case 51. Hodgkin's disease, disseminated, involving the bone marrow, bone marrow smears. (Wright's stain; ×950.)

Bone marrow differential count

Cell	Percent		Cell	Percent	
Myeloblasts		1.1	Segmented (total)		25.8
Progranulocytes		0.5	Neutrophils	24.0	
Myelocytes		11.0	Eosinophils	1.8	
Metamyelocytes (total)		14.0	Lymphocytes		7.1
Neutrophilic	11.0		Pronormoblasts		2.5
Eosinophilic	3.0		Basophilic normoblasts		4.5
Band cells (total)		21.0	Polychromatophilic normoblasts		4.8
Neutrophilic	19.0		Orthochromic normoblasts		2.7
Eosinophilic	2.0		Reticulum cells		5.0

Many mature and immature Reed-Sternberg cells present

History and physical examination: The diagnosis of Hodgkin's disease had been established 12 years previously in this 36-year-old white male. He had been well controlled by x-ray therapy to lymph nodes as they became enlarged, but during the year before this final admission there were bouts of fever, weight loss, and malaise. Three weeks before admission there was onset of jaundice and peripheral edema. Physical examination showed that he was jaundiced, febrile, and acutely ill. There were marked hepatomegaly and splenomegaly, ascites, and pitting edema, but no lymphadenopathy.

Laboratory data: There were at first moderate anemia and normal leukocyte, differential, and platelet counts. The total serum bilirubin was 4.2 mg/dl, with 3.6 mg/dl in the direct reacting fraction, and this and other findings pointed to the jaundice being of the obstructive type. However, there soon developed a severe anemia thought to be of the hemolytic type because of decreased erythrocyte survival (half-life of 7.5 days). The direct antiglobulin test was negative.

Discussion: He was treated with prednisone, nitrogen mustard, and later Valban, as well as numerous blood transfusions. He seemed to improve for a short time, but the chemotherapy was complicated by a severe leukopenia and thrombocytopenia. Terminally he developed a *Staphylococcus aureus* bacteremia. Necropsy confirmed involvement with Hodgkin's infiltrate of the spleen, liver, and lymph nodes.

This case does not present a problem in diagnosis, since the patient was known to have had Hodgkin's disease for the previous 12 years. It is presented because the involvement of the bone marrow is striking. Reed-Sternberg cells in the bone marrow are as characteristic as they are in tissue sections. In fact, I believe that these are subtle changes, in the form of atypical reticulum cells, sometimes seen more easily in bone marrow smears than in paraffin sections.

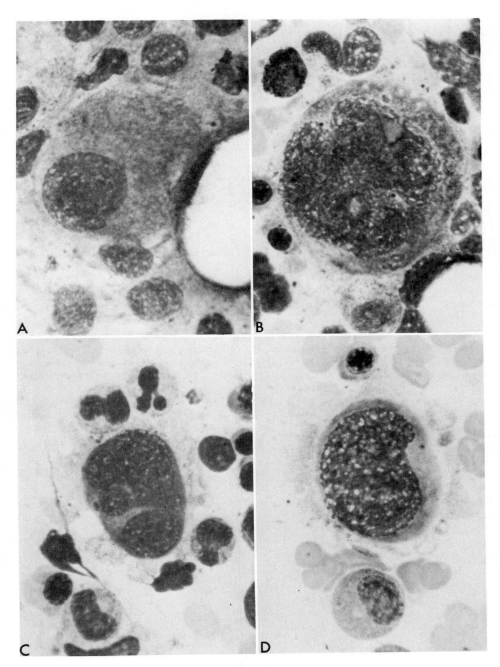

Fig. 5-77

Fig. 5-78. Case 52. Bronchogenic carcinoma metastatic to the bone marrow, bone marrow smears. (Wright's stain; ×950.)

Bone marrow differential count

Cell	Percent		Cell	Percent	
Myeloblasts		1.6	Segmented (total)		11.6
Progranulocytes		0.4	Neutrophils	10.8	
Myelocytes (total)		11.2	Eosinophils	0.8	
Neutrophilic	11.2		Lymphocytes		10.0
Metamyelocytes (total		15.6	Plasmacytes		0.4
Neutrophilic	15.2		Basophilic normoblasts		4.0
Basophilic	0.4		Polychromatophilic normoblasts		3.6
Band cells (total)		27.6	Orthochromic normoblasts		8.8
Neutrophilic	27.2		Unidentified		5.2
Eosinophilic	0.4				

History and physical examination: This 71-year-old man was admitted to the hospital with a presumptive diagnosis of pulmonary tuberculosis. He had complained of increasing weakness, anorexia, weight loss, and occasional hemoptysis and night sweats. He was pale and poorly nourished. The left chest showed dullness to percussion, tubular breathing, and coarse rales. Roentgenograms revealed almost complete consolidation of the left lung.

Laboratory data: Hb 9.2 Gm/dl of blood, RBC 3.4 million/mm³ (3.4×10^{12}/l), WBC 19,200/mm³ (19.2×10^9/l); leukocyte differential count: 26% band neutrophils, 58% segmented neutrophils, 9% lymphocytes, and 7% monocytes. Peripheral blood smear showed 2 normoblasts per 100 leukocytes and occasional macrocytic erythrocytes.

Discussion: No acid-fast bacilli were found in specimens of sputum and gastric lavage. The bone marrow aspiration was done to obtain material for culture, but routine smears revealed the presence of tumor cells. The patient died 2 weeks later, and necropsy confirmed the diagnosis of bronchogenic caricinoma of the left lung.

One other point of interest is presented by this case, and that is the missed significance of the peripheral blood findings. We have noted, as have others, that bone marrow invasion by neoplasms often results in the presence of macrocytic erythrocytes and normoblasts in the peripheral blood. Miliary tuberculous involvement of the bone marrow might give rise to the same findings, but in either case a bone marrow aspiration is strongly indicated when such a peripheral blood picture is encountered.

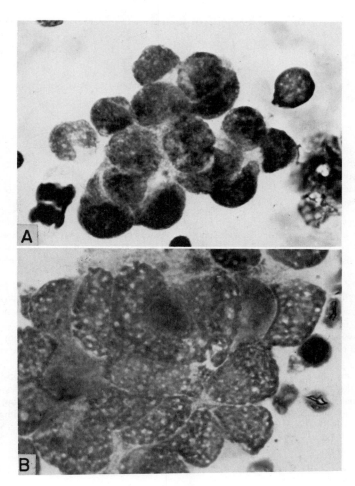

Fig. 5-78

Fig. 5-79. Case 53. Metastatic tumor to bone marrow (carcinoma of prostate). **A-C,** Bone marrow smear. (×950.) **D,** Prostate. (Hematoxylin-eosin stain; ×66.)

Bone marrow differential count

Cell	Percent	Cell	Percent
Myeloblasts	1.0	Segmented	13.6
Progranulocytes	3.0	Lymphocytes	9.2
Myelocytes	8.9	Monocytes	1.0
Metamyelocytes	12.0	Plasmablasts	0.6
Band cells	18.9	Normoblasts	30.7

History and physical examination: This was a 69-year-old white male. One year before this admission he had a surgical repair of a ruptured abdominal aneurysm. Recovery was uneventful, and the peripheral blood picture was then normal. The present admission was for the purpose of evaluating a leukopenia and thrombocytopenia discovered in the course of routine follow-up. He had been feeling well, and physical examination revealed nothing of note.

Laboratory data: The peripheral blood showed the Hb concentration to be 14.4 Gm/dl, hematocrit 45%, WBC 2,650/mm³ (2.65 × 10⁹/l), and the platelet count 21,000/mm³ (0.021 × 10¹²/l). The leukocyte differential count showed segmented neutrophils 28%, band neutrophils 5%, metamyelocytes 1%, monocytes 4%, and lymphocytes 62%. Erythrocytes were morphologically normal.

Discussion: Two samples of marrow were obtained, one from the sternum and one from the ilium. Both revealed clumps of tumor cells. When this finding was reported, an intensive search for the primary site was instituted.

For the next 6 months he remained asymptomatic, but a second marrow aspiration biopsy again showed clumps of abnormal cells interpreted as metastatic. There was at no time evidence of a primary tumor. About 6 months after the first marrow biopsy he died rather suddenly with cardiac failure. At necropsy there was no obvious primary tumor, and routine sections did not show tumor either. However, on resectioning prostatic tissue a small nodule of carcinoma was found, **D.**

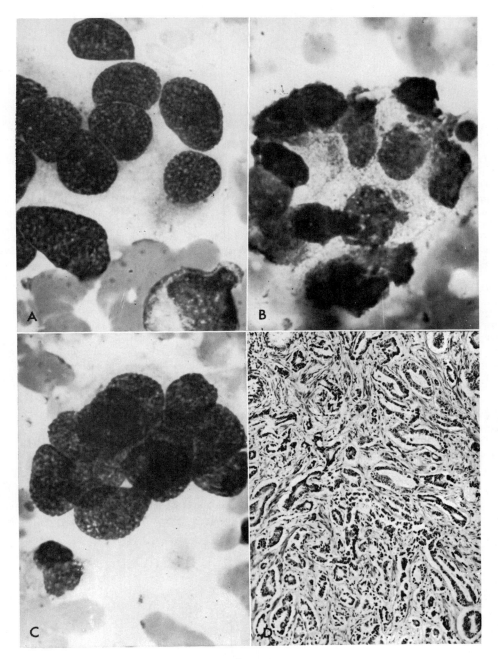

Fig. 5-79

Fig. 5-80. Case 54. Normoblastosis of peripheral blood associated with carcinoma metastatic to bone marrow. **A-C,** Peripheral blood. (Wright's stain; ×950.) **D,** Peripheral blood. (Wright's stain; ×100.)

History and physical examination: This 60-year-old woman had radical breast surgery 2 years previously for carcinoma of the breast, metastatic to axillary lymph nodes. Subsequently she developed evidence of metastases to the pelvis, hips, and cervical nodes. She was admitted because of fever and inability to take food and fluids.

On physical examination she was chronically ill and febrile (100° F, 37.78° C). Positive findings were as follows: dehydration, exophthalmos of right eye, liver enlarged 3 fingerbreadths below the costal margin, and nodular, cervical nodes enlarged and hard bilaterally, enlarged nodes in axillae and groin. There was no icterus.

Laboratory data: The peripheral blood picture and the bone marrow findings are pertinent to this presentation. On admission the peripheral blood showed the following: Hb 10.0 Gm/dl, hematocrit 32%, WBC 58,200 (58.2 × 10⁹/l), corrected to 4,127/mm³ (4.127 × 10⁹/l), nucleated red cells 1,310/100 WBC; leukocyte differential count: segmented neutrophils 41%, stab neutrophils 17%, metamyelocytes 8%, myelocytes 6%, lymphocytes 22%, monocytes 1%, eosinophils 3%, and basophils 2%; platelets appeared decreased. There was moderate basophilic stippling, polychromasia, and 4+ anisocytosis. Reticulocyte count was 4.9%. Total serum bilirubin concentration was 1.9 mg/dl. Aspiration biopsy of the bone marrow showed metastatic tumor.

It is interesting that 1 month previously there was only moderate normoblastosis of the peripheral blood, the WBC being 5,900/mm³ (5.9 × 10⁹/l), corrected to 4,250/mm³ (4.25 × 10⁹/l) with 38 nucleated RBC/100 WBC.

Discussion: The patient's course was rapidly downhill, and she died 10 days after admission. The terminal events were localized and then generalized convulsions, supposedly from brain metastases, and terminal pneumonia occurred. Permission for necropsy was refused, so the extent of bone marrow involvement is not known. Judging, however, from the clinical and roentgenographic signs during life, it can be assumed that it was extensive.

The degree of normoblastosis in the peripheral blood is extreme and resembles that seen in isoimmune hemolytic disease of the newborn. While hemolytic disease is not completely ruled out in the case presented here, it must be assumed that it is not present, since there was no icterus and the serum bilirubin concentration was not significantly elevated. If this is so, then the reaction is of the leukemoid type associated with the invasion of the bone marrow by carcinomatous tissue.

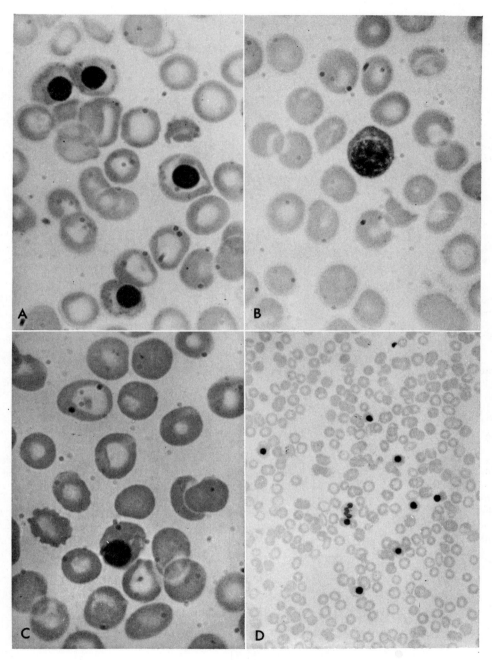

Fig. 5-80

Fig. 5-81. Case 55. Neuroblastoma metastatic to the bone marrow, bone marrow smears. (Wright's stain; ×950.)

Bone marrow differential count

Cell	Percent		Cell	Percent
Myeloblasts		2.6	Segmented (total)	6.4
Progranulocytes		2.8	Neutrophils	5.4	
Myelocytes (total)		8.0	Eosinophils	1.0	
Neutrophilic	7.0		Lymphocytes	26.2
Eosinophilic	1.0		Monocytes	0.6
Metamyelocytes (total)		9.4	Plasmacytes	0.6
Neutrophilic	8.0		Pronormoblasts	2.0
Eosinophilic	1.4		Basophilic normoblasts	9.6
Band cells (total)		13.0	Polychromatophilic normoblasts	8.2
Neutrophilic	12.0		Orthochromic normoblasts	2.2
Eosinophilic	1.0		Tumor cells	8.4

History and physical examination: This 4-year-old girl was taken to a pediatrician because the mother thought the child was pale. When a blood count revealed an Hb of 5 Gm/dl of blood and an RBC of 2.29 million/mm³ (2.29×10^{12}/l), she was admitted to the hospital for further studies. On physical examination the only positive finding was diffuse slight lymphadenopathy.

Laboratory data: Hb 5.2 Gm/dl of blood, RBC 2.08 million/mm³ (2.08×10^{12}/l), WBC 8,600/mm³ (8.6×10^9/l); leukocyte differential count normal. On peripheral blood smear the erythrocytes showed 1+ hypochromia, and there were 4 normoblasts per 100 leukocytes. Platelet count was 327,000/mm³ (0.327×10^{12}/l).

Discussion: Bone marrow aspiration from a spinous process was done in the investigation of the anemia. It revealed typical neuroblastoma cells as illustrated. Later, a roentgenographic survey of the skeleton revealed diffuse destructive changes. The primary tumor was localized in the left adrenal. The diagnosis of neuroblastoma is not difficult when pseudorosettes are found, but the identification of single neuroblastoma cells is often difficult. The single cells resemble immature blast forms and may be mistaken for lymphoblasts or myeloblasts. It may be helpful to remember that neuroblastoma cells have a highly fragile nuclear membrane, so that the cytoplasm may be indistinct or the smear may present many naked nuclei. Such cells are found occasionally in peripheral blood.

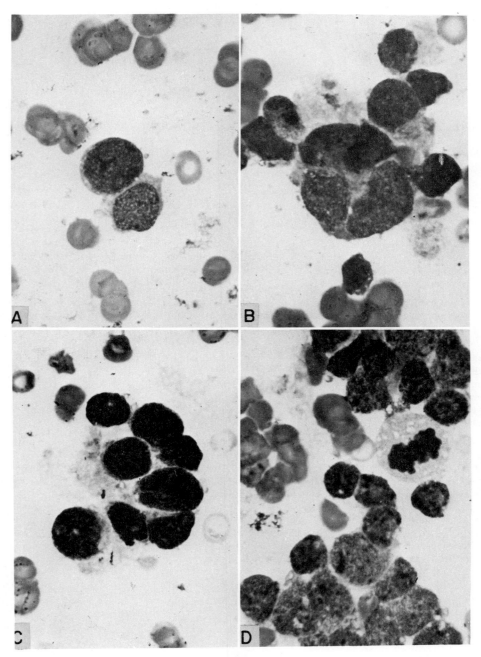

Fig. 5-81

Fig. 5-82. Case 56. Infectious mononucleosis. **A** and **B,** Peripheral blood smears. (Wright's stain; ×1,450.) **C,** Bone marrow smear. (Wright's stain; ×1,450.) **D,** Paraffin section of marrow. (Hematoxylin-eosin stain; ×200.)

Bone marrow differential count

Cell	Percent	Cell	Percent
Myeloblasts	0.8	Monocytes	1.6
Progranulocytes	1.0	Plasmacytes	1.4
Myelocytes	2.4	Pronormoblasts	0.8
Metamyelocytes	2.6	Basophilic normoblasts	3.0
Band cells	18.2	Polychromatophilic normoblasts	11.0
Segmented cells	4.2	Orthochromic normoblasts	13.0
Lymphocytes	40.0		

History and physical examination: This 18-year-old male, a college student, became ill while in school. Onset was moderately acute and characterized by fever and sore throat. There was cervical lymphadenopathy but no splenomegaly.

Laboratory data:

Day of illness	Heterophil titer	WBC	Seg.	Stab	Lymph	Mon.	Eos.	Baso.
Third	1:7	5,500	57	12	28	3	—	—
Seventh	—	8,700	32	16	44	3	5	—
Eleventh	1:28	14,000	13	10	70	5	2	—
Twelfth	1:56	18,000	6	7	84	1	0	1

On the thirteenth day of his illness the following data were obtained: Hb 14.5 Gm/dl of blood, hematocrit 48%, RBC 5.52 million/mm^3 (5.52 × 10^{12}/l), WBC 20,500/mm^3 (20.5 × 10^9/l); leukocyte differential count: 14% segmented neutrophils, 5% stab neutrophils, 79% lymphocytes, and 2% monocytes. Almost all lymphocytes were of the virocyte type. Platelet count was 212,000/mm^3 (0.212 × 10^{12}/l); heterophil titer 1:112, not absorbed by guinea pig kidney (titer 1:112) and completely absorbed by beef erythrocytes (titer 0).

Discussion: A complete study was done in this case because of the referring physician's concern over the rise in leukocyte count, the lymphocytosis, and the lymphadenopathy in the presence of a low heterophil titer. Actually the results of the differential absorption study were diagnostic of infectious mononucleosis. I suspect that a diagnostic pattern would have been seen when the screening titer was even lower. The lymphocytosis in the bone marrow is striking, the cells exhibiting the same morphology as those in the peripheral blood.

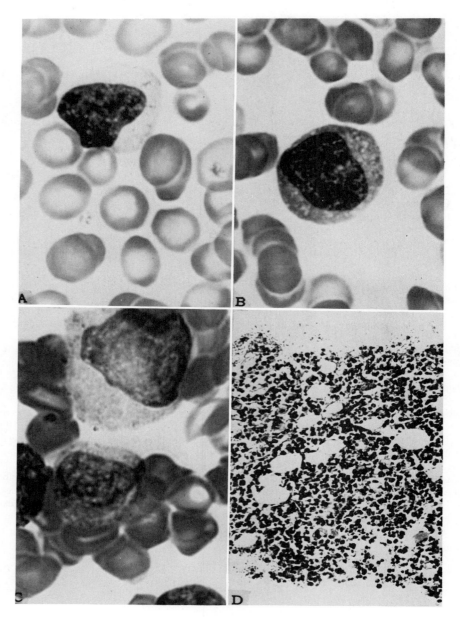

Fig. 5-82

Fig. 5-83. Case 57. Miliary tuberculosis involving the bone marrow. **A,** Bone marrow. (Hematoxylin-eosin stain; ×120.) **B** and **C,** Liver. (Hematoxylin-eosin stain; ×120.)

Bone marrow differential count

Cell	Percent	Cell	Percent
Blasts	1.5	Lymphocytes	2.0
Progranulocytes	4.5	Plasmacytes	2.0
Myelocytes	5.0	Pronormoblasts	3.0
Metamyelocytes	9.5	Basophilic normoblasts	9.0
Bands	8.0	Polychromatophilic normoblasts	36.0
Segmented	6.0	Orthochromic normoblasts	11.0
		Reticulum cells	2.5

History and physical examination: A 77-year-old retired coal miner was brought to the hospital by the police because he was unable to care for himself. He had been well up to 6 months previously, at which time he began to feel tired, weak, and noted low backache and pain in his legs. He felt better when in bed and had therefore remained in bed except for going to the bathroom. For 2 months before admission he had eaten practically no solid food. One week before admission he noted, for the first time, a dry barking cough.

Physical examination showed a febrile, acutely ill, emaciated man. BP was 100/60; temperature was 102° F (38.89° C). Positive findings were bilateral induration of the epididymis, dry crackling rales in both lung fields, and choroidal tubercles on ophthalmoscopic examination.

Laboratory data: Blood Hb 11.2 Gm/dl, hematocrit 36.5%, WBC 4,600/mm³ (4.6 × 10⁹/l); leukocyte differential count: segmented neutrophils 70%, stab neutrophils 18%, lymphocytes 10%, and monocytes 2%. Urinalysis showed 15 to 25 WBC/hpf and many bacteria, which on culture were shown to be *Escherichia coli*. Sputum, gastric washings, and urine were positive for *Mycobacterium tuberculosis*. Roentgenograms of the chest showed bilateral miliary lesions with some confluence of densities suggestive of silicotuberculosis. Bone marrow tissue obtained by aspiration biopsy from the sternum showed granulomatous lesions, as did the tissue from a liver biopsy.

Discussion: While the diagnosis of disseminated infection with *Mycobacterium tuberculosis* was easily established in this case, there are many reports attesting to the value of bone marrow biopsy when the disease is not otherwise apparent. In some instances, granulomatous involvement of the bone marrow presents as an anemia, leukopenia, thrombocytopenia, or even as a leukemoid reaction. In this case the marrow showed a moderate decrease in the myeloid series. The granulomatous lesions are shown in the illustration.

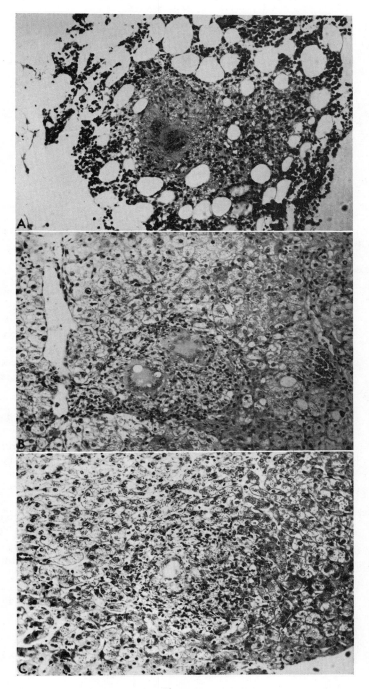

Fig. 5-83

The blood

INTRODUCTION
THE BLOOD
  Embryonic development
  Composition of blood
  Changes in drawn blood
RHEOLOGY AND VISCOSITY OF BLOOD
SEDIMENTATION RATE
  Factors that affect sedimentation rate
    Aggregation of erythrocytes
    Effect of changes in plasma composition
    Number of erythrocytes
      Corrections for anemia
    Size of erythrocytes
    Number of leukocytes
    Caliber and length of tube
    Position of tube
    Anticoagulant used
    Effect of temperature
    Effect of delay in performing test
  Clinical correlation
HEMATOCRIT
  Definitions
  Conditions of centrifugation
  Amount of trapped plasma
  Use of hematocrit data
  Microhematocrit methods
  Calculated hematocrit (Coulter S and Hemac apparatus)
  Normal values
  Clinical correlation
  Distribution of blood cells on centrifugation
BLOOD VOLUME, PLASMA VOLUME, AND ERYTHROCYTE MASS
  Clinical correlation
  Methods
  Normal values

INTRODUCTION

Because of its dramatic importance to life and ready accessibility, blood has occupied the attention of scientists for hundreds of years. Their observations were at first crude and their interpretations were somewhat colored by folklore. Eventually developments in the fields of biochemistry, immunology, enzymology, and morphologic hematology revealed the infinite complexity of blood. It also came to be appreciated that many disease states produce typical changes in the composition of blood. Some of these changes affect the blood cells, others the chemical composition of the plasma, and still others the gross properties of blood as a fluid. Those measurements of blood as a whole that are most useful in clinical medicine are described in this chapter.

THE BLOOD
Embryonic development

The establishment of blood as a distinct somatic component occurs early in embryonic life. By the end of the first month of embryonic development, primitive endothelium-lined vascular spaces are well defined. At this time blood is static and consists of primitive erythroblasts suspended in plasma derived from extravascular spaces. Later, circulation is established. Blood then becomes a circulating fluid that will flow in the vascular system throughout life.

Composition of blood

Any single measurement of cellular and noncellular blood components represents only a momentary glimpse of an ever-changing state. It is well to emphasize this dynamic state, for one observation does not necessarily define the situation as it was a few hours before or will be a few hours hence. Some equilibriums shift rapidly and others slowly.

Circulating blood consists of formed elements suspended in fluid. The formed elements are *blood cells* (erythrocytes, leukocytes, and platelets). The fluid is *native plasma*, a highly complex liquid whose composition is determined by equilibriums between it and the extravascular fluid.

Changes in drawn blood

Although there have been some observations of blood within the intact vascular system (Knisley, 1960), most studies are perforce done on blood removed from its normal habitat. Significant changes are known to take place, and there may be others that we do not yet appreciate.

In the first place, unless an anticoagulant is added, normal blood withdrawn from the circulation inevitably gels and forms a clot. This deceptively simple physical change is caused by the polymerization of the plasma protein *fibrinogen* into *fibrin*. When whole blood coagulates, the formed elements are trapped in the fibrin network. On standing, the clot retracts, expressing a fluid, *serum,* which differs from plasma chiefly in that it contains no fibrinogen. Other known differences between plasma and serum concern changes that take place in the blood clotting factors. Blood coagulation may be inhibited by the addition of various anticoagulant substances, and *plasma* may then be obtained by centrifugation or sedimentation. This plasma differs from native plasma in that it contains an anticoagulant.

Both plasma and serum undergo changes on standing. If they remain in contact with erythrocytes, there is a constant shift of electrolytes between fluid and cells, accompanied by a rise in pH because of loss of carbon dioxide into the atmosphere. Plasma and serum standing in an uncapped tube will also have a shift of the pH to the alkaline side. Ionic shifts may be so great as to invalidate certain chemical determinations. Other changes that take place are a result of the inherent chemical or physical instability of substances such as glucose, the enzymes, etc., and they vary in proportion to the time elapsed and the storage temperature.

RHEOLOGY AND VISCOSITY OF BLOOD

Rheology is the science dealing with the behavior of flowing liquids. The behavior of blood as it flows through normal and sometimes abnormal blood vessels has received some attention. Considering the importance of understanding the factors involved in vivo, however, the subject has been only superficially explored. There are recorded observations of the behavior of blood flowing through vessels in vivo, notably Knisley's (1960) work on *sludging,* but blood is generally studied in vitro and the observations extrapolated, with sometimes questionable justification, to its abnormalities in vivo. It seems obvious that more attention should be paid to in vivo phenomena.

The study of blood flow through vessels has more recently been called "hemorheology," defined as the study of the flow of blood and its relation to the vessel in which it is contained, particularly the vessel wall. From a modest experiment in flow dynamics, the science of hemorheology has assumed increasing importance. It involves not only the question of blood viscosity (discussed briefly in this section) but also fundamental liquid-surface interface reactions that regulate normal hemostasis and that are involved in thrombus formation in pathologic circumstances.

The student interested in this newly developing science is referred to the *Proceedings of the First International Conference on Hemorheology,* edited by Copley (1968), and to the *Conference on Moving Blood* (Varco, 1971).

As a flowing liquid, blood is considered a suspension of particles (erythrocytes, leukocytes, and platelets) in a newtonian solution, the native plasma. A newtonian solution is one that, flowing through a cylindric tube, obeys Poiseuille's law:

$$\text{Volume rate of flow} = \frac{\pi \, PR^4}{8 \, \eta}$$

where

P = Pressure gradient per unit tube length
R = Tube radius
η = Newtonian coefficient of viscosity

For a newtonian fluid, the pressure-flow plot is a straight line passing through the origin, and the coefficient of viscosity at a given constant temperature is inversely proportional to the slope of the pressure-flow line.

Whole blood, however, has a nonlinear pressure-flow relationship and, as a result, does not possess a unique newtonian coefficient of viscosity. The nonlinearity is induced by the presence of suspended cells, the effect being related primarily to the number and properties of the erythrocytes. Furthermore, the flow of blood in vivo is along very different gradients of pressure (from about 130 mm Hg in the large arteries to 5 mm Hg in the veins) and along vessels of varying diameter (from 2.5 cm to 8 μ). Two additional factors complicate the physical definition of the behavior of flowing blood: (1) the flow induced by cardiac systole is pulsatile and (2) the vessels are elastic rather than rigid (Rubinow and Keller, 1972). A discussion of the fluid characteristics of blood flow in capillaries is presented by Lin et al (1973).

Theoretically, other expressions of the viscosity of whole blood can be derived from in vitro data (Haynes, 1960, 1962). Practically, however, the measurement of viscosity is limited to determining "relative viscosity" or "apparent viscosity." This is defined as the ratio of the volumes of water and blood that flow under standard conditions of temperature and pressure per unit time. Instruments, such as the Ostwald Viscometer, designed to measure relative viscosity are commercially available.

It should be obvious that in vitro measurement of relative viscosity is far removed from the physiology of blood in the vascular tree. Nevertheless, some interesting data are available and may be summarized as follows:

1. The relationship between relative viscosity of blood and hematocrit is nearly linear for hematocrit values below 40%. Above 40% the relative viscosity becomes progressively greater.
2. The relative viscosity of blood is affected by the size of the erythrocytes. At a given level of erythrocyte count, microcytosis decreases and macrocytosis increases the relative viscosity.
3. The relative viscosity seems directly proportional to erythrocyte mass (Strumia and Phillips, 1963).
4. Relative viscosity is also affected by the protein composition of the plasma. For example, Jasin et al (1970) present two rheumatoid arthritis patients with "hyperviscosity syndrome" (HVS) characterized by hyperproteinemia and an increased concentration of IgG complexes. Tuddenham et al (1974a) report four cases of IgA myeloma with increased plasma and whole blood viscosity and the hyperviscosity syndrome. They recommend plasmapheresis for patients with HVS to improve the symptoms of the syndrome.
5. The average plasma viscosity of joggers is 9% lower than that of nonjoggers (Charm et al, 1979).
6. The relationship of increased blood viscosity to cardiovascular, hypertensive, and renal disease is discussed by Dintenfass (1977a, 1977b) and Dintenfass and Davis (1977).

SEDIMENTATION RATE

If blood is drawn and mixed with an anticoagulant so that it remains fluid, the erythrocytes will gradually settle to the bottom of the container. In most normal persons, sedimentation takes place slowly, but in a variety of disease states the rate is rapid and in some cases proportional to the severity of the disease. Measurement of the sedimentation rate has become a helpful laboratory test in diagnosing occult disease or confirming and following the course of manifest disease. The sedimentation rate is expressed as the distance (in millimeters) that erythrocytes fall per unit of time (usually 1 hour, although interval measurements show that the rate of sedimentation is not constant throughout the 1-hour period) (Puccini et al, 1977).

The erythrocyte sedimentation rate (ESR) was adopted by modern medicine in 1918 when Fåhraeus published his observations on the ESR in pregnancy. He at first proposed it as a test for pregnancy, but in 1921 he wrote a more detailed report in which the phenomenon was related to many factors other than pregnancy (historical background given by Jorpes, 1969). Historically, the sedimentation of drawn blood was one of the principles on which ancient Greek medicine was based. The ancients held that by observing blood drawn by venesection certain "humours" of the body could be distinguished. They noted that some bloods sedimented quickly, so that a slowly forming clot produced a whitish, mucoid "crust" on the surface, the "crusta inflammatoria" or "crusta phlogistica." For over 2,000 years the "phlegm" that formed the "crust" was considered a "humour" responsible for disease, the remedy for which was repeated venesection. Blood let by the ancient technic of venesection did, of course, clot, so that the actual sedimentation of erythrocytes was not measured; the mass of red cells at the bottom of the clot was called the "black gall." (See also the discussion of the history of blood transfusion on p. 524.)

Factors that affect sedimentation rate

Investigation into the mechanism concerned in the sedimentation of erythrocytes has revealed a complex interplay of several factors, some of theoretical interest only and others having practical implications. While these factors are discussed individually, we must remember that they act together to produce the observed sedimentation rate.

In general the sedimentation rate is affected by properties of the erythrocytes, by properties of the plasma, and by mechanical or technical factors.

Aggregation of erythrocytes

The spontaneous sedimentation velocity of a single *spherical* body falling freely through a simple fluid may be expressed by the Stokes equation as follows:

$$V = \frac{2r^2 (d_1 - d_2) g}{9 \eta}$$

where

V = Sedimentation velocity
r = Radius of the sphere
d_1 = Density of the sphere
d_2 = Density of the fluid
g = Force of gravity
η = Viscosity of the fluid

By substituting ac for r^2 and changing the denominator to 7.65 η, the preceding equation can be made to apply to a disk-shaped body, having a radius "a" and thickness "c," falling through plasma (Ponder, 1948). The expression then reads as follows:

$$V = \frac{2ac (d_1 - d_2) g}{7.65 \eta}$$

This formula, although not directly applicable to the determination of the sedimentation velocity of erythrocytes in plasma, expresses several pertinent relationships. It will be noted, for example, that sedimentation velocity is directly proportional to the mass of the sedimenting particle and to the difference in density between the particle and the fluid. It is inversely proportional, however, to the viscosity of the fluid.

In normal blood, erythrocytes suspended in plasma form few if any aggregates. The mass of the sedimenting particle is therefore small, and the sedimentation velocity tends to be low. In abnormal blood, rouleau formation or erythrocyte agglutination may take place, increasing the particle mass and the sedimentation velocity. Rouleau formation depends on the protein composition of the plasma, particularly with regard to fibrinogen and globulin. True agglutination is caused by specific changes in the erythrocyte surface as when there is autoagglutination or other immune interactions. In either case, there will be an increase in sedimentation velocity because of the larger particle size (Fig. 6-1).

When the shape of the erythrocytes is such as to make rouleau formation impossible, a low sedimentation rate can be expected. In sickle cell disease the irregularly shaped erythrocytes cannot form rouleaux. The sedimentation rate will therefore be low when sickling is severe. Acanthocytosis and severe anisocytosis also interfere with rouleau formation. In hemolytic anemias, also, the spherocytic red blood cells cannot form rouleaux, and unless there is autoagglutination, the sedimentation rate is low. Since it is impossible to quantify the effect of these cellular malformations, measurement of the sedimentation rate is of little value in these conditions. Severe anemia is another complicating factor frequently found in these cases.

Effect of changes in plasma composition

Erythrocytes are negatively charged and normally repel each other. The negative charge is expressed as the *zeta potential,* a function of the negatively charged sialic acid groups on the erythrocyte membrane, the pH of the medium, the ionic strength of the medium, and the dielectric effect (the force of attraction between two charges at a given distance from each other) of protein molecules in the surrounding medium. All protein molecules and other macromolecules (Chien, 1976; Pittz et al, 1977) decrease the zeta potential, but the greatest effect is exerted by asymmetric molecules (Pollack et al, 1965) such as fibrinogen and immunoglobulin. Thus when the plasma concentration of fibrinogen and immunoglobulin is increased, the zeta potential of the erythrocytes is decreased and rouleau formation is increased. It is predictable, therefore, that the sedimentation rate should be increased in those diseases characterized by

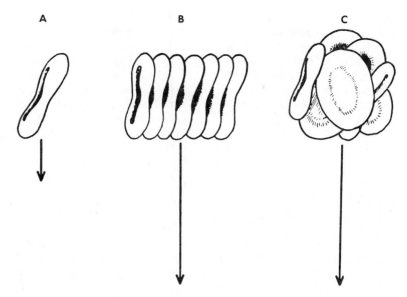

Fig. 6-1. Relationship of mass to sedimentation velocity. The length of the arrows indicates relative sedimentation velocities of, **A,** a single erythrocyte, **B,** a rouleau of erythrocytes, and, **C,** a clump of agglutinated erythrocytes.

hyperfibrinogenemia (tissue necrosis, infection, pregnancy) or elevated immunoglobulins (multiple myeloma and other immunoglobulinopathies).

The greatest effect is exerted by fibrinogen, as shown by Myers et al (1953):

Sedimentation rate =

$$\left[\frac{P}{C}(6.060 \text{ Fib.} + 0.866 \text{ }\gamma\text{-glob.} + 0.326 \text{ }\beta\text{-glob.} + 2.091 \text{ }\alpha_2\text{-glob.} + 0.183 \text{ }\alpha_1\text{-glob.} = 1.958) - 1.327\right]\frac{H}{25}$$

where

$\frac{P}{C}$ = Plasma-to-cell ratio

H = MCHC − Total protein (Gm/dl)

Sedimentation rates calculated by this formula show a coefficient of correlation with the observed rates of 0.982 ± 0.004. Fibrinogen exerts an effect 33 times greater than α_1-globulin, 18 times greater than β-globulin, and 3 times greater than α_2-globulin. Albumin apparently exerts very little effect. Although the effect of various protein fractions can be measured experimentally, the sedimentation rate is determined by a complex interrelationship of the various proteins and cannot be used to estimate increases or decreases in any given fraction. It is also interesting to note that there exists a direct relationship between the concentration of serum haptoglobin and the sedimentation rate. When one is increased, the other usually is also. This is not surprising since the serum haptoglobin concentration is increased when there is chronic infection, malignancy, etc. (p. 464).

Centrifugation of blood overcomes the mutually repelling negative charge of individual erythrocytes, and in many immunohematologic tests where agglutination is the end point, centrifugation under controlled conditions is used to enhance agglutination. Bull and Brailsford (1972) have adopted the same principle to modify the standard sedimentation rate procedure. They have shown that under controlled conditions of centrifugation, the degree of packing—the ZSR (zeta sedimentation ratio)—is the same in men and women, is unaffected by anemia, and is directly proportional to changes in plasma protein composition. A special centrifuge is required (Zetafuge) and the special capillary tube is subjected to four short centrifugation cycles. In spite of the advantage of requiring less time there are serious drawbacks: (1) special apparatus is required, (2) a new set of normals must be used (51% to 54% for normal individuals), and (3) the hematocrit must be determined as a separate step to calculate the ZSR. Admitting the crudeness of the standard sedimentation rate measurement, there is no evidence that this ingenious modification gives data that are clinically more significant.

Number of erythrocytes

When the number of erythrocytes per unit volume of blood is greater or less than normal, the true sedimentation velocity is modified. In severe anemia the sedimentation rate is very rapid, supposedly because of the greater ease of settling of a small number of particles in a large volume of fluid. The converse is true in polycythemia. By analogy it has been reasoned that the increased crowding of the settling particles tends to retard their fall. Although this explanation is vivid and useful, it is only conjectural.

CORRECTIONS FOR ANEMIA. Several methods have been proposed to "correct" for the effect of the anemia.

One of these is based on a series of studies by Wintrobe and Landsberg (1935) in which the cell content of normal blood was adjusted to various hematocrit levels. After the observed sedimentation rates were plotted, a series of "smoothed" curves were drawn. By means of this chart the sedimentation rate of blood with an abnormally low hematocrit can be "corrected" to predict what the true sedimentation rate would be if the hematocrit were normal.

There are serious objections to this method of correction, the most important being that in abnormal blood the curves obtained are less regular. While the Wintrobe-Landsberg chart is probably accurate in correcting for anemia caused by acute hemorrhage, it does not apply to every anemia. Hynes and Whitby (1938), in studies similar to Wintrobe's, used blood from various anemias. Their results demonstrate a striking difference between normal and abnormal bloods at the same hematocrit level.

It is now generally agreed that there is little merit to reporting corrected sedimentation rates.

Size of erythrocytes

Macrocytes fall more rapidly and microcytes less rapidly than normal erythrocytes. The effect is significant only in extreme cases. The use of any correction chart in extreme microcytosis will tend to overcorrect for the anemia.

Number of leukocytes

There is no effect of leukocytes on the sedimentation rate except in cases of extreme leukocytosis. Glass (1971) reports an instance of false low sedimentaion rate in a case of chronic lymphocytic leukemia having a white blood cell count of 700,000/mm^3 (700 $\times$ 10^9/l).

Caliber and length of tube

The different normal values given for various methods are caused by variations in the caliber of the tube and the height of the column of blood. The taller the column of blood (given the same tube bore), the more rapid will be the first phase of sedimentation because of delayed packing of cells at the bottom of the tube. Rapid sedimentation occurs in large-bore tubes. When normal values are determined for tubes of various bores and lengths, there are no important reasons for choosing one design over another. Ease of handling and the convenient rack made the Westergren tube a favorite among technologists. For infants, micromethods have been devised. To reduce the volume of blood needed, the bore of the tube is necessarily smaller than in standard tubes. A different set of normal values is then required. A comparison of the various tubes and the normal values for each are given in Table 6-1.

Position of tube

In all methods it is important to keep the tube exactly perpendicular. Minor degrees of tilting have a marked accelerating effect on the sedimentation rate. This is thought to be caused by the settling of cells to one side of the tube, affording the plasma easier displacement upward. Whatever the reason, larger technical errors occur through inclination of the tube than from any other factor. The use of special racks that keep the tubes exactly perpendicular is essential.

Anticoagulant used

It is possible for the anticoagulant to affect the size of the erythrocytes sufficiently to alter the sedimentation rate. For example, dry sodium or potassium oxalate can shrink the erythrocytes as much as 11%. The Heller and Paul (1934) mixture is better but still causes a little cell shrinkage. Heparin causes negligible cell shrinkage but produces false elevation of the sedimentation rate (Jeannet and Hässig, 1964). We now use dry EDTA, the anticoagulant recommended by Gambino et al (1965); there is little or no cell shrinkage even after some hours and the blood sample can be used in elec-

Table 6-1. Comparison of various sedimentation tubes and normal values applying to each method*

Method	Length of tube (mm)	Bore (mm)	Amount of blood (ml)	Normal values (mm/1 hr)		SD of method
Westergren† (1924)	300	2.5	2.0	Men	0-15	±1 mm
				Women	0-20	
				Children	0-10	
Cutler (1929)	70	5.0	1.0	Men	0-8	±2 mm
				Women	0-10	
				Children	4-13	
Wintrobe and Landsburg (1935)	100	2.5	1.0	Men	0-9	±1.5 mm
				Women	0-20	
				Children	0-13	
Landau (1933) (micromethod)	120	1.0	0.25	Men	1-6	±2 mm
				Women	1-9	
				Children (0-2 yr)	1-6	
				Children (2-14 yr)	1-9	
Smith (micromethod) (1936)	50	2.5	0.25	Children (12 days-14 yr)	3-13	

*See also effects of advanced age, p. 355.
†Westergren's original technic specified sodium citrate as the anticoagulant: 4 parts of venous blood to 1 part of 3.7% sodium citrate. Normal values are then 0 to 5 mm for men and 0 to 12 mm for women. The normal values given in the table are for a blood collected in dry EDTA. (See appendix.)

tronic cell counters. EDTA-anticoagulated blood is also suitable for white and red cell counts, even after 48 hours of storage at room temperature (Lampasso, 1968). We do not use the liquid sodium citrate anticoagulant (see footnote to Table 6-1) mainly because we do not like to draw additional blood for only one test.

Effect of temperature

Minor variations in room temperature do not greatly affect the sedimentation rate. However, when large daily or seasonal variations in temperature occur, the sedimentation rate is affected significantly. The nomogram constructed by Manley (1957) (Fig. 6-2) can be used to correct the observed rate to 65° F. It will be noted that the need for correction is greater when the observed rate is high than when it is normal. It has been shown that if the blood is at refrigerator temperature, the sedimentation rate is significantly decreased, probably because of the increase in plasma viscosity. It is important, therefore, to allow refrigerated blood to return to room temperature before performing the test.

Effect of delay in performing test

The sedimentation rate remains unchanged for up to 12 hours if the blood has been drawn in dry EDTA, but an appreciable reduction will be found if the test is done after more than 3 hours with blood drawn in double oxalate anticoagulant.

Clinical correlation

The sedimentation rate remains fairly constant in healthy persons, and although the normal ranges given in Table 6-1 include a maximum, the values observed in most normals are in the lower ranges. In newborn infants the sedimentation rate is seldom over 2 mm/hour, perhaps because of a high hematocrit. The sedimentation rate of blood from the unbilical cord is also very low. Children usually have a lower sedimentation rate than adults and the middle-aged a lower rate than the elderly (Böttiger and Svedberg, 1967). The sedimentation rate in elderly, apparently healthy persons is frequently higher than the values given for normal adults. Weinsaft and Haltaufderhyde (1965) give the following normal values (mm/hour, Wintrobe method) for the 69- to 94-year-old age group; 0 to 10 in 3.9%, 11 to 20 in 25.6%, 21 to 30 in 21.8%, and 41 to 50 in 20.5%. Using the preferred Westergren method, Gilbertsen (1965) confirmed that the sedimentation rate normally increases with advancing age; men 65 to 79 years, 0 to 38 mm/hour (90% range); women 65 to 79 years, 1 to 53 mm/hour (90% range).

There is a significant difference between the sedimentation rate of normal men and women regardless of age, women showing a higher rate than men. It has been suggested that the sex difference is related to the concentration of androgenic steroids—castration of the male produces a rise in the sedimentation rate (Hamilton et al, 1964) and administration of testosterone to eunuchs lowers the sedimentation

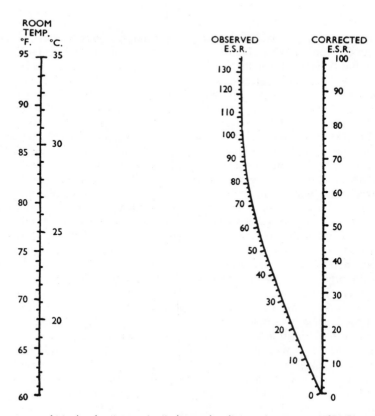

Fig. 6-2. Nomogram of Manley for "correcting" observed sedimentation rate to 65°F. (From Manley, 1957.)

Table 6-2. Clinical correlation of sedimentation rate

I. Sedimentation rate markedly increased (100 mm more per hour)
  A. Multiple myeloma and Waldenström's macroglobulinemia
  B. Malignant lymphoma
  C. Leukemia
  D. Severe anemia
  E. Carcinoma
  F. Sarcoma
  G. Acute severe bacterial infection
  H. Collagen diseases
  I. Active portal or biliary cirrhosis
  J. Ulcerative colitis
  K. Severe renal disease
  L. Viral pneumonitis (early)
II. Sedimentation rate moderately increased
  A. Acute and chronic infectious diseases
  B. Acute localized infections
  C. Reactivation of a chronic infection
  D. Rheumatic fever
  E. Rheumatoid arthritis
  F. Myocardial infarction
  G. Malignant tumors with necrosis
  H. Hyperthryoidism
  I. Hypothyroidism
  J. Lead and arsenic intoxication
  K. Nephrosis
  L. Internal hemorrhage
  M. Acute hepatitis (viral)
  N. Unruptured ectopic pregnancy after third month
  O. Ruptured ectopic pregnancy
  P. Menstruation
  Q. Normal pregnancy after third month
  R. Ingestion of oral contraceptives
  S. Tuberculosis
  T. Postcommissurotomy syndrome
  U. Intravenous dextran (high molecular weight)
  V. Anaphylactoid purpura (Henoch-Schönlein)
  W. Acute glomerulonephritis
  X. Advanced age
  Y. Hyperlipidemia
III. Sedimentation rate usually normal
  A. Early acute appendicitis (within first 24 hours)
  B. Early unruptured ectopic pregnancy
  C. Malarial paroxysm
  D. Cirrhosis of liver
  E. Degenerative arthritis
  F. Infectious mononucleosis (uncomplicated)
  G. Acute allergies
  H. Uncomplicated virus diseases
  I. Peptic ulcer
  J. Typhoid fever
  K. Undulant fever
  L. Rheumatic carditis with cardiac failure
  M. Pertussis
  N. Rickettsial diseases
  O. Toxoplasmosis
IV. Sedimentation rate usually low or "zero"
  A. Polycythemia vera
  B. Sickle cell anemia
  C. Hb C disease
  D. Spherocytosis

rate to normal male levels. In pregnancy the sedimentation rate begins to increase at about the third month and remains elevated until about 3 weeks after delivery. Since there is a 20% to 25% increase in blood volume during pregnancy, with a greater increase in plasma volume than in erythrocyte mass, this effect is, at least in part, caused by a change in the ratio between plasma and cell volume. A moderate elevation is commonly found just before and during menstruation.

Indications for determining the sedimentation rate are varied. It is useful in detecting occult organic disease. In some cases it confirms the presence of disease diagnosed by other means. It may also serve as a guide in following the course of a disease and marking a point of change. In general one can expect the sedimentation rate to be high when there is an infectious disease or a significant amount of tissue necrosis.

Typical changes in the sedimentation rate are listed in Table 6-2. It is particularly important to know the special situations in which the sedimentation rate does not conform to what is expected; e.g., early in the course of an uncomplicated virus infection the ESR is usually normal; it may rise later if there is superimposed bacterial infection. Early in acute appendicitis, within the first 24 hours, the ESR is not elevated, but during the early stage of acute pelvic inflammatory disease or of ruptured ectopic pregnancy, it is elevated. Such differences help to differentiate between conditions that present similar clinical findings; e.g., the ESR is elevated in established myocardial infarction but

normal in angina pectoris; it is elevated in rheumatic fever, rheumatoid arthritis, and pyogenic arthritis but not in osteoarthritis; it is generally normal in cirrhosis of the liver but may be elevated in carcinoma of the liver, particularly if there is extensive necrosis of tumor tissue. In an acute febrile illness a normal sedimentation rate usually excludes a systemic infectious process; an exception is malaria, which is notably accompanied by a normal ESR.

Elevation of the sedimentation rate in rheumatic fever is usually parallel to the severity of the infection, but here again there are some important variations. It is well established that when cardiac failure occurs in rheumatic fever the ESR will drop; it may become normal in spite of severe underlying rheumatic carditis (Harris et al, 1957). It has also been noted that the ESR becomes low or normal in the course of massive salicylate therapy and following ACTH or cortisone therapy. On the other hand, prophylactic administration of penicillin to patients with inactive rheumatic fever is reported to cause an elevation in the sedimentation rate.

Some years ago the sedimentation rate was considered the most reliable index of the activity of pulmonary tuberculosis. More recently, many have noted that with early diagnosis and a generally less virulent disease, many patients with proved tuberculosis have a normal ESR. When the sedimentation rate is elevated, it often falls promptly after the inception of antituberculosis chemotherapy, often well before the roentgenograms show improvement. A rising ESR, on the other hand, usually indicates progression of the disease or some complication such as pleural effusion.

Zacharski and Kyle (1967) present some interesting data from 263 patients who showed a sedimentation rate of 100 mm or more per hour (Westergren method). They found that 58% had malignancy, 25% had inflammatory disease (infection or collagen disease), while 8% had renal disease. In 14 patients, no explanation was found for the very high sedimentation rate. In the malignancy group, multiple myeloma, lymphoma, and metastatic carcinoma have always been known to produce a very high sedimentation rate. In general, however, there is little correlation between the degree of elevation of the sedimentation rate and the prognosis in any one given case.

In general no direct correlation exists between fever and the ESR. It should also be noted that the ESR in sickle cell anemia is unpredictable and totally unreliable. The results are affected not only by the severe anemia but also by a failure of the abnormally shaped erythrocytes to form rouleaux.

HEMATOCRIT

The term "hematocrit" (*hemato* = blood + *kritēs* = to judge) is defined in Webster's *New International Dictionary* as "an instrument for determining the relative amounts of plasma and corpuscles in blood." When the term is used in this sense, the measurement proper would be the "volume of packed erythrocytes" or, more correctly, the "volume of packed erythrocytes per dl of blood."

Common usage and convenience have led us to use the term "hematocrit" as synonymous with "volume of packed erythrocytes per dl of blood" rather than to limit its meaning to the name of the instrument.

Definitions

Hematocrit is defined as the volume occupied by erythrocytes in a given volume of blood and is usually expressed as volume of erythrocytes per dl of blood. The hematocrit of venous blood is called the *venous hematocrit*. This represents the hematocrit of peripheral blood and (as discussed later) does not indicate the proportion of erythrocytes to plasma in the entire circulation. The ratio of total erythrocyte mass to total blood volume is the *body hematocrit* and is calculated by a different method. Both measurements are of value, but the most commonly used is the venous hematocrit.

Conditions of centrifugation

To determine the hematocrit, the process of spontaneous sedimentation is accelerated by centrifuging a specimen of venous blood to which an anticoagulant has been added. After centrifugation the erythrocytes will be packed in the bottom of the tube. Above them is a layer of leukocytes and platelets (the buffy coat) and above this the relatively cell-free plasma.

If this measurement is to be meaningful, we must first define what is meant by "packed erythrocytes." Packing can be achieved at various centrifugal speeds maintained for various periods of time. It has been stated that the criterion for complete packing is centrifugation to a constant volume.

Millar's (1925) work, however, showed that, although it is possible to pack erythrocytes to a constant volume at different speeds, the packed volume is not the same for each speed; e.g., centrifugation at 2,000 rpm may yield a hematocrit of 49, whereas centrifugation at 10,000 rpm may yield a hematocrit of 42. In neither case does further centrifugation affect the values; therefore a constant volume has been achieved. Neither value need represent maximal or complete packing.

A given hematocrit therefore expresses only the volume of erythrocytes packed under certain conditions of centrifugation. These are (1) the radius of the centrifuge, (2) the speed of centrifugation, and (3) the duration of centrifugation.

The radius of the centrifuge is measured from the center of the shaft to the bottom of the centrifuge tube when the tube is in a horizontal position. The speed of centrifugation is measured in revolutions per minute. Since the speed varies with different loads, mechanical condition of the centrifuge, and fluctuation of the line voltage, it should be measured with a tachometer. The radius of the centrifuge and the speed of centrifugation determine the centrifugal force applied, according to the formula:

$$F = M\, r\, w^2$$

in which F is the force in dynes, M the mass in grams, r the radius of centrifugation in centimeters, and w the angular velocity in radians per second.

The expression w^2 can be converted to rpm^2 (or n^2) by multiplying by $\dfrac{(2\pi)^2}{60^2}$. This gives the constant 0.01096. The formula then becomes:

$$F = M \times r \times 0.01096 \times n^2$$

Since the force of gravity exerted on a 1 Gm mass at 45° lat. is 980.616 dynes, the formula can be modified to express F in grams rather than dynes:

$$F \text{ (in grams)} = M \times r \times \frac{0.01096}{980.616} \times n^2$$
$$= M \times r \times 0.00001118 \times n^2$$

Since we are seldom interested in the actual force exerted in grams, but only in the relative centrifugal force regardless of the mass, grams can be canceled out of both sides of the equation. The resulting expression for *relative centrifugal force* (RCF in number × g, where r is in *centimeters*) is:

$$\text{RCF or } g = 0.00001118 \times r \times n^2$$

The RCF *(g)* for a given set of conditions can be determined by knowing the radius of centrifugation and the revolutions per minute (n). A nomograph to simplify the computation of RCF (Fig. 6-3) has been constructed by a manufacturer.*

It is obvious that the greater the radius of centrifugation, the greater will be the value of RCF. Likewise, the greater the speed, the greater will be the force applied, RCF varying with the square of the revolutions per minute. The total effect is determined by the length of time that force is

---

*International Equipment Co., Boston, Mass.

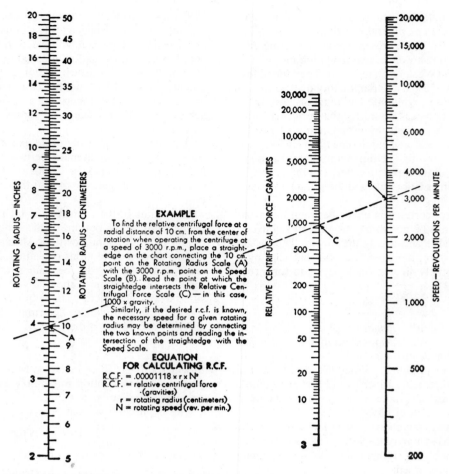

Fig. 6-3. Nomograph for computing relative centrifugal force (RCF). (Courtesy International Equipment Co., Boston, Mass.)

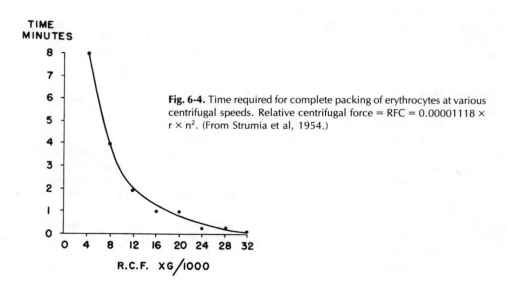

Fig. 6-4. Time required for complete packing of erythrocytes at various centrifugal speeds. Relative centrifugal force = RFC = $0.00001118 \times r \times n^2$. (From Strumia et al, 1954.)

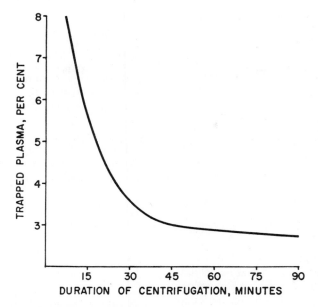

Fig. 6-5. Amount of plasma trapped in the erythrocyte column in relation to the duration of centrifugation at 3,500 rpm, centrifuge radius 15 cm, 2,050 g. (From Bernstein, 1955.)

exerted on a unit mass. In respect to packing erythrocytes, the relationship between time and RCF is not linear (Fig. 6-4), the time required for maximum packing at low RCF values being relatively greater than at high RCF values. Many different speeds and various periods of centrifugation have been suggested, from 2,500 rpm to ultracentrifugal speeds and from 2 hours to 1 minute. For each set of conditions the erythrocytes can be packed to constant volume. At the lower speeds, hematocrits are higher, probably because of the greater volume of trapped plasma.

Amount of trapped plasma

The ability to centrifuge blood to different constant volumes of packed erythrocytes under various conditions is almost entirely a result of differences in the amount of plasma trapped among the packed erythrocytes. The amount of trapped plasma may be determined experimentally by adding to the blood a substance that remains in the plasma and is not attached to the erythrocytes—Evans blue dye (T-1824) or radioiodinated (^{131}I) albumin. After centrifugation the supernatant plasma is carefully removed, and the amount of trapped plasma in the erythrocyte column is determined by appropriate procedures.

Quoted data on trapped plasma are meaningless unless account is taken of the conditions of centrifugation. Values given vary from 2% to as high as 8.5%. According to England et al (1972) the amount of trapped plasma may be 5% to 6% in microcytosis and 20% or more in both sickle cell anemia and sickle cell trait, the latter depending on the degree of sickling in the blood sample. In their study the amount of plasma trapping in normal subjects was slightly over 3%. If correction for trapped plasma is required, either for the calculation of erythrocyte indices or for blood volume studies, a figure applicable to the conditions of centrif-

ugation must be applied rather than one chosen at random from other studies.

Fig. 6-5 illustrates that, at a given RCF, the amount of trapped plasma varies with the duration of centrifugation. It will be noted that the amount of plasma trapped after 30 minutes of centrifugation under the stated conditions is about 3.6% and after 45 minutes of centrifugation about 3.0%. These figures do not apply when the erythrocytes are hardened by fixative and are therefore not deformable (Chien et al, 1968).

Use of hematocrit data

It is necessary to define what information is wanted from the hematocrit in order to establish the best method of obtaining the data and its reliability in view of the variables just discussed.

The hematocrit is used in determining erythrocyte indices, calculating blood volume and total erythrocyte mass, and establishing whether or not the patient is anemic. In calculating the erythrocyte indices by Wintrobe's method and formulas, the hematocrit is determined by centrifugation at 3,000 rpm for 30 minutes in a centrifuge having a sufficient radius to produce a relative centrifugal force (RCF) of 2,250 g. It is clear that these conditions achieve *optimal* rather than *complete* packing of the erythrocytes, in the sense that the indices calculated with this hematocrit correspond to erythrocyte measurements by other methods. These conditions of centrifugation are therefore justified for determining the erythrocyte indices.

In blood volume calculations it is possible to make a correction for trapped plasma, provided that the correction factor is determined for the conditions actually used (Fig. 6-5). It has also been shown that the amount of plasma that is trapped varies with the height of the packed cell volume and is not the same at all levels of the erythrocyte column. In addition, it is generally agreed that venous hematocrits are normally about 9% higher than total body hematocrit. Direct application of this correction factor is not always justified since in heart failure or shock the difference between the venous hematocrit and the body hematocrit may be smaller than 9%.

Finally, the hematocrit gives a rough indication of anemia inasmuch as a low hematocrit indicates that the concentration of erythrocytes is reduced. Both the erythrocyte count and the hematocrit measure concentration of erythrocytes, but neither measures the total volume of erythrocytes present in the blood nor its oxygen-carrying capacity. Both must be related to blood volume data to have any significance.

Since the inherent error of erythrocyte counting (Chapter 7) may be as high as 7% for manual methods and 2% for electronic particle counting apparatus and that of the hematocrit about 1%, some have recommended that hematocrits be substituted for erythrocyte counts in routine hematologic studies. This has become easier to justify with the perfection of microhematocrit methods that require a very short time. However, hematocrit cannot completely replace erythrocyte counts since the latter are needed to calculate some of the erythrocyte indices.

For *normal* blood, hemoglobin and erythrocyte counts may be estimated from the microhematocrit reading according to the following formulas:

(1)   1 hematocrit point = 0.34 Gm hemoglobin per dl of blood

(2)   1 hematocrit point = 107,000 erythrocytes per cubic millimeter of blood

Microhematocrit methods

Microhematocrit methods have several advantages. Centrifugation in capillary tubes at 16,500 rpm for 2 minutes (11,000 g) or at 28,000 g for 1 minute, as recommended by Strumia et al (1954) produces maximal packing that is about 2.8% lower than that obtained by Wintrobe's method. Under these conditions the value for trapped plasma is probably negligible. With regard to calculation of corpuscular constants, mean corpuscular volume will be a little lower and mean corpuscular hemoglobin concentration a little higher if capillary hematocrit values are used. The difference is probably not significant since the normal range is greater than the difference between hematocrit methods. The short time required for microhematocrit determinations makes the method very valuable from the clinical standpoint. Microhematocrit methods make this determination possible in patients in whom a venipuncture is difficult or undesirable, such as in patients with severe burns or in infants. Another important advantage of microhematocrit methods is that, while the centrifuges differ in design and operation, they have similar performance characteristics. The accuracy of the microhematocrit method (when replicates are read by the same observer), as determined in our laboratory, is ± 0.21%. There is however, a significant observation error, about 2% variation, when different technologists read the same microhematocrit preparation.

Calculated hematocrit (Coulter S and Hemac apparatus)

The erythrocyte indices (MCV, MCH, MCHC—Chapter 7) are useful expressions of the average size and hemoglobin content of the erythrocyte. Wintrobe's formulas are based on the calculation of the indices from observed values for hemoglobin concentration, erythrocyte count, and hematocrit.

The Coulter cell counter (Model S) and the Hemac laser cell counter are designed to give a direct measurement of mean corpuscular volume (MCV) and erythrocyte count; from these the hematocrit can be calculated, for if:

$$MCV = \frac{Hematocrit \times 10}{Erythrocyte\ count\ (millions/mm^3)}$$

then

$$Hematocrit = \frac{MCV \times Erythrocyte\ count}{10}$$

As in the calculation of the cell indices, the significance of the calculated value depends on the significance of the measured values. If the instrument is calibrated accurately for the measurement of MCV and erythrocyte count, calculated hematocrit should be comparable to independent hematocrit measurements. However, note that the measured microhematocrit includes trapped plasma, whereas the calculated hematocrit does not. In a comparative study performed in our laboratory we found the calculated hematocrit to be 2% lower than the microhematocrit at the 40% level. England et al (1972) suggest that this difference should be eliminated by adjusting the hematocrit reading on the Coulter S counter, but since the difference between measured and calculated hematocrit is not constant for different types of anemia this is not a very practical suggestion. It is important to note that in a severe microcytic hypochromic anemia the calculated hematocrit is significantly lower than the measured hematocrit and that the red cell indices may then be higher than the true values. Penn et al (1979) compared microhematocrit and calculated hematocrit values in newborns and adults and found the calculated hematocrit values were generally lower than the microhematocrit values. Fairbanks (1980) emphasized the difference between the calculated hematocrit values and those obtained by the Wintrobe tube method.

Normal values

Normal values for blood microhematocrit are given in Table 6-3 and in Figs. 6-6 to 6-8.

The hematocrit is high in the newborn infant, drops to its lowest point at about 1 year of age, and then gradually climbs to the adult values. There is a tendency toward lower values in both men and women after 50 years of age, corresponding to lower values for erythrocyte counts in this age group. Hematocrits for normal pregnant women are slightly lower than for nonpregnant women.

Changes in blood volume affect the hematocrit. Immediately following an acute hemorrhage the hematocrit and erythrocyte counts may be normal in spite of the markedly reduced blood volume. During the recovery phase, restitu-

Table 6-3. Normal microhematocrit values*

Age	Average normal	Minimal normal
Children—both sexes		
At birth	56.6	51.0
First day	56.1	50.5
End of first week	52.7	47.5
End of second week	49.6	44.7
End of third week	46.6	42.0
End of fourth week	44.6	40.0
End of second month	38.9	35.1
End of fourth month	36.5	32.9
End of sixth month	36.2	32.6
End of eighth month	35.8	32.3
End of tenth month	35.5	32.0
End of first year	35.2	31.7
End of second year	35.5	32.0
End of fourth year	37.1	33.4
End of sixth year	37.9	34.2
End of eighth year	38.9	35.1
End of twelfth year	39.6	35.7
Men		
End of fourteenth year	44	39.6
End of eighteenth year	47	42.3
18-50 yr	47	42.3
50-60 yr	45	40.5
60-70 yr	43	38.7
70-80 yr	40	36.0
Nonpregnant women		
14-50 yr	42	36
50-80 yr	40	36
Pregnant women		
End of fourth month	42	30
End of fifth month	40	30
End of sixth month	37	30
End of seventh month	37	30
End of eighth month	39	30
End of ninth month	40	30

*Courtesy Dr. M. Strumia and The Drummond Scientific Co., Broomall, Pa.

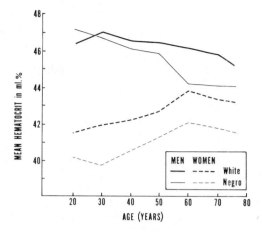

Fig. 6-6. Mean hematocrit in adults, by age, race, and sex, in the United States (1960-1962). (Data from National Center for Health Statistics, 1967.)

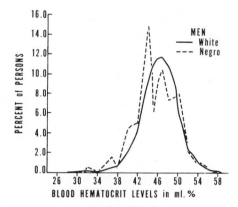

Fig. 6-7. Frequency distribution of hematocrit values in adult males, white and black, in the United States (1960-1962). (Data from National Center for Health Statistics, 1967.)

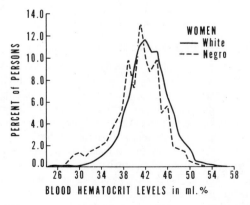

Fig. 6-8. Frequency distribution of hematocrit values in adult females, white and black, in the United States (1960-1962). (Data from National Center for Health Statistics, 1967.)

tion of blood volume is produced by an increase in plasma volume, and both the hematocrit and erythrocyte counts will be reduced markedly. This may occur even while whole blood is being administered. Dehydration, on the other hand, will produce high hematocrit and erythrocyte counts, perhaps obscuring a preexisting anemia. The correction of dehydration may reveal or accentuate anemia. When the results of fluid or transfusion therapy appear paradoxical, blood volume determinations should be done.

Diurnal variation in hematocrit values is usually ignored, but in some individuals it can be significant. Finlayson et al (1964) have shown that the hematocrit may be as much as 10% lower in the evening than in the morning. This is secondary to clinical variation in plasma volume.

Clinical correlation

As noted earlier, the relationship between the relative viscosity of blood and the hematocrit is nearly linear for hematocrit values below 40%; above 40% the relative viscosity becomes progressively greater. Burch and DePasquale

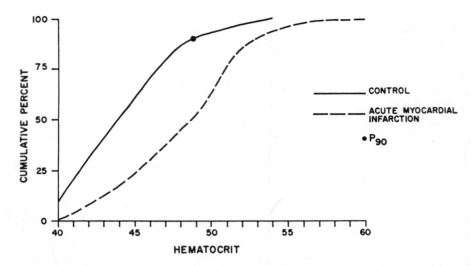

Fig. 6-9. Cumulative distribution of hematocrit for 100 control subjects and 100 patients with acute myocardial infarction. (From Burch and DePasquale, 1962.) Contradicting data are presented by Conley et al, 1964.

(1961) suggested that increased blood viscosity caused by a high hematocrit might be an etiologic or otherwise related factor in coronary thrombosis (Fig. 6-9). Conley et al (1964), however, concluded from their data that a high hematocrit value is not by itself a significant factor in predisposition to coronary thrombosis. Others (Bergentz et al, 1963; Ditzel, 1959; Gelin, 1965) believe that increased viscosity is only coincidentally related to the increased hematocrit, reflecting rather a response to tissue injury and secondary to increased concentrations of fibrinogen and α_2-globulin.

The significance of the relationship of hematocrit to predisposition to coronary thrombosis is probably negligible. Hershberg et al (1972) correlated the hematocrit values of 190 patients on admission to a coronary care unit with their ultimate clinical course. They showed that the hematocrit for the infarction group (mean:42.1%) was not significantly higher than that for a control group (mean:39.8%) of the same age distribution. One point made by these investigators should be of great interest to both clinicians and pathologists, that the amount of blood drawn for diagnostic laboratory studies during a 3-day stay in the coronary care unit ranged from 100 to 250 ml in 28 of 30 patients.

Distribution of blood cells on centrifugation

Since the sedimentation velocity is dependent in part on the particles, centrifugation of whole blood produces predictable differential separation of blood cells. Centrifugation at slow speed produces sedimentation of the erythrocytes and leukocytes, the latter in the upper portion of the erythrocyte column. Platelets remain in the supernatant plasma, except for a very few trapped in the lightly packed erythrocytes. Prolonged centrifugation at high speed produces a distinct layer of leukocytes and platelets at the top of the erythrocte column. This layer, the "buffy coat," is composed of a mixture of leukocytes and platelets. The concentration of each varies at different levels; the top portion is rich in platelets, while the portion adjoining the erythrocyte column in almost entirely composed of leukocytes.

When the platelet count is high, it is sometimes possible to see a grayish platelet zone that is fairly distinct from the creamy leukocyte layer.

Somewhat surprising are the results of studies on the distribution of erythrocytes within the column of packed cells. Bromberg et al (1956) have shown that when blood from a newborn infant is centrifuged the concentration of fetal hemoglobin is higher at the bottom of the packed erythrocyte column than at the top. The cells at the bottom are also larger and have a higher mean corpuscular volume than those at the top. Microcytes are more numerous in the top portion of the column, as are erythrocytes containing malarial parasites and, suprisingly, nucleated erythrocyte precursors. Reticulocytes also are distributed into the upper portion of the column. Davidson (1960) presents data indicating that the erythrocytes most fragile to hypotonic solutions tend to concentrate in the lower part of the packed red cell column.

BLOOD VOLUME, PLASMA VOLUME, AND ERYTHROCYTE MASS
Clinical correlation

Blood is made up of two components, the blood cells and the plasma. Since the volume occupied normally by leukocytes and platelets is negligible, we can consider only two components, the total mass of erythrocytes and the volume of plasma. The total blood volume is maintained normally within fairly small extremes, since the erythrocyte mass is replaced at a rate equal to the rate of erythrocyte destruction and the fluid compartment is in a steady-state equilibrium with extravascular compartments. When the balances are disturbed, the total blood volume may be altered by increases or decreases in the two chief components.

Measurements of blood volume and compartments are applicable to the interpretation of several hematologic parameters. Erythrocyte counts and hematocrits do not always reflect deficits or excesses. For example, in acute hemorrhage the concomitant loss of erythrocytes and plasma can reduce the total blood volume and, more importantly, the total erythrocyte mass to near fatal levels without any abnormality reflected in the erythrocyte count and hematocrit. Erythrocyte counts and hematocrits may be equally misleading when there are acute shifts in body fluids between intravascular and extravascular space, as for example in cardiac decompensation or in shock. In some situations such as the last trimester of pregnancy there is a physiologic increase in plasma volume (Rominger, 1964; Chesley et al, 1972) so that the reduced erythrocyte count and hematocrit alone may indicate a mild anemia in a normal woman or a severe anemia in a mildly anemic woman. The same exaggeration is seen in other situations where there is an increase in plasma volume, as in toxemia of pregnancy (Rominger, 1964) or uremia (Berlin et al, 1952).

The determination of erythrocyte mass is a useful adjunct in the differential diagnosis of the polycythemias (Chapter 16). In polycythemia vera there is usually an increase in erythrocyte mass and in plasma volume and total blood volume, the increase in plasma volume being proportionately smaller than that in the erythrocyte mass. In erythrocytosis, on the other hand, there is usually an increase in erythrocyte mass and a normal plasma volume. In one special type of erythrocytosis, the red cell mass is normal but there is a decrease in the plasma volume producing a high erythrocyte count and hematocrit.

Plasma volume and erythrocyte mass measurements can be useful guides to proper transfusion therapy. As discussed in Chapter 12, whenever transfusion therapy is contemplated, the transfusion material chosen should be that which best supplies what is needed. If the deficit is primarily one of erythrocytes, then packed erythrocytes alone are sufficient. In most cases the decision can be made on the basis of clinical information, but at times the measurement of blood compartments can clarify a questionable situation. Blood volume measurements also guide the amount of fluid to be given. A young or middle-aged patients's vascular bed can take a good bit of abuse and overcome it by efficient physiologic adjustments, but children and elderly persons may not be able to compensate rapidly enough if too large a volume of fluid is transfused and may be thrown into cardiac failure.

Determinations of plasma volume, erythrocyte mass, and erythrocyte survival have been performed on astronauts before and after Gemini IV, V, and VII orbital flights (Fischer et al, 1967). There was a decrease in plasma volume that was compensated for during the longer Gemini VII flight. In the astronauts involved in the Gemini V and VII flights there was also a decrease in erythrocyte mass accompanied by decreased RBC survival and no evidence of blood loss. None of the changes was so severe as to affect the safety of the astronauts.

Methods

Specific methodology and appropriate references are given by Silver (1968)and in a later report (Report by the International Committee, 1973). All methods are based on the principle that the degree of dilution by the blood of a measurable substance is proportional to the volume of the diluent. Specifically, several approaches are possible:

1. Use of a substance that, because of its affinity for plasma but not for erythrocytes, can be used to measure plasma volume. The oldest of these is Evans blue dye (T-1824), now generally replaced by isotopic tracers such a radioiodinated human serum albumin (RISA), isotopically labeled chromic chloride ($^{51}CrCl_3$) (Nadler et al, 1962) or pertechnetate-labeled human serum albumin (Yant, et al, 1978).

2. Use of a substance that, because of its affinity for erythrocytes but not for plasma, can be used to measure erythrocyte mass. Several radionuclides satisfy this criterion, some of which combine with erythrocytes in vivo as part of the metabolic activity of the erythrocyte (^{55}Fe, ^{59}Fe, ^{15}N, ^{14}C), others combine readily in vitro (^{32}P, ^{86}Rb, ^{42}K, ^{51}Cr as sodium chromate $Na_2{}^{51}CrO_4$). Price et al (1976) describe the use of nonradioactive cesium labeling of erythrocytes, quantified by fluorescent excitation analysis (FEA). Sodium pertechnetate is another useful red cell label (Shmidt et al, 1976).

3. When only one compartment (plasma volume or erythrocyte mass) is measured, the other is calculated from the hematocrit, including multipliction by the factor 0.914 to correct for trapped plasma in the peripheral hematocrit.

4. Simultaneous but independent measure of erythrocyte mass and plasma volume, in which case the total blood volume is the sum of the two and no correction is made for trapped plasma in the hematocrit. This is without doubt the best and most accurate method.

Normal values

Since plasma volume and erthrocyte mass measurements are used to determine deficits and excesses, they must be compared to what is considered normal for a given patient.

Normal values vary with the method used. Table 6-4 gives normal values for the ^{51}Cr method. Normal values for total blood volume and plasma are higher for ^{32}P methods (Wasserman and Mayerson, 1955; Berlin et al, 1956). Body habitus, varying with age, muscular development, sex, degree of obesity, and type of skeletal frame (large, medium, or small) dictates significant differences among normal individuals. Body height is a commonly used parameter for defining these differences (Fig. 6-10), and correlation with surface area is even better (Fig. 6-11) (Inkley et al, 1955; Morse, 1978). In most laboratories, the data used for normals are those of Nadler et al (1962) shown in Table 6-5. Huff and Feller (1956) state that the amount of blood associated with fatty tissue is about two-thirds of that with lean

Table 6-4. Blood, plasma, and erythrocyte volumes in normal adult males and females (^{51}Cr method)*†

Measurement	Men	Women
Blood volume (ml/kg)	61.54 ± 8.59	58.95 ± 4.94
Erythrocyte volume (ml/kg)	28.27 ± 4.11	24.24 ± 2.59
Plasma volume (ml/kg)	33.45 ± 5.18	34.77 ± 3.24

*After Huff and Feller, 1956.
†Observations on 42 normal men and 20 normal women. The figures given are averages ±2 SD. The erythrocyte volume is measured (sodium radiochromate); the others are calculated from the venous hematocrit. No correction is made for trapped plasma.

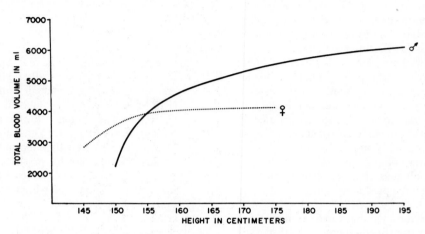

Fig. 6-10. Relation between total blood volume and body height. (From Gibson and Evans, 1937.)

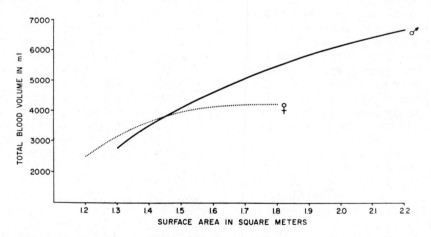

Fig. 6-11. Relation between total blood volume and surface area. Computed from the nomogram of Boothby and Sandiford. (From Gibson and Evans, 1937.)

Table 6-5. Table of predicted normal blood volumes in men and women, ^{131}I HSA method*

Weight (lb)	Volume (ml) by height (in.)							
	60	62	64	66	68	70	72	74
Men								
100	3,365	3,500	3,643	3,795	3,957	4,129	4,311	4,503
110	3,512	3,646	3,789	3,941	4,103	4,275	4,457	4,649
120	3,658	3,792	3,935	4,088	4,250	4,422	4,603	4,796
130	3,804	3,938	4,082	4,234	4,396	4,568	4,750	4,942
140	3,951	4,085	4,228	4,380	4,542	4,714	4,896	5,088
150	4,097	4,231	4,374	4,527	4,689	4,860	5,042	5,235
160	4,243	4,377	4,521	4,673	4,835	5,007	5,189	5,381
170	4,389	4,524	4,667	4,819	4,981	5,153	5,335	5,527
180	4,536	4,670	4,813	4,966	5,128	5,299	5,481	5,673
190	4,682	4,816	4,959	5,112	5,274	5,446	5,627	5,820
200	4,828	4,963	5,106	5,258	5,420	5,592	5,774	5,966
210	4,975	5,109	5,252	5,405	5,566	5,738	5,920	6,112
220	5,121	5,255	5,398	5,551	5,713	5,885	6,066	6,295
230	5,267	5,402	5,545	5,697	5,859	6,031	6,213	6,405
240	5,414	5,548	5,691	5,843	6,005	6,177	6,359	6,551
250	5,560	5,694	5,837	5,990	6,152	6,323	6,505	6,698
260	5,706	5,840	5,984	6,136	6,298	6,470	6,652	6,844
270	5,852	5,987	6,130	6,282	6,444	6,616	6,798	6,990
280	5,999	6,133	6,276	6,429	6,591	6,762	6,944	7,136
290	6,145	6,279	6,423	6,575	6,737	6,909	7,091	7,283
300	6,291	6,426	6,569	6,721	6,883	7,055	7,237	7,429
310	6,438	6,572	6,715	6,868	7,030	7,201	7,383	7,575
Women								
80	2,646	2,776	2,915	3,063	3,220	3,387	3,564	3,750
90	2,796	2,927	3,066	3,214	3,371	3,537	3,714	3,901
100	2,947	3,077	3,216	3,364	3,521	3,688	3,864	4,052
110	3,097	3,227	3,366	3,514	3,671	3,838	4,015	4,201
120	3,247	3,378	3,517	3,665	3,822	3,989	4,165	4,352
130	3,398	3,528	3,667	3,815	3,972	4,139	4,315	4,502
140	3,548	3,678	3,817	3,965	4,123	4,289	4,466	4,652
150	3,698	3,829	3,968	4,116	4,273	4,440	4,616	4,803
160	3,849	3,979	4,118	4,266	4,423	4,590	4,766	4,953
170	3,999	4,129	4,268	4,416	4,574	4,740	4,917	5,103
180	4,150	4,280	4,419	4,567	4,724	4,891	5,067	5,254
190	4,300	4,430	4,569	4,717	4,874	5,041	5,217	5,404
200	4,450	4,581	4,719	4,867	5,025	5,191	5,368	5,554
210	4,601	4,731	4,870	5,018	5,175	5,342	5,518	5,705
220	4,751	4,881	5,020	5,168	5,325	5,492	5,669	5,855
230	4,901	5,032	5,171	5,318	5,476	5,642	5,819	6,005
240	5,052	5,182	5,321	5,469	5,626	5,793	5,969	6,156
250	5,202	5,332	5,471	5,619	5,776	5,943	6,120	6,306
260	5,352	5,483	5,622	5,770	5,927	6,093	6,270	6,457
270	5,503	5,633	5,772	5,920	6,077	6,244	6,420	6,607
280	5,653	5,783	5,922	6,070	6,227	6,394	6,571	6,757
290	5,803	5,934	6,073	6,221	6,378	6,544	6,721	6,908

*From Nadler et al, 1962.

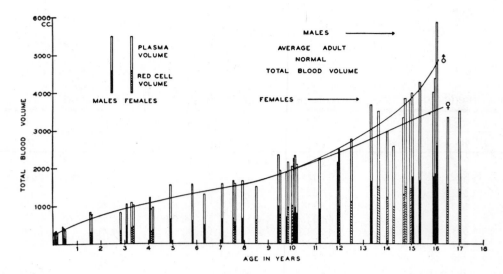

Fig. 6-12. Plasma, erythrocyte, and total blood volumes in normal infants and children. Solid lines represent the averages for total blood volume for the entire group. (From Brines et al, 1941.)

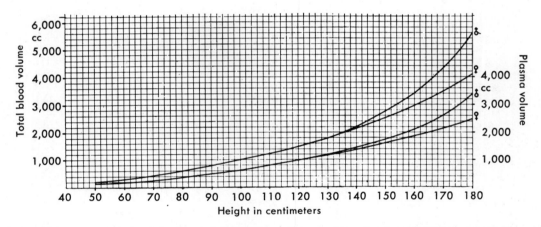

Fig. 6-13. Nomogram for predicting normal plasma and total blood volumes in infants and children. Lower lines represent plasma, and upper lines represent total blood volume. (From Brines et al, 1941.)

tissue. When dealing with obese individuals, the normal value for that individual will be smaller than that for a lean individual of the same weight. Likewise, if there has been marked loss of weight within a short time, the normal value for that individual will be larger then that for a lean individual of the same weight. Blood volume determinations in infants and children show the total blood volume at birth to be about 300 ml. Normal values can be defined either by age (Fig. 6-12) or by body height (Fig. 6-13). The difference between males and females is first apparent at about 10 years of age.

While not usually taken into account, blood volume may be as much as 16% higher in the evening than in the morning (Finlayson et al, 1964).

7

Application of statistics and quality assurance in hematology

INTRODUCTION
INTERPRETATION OF QUANTITATIVE DATA IN HEMATOLOGY
  Introduction to statistical analysis
  Principles of statistics
    Standard deviation (SD, sigma, σ)
    Probable error (PE)
    Coefficient of variation (CV)
ERROR OF THE ERYTHROCYTE COUNT
  Hemocytometer method
    Inherent errors
    Technical and human errors
    Calculation of SD from control data—standard method
    Calculation of SD from control data—duplicate analysis
      method
  The Coulter cell counter
  The Hemac laser cell counter
SIGNIFICANCE OF SUCCESSIVE CELL COUNTS
  Significant difference between successive hemocytometer counts
  Significant difference between successive electronic cell counts
NORMAL HEMATOLOGIC VALUES (RED BLOOD CELLS)
  Statistical determination of normal values
  Normal values
  Physiologic variations
    Posture
    Exercise or excitement
    Dehydration
    Age
    Sex
    Altitude
  Erythrocyte indices
    Mean corpuscular volume (MCV)
    Mean corpuscular hemoglobin (MCH)
    Mean corpuscular hemoglobin concentration (MCHC)
    Use of erythrocyte indices
    Erythrocyte indices calculated by electronic counters
QUALITY ASSURANCE IN HEMATOLOGY
  Introduction
  Coulter Model S
  Blood hemoglobin
  Microhematocrit
  Leukocyte differential counts
  Platelet counts
    Phase contrast microscopy method
    Semiautomated platelet counts
  Prothombin time
  Partial thromboplastin time
ADOPTION OF SI UNITS

INTRODUCTION

Much of the material in the chapters that follow will deal with quantitative hematologic data. To interpret such data intelligently it is necessary to discuss the statistical basis for its interpretation and the reliability of the data with regard to precision, accuracy, and quality assurance.

INTERPRETATION OF QUANTITATIVE DATA IN HEMATOLOGY
Introduction to statistical analysis

Laboratory observations deal with qualitative and quantitative data. Qualitative data are descriptive and depend on the use of words to transmit information concerning the nature and properties of the object being examined. Quantitative data depend on numbers to tell *how many* objects there are or *how much* of a substance is present.

Most will admit that words are "tricky," the meaning of some being subject to various interpretations and dependent on what other words precede or follow. Professions such as law and theology have grown out of the need for interpreting the meaning of words. On the other hand, numbers are often accepted as having an almost magical quality, implying certainty, which may be the reason for their attractiveness to uncertain persons in uncertain situations.

We need not dwell on the necessity for caution and accuracy in using descriptive terms. Everyone is aware of this necessity and usually makes an effort to say exactly what he or she means. If one word is not enough, several are used, giving us such gems of medical terminology as "chronic febrile relapsing suppurative panniculitis" and "megaloblastoid normoblasts." However, when a number is used, especially if very small or very large, it has such a sincere sound to it that one is tempted to accept it as absolute, without any hesitation or mental reservation, an assumption that is completely unwarranted. The significance of quantitative data can only be determined after considering the harsh reality of statistical laws.

The significance of quantitative laboratory data depends also on factors such as accuracy of methodology and observation. In most laboratories stringent control measures are taken to ensure that variations caused by technical factors are minimal. Granted such vigilance, exercised to the highest degree by all persons concerned, variations still remain that are not caused by avoidable technical difficulties. These variations cannot be controlled by the analyst. Statistical analysis is the study of all such variables. If laboratory data are to be used intelligently, the physician must evaluate them from the standpoint of statistical reliability. Technical variables are measured by *precision* (the variation introduced by methodology in replicate analyses of the same sample) and by *accuracy* (variation from the "true" value). Biologic variables include, of course, the effect of technical variables.

Principles of statistics

This section is necessarily limited to the application of statistics for the interpretation of hematologic data. The physician needs to decide whether a given value is normal or abnormal for that patient or for a given population. In serial determinations the physician needs to decide whether the values represent a statistically significant difference from previous values. The first decision is based on the definition of "normality." The second can be approached by a variety of tests of significant difference. In both cases significance is almost never absolute but rather is expressed as the *degree of statistical probability*. The book by Barnett (1979) discusses in detail the application of statistics to all types of laboratory data.

A coin flipped enough times will eventually and inevitably show an equal number of "heads" and "tails." Since there are only two possibilities, heads or tails, the laws of chance for one occurrence or the other are equal. If a coin is flipped just once, we can say that the chances are even (1:1) that it will come down either heads or tails. A single flip

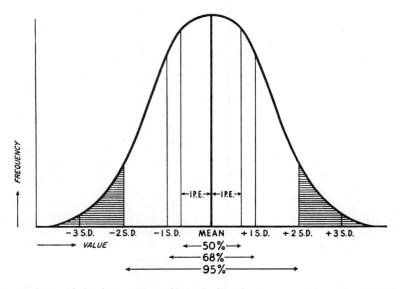

Fig. 7-1. Theoretical normal distribution curve obtained when the percent incidence is plotted for a series of values on either side of the mean. SD = standard deviation; PE = probable error.

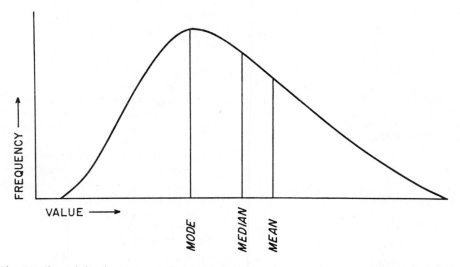

Fig. 7-2. Skewed distribution curve showing the difference between the mean, mode, and median.

resulting in heads cannot be interpreted as meaning that all other flips will result in heads. Similarly, the uncontrollable variables encountered in obtaining laboratory data limit the significance of a single determination. Any result must be interpreted with the aid of two separate statistical principles, one applying to the distribution of values for a sufficiently large number of normal persons and the other to the distribution of values when many determinations are done on the same specimen.

In either case if a large number of determinations are plotted according to their value and frequency, a *distribution curve* is obtained. The *normal* or *gaussian distribution curve* is symmetric (Fig. 7-1), an equal number of determinations falling on either side of the average value *(arithmetic mean)*. The *mean* also coincides with the *median* (the middle value when the samples are given in order of magnitude) and with the *mode* (the value that occurs most frequently). An excess or deficit of observations at the upper and lower portions of the normal curve widens or narrows the base, and this is known as *kurtosis*. If more determinations fall on one side of the mean than on the other, the curve is said to be "skewed" (Fig. 7-2).

Biologic data sometimes fall into a normal distribution, sometimes not. Whether they do or not must be determined either from an actual plot of frequency distribution or by using technics outlined in the sections that follow and given in detail in standard tests on statistical analysis. The concept of the *standard deviation from the arithmetic mean* is applicable only to a normal distribution. If this caution is ignored and the assumption of a normal distribution does not hold, then bizarre statistical analyses result.

When the curve is skewed, so that the data are distributed on the *geometric* mean, the distribution is usually *lognormal*. This is defined as a distribution that assumes the "normal" configuration after log transformation of the data. Such data are not analyzable in terms of standard deviation. Skewed distributions are not necessarily lognormal; they may be biphasic or other.

Quantitative data relating to normal and abnormal values will be presented frequently in this and following chapters. It can be assumed that data presented in terms of mean value and standard deviation are derived from normal distribution curves. When distribution is lognormal or not known, different calculations have been employed, or the 95% range will be presented. Special circumstances dealing with the group from which data are derived will be discussed when appropriate.

Standard deviation (SD, sigma, σ)

The shape of the gaussian curve gives a rough estimate of the degree of variation. A narrow, high curve suggests that the variation is small and the range narrow, whereas a wide, low curve indicates a wide variation. A more exact analysis can be made on the basis of the standard deviation (SD, sigma, or σ):

(1)
$$SD = \sqrt{\frac{\Sigma\ (\overline{X} - X)^2}{n - 1}}$$

where

SD = Standard deviation (sigma, σ)
$\overline{X}$ = Mean value
X = Individual value
N = Number of measurements

In other words, SD is equal to the square root of the sum of the squares of the differences between the mean and individual values, divided by one less than the total number of observations. In a normal distribution, ± 1 SD includes 68.27%, ± 2 SD includes 95.45%, and ± 3 SD includes 99.73% of all values. Therefore, if an observed value is within 2 SD of the mean, the chances for its occurrence are 19 out of 20. This is usually accepted as a reasonable measure of significance, so that most laboratory data are evaluated on the basis of a ± 2 SD provided that they fall on a normal distribution curve. Fewer normals will be excluded if the 3 SD range is used.

It cannot be emphasized too strongly that the concept of SD of the mean *applies only to normal distributions*. When

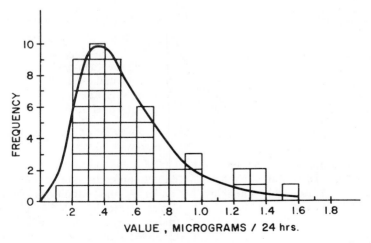

Fig. 7-3. Frequency distribution of values for urinary excretion of folinic acid in normal adults. (Data from O'Brien, 1960.)

applied to values distributed lognormally, weird and misleading conclusions will be drawn. Examples of this can be found in highly respected medical journals. Note the following striking misapplication of statistical analysis. The author measured the urinary excretion of folinic acid in the urine of normal adults and gave the following results: Range 0.19 to 1.60 μg/24 hours, mean 0.59 μg/24 hours, and 1 SD 0.47 μg. Now it is obvious that something is wrong, for 2 SD less than the mean gives a minus value. What is wrong is readily apparent if one plots the author's data for frequency distribution (Fig. 7-3). The curve is skewed to the left and of the lognormal type, and the analysis for SD does not apply.

Probable error (PE)

The expression probable error (PE) is also used and is defined as the value that, if added to or subtracted from the result obtained, will give a range of values such that the chances are even (1:1) that the range will include the true result. Since 1 PE includes 50% of the values, this corresponds to about ±0.67 SD (Fig. 7-1), and the relationship between PE and SD is

(2) $$1 \text{ PE} = 0.67449 \text{ SD}$$

Coefficient of variation (CV)

The coefficient of variation (CV) expresses the error in percent, according to the following formula:

(3) $$CV = \frac{SD}{\overline{X}} \times 100$$

where

CV = Coefficient of variation
SD = Standard deviation
$\overline{X}$ = Mean value

The CV expresses the error in percent of a set of values and is therefore useful when comparing the error or variation of two sets of dissimilar observations; e.g., it is difficult to compare the SD of "weight of adult males" and "erythrocyte count of normal males" since the first is expressed in pounds and the second in cells per cubic millimeter of blood. However, if the two CVs are compared, it is possible to decide which one of the two sets of data shows the greater variation of values.

ERROR OF THE ERYTHROCYTE COUNT
Hemocytometer method

The error of the erythrocyte count refers to the precision of the method, the variation obtained between counts performed on the same specimen of blood. Even though I suspect that there are now very few laboratories that depend on the hemocytometer method for blood cell counts, this discussion illustrates several statistical principles that bear on the interpretation of quantitative data. The inability to reproduce hemocytometer counts exactly is caused by variables introduced by human and technical errors.

Inherent errors

Errors inherent in the method are (1) the *field error*, (2) the *pipet error*, and (3) the *chamber error*.

The field error is unavoidable. It is caused by the random settling of cells when the specimen is placed in the hemocytometer. In settling the number of cells falling into each square varies. The magnitude of the field error may be reduced by counting more cells, but it cannot be eliminated. When 500 cells are counted, variations in distribution introduce a possible error of ±4%. Counting 1,000 cells reduces the variation to ±2.9%. Other errors inherent in the method are caused by inaccuracy of pipets and hemocytometers. It goes without saying that the best equipment possible must be used. Inexpensive pipets are often very inaccurate, and their use makes large errors unavoidable. I feel a guaranteed calibration of ±1% is the least that should be expected. Hemocytometers also vary in quality, but most have only small errors, particularly if the best quality coverslips are used.

The magnitude of the inherent errors was determined by Berkson et al (1940). They found that the three variables discussed added up to ±7% under the "standard" laboratory conditions existing at that time. The error could be estimated by:

(4) $$CV = \sqrt{\frac{(0.92 \times 100)^2}{n_b} + \frac{(4.6)^2}{n_c} \times \frac{(4.7)^2}{n_p}}$$

where

n_b = Cells *counted* (not the calculated count)
n_c = Number of chambers used
n_p = Number of pipets used
CV = Coefficient of variation

When one pipet is used to fill one side of the hemocytometer and the cells in ⅕ mm² are counted, 7% is obtained.

This formula indicates how the inherent errors may be minimized. It is obvious that the total error can be reduced by counting more cells, by using more than one pipet, and by counting the cells in more than one chamber; e.g., the error can be reduced by one or more of the following: (1) sampling in duplicate pipets, (2) filling two chambers separately with each, and (3) doubling the number of cells counted.

Technical and human errors

In addition to errors inherent in the method, errors are possible in sampling, in diluting and mixing the blood, and in filling the chamber from the pipet. There are also errors caused by human failure such as inaccuracy in counting or from unconscious bias. These errors may be considerable if the technical staff is unskilled.

Calculation of SD from control data—standard method

Table 7-1 shows the data and calculations necessary for determining the SD of the erythrocyte count performed under specified conditions. The data were obtained and analyzed as a class exercise in a course in clinical pathology given to sophomore medical students. The students had received about 2 weeks' training in hemocytometer counts. The equipment used represents a fair cross section of standard brands of pipets and hemocytometers.

Table 7-1. Calculation of SD for hemocytometer erythrocyte counts performed by medical students*

Count no.	Count (million)	Difference $(\overline{X} - X)$	Difference^2 $(\overline{X} - X)^2$
1	4.74	0.263	0.069169
2	4.23	0.247	0.061009
3	4.19	0.287	0.082369
—	—	—	—
—	—	—	—
—	—	—	—
—	—	—	—
50	4.18	0.297	0.088209
AVERAGE	4.477	TOTAL	3.30025

Calculation

1. The mean of 50 counts $(\overline{X})$ is 4.447 million.
2. The difference between each count and the mean is given in the third column $(\overline{X} - X)$.
3. Each difference is squared in the last column $(\overline{X} - X)^2$.
4. The sum of the squared differences is 3.30025.
5. Therefore:

$$SD = \sqrt{\frac{\Sigma (\overline{X} - X)^2}{n - 1}}$$

$$SD = \sqrt{\frac{3.30025}{49}} = \sqrt{0.067148} = 0.2591 \text{ million}$$

6. 1 SD = 259,100 cells/mm^3; 2 SD = 518,200 cells/mm^3.

*Class exercise in clinical pathology laboratory. Fifty counts were performed independently on the same specimen of oxalated blood by inexperienced sophomore medical students. Each used a different pipet and counting chamber. In each case cells were counted in five small squares ($\frac{1}{5}$ mm^2).

It will be noted that, with this inexperienced group, 1 SD amounts to 259,000 cells/mm^3 ($0.259 \times 10^{12}/1$). In other words, 67% of the counts fall within $\pm259,000$ cells of the mean (4,217,900 to 4,736,100), while 95% fall within $\pm518,200$ (3,959,000 to 4,995,000). Considering that these results include all errors from the initial sampling to the final counting and that the group was inexperienced, it seems justified to conclude that this is the degree of accuracy that can be expected under the least ideal conditions.

In order to compare this result with the $\pm7\%$ variation expected according to the formula of Berkson et al (1940) the CV can be calculated as follows using formula 3:

$$CV = \frac{SD}{\overline{X}} \times 100$$

where

CV = Coefficient of variation (in %)
SD = Standard deviation (σ)
$\overline{X}$ = Mean value

therefore

$$CV = \frac{0.259}{4.477} \times 100 = 5.8\%$$

When the same study was done using a group of skilled technologists, the results were significantly better. An SD of 167,000 cells was obtained, and the CV was $\pm3.7\%$. Blood-diluting pipets with a guaranteed calibration of 91%

were used since these are standard equipment in our laboratory. We feel that this SD and CV represent the actual accuracy of hemocytometer erythrocyte counts in our hematology laboratory.

Calculation of SD from control data—duplicate analysis method

A method has been advocated by Copeland (1957) that, although not as accurate as the standard, may be valuable because it is adaptable to the usual laboratory conditions and does not require elaborate planning. This method of "duplicates" requires only that duplicate counts or analyses be run on at least 20 routine specimens. The difference between the first and second of each pair of determinations is obtained, and the SD is calculated according to the following formula:

(5) $$SD = \sqrt{\frac{\text{Sum (differences)}^2}{2 \times \text{No. of pairs}}}$$

The chief disadvantage of this method is that the SD obtained is for the average value of the determinations, being somewhat higher than the true SD for the low values and lower for high ones; e.g., 20 different blood specimens may range from 68 to 176 mg of glucose per dl of blood. If the SD calculated by this method is 1.4, this is a little high when applied to values near 68 mg and low for values near 175 mg of glucose. The standard method also has a shortcomming in that the SD obtained applies only to the mean value and is different at values significantly higher or lower than the mean. The duplicate method of calculating SD is most useful therefore when the range of values is narrow.

The Coulter cell counter

There is no doubt that the development of electronic particle-counting instruments has restored the reputation of erythrocyte and leukocyte counts. Analysis of the performance of the Coulter counter indicates that errors can be reduced to a minimum. The apparatus is designed to count individual cells as they stream through a tiny opening. Information and instruction in use of the instrument is available from the manufacturer, and detailed studies of the performance of the system are reported by several authors (Mattern et al, 1957; Richar and Breakell, 1959; Brittin et al, 1968; Pinkerton et al, 1970; Bull et al, 1974).

To evaluate the accuracy with which the Coulter counter enumerates erythrocytes and leukocytes in our laboratory, a sample of normal venous blood was obtained by venipuncture, was anticoagulated and after thorough mixing, was divided into 10 portions. Using the Coulter counter, 20 erythrocyte counts and 20 leukocyte counts were done on each of the 10 samples, a total of 200 counts of each. Forty parallel chamber counts were also done. In order to evaluate the method under standard laboratory conditions, the samples were counted by various technologists, and a different pipet and dilution were used for each count.

The mean erythrocyte count using the Coulter method was 5.12 million/mm^3 ($5.12 \times 10^{12}/1$), range 4.87 to 5.35 million/mm^3 (4.87 to $5.35 \times 10^{12}/1$), and the SD 102,800 cells/mm^3 ($0.1028 \times 10^{12}/1$) of blood. The chamber counts showed a mean of 5.39 million/mm^3 ($5.39 \times 10^{12}/1$), range

Table 7-2. Precision of measurements with Coulter Model S*

Determination	Mean	±1 SD	CV (%)
Normal control			
Leukocyte count (cells/mm³)†	7,577	108	1.43
Erythrocyte count (cells/mm³)‡	4,798,790	41,000	0.85
Hemoglobin (Gm/dl)	13.62	0.1	0.73
Hematocrit (%)	40.2	0.34	0.85
MCV (fl)	83.8	0.43	0.51
MCH (pg)	28.34	0.25	0.88
MCHC (%)	33.68	0.31	0.92
Abnormal control			
Leukocyte count (cells/mm³)†	13,791	198	1.44
Erythrocyte count (cells/mm³)‡	3,091,090	29,859	0.97
Hemoglobin (Gm/dl)	8.86	0.07	0.79
Hematocrit (%)	26.09	0.27	1.03
MCV (fl)	83.85	0.52	0.62
MCH (pg)	28.90	0.43	1.49
MCHC (%)	33.98	0.38	1.12

*100 replicate measurements each on normal and abnormal hematology control material (Dade Reagents, Inc.).
†To convert to SI units: cells in thousands × 10⁹/1.
‡To convert to SI units: cells in millions × 10¹²/1.

Table 7-3. Precision of measurements with the Hemac Laser hematology counter*

Determination	Mean	±1 SD	CV (%)
Normal control			
Leukocyte count (cells/mm³)†	6,537	131.3	2.01
Erythrocyte count (cells/mm³)†	4,847,000	68,200	1.41
Hemoglobin (Gm/dl)	17.59	0.183	1.04
Hematocrit (%)	49.97	0.9	1.8
MCV (fl)	103.12	0.77	0.75
MCH (pg)	36.39	0.62	1.70
MCHC (%)	35.29	0.40	1.13
Abnormal control			
Leukocyte count (cells/mm³)†	14,406	195	1.35
Erythrocyte count (cells/mm³)†	2,998,000	38,700	1.29
Hemoglobin (Gm/dl)	10.02	0.10	1.0
Hematocrit (%)	30.55	0.447	1.46
MCV (fl)	101.6	0.72	0.71
MCH (pg)	33.36	0.53	1.59
MCHC (%)	32.8	0.57	1.74

*1,200 determinations, 100 per day, of Dade Reagents, Inc., normal and abnormal controls.
†See footnotes, Table 7-2.

of 4.49 to 5.75 million/mm³ (4.49 to 5.75 × 10¹²/1), and an SD of 195,000 cells/mm³/(0.195 × 10¹²/1) of blood. It should be noted that the difference between the lowest and highest count in the Coulter series is 0.48 million/mm³ (0.48 × 10¹²/1); in the hemocytometer series it is 1.36 million/mm³ (1.36 × 10¹²/1). The CV for erythrocyte counts performed with the Coulter counter is 2%.

The reproducibility of leukocyte counts was found to be affected by the quality and concentration of the saponin used. Under our conditions the mean value was 7,800 leukocytes/mm³ (7.8 × 10⁹/1) of blood; 1 SD was ±218 cells. This represents a CV of 2.8%. Note that it is slightly higher for the leukocyte count than for the erythrocyte count. However, both are well below coefficients derived from hemocytometer counts.

The accuracy and reproducibility of cell counts performed with the Coulter Model S were determined from 102 replicate successive counts on the same blood specimen. Analysis of the data is presented in Table 7-2.

The Hemac laser cell counter

The Hemac laser hematology counter (Ortho Instrument Division) is an electronic particle-counting apparatus that measures by direct count the red blood cell count and the white blood cell count. The blood hemoglobin concentration is determined spectrophotometrically as cyanmethemoglobin. The mean corpscular volume (MCV) is measured by an integrated threshold circuit. Like the Coulter S counter, the hematocrit, MCH, and MCHC are calculated automatically from the measured parameters. Unlike the Coulter S counter that counts particles as they move past a fixed aperture, the Hemac counts particles as they flow in a monolayer past a narrow laser beam.

We have evaluated the original Hemac apparatus with respect to precision, accuracy, sample interaction, and linearity. Later models of the Hemac are now available (Ortho ELT-8).

Precision was determined by performing 100 replicates of the same lot of normal and abnormal hematology control cells (Dade Reagents, Inc.) daily on 60 different days. The results are shown in Table 7-3. Precision is acceptable and is well within a CV of 2% generally considered acceptable for automated cell counters.

Accuracy was determined by simultaneously analyzing blood from 1,200 hospital patients by three methods: (1) by the Hemac cell counter, (2) by the Coulter S counter, and (3) by independent measurements (Coulter ZBI counter, manual microhematocrit, and manual hemoglobin by the standard cyanmethemoglobin method). The correlation coefficients in the WBC count comparing methods against each other were: (1) Hemac vs Coulter S: 0.994; (2) Hemac vs ZBI: 0.995; and (3) Coulter S vs ZBI: 0.996. For the RBC count the correlation coefficients were: (1) Hemac vs Coulter S: 0.994; (2) Hemac vs ZBI: 0.992; and (3) Coulter S vs ZBI: 0.997. For hemoglobin concentration the correlation coefficients were: (1) Hemac vs Coulter S: 0.997; (2) Hemac vs manual method: 0.994; and (3) Coulter S vs manual determination: 0.995. For hematocrit values the correlation coefficients were: (1) Hemac vs Coulter S: 0.975; (2) Hemac vs manual microhematocrit: 0.964; and (3) Coulter S vs manual microhematocrit: 0.991. For MCV determinations the correlation coefficient of Hemac vs Coulter S was 0.930. The various methods agree acceptably well with each other.

Sample interaction (carry-over) was determined using EDTA-anticoagulated fresh blood drawn from five donors with a known high hematocrit value (49% to 55%). For each, a low hematocrit sample was prepared (26% to 29%) by adding autologous plasma to whole blood, and the high hematocrit (H) and low hematocrit (L) samples were introduced into the Hemac counter. A sequence of H, H, H, H, H, L, L, L, L, L, H, H, H, H, H, etc. was followed until 55 values were obtained for each of the 5 blood samples. For the parameters (1) WBC, (2) RBC, (3) hemoglobin, and (4) hematocrit, the first high sample after the last low sample showed a maximum reduction of 0.04%, while the first low sample after the last high sample showed a maximum increase of 1%.

Linearity for RBC, hemoglobin, and hematocrit was determined by preparing 1:2, 1:4, and 1:8 dilutions of red blood cells with homologous plasma, using blood from five donors. Linearity of the WBC count was determined by making 1:2, 1:4, and 1:8 dilutions of donor bloods with group AB plasma. Plots of the results showed the data to be linear over the following ranges: WBC, 7,160 to 51,100/mm^3 (7.16 to 51.1. $\times 10^9/l$); RBC, 700,000 to 5,500,000/mm^3 (0.7 to 5.5 $\times 10^{12}/l$); hemoglobin, 2.45 to 20.51 Gm/dl; hematocrit, 6.5% to 48%.

SIGNIFICANCE OF SUCCESSIVE CELL COUNTS

The discussion so far has dealt with the significance of an erythrocyte count based on the total error of the determination. Of equal, if not greater, importance is a consideration of how to determine whether a second count, performed on the patient later, is significantly different from the first.

A useful rule of thumb is that the second count is probably significantly different if it differs by at least 2 SD; e.g., if the SD for erythrocyte counts in a given laboratory is 200,000, then the second erythrocyte count must be at least 400,000 greater or less than the first to be significant. A difference of 2 SD implies that the chances of the second being significantly different are about 20:1. The greater the difference, the nearer one approaches certainty.

The rule is probably sufficient for most purposes, requiring only that the laboratory make available to the physician the *determined* SD for a given procedure. It must be remembered that the SD is not the same for the full range of high to low values, being smaller when values are low and greater when values are high.

A more exact comparison of two values can be made if the SD of each is known. One of the probability theorems states that the SD *of the difference* (SD_{Diff}) between two independent values is equal to the square root of the sum of the squares of the individual SDs, as follows:

$$\text{(6)} \qquad SD_{Diff} = \sqrt{(SD_1)^2 + (SD_2)^2}$$

It has also been determined that the ratio $\dfrac{\text{Deviation}}{SD_{Diff}}$ expresses the probability of occurrence of such a deviation (or difference) between two values. According to Table 7-4 a ratio of 2.0 means that the odds are 20.98:1 against the occurrence of a difference as great as, or greater than, the one observed.

Significant difference between successive hemocytometer counts

The following formula can be applied to evaluate the significance of the difference between two successive cell counts when the hemocytometer is used:

$$\text{(7)} \qquad \frac{\text{Deviation}}{SD_{Diff}} = \frac{\text{Cells counted}_1 - \text{Cells counted}_2}{\sqrt{(SD_1)^2 + (SD_2)^2}}$$

Then, since the SD of each determination can be approximated by

$$\text{(8)} \qquad SD = \sqrt{n}$$

where n is the number of cells *counted* (not the calculated count), substitution of $\sqrt{n}$ for SD in formula 7 gives:

$$\text{(9)} \qquad \frac{\text{Deviation}}{SD_{Diff}} = \frac{\text{Cells counted}_1 - \text{Cells counted}_2}{\sqrt{\text{Cells counted}_1 + \text{Cells counted}_2}}$$

Note that in this calculation only the actual number of cells counted may be used, not the calculated count. Also, when two counts are compared, it is necessary to compare the cells counted in areas of identical size.

Example 1: A patient's erythrocyte count on admission was 4,000,000/mm^3 ($4.0 \times 10^{12}/l$) (400 cells counted). The next day a second erythrocyte count was 3,600,000 ($3.6 \times 10^{12}/l$) (360 cells counted). Has there been a significant change between the first and the second count?
Calculation:

$$\frac{\text{Deviation}}{SD_{Diff}} = \frac{400 - 360}{\sqrt{400 + 360}} = \frac{40}{\sqrt{760}} = \frac{40}{27.56} = 1.45$$

Therefore (from Table 7-4) the odds are only about 6:1 that the difference is not caused by chance. Since we have established a ratio of at least 2.0 (and odds of 20:1) as the minimum that is significant, we can say that the drop from 4,000,000 to 3,600,000 cells is probably not significant.

Example 2: A patient with an erythrocyte count of 3,500,000/mm^3 ($3.5 \times 10^{12}/l$) is given antianemic therapy and a few weeks later the count is 4,000,000/mm^3 ($4.0 \times 10^{12}/l$). Does this mean that the patient is definitely being helped by the prescribed therapy?
Calculation:

$$\frac{\text{Deviation}}{SD_{Diff}} = \frac{400 - 350}{\sqrt{400 + 350}} = \frac{50}{\sqrt{750}} = \frac{50}{27.38} = 1.82$$

Although the odds are about 13:1 that this is a significant change, it is not quite within the limits of 20:1.

Example 3: A patient with acute abdominal pain is admitted to the hospital with a leukocyte count of 12,000/mm^3 ($12 \times 10^9/l$). It is decided to wait and see if the leukocyte count rises before operating. A few hours later the leukocyte count is repeated and is then 13,500/mm^3 ($13.5 \times 10^9/l$). Is this a significant rise?
Calculation:

$$\frac{\text{Deviation}}{SD_{Diff}} = \frac{270 - 240}{\sqrt{270 + 240}} = \frac{30}{\sqrt{510}} = \frac{30}{22.58} = 1.33$$

The odds are only about 4:1; therefore the rise in the leukocyte count is probably not significant.

Example 4: A patient with thrombocytopenic purpura has a platelet count of 50,000/mm^3 ($0.05 \times 10^{12}/l$) (50 platelets counted

Table 7-4. Probability of occurrence of statistical deviations given the ratio $\dfrac{\text{Deviation}}{\text{SD}_{\text{Diff}}}$ of different magnitudes*†

$\dfrac{\text{Deviation}}{\text{SD}_{\text{Diff}}}$	Probable occurrence of deviation as great or greater than one designated (%)	Odds against occurrence of deviation as great or greater than one designated
0.67449	50.00	1.00:1
0.7	48.39	1.07:1
0.8	42.37	1.36:1
0.9	36.81	1.72:1
1.0	31.73	2.15:1
1.1	27.13	2.69:1
1.2	23.01	3.35:1
1.3	19.36	4.17:1
1.4	16.15	5.19:1
1.5	13.36	6.48:1
1.6	10.96	8.12:1
1.7	8.91	10.22:1
1.8	7.19	12.92:1
1.9	5.74	16.41:1
2.0	4.55	20.98:1
2.1	3.57	26.99:1
2.2	2.78	34.96:1
2.3	2.14	45.62:1
2.4	1.64	60.00:1
2.5	1.24	79.52:1
2.6	0.932	106.3:1
2.7	0.693	143.2:1
2.8	0.511	194.7:1
2.9	0.373	267.0:1
3.0	0.270	369.4:1

*From Pearl, 1941.

†The probability of occurrence, in percent, expresses the probability that a greater deviation will occur, and from this are calculated the odds against the occurrence; e.g., if the ratio $\dfrac{\text{Deviation}}{\text{SD}_{\text{Diff}}}$ is 2.0, a greater deviation can be expected to occur only 4.55% of the time, and the odds against such an occurrence are 20.98:1.

in two chambers). Following ACTH therapy the platelet count rises to 100,000/mm³ (0.10×10^{12}/1) (100 platelets counted). Is this a significant rise?

Calculation:

$$\frac{\text{Deviation}}{\text{SD}_{\text{Diff}}} = \frac{100 - 50}{\sqrt{100 + 50}} = \frac{50}{\sqrt{150}} = \frac{50}{12.24} = 4.1$$

Therefore the rise in the platelet count is significant.

These examples will serve to illustrate how formula 9 can be used to approximate the statistical significance of the difference between two hemocytometer counts. The calculation is not difficult, but for convenient reference the significant differences for erythrocyte counts, leukocyte counts, and platelet counts, as calculated by this method, are given in Tables 7-5 to 7-7. Note that the values given are for counts performed with a hemocytometer chamber and for which a specified area is counted. If the area counted is larger, the number of cells counted is also greater, and the required significant difference between two counts is then smaller.

Significant difference between successive electronic cell counts

Since formulas 7 to 9 are based on the number of cells counted in a chamber, they cannot be applied to electronic counts. For electronic counts an approximation of the sig-

nificant difference between two counts can be made by using the measured SD of the method, i.e., a count should be larger or smaller than the first by two standard deviations to be significantly different. The range of ± 2 SD is narrower for the Coulter S and Hemac counters (Tables 7-2 and 7-3) so that the estimated significant difference between successive counts is smaller. For example, if the first WBC count determined by the Hemac counter is 14,406/mm³ (14.4×10^9/1), the second is significantly different (odds of 20:1) if it is less than 14,000/mm³ (14×10^9/1) or greater than 14,800/mm³ (14.8×10^9/1).

NORMAL HEMATOLOGIC VALUES (RED BLOOD CELLS)

Some philosophers have argued that the concept of "good" would be meaningless unless contrasted to the concept of "evil." In laboratory medicine, likewise, there is no way to define "abnormal" without reference to the "normal." The definition of the limits of normality is essential for the interpretation of all data derived from the laboratory and the better the definition the more valid the physician's decision that disease is or is not present. Two questions concern us. First, we want to be reasonably certain that the laboratory data indicate that disease is present and, second, we want to be reasonably sure that we do not diagnose nondisease as disease (Miale, 1971).

The establishment of the normal for a given measurement

Table 7-5. Significant difference (20:1 odds) between two successive hemocytometer leukocyte counts based on cells counted in four large squares (4 mm^2; dilution 1:20)*

If first count is (thousand/mm^3)	Second count to be significantly different must be	
	Higher than (thousand/mm^3)	Lower than (thousand/mm^3)
1.0	1.8	0.5
1.4	2.3	0.75
1.8	2.75	1.0
2.2	3.25	1.38
2.6	3.7	1.65
3.0	4.2	2.0
3.4	4.7	2.35
3.8	5.15	2.65
4.2	5.65	3.0
4.6	6.3	3.25
5.0	6.6	3.65
5.4	7.2	4.0
5.8	7.5	4.4
6.2	7.95	4.7
6.6	8.4	5.2
7.0	8.8	5.4
7.4	9.25	5.75
7.8	9.7	6.1
8.2	10.15	6.5
8.6	10.75	6.9
9.0	11.0	7.2
9.4	11.45	7.5
9.8	11.95	7.9
10.2	12.4	8.25
10.6	12.85	8.6
11.0	13.2	9.0
12.0	14.3	9.9
13.0	15.3	10.0
14.0	16.6	11.8
16.0	18.7	13.5
20.0	23.0	17.2
25.0	28.4	22.0
30.0	33.8	26.5
40.0	44.0	36.0

*Calculations based on formula 9, p. 373.

Table 7-6. Significant difference (20:1 odds) between two successive hemocytometer erythrocyte counts based on cells counted in 80 small squares (1/5 mm^2; dilution 1:200)*

If first count is (million/mm^3)	Second count to be significantly different must be	
	Higher than (million/mm^3)	Lower than (million/mm^3)
1.0	1.31	0.73
1.2	1.53	0.9
1.4	1.76	1.08
1.6	1.98	1.26
1.8	2.2	1.43
2.0	2.42	1.62
2.2	2.65	1.7
2.4	2.85	1.98
2.6	3.1	2.15
2.8	3.3	2.35
3.0	3.5	2.52
3.2	3.72	2.7
3.4	3.95	2.9
3.6	4.18	3.08
3.8	4.38	3.25
4.0	4.6	3.45
4.2	4.8	3.65
4.4	5.0	3.8
4.6	5.25	4.0
4.8	5.45	4.2
5.0	5.65	4.38
5.2	5.87	4.58
5.4	6.1	4.75
5.6	6.4	4.95
5.8	6.55	5.13
6.0	6.75	5.3

*Calculations based on formula 9, p. 373.

Table 7-7. Significant difference (20:1 odds) between two successive platelet counts based on cells counted in two chambers (2 mm^2; dilution 1:200; phase microscopy)*

If first count is (platelets/mm^3)	Second count to be significantly different must be	
	Higher than (platelets/mm^3)	Lower than (platelets/mm^3)
10,000	20,000	8,400
20,000	35,000	10,000
40,000	60,000	24,000
60,000	84,000	40,000
100,000	130,000	73,000
150,000	188,000	118,000
200,000	243,000	160,000
250,000	297,000	208,000
300,000	352,000	252,000
350,000	407,000	298,000
400,000	458,000	343,000
500,000	568,000	440,000
600,000	675,000	530,000

*Calculations based on formula 9, p. 373.

depends on the accuracy and precision of the methodology and on the criteria used to define a healthy normal person. When the precision and accuracy of the methodology are not good, the range of normal values for a normal population will be greater than it would be if determined by a more precise and accurate method. For example, the range of the normal erythrocyte count is wider when established by hemocytometer counts having a CV of about 7% than when established by properly calibrated electronic cell counters having a CV of about 2%. Likewise the range of normal for blood hemoglobin concentration is narrower since the adoption of the cyanmethemoglobin standard. For these reasons summaries of normal values, some determined as long ago as the 1940s and found in the *Handbook of Clinical Laboratory Data* (Faulkner et al, 1968), the *Biology Data Book* (Altman and Dittmer, 1964), and in *Standard Values in*

Blood (Albritton, 1940), are chiefly of historical interest. An additional technical variable is whether the venous blood samples are collected with or without stasis, since stasis produces hemoconcentration and higher hematologic values (Garby, 1970).

The definition of a "healthy normal" person should also be considered carefully. Most investigators use "random, apparently healthy subjects." Some use subjects who either have been on supplementary iron (Garby et al, 1969; Garby, 1970) or who are shown to be adequately nourished from the erythropoietic point of view based on the serum iron concentration, saturation of transferrin, and serum folate and vitamin B_{12} concentration (Viteri et al, 1972). Normal values derived from the latter group, using acceptable methodology, are undoubtedly the most valid.

Statistical determination of normal values

When I was a house officer many years ago, our most prized possession was a pocket loose-leaf notebook containing, for example, "routine orders," "special procedures,"

and "normal values." These were diligently copied by new interns and eventually passed on like a legacy to incoming house officers. In later years, as I became involved in laboratory medicine, both practicing and teaching, I found students receptive to a redefinition of "normality." This change was encouraged to a great extent by the inclusion in the medical curriculum of a designated course in laboratory medicine and especially by laboratory exercises. In recent years the vogue in designing "new" medical curricula has effectively eliminated from most medical schools structured instruction in the interpretation of laboratory data. The new house officer learns it from his seniors, not unlike the loose-leaf notebook of my time. Unfortunately, this is sometimes the proctorship of the unlearned to those only somewhat more knowledgeable. Furthermore, tests are "ordered," as one would order groceries, and this fosters the attitude that abnormal results should be "flagged" so that the clinician does not overlook them.

It is generally agreed that each laboratory shall, except for highly specialized procedures, determine its own normal

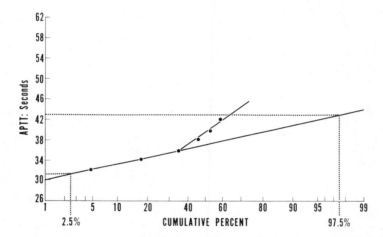

Fig. 7-4. The use of normal probability paper to determine the mean and the upper and lower 2.5% limits for a set of data. The data plotted here are the same as for Fig. 7-5.

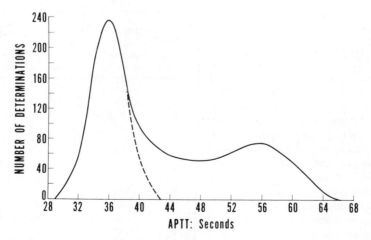

Fig. 7-5. Frequency distribution curves for 1,393 consecutive APTT values obtained on hospitalized patients. The strikingly skewed distribution is attributed to values from patients receiving therapy. The normal curve is fitted by eye.

values. The pathologist in charge can plead the need for time and personnel assigned to this function, but it is a function that rarely receives special support, even though such data are needed to interpret test data and thus to provide good medical care. In fact, I estimate that about 5% of overall laboratory function assigned to this activity is barely sufficient. If an additional 10% or more is dedicated to quality control programs, we see that special provisions must be made—time, space, and funds—lest these necessary functions be slighted in favor of "getting the work out."

Selection of the method for calculating normal values depends in part on the selection of the population. Ideally the values should be determined for a population as "normal" as possible and as homogeneous as possible with regard to age, sex, and any other parameters that can affect the test in question. It is probably not realistic to aim for sets matched completely for all the variables and yet any compromise is open to criticism. If a group of supposedly ambulatory subjects is used, it can be argued that some of their values do not apply to hospitalized patients (Barnett, 1966) or to patients seen in a busy clinic or emergency room. If one analyzes data from hospitalized patients, it is difficult to consider these subjects as normal, regardless of how the data are manipulated. Each approach is useful, nevertheless.

If normal values are determined for an apparently healthy, normal ambulatory population, either encompassing a broad age group or, if possible, subdivided into subgroups according to age and sex, each group should consist of no less than 40 subjects. The statistical analysis is simple. First, determine by plotting a frequency distribution curve whether the curve is symmetric (normal) or skewed (lognormal) (p. 369). If it is approximately symmetric, the standard deviation is calculated according to formula 1 (p. 368). Values falling within $+2$ and -2 SD represent 95.45% of the population, and the highest and lowest 2.27% are excluded. If the range of $+3$ to -3 SD is used, then 99.73% of the values are included. If we use ± 2 SD as the normal range, 5% of normal individuals will fall outside the range, whereas using a range of ± 3 SD excludes only 0.36% of the highest or lowest values. Barnett (1979) recommends establishing the ± 3 SD range, recalculating the SD of these values, and then taking as the normal range ± 2 SD of the recalculated values.

If the curve is skewed, and unfortunately, most biologic data give a skewed plot (Flynn et al, 1974), four approaches are possible. The simplest approach is to eliminate the upper and lower 2.5% of values and to take the 95% range as being normal (Golob, 1960). This approach is not valid if the curve is markedly skewed but is applicable to curves that are slightly skewed. The second approach is to assume that the distribution is lognormal, although a skewed curve need not be lognormal, and to use a lognormal transformation whereby values are arranged by classes, each having the same range of values and the log of the midpoint of each class plotted on plain paper. After the transformation the plot is treated as a normal curve. The third method is probably the best, since it does not assume a lognormal distribution. This uses normal probability graph paper, as shown in Fig. 7-4. The fourth analysis described by Hoffman (1971) is very useful when determining normal values using data obtained

from hospitalized patients. Frequency distribution plots of such data are usually skewed markedly to the right or biphasic, indicating two populations, one normal and one abnormal. A normal curve can be fitted to the plot, and then the normal range can be established from the normal curve (Fig. 7-5). In the sample shown here for the activated partial thromboplastin time (APTT) test, the values obtained from the fitted curve correspond with those obtained in a separate study from normal laboratory personnel and students. This method is useful in a hospital setting, particularly when a computer is available, because it is recommended that at least 600 determinations be used for each plot. It has the added advantage that the statistical analysis can be performed for subgroups, for example, segregated as to age or sex, provided that each group consists of at least 600 determinations.

Normal values

Normal values from our laboratory are given in Table 7-8. In general there is good agreement among laboratories using electronic cell counters and the cyanmethemoglobin standard for the determination of hemoglobin concentration (Dallman and Siimes, 1979). It should be noted that the 95% range, equivalent to ± 2 SD if the distribution is normal, still excludes 5% of normal individuals. The probability of abnormality is increased if a given value falls between the second and the third SD (Schoen and Brooks, 1970; Dutcher, 1971; Miale, 1971).

As Viteri et al (1972) point out, there is probably no significant difference in normal values for persons residing in tropical areas. The question of differences because of race probably depends on the definition of "normal." Our original survey of hematologic values in the southern Florida area showed a significant difference between Whites and Blacks, the latter averaging about 500,000 red cells/mm³ less than the Whites. A like difference between Whites and Blacks in North Carolina was found by Barkley et al (1965), but the same authors found no significant difference in the hemoglobin level between Black soldiers and White soldiers, both levels being higher in fact than for nonmilitary men and women. It is likely that subclinical nutritional deficiencies account for the racial differences, in which case such persons cannot be considered hematologically normal. The data of Schmaier et al (1974) and of Dallman et al (1978b) show that apparently normal Black children have somewhat lower values for erythrocyte parameters than those given in Table 7-8. However, I know of no study in which a racial difference has been found in hematologicallly normal persons as defined by Viteri et al (1972). It goes without saying that one cannot assume that "apparently normal" individuals are hematologically normal. It might be expected that young ahtletes participating in the Olympic games would be hematologically normal, and yet Clement et al (1977) have shown that both male and female athletes participating in the 1976 Olympics had hemoglobin levels lower than those for the general Canadian population.

Physiologic variations

It has been said that erythrocyte counts show certain physiologic variations such as diurnal fluctuation and variations

Table 7-8. Normal values for the red blood cell compartment of "apparently healthy" subjects, White and Black*

Subjects	HGB (Gm/dl)	RBC (millions/mm³†)	HCT (%)	MCV (fl‡)	MCH (pg§)	MCHC (%)
Adult men	15.1 (13.9-16.3)	5.1 (4.3-5.9)	47 (39-55)	90 (80-100)	30 (25.4-34.6)	34 (31-37)
Adult women	13.5 (12.0-15.0)	4.5 (3.5-5.5)	42 (36-48)	88 (79-98)	30 (25.4-34.6)	33 (30-36)
Boys						
Birth	20.0 (18.5-21.5)	5.6 (5.0-6.3)	59 (53-65)	105 (95-115)	36 (30-42)	33 (32-34)
1 month	17.0 (15.5-18.5)	5.2 (4.7-5.9)	50 (44-56)	101 (92-110)	36 (30-42)	32 (31-33)
3 months	15.0 (13.5-16.5)	4.5 (3.8-5.2)	45 (39-52)	100 (92-110)	33 (28-38)	33 (32-34)
6 months	14.0 (13.0-16.0)	4.6 (3.8-5.1)	46 (39-51)	100 (92-109)	30 (27-34)	30 (29-31)
9 months	13.0 (12.0-14.0)	4.6 (3.7-5.2)	45 (39-52)	97 (90-104)	28 (24-32)	28 (27-30)
1 year	12.1 (10.0-14.0)	4.2 (3.5-4.9)	41 (37-45)	95 (87-98)	27 (24-32)	29 (28-30)
2 years	12.3 (10.5-14.2)	4.2 (3.5-5.9)	40 (36-47)	88 (80-95)	28 (24-32)	30 (28-31)
4 years	12.6 (11.2-14.3)	4.2 (3.7-5.0)	37 (30-44)	89 (80-96)	28 (24-32)	28 (27-29)
8 years	13.4 (12.0-14.8)	4.6 (4.0-5.1)	41 (37-45)	87 (80-94)	29 (23-34)	29 (28-30)
14 years	14.0 (12.5-15.0)	4.7 (3.9-5.3)	41 (36-46)	88 (80-95)	29 (23-34)	30 (29-31)
Girls						
Birth	19.5 (18.0-21.0)	5.6 (5.0-6.3)	58 (51-65)	103 (94-114)	34 (28-40)	34 (33-35)
1 month	17.0 (15.8-18.9)	5.2 (4.7-6.0)	49 (42-56)	102 (92-112)	36 (30-42)	32 (31-33)
3 months	14.8 (13.3-16.4)	4.4 (3.8-5.2)	44 (39-51)	104 (92-112)	33 (27-39)	33 (32-34)
6 months	13.8 (12.8-14.8)	4.2 (3.5-4.9)	44 (39-50)	100 (91-109)	30 (25-35)	32 (31-33)
9 months	12.8 (11.7-13.9)	4.2 (3.5-4.9)	43 (37-50)	98 (90-105)	28 (23-34)	30 (29-31)
1 year	12.2 (10.0-14.0)	4.2 (3.4-5.0)	43 (37-49)	95 (87-100)	27 (22-30)	30 (29-31)
2 years	12.2 (10.5-14.2)	4.2 (3.5-5.0)	43 (36-50)	94 (86-101)	27 (22-30)	30 (29-31)
4 years	12.7 (11.3-14.2)	4.4 (3.8-5.2)	43 (36-51)	88 (80-95)	28 (23-31)	28 (27-29)
8 years	13.0 (11.5-14.5)	4.5 (3.9-5.1)	40 (36-46)	89 (80-96)	29 (23-33)	28 (27-29)
14 years	13.2 (11.6-14.8)	4.5 (3.8-5.2)	40 (36-47)	87 (80-94)	29 (23-33)	29 (28-30)

*Values represent the mean and 95% range. Data from Coulter S or Hemac cell counters.
†To convert to SI units: millions × $10^{12}/1$.
‡fl is new symbol for cubic microns (μ^3).
§pg is new symbol for micromicrograms ($\mu\mu$g). To convert to SI units (fmol): pg × 0.0155.

after food intake. Statistical analysis of the data from which these conclusions were drawn shows that the differences observed are probably not significant. Actually only six factors have a *statistically* significant effect on the erythrocyte count: (1) posture, (2) extreme physical exercise or excitement, (3) severe dehydration, (4) age, (5) sex, and (6) altitude.

Posture

Several investigators have found that values for some blood constituents are significantly lower if blood is drawn after the subject has been in a recumbent posture. Tombridge (1968) found hemoglobin and hematocrit values to be 5.7% lower in the recumbent position than in the upright position. The difference in anemic subjects is even larger.

Exercise or excitement

Although moderate mental and physical activity has no significant effect on the erythrocyte count, extreme physical exertion or excitement does produce counts significantly higher than those obtained under basal conditions. Counts obtained under conditions of extreme excitement may be of doubtful clinical value. Although excitement is seldom an important factor in adults, it is important in children.

Dehydration

Severe hemoconcentration can produce erythrocyte counts that are higher than the true one. In adults this is seen

only in extreme conditions such as severe burns, untreated intestinal obstruction, severe vomiting, or persistent vomiting in pregnancy. In children, on the other hand, fluid and electrolyte balance is easily upset, and hemoconcentration is not an uncommon phenomenon. Hemoconcentration may obscure a significant anemia.

Age

The normal erythrocyte count of the newborn infant is higher than that of the adult. The average erythrocyte count in newborn infants is 5.7 million/mm³ ($5.7 \times 10^{12}/1$), but counts above 6 million are not unusual. The count drops rapidly after birth, reaching its lowest values between the second and fourth months of life. A gradual rise is then noted, the normal adult level being reached at 14 years of age. This level is maintained until old age, at which time there is usually a gradual drop (Vellar, 1967) caused in part by deficient iron intake.

Sex

Women have a lower erythrocyte count than men, but there is no significant difference before puberty or in old age. It is possible that the difference reflects the inhibitory effect of estrogen on erythropoiesis (Chapter 1).

Altitude

Residents at high altitudes normally have higher erythrocyte counts and hemoglobin levels than those at sea level.

There is a moderate but significant difference between normal persons residing at an altitude of 0 to 750 m as compared to the group residing at 751 to 1,500 m. The higher the altitude, the less will be the oxygen tension; the resultant hypoxia stimulates erythropoiesis (Rørth, 1974). If a resident at sea level quickly ascends to a high altitude, he may at first suffer from hypoxia, with symptoms such as dizziness, weakness, and shortness of breath. Within a few days reticulocytosis is noted, followed by a gradual increase in the erythrocyte count and hemoglobin concentration. After a few months the count may reach polycythemic levels. This type of polycythemia is secondary to hypoxia and is more properly called *erythrocytosis,* as distinguished from the primary disease *erythremia* or *polycythemia vera,* which is not caused by residence at a high altitude.

Pugh (1964) studied a group of subjects at sea level and, later, after a stay at altitudes varying from 13,000 to 19,000 feet. At first he found a mean reduction in blood volume of 9%, but later the blood volume returned to normal or higher than normal values. The hemoglobin concentration showed a progressive rise to a mean of 49% above the sea level values. Erythrocytosis caused by high altitude is accompanied by an increased total erythrocyte mass. Within about a month after returning to sea level, a patient with this type of erythrocytosis will usually show a return to the normal erythrocyte count.

Erythrocytosis at high altitudes is due to the stimulatory effect of hypoxia on erythropoietin (Chapter 1). There also occurs an increase in red cell 2,3-DPG (Lenfant et al, 1968). It has been suggested that the observed shift to the right of the oxygen dissociation curve is not entirely because of the 2,3-DPG effect, but also because of alkalosis (Lenfant et al, 1971).

Erythrocyte indices

The values for erythrocyte count, hemoglobin concentration, and hematocrit can be used to obtain certain erythrocyte indices that define the size and hemoglobin content of the erythrocyte and are useful as indices for a preliminary evaluation of anemia, primarily that secondary to iron deficiency (Griner and Oranburg, 1978).

A number of ratios have been proposed, such as color index (CI) and saturation index (SI). These are based on an arbitrary figure for normal hemoglobin and erythrocyte counts and have been responsible for the erroneous concept that erythrocytes may be hyperchromic. On the other hand, there is some merit to the short-cut method of calculating color index for rapid evaluation of a given erythrocyte count and hemoglobin value.

$$(10) \qquad CI = \frac{Hb \ (Gm/dl)}{RBC \ (in \ millions) \times 3}$$

This is merely an estimate based on the formula for mean corpuscular hemoglobin. The normal color index is 0.9 to 1.1.

Wintrobe's (1934) indices, *mean corpuscular volume* (MCV), *mean corpuscular hemoglobin* (MCH), and *mean corpuscular hemoglobin concentration* (MCHC), have generally replaced the other ratios. The range of normal values given by Wintrobe was based on a relatively small number of samples and on methodology (measurement of hemoglobin concentration, determination of hematocrit, and erythrocyte counting) that has been changed and refined in more recent years. This subject is reviewed by Dutcher (1971), and the normal values given in Table 7-8 generally agree with those proposed by him and by Silver and Frankel (1971).

Mean corpuscular volume (MCV)

For many years intensive efforts were made to describe the erythrocyte regarding size. The various methods were discussed in Ponder's monograph (1948), but most of them are too elaborate and time-consuming to be used routinely. Recent advances in electronic sizing answer this criticism. When the diameters of a large number of erythrocytes are determined and plotted as to frequency, a typical distribution curve is obtained (Price-Jones distribution curve). The mean diameter measured from dried smears is 7.3 to 7.5 μ. If there is microcytosis or macrocytosis, the distribution curve is shifted to one side or the other, with a corresponding shift in the mean diameter. In cases in which there is a marked difference in the size of the erythrocytes (anisocytosis), the curve has a broader base than normal. When two peaks are found, they indicate a population of two kinds of erythrocytes.

According to Wintrobe, the MCV may be estimated by applying the following formula:

$$(11) \qquad MCV = \frac{Hematocrit \times 10}{Erythrocyte \ count \ (millions/mm^3)}$$

The result expresses the mean volume in cubic microns. Normal erythrocytes have a mean MCV of 90 fl (new symbol for μ^3), 1 SD = 5. Results below 80 (2 SD) and 75 (3 SD) indicate a smaller than normal MCV, i.e., the erythrocytes are, on an average, *microcytic.* Similarly, an MCV above 100 (2 SD) and 105 (3 SD) indicates that the erythrocytes are *macrocytic.*

It is imperative to interpret the value for MCV along with a careful inspection of the peripheral blood smear since the MCV is only a *mean* volume measurement. It is possible, for example, to have a wide variation in cell size, from cells that are microcytic to some that are macrocytic, and still have an MCV within the normal range. This may be true if there is a large number of reticulocytes in the peripheral blood, since reticulocytes usually have a larger volume than adult cells. At times erythrocytes should also be examined in the fresh state, for only then can abnormal forms be readily identified. In sickle cell and other anemias characterized by an abnormal erythrocyte shape, the MCV is of doubtful value since the hematocrit is not reliable. The MCV is usually higher than normal in the newborn and infant (Table 7-8).

Mean corpuscular hemoglobin (MCH)

The MCH is an expression in absolute units of the average weight of hemoglobin contained in an erythrocyte. It is calculated according to the following formula:

$$(12) \qquad MCH = \frac{Hb \ (Gm/dl) \times 10}{Erythrocyte \ count \ (millions/mm^3)}$$

The result gives the average content of hemoglobin per erythrocyte in picograms, pg (replaces the old units, micro-micrograms, or Gm $\times 10^{-12}$). It is higher in newborns and infants since their MCV is generally higher than in adults. For the same reason high MCH values are obtained in uncomplicated macrocytic anemias. At times macrocytic anemia will be accompanied by deficient hemoglobin synthesis, in which case normal, or even low, values for the MCH may be obtained. This may be seen in pernicious anemia after treatment when, as the erythrocyte count rises, hemoglobin synthesis may not be sufficient to keep up with the rapid formation of erythrocytes. The result will be erythrocytes, deficient in hemoglobin, that are both macrocytic (high MCV) and hypochromic (low MCH). MCH values are consistently below normal in anemias of the iron-deficiency type and may be as low as 20 pg.

Mean corpuscular hemoglobin concentration (MCHC)

Whereas mean corpuscular hemoglobin represents the mean weight of hemoglobin per erythrocyte, MCHC expresses the mean *concentration* of hemoglobin in each erythrocyte. It is calculated according to the following formula:

(13) $$\text{MCHC} = \frac{\text{Hb (Gm/dl)} \times 100)}{\text{Hematocrit}}$$

The result is in percent. Values in the newborn and other infants are not significantly higher than normal, even though the MCV and MCH are usually higher than normal. The normal erythrocyte already contains all the hemoglobin molecules it can, making a higher than normal hemoglobin concentration impossible. On the other hand, regardless of erythrocyte size, the cell may have a low hemoglobin concentration, indicating that such a cell is *hypochromic*.

Use of erythrocyte indices

The erythrocyte indices, in conjunction with the appearance of the erythrocytes on fixed smears, yield an accurate picture of erythrocyte morphology.

Example 1: Erythrocytes 4.5 million/mm³ (4.5 $\times 10^{12}$/1), Hb 13.5 Gm/dl, hematocrit 40%

$$\text{MCV} = \frac{40 \times 10}{4.5} = 89 \text{ fl}$$

$$\text{MCH} = \frac{13.5 \times 10}{4.5} = 30 \text{ pg}$$

$$\text{MCHC} = \frac{13.5 \times 100}{40} = 33.8\%$$

Therefore the erythrocytes are normal in size (*normocytic*) and contain a normal concentration of hemoglobin (*normochromic*).

Example 2: Erythrocytes 4.5 million/mm³ (4.5 $\times 10^{12}$/1), Hb 11.5 Gm/dl, hematocrit 40%

$$\text{MCV} = \frac{40 \times 10}{4.5} = 89 \text{ fl}$$

$$\text{MCH} = \frac{11.5 \times 10}{4.5} = 25.5 \text{ pg}$$

$$\text{MCHC} = \frac{11.5 \times 100}{40} = 28.8\%$$

Therefore the erythrocytes are normal in size (*normocytic*) but contain less hemoglobin than normal. The low MCHC shows them to be *hypochromic*.

Example 3: Erythrocytes 4.5 million/mm³ (4.5 $\times 10^{12}$/1), Hb 10 Gm/dl, hematocrit 32%

$$\text{MCV} = \frac{32 \times 10}{4.5} = 71 \text{ fl}$$

$$\text{MCH} = \frac{10.0 \times 10}{4.5} = 22.2 \text{ pg}$$

$$\text{MCHC} = \frac{10.0 \times 100}{32} = 31.2\%$$

Therefore the erythrocytes are smaller than normal (*microcytic*) and contain less than the normal weight of hemoglobin. Since the MCHC is low, they are also *hypochromic*.

Example 4: Erythrocyte count 2.2 million/mm³ (2.2 $\times 10^{12}$/1), Hb 7.5 Gm/dl, hematocrit 25%

$$\text{MCV} = \frac{25 \times 10}{2.2} = 114 \text{ fl}$$

$$\text{MCH} = \frac{7.5 \times 10}{2.2} = 34 \text{ pg}$$

$$\text{MCHC} = \frac{7.5 \times 100}{25} = 30\%$$

Therefore the erythrocytes are larger than normal (*macrocytic*). Although they contain a larger than normal weight of hemoglobin, the MCHC is normal. The cells are therefore *normochromic*.

Example 5: Erythrocyte count 2.2 million/mm³ (2.2 $\times 10^{12}$/1), Hb 5 Gm/dl, hematocrit 25%

$$\text{MCV} = \frac{25 \times 10}{2.2} = 114 \text{ fl}$$

$$\text{MCH} = \frac{5 \times 10}{2.2} = 22.8 \text{ pg}$$

$$\text{MCHC} = \frac{5 \times 100}{25} = 20\%$$

As in example 4, these erythrocytes are *macrocytic*. However, the MCHC is lower than normal; therefore they are also *hypochromic*.

In summary, the determination of the MCV, MCH, and MCHC gives valuable information that helps to characterize erythrocytes. According to the MCV, erythrocytes may be classified as normal (normocytic), small (microcytic), or large (macrocytic). According to the MCHC erythrocytes may be normal (normochromic) or deficient (hypochromic). A higher than normal hemoglobin concentration does not occur except in some cases of hereditary spherocytosis. MCH expresses only the mean weight of hemoglobin per erythrocyte.

Erythrocyte indices calculated by electronic counters

The Coulter Model S counter and the Hemac laser counter measure RBC, hemoglobin, and MCV and from these measurements calculate hematocrit, MCH, and MCHC. The accuracy of the calculated indices obviously depends on the accuracy of the primary measurements.

QUALITY ASSURANCE IN HEMATOLOGY
Introduction

The term "quality control," in common usage, means a system of internal control on the quality of a product, whether it be a manufactured product or an analytic result. In fact, it is better to think in terms of "quality assurance." For example, a very elaborate system of quality control can be set up, with a faithful and detailed record of control data, but unless these data are used to guarantee that a bad product is not given to the consumer, a quality control program is no more than an exercise in record keeping. Quality assurance, then, is derived from quality control programs when quality control data are applied properly.

It follows, then, that a good and effective program consists of two essential parts: the quality control systems proper from which data are derived indicating whether the procedure is "in control" or "not in control," and the prompt action taken when the procedure is "not in control" to prevent the erroneous results from being reported and the steps taken to correct the problem. Implicit in the total program is an immediate, almost minute-by-minute, availability of control data in the area or at the instrument where the analysis is being performed, which provides both a prompt estimate of "in control" or "not in control" and the assignment of responsibility for taking appropriate action. An unacceptable program is one in which an acceptably complete program generates data duly recorded but not evaluated promptly so that appropriate action is not taken as soon as it should be.

It should be self-evident, then, that when an analysis is found to be "not in control," the results obtained after the last "in control" status are void and the problem must be identified and corrected before the results are again considered valid. This guarantees that the quality control program provides quality assurance.

Every laboratory procedure should be quality controlled. In this section only the more commonly used tests are discussed. Detailed discussions of many aspects of quality control in hematology can be found in Lewis and Koster (1975) and Barnett (1979).

It must be noted also that in addition to programs designed to check specific instruments, all laboratory equipment should be checked periodically to ensure proper performance. Examples are: (1) the temperature of all refrigerators should be maintained at $4° \pm 2°\,C$, (2) the rotation velocity of all centrifuges should be checked with a stroboscope, (3) the temperature of water baths should be within $\pm 1°\,C$ of the desired temperature, and (4) reagents and solutions should be labeled as to date of purchase or preparation, expiration date if applicable, initialled by the technologist who prepared them, and stored under appropriate conditions. Of a different category, but of great importance, is clerical quality control to ensure proper identification of specimens, proper processing, and accurate reporting and charting of results.

Quality control programs are sometimes said to be "expensive," but in the long run quality assurance guarantees, as far as is humanly possible, that an erroneous result does not leave the laboratory, for this is potentially an even more expensive, if not dangerous, situation for the patient.

Coulter Model S

1. Instrument maintenance is important. The procedures for preventive maintenance, proper use of the instrument, and troubleshooting are detailed fully by the manufacturer and need not be repeated here.
2. Calibration
   a. Ideally, the instrument should be calibrated with fresh whole blood collected in dry EDTA anticoagulant, the values being determined by independent manual or automated technics.
      (1) RBC, counted in the Coulter ZBI
      (2) WBC, counted in the Coulter ZBI
      (3) Hemoglobin, manually, replicate measurements using the cyanmethemoglobin method
      (4) Hematocrit, manually, using the microhematocrit technic. Note that the hematocrit from the Coulter S is lower than the manual microhematocrit by a factor of 0.94 (Coulter S hematocrit = 0.94 × microhematocrit). The "corrected" hematocrit figure is used for calibrating the Coulter S. The manual hematocrit figure cannot be used without correction, because this would give false values for the red cell constants.
   b. If a ZBI instrument is not available for independent measurement of WBC and RBC counts, the instrument is calibrated with the manufacturer's 4C Hematology Control for the cell counts and with manual hemoglobin and hematocrit measurements as in *a* above. Hemocytometer cell counts are not used for calibration because the inherent error of 5% to 7% is too large for a calibration method.
      (1) After the instrument is operating per manufacturer's recommendations, the instrument is cycled 4 times with Isoton.
      (2) A random blood sample is run through 4 to 6 times to prime the instruments. These values are discarded.
      (3) The bottle of 4C Control is brought to room temperature, if necessary, and rotated on the Ames aliquot mixer for 10 minutes. Several times during this mixing, the bottle is removed from the mixer and rotated briskly between the palms of both hands to ensure that no cells adhere to the sides of the bottle.
      (4) A sample of the well-mixed 4C Control is run through, and the values given by the manufacturer are used to calibrate for WBC, RBC, hemoglobin, and hematocrit.
      (5) The calibration of hemoglobin and hematocrit is checked by comparing them with manual methods.
3. Day-to-day quality control
   a. After the instrument is operating in the morning, 4 samples of Isoton are run through. At the fourth sample, the results are recorded to check the RBC and WBC background count.
   b. Background counts of no more than 20,000 RBC and 400 WBC are acceptable. If background counts exceed these values, clean with Clorox reagent and

repeat washing with Isoton until acceptable values are obtained. If high background values persist, it is probably because of foreign particles in the Isoton.

c. The instrument is primed by running a blood sample through 4 times. These values are not recorded.

d. Several assayed blood samples, saved from the previous day and brought to room temperature, are run through. The values are recorded and compared with the previous day's values. If these check, proceed to check calibration with 4C Control. If only one parameter does not check and no problem is detected by visual inspection of the chambers and tubing, the 4C Control is run through and the one parameter recalibrated according to the 4C value. If several parameters do not check, the entire initial calibration procedure must be performed again.

e. The 4C Control is run through and the results recorded. With each lot the manufacturer supplies the mean value, the standard deviation, the CV, and the acceptable range. If the obtained values for the 7 parameters fall within the recommended acceptable limits, the instrument is in control and patient samples can be run through.

f. Within a day's run the instrument is checked two to three times by one or both of the following procedures: (1) check values of 4C Control or (2) check assayed blood samples saved from earlier in the day. If either or both of these items give acceptable checks the instrument is still "in control."

g. At any time that the instrument has been shut off, cleaned, or rinsed with Isoton, a blood sample is run through 4 times to "prime" the instrument before the first patient or control sample is counted.

h. The hemoglobin and hematocrit calibration is checked daily by replicate manual methods.

i. WBC counts below $4,000/mm^3$ ($4 \times 10^9/l$) and above $30,000/mm^3$ ($30 \times 10^9/l$) are rechecked as recommended by the manufacturer. WBC counts are unreliable in cases of chronic lymphocytic leukemia or in other types of lymphocytosis characterized by an increase in small lymphocytes. Whenever these abnormalities are detected on the blood smear, the WBC count is performed manually.

j. The report card is given to the technologist who does the differential leukocyte count, and the values are compared with both red cell morphology on the smear and the number of WBC and platelets estimated from the smear. This will usually detect gross errors.

k. "Drift" is detected from an analysis of quality control data (from 4C determinations) over several days. Drift is best determined from a plot of daily data, the points being plotted on a graph showing the mean values and acceptable upper and lower limits. Unacceptable drift is usually caused by an instrument problem that must be corrected.

l. An alternate method of detecting drift is to record the differences daily between that day's results and the results of the previous day's bloods used for the instrument check. Normally, with no drift, there will

be approximately the same number of positive and negative differences. A preponderance of one or the other indicates drift. More sensitive but more complicated methods for determing drift are given by Bull (1975) and by Korpman and Bull (1976).

m. In spite of claims of reliability by the manufacturers of hematology control materials, they are difficult to prepare and in our experience all may have unsatisfactory lots from time to time. Note that fixed controls do not behave in the same manner as unfixed controls. Those currently available are listed in Table 7-9.

n. The efficiency of the lysing agent is checked when a new lot number is put into use or when a problem exists in the WBC parameter. This is done by adding 1 ml of lysing agent to 9 ml of a 1:224 dilution of whole blood made in Isoton. The solution is observed for complete clearing in 15 to 18 seconds. This time should not be exceeded. Alternately, a drop can be put on a slide, covered with a coverslip, and examined with a microscope to determine if any red cells are not lysed. Here, also, the time limit of 15 to 18 seconds should not be exceeded.

o. The presence of cold agglutinins causes a spurious low erythrocyte count and correspondingly spurious high MCV, MCH, and MCHC (Hattersley et al, 1971a and b; Petrucci et al, 1971).

p. Hyperlipidemia can produce spurious high values for hemoglobin.

Blood hemoglobin

The reference method is based on the conversion of hemoglobin to cyanmethemoglobin. The standard curve and test results are determined using the Coleman spectrophotometer.

1. The standard curve is prepared by making dilutions of the Cyanmethemoglobin Standard (Hycel) equivalent to 5, 10, 15, and 20 Gm/dl of hemoglobin. Dilutions are made with certified 5 ml volumetric pipets: 5 ml of undiluted standard (20 Gm/dl) + 5 ml of diluent = 10 Gm/dl; 5 ml of 10 Gm/dl solution + 5 ml of diluent = 5 Gm/dl; 5 ml of undiluted standard (20 Gm/dl) + 5 ml of 10 Gm/dl solution = 15 Gm/dl.

2. Dilutions are read in the Coleman spectrophotometer, at 540 mμ, after the didymium filter is used to check the wavelength accuracy of the instrument. OD is plotted against concentration on arithmetic graph paper, or %T against concentration on semilog graph paper.

3. Standard curve is determined weekly and compared with previous curves.

4. A check of wavelength with the didymium filter should be performed monthly of whenever successive standard curves do not agree.

5. The cuvettes used should be matched to give the same OD when a 10 Gm/dl dilution of the standard is read in the spectrophotometer.

6. Blood hemoglobin is measured by adding 0.02 ml of blood to 5 ml of reagent. The 0.02 ml pipets should be certified to an accuracy of ± 1%. The reagent should be dispensed with certified 5 ml volumetric pipets. If an auto-

Table 7-9. Commercially available hematology controls

Manufacturer	Brand name	Type of red cells	Type of white cells	Parameters	Levels available	Expiration dating
General Diagnostics	CBC-trol	Unfixed human RBCs	Fixed avian RBCs	HgB, HCT, RBC, WBC, MCV, MCHC, MCH	Normal Abnormal Abnormal II	30 days
Coulter	4C 4C Plus	Fixed human RBCs	Fixed human RBCs	HgB, HCT, RBC,* WBC, MCV, MCHC, MCH, PLT, RDW	Normal Abnormal low Abnormal high	30 days
(Scientific Products) Dade	CH-60	Modified human RBCs	Fixed avian RBCs	HgB, HCT, RBC,* WBC, MCV, MCHC, MCH, PLT	Three levels	60 days
Baker Diagnostics	HAEM-C	Fixed human RBCs	Fixed human RBCs	HgB, HCT, RBC, WBC, MCV, MCHC, MCH	Normal Abnormal high Abnormal low	60 days
Fisher Diagnostics	Hematall-C	Stabilized human RBCs	Fixed avian RBCs	HgB, HCT, RBC, WBC, MCV, MCHC, MCH	Normal Low abnormal High abnormal Abnormal	30 days
Diagnostic Technology	Count-A-Part Complete (calibrator)	Human RBCs	Simulated white cells of animal origin	HgB, HCT, RBC, WBC, MCV, MCHC, MCH	Two levels	2 weeks
Diagnostic Technology	Counter-check	Unfixed human RBCs	Unspecified animal cells	HgB, HCT, RBC,* WBC, MCV, MCHC, MCH, PLT	Three levels	30 days
Diagnostic Technology	Laser-check	Unfixed RBCs	Unspecified animal cells	HgB, HCT, RBC, WBC, MCH, MCV, MCHC	Three levels	30 days
Streck	Para-8 Para-7	Unfixed RBCs	Avian RBCs	HgB, HCT, RBC,* WBC, MCV, MCHC, MCH, PLT	Three levels	6 months
BHP	Quanticel HHR + Quanticel-HHR	Unfixed RBCs	Human leukocytes	HgB, HCT, RBC,* MCH, WBC, MCV, MCHC, PLT	Three levels	60 days
Interscience	IHC	Unfixed RBCs	Fixed RBCs	HgB, HCT, RBC, WBC, MCH, MCV, MVHC	Three levels	60 days
Hy-Cel	Tri Cell	Unfixed human RBCs	Fixed avian RBCs	HgB, HCT, RBC, WBC, MCH, MCV, MCHC	Three levels	30 days
Ortho	Hematology Control	Stabilized human RBCs	Human RBCs	WBC, RBC, HgB, HCT, MCV, MCH, MCHC	Normal Abnormal low Abnormal high	6 weeks
R & D Systems	CBC-PLT-4	Stabilized human RBCs	Avian	WBC, RBC, HgB, HCT, MCV, MCH, MCHC, RDW, PLT, MPV, PCV	Low Normal High	30 days

*Seven, eight, or nine parameters.

matic pipet is used to dispense 5 ml of reagent, the accuracy of the dispensed volume should be checked weekly by dispensing 10 aliquots into an accurate 50 ml volumetric flask. The automatic pipet should be adjusted if the volume is smaller or larger than 50 ml.

7. The cyanmethemoglobin reagent (Hyland) prepared by dissolving the preweighed powder to make 1,000 ml with distilled water usually fails to completely lyse red cells containing Hb S or Hb C and sometimes the platycytes of liver disease. For this reason we make up the reagent to double the volume, 2,000 ml.

8. Hyperlipemia, specifically the increase in chylomicra in hyperlipoproteinemia types I or V, produces false high values for hemoglobin when measured in the Coulter Model S (Shah et al, 1975; Gagné et al, 1977). Corresponding values for MCH are then also higher than the true value.

Microhematocrit

1. The chief advantage of microhematocrit methods is the achievement of maximum packing of red cells at high g values within a very short time.

2. The available microhematocrit centrifuges have been checked carefully by the manufacturer and perform according to specifications. After some time, however, there may be a loss of rotational velocity, which is responsible for suboptimum packing. Check rpm weekly with stroboscope.

3. Microhematocrit sample tubes should be set up in quadruplicate, spun for the time specified by the manufacturer, read in the hematocrit reader, and then spun again for 1 additional minute. If there is additional packing of more than 1% with the second centrifugation, the longer centrifugation time should be used.

4. Microhematocrit values can also be checked against Coulter S or Hemac hematocrits, but this is not profitable except in the detection of gross disparities.

5. While the precision of the microhematocrit when replicates are read by the same observer is excellent (± 0.21%), we find the observation error to be about 2% when different technologists read the same microhematocrit.

6. As noted on p. 360, the calculated hematocrit from

the Coulter electronic counter is more accurate than spun hematocrits.

Leukocyte differential counts

1. Quality assurance of leukocyte differential counts begins with a properly prepared smear. An acceptable smear prepared manually should cover about half the area of a slide, should not extend to the edges, should not have ridges, and should have about one third of the area at the thin edge in which the red cells are not touching. These criteria are met without difficulty if one begins with a very small drop of blood on the slide. Instruments for automated differential counting have attachments to make blood smears automatically. "Spun" smears are uniformly good with an even distribution of leukocytes. "Wedge" smears almost always have unacceptable margination of white cells, giving inaccurate differentials.

2. Smears made from anticoagulated blood (EDTA) usually show no artifacts if made within 1 to 2 hours after the blood is obtained. Delays of many hours will produce cellular artifacts.

3. If abnormalities of red cell shape or leukocytic morphology are noted on a smear made from anticoagulated blood, fresh smears made from capillary blood should be obtained and studied.

4. A properly prepared and aged Wright's or Wright-Giemsa stain will perform well if the smear is properly made. The quality of the stain cannot be judged from a thick smear. The most reliable criterion of the stain quality and staining procedure is the way monocytes are stained. We prefer to check the stain with a thin smear made with an infant's blood because one can expect a good number of monocytes to be present. The nucleus should show the delicate vesicular structure, and the cytoplasm should show the very fine pink granules. If the granules of a monocyte are coarse and purplish, either the stain or the staining procedure is at fault.

5. The popularity of automatic staining devices may be justified on the basis of time-saving mass production but certainly not on the basis of quality of staining. I prefer a manually stained Wright-Giemsa smear.

6. Given well-stained thin smears, it is essential that the technologists performing the differential count be well trained in cell morphology. The criteria for cell identification should be uniform within a laboratory and, ideally, among all hematologists. In fact there is still an unresolved controversy in the classification of stab and segmented neutrophils (Koepke, 1978). In my opinion no cell should be classified as a segmented form unless a thin filament is visible.

7. The number of cells counted is dictated by the WBC count: 100 cells for a normal count, 300 for a count between 20,000 and 50,000/mm³ (20 to 50 × 10⁹/1), and 400 to 500 cells for counts above 50,000/mm³ (50 × 10⁹/1).

8. Differential counts are done beginning at the thin edge of the smear, under oil immersion, moving sequentially from one edge of the smear to the other. In thick smears the leukocytes are rounded up, overstained, and difficult to classify.

9. Differential counts should include a description of red cell morphology and an estimate of the platelet number (low, normal, or high). The estimation of platelets is made more reliably from a smear of fresh capillary blood.

10. In addition to the points above, quality control within the laboratory can be done by putting aside a collection of normal and abnormal smears that have known differential counts or identified abnormalities. These can be used as unknowns periodically and also to check out newly employed technologists. Exact duplication is not possible, but there should be reasonable agreement with known values, and morphologic abnormalities should not be missed.

11. In our laboratory all abnormal differentials and smears that show immature or abnormal cells or morphologic abnormalities of the red cells are checked by the supervisory technologist and, if necessary, by the pathologist.

12. A number of automated differential cell counting instruments are available. An evaluation of the Larc, the Coulter diff3, Hematrak and the Technicon Hemalog D is given in Koepke (1978).

Platelet counts

The reference method for platelet counts is by phase contrast microscopy using the hemocytometer. The precision of this method has been found to have a CV of about 8% and in a normal population the mean value for the platelet count is 258,800/mm³ ($0.258 \times 10^{12}/1$), 95% range 145,000 to 375,000/mm³ (0.145 to $0.375 \times 10^{12}/1$). The adoption of a method that is semiautomated should be based on a comparison of the instrument with the reference method.

Phase contrast microscopy method

1. The diluent is 1% ammonium oxalate. This solution is prepared in 200 ml amounts and stored in the refrigerator. When checked, a small amount is filtered through fine, hard filter paper (Whatman No. 50) just before use. The filtered solution should be allowed to come to room temperature before use.

2. Capillary blood is obtained by making a deep clean puncture with a No. 11 Bard-Parker surgical blade. The first drop of blood is wiped away with a dry sponge and the diluting pipet is filled from the second drop. This method of collection should be adhered to, for the platelet count will be smaller in subsequent drops of blood. The blood is used to prepare a 1:200 dilution in a RBC diluting pipet certified to have a ± 1% or less error. Thorough shaking in a mechanical shaker for 3 minutes is essential.

3. Both sides of the hemocytometer chamber are filled and the hemocytometer is allowed to stand in a covered Petri dish lined with moist filter paper for no less than 10 and no more than 20 minutes.

4. The platelets in the center 1 mm² square are counted on both sides of the chamber. A fresh chamber is prepared, preferably from a different blood sample, if (a) some platelet clumping is seen or (b) there is poor agreement (greater than a 5% difference) between the counts from the two sides of the hemocytometer.

5. Attention to these technical details is probably the most effective approach to quality control of manual platelets counts. Suspensions of fixed platelets to be used as reference reagents are available commercially. They are most useful when used weekly as an independent check of the

performance of an electronic platelet-counting instrument. They are not suitable as primary standards because the result of the instrument count depends on the threshold chosen. All the commercial products I have looked at have small fragments that are excluded in an instrument count. The presence of a wide range of sizes also makes commercial suspensions of fixed platelets unsuitable as a reference for phase counts.

6. We maintain a record of all platelet counts and, if a second platelet count differs significantly from the previous count, a new blood sample is used to repeat the count. If a blood smear is available, this is sometimes helpful to detect gross instrument errors in cases of extreme differences between the successive platelet counts.

Semiautomated platelet counts

We have evaluated and use two electronic platelet-counting instruments, the Technicon Autocounter and the Coulter Model F. Each instrument correlates well with the reference method. Because there are some differences in the way the two are used, the quality control programs for the two are somewhat different.

1. The Technicon Autocounter
   a. Venous blood is collected in EDTA anticoagulant, and the instrument counts platelets in whole blood. A microhematocrit is determined for each blood sample and is used to calculate the corrected platelet count.
   b. The instrument is calibrated with platelet counts performed by phase or with the commercial preparation of fixed platelets.
   c. The quality control program consists of checking the calibration with the reference material several times in the course of the day's run and, testing random specimens during the day, comparing the instrument counts with manual counts using the reference phase contrast method. A third comparison is made by saving some of assayed blood samples and running them again later in the day. This can be done because the platelet count in EDTA blood remains unchanged for at least 8 hours and probably for as long as 12 hours.
   d. Our criterion for deciding that the system is in control is that the counts obtained by the three sets of comparison data should vary by no more than 5% within a day's run.
2. The Coulter Model F
   a. This instrument performs platelet counts on platelet-rich plasma and also requires correction according to the microhematocrit.
   b. The preparation of the platelet-rich plasma sample is critical, for the sample should be free of red and white cells without any loss of platelets. This can be done by carefully controlled sedimentation or centrifugation.
   c. We have evolved a standard centrifugation technic that we think is superior to the other methods for preparing the plasma sample. We use a specially machined adapter for the centrifuge cups of a Serofuge centrifuge and prepare the plasma sample by carefully controlled centrifugation. Since the speed

of rotation in the Serofuge is constant, sedimentation is a function only of the duration of centrifugation. This was established by centrifuging aliquots of blood for various times until one was found that constantly gave platelet counts of the platelet-rich plasma that matched the results obtained on the same blood by the reference phase contrast method.
   d. The only quality control scheme applicable with this system is a weekly check of the comparison of instrument results with those obtained with the reference method. It is possible to use the reference material supplied by the manufacturer, but this is of little value except to determine the stability of the instrument as a particle counter, for without the hematocrit correction it is impossible to compare the count in the platelet-rich plasma with the count in the reference material.
   e. When a blood smear is available for the blood in which the platelets are counted, a comparison of the instrument count with the estimated number of platelets on the smear is sometimes useful in detecting gross errors.

Prothrombin time

Assurance of good quality in this and other coagulation tests is based primarily on the adoption and use of an acceptable technic at all steps of the procedure. When this technical excellence is adhered to, the importance of the day-to-day quality control program becomes minor. In our experience reagent problems almost never are the cause for the test system being out of control.

Whether the test is performed manually or by one of several instruments, the following criteria should be met:

1. Blood should be collected in 3.2% (0.109M) sodium citrate solution, 9 parts blood to 1 part anticoagulant, with prompt mixing.
2. The tube of blood is stoppered if an open system is used. If the vacutainer system is used, the stopper is left in. The blood is centrifuged, and it does not matter if the plasma is platelet rich or platelet poor. Grossly hemolyzed samples should not be used.
3. There is no general agreement as to how the sample should be handled after centrifugation. The most important consideration is to avoid a rise in pH as the specimen stands. This is accomplished by leaving the tube stoppered, whether it is refrigerated or kept at room temperature. We have shown that very little pH change occurs in stoppered vacutainer tubes over a period of 12 hours (Miale and Kent, 1979). If the plasma is aspirated into a separate tube, this tube should be stoppered.
4. Some feel that blood or plasma should not be refrigerated, since factor VII is activated slightly at refrigerator temperatures. I believe this effect to be so small as to be unimportant, but there is no objection to maintaining the plasma at controlled room temperature. In a hot climate and in the absence of air conditioning, I recommend refrigeration.
5. Whether the end point is read visually or in an instrument, the temperature of the reaction mixture should

Table 7-10. Comparison of traditional and SI units for hematologic data*

Test	Normal values			
	Present units	**Factor**	**SI units**	
Platelet count	150,000-400,000/μl	10^6	$0.15\text{-}0.40 \times 10^{12}$/l	
Reticulocyte count	0.5-1.5%	0.01	0.005-0.015	
	25,000-75,000 cells/μl	10^6	$25\text{-}75 \times 10^9$/l	
Sedimentation rate (ESR)				
Men				
Under 50 yr	< 15 mm/hr	1	< 15 mm/hr	
Over 50 yr	< 20 mm/hr		< 20 mm/hr	
Women				
Under 50 yr	< 20 mm/hr		< 20 mm/hr	
Over 50 yr	< 30 mm/hr		< 30 mm/hr	
Complete blood count (CBC)				
Hematocrit				
Male	40-54%	0.01	0.40-0.54	
Female	38-47%		0.38-0.47	
Hemoglobin				
Male	13.5-18.0 Gm/dl	0.155	2.09-2.79 mM/l	
Female	12.0-16.0 Gm/dl		1.86-2.48 mM/l	
Erythrocyte count				
Male	$4.6\text{-}6.2 \times 10^6$μl	10^6	$4.6\text{-}6.2 \times 10^{12}$/l	
Female	$4.2\text{-}5.4 \times 10^6$/μl		$4.2\text{-}5.4 \times 10^{12}$/l	
Leukocyte count	4,500-11,000/μl	10^6	$4.5\text{-}11.0 \times 10^9$/l	
Erythrocyte indices				
Mean corpuscular volume (MCV)	82-98 μ³	1	82-98 fl	
Mean corpuscular hemoglobin (MCH)	27-31 pg	0.0155	0.42-0.48 fmol	
Mean corpuscular hemoglobin concentration (MCHC)	32-36%	0.01	0.32-0.36	

	Mean %	**Range of absolute counts**		**Mean fraction**	**Range of absolute count**
Leukocyte differential					
Segmented neutrophils	56	1,800-7,000/μl	10^6	0.56	$1.8\text{-}7.0 \times 10^9$/l
Bands	3	0-700/μl	10^6	0.03	$0\text{-}0.7 \times 10^9$/l
Eosinophils	2.7	0-450/μl	10^6	0.027	$0\text{-}0.45 \times 10^9$/l
Basophils	0.3	0-200/μl	10^6	0.003	$0\text{-}0.2 \times 10^9$/l
Lymphocytes	34	1,000-4,800/μl	10^6	0.34	$1.0\text{-}4.8 \times 10^9$/l
Monocytes	4	0-800/μl	10^6	0.04	$0\text{-}0.8 \times 10^9$/l

Test	Present units	Factor	SI units	
Blood volume				
Male	69 ml/kg	0.001	0.069 1/kg	
Female	65 ml/kg		0.065 1/kg	
Plasma volume				
Male	39 ml/kg	0.001	0.039 1/kg	
Female	40 ml/kg		0.040 1/kg	
Coagulation tests				
Bleeding time (Ivy)	1-6 min	1	1-6 min	
Bleeding time (Duke)	1-3 min	1	1-3 min	
Clot retraction	50% of the original mass in 2 hr	0.01	0.5 of the original mass in 2 hr	
Partial thromboplastin time (PTT)	60-70 sec	1	60-70 sec	
Partial thromboplastin time, kaolin activated	35-50 sec	1	35-50 sec	
Prothrombin time	12-14 sec	1	12-14 sec	

*Modified from Lehmann, 1976. The normal values given in this table are not necessarily those given in this text.

be maintained as closely as possible at 37° C. For the manual technic this is best accomplished by leaving the tube in a transparent 37° C water bath and reading the end point with a wire loop. Automatic end point reading devices should be checked with a sensitive temperature-measuring device not only with respect to the temperature of the reaction chamber or well, but also with respect to the actual reaction temperature during the test. The latter cannot be done for a plasma-thromboplastin-calcium mixture because clotting may occur too quickly, but it can be done if defibrinated plasma is used instead of normal plasma.

6. The plasma should be warmed to 37° C just before it is used, but prolonged holding at this temperature should be avoided.

7. Quality control program
   a. At the beginning of each day, or when a new bottle of thromboplastin is put into use, check the system using commercial control plasmas (Verify Normal and Verify Abnormal citrate, level II). The Verify Abnormal control is tested after each group of 10 patient samples. Vials of control plasma are refrigerated or kept on ice during the working day.
   b. The temperature of water baths is checked daily. The temperature of instruments is checked weekly. An occasional check of instrument temperature during a working day is recommended to detect overheating of the instrument on prolonged use.
   c. Reconstitution and storage of control plasmas and thromboplastin should follow the recommendations of the manufacturer.
   d. We do not routinely perform prothrombin time tests on a patient's plasma in duplicate, but abnormal results are checked by a duplicate test. Note the precaution against prolonged incubation of plasma.

Partial thromboplastin time

The technical pecautions are the same as for the prothrombin time test, with some special considerations.

1. The reagent we use (APTT, General Diagnostics) is stable, when reconstituted, for 1 week. If a vial is used for more than 1 day, it should be labeled with the date and time it was reconstituted. The reagent is stored in the refrigerator when not in use.
2. Some partial thromboplastin reagents use a particulate activator that settles out quickly. When using these it is essential that the activator be evenly suspended before the reagent is pipetted and just before it is mixed with the test plasma.

ADOPTION OF SI UNITS

In a recent publication Lehmann (1976) discusses the evolution of the standardized unit nomenclature shown as "SI units" (Système international d'unites). Recognizing the importance of standardizing a mode of communication so that it can be understood internationally, this is a much-needed reform, especially in clinical chemistry. Extensive conversion tables are given by Sax (1979) and Lippert and Lehmann (1978). There has not been uniformly enthusiastic acceptance of the change (Gibson [1980] writes a humorous but scathing critique), but SI units have been adopted by many foreign journals. The Editorial Board of the American Journal of Clinical Pathology recommends that quantitative measurements in conventional units be followed by SI units in parentheses. This convention has been followed in this edition, except for unintentional oversights.

I do regret, however, some of the unit changes for hematology values (Table 7-10). Since there has never been a confusion of unit systems in hematology, like that in clinical chemistry, most of the recommended changes are meant only to conform to the overall SI system. They do not make the values easier to interpret; in fact I find the opposite. Reporting the platelet count as a number $\times 10^{12}/1$, the WBC count as a number $\times 10^9/1$, the RBC count as a number $\times 10^{12}/1$, or the hemoglobin concentration in mM/1, for example, seems sheer folly. I find it necessary to have the conversion table available at all times. We have not yet faced the problem of communicating with the recipients of our laboratory data nor the problems of changes necessary in instruments having printout capabilities. .

8

"In malignant fevers, with the blood vessels so gorged with blood that they are about to burst, and the blood about to rush to the brain, and the body filled with bile and various other fermenting substances, all of them poisonous to the organism, it is plain to common sense that bleeding is necessary."

Voltaire

Oxygen transport and delivery: iron-deficiency anemia

INTRODUCTION
OXYGEN TRANSPORT AND DELIVERY
  Hypoxia
  Normal oxygen transport
  Role of 2,3-DPG
    Synthesis and degradation
    Interaction with hemoglobin
  Adaptations to hypoxia at high altitude
  Adaptations to anemic hypoxia
PATHOGENESIS OF ANEMIA
  Classification according to pathogenesis
  Anemia due to increased plasma volume
IRON
  General considerations
  Iron metabolism
    Use of radioactive iron
    Distribution
    Dietary iron
    Iron absorption
    Iron transport
    Iron storage
    Iron loss and excretion
    Iron requirements
    Iron utilization
COPPER
COBALT
ZINC
IRON-DEFICIENCY ANEMIA
  Classification
  Clinical picture
  Laboratory diagnosis
    Degree of anemia
    Red cell morphology
    Red cell indices
    Reticulocytes
    Leukocytes
    Platelets
    Bone marrow
    Osmotic fragility of red cells
    Evaluation of iron metabolism
      Serum ferritin concentration
      Serum iron concentration
      Serum iron-binding capacity
      Estimation of iron stores

      Free erythrocyte protoporphyrin
      Other studies of iron metabolism
    Detection of blood loss
  Summary of iron-deficiency anemias
    Sideropenic iron-deficiency anemias
      Nutritional iron deficiency
      Anemia due to poor iron absorption
      Anemia due to physiologically increased iron requirements
      Anemia due to blood loss
    Sideroachrestic anemias
      Anemia of chronic disorders
      Sideroblastic anemias
      Hereditary iron-loading anemia
    Anemia in transferrin deficiency

INTRODUCTION

The laboratory diagnosis of anemia is based on the detection of a lower than normal red blood cell count or blood hemoglobin concentration. These are practical but indirect assays of the oxygen-carrying capacity of blood; clinical symptoms develop when, for various reasons, the oxygen-carrying capacity of blood is decreased relative to the body's need. For example, hypoxic symptoms can develop when a person who is moderately anemic but asymptomatic in the course of normal activity undertakes strenuous exercise. Also, the red blood cell count and hemoglobin concentration do not in some cases correlate with the oxygen-carrying or oxygen-exchanging capacity of the red blood cell as modified by structurally abnormal hemoglobin or deficient systems, such as 2,3-DPG, that regulate the function of the hemoglobin molecule.

OXYGEN TRANSPORT AND DELIVERY
Hypoxia

Whatever the mechanism by which anemia is produced, the symptoms and harmful effects are the result of the decreased red blood cell mass, the decreased oxygen-carrying capacity of the blood (Fig. 8-1), and tissue hypoxia. While tissue hypoxia can also be produced by a reduction in the oxygen content of inspired air or decreased alveolar–capillary oxygen exchange (pulmonary fibrosis, emphysema, etc.), this is not pertinent to this discussion, for it does not produce anemia but rather erythrocytosis (Chapter 16). A third mechanism by which tissue hypoxia is produced is a defect in the erythrocytic oxygen transport system, either by abnormal hemoglobin function or inappropriate concentration of erythrocytic 2,3-DPG (Harkness, 1971).

Erythrocytes have three major functions: (1) they make up about 40% of the blood volume, (2) they carry oxygen to the tissues, and (3) they transport CO_2 away from the tissues and, in doing so, not only eliminate this waste product, but act as an important pH buffer. Our concern here is with oxygen transport.

Hypoxia at the organ and cellular level can result from many causes, but we are concerned here with anemic hypoxia caused by a reduction in red cell mass, with hypoxia due to deficient transport caused by abnormal hemoglobin structure, and with hypoxia resulting from deficient oxygen transport caused by intraerythrocytic enzymatic deficiency.

Normal oxygen transport

The structure of the hemoglobin molecule and the relationship between structure and function are discussed in Chapter 14 (p. 607).

The affinity of hemoglobin for oxygen varies with different partial pressures of oxygen (Po_2) so that a plot of the oxygen content against Po_2 does not give a straight line but rather a sigmoid curve (Fig. 8-1). The sigmoid shape is an expression of heme-heme interaction, i.e., the combination of oxygen with one heme group changes the affinity for oxygen of the heme group in the neighboring chain. It is thought that the configuration of the hemoglobin molecule changes from deoxy- to oxy- when the third heme is oxy-

genated (Gibson, 1970; Thomas et al, 1974). As though by design, the sigmoid shape indicates a more efficient system of oxygen transport than would be the case if the relationship between oxygen content and Po_2 were linear. One obvious advantage is that at the venous Po_2 of 40 mm Hg the dissociation curve is very steep so that the amount of oxygen released is relatively large when the change in Po_2 is small. This provides for maximum delivery to the tissues. Oxygen affinity is also dependent on temperature, not an important factor in human physiology, and on hydrogen ion concentration. The change in oxygen affinity related to pH is called the *Bohr effect* (Bohr, 1904), the shift to the right of the curve with decreasing pH. This is due to the greater proton binding of deoxyhemoglobin as compared with oxyhemoglobin. The shift to the right at the more acid pH of the tissues results in a decreased affinity of hemoglobin for oxygen and this facilitates release of oxygen to the tissues. By convention, the position of the curve can be defined at the P_{50} point, the Po_2 at which hemoglobin is 50% saturated under a given set of conditions (normal about 27 mm Hg). The P_{50} value can be derived from measured oxyhemoglobin concentration and Po_2 according to the Hill equation (Hill, 1910):

$$\frac{\% \text{ Saturation}}{100 - \% \text{ Saturation}} = K\,(Po_2)^n$$

where $n = 2.7$ for normal blood, but only in the range of 40% to 60% saturation (Valeri, 1974a).

Oxygenation of reduced hemoglobin produces a shift from a weaker to a stronger acid and adds hydrogen ions, whereas the change from oxyhemoglobin to deoxyhemoglobin is in the opposite direction, tending to remove hydrogen ions. This produces an important and powerful buffer system that makes it possible to transport large amounts of acid carbon dioxide without a change in pH. Such a system is called *isohydric*. For each mM of oxyhemoglobin converted to deoxyhemoglobin, 0.7 mM of hydrogen ions can be added without a change in pH.

An excess of hydrogen ion shifts the oxygen dissociation curve to the right, toward the deoxyhemoglobin conformation. This is due to changing some amino acids to weaker acids. The hemoglobin ligand, carbon dioxide, also decreases oxygen affinity by its influence on pH and by combining with the four *N*-terminal amino acids to form carbamino compounds. Acidosis therefore decreases oxygen affinity, but this is quickly compensated for by the inhibition of 2,3-DPG synthesis, which shifts the oxygen dissociation curve to the left. An understanding of these opposing mechanisms is important in the clinical management of acid-base disturbances. For example, a patient in diabetic ketoacidosis with a low blood pH usually has a normally positioned dissociation curve due to a low concentration of 2,3-DPG, but if the acidosis is corrected too vigorously the effect of low 2,3-DPG combined with a normal or alkaline pH can shift the dissociation curve to the left of normal and thus decrease the efficiency of oxygen unloading (Bellingham et al, 1971).

The delivery of oxygen to the tissues is dependent on the difference between the Po_2 of the blood arriving at the tissue

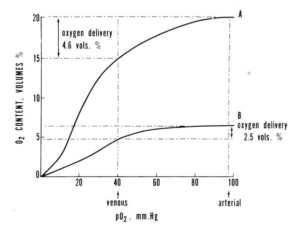

Fig. 8-1. Oxygen dissociation curves of a normal subject (Hb 15 Gm/dl), **A,** and of a subject with severe anemia (Hb 5.7 Gm/dl), **B,** at pH 7.4, 37° C. The P_{O_2} of venous blood is taken as 40 mm Hg, that of arterial blood as slightly less than 100 mm Hg. The difference between the oxygen content of venous blood and arterial blood for each curve is the amount of oxygen that can be delivered to the tissues, roughly half of the normal in the anemic subject. (Data from Bellingham, 1973).

and the lower P_{O_2} at the unloading point. This relationship is expressed by Fick's equation:

$$\text{Cons. } O_2 = BF (O_2a - O_2b)$$

where

    Cons. O_2 = Oxygen consumption
        BF = Cardiac output
      O_2a = Arterial oxygen content
      O_2b = Venous oxygen content

Oxygen delivery is also a function of blood flow, and this can be increased as one of the compensatory mechanisms. Foremost, however, is the oxygen-binding capacity of the blood, and this is regulated by three allosteric (competing spatially) ligands of hemoglobin: (1) protons, (2) carbon dioxide, and (3) 2,3-diphosphoglycerate (2,3-DPG) (Rørth, 1974).

Because oxyhemoglobin is a stronger acid than deoxyhemoglobin, protons bind preferentially to deoxyhemoglobin and by so doing tend to decrease the oxygen affinity of hemoglobin. Oxygen-linked proton binding involves the amino- and imidazole-amino acid residues whose pK value changes with the change in oxygenation of the hemoglobin molecule (Kilmartin and Rossi-Bernardi, 1973). Carbon dioxide decreases the affinity of hemoglobin for oxygen by reacting with uncharged amino groups ($-NH_2$) at the N-terminals of the globin chains, forming carbamino groups (Rossi-Bernardi and Roughton, 1967). The third ligand, 2,3-DPG, is interrelated with the other two insofar as it is pH dependent, and in this sense can be considered the key mechanism regulating the position of the oxygen dissociation curve and thus the transport and delivery of oxygen. It should be noted that fetal hemoglobin (Hb F) does not bind 2,3-DPG to the same degree as adult hemoglobin (Hb A) (Oski, 1972). Because of this, the oxygen dissociation curve of the blood of a newborn infant, or of any blood containing a high concentration of Hb F, is shifted to the left. Hypoxic symptoms in anemic premature infants are related to both the hemoglobin concentration and the high oxygen affinity of the blood (Wardrop et al, 1978).

Role of 2,3-DPG

The oxygen dissociation curve is shifted to the right when the concentration of the intraerythrocytic organic phosphate 2,3-DPG is increased (Chanutin and Curnish, 1967; Benesch and Benesch, 1967). The opposite, a shift to the left, is produced when the concentration of 2,3-DPG is decreased.

2,3-DPG is an intermediate in the anaerobic (Embden-Meyerhof) glycolytic pathway. About 25 years ago, Rapoport and Luebering (Rapoport and Luebering, 1951, 1952; Rapoport, 1968) discovered that 2,3-DPG is derived from 1,3-DPG, a reaction dependent on diphosphoglycerate mutase, and is degraded to 3-PG by 2,3-diphosphoglycerate phosphatase (Fig. 8-2). This detour in the glycolytic pathway is known as the *Rapoport-Luebering cycle*. 2,3-DPG accounts for about two-thirds of the total organic phosphate of the human red blood cell, an amount in great excess of the first role assigned to it, that of a cofactor for phosphoglycerate mutase (Sutherland et al, 1949). We appreciate now

that 2,3-DPG is probably the most important regulator of oxygen transport and delivery. As such it is intimately involved in adaptive responses (anemic hypoxia, high altitude hypoxia, etc.). Under most conditions of storage, red blood cells lose 2,3-DPG, and this becomes an important consideration in blood transfusion therapy (Chapter 12).

Synthesis and degradation

The rate of synthesis of 2,3-DPG is dependent primarily on the concentration of 1,3-DPG and this in turn is dependent on phosphofructokinase (PFK, enzyme 1 in Fig. 8-2), the major rate-limiting enzyme in glycolysis. The synthesis of 1,3-DPG is under the immediate control of GAPDH

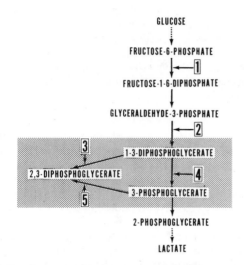

Fig. 8-2. The Rapoport-Luebering pathway for synthesis and degradation of 2,3-DPG (reactions in shaded area). Pertinent enzymes are numbered: **(1)** phosphofructokinase (PFK), **(2)** glyceraldehyde-3-phosphate dehydrogenase (GAPDH), **(3)** diphosphoglycerate mutase, **(4)** phosphoglycerate kinase (PGK), and **(5)** 2,3-diphosphoglycerate phosphatase.

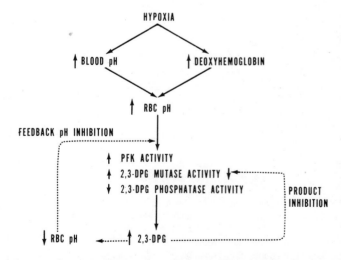

Fig. 8-3. The concentration of 2,3-DPG in red blood cells is regulated by hypoxia, a shift in RBC pH, and two feedback mechanisms.

(glyceraldehyde-3-phosphate dehydrogenase, enzyme 2 in Fig. 8-2). The degradation of 2,3-DPG to 3-PG is controlled by 2,3-DPG phosphatase, and this enzyme is influenced strongly by pH, a decrease in intracellular pH leading to accelerated breakdown of 2,3-DPG whereas an increase in intracellular pH leads to accumulation of 2,3-DPG. In vitro, incubation of red blood cells with inosine, inorganic phosphate, and pyruvate induces rapid synthesis of 2,3-DPG (Duhm and Gerlach, 1974; Zacara, 1977). Restoration of erythrocytic 2,3-DPG is of great importance in blood storage and transfusion therapy (Chapter 12).

Regulation of the intraerythrocytic concentration of 2,3-DPG is effected chiefly by pH and Po_2. A rise in pH increases the activity of PFK and 2,3-DPG mutase and decreases the activity of 2,3-DPG phosphatase. The result is an increase in 2,3-DPG concentration (Rapoport et al, 1972; Gerlach and Duhm, 1972a). As the concentration of 2,3-DPG rises at the higher pH, less of it is bound to hemoglobin, the concentration of unbound 2,3-DPG increases, and new synthesis of 2,3-DPG is inhibited, either by inhibition of DPG mutase (Gerlach and Duhm, 1972b) or by a fall in intracellular pH (Astrup et al, 1970). In vivo, the effect of pH may be of lesser importance (Duhm and Gerlach, 1971).

Hypoxia causes an increase in 2,3-DPG probably because the increased intracellular concentration of deoxyhemoglobin is accompanied by a rise in pH, which in turn stimulates synthesis of 2,3-DPG through mechanisms discussed above. Hypoxia produces a shift of 2,3-DPG toward the bound form of deoxyhemoglobin with resulting decrease in the unbound form, which in turn decreases inhibition of 2,3-DPG mutase and increases synthesis of 2,3-DPG. This second mechanism for 2,3-DPG stimulation by hypoxia is thought to be of little importance (Rapoport et al, 1972). Fig. 8-3 summarizes the factors influencing the synthesis of 2,3-DPG.

Interaction with hemoglobin

The shift to the right of the oxygen dissociation curve found in anemic hypoxia (Fig. 8-1) is the result of the interaction of 2,3-DPG with the hemoglobin molecule.

The hemoglobin molecule is a tetramer of two pairs of unlike polypeptide chains, each nestling a heme group (see Chapter 14). The elegant studies of Perutz (1970a, 1970b) gave us a definitive model of the tetramer. The tetramer is held together by bonds between unlike chains. The remarkable feature is that some of the bonds are broken when a ligand such as oxygen attaches to the molecule, and this causes a spatial rearrangement within the tetramer. The molecule of oxyhemoglobin then is either tight or loose, and the

central cavity contracts or enlarges, as though the molecule itself is "breathing in and out" in a respiratory movement. In the deoxyconfiguration the central cavity is sufficiently large (7 Å larger than in oxyhemoglobin) to allow the acidic groups of a molecule of 2,3-DPG to attach to specific residues of the β-chains (Noble and Ranney, 1974) and to stabilize the conformation. According to Perutz (1970a), the 2,3-DPG molecule fits into the central cavity of deoxyhemoglobin in such a way that its five anionic groups bind with positively-charged residues in each of the two β-chains, histidyl 143 and N-terminal valine of one chain and histidyl 143, N-terminal valine, and lysine 82 of the other (Arnone, 1972). Upon oxygenation there is a change in the conformation of the central cavity such that the distance between the N-terminal group of the two β-chains increases so that 2,3-DPG cannot bind to both and is therefore released.

In the deoxy- conformation with attached 2,3-DPG, the oxygen affinity is reduced. On the other hand, in the oxy-conformation there is no binding of 2,3-DPG and the oxygen affinity is increased. In a very simplistic model we can say that 2,3-DPG and oxygen are competitive ligands (Fig. 8-4), the attachment of one inhibiting the attachment of the other. The preferential binding of 2,3-DPG to deoxyhemoglobin, 1 mole to 1 mole (Arnone, 1972), is the basis for understanding the compensatory changes that occur in anemic and other types of hypoxia.

Adaptations to hypoxia at high altitude

Hypoxia occurs at high altitudes because, although the atmosphere contains a constant 20.93% oxygen up to 110,000 feet, the oxygen at a high altitude is at a lower partial pressure than at sea level as a result of the reduced barometric pressure (Frisancho, 1975). At sea level barometric pressure is 760 mm Hg, and partial pressure of oxygen (Po_2) is 159 mm Hg: at 3,500 m (11,840 feet) the Po_2 is 103 mm; and at 4,500 m the Po_2 is 91 mm Hg. The lower the Po_2 of inspired air, the lower the oxygen saturation of arterial blood and the oxygen available at the tissue level. Whether or not symptoms develop or are severe depends on how much the Po_2 is decreased, on the level of physical activity, and on the adaptations that take place to compensate for the hypoxia.

A distinction should be made between adaptive changes occurring in a resident at sea level who moves to a high altitude and one who is a native at a high altitude. For example, natives at high altitudes have a greater lung volume and a greater alveolar surface area than matched controls born and raised at sea level (Frisancho et al, 1973). this enables natives at high altitude to have a relatively high pulmonary-diffusing capacity. In contrast, lowland natives acclimatized as adults do not have an increase in alveolar surface, and other adaptations are made. One adaptation is an increase in the red blood cell count and hemoglobin level in response to stimulation of erythropoiesis by erythropoietin. Another change is an increase in red blood cell 2,3-DPG, as a result of which the oxygen dissociation curve is shifted to the right, and there is improved release of arterial oxygen. The lowland native moving to a high altitude also experiences an increase in pulse rate and cardiac output and an increase in

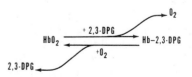

Fig. 8-4. The competition between two ligands, oxygen and 2,3-DPG, for the hemoglobin molecule.

the rate and depth of respiration. These adaptive changes improve the delivery of oxygen to the tissues.

Adaptations to anemic hypoxia

The symptoms of anemia and the intensity of adaptive changes are determined not only by the severity of the hemoglobin deficit but also by the degree of physical activity. The demand for oxygen at rest is relatively lower than that during physical exertion and might be met without symptoms when the hemoglobin concentration is lower than normal. At the same hemoglobin concentration, however, exertion can exceed the oxygen-delivering capacity and a spectrum of symptoms appear, roughly proportional to the oxygen deficit. In addition, a moderately severe anemia of acute onset, as from hemorrhage, can be accompanied by severe symptoms whereas the same degree of anemia developing very gradually might be asymptomatic due to gradual compensatory changes.

Because of this, it is not possible to exactly correlate symptoms with hemoglobin concentration. From mild to severe, the symptoms are: tachycardia, dyspnea on exertion, headache, dizziness, palpitations, weakness, anorexia, dyspnea at rest, fever, cardiac failure, and coma. Some of these are primary symptoms of hypoxia, others reflect cardiorespiratory compensation.

Cardiovascular compensation consists first of an increase in stroke volume without acceleration of rate (Duke and Abelmann, 1969). After some time the heart rate increases, and in chronic anemia there may be cardiac enlargement and the development of murmurs.

In contrast to these adaptive changes, the concentration of 2,3-DPG is extremely sensitive to the anemia (Bellingham, 1974) and increases as soon as the hemoglobin concentration decreases. Some feel that 2,3-DPG response is regulated more by the reduction in red cell mass than by the drop in hemoglobin concentration or hematocrit (Valeri and Fortier, 1969). This is particularly the case in iron-deficiency anemia (Slawsky and Desforges, 1972) and in hereditary spherocytosis (Palek et al, 1969). In any case, the increase in 2,3-DPG reduces oxygen affinity and improves the unloading of oxygen at the cellular level. While there is no doubt that there is an inverse relationship between the hemoglobin concentration and that of 2,3-DPG (Brewer and Eaton, 1971), it has been suggested (Rørth, 1974) that the change in oxygen affinity regulates erythropoietin production, stimulating in increased affinity and inhibiting in decreased affinity.

There are situations in which changes in 2,3-DPG concentration are not the result primarily of anemic hypoxia. As shown in Fig. 8-2, 2,3-DPG is an intermediate in the glycolytic pathway, of which the Rapoport-Luebering shunt is a part, so that defects in the pathway other than in the shunt can affect the concentration of 2,3-DPG. Enzyme deficiencies proximal or distal to the shunt can affect the synthesis of 2,3-DPG. Hexokinase acts proximally to the shunt, converting glucose to glucose-6-phosphate, and in congenital deficiency of hexokinase there is impaired synthesis of 2,3-DPG (Oski and Delivoria-Papadopoulos, 1970), reduced levels of red cell 2,3-DPG, increased oxygen affinity, and, in some cases, a low blood hemoglobin. In a lesion distal to the shunt, pyruvate kinase deficiency, there is an increase in

2,3-DPG, reduced oxygen affinity (Bellingham, 1974), and, in some cases, an increased red cell mass. It is to be expected that other congenital enzymatic defects occurring proximally to the shunt (phosphohexose isomerase, phosphofructokinase, and possibly aldolase) may also diminish red cell 2,3-DPG, but to my knowledge this has not been documented. Enzymatic deficiencies outside the shunt may also interfere with the expected response to hypoxia.

There are also some complex clinical situations where several factors interact. For example, the increased concentration of 2,3-DPG in uremia is due to both the anemia (Torrance et al, 1970) and to the increase in plasma inorganic phosphate (Hurt and Chanutin, 1964). In cirrhosis of the liver the increase in 2,3-DPG may be due both to the anemia and, when present, to metabolic alkalosis (Astrup and Rørth, 1973). Androgens stimulate erythropoiesis (Chapter 1) but also increase 2,3-DPG (Parker et al, 1972). The role of thyroid hormone is less clear (Snyder and Reddy, 1970).

PATHOGENESIS OF ANEMIA

Under normal conditions, peripheral blood values for erythrocytes and hemoglobin are maintained at a constant level. This is accomplished by a balance between the rate of erythrocyte production and the rate of destruction. Anemia can occur if the rate of erythrocyte production is decreased while the rate of destruction remains normal or as a result of accelerated erythrocyte destruction (decreased survival) with normal rate of production. From the standpoint of pathogenesis, therefore, the anemias fall into two major categories: (1) those primarily caused by diminished or deficient erythropoiesis and (2) those primarily caused by accelerated destruction of erythrocytes. Also, since the laboratory diagnosis of anemia is based on the erythrocyte count and hemoglobin concentration, anemia may be the result of an increased plasma volume, with no reduction in absolute red cell mass but reduction in the erythrocyte and hemoglobin concentration, rather than of decreased production or increased destruction. Thus the third category, anemia caused by increased plasma volume, is added to the etiologic classification and deserves a short discussion.

Anemias on the basis of iron deficiency are discussed later in this chapter. Anemias caused by deficiency of vitamin B_{12} or folate are covered in Chapter 9. Anemias caused by decreased erythrocyte survival, the hemolytic anemias, are discussed in Chapters 13 and 14.

Classification according to pathogenesis

Anemia has been classified on the basis of the morphology of the erythrocytes into *microcytic anemia, normocytic anemia,* and *macrocytic anemia.* While the study of erythrocyte morphology is an important laboratory procedure, a classification based on morphology alone leaves much to be desired. The chief drawback is that, except by inference, it tells us nothing about the pathogenesis or etiology. To use an analogy, while it is not difficult to sort potatoes into two sizes, large and small, the ability to do so requires no knowledge of farming in general or potatoes in particular.

The classification given in Table 8-1 divides anemias into various categories according to pathogenesis. In spite of shortcomings because of incomplete knowledge of the basic

Table 8-1. Etiologic classification of anemia

I. Anemia caused by increased plasma volume
  A. Pregnancy
  B. Hyperproteinemia
  C. Simple splenomegaly
  D. Iatrogenic hyperhydration (intravenous fluids)
II. Hypochromic anemia caused by iron deficiency (*sideropenic*)
  A. Low iron intake (nutritional)
  B. Diminished iron absorption
    1. Achlorhydria (?)
    2. Sprue
    3. Idiopathic steatorrhea
    4. Celiac disease
    5. Chronic dysentery
    6. "Dumping syndrome"
    7. Pica
  C. Increased iron requirements
    1. Pregnancy
    2. Infancy
    3. Prematurity
  D. Excessive iron loss
    1. Chronic hemorrhage
    2. Hookworm infection
III. Hypochromic anemia not caused by iron deficiency (inadequate utilization of iron; *sideroachrestic*)
  A. Infection
  B. Thalassemia (and other hemoglobinopathies)
  C. Sideroblastic anemia
    1. Primary
      a. Acquired sideroblastic anemia
      b. Sex-linked sideroblastic anemia
    2. Secondary
      a. Associated with various diseases
      b. Drug induced (antituberculosis drugs)
      c. Lead poisoning
      d. Pyridoxine deficiency
  D. Hypochromic anemia responsive to crude liver extract
  E. Congenital and acquired transferrin deficiency
  F. Hereditary iron-loading anemia
    1. Byrd-Cooper type
    2. Shahidi-Nathan-Diamond type
  G. Chronic renal disease
IV. Hypochromic anemia of unknown pathogenesis
  A. Anemia of diaphragmatic hernia
  B. Rheumatoid arthritis
  C. Disseminated lupus erythematosus
  D. Associated with mesenteric lymphoid hamartoma
V. Anemia caused by deficiency of vitamin B_{12} or folic acid
  A. Viatmin B_{12} deficiency
    1. Classic pernicious anemia
      a. In the adult
      b. In childhood
    2. *Dibothriocephalus latus* infection
    3. Gastrectomy
    4. Nutritional deficiency
    5. Abnormalities of small intestine
  B. Folic acid deficiency
    1. Megaloblastic anemia of pregnancy
    2. Megaloblastic anemia of infancy
    3. Sprue
    4. Macrocytic anemia of scurvy
    5. Tropical macrocytic anemia
    6. Idiopathic steatorrhea (nontropical sprue)
    7. Celiac disease
    8. Alcoholism and cirrhosis of liver

  C. Deficiency not definitely known; may be due to combined or partial deficiencies of various factors
    1. Macrocytic anemia of liver disease
    2. Nutritional macrocytic anemia
    3. "Refractory megaloblastic anemia"
    4. "Achrestic anemia"
    5. Macrocytic anemia of rapid blood regeneration
    6. Macrocytic anemia associated with neoplastic infiltration into bone marrow
    7. Macrocytic anemia after administration of antimetabolic drugs
VI. Anemia caused by decreased erythrocyte survival—hemolytic anemias (see Chapters 13 and 14 for complete classification)
  A. Decreased erythrocyte survival due to intrinsic defects in erythrocyte
    1. Hereditary spherocytosis
    2. Congenital nonspherocytic hemolytic anemia (G-6-PD and other enzymatic deficiencies)
    3. Paroxysmal nocturnal hemoglobinuria
    4. Hereditary elliptocytosis
    5. Porphyria erythropoietica
    6. Pernicious anemia
    7. Acanthocytosis
    8. Hemoglobinopathies (Chapter 14)
  B. Decreased erythrocyte survival due to extracorpuscular factors
    1. Acquired autoimmune hemolytic anemia
    2. Acquired isoimmune hemolytic anemia
    3. Caused by bacterial agents and protozoal parasites
    4. Caused by chemical agents
    5. Caused by physical agents (vascular prosthesis, march hemoglobinuria)
    6. Burns
VII. Anemia caused by abnormal bone marrow function—"aplastic" or "aregenerative" anemia and "myeloproliferative syndromes"
  A. Bone marrow injury due to chemical or physical agents
    1. Ionizing radiation
    2. Chemical agents (partial list)
      a. Benzol
      b. Gold sodium thiosulfate
      c. Arsenicals (organic)
      d. Nitrogen mustards
      e. Thiourea compounds
      f. Sulfa drugs
      g. Chloramphenicol
      h. Phenylbutazone
      i. Bismuth salts
      j. Colloidal silver
      k. Mercury salts
      l. Dinitrophenol
      m. Trinitrotoluene
      n. Hair dyes (paraphenylenediamine)
      o. Streptomycin
      p. Tridione
      q. Mesantoin
      r. Thiantoin
      s. Atabrine
      t. Thorium dioxide
  B. Inhibition of bone marrow erythropoiesis
    1. "Myelophthisic anemia" due to the presence of abnormal tissue in bone marrow
      a. Metastatic neoplasm
      b. Lymphomas
      c. Leukemias

Continued.

Table 8-1. Etiologic classification of anemia—cont'd

d. Multiple myeloma
e. Storage diseases (Gaucher's disease, Niemann-Pick disease, and Schüller-Christian disease)
f. Tuberculosis and other granulomas
g. Myelofibrosis and myelosclerosis
h. Osteopetrosis
2. Metabolic inhibition of bone marrow erythropoiesis
  a. Malignancy
  b. Infection
  c. Chronic renal disease
	d. Hypopituitarism
	e. Hypothyroidism
	f. Chronic liver disease
	C. Bone marrow erythropoiesis deficiency, cause unknown
	  1. "Idiopathic aplastic anemia"
	  2. "Familial aplastic anemia"
	  3. Associated with myasthenia gravis and thymic tumors
	  4. "Physiologic anemia" of premature babies and infants (? erythropoietin deficiency)

mechanisms, a classification based on pathogenesis is basic to the honest treatment of anemia. It points up the etiology and helps in the selection of specific therapy.

Anemia due to increased plasma volume

There are limits beyond which a normal plasma volume cannot be expanded without causing obvious circulatory failure. Because of this, it is unlikely that a severe anemia would be produced by increased plasma volume alone. However, an increase in plasma volume can produce sufficient hemodilution to convert a low normal hemoglobin concentration into an anemic level or to convert a mild anemic state into a more severe one.

Normal pregnancy is a good example of this. During the last trimester of pregnancy there may be a 25% increase in blood volume, most of it an increase in plasma volume. This could account for a decrease in blood hemoglobin concentration of as much as 2 Gm/dl. Since the increased requirements for iron during pregnancy sometimes produce an iron-deficiency state and iron-deficiency anemia, the increase in plasma volume would accentuate the anemia. After delivery there is a prompt return of the plasma volume to normal.

An increase in plasma volume is to be expected in hyperproteinemia, particularly macroglobulin abnormalities. An experimental model of this is to be found in mice implanted with plasma cell tumors that produce large amounts of myeloma protein.

The increased plasma volume in some cases may be relative rather than absolute, as in simple splenomegaly. The spleen is capable of sequestering a good deal of blood relatively rich in erythrocytes. In the splenomegaly that is part of a myeloproliferative disorder, the ratio of body hematocrit to venous hematocrit is sometimes 1.0 or higher, as compared to the normal value of about 0.9. There are reports (Hess et al, 1976) to indicate that an increase in the ratio of body hematocrit to venous hematocrit is to be found in splenomegaly regardless of etiology. When splenomegaly accompanies a disorder that by itself produces anemia, the increased plasma volume can be expected to make the anemia more severe.

IRON
General considerations

Iron was the first metal used for fashioning tools and weapons, and the use of iron compounds to cure a variety of illnesses dates almost as far back (Fairbanks, et al, 1971). The therapeutic effectiveness of iron compounds in as diverse a group of conditions as acne, hemorrhoids, and diarrhea, not to mention falling hair, was summarized by Caius Plinus (the Elder) in the first century and repeated essentially unchanged in the sixteenth century by the Spanish physician Monardes.

Iron therapy achieved respectability in the 1800s when Pierre Blaud showed it to be effective in chlorosis, the "green sickness." This now nonexistent disease was prevalent in young women during a span of over 200 years and then disappeared with the onset of this century. The disease was characterized by a greenish pallor and many of the symptoms we now ascribe to anemia. It was held to be a disease of young virgins (*morbus virgineo*, the "sickness of virgins"), related somehow to their chaste state, with many references to scanty menses as well as to the beneficial effects of stopping the menstrual flow. In fact in 1554, Lange (Major, 1945) stated "I therefore say, I instruct virgins afflicted with this disease, that as soon as possible they live with men and copulate, if they conceive they recover."

We cannot judge whether this advice was responsible for a significant decrease in the number of virgins nor what role it may have played in the disappearance of chlorosis. Certainly, the disease seems to have had a romantic mystique, for it was also known as the "love-sickness," which may have contributed to it achieving almost epidemic proportions. However, Blaud (1832) reported that chlorosis could be cured by administering ferrous sulfate ("Blaud's Pills" contained ferrous sulfate and potassium carbonate) and many others confirmed his findings so that the administration of iron compounds became the standard treatment of chlorosis. It was not until the late 1800s that physicians had the laboratory tools to study anemia, and with the availability of blood cell counts and chemical analyses of the blood for iron, the true relationship of iron to anemia became apparent. In the 1900s anemia became the object of extensive investigations, so that in our time iron deficiency is recognized as only one of many pathogenetic mechanisms leading to anemia.

The disappearance of chlorosis has never been explained adequately (Fowler, 1936). There is no doubt that when it was most prevalent it included severe anemias related to tuberculosis, malignancies, and malabsorption syndromes as well as anemias of other etiology, such as pernicious anemia. Some have expressed the opinion that the modern diet is less likely to be deficient, but there is little evidence to support the implication that diets during the height of the chlorosis era were severely deficient in iron. It is more probable that the availability of better medical care and the emphasis on preventive medicine has been responsible for detecting anemias in the early stages, before "chlorosis" develops. In any case, the disease is now seen as the yellowing of some plants when the nutrients are iron deficient, for an iron-containing protein (ferrodoxin) (Arnon, 1965) as well as iron-containing enzymes (cytochromes) are necessary for photosynthesis. The current fad that plants thrive if one speaks lovingly to them may imply something else in common between chlorosis of plants and the love sickness of virgins.

The anemias classified as being caused by iron deficiency are not all the result of excessive iron loss or deficient iron intake. Iron deficiency is also defined as a lack of available iron and, in some instances, as the failure to utilize heme for the synthesis of hemoglobin. While the end result of iron loss, deficient intake of iron, lack of available iron, or lack of heme utilization is the same—an anemia characterized by hypochromic red cells—therapy with iron is effective only in those situations in which iron is depleted and there is no defect in its utilization.

Iron metabolism

Use of radioactive iron

The use of radioactive iron (^{59}Fe) to study iron kinetics and to evaluate erythropoiesis has provided the most accurate measurements of iron metabolism in normal and in anemic persons (Cavill et al, 1977). Radioactive iron studies require expert technic and interpretation and should be performed only in centers having these qualifications. Most iron-deficiency anemias can be managed by simpler approaches as outlined in the following sections. However, radioactive iron studies provide an intricate look at the role of iron in erythropoiesis.

Absorbed iron is bound to transferrin; one possible measurement is that of radioactive iron bound to transferrin and circulating in the plasma. After a standard dose of radioactive iron is given intravenously, most of it disappears from plasma within 60 to 90 minutes; by the end of one day 99% of the radioactive iron has been cleared from the plasma. The clearance curve (plasma iron turnover, PIT) is complex because of the return to the plasma of radioactive iron from interstitial fluid and from ineffective erythropoiesis, but it can be analyzed if reflux radioactive iron is taken into account (Cavill et al, 1976).

Radioactive iron entering the bone marrow is incorporated into hemoglobin-synthesizing erythroid cells and later appears as a label on circulating mature red blood cells. This is the red cell radioactive iron uptake. Suitable analysis of these data (Ricketts et al, 1975) provides an estimate of total erythropoiesis (marrow iron turnover, MIT), effective erythropoiesis (red cell iron turnover, RCIT), ineffective erythropoiesis (ineffective iron turnover, IIT), and even mean red cell life span (MRCL).

Distribution

Iron is indispensable to three vital processes: the synthesis of hemoglobin, the synthesis of iron-containing enzymes, and the synthesis of myoglobin.

The body of an adult contains about 4 Gm of iron, about

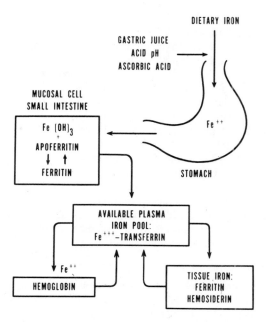

Fig. 8-5. Pathways of iron absorption and utilization.

70% in hemoglobin, 4% in myoglobin, 25% as storage iron (ferritin and hemosiderin) and labile iron pool, and the rest in various somatic cells chiefly in iron-containing enzymes. Myoglobin and enzyme iron can be considered essentially unavailable for hemoglobin synthesis. Hemoglobin synthesis utilizes storage and labile iron pool, as shown in Fig. 8-5.

Dietary iron

A normal diet in the United States supplies about 17 mg of iron per day. A hematologically normal person absorbs about 10% of this dietary iron, and 1.7 mg/day is usually adequate to satisfy the body's needs. The amount of iron ingested varies, depending on the type of food eaten (foods relatively rich in iron are meat, eggs, legumes, and leafy vegetables; foods relatively poor in iron are milk, rice, fruit, and potatoes), but actually it is affected most by the type of container used in cooking. It is now appreciated that the old-fashioned, cast-iron skillet or Dutch oven adds considerable amounts of iron to the food cooked in it. For example, spaghetti sauce simmered in a glass dish contains 3 mg of iron/100 Gm; when cooked in an iron pot, it contains 87.5 mg/100 Gm. In countries where iron cooking utensils are used, the intake of dietary iron is very high and bears little relation to the iron content of the food used, as calculated from dietary tables. Indeed, among the Bantu, who use iron pots both for cooking and for brewing their version of home brew, the dietary iron intake is extremely high, and the incidence of secondary hemochromatosis is also high.

Foodstuffs vary a great deal in their content of iron. A tabulation of the iron content of various foods is given by Sunderman and Boerner (1950). There are not many foods that are as low in iron as milk (0.07 mg/100 Gm dry weight) and yet the dairy industry touts milk as the "perfect food." In fact, it is the most expensive way of buying drinking water and the other ingredients that milk contains. In comparison with milk, cheese contains about 8 times as much iron, meat 36 times as much, liver 170 times as much, eggs 120 times as much, spinach 43 times as much, fish 20 times as much, fresh oysters 100 times as much, and potatoes 10 times as much. Red wine averages 33 mg/liter of iron (Perman, 1967), should any justification be needed for enjoying the juice of the grape. The absorption of iron from meat is about 3 times as much as from vegetables.

Two facors modify these data. The first is the effect of cooking, which generally moderately reduces the amount of available iron. The second is the variable availability of iron in different foods. For example, meat iron is about 60% available, as compared with about 17% for milk. Inorganic iron salts are absorbed more efficiently than food iron (Callender and Warner, 1968), and the composition of the diet influences the availability of supplemental iron added to bread and other foods (Layrisse et al, 1973).

Iron absorption

Dietary iron usually consists of ferrous and ferric organic iron complexes. Favored by an acid pH in the stomach, these complexes are broken down to simpler inorganic salts and ultimately reduced to the ferrous form. In the small intestine, an alkaline pH favors the formation of ferrous hydroxide, the form in which dietary iron is absorbed. Ferrous hydroxide enters the mucosal cells in the small intestine, where it is changed to ferric hydroxide. This combines with an intracellular protein, *apoferritin,* to form the compound *ferritin.* Still within the mucosal cell, the ferric iron in ferritin is again reduced to the ferrous state; in this form it diffuses out of the cell into the portal circulation.

It was once thought that apoferritin in the mucosal cell served as a regulatory mechanism for iron absorption. According to this concept, only as much iron can be absorbed as there is apoferritin to combine with it and pass it on, i.e., when apoferritin is saturated with iron and the mucosal cell is pregnant with ferritin, no more absorption can take place. Thus, according to the "mucosal block" theory (Granick, 1946), the rate and amount of iron absorption depend on the oxidation–reduction capacity of the mucosal cell. If ferric iron in ferritin is not reduced to the ferrous state, all the apoferritin remains in the combined form, and none is available for further iron absorption. Conversely, when intracellular conditions favor reduction of ferric to ferrous iron, the rate of dissociation of ferritin is accelerated, a constant supply of apoferritin is provided, and absorption of iron from the intestinal lumen is facilitated.

It seems a shame to abandon such a tidy theory, but all the evidence indicates that no such mucosal block mechanism regulates the absorption of iron. True, apoferritin and ferritin are involved, but the rate and degree of iron absorption are regulated by other factors. Of these, the most obvious are (1) the state of body stores of iron, (2) the degree of hemopoietic activity, and (3) how much iron is ingested. In general, when iron stores are depleted, iron absorption is increased; when there is active erythropoiesis, iron absorption is also increased; and when large amounts of iron are given by mouth, large amounts of iron are absorbed regardless of body stores and erythropoietic activity.

Regarding the last point, it is true that a larger *percent* of a small dose of iron and a smaller *percent* of a large dose are absorbed; nevertheless, the *amount* absorbed is greater when the larger dose is given. There are much data substantiating this conclusion. For example, when normal subjects are given oral iron, either 1 μg or 1,000 μg, 62% of the small dose is absorbed as compared with 11% of the large dose. However, the amount of iron absorbed is 0.62 μg of the smaller dose as compared with 110 μg of the larger (Bonnet et al, 1960). Iron absorption is enhanced in anemias (Haurani et al, 1965) excepting those secondary to infection or malignancy. The application of these data to any individual case is complicated by the variability in absorption of a standard dose in healthy subjects (Cook and Lipschitz, 1977).

While the classic concept of a mucosal block has been largely discarded, in the sense that the mucosal cell of the intestine exerts rate-regulating control over the amount of iron absorbed, the cell does exert some control over the amount of iron absorbed. The evidence is that the cell receives instruction, in a manner still not understood, as to the amount of iron needed, or else there would be no variation in iron absorption in proportion to the amount of storage iron. Conrad and Crosby (1963) propose that absorption is regulated by the amount of ferritin, derived from body stores, that is incorporated into newly formed mucosal cells. It is obvious that when extremely high doses of iron are ingested the regulatory system is overwhelmed or ignored, but this does not disprove the concept that under physiologic conditions an absorption-regulating mechanism is operative. In fact, the evidence indicates two very different mechanisms of absorption, depending on the dose of iron. The physiologic system depends on a carrier mechanism (Moore et al, 1964), while absorption when massive doese are given depends on the concentration of iron in the lumen of the bowel (Smith and Pannacciulli, 1958).

Table 8-2 summarizes the factors that increase or decrease the absorption of a standard dose of iron from the gastrointestinal tract. All iron compounds must be reduced to the ferrous form before absorption can occur (Moore et al, 1939).

Table 8-2. Factors that increase or decrease absorption of a standard dose of iron from intestine

A. Increased iron absorption
  1. Anemia of any type
  2. Iron-deficiency state
  3. Increased erythropoiesis with or without anemia
  4. Anoxia
  5. Cobalt administration
  6. Ascorbic acid
  7. Succinate
  8. Ethionine
  9. Inosine
  10. High altitude
B. Decreased iron absorption
  1. Malabsorption diseases
  2. Transfusion polycythemia
  3. Increased iron stores
  4. Phytates
  5. Oral administration of alkali
  6. Fever

Ascorbic acid and foods containing high concentrations of asorbic acid enhance absorption of iron in both normal and iron-deficient persons (Moore, 1961). Ascorbic acid may also be involved in the transfer of iron from the pool to body stores. The facilitation of the absorption of iron by *gastric juice* is not entirely because of the hydrochloric acid it contains. In patients with achlorhydria the addition of dilute hydrochloric acid to the food does not produce improved absorption of ^{59}Fe from food. It would appear that gastric hydrochloric acid plays only a very minor, if any, role in ferrous iron absorption and yet gastric juice contains a substance or substances that enhance the absorption of iron (Jacobs and Miles, 1969). Also, iron is absorbed better when instilled into the stomach than when instilled directly into the small bowel (Rhodes et al, 1968). This raises some doubt as to the advisability of administering iron in enteric-coated tablets that pass through the stomach before dissolving.

Phosphates retard iron absorption (Hegsted et al, 1949), thus iron in phosphate-poor foods is absorbed more readily than that in phosphate-rich foods. *Phytates* (from cereals) also retard absorption of iron salts (Sharpe et al, 1950) but not of hemoglobin iron. From this it has been postulated that the two forms of iron are absorbed by different mechanisms. Oral administration of alkali retards absorption by the formation of insoluble iron hydroxides. Succinate, fructose (Pollack et al, 1964), and amino acids (Kroe et al, 1963) enhance the absorption of iron. The influence of a too brief period of breast-feeding on iron deficiency in infancy is discussed by Dallman (1980).

Compulsive eating of unusual materials sometimes accompanies iron deficiency. *Pica,* a craving for unnatural materials, takes many forms (Cooper, 1957). *Pagophagia* (compulsive eating of ice), *geophagia* (compulsive eating of earth or clay), and *amylophagia* (compulsive eating of cornstarch or laundry starch) have been attributed to various emotional, cultural, and medicinal factors. In 1835 Craigin described a debilitating disease affecting blacks living in tropical countries who were in the habit of eating earth. He named the disease "cachexia Africana." Geophagia and amylophagia are encountered in black women, particularly in southern states. Black women living in northern states have been known to have red clay sent to them from their home state. The practice is apparently handed down from the elders as beneficial, particularly during pregnancy, and then becomes a habit. Pica is associated with iron deficiency either because the material (clay) interferes with iron absorption (Minnich et al, 1968) or because an iron-poor food (laundry starch) is substituted for a normal diet. Geophagia is not limited to the United States. Bateson and Lebroy (1978) report on clay eating in Australia and point out that it can have serious complications, such as intestinal obstruction and perforation of the colon. Habitual ingestion of clay has also been found in combination with a syndrome of dwarfism, hepatomegaly, anemia, and hypogonadism (Prasad et al, 1961), probably related to combined iron and zinc deficiency (Halsted, 1968) (p. 405).

The generally disturbed absorption in malabsorption syndromes (Chapter 9) usually includes malabsorption of iron (Giuliani et al, 1961) even when there is severe iron deficiency. In celiac disease and tropical sprue, absorption of iron, and vitamin B_{12} as well, is improved when wheat germ is excluded from the diet (gluten-free diet), though it is not known how gluten affects absorption. The primary failure appears to be in the mucosal cell since iron absorption can be restored to normal by steroid therapy even when gluten is not excluded from the diet. Malabsorption of iron is also seen in chronic diarrhea and hypermotility of the bowel, regardless of etiology. Malabsorption of iron is also a feature of immunoglobulin deficiency associated with atrophy of intestinal mucosa (Johnson et al, 1967) and has been reported in high fever caused by infection (Beresford et al, 1971) and in inflammation (Hershko et al, 1974).

The opposite situation, excessive absorption of iron, is seen in hemochromatosis. Here the mucosal cell is a veritable glutton, unable to stop absorbing iron though the body stores are overloaded with it. The serum iron concentration is usually increased, and the serum iron-binding capacity is saturated but only slightly increased. This may again reflect a biochemical failure of the mucosal cell, but there is no agreement on the nature of the defect. There is strong evidence for a genetic defect inherited as an autosomal recessive trait (Cartwright et al, 1979). There is a strongly familial incidence, and a significant number of family members having no evidence of liver damage have increased levels of serum iron and an abnormal accumulation of iron in the liver (Debré et al, 1952). Homozygotes have increased levels of serum ferritin, whereas heterozygotes usually do not (Beaumont et al, 1979). Because an increase in storage iron in the liver is found in about 20% of patients with portal or alcoholic cirrhosis (Zimmerman et al, 1961), some have implicated alcoholism as the culprit in idiopathic hemochromatosis, but the incidence of alcoholism in these cases is probably of the same order as in Laennec's cirrhosis. In any case, the iron deposits in hemochromatosis are found in all organs and tissues, and this is not the case in portal cirrhosis. At the cellular level, there is evidence that xanthine oxidase regulates the release of iron from ferritin (Mazur et al, 1958), but the attractive hypothesis that excess iron accumulates because of a deficiency of hepatic xanthine oxidase has little support (Ayvazian, 1964; Seegmiller et al, 1964).

Iron transport

After entering the blood, ferrous iron combines with a plasma protein called *transferrin*. This is a β_1-globulin that, at a normal blood pH of 7.4, combines avidly with ferrous ions. After combining with transferrin, the iron is again converted to the ferric state. It enters the *available plasma iron pool* in this form. Iron from the plasma iron pool is utilized mostly for hemoglobin synthesis, but it also satisfies the need for the synthesis of iron-containing enzymes. The concentration of iron in plasma is measured as serum iron, whereas the capacity of plasma to combine with iron is measured as the serum iron-binding capacity. Serum iron concentration is roughly one-third of the total serum iron-binding capacity.

Transferrin is the specific iron-binding β-globulin, 1 mg of transferrin binding 1.25 μg of iron. It is sometimes reduced or lacking. Transferrin bands are readily identified on starch gel electrophoretic slabs (Fig. 8-6) either by rou-

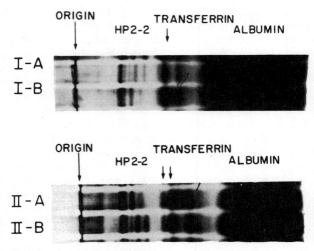

Fig. 8-6. Human transferrins, starch gel electrophoresis, Amidoschwarz stain. **I-A,** Type C transferrin, human serum, type 2-2 haptoglobin, no hemoglobin added. **I-B,** Same as **I-A** but with hemoglobin added. **II-A,** Type CD transferrin, human serum, haptoglobin type 2-2, with hemoglobin added. **II-B,** Same as **II-A** but without hemoglobin.

tine protein staining or, better, by tagging with radioiron. Transferrins migrating at different rates were first identified by Smithies (1957), and later studies have led to the conclusion that, like other genetically determined serum proteins, transferrins are controlled by alleles at a single locus and inherited as an autosomal system without dominance (Smithies and Hiller, 1959; Giblett, 1969).

The most common transferrin is designated C (another recently proposed nomenclature is Tf^c, Tf for transferrin and the superscript for the type). Those transferrins migrating more slowly than C toward the anode are type D, and those migrating faster than C are type B (Fig. 8-7). A given person may be homozygous for one of the transferrins, in which case only one band is present, or heterozygous, showing two transferrin types (about 1% of whites are type B_2C). The high frequency of type C (about 99% of the white population) makes this not only the most common type but also usually homozygous. The remaining variants may, in other ethnic groups, occur in greater frequency than in whites; e.g., type B_{0-1} in Navajo Indians, D_1 in American blacks (about 10% incidence) and Australian aborigines (more than 10%), and D_{chi} in the Chinese. In these special populations, one of the rarer types is occasionally found in the homozygous form.

The different variants of transferrin are of great genetic importance and interest, but they do not differ in their avidity for iron, in their transfer function, or in their immunology (Fig. 8-8). Transferrin has been shown to be the heat-stable bacteriostatic substance in serum. Rifkind et al (1961) described the loss of large amounts of transferrin in the urine of persons with nephrosis. This accounted for the loss of as much as 1,000 μg daily and would contribute to the iron-deficiency state in the nephrotic syndrome (both the serum iron and total iron-binding capacity are below normal).

Serum iron concentration (as transferrin) normally shows diurnal and individual variation. The serum iron concentration is about 30% higher in the morning than in the evening and about 30% lower at the onset of menstruation (Speck, 1968; Zilva and Patston, 1966). Our normal values are: mean, 105 μg/dl; range 65 to 185 μg/dl. This is in agreement with other published results. High serum iron levels are found in acute liver disease.

The total iron-binding capacity of serum (TIBC) is remarkably constant. Our normal values are: mean, 360 μg/dl; range, 250 to 440 μg/dl. Even after maximum saturation with iron, serum is seldom able to contain more than 450 μg/dl. This suggests that the plasma pool is of limited capacity, containing at most a total of 0.1 Gm of iron. Oral contraceptives increase TIBC by increasing the concentration of transferrin, the increase being of the same magnitude as is found in the second half of pregnancy (Jacobi et al, 1969).

The iron in the plasma pool undergoes a constant turnover. A fairly constant level is maintained by a balanced redistribution, iron coming into the pool from dietary sources and from hemoglobin catabolism and leaving the pool to be stored or used for the synthesis of new hemoglobin. The plasma iron turnover rate (PITR) has been measured by means of tracer doses of ^{59}Fe (Bothwell et al, 1956, 1957). In normal persons, 38 mg of iron enter and leave the plasma pool each day. The use of ^{59}Fe as a tracer also allows an estimation of the rate of incorporation of iron into erythrocytes (RBC PITR); 70% to 100% of injected radioiron is incorporated into erythrocytes within 7 to 14 days.

Intake of excessively large doses of iron, either by accidental poisoning or in experimental animals, produces a very high serum iron concentration (3,000 μg/dl and higher) (Jacobs et al, 1965). There is usually a moderate increase in iron-binding capacity and a high transferrin saturation, but when the serum iron level is very high most of it is free in the sense that it is not bound to transferrin. In humans and experimental animals, iron intoxication is reported to cause leukocytosis (Covey, 1964), thrombocytopenia, fibrinogenopenia, altered clotting reactivity of the fibrinogen, and a prolonged venous coagulation time (Wilson et al, 1958).

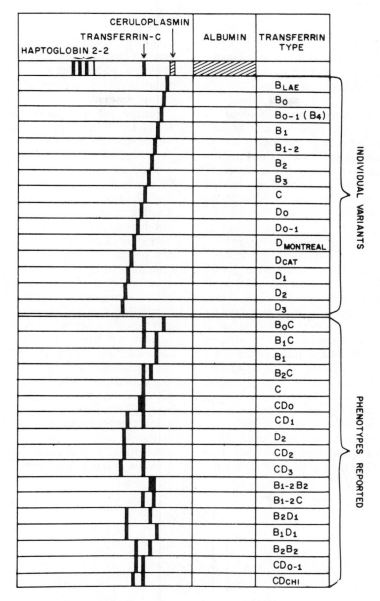

Fig. 8-7. Human transferrins (schematic).

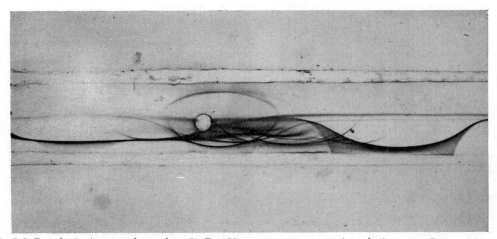

Fig. 8-8. Transferrin, immunoelectrophoresis. *Top,* Human serum versus antitransferrin serum. *Bottom,* Human serum versus polyvalent serum.

The clinical picture of acute iron intoxication is characteristic (Henderson et al, 1963; Westlin, 1966). There is usually vomiting, sometimes blood-tinged, and evidence of severe shock with grayish cyanosis. Deepening coma leads to death within 4 hours in about one-fourth of the cases. Those surviving may show a temporary improvement followed by progressively severe neurologic signs (convulsions or flaccidity), evidence of pneumonitis, and deepening coma. There may be metabolic acidosis and sometimes hyperbilirubinemia and jaundice. Most cases showing this combination of findings have a fatal outcome. Most patients survive if early treatment with gastric lavage and deferrioxamine (Whitten et al, 1966) is instituted.

Iron storage

The ability of plasma to bind and transport iron is limited. Normally the iron content of plasma, measured as *serum iron,* and the capacity of plasma to bind iron, the *iron-binding capacity,* are fairly constant.

A distinction should be made between *latent iron-binding capacity* and *total iron-binding capacity* (TIBC). The first is a measure of how much iron the serum can bind, in addition to what it already contains. This, then, is the measure of the unsaturated iron-binding capacity (UIBC). The *total* binding capacity is the sum of iron already bound plus the latent capacity (Fig. 8-9).

Excess iron, whether from increased absorption or increased hemoglobin catabolism, is stored in the liver, spleen, bone marrow, and other tissues. Stored iron normally represents about 25% of the total iron in the body. It is stored in the form of *ferritin* and *hemosiderin,* under normal conditions mostly as ferritin. The physical properties of the iron in hemosiderin closely resemble those of the iron core of ferritin (Fishback et al, 1971), supporting the concept that hemosiderin is derived from ferritin (Wapnick et al, 1970).

Ferritin, the same compound active in the mucosal mechanism for absorption, is composed of clusters of ferric hydroxyphosphate molecules bound to the protein apoferritin. It is probable that the mechanism for storage and release is based on reversible oxidation and reduction of iron, as in the mucosal cell. Ferritin is water soluble and is not visible microscopically, nor can it be demonstrated by iron stains, possibly because of the small size of the molecule and its fine dispersion throughout the cell. By electron microscopy, ferritin has a characteristic appearance of tetrads of octahedral particles (Bessis and Breton-Gorius, 1960). The concentration of ferritin in serum is proportional to total iron stores and to the amount of mobilizable iron (Jacobs et al, 1972). Hemosiderin, on the other hand, is seen readily in unstained tissue sections as irregular coarse golden brown granules and is identified by means of special stains for ferric iron. It is found normally in phagocytic reticuloendothelial cells in the bone marrow and in cases of iron overload in the spleen, liver, and other organs. Hemosiderin is sometimes found in plasma cells (Goodman and Hall, 1966). It probably consists of several iron-congeners having insolubility in water in common (Granick, 1949). Whereas the amount of iron that can be stored as ferritin is limited, extremely large amounts can be stored as hemosiderin. In either form, iron is available when needed.

When iron is given intravenously, some is bound to trans-

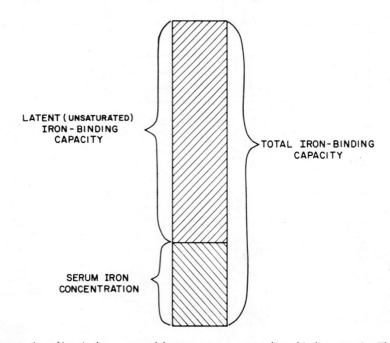

Fig. 8-9. Concentration of iron in the serum and the two measurements of iron-binding capacity. The normal ratio of serum iron concentration to total iron-binding capacity (transferrin saturation) is about 0.3 calculated according to the formula:

$$\text{Transferrin saturation} = \frac{\text{Serum iron } (\mu g/dl) \times 100}{\text{Total iron-binding capacity } (\mu g/dl)}.$$

ferrin to the limit of the iron-binding capacity. The excess is first taken up by reticuloendothelial cells throughout the body and is later concentrated in the liver. This sequence occurs when either ionizable or colloidal iron is given. It is thought that in the ionizable form, iron acts as a toxic ion, but that colloidal iron is not toxic. In either case, when the iron overload is sufficiently severe, the deposition of iron in the tissues is extensive, producing *siderosis (hemosiderosis)*. Siderosis of the liver, spleen, and other tissues is commonly seen in chronic hemolytic anemias, the continuous and increased hemolysis necessitating the disposal by storage of large quantities of hemoglobin-derived iron. Siderosis can also result from repeated blood transfusions. The iron is then derived from donor erythrocytes. It is important to remember that each "pint" of blood given contains between 200 and 250 mg of iron, and that only 16 transfusions are required to double the total iron content of the body.

Idiopathic pulmonary hemosiderosis is not a generalized iron storage disease, but rather is a syndrome of chronic bleeding into lung tissue resulting in the accumulation of hemosiderin in the lungs alone (Fuleihan et al, 1968). The disease is seen predominantly in children and young adults. The serum iron concentration is low, and serum iron-binding capacity is normal. There is chronic anemia of the hypochromic microcytic type, pulmonary insufficiency, occasional eosinophilia, and no laboratory evidence of a hemorrhagic diathesis. Identification of iron-laden macrophages in the sputum is helpful in establishing the diagnosis. *Goodpasture's syndrome* is characterized by the association of progressive glomerulonephritis and recurrent pulmonary hemorrhage with pulmonary hemosiderosis (Bergdahl et al, 1969). In contrast to idiopathic pulmonary hemosiderosis, Goodpasture's syndrome is found predominantly in older adults.

Vitale et al (1969) described an unusual iron storage disease that they call *congenital and familial iron overload*. The subjects were two infants with hypotonia and a marked increase in iron stored in the liver, bone marrow, and kidney. There was no evidence of hemolytic disease or of excessive iron intake. They postulate there was a genetically determined disturbance of iron transfer in utero. Another abnormality of iron metabolism has been described as *iron-deficiency anemia associated with an error of iron metabolism* by Shahidi et al (1964). The two syndromes have some similarities but differ in that the patients described by Shahidi et al had no iron deposits in the bone marrow.

Iron stores may be adequate or even excessive, without iron being available for hemoglobin synthesis; e.g., iron-deficiency anemia due to chronic infection characteristically shows increased amounts of storage iron. In spite of an acute need, the stored iron is not available. This iron starvation in the face of plenty emphasizes the physiologic importance of the concept of *available iron* rather than *total iron*.

Normal and abnormal values for iron are given in Table 8-6.

Iron loss and excretion

Iron is one of the most carefully conserved substances. Under normal conditions so little iron is lost that for all practical purposes iron loss is negligible. This jealous conservation has one drawback—the inability to eliminate excess iron. A little iron is eliminated when epithelial cells, mucosal cells, and epidermal derivatives such as hair and nails are shed. Some may be lost in bile. The total loss per day in a normal adult male has been estimated to be less than 1 mg (Green et al, 1968). It is probable that a given atom of iron participates in many cycles of hemoglobin synthesis and catabolism (Saito et al, 1964).

Iron can be lost as the result of bleeding. Hemoglobin contains about 0.34% by weight of iron; with each milliliter of blood lost, about 0.5 mg of iron is also lost. A normal menstrual loss averages 34 ml of blood (Hallberg et al, 1966), equivalent to a loss of about 17 mg of iron, while 80 ml of blood, equivalent to 40 mg of iron, is considered the upper limit of normal menstrual blood loss (Haynes et al, 1977). When menstrual bleeding is profuse or prolonged, iron loss may be sufficient eventually to produce an iron deficiency. One of the subjects described in the study of Rankin et al (1962) as having a heavy flow during the menstrual period lost 970 ml of blood each month, which is equivalent to an iron loss of about 485 mg. Pregnancy and lactation account for additional loss of iron, about 400 mg going to the fetus, 150 mg to the placenta, 200 ml lost at delivery, and 0.5 mg/day lost in milk.

The question of occult blood loss from the gastrointestinal tract as the result of aspirin ingestion deserves some discussion. While there is no doubt that the ingestion of aspirin increases the amount of occult blood in the stool (Matsumoto and Grossman, 1959) and that aspirin can cause gross bleeding from preexisting ulcerative lesions (Muir and Cossar, 1959), there is no convincing evidence that chronic ingestion of aspirin by normal persons eating a normal diet and having no other cause to lose iron can lead to iron deficiency on the basis of chronic blood loss. By the most accurate technic—measurement of loss of labeled red cells—normal individuals not ingesting aspirin lose an average of about 0.8 ml of blood per day; high-dose aspirin ingestion (3 Gm/day) is accompanied by a fecal blood loss of 2 to 3 ml/day (Grossman et al, 1961; Beeken, 1968) or about 1.5 mg of iron per day.

In cases of iron overload, iron excretion can be accelerated by using *chelating* agents that have an affinity for iron and are then excreted together with iron in the urine (Cleton et al, 1963; Cumming et al, 1969; Fairbanks et al, 1971; Propper et al, 1976). These agents make possible the excretion of large amounts of iron (10 to 20 mg/day, depending on the chelating agent used and the intensity of treatment), but it has been pointed out (Fairbanks et al, 1971) that phlebotomy of 500 ml of blood twice weekly is 3 times as effective in reducing body iron.

Iron requirements

Normal dietary requirements (assuming 10% absorption) are as follows: (1) adult men and nonmenstruating women, 10 mg/day, (2) adult women, 20 mg/day, and (3) pregnant women, 35 mg/day. The iron requirement of infants and children is slightly greater than that of adults. In addition to the basic iron requirements, an infant must have sufficient iron for a thirtyfold increase in the total erythrocyte mass from infant to adult values. Special care must be taken to avoid the development of iron deficiency in premature infants, since they begin life with less available iron than the full-term infant (Schulman, 1961).

A normal diet supplies the adult with about 10 to 15 mg of iron per day. Normally about 10% is absorbed so that if there are not unusual requirements, a normal diet supplies all the necessary iron. In geographic areas where the soil is poor in iron (Natvig, 1963), the diet may supply only about one-third of the optimum. Poverty diets and food fads can also fail to satisfy the normal dietary requirements for iron. During pregnancy a normal diet is not sufficiently rich in iron to supply the daily requirement (35 mg). Cow's milk contains about 0.07 mg of iron/100 ml, an insufficient amount to supply, by itself, the requirements of the growing infant. Human milk contains a little more iron than does cow's milk, but is it still a poor source of dietary iron for the infant.

Iron utilization

There remains the question of how iron from the plasma pool is transferred across the cellular membrane of the developing normoblast.

The chief mechanism involves the binding of iron-transferrin to receptor sites at the surface of immature erythroid cells (polychromatophilic normoblasts and orthochromic normoblasts) (Katz, 1965; Aisen, 1974). The receptors are a property of the cell membrane, since they can be removed by trypsin. The transferrin bound to the membrane gives up the iron but it is not established whether the iron alone passes through the membrane or whether the entire iron–transferrin complex enters the cell (Morgan and Appleton, 1969). Appreciating the rapid rate at which hemoglobin molecules are synthesized (Chapter 10), it should be expected that the delivery system for iron needs to be very efficient. Indeed, it has been calculated that about 50,000 atoms

of iron are delivered to the erythropoietic cell per minute. Having entered the cell, iron is utilized by mitochondria for the synthesis of heme from protoporphyrin and iron. Any abnormality in this final step (lead poisoning, sideroachrestic anemias) causes an accumulation of iron on the surface of the mitochondria and the formation of *siderotic granules* in erythroid cells classified as *sideroblasts* (p. 408).

A second mechanism exists for utilizing iron in hemoglobin synthesis. Bessis and Breton-Gorius (1961) have shown that normoblasts tend to encircle an iron-containing reticulum cell, from which ferritin supposedly is transferred to the normoblasts. The transfer is effected by the pinocytotic process of "ropheocytosis," an invagination of the cytoplasmic membrane of the normoblast by which ferritin particles are suckled by the normoblast from the "nurse cell." Unfortunately, this vivid concept is of very minor importance quantitatively. Indeed some believe that the reticulum cell is removing from rather than giving iron to the normoblasts (Zail et al, 1964), while others (Tanaka and Brecher, 1971) suggest that ferritin is synthesized de novo at the membrane of the normoblast.

Once hemoglobin is synthesized, iron remains in the erythrocytes until cellular disintegration takes place, at which time it is frugally returned to the plasma pool for subsequent reutilization.

Some evidence exists that iron by itself exerts a stimulating effect on erythropoiesis other than hemoglobin synthesis. When iron is administered to a patient with iron-deficiency anemia, not only does it produce the expected increase in corpuscular hemoglobin concentration but also two other striking effects occur: (1) a rise in reticulocytes, indicating an increase in erythropoiesis and (2) a rise in the total number of erythrocytes. This is illustrated in Fig. 8-10. The microcytosis in iron-deficiency anemia cannot be

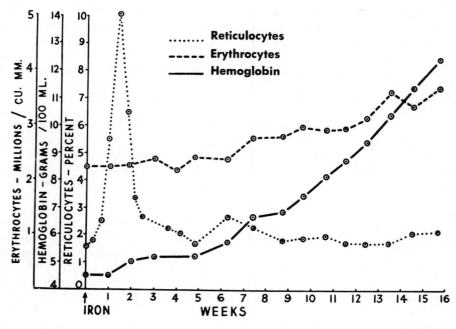

Fig. 8-10. Reticulocyte response following administration of iron alone in iron-deficiency anemia.

explained on the basis of hypochromia. In fact, there are reports that hypochromic microcytic erythrocytes have a shortened survival time (Loria et al, 1967).

COPPER

Copper qualifies as a trace element since the body of an adult contains only about 100 to 150 mg of copper. There is good evidence that copper is essential for normal erythropoiesis in animals (Lee et al, 1968a), but its role in erythropoiesis in humans is not yet clear. In crustaceans (such as the Florida lobster) the oxygen-carrying function of the blood is performed by copper-containing hemocyanin rather than iron-containing hemoglobin, showing that copper and iron have similar chemical affinities for oxygen.

Copper deficiency in pigs produces a hypochromic microcytic anemia that does not respond to iron alone. This anemia is characterized by a decreased erythrocyte survival time, while the rate of incorporation of iron into hemoglobin is proportionately decreased. Nutritional copper deficiency can occur in children (Cordano et al, 1964; Al-Rashid and Spangler, 1971) and is characterized by anemia, neutropenia, and osteoporosis. The anemia does not respond to iron administration unless copper is also given. A more severe copper deficiency in infants is the "kinky hair syndrome" (Menkes et al, 1962). This is a sex-linked recessive syndrome, the features being kinky, depigmented hair and focal cerebral and cerebellar degeneration causing seizures and death in the early years of infancy. Danks et al (1972 and 1973) defined other features of this syndrome: elongated, tortuous, and supernumerary cerebral and mesenteric arteries, excessive copper concentration in the cells of the intestinal mucosa, and increased concentration of copper in the brain and other organs.

The combination of iron and copper deficiency in infants nourished exclusively on milk also has the component of hypoproteinemia (Schubert and Lahey, 1959; Wilson et al, 1961). In addition to the low iron and copper content of milk, cow's milk contains a thermolabile factor that in some infants causes gastrointestinal bleeding and aggravates the iron deficiency (Wilson et al 1964). Copper relates to iron metabolism and anemia in two ways: (1) ceruloplasmin is required for normal release of storage iron (Roeser et al, 1970) and (2) ceruloplasmin is required for proper utilization of iron by normoblasts for synthesis of hemoglobin, probably by influencing mitochondrial uptake of iron (Williams et al, 1973) through its role in the oxidation of ferrous to ferric iron. Because of this enzymatic role in iron metabolism, ceruloplasmin is now called *ferroxidase*. Except in the case of the "milk anemia" discussed above, it is doubtful that these functions of copper are of great importance.

Copper metabolism in humans is reviewed by Dowdy (1969). Experiments with ingested ^{64}Cu reveal that soon after absorption, copper is found in the serum albumin fraction, but within 24 hours most of it has become bound to an α_2-globulin called *ceruloplasmin* or *ferroxidase* (Morell et al, 1964), Fig. 8-11. This is found in Cohn's fraction IV-1 and has a molecular weight of about 160,000 and a copper content of 0.32%. There are 7 atoms of copper per molecule. In blacks, but rarely in whites, there is polymorphism on a genetic basis. Three electrophoretic variants have been described, CpA (fast), CpB (intermediate), and CpC (slow). It is probable that the A and B forms are controlled by a pair of allelic genes, Cp^A, and Cp^B, while the C form may be controlled by another allele, Cp^C, at the same locus (Shreffler, 1967).

In vivo, copper is incorporated into the ceruloplasmin molecule at the time the protein moiety, *apoceruloplasmin*, is synthesized. In humans, 93% of the copper is bound to ceruloplasmin ("firmly bound copper"), and 7% is loosely bound to albumin or other proteins. The loosely bound copper is also called "direct-reading copper" because it reacts directly with sodium diethyldithiocarbonate without prior acid treatment of the plasma. Ceruloplasmin, an oxidative enzyme, supposedly accounts for the oxidative properties of plasma regarding various substrates, acting as a polyphenol oxidase, serum catecholase, monoamine oxidase, and possibly an ascorbic acid oxidase (Humoller et al, 1960). Normal serum ceruloplasmin concentration in adults is 33 mg/dl (95% range, 27 to 47 mg/dl). In newborn infants the plasma ceruloplasmin concentration ranges from 5 to 18 mg/dl, the mean being 8 mg/dl (Buffone et al, 1979). The major pathway of copper excretion is the bile. Small amounts are

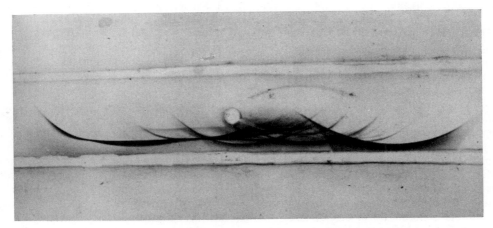

Fig. 8-11. Ceruloplasmin, immunoelectrophoresis. *Top,* Human serum versus anticeruloplasmin serum. *Bottom,* Human serum versus polyvalent serum.

Table 8-3. Total serum copper concentration in various conditions

Condition	Mean ± SD (μg/dl)	Range (μg/dl)
Normal adults*	116	68-161
Males†	110 ± 15.7	68-161
Females†	120 ± 17.8	83-165
Newborn infants*	75	45-110
Nephrotic syndrome*	64	20-96
Wilson's disease†	61 ± 20.8	34-116
Portal cirrhosis of liver‡	141 ± 38.6	72-225
Sprue, relapse§	87 ± 33	19-157
Sprue, remission§	114 ± 33	24-186
Megaloblastic anemia of pregnancy§	159	105-242
Pernicious anemia*	121 ± 36	
Pregnancy (normal)*	222 ± 38	
Acute leukemia*	236 ± 79	
Hemochromatosis*	134 ± 24	

*From Gubler, 1956.
†From Cartwright et al, 1960.
‡From Gubler et al, 1957.
§From Butterworth et al, 1958.

Table 8-4. Normal values for various parameters of copper metabolism*

Fraction	Mean	95% range
Total serum copper/dl		
Men	109 μg	81-137 μg
Women	120 μg	87-153 μg
Serum copper/dl (direct reading)	7 μg	0-20 μg
Ceruloplasmin/dl		
Men	31 mg	25-37 mg
Women	36 mg	25-47 mg
Newborn†	6.5 mg	1.8-13.1 mg
Erythrocyte copper/dl of packed RBCs	89 μg	66-112 μg
Erythrocuprein/dl of packed RBCs	16 mg	10-22 mg
Urinary copper/day	15 μg	5-25 μg
Spinal fluid copper/dl	6 μg	2-11 μg

*From Cartwright and Wintrobe, 1964.
†Data from Scheinberg et al, 1954.

excreted in the urine. Ceruloplasmin can be demonstrated not only in the urine but also in ascitic, synovial, and cerebrospinal fluid.

Since most of the copper in serum is bound to ceruloplasmin, values for both are correspondingly high, low, or normal in various disease states (Table 8-3). In adults hypercupremia is found in pregnancy (especially during the third trimester) and in such a diverse group of diseases as to be of little significance. Serum copper concentration is elevated in uncomplicated iron-deficiency anemia. Acute copper intoxication has been described following ingestion or absorption through the skin of copper salts. The manifestations are jaundice, hemolytic anemia, oliguria, and a striking increase in the serum ceruloplasmin concentration (Fairbanks, 1967). Serum copper concentration is low in Wilson's disease (Dobyns et al, 1979), a syndrome characterized by cirrhosis of the liver, degeneration of the lenticular nucleus in the brain, and pigmentation of the cornea in the form of a smoky brown or gray-green ring (the Kayser-Fleischer ring). The corneal ring is always present and is an even more reliable diagnostic sign than hypocupremia. The syndrome is one of the inborn errors of metabolism and is inherited as an autosomal recessive trait. Hoagland and Goldstein (1978) found leukopenia and thrombocytopenia in 54% of the patients with Wilson's disease. There are several theories as to the nature of the defect, including: (1) overabsorption of copper from the upper gastrointestinal tract, (2) a deficiency of ceruloplasmin, (3) an increased avidity of proteins for copper resulting in increased deposition in the liver, cornea, kidney, and basal ganglia of the brain, and (4) defective transfer of serum copper to ceruloplasmin, possibly because of some abnormality in apoceruloplasmin. In any case, a measurable abnormality in this disease is a decreased concentration of ceruloplasmin in the serum. As a result, the proportion of bound copper in the serum is decreased, while body stores and excretion of copper in the urine are increased. Hypocupremia is also found in nephrosis, idiopathic hypoproteinemia, kwashiorkor, celiac disease, and tropical sprue. It is possible to attribute the hypocupremia in each of these to a deficiency of ceruloplasmin caused by the disordered protein metabolism.

Copper is also found within the erythrocytes. The concentration is roughly equal to that in the serum. Here, also, it is bound to protein, forming the copper compound *erythrocuprein* (Hartz and Deutsch, 1969). This compound differs markedly from ceruloplasmin. Erythrocuprein has a molecular weight of about 33,000 and has 2 copper atoms per molecule. The two copper-binding proteins are also immunologically different. The concentration of copper in erythrocytes is 93 to 114 μg/dl of washed packed cells, that of erythrocuprein 30 to 36 mg, and that of erythrocuprein copper 94 to 108 μg/dl (Markowitz et al, 1959). It would seem that most, if not all, of the copper in erythrocytes can be accounted for as erythrocuprein bound. Pagliardi et al (1958) report slightly different normal values for erythrocyte copper in Italian subjects: males, 123 ± 36 μg/dl (range 70 to 200 μg/dl) and females, 139 ± 23 μg/dl (range 80 to 180 μg/dl). Normal values for the various copper parameters are given in Table 8-4.

COBALT

Cobalt is normally incorporated into the molecue of cyanocobalamin (vitamin B_{12}), but there is no evidence that cobalt deficiency produces a hemopoietic factor deficiency. Ruminants pastured in areas where the soil is poor in cobalt develop anemia and emaciation, but nonruminant herbivorous animals are not affected. It is doubtful whether a cobalt deficiency can develop in human beings. Nevertheless, the administration of cobalt salts in experimental animals has resulted in polycythemia. We now know that cobalt does stimulate the elaboration of erythropoietin and that its activity is entirely a result of this effect (Chapter 1).

Table 8-5. Classification of iron-deficiency anemia

I. Anemia due to quantitative iron deficiency (*sideropenic anemias*)
  A. Low iron intake (nutritional)
  B. Diminished iron absorption
    1. Achlorhydria (?)
    2. Malabsorption syndromes
    3. Gastrectomy
    4. Chronic dysentery
    5. Pica
    6. Infection and hyperpyrexia
  C. Physiologically increased iron requirements
    1. Pregnancy and lactation
    2. Infancy
    3. Prematurity
  D. Excessive iron loss
    1. Chronic hemorrhage
    2. Hookworm infection
  E. Iron and zinc deficiency with dwarfism and hypogonadism
II. Anemia due to inadequate utilization of iron (*sideroachrestic anemias*)*
  A. Chronic disorders
    1. Infections (bacterial, mycotic)
    2. Rheumatoid arthritis
    3. Rheumatic fever
    4. Systemic lupus erythematosus
    5. Other collagen diseases
    6. Carcinoma
    7. Lymphoma
    8. Leukemia
  B. Thalassemia (and other hemoglobinopathies) (Chapter 14)

  C. Sideroblastic anemia
    1. Primary
      a. Idiopathic refractory sideroblastic anemia
      b. Pyridoxine-responsive sideroblastic anemia
    2. Acquired
      a. In systemic disease
        (1) Rheumatoid arthritis
        (2) Periarteritis nodosa
        (3) Disseminated lupus erythematosus
        (4) Leukemia
        (5) Lymphoma
        (6) Carcinoma
        (7) Mulitple myeloma
        (8) Myeloproliferative disorders
        (9) Megaloblastic anemias
        (10) Myxedema
        (11) Thyrotoxicosis
        (12) Uremia
        (13) Porphyria
        (14) Associated with mesenteric lymphoid hamartoma
      b. Caused by drugs
        (1) Lead
        (2) Chloramphenicol
        (3) Alcohol
        (4) Antituberculosis drugs
        (5) Drugs used in cancer chemotherapy
  D. Hereditary iron-loading anemia
    1. Shahidi-Nathan-Diamond type
    2. Vitale type
III. Anemia due to transferrin deficiency
  A. Congenital
  B. Acquired

*From the Greek *achrēstia*, the nonutilization of something.

ZINC

Except in the dwarf syndrome described by Prasad et al (1961), zinc deficiency does not play a role in the etiology of anemia. Zinc deficiency causes a lethal inherited disease called *acrodermatitis enteropathica* (Moynahan, 1974; Walravens, 1980).

IRON-DEFICIENCY ANEMIA
Classification

Iron deficiency should be thought of as the unavailability of iron for hemoglobin synthesis. Iron may be unavailable because it is in short supply, because it is present in adequate, even excessive, amounts but it is not available to the normoblast for hemoglobin synthesis, or because the normoblast is pathologically unable to utilize it. The concept, then, of *available iron* is more important than that of *total iron*. It follows that correct diagnosis and appropriate and effective treatment depend on determining not only that an anemia is of the iron-deficiency type but also the reason iron is not available.

The classification given in Table 8-5 divides iron deficiency anemia into three categories. The *sideropenic* iron deficiency anemias are those in which there is an insufficient supply of iron. The *sideroachrestic* anemias are those in which the supply of iron is adequate or excessive but there is deficient utilization of it. The third category, *transferrin deficiency,* has some features that seem to set it apart from the other two.

Clinical picture

It has been estimated that iron deficiency is not only the most common cause of anemia (Prager, 1972; Woodruff, 1977) but also the most common deficiency of an essential nutrient. Iron deficiency would be considered even more common if one includes "latent" iron deficiency, i.e., persons with low serum iron and depleted storage iron but not yet anemic (Verloop, 1970). Iron deficiency is about five times more common in women than in men and the distribution of incidence according to age is almost symmetrical between 10 and 70 years of age (Beveridge et al, 1965), with the highest incidence in middle adult life.

The general symptoms of anemic hypoxia are discussed on p. 392. Some special features of iron deficiency should be noted. Fatigue occurs in latent iron deficiency and in the absence of anemia (Beutler et al, 1960; Morrow et al, 1968). In these two reports iron therapy not only led to improvement of the symptom in about two-thirds of the women but also the blood hemoglobin level increased an average of 1.7

Gm/dl. Iron deficiency is accompanied by depletion of iron-containing compounds that may contribute to the symptomatology (Dallman et al, 1978a; Oski, 1979). There are three categories of these compounds: (1) heme iron compounds whose structure is similar to that of hemoglobin (the cytochromes, catalase, and peroxidase), (2) iron-containing compounds not in the heme conformation (NADH dehydrogenase, succinic dehydrogenase, and xanthine oxidase), and (3) compounds that do not contain iron but require heme or iron as a cofactor (aconitase and tryptophan pyrrolone). In addition, there are some enzymes presumed to contain iron in which the form of iron is uncertain (α-d-glycerophosphate dehydrogenase and ribonucleotide reductase). It seems that iron deficiency may cause subtle but significant metablic abnormalities. For example, the neutrophils of subjects with severe iron deficiency have normal phagocytic but diminished bactericidal activity and are defective in the reduction of nitroblue tetrazolium (NBT). The defect is corrected by the administration of iron; it is tempting to assume that the abnormal neutrophils are deficient in the iron-containing myeloperoxidase.

Iron-deficiency anemia is accompanied by characteristic, not necessarily diagnostic, tissue changes. The fingernails are brittle, ridged, and flattened or concave and "spoon-shaped" *(koilonychia)* (Witts, 1969). This is a finding in about one-third of adults, but is occasionally seen in infants (Hogan and Jones, 1970). The oral mucosa may be atrophic, with an increase in keratinization. The atrophy may involve the tongue, which becomes smooth with loss of papillae (Jacobs and Cavill, 1968), and may simulate the glossitis of pernicious anemia. Difficulty in swallowing, known as the Plummer-Vinson syndrome or, more properly, as the Paterson-Kelly syndrome (Waldenström and Kjellberg, 1939; Jacobs and Kilpatrick, 1964), is called *sideropenic dysphagia* because of its association with iron-deficiency anemia. The lesion consists of web-like obstructions in the upper part of the esophagus, and occasionally progresses to carcinoma. The mucosa of the gastrointestinal tract is also involved, as evidenced by gastritis (Ikkala et al, 1970), reduced gastric

secretion, and hypochlorhydria in about 40% of anemic patients (Beveridge et al, 1965). Antibodies against gastric parietal cells can be demonstrated in the serum (Wright et al, 1966) in about one-third of the patients. All of these epithelial changes strongly suggest that iron deficiency is responsible for a variety of cellular dysfunctions, only one of which results in anemia.

Laboratory diagnosis
Degree of anemia

In latent iron deficiency there may be no anemia, but, as noted, many of these patients respond to iron therapy with a significant increase in the blood hemoglobin concentration. In established iron-deficiency anemia the severity varies from mild to severe depending on duration and etiology. We find that iron-deficiency anemia in infants sometimes presents with a normal to slightly reduced erythrocyte count and a markedly reduced blood hemoglobin concentration.

Red cell morphology

In the typical example of iron-deficiency anemia, as caused by chronic bleeding, the peripheral blood smear will show hypochromic microcytic erythrocytes (Fig. 8-12) and moderate anisocytosis and poikilocytosis. The degree of microcytosis and hypochromia depends in general on the severity of the anemia, but these measurements are subjective to some degree and the severity of the anemia is not always reflected in the interpretation of red cell morphology (Fairbanks, 1971). Another difficulty is that the clinical stage of the anemia may be such that not all the red cells are hypochromic and microcytic. There may be a mixture of hypochromic and normal red cells, a dimorphic picture that complicates the grading of the abnormality. Depending on whether or not there is increased erythropoiesis, the smear may show polychromatophilic red cells in proportion to the reticulocytosis. When reticulocytosis follows the administration of iron, the smear may show a mixture of microcytes, normocytes, and macrocytes (Bessman, 1977). An occa-

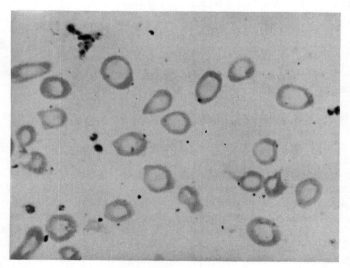

Fig. 8-12. Peripheral blood smear, iron-deficiency anemia. Note hypochromia, microcytosis, anisocytosis, and poikilocytosis. (Wright's stain; ×950.)

sional target cell and stippled erythrocyte may be found, but these are few in comparison with the number seen in other anemias.

This morphologic picture is characteristic of the anemias in category I, Table 8-5. The anemias in category II have, as a common denominator, the poor utilization of iron that is present in more than adequate amounts; the red cell morphology is sometimes characteristic. For example, the anemias of thalassemic syndromes and some other hemoglobinopathies show hypochromic red cells but there are also many target cells. Poikilocytosis and anisocytosis are striking. Stippled erythrocytes, normoblasts, and Howell-Jolly bodies are present, and, because there is usually an increase in reticulocytes, polychromatophilic red cells are found easily. In the sideroblastic anemias the hypochromia of the red cells is usually moderate, and the presence of hypochromic red cells and normal red cells (dimorphism, Fig. 8-13) is common. In all of the sideroblastic anemias a few basophilic stippled erythrocytes can be found, but in the sideroblastic anemia of lead intoxication, basophilic stippling may be striking. The sideroblastic anemias show typical bone marrow findings (p. 413).

Red cell indices

In iron-deficiency anemia, the reduction in the hemoglobin concentration is proportionately greater than the reduction in the erythrocyte count. As noted above, there is also microcytosis. Accordingly, the mean corpuscular volume (MCV) is smaller than normal, usually in direct proportion to the severity of the anemia. In mild anemias the MCV may be close to normal. In interpreting any of the values for the red cell indices it must be remembered that they represent *average* values and as such must be correlated with the appearance of the red cells on the blood smear. The MCV will be otherwise misleading when there is a dimorphic population or, as is sometimes the case in sideroblastic anemias, the simultaneous presence of microctyes, normal red cells, and some macrocytes. The same considerations apply to the interpretation of MCH values that range from normal in mild cases to significantly reduced in severe iron-deficiency anemia. The MCHC is usually less abnormal than the other indices, even in a severe anemia.

Reticulocytes

The reticulocyte count is not helpful in the initial diagnosis of iron-deficiency anemia, but we always perform one in the study of anemia as an index of the degree of red blood cell production and release. In iron-deficiency anemia the reticulocyte count is usually normal to slightly elevated, whereas it is low in aplastic anemia and increased in hemolytic anemias. When a severe iron-deficiency anemia is treated adequately, a significant reticulocytosis occurs within a few days (Fig. 8-10).

Leukocytes

The leukocyte count and morphology are usually normal. There may be a neutrophilic leukocytosis when a significant amount of blood is present in the gastrointestinal tract or when there has been massive hemorrhage. Neutropenia has been described in severe chronic iron-deficiency anemia (Voigt et al, 1967).

Platelets

Moderate thrombocytopenia is not uncommon in severely anemic infants and children (Gross et al, 1964) and is corrected by iron therapy. Both thrombocytopenia and throm-

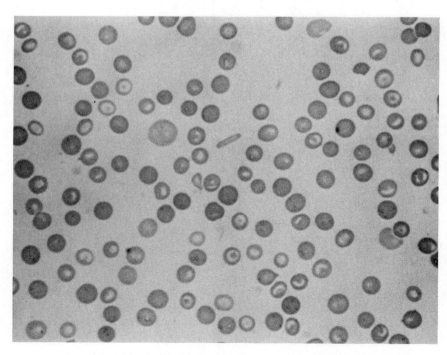

Fig. 8-13. Dimorphism of red blood cells in sideroblastic anemia, peripheral blood. Note the two populations, one of normochromic red cells, the other hypochromic with target cell formation. (Wright's stain; ×350.)

bocytosis are recorded (Dinçol and Aksoy, 1969), but thrombocytosis may be caused by blood loss rather than being a feature of iron deficiency.

Bone marrow

The chief indication for performing a biopsy of the bone marrow is to estimate the amount of storage iron. In sideropenic iron-deficiency anemia the morphology of the erythroid cells is usually normal and the degree of erythroid hyperplasia depends on the degree to which the anemia is being compensated for. Occasionally the polychromatophilic and orthochromic normoblasts appear to have scanty, frayed, and poorly hemoglobinated cytoplasm, but this is not a feature diagnostic of any one type of anemia.

In sideroblastic anemias bone marrow smears stained for iron reveal many iron-containing inclusions in the erythrocytes and normoblasts. Cartwright and Deiss (1975) classify the iron-containing cells into three types: *sideroblasts, reticulated siderocytes,* and *siderocytes.*

Sideroblasts are normoblasts that contain one or a few iron-containing granules. These represent aggregates of ferritin in the cytoplasm not associated with mitochondria. Since this is ferritin on the way to mitochondria to be used for heme synthesis, this type of inclusion is normal; in fact, 30% to 50% of the normoblasts in normal marrow contain this type of inclusion (Bainton and Finch, 1964; Bessis, 1973b). The number of sideroblasts of this type is directly proportional to the transferrin saturation, so that only a few or none are present in sideropenic states.

Ringed sideroblasts (Fig. 8-14) differ from the normal sideroblasts in that the inclusions are numerous and form a ring around the nucleus, and the iron is associated with mitochondria. Since the mitochondria usually lie in a perinuclear ring (Bowman, 1961), the ring pattern is retained when they become overloaded with iron. Ringed sideroblasts are characteristic of sideroblastic anemias (Hall and Losowsky, 1966; Goodman and Hall, 1967; Hines and Grasso, 1970). As many as 70% of the normoblasts are ringed sideroblasts in idiopathic sideroblastic anemia and are usually less numerous in drug-induced sideroblastic anemia (MacGibbon and Mollin, 1965). By electron microscopy the iron-laden mitochondria are distorted, swollen, and may be disrupted (Hammond et al, 1969). The destruction of most, or all, of the mitochondria renders the normoblast ineffective in hemoglobin synthesis.

Reticulated siderocytes are produced by extrusion of the nucleus of a normal sideroblast. They contain reticulum as well as siderotic granules and are still metabolically active in the synthesis of hemoglobin. The presence of both reticulum and siderotic granules distinguishes them from *reticulocytes,* containing only reticulum, and from *siderocytes,* containing only granules. Reticulated siderocytes are normally not found in the peripheral blood, but during hyperactive erythropoiesis both reticulated siderocytes and reticulocytes may be released from the bone marrow into the peripheral blood. Siderocytes are found in the peripheral blood only in sideroblastic anemias, and then only in small numbers (Kurth et al, 1969). Siderocytes are more numerous in splenectomized subjects (p. 64).

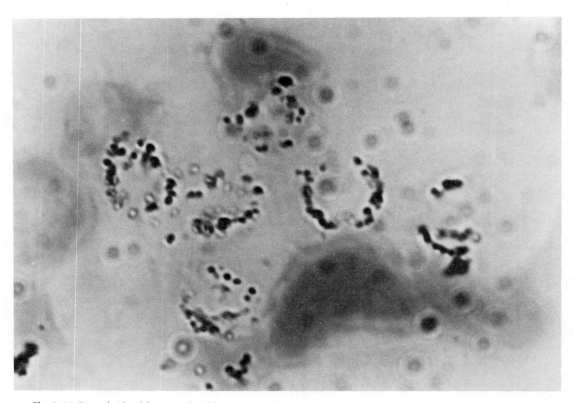

Fig. 8-14. Ringed sideroblasts in sideroblastic anemia, bone marrow. Note the perinuclear arrangement of coarse iron-containing inclusions. (Iron stain; ×1,000.)

Osmotic fragility of red cells

Moderately decreased osmotic fragility (increased resistance to hypotonic lysis) is encountered at times in anemias caused by a deficiency of iron (Reimann and Arkun, 1956), while markedly decreased osmotic fragility is characteristic of thalassemia (p. 649). This test is useful in the diagnosis of some of the hemolytic anemias (p. 582) but is of no value in iron-deficiency anemia and of limited value in the diagnosis of thalassemia. Decreased osmotic fragility also has been reported in the anemia of lead poisoning (Griggs, 1964). These findings indicate a mild membrane defect, but there are also reports of moderately decreased red cell survival in iron-deficiency anemia of chronic disorders (Cartwright, 1966).

Evaluation of iron metabolism

An evaluation of the state of iron metabolism is basic to the investigation of iron-deficiency anemia. It is now generally agreed that the most sensitive and discriminatory measurement of iron deficiency is the concentration of serum ferritin. However, ferritin in serum is present in minute quantities, and the determination of ferritin concentration is based on radioimmunometric technics that allow quantification in nanogram quantities (Saab et al, 1978; Sheehan et al, 1978). Not all laboratories have the capability to perform radioimmunometric assays, so that in this section the more traditional tests (serum iron concentration, total iron-binding capacity, and estimation of bone marrow iron stores) are also discussed.

SERUM FERRITIN CONCENTRATION. Storage iron is mostly in the form of ferritin (Harrison, 1977). Assuming that the body contains a total of 4.5 Gm of iron, this is distributed chiefly between hemoglobin (3.15 Gm) and ferritin (0.9 Gm). The remainder is in myoglobin, iron-containing enzymes, and hemosiderin. Ferritin is stored in reticuloendothelial cells (Alfrey et al, 1967), and the serum concentration is directly proportional to storage iron (Lipschitz et al, 1974; Ali et al, 1978) (Table 8-6). It must be assumed that the ferritin in serum is in equilibrium with storage iron; thus when iron stores are low, so is the concentration of ferritin in serum. This concept is supported by studies showing that serum ferritin levels are low when storage iron is decreased early in the state of iron deficiency before anemia develops (Walters et al, 1973). With advancing deficiency of iron the serum iron concentration is low, and the iron-binding capacity is high. In fully developed iron-deficiency (sideropenic) anemia the ferritin level in serum is in the range of 0.6 to 12.0 ng/ml, serum iron concentration is in the range of 7 to 60 μg/dl, the iron-binding capacity is increased to 450 to 500 μg/dl, and there is a complete absence of storage iron in the bone marrow.

In the sideroachrestic anemias (Table 8-5) where there is ineffective erythropoiesis due to failure to utilize iron, it will be found that bone marrow iron stores and the ferritin concentration in serum are high. A striking increase in storage iron is seen in iron overload states (hemochromatosis, siderosis), and these are also characterized by very high serum ferritin concentrations (Lipschitz et al, 1974; Halliday et al, 1977).

The serum ferritin concentration reaches normal levels within a few days when iron therapy is instituted in iron-deficiency (sideropenic) anemia, so that the test has no diagnostic value if the patient is taking iron. Normal or elevated serum ferritin levels are found in conjunction with absent bone marrow iron in the anemia of leukemia, Hodgkin's disease, lymphoma, myeloma, and liver disease (Jacobs and Worwood, 1975; Krause and Stolc, 1979). Serum ferritin levels are high in hemochromatosis (Beamish et al, 1974) and can be reduced to normal levels by repeated phlebotomies. Family members with latent familial hemochromatosis have normal serum ferritin levels in spite of high levels of serum iron and high transferrin saturation (Lipschitz et al, 1974).

SERUM IRON CONCENTRATION. All sera contain some iron that is in free hemoglobin, derived from physiologic breakdown of red cells. This amounts to 0.16 to 0.58 mg/dl (mean 0.31 mg/dl) (Hanks et al, 1960). Transport iron is bound to transferrin, and in the determination of transport iron, the iron is split away from the transferrin by technics that do not liberate hemoglobin iron. For this reason transport iron has been called "loosely bound iron" to distinguish it from hemoglobin iron.

Over the years many methods have been used to measure transport iron. Many of these methods leave much to be desired from the standpoint of precision and accuracy. Also, different methods have yielded different results, resulting in high interlaboratory variance. An Expert Panel (International Committee for Standardization in Hematology, 1978a, 1978b) has recommended a standard method for serum iron and for total and unsaturated iron-binding capacity. Blood samples for iron studies should be drawn in the morning because later samples can show a significant physiologic decrease in iron concentration (Statland and Winkel, 1977). Serum iron is lower during menstruation than in the intermenstrual phase (Zilva and Patston, 1966) regardless of whether or not the subject is using an oral contraceptive.

SERUM IRON-BINDING CAPACITY. The third parameter of iron metabolism is the measurement of transferrin as an indication of the iron transport capability. Since transferrin is a protein present in surprisingly high concentration in serum (200 to 400 mg/dl), it can be quantified directly by electroimmunoassay (Olesen and Terp, 1968; Laurell, 1972) or by immunoprecipitation (Ritchie, 1971). These direct methods will undoubtedly be used more widely in the future, for chemical methods are not only subject to technical variables but are also time-consuming. For the present, most laboratories measure the TIBC, by adding an excess of iron, eliminating what is not bound, and then measuring the iron concentration of the sample. This measures the sum of previously bound iron and the additional iron bound by the excess transferrin and thus does in fact represent the total binding capacity. Previously unbound transferrin can be calculated by subtracting the serum iron concentration from the value for TIBC (Fig. 8-9), this fraction being the labile iron-binding capacity (LIBC). The proportion of transferrin bound to iron in the unmodified serum, the *transferrin saturation*, is then:

$$\text{Transferrin saturation (\%)} = \frac{\text{Serum iron (μg/dl)} \times 100}{\text{TIBC (μg/dl)}}$$

In normal subjects the transferrin saturation is about 30% (normal range, 20% to 45%). In the sideropenic iron-defi-

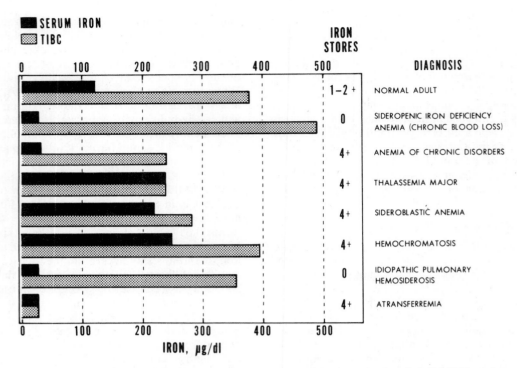

Fig. 8-15. Serum iron and serum TIBC in states of disturbed iron metabolism. Reticuloendothelial (RE) iron stores are graded 0 to 4+ on the basis of stainable iron in bone marrow sections.

ciency anemias, the transferrin saturation is lower than 16% (Bainton and Finch, 1964) and in a severe case may be very low. For example, in a young woman severely anemic (hemoglobin, 6.1 Gm/dl) the serum iron concentration measured 24 μg/dl and the TIBC, 470 μg/dl, so that the transferrin concentration was 5.1%.

The pattern of low serum iron concentration and high TIBC is characteristic of sideropenic anemia as from chronic blood loss (Fig. 8-15). Low serum iron with a low value of TIBC is characteristic of the anemias accompanying chronic disorders (chronic bacterial and fungal infection, rheumatoid arthritis, systemic lupus erythematosus, carcinomas and lymphomas, nephrotic syndrome). However, these patterns are sometimes not so distinct; e.g., an occasional patient with iron deficiency showing a low TIBC or one with anemia of chronic disorders showing a high TIBC. The pattern of low serum iron and high TIBC is also characteristic of idiopathic pulmonary siderosis, but since these patients usually have obvious pulmonary disease there should be no confusion with other causes of sideropenia.

High transferrin saturation (60% to 100%) is characteristic of thalassemia, sideroblastic anemias, hemochromatosis, and congenital iron-loading anemia. In atransferremia both the serum iron concentration and the TIBC are very low.

ESTIMATION OF IRON STORES. It might seem that the measurement of serum iron together with the iron-binding capacity should be sufficient to classify most abnormalities. In fact, the laboratory investigation requires one additional parameter, the estimation of storage iron. This is done most conveniently from biopsied bone marrow tissue, either from an unstained smear, in which hemosiderin appears as coarse refractile golden yellow pigment, or from smears or sections stained for iron (Lundin et al, 1964). The pigment is usually found in phagocytic histiocytes but in severe iron overload it is sometimes found outside presumably ruptured cells. There is better correlation between iron in histologic sections of marrow obtained by trephine biopsy or of sectioned marrow particles and iron in bone marrow particle smears than between sections and thin smears (Rywlin, 1976; Krause et al, 1979). However, thin smears are far superior to particle smears for studying the morphology of cells, and I prefer to use thin smears for differential counts and histologic sections of marrow particles for estimation of iron. Thin smears stained for iron are excellent for demonstrating sideroblasts, and better for this purpose than marrow sections. Bone marrow tissue should be fixed in neutral formalin since, in unbuffered formalin, some of the hemosiderin may be lost. Iron stores are usually graded 0 to 4 +, but rigid criteria are difficult to establish; the useful decision that must be made is whether iron is markedly reduced, normal, or increased.

Using the three parameters of serum iron, TIBC, and marrow iron, most iron-deficiency anemias show typical patterns (Fig. 8-15 and Table 8-6). An atypical pattern may be encountered when more than one etiologic factor is present, as in chronic bleeding and carcinoma or lymphoma, or when malabsorption or hypoproteinemia are superimposed. It should be noted also that in latent iron deficiency the concentration of serum iron is maintained at a fairly normal level by drawing on storage iron, so that there may be absence of significant anemia, normal serum iron, and normal TIBC but depleted marrow iron.

FREE ERYTHROCYTE PROTOPORPHYRIN. Protoporphyrin is normally bound to iron to construct the heme moi-

Table 8-6. Laboratory measurements of iron metabolism

Disease	Serum ferritin (ng/ml)	Serum iron (μg/dl)	Iron-binding capacity (μg/dl)	Transferrin saturation* (%)	Free erythrocyte protoporphyrin (μ/dl of cells)	Tissue iron stores
Normal	20-300†	65-185‡	250-440	30	12-79	N§
Iron depletion, early; no anemia	↓	N	N	N	N	↓
Iron depletion, intermediate; no anemia	↓	↓	↑	↓	↑	↓
Iron-deficiency anemia	↓	↓	↑	↓	↑	↓
Anemia of chronic infection	↑	↓	↓	N	↑	↑
Thalassemia	↑	↑	↑	↑	↑	↑
Hemochromatosis	↑	↑	↑	↑	N	↑
Lead poisoning	N	N	N	↑	↑	N

*Varies with age. Averages 38% at birth, 23% at 1 year (Koerper and Dallman, 1977; Saarinen and Siimes, 1977).
†Varies with age and sex. Average for newborn, 100 ng/ml; average at age 1 month, 350 ng/ml; adult women, averages 28.8 to 44, ranges 2 to 175 ng/ml; adult men, averages 52 to 140, ranges 6 to 329 ng/ml (Addison et al, 1972; Jacobs et al, 1972; Walters et al, 1973; Cook et al, 1974; Siimes et al, 1974).
‡Varies with age. Averages 120 μg/dl at 1 month; 77 μg/dl at 6 months to 1 year (Koerper and Dallman, 1977; Saarinen and Siimes, 1977).
§N, normal; ↓, decreased; ↑, increased.

ety of hemoglobin. If iron is not available, free protoporphyrin accumulates in the red blood cells (Gutniak et al, 1971; Langer et al, 1972). Measurement of free erythrocyte protoporphyrin (FEP) (Table 8-6) is therefore an indirect index of iron availability. An inverse relationship exists between the hemoglobin concentration in sideropenic iron-deficiency anemia and FEP (Koller et al, 1978). It should be noted that this is valid only when protoporphyrin synthesis is normal, and FEP will be high when there is a failure to incorporate iron into the protoporphyrin molecule, as in lead intoxication (p. 455) (Chisolm, 1964; Koenig, 1976) or in erythropoietic protoporphyria (DeGoeij et al, 1977). Some authors believe that FEP measurements can detect rapid changes in the balance between the demand and supply of iron to the erythron before there is a significant change in serum ferritin (Thomas et al, 1977; Koller et al, 1978).

OTHER STUDIES OF IRON METABOLISM. Radioactive iron (^{59}Fe) has been used to follow the metabolism of iron injected intravenously, particularly the rate of clearance from the plasma and the rate of incorporation into hemoglobin. The application of radioactive iron studies to iron-deficiency anemia raises more questions than it solves. For example, plasma iron turnover is said to be normal, as is the supply of iron to the bone marrow (Cavill et al, 1977). There is evidence to indicate an increase in ineffective erythropoiesis and a decrease in red blood cell survival.

Detection of blood loss

Most of the sideropenic iron-deficiency anemias are due to chronic bleeding, most commonly menorrhagia in women, gastrointestinal bleeding in men and women, and bleeding from a Meckel's diverticulum in children. When there is gross bleeding, the problem is relatively simple, but it is sometimes difficult to estimate the amount of blood lost. For example, in obtaining a menstrual history one may find that some women have no concept of what is a "normal" menstrual period. It is best to ask specifically the frequency of periods, duration, and the number of pads or tampons used each day, but this is not an entirely reliable estimate of blood loss. Haynes et al (1977) define normal menstrual blood loss as less than 80 ml. Copious gastrointestinal bleeding high in the tract produces obviously black stools, and bleeding from the lower tract may produce obviously bloody stools, but sometimes a bleeding hemorrhoid may only coat the stool with bright red blood. One author (Beychok, 1978) uses the word "hematochezia" for severe bleeding from the rectum. I did not know what the report was about until I looked up the word in the medical dictionary!

The detection of occult blood loss from the gastrointestinal tract is both simple and difficult. Simple because a variety of methods is available all of which detect occult blood; difficult because the methods range from some that are extremely sensitive and yield a high number of false positive results to some that are sensitive only to high concentrations of blood and thus may yield a large number of false negatives (Irons and Kirsner, 1965; Paver and Goldman, 1966; Humphrey and Goulston, 1969). In my laboratory we have at one time or another evaluated and compared these tests and have formed the following opinions: (1) the tests using orthotolidine, such as Hematest, are so sensitive as to be of little use, (2) the tests using benzidine have the same flaw and because of alleged carcinogenicity (Ferretti et al, 1977), benzidine should be handled with care, and (3) the test using a solution of guaiac is recommended. The guaiac test is not affected if the patient is on oral iron medication (Brayshaw et al, 1963) but is occasionally positive if the patient has eaten meat. For critical evaluation of occult blood loss in stools the patient should be on a meat-free diet for the preceding 4 days and several specimens should be examined to detect intermittent bleeding. Oral intake of vitamin C in high doses (over 750 mg) can cause false negative results with all of the tests for occult blood (Jaffe et al, 1975).

Blood loss can be quantified very accurately by using ^{51}Cr-tagged red cells, but this is not recommended for routine use.

The discovery of gastrointestinal bleeding, whether gross or occult, calls for a thorough investigation to determine the site and nature of the bleeding lesion. The most common lesions are peptic ulcer, diaphragmatic hernia, malignancy, diverticulosis, and diverticulitis (Beveridge et al, 1965). Endemic hookworm infection, hematobium infection, and *Trichuris* infection are common causes of iron-deficiency anemia (Gilles et al, 1964). It is possible for chronic hemorrhoidal bleeding to result in iron-deficiency anemia but this is uncommon in our time, and one should guard against accepting such an obvious source of bleeding while missing another more serious gastrointestinal lesion.

Summary of iron-deficiency anemias

Iron-deficiency anemias are classified in Table 8-5.

Sideropenic iron-deficiency anemias

NUTRITIONAL IRON DEFICIENCY. Iron deficiency only on the basis of inadequate dietary iron is rare in the United States and other developed countries, but may account in part for a negative iron balance in underdeveloped areas where the diet is poor in iron, during wartime restrictions (Davidson et al, 1943), in infants and children fed only unsupplemented milk (Woodruff et al, 1972), or in women during the menstrual years. Many staple foods (baby foods, cereals, pasteurized milk, bread) now contain supplemental iron. This may help in general to reduce the possibility of nutritional iron deficiency, but it is true that iron from some foods, such as when added to bread, is not absorbed well (Callender and Warner, 1968).

ANEMIA DUE TO POOR IRON ABSORPTION. It is extremely improbable that a selective defect that decreases only the absorption of iron can occur. Diminished absorption does occur after gastrectomy (Baird et al, 1959; Adams, 1968), in malabsorption syndromes (Kilpatrick and Katz, 1969), and in pica. Histamine-fast achlorhydria, found in a high percentage of iron-deficient subjects (Beveridge et al, 1965) is probably the result rather than the cause of iron deficiency (Jacobs et al, 1966). Malabsorption is a feature of immunoglobulin deficiency associated with atrophy of the intestinal mucosa (Johnson et al, 1967). There is diminished iron absorption in high fever caused by infection (Beresford et al, 1971) and in inflammation (Hershko et al, 1974), but these two conditions are of limited duration. Some physicians assume that an anemic subject who does not respond to oral iron has an absorption defect and resort to injectable preparations. This assumption is valid only when the anemia has been shown to be of the sideropenic type and the several causes of malabsorption have been ruled out. The characteristics of injectable iron preparations are reviewed by Fairbanks et al (1971).

ANEMIA DUE TO PHYSIOLOGICALLY INCREASED IRON REQUIREMENTS. The three conditions in which the need for iron is physiologically increased are pregnancy and lactation, infancy, and prematurity.

In the course of a full-term pregnancy the mother supplies about 400 mg of iron to the fetus. An additional 150 mg is needed for the growing placenta and enlarging uterus. There is also the need to increase the red cell mass of the fetus, requiring an additional 300 to 400 mg. Iron lost in milk

during lactation amounts to about 30 mg/month. The drain on iron stores is greatest during the last trimester when iron-deficiency anemia may become manifest (De Leeuw et al, 1966). In developed countries it is almost universal practice to prescribe iron supplement in pregnancy, but where this is not done, repeated pregnancies are a major cause of iron deficiency. Anemia may be intensified by the increase in plasma volume, which is proportionately greater than the increase in red cell mass, for hemodilution by itself can produce a drop of up to 2 Gm/dl in the blood hemoglobin concentration.

The increased requirement for iron in a normal full-term infant is dictated by the need for expanding the red cell mass as the infant grows. During the first 6 months of life, about 50 Gm of new hemoglobin must be synthesized, and additional iron is needed for myoglobin and for other tissue iron. Iron stores at birth are relatively small, about 30 mg, and are soon depleted unless supplemental iron is given. Milk is a poor source of iron and if used exclusively will not supply the iron needed by the developing infant. Although there is some difference of opinion, it is probable that the state of iron balance in the mother does not affect the amount of storage iron in the newborn (Lanzkowsky, 1961). However, premature clamping of the umbilical cord at birth, trapping a large volume of blood in the placenta, is responsible for the infant beginning life with a red cell deficit (Yao et al, 1969).

Infants born prematurely have a greater need for iron than full-term infants. First, the body store of iron is smaller and, second, the rate of growth is relatively greater so that a proportionately greater increase in red cell mass must be provided for.

ANEMIA DUE TO BLOOD LOSS. The iron economy of the body is so efficient that normally only minute amounts of iron are lost by excretion. However, when there is loss of red blood cells by bleeding not only are considerable amounts of iron lost, but the iron needed to synthesize new hemoglobin must be provided from iron stores and the labile iron pool, which are in turn replenished by food or medicinal iron. In chronic bleeding, whatever the source, a negative iron balance is established that sooner or later produces sideropenia and sideropenic iron-deficiency anemia.

Chronic blood loss is the most common cause of sideropenic iron-deficiency anemia, although a massive hemorrhage not replaced by transfusion can exhaust iron stores as the red cell mass is regenerated. In men, lesions of the gastrointestinal tract account for most of the anemias in this category, while in women excessive menstrual bleeding is the most common etiology. The gastrointestinal lesions most likely to produce chronic blood loss are peptic ulcer, diaphragmatic hernia, malignancy, diverticulosis, and diverticulitis. Bleeding, sometimes massive, may occur from a telangiectatic lesion of congenital hemorrhagic telangiectasia (Chapter 17), and these lesions are not demonstrable by roentgenographic studies.

Infection with hookworm, particularly when accompanied by pregnancies and an inadequate diet, causes iron deficiency because the worm feeds on the host's blood. The amount of blood consumed is directly proportional to the number of worms, which can be considerable. It is obviously important to eliminate the parasites, but it is interesting to note that the anemia responds well to oral iron therapy even when the parasites are not eliminated.

Blood loss from any other site or by any other mechanism can cause iron-deficiency anemia. Menstrual blood loss may be in fact due to uterine fibromyomata or cancer of the uterus, emphasizing the importance of discovering the cause of the bleeding. Considerable amounts of iron can be lost in the urine in paroxysmal nocturnal hemoglobinuria and other hemolytic diseases (Sears et al, 1966). Hemosiderin in the urinary sediment can be demonstrated by the iron stain. Hemoptysis can account for considerable blood loss, but it is such an alarming symptom that it is unlikely to be ignored for very long. A considerable amount of blood is inevitably swallowed, and this can give a positive test for blood in the stool. Intrapulmonary hemorrhage in idiopathic pulmonary hemosiderosis and in Goodpasture's syndrome (pulmonary hemorrhage with progressive glomerulonephritis) are not likely to be overlooked by the physician who conscientiously searches for the etiology of the iron deficiency.

An unusual type of blood loss is sometimes seen when one of a pair of monozygotic twins is born anemic and the other polycythemic (Hodapp, 1962). Here a fetus-to-fetus transfusion of blood takes place, probably through vascular anastomoses in the monochorionic placenta. The apt term "red and white twins" has been used to describe the appearance of the babies at birth. Another type of intrauterine blood loss is feto-maternal transfusion (Pearson and Diamond, 1959), which can vary from small to large. It is likely that a newborn with sideropenic iron-deficiency anemia has suffered from repeated feto-maternal transfusions (Eshaghpour et al, 1966).

Sideroachrestic anemias

We use the term "sideroachrestic" for those anemias characterized by iron deficiency on the basis of inadequate utilization. A working subclassification is given in Table 8-5. The anemias of some chronic disorders seem to have, as common denominators, hypoferremia and increased iron stores. In thalassemia, as an example of some of the hemoglobinopathies, there is a failure of globin synthesis so that hemoglobin synthesis is deficient in spite of increased iron stores. In the sideroblastic anemias, the characteristic findings, in addition to high serum iron and increased iron stores, are the accumulation of iron in the mitochondria of normoblasts forming "ringed sideroblasts" and a dimorphic population of red cells.

ANEMIA OF CHRONIC DISORDERS. Anemia in chronic disorders such as chronic infections, rheumatoid arthritis, rheumatic fever, chronic renal failure, disseminated lupus erythematosus and other collagen diseases, carcinomas, lymphomas, and leukemias is also of the iron-deficiency type, but characteristically serum iron is low, TIBC decreased, iron stores increased, and marrow sideroblasts decreased. Also characteristic is the usual experience that the anemia in chronic disorders is seldom as severe as some of the sideropenic anemias unless complicated by additional factors such as hemolysis or hemorrhage. Chronic disorders enter into the differential diagnosis of any iron-deficiency anemia and in fact the discovery of anemia often leads to a

more important underlying disease. As noted, there is inadequate utilization of iron and this pathogenesis seems sufficient, even though there may be other contributing factors that are just as likely to be the result rather than the cause of the abnormal iron metabolism or underlying chronic disease. These are decreased red cell survival (Cartwright and Lee, 1971) and low erythropoietin levels (Ward et al, 1971). In some chronic disorders a characteristic sideroblastic picture is seen. There is evidence favoring an inhibitor of erythropoiesis in the blood of patients in chronic renal failure (Wallner et al, 1976, 1978). Campbell et al (1978) found only one enzyme active in heme synthesis to be elevated: coproporphyrinogen oxidase.

SIDEROBLASTIC ANEMIAS. The most characteristic finding is the presence of "ringed sideroblasts" in the bone marrow. The serum iron concentration is high, the TIBC moderately decreased, and the transferrin saturation high. The peripheral blood shows moderate to severe anemia and the red cell population is usually dimorphic, a mixture of normal or macrocytic and microcytic hypochromic cells. This is true dimorphism, as evidenced by a difference in the Xg^a antigen in the two types of red cells and also in free erythrocyte protoporphyrin (FEP), low in the microcytic and normal in the normocytic cells (Lee et al, 1968b). The peripheral blood also contains some heavily stippled red cells, not only in sideroblastic anemia secondary to lead intoxication but in the others as well. Monocytosis is common (Kushner et al, 1971) and the monocytes may appear atypical, with coarseness of the nuclear chromatin and vacuolization of the cytoplasm.

Sideroblastic anemias are divided into two groups, the primary and the secondary. Subclassification within the primary group is not satisfactory, and the distinction between sideroblastic anemia refractory to treatment and that responsive to pyridoxine is difficult to justify, since the response to pyridoxine within the pyridoxine-responsive group, and even in the same patient, is variable and unpredictable (Bourne et al, 1965; Losowsky and Hall, 1965). It is true, however, that some patients are refractory to all therapy. Nevertheless, the distinction based on response to therapy makes one uncomfortable.

Some classifications emphasize the hereditary and familial features of the anemia, primary refractory anemia affecting older persons with no clear sex predominance (Kushner et al, 1971), or showing a predominantly X-linked recessive trait (Elves et al, 1966) or even an autosomal inheritance pattern (Cotton and Harris, 1962). It has even been proposed that primary refractory anemia is a malignant, preleukemic disease (Dameshek, 1965; Lewy et al, 1979). Review of the literature on sideoblastic anemia is confusing and somewhat frustrating. A classification can be accurate only if it is based on sound criteria, and it seems to me that acceptable criteria are not yet available.

Secondary sideroblastic anemia is more easily classified in that it is associated with systemic diseases (Hines and Grasso, 1970; Williams et al, 1972; Wintrobe et al, 1974) and, quite clearly, with the ingestion of some drugs (Table 8-5). A cause-and-effect relationship in systemic disease is not always easy to accept, since in a given disease only some patients develop sideroblastic anemia. In the case of

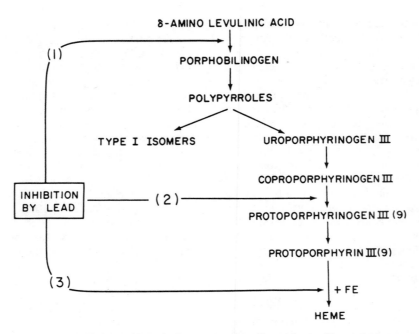

Fig. 8-16. Inhibition by lead of various steps in the synthesis of hemoglobin.

drugs, however, the causal relationship is clearer although not all subjects develop sideroblastic anemia. The most common are lead (Goldberg, 1968), drugs used in cancer chemotherapy (Melphalan [Khaleeli et al, 1973], azathioprine [Dacie and Molin, 1966], nitrogen mustard [Bowman, 1961]), antituberculosis drugs, singly or in combination (INH, cycloserine, pyrazinamide [Haden, 1967]), chloramphenicol (Beck and Lüdin, 1967), and alcohol (Hines and Cowan, 1970). Two cases are reported in which the sideroblastic anemia was antibody mediated (Zervas et al, 1974; Ritchey et al, 1979).

Judging from what is known, it is likely that a variety of different biochemical lesions in the heme synthetic pathway can produce the same end result of sideroblastic anemia.

In the case of lead intoxication the synthesis of heme in mitochondria is disturbed at three points (Fig. 8-16). The first block is in the conversion of δ-aminolevulinic acid to porphobilinogen. Accordingly, large amounts of δ-aminolevulinic acid are excreted in the urine. The second block is in the conversion of coproporphyrinogen to protoporphyrinogen, so that coproporphyrinogen is increased in the erythrocytes and may be excreted in the urine. The third block is in the incorporation of iron into protoporphyrin to form heme. As a result of this block, not only is there accumulation of protoporphyrin in the red cells (Table 8-6) but also defective hemoglobin synthesis. The accumulation of coproporphyrinogen and protoporphyrin in the red cells causes them to fluoresce strongly under ultraviolet light (fluorescytes). Coarse basophilic stippling is common, represents aggregated ribosomes and probably, degenerating mitochondria. The accumulation of mitochondrial iron produces ringed sideroblasts.

In pyridoxine-responsive sideroblastic anemia, the metabolic block is in the formation of δ-aminolevulinic acid

within the mitochondria from glycine and succinyl-CoA (Harris, 1964). This step requires pyridoxal-6-phosphate, the active coenzyme form of pyridoxine, and ALA synthetase so that lack or inhibition of the enzyme or coenzyme seems to explain the pathogenesis of this anemia (Vogler and Mingioli, 1968) and is in line with the finding of low porphyrin concentration in the red cells. This is also in agreement with studies on the animal model of sideroblastic anemia. However, in some cases, erythrocyte protoporphyrin is found to be normal or even high and this would not follow if the only metabolic lesion were inhibition of δ-aminolevulinic acid. It must be supposed that these are cases that respond poorly or not at all to the administration of pyridoxine and that the metabolic lesion is distal to δ-aminolevulinic acid.

In many cases of sideroblastic anemia the bone marrow is either frankly megaloblastic or contains intermediate megaloblasts. This reflects the interrelationship of folate and pyridoxine (Solomon and Hillman, 1979), and in fact some patients with sideroblastic anemia respond to the two together or in sequence when they respond poorly to pyridoxine alone (MacGibbon and Molin, 1965).

Finally, there is evidence that the red cell membrane is also abnormal in sideroblastic anemia, as evidenced by the increased agglutinability of these red cells by cold antibodies of anti-i specificity (Cooper et al, 1968).

HEREDITARY IRON-LOADING ANEMIA. In our classification this term is reserved for the cases described by Shahidi et al (1964) and by Vitale et al (1969), p. 401. Their occurrence in infants and the unusual distribution of storage iron sets them apart from other sideroachrestic anemias. The "iron-loading anemia" described by Byrd and Cooper (1961) fits more properly in the primary sideroblastic anemia group.

Anemia in transferrin deficiency

Only three instances of congenital absence of transferrin (*atransferremia*) have been reported (Heilmeyer et al, 1961; Cáp et al, 1968; Goya et al, 1972). There is severe hypochromic microcytic anemia, very low serum iron and TIBC with complete saturation, marked hemosiderosis of liver and spleen with absent bone marrow iron, and no demonstrable serum transferrin by immunologic methods. By its very nature and effect on iron metabolism it is unlikely that congenital atransferremia would be detected first in older individuals. However, acquired atransferremia has been reported in association with the nephrotic syndrome (Oliva et al, 1968), probably explainable on the basis of loss of transferrin, along with other protein, in the urine (Hancock et al, 1976). The case of atransferremia associated with erythroleukemia (Hitzig et al, 1960) defies explanation.

9

"Friend Sancho, reply'd Don Quixote,
know 'tis any easy matter for Necromancers to change
the Shapes of Things as they please. . . ."

Cervantes: *Don Quixote*

Folic acid, vitamin B₁₂, and macrocytic anemia

FOLIC ACID AND VITAMIN B₁₂
  Historical background
  Folic acid
    Chemistry
    Metabolic function
      Overview
      Role of folates and B₁₂
      Biochemical basis of megaloblastic dyspoiesis
    Folate in foods
    Assay of serum and red cell folate
    Excretion of formiminoglutamic acid
  Vitamin B₁₂
    Source
    Chemical structure
    Metabolic role
      Cobamide coenzymes
      Methylmalonyl CoA isomerase
      Synthesis of methionine methyl
      DNA synthesis
    Absorption
    Dietary vitamin B₁₂
    Intrinsic factor (IF)
    Transport
    Storage
  Interrelation of folate and vitamin B₁₂
ANEMIA DUE TO DEFICIENCY OF VITAMIN B₁₂ OR FOLIC ACID
  Classification
  Macrocytosis
  Concept of megaloblastic dyspoiesis
MEGALOBLASTIC ANEMIAS
  Due to deficiency of vitamin B₁₂
    Inadequate intake
    Pernicious anemia in the adult
      Pathogenesis
      Clinical features
      Laboratory diagnosis
        Peripheral blood
        Gastric analysis
        Bone marrow
        Excretion of labeled vitamin B₁₂ (Schilling test)
        Assay of vitamin B₁₂
        Excretion of methylmalonic acid in urine
        Reticulocyte response after therapeutic trial
        Erythrocyte survival
        Urine and renal function
        Iron metabolism
        Pigment excretion

        Biochemical findings
        Deoxyuridine suppression test
    Pernicious anemia in infants and children
    After gastrectomy
    Due to biologically inert intrinsic factor
    Due to disease of small intestine
    Familial selective vitamin B₁₂ malabsorption
    Deficiency of transcobalamin II
    Drug-induced malabsorption
    In the Zollinger-Ellison syndrome
    Increased requirements for vitamin B₁₂
  Due to deficiency of folate
    Dietary deficiency
    Megaloblastic anemia of pregnancy
    Megaloblastic anemia of infancy
    Caused by increased cellular proliferation
    Due to malabsorption of folate
      Congenital folate malabsorption
      Drug-induced folate malabsorption
      In the steatorrheas
    Defective folate interconversion
  Of uncertain etiology
    In hemochromatosis
    In Di Guglielmo's syndrome (erythroleukemia)
    In sideroblastic anemias
    The OSLAM syndrome

FOLIC ACID AND VITAMIN B₁₂

In the preceding chapter we discussed the necessity for iron in the synthesis of hemoglobin and therefore for the formation of erythrocytes that contain a normal amount of the oxygen-carrying pigment. With perhaps minor reservations it may be said that iron is not required for the normal maturation of erythroid precursors. Normal maturation is dependent on two classes of hemopoietic factors—the vitamin B₁₂ coenzymes and the folates. Macrocytic anemia and megaloblastic dyspoiesis occur when one or the other is deficient. This reflects the biochemical role played by these factors at the cellular level.

Historical background

Since it was not until the late 1920s that the pathogenesis of pernicious anemia began to be understood, it is difficult to be sure which prior descriptions referred specifically to this disease. In the prior hundred years one finds descriptions of severe "idiopathic" anemias, in children as well as in adults, that seemed to "resist all remedial efforts and sooner or later terminated fatally." We can feel fairly certain that some of these patients had what we now define as pernicious anemia; we can be just as certain that others did not. Since treatment was primitive and empirical, the lack of response to treatment is not by itself a helpful criterion.

In 1855 Addison introduced his discussion on disease of the suprarenal capsule with a vivid description of an idiopathic anemia ("cases in which there had been no previous loss of blood, no exhausting diarrhea, no chlorosis, no purpura, no renal, splenic, miasmatic, glandular, strumous, or malignant disease") that progressed inexorably to death. He usually is credited with the first accurate clinical description of pernicious anemia, hence the term "addisonian anemia" of the older literature. The term "pernicious anemia" was first used by Biermer in 1872 in describing 15 cases of progressive anemia. However, it is certain that not all, and indeed perhaps none, had pernicious anemia in the modern sense, for some of the anemias were related to pregnancy, some possibly to malabsorption, and some may have been of the aplastic type secondary to exposure to aniline dyes (see summary of Biermer's cases given by Huser, 1966). Some have preferred the eponym "Biermer's" anemia to "addisonian."

Neither Addison nor Biermer was able to characterize the anemia on the basis of cell morphology. What is more disappointing is that neither mentions the numbness and tingling of the extremities or other neurologic disturbances. The neurologic symptoms were noted by Osler and Gardner in 1877 and the spinal cord involvement was noted by Lichtheim in 1877. The major morphologic contributions came in 1880 when Ehrlich described the megaloblast and in 1923 when Naegeli described hypersegmentation of neutrophils in the peripheral blood smear.

In 1925 Whipple (Whipple and Robscheit-Robbins, 1925) reported that the addition of liver to the diet had a beneficial effect on erythrocyte regeneration in dogs made anemic by repeated phlebotomy. This experimental observation led Minot and Murphy (1926) to the trial use of raw liver by mouth in pernicious anemia. Improvement was dramatic and lifesaving and initiated a new era in the study of not only pernicious anemia but other anemias as well. The award of the 1934 Nobel Prize for Medicine to Minot, Murphy, and Whipple gave recognition to their contributions.

In a series of reports beginning in 1929 (Castle, 1953) Castle showed that feeding ground beef that had been preincubated with normal gastric juice induced a remission in eight out of ten patients with pernicious anemia. Beef by itself was ineffective. Castle concluded that there was an interaction between a factor present in normal gastric juice and absent in pernicious anemia, *intrinsic factor,* and the hemopoietic factor in meat, *extrinsic factor.* We now know that intrinsic factor is required for absorption of vitamin B$_{12}$ from the diet. It should be noted that, in retrospect, the beneficial effects of oral liver in Minot and Murphy's cases were caused as much by folic acid, which does not require intrinsic factor, as by vitamin B$_{12}$.

It seemed logical to progress from therapy with raw liver by mouth to parenteral injections of crude liver extracts and then to progressively more purified extracts. It was expected that progressive purification would ultimately produce a pure concentrate of what may be thought to be one hemopoietic anti–pernicious anemia factor. Interestingly enough, it is now apparent that the anti–pernicious anemia factor is B$_{12}$, that liver is relatively poor in folic acid but rich in B$_{12}$, and that folic acid is the hemopoietic factor lacking in folic acid deficiency. The discovery of folic acid as a growth factor for certain bacteria did not at first seem to have any relationship to anemia.

The isolation of folic acid and its application to the study and treatment of macrocytic anemias are milestones in the history of anemia; its discovery makes one of the most interesting stories in the field of research. In 1889 Hopkins studied the yellow pigment of butterfly wings and noted its chemical similarity to uric acid. In 1925 Wieland isolated the butterfly pigment in pure crystalline form, determined its structural formula, and called it "xanthopterin" (from the Greek, meaning "yellow wings"). Neither of these observations would appear to have much significance, but they were to play an important role in future developments.

In 1936 it was found that xanthopterin would cure experimental macrocytic anemia in rats and, in 1941, nutritional macrocytic anemia in Chinook salmon. Snell and Peterson (1940), while studying the nutritional growth requirements of bacteria, found that their test organism, *Lactobacillus casei,* grew faster when yeast extract was added to the medium. After adsorption of yeast extracts with norite and subsequent elution, the growth factor was found in the eluate and was called the norite-eluate factor. A substance having similar activity was later isolated from liver.

Mitchell et al (1941) found that another test organism, *Streptococcus lactis R,* grew better when leaf juice was added to the media. From several tons of spinach they were able to extract 1 Gm of the active material. This was called folic acid because of its source from leaves and was found to have a chemical structure similar to that of xanthopterin. The development of this important therapeutic agent owes much to the original studies on the yellow pigment of butterfly wings. Even the synthesis of folic acid from commercially available guanidine was based on the original determination of the molecular structure of xanthopterin (Waller et al, 1948).

Within the last few years we have seen the development of the concept that pernicious anemia is a genetically determined autoimmune disease. It is felt that antibodies against parietal cells and intrinsic factor are responsible for the absorptive and anatomic lesion in the stomach. These in turn produce the classic disease. There is no doubt that these studies mark yet another important milestone in the history of this disease.

Folic acid

Chemistry

Folic acid is pteroylmonoglutamic acid (Fig. 9-1), a condensation product of pteroic acid (a pteridine residue plus para-aminobenzoic acid) and one glutamic acid residue.

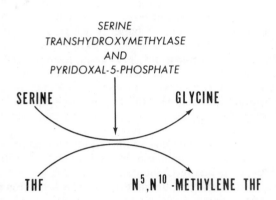

Fig. 9-1. Pteroylmonoglutamic acid (folic acid) showing the convention for numbering the atoms where some substitutions occur. Additional glutamic acid residues are added by linking the amino group to the terminal carboxyl group.

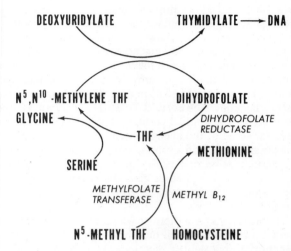

Fig. 9-2. The transfer of two single carbon methylene units in the conversion of serine to glycine.

Fig. 9-3. Metabolic role of folates and the interrelation of folate and vitamin B_{12}. (See Fig. 9-4 for expansion of the final pathway for DNA synthesis.)

This is the parent compound of a large number of derivatives known as the *folates*, which differ in the number of glutamic acid residues (e.g., pteroyldiglutamate and pteroyltriglutamate), in the degree of reduction (e.g., dihydrofolates and tetrahydrofolates), and in other substitutions (e.g., formimino, CHNH; formyl, CHO; methyl, CH_3; and methylene, CH_2) at specified loci, usually N^5 or N^{10}. For example, N^{10}-formylpteroylglutamic acid has a formyl residue at N^{10}.

Metabolic function

OVERVIEW. The metabolically active folates are tetrahydrofolates (H_4 folate or FH_4), and these act as coenzymes in the transfer of "single carbon" units from a donor to a recipient compound. A typical reaction is the serine $\rightleftharpoons$ glycine system (Fig. 9-2), in which FH_4 is the coenzyme of serinehydroxymethyltransferase in the transfer of two methylene units, one to N^5 and one to N^{10}.

Folates act as growth factors by regulating the transfer of single carbon units in microbial systems as well as for many other biologic systems (Stokstad and Koch, 1967; Huennekens, 1968; Scott and Weir, 1976). Pertinent to our subject is the role of folates in the synthesis of DNA. This depends on the action of folates, so that a deficiency of folates leads to impaired DNA synthesis in erythroid cells, one of the features of megaloblastic erythropoiesis (dyserythropoiesis).

Table 9-1. Drugs that interfere with folate metabolism*

Inhibitors of dihydrofolate reductase†	Mechanism not certain‡
Methotrexate	Diphenylhydantoin
Aminopterin	Primidone
Pyrimethamine	Barbiturates
Triamterene	Oral contraceptives
Trimethoprim	Alcohol
Pentamidine	Isoniazid
	Cycloserine
	Metformin

*Modified from Stebbins and Bertino (1976).
†In order of decreasing effect and likelihood of causing megaloblastosis.
‡Impaired absorption or utilization of folate.

Impaired DNA synthesis and megaloblastic dyserythropoiesis can also result from a deficiency of vitamin B_{12}. Folate and B_{12} metabolic reactions are interrelated, probably through a late step in DNA synthesis (p. 419).

ROLE OF FOLATES AND B_{12}. The precursor of DNA is thymidylate (pyrimidine nucleotide). This is derived from deoxyuridylate, the rate of the reaction being regulated by the conversion of N^5, N^{10}-methylene tetrahydrofolate to dihydrofolate (Fig. 9-3). Dihydrofolate is reduced to tetra-

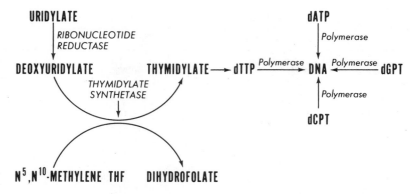

Fig. 9-4. Final pathway for the synthesis of DNA. Preceding pathways that are dependent on folate and B_{12} are shown in Fig. 9-3. **dTTP** = deoxythymidine triphosphate; **dATP** = deoxyadenosine triphosphate; **dGPT** = deoxyguanosine triphosphate; **dCPT** = deoxycytidine triphosphate. (Modified from Edenberg and Huberman, 1975).

hydrofolate (THF) by the action of the enzyme dihydrofolate reductase, providing a new supply of THF for the de novo synthesis of more N^5, N^{10}-methylene THF. Additional THF is generated from N^5-methyl THF as homocysteine is converted to methionine. This conversion requires methyl B_{12} (methylcobalamin). Therefore deficient synthesis of DNA, manifested as megaloblastic dyserythropoiesis, can be the direct result of folate deficiency or of folate deficiency caused indirectly by deficiency of B_{12}.

The disturbance of folate metabolism caused by a deficiency of B_{12} has been called the "folate trap" or "methyl folate trap", the accumulation of N^5-methyl THF that is not converted to THF in the folate cycle. As expected, the concentration of N^5-methyl THF in the serum of patients who are B_{12} deficient is about twice the normal and falls to normal following adequate therapy with B_{12} (Herbert and Zalusky, 1962). Vitamin B_{12} acts in conjunction with an apoenzyme, and Arakawa (1970) has reported a case of megaloblastic anemia in a Japanese child congenitally deficient in the apoenzyme methylfolate transferase. The anemia did not respond to vitamin B_{12}, and the elevated level of N^5-methyl THF in the serum supports the concept of the folate trap when there is failure to convert N^5-methyl THF to THF.

Some drugs used in cancer chemotherapy, such as methotrexate and aminopterin, are classified as antifolates because they inhibit dihydrofolate reductase. As a consequence, DNA synthesis is impaired. Other drugs act as antifolates but have weaker antienzymatic activity (e.g., pyrimethamine, an antimalarial; triamterene, a diuretic; and trimethoprim, an antibacterial) (Stebbins and Bertino, 1976). Other drugs interfere with folate metabolism (Table 9-1), but the mechanism is not certain.

BIOCHEMICAL BASIS OF MEGALOBLASTIC DYSPOIESIS. Megaloblastic dyspoiesis is the result of reduced DNA synthesis. Hoffbrand et al (1976) discuss the several possibilities to account for the reduced synthesis of DNA and conclude that it is caused by an insufficient supply of one or more deoxyribonucleoside triphosphate precursors or by inhibition of one or more DNA polymerases. The first mechanism is operative in folate or vitamin B_{12} deficiency, since these lead to a reduction of the key deoxythymidine triphosphate (dTTP) (Fig. 9-4). Reduction of dTTP also follows inhibition of dehydrofolate reductase by methotrexate, pyrimethamine, or trimethoprim, and megaloblastosis is common as a consequence of chemotherapy with these antifolate drugs. Other chemotherapeutic agents act by inhibition of other metabolic steps. For example, 5-fluorouracil inhibits thymidylate synthetase, and 6-mercaptopurine, hydroxyurea, and azaserine inhibit synthesis of dAPT and dGPT. Azauridine inhibits both dTTP and dCPT, the same synthetic defect present in orotic aciduria. Cytosine arabinoside inhibits DNA polymerase.

The reduced supply of one or more of the four triphosphates, whatever the cause, impairs the cell's ability to elongate newly formed DNA fragments. This prolongs the synthetic phase, and the premitotic interval is longer than normal. The result is that the nucleus is large, and, since there is active protein synthesis during the prolonged premitotic phase, there is an abnormally high amount of cytoplasmic RNA and early synthesis of hemoglobin. Furthermore, many cells never undergo mitosis and break down in the bone marrow, accounting for the high serum level of lactic dehydrogenase in megaloblastic anemias. The same explanation may apply to the genesis of abnormalities in the nuclei of leukocytes and other cells.

Folate in foods

The folate content of feces is high, from microbial synthesis, but this is not available for the body's needs since there is no absorption of folate from the colon. Folate from food is absorbed preferentially from the upper part of the small bowel; the requirements must be supplied by ingested food. In natural foods, folates exist as polyglutamates of THF. These are unstable when exposed to oxygen, ultraviolet light, and heat. Oxidative reduction can be inhibited by ascorbate. Polyglutamates must be reduced to monoglutamates, after which they are readily absorbed (Whitehead et al, 1972; Rosenberg, 1975).

The folate content of foods can be measured as either

Table 9-2. Folate content of various foods (μg/100 Gm wet weight, *L. casei* assay)*

Food	Folate content	Food	Folate content
Beef steak	9.2	Spinach	75
Beef liver	294	Apples	2
Ham	10.6	Avocados	30
Eggs	5.1	Bananas	9.7
Cow's milk, pasteurized	5.1	Grapefruit	2.8
Cheese (cheddar)	12.2-15.0	Dates	24.7
Cheese (cottage)	25.3-51.7	Raisins	10
Asparagus	109	Bread	15
Beans	27-38	Almonds	45
Brussels sprouts	49	Walnuts	77
Lettuce	21	Peanuts	56.5
Mushrooms	24	Chocolate	99
Potatoes	6.8	Brewer's yeast	2,022

*Data from Herbert, 1963.

Table 9-3. Folate analogues and their microbiologic activity with assay bacteria*

Folate	P. cerevisiae	Str. faecalis	L. casei
PteGlu†	−	−	+
PteGlu$_2$	−	+	+
PteGlu$_3$	−	−	+
10-Formyl PteGlu	−	+	+
10-Formyl PteGlu$_3$	−	−	+
H$_2$ PteGlu	−	+	+
10-Formyl H$_2$ PteGlu	−	+	+
H$_4$ PteGlu	+	+	+
5-Formyl H$_4$ PteGlu	+	+	+
10-Formyl H$_4$ PteGlu	+	+	−
5-Methyl H$_4$ PteGlu	−	−	+
5-Formyl H$_4$ PteGlu$_2$	+	+	+
5-Formyl H$_4$ PteGlu$_3$	+	−	+

*Modified from Johns and Bertino, 1965; and Baugh and Krumdieck, 1971.
†PteGlu = pteroylglutamic acid.

"free folate," folate available without enzymatic (conjugase) digestion, or as "total folate" after enzyme treatment. The polyglutamate forms must be treated with conjugase (Baugh et al, 1975) to make them available for microbiologic assay. Some representative foods and folate contents are given in Table 9-2. A diet calculated to provide adequate folate may in fact be folate deficient because a variable but high loss occurs in cooking. An average diet supplies about 50 to 100 μg of folate daily. According to Chung et al (1961) a "high-cost" diet provides 193 μg of folate daily, a "low-cost" diet provides 157 μg daily, and a "poor diet" supplies 47 μg daily. Chanarin (1969) found the mean folate content in a normal diet to be 160 μg/24 hours. The minimum requirement of about 50 μg/day (as folic acid) is equivalent to about 100 to 200 μg of food folate. The recommended daily folate intake is 40 to 60 μg for infants, 100 μg for children, 200 μg for adults, and 400 μg for pregnant women (WHO Techn Rep, 1970).

Body stores of folate are rather small, about 5 to 10 mg total, and megaloblastic anemia will develop after about 4 months of a severely folate-deficient diet (Herbert, 1962).

This is in contrast to the slow rate at which body stores of vitamin B$_{12}$ are depleted (p. 426). Folate is stored in the liver, which is also the site of reduction and methylation reactions. Folate in serum is found both free and bound to various proteins (Elsborg, 1972; Markkanen et al, 1972; Waxman and Schreiber, 1973b). There is some evidence that serum and cells contain a specific folate-binding protein (Waxman, 1975; Rothenberg and DaCosta, 1976) that may play a role in folate absorption. Increased serum folate-binding capacity (FABC) has been found in a few supposedly normal persons and in various conditions: folate deficiency (Waxman and Schreiber, 1973a); pregnancy or intake of oral contraceptives (DaCosta and Rothenberg, 1974); anticonvulsant drug intake (Markkanen et al, 1973; multiple myeloma (Markkanen et al, 1973); pernicious anemia (Markkanen et al, 1974); cirrhosis of the liver (Colman and Herbert, 1974); azotemia (Colman and Herbert, 1974); and as a familial trait (Muckerheide et al, 1977). Serum folate is mainly 5-MeFH$_4$, and when folic acid is given orally some is absorbed as folic acid and some is converted to 5-MeFH$_4$ by the mucosal cells of the jejunum (Olinger et al, 1973). Unaltered folic acid is methylated in the liver.

Assay of serum and red cell folate

The classic method for folate assay is based on the growth requirement of some microorganisms for folate. As shown in Table 9-3, the three microorganisms that have been used for the microbiologic assay of folate have different requirements for folate analogues. The organism of choice is *L. casei* since it is sensitive to most analogues, particularly 5-MeH$_4$, the folate in serum. The method of Goulian and Beck (1966) is recommended. The assay is time-consuming and requires meticulous technic. Erroneous results may be caused by bacterial contamination of the serum and interference by antibiotics (Beard and Allen, 1967) or antifolates.

Ligand radioassay methods are receiving increasing attention (Rothenberg et al, 1972a; Waxman and Schreiber, 1973a; Schreiber and Waxman, 1974). These are based on the use of commercially available β-Lactoglobulin as the folate binder and labeled folic acid (^{3}H-PGA). The radioassay method is more rapid than the microbiologic methods

Table 9-4. Concentration of serum folate and erythrocyte folate in normal persons

Reference	Serum folate (ng/ml)*		Erythrocyte folate (ng/ml)	
	Range	Mean	Range	Mean
Toennies et al, 1956	2.6-10.5	5.5	24-300	120
Hansen and Weinfeld, 1962	3.7-9.3	5.4	51-204	105
Grossowicz et al, 1962	3.2-15.0	8.3	104-330	197
Cooper and Lowenstein, 1964	4.0-18.0	8.1	175-875	422
Grzesinkowicz et al, 1965	6.7-14.6	9.2	325-470	407
Vanier and Tyas, 1966	7.0-20.0	13.1	100-837	454
Magnus, 1967	3.0-11.0	5.7	78-245	144
Hoffbrand and Newcombe, 1967	6.5-19.6	9.8	165-600	336
Schreiber and Waxman, 1974†	—	—	200-875	—
Waksman and Schreiber, 1973a†	>6	—	—	—
Jones et al, 1979	5.0-18.0	3.81	147-555	—
		3.68†		
Vatanavicharn et al, 1979	2.8-16.65	8.87	278-655	436

*ng = nanograms = millimicrograms (Gm × 10^{-9}).
†Radioassay method.

and is not subject to interference by antibiotics. Results are generally comparable to *L. casei* assays. Mortensen (1976) and Kubasik et al (1979) point out that the radioassay method is subject to technical variables such as duration of storage, hemolysis, presence of ascorbic acid, and pH control at the time of extraction and in the final mixture.

As shown in Table 9-4, erythrocytes contain much more folate than serum. Significant folate deficiency is indicated by a serum folate concentration of less than 3 ng/ml (Table 9-5) and a red cell folate concentration of less than 140 ng/ml (Rothenberg and DaCosta, 1976), depending on the normal values for the given laboratory. In severe, fully developed folate deficiency, serum and red cell folate values may be very low. Since folate body stores can be depleted rapidly (p. 420), low serum folate assays can precede evidence of hematologic abnormalities, or may be accompanied only by hypersegmentation of neutrophil leukocytes (Halsted et al, 1973; Lindenbaum and Nath, 1980) and slight macrocytosis. In vitamin B$_{12}$ deficiency folate levels in serum are usually increased (Baker et al, 1959) while red cell folate is usually decreased.

Excretion of formiminoglutamic acid

Formiminoglutamic acid (FIGLU) is an intermediate in the metabolism of histidine. The transformation of formiminoglutamic acid to glutamic acid (Fig. 9-5) involves the transfer of the formimino group to tetrahydrofolic acid, forming 5-formiminotetrahydrofolic acid and glutamic acid. Thus, if tetrahydrofolic acid is deficient, transfer of the formimino group is also deficient, and FIGLU accumulates and is excreted in the urine in larger than normal amounts. Increased excretion of FIGLU also occurs if there is a deficiency of the formimino-transferring enzyme (formiminotransferase).

It has been shown that after a standard dose of oral histidine (15 Gm of L-histidine hydrochloride in orange or apple juice), patients with folic-acid deficiency excrete from 40 to 200 times the normal amount of FIGLU. The normal range of FIGLU in the urine after histidine loading is 1 to 17

Table 9-5. Serum folate levels in various megaloblastic disorders*

Diagnosis	Serum folate (ng/ml)†
Normal	7.5-24
Vegan	8‡
Pernicious anemia	9-22§
Alcoholic cirrhosis	0.75
Infancy	2.4-3.3
Pregnancy	2.9-4.5
Steatorrhea	1.2-4.8

*Representative examples from Herbert et al, 1960.
†*L. casei* assay.
‡Serum vitamin B$_{12}$ = 49 pg/ml.
§Serum vitamin B$_{12}$ = 15 to 110 pg/ml.

mg/24 hr. In folate-deficiency states, FIGLU excretion is 185 to 2,047 mg/24 hr. This has been found to be true for any of the folic-acid deficiency states, with only an occasional patient showing an unexplained normal excretion. In pernicious anemia one would expect FIGLU excretion to be increased also, and indeed it is in most cases. Usually the amount of FIGLU excreted is less than in folate deficiency but on occasion, particularly in severely anemic patients, it may be very high. Thus FIGLU excretion is a measure of folic acid deficiency only when there is no deficiency of vitamin B$_{12}$. FIGLU excretion is increased also in liver disease.

Vitamin B$_{12}$

Vitamin B$_{12}$ was isolated at about the same time by Smith (1948) in England and by Rickes et al (1948) in this country. It is a coincidence that this, the most powerful hemopoietic factor, is a red compound. Its activity is fantastic. Clinically, it is effective in microgram doses while organisms that require B$_{12}$ for growth need only a few molecules of the vitamin for normal metabolic activity. Together with folates, vitamin B$_{12}$ is involved in the activation of many

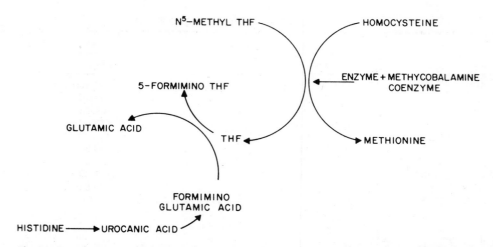

Fig. 9-5. Transformation of formiminoglutamic acid (FIGLU) to glutamic acid is tetrahydrofolate (THF) and vitamin B_{12} dependent, whereas transformation of homocysteine to methionine is a vitamin B_{12}-dependent reaction.

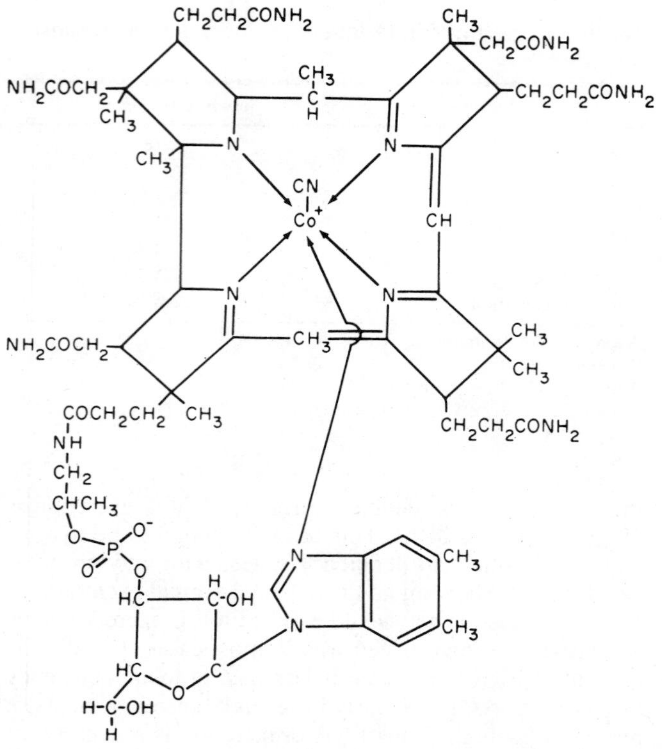

Fig. 9-6. Formula of cyanocobalamin (vitamin B_{12}).

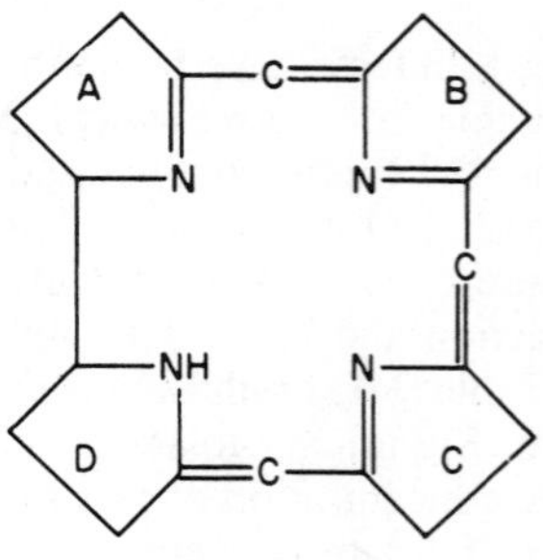

Fig. 9-7. Corrin ring.

biochemical systems. We are concerned here with its role in erythropoiesis, its interrelation with folate, and its effects in the deficiency states.

Source

Vitamin B_{12} differs from most other vitamins in that it is synthesized by only certain microorganisms. It is not synthesized by plant or animal cells and its presence in foods is a reflection of a synthesis by microorganisms somewhere

back in the biologic cycle. Carnivores depend on vitamin B_{12} stored in the meat they eat, herbivores depend on contamination with vitamin B_{12}-synthesizing bacteria, and oysters extract it from water in which it is present by bacterial action. Vitamin B_{12} is synthesized in the gastrointestinal tract of humans and other higher species by bacterial action but none of this is adsorbed. Relatively large amounts can be recovered from sludge.

Most microorganisms synthesize minute amounts of vitamin B_{12}; a few are veritable metabolic factories that produce it in large amounts (*Propionibacterium shermanii, Streptomyces griseus,* and *Streptomyces aureofaciens*). Some microorganisms are unable to synthesize it, and for their optimal growth and metabolism the vitamin must be derived from exogenous sources. These microorganisms (*Lactobacillus lactis, Lactobacillus leichmannii,* and *Euglena gracilis*) are therefore suitable organisms for assaying this vitamin.

Chemical structure

The molecule of vitamin B_{12} ($C_{63}H_{88}O_{14}N_{14}$—PCo; mol wt 1,355) is made up of a *planar* group and a *nucleotide* group attached to the cobalt atom and lying perpendicular to the planar group (Stadtman, 1971). The stereochemical configuration resembles an open umbrella. The planar group is

Table 9-6. Nomenclature of vitamin B$_{12}$ and related compounds*

| Trivial name | Semisystematic name | Ligands of cobalt | | Systematic name |
		Above plane	Below plane	
Vitamin B$_{12}$	Cyanocobalamin	CN—	5,6-Dimethylbenzimidazole	-(5,6-Dimethylbenzimidazolyl) cyanocobamide
Vitamin B$_{12a}$	Hydroxocobalamin	OH—	5,6-Dimethylbenzimidazole	-(5,6-Dimethylbenzimidazolyl) hydroxocobamide
Vitamin B$_{12b}$	Aquocobalamin	H$_2$O	5,6-Dimethylbenzimidazole	-(5,6-Dimethylbenzimidazolyl) aquocobamide
None	Diaquocobalamin	H$_2$O	H$_2$O	-(5,6-Dimethylbanzimidazolyl) diaquocobamide
Vitamin B$_{12c}$	Nitrocobalamin	NO$_2$—	5,6-Dimethylbenzimidazole	-(5,6-Dimethylbenzimidazolyl) nitrocobamide
Pseudovitamin B$_{12}$	—	CN—	Adenine	-(Adenyl) cyanocobamide
Factor B	Aetiocobalamin	CN—	H$_2$O	Cyanocobinamide
Factor B ribose phosphate	Aetiocobalamin	CN—	H$_2$O	Cyanocobamide

*After Beck, 1962.

a tetrapyrrole, basically the same structure as the porphyrin ring of hemoglobin. It has four reduced pyrrole rings linked to a central cobalt atom whose two remaining coordination bonds are occupied by a CN—group above the plane and a dimethylbenzimidazole below the plane (Fig. 9-6). There are three important structural differences between the planar group of vitamin B$_{12}$ and the porphyrin rings of hemoglobin: (1) in vitamin B$_{12}$ the alpha carbons of rings A and D are linked directly rather than by a methene bridge (compare with Fig. 10-3, p. 448), (2) the pyrrole rings in vitamin B$_{12}$ are strongly reduced and extensively substituted with methyl, acetamide, and propionamide groups, and (3) the central atom in vitamin B$_{12}$ is cobalt, whereas in hemoglobin it is iron.

By international agreement, the macro ring is called the *corrin* ring (Fig. 9-7). Derivatives are called *corrinoid* compounds. The nucleotide derivatives are given systematic names by adding a -yl ending to the nucleotide; e.g., vitamin B$_{12}$ is α-(5,6-dimethylbenzimidazolyl) cyanocobamide (Table 9-6). The trivial and semisystematic names, proposed before the chemical structure of the compound was defined, are in common usage. Thus the term "cobalamin" was introduced before the chemical structure of vitamin B$_{12}$ was clarified and is sometimes applied to the vitamin B$_{12}$ molecule minus the cyanide group. Accordingly, vitamin B$_{12}$ is cyanocobalamin.

Metabolic role

COBAMIDE COENZYMES. Studies on the fermentation of glutamate by *Clostridium tetanomorphum* first revealed the coenzyme form of vitamin B$_{12}$. It was shown that the enzymatic conversion, by glutamate isomerase, of glutamate to β-methylaspartate requires a coenzyme form of vitamin B$_{12}$. Vitamin B$_{12}$, not in the coenzyme form, is inactive, and it may be generalized that (1) the biologic activity of vitamin B$_{12}$ resides in the coenzyme form and (2) the cyanocobalamins, including vitamin B$_{12}$, do not occur natural-

ly, and therapeutically administered cyanocobalamin must be converted to 5′-adenosylcobalamin and methylcobalamin.

The participation of cobamide coenzyme in an impressively large number of metabolic conversions suggests that these enzymes, plus the folate coenzymes, occupy a key position in cellular metabolism.

METHYLMALONYL COA ISOMERASE. The utilization of propionic acid in animal tissues requires the intermediate methylmalonyl CoA (Fig. 9-8). Several aspects of these reactions, particularly the conversion of methylmalonyl CoA to succinyl CoA, implicate a contribution by cobamide coenzyme. First, it was shown that propionic acid metabolism is abnormal in tissues deprived of vitamin B$_{12}$. These tissues show decreased methylmalonyl CoA isomerase activity. Next, it was found that cobamide coenzymes participate in the isomerization of methylmalonyl CoA. Finally, it was found that there is increased excretion in the urine of methylmalonic acid (Fig. 9-9) in pernicious anemia and other vitamin B$_{12}$ deficiency states (Cox and White, 1962). The quantification of methylmalonic acid in the urine has therefore been proposed as a diagnostic aid in vitamin B$_{12}$-deficient states (Kahn et al, 1965). It is noteworthy that methylmalonic acid excretion in urine is not increased in folic acid deficiency, nor is it affected by folic acid therapy in vitamin B$_{12}$ deficiency.

SYNTHESIS OF METHIONINE METHYL. The amino acid, methionine, is essential as a source of sulfur and methyl groups. When methionine is deficient, other methyl-containing compounds (choline and betaine) replace it in part, acting to convert homocysteine to methionine. Methionine is activated to *S*-adenosylmethionine, which then acts, by transmethylation, in the transfer of methionine methyl groups to acceptors such as norepinephrine and nicotinamide. It has been shown that homocysteine will replace the requirement for methionine in a methyl-free diet provided that vitamin B$_{12}$ and folic acid are supplied. Thus in the

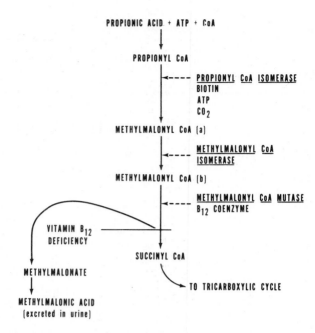

PROPIONIC ACID + ATP + CoA

↓

PROPIONYL CoA

↓ ←---- <u>PROPIONYL CoA ISOMERASE</u>
BIOTIN
ATP
CO_2

METHYLMALONYL CoA (a)

↓ ←---- <u>METHYLMALONYL CoA
ISOMERASE</u>

METHYLMALONYL CoA (b)

↓ ←---- <u>METHYLMALONYL CoA MUTASE</u>
B_{12} COENZYME

VITAMIN B_{12}
DEFICIENCY

METHYLMALONATE

↓

METHYLMALONIC ACID
(excreted in urine)

SUCCINYL CoA

↘ TO TRICARBOXYLIC CYCLE

Fig. 9-8. Vitamin B_{12}–dependent conversion of methylmalonyl CoA to succinyl CoA and excretion of methyl-malonic acid in vitamin B_{12} deficiency. The B_{12} coenzyme is deoxyadenosylcobalamin.

Fig. 9-9. Excretion of methylmalonic acid in the urine in pernicious anemia (paper chromatography). Light spot is methylmalonic acid.

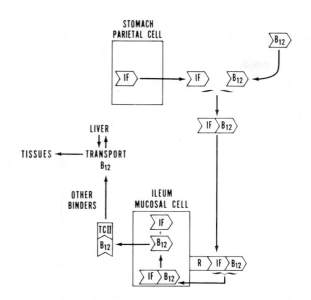

Fig. 9-10. Absorption, transport, and storage of vitamin B$_{12}$. **IF** = intrinsic factor; **R** = tissue binders; **TC II** = transcobalamin II.

Table 9-7. Content of vitamin B$_{12}$ in various foods*

Food	Vitamin B$_{12}$ content (μg/100 Gm wet weight)
Steak	1.93
Kidney (beef)	38.3
Liver (beef)	116.0
Cheese (cheddar)	2
Cheese (cottage)	0.58
Milk	
Pasteurized cow's	0.36
Human	0.01-0.15
Eggs	3.13
Chicken	0.38
Oysters	21.4
Shrimp	0.9

*Data from Lichtenstein et al, 1961.

presence of these two vitamins there is a de novo synthesis of methyl groups (Sauer and Wilmanns, 1977). The basic reaction is shown in Fig. 9-3.

DNA SYNTHESIS. The role of vitamin B$_{12}$, and its interrelation with folates, is discussed on p. 418.

Absorption

Human beings depend entirely on dietary sources of vitamin B$_{12}$. In order for the vitamin to be utilized, it is necessary that it be absorbed and then transported to final destinations (Fig. 9-10). An understanding of the absorption mechanism is basic to an application of the pathogenesis of vitamin B$_{12}$ deficiency.

Dietary vitamin B$_{12}$

A normal diet supplies an excess of the minimum daily requirement for vitamin B$_{12}$, and even a "low-cost" diet

supplies an excess. The daily requirement is 5 μg for adults and 1 to 2 μg for children (Heyssel et al, 1966). Assuming that about 20% of dietary vitamin B$_{12}$ is absorbed, the daily requirement of an adult can be met by a daily intake of 25 μg, which can be easily supplied by any diet other than one that consists exclusively of vegetable foods. The vitamin B$_{12}$ content of common foods is given in Table 9-7. According to Herbert and Jacob (1974) the ingestion of large doses of ascorbic acid (vitamin C) destroys a significant amount of dietary vitamin B$_{12}$.

Intrinsic factor (IF)

Vitamin B$_{12}$ requires intrinsic factor in the gastric juice for absorption. In man intrinsic factor is secreted by the parietal cells of the mucosa in the fundus region of the stomach. Normally the gastric juice will have a low pH due to secreted hydrochloric acid, and at the low pH the vitamin B$_{12}$ that is split away from dietary protein combines avidly with IF, and the IF-B$_{12}$ complex is stable. The IF-B$_{12}$ complex consists of two molecules of IF monomer and two molecules of vitamin B$_{12}$ (Corcino et al, 1970). The complex then moves down the gastrointestinal tract. Unabsorbed until it reaches the ileum (Okuda, 1972), the IF-B$_{12}$ complex attaches to specific receptor sites at the surface of the mucosal cell, probably at one of the two specific reactive sites of IF, the other being occupied by vitamin B$_{12}$ (Herbert, 1959).

Passage through the mucosal cell probably involves absorption of the entire IF-B$_{12}$ complex, since IF and vitamin B$_{12}$ can be shown to be components of mitochondria (Rothenberg et al, 1972b). Mitochondria have an affinity for various cobalamin analogues (Peters and Hoffbrand, 1970), but it is not known what role the mitochondria play in the processing of vitamin B$_{12}$.

Transport

Release from the mucosal cell and transport in the blood to tissues depends on at least two specific globulin proteins called *transcobalamins* (Finkler et al, 1970; Hall, 1971; Stenman, 1976; Hall, 1979). *Transcobalamin II*, a small protein (mol wt 38,000) is required for the release of vitamin B$_{12}$ and acts as the vitamin acceptor and principal carrier to the liver and other tissues. There is evidence that transcobalamin II also stimulates vitamin B$_{12}$ uptake by reticulocytes (Retief et al, 1967). Carmel et al (1977) report on a subject who developed an antibody to transcobalamin II, causing retention of vitamin B$_{12}$ in the blood.

The second carrier, *transcobalamin I*, has a higher molecular weight (121,000) and probably serves only as a backup transport system for endogenous B$_{12}$. It is not needed for the release of vitamin B$_{12}$ from the mucosal cell. Recent studies (England et al, 1973) show that, contrary to previous data, the clearance of vitamin B$_{12}$-transcobalamin complexes is the same for all the transcobalamins. Whereas a deficiency of transcobalamin II leads to vitamin B$_{12}$ deficiency, a deficiency of transcobalamin I does not. Bloomfield and Scott (1972) and Carmel (1972) have reported a third binder named *transcobalamin III*, found both in normal persons and in some patients with leukocytosis, which is derived from granulocytes and other body cells. According to

England et al (1973) and Stenman (1976), transcobalamins I and III exist as a complex showing immunologic identity with other binders in tissue fluids (R binders). Hall and Begley (1977) describe a congenital deficiency of R-type binding proteins. The vitamin B₁₂ binder associated with hepatocellular carcinoma is also of the R type (Waksman and Gilbert, 1974). A fourth globulin vitamin B₁₂ binder of the R type has been identified in the plasma of patients with polycythemia vera (Hall and Finkler, 1969) and is called *PV binder*. A small portion of vitamin B₁₂ is bound to macroglobulin *(transcobalamin O)* (Hom, 1967).

Storage

Of the total storage vitamin B₁₂ (about 5,000 μg), about one-third is stored in the liver (Heinrich, 1964; Stahlberg et al, 1967). Assuming an average loss of about 5 μg/day (Adams and Boddy, 1968) it would take about 1,000 days to develop a total deficiency if no additional vitamin B₁₂ is ingested or absorbed. This total lack of vitamin B₁₂ intake is not likely to occur except in exclusively vegetable diets or when there is a complete lack of intrinsic factor.

Interrelation of folate and vitamin B₁₂

The interrelation of folate and vitamin B₁₂ is discussed on p. 418. We know that each is capable of effecting normoblastic conversion of a megaloblastic marrow. We also know that conversion of a megaloblastic marrow does not, by itself, mean that each can fully correct a deficiency of the other; e.g., folic acid can produce a hematologic response in pernicious anemia but does not affect, and indeed may be detrimental to, the spinal cord degeneration.

ANEMIA DUE TO DEFICIENCY OF VITAMIN B₁₂ OR FOLIC ACID
Classification

The anemia resulting from a deficiency of either vitamin B₁₂ or folic acid is characteristically macrocytic and normochromic.

Table 9-8. Morphologic classification of macrocytic anemias*

I. Macrocytosis plus megaloblastic dysplasia (true macrocytosis)
  A. Pernicious anemia
  B. Tropical sprue
  C. Idiopathic steatorrhea
  D. Celiac disease
  E. Infection with *Dibothriocephalus latus (Diphyllobothrium latum)*
  F. Megaloblastic anemia of pregnancy and puerperium
  G. Megaloblastic anemia of infancy
  H. Erythroleukemia (Di Guglielmo)
  I. Advanced liver disease
  J. Nutritional deficiency (tropical macrocytic anemia)
  K. Gastrectomy or gastric disease
  L. Strictures and anastomoses of small intestine
  M. Neoplastic infiltration of bone marrow
  N. Following therapy with folic acid antagonists
  O. Idiopathic refractory megaloblastic anemia
  P. Aregenerative anemias
  Q. Hemolytic anemias
  R. Following therapy with anticonvulsant drugs
  S. Hemochromatosis
  T. Scurvy (rare)
II. Macrocytosis without megaloblastic dysplasia (pseudomacrocytosis)
  A. Scurvy
  B. Myxedema
  C. Liver disease
  D. Obstructive jaundice
  E. "Physiologic" macrocytosis of newborn infant
  F. Caused by presence of large numbers of reticulocytes
  G. Postsplenectomy
  H. The 5q-syndrome

*Macrocytic anemia, thrombocytosis, and nonlobulated megakaryocytes (Mahmood et al, 1979).

Table 9-9. Classification of anemia caused by deficiency of vitamin B₁₂ or folate

I. Vitamin B₁₂ deficiency
  A. Caused by deficient intake (vegans)
  B. Resulting from lack of intrinsic factor
    1. Classic pernicious anemia
     a. In adults
     b. In children
    2. After gastrectomy
    3. After destruction of gastric mucosa
    4. Because of biologically inert intrinsic factor
  C. Due to disease of small intestine
    1. Blind loop syndrome
    2. Diseased or resected ileum
    3. In *Dibothriocephalus latus* infection
    4. Pancreatic dysfunction
  D. Familial selective vitamin B₁₂ malabsorption (Imerslund's syndrome)
  E. Deficiency of transcobalamin II
  F. Drug-induced malabsorption
  G. Zollinger-Ellison syndrome with steatorrhea
  H. Increased requirements
II. Folate deficiency
  A. Dietary deficiency
  B. Increased folate requirements
    1. Pregnancy (megaloblastic anemia of pregnancy)
    2. Infancy (megaloblastic anemia of infancy)
    3. Increased cellular proliferation (leukemia, hemolytic anemia)
  C. Due to malabsorption of folate
    1. Congenital folate malabsorption
    2. Drug-induced folate malabsorption
    3. Steatorrheas
  D. Due to defective folate interconversion
III. Megaloblastic anemia of uncertain etiology
  A. In hemochromatosis
  B. In Di Guglielmo's syndrome (erythroleukemia)
  C. Pyridoxine-responsive megaloblastic anemia

If one deals only with morphologic features, the macrocytic anemias can be classified into those that are accompanied by megaloblastic dysplasia and those that are not (Table 9-8). This is a useful classification, but aside from the failure to deal with pathogenesis, it has one other serious shortcoming: it is based on a purely morphologic definition of megaloblastic dysplasia. In its fully manifest form, megaloblastic dysplasia is striking and characteristic. As we will note, however, morphologic variants intermediate between florid megaloblastosis and normal normoblastosis are encountered. If we classify these intermediate forms as megaloblastic, as I feel we should, some of the macrocytic anemias thought to be normoblastic classically would be shifted out of this group. Also, if one finds macrocytic erythrocytes in the peripheral blood, one wonders how they can be derived from perfectly normal normoblasts and thus whether the morphologic distinction between megaloblasts and normoblasts is a full and adequate reflection of cellular function at the precursor level.

The etiologic classification in Table 9-9 is based on which factor is deficient, when the deficiency is known, and the pathogenesis of the deficiency. An etiologic classification has the important advantage of serving as a guide to therapy, for in this group of anemias, specific therapy is extremely important.

Macrocytosis

Two types of macrocytosis of the red blood cells should be distinguished, *true macrocytosis* and *pseudomacrocytosis*.

True macrocytosis accompanies megaloblastic dysplasia and reflects the megaloblastic nature of the red cell precursors and the abnormal nucleic acid metabolism. True macrocytes as observed in a blood smear are 1½ to 2 times larger, usually ovoid, and lacking a central pallor. The cell indices correspond to the morphology, with an increase in MCV and MCH but a normal MCHC.

On the other hand, erythrocytes may appear larger than normal in a blood smear, but this type of pseudomacrocytosis is the result of an exaggerated flattening, the so-called *leptocyte*. These cells are usually not as ovoid as true macrocytes, and because they are flattened the central pallor is obvious. Target cells (codocytes) are leptocytes that have a central thickening. In pseudomacrocytosis there is no increase in MCV or MCH. Pseudomacrocytosis is common in cirrhosis (Bingham, 1959; Hattersley, 1964), in obstructive jaundice, and in postsplenectomy—conditions that affect the nature of the red cell membrane (Chapter 13). Reticulocytes are normally larger than mature red cells but are not leptocytes.

Concept of megaloblastic dyspoiesis

The morphology of megaloblastic cells is described and illustrated in Chapters 4 and 5. The description of the morphologic differences between megaloblasts and normoblasts is one of the major contributions made by morphologists.

Large cells that had a nucleus showing an open chromatin network were described by Ehrlich, who found them in the peripheral blood of some patients with severe anemia. He concluded that this type of immature erythroid cell was characteristic of "pernicious anemia." Later, cells having this characteristic morphology were found in the bone marrow tissue of persons having pernicious anemia. Subsequent studies confirmed the intimate relationship between megaloblastic erythropoiesis and a deficiency of folate or vitamin B$_{12}$. These deficiencies affect the morphology of myeloid and megakaryocytic cells as well. There appears to be an abnormality of maturation in all cell types, a *dyspoiesis*. Because of the prominence of megaloblastosis, this is also called *megaloblastic dyspoiesis*. While the most striking changes are seen in hemopoietic cells, there is a generalized change in other cells, such as the squamous cells from the buccal mucosa (Farrant, 1960).

The severity of dyspoiesis found in the bone marrow is in proportion to the deficiency of hemopoietic factors. In the most severe form of deficiency—pernicious anemia in relapse—the bone marrow will show extreme megaloblastosis, giant metamyelocytes, and large hypersegmented megakaryocytes. In milder deficiencies the changes are more subtle, there being fewer megaloblasts, some not typical, and less obvious evidence of abnormal maturation in the myeloid and megakaryocytic series. Intermediate degrees of deficiency show intermediate degrees of morphologic abnormality.

The fully developed variant can usually be recognized without difficulty (Fig. 9-11 and Plates 20 to 23). Promegaloblasts, basophilic megaloblasts, polychromatophilic megaloblasts, and orthochromic megaloblasts are present in large numbers. A few normoblastic cells are found in even the most severe deficiencies. The young granulocytes are large and poorly granulated and show evidence of an asynchronism between nuclear and cytoplasmic maturation. Adult segmented neutrophils are also larger than normal, with their nuclei hypersegmented into six or more lobes. The megakaryocytes are sometimes hypersegmented and may be more numerous than usual.

The bone marrow in partial deficiencies may show erythroid cells that are intermediate in morphology between megaloblasts and normoblasts (Fig. 9-12). They may be large or small. The nucleus still shows the stippled chromatin structure of megaloblasts, but it has a coarseness between that of the typical megaloblast and that of a normoblast (Fudenberg and Estren, 1958). These intermediate forms have been called megaloblastoid normoblasts, a bastard designation that fails to recognize them as basically megaloblastic. Occasionally the presence of typical large orthochromic megaloblasts helps to identify correctly the intermediate forms of earlier cells. It is important to note that in some megaloblastic anemias, particularly those caused by folic acid deficiency, the abnormalities of the granulocytes may be typical and therefore diagnostic, even when megaloblastosis is minimal.

Intermediate degrees of megaloblastic dyspoiesis can also be seen when a patient having an otherwise typical megaloblastic anemia receives suboptimal doses of vitamin B$_{12}$ or folic acid (Frolich, 1958). The question as to whether vitamin supplements containing folic acid can mask pernicious anemia has given rise to some difference of opinion. It is true that federal law prohibits more than 0.2 mg of folic acid per nonprescription vitamin capsule, and it is also accepted

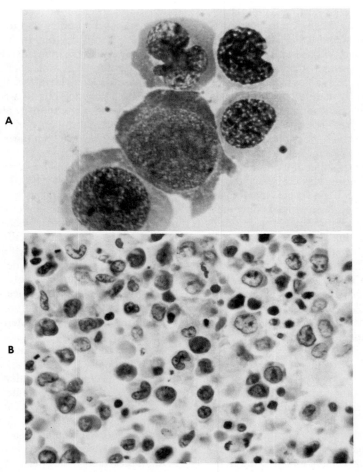

Fig. 9-11. Megaloblastic dyspoiesis. **A,** Bone marrow smear, pernicious anemia. Cell in the center is a basophilic megaloblast; others are polychromatophilic megaloblasts. (Wright's stain; ×950.) **B,** Paraffin section, bone marrow, pernicious anemia. Megaloblasts and giant stabs are easily recognized. (Hematoxylin-eosin stain; ×400.)

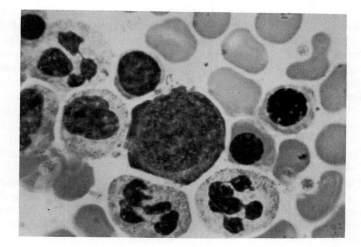

Fig. 9-12. Intermediate megaloblast. Bone marrow smear, pernicious anemia, shortly after treatment was initiated. Note macrocytosis, large hypersegmented neutrophils, and two normoblasts to right of intermediate megaloblast. (Wright's stain; ×950.)

that daily intake of this amount of folic acid will not affect a vitamin B$_{12}$ deficiency. However, cases are reported in which the intake of vitamin capsules is not limited to one per day, in which case the amount of folic acid would be sufficient to mask the hematologic picture while allowing the neurologic lesions to progress. In other cases of pernicious anemia, hematinic preparations containing significantly large amounts of folic acid have been used, with serious sequelae (Ellison, 1960).

MEGALOBLASTIC ANEMIAS

Although megaloblastic dyspoiesis is of varied etiology (Table 9-9), the megaloblastic anemias that result have many common features. Pernicious anemia can be taken as the classic example. Special features of the other anemias will be discussed in the sections that follow. The discussion of anemias caused by deficiencies of vitamin B$_{12}$ or folate follows the order presented in Table 9-9.

Due to deficiency of vitamin B$_{12}$
Inadequate intake

Persons who are strict vegetarians (vegans) often develop a deficiency of vitamin B$_{12}$ (Hines, 1966). A deficiency does not develop if a vegetarian diet is supplemented with eggs, cheese, or milk. Vitamin B$_{12}$ deficiency may develop in old persons living under poor economic circumstances (Ellis, 1974). Higginbottom et al (1978) report the occurrence of megaloblastic anemia in a breast-fed infant of a strict vegetarian.

Pernicious anemia in the adult

Pernicious anemia characteristically occurs in older persons, and the classic descriptions, clinical and pathogenetic, refer to this disease entity. However, pernicious anemia in childhood was described by Pohl in 1940, and other cases, totaling about three dozen, have been described since then. At first these cases were thought to be curiosities, a disease of the elderly occurring occasionally in childhood. There is now good reason to think that there are fundamental differences between pernicious anemia occurring in the adult and that seen in the child. Accordingly, they are described separately.

The incidence of pernicious anemia in the adult is highest among the people of northern Europe, particularly Great Britain and the Scandinavian countries (Friedlander, 1934). In the United States the incidence among whites is several times that among blacks (Hart and McCurdy, 1971). The incidence among women is slightly higher than among men (Chanarin, 1969). About 80% of the cases occur in the 40- to 70-year-old group (Chanarin, 1969). There is a significant familial incidence, as high as 30% in some series (Wangel et al, 1968; Chanarin, 1969), and a high familial incidence of achlorhydria, decreased serum vitamin B$_{12}$ levels, and immunologic abnormalities (Whittingham et al, 1969), although studies of identical twins have shown that in some pairs one develops pernicious anemia while the other does not (Balcerzak et al, 1968b). It is noteworthy that there is a high incidence of carcinoma of the stomach in subjects with pernicious anemia and in family members as well (Zamchek et al, 1955; Rousso and Cruchaud, 1966). Hoffman (1970),

however, believes that there is no causal relationship between pernicious anemia and carcinoma of the stomach, pointing out that the incidence of carcinoma of the stomach has been decreasing, whereas the incidence of pernicious anemia has remained constant.

PATHOGENESIS. The fundamental defect is a lack of intrinsic factor. Without it, vitamin B$_{12}$ cannot be absorbed. This leads to a deficiency of vitamin B$_{12}$, disordered nucleic acid metabolism, abnormal (megaloblastic) erythropoiesis and dyspoiesis, abnormal production and maturation of erythrocytes, and anemia. It is well recognized, also, that leukocytes, platelets, and squamous and columnar epithelial cells are morphologically abnormal.

Finch et al (1956) have studied erythrokinetics in pernicious anemia. They have shown that in untreated pernicious anemia the rate at which radioiron is incorporated into hemoglobin and the time it takes to appear in circulating erythrocytes are approximately normal. Erythropoietic activity in the bone marrow is increased to about three times the normal, but the rate of release of erythrocytes into the blood is not increased and erythropoiesis is said to be "ineffective." In part this is caused by arrest of DNA synthesis, an accumulation of cells in the premitotic stage that probably die before reaching maturity (Wickramasinghe et al, 1969).

This alone would not produce the severe anemia. Actually, the relative reticulocyte count is normal in untreated pernicious anemia, while the absolute reticulocyte count (percent reticulocytes × erythrocyte count) is low, indicating reduced release of reticulocytes from the bone marrow. This is supported by the long known, but usually ignored, observation that in pernicious anemia the bone marrow is filled with reticulocytes. In addition, there is a strong element of decreased erythrocyte survival, as Dock (1938) pointed out many years ago. Erythrocytes from patients with pernicious anemia show decreased survival when transfused into normal recipients, indicating an intrinsic erythrocyte defect.

Indirect evidence for decreased erythrocyte survival is provided by hyperbilirubinemia, mild as measured chemically but indicative of severe hemolysis when related to the low total circulating hemoglobin. There is increased excretion of urobilinogen in urine and feces, which again, when calculated on the basis of total circulating hemoglobin, indicates a high degree of hemolysis. Some of the urobilinogen (about 40%) has been shown to come from sources other than circulating erythrocytes, an observation that led to the concept of a "shunt" in hemoglobin synthesis whereby that percent of the final product is going to waste (London and West, 1950). Actually, the wastage probably takes place in the bone marrow, by hemolysis of reticulocytes and erythrocytes before they can be released. Finally, the almost immediate reversal of decreased erythrocyte survival occurring after vitamin B$_{12}$ is given, speaks for an antihemolytic effect of vitamin B$_{12}$ that precedes its effect on megaloblastic erythropoiesis in the bone marrow.

There is now strong evidence in favor of the concept that pernicious anemia develops as the result of genetically determined autoimmune disease (Chanarin, 1972; Chanarin and James, 1974). The first serum antibody discovered was active against intrinsic factor, and this is found in 30% to

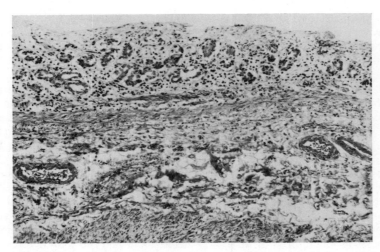

Fig. 9-13. Atrophy of gastric mucosa in pernicious anemia. The characteristic findings are the thin, gland-poor mucosa and infiltration with inflammatory cells.

40% of cases. It is now thought that intrinsic factor antibody has two components, one a *binding* antibody and one a *blocking* antibody (Taylor, 1976). Marcoullis et al (1979) identified blocking and binding antibodies to intrinsic R-type binding proteins in one patient with treated pernicious anemia. The blocking antibody prevents the complexing of vitamin B_{12} with intrinsic factor; the binding antibody reacts with the IF-B_{12} complex. In either case, there is inhibition of absorption of vitamin B_{12}. Two additional antibodies have been detected, one active against a saline extract of gastric fundus mucosa and the other against parietal cells of the gastric mucosa (the latter present in 87% of the cases). It has also been shown by te Velde et al (1964) that parietal cell antibody is present in 20% of the relatives of patients with pernicious anemia. They suggest that the development of the antibody is controlled by a dominant autosomal gene. Antibodies against intrinsic factor usually are not found in diseases other than pernicious anemia, but can be detected in a small percentage of normal elderly persons and in persons with thyroid disease (Irvine, 1965). Parietal cell antibodies are found not only in pernicious anemia but also are common in thyroid disease (32% of cases of myxedema and 28% of cases of Graves' disease) and in Addison's disease (23%). The association of thyroid and parietal cell antibody is in line with the observation that pernicious anemia occurs more frequently in patients with thyroid disease than in euthyroid patients (Ardeman et al, 1966). Pirofsky and Vaughn (1968) emphasized that a moderately strong positive antiglobulin test (Coombs') is not uncommon in untreated pernicious anemia; it usually becomes negative after adequate therapy. Corticosteroid administration is sometimes strikingly beneficial, probably acting by suppressing antibodies against intrinsic factor. Good reticulocyte responses, up to 15%, are reported following corticosteroid therapy alone (Doig et al, 1957).

Serum antibodies may in fact be of less importance than antibodies in the gastric secretion (Schade et al 1966). Rose and Chanarin (1971) found the most severe malabsorption of vitamin B_{12} in subjects having both serum and gastric juice antibodies against intrinsic factor. Twomey et al

(1969) reported ten subjects with pernicious anemia with IgG deficiency and absence of serum antibodies that preceded the onset of pernicious anemia and suggested that the immunoglobulin deficiency may be the primary cause of the gastric atrophy. Ginsberg and Mullinax (1970) reported on a subject with IgA deficiency and pernicious anemia who had serum antibodies to intrinsic factor and a monoclonal IgG peak.

Serum antibodies are of the IgG type and heterogeneous with respect to light chains (Bernier and Hines, 1967). Antibodies in gastric juice may be either of the IgG or the secretory IgA type (Goldberg and Bluestone, 1970). Transplacental passage of antibody is possible (Bar-Shany and Herbert, 1967; Goldberg et al, 1967).

While there is no doubt that autoantibodies to parietal cell cytoplasm and intrinsic factor do inhibit absorption of vitamin B_{12}, there is still the question of what is the sequence of events that terminates in the classic picture of pernicious anemia.

The simplest scheme begins with a fundamental genetic defect that allows the formation of autoantibodies against parietal cells. The antibodies attack and destroy most or all of the parietal cells and, in the most severe situation, damage the chief cells as well, leading to atrophy of the gastric mucosa (Fig. 9-13). Exfoliated surface cells are larger than normal and may be sufficiently atypical to suggest malignancy (Nieburgs and Glass, 1963; Boddington and Spriggs, 1969). Loss of parietal cells then leads to a failure to secrete intrinsic factor, HCl, and enzymes. Lack of intrinsic factor leads to impaired absorption of vitamin B_{12}.

A second scheme assumes that there is a primary atrophic gastritis, followed by the development of antibodies. Neither of these hypotheses, for that is what they are, is completely satisfactory, leaving one with the uneasy feeling that we can with unfailing success cure a disease whose etiology and pathogenesis is still somewhat obscure. It might be argued that this is preferable to a complete understanding of etiology and pathogenesis of a disease for which there is no known cure.

CLINICAL FEATURES. The onset is gradual and insidi-

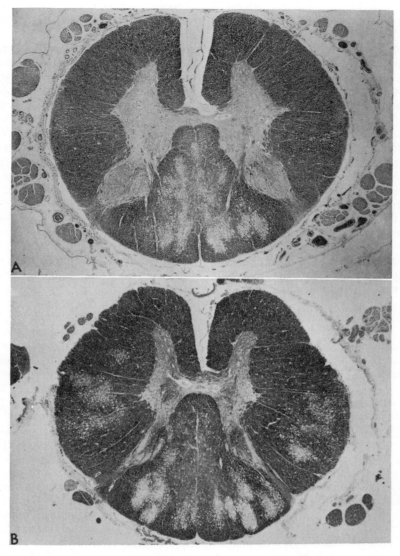

Fig. 9-14. Spinal cord, pernicious anemia. Pale-staining areas represent degeneration and demyelination of posterior and lateral fasciculi. (**A,** Hematoxylin-eosin stain; **B,** myelin stain.)

ous, and it is not uncommon to encounter a person with severe anemia and almost no symptoms. I have seen one case, an elderly male, with an erythrocyte count of 750,000/ mm^3 (0.75 × 10^{12}/l), and only moderate dyspnea as a symptom. Since the anemia develops over a long period, there is time for surprisingly efficient cardiovascular compensation, and symptoms referable to anemia (Chapter 8) are milder than expected. Sometimes the disease is discovered because the patient complains of neurologic disturbances (numbness, tingling, and weakness of the extremities) or of a sore tongue. There is often loss of appetite and moderate loss of weight. Diarrhea, sometimes alternating with constipation, can suggest a malabsorption syndrome. Mental disturbances are common but are usually mild and of such a nature (irritability, unreliable memory, and depression) that their significance can easily be missed when the patient is elderly. Mental disturbance is sometimes severe and has aptly been called "megaloblastic madness" (Smith and Oliver, 1967).

Rarely the sign calling attention to the disease is fever of unknown origin, and I have seen one patient with fever ranging between 102° and 104° F as the presenting feature. It is interesting to note that in 1871 Biermer described fever as one of the features of "progressive pernicious anemia" (Huser, 1966). Glossitis (painful, smooth beefy red tongue) is seen in about half the cases.

The neurologic damage resulting from a deficiency of vitamin B$_{12}$ is certainly the most severe and most dangerous of the clinical symptoms. It has been estimated that neurologic symptoms are the initial complaints in about one-fourth of the cases of pernicious anemia, but can be encountered in any type of vitamin B$_{12}$ deficiency (Richmond and Davidson, 1958). The diagnosis of pernicious anemia is now being made earlier, and therapy is more prompt than it was some years ago, so that neurologic symptoms tend to be less frequent and less severe. The signs and symptoms are referable to peripheral nerve degeneration, degeneration of the posterior columns of the spinal cord (Fig. 9-14), or both (combined system disease). The peripheral nerve damage accounts for numbness, hypoesthesia, or hyperesthesia. The degeneration of the posterior columns accounts for loss of reflexes, proprioception, incoordination, and loss of vibratory sense. Degeneration of the lateral columns as well leads to spasticity, hyperactive reflexes, and a plantar extension response (positive Babinski's test).

There has been much speculation about the pathogenesis of the neurologic lesions (Reynolds, 1976). Although deficiencies of B_{12} or folate interfere with DNA synthesis, this cannot be a factor in degenerative disease of the nervous system because (1) nerve cells do not undergo mitosis and therefore are not dependent on DNA synthesis and (2) the neurologic lesion is demyelination, and no acceptable connection can be made between the integrity of myelin and a deficiency of B_{12}.

LABORATORY DIAGNOSIS. The diagnosis of pernicious anemia can be established unequivocally only by laboratory studies. Those directly pertinent and specific are the following:

1. Study of the peripheral blood cells, quantitative and qualitative.
2. Achlorhydria after histamine
3. Megaloblastic dysplasia of the bone marrow
4. Low excretion of radioactive (^{60}Co- or ^{57}Co-) vitamin B_{12} (Schilling test)
5. Low concentration of vitamin B_{12} in the serum
6. Increased excretion of methylmalonic acid in the urine
7. Reticulocyte response after proper therapeutic trial

Other laboratory findings that are of interest but that are not specific for pernicious anemia are the following:

1. Increased excretion of FIGLU after the administration of histidine (seen in both vitamin B_{12} and folic acid deficiency)
2. Increased concentration of bilirubin in the serum and increased excretion of urobilinogen and coproporphyrin in urine and feces (seen in any hemolytic anemia)
3. Elevated serum iron concentration
4. Urine abnormalities (low and fixed specific gravity, albuminuria, and cylindruria)
5. Low erythrocyte and whole-blood cholinesterase activity (in relapse)
6. High serum lactic dehydrogenase activity
7. Low serum haptoglobin concentration
8. Low serum alkaline phosphatase
9. Low serum uric acid

PERIPHERAL BLOOD. The erythrocyte count and the hemoglobin concentration may vary from very low values to moderately low, depending on the stage of the disease. In relapse the erythrocyte count and the hemoglobin concentration are surprisingly low; counts of 500,000 to 750,000 erythrocytes/mm^3 (0.5 to 0.75×10^{12}/l) are not unusual. If suboptimal therapy has been given, the erythrocyte count may be only moderately low.

The MCV will be greater than normal, usually well above 100 fl. The MCV returns to normal after adequate therapy, rapidly at first as macrocytes with short life spans disappear

and more slowly later as the red population is replaced with new normocytes (Patel and Chanarin, 1975). The MCH is usually higher than the normal value of 27 to 31 fmol but the MCHC never goes above 36%. As a result of treatment, erythrocyte regeneration may outstrip the rate of hemoglobin synthesis, and the MCH will become normal or even lower than normal. The MCHC will also fall.

The stained blood smear usually presents a typical picture. There is obvious *macrocytosis* of some cells, whereas others will be normal or smaller than normal. The red blood cells are more ovoid than normal and are normally hemoglobinated. This *anisocytosis* is usually extreme in degree. *Poikilocytosis* is also striking, the erythrocytes varying from oval to pear or tennis racquet–like shapes (Fig. 9-15) and in severe cases may have bizarre shapes. The erythrocyte abnormalities are most severe when the anemia is severe. *Hypersegmented neutrophils* with six or more lobes are characteristic (Fig. 9-16) and the average lobe count is 4 to 5 or higher rather than the normal average of about 3. Many neutrophils have 6 to 10 lobes, and I have seen one with 13 lobes (Plate 23). These cells also tend to be larger than normal and are called *macropolycytes*. These cells are not hyperlobulatd because they are older and more mature, as was once thought, but because granulocytopoiesis is abnormal. Hypersegmented neutrophils can be found for 2 weeks or longer after treatment of uncomplicated megaloblastic anemia (Nath and Lindenbaum, 1979). *Orthrochromic megaloblasts* may be found (Fig. 9-17), but they are uncommon. Evidence of erythrocyte regeneration is seen in the *polychromatophilia, diffuse basophilia,* or *punctate basophilia* of some of the erythrocytes. These tinctorial features, noted in Romanowsky-stained smears, indicate the presence of basophilic reticulum within the immature erythrocytes, *reticulocytes*. In an untreated patient, the reticulocyte count is seldom higher than 2% even though the reticulocyte content of the marrow is high. Erythrocyte inclusions such as Howell-Jolly bodies and Cabot rings can usually be found (Fig. 9-18).

Leukopenia is common in the untreated patient. A leukocyte count of 4,000 to 5,000/mm^3 (4 to 5 $\times 10^9$/l) is the rule, but a higher count does not exclude pernicious anemia. The differential leukocyte count usually shows both relative and absolute neutropenia and relative lymphocytosis. A mild shift to the left is not unusual. The band neutrophils may appear large and poorly granulated. The hypersegmentation of the polymorphonuclear neutrophils has already been mentioned. Occasional patients show a moderate eosinophilia.

The patient with a severe untreated anemia usually shows thrombocytopenia in addition to anemia and leukopenia, a triad suggestive of an aplastic anemia. Usually neither the leukopenia nor the thrombocytopenia is severe enough to confuse the diagnosis seriously. Platelet counts under 50,000/mm^3 (0.05×10^{12}/l) are unusual. The thrombocytopenia may be enhanced following transfusion of packed or washed erythrocytes (Fillet et al, 1977). Purpura is uncommon, and abnormal bleeding rarely is encountered. As in all thrombocytopenic states, the platelet morphology on stained smears may be abnormal, with giant platelets a prominent feature. Riddle et al (1960) have shown by electron micros-

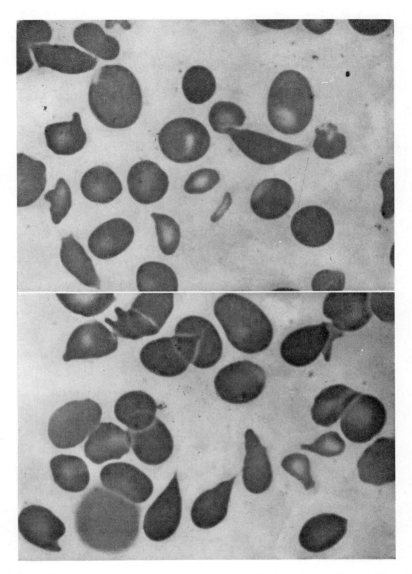

Fig. 9-15. Peripheral blood, pernicious anemia. Note macrocytosis, 4+ anisocytosis, and 4+ poikilocytosis. (Wright's stain; ×950.)

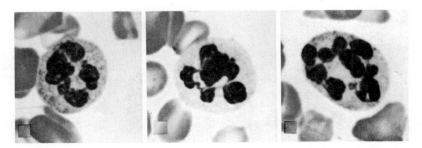

Fig. 9-16. Hypersegmented neutrophils, pernicious anemia, peripheral blood. (Wright's stain; ×950.)

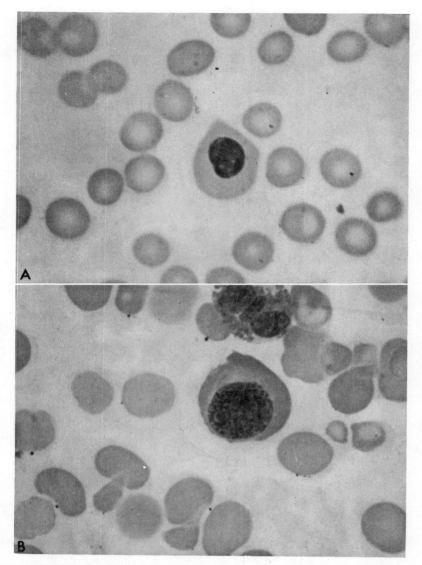

Fig. 9-17. Peripheral blood, pernicious anemia. **A,** Orthochromic megaloblast. **B,** Late polychromatophilic megaloblast. (Wright's stain; ×950.)

copy that the platelets in pernicious anemia have an abnormal structure and that this does not change when vitamin B$_{12}$ is given.

GASTRIC ANALYSIS. In spite of isolated reports to the contrary, it is generally agreed that for a positive diagnosis of pernicious anemia of the adult type there must be an absence of free hydrochloric acid in the gastric juice *(achlorhydria)* after histamine stimulation. In pernicious anemia in childhood there is a deficiency of intrinsic factor secretion without failure to secrete acid. When the onset of the disease occurs early in adult life, the gastric juice may contain free acid. In the usual case of adult pernicious anemia the dysfunction in gastric secretion is reflected not only in the achlorhydria but also in the reduced volume of gastric juice and in the absence or marked reduction of pepsin and rennin *(achylia)*. While the presence of achlorhydria confirms the diagnosis of pernicious anemia, it should be noted that achlorhydria is not uncommon in iron-deficiency anemias or even in healthy elderly persons.

The standard intubation method should be used. The so-called "tubeless" gastric analysis method (Diagnex blue test) is not recommended because (1) abnormalities of absorption from the small intestine will yield false low values, (2) liver dysfunction will yield false low values, (3) renal disease or incomplete emptying of the bladder at the beginning of the test yields false low values, and (4) the test is not reliable when only a small amount of free acid is present in the stomach.

BONE MARROW. Most of the hyperplasia is caused by proliferation of the erythroid cells. In most cases, normoblasts and megaloblasts are found in about equal number. Marrow megaloblasts show intense nonspecific esterase activity using α-naphthyl acetate as substrate (Kass and Peters, 1977). This reaction is blocked by fluoride. It is not

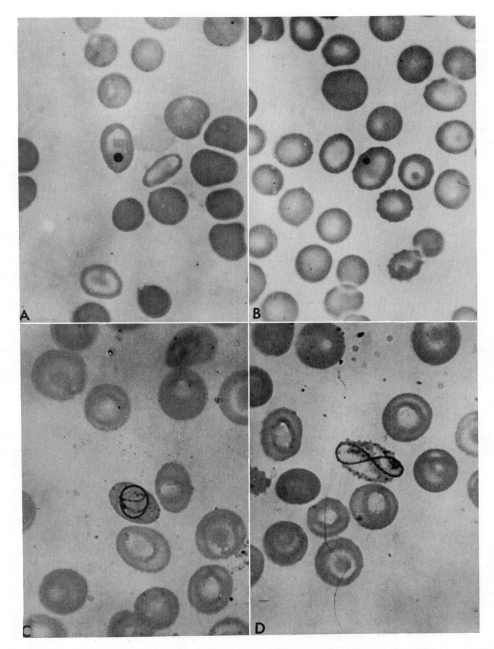

Fig. 9-18. Peripheral blood, pernicious anemia. **A** and **B,** Howell-Jolly bodies. **C** and **D,** Cabot rings. (Wright's stain; ×950.)

specific for megaloblasts in pernicious anemia, since this nonspecific esterase activity is found in chronic erythremic myelosis as well as in normoblasts in untreated iron-deficiency anemia. There is no obvious explanation for this esterase positivity or for the report that megaloblasts in untreated pernicious anemia show PAS positivity (Kass, 1977b).

In partially treated patients, megaloblastic features may be minimal, but it is unusual not to find at least a few typical megaloblasts, usually of the polychromatophilic or orthochromic variety. Within 24 to 48 hours after optimal therapy

is started, only normoblastic cells will be found. Partial reversion of a megaloblastic marrow to a normoblastic marrow can be produced by blood transfusions. Recognition of suboptimally treated pernicious anemia is at times extremely difficult.

The morphologic alterations in leukocytes and megakaryocytes are just as diagnostic as the presence of megaloblasts. There is an asynchronism in granulocytes between nuclear and cytoplasmic maturation, producing myelocytes poor in granules. The metamyelocytes and band forms are two to three times larger than normal and have large nuclei

Table 9-10. Pattern of results of Schilling test when there is a vitamin B_{12} deficiency state

I. Normal Schilling test
  A. Dietary deficiency of vitamin B_{12}
II. Malabsorption pattern (abnormal with no change after intrinsic factor is given)
  A. Malabsorption syndrome (tropical sprue, celiac disease, idiopathic steatorrhea)
  B. Malabsorption secondary to intestinal abnormalities
    1. Regional enteritis
    2. Stricture of small intestine
    3. Shunting anastomoses of small intestine
    4. Multiple diverticula of small intestine
    5. Resection of ileum
    6. Pancreatic dysfunction
    7. *Dibothriocephalus* infection
    8. Deficiency of transcobalamin II
III. Pernicious anemia pattern (abnormal standard test, normal excretion after intrinsic factor is given)
  A. Pernicious anemia (adult and juvenile)
  B. Gastrectomy
  C. Hypothyroidism
  D. Intrinsic factor inhibitor in gastric juice

Table 9-11. Serum vitamin B_{12} concentration in normal persons and in patients with pernicious anemia in relapse (*L. leichmannii* assay)

Reference	Normals (pg/ml)*		Pernicious anemia (pg/ml)	
	Range	Mean	Range	Mean
Spray and Witts, 1958	150-1,000	450	10-170	64
Kristensen and Gormsen, 1958	165-1,135	392	20-165	—
Halstead, 1959	155-1,187	476	16-104	37
Brandt and Metz, 1961	214-1,150	682	10-160	54
Matthews, 1962	120-1,150	480	50-125	—

*pg = picogram = $\mu\mu$g (Gm $\times$ 10^{-12}).

and deficient cytoplasmic granulation. There are occasional large polymorphonuclear neutrophils, with hypersegmentation of the nucleus into six or more lobes.

Megakaryocytes may be many or few. They are often very large. The granulation of the cytoplasm is sometimes deficient. The nucleus is even more bizarre than usual, showing numerous distinct and unattached lobes that give the cell an "exploded" appearance. These abnormal megakaryocytes are similar in some respects to the abnormal forms described in immune thrombocytopenia, but the excessive nuclear malformation is typical of pernicious anemia. As a rule, there is an increase in the number of reticulum cells, many of which are phagocytic.

EXCRETION OF LABELED VITAMIN B_{12} (SCHILLING TEST). The availability of tagged vitamin B_{12} has made possible a specific technic for measuring the absorption of the vitamin (Chanarin, 1976). By giving a standard dose of ^{57}Co-vitamin B_{12} (preferred over ^{60}Co-vitamin B_{12} because the latter has a longer half-life) by mouth and then measuring the amount excreted in the urine (Schilling test) or the amount picked up by the liver, it is possible to estimate whether or not absorption is normal. If absorption is impaired, the test is repeated, with the addition of intrinsic factor (60 mg of hog intrinsic factor). This allows distinction between simple malabsorption on the basis of gastrointestinal dysfunction and malabsorption caused by lack of intrinsic factor.

The actual performance of the test depends on saturating the capacity of the serum to bind vitamin B_{12} so that the tagged vitamin B_{12} will be excreted in the urine. Accordingly, the tagged vitamin B_{12} is given orally, and within 2 hours 1,000 μg of ordinary vitamin B_{12} is given intramuscularly. The urine excreted during the next 24 hours is collected and its radioactivity measured and compared to a suitable standard.

The results of the test will vary with the amount of tagged vitamin B_{12} used as a test dose. Various technics call for the administration of 0.5 to 2.0 μg, but the smaller dose produces a higher percent excretion than that produced by the larger dose. With a test dose of 0.5 μg, the excretion during the 24-hour collection period is normally greater than 7% to 8% of the test dose. If excretion is below these levels, there is evidence that the radioactive vitamin B_{12} has been poorly absorbed. If absorption is still abnormal after intrinsic factor is given, the defect is in the absorptive process and unrelated to intrinsic factor. If intrinsic factor causes normal excretion, then malabsorption is related to lack of intrinsic factor, the pattern expected in pernicious anemia (Table 9-10).

The value of the Schilling test in the diagnosis of pernicious anemia is well documented (Persson and Hansen, 1963). In the differential diagnosis of megaloblastic anemia, the test does, however, have some shortcomings. The "flushing" dose of 1,000 μg of vitamin B_{12} will interfere with any subsequent diagnostic tests or therapeutic trials. This is particularly important when the investigation proceeds from the bone marrow examination directly to the Schilling test. If the disease is pernicious anemia, no harm is done, but if the disease is instead a folic acid deficiency, the large dose of vitamin B_{12} will produce a reticulocyte response even though the deficiency is not vitamin B_{12}. It would be better, given a typical clinical picture, peripheral blood, bone marrow, and gastric analysis, first to perform a proper therapeutic trial (discussed subsequently) with folic acid and vitamin B$_{12}$, preferably after measuring serum folate and vitamin B$_{12}$ levels, and to use the Schilling test only after the defect is shown to be in vitamin B$_{12}$ and in the presence of normal serum folate concentration. It seems to me that after all this evidence is at hand the Schilling test is probably unnecessary. It seems obvious, but is sometimes forgotten, that the Schilling test is of little value when there is severe renal disease, since it is based on normal glomerular function. It is also obvious that there should be a complete collection of the 24-hour urine sample.

ASSAY OF VITAMIN B$_{12}$. Several microorganisms can be used for the microbiologic assay, including *Lactobacillus lactis*, *Lactobacillus leichmannii*, *Euglena gracilis*, *Ochromonas malhamensis*, and *Escherichia coli*. The two most commonly in use are *Euglena gracilis* and *Lactobacillus leichmannii*. The sensitivity of the two organisms is the same, but *Euglena gracilis* has such strict requirements of temperature and exposure to light that special and involved apparatus is required. On the other hand, assay with *Lactobacillus leichmannii* requires the same simple equipment needed for the assay of folate. *Lactobacillus leichmannii* is therefore the organism of choice.

Even with the most meticulous technic, replicate analyses of the same sample show a variation of about 15%. Factors that can introduce large errors are dirty glassware, antibiotics in the serum (penicillin inhibits growth, but most of the others do not), or a sluggish stock culture of the organism.

Normal values and assays in patients with pernicious anemia in relapse are given in Table 9-11. Vitamin B$_{12}$ levels may be subnormal in folate deficiency. As for folate assays, the normal values vary widely among different laboratories, and each should establish its own normals. Since there is some overlap between the highest values found in pernicious anemia and the lowest ones in normal persons, assay values should not be considered the final proof that a vitamin B$_{12}$ deficiency state exists. In general, it is reasonable to use a value of 160 pg/ml as the low limit of normal and a value of between 120 and 160 pg/ml as of doubtful significance. Factors to be taken into account are age (Gaffney et al, 1957), diet (a vegetarian diet is normally accompanied by low vitamin B$_{12}$ assay values), and pregnancy (the vitamin B$_{12}$ concentration in serum normally falls throughout pregnancy to a low at term). In general, low assay values are found in almost all cases of pernicious anemia in relapse (mean 37 pg/ml, range 16 to 104 pg/ml) and in a high percentage of other diseases that may be accompanied by megaloblastic dyspoiesis (total gastrectomy, steatorrheas, anticonvulsant drug therapy, and infection with tapeworm). It should be noted that the serum vitamin B$_{12}$ level is often low in patients having a pure deficiency of folate. Low levels are not uncommon in multiple myeloma. Low serum levels are also reported after massive hemorrhage.

High serum concentrations of vitamin B$_{12}$ and of B$_{12}$-binding proteins are found sometimes in chronic and acute myelocytic leukemia (Hall and Finkler, 1966), in the myeloproliferative disorders (Mollin and Ross, 1955), and when there is acute necrosis of parenchymal liver cells. However, the application of elevated levels in the differential diagnosis of these conditions (Herbert, 1968) is limited by the finding that simple leukocytosis can also be accompanied by increased serum vitamin B$_{12}$ concentration (Carmel and Coltman, 1971; Carmel, 1972).

In addition to other defects in pernicious anemia, the binding capacity of serum for vitamin B$_{12}$ is reduced. Normality is reestablished by treatment. A high binding capacity and high serum concentrations of vitamin B$_{12}$ have been found in liver disease (acute hepatitis but not cirrhosis), myeloproliferative disorders, and chronic myelocytic leukemia.

Folate and vitamin B$_{12}$ should be assayed at the same time. It is then usual to find an increase in folate concentration in serum and a decrease in folate concentration in red blood cells. Accumulation of folate in serum reflects an accumulation of 5-methyl-TH$_4$.

The use of radioimmunoassay using isotope-labeled vitamin B$_{12}$ and various binding agents promises to replace microbiologic assay technics (Rothenberg, 1973). In general, assays by the radioisotope method tend to yield higher values than do the microbiologic technics (Raven et al, 1971). Cooper and Whitehead (1978) determined serum B$_{12}$ levels by both microbiologic assay and radioimmunoassay in 43 patients with classic pernicious anemia and found that the radiodilution assay was not as reliable as the *E. gracilis* assay. Potential inaccuracies of the radioligand methods are also discussed by Kolhouse et al (1978) and by Rothenberg and Lawson (1979).

EXCRETION OF METHYLMALONIC ACID IN URINE. As discussed on p. 423, an increased excretion of methylmalonic acid is an absolute index of vitamin B$_{12}$ deficiency. The only exception is congenital methylmalonic aciduria (Rosenberg et al, 1969; Levy et al, 1970), a defect not accompanied by macrocytic anemia or megaloblastic dysplasia. There has been some reluctance to use this test routinely because it requires chromatography on paper or other vehicles, but in fact the technic is not difficult. It is more specific than the other tests in the sense that the correlation between the serum concentration of vitamin B$_{12}$ and the bone marrow morphology depends in part on the status of folate metabolism and in part on the exhaustion of tissue stores of vitamin B$_{12}$. The excretion of methylmalonic acid, on the other hand, is independent of folate metabolism and there is no increased excretion in folate deficiency.

RETICULOCYTE RESPONSE AFTER THERAPEUTIC TRIAL. If one gives sufficiently large doses of either folic acid or vitamin B$_{12}$, a reticulocyte response will be produced regardless of which deficiency state exists; e.g., patients with folic acid deficiency will respond to 500 μg of B$_{12}$ daily, and patients with vitamin B$_{12}$ deficiency states will respond to 400 μg of folic acid daily. A proper therapeutic trial should utilize the minimum effective dose of the vitamin to produce a specific response. If vitamin B$_{12}$ deficiency is suspected, 1 μg of vitamin B$_{12}$ is given daily, and if there is a reticulocyte response in 5 to 7 days, the deficiency is in vitamin B$_{12}$ (Sullivan and Herbert, 1965). This small dose of vitamin B$_{12}$ will not produce reticulocytosis if the deficiency is in folic acid. Likewise, parenteral folic acid in daily doses of 100 to 200 μg is used for a therapeutic trial when folic acid deficiency is suspected. This will not produce a reticulocyte response in pernicious anemia.

With optimum and specific therapy, the reticulocyte response is proportional to the severity of the anemia. Regardless of the severity of the anemia, the erythrocyte count reaches normal values after 8 to 12 weeks of optimum therapy. The hemoglobin concentration increases at a somewhat slower rate. With rapid erythrocyte generation, one often encounters iron deficiency and hypochromia of the red blood cells unless supplemental iron therapy is given as well.

ERYTHROCYTE SURVIVAL. The icterus, hyperbilirubinemia, increased excretion of hemoglobin pigments, and reduced concentration of serum haptoglobin point to a decreased erythrocyte survival. Direct measurements have shown that erythrocytes in pernicious anemia have one-fourth to one-half the survival rate of normal erythrocytes. The defect is intrinsic since erythrocytes from a patient with pernicious anemia have a short survival when transfused into a normal recipient. The survival rate can be restored to normal by the administration of adequate amounts of vitamin B_{12}. Hamilton et al (1958) have calculated that the decreased erythrocyte survival can by itself account for the development of anemia. Recent studies with ^{51}Cr-tagged erythrocytes have shown that decreased survival is also found in megaloblastic anemia of pregnancy; decreased survival in this case is partially improved by folic acid therapy.

URINE AND RENAL FUNCTION. Low and fixed specific gravity, albuminuria, and cylindruria have been described. The most typical urinary finding is an increased amount of urobilinogen and urobilin. In relapse, urobilinogen and coproporphyrin I excretion is several times normal. When full therapy is instituted, urinary urobilinogen excretion returns to normal within a few hours, preceding the reticulocyte response. Mild elevation of blood nonprotein nitrogen concentration and reduced urea clearance values have been described. The renal function often returns to normal when the anemia improves.

IRON METABOLISM. There is almost always an elevation of the serum iron concentration when the disease is in relapse. The serum iron-binding capacity is normal or slightly decreased. Serum copper values are also normal, and in the untreated patient, erythrocyte protoporphyrin is not significantly different from normal. Rather sharp differences are found after treatment is begun, such as a drop in serum iron concentration to normal, or lower than normal, levels and a sharp rise in erythrocyte protoporphyrin. This sharp drop in serum iron concentration may be helpful in diagnosing the disease in patients who have been partially treated or in those who do not show a typical peripheral blood and bone marrow picture.

PIGMENT EXCRETION. The characteristic lemon-yellow tint of the skin is seen only in patients with very low erythrocyte counts. It is in these patients that the hemolytic element is most striking. The serum bilirubin concentration is increased but is seldom above 4 mg/dl, the major portion being indirect-reacting bilirubin. A high concentration of urobilinogen and coproporphyrin I is found in the urine. When specific therapy is given there is an immediate reversion to normal.

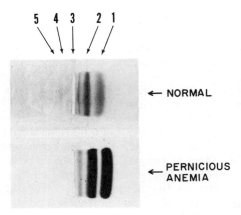

Fig. 9-19. Increased serum LDH activity in pernicious anemia. Electrophoresis on agar. Note striking increase in fractions 1 and 2 (international nomenclature of LDH isoenzymes). Note that LDH-2 is normally greater than LDH-1, but in megaloblastic anemias the pattern is reversed, LDH-1 being greater than LDH-2. (Courtesy Dr. Jon V. Straumfjord.)

BIOCHEMICAL FINDINGS. *Erythrocyte cholinesterase* is low during relapse and returns to normal after therapy. The *serum cholesterol* concentration is usually moderately low before treatment. After treatment it rises to levels higher than normal, a rise that is most marked at the peak of the reticulocyte response. The concentration of *uric acid* becomes greater during treatment, at which time there is also an increase in the amount of uric acid excreted in the urine. Both remain increased as long as rapid erythrocyte regeneration takes place, 10 Gm of endogenous uric acid being excreted for each increment of 1 million erythrocytes in the peripheral blood count. There have been reports of acute gouty arthritis occurring during this phase. *Muramidase* in urine is usually increased.

One of the intriguing biochemical findings in pernicious anemia is the very high activity of *lactic dehydrogenase* (LDH) in the serum (Anderssen, 1964), the increase being in fractions 1 and 2 (Winston et al, 1970) (Fig. 9-19). Since this was first reported, other reports of increased LDH activity in pernicious anemia have appeared. The highest activity so far reported is 28,125 units. LDH activity drops at about the time the reticulocyte response begins. Heller et al (1960) have found increased LDH activity in megaloblastic marrow tissue, and it is assumed that this is the source of the high activity of LDH in serum. In the megaloblastic anemias, high LDH levels have also been reported in *Dibothriocephalus latus* infection and in megaloblastic anemia of pregnancy. High LDH levels are also found in a variety of hemolytic anemias but the increase is usually moderate.

Other biochemical findings, some important when treatment is instituted, are: (1) a low serum alkaline phosphatase activity increasing after treatment (van Dommelen et al, 1964a), (2) depressed serum uric acid level rising immediately after treatment (Riddle, 1929), and (3) an immediate decrease in serum potassium (Lawson et al, 1970), sometimes responsible for symptoms and signs of hypokalemia.

DEOXYURIDINE SUPPRESSION TEST. The deoxyuridine

(dU) suppression test measures the incorporation of tritiated thymidine into DNA-thymine. Preincubation of normal bone marrow cells with deoxyuridine suppresses incorporation, but in megaloblastic marrow there is less suppression (Herbert et al, 1973). It is said to be useful when the morphologic findings and the serum vitamin B$_{12}$ or folate levels are equivocal. Wickramasinghe and Saunders (1977) found the test positive in all patients with folate or B$_{12}$ deficiency, in some patients receiving drugs that inhibit dihydrofolate reductase, in 4 of 19 patients with epilepsy receiving anticonvulsants, and in 2 of 21 patients with iron-deficiency anemia. However, other patients with megaloblastosis from various causes (e.g., sideroblastic anemia, erythremic myelosis) with subnormal folate of B$_{12}$ serum levels had a normal dU suppression.

Pernicious anemia in infants and children

Classic pernicious anemia is rare before 18 years of age. Megaloblastic anemias caused by vitamin B$_{12}$ deficiency in infants and children can be divided into a number of possibly overlapping categories.

It was once thought that "juvenile pernicious anemia" consisted of a homogeneous group characterized by the lack of intrinsic factor but having normal acid and enzyme secretion in the gastric juice and a normal gastric mucosa. McIntyre et al (1965) summarized 26 cases and found that they divided into two groups, 20 showing absence of intrinsic factor, normal gastric secretion, and absence of antibodies against parietal cells and intrinsic factor, while six cases showed absence of intrinsic factor, deficiency of gastric secretion, atrophic gastric mucosa, and demonstrable antibodies against intrinsic factor and parietal cells. These two groups are included in the general category of "congenital deficiency of intrinsic factor" (Table 9-12). This group also includes the case reported by Katz et al (1972) as caused by biologically inert intrinsic factor.

The second major category, congenital vitamin B$_{12}$ malabsorption, includes Imerslund's syndrome and congenital absence of transcobalamin II. In these cases there is no deficiency of intrinsic factor and no antibodies to intrinsic factor of parietal cells.

The third category includes cases of vitamin B$_{12}$ deficiency in the infant born to a vitamin B$_{12}$-deficient mother (Jadhav et al, 1962; Goldberg et al, 1967; Srikantia and Reddy, 1967) sometimes complicated by transplacental transfer of antibodies to intrinsic factor and parietal cells.

After gastrectomy

The patient who undergoes gastrectomy may develop an iron-deficiency anemia in the first year and a megaloblastic anemia several years later (Shafer et al, 1973). Iron deficiency is common (Weir and Gatenby, 1963; Hines et al, 1967), caused in part by both an impaired absorption of food iron and a preoperative deficiency. Almost all have impaired absorption of vitamin B$_{12}$ caused by deficiency of intrinsic factor and about 18% develop megaloblastic anemia (Hines et al, 1967). The more extensive the resection, the more severe the deficiency of intrinsic factor. Neurologic symptoms are the same as in classic pernicious anemia and are present in the same frequency (Weir and Gatenby, 1963). Occasionally the megaloblastic anemia is caused by

Table 9-12. Classification of vitamin B$_{12}$ deficiency in infancy and childhood

I. Congenital deficiency of intrinsic factor
  A. Juvenile pernicious anemia
  B. Pernicious anemia of childhood with atrophy
  C. Due to biologically inert intrinsic factor
II. Congenital vitamin B$_{12}$ malabsorption
  A. Familial selective vitamin B$_{12}$ malabsorption (Imerslund's syndrome)
  B. Congenital deficiency of transcobalamin II
III. Transplacental transfer of antibody to intrinsic factor

deficiency of folate (Gough et al, 1965). Folate deficiency may become manifest during the first year, but megaloblastic anemia due to vitamin B$_{12}$ deficiency may not develop for many years.

The etiology of postgastrectomy anemia should be established by laboratory studies. If iron deficiency is present there may be only hypochromia of the red cells. Later, hypochromic red cells and macrocytes are present. Determination of serum folate and vitamin B$_{12}$ concentrations is indicated and usually both will be depressed in contrast with pernicious anemia in which folate is normal or increased. Since the spleen is usually excised as well, the peripheral blood smear may show numerous Howell-Jolly bodies (p. 64).

Loss of gastric mucosa following ingestion of acid is equivalent to gastrectomy and may cause megaloblastic anemia (Alsted, 1937).

Due to biologically inert intrinsic factor

One case is reported (Katz et al, 1972) of megaloblastic anemia in a 13-year-old child in which the gastric secretion contained immunologically reactive intrinsic factor but deficient vitamin B$_{12}$ absorption. The abnormal intrinsic factor was shown to bind vitamin B$_{12}$ normally, and the abnormality was assumed to be at the site of binding to the ileal mucosal cell. Katz et al (1974) concluded that the patient was homozygous and that the father, mother, and sister were heterozygous for a structurally abnormal intrinsic factor with markedly decreased affinity to ileal IF-B$_{12}$ complex receptors.

Due to disease of small intestine

Since vitamin B$_{12}$ is absorbed only in the lower ileum, various diseases of the small intestine can produce a deficiency. Resection of the terminal ileum (Allcock, 1961; Fone et al, 1961), regional ileitis (Steinberg, 1961), strictures and anastomoses (Ainley and Lamb, 1961; Donaldson, 1965), multiple jejunal diverticulosis (Carter and Hocking, 1967), and scleroderma involving the small intestine (Salen et al, 1966) have been responsible for vitamin B$_{12}$ deficiency. Except in the case of surgical resection of the ileum, a major contributing cause is the competition of proliferating bacteria, not normally present in the ileum, for vitamin B$_{12}$ (Dellipiani et al, 1968). When there is stasis and multiplication of bacteria the term "blind loop syndrome" is used, but this hardly applies to all abnormalities of jejunal absorption.

Competition for vitamin B_{12} is also a feature of *Dibothriocephalus* infection, particularly in Finland (Nyberg and Saarni, 1964). Many parasites lodged in the ileum avidly take up vitamin B_{12}, and in fact it can be shown that the worms are rich in vitamin B_{12} (Nyberg, 1952). The laboratory diagnosis is based on finding the ova in the feces.

It should be noted that structural and functional abnormalities of the jejunal mucosa are a feature of untreated pernicious anemia (Peña et al, 1972). These include shortening of the villi with diminished surface area, megalocytic changes of the epithelial cells, increased inflammatory infiltrate, and depression of disaccharidase activity.

Veeger et al (1962) and Toskes and Deren (1973) have shown that there is impaired absorption of vitamin B_{12} when the exocrine secretion of the pancreas is deficient. Megaloblastic anemia is rare in pancreatic disease, but this may be because of the long period of time required to deplete the body of its stores of vitamin B_{12}.

Familial selective vitamin B_{12} malabsorption

The lesion in the cases reported by Imerslund (1960) and by Gräsbeck et al (1960), sometimes called the Imerslund or Imerslund-Gräsbeck syndrome, was thought to be a lack of the ileal receptors for the IF-B_{12} complex. Mackenzie et al (1972) have proposed that the abnormality occurs after attachment of the IF-B_{12} complex but before binding to transcobalamin II. Gastric secretion is normal and there are no antiparietal cell antibodies. Characteristically the affected children show severe proteinuria, which persists after the anemia is corrected by the administration of vitamin B_{12}.

Deficiency of transcobalamin II

Hakami et al (1971) have reported the occurrence of megaloblastic anemia in two female siblings congenitally lacking transcobalamin II. Similar cases are reported by Scott et al (1972), by Gimpert et al (1975), and by Burman et al (1979). An ineffective abnormal transcobalamin II, transcobalamin Cardeza, caused megaloblastic anemia in the case reported by Haurani et al (1979). These cases lend support to the concept that transcobalamin II is the primary receptor of vitamin B_{12} from the ileal cell. Carmel and Herbert (1969) documented a deficiency of transcobalamin I in two brothers, not accompanied by anemia. Nexø et al (1975) report on a patient with hepatocellular carcinoma, undetectable amounts of transcobalamin II, markedly increased transcobalamin I, and megaloblastic anemia.

Drug-induced malabsorption

Moderate interference with vitamin B_{12} absorption has been noted after long-term ingestion of some drugs: para-aminosalicylic acid (Toskes and Deren, 1972), neomycin (Jacobson et al, 1960), ethyl alcohol (Lindenbaum and Lieber, 1969), colchicine (Webb et al, 1968), and phenformin (Jounela et al, 1974). A complete list of drugs that interfere with absorption of folate or vitamin B_{12} is given by Waksman et al (1970).

In the Zollinger-Ellison syndrome

The Zollinger-Ellison syndrome is characterized by massive hypersecretion of gastric juice, widespread ulceration in the gastrointestinal tract, and noninsulin-producing islet cell tumors of the pancreas. One consequence of the massive hypersecretion of acid gastric juice is a low intestinal pH that interferes with the binding of vitamin B_{12} to intrinsic factor or with the binding of IF-B_{12} complex to ileal receptors (Shimoda et al, 1968; Shum et al, 1971). Steatorrhea is common and there are multiple absorption defects, including malabsorption of iron, but frank megaloblastosis does not occur.

Increased requirements for vitamin B_{12}

While body stores of folate are easily depleted by increased requirements, it is rare for increased requirements to deplete the stores of vitamin B_{12}. Depletion of vitamin B_{12} is reported in Waldenström's macroglobulinemia (van Dommelen et al, 1964b) and in myeloproliferative disorders (Wellington and Whitcomb, 1960); but if these are examples of depletion of vitamin B_{12} by increased requirements, some mechanism must be operative that sets them apart from other proliferative diseases.

Due to deficiency of folate
Dietary deficiency

A dietary deficiency of folate in the adult is extremely rare in this country, possible only in persons having most unusual dietary habits, as in chronic alcoholics (Eichner and Hillman, 1971; Eichner and Hillman, 1973) as the result of low folate intake, the interference of alcohol with folate metabolism, and malabsorption (Lieber, 1980; Lindenbaum, 1980). Chanarin (1979) emphasizes the difference between the chronic skid-row alcoholic and the alcoholic who drinks a great deal but who also eats a normal diet. Kaunitz and Lindenbaum (1977) point out that folic acid can be added to wine, from which it is readily absorbed. Megaloblastic anemia caused by folate deficiency is found in about 20% of patients having alcoholic cirrhosis (Kimber et al, 1965) and an even greater percentage have low folate levels with macrocytosis and hypersegmentation of the neutrophils without frank megaloblastosis (Herbert et al, 1963). The folate deficiency in cirrhosis is due in part to dietary deficiency and in part to inadequate storage in the liver (Cherrick et al, 1965) and to excessive loss of folate in the urine (Retief and Huskisson, 1969). Folate absorption is normal (Halsted et al, 1971). Alcohol has a toxic effect on erythroid precursors, as evidenced by vacuolization of the cytoplasm of normoblasts in acute alcoholism (McCurdy and Rath, 1980). It should be noted that macrocytosis without megaloblastosis is common in cirrhosis.

Megaloblastic anemia of pregnancy

Most true anemias that occur during pregnancy are of the iron-deficiency type. It should be noted that the increase in plasma volume that occurs normally as pregnancy progresses accounts for some decrease in the red cell count and hemoglobin concentration. Occasionally macrocytic anemia with megaloblastic dysplasia of the bone marrow is encountered, caused by a deficiency of folate. Because of its similarity to classic pernicious anemia, it is often incorrectly referred to as "pernicious anemia of pregnancy." Classic pernicious anemia may occur in a pregnant woman (Martin et al, 1967), but it should not be confused with megaloblastic anemia of pregnancy. The differentiation is important since megaloblastic anemia of pregnancy is a self-limiting disease, whereas classic pernicious anemia represents a life-long deficiency state.

The differential diagnosis depends on both clinical and laboratory evidence. In a young pregnant woman, macrocytic anemia is almost certainly related to the pregnancy. If macrocytic anemia occurred during a previous pregnancy and there was a spontaneous remission after delivery, this strongly favors the diagnosis of megaloblastic anemia of pregnancy. The hematologic findings are usually less abnormal than in pernicious anemia. In megaloblastic anemia of pregnancy, achlorhydria after the administration of histamine is unusual. However, it should be remembered that hypochlorhydria is not uncommon in pregnancy and that achlorhydria unrelated to the macrocytic anemia may also be seen. If achlorhydria is present, it often disappears after delivery. Careful and complete hematologic studies are indicated whenever anemia develops during pregnancy. The presence of even occasional macrocytes and hypersegmented neutrophils is indication for a bone marrow study because megaloblastic anemia of pregnancy can progress very rapidly and endanger the life of both the mother and the fetus. Rarely, the onset is acute with minimal abnormalities in the peripheral blood but severe megaloblastic change in the bone marrow (Chanarin and Davey, 1964).

Folic acid usually produces an excellent response. Vitamin B$_{12}$, on the other hand, is seldom effective. The pathogenesis of the deficiency remains obscure. Because of the profound metabolic changes that accompany pregnancy, it is not unlikely that several factors combine to produce this deficiency. One factor is an increased requirement for folate (Chanarin et al, 1968; Daniel et al, 1971). In some cases, intercurrent acute pyelonephritis seems responsible for an unusual acute onset (Martin et al, 1967). The important role of hemolysis in megaloblastic anemia of pregnancy has been emphasized by Hollingsworth and Adams (1955).

Megaloblastic anemia of infancy

This macrocytic anemia of infancy occurs most commonly in premature infants (Strelling et al, 1966) or between 6 and 12 months of age, and is caused by a folic acid deficiency, conditioned or accentuated by a concomitant vitamin C deficiency. The few acceptable reports of classic pernicious anemia in older children suggest that, in infancy and childhood, macrocytic anemia with megaloblastic dysplasia of the bone marrow is usually caused by nutritional deficiency accentuated by malnutrition, chronic infections, and prematurity (MacIver and Back, 1960). In tropical countries megaloblastic anemia secondary to kwashiorkor is frequent (Spector and Metz, 1966). It is now thought that the "goat's milk anemia" of infancy described in older reports is identical to megaloblastic anemia of infancy caused by folate deficiency. Goat's milk per se does not contain an anemia-producing factor, but a diet of goat's milk favors the development of folic acid and ascorbic acid deficiencies.

Clarification of the clinical and hematologic features of this anemia followed the detailed studies of Amato (1946) in Italy and Zuelzer and Ogden (1946) in this country. Although the disease is not common, these investigators reported a large number of cases and suggested that mega-

loblastic anemia of infancy may easily be overlooked by one who is not completely familiar with the hematologic criteria. It is true, however, that only a small percentage of anemias in infants fall into this category.

The importance of emphasizing this hematologic picture is that definitive descriptions by these investigators, especially Zuelzer and Ogden, lend support to the concept that megaloblastic dysplasia of the bone marrow is not an all-or-none response. A spectrum of various degrees of megaloblastic dysplasia is seen when all the macrocytic anemias are studied as a group, ranging from the typical megaloblastosis of pernicious anemia in relapse to the partial dysplasia sometimes seen in megaloblastic anemia of infancy.

The peripheral blood smear shows macrocytosis, anisocytosis, poikilocytosis, and occasional hypersegmented neutrophils, but these morphologic abnormalities are seldom as severe as in pernicious anemia in relapse. The bone marrow shows megaloblastic dyspoiesis, varying in degree from mild to severe. Occasionally only "transitional" or "intermediate" megaloblasts are present, but the atypical morphology of granulocytes is constant and diagnostic. After therapy with folic acid and vitamin C, there is a typical reticulocyte response similar to that seen in pernicious anemia.

Caused by increased cellular proliferation

Rapid proliferation of hemopoietic cells quickly depletes folate stores and various degrees of folate deficiency may be encountered, from macrocytosis and hypersegmentation of neutrophils to early megaloblastic dyspoiesis to frank megaloblastosis. The most common example is seen in hemolytic anemias of all types, i.e., sickle cell anemia (Alperin, 1967), hereditary spherocytosis (Komninos et al, 1965), and thalassemia (Robinson and Watson, 1963). Various degrees of folate deficiency are also encountered in leukemias and lymphomas (Rose, 1966), in multiple myeloma (Hoffbrand et al, 1967), and in sideroblastic anemias.

Due to malabsorption of folate

CONGENITAL FOLATE MALABSORPTION. This rare condition is reported in only three patients (Lanzkowsky, 1970). Waksman (1975) speculates that the defect may lie in a dysfunction of folate-binding protein (FABP) in serum. A congenital defect in folate intake at the cellular level is reported by Branda et al (1978a).

DRUG-INDUCED FOLATE MALABSORPTION. Some drugs cause megaloblastic anemia by inhibiting folate absorption or utilization (Stebbins and Bertino, 1976). The folate deficiency that often accompanies ingestion of anticonvulsant drugs (Dilantin, Mysoline, phenobarbital) (Fig. 9-20) is attributed to a drug-induced absorption defect (Reynolds et al, 1965; Miller, 1968). Folate deficiency is common and severe megaloblastic anemia is a serious complication (Reynolds et al, 1966). Folate deficiency is a rare complication of oral contraceptive intake (Wood et al, 1972). Chemotherapy with antifolates is effective by inducing a deficiency of folate (Bertino et al, 1964) by inhibiting dihydrofolate reductase. Folate deficiency following long-term tetracycline therapy is reported by Jones (1973).

IN THE STEATORRHEAS. There are three gastrointestinal diseases that have in common the predominance of gastro-

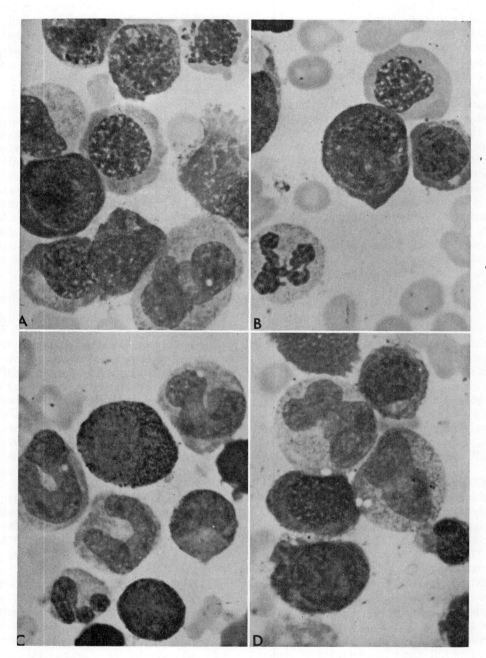

Fig. 9-20. Megaloblastic anemia following therapy for epilepsy with hydantoin, bone marrow smear. **A** shows megaloblasts and giant metamyelocyte in the right lower corner. **B** shows megaloblasts and macropolycyte. **C** shows three giant metamyelocytes. **D** shows megaloblasts and two giant metamyelocytes. (Wright's stain; ×950.)

intestinal symptoms and the passage of bulky stools rich in fat. The fatty stools account for the general classification of these diseases as *steatorrheas*. The group is usually subdivided into *tropical sprue, idiopathic steatorrhea (nontropical sprue),* sometimes called adult celiac disease, and *celiac disease,* even though differentiation within the group is sometimes difficult. Nontropical sprue and celiac disease are now called *gluten-sensitive enteropathies* since both are characterized by an abnormal reaction of the intestinal tract to gluten, a water-insoluble component of wheat and other grains (Alarcón-Segovia et al, 1964). The first two diseases are usually associated with macrocytic anemia and megaloblastic dysplasia of the bone marrow. The third is usually accompanied by a hypochromic microcytic anemia and normoblastic bone marrow, but it has been included because very occasionally megaloblastic macrocytic anemia is found (Dormandy et al, 1963). Wruble and Kalser (1964) have added *diabetic steatorrhea* to this group. From current reports, this type of steatorrhea is not accompanied by anemia even though there is evidence for a concomitant deficiency of folic acid.

The pathogenesis of the steatorrheas is basically a matter of defective intestinal function. A metabolic failure of phosphorylation seems likely, and it is noteworthy that the phosphorylating enzymes are, in their active form, associated with various B-complex vitamins. In the absence of adequate phosphorylation, fatty acids, glycerol, and sugars are incompletely absorbed. The stools are fatty and, as a result of abnormal intestinal fermentation, become bulky, gaseous, and foul. Fecal fat may make up as much as 60% to 70% of their weight (Pimparkar et al, 1961). A simple microscopic examination for neutral fats and split fats may be a useful screening procedure (Drummey et al, 1961). Oral glucose tolerance tests give a flat curve because of poor intestinal absorption, and hypocalcemia is produced by loss of calcium in the stools. Hypoproteinemia is common because of a combination of inanition and poor absorption.

The metabolic dysfunction is profound, affecting fats, carbohydrates, and proteins. It is likely, therefore, that the anemia is not caused entirely by a failure to absorb folate. There is a difference of opinion as to whether vitamin B$_{12}$ and folic acid are absorbed normally. Most agree that there is no impairment of vitamin B$_{12}$ absorption, but occasionally the deficiency seems to relate to both vitamin B$_{12}$ and folic acid. Malabsorption of vitamin B$_{12}$ is reported in some cases of tropical sprue (Baker, 1972) while Klipstein (1972) demonstrated a failure to absorb folate. Baker et al (1964a), using an oral folic acid tolerance test, provided data showing that in nontropical sprue there is defective folic acid absorption, presumably on the basis of an intestinal enzymatic defect in conjugating synthetic folic acid and in deconjugating natural folates to the glutamyl form that is easily absorbed. One other factor, the consumption of hemopoietic substances by the abnormal bacterial flora, is almost certainly of equal importance in producing a deficiency state. The anemia is intensified by hypoproteinemia and failure to absorb dietary iron. One additional factor may be bacterial inhibition of intestinal conjugase.

It is not surprising that the result of therapy in these diseases is unsatisfactory and somewhat confusing. It is assumed that the dyspoiesis is usually caused by a folic acid deficiency, but some patients who are helped by folic acid later suffer a relapse and subsequently respond to vitamin B$_{12}$. Others will not respond to folic acid alone but do respond to vitamin B$_{12}$ or to a combination of folic acid and vitamin B$_{12}$. Also important, is the small group of patients in whom folic acid improves the intestinal symptoms but has little effect on the anemia.

When fully developed, these diseases are seldom diagnostic problems. Sometimes, however, the intestinal disturbance is minimal, and one is presented with a macrocytic anemia that is difficult to classify.

One rare but interesting type of steatorrhea is seen in IgA heavy chain (α-chain) disease (p. 748) (Seligmann et al, 1968b; Seligmann and Rambaud, 1969) associated with intestinal lymphomatosis. Immunoelectrophoresis of serum shows an increased concentration of IgA α-chains (Seligmann et al, 1969).

Aside from the typical stool findings, other laboratory findings aid in the differential diagnosis of the steatorrheas and pernicious anemia. Macrocytic anemia is seldom as severe in the steatorrheas as in pernicious anemia, and achlorhydria is present in only a small percentage of cases. Sprue accompanied by achlorhydria occasionally gives some difficulty but fortunately is uncommon. This achlorhydria will sometimes disappear after therapy, unlike the persistent achlorhydria of pernicious anemia. In doubtful cases, particularly those in which the intestinal symptoms are less marked, determinations of fecal fat while the patient is on a diet of known fat content may give definitive information.

Bone marrow studies may reveal all gradations of megaloblastic dysplasia, from one that indicates a severe deficiency to one in which megaloblastosis is minimal. The cytology of the latter is that of a partial deficiency in which transition forms of megaloblasts should not be overlooked. Frequently orthochromic megaloblasts are the only abnormal erythroid cells with coexisting abnormalities in the leukocytes and megakaryocytes. This picture of partial deficiency must not be dismissed.

Accessory laboratory findings that favor the diagnosis of steatorrhea are (1) hypoprothrombinemia, more common in severe steatorrhea than in pernicious anemia, (2) hypocalcemia, unusual in pernicious anemia, (3) severe hypoproteinemia, which, if present in pernicious anemia, is generally mild, (4) typical roentgenologic findings when the small intestine is studied by means of a barium meal, and (5) pseudoicterus of the serum caused by carotinemia.

Defective folate interconversion

Defective folate interconversion caused by congenital deficiency of converting enzymes (glutamate formiminotransferase, dihydrofolate reductase, and possibly others) has been reported in isolated cases (Erbe, 1975). Megaloblastic anemia is sometimes present (Tauro et al, 1976). Some of the cases have had serious neurologic dysfunctions.

Of uncertain etiology

In hemochromatosis

Fully expressed megaloblastic anemia in hemochromatosis is rare but has been reported (Granville and Dameshek, 1958), and we have seen a typical example of it (Fig.5-48). It responds to folic acid therapy (Greenberg and Grace, 1970). It is tempting to ascribe the folate deficiency to the cirrhosis, but the rarity of this type of anemia in hemochromatosis suggests that other factors are operative.

In Di Guglielmo's syndrome (erythroleukemia)

In erythroleukemia (p. 711), the bone marrow and sometimes the peripheral blood contain erythroid precursors that have megaloblastic features (Crossen et al, 1969). Serum vitamin B_{12} and folate levels are normal and treatment with either or both is ineffective.

In sideroblastic anemias

In sideroblastic anemias (p. 413) there is sometimes a megaloblastic bone marrow (Horrigan and Harris, 1964), presumably on the basis of folate deficiency, since in some there is improvement of the anemia when folic acid is administered (MacGibbon and Mollin, 1965). However, treatment of the sideroblastic anemias is notably frustrating.

The OSLAM syndrome

The OSLAM syndrome (osteosarcoma, limb anomalies, erythroid macrocytosis, and megaloblastic bone marrow) is described by Mulvihill et al (1977) in three of nine children in an Oneida Indian family. In spite of extensive investigation, no relationship could be established between the macrocytosis and megaloblastosis and the other abnormalities.

10

"The body, as we know, contains four fluids—blood, phlegm, choler, and melancholy. In Mooney, these had become so mingled as to produce a morbid state, so adulterated with the vapors of disappointment and defeat as to produce a fatal toxicity."

E.B. White: *The Seven Steps To Heaven*

The erythrocyte: porphyrin and hemoglobin metabolism

PROTOPORPHYRIN AND PORPHYRIN METABOLISM
History: porphyria, a "royal malady"
Chemical structure of the porphyrins
Biosynthesis of the porphyrins and heme
The porphyrias
  Classification
  Congenital erythropoietic porphyria (Günther's disease)
  Congenital erythropoietic protoporphyria
  Erythropoietic coproporphyria
  Hepatic porphyria
    Intermittent acute porphyria
    Hereditary coproporphyria
    Variegate porphyria
    Porphyria cutanea tarda
  Acquired porphyria
    Secondary to hexachlorobenzene
    Secondary to griseofulvin
    Secondary to hepatoma
    Other acquired porphyrias
HEMOGLOBIN
Abnormal hemoglobin pigments
  Carboxyhemoglobin
  Methemoglobin
    Hereditary methemoglobinemia: Hb M variants
    Hereditary methemoglobinemia: deficient reducing systems
    Hereditary methemoglobinemia: excessive oxidative activity
    Acquired methemoglobinemia
  Sulfhemoglobin
  Methemalbumin
  Spectroscopic identification
Haptoglobin
Hemoglobin catabolism
  Formation of bilirubin
  Hyperbilirubinemia
    Neonatal hyperbilirubinemia
    Hereditary hyperbilirubinemia in rats (Gunn strain)
    Hereditary hyperbilirubinemia in sheep
    Hemolytic disease
    Unconjugated hyperbilirubinemia in ineffective erythropoiesis
    Obstructive jaundice
    Constitutional hepatic dysfunction (Gilbert's syndrome)
    Chronic idiopathic jaundice (Dubin-Johnson syndrome)
    Congenital nonhemolytic jaundice (Crigler-Najjar syndrome)
    Familial nonhemolytic jaundice (Rotor's syndrome)

PROTOPORPHYRIN AND PORPHYRIN METABOLISM
History: porphyria, a "royal malady"

Many diseases are familial. When such a disease affects a prominent family or person, it is unavoidably of greater interest. When the affected family is royal, as in some familial hemophilias (Chapter 17) and porphyrias, our interest is even keener. The average person's nature is such as to require a focus for political interest, regardless of whether the focus is provided by succession or election. When such a disease affects a series of rulers whose actions, good and bad, affect the course of history, we cannot help but take special notice.

Such a disease is porphyria. It affected members of the Houses of Stuart, Hanover, and Prussia (Fig. 10-1) and was called a "royal malady" in two classic and scholarly papers by Macalpine and Hunter (1966) and by Macalpine et al (1968). Porphyria directly caused at least two major national crises. The first was the Regency Crisis in 1788 when George III had his severest attack, the second was the death of Princess Charlotte and her baby during childbirth in 1817.

Historians have told us that George III was the victim of mental disease, a "manic-depressive psychosis caused by an underlying conflict exacerbated by violent frustrations, annoyances, and emotions." In fact, while he did have mental symptoms such as excitement, depression, and confusion, his physical symptoms were much more severe. However, it was the King's "mental" state that concerned the Court and the nation, since this reflected on his competence to rule. The Court physicians did the best they could under the circumstances. Medicine was still primitive, limited by the lack of the stethoscope, clinical thermometer, and knee-jerk hammer. Laboratory tests were not available, and the "piss-doctors" were limited to examination of the urine by inspection. Surprisingly, only a few observations about the color of the urine are to be found—"bilious," "bluish," and "bloody." The physicians were further limited by protocol, for unless the King spoke first, they were not allowed to ask pertinent questions, as shown by the following report

445

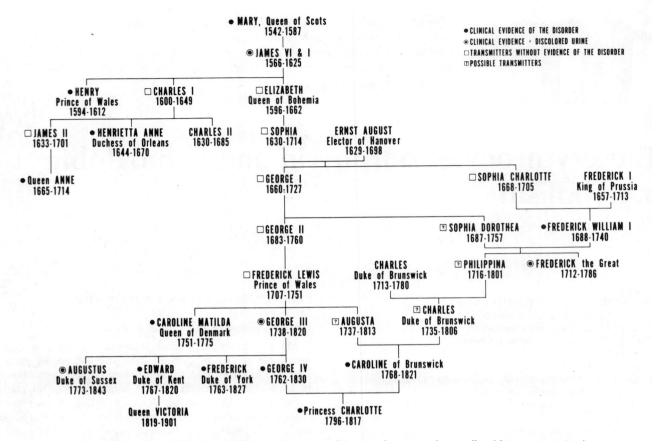

Fig. 10-1. Members of the Houses of Stuart, Hanover, and Prussia who seem to have suffered from or transmitted porphyria. (From Macalpine and Hunter, 1966.)

to the Queen's Council (January 8, 1812): "His Majesty appears to be very quiet this morning, but not having been addressed, we know nothing of His Majesty's condition of mind or body than what is obvious in his external appearance." Finally, there was nothing private about a king's illness, and nothing privileged, so that the daily bulletins had to be both informative and reassuring, for their content in fact reflected on the state of the government. The physicians were not only responsible for the King's health but also indirectly for whether he was well enough to attend Parliament and perform other official duties.

George III's illness took the form of five major, and several minor, attacks. They presented a puzzling combination of physical and mental symptoms: abdominal pain, tachycardia, constipation, weakness and stiffness of the limbs, hoarseness, hyperesthesia, hypoesthesia, tremor, agitation, confusion, and hallucinations. The physicians were puzzled, and soon the various opinions sorted themselves into two equally nonsensical groups. The physicians did the best they could to explain the illness on an organic basis:

The cause to which they all agree to ascribe it, is the force of a humor which was beginning to show itself in the legs, when the King's imprudence drove it from thence into the bowels; and the medicines which they were there obliged to use for the preservation of his life, have repelled it upon the brain. The physicians are now endeavoring to bring it down again into the legs, which nature had originally pointed out as the best mode of discharge.

The neurologic and mental symptoms were, prophetically, thought to be the result of the King's baffling malady. On the other hand, the Court and the public cared little, in the political sense, for the King's physical suffering, but his "madness" was something else, since this affected his ability to rule. This, plus the notable lack of therapeutic success, caused Parliament to call in the "mad-doctors" of the infant discipline of psychiatry to take charge of the case. These doctors merely introduced a new system of mumbo jumbo and argued that the madness was neither "mania" nor "delirium," but something in between. The people were reassured that "although the disorder has deranged the head, it is not, as was once dreaded, a mental incapacity called Insanity, for that calamity will not admit of a sudden and effectual cure." The physical symptoms were conveniently ignored; it was even suggested that the King was, through physical suffering, attempting to delude himself and his country into viewing the illness as anything but insanity. Nine months after the acute onset of the disease that we now appreciate as acute porphyria, George III recovered in spite of the physicians and "mad-doctors." There was much rejoicing and public thanksgiving. One of his physicians (Willis), much disliked by the King, took an inordinate amount of credit for the recovery; he had a medal struck, one side of which bore his own name and likeness and the other the inscription "Britons Rejoice, Your King's Restored." George III remained well for the next 12 years only to die of an acute episode at the age of 72 years.

George III's illness spawned years of great political significance for Great Britain. It was his insistence that Parliament had the right to levy taxes against the American colonies that triggered the Revolution and, some say, his inept handling of the revolt that made the Revolution successful. His second to the last acute episode caused a parliamentary crisis, the Regency Crisis, over how much power the Regent Prince of Wales should have while his father, whom he detested and ridiculed for his "madness," hovered between life and death.

George III passed the disease on to his sons, one of whom became George IV. The death in childbirth of Princess Charlotte, the daughter of George IV and granddaughter of George III, was a disaster in that she and the child represented the next two successions to the throne. In retrospect, there is little doubt that she had porphyria, that she had suffered from its effects all her life, and that death can be attributed to an acute attack at the time of delivery. It was not until the birth of Victoria in 1819, two years after Charlotte's death, that the Hanoverian succession was assured. There is no evidence that Queen Victoria either inherited or transmitted the disease. Still, most of the royal houses of Europe in the eighteenth and nineteenth centuries trace their origin to Mary, Queen of Scots, and her son James I: the House of Hanover, the House of Stuart, the House of Prussia, and the House of Savoy. The name "royal malady" is apt.

The first case of porphyria was described in 1874 as "pemphigus leprosus." The patient had photosensitivity and liver disease and was found to excrete a urinary pigment called *urorubrohematin*, probably the compound now known as uroporphyrin. In 1883 McMunn described five patients suffering from "subacute rheumatism," or "idiopathic pericarditis," whose urine contained a red pigment that he named *urohematin*, probably coproporphyrin in modern terminology. In 1871 Hoppe-Seyler prepared *hematoporphyrin* from hemoglobin. In 1888 Nenchi and Sieber identified hematoporphyrin as a derivative of heme, and it seemed logical to conclude that urinary porphyrins are derived from hemoglobin breakdown. It was not until 1925 that H. Fischer described significant structural differences between hematoporphyrin, i.e., the compound prepared by degradation of hemoglobin, and the porphyrins found in urine. Even more significant was the discovery of several isomeric forms of the basic tetrapyrrole nucleus and the demonstration that at least some of the porphyrins had an isomeric orientation different from that of heme and therefore could not be derivatives of hemoglobin.

These and other considerations led Fischer to propose that type I isomers of congenital porphyria are synthesized separately, but parallel with hemoglobin in the erythroid cells of the bone marrow. According to him, this was a biochemical recapitulation of ontogeny. Later, it became apparent that this hypothesis did not explain the findings in both acute porphyria and porphyria cutanea tarda. Waldenström, in 1934, suggested that not only are there fundamentally different defects in different types of porphyria but also that porphyrins are synthesized in tissues other than bone marrow. Further studies pointed to the liver as the culprit in porphyrias other than the congenital erythropoietic type.

This led Watson (1960) to propose the basic classification of porphyria into two main types, the *congenital erythropoietic* and the *hepatic*.

Chemical structure of the porphyrins

From the standpoint of comparative biochemistry, the porphyrins are widely distributed in nature and, in combination with various metallic ions, form pigments and enzymes that are indispensable to both animal and vegetable life. In plants the pigment is *chlorophyll*, a magnesium porphyrin, essential for the utilization of light energy in the synthesis of carbohydrates (Gibson et al, 1961). The vanadium porphyrins found in petroleum deposits are thought to be the ghosts of prehistoric sea squirts, since the modern sea squirt is able to extract vanadium from seawater. In crustaceans, copper porphyrin (hemocyanin) is in solution in the blood and serves the animal's oxygen-carrying needs. In higher species the respiratory pigment is an iron-porphyrin-globin compound, *hemoglobin*. The porphyrin nucleus is found in other important compounds such as *myoglobin* and the *respiratory enzymes* (cytochromes, peroxidase, catalases, etc.) responsible for the superb efficiency of internal respiration. Teleologically, the porphyrin structure may well be the most important chemical configuration evolved, for without chlorophyll, an oxygen-containing atmosphere would not have developed, and the earth would have retained its primitive atmosphere of hydrogen, methane, and carbon dioxide. Porphyrin pigments have been found in meteorites and it has been shown that porphyrin structure can be synthesized under conditions reflecting the prebiotic primitive atmosphere (Simionescu et al, 1978).

Our knowledge of the porphyrins is based on studies of cases in which a derangement of porphyrin metabolism leads to the disease known as *porphyria* and on chemical studies of degradation products of hemoglobin. The basic structure is four pyrrole rings (Fig. 10-2, *A*) joined together by methene bridges ($= CH-$), forming the tetrapyrrole structure (Fig. 10-2, *B*). A series of compounds is possible, depending on the radical or combinations of radicals substituted for hydrogen at the eight available loci. These points are numbered 1 through 8 in a clockwise manner, and the four methene bridges are numbered in a like manner by the Greek letters, alpha, beta, gamma, and delta (Fig. 10-2, *C*). The simplest substitution of four methyl and four ethyl radicals produces a tetramethyl-tetraethyl porphyrin called *aetioporphyrin*. Four isomers of this compound are theoretically possible, depending on the arrangement of methyl and ethyl groups. They are designated as types I, II, III, and IV. All four types have been identified, but only type I (methyl group at 1, 3, 5, and 7) and type III (methyl group at 1, 3, 5, and 8) occur in nature (Fig. 10-3).

Substitution of vinyl groups ($-CH = CH_2$) at positions 2 and 4 and of propionic acid groups ($-CH_2-CH_2-COOH$) at positions 6 and 7 produces *protoporphyrin type III*, isomer 9 of 15 possible isomers (Fig. 10-3).

It is this compound into which one atom of iron is incorporated to form the iron-containing porphyrin *heme* (Fig. 10-3). Heme is capable of combining with nitrogenous compounds to form hemochromes. When it combines with the protein *globin*, it forms *hemoglobin*. In different molecular arrangements and combinations, heme is a constituent of

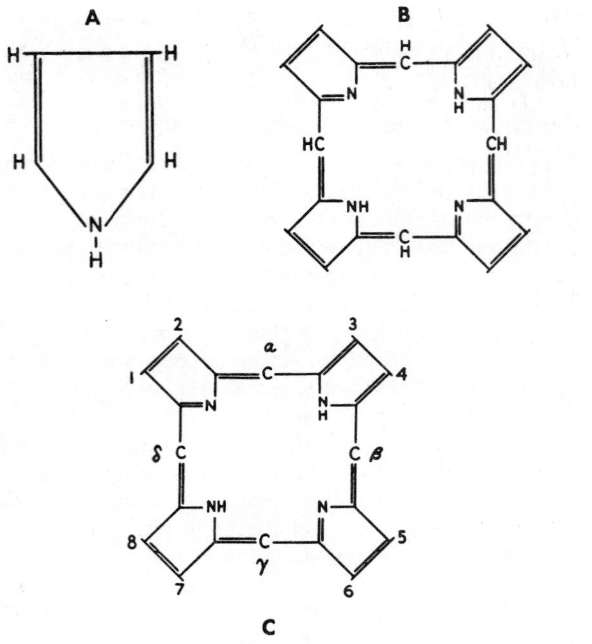

Fig. 10-2. Structure of the porphyrins. **A,** Pyrrole ring. **B,** Basic structure of porphyrin. **C,** Designation of isomeric loci and methene bridges.

other important hemochromes such as myoglobin and the enzymes cytochrome, peroxidase, and catalase.

Biosynthesis of the porphyrins and heme

The biosynthesis of porphyrins and heme is outlined in Fig. 10-4.

The first basic reaction is the formation of α-amino-ketoadipic acid from succinyl CoA, derived from the tricarboxylic acid cycle, and the pyridoxal phosphate derivative of glycine. By decarboxylation catalyzed by synthetase, α-amino-ketoadipic acid is converted to δ-aminolevulinic acid (ALA) (Kikushi et al, 1958). δ-Aminolevulinic synthetase (ALA synthetase) is the key enzyme in the biochemical sequence (Kappas et al, 1968), and an increase in this "inducible" enzyme is characteristic of both primary porphyric syndromes and of secondary porphyrinuria in liver disease. Induction of the enzyme is inhibited by carbohydrate administration (Tschudy et al, 1964), the "glucose effect," attributed by Kappas and Granick (1968) to conjugation of the inducer with glucuronide. ALA synthetase is stimulated by stilbesterol, estradiol, and steroids having the 5-beta configuration (etiocholane and pregnane derivatives) (Levit et al, 1957; Levere, 1966; Perlroth et al, 1965). Barbiturates are probably the most potent inducers of this enzyme (DeMatteis, 1968).

δ-Aminolevulinic acid is transformed to porphobilinogen

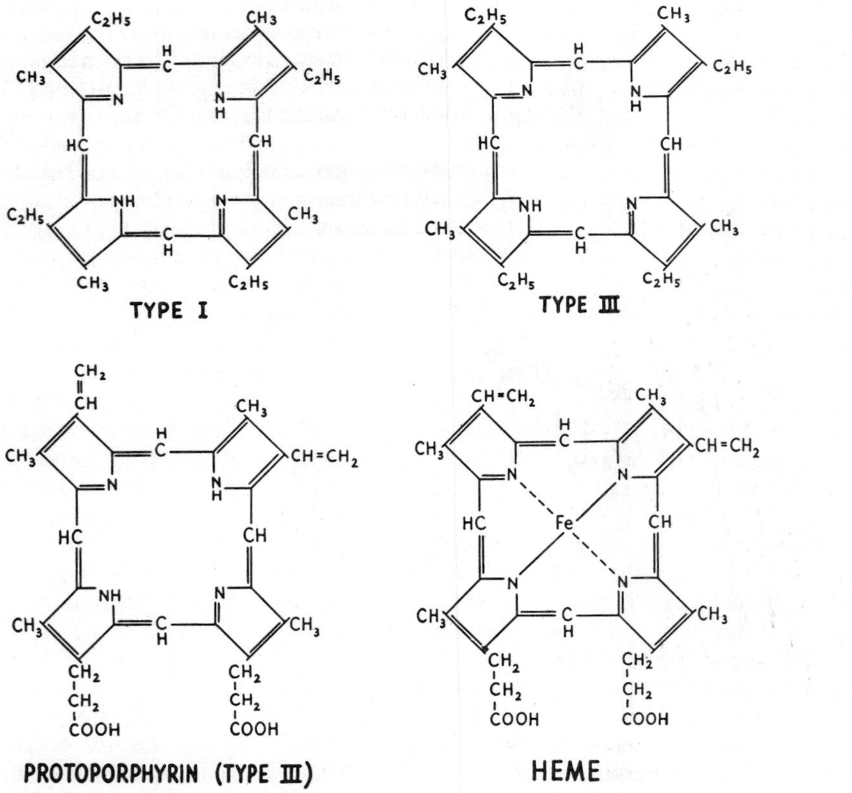

Fig. 10-3. Structure of porphyrin compound: types I and III isomers, protoporphyrin (type III), and heme.

by condensation. Porphobilinogen is the monopyrrole precursor of the porphyrins. Deaminating reactions, induced by one or more deaminase enzymes, form dipyrroles and tetrapyrroles (Radmer and Bogorad, 1972). It is probable that the conversion of porphobilinogen to uroporphyrins I and III involves two enzymatic steps—uroporphyrinogen I synthetase being responsible for the formation of intermediate polypyrrylmethane compounds, and uroporphyrinogen III cosynthetase being responsible for driving the reaction toward the formation of the normal uroporphyrinogen III isomer, the precursor for the synthesis of heme. Type I isomers are not used in the synthesis of heme.

Uroporphyrin III is probably synthesized within normoblasts in the bone marrow, followed by further intracellular transformation to coproporphyrin III and protoporphyrin III. Protoporphyrin III is finally converted to heme by the insertion of an iron atom into the porphyrin ring, a reaction dependent on the enzyme *heme synthetase,* also called *ferrochelatase* (Lockhead et al, 1963). This reaction, as well as the synthesis of δ-aminolevulinic acid, takes place on or in the mitochondria of normoblasts (Jones and Jones, 1969), whereas intermediate reactions are extramitochondrial. As expected, the loss of mitochondria in maturing erythrocytes is accompanied by an inability to synthesize ALA and heme.

Primitive erythroblasts in the embryo contain uroporphyrin, justifying the concept that uroporphyrin is synthesized before protoporphyrin. Reticulocytes are rich in protoporphyrin and, when viewed by ultraviolet light, may show marked fluorescence, as will all other cells containing fluorescent protoporphyrin. Erythrocytes that fluoresce have been called *fluorescytes.*

Adult erythrocytes contain a small amount of *free erythrocyte coproporphyrin* (FEC) (0.5 to 1.5 μg/dl of packed cells) and larger amounts of *free erythrocyte protoporphyrin* (FEP) (25 to 75 μg/dl of packed cells) (Marver and Schmid, 1972). FEP values are increased in hemolytic anemia, in iron-deficiency anemia (Dagg et al, 1966), in the anemia of chronic infection, in lead intoxication, and in some sideroblastic anemias—conditions characterized by ineffective utilization of protoporphyrin for heme synthesis. FEC values are directly proportional to the number of reticulocytes in the peripheral blood and, in hemolytic anemias, are proportionally greater than those for FEP (Watson, 1950).

The porphyrias
Classification

The classification of disorders of porphyrin metabolism, the porphyrias, has changed over the years. As new and sophisticated methods were applied to the study of heme and porphyrin synthesis, many of the old concepts and much confusing terminology were assigned to historical limbo. The most recent authoritative review of porphyrin metabolism and the porphyrias is given by Meyer and Schmid (1978). Most pertinent references (721) are given in that publication.

The current classification of the porphyrias is given in Table 10-1. Only one, erythropoietic porphyria, causes a

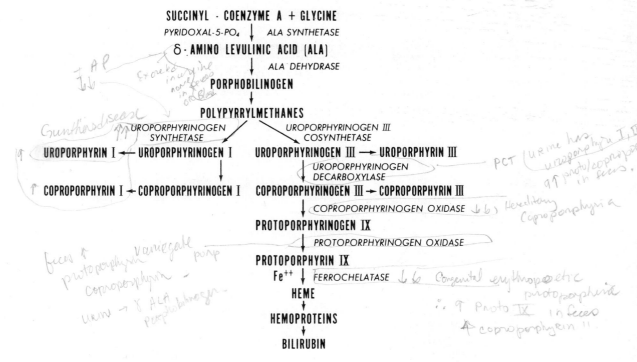

Fig. 10-4. Biosynthesis of porphyrins and heme. The conversion of porphobilinogen to type I and type III porphyrins requires an interaction of synthetase and cosynthetase, which is poorly understood, but probably involves cooperative action on an intermediate polypyrrylmethane compound (Higuchi and Bogorad, 1975). Feedback inhibition of ALA synthesis, not shown in this diagram, is discussed on p. 454.

Table 10-1. Classification and characteristics of the congenital porphyrias

Disease	Enzymatic defect	Metabolites present in excess		
		Urine	Feces	Erythroid cells
Congenital erythropoietic porphyria	Uroporphyrinogen I synthetase and uroporphyrinogen III cosynthetase	Uroporphyrin I ++++ Coproporphyrin I ++	Coproporphyrin I ++++ Uroporphyrin I ++	Uroporphyrin I ++++ Coproporphyrin I ++
Congenital erythropoietic protoporphyria	Ferrochelatase	Normal	Protoporphyrin ++++ Coproporphyrin +	Protoporphyrin ++++ Coproporphyrin +
Erythropoietic coproporphyria	?	Normal	Normal	Coproporphyrin III ++++ Protoporphyrin + Uroporphyrin +
Hepatic porphyria				
Intermittent acute	Uroporphyrinogen I synthetase	δ-aminolevulinic acid ++++ Porphobilinogen ++++	Normal	Normal
Hereditary coproporphyria	Coproporphyrinogen synthetase	Coproporphyrin III +++	Coproporphyrin III ++++ Protoporphyria +	Normal
Variegate porphyria	Protoporphyrinogen oxidase	δ-aminolevulinic acid ++ Porphobilinogen ++	X-porphyrin ++++ Protoporphyrin ++++ Coproporphyrin ++++	Normal
Cutanea tarda	Uroporphyrinogen decarboxylase	Uroporphyrin I and III ++++	Protoporphyrin N to ++ Coproporphyrin N to ++	Normal

Table 10-2. Values for porphyrins excreted in urine and feces of healthy subjects

I. Urine
  A. Coproporphyrin
    Adult males: 75-225 μg/24 hr*; 100-300 μg/24 hr†
    Adult females: 50-200 μg/24 hr*; 75-275 μg/24 hr†
    All adults: 0-175 μg/1‡
    Boys (40-170 lb): 38-66 μg/24 hr*
    Girls (60-110 lb): 76-113 μg/24 hr*
  B. Uroporphyrin
    Adults: 5-30 μg/24 hr*; 10-40 μg/24 hr†; 0-15 μg/1‡
  C. δ-Aminolevulinic acid
    Adults: 2.5 mg/24 hr*; 1.9 ± 0.6 mg/Gm of creatinine‡
    Children: 3.7 ± 1.4 mg/Gm of creatinine‡
  D. Porphobilinogen
    Adults: Less than 1 mg/24 hr*; 0.7 ± 0.4 mg/Gm of creatinine‡
    Children: 0.6 ± 0.3 mg/Gm of creatinine‡

II. Feces
  A. Coproporphyrin
    Adult males: 0.20 μg/Gm (dry wt)*
    Adult females: 0.36 μg/Gm (dry wt)*
    All adults: < 20 μg/Gm (dry wt)§; 0.27 μg/Gm (dry wt)¶
    Children: 0-14 μg/Gm (dry wt)#
  B. Protoporphyrin
    Adult males: 0-30 μg/Gm (dry wt)*
    Adult females: 0-113 μg/Gm (dry wt)*
    All adults: < 30 μg/Gm (dry wt)§; 15 ± 12 μg/Gm (dry wt)‖; 2-99 μg/Gm (dry wt)¶
    Children: 5-51 μg/Gm (dry wt)#

*Barnes, 1963.
†Zieve et al, 1953.
‡Haeger, 1958.
§Holti et al, 1958.
‖Haeger-Aronsen, 1962.
¶Eales, 1960.
#Barnes, 1958.

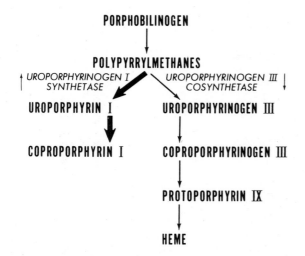

PORPHOBILINOGEN

POLYPYRRYLMETHANES

UROPORPHYRINOGEN I SYNTHETASE   UROPORPHYRINOGEN III COSYNTHETASE

UROPORPHYRIN I   UROPORPHYRINOGEN III

COPROPORPHYRIN I   COPROPORPHYRINOGEN III

PROTOPORPHYRIN IX

HEME

Fig. 10-5. Porphyrin synthesis in congenital erythropoietic porphyria. The activity of the uroporphyrinogen I synthetase is increased, and as a result, isomers of type I are formed preferentially.

significant abnormality of erythropoiesis. However, the diagnosis depends in part on the interpretation of the patterns of porphyrin excretion, requiring at least some familiarity with the findings in the other types of porphyria. Normal values are given in Table 10-2.

Congenital erythropoietic porphyria (Günther's disease)

Congenital erythropoietic porphyria, sometimes called Günther's disease, is the rarest of the congenital porphyrias, there being no more than 100 reported cases. It is inherited as an autosomal recessive trait, usually manifests early in life, and has a wide racial distribution.

The metabolic defect is localized in the nuclei of erythroid cells in the bone marrow. The biochemical lesion is an increase in the enzyme uroporphyrinogen I synthetase relative to uroporphyrinogen III cosynthetase, resulting in overproduction of uroporphyrin I and, to a lesser degree, coproporphyrin I (Fig. 10-5). These porphyrins accumulate in the red blood cells, are released into the blood, and are excreted in the urine and feces (Table 10-1).

A characteristic sign that may be noted at birth or early infancy is wine-red urine, but the amount of porphyrin excreted varies from time to time so that some patients have shown cyclic variations, whereas others consistently excrete strongly colored urine. The daily excretion of uroporphyrin is increased from the normal measured in *micrograms* to several hundred *milligrams*.

Clinically there is photosensitivity, discoloration of the teeth, splenomegaly, hemolytic anemia, and hypertrichosis. Illis (1964) suggested that the legendary werewolf may in fact have been a person who, suffering from porphyria, had stained teeth and a hairy disfigured face and preferred to go about at night to avoid exposure to sunlight. The porphyrins are photosensitizing agents, and the increased concentration in the blood and subsequent diffusion into the skin prepare this tissue for the destructive effects of sunlight. The photo-

sensitivity produces bullous or vesicular skin lesions *(hydroa aestivale)* that progress to ulcerations, scarring, and severe mutilation, commonly of the hands and face (Fig. 10-6, *A*). Photosensitivity is a feature of other porphyrias but is seldom so severe. The teeth are discolored (Fig. 10-6, *A*), and although the discoloration is called *erythrodontia*, the teeth are yellow, brownish pink, or brownish purple rather than red. Under ultraviolet light they show startling fluorescence. Splenomegaly is found in all cases and becomes more pronounced as the disease progresses. Anemia is present in most cases, but it may be mild or cyclic; when present, it is of the hemolytic type, with decreased red cell survival, reticulocytosis, and the presence of normoblasts in the blood. Anemia is accompanied by normoblastic hyperplasia of the bone marrow. The defect is intrinsic in the erythrocytes, because normal erythrocytes transfused into an affected person have a normal life span. Although the erythrocytes are rich in uroporphyrin and coproporphyrin, there is no obvious relationship to decreased survival. It is interesting that the erythrocytes in this disease show increased photohemolysis in vitro (Harber et al, 1964).

On routinely stained smears of aspirated bone marrow the nuclei of some normoblasts contain pale inclusions (Fig. 10-7) that take the benzidine stain (Schmid et al, 1955); 30% to 70% of the normoblasts show intense nuclear fluorescence (Fig. 10-6, *B*), indicating a high concentration of porphyrin (probably uroporphyrin) in the nucleus. Electron microscopy shows that the inclusions have the same density as the cytoplasm (Fig. 10-8). A few fluorescent erythrocytes can be seen in the blood and bone marrow. There is little doubt that the normoblasts in the bone marrow have gone metabolically awry and are responsible for the overproduction of uroporphyrin. At the same time, there is no deficiency of heme synthesis, probably because uroporphyrinogen III cosynthetase is still sufficient for heme synthesis, but other explanations are possible (Meyer and Schmid, 1978).

Congenital erythropoietic protoporphyria

Congenital erythropoietic protoporphyria, the second type of erythropoietic porphyria, was recognized as a distinct entity by Magnus et al (1961). More than 300 cases have been reported. It is inherited as an autosomal dominant trait. In most cases photosensitivity is mild but may be severe (Fig. 10-9). Exposure to sunlight causes itching and erythema, with scar formation as the exception. In one young woman studied in my laboratory, only the hands showed actinic dermatitis.

The erythrocytes and feces contain markedly increased amounts of protoporphyrin IX and slightly increased coproporphyrin, while the urine is normal in cases not complicated by hepatic disease. The enzymatic lesion is diminished ferrochelatase activity, causing an accumulation of protoporphyrin IX in the erythroid cells of the bone marrow. These show intense cytoplasmic fluorescence, in contrast with the nuclear fluorescence in erythropoietic porphyria. Young red blood cells and reticulocytes also fluoresce, and fluorescent red blood cells exhibit photohemolysis.

Because the liver is also rich in protoporphyrin and because cirrhosis and gallstones rich in protoporphyrin are

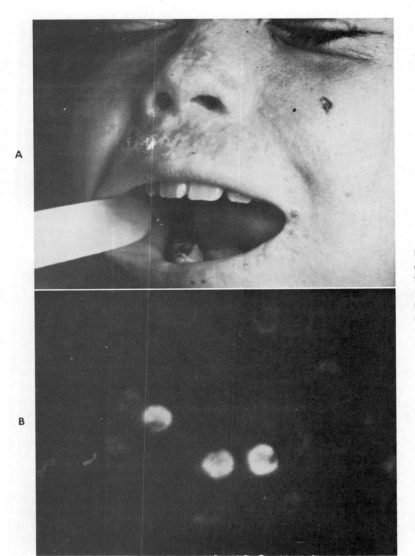

Fig. 10-6. Congenital erythropoietic porphyria. **A,** Erythrodontia, particularly noticeable near the gingival margin, fresh and scarred skin lesions due to exposure to sunlight. **B,** Unstained bone marrow smear viewed by ultraviolet microscopy. Three normoblasts showing striking cytoplasmic fluorescence. (×800.) (From Winterhalter, 1964.)

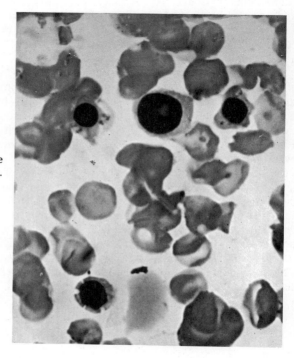

Fig. 10-7. Normoblasts in porphyria erythropoietica. (Wright's stain; ×900.) The large normoblast (top center) contains porphyrin, seen as a pale area (see Fig. 10-8). (Courtesy Dr. R. Schmid.)

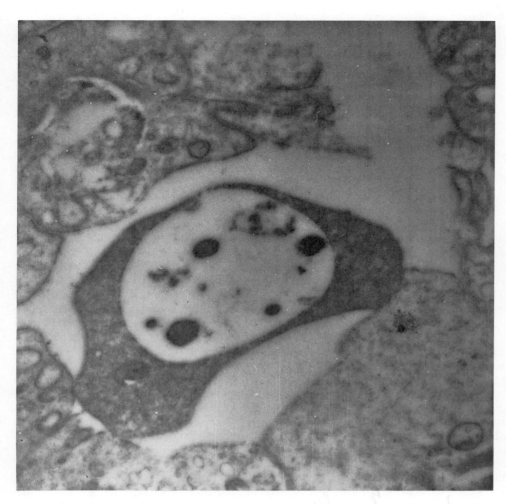

Fig. 10-8. Normoblast in erythropoietic porphyria. The nucleus is dark and contains a large electron-transparent (light) inclusion. (Electron microscopy; ×32,000.) (From Gross et al, 1965.)

Fig. 10-9. Skin lesions of the photosensitivity type in erythropoietic protoporphyria in a 6-year-old boy. (From Porter and Lowe, 1963.)

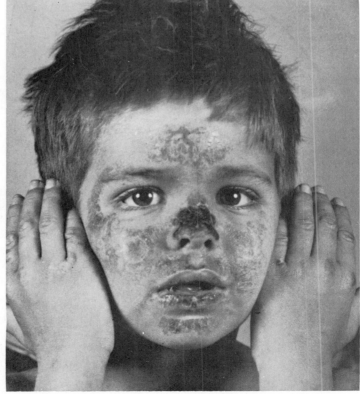

serious complications, there is some doubt as to whether this porphyria is strictly erythropoietic or whether it affects the liver as well. However, the pigment in the liver and its excretion in the bile can be explained by assuming hyperproduction of protoporphyrin in normoblasts and secondary deposition in the liver.

In spite of the reduced activity of ferrochelatase, there is no obvious deficiency in heme synthesis and no anemia.

Erythropoietic coproporphyria

Erythropoietic coproporphyria, the third type of porphyria involving erythroid cells, is probably the rarest of the three (Heilmeyer and Clotten, 1964; Goldberg et al, 1967). The red cells contain a markedly increased amount of coproporphyrin III and slightly elevated levels of protoporphyrin and uroporphyrin. However, there is no increase in urinary or fecal porphyrins. The enzymatic defect has not been identified. Meyer and Schmid (1978) suggest that this porphyria is a variant of congenital erythropoietic porphyria.

Hepatic porphyria

The hepatic porphyrias are so named because the site of abnormal porphyrin synthesis is the liver. There is no involvement of erythropoietic tissue and no anemia. There is no obvious explanation for normal heme synthesis in the hepatic porphyrias, given the various enzymatic deficiencies that should affect the subsequent synthetic sequences. It has been postulated that the enzymatic block is not complete and that some enzymes, such as uroporphyrinogen III cosynthetase, are present in excess concentration. A more likely explanation involves feedback inhibition of ALA synthetase by heme. Under normal conditions, ALA synthetase is the key enzyme regulating the rate of subsequent steps in the biosynthetic pathway. Heme, for example, inhibits ALA synthetase at a very low concentration, so that as heme is synthesized normally, the inhibition of ALA synthetase regulates the rate of synthesis along the entire pathway. On the other hand, a deficiency of heme synthesis stimulates ALA synthetase, and the rate of biosynthesis is increased. It can be assumed, then, that in the hepatic porphyrias a break in the synthetic pathway does reduce heme synthesis only temporarily, because the increase in ALA synthetase activity quickly increases the rate of biosynthesis and compensates for the early defect in heme synthesis.

INTERMITTENT ACUTE PORPHYRIA. Intermittent acute porphyria is sometimes called the Swedish type of porphyria because of the pioneer studies of Waldenström (1957). The symptoms are intermittent and characterized in the acute phase by abdominal pain, neurologic involvement of the central or peripheral nervous system, and psychiatric dysfunction. Acute attacks are precipitated by estrogens and are sometimes related to the menstrual cycle or pregnancy. Hyponatremia, hypomagnesemia, and other biochemical or hormonal abnormalities may be present. The disease is frequently familial, and the inheritance is autosomal dominant. There is no photosensitivity. Lamon et al (1979) have shown that latent intermittent acute porphyria can be identified by determining the activity of red blood cell uroporphyrinogen I synthetase.

The enzymatic lesion is a deficiency of uroporphyrinogen I synthetase. During the acute attack porphobilinogen and δ-aminolevulinic acid are excreted in large amounts in the urine, whereas feces and red blood cells do not contain excess porphyrins.

HEREDITARY COPROPORPHYRIA. The clinical picture for hereditary coproporphyria is similar to that in intermittent acute porphyria, with abdominal pain and neuropsychiatric symptoms in the acute phase. It is distinguished from the other porphyrias in that the enzymatic deficiency is of coproporphyrinogen synthetase. As a result, large amounts of coproporphyrin III are excreted in the feces and urine. There is no involvement of erythroid cells.

VARIEGATE PORPHYRIA. Variegate porphyria is sometimes called the South African type because it was first identified in a large group of Afrikaner individuals in that country. Clinically it resembles intermittent acute porphyria, but in addition to causing abdominal and neuropsychiatric symptoms, variegate porphyria shows photosensitivity of the skin exposed to sunlight as well as excessive mechanical fragility of the skin. Acute attacks are precipitated by the ingestion of various drugs: barbiturates, sulfonamides, general anesthetics, or alcohol. The disease is familial, and the inheritance is autosomal dominant.

The enzymatic defect is probably of protoporphyrinogen oxidase. The feces contain large amounts of protoporphyrin and coproporphyrin as well as poorly identified ether-insoluble porphyrins (X-porphyrins), even when the subject is in clinical remission. During an acute attack the urine contains large amounts of δ-aminolevulinic acid and porphobilinogen.

PORPHYRIA CUTANEA TARDA. Porphyria cutanea tarda is a type of hepatic porphyria that does not exhibit the abdominal or neuropsychiatric symptoms of the other hepatic porphyrias, and the major manifestations are limited to the skin. It is familial, and the inheritance is autosomal dominant. It has been reported from many parts of the world, but the highest incidence is among the Bantus in South Africa.

The enzymatic defect is a deficiency of uroporphyrinogen decarboxylase. This defect apparently can remain dormant until activated by superimposed liver injury or hepatic siderosis, by excessive intake of alcohol, with or without cirrhosis, and sometimes by estrogens.

The onset is usually marked by the presence of red or brownish urine, increased fragility of skin areas exposed to sunlight, pigmentation, and scarring. There is often hypertrichosis of the face and forearms.

The urine contains a large amount of uroporphyrin types I and III. Fecal porphyrin content is variable, from normal to high, consisting primarily of protoporphyrin and coproporphyrin. Abnormally high avidity for iron results in high serum iron levels and siderosis of the liver and bone marrow. There is no involvement of erythroid cells.

Acquired porphyria

SECONDARY TO HEXACHLOROBENZENE. A disease resembling porphyria cutanea tarda (skin lesions of the photosensitive type, hyperpigmentation, hypertrichosis, and cachexia) was prevalent in southeastern Turkey and was shown to be caused by ingestion of hexachlorobenzene, which was used as a preservative for wheat (Schmid, 1960). The wheat was given to the farmers by the Turkish government and was intended to be used as seed. Hexachlorobenzene had been used to prevent molding. However, instead of planting the wheat, the farmers used it to make flour and bread, with disastrous consequences. The human disease can be reproduced in rats fed hexachlorobenzene (Stonard, 1974). The pattern of porphyrin excretion is similar to that in porphyria cutanea tarda, and the enzymatic deficiency is in uroporphyrinogen decarboxylase.

SECONDARY TO GRISEOFULVIN. Griseofulvin is a fungicidal antibiotic. Intake of this drug causes massive excretion of coproporphyrin and protoporphyrin in the feces, followed by increased urinary excretion of δ-aminolevulinic acid, porphobilinogen, and coproporphyrin. Since there is also an increase in protoporphyrin in erythroid cells, this porphyria resembles congenital erythropoietic protoporphyria. The enzymatic defect is in ferrochelatase.

SECONDARY TO HEPATOMA. Acquired cutaneous porphyria secondary to a porphyrin-producing hepatoma was described by Tio et al (1957). The patient was an 80-year-old woman who developed bullous cutaneous lesions and showed markedly increased excretion of porphyrins in the urine and feces. The urine contained large amounts of uroporphyrin, and the feces contained large amounts of coproporphyrin and protoporphyrin. The excised tumor was rich in uroporphyrin III, protoporphyrin, and coproporphyrin I. After the hepatoma was excised, all clinical and chemical evidence of porphyria disappeared.

OTHER ACQUIRED PORPHYRIAS. Secondary porphyrinuria is common in all types of parenchymal liver disease.

The excreted metabolite is principally coproporphyrin. In cirrhosis an elevation in coproporphyrin excretion is found in almost all cases. It has been shown that in cirrhosis there is an increase in liver δ-aminolevulinic acid synthetase, the same enzyme increased in the primary porphyrias (Levere, 1967). In acute (infectious) hepatitis, coproporphyrin excretion is increased and remains high even after other liver function tests return to normal. In infectious mononucleosis, excretion of coproporphyrin parallels the degree of liver involvement.

Intake of alcohol, in both normal persons and in those suffering from cirrhosis of the liver, produces increased excretion of coproporphyrin in the urine (Waldenström and Haeger-Aronson, 1967).

One of the important effects of lead intoxication (plumbism) in humans is a disturbance in the synthesis of heme. In the course of the inhibited synthesis of heme, two of its precursors, δ-aminolevulinic acid and coproporphyrin, are excreted in large quantity in the urine, while there is an increase in free erythrocyte coproporphyrin and protoporphyrin. These compounds cause the erythrocytes to fluoresce (fluorescytes) under fluorescent light. Normally only about 1% of the erythrocytes fluoresce. In lead poisoning, fluorescence is seen in 10% or more of the erythrocytes. In spite of the fact that lead intoxication is often accompanied by decreased erythrocyte survival, indicating hemolytic disease, the excretion of porphyrins is, of course, not related to erythrocyte destruction and hemolytic breakdown. Rather, several blocks in the biosynthesis of heme interfere with the normal utilization of heme precursors and account for the accumulation or excretion of porphyrin compounds to a

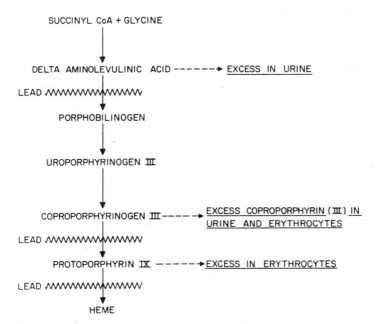

Fig. 10-10. Effect of lead on heme synthesis. The first block in the pathway of heme synthesis occurs at the conversion of ALA to porphobilinogen, probably by inhibition of ALA dehydrase (Nakao et al, 1968), with accumulation and increased excretion in the urine of ALA. The second block occurs at conversion of coproporphyrinogen to protoporphyrin, probably by inhibition of oxidase, resulting in excess coproporphyrin in the urine and in erythrocytes. The third block is in the synthesis of heme from protoporphyrin and iron, both of which accumulate in erythrocytes and precursors.

pathologic degree. The effects of lead intoxication on the normal pathway of heme synthesis are shown in Fig. 10-10.

We now have a better understanding of the nature of the *basophilic stippling* or *punctate basophilia* seen in many of the erythrocytes in plumbism. The basophilic stippling consists of mitochondria, normally absent in mature erythrocytes, ribonucleic acid, and iron. Iron accumulates because of the block in heme synthesis and is stainable. Accumulation of mitochondria-associated iron in normoblasts gives rise to sideroblasts, sometimes ringed, and some authors classify the anemia of lead intoxication with the sideroblastic anemias. Since the synthesis of δ-aminolevulinic acid and of protoporphyrin is also dependent on mitochondria-associated enzymes, these abnormal erythrocytes are capable of synthesizing these substances. The fluorescence of erythrocytes when viewed by ultraviolet microscopy, as well as the increased excretion of coproporphyrin in the urine, is a sensitive indicator of lead intoxication even in the absence of anemia and clinical signs and symptoms. These tests are more sensitive than the finding of punctate basophilia in routine blood smears.

HEMOGLOBIN

The synthesis of hemoglobin from heme and the tetramer of polypeptide chains that make up the globin portion is discussed in Chapter 14. We are concerned here with some special reactions of hemoglobin and with its catabolic fate.

Abnormal hemoglobin pigments

In its role as a respiratory pigment, hemoglobin combines with oxygen to form oxyhemoglobin. The oxygenation of hemoglobin in the lungs is an extremely efficient process, and at the partial pressure of oxygen in alveolar air (100 mm Hg), almost all hemoglobin is converted to oxyhemoglobin. In addition, a small amount of oxygen goes directly into solution in the blood. The diffusion of oxygen through the red cell membrane is rapid, and the total surface of erythrocytes exposed to this exchange in the lungs is about 80 square meters each second. Oxygen is given up in the tissues, and oxyhemoglobin becomes reduced hemoglobin, effecting a release of base that binds incoming carbon dioxide. Carbon dioxide is also bound at the free amino groups, forming a carbamate compound. The third manner of carbon dioxide transport is by diffusion of CO_2 from plasma into the erythrocyte where, catalyzed by the enzyme carbonic anhydrase, it quickly combines with water to form carbonic acid. On dissociation into $(H)^+$ and $(HCO_3)^-$ the hydrogen ions are buffered in part by the oxyhemoglobin and in part by other intracellular buffers. The $(HCO_3)^-$ then diffuses into the plasma, being replaced by a shift of chloride ions into the cell, a process known as the "chloride shift." When venous blood is returned to the lungs and oxygen again diffuses into the cell, the process is reversed and another internal respiratory cycle is begun.

The efficiency of this mechanism is reduced when an abnormal hemoglobin with altered oxygen affinity is present (Chapter 14) or when hemoglobin is converted to abnormal hemoglobin pigments that are not capable of transporting oxygen. The ones of clinical importance are *carboxyhemoglobin, methemoglobin,* and *sulfhemoglobin.* A high concentration of any one may produce hypoxia or cyanosis. *Hypoxia* is proportional to the diminished concentration of hemoglobin, and *cyanosis* is proportional to the concentration of abnormal hemoglobin pigment. For each compound there is a critical concentration at which cyanosis is produced—carboxyhemoglobin, 5 Gm/dl; methemoglobin, 1.5 Gm/dl; sulfhemoglobin, 0.5 Gm/dl.

Carboxyhemoglobin

Carboxyhemoglobin is formed when hemoglobin is exposed to carbon monoxide. The affinity of hemoglobin for carbon monoxide is 218 times greater than for oxygen at 37°C and is not affected if helium is substituted for nitrogen as the inert gas (as in prolonged underwater diving). If toxic levels of carbon monoxide are present in the air and carboxyhemoglobin is formed, the amount of oxyhemoglobin is decreased. Since carboxyhemoglobin is not capable of transporting oxygen, hypoxia results. If the concentration of carboxyhemoglobin is very high, death may result from anoxia and irreversible tissue changes. Carboxyhemoglobin produces a cherry-red color of the blood, both the patient's skin and the blood obtained by venipuncture showing this typical color. At times the color is noted to have a violet tinge because of the simultaneous presence of moderate quantities of reduced hemoglobin.

Carboxyhemoglobin can be identified and quantified by a variety of methods—spectroscopic, chemical, spectrophotometric, gas chromatographic (Collison et al, 1968; Malenfant et al, 1968). Blood normally contains a little carboxyhemoglobin derived from carbon monoxide from porphyrin catabolism (Landaw et al, 1970). The concentration of carboxyhemoglobin in blood depends primarily on whether the subject is a smoker or nonsmoker and on the environment in which he or she lives (Seppänen and Uusitalo, 1977; Wald et al, 1978). Nonsmokers living in the country have blood concentrations in the range of 0.1% to 0.4% whereas smokers living in the country range from 0.26% to 1.2% (Henry, 1968). These figures do not apply to persons living in large cities. Stewart et al (1973) sampled persons living in four large cities (Chicago, Los Angeles, New York, and Milwaukee) and found the carboxyhemoglobin concentration in the blood of nonsmokers to range from 0.4% to as high as 6.9%, while cigarette smokers ranged from 0.9% to 11.9%. Not surprisingly, persons exposed to combustion fumes, as in the case of passengers, taxicab drivers, and other workers in busy airports, had the highest concentrations.

Methemoglobin

Methemoglobin differs from oxyhemoglobin in that it contains ferric rather than ferrous iron, the O_2 being replaced by —OH. Methemoglobin is therefore oxidized hemoglobin, or ferrihemoglobin. Because it is unable to act as an oxygen carrier, methemoglobin in sufficiently high concentration causes hypoxia and cyanosis. The symptoms of hypoxia are usually not so severe as in carboxyhemoglobinemia, nor is methemoglobinemia as dangerous. Methemoglobin is present in small amounts in normal blood, 0.3% to 3.1% of the total blood pigment. Kravitz et al (1956) give

Table 10-3. Classification of methemoglobinemia

I. Hereditary
  A. Associated with abnormal methemo-globins (Hb M variants)
  B. Associated with deficient reducing system
  C. Associated with excessive oxidative activity
II. Acquired
  A. Chemical
    1. Acetanilid
    2. Acetophenetidin
    3. Alpha naphthylamine
    4. Aminophenol
    5. Ammonium nitrate
    6. Amyl nitrite
    7. Aniline
    8. Anilinethanol
    9. Antipyrine
    10. Arsine
    11. Benzocaine
    12. Bismuth subnitrate
    13. Chloronitrobenzene
    14. Dimethylamine
    15. Dinitrophenol
    16. Dinitrotoluene
    17. Hydroquinone
    18. Hydroxylacetanilid
    19. Hydroxylamine
    20. Lidocaine
    21. Methylacetanilid
    22. Monochloroaniline
    23. Nitrites
    24. Nitrobenzene
    25. Nitroglycerin
    26. Nitrophenol
    27. Nitrosobenzene
    28. Para-aminopropiophenone
    29. Para-bromoaniline
    30. Paranitroaniline
    31. Phenacetin
    32. Phenylenediamine
    33. Phenylhydrazine
    34. Phenylhydroxylamine
    35. Plasmoquin
    36. Potassium chlorate
    37. Propitocaine
    38. Pyridium
    39. Pyrogallol
    40. Resorcinol
    41. Sulfonal
    42. Sulfonamides
    43. Toluenediamine
    44. Toluylhydroxylamine
    45. Trichlorocarbonilide (TCC)
    46. Trinitrotoluene
    47. Trional
  B. Other
    1. Intestinal obstruction
    2. *Clostridium welchii* sepsis
    3. Contaminated well water (nitrates and nitrites)
    4. Ingestion of colored wax crayons or chalk
    5. Exposure to ionizing radiation

the following values for methemoglobin in normal subjects: premature infants, 2.2%; infants up to 1 year of age, 1% to 1.5%; and older children and adults, up to 1%. The formation of methemoglobin is a normal process, kept within bounds by a normal intraerythrocytic system capable of reducing methemoglobin to hemoglobin again.

Methemoglobinemia is classified into two major groups, hereditary and acquired (Table 10-3). The hereditary methemoglobinemias are further divided into three types, the one associated with Hb M being characterized by a type of methemoglobin that differs spectroscopically from all the others. This important difference can lead to serious analytic errors if the Evelyn and Malloy technic is used to quantify this type of methemoglobin.

The Hb M variants are actually variants of normal hemoglobin and are part of the family of genetically determined abnormal hemoglobins (Chapter 14). Clinically the presence of an Hb M variant does not produce hemolytic disease. From the standpoint of therapy, methemoglobinemia can be divided into (1) the type that does not respond to treatment with methylene blue or ascorbic acid (that associated with Hb M pigments) and (2) all others that do respond to these agents.

HEREDITARY METHEMOGLOBINEMIA: HB M VARIANTS. The hemoglobins designated M are variants that, because of a substitution of an amino acid in either the α- or the β-chain, have altered heme-globin binding. They are discussed here rather than in Chapter 14 because they account for one of the forms of methemoglobinemia and are only rarely associated with diminished erythrocyte survival.

A methemoglobin differing spectroscopically from "normal" methemoglobin was described by Hörlein and Weber (1948) and the designation of this hemoglobin as M was

later suggested by Singer (1955). Some years later Shibata et al (1960) reported that in the disease known as hereditary nigremia or Kuroko (black child), known to have occurred in a village of the Iwate province in Japan for almost two centuries, there was an abnormal methemoglobin designated as Hb M Iwate. Since that time many Hb M variants have been described, but structural studies show that there are in fact only five or six (Table 10-4).

In four of the variants, the substitution involves the proximal or distal histidines of the globin polypeptide chains. The α58 and β63 histidines lie opposite the heme iron but are not linked to it. These are the distal histidines. The α87 and β92 histidines are linked to the heme iron. The substitution of tyrosine for these histidines brings about the stabilization of the heme iron in the ferric state. In this state hemoglobin is unable to bind oxygen reversibly. When the heme iron is in the ferric form, methemoglobin, sometimes also called hemiglobin, is the respiratory pigment that is formed. The substitution in Hb M Milwaukee does not involve the histidine interaction. Instead, the glutamate binds the sixth coordination valence of heme iron (Perutz et al, 1972).

The cyanmethemoglobin (cyanferrihemoglobin) forms of some of the Hb M pigments have spectral absorption curves that differ from that of normal cyanmethemoglobin (Shibata et al, 1967). This is seen with Hb M Boston and Hb M Iwate, with maxima at 602 and 610 nm, respectively. Because of this anomalous reaction with cyanide, the Evelyn and Malloy technic for quantifying methemoglobin is not applicable to the Hb M variants. This technic is based on the difference in absorption at 632 nm after the methemoglobin is converted to cyanmethemoglobin by cyanide. The conversion applies only when methemoglobin reacts normally, as in the acquired methemoglobinemias. By the same

Table 10-4. Classification of hemoglobin M

Hemoglobin	Substitution	Absorption maxima, cyanferrihemoglobin (nm)*
Substitution involves proximal or distal histidine		
Hb M Boston†	α58 His → Tyr	495;602
Hb M Iwate‡	α87 His → Tyr	490;610
Hb M Saskatoon§	β63 His → Tyr	492;602
Hb M Hyde Park‖	β92 His → Tyr	—
Substitution does not involve proximal or distal histidine		
Hb M Milwaukee	β67 Val → Glu	500;622

*Absorption maxima for "normal" methemoglobin: 502;632.
†Same as Hb M Gothenberg, Hb M Osaka, Hb M Kiskunhalas.
‡Same as Hb M Kankakee, Hb M Oldenberg.
§Same as Hb M Århus, Hb M Chicago, Hb M Emory, Hb M Hamburg, Hb M Hida, Hb M Kurume, Hb M Radom, Hb M Leipzig, Hb M Novi sad, Hb M Erlangen.
‖Same as Hb M Akita.

token, the characteristic absorption band of normal methemoglobin seen spectroscopically at 632 nm cannot be used to identify the Hb M variants.

Clinically, affected persons show bluish slate-gray or brown cyanosis of the skin, lips, and nail beds. Transmission is autosomal dominant. Affected persons are heterozygous and the homozygous state is probably lethal in utero. The cyanosis is present from birth in the α-chain variants, whereas in the β-chain variants it may not appear until some months later. Affected individuals lead normal lives, the only danger being that the etiology of the cyanosis may be misdiagnosed. There is no hemolytic disease. Pisciotta et al (1959) have reported instances of an Hb M and Hb C in the same person, producing mild hemolytic disease. The cyanosis caused by Hb M variants does not respond to therapy with methylene blue or ascorbic acid.

The diagnosis of Hb M variants should present no problem. Cyanosis at birth may be caused by congenital cardiac anomalies, but the presence of Hb M should be ruled out before undertaking cardiovascular investigations (Stamatoyannopoulos et al, 1976). The cyanosis of methemoglobinemia is usually not the pure violaceous color of that caused by pure hypoxia. Gross observation of drawn blood gives an important clue, the blood being brownish-green or brownish-gray even after exposure to air. Electrophoresis is not a reliable diagnostic help, Hb M Iwate and Hb M Saskatoon being the only ones that show minor differences in mobility, but the bands seen are greenish or gray rather than the normal brown. Spectral absorption curves provide the most definitive characterization (Tönz, 1968). Kohne et al (1977) identified a second occurrence of Hb M Milwaukee, this time in a German family, by identifying the characteristic amino acid substitution in the abnormal β-chain.

HEREDITARY METHEMOGLOBINEMIA; DEFICIENT REDUCING SYSTEMS. Human erythrocytes metabolize glucose to pyruvate and lactate by the major glycolytic (anaerobic) pathway, the Embden-Meyerhof pathway. An aerobic pathway also exists, the hexose monophosphate shunt, Fig. 10-11. In a normal subject the maintenance of the concentration of methemoglobin at a low level (0.2% to 1% of

total hemoglobin [Tönz, 1968]) is dependent on the activity of enzymes known trivially as reductases. These act to reduce methemoglobin to hemoglobin. They are dependent on NADH generated in the anaerobic pathway or on NADPH generated in the shunt pathway (Keitt, 1972). It is difficult to judge the independence or interdependence of the two enzyme systems, but it is likely that NADH-methemoglobin reductase is of the greater importance in vivo, whereas NADPH-methemoglobin reductase activity is minor except in the response to therapy with methylene blue.

The abnormal function of the M hemoglobins can be related to the effect of the amino acid substitution on the R (relaxed) or T (tense) conformation of the hemoglobin molecule (Winslow and Anderson, 1978). In all the M hemoglobins the insertion of a new amino acid group stabilizes the heme groups and holds the iron in the ferric state. In M hemoglobins with α-chain substitutions (Boston and Iwate) the R-T equilibrium is forced to the T state so that oxygen affinity is low and the Bohr effect is absent. In two of the β-chain–substituted M hemoglobins (Saskatoon and Hyde Park) a T-R transition does occur and a Bohr effect is present. In the other M hemoglobin having a β-chain substitution (Milwaukee) the ferric β-subunits do undergo a change in their tertiary structure on oxygenation of the α-chains, but this is a late event, and a Bohr effect is seen. In effect, all the M hemoglobins have only two oxygen-binding sites per hemoglobin tetramer.

Methemoglobinemia caused by a deficiency of NADH-methemoglobin reductase within the red cells is an inherited disease transmitted as an autosomal recessive trait (Jaffé, 1966; Schwartz and Jaffé, 1978). A number of genetic variants of NADH-methemoglobin reductase have been reported (Hsieh and Jaffé, 1971). Kaplan et al (1974) report a homozygous deficiency of a variant NADH-methemoglobin reductase associated with complete deficiency of cytochrome-B5-reductase and suggest that the two reductases are involved in the pathogenesis of both the methemoglobinemia and the mental retardation. Affected infants are cyanotic at birth, in contrast to the cyanosis of some of the Hb M

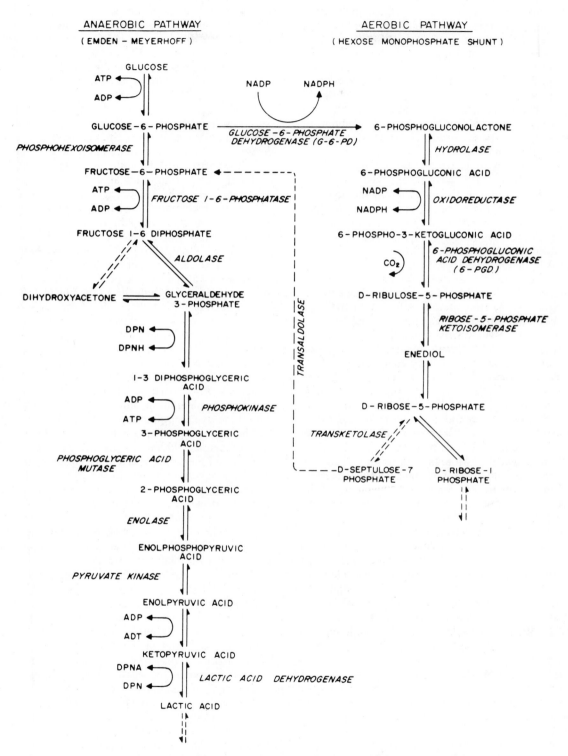

Fig. 10-11. Aerobic and anaerobic pathways of glucose metabolism in the erythrocyte.

variants that develops during the first year of life. There is mental retardation sometimes (Fialkow et al, 1965), but generally the disease is benign. The methemoglobinemia responds dramatically to treatment with methylene blue and, less quickly, with ascorbic acid. Methylene blue should not be administered to an infant if there is a deficiency of glucose-6-phosphate dehydrogenase (Hibbard et al, 1978). A 1% solution of methylene blue is given slowly intravenously, the dose depending on weight and age (adults, 1 mg/kg; children 1.5 mg/kg; infants 2 mg/kg). Methylene blue can be used as a rapid in vitro diagnostic test; the addition of methylene blue to the typically brown blood of reductase deficiency causes a rapid change to red. This color change is not seen in the blood with an Hb M abnormality.

Kleihauer and Betke (1963) have described an elution procedure to demonstrate the distribution of methemoglobin in erythrocytes from blood smear preparations. In diaphorase deficiency the distribution is heterogeneous, indicating that methemoglobin accumulates in only some of the red blood cells (Keitt et al, 1966), just as Hb F is heterogeneously distributed in the thalassemias.

An interesting kindred with methemoglobinemia caused by a deficiency of diaphorase was reported by Cawein et al (1962). The patient had emigrated from France in 1820 and established his family in eastern Kentucky on the banks of Troublesome Creek. By 1958 the kindred numbered more than 150, and in that year the propositus, Luke Combs, took his wife to the University of Kentucky Hospital in Lexington, Kentucky. It was the husband and not the wife who startled the doctors. "Luke was just as blue as Lake Louise on a cool summer day," said one of the doctors. Many members of the kindred were found to have methemoglobinemia secondary to diaphorase deficiency. The two families showing the trait came to be known as the "blue Combses" and the "blue Fugates." Mountain superstition claimed they were hexed, and the Combses and the Fugates stayed away from the townspeople. Some male members of the "blue" families were rejected by the military because of the color of their skin.

HEREDITARY METHEMOGLOBINEMIA: EXCESSIVE OXIDATIVE ACTIVITY. The existence of this third group rests on Fishberg's (1948) report describing a patient with cyanosis, methemoglobinemia, and ascorbic acid deficiency. The patient excreted large amounts of benzoquinone acetic acid in the urine. Ascorbic acid rapidly abolished both the methemoglobinemia and the excretion of benzoquinone acetic acid. Fishberg suggests that the methemoglobinemia was a result of the oxidation of hemoglobin by benzoquinone acetic acid.

ACQUIRED METHEMOGLOBINEMIA. Most cases of methemoglobinemia fall into the acquired group. Only a dozen cases of the Hb M type and about a hundred of the enzyme-deficient type have been described. Cases described prior to recognition of the two major types of hereditary methemoglobinemia are difficult to classify.

The most common cause of methemoglobinemia is the toxic effect of drugs such as aniline dyes, aniline derivatives, sulfonamides, nitrates and nitrites, acetanilid, acetophenetidin, and chlorates (Bodansky, 1951; Cohen et al, 1968). The exposure to these agents is sometimes not obvious (Singley, 1962). For example, methemoglobinemia has been described as the result of eating Polish sausage (kiszka), which is rich in nitrite and nitrate (Bakshi et al, 1967). There may also be absorption of nitrate from silver nitrate used to treat extensive burns (Cushing and Smith, 1969). Methemoglobinemia can be produced by exposure to ionizing radiation; given moderate doses of radiation, the degree of methemoglobinemia is directly proportional to the dose (Dowben and Walker, 1955).

Methemoglobinemia presents a special problem in pediatric practice. Because Hb F is more readily converted to methemoglobin than Hb A, infants are susceptible to methemoglobinemia when exposed to toxic agents in doses that would not affect an older child or an adult (Fisch et al, 1963; Goluboff, 1958; Johnson et al, 1963; Peterson, 1960). Furthermore, the erythrocytes of newborn infants are relatively deficient in methemoglobin-reducing enzymes. An example is the methemoglobinemia of infants caused by the ingestion of well water having a high nitrate or nitrite content (Ewing and Mayon-White, 1951). Water having a high nitrate content from surface contaminants is a common offender. When such water is used to prepare an infant's formula, the nitrate is converted to nitrite in the bowel and causes methemoglobinemeia. Methemoglobinemia has developed in children who have eaten wax crayons or chalk colored with aniline dyes; but it is now illegal to use aniline dye in the manufacture of crayons. However, children will generally eat or drink anything within their reach; e.g., marking ink, furniture polish, and other products containing nitrobenzene. Ramsay and Harvey (1959) reported an outbreak of methemoglobinemia in infants attributed to the absorption of aniline dye from the marking ink used on diapers.

The methemoglobin concentration in hereditary methemoglobinemia seldom exceeds 40%, but the concentration in acquired methemoglobinemia may be very high if there has been severe exposure to the toxic agent. Cyanosis is manifest at a concentration of about 15%. Symptoms of hypoxia occur at a concentration of 60% and higher. Although it is remarkable to see how quickly cyanosis disappears when the offending agent is eliminated, if there are symptoms of hypoxia acquired, methemoglobinemia should be treated with methylene blue.

Toxic dyes may produce other hematologic disturbances that are of greater clinical significance than the methemoglobinemia. Hemolytic anemia caused by a toxic effect of the drug or dye on the erythrocytes is not uncommon. At times hemolysis is mild, producing only slight anemia, reticulocytosis, and moderately increased serum bilirubin concentration. It may be severe, however, producing severe anemia, markedly elevated serum bilirubin, and striking Heinz body formation in the erythrocytes. Compensatory polycythemia may follow prolonged anoxia. Either of these syndromes may be striking enough to overshadow a minimal methemoglobinemia.

One uncommon finding in some cases of methemoglobinemia, particularly those caused by sulfonamides (Hayes and Feltz, 1964), is an increased excretion of porphyrins. In these cases, methemoglobinemia may be transient, porphyria may be the dominant sign, and anemia may develop without any rise in serum bilirubin.

Sulfhemoglobin

Sulfhemoglobin is a stable compound of hemoglobin and sulfur. Its structure is not known. *Sulfhemoglobinemia* often accompanies methemoglobinemia (Finch, 1948; Gibson, 1954), and the symptoms are those of anoxia (Begg, 1955; Fichter, 1954). Sulfhemoglobinemia is a complication of exposure to trinitrotoluene or acetanilid (Reynolds and Ware, 1952). It has also been reported as a complication of exposure to the fungicide zinc ethylene bisdithiocarbamate (Pinkhas, 1963). Sulfhemoglobin, once formed, is so stable that it disappears from the circulation only after the erythrocytes containing it are naturally destroyed. Since this reaction cannot be reversed, therapy is usually directed toward the accompanying methemoglobinemia, the sulfhemoglobinemia being allowed to pass off by itself. Erythrocytes containing sulfhemoglobin have normal survival and osmotic fragility.

The cyanosis of sulfhemoglobinemia is clinically indistinguishable from that of methemoglobinemia. It does not respond to treatment with ascorbic acid or methylene blue. Miller (1957) has reported familial and congenital sulfhemoglobinemia in a newborn infant. An absorption band at 618 nm can be seen when sulfhemoglobin is examined spectroscopically. The position of the band does not shift when cyanide is added.

The normal concentration of sulfhemoglobin in blood is 0% to 2.2% of total hemoglobin.

Methemalbumin

Methemalbumin (Fairley's pigment), consists of hematin bound to serum albumin. It has been found in various hemolytic diseases, hemoglobinuria, liver disease, and pernicious anemia. Methemalbumin is formed after the haptoglobin binding capacity for free hemoglobin is exceeded. However, Northam et al (1963) found methemalbumin in the serum from patients with acute hemorrhagic pancreatitis with haptoglobin still present in the serum. One important difference between methemalbumin and other hemoglobin compounds is that methemalbumin is found only in the plasma or serum.

Spectroscopic identification

Hemoglobin and hemoglobin compounds absorb light in the visible spectrum (Martinek, 1965). In general, absorption of light of short wavelengths is more intense than absorption at longer wavelengths. Each compound characteristically absorbs light of different wavelengths (Table 10-5), accounting for the characteristic color of some of the compounds and for the specific absorption bands observed with the spectroscope and the recording spectrophotometer (Figs. 10-12 to 10-18). The bands represent zones of maximum absorption, determined by the valence of the iron molecule and the type of chemical bonds. *Ferric* compounds with *paramagnetic ionic bonds* (hemin, hematin, and methemoglobin) have absorption bands in the red portion of the spectrum, *ferric* compounds with *diamagnetic covalent bonds* (cyanmethemoglobin and hemichromes) have bands in the green portion, and *ferrous* compounds with *diamagnetic covalent bonds* (heme, oxyhemoglobin, and carboxyhemoglobin) have two intense bands in the yellow-green portion of the spectrum. The degradation products of hemoglobin that contain neither iron nor globin also have characteristic absorption spectra.

Spectroscopic analysis affords a simple method for identifying various compounds. Optimum results depend on a systematic approach to the analysis, utilization of known chemical reactions, and experience in the use of the instrument. Particular care must be paid to the slit width, the light source, and the concentration of the solution tested. Since abnormal pigments are usually present in mixtures with oxy-

Table 10-5. Wavelengths of maxima of absorption bands of hemoglobin and related compounds*

Compound	Alpha	Beta	Gamma	Delta
Oxyhemoglobin (HbO$_2$)	578	540		
Reduced hemoglobin (Hb)	556			
Carboxyhemoglobin (HbCO)	572	535	(540)	
Sulfhemoglobin	618	(578)	540	500
Methemoglobin	630	578		
Cyanmethemoglobin	540			
Methemalbumin	623	540	500	
Acid hematin				
In ether	638	582	540	505
In N/10 HCl	662			
In acetic acid	630			
Alkaline hematin	610			
Protoporphyrin				
Alkaline N/10 NaOH	645	591	540	504
Acid, 25% HCl (w/v)	602	557		
Uroporphyrin				
Alkaline, N/10 NaOH	612	560	539	504
Acid, 25% HCl (w/v)	596	577	554	
Coproporphyrin				
Alkaline, N/10 NaOH	612	568	538	504
Acid, 25% HCl (w/v)	594	574	551	

*After Sunderman et al, 1953.

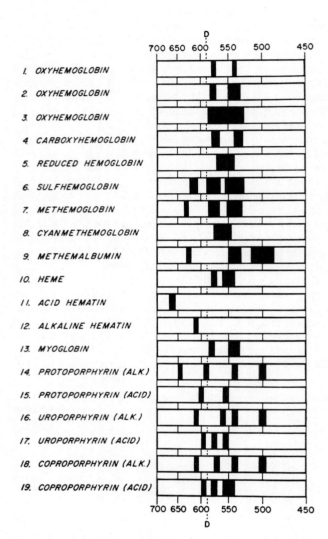

Fig. 10-12. Characteristic absorption spectra of hemoglobin derivatives. The three spectra for oxyhemoglobin at the top represent increasing concentrations of oxyhemoglobin.

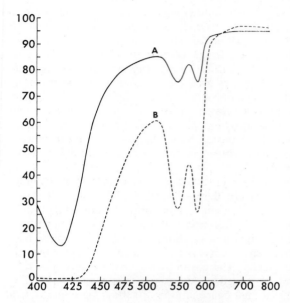

Fig. 10-13. S-T curve of oxyhemoglobin. **A,** Dilute; **B,** concentrated.

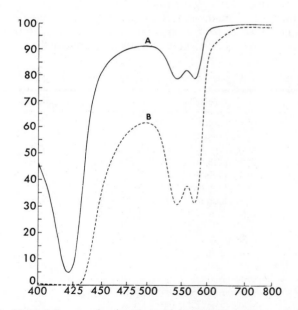

Fig. 10-14. S-T curve of carboxyhemoglobin. **A,** Dilute; **B,** concentrated.

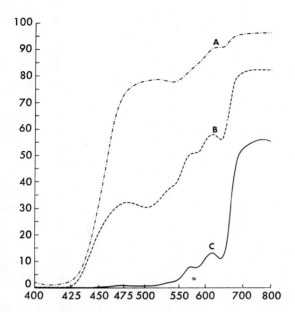

Fig. 10-15. S-T curve of neutral methemoglobin. **A,** Most dilute; **C,** most concentrated.

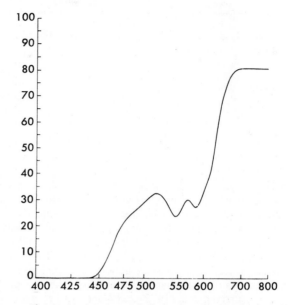

Fig. 10-16. S-T curve of alkaline methemoglobin.

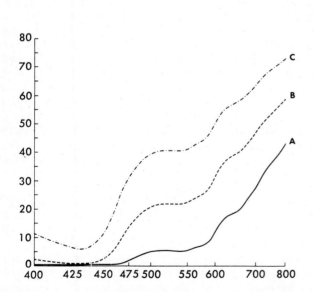

Fig. 10-17. S-T curve of sulfhemoglobin. **C,** Most dilute; **A,** most concentrated.

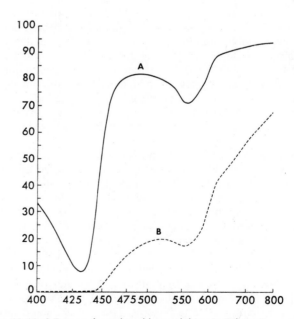

Fig. 10-18. S-T curve for reduced hemoglobin. **A,** Dilute; **B,** concentrated.

Table 10-6. Limit of sensitivity and relative intensity of absorption bands for hemoglobin and hemoglobin compounds (alpha band of oxyhemoglobin = 100)*

Compound	Color of dilute solution	Limit of sensitivity† (mg/dl)	Relative intensity of band		
			Alpha	Beta	Gamma
Oxyhemoglobin	Pale yellow	5.0	100	57	
Carboxyhemoglobin	Pink-straw	7.9	63	45	
Reduced hemoglobin	Pale red-brown	48	10		
Methemoglobin	Yellow-brown	57	9	5	7
Sulfhemoglobin	Green-yellow	50	10	35	16
Acid hematin	Brown	67	7	2	6
Alkaline hematin	Green-brown	165	3		

*After Bloem, 1933; Sunderman et al, 1953.
†For alpha band.

hemoglobin, their bands may be obscured by those of oxyhemoglobin; e.g., the bands for carboxyhemoglobin and myoglobin usually cannot be distinguished from those of oxyhemoglobin unless a mercury arc lamp is used. Another limiting factor is the concentration of the abnormal compound and the intensity of its absorption bands (Table 10-6). Methods for preparing known fractions of hemoglobin pigments and for quantitative determinations are given by Siggaard-Andersen et al (1972) and Nørgaard-Pedersen et al (1972).

Haptoglobin

The term "haptoglobin" (Fig. 10-19) is applied to a polymer family of plasma proteins that have the property of combining with free hemoglobin, the binding site being probably on the α-polypeptide chain of globin. On electrophoresis, haptoglobin migrates with the α_2-globulins, the haptoglobin-hemoglobin complex migrates with the β_1-fraction, and free hemoglobin falls between the β- and γ-fractions. This differential migration can be used to measure the concentration of hemoglobin-binding protein in the blood. The complex of haptoglobin and hemoglobin also has peroxidase activity, thus providing a second method of estimating haptoglobin.

Smithies (1955) showed that, with starch electrophoresis, the sera of normal human subjects fall into three groups. Since the difference concerns haptoglobin, Smithies and Walker (1956) later proposed that the three groups should be termed haptoglobin phenotypes 1-1, 2-1, and 2-2. It was first suggested that a single pair of genes, Hp^1 and Hp^2, inherited in a regular manner, are responsible for the three genotypes (Hp^1/Hp^1, Hp^1/Hp^2, and Hp^2/Hp^2). This does not account for the observation that a small percentage of normal adults have no haptoglobin. The frequency of ahaptoglobinemia in normal adults varies from 1% in Denmark and 2% in Britain to 32% in Nigeria. These observations have led to the postulation of an Hp^0 gene responsible for the absence of haptoglobin. Giblett and Steinberg (1960) postulated three alleles at the haptoglobin locus: Hp^1, Hp^2, and Hp^{2m}, the last a "modified" Hp^2 (Figs. 10-20 and 10-21) occurring predominantly, but not exclusively, in American blacks. They suggest that allele Hp^{2m}, in combination with Hp^1, produces either $Hp^{2-1(m)}$ or ahaptoglobinemia. There

are, in addition, rare mutants. One of these is type "Johnson," originally described by Giblett (1960) in two members of a black family in Seattle and since described in a family in Urmia, Persia, and in a family studied in my laboratory in Miami (Fig. 10-22). The other, originally Hp G but now called Hp Carlsburg (Giblett, 1969), is a rare variant described by Galatius-Jensen (1958). It is thought to be a variant of haptoglobin type 2-1.

Smithies et al (1966) have shown that haptoglobin subjected to reductive cleavage by urea and mercaptoethanol is separable by electrophoresis into two polypeptide chains, α and β. The β-chain is apparently the same in all the haptoglobin variants, but the α-chain is modified as an expression of haptoglobin genes. Five different α-polypeptides have been identified: hp 1F, hp 1S, hp 2, hp J, and hp 2M. These account for a number of subtypes: subtypes 1S-1S, 1S-1F, and 1F-1F of Hp 1-1; subtypes 2-1S and 2-1F of Hp 2-1. Other subtypes are dependent on α-chain and β-chain substitutions or quantitative variants when the polypeptide chain is qualitatively normal but quantitatively suppressed. It is now thought that these five polypeptides are the expression of five alleles, Hp^{1F}, Hp^{1S}, Hp^2, Hp^{2J}, and Hp^{2M}. Of the 15 possible genotypes, at least 10 phenotypic expressions have been identified (Table 10-7). The frequency of haptoglobin types, haptoglobin subtypes, and gene frequency for three racial groups in Seattle, Washington, are given in Tables 10-8 and 10-9. Atypical segregation is sometimes explained by assuming an inert allele, Hp^0, or an independent suppressor with complete penetrance.

The three most common alleles, Hp^{1F}, Hp^{1S}, and Hp^2, determine the three most common haptoglobin types (1-1, 2-1, and 2-2) and the corresponding phenotypes (1F-1F, 1F-1S, 1S-1S, 2-1F, 2-1S, 2-2, and 2-2M) (Table 10-7). Family studies have shown no exceptions to the predicted inheritance pattern, and it has been suggested that the haptoglobin system adds one additional serologic factor to the study of disputed parentage. Predicted inheritance patterns are given in Table 10-10. Data on the observed inheritance of the less common types are still scarce and probably insufficient to apply to medicolegal studies.

Haptoglobin is synthesized in the liver. Merrill et al (1964) describe a remarkable case that illustrates this point. A patient scheduled for a liver transplant was found to have

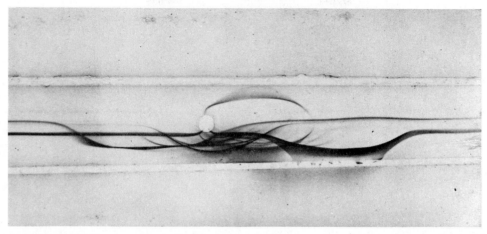

Fig. 10-19. Haptoglobin as demonstrated by immunoelectrophoresis. Top, Human serum versus antihaptoglobin serum. Bottom, Human serum versus polyvalent antiserum.

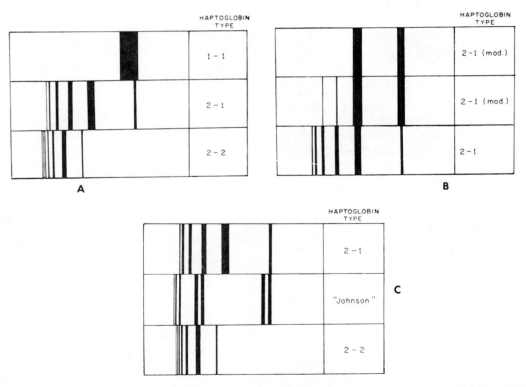

Fig. 10-20. Haptoglobin types. **A,** Types 1-1, 2-1, and 2-2. **B,** Type 2-1 and two forms of type 2-1 (modified). **C,** Haptoglobin type "Johnson." (From Giblett, 1960.)

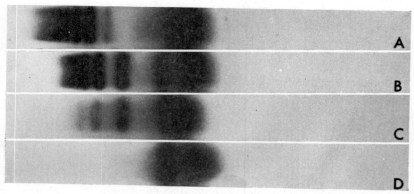

Fig. 10-21. Human haptoglobin types. Vertical starch gel electrophoresis, Amidoschwarz stain. **A,** Type 2-2. **B,** Type 2-1. **C,** Type 2-1 (modified). **D,** Type 1-1.

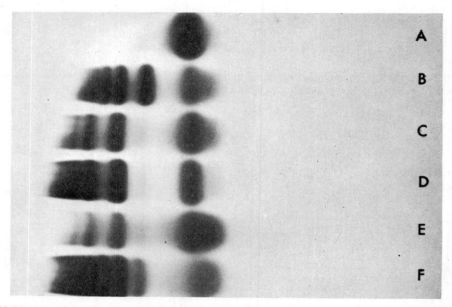

Fig. 10-22. Haptoglobin "Johnson" compared to the standard types. **A,** Type 1-1. **B,** Type 2-1. **C-E,** Mother, son, and grandson, type "Johnson." **F,** Type 2-2.

Table 10-7. Haptoglobin types and subtypes

Haptoglobin type (phenotype)	Haptoglobin subtypes	Haptoglobin type (phenotype)	Haptoglobin subtypes
I. Common phenotypes		Hp 1H	None
Hp 1-1	hp 1S-1S	Hp 1-1 Marburg	None
	hp 1S-1F	Hp 2-1 Modified	None
	hp 1F-1F	Hp 2-1 Bellevue	None
Hp 2-1	hp 2-1S	Hp 2-1D	None
	hp 2-1F	Hp 2-1 Haw	None
Hp 2-2	hp 2-2	Hp 2-1 Marburg	None
	hp 2-2M	Hp 2-1 Trans	None
Hp 0	None	Hp 2B	None
II. Rare phenotypes		Hp 2-P	None
Hp 1 (Johnson)	hp 1 (J)F	Hp 2-H	None
	hp 1 (J)S	Hp 2-L	None
Hp 1B	None	Hp AG	None
Hp 1P	None	Hp Carlsberg	None
		Hp 2J	None

Table 10-8. Frequency (percent) of haptoglobin types and subtypes in 2,560 blood donors of three racial groups*

Ethnic group	Haptoglobin types					Gene frequency		
	1-1	2-2	2-1	2-1 (mod.)	0	Hp^1	Hp^2	Hp^{2m}
White (409)	13.2%	36.4%	50.3%	—	—	0.384	0.616	—
Black (1,657)	28.5%	18.5%	38.7%	10.9%	3.4%	0.552	0.349	0.099
Oriental (494)	6.9%	54.7%	38.4%	—	—	0.261	0.739	—

*Data from Giblett and Brooks, 1963.

Table 10-9. Haptoglobin subtypes of 368 selected donors of three racial groups (gene frequency calculated by applying subtype proportion to respective Hp^1 frequencies)*

Ethnic group	No.	Haptoglobin subtypes (No. of cases)							Gene frequency	
		1S-1S	1F-1F	1S-1F	2-1S	2-1F	2M-1S	2M-1F	Hp^{1F}	Hp^{1S}
White	66	4	0	5	36	21	0	0	0.133	0.251
Black	222	26	20	49	61	55	6	5	0.259	0.293
Oriental	80	14	0	1	64	1	0	0	0.005	0.256

*Data from Giblett and Brooks, 1963.

Table 10-10. Predicted inheritance of three common haptoglobin types and six corresponding subtypes, based on three allelic genes (X indicates offspring expected, O indicates offspring not possible; underlined matings and offspring have been reported)*

Mating		Expected offspring						
Hp type	Hp subtype	1F-1F	1F-1S	1S-1S	2-1F	2-1S	2-2	Hp type
1-1 X 1-1	1F-1F X 1F-1F	X	O	O	O	O	O	1-1
	1F-1F X 1F-1S	X	X	O	O	O	O	1-1
	1F-1F X 1S-1S	O	X	O	O	O	O	1-1
	1F-1S X 1F-1S	X	X	X	O	O	O	1-1
	1F-1S X 1S-1S	O	X	X	O	O	O	1-1
	1S-1S X 1S-1S	O	O	X	O	O	O	1-1
2-1 X 1-1	2-1F X 1F-1F	X	O	O	X	O	O	2-1 or 1-1
	2-1F X 1F-1S	X	X	O	X	X	O	2-1 or 1-1
	2-1F X 1S-1S	O	X	O	O	X	O	2-1 or 1-1
	2-1S X 1F-1F	O	X	O	X	O	O	2-1 or 1-1
	2-1S X 1F-1S	O	X	X	X	X	O	2-1 or 1-1
	2-1S X 1S-1S	O	O	X	O	X	O	2-1 or 1-1
2-1 X 2-1	2-1F X 2-1F	X	O	O	X	O	X	2-1, 2-2, or 1-1
	2-1F X 2-1S	O	X	O	X	X	X	2-1, 2-2, or 1-1
	2-1S X 2-1S	O	O	X	O	X	X	2-1, 2-2, or 1-1
2-1 X 2-2	2-1F X 2-2	O	O	O	X	O	X	2-1 or 2-2
	2-1S X 2-2	O	O	O	O	X	X	2-1 or 2-2
2-2 X 1-1	2-2 X 1F-1F	O	O	O	X	O	O	2-1
	2-2 X 1F-1S	O	O	O	X	X	O	2-1
	2-2 X 1S-1S	O	O	O	O	X	O	2-1
2-1 X 2-2	2-2 X 2-2	O	O	O	O	O	X	2-2

*From Smithies et al, 1962.

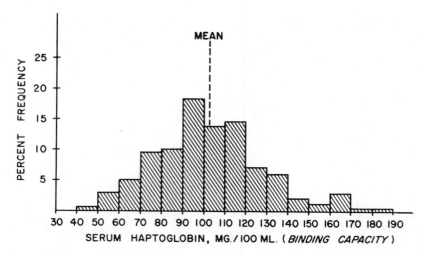

Fig. 10-23. Distribution of serum haptoglobin concentration in 213 normal adults, electrophoresis method.

haptoglobin type 2-1. The transplanted liver was from a donor of haptoglobin type 2-2. Following the transplant, the recipient showed type 2-2 haptoglobin in her serum.

Haptoglobin can be demonstrated in only about 10% of newborns (cord blood) (de Azavedo et al, 1974). It has been assumed that the liver of the newborn does not synthesize haptoglobin at a normal rate, but there is also evidence that the blood of the newborn contains haptoglobin that is not active in the binding of hemoglobin and thus cannot be measured by technics based on reactions of the haptoglobin-hemoglobin complex.

The measurement of serum haptoglobin concentration depends on two characteristics of the hemoglobin-haptoglobin complex. The first is the differential mobility of hemoglobin and the haptoglobin-hemoglobin complex when subjected to electrophoresis (Valeri et al, 1965). The second is the peroxidase activity of the hemoglobin-haptoglobin complex. Both methods measure haptoglobin indirectly, as a function of its capacity to bind hemoglobin. Neither method should be considered entirely satisfactory. The electrophoretic method, used in our laboratory, is more direct and simple, but because the exact ratios of molecular binding between haptoglobin polymers and hemoglobin are not perfectly understood, it is a better measure of hemoglobin-binding capacity than it is of haptoglobin per se. The electrophoretic method assumes a hemoglobin-haptoglobin binding ratio of 1:1, and yet the molecular weight of haptoglobin varies according to type (type 1-1, mol wt 100,000; type 2-1, mol wt 220,000; type 2-2, mol wt 400,000). However, the binding capacity in sera containing haptoglobin of various types does not vary as much as the molecular weight (see the following normal values). Methods based on peroxidase activity are subject to variations in temperature and time; in addition, it is possible for haptoglobin to be altered so that its hemoglobin complex has little peroxidase activity; e.g., purified haptoglobin (method of Connell and Smithies, 1959) retains its electrophoretic properties but loses peroxidase activity.

In spite of these shortcomings, both methods yield measurements that are clinically significant. Electrophoresis

demonstrates that the mean serum haptoglobin concentration is 102 mg/dl (in terms of binding capacity for hemoglobin), SD 22.5, and 95% range 57 to 147 mg (Fig. 10-23). The difference among the three main types is slight: type 1-1, mean 110.5, SD 29.7; type 2-1, mean 101, SD 22.5; type 2-2, mean 101, SD 21.5. The difference in normal values among the various types probably reflects the difference in molecular weights (Javid, 1965).

Because haptoglobin specifically binds hemoglobin, when there is intravascular hemolysis there is a direct relationship between the binding capacity of serum and the appearance of hemoglobin in the urine. It has long been known that hemoglobinuria occurs only when the serum hemoglobin concentration exceeds 100 to 135 mg/dl. This was called the minimal renal threshold by Lichty et al (1932) who also noted that the threshold could be lowered by repeated intravenous administration of hemoglobin. It is now clear that hemoglobin given intravenously is bound to haptoglobin, the complex being very stable. Hemoglobinuria occurs only after the hemoglobin-binding capacity of plasma is saturated (Allison, 1957). If a sufficiently large amount of hemoglobin is given or liberated by intravascular hemolysis, the haptoglobin concentration drops rapidly, reaching 0 in 8 to 12 hours. The hemoglobin-haptoglobin complex is not excreted in the urine. Low haptoglobin levels are therefore characteristic of acute and chronic hemolytic anemia and in hemolytic transfusion reactions (Fink et al, 1967). It is interesting to note that little or no haptoglobin is found in the serum of patients with untreated pernicious anemia (see discussion of the hemolytic nature of pernicious anemia in Chapter 9).

Human haptoglobin binds not only human hemoglobin but also hemoglobin of other species (monkey, rabbit, horse, cow, dog, and mouse). Human hemoglobins A_1, A_2, F_1, Lepore, C, and S are bound equally by human haptoglobin. Hemoglobins H and Bart's are not bound by human haptoglobin (Nagel and Ranney, 1964). Note that these two variants contain no α-chains (Chapter 14). Haptoglobin does not combine with heme or myoglobin.

Serum haptoglobin levels are high in a number of diseases

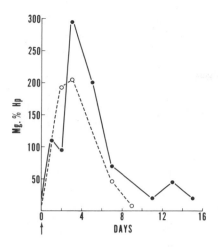

Fig. 10-24. Stimulation of serum haptoglobin production in two rabbits by a turpentine abscess. (Redrawn from Miale and Kent, 1962.)

characterized by inflammation (Fig. 10-24) or destruction of tissue (pyogenic infection, rheumatic fever, rheumatoid arthritis, and some cancers). High haptoglobin levels are reported in chronic alcoholics (Lamy, 1973). The suggestion has been made (Jayle and Boussier, 1955) that haptoglobins are of connective tissue origin and may contribute to the increase in the serum glycoprotein fraction that is characteristically elevated in rheumatoid arthritis.

Although hemoglobin binding is almost exclusively dependent on haptoglobin, other serum proteins are involved in binding the catabolic products of hemoglobin. A β-globulin that binds heme (heme-binding globulin) and the albumin-binding of heme have been described. Albumin and heme combine to form methemalbumin. A protein of the β_1-type with an affinity for heme has been named *hemopexin* (Müller-Eberhard, 1970; Morgan, 1976; Myrhed et al, 1976). The normal range of serum hemopexin concentration is 40 to 122 mg/dl (Zinkham et al, 1979a).

Hemoglobin catabolism
Formation of bilirubin

When erythrocytes come to the end of their life span, normally about 120 days but less in hemolytic disease, they are removed from the bloodstream by reticuloendothelial cells. The chief site of phagocytosis is the spleen, but in hemolytic disease the liver and bone marrow also assume this function (Harris, 1963). Within the reticuloendothelial cells, hemoglobin is degraded to *bilirubin* by a series of degradations that first involve the splitting of globin from the heme (Schmid, 1972; Schmid and McDonagh, 1978; Schmid, 1978), followed by the opening of the porphyrin ring at the α-methene bridge, yielding biliverdin and carbon monoxide (Landaw et al, 1970). The globin is returned to the plasma protein and aminoacid pool, and the heme iron is returned to the plasma iron pool (Fig. 10-25).

The conversion of hematin to biliverdin is an enzymatic step dependent on the activity of microsomal *heme oxygenase,* and the conversion of biliverdin to bilirubin is dependent on the enzyme *biliverdin reductase* (Tenhunen et al, 1970). Splenic tissue is rich in these enzymes, but heme

oxygenase activity is also present in bone marrow, liver, brain, kidney, and lung (Schmid, 1972).

The formation of bilirubin is an intracellular process. Bilirubin then passes out of the cell into the blood where it is bound to albumin (Ostrow and Schmid, 1963). In this form the bilirubin is *unconjugated* and *indirect reacting.* Unconjugated bilirubin is cleared rapidly from the blood by the parenchymal cells of the liver where it is conjugated with glucuronic acid. In this form the bilirubin is *conjugated* and *direct reacting.* The preferred usage is to call the unconjugated form simply *bilirubin* and the conjugated form *conjugated bilirubin.* The glucuronic acid donor is uridine diphosphoglucuronic acid (Fig. 10-26). The enzyme *glucuronyl transferase* is required for conjugation. In the conjugated form it is secreted into the bile ductules of the liver and passes into the small intestine by way of the common bile duct.

Most of the conjugated bilirubin in human beings is in the form of the diglucuronide (Billing et al, 1957) with a minor component as the monoglucuronide (Billing and Lathe, 1958). A minor fraction is also conjugated with sulfate rather than with glucuronide (Gregory and Watson, 1962). Some drugs, notably the barbiturates, are active in inducing transferase activity and enhancing conjugation of bilirubin (Remmer and Merker, 1963).

In normal serum the total bilirubin concentration is 0.1 to 1.0 mg/dl. Of this it is common to find normally 0 to 0.2 mg/dl of the direct-reacting pigment. The chemical partition into direct reacting and indirect reacting using the van den Bergh reaction (Hijmans van den Bergh and Mueller, 1916) is only an approximation of the conjugated and unconjugated fractions. The glucuronide is water soluble and does not need to be made soluble by alcohol to react with the diazo reagent. This reaction is therefore direct. In a normal person, the direct-reacting fraction is not bilirubin glucuronide, but bilirubin solubilized by serum substances such as bile acids and urea. The unconjugated bilirubin is not water soluble and hence requires alcohol (or some other suitable solvent) to react with the diazo reagent.

If no block exists in the bile duct system, bilirubin glucuronide is excreted into the duodenum through the ampulla of Vater. In the intestine it is reduced by bacterial action to the colorless compound *mesobilirubinogen.* Urobilinogen, stercobilinogen, and other related compounds are formed from mesobilirubinogen and excreted in both urine and feces. Urobilinogen is partially absorbed from the colon into the blood. A little is excreted in the urine, and 35% to 70% of it is returned to the liver by the portal circulation. It is then reexcreted by the liver cells. When parenchymal liver damage exists, absorbed urobilinogen cannot be excreted by the liver cells, is rejected, and remains in the bloodstream. It then appears in the urine in large amounts. On the other hand, sterilization, even partial, of the bacterial flora of the gastrointestinal tract by antibiotics reduces the conversion of bilirubin to urobilinogen, resulting in low fecal and urinary urobilinogen excretion (Dearing et al, 1958). Table 10-11 gives the color reactions (Ehrlich's aldehyde and others) of urobilinogen, porphobilinogen, and other indoles.

The final step, oxidation of urobilinogen and stercobilinogen to *urobilin* and *stercobilin,* probably occurs chiefly when excreta are allowed to stand. It is important that exam-

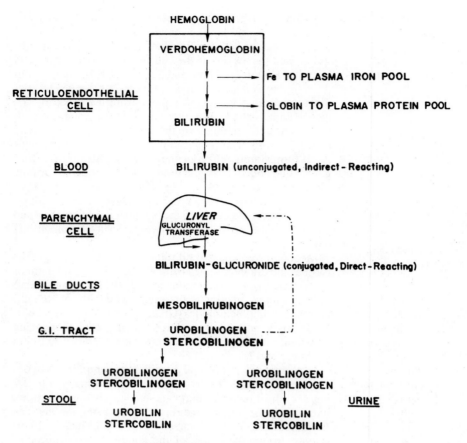

Fig. 10-25. Catabolic pathways of hemoglobin.

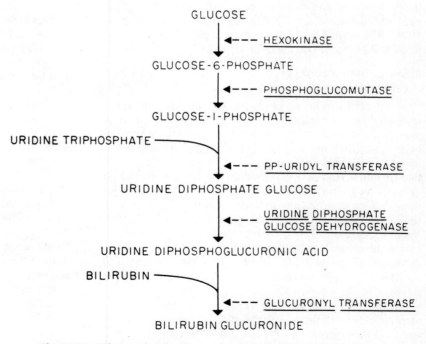

Fig. 10-26. Pathway of enzymatic conjugation of bilirubin with glucuronide.

Table 10-11. Ehrlich's reaction and other characteristics of some naturally occurring indoles compared with urobilinogen (UBG) and porphobilinogen (PBG)*

Indole (dissolved in normal urine)	Ehrlich reaction				Color with 22% hydrochloric acid	Paper chromatography (R_f) (butanol 63:acetic acid 10:water 27)
	Primary color	After sodium acetate	Immediate chloroform extract	Butanol extract after chloroform†		
Indican	Brown-yellow	Red-orange	Orange-yellow	Negative	Negative	0.43-0.48
Indoxyl acetate	Brown-yellow	Red-orange	Orange-yellow	Negative	Negative	—
Indoleacetic acid	Pink-violet	Pink-violet, fading	Fades	Negative	Pink or red with urine containing nitrite	0.86-0.92
Indoleacetamide	Pink-violet	Pink-violet, fading	Fades	Negative	—	0.84-0.90
5-HIAA	Delayed blue	Delayed blue	Negative	Negative	Negative	0.72-0.78
Indole	Pink	Bluish	Pink	Negative	Yellow	0.92-0.96
Skatole	Violet-blue	Blue	Blue, fades	Negative	Light yellow	0.94-0.98
5,6-Dihydroxy-indole	Yellow-orange	Blue	Negative	Blue	Lilac (chloroform insoluble, butanol soluble)	Not done
UBG	Faint pink	Strong red-violet	Red	Negative	Negative	1.0
PBG	Red	Slight intensification; red-violet	Negative	Negative	Negative	0.45-0.50

*From Watson et al, 1964b.

†In all instances indicated as negative in this column the solution had first been shaken with chloroform and all color removed. Butanol would have served equally well to extract the aldehyde compound.

inations for urobilinogen and stercobilinogen be carried out on freshly passed specimens.

Hyperbilirubinemia

Hyperbilirubinemia is the result of an increased concentration in the blood of either, or both, bilirubin fractions (Schmid and McDonagh, 1978). Based on pathogenesis, hyperbilirubinemia is of three types. The first is caused by accelerated breakdown of hemoglobin, typically as in hemolytic disease. The second is caused by a deficiency of glucuronyl transferase, as in some of the congenital hyperbilirubinemic syndromes. The third is caused by obstruction of the bile ducts. Each type shows characteristic patterns of bilirubin accumulation.

When there is accelerated breakdown of hemoglobin, bilirubin formation may exceed the capacity of the liver to clear it from the blood and to conjugate it. Typically there is an increase in bilirubin (unconjugated) and, assuming normal liver function, an increase in the conjugated fraction as well, though the increase in unconjugated bilirubin is proportionately greater. In chronic hemolytic disease the excessive pigment load over a long time may produce cholestasis, blockage of the small bile ducts by inspissated pigment, and the obstructive element may be reflected in a proportionately greater increase in the conjugated bilirubin fraction.

Syndromes characterized by absence or reduction of glucuronyl transferase show an increase in unconjugated bilirubin.

Obstruction of the bile ducts leads to accumulation of conjugated bilirubin that has left the hepatic cell but is prevented from going into the intestine by the blockage of the bile ducts. It is assumed that there is regurgitation into the blood through the lining of the bile ducts and this type of hyperbilirubinemia is commonly called *regurgitation jaundice.*

Hyperbilirubinemic syndromes are not always so classic in their pathogenesis and manifestations. For example, hyperbilirubinemia of infancy is the result of accelerated hemoglobin breakdown plus a partial deficiency of transferase. In liver disease, the jaundice may be caused by damage of parenchymal cells, intrahepatic obstruction, or a combination of both. In addition there is often decreased red cell life span. A primary deficiency of liver storage has been described by Dhumeaux and Berthelot (1975). The defective uptake or storage of bilirubin results in accumulation of conjugated bilirubin in the blood. Cyclic premenstrual hyperbilirubinemia (Yamaguchi et al, 1975) is of uncertain etiology.

Accumulation of unconjugated bilirubin is a potentially dangerous situation in the infant (Table 10-12). Unconjugated bilirubin has an affinity for the basal ganglia of the brain, and damage to the ganglia (kernicterus) results in convulsions and, if the infant survives, severe neurologic damage. Conjugated bilirubin does not cross the blood-brain barrier (Diamond and Schmid, 1966).

NEONATAL HYPERBILIRUBINEMIA. The bilirubin produced in utero by the fetus passes into the maternal circulation, where it is conjugated and excreted by the mother's liver. When the umbilical cord is severed at birth, the newborn infant is deprived of the maternal mechanism and must depend on its own liver to conjugate and excrete bilirubin. The mechanism for conjugating bilirubin, however, is poor-

Table 10-12. Classification of hyperbilirubinemia*

I. Neonatal hyperbilirubinemia
  A. Increase in the unconjugated fraction
    1. Physiologic jaundice (icterus neonatorum)
    2. Exaggeration or prolongation of physiologic jaundice
      a. Prematurity
      b. Respiratory distress and hypoxia
      c. Disturbed metabolism
        (1) Babies born to diabetic mothers
        (2) Galactosemia
        (3) Pyloric stenosis
        (4) Intestinal obstruction
        (5) Dehydration
        (6) Cretinism
        (7) Mongolism
        (8) Pyknocytosis
      d. Drugs, given to mother or infant (particularly vitamin K)
        (1) Causing hemolysis
        (2) Causing hepatocellular damage
        (3) Progesterone and derivatives
        (4) Drugs competing for glucuronide (antibiotics, sulfonamides, tranquilizers)
      e. Viral (particularly cytomegalic inclusion disease), bacterial, or protozoal (leptospirosis infection)
      f. Hematoma, in infant or placenta
    3. Genetic errors in bilirubin metabolism
      a. Crigler-Najjar syndrome
      b. Transient familial hyperbilirubinemia
      c. Cyclic premenstrual hyperbilirubinemia
    4. Increased hemolysis
      a. Isoimmune hemolytic disease
      b. Sepsis
      c. Congenital hemolytic anemia due to G-6-PD, pyruvate kinase, and other enzymatic deficiencies
      d. G-6-PD deficiency without anemia
  B. Increase in conjugated bilirubin
    1. Hepatocellular damage
    2. Biliary tract obstruction
    3. Hepatic storage disease
II. Hyperbilirubinemia of adolescents and adults
  A. Increase in the unconjugated fraction
    1. Genetic errors in bilirubin metabolism
      a. Crigler-Najjar syndrome
      b. Gilbert's syndrome
      c. "Shunt" hyperbilirubinemia
    2. Hemolytic disease
    3. Idiopathic dyserythropoietic jaundice
  B. Increase in the conjugated fraction
    1. Genetic errors in bilirubin metabolism
      a. Dubin-Johnson syndrome
      b. Rotor's syndrome
    2. Hepatocellular damage
    3. Biliary tract obstruction
    4. "Recurrent idiopathic jaundice of pregnancy"
    5. Intake of oral contraceptives

*Modified from Aponte. In Sunderman and Sunderman, 1964.

ly developed at birth and even less developed in premature infants. As a result, there is transient hyperbilirubinemia (Odell, 1967). It has been estimated that the ability of the newborn infant to conjugate bilirubin is about 1% that of the adult. This inadequacy may reflect a deficient synthesis of uridine diphosphate glucuronic acid as well as a deficiency of the glucuronyl transferase system. After birth at term, glucuronide formation quickly improves and in a few days reaches normal adult activity. (Weech, 1947; Brown and Zuelzer, 1958). Should there be hyperbilirubinemia as the result of hemolytic disease plus the conjugation defect, the infant can be seriously affected. Since bilirubin is bound to serum albumin, hypoalbuminemia predisposes to kernicterus by allowing more bilirubin to be unbound.

HEREDITARY HYPERBILIRUBINEMIA IN RATS (GUNN STRAIN). In 1938 Gunn described a mutant strain of Wistar rats exhibiting jaundice as an inherited recessive trait. Two years later, Malloy and Lowenstein (1940) predicted that the genetic defect would be found to consist of a lack of the normal mechanism for producing direct-reacting bilirubin. Recent studies have shown this to indeed be so; we find the primary defect in affected rats to be a failure of the glucuronyl transferase system, without which all plasma bilirubin is of the unconjugated type (Carbone and Grodsky, 1957). No bilirubin is excreted in the urine, and there is frequent evidence of central nervous system damage.

HEREDITARY HYPERBILIRUBINEMIA IN SHEEP. Congenital hyperbilirubinemia in sheep is similar to the unconjugated hyperbilirubinemia in Gunn rats (Cornelius et al, 1968). These animals show a severe photosensitivity.

HEMOLYTIC DISEASE. In acute hemolytic disease uncomplicated by liver dysfunction, hyperbilirubinemia simply reflects the formation of large quantities of bilirubin. Although there is usually no abnormality of conjugation, there may be an accumulation of bilirubin in serum when the capacity of the liver to conjugate bilirubin is exceeded. Therefore the serum contains a high concentration of bilirubin. In chronic hemolytic disease it is common to find also a moderate to marked increase in the concentration of conjugated bilirubin. This is a reflection of superimposed obstructive jaundice as a result of intrahepatic obstruction or early cirrhosis.

UNCONJUGATED HYPERBILIRUBINEMIA IN INEFFECTIVE ERYTHROPOIESIS. Unconjugated hyperbilirubinemia is a feature of ineffective erythropoiesis (Verwilghen et al, 1969).

OBSTRUCTIVE JAUNDICE. When there is simple obstruction in the biliary duct system, bilirubin is converted normally to conjugated bilirubin. However, obstruction to the flow of bile causes the conjugated pigment to be regurgitated into the bloodstream. As a result, there is progressive hyperbilirubinemia, in which most of the pigment is of the conjugated type. In chronic obstruction of the biliary system there is a secondary failure of liver function, with some accumulation of unconjugated bilirubin.

CONSTITUTIONAL HEPATIC DYSFUNCTION (GILBERT'S SYNDROME). The familial or congenital syndromes described in Table 10-13 are characterized by jaundice of the nonhemolytic type. Although some syndromes are satisfactorily defined, others are not. As the number of cases

Table 10-13. Comparison of some important features of four familial nonhemolytic jaundice syndromes

	Gilbert	Dubin-Johnson	Crigler-Najjar	Rotor
Serum				
Bilirubin	Increased	Increased	Increased	Increased
Conjugated bilirubin	Normal*	Increased	Normal†	Increased
Urine				
Bile	Negative	Positive	Negative	Positive
Urobilinogen	Normal	Increased	Decreased	Normal
Pigment in liver	Absent	Present	Absent†	Absent
Liver function tests				
Bilirubin clearance	Diminished	Diminished	Diminished	Diminished
BSP retention	Normal	Slightly increased	Normal	Increased
Cephalin flocculation	Normal	Normal or increased	Normal	Normal or increased
Thymol turbidity	Normal	Normal or increased	Normal	Normal
Serum alkaline phosphatase	Normal	Normal	Normal or sl. increased	Normal

*Less than 10% of total serum bilirubin.
†Inspissated bile in canaliculi.

reported has increased, so have the synonyms. As a result, there is no general agreement as to terminology, and it is necessary to define each by continuing to use the investigator's name.

In 1907 Gilbert et al described some cases of congenital icterus with elevation of indirect-reacting bilirubin. As often happens, there is some doubt whether Gilbert's cases were identical to some described later that had the benefit of better investigative methods (Schmid, 1972). Similar cases have been called hereditary nonhemolytic bilirubinemia (Alwall, 1946), familial nonhemolytic jaundice (Dameshek and Singer, 1945), and constitutional hepatic dysfunction (Comfort, 1935).

Clinically, jaundice may be present from birth but is usually noted later in life. It is more common in males and is seen frequently in physicians and medical students. Icterus is chronic, usually fluctuating in severity, and is aggravated by emotional upsets, fatigue, alcohol, and infectious diseases. There is no hepatomegaly or splenomegaly. There is a definite familial incidence, probably inherited as an autosomal dominant trait (Powell et al, 1967). The disease is clinically benign. Cartei and Dini (1975) found the coexistence of β-thalassemia trait and Gilbert's syndrome in three subjects. There was mild unconjugated hyperbilirubinemia (1.6 to 2.1 mg/dl) with normal erythrocyte life span, and the hyperbilirubinemia was ascribed to the Gilbert's syndrome rather than to the thalassemia trait. The combination was clinically benign.

Investigation reveals hyperbilirubinemia, usually about 6 mg% and seldom higher than 12 mg% (one case reported had 18.8 mg%). Most of the bilirubin is unconjugated. The urine contains no bile or melanin, and the urobilinogen excretion is normal. Uroporphyrin excretion is normal, but half the subjects excrete increased amounts of coproporphyrin. Liver function tests other than bilirubin clearance are normal. Liver tissue obtained by needle biopsy is normal in routine paraffin sections, but electron microscopy shows some abnormalities of the liver cell membranes (Simon and Varonier, 1963). Bilirubin clearance is impaired (Okolicsanyi et al, 1978). While there is no doubt that the icterus is caused by a failure of bilirubin conjugation, the basic defect

is not clear. Arias and London (1957) studied the conjugating activity of liver tissue from two persons who had this disease. Using bilirubin as the substrate and normal rat liver extract as the source of uridine diphosphoglucuronic acid, they showed a lack of conjugation when there is a deficiency of glucuronyl transferase. Because this approach cannot be used when a small piece of liver tissue from needle biopsy is all that is available, a micromethod was devised in which 4-methyl-umbelliferone was used as the substrate instead of bilirubin. With this technic, six out of seven patients showed deficient glucuronide conjugation. If it is assumed that glucuronyl transferase is the active enzyme in each system, it can be concluded that the basic defect in Gilbert's syndrome is a failure of this enzyme system. However, this assumption may not be valid, for conjugation of 4-methyl-umbelliferone with glucuronic acid forms an ether linkage, whereas conjugation of bilirubin with glucuronic acid forms an ester (acyl) linkage. When glucuronic acid excretion is studied by administering substances that are normally excreted as glucuronides (salicylamide, menthol, acetyl-paraminophenol, or anisic acid), no abnormality is found. Unfortunately, none of these form acyl glucuronides, either.

CHRONIC IDIOPATHIC JAUNDICE (DUBIN-JOHNSON SYNDROME). This syndrome was reported by Dubin and Johnson (1954) and by Sprinz and Nelson (1954). Though the reports appeared almost simultaneously, the disease is most often called the Dubin-Johnson syndrome.

The disease is usually familial and affects children and young adults. Though both sexes are affected, there is a preponderance of affected males. Clinically, there is chronic intermittent jaundice, often precipitated by pregnancy, surgery, exercise, alcohol, or infectious disease. About half the affected persons have hepatomegaly, and some complain of weakness and abdominal pain.

When there is hyperbilirubinemia, both unconjugated and conjugated bilirubin are increased. The total bilirubin concentration ranges up to 19 mg%, but in slightly more than half the patients the total serum bilirubin is below 6 mg%. Conjugated bilirubin makes up about 60% of the total, ranging from 25% to 86%. Bilirubin clearance is decreased; there is occasionally a moderate increase in BSP retention,

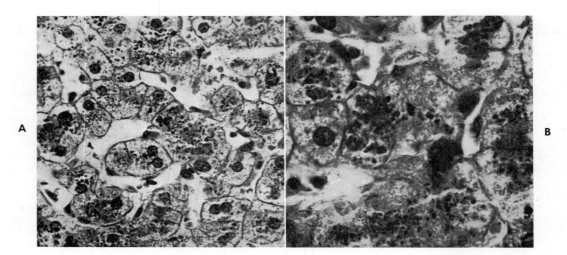

Fig. 10-27. Histopathology of liver in Dubin-Johnson syndrome. (Hematoxylin-eosin stain; **A,** ×600; **B,** ×900.)

and at times a positive flocculation test. Other tests of liver function show no abnormality. The urine contains bile and a normal amount of coproporphyrin with an absolute increase in the type I isomer. In one instance the urine was reported to contain melanin.

In addition to the presence of both unconjugated and conjugated bilirubin in the serum, this syndrome can be identified by a characteristic pigment in the liver. Grossly, the liver tissue is dark gray or green-black. Microscopically, the parenchymal cells contain an abundance of coarse dark-brown pigment (Fig. 10-27), particularly in the centrolobular zone. The Kupffer cells may contain some pigment when involvement is severe. Apparently, pigmentation may be minimal in some cases and could conceivably be overlooked (Schmid, 1972). The nature of the pigment is not known. It does not have the characteristics of hemosiderin, bile, or hematin. It stains with performic acid–Schiff or periodic acid–Schiff. It is argentophilic and not acid fast. It has some properties of a lipid, staining with oil red O and Sudan black B in a fresh frozen section but not with Sudan IV. No solvent has yet been found that will affect it. The suggestion that this pigment belongs in the lipofuscin group (Brown and Shnitka, 1956) is not accepted by all. As yet, nothing is known of the underlying abnormality responsible for the jaundice and pigmentation.

CONGENITAL NONHEMOLYTIC JAUNDICE (CRIGLER-NAJJAR SYNDROME). This syndrome, described by Crigler and Najjar (1952) is remarkably similar to Gilbert's syndrome and to hereditary hyperbilirubinemia in the Gunn strain of rat. It is not always possible to distinguish the Crigler-Najjar syndrome from Gilbert's syndrome, though the former is usually severe and the latter asymptomatic.

Clinically, jaundice is usually severe. In most instances it is discovered on the first or second day of life. The hyperbilirubinemia is caused by the retention of unconjugated bilirubin and is severe enough to cause damage to the central nervous system. There is indirect evidence that the underlying defect is a failure of bilirubin conjugation. This is reviewed in the section on Gilbert's syndrome and murine icterus. The liver is histologically normal except for the inconstant finding of inspissated bile in the bile canaliculi (Crigler and Najjar, 1952).

Schmid and McDonagh (1978) distinguish between two types of this disease. In type I there is evidence of complete lack of bilirubin conjugation, since there is no improvement after therapy with phenobarbital. The type I disease is seen in young infants, and there is damage to the central nervous system. In type II there is presumed to be only a partial lack of bilirubin conjugation, and the serum bilirubin can be reduced by therapy with phenobarbital. The type II disease is mild and is seen in older subjects.

FAMILIAL NONHEMOLYTIC JAUNDICE (ROTOR'S SYNDROME). A possible fourth variant of familial nonhemolytic jaundice has been described in a Filipino family by Rotor et al (1948); in Italians by Dagnini and Moreschi (1957), by Canali (1957), by Cinotti et al (1957); and in a Japanese woman by Schiff et al (1959). Young adults are affected by this jaundice, which is chronic and fluctuating. Except for occasional abdominal pain, the condition is asymptomatic. The serum bilirubin concentration is only moderately increased, and there is both unconjugated and conjugated bilirubin. The liver is histologically normal. BSP retention is increased and bilirubin clearance is impaired, whereas other liver function tests are usually normal. Urinary porphyrin excretion is increased in the form of coproporphyrin I and III.

11

"Let me count the ways. . . ."

Elizabeth Barrett Browning: *Sonnets From the Portuguese, XLIII*

The erythrocyte: abnormal forms and immunology

ABNORMAL FORMS OF THE ERYTHROCYTE
  Abnormalities in size
    Anisocytosis
    Microcytosis
    Macrocytosis
  Abnormalities in shape
    Introduction
    The discocyte
    The echinocyte
    The stomatocyte
    The acanthocyte
    The codocyte
    The dacryocyte
    The drepanocyte
    The elliptocyte
    The keratocyte and the schizocyte
    The leptocyte
    The megalocyte
    The spherocyte
    The knizocyte
  Erythrocytic inclusions
    Reticulocytes, diffuse basophilia, polychromatophilia,
      basophilic stippling
    Howell-Jolly bodies
    Cabot rings
    Heinz bodies
    Siderotic granules
IMMUNOLOGY OF THE ERYTHROCYTE
  Introduction
  Paleoimmunohematology
  Fundamentals of immunogenetics
  A-B-O blood group system
    Genetics
    Inheritance
    Blood group "cis-AB"
    Origin of isoagglutinins
    Missing isoagglutinins
    Lectins
    Agglutinins from snails and other animals
    Chemistry of blood group substances
    Subgroups of A
    Subgroups of B
    Acquired B (pseudo B)
    A^b group
    Blood group O and the H substance

    Bombay (O_h) blood group
    Blood factors A_1 and A
    Blood factor C
    Secretion of group-specific substances in saliva
    Summary of serologic characteristics of A-B-O system
  M-N-S-s blood group system
    Basic composition
    Medicolegal application
    Variants and related factors
  P blood group system
  Rh-Hr blood group system
    Basic genetics and serology
    Additional Rh-Hr factors
    C-D-E "nomenclature" versus Rh-Hr serology
    The Rosenfield numerical notation
    Rh_{null} type
    Rh antibodies
  Lewis blood group system
  Lutheran blood group system
  Kell blood group system
  Duffy blood group system
  Kidd blood group system
  I-i blood group system
  Diego blood group system
  Sex-linked blood group system Xg
  **"Private" (low-incidence) and "public" high-incidence)
    blood factors**
SEROLOGIC TESTS IN DISPUTED PARENTAGE
  Exclusion of paternity or maternity
    Types of exclusion
      Exclusion of nonfather
      Exclusion of nonmother
      Importance of genetic mutation
  The likelihood of paternity
  Use of individual systems
    A-B-O (A_1-A_2-B-O) blood group system
    The Rh blood group system
    The M-N-S-s blood group system
    The Kell blood group system
    The Duffy blood group system
    The Kidd blood group system
    The HLA system
      Exclusion of paternity
      Likelihood of paternity

Procedures and forms relating to the introduction of evidence
The initial request
Identification of parties
Identification of specimens
Guidelines for the expert
Report of the expert
CODING OF PHENOTYPES

ABNORMAL FORMS OF THE ERYTHROCYTE

Abnormalities of erythrocyte morphology fall into three categories: abnormalities in size, abnormalities in shape, and erythrocytic inclusions.

Abnormalities in size
Anisocytosis

A moderate variation in size is normal. In normal blood, the distribution curve for size frequency on fixed smears follows a normal curve (Price-Jones curve) with extreme limits of 6.2 to 8.2 μ in diameter and a mean diameter of 7.2 μ. The distribution is such that on a routine blood smear most of the cells appear to vary only slightly in size from 6.8 to 7.5 μ. *Anisocytosis* refers to a variation in cell diameters in a stained smear outside the normal limits. It is arbitrarily graded 1+ to 4+ (Figs. 11-1 and 11-3).

Significant anisocytosis can be found in a variety of situations: a range in diameter from normal to small, from large to normal, from large to small, or when two distinct populations exist (typical of sideroblastic anemias, Fig. 8-13, p. 407). In general the more severe anemias are accompanied by the most severe anisocytosis. It should be obvious that the MCV need not reflect a variation in size, since the MCV represents the mean size and not the size distribution.

Microcytosis

Microcytosis is usually accompanied by an MCV below 75 fl, but when only a few cells are microcytic the MCV may not be affected. Microcytes are less than 6 μ in diameter and characteristically are found in iron-deficiency anemias and thalassemias. In these situations the red blood cells are also poor in hemoglobin so that the cells are both microcytic and hypochromic (Fig. 11-2). Microcytic cells that are not poor in hemoglobin are seen in some hemolytic anemias.

Macrocytosis

Red blood cells are macrocytic if they have a diameter greater than 8.5 or 9 μ (Fig. 11-3). If only a few such cells are present the MCV will be within normal limits, but in most untreated megaloblastic anemias the MCV is usually above 105 fl. Macrocytosis is seen normally in the newborn and infant. Because reticulocytes are usually larger than adult cells, macrocytes may be seen on the peripheral blood smear when a large number of reticulocytes is present. Reticulocytes can be distinguished from mature macrocytes by their polychromatophilic or diffusely basophilic staining. In general macrocytosis is characteristic of folate or vitamin B₁₂ deficiency. The increased cell diameter is caused in part by flattening of the cells on smearing. The macrocytes in pernicious anemia are usually ovoid.

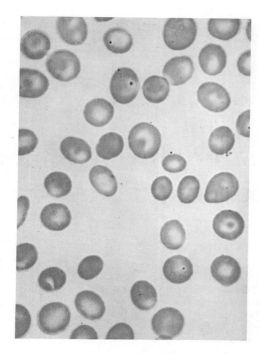

Fig. 11-1. Anisocytosis.

Abnormalities in shape
Introduction

"Poikilocytosis" is a general term that indicates the presence of red blood cells varying from the normal ovoid smooth shape. Poikilocytosis can be graded 1+ to 4+, as for anisocytosis, but the grading here is of lesser significance because it is the shape assumed by individual cells that is important.

The elegant application of scanning electron microscopy to the study of red cell shape by Bessis and others (Bessis, 1973b, 1973c; Bessis et al, 1973) makes it necessary to expand and standardize the nomenclature applied to variously deformed erythrocytes. The scanning electron microscope reveals details of red cell shape in three dimensions and in greater detail than the standard optical microscope. These revealing images, related to what we usually see on routine smears, make possible a better understanding of various abnormalities of red cell shape.

The proposed new nomenclature (Bessis, 1973c; Brecher, 1973) is given in Table 11-1 and has been adopted in this text. Some of the shapes are artifactual in the sense that they result from in vitro alterations of the cell environment and may not have exact counterparts on routine smears.

The discocyte

A discocyte (Fig. 11-4) is the normal, biconcave disk-shaped erythrocyte. This is a stable structure that provides the maximum surface area for the volume of the cell (Ponder, 1948) and corresponds to the shape of minimum electrostatic energy (Adams, 1973). The shape is not rigid, however, and in passing through small capillary vessels the cell assumes a cup shape that, in effect, reduces the cell diameter (Skalak and Branemark, 1969).

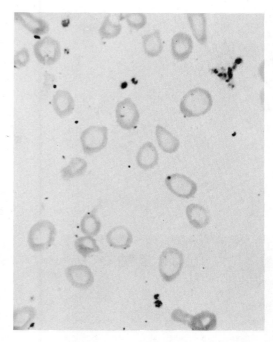

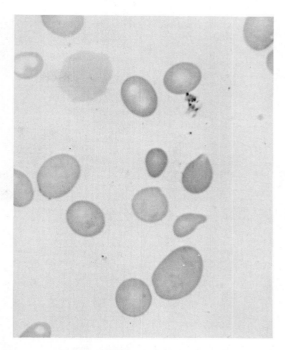

Fig. 11-2. Microcytosis and hypochromia, blood smear, from a child with severe iron-deficiency anemia. The erythrocytes are both smaller than normal and deficient in hemoglobin. (Wright's stain.)

Fig. 11-3. Macrocytosis and anisocytosis, blood smear, pernicious anemia. Many cells are larger than normal and the anisocytosis is graded 4+ because of the marked difference in size between the largest and the smallest cells.

Table 11-1. Nomenclature of red cell shapes*

New name†	Meaning of Greek stem	Old name
Discocyte	Disk	Biconcave disk
Echinocyte (I, II, III)	Sea urchin	Crenated cell
Stomatocyte (I, II, III)	Mouth	Stomatocyte
Acanthocyte	Spike	Acanthocyte
Codocyte	Bell	Target cell
Dacryocyte	Teardrop	Teardrop cell
Drepanocyte	Sickle	Sickle cell
Elliptocyte	Oval	Elliptocyte (ovalocyte)
Keratocyte	Horn	—
Schizocyte	Cut	Burr cell, spur cell, irregularly contracted erythrocyte
Leptocyte	Thin	—
Megalocyte	Giant	Oval macrocyte
Spherocyte	Sphere	Spherocyte

*Modified from Bessis, 1973c.
†May be combined with various prefixes, i.e., micro-, macro-, etc.

The echinocyte

An echinocyte is a red cell whose surface shows crenations (Fig. 11-5). The transformation of a discocyte into an echinocyte is reviewed by Brecher and Bessis (1973). Many years ago Ponder (1948) showed that an erythrocyte exposed to a lytic agent undergoes a predictable series of changes in outline, passing through a "crenated disk" to a "crenated sphere," then losing the crenations to form the "prolytic sphere" and finally hemolyzing to end up a red cell "ghost." The process is reversible prior to the forma-

tion of the prolytic sphere. The transformation of discocyte to echinocyte can be produced by suspending erythrocytes in saline between a glass slide and coverslip (not between plastic slide and coverslip) as well as by the action of various lytic agents such as saponin, bile salts, soaps, ionic detergents, or lecithin (Weed and Chailley, 1972).

The scanning electron microscope allows a more critical definition of this sequence of changes in normal erythrocytes (echinocyte I, echinocyte II, echinocyte III) and in abnormal erythrocytes (echino-acanthocyte, drepanoechino-

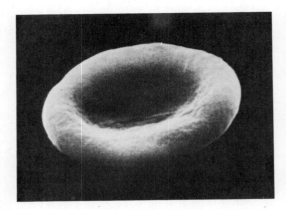

Fig. 11-4. The discocyte, a normal erythrocyte. Scanning electron microscope photograph. (Courtesy Dr. M. Bessis.)

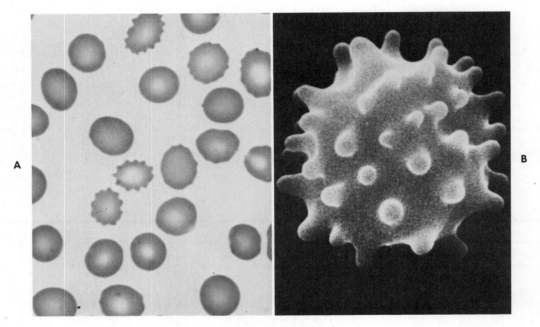

Fig. 11-5. The echinocyte (crenated erythrocyte). **A,** Peripheral blood smear. (Wright's stain.) **B,** Scanning electron microscope photograph. (Courtesy Dr. M. Bessis.)

cyte, etc.). No such distinctions are possible from fixed smears, the most common echinocyte being the crenated red cell, with evenly distributed, rounded, short "goose bumps" on the surface, seen most often when anticoagulated blood is smeared after standing for some hours. The use of the term "spicules" in connection with the transformation of normal discocytes into echinocytes is unfortunate, for spicules (sharp, pointed projections) observed on routine fixed smears indicate pathologic erythrocytes. At this time, at least, not all the changes revealed by the scanning electron microscope can be related to what is seen in fixed smears.

The stomatocyte

The stomatocyte (Fig. 11-6) is a cup-shaped erythrocyte that, in a fixed smear, shows an elongated area of central pallor—mouth-like given enough imagination. While the transformation of discocyte into stomatocyte can be produced in vitro by phenothiazine, chlorpromazine, or very low pH (Weed and Bessis, 1973), detection of stomatocytes on routine smears is characteristic of the hemolytic anemia called *hereditary stomatocytosis* (Chapter 13). Stomatocytes are occasionally seen in acute alcoholism but, in contrast to the hereditary hemolytic anemia, their appearance is transient. Stomatocytosis is sometimes a feature of Rh_{null} disease.

The acanthocyte

The term "acanthocyte" is not new. Bassen and Kornzweig (1950) described a girl with steatorrhea and atypical retinitis pigmentosa whose erythrocytes showed a striking degree of thorny crenation. Malformed cells were also found in a younger brother. The parents were cousins. Singer et al (1952) proposed the term "acanthrocytosis" for the

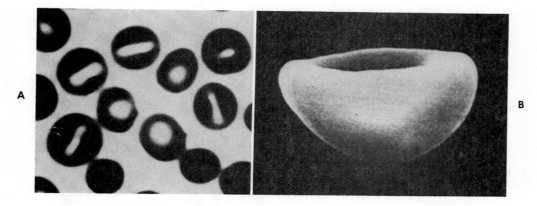

Fig. 11-6. The stomatocyte. **A,** Blood smear. (Wright's stain.) **B,** Scanning electron microscope photograph. (Courtesy Dr. M. Bessis.)

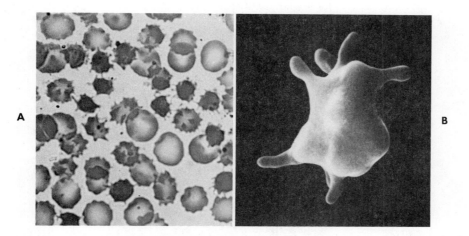

Fig. 11-7. The acanthocyte. **A,** Blood smear. (Wright's stain.) **B,** Scanning electron microscope photograph. (**A** courtesy Dr. K. Singer; **B** courtesy Dr. M. Bessis.)

abnormal shape of the red cells, but the more correct term for the shape abnormality is "acanthocytosis." Sometimes the term "acanthocytosis" is used to describe the disease syndrome, but more correct is the term "abetalipoprotein-emia" (Fredrickson et al, 1978; Herbert et al, 1978).

The acanthocyte is characteristic of abetalipoproteinemia. Almost all the erythrocytes show irregularly spaced pointed spicules, varying in length and in the number seen in each cell (Fig. 11-7). The involvement of the majority of the red cells is an important differential from other abnormalities that show only a few spiculated cells scattered among normal ones. While it is true that abetalipoproteinemia is always accompanied by acanthocytosis, the reverse is not always true. Acanthocytes may be seen in alcoholic cirrhosis with hemolytic anemia (Smith et al, 1964; Silber et al, 1966), in some cases of hemolytic anemia caused by pyruvate kinase deficiency (Oski et al, 1964; Nathan et al, 1965), in hepatitis of the newborn (Tchernia et al, 1968), after administration of heparin (Silber, 1969), and after

splenectomy (Brecher et al, 1972). It is distinctly unusual, however, for these cases to show as many acanthocytes as are usually seen in abetalipoproteinemia. Also in these cases, the β-lipoproteins are normal.

The etiology of abetalipoproteinemia and the mechanism of acanthocyte formation remain unclear (Fredrickson et al, 1978; Herbert et al, 1978). A number of biochemical abnormalities are present in addition to the total absence of β-lipoproteins: low serum total lipids, low serum phospholipids, low serum cholesterol, increased tolerance to carbohydrates, and low plasma vitamins A and E concentrations. The most likely mechanism is that a disproportion in the ratio of unesterified cholesterol to phospholipid in the plasma causes an increase in the cholesterol/phospholipid ratio in some areas of red cell membrane, followed by the shape change (Cooper et al, 1974, 1975).

Although unusual, hemolytic disease can be seen in abetalipoproteinemia, and Dodge et al (1967) have shown that hemolysis of acanthocytes occurs as the result of lipid per-

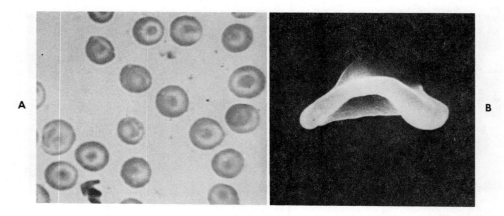

Fig. 11-8. The codocyte (target cell). **A,** Blood smear. (Wright's stain.) **B,** Scanning electron microscope photograph. (Courtesy Dr. M. Bessis.)

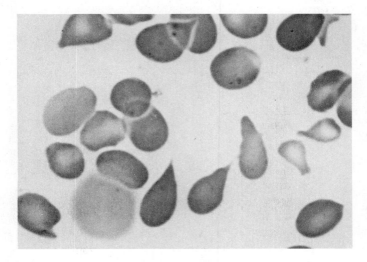

Fig. 11-9. The dacryocyte (pointed cells, center bottom). Blood smear, pernicious anemia. (Wright's stain.)

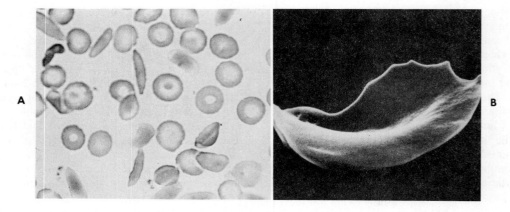

Fig. 11-10. The drepanocyte (sickle cell). **A,** Blood smear, sickle cell anemia. (Wright's stain.) **B,** Scanning electron microscope photograph. (Courtesy Dr. M. Bessis.)

oxidation. Formation of peroxide in vivo (from infection with *Mycoplasma* [Cohen and Somerson, 1967] or ingestion of 8-aminoquinoline antimalarials, menadione, aspirin, phenacetin, or sulfonamides) can theoretically precipitate hemolysis of acanthocytes.

The codocyte

Bessis (1973b, 1973c) has shown that cells that have the "target" or "Mexican hat" appearance on fixed smears are thin and bell-shaped in the wet state and then do not show the central dimple. When these codocytes are flattened in a smear preparation they assume the familiar target appearance, dark in the center and around the periphery with a lighter ring in between (Fig. 11-8). Codocytes are common in thalassemia, Hb C disease, sickle cell anemia, sickle cell–Hb C disease and sickle cell–thalassemia. They are characteristic of the postsplenectomy blood picture. Codocytes are sometimes found in iron-deficiency anemia and in liver disease with or without jaundice.

Codocytes in the blood smear are a feature of familial lecithin-cholesterol acyltransferase (LCAT) deficiency, in which there is hyperlipidemia, high levels of unesterified cholesterol and lecithin, and low levels of cholesteryl ester and lysolecithin in the serum (Norum et al, 1972; Gjone et al, 1978). In the formation of both acanthocytes and codocytes there are abnormalities in blood lipids that probably alter the lipid composition of the red cell membrane, but the nature of the interaction is not clear.

Codocytes are sometimes found to be artifacts. This is not uncommon when blood smears are made in humid climates. The artifact can sometimes be produced by blowing on a freshly made, and still wet, blood smear. The artifact can be suspected when target cells are seen in only one portion of the blood smear.

The dacryocyte

A dacryocyte is a teardrop-shaped red blood cell (Fig. 11-9). No one knows what causes this shape abnormality. In the myeloproliferative syndromes almost every oil immersion field will show at least one dacryocyte. They are somewhat less common in pernicious anemia and thalassemia.

The drepanocyte

Drepanocytes (sickle cells) are usually red blood cells that contain Hb S but may be induced in some other hemoglobinopathies. If an erythrocyte contains Hb S, it will undergo bizarre shape changes if the oxygen tension or pH is reduced. The tendency is to form crescent-shaped, i.e., sicklelike, forms (Fig. 11-10), but usually irregular spines, filaments, and a holly-leaved appearance are noted when the cells are exposed to powerful reducing agents. I have seen drepanocytes in vaginal smears from women with sickle cell anemia. Bessis (1973c) illustrates various forms of drepanocytes (drepano-discocyte, drepano-echinocyte, and drepano-stomatocytes) in wet preparations, which are presently of only theoretical interest. Drepanocytes often form "myelin bodies" (Bessis, 1973b), representing filamentous extrusions from the cell membrane. Ward et al (1979) describe the occurrence of myelin bodies in a routinely prepared and stained blood smear from a patient having both sickle cell anemia and cold agglutinins. Presumably the immunologic damage to an already labile membrane produced the unusual occurrence in the blood smear. I doubt, however, that this old phenomenon deserves the suggested name of "erythrocytic ecdysis."

Drepanocytes show a decreased osmotic fragility, usually moderate in degree but at times striking. Mechanical fragility is increased, and it has been proposed that intravascular hemolysis may be caused by abnormal mechanical fragility. Because of their abnormal shape, they do not form rouleaux, and therefore the sedimentation rate is low, even when anemia is severe.

The elliptocyte

Elliptocytosis (Fig. 11-11) is a congenital abnormality of erythrocytes transmitted as an autosomal dominant with complete penetrance. On blood smears these cells appear oval in outline. When viewed in the fresh state, the cells are seen to be ellipsoidal and biconcave. Using electron microscopy and a shadow-casting technic, Rebuck and Van Slyck (1968) have shown that the human elliptocyte is a biconcave, dumbbell-shaped structure in one plane and an ellipse in another, with bipolar massing of hemoglobin. They can

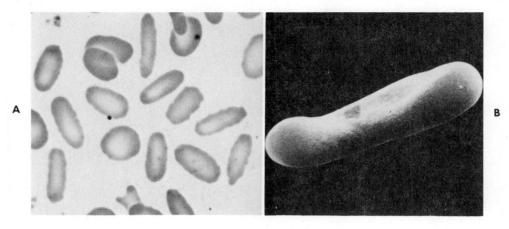

Fig. 11-11. The elliptocyte. **A,** Blood smear, hereditary elliptocytosis. (Wright's stain.) **B,** Scanning electron microscope photograph. (Courtesy Dr. M. Bessis.)

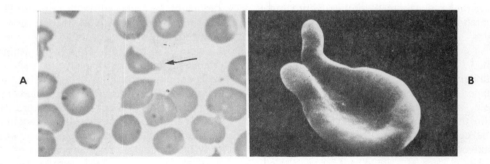

Fig. 11-12. The keratocyte. **A,** Blood smear. (Wright's stain.) **B,** Scanning electron microscope photograph. (Courtesy Dr. M. Bessis.)

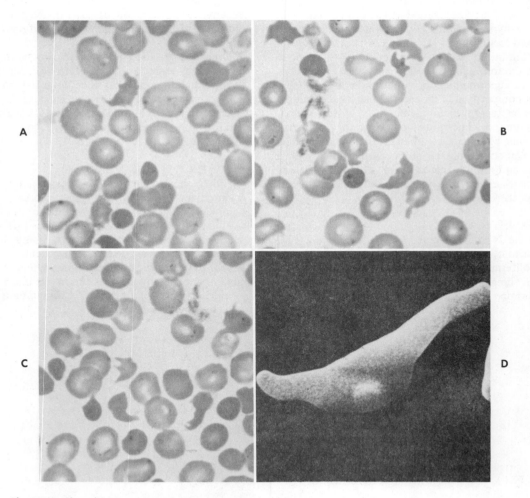

Fig. 11-13. The schizocyte. **A-C,** Blood smears. (Wright's stain.) **D,** Scanning electron microscope photograph. (Courtesy Dr. M. Bessis.)

form typical rouleaux. The shape varies from slightly oval to rod or sausage forms. Ponder (1948) has shown that elliptocytes undergo the same shape transformations in vitro as normal cells.

As in congenital spherocytosis, the elliptocyte precursors, including the early reticulocytes, are usually normal in shape, but Löffler and Hansen (1967) report one case in which the normoblasts in the bone marrow were elliptical. The transformation of elliptocytes is a complete mystery. It is noteworthy that, in an effected person, only a few elliptocytes are present at birth, the number increasing with age. Elliptocytosis is at times prominent in thalassemia, sickle cell trait, and Hb C trait, conditions usually characterized by codocytes. Aksoy (1963a) and Perillie and Chernoff (1965) report the combination of hereditary elliptocytosis with heterozygous β-thalassemia. It may, in minor degrees, also accompany anemias other than the hemolytic type. Özer and Mills (1964) have reported the coincidence of elliptocytic hemolytic anemia with cirrhosis, with decreased erythrocyte glutathione, and with glucose-6-phosphate deficiency. One case has been reported in which elliptocytosis was associated with hereditary hemorrhagic telangiectasia (Penfold and Lipscomb, 1943). In asymptomatic cases (heterozygous), elliptocytes have a normal or slightly increased osmotic fragility, but in elliptocytic hemolytic anemia (Chapter 13) the osmotic fragility is increased. The erythrocytes of the llama are normally elliptocytic, but they do not have bipolar aggregation of hemoglobin and do not lyse in distilled water (Rebuck and Van Slyck, 1968).

The keratocyte and the schizocyte

These terms apply to erythrocytes that are distorted because of fragmentation. A keratocyte (Fig. 11-12) is a damaged cell, deformed because of an incomplete cut so that there is no loss of a hemoglobinated fragment. On a routine fixed blood smear the cell may appear slightly irregular at one end. Fragmentation into two or more pieces produces irregularly shaped hemoglobinated fragments, the schizocyte. In a smear these are the "irregularly contracted erythrocytes" (Fig. 11-13), sometimes called "schistocytes," "helmet cells," "burr cells," or "spur cells," terms that should no longer be used. Of the two types of distortion, the schizocyte is the more important.

The studies of Bull et al (1968) and Bull and Kuhn (1970) showed that one mechanism for producing schizocytes involves the clothesline effect of a fibrin strand on a passing red cell. The cell can be partially deformed but not cut (a keratocyte), or it can be cut in two. In the latter situation the larger fragment is the irregularly shaped schizocyte. This mechanism applies in situations in which there is intravascular deposition of fibrin, as in diffuse intravascular coagulation (DIC) or microangiopathic hemolytic anemia. The formation of schizocytes in patients with prosthetic heart valves or even with untreated valvular stenosis and in some cases of hypertension implies fragmentation by mechanical trauma alone. In other conditions there is no obvious mechanical injury—uremia, extensive burns without DIC (Fig. 11-14), bleeding peptic ulcer, aplastic anemia, pyruvate kinase deficiency (Oski et al, 1964), or the normal newborn (Tuffy et al, 1959).

Tuffy et al (1959) point out that a significant number of schizocytes are found in smears from normal premature and newborn infants. These authors also describe 11 infants with severe hemolytic anemia and up to 50% occurrence of schizocytes in the peripheral blood. They proposed the term "infantile pyknocytosis" for this syndrome. It must be assumed that in these situations the red cell membrane is damaged either by antigen-antibody complexes or by the severe hyperbilirubinemia (Ackerman, 1969).

Schizocytes should be distinguished from echinocytes, which have short, blunt projections and from acanthocytes, which have many long, spiny projections. It may be helpful to note that in conditions leading to schizocyte formation relatively few of the cells will be abnormal, whereas in acanthocytosis and in echinocyte transformation on storage most of the red cells will be malformed. Schizocytes should also be distinguished from *selenoid bodies,* half-moon–shaped red cell ghosts. Cuadra (1958) showed that they are produced by the mechanical shear of smearing when the erythrocytes are abnormal or young and when the plasma is lipid rich.

The leptocyte

The leptocyte is a thin, flat red blood cell (Fig. 11-15). The diameter is increased but the volume is normal. They appear hypochromic on fixed smears. Codocytes are also flat but have the characteristic central dimple. Leptocytes are seen in liver disease (Werre et al, 1970), in iron-deficiency anemia, and in thalassemia. In liver disease and thalassemia a variable number of leptocytes form codocytes.

The megalocyte

The term "megalocyte" refers specifically to the large oval erythrocytes (Fig. 11-16) seen in megaloblastic anemias (Chapter 9).

The spherocyte

When the discocyte assumes a spheroid shape it is called a spherocyte. Depending on what causes this shape, the cells either have a normal volume or they may be small as well as spherocytic, the *microspherocyte* characteristic of hereditary spherocytosis (Fig. 11-17). In the wet state they often appear as stomatospherocytes.

The transformation of discocyte into spherocyte occurs in vitro as a result of prolonged storage, as in stored bank blood. Blood smears from patients who have received stored blood may show a double population, the patient's own red cells and spherocytes from the transfused blood. The transformation of discocyte into spherocyte in vitro can be produced by various lytic agents such as saponin, bile salts, soaps, ionic detergents, some dyes, lecithin, or hemolysin, the last requiring complement. Normal blood contains a substance, absorbed by glass, that inhibits the formation of spherocytes.

In vivo, spherocytes are characteristic of congenital spherocytosis, isoimmune hemolytic anemia, and other hemolytic anemias (Chapter 13). The mechanism of spherocyte formation in vivo is discussed on p. 567.

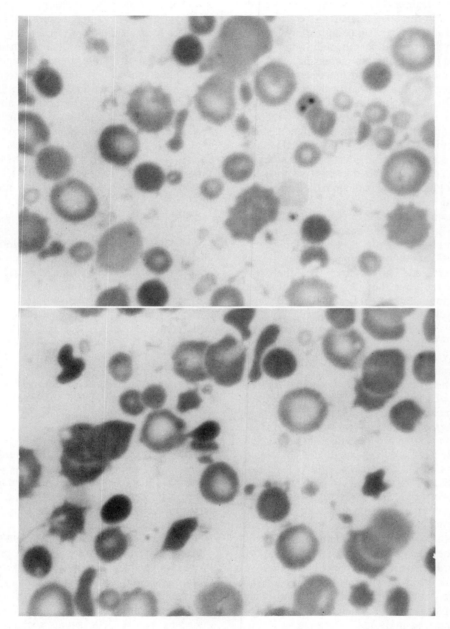

Fig. 11-14. Schizocytes. Blood smear from a 3-year-old child who expired 3 hours after suffering extensive burns in a gas explosion. (Wright's stain.)

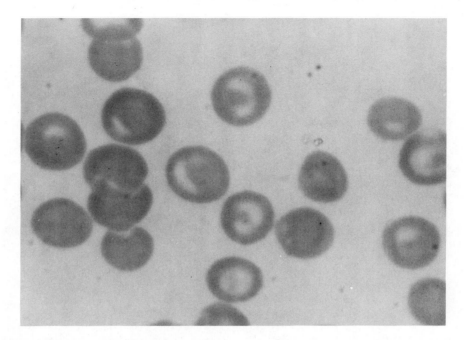

Fig. 11-15. The leptocyte. Thin, flat red blood cells from a patient with cirrhosis of the liver. Some of the cells have a central thickening and resemble codocytes.

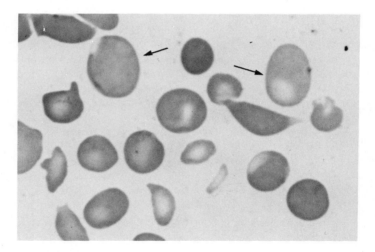

Fig. 11-16. The megalocyte. Blood smear, pernicious anemia. (Wright's stain.)

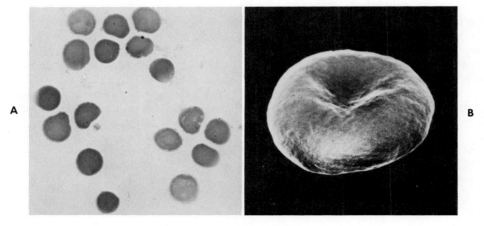

Fig. 11-17. The microspherocyte. **A,** Blood smear from patient with hereditary spherocytosis. (Wright's stain.) **B,** Scanning electron microscope photograph. (Courtesy Dr. M. Bessis.)

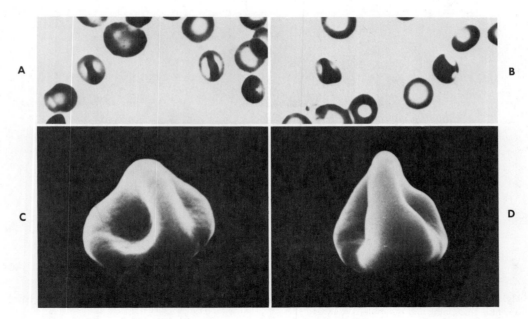

Fig. 11-18. The knizocyte. **A** and **B,** Blood smears. **C** and **D,** Scanning electron microscope photographs. (Courtesy Dr. M. Bessis.)

The knizocyte

The knizocyte (Fig. 11-18) derives its name from its similarity to a pinch bottle. It is sometimes seen in various hemolytic anemias, including hereditary spherocytosis.

Erythrocytic inclusions

Reticulocytes, diffuse basophilia, polychromatophilia, basophilic stippling

After the orthochromic normoblast loses its nucleus, a small amount of the basophilic substance characteristic of immature forms remains in the cytoplasm. This vestige of cellular maturation is composed of RNA and protoporphyrin, the latter being responsible for the fluorescence of some erythrocytes when viewed by ultraviolet light (fluorescytes). In an unfixed cell the basophilic substance is distributed evenly throughout the cell, but after fixation it may form basophilic aggregates. In a Wright-stained smear the basophilic substance may be evenly distributed throughout an erythrocyte—*diffuse basophilia*—giving the cell an overall bluish tinge. It may also have a patchy distribution, the cell appearing mottled, with orange (hemoglobin) and bluish (basophilic substance) areas. This is known as *polychromatophilia*. At other times a stained cell may show punctate aggregations of the basophilic substance in the form of a large number of fine or coarse blue granules. This is *punctate basophilia* or *basophilic stippling*. Jensen et al (1965) have shown that stipple formation is dependent on the desiccation of cells. In lead intoxication, in which basophilic stippling may be striking, the stippling reflects both an abnormality in ribosomal aggregates and iron-laden mitochondria.

Probably the most familiar form taken by the basophilic substance is that of granular and filamented aggregates, demonstrable when the young cell is exposed to dyes such as

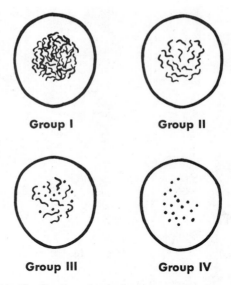

Group I **Group II**

Group III **Group IV**

Fig. 11-19. Classification of reticulocytes according to age. Group I cells are the least mature, and group IV cells are the most mature.

brilliant cresyl blue, Nile blue sulfate, or new methylene blue (CI 927). This cell is then called a *reticulocyte*. The reticulum may be abundant or sparse, depending on the stage of development (Fig. 11-19), and it may appear coarse or fine, depending on the strength and pH of the stain used, the rapidity of fixation, and the strength of the fixative. *Reticulum is poorly stained, or not at all, if glucose is present in high concentrations.*

Normally about 0.5% to 1.5% of all erythrocytes in adults

are reticulocytes. Normal values at birth range from 2.5% to 6.5%, falling to the normal adult level by the end of the second week.

The most mature reticulocytes (group IV) present the greatest technical problem in identification (Gilmer and Koepke, 1976). Since they make up about 60% of the reticulocytes in normal blood (Lowenstein, 1959), it should be agreed that a reticulocyte in group IV should have at least two distinct blue granules, not in proximity to the cell membrane. Fortunately, younger reticulocytes are predominant when the reticulocyte count is increased, but even then enough group IV cells remain to cause significant differences among observers.

The degree of reticulocytosis is proportional to erythropoietic activity. Reticulocyte counts above normal indicate that erythropoiesis is increased. Acute hemorrhage is usually followed by reticulocytosis, indicating accelerated erythropoiesis. The reticulocytosis usually is expected by the third or fourth day, but may occur earlier in massive hemorrhage. Also, in the usual case the reticulocyte level is seldom higher than 5%, but it may be 10% or higher in massive hemorrhage. Chronic hemorrhage is also followed by reticulocytosis, though not as high as in acute hemorrhage. In thalassemia major and chronic iron-deficiency anemia the reticulocyte count may be low. The response to treatment with oral iron in iron-deficiency anemia is shown in Fig. 8-10, p. 402. The degree of reticulocytosis is proportional to the severity of the anemia, but in the usual case it ranges between 5% and 10%. In chronic hemolytic anemias, persistent reticulocytosis (5% to 10%) is the result of a constant demand for new erythrocytes, and acute hemolytic episodes are generally followed by a sudden rise in reticulocytes to even higher levels.

In untreated megaloblastic anemias such as pernicious anemia the reticulocyte count is normal or low. Following treatment with hemopoietic substances a striking reticulocyte response occurs. The degree of reticulocytosis is proportional to the amount of folate or vitamin B_{12} supplied and its utilization, to the initial severity of the anemia, and to the reactivity of the bone marrow. This response is so characteristic that it is used not only in clinical diagnosis but also in the assay of hemopoietic preparations. Under optimum conditions the reticulocyte count begins to rise by the fourth day after therapy is begun and reaches a maximum on the eighth or ninth day. It usually returns to normal by the end of the second week of therapy. The magnitude of the response is roughly proportional to the severity of the anemia, i.e., inversely proportional to the erythrocyte count before therapy is begun. Formulas have been devised whereby the expected reticulocyte response can be predicted, but in a given case it may be difficult to evaluate all the factors that may produce a submaximal response. Failure to obtain a satisfactory response should lead the physician to look for localized or systemic infection, which is known to interfere with the efficacy of antianemic therapy, or to consider the possibility that the therapy used is inadequate. If a suboptimal response is caused by inadequate dosage, increasing the dosage after the first reticulocyte response has subsided will produce a second reticulocytosis. This method is used sometimes for comparing the potency of an unknown to a standard preparation. As a corollary, if a patient has been on suboptimal therapy for some time, possibly without knowledge of the physician, the reticulocyte response will not reach the predicted maximum when definitive therapy is given. The following formula, proposed by Isaacs and Friedman (1938), may be used to calculate the reticulocyte response expected in pernicious anemia, based on the erythrocyte count (in millions) before treatment.

$$\text{Reticulocytes (\%)} = \frac{82 - (22 \times \text{Initial erythrocyte count})}{1 + (0.5 \times \text{Initial erythrocyte count})}$$

In round figures the following values can be expected:

Initial count (million)	Expected reticulocytes (%)
0.5	60
1.0	40
1.5	30
2.0	20
2.5	10
3.0	5

Following a satisfactory reticulocyte response, the erythrocyte count should reach normal levels in about 8 weeks.

In general, then, an elevated reticulocyte count indicates that erythropoiesis is hyperactive. The discovery of reticulocytosis may lead to the recognition of an otherwise occult disease such as hidden hemorrhage or unrecognized hemolysis. Persistently low reticulocyte counts, particularly in the presence of anemia, usually suggest markedly defective erythropoiesis. Persistent absence of reticulocytes from the peripheral blood in aplastic anemias generally indicates a poor prognosis. A persistently elevated reticulocyte count is the rule in chronic hemolytic anemia, a drop to very low values indicating marrow failure (the so-called aplastic crisis).

Before leaving the subject of reticulocytes, a word about the error of the reticulocyte count is in order. Aside from technical factors, the reticulocyte count has certain inherent statistical errors that determine the limits of significance. The error is greater in low counts than in high ones. Part of the statistical error is the result of random distribution of the reticulocytes among adult erythrocytes. Statistical data from our laboratory are presented in Table 11-2.

Table 11-2. Statistical error of reticulocyte count

% Reticulocytes	SD (% reticulocytes)	95% range (% reticulocytes)	Significant difference (%) between 2 reticulocyte counts at given level
1	0.5	0-2	1.0
5	1.1	2.8-7.2	2.2
10	1.4	7.2-12.8	2.8
20	2.0	16-24	4.0
30	2.4	25.2-34.8	4.8
40	3.3	33.4-46.6	6.6
50	3.5	43.0-57.0	7.0

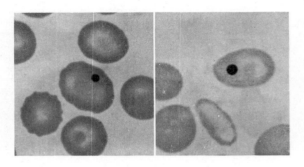

Fig. 11-20. Howell-Jolly bodies. (Wright's stain; ×1,600.)

Table 11-3. Differential features of erythrocytic inclusions

Inclusions	Preparation or stain					
	Supravital staining	Wet preparation	Phase microscopy	Wright's stain	Iron stains	Feulgen reaction
Reticulocytes	Yes	No	Yes	No	No	Negative
Basophilic stippling	Yes	No	Yes	Yes	No	Negative
Howell-Jolly bodies	Yes	Yes	Yes	Yes	No	Positive
Cabot rings	No	No	No	Yes	No	Negative
Heinz bodies	Yes	Yes	Yes	No	No	Negative
Siderotic granules	No	No	No	Yes	Yes	Negative

Howell-Jolly bodies

Howell-Jolly bodies (Fig. 11-20) are remnants of nuclear material after the normoblast nucleus is extruded. Howell-Jolly bodies are thought to represent nuclear or chromosomal remnants because they are stained by specific chromatin stains such as methyl green. They are also Feulgen positive, indicating the presence of DNA. On Wright-stained smears they appear as single, at times double, spherical bluish bodies within the erythrocytes. They are also visible in unstained and unfixed cells by phase microscopy. Howell-Jolly bodies can be distinguished from superimposed granules because they are not refractile. The differentiation from other inclusions is given in Table 11-3.

Howell-Jolly bodies are common in pernicious anemia and in various hemolytic anemias, but they are seldom seen in iron-deficiency anemia. They are frequently found after splenectomy; a discussion of the role of the spleen in removing erythrocytic inclusions is given on p. 64.

Cabot rings

Cabot rings (Fig. 11-21) are also thought to represent nuclear remnants, but they may be merely artifacts. They are not composed of chromatin, being Feulgen negative, and are not visible by phase microscopy. Schleicher (1942) has been able to produce them as artifacts and considers them to represent denatured protein following cell degeneration. Kass (1975a) identified arginine-rich histone and non-hemoglobin iron in Cabot rings found in pernicious anemia and suggested that the inclusions are a reflection of abnormal histone biosynthesis. They are seen in anemia, particularly pernicious anemia, and in lead poisoning. In a Wright-stained smear they are fine ringlike purple structures, usually single, but at times double. They are distinguished from

the ring forms of *Plasmodium* by their larger size and by the absence of a red chromatin mass.

Heinz bodies

Heinz bodies (Heinz-Ehrlich bodies) are small round inclusions (Fig. 11-22) thought to consist of denatured hemoglobin, probably preceded by methemoglobin accumulation. They are prominent in hemolytic anemias produced by agents toxic to the erythrocytes. They are single or multiple, refractile, round, oval, or irregular bodies and are never found in reticulocytes. They are invisible in Wright-stained preparations but are easily seen in reticulocyte preparations as well as in unfixed and unstained smears. *They disappear after fixation with ethyl or methyl alcohol.* Their presence is indicative of erythrocyte injury and may occasionally indicate an unsuspected hemolytic anemia (see Chapters 13 and 14 for discussion). Table 11-3 compares the features distinguishing Heinz bodies from other structures within the erythrocyte.

Siderotic granules

Siderotic granules are iron-containing structures. The erythrocytes containing them are called *siderocytes.* The granules are usually multiple, but they may be single. In Wright-stained cells they appear as very faint bluish granules (Pappenheimer bodies). They represent ferric iron aggregates and are specifically demonstrated by iron stains such as Perls' Prussian blue reaction. Siderotic granules can be found in developing normoblasts, in some of the reticulocytes, and in a small number of normal adult erythrocytes. They probably represent intraerythrocytic iron in excess or not yet incorporated into hemoglobin. Electron microscopy shows that siderotic granules are composed, in part at least,

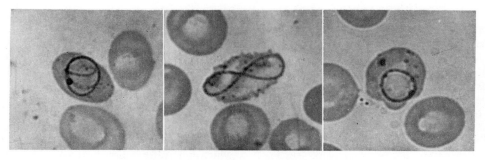

Fig. 11-21. Cabot rings. (Wright's stain; ×1,600.)

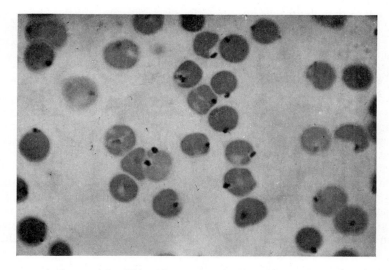

Fig. 11-22. Heinz bodies, peripheral blood from a man who drank liquid shoe polish. (Brilliant cresyl violet stain; ×950.)

of iron-laden mitochondria. They are found in large numbers when hemoglobin synthesis is impaired (the sideroblastic anemias, Chapter 8) and are absent in iron-deficiency states. They also appear in large numbers after splenectomy.

IMMUNOLOGY OF THE ERYTHROCYTE
Introduction

The blood group *antigens* of the erythrocyte are contained in both the stromal network throughout the cell and the surface ultrastructure. At the surface, antigenic groups are exposed and are available to react with specific antibodies. When we consider the spatial features of relatively small antigenic groups exposed at the surface, we realize that each erythrocyte can have a large number and variety of surface antigens without having them crowded. It is probable that blood group antigens first make their appearance in late normoblasts. Pisciotta and Hinz (1956) have shown that the normoblasts from a patient with autoimmune hemolytic anemia are agglutinated by autoagglutinins and react with antiglobulin serum.

With respect to blood group antigens and antibodies, two situations exist in human blood. In one, of which the A-B-O system is an example, the erythrocytes contain *specific group substances,* and the serum contains *naturally occurring antibodies.* These antibodies, of course, do not react with the antigen of the red cells in the same blood, as will be discussed later. In the second situation, comprising almost all other blood group systems, the serum does not normally contain antibodies; antibodies, when present, must result from artificial (iso- or auto-) immunization and are therefore *acquired antibodies* (a discussion of the nature and reactions of antibodies is found in Chapter 13).

Our knowledge of blood group antigens and antibodies began with Landsteiner's demonstrations in 1900 and 1901 that human blood could be classified into three groups (A, B, and O). In 1902, DeCastello and Sturli discovered the fourth group in this system, AB. Still other blood group systems were discovered, and the knowledge was applied to blood transfusion and other problems in immunohematology. The accumulation and application of such knowledge have not only contributed significantly to the development of diagnostic and therapeutic methods but also have stimulated as well as benefited by studies of general and special genetics.

Once established, the erythrocyte antigens are immutable

and thus a person's blood groups do not change. There are a few reports of a change in various blood groups secondary to leukemia or other neoplastic disease, but it is probably wiser to question the validity of the reports than to accept the occurrence of such a marked antigenic change. We can, however, agree that disease may alter the reactivity, which in turn might be interpreted as a change in the blood group. Note also the role of "acquired **B**" (p. 497).

Paleoimmunohematology

The present-day distribution and population frequencies of the blood groups has evolved over many centuries. Two categories of changes are involved. The first deals with the phylogenetic evolution of the present-day blood groups; the second, with the influence of population migrations to produce the modern distribution.

It is not possible to describe categorically how man's erythrocytes developed the various blood group characteristics. The various hypotheses that have been proposed read very well and are quite believable. The one that seems to provoke the least objections states that "once upon a time" there evolved a primitive blood group substance of H specificity from which, by mutations, there developed blood group substances A and B and supposedly other groups and subgroups. It is also probable that in the course of mutation three different races developed, one with group A, one with group B, and one with group O, in Europe, Asia, and America, respectively. As is the case regarding the present-day distribution of the hemoglobinopathies (Chapter 14), migration caused a mixture of the original populations.

This hypothesis undoubtedly oversimplifies the situation. The work of Wiener (1963), Wiener and Moor-Jankowski (1965, 1969), and Wiener et al (1963, 1964a, 1964c, 1965) on the blood groups of nonhuman primates is very pertinent to this question. The basic concept of local mutations followed by migration is probably valid. Even today, certain blood groups are more common in some regions than in others. It is probable that the early Europeans were Rh_0 negative and may have derived the Rh_0-positive gene from Mongolia. In the East, Rh_0 positivity is high, while rh is rare. American Indians also show a high incidence of Rh_0 positivity, and it has been suggested that they migrated originally from Mongolia via the Bering Strait to the American continent. The same derivation is postulated for the Diego factor. The Indians of Latin America are almost always Rh_0 positive. The American Indians are predominantly of group A or O, agglutinogen B being extremely rare.

Fundamentals of immunogenetics

To one interested both in blood group serology and blood coagulation, the similarity of the problem basic to both is striking. In both fields the investigator can with remarkable, even misleading, ease make something happen in vitro. In blood grouping, a mixture of erythrocytes and antiserum will either clump or not; in blood coagulation, a mixture of plasma and specially prepared blood or tissue products will either clot or not. In both instances, independent observers would agree that agglutination, or clotting, has or has not occurred, and if it has, that it occurred with a measurable intensity or rate. Agreement in the end-point measurement

indicates simply that the phenomenon can be observed objectively.

The problem in both fields is the deduction of what is the fundamental significance of the observed end point phenomenon. Because the significance of the phenomena is largely deductive, one would think that a degree of restraint would be in order in supporting any one deduction in favor of another. Certainly it could be predicted that the observed data, always valid, would be subject to reinterpretation as to significance with a frequency proportional only to the rate at which new information becomes available—obvious, and yet so frequently ignored. It would seem as if there is no limit to the number of scientific bloody noses we can receive and still not learn anything thereby.

In distinguishing shadow from substance, then, the virtues of objectivity, restraint, openmindedness, and even a sense of humor can help us to reevaluate data and to come as close to scientific truth as we can get at a given time.

As for immunohematology, specifically, the ideal understanding involves questions of serology and genetics applied to transfusion therapy, isoimmune hemolytic disease, and medicolegal problems. In the last application particularly, scientific accuracy is absolutely essential and expediency and simplification have no place.

The basic problems of serology and genetics are closely related, but perhaps the key to understanding immunogenetics as applied to blood grouping is the question of the relationship between *genes,* gene products *(agglutinogens),* and the serologic attributes of agglutinogens *(blood factors).* The simplest relationship is one in which one gene produces only one product, the one-to-one relationship between agglutinogens and antibodies. But the truth is by no means so simple, and in areas other than blood grouping it has come to be recognized that the relationship between antigen and antibody is not always one-to-one. Indeed, in most situations an antigen is able to form a whole spectrum of related antibodies. If one adheres to the one-to-one concept, then for every demonstrable serologic variant, a corresponding agglutinogen and determining gene must be postulated. On the other hand, if it is assumed that a gene determines an agglutinogen that in turn can determine a number of serologic factors, there is no need to postulate a large number of genes to match the many serologic specificities (factors) that have been discovered.

In his many publications, Wiener and associates have presented cogent arguments against the one-to-one concept and in favor of a clear distinction between genes, agglutinogens, and blood factors. It must be pointed out that while the problem is primarily a serologic one, extrapolation to gene action involves basic questions of genetics and inheritance of blood groups.

As far as notation is concerned, the following usage is adopted:

1. *Agglutinogens* and *phenotypes* are designated by regular type; e.g., A_1, A_2, etc.
2. *Genes* are designated by italics; e.g., *R, r,* etc.
3. *Blood factors* (serologic specificities) and corresponding antisera are designated by boldface type e.g., **A, A_1, C,** etc.

A-B-O blood group system

In Chapter 4 it was noted that the nucleus of the somatic cell in human beings contains 23 pairs of chromosomes or 46 individual chromosomes. Of each pair, one is derived from the mother and one from the father. Each of the chromosomes derived from the same parent is different from the others; the 23 chromosomes constitute a *chromosome set*. Each chromosome is composed of DNA molecules, and it may be assumed that the molecule or molecules at a given point (locus) determine specific properties of the cell, particularly the substances synthesized by the cell. It may also be assumed that such a locus is identical with the concept of the *gene*.

It is possible, especially in *Drosophila* having giant salivary chromosomes, to see individual bands or nodules in the chromosome that can be shown to be related to certain somatic features. The existence of a given gene is inferred from properties demonstrable in the cell (antigens, enzymes, etc.) or in the individual. As in Plato's famous example, we see the shadows on the wall (cellular or humoral constituents) and infer that they are produced by structures we do not see (genes). Hence it is necessary to distinguish clearly between the *factors* responsible for certain demonstrable features of erythrocytes and the *genes* presumed to be responsible for the factors.

In a pair of chromosomes, one derived from the mother and the other from the father, the loci (or genes) that are opposite each other in a pair are called *allelomorphic genes* or *alleles*. Alleles may be the same or different with respect to what they induce. When they are the same, their existence can only be inferred. When they are different, like the alleles determining the blood groups, their difference is detectable from the different properties they produce and from the variety of combinations. Since we are dealing with paired chromosomes, corresponding loci are the site of only one allele. If more than one pair of alleles is postulated, then more than one pair of loci must be postulated. It is possible for different alleles to occupy a given locus, these being *alternate alleles*, but in any case there can be only one pair of alleles at one time and at corresponding loci.

It is customary to denote genes by italicized capital letters. The letter may be chosen arbitrarily or may have a specific connotation; e.g., we used the notation *Hp* for haptoglobin alleles. With respect to blood group genes, the symbol *I* (for isoagglutinogen) can be used, with the addition of some distinguishing notation for alleles such as I^O and I^A, or *O* and *A*, or *R* or *r* for the Rh notation. The use of capital and small letters (as in *R* and *r*) implies that *R* is dominant and *r* recessive. The designation *OO* indicates that the individual is homozygous with respect to the gene *O*, or *phenotype* group O, and *genotype OO*. An individual of genotype *AO* is heterozygous with respect to each gene, and his phenotype depends on which of the two is dominant; in this example, *A* is dominant over *O*, and the individual is of phenotype group A. The A-B-O blood group can be used to illustrate another relation between alleles, that of *codominance*. While *A* is dominant over *O*, and *B* is also dominant over *O*, in combination with each other neither *A* nor *B* is dominant; they are instead co-dominant, and the blood group corresponding to genotype *AB* is AB.

The dominance is, in modern terms, an expression of how allelic genes produce enzymes that modify a common substrate to produce a variety of "gene products." For example, when a strong and weak gene (such as *B* and A^2, respectively, of subgroup A_2B) compete for the same substrate, agglutinogen B will be strong and agglutinogen A_2 weak. This may result in misgrouping A_2B cells as B if a weak anti-A serum is used. This characteristic of A_2B cells is important in paternity litigation but relatively unimportant in matching blood for transfusion since recipients of blood group B given A_2B blood will show only slight hemolysis. Note also that when A^2 and *O* compete for the same substrate (as in a person of genotype A^2O), the serologic expression of gene A^2 will be strong since it competes with the "amorph" (inactive) gene *O*.

Genetics

It was first thought that an individual's blood group (A-B-O) was determined by two pairs of genes as two independent loci. When data using the methods of population genetics made this assumption untenable, Bernstein, in 1925, proposed instead the existence of three multiple alleles. *A, B,* and *O*.

As distinct from systems involving only two varieties of a gene at a given locus (i.e., alleles), *multiple alleles* are closely related group of more than two that, it is implied, govern the same general type of response. Multiple alleles obey the same rules of transmission as paired alleles, since in spite of multiple possibilities, transmission necessarily involves only the two occupying the locus at that time. Multiple alleles make possible a large number of genotypes since the number of possible combinations is larger. When a gene has only two alleles, only three genotypes are possible (two homozygous and one heterozygous). The number of possible genotypes can be calculated as follows:

$$(1) \qquad g = \tfrac{1}{2}n\,(n+1)$$

where n is the number of alleles. If there are three multiple alleles, as in the basic A-B-O group, the number of possible genotypes is six.

Assuming triple alleles for the A-B-O group, the theoretical frequency of each can be calculated by the system of allele frequency analysis outlined by Stern (1960). Table 11-4 shows the theoretical frequency of the genotypes and phenotypes in the A-B-O blood group.

Table 11-4. Theoretical frequency of genotypes in A-B-O blood group according to theory of three multiple alleles*

Blood group	Genotype	Frequency	
		Genotype	Genotypes in group
O	OO	r^2	r^2
A	AA	p^2	$2pr + p^2$
	AO	$2pr$	
B	BB	q^2	$2qr + q^2$
	BO	$2qr$	
AB	AB	$2pq$	$2pq$

*r = frequency of gene *O*; p = frequency of gene *A*; q = frequency of gene *B*.

The frequency of the three allelic genes must total 1. The theoretical frequencies can be calculated and compared with the observed frequency of occurrence as obtained from blood grouping tests.

Since the frequency $\overline{O}$ of individuals of group O is r^2 and the frequency $\overline{A}$ of individuals of group A is $p^2 + 2pr$. the frequency of $\overline{O}$ plus $\overline{A}$ is as follows:

(2)
$$\overline{O} + \overline{A} = r^2 + p^2 + 2pr$$

or

(3)
$$\overline{O} + \overline{A} = (p + r)^2$$

or

(4)
$$p + r = \sqrt{\overline{O} + \overline{A}}$$

Likewise:

(5)
$$\overline{O} + \overline{B} = q^2 + 2qr + r^2$$

or

(6)
$$\overline{O} + \overline{B} = (q + r)^2$$

or

(7)
$$q + r = \sqrt{\overline{O} + \overline{B}}$$

Formulas 4 and 7 can be simplified by substituting $\sqrt{\overline{O}}$ for r, since if:

$$r^2 = \overline{O}$$

then

(8)
$$r = \sqrt{\overline{O}}$$

Accordingly:

(9)
$$p = \sqrt{\overline{O} + \overline{A}} - \sqrt{\overline{O}}$$

and

(10)
$$q = \sqrt{\overline{O} + \overline{B}} - \sqrt{\overline{O}}$$

We can now express the sum of the three frequencies, p, q, and r, according to formulas 8 to 10, as follows:

(11) $p + q + r = \sqrt{\overline{O} + \overline{A}} - \sqrt{\overline{O}} + \sqrt{\overline{O} + \overline{B}} - \sqrt{\overline{O}} + \sqrt{\overline{O}}$

and since the sum of the frequencies is 1, then:

(12)
$$\sqrt{\overline{O} + \overline{A}} + \sqrt{\overline{O} + \overline{B}} - \sqrt{\overline{O}} = 1$$

The validity of this derivation can be tested against observed frequencies (Table 11-5). The observed sum of the frequencies in each group is close enough to 1 to indicate that the theory of three alleles for the A-B-O blood group is correct.

Inclusion of the subgroups of A increases the number of genotypes and phenotypes that are possible. Table 11-6 includes the important A^1 and A^2 alleles. The other subgroups of A are very rare.

The A-B-O classification is based on the presence in the erythrocyte of either, neither, or both of two antigenic and type-specific polysaccharide substances, A and B. Group O cells have neither, group A cells only A, group B cells only B, and group AB cells have both. When cells of a given group are injected into a recipient of a different group or into an animal, specific antibodies are produced, anti-**A,** anti-**B,** or both, depending on the antigen injected. These antibodies are capable of specifically agglutinating erythrocytes having the corresponding antigen. The antibody is therefore called an *agglutinin* and the specific antigen in the erythrocyte an *agglutinogen.*

Human blood normally contains isoagglutinins of the A-B-O system, but fortunately they are not specific for the erythrocytes present in the same blood. The agglutinogens appear at an earlier age than the isoagglutinins. Group O cells are accompanied by anti-**A** and anti-**B** agglutinins in the serum, group A cells by anti-**B** agglutinins, group B cells by anti-**A** agglutinins, and group AB cells by no agglutinins. It will be noted that autoagglutination is avoided by this combination of agglutinins and agglutinogens. The basic relationships of the A-B-O blood groups are shown in Table 11-6. *The blood group is determined by the agglutinogen of the erythrocytes.*

In further study of the agglutination reactions it becomes apparent that A cells do not always react similarly with anti-**A** sera. It has been discovered that subgroups of A exist, and these have been designated as A_1 and A_2. Subgroups A_3, A_4, A_5, and A_0 have also been identified, but they are weak reactors and rare. A_0 can not be detected with potent anti-**A** sera but is detected readily with group O sera.

Subgroups of B (B_w, B_x, B_z, and "weak" B) have been described but have not been applied to either blood banking or medicolegal problems. However, the existence of subgroups A_1 and A_2 increase the possible combinations in group AB by producing subgroups such as A_1B, A_2B, etc. The major phenotypes in the A-B-O system are O, A_1, A_2, B, A_1B, and A_2B. The genotype is determined by the combinations of allelic genes O, A^1, A^2, and B (Table 11-6).

Inheritance

The inheritance pattern depends on four sets of allelic genes: O, A^1, A^2, and B, as shown in Table 11-7. One can predict the possible phenotypes of the children if the mother's and father's phenotypes are known. Blood group systems other than A-B-O also follow a definite inheritance pattern. The rules governing the inheritance of blood groups have been applied in cases of disputed parentage. Regarding the basic A-B-O system, these rules may be summarized as follows:

Rule 1: Agglutinogens A or B cannot be present in the blood of a child unless present in the blood of one or both parents.

Rule 2: A parent with group AB must transmit to the child either A or B and therefore cannot be the parent of a child with group O.

Rule 3: A person with group O cannot be the parent of a child with group AB.

Rule 4: The agglutinogen A_1 cannot appear in the child unless it is present in at least one of the parents. An A_1 parent of genotype A^1A^2 can have an A_2 child.

Table 11-7 shows the inheritance pattern of the basic A-B-O groups and Table 11-8 extends the rules of inheritance to the A_1A_2 subgroups. The discovery of subgroups A_1 and A_2 does not alter the validity of the three basic laws of inheritance, but it is necessary to extend them by postulating an

Table 11-5. Representative data on racial distribution of A-B-O blood groups: statistical test of Bernstein's theory*

Race	No. of people	Frequencies of groups				p	q	r	p+q+r
		O	A	B	AB				
English	500	0.464	0.434	0.072	0.031	0.268	0.052	0.681	1.001
French	500	0.432	0.426	0.112	0.030	0.262	0.074	0.657	0.993
Italian	500	0.472	0.380	0.110	0.038	0.237	0.077	0.687	1.001
Serbian	500	0.380	0.418	0.156	0.046	0.268	0.107	0.516	0.991
Greek	500	0.382	0.416	0.162	0.040	0.262	0.107	0.618	0.987
Bulgarian	500	0.390	0.406	0.142	0.062	0.271	0.108	0.624	1.003
Arab	500	0.432	0.324	0.190	0.050	0.209	0.129	0.660	0.998
Turk (Macedonia)	500	0.368	0.380	0.186	0.066	0.256	0.136	0.607	0.999
Russian	1,000	0.407	0.312	0.218	0.063	0.210	0.152	0.638	1.000
Hindu	1,000	0.313	0.190	0.412	0.085	0.149	0.291	0.560	1.000

*From Wiener and Wexler, 1958.

Table 11-6. Relationship between agglutinogens and agglutinins in complete A-B-O system*

Blood group (phenotype) and frequency	Genotype and frequency	Agglutinogens on erythrocytes	Agglutinins in serum	Serum agglutinates erythrocytes of blood groups					
				O	A_1	A_2	B	A_1B	A_2B
O (45.00%)	OO (45.00%)	O	Anti-A_1 Anti-**A** Anti-**B**	−	+	+	+	+	+
A_1 (31.39%)	A^1A^1 (3.53%) A^1A^2 (2.56%) A^1O (25.30%)	A_1	Anti-**B** (Anti-**H**)†	−	−	− (+)†	+	+	+
A_2 (9.61%)	A^2A^2 (0.46%) A^2O (9.15%)	A_2	Anti-**B** (Anti-A_1)†	−	− (+)†	−	+	+	+
B (10.00%)	BB (0.72%) BO (9.28%)	B	Anti-A_1‡ Anti-**A**‡	−	+	+	−	+	+
A_1B (2.94%)	A^1B (2.94%)	A_1;B	None (Anti-A_2)†	−	−	(+)†	−	−	−
A_2B (1.06%)	A^2B (1.06%)	A_2;B	None (Anti-A_1)†	−	(+)†	−	−	−	−

*Frequency data for white persons in the United States from Albritton, 1952.
†Occasionally serum from group A_1 or A_2 blood will agglutinate cells of the other subgroup (A_2 or A_1, respectively). These rare agglutinins rare probably of anti-**H** and anti-A_1 specificities, respectively.
‡Most anti-**A** sera show a higher titer for A_1 than for A_2 and react very weakly with the rare A_3 cells.

additional law (rule 4). In applying this law the genotype must be taken into account; e.g., phenotype A_1 may be genotype A^1A^1, A^1A^2, or A^1O (Table 11-8).

Regarding medicolegal application of immunohematology (discussed on p. 514), it might be well to point out that, in general, the blood groups are well established at the time of birth, and blood grouping can be done from cord blood or anytime thereafter. It must be noted, however, that there are some blood factors that may be incompletely developed at birth. These are A_1, **H, I,** and **Le.** The isoagglutinins of the

A-B-O system can be detected with confidence at the age of 3 to 6 months; the titer reaches a maximum in the 5- to 10-year age group. The Rh factors present no problem.

Blood group "cis-AB"

There is a rare exception to the usual inheritance of the A-B-O groups as outlined below. It has been found that in over a dozen persons in several families group AB is transmitted as if by a single allele from a single parent so that in the mating, AB and O children of group O are possible, contrary to expectation (Tables 11-7 and 11-8). This very rare situation has resulted in a blood group called the "cis-AB" group (Reviron et al, 1968) (sometimes called AB*). Persons having this rare allele can be either cis-A_1B or cis-A_2B. The reactions with anti-**A** are typical but are weak with the usual anti-**B** antisera. The reaction is stronger when anti-**B** from group A_2 individuals is used. The serum of a person of group cis-AB contains an anti-**B** isoagglutinin that clumps group B or AB red cells but not cis-AB cells.

The most recent study (Badet et al, 1978; Sabo et al, 1978) indicate that the gene *AB* causes a mutation of a transferase so that it is active in transferring both galactose and *N*-acetylgalactosamine.

The possibility of having a parent with cis-AB group must be taken into account whenever the exclusion of paternity is based on the rule that a person with a group AB cannot be the parent of a child with group O.

Origin of isoagglutinins

We have already spoken of the isoantibodies of the A-B-O blood group as "natural" and pointed out that the com-

Table 11-7. Inheritance pattern of basic A-B-O blood groups*

Phenotypes of parents	Phenotypes possible in children	Phenotypes not possible in children
O and O	O	A, B, AB
O and A	A, O	B, AB
O and B	B, O	A, AB
A and A	A, O†	B, AB
A and B	AB, O,‡ A,§ B†	None
B and B	B, O§	A, AB
O and AB	A, B	O, AB
A and AB	A, AB, B†	O
B and AB	B, AB, A§	O
AB and AB	A, B, AB	O

*From Albritton, 1952.
†Not possible if either parent is genotype *AA*.
‡Possible if one parent is genotype *AO* and the other *BO*.
§Not possible if one parent is genotype *BB*.

Table 11-8. Inheritance pattern of A_1-A_2-B-O blood groups*

Phenotypes of parents	Phenotypes possible in children	Phenotypes not possible in children
A_1 and O	O,† A_1, A‡	B, A_1B, A_2B
A_1 and A_1	O,† A_1, A_2§	B, A_1B, A_2B
A_1 and A_2	O, A_1, A_2	B, A_1B, A_2B
A_1 and B	O, A_1, A_2,‡ B, A_1B, A_2B‡	None
A_1 and A_2B	A_1, A_2,‡ B, A_1B, A_2 B	O
A_1B and O	A_1, B	O, A_2, A_1B, A_2B
A_1B and A_1	A_1, B, A_1B, A_2B‡	O, A_2
A_1B and A_2	A_1, B, A_2B	O, A_2, A_1B
A_1B and A_2B	A_1, B, A_1B, A_2B	O, A_2
A_1B and B	A_1, B, A_1B	O, A_2, A_2B
A_1B and A_1B	A_1, B, A_1B	O, A_2, A_2B
A_2 and O	O, A_2	A_1, B, A_1B, A_2B
A_2 and A_2	O, A_2	A_1, B, A_1B, A_2B
A_2 and B	O, A_2, B, A_2B	A_1, A_1B
A_2B and O	A_2, B	O, A_1, A_1B, A_2B
A_2B and A_2	A_2, B, A_2B	O, A_1, A_1B
A_2B and B	A_2, B, A_2B	O, A_1, A_1B
A_2B and A_2B	A_2, B, A_2B	O, A_1, A_1B

*From Albritton, 1952.
†Possible if parent A_1 is of genotype A^1O.
‡Possible if parent A_1 is of genotype A^1A^2.
§Possible if one parent is genotype A^1A^2 and the other is A^1A^2 or A^1O.

bination of agglutinogens on the erythrocytes and the isoantibodies in the serum are such that there is no mutual specificity and thus no autoagglutination. There have been a number of suggestions as to how this situation comes about. If we accept that the origin of isoantibodies is genetically determined (as inferred from a comparison of titers of isoagglutinins in monovular twins with those from biovular twins and other observations) and also that they are the result of antigenic stimulation (intrinsic or extrinsic), then several explanations are possible.

It has been suggested (Wiener, 1951) that natural isoantibodies are "cryptogenic" in the sense that they are formed in response to an exogenous antigen such as food. Some experiments with germ-free and conventional chickens (Springer et al, 1959) suggest that isoagglutinins are heteroantibodies (i.e., the antigenic stimulus is exogenous) that cross-react with the A-B-O blood group agglutinogens. Another theory supposes that, early in fetal life, the agglutinogens stimulate the production of isoagglutinins, which are selectively absorbed so as to bring about the adult situation. More in accordance with modern concepts is the hypothesis that the clones of immunocytes that produce an isoagglutinin (e.g., anti-**B**) are not eliminated in a person of corresponding blood group A, while those that produce anti-**A** are destroyed.

Missing isoagglutinins

The absence of isoagglutinins in a person over 1 year of age indicates four possibilities: (1) most commonly, a congenital or acquired agammaglobulinemia, (2) the presence of a very weakly reacting homologous receptor (e.g., in one case the patient was thought to have group O but, lacking anti-**A** isoagglutinins, proved to have group A_4), (3) the presence of a blood chimera, or (4) a person with the rare blood group A_{el}.

Since isoagglutinins are immunoglobulins of the gamma type, their absence (or presence in very low titer) is characteristic of children with congenital types of agammaglobulinemia and of some adults with acquired agammaglobulinemia. Before specific immunoelectrophoretic technics became available, the absence of isoagglutinins in the serum of a child was presumptive or confirmatory evidence that the child had agammaglobulinemia. In the adult, acquired agammaglobulinemia caused by diseases such as syphilis, leukemia, lymphoma, etc., will also be manifest by reduced or undetectable titers of isoagglutinins.

A number of cases of blood chimera (from the Greek *khimaira*, in mythology a frightful monster made up of parts of different animals—therefore a mixture of blood cells of different groups) have been reported. Chimeras are produced in biovular twins when, because vascular anastomoses are present, normoblasts from one twin lodge in the bone marrow of the second and produce erthrocytes that are of the blood group of the donor twin; if the twins are of different blood groups, then the recipient twin will have a mixed population of erythrocytes. The "foreign" erythrocytes may be in the minority, but there are cases reported where they are in the majority. Chimera of blood cells was described first in cattle (Owen, 1945) but has been found also in sheep and human beings. Beattie et al (1964)

describe one interesting case in which one population of erythrocytes was group A and sickled, whereas the other was group B and did not sickle. Blood chimerism may also be an expression of chromosomal mosaicism in hermaphrodites. Chimerism can be demonstrated by differential agglutination. The technic of differential immunofluorescence is particularly impressive (Matej, 1962; Prokop and Uhlenbruck, 1969).

It also should be noted that there is a reduction in the titer of isoagglutinins with advancing age. In the elderly (70 to 80 years of age or more) there is a surprisingly low titer. This may account for the impression that transfusion reactions seldom occur in elderly recipients.

Lectins

The ability of lectins (extracts of some plant seeds, leaves, or roots) to agglutinate erythrocytes was recognized many years before the discovery of blood groups. Many lectins with various specificities are now recognized, and a complete discussion can be found in Prokop and Uhlenbruck (1969) and Gold and Balding (1975). The lectins in more common use and their specificity and application can be summarized as follows:

1. Lectins of anti-**H** specificity such as from *Ulex europaeus*—can also be used to detect **H** in body secretions.
2. Lectins of anti-**H** and anti-**B** specificity such as *Evonymus europaeus*.
3. Lectins of anti-**A** specificity such as *Dolichos biflorus*—useful as an anti-A_1 reagent.
4. Lectins with anti-**B** specificity such as *Evonymus sieboldianus*.
5. Lectins of anti-**B** plus anti-**A** (anti-**C**) activity such as *Sophora japonica*—other lectins have stronger specificity against **B** than **A** and vice versa.
6. Lectins of anti-**N** specificity such as *Vicia graminea*, *Vicia unijuga*, certain species of *Bauhinia*, and *Molucella laevis*.
7. Lectins of anti-**M** specificity such as *Iberis amara* have been described but, according to Wiener (personal communication), do not work.

Agglutinins from snails and other animals

Prokop et al (1965) have described a new type of antibody-like substance derived from the garden snail *(Helix hortensis)* that identifies a specificity of human group A (and animal) erythrocytes called A_{hel}. They found the snail to have a blood group system of B substance in the tissues with anti-**A** in the albumin gland, the latter called anti-A_{hel}. The antibody has been localized to the albumin gland of the sexual apparatus of the snail. They believe that in the snail the antibody protects the eggs during their exposure to open air. Snail *(Helix)* agglutinins and similar antibody-like substances from eggs of other animals are, for this reason, also called "protectins."

Snail agglutinin from *Otala lactea* is useful in that it specifically agglutinates erythrocytes of groups A_1, A_2, A_1B, and A_2B. It also agglutinates erythrocytes of groups A_3 and A, is specifically absorbed by these erythrocytes, and the eluates show anti-**A** activity.

Some snails and bacteria contain enzymes that specifically destroy individual blood group substances. Extracts of *Helix pomatia* contain **A**-destroying enzyme.

Chemistry of blood group substances

Blood group substances act as antigens and, together with corresponding antibody, define the various blood group systems.

Blood group substances can be classified into four categories:

1. Glycoproteins (secreted A-B-H substances, secreted Lewis substances, erythrocyte M-N-S and I mucoids, and P_1-active mucoids derived from hydatid cysts). These are glycoproteins having a high carbohydrate content and are water soluble.
2. Glycolipids (A and B substances derived from erythrocytes). These are composed of sphingosine, fatty acids, and carbohydrate and are relatively insoluble in water.
3. Polysaccharides, blood group–active substances derived from plants (not phytohemagglutinins), some bacteria, and molluscs.
4. Lipopolysaccharides (from *Salmonella* and *Escherichia*).

It has been found that **A-B-H** and **M-N-S** blood group substances are very stable. They are resistant to heat and drying and can be demonstrated in mummies.

New technics for studying the chemical structure of the antigenic determinants of **A, B, H, Le₁,** and **Le^H** substances have shown that, by degradation, the derived oligosaccharides have blood group activity (Lloyd and Kabat, 1968; Prokop and Uhlenbruck, 1969; Watkins, 1967). It has been shown that blood group substances all contain 15 common amino acids and the same five sugars; L-fucose, D-galactose, *N*-acetylglucosamine, *N*-acetylgalactosamine, and *N*-acetylneuraminic acid. The general structure is probably that of a long polypeptide chain with short sugar side chains. Additional evidence for the concept that specific blood group substances are derived from a "precursor substance" is found in the observation that nonsecretors of **A-B-H** and **Lewis** substance have a glycoprotein of very low fucose content in their saliva. This is thought to be the "precursor substance" that, by specific gene action, is converted to specific blood group substances. The precursor substance cross-reacts with type XIV pneumococcal antiserum; after degradation the group-specific substances also acquire this characteristic. The serologic specificity of the blood group substances resides in the one sugar that seems responsible for immunologic specificity, hence the "immunodominant sugar." These are as follows:

A substance	*N*-Acetyl-D-galactosamine
B substance	D-Galactose
H substance	L-Fucose
Le^a substance	L-Fucose

The cross-reactivity with pneumococcal antiserum of precursor substance and of **A-B-H** and **Le^a** substance has been traced to the common component β-galactosyl(1-4)-*N*-acetylglucosamine.

Several specificities are built into the macromolecule of glycoprotein, although the manifest specificity is the result of a characteristic linkage of the subunits. For example, in a group AB person both A and B specificity are carried on the same macromolecule; some of the carbohydrate chains are assembled as **A**-active and others as **B**-active structures. The same macromolecule has also **H**-active and **Le^a**-active structures. Individual specificities can be enhanced by destroying the others, i.e., treatment of **A** substance with A-destroying enzyme (from *Treponema foetus* or *Helix pomatia*) liberates *N*-acetylgalactosamine and the residue has enhanced **H** activity. Treatment of **B** substance with B-destroying enzyme (from *Treponema foetus, Clostridium maebashi*, or with coffee-bean α-galactosidase) liberates galactose and the residue has enhanced **H** activity. Treatment of **H** substance with H-destroying enzyme liberates L-fucose and, in some instances, the residue develops activity. Treatment of **Le^a** substance similarly leaves a residue that only reacts with type XIV pneumococcal antiserum.

The observations indicate that **H** substance is the precursor to the formation of **A, B,** and **Lewis (Le)** substances. **Le** substance is, in turn, derived from a "precursor substance." The formation of **H** substance is a prerequisite for the formation of the other blood group substances; the enzymes controlled by genes *A* and *B,* for instance, can all effect the addition of *N*-acetylgalactosamine (for **A** substance) or D-galactose (for **B** substance) if the fucosyl group (in **H** substance) is already added to the terminal galactose unit of the precursor substance. The *H* gene controls the addition of fucose to the precursor substance, but this can take place only if the person is a secretor (genotype *SeSe* or *Sese*). In the absence of the secretor gene, **A, B,** and **H** substances cannot be formed.

Subgroups of A

Subgroups of A were first recognized in 1911 when von Dungern and Hirszfield described two different agglutinins of A specificity in the serum of persons with group B or O blood. The subgroups of A were at first called "A" and "a" but later were called A_1 and A_2. Antisera called anti-**A** are derived from persons with blood group O and contain a mixture of antibodies of closely related specificities. Most antisera called anti-A will agglutinate A_1 cells strongly and A_2 cells weakly. Some will fail to agglutinate A_2 cells. If such an antiserum is adsorbed with erythrocytes of group A_2, the adsorbed serum has only anti-A_1 specificity (called adsorbed anti-A serum) and can be used to distinguish blood group A_1 from A_2 and A_1B from A_2B. A useful reagent for distinguishing A_1 from A_2 is the phytohemagglutinin extracted from the seeds of *Dolichos biflorus*. This phytohemagglutinin has specific anti-A_1 activity when properly diluted. The concentrated extract is said to agglutinate A_1B and A_2B cells but not A_3B cells.

There are several other subgroups of A (Table 11-9). The only one of any importance is A_3, usually recognized when a mixed field agglutination reaction is observed with anti-**A** antiserum. However, at times the degree of agglutination is so slight that it will be missed. Rarer subgroups may, in instances when there is no agglutination by anti-**A** antiserum but agglutination by the serum of group O blood, represent blood group C (Wiener and Ward, 1966). As noted in Table 11-9, a transfusion reaction due to A_x has been reported.

Table 11-9. Subgroups of A

Subgroup	Comments	Subgroup	Comments
A_1	The major subgroup; reacts strongly with anti-**A** serum	A_i	So-called "intermediate"; agglutinated by both anti-A_1 and anti-**H**
A_2	Reacts weakly with most anti-**A** sera and with some not at all	A_x	Very rare; incidence about 1 in 500,000 (Gammelgaard, 1944; Glover and Walford, 1958); can cause transfusion reaction if recipient has high titer of anti-**A** (Schmidt et al, 1959)
A_3	Incidence 1 in 1,000; reacts very weakly with mixed field agglutination or not at all with anti-**A** sera; serum contains no anti-**A** but may contain anti-A_1; in routine typing, persons of A_3B may be called group B; the lectin from *Phaseolus lunatus* agglutinates A_1B, A_2B, or A_3B cells; concentrated extracts of *Dolichos biflorus* agglutinate only A_1B and A_2B cells (Friedenreich, 1936; Wiener and Silverman, 1941)	A_m	Very rare (Wiener and Gordon, 1956; Junquiera et al, 1957)
		A_o	Very rare (Grove-Rasmussen et al, 1952; Ellis and Crawley, 1957)
		A_{end}	Very rare (Moore et al, 1961)
		A_{el}	Very rare (Sturgeon et al, 1964)

Table 11-10. Serologic reactions in group A and subgroups

Phenotype	Direct grouping (cells)					Reverse grouping (serum)			
	Anti-**A**	Anti-**B**	Anti-A_1*	Group O serum	Anti-**H**†	A_1 cells	A_2 cells	B cells	O cells
A_1	+	−	+	+	+ to −§	−	−	+	−
A_i	+ to ±	−	±	+	+	−	−	+	−
A_2	+ to ±	−	−	+	+	−	−	+	−
A_3	±	−	−	±	+	−	−	+	−
A_x	± to −	−	−	+	+	+ to −	−	+	−
A_m	−	−	−	+	−	−	−	+	−
A_{end}	−	−	−	±	+	−	−	+	−
A_{el}	−	−	−	−	+	−	−	+	−

*Adsorbed anti-**A** or *Dolichos biflorus* lectin.
†*Ulex europaeus* lectin.
§Most reactions are weak, some are very strong, and about 20% are negative.

The serologic reaction in group A and subgroups are given in Table 11-10.

Weak or nonreacting subgroups of A can be confirmed by detecting the **A** substance in the saliva if the person is a secretor. Also, if the erythrocytes are exposed to anti-**A** serum, the eluate will contain anti-**A**, indicating the cell was capable of adsorbing anti-**A** even though not agglutinated by it.

Subgroups of B

Group B cells are, as noted for group A cells, variable in the intensity with which they are agglutinated by anti-**B** serum. Strongly agglutinated cells are designated B_1 and weakly agglutinated cells are designated B_2. Other weakly reacting variants of B have been described; B_3 (Wiener and Cioffi, 1972), B_v, B_w, B_x, and B_m (Dunsford et al, 1956; Kitahama et al, 1957; Erskine and Socha, 1978). Simmons and Twaitt (1975) report on a family in which five members had a weak B variant with normal levels of **B** and **H** substances in the saliva of the secretors. An additional and important weakly reacting B, acquired B, is discussed in the following section.

Acquired B (pseudo B)

Cameron et al (1959) described seven instances of patients with blood group A_1 who developed a B-like red cell antigen. This is an acquired characteristic that is related to concurrent disease such as carcinoma of the colon, carcinoma of the cervix, gangrene, or various infections. All of the reports to date show that only persons of group A_1 or A_2 are susceptible to this acquired characteristic. Many organisms, usually gram-negative, produce soluble B-like antigens in culture. It has been shown that polysaccharides from gram-negative bacilli, notably *Escherichia coli* O_{86}, can be adsorbed in vitro by erythrocytes of group A or O. It is presumed that the same phenomenon occurs in vivo, bacterial and possibly other substances that act like B antigens being adsorbed onto the surface of the group A erythrocyte. Marsh (1960) believes that the product of bacterial growth acts as an enzyme that modifies the basic nonspecific group substance within the erythrocyte. While most of the reactions with anti-**B** are weak, some are sufficiently strong to produce an apparent change in blood group from A to AB. There is evidence also that at times the acquired B has sufficient avidity for the isoagglutinin anti-**B** in the serum of a group A patient to produce autohemolysis.

The possibility of an acquired B should be considered in patients with gastrointestinal carcinoma and bacterial infections, particularly those due to gram-negative bacteria. It should be suspected when, in an apparent A_1B person, the reaction with anti-**B** is weak and when the serum contains isoagglutinin anti-**B**.

Another acquired characteristic, the Thomsen phenomenon, or T transformation, might be mentioned here, although the transformation is not the acquisition of a group specificity but rather panagglutination (Prokop and Uhlenbruck, 1969). It can occur when the surface of the erythrocyte is altered by viruses, bacteria, or their enzymatic products. It is thought that all erythrocytes have the T receptor but that this is latent and therefore the erythrocytes are not agglutinated by the anti-T normally present in adult serum. Following "activation" or "transformation" by microbial action, however, the cells become panagglutinable by all adult sera, including the patient's own. Anti-T is not present in the serum of the newborn, usually appearing at about the age of 6 months. Therefore erythrocytes exhibiting the T transformation will not be agglutinated by cord blood serum.

A^b group

This is a rare blood type described by Anderson (1960) that behaves somewhat like an acquired B but is different in that (1) it has been found in healthy persons, (2) it is inherited, (3) it may take the form of either A_1^b or A_2^b, but the latter is more common, and (4) the b characteristic is not absorbed onto group O cells.

Blood group O and the H substance

Shortly after Bernstein proposed the theory of multiple allelic genes for the A-B-O blood group, it was found that some sera agglutinated cells of group O. At first it was thought that the reaction was with an agglutinogen on group O cells and that, analogous to genes A and B determining agglutinogens A and B, the O agglutinogen resulted from the action of gene O. Later it became obvious that the agglutination was not detecting the product of gene O but rather another and quite different substance. This was called **H** substance because the problem was clarified in part by the use of anti-*Shigella* serum and the antibody was therefore thought to be "heterogenetic." The antiserum that detects the **H** substance is then called anti-**H**. The **H** substance is the product of gene *H*, a gene widely prevalent in humans and in animals. Anti-**H** reacts preferentially with group O and group A_2 cells. Erythrocytes of group A_1 show a spectrum of agglutinability by anti-**H** ranging from complete clumping to no agglutination, most of the reactions being weak (or negative in 20% of the cases). The **H** substance also occurs in secreted fluids. Erythrocytes of the Bombay blood group (see following discussion) have no **H** substance and are not agglutinated by anti-**H**. Eel serum and the lectin from *Ulex europaeus* have specific anti-**H** activity.

It is generally agreed that the genes *A*, *B*, and *O* and genes *H* and *h* compete for the same blood group precursor substance. These genes, in turn, are influenced by gene *X*, which is necessary to convert the blood group precursor substance to a form susceptible to the action of the *A*, *B*, and *H* genes. Genes *X*, *A*, *B*, and *H* then act in conjunction with each other and are called "epistatic." Characteristically, both of a set of epistatic genes must be present for the result of gene action to appear. The concept of epistatic genes applies to (1) the basis for the Bombay (O_h) blood group and (2) the basis for the A-B-H and Lewis secretor types (Fig. 11-23).

Bombay (O_h) blood group

The Bombay blood group was described in 1951 by Bhende et al (1952). Characteristic are the following reactions: (1) the erythrocytes are not agglutinated by anti-**A**, anti-**B**, or anti-**H** (note that unless anti-**H** is used the cells would be classified as group O), (2) the serum contains anti-**A**, anti-**B**, and anti-**H**, and (3) the saliva contains neither **A** nor **B** nor **H** substance. As the name indicates, the group was first discovered in Bombay, and although relatively rare in India (1 in 13,000) and even more rare in other countries, it can present problems in transfusion practice. It is recommended that testing with anti-**H** be done on the blood of all persons of Indian derivation. Genetically, persons of group O_h lack the gene *X* and are of genotype *xx*. Lacking *X* they cannot produce **A-B-H** substances from the blood group precursor substance.

Blood factors A_1 and A

The observation that group A cells are agglutinated by anti-**A** serum led to the postulation of agglutinogen A. With the discovery of subgroups of A, it was observed that A_1 cells are agglutinated by both anti-**A** and anti-A_1, and the A_2 cells do not react with anti-A_1 serum.

It might be assumed, then, that subgroup A_1 cells have two agglutinogens, A and A_1. However, if this were so, then in the mating $A_1 \times O$, half of the children should be of genotype A_1O and half of genotype AO. Instead, in some families all the children are A_1, in others half are A_1 and half are O, while in occasional families half of the children are A_1 and half are A_2. Thus, rather than a one-to-one relationship, gene A_1 gives rise to the agglutinogen A_1, having two serologic manifestations (or blood factors) A_1 and A (Table 11-11).

Blood factor C

Another blood factor in the A-B-O group is factor **C**. The serum of group O individuals agglutinates cells of groups A, B, and AB but not cells of group O, since it contains both anti-**A** and anti-**B**. Two observations indicate that the system is not quite so simple: (1) adsorption of group O serum with A cells reduces the titer of anti-**A** as expected but in addition often reduces the titer of anti-**B** as well and (2) transfusion of group A blood into a group O recipient raises the titer of anti-**A** in the recipient as expected but also often raises the titer of anti-**B**. Again, adsorption of this serum with group A cells reduces the titer of both anti-**A** and anti-**B**. While it is possible to propose several possible explanations for these observations, the one consistent with other serologic attributes of the erythrocyte is that erythrocytes of group A and group B share a common serologic attribute designated blood factor **C** (Wiener, 1953; Wiener and Ward, 1966; Socha and Wiener, 1973) and that serum from a group O individual contains not only anti-**A** and anti-**B** but anti-**C** as well.

On the basis that only group O individuals can produce anti-**C**, Wiener and Unger (1955) proposed an explanation for the relatively high incidence of A-B-O hemolytic disease in which the mother is group O and the baby group A or B and the extremely low incidence in other A-B-O combinations. He proposes that it is anti-**C** that is produced in the mother and that crosses the placental barrier to induce hemo-

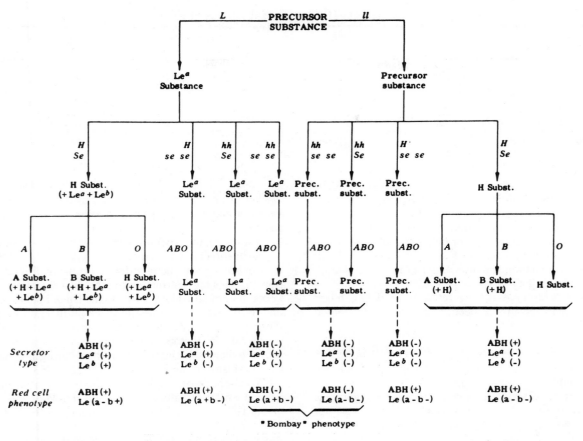

Fig. 11-23. Suggested genetic pathways for the biosynthesis of blood group **A, B, H, Le^a**, and **Le^b** substances. (From Watkins, 1967.)

Table 11-11. Blood cell factors and naturally occurring antibodies in A-B-O blood group*

Phenotype	Agglutinogen	Blood factors	Antibodies in serum
O	None	None	Anti-**A**, anti-**A₁**, anti-**B**, anti-**C**
A₁	A₁	**A, A₁, C**	Anti-**B** (and anti-**H**†)
A₂	A₂	**A, C**	Anti-**B** (and anti-**A₁**†)
B	B	**B, C**	Anti-**A** and Anti-**A₁**
A₁B	A₁ and B	**A, A₁, C, B**	(Anti-**H**†)
A₂B	A₂ and B	**A, C, B**	(Anti-**A₁**†)

*From Wiener, 1961.
†Present only in a few individuals.

lytic disease in the newborn. With regard to combining sites, Jones and Kaneb (1960) have shown that in agglutinogen A the combining sites for anti-**A** and anti-**C** are the same or overlap, as are those for anti-**B** and anti-**C**. From this it follows that because of a large number of overlapping combinations there may be multiple serologic attributes of a given agglutinogen.

Secretion of group-specific substances in saliva

A-B-O blood group substances are found in the body in two forms, one soluble in alcohol (found in the erythrocytes and body cells of all individuals with the appropriate blood group) and the other as water-soluble mucopolysaccharides.

The soluble form is not found in all individuals, only 75% of Caucasoids having it in their body. These are called *secretors*, as contrasted to the 25% *nonsecretors*. The watersoluble mucopolysaccharides occur in highest concentration in the secretory organs (salivary glands, intestinal mucosa, pancreas, and seminal vesicles). Saliva is a ready fluid for their detection. Immediately after collection, the saliva specimens should be heated for 20 minutes in a boiling water bath to destroy bacteria and blood group enzymes (Weiner and Socha, 1976).

The test for secretors is based on the ability of saliva to inhibit specific agglutination reactions (Table 11-12). Saliva from secretors of all blood groups inhibits the agglutination

Table 11-12. Inhibition test to detect presence of A-B-O group substances in saliva*

Saliva of	Anti-**A** serum + A$_2$ cells + saliva	Anti-**B** serum + B cells + saliva	Anti-**H** lectin + O cells + saliva
Secretor group O	+	+	0
Secretor group A	0	+	0
Secretor group B	+	0	0
Secretor group AB	0	0	0
Nonsecretor, all groups	+	+	+

*+ = agglutination; 0 = no agglutination.

of group O cells by anti-**H** serum and lectins (*Ulex europaeus*), having anti-**H** activity. The secretor status is genetically determined by a pair of allelic genes *Se* and *se*. Secretors may be homozygous *SeSe* or heterozygous *Sese*. Nonsecretors are always homozygous *sese*. In family studies it has been shown that transmission of genes *Se* and *se* is independent of the A-B-O genes.

The relationship of A-B-H secretion to the Lewis blood group is discussed in the section on the Lewis blood group.

Summary of serologic characteristics of A-B-O system

1. Antibodies are "naturally occurring" isoagglutinins or "immune" isoagglutinins.
2. Naturally occurring antibodies are saline agglutinins active in the cold and usually nonreactive at 37° C. They do not cross the placenta and are IgM immunoglobulins.
3. Immune antibodies are more active at 37° C than in the cold and react in high-protein media. They do cross the placenta and are IgG immunoglobulins.
4. Naturally occurring anti-**A**, found in the serum of group O or group B persons, has two major specificities: anti-**A**, which reacts only with A$_1$ and A$_2$ cells, and anti-**A$_1$**, which reacts only with A$_1$ cells.
5. Adsorption of anti-**A** serum with A$_2$ cells yields "adsorbed anti-**A**" serum of anti-**A$_1$** specificity.
6. The lectin from *Dolichos biflorus* has anti-**A$_1$** specificity.
7. The serum of group O individuals contains not only anti-**A** and anti-**B** but cross-reacting anti-**C** as well.
8. Group O cells have the greatest amount of **H** substance, followed in decreasing order by cells of group A, A$_2$B, B, A$_1$, and A$_1$B.
9. Anti-**H** is found in some group A$_1$, A$_1$B, and B sera in which the erythrocytes have very little **H**.

M-N-S-s blood group system
Basic composition

In addition to the A-B-O agglutinogens, the erythrocyte carries a second set of agglutinogens that make up the M-N-S-s system. The two are independent of each other, so that the erythrocytes of a given person can be classified according to both systems (Table 11-13). Accordingly, erythrocytes may be of group OM, ON, OMN, etc. Erythrocytes agglutinated by anti-**M** serum are designated **M**, etc. The biochemical genetics of the MN system according to

Walker et al (1977) are postulated to involve an effect of genes *M* and *N* on the protein portion of the group glycopeptide.

By testing human beings with anti-**M** and anti-**N** serum, it is possible to classify each as phenotype M, N, or MN. The distribution varies among different people in different countries, as does the distribution of other blood groups. Roughly one-half of all white persons in the United States are MN, one-fourth are M, and one-fourth are N. In addition, each of these must have either the **S** or the **s** or both factors. As is the case for the Rh factors, the rare presence of antibodies in the serum indicates immunization, either during pregnancy or by transfusion (Gagliardo and Curiano, 1963; Winn et al 1975), although occasional individuals have been shown to have low titers of naturally occurring anti-**M** or anti-**N** (Kao et al, 1978). The M-N-S-s agglutinogens are fortunately extremely weak antigens for human beings, and the determination of phenotype and genotype in this group is chiefly of medicolegal or anthropologic importance.

Medicolegal application

From the medicolegal standpoint tests are usually performed with anti-**M**, anti-**N**, and anti-**S** sera because of the scarcity and variability of anti-**s** serum. The inheritance pattern for M, N, and MN phenotypes is given in Table 11-14. Table 11-41 is extended to include reactions with anti-**S**. Wiener and Socha (1976) recommend the use of anti-**N** lectins (*Vicia graminea* or *Vicia unijuga*) to check the results obtained with commercial anti-**N** anti-serum. It will be obvious that a greater degree of certainty and a large number of exclusions in cases of disputed parentage would be possible if anti-**s** were available, for then one could distinguish between the homozygous and heterozygous with respect to **S**. The inheritance pattern is based on the supposition that the child must receive one gene from each parent. Therefore two additional rules of inheritance are as follows:

Rule 5: A parent M cannot have a child N, nor can a parent N have a child M.

Rule 6: A child cannot be MN unless M and N are combined in one parent or available, one from each parent.

Variants and related factors

Wiener et al (1953) described a fatal hemolytic transfusion reaction caused by sensitization to a new factor, U. Greenwalt et al (1954) have shown that individuals whose cells do not react with anti-**U** also fail to react with anti-**S**

Table 11-13. M-N-S blood group system and reactions between erythrocytes and antisera*

Blood group (phenotype)	Aggutinogens of erythrocytes	Agglutination of erythrocytes by antisera		
		Anti-M	Anti-N	Anti-S
M (28.53%)				
Ms (7.74%)	M and s	+	−	−
MS (20.79%)	M, S, and s or M and S	+	−	+
N (21.68%)				
Ns (14.78%)	N and s	−	+	−
NS (6.90%)	N, S, and s or N and S	−	+	+
MN (49.80%)				
MNs (21.45%)	M, N, and s	+	+	−
MNS (28.35%)	M, N, S, and s or M, N, and S	+	+	+

*Frequency data for white persons in England from Albritton, 1952. See also Tables 16 to 18 in Mourant, 1954.

Table 11-14. Inheritance pattern of **M** and **N** factors without regard to **S** or **s**

Phenotypes of parents	Phenotypes possible in children	Phenotypes not possible in children
M and M	M	N, MN
M and N	MN	M, N
M and MN	M, MN	N
N and N	N	M, MN
N and MN	N, MN	M
MN and MN	M, N, MN	None

and anti-s. A third *Ss* allele, *S*^{u}, has been proposed. Anti-**U** has not been found in whites and has been found in only a few blacks. The blood of all whites and that of all but a rare (1 in 359) black react with anti-**U**. The antibody is best identified by the antiglobulin technic at 37° C. It has caused both isoimmune hemolytic disease of the newborn and hemolytic transfusion reactions.

A weakly reacting variant of **N**, called **N₂**, is agglutinated weakly or not at all by some anti-**N** sera. Variant **M₂** differs in its reactivity with rabbit and human anti-**M** sera. Variant **M₁** differs qualitatively from **M** in that anti-**M₁** has been found only in human anti-**M** sera. No anti-**M₁** activity is found in rabbit or horse anti-**M** sera. Variant **M**^{c} reacts only with some anti-**M** and anti-**N** sera. Factor **Vw** (Verwyst) has a low incidence (1 in 2,000) but has caused hemolytic disease of the newborn. Factor **Mi**^{a} (Miltenberger) is closely related to **Vw** as well as the M-N-S system. The incidence of **Mi**^{a} is 1 in 715 whites and 1 in 305 blacks. **Mi**^{a} has been found to occur without **Vw**, but when **Vw** is present, **Mi**^{a} is always present also. Anti-**Mi**^{a} and anti-**Vw** may occur as natural antibodies reacting in saline solution at room temperature or as incomplete antibodies reacting at 37° C. Both have caused hemolytic disease of the newborn. Factor **Vr** (van der Hart) has an incidence of 1 in 400 Dutch.

Two factors found principally in blacks are **Hu** (Hunter) and **He** (Henshaw). The antibodies anti-**Hu** and anti-**He** are produced when the subject's erythrocytes are injected into rabbits. No human serum containing these antibodies has been found to date. Rabbit anti-**Hu** reacts with cells of 21.7% of American and West African blacks. Rabbit anti-

He reacts with cells of 2.7% of West African blacks. Factor **M**^{e} is related to **He** in that it is found in blood having either the **M** or **He** factor or both. Anti-**M**^{e} reacts with all types of **M** cells but also with **N**, **He**-positive cells.

The rare factor **M**^{g} described by Allen et al (1958) has some importance in blood grouping in cases of disputed parentage. Cells having **M**^{g} react neither with anti-**M** nor with anti-**N** sera but are agglutinated by anti-**M**^{g}. In a situation in which the putative father is excluded by MN grouping it may be important to test for **M**^{g}; e.g., in a litigation referred to me the mother was **N**, the child was **N**, and the putative father was **M**. Exclusion seemed certain, but there was the possibility that the father had factors **M** and **M**^{g} (**M**^{g} not reacting with anti-**N** or anti-**M**), in which case, if the child had factors **N** and **M**^{g}, exclusion would not have been possible. We did find all three to be **M**^{g} negative and so the exclusion held.

P blood group system

Factor **P** was originally described by Landsteiner and Levine (1927). In preparing the first anti-**M** and anti-**N** rabbit antisera, they also obtained an antiserum that agglutinated erythrocytes independently of A-B-O or MN reactivity. Serum of anti-**P** specificity has been found in some normal persons, in animals, and in immunization following blood transfusion. **P** is very common in blacks (98%), less common in whites (79%), and still less common in the Japanese (30%). It is inherited as a simple mendelian dominant. Anti-**P** has the properties of a cold agglutinin. Cameron and Stavely (1957) found that an occasional person with hydatid disease had strong inhibition of anti-**P** antibodies in the serum and then found strong inhibition of anti-**P** by the cyst fluid. This evidence that the scolices from hydatid cysts contain a great deal of **P** led investigators to attempt the production of anti-**P** by using cyst fluid as the antigen. Some of these attempts have been successful. Wiener feels that anti-**P** agglutinins are, as discussed on p. 494), of heterogenetic origin. Severe transfusion reactions due to anti-**P** have been reported.

Levine et al (1951) found a serum from a patient whose name was Mrs. Jay that agglutinated the erythrocytes of 3,000 unselected group O samples but did not agglutinate Mrs. Jay's erythrocytes nor those of her three siblings.

Table 11-15. P blood group system according to Matson et al, 1959

Phenotype	Antigens in erythrocytes	Antibodies in serum	Genotype
P_1	P and P_1	None	P^1P^1 P^1P^2 P^1P^k P^1p
P_2	P	Anti-P_1 Anti-P^k	P^2P^2 P^2P^k P^2p
P^k	P^k	Anti-P	P^kP^k P^kp
p	None	Anti-P Anti-P_1 Anti-P^k	pp

Table 11-16. P blood group system according to Wiener*†

Phenotype	Reactions of cells with		Isoantibodies in serum
	Anti-P	Anti-p′	
p	−	−	Anti-P and anti-p′
p′	−	+	Anti-P
P	+	−	Anti-p′
P_1	+	+	None

*From Wiener, 1968a.
†Anti-p′ corresponds to the original anti-P; anti-P corresponds to the original anti-Tjᵃ.

Erythrocytes were hemolyzed by fresh serum but not by serum that had been inactivated. The patient had an adenocarcinoma of the stomach, and from the presence of the tumor and the patient's last name the factor detected by the serum was called **Tj** and the antibody anti-**Tj**. Other anti-**Tj** sera were soon found in various countries and in most of these the cells were Tj negative when the serum contained anti-**Tj**.

When Sanger (1955) showed that Tj-negative persons with anti-**Tj** in their serum were also **P** negative, it seemed probable that there was a relationship between Tj and P. She postulated three genes at the P locus—P^1, which determined agglutinogen P_1 and blood factors **P** and **Tjᵃ**; P^2, which determined agglutinogen P_2 and blood factor **Tjᵃ** only; and p, which determined agglutinogen p and presumably has no associated factors. When it was found that the classic anti-**P** serum reacts with two different erythrocyte receptors, **P** and **Pᵏ**, Matson et al (1959) concluded that factor **Pᵏ** is probably the product of gene P^k and is present if genes P^1 and P^2 are present, i.e., the person is genotype P^kp or P^kp^k (Table 11-15).

Wiener (1968a) has criticized this scheme and proposes instead a system of only two isoantibodies, anti-**P** and

anti-**p′**, feeling that the evidence for the antigen pᵏ is weak. His scheme is shown in Table 11-16.

Rh-Hr blood group system
Basic genetics and serology

Our present awareness of the significance of the Rh blood group and its clinical application is the result of a synthesis of many studies. Historically, precedence belongs to Landsteiner and Wiener (1940) who injected erythrocytes from a rhesus monkey into rabbits and produced an antirhesus (or anti-**Rh**) serum. This serum reacted specifically with the M agglutinogen of human erythrocytes. In addition, they found that after the anti-**M** agglutinin was absorbed in some of the sera there remained an antibody that would agglutinate human erythrocytes in about 85% of the population. They therefore divided human blood into two groups, the 85% that were agglutinated by antirhesus serum (Rh+) and the 15% that were not (Rh−). According to present nomenclature, this reflected the presence of the factor called **Rh₀**.

The situation seemed simple, for a single pair of allelic genes (tentatively, *Rh* and *rh*) could be postulated. Gene frequency analysis showed that the expected frequency of Rh-positive and Rh-negative blood corresponded to the observed frequency as follows: (1) Observed frequencies are Rh positive = 84.6% and Rh negative = 15.4%. (2) Since *Rh* is dominant over *rh*, then gene frequencies are as follows:

(a)
$$q^2 = \overline{\text{Rh neg}}$$

and

$$q = \sqrt{\overline{\text{Rh neg}}} = \sqrt{0.154} = 39.2\%$$

where

$$q = \text{Frequency of } rh$$
$$\overline{\text{Rh neg}} = \text{Frequency of Rh-negative individuals}$$

as in the calculations of gene frequencies of the A-B-O group.

(b) $p = 1 - q = 100 - 39.2 = 60.8\%$

(c) Rh-positive genotype $RhRh = (0.608)^2 = 37.0\%$

Rh-positive genotype $Rhrh = 2(0.608 \times 0.392) = 47.6\%$

Rh-negative genotype $rhrh = (0.392)^2 = 15.4\%$

Wiener and Peters (1940) and Wiener (1941) described an agglutinin in the serum of patients with hemolytic reactions following transfusion of blood of the same A-B-O blood group. At about the same time Levine et al (1941) demonstrated that cases of erythroblastosis fetalis were caused by isosensitization to the Rh factor in pregnancy. These two reports clarified the role of the Rh factor in both transfusion reactions and erythroblastosis fetalis. Wiener (1941) showed that the agglutinin in one of his patients reacted with the erythrocytes of about 70% of white persons, in contrast to the 85% incidence for the rhesus blood factor. The problem arose as to the relationship of the original *factor* (**Rh₀**) and the new *factor* (**rh′**). Wiener postulated the existence of two blood factors, **Rh₀** and **rh′**, corresponding to the *agglutinins* anti-**Rh₀** and anti-**rh′**.

Table 11-17. Status of Rh system considering only first two antisera*

Pheno-type	Reaction with serum		Possible genotypes
	Anti-Rh_0	Anti-rh'	
rh	−	−	rr
rh′	−	+	$r'r$ and $r'r'$
Rh_0	+	−	R^0r and R^0R^0
Rh_1	+	+	R^1r, R^1R^0, R^0r', R^1R^1, and R^1r'

*From Wiener and Wexler, 1958.

Table 11-18. Eight Rh phenotypes distinguished by reactions with three antisera*

Phenotype	Reaction with		
	Anti-Rh_0	Anti-rh'	Anti-rh''
Rh negative			
rh	−	−	−
rh′	−	+	−
rh″	−	−	+
rh′rh″	−	+	+
Rh positive			
Rh_0	+	−	−
Rh_1	+	+	−
Rh_2	+	−	+
Rh_1Rh_2	+	+	+

*From Wiener and Wexler, 1958.

It must be kept clearly in mind that Wiener distinguishes sharply between the terms "blood factor" and "agglutinogen." The *agglutinogen* is the substance in or on the erythrocyte, whereas the *factors* are the serologic specificities by which the agglutinogen is characterized. Another basic concept is that an agglutinogen can be characterized by more than one blood factor. By the same token, one gene can determine one agglutinogen with more than one factor. We will see that this basic concept of the relationship betweeen antigen and antibody is one of the basic differences between the multiple allele theory of Wiener and the linked allele theory of the British workers.

With the discovery of the factor **rh′**, Wiener postulated the existence of four allelic genes; r, giving rise to an agglutinogen lacking both factors **Rh_0** and **rh′**; r', giving rise to an agglutinogen having only factor **rh′**; R^0, giving rise to an agglutinogen having only factor **Rh_0**; and R^1, giving rise to an agglutinogen characterized by both factors **Rh_0** and **rh′** (Table 11-17). Accordingly, four phenotypes can be distinguished on the basis of the two sera, anti-**Rh_0** and anti-**rh′**, and there are 10 possible genotypes.

It is important to note that Wiener postulated the situation thus rather than consider a superficially simpler explanation that was not compatible with the observed frequencies; e.g., given the two factors **Rh_0** and **rh′**, the simplest relationship would be to assume only two agglutinogens, Rh_0 and rh′, with factor and agglutinogen corresponding on a one-to-one basis. If this were so, four phenotypes would be possible. Rh_0rh′, Rh_0, rh′, and Rh negative, with two corresponding genes, R^0 and r'. If these genes are allelic, then the frequency of genotype R^0r', and therefore of individuals whose blood cells react with both anti-**Rh_0** and anti-**rh′**, would have to be 50% or less; actually, the observed frequency was 72%.

Wiener and Sonn (1943) described a third antiserum that agglutinated the erythrocytes of 30% of the white population. This serum was designated anti-**rh″**. Tests with the three antisera could then identify eight phenotypes (Table 11-18). The assumption of six multiple allelic genes was tested by gene frequency analysis and found to agree very well with the observed frequencies, their sum being 99.8%. Later, two additional genes were added to account for certain rare familial patterns. These are r^y, which determines agglutinogen rh$_y$ and has factors **rh′** and **rh″** but not **Rh_0**, and R^z, which determines agglutinogen Rh$_z$ and has factors **Rh_0**, **rh′**, and **rh″**.

Levine and Javert (1941) described an antibody, encoun-

tered in the serum of a sensitized mother, that reacted with the blood of white individuals in about 30% of the cases. The factor detected by this serum was named **Hr** since all Rh-negative blood gave a positive reaction when tested with the serum. Wiener designated it **hr′** to indicate a reciprocal relationship to **rh′**, i.e., blood must be either rh′ positive or hr′ positive. He also pointed out that the correct frequency of hr′ was 80% instead of 30%. No modification in the eight basic genes was necessary since **hr′** was a factor that could be assigned to a previously designated agglutinogen. In 1944 Fisher (quoted by Race, 1944) predicted that two additional Hr factors would be found if his theory of linked genes were correct. The factors he predicted were e (**hr″**) and d. Serum containing anti-**hr″** was indeed found the following year by Mourant, but d has been described only twice, in reports that have been seriously questioned. This weakens the status of the Fisher-Race linked-gene hypothesis (Fisher and Race, 1946) because theoretically the frequency of d in white persons is high.

Additional Rh-Hr factors

Other factors must be added before the list of basic reactions is complete. The first, **rh^w**, was described by Callender and Race (1946). The patient, phenotype Rh_1Rh_1, had received many transfusions and had become sensitized to **hr′, N,** and the new factor **rh^w**. The incidence of **rh^w** is low, and persons having **rh^w** also possess factor **rh′**. The discovery of this new factor made it necessary to add genes R^{1w} and r'^w, bringing the total number of basic genes to 10. Later Rosenfield et al (1953) described an antibody they called anti-f and that Wiener called anti-**hr**. This factor is found in persons having the genes r and R^0 (according to the Fisher-Race scheme, anti-f is present only when c and e occur in the same chromosome) and distinguishes between individuals who are phenotype rh′rh″ or rh$_y$rh, and between individuals who are phenotype Rh_1Rh_2 or Rh_2rh (see Table 11-23).

Factor **hr^v** was described by deNatale et al (1955). It is rare among whites (0.5%) but common in New York City blacks (27%) and in African blacks (40%). Individuals possessing the **hr^v** factor have one or both r and R^0 genes, so that **hr^v** has the same relationship to **hr** that factor **rh^w** bears to factor **rh′**.

Table 11-19. Ten basic Rh genes and agglutinogens and corresponding blood factors identifiable by seven antisera: anti-**Rh₀**, anti-**rh'**, anti-**rhʷ**, anti-**rh″**, anti-**hr'**, anti-**hr″**, anti-**hr***

Genes	Frequency among whites (%)	Corresponding agglutinogens	Blood factors present
r	38.0	rh	hr', hr″, hr
r'	0.6	rh'	rh', hr″
r'ʷ	0.005	rh'ʷ	rh', rhʷ, hr″
r″	0.5	rh″	rh″, hr'
rʸ	0.01	rhʸ	rh', rh″
R⁰	2.7	Rh₀	Rh₀, hr', hr″, hr
R¹	41.0	Rh₁	Rh₀, rh', hr″
R¹ʷ	2.0	Rh₁ʷ	Rh₀, rh', rhʷ, hr″
R²	15.0	Rh₂	Rh₀, rh″, hr'
Rᶻ	0.2	Rh_z	Rh₀, rh', rh″

*From Wiener and Wexler, 1958. To calculate genotype frequencies: (1) with two like genes the genotype frequency is the square of the gene frequency; (2) with two unlike genes the genotype frequency is twice the product of the two frequencies; e.g., the frequency of genotype $R^2R^2 = (0.15)^2 = 2.25\%$; the frequency of genotype $R^1R^2 = 2(0.41 \times 0.15) = 0.123\%$.

The symbol $\mathcal{R}h_0$ is used by Wiener (1944a) to identify a group of variants of Rh_0 characterized by variable reactivity when tested with anti-Rh_0 serum. Characteristically, the Rh_0 variants do not react with anti-**Rh₀** in the saline media but react with univalent anti-**Rh₀** serum if the ficin or the antiglobulin technic is used. These variants are relatively rare among whites and occur not infrequently in blacks. Weakly reacting variants may lead to erroneous grouping and to sensitization by blood transfusion. Factor $\mathcal{R}h_0$ is considered analogous to D^u. On the other hand, factors Rh^A, Rh^B, Rh^C, and Rh^D are additional specificities of Rh_0-positive erythrocytes (Unger and Wiener, 1959) and not variants in the same sense as $\mathcal{R}h_0$. In rare Rh-positive individuals, one or more of these specificities may be missing and such a person can be sensitized to the missing factor. Rh_0-positive blood lacking factor Rh^A is extremely rare in whites but occurs in about 1 in 200 blacks.

Race et al (1950) discovered, in the serum of a mother who had given birth to an erythroblastotic infant, an antibody that agglutinated all blood specimens studied. The subject's erythrocytes were agglutinated by anti-**Rh₀** but

Table 11-20. Rh-Hr blood group system, extended to include rare genes*

Genes	Corresponding agglutinogens (antigens)	Rh blood factors				Hr blood factors		
		Rh₀	rh'	rh″	rhʷ	hr'	hr″	hr
r	rh	−	−	−	−	+	+	+
r'	rh'	−	+	−	−	−	+	−
r'ʷ	rh'ʷ	−	+	−	+	−	+	−
r″	rh″	−	−	+	−	+	−	−
rʸ	rhʸ	−	+	+	−	−	−	−
(rʸʷ)	(rhʸʷ)	−	+	+	+	−	−	−
R⁰	Rh₀	+	−	−	−	+	+	+
R¹	Rh₁	+	+	−	−	−	+	−
R¹ʷ	Rh₁ʷ	+	+	−	+	−	+	−
R²	Rh₂	+	−	+	−	+	−	−
Rᶻ	Rh_z	+	+	+	−	−	−	−
(Rᶻʷ)	(Rh_zʷ)	+	+	+	+	−	−	−
(R̄⁰)	(R̄h₀)	+	−	−	−	+	−	+
(R̿⁰)	(R̿h₀)	+	−	−	−	−	−	−
(R̄ʷ)	(R̄hʷ)	+	−	−	+	−	−	−
$\mathcal{R}^0$	$\mathcal{R}h_0$	±	−	−	−	+	+	+

*From Wiener, 1968b.

Table 11-21. Representative data on racial distribution of eight Rh types*

Ethnic group	Approximate frequency (% of blood types)							
	rh	rh'	rh″	rh'rh″	Rh₀	Rh₁	Rh₂	Rh₁Rh₂
Whites (New York City)	13.5	1.0	0.5	0.02	2.5	53.0	15.0	14.5
Blacks								
New York City	7.5	1.5	0	0	45.0	25.0	15.5	5.5
Africa	3.75	0.75	0	0	70.0	15.0	9.0	1.5
Puerto Ricans	10.1	1.7	0.5	0	15.1	39.1	19.6	14.0
Chinese	1.5	0	0	0	0.9	60.6	3.0	34.4
Japanese	0.6	0	0	0	0	51.7	8.3	39.4
Filipinos	0	0	0	0	0	87.0	2.0	11.0
Mexican Indians	0	0	0	0	1.1	48.1	9.5	41.2

*Slightly modified from Wiener and Wexler, 1958.

lacked both factors of the pairs **rh'-hr'** and **rh''-hr''**. Once considered an example of "gene deletion," this situation is now thought to represent the presence on the erythrocytes of a special factor, $\overline{\overline{Rh}}_0$, having increased reactivity with anti-**Rh₀** so that reactivity with other antisera is "crowded out." Another allelic gene, R^0, is postulated. The presence of $\overline{\overline{Rh}}^0$ is detected by the agglutination of the person's erythrocytes with univalent anti-**Rh₀** in a saline medium. Gunson and Donohue (1957) described another "super" factor, $\overline{\overline{Rh}}^W$. The corresponding gene is designated $\overline{\overline{R}}^W$.

Summarizing Wiener's scheme, there are 10 basic Rh genes, each of which is associated with more than one blood factor (Table 11-19). The extended system, including rare genes, is given in Table 11-20. The racial distribution of eight Rh types is given in Table 11-21. A comparison of the two nomenclatures is given in Table 11-22. The reactions with one, four, and seven antisera and the corresponding phenotypes and genotypes are given in Table 11-23.

C-D-E "nomenclature" versus Rh-Hr serology

It will be apparent that Wiener's genetic analysis is believed correct. The reasons for this conclusion are as follows.

Analysis of the data led Fisher (quoted by Race, 1944) to postulate three pairs of linked genes determining six antigens. The genes and antigens were given the same letter designation: D, d; C, c; E, e. The basic difference between Wiener's and Fisher's concepts is that Fisher considers a one-to-one relationship between a gene and a specificity, whereas Wiener considers a blood factor one of several serologic attributes of the agglutinogen determined by the gene. Fisher assumed the three pairs of genes to be linked. Recent-

ly, adherents of this theory have assumed the genes to be very closely linked. Oviously the more closely linked the genes, the more closely this concept approaches that of multiple alleles.

Fisher's analysis predicates three things: the existence of anti-d antibodies, the existence of anti-e antibodies, and the crossing over of linked genes. It is necessary to examine each.

Mourant's discovery (1946) of an antiserum behaving like the predicted anti-e supported Fisher's hypothesis. Other investigators have independently confirmed this finding. Anti-d, however, has been reported only a few times at best, even taking the reports at face value. There is considerable doubt as to the validity of the reports, and it is fair to say the existence of antisera of anti-d specificity has not been confirmed. As for crossovers, this concept too can be seriously questioned. It is possible to support crossovers with data for certain ethnic groups and refute it with data for others.

There are two other perhaps more serious objections. The first involves the discovery of the antiserum anti-f (anti-**hr**). To conform with the linked-gene hypothesis, two additional genes must be postulated, F and f, but serum of anti-F specificity has not been discovered. This is the second antiserum postulated by the linked-gene theory that has not been found. Finally, the "intermediate" factors (such as c^w of Race et al, 1950) are difficult to place in the linked-gene scheme unless we assume that C and C^w are multiple alleles. If this is done with factors but recently described, such as the variants of **Rh₀**, the position of the linked-gene hypothesis becomes very weak, and the hypothesis is so altered that it must be redefined or abandoned.

It is clear, then, that I believe the serologic and genetic principles implicit in Wiener's nomenclature to be correct. It should also be clear that *the choice is not between nomenclatures* but in favor of principles that are believed to be serologically and genetically correct. It would be presumptuous for me to anticipate that the arguments presented will convince those who do not want to be convinced.

To summarize the arguments, then, the following must be pointed out:

1. Implicit in the C-D-E nomenclature is the concept of a one-to-one relationship between gene, agglutinogen, and antibody. Each new serologic reaction, and there is no doubt that there are still some to be discovered, must be the product of a new gene. While this is not, by itself, impossible, it does require a most improbable genetic system.

2. The Fisher-Race linked-gene hypothesis originally proposed three loci for allelic genes Dd, Cc, and Ee. The discovery of factor **hr** (f) and factor **hr^v** (V) has dictated extending the number of loci to five to accommodate gene pairs Ff and Vv. Of the 10 postulated antisera, two are yet to be found, anti-d and anti-F.

3. When translating the results of serologic tests into phenotypes and genotypes with the C-D-E notation, one is sometimes forced to designate the "most likely" genotype on the basis of frequency rather than the actual genotype. This is primarily due to the nonexistence of anti-d serum. In the Wiener system, conclusions as to genotype are not based on probability.

4. Implicit in the Fisher-Race analysis is the concept that the rarer gene combinations result from crossovers of the

Table 11-22. Comparison of Fisher-Race CcDdEe notation and Wiener's Rh nomenclature*†

Wiener	Fisher-Race
Genes	
r	cde
r'	Cde
R'^w	C^wde
r''	cdE
r^y	CdE
R^0	cDe
R^1	CDe
R^{1w}	C^wDe
R^2	cDE
R^z	CDE
Antisera	
Anti-**rh'**	Anti-C
Anti-**Rh₀**	Anti-D
Anti-**rh''**	Anti-E
Anti-**rh^w**	Anti-C^w
Anti-**hr'**	Anti-c
Anti-**hr''**	Anti-e
Anti-**hr**	Anti-f

*The two are not interchangeable since they represent totally different serologic and genetic concepts (see text).

†We purposely omit Rosenfield's numbered notation, a nonsense system that few have taken seriously (p. 508).

Table 11-23. Rh-Hr blood group system; determination of phenotype by one, four, and seven antisera

One antiserum		Four antisera					Reactions with antisera and phenotypes — Seven antisera								Genotype	Frequency (%)
Anti-Rh₀	Phenotype	Anti-Rh₀	Anti-rh'	Anti-rh"	Anti-rhʷ	Phenotype	Anti-Rh₀	Anti-rh'	Anti-rh"	Anti-rhʷ	Anti-hr'	Anti-hr"	Anti-hr	Phenotype		
Negative	Rh₀ negative (Rh negative)	−	−	−	−	rh	−	−	−	−	+	+	+	rh	rr	14.4
		−	+	−	−	rh'	−	+	−	−	+	+	+	rh'rh	r'r	0.46
							−	+	−	−	−	+	−	rh'rh'	r'r'	0.0036
		−	+	−	+	rh'ʷ	−	+	−	+	+	+	+	rhʷrh	rʷr	0.004
							−	+	−	+	−	+	−	rhʷrh'	r'ʷr', r'ʷrʷ	0.00006
		−	−	+	−	rh"	−	−	+	−	+	+	+	rh"rh	r"r	0.38
							−	−	+	−	+	−	−	rh"rh"	r"r"	0.0025
		−	+	+	−	rhʸ	−	+	+	−	+	+	−	rh'rh"	r'r"	0.006
							−	+	+	−	+	+	+	rhʸrh	rʸr	0.008
							−	+	+	−	−	+	−	rhʸrh'	rʸr'	0.0001
							−	+	+	−	+	−	−	rhʸrh"	rʸr"	0.0001
							−	+	+	−	−	−	−	rhʸrhʸ	rʸrʸ	0.000001
		−	+	+	+	rhʸʷ	−	+	+	+	+	+	−	rh'ʷrh"	r'ʷr"	0.00005
							−	+	+	+	−	+	−	rhʸʷrh'	rʸʷrʸ	0.000001
+		+	−	−	−	Rh₀	+	−	−	−	+	+	+	Rh₀	R⁰r, R⁰R⁰	2.05, 0.073
+		+	+	−	−	Rh₁	+	+	−	−	+	+	+	Rh₁rh	R¹r, R¹R⁰, R⁰r'	31.2, 2.2, 0.03
							+	+	−	−	−	+	−	Rh₁Rh₁	R¹R¹, R¹r'	16.8, 0.5
							+	+	−	+	+	+	+	Rh₁ʷrh	R¹ʷr, R¹ʷR⁰	1.5, 0.11

Genotype	Phenotype							Frequency (%)
R^wR R^1r' $R^{1w}r'$ $R^{1w}R^{1w}$ $R^{1w}r'w$	$Rh_1^w Rh_1$	−	+	−	+	−	+	1.6 0.004 0.02 0.04 0.0001
R^2r R^2R^0 R^0r''	$Rh_2 rh$	+	+	+	−	+	+	11.4 0.8 0.027
R^2R^2 R^2r''	$Rh_2 Rh_2$	−	−	+	−	+	+	2.25 0.15
R^1R^2 R^1r'' R^2r'	$Rh_1 Rh_2$	−	+	+	−	+	+	12.3 0.4 0.2
R^zr R^zR^0 R^0r^y	$Rh_z rh$	+	+	+	−	+	+	0.15 0.01 0.0005
R^zR^1 R^zr' R^1r^y	$Rh_z Rh_1$	−	+	−	−	+	+	0.16 0.02 0.008
R^zR^2 R^zr'' R^2r^y	$Rh_z Rh_2$	−	−	+	−	+	+	0.06 0.002 0.003
R^zR^z R^zr^y	$Rh_z Rh_z$	−	−	−	−	+	+	0.0004 0.00004
$R^{1w}R^2$ $R^{1w}r''$ $R^2r'w$	$Rh_1^w Rh_2$	−	+	+	+	+	+	0.6 0.02 0.0015
$R^{1w}R^z$ $R^{1w}r^y$ R^zr^{1w}	$Rh_z^w Rh_1$	−	+	−	+	+	+	0.008 0.0004 0.0002

Rh$_1^w$ + − + +

Rh$_2$ − + − +

Rh$_z$ − + + +

Rh$_z^w$ + + + +

Rh$_o$ positive (Rh positive)

Positive

standard C-D-E-F-V linear arrangement. Analysis of various population groups indicates that the concept can be substantiated for some groups but not for others.

5. With standard methods of genetic analysis, the data fit the multiple allele concept of Wiener and do not fit the linked-gene concept of Fisher and Race.

6. The weakly reacting variants of Rh_0 and the specificities Rh^A, Rh^B, Rh^C, and Rh^D can, when considered as blood factors, be quite readily fitted into the existing scheme, since they are then additional serologic attributes of one agglutinogen. Wiener and Unger (1962) suggest that blood of Rh_0-positive individuals usually has all the associated cognate blood factors, but that occasionally one factor is absent, making that individual susceptible to immunization to the missing factor. According to the Fisher-Race concept, weakly reacting anti-D is called anti-D^u, a D^u gene is postulated, and by definition only one kind of anti-D^u antibody can be produced.

7. The discovery of bloods that have factor Rh_0 (D) but lack both members of the pairs rh'-hr' (C-c) and rh''-hr'' (E-e) has been cited as support for the Fisher-Race concept in that the resulting configuration $D - -/D - -$ has been called an example of gene deletion. The blood type $DC^w -/DC^w -$ has also been described. In general, gene deletions are accompanied by other defects, particularly when the deletion is of the homozygous configuration. The individuals with these rare serologic manifestations seem, however, to be otherwise normal. The significance of these rare cases is certainly not clear at the present time.

It is to be hoped that as time goes on the C-D-E nomenclature will be discarded. At the very least it should be unacceptable for medicolegal reports. Manufacturers of typing sera will probably continue to use both the Wiener and the C-D-E nomenclature on the label, and I suppose they have no other choice until the Division of Biologic Standards of the FDA outlaws the C-D-E designation on labels. I can think of no good reason for retaining it. At a special meeting on Rh-Hr nomenclature held at the New York Academy of Sciences in April 1967 we again recommended that the Division of Biologic Standards require that antisera be labeled properly, using Wiener's Rh nomenclature and eliminating the C-D-E symbols. So far this recommendation has been ignored. It is nevertheless my opinion that, aside from other cogent arguments, the C-D-E system is unacceptable for medicolegal purposes. There are, of course, respected serologists who disagree with this view. As for the C-D-E notation being simpler, so is the Galenic concept of "humours" as a cause of disease, and we well know that nature is not obliged, or even predisposed, to make things simple just because we would find it convenient. Table 11-24, giving the reactions and genotypes according to the Fisher-Race theory, is retained for the sake of those who are not swayed by my argument.

The Rosenfield numerical notation

In spite of personal preference for either the C-D-E or the Wiener nomenclature, most immunohematologists are conversant with both, and in routine blood banking the difference in the two genetic concepts does not come into play. In medicolegal cases, however, genetic principles must be tak-

en into account and, not infrequently, these must be defended in a court of law.

Rosenfield et al (1962) suggested a third nomenclature based on assigning a number to each Rh antigen (Table 11-25). Positive reactions with a given antiserum are recorded by the number assigned to the antiserum; negative reactions are recorded as the minus number. The two proposed advantages are (1) avoidance of a commitment to either genetic system and (2) the ability to report serologic data that indicate not only positive reactions but also the negative ones obtained.

These proposed advantages are in fact the very weaknesses of the numerical rotation. For example, the numerical nomenclature must be translated back to either the C-D-E or the Wiener systems when genetics must be taken into account, as in cases of disputed parentage. Nor is there any obvious practical advantage in reporting serologic reactions. If a person is found to be phenotype Rh_1rh by testing with standard antisera, reporting the phenotype as Rh1, 2, −3, 4, 5, 6 does not seem very constructive.

Rh_{null} type

It is appropriate to discuss here the "minus-minus" phenotypes, since the interpretation of these situations depends on principles of immunogenetics. Occasional individuals have been encountered whose erythrocytes appear to lack one or more antigens of a given blood group, as revealed by nonagglutinability of these cells in the presence of specific antisera; e.g., the "Bombay" type of blood has erythrocytes that do not react with anti-A, anti-B, or anti-H. Other examples have been reported in the Rh system (Hr_0-; $C-c-E-e-D+$; $C-c-E-e-D-$), the M-N-S system ($S-s-U-$), the Lewis system ($Le[a-b-]$), the Duffy system ($Fy[a-b-]$), the P system ($P-Tj[a-]$), the Kell system ($K-k-Kp[a-b-]Ku-$), the Kidd system ($JK[a-b-]$), and the Lutheran system ($Lu[a-b-]$). If it is assumed that one gene is responsible for one serologic attribute, then these are examples of gene "deletion," complete or partial, or gene suppression of various types. If one is not limited by the one-to-one concept, then it is more logical to suppose that it is suppression of the serologic expression of a gene rather than deletion, the latter being a drastic alteration.

For example, Vos et al (1961) described a blood lacking all Rh factors. Levine et al (1964) described another like it and called it Rh_{null}. These and the other examples given have been cited as examples of "gene deletions," but there is a more acceptable explanation. Family studies have shown that Rh_{null} blood can result from the effect of a suppressor gene when the person is homozygous for that gene. In this situation the blood is designated as $\overset{\circ}{r}h$. Rh_{null} can also result from homozygosity for another allelic gene—genetic designation rr, blood group rh (Ishimori and Hasekura, 1967). It has been estimated that the incidence of Rh_{null} individuals is one in six million (Seidl et al, 1972).

Individuals of type Rh_{null} show some interesting serologic and hematologic anomalies (Nagel et al, 1972; Levine et al, 1973). There is presumably an abnormality of the erythrocyte membrane that produces a mild hemolytic anemia, reticulocytosis, spherocytosis, and stomatocytosis. The

Table 11-24. Rh blood group system according to Fisher-Race nomenclature

Reactions with antisera							Genotype	Frequency (%)
Anti-D	Anti-C	Anti-E	Anti-c^w	Anti-c	Anti-e	Anti-f		
−	−	−	−	+	+	+	cde/cde	14.4
−	+	−	−	+	+	+	Cde/cde	0.46
				−	+	−	Cde/Cde	0.0036
−	+	−	+	+	+	+	C^{w}de/cde	0.004
				−	+	−	C^{w}de/Cde, C^{w}de/C^{w}de }	0.00006
−	−	+	−	+	+	+	cdE/cde	0.38
				+	−	−	cdE/cdE	0.0025
−	+	+	−	+	+	−	Cde/cdE	0.006
				+	+	+	CdE/cde	0.008
				−	+	−	CdE/Cde	0.0001
				+	−	−	CdE/cdE	0.0001
				−	−	−	CdE/CdE	0.00001
−	+	+	+	+	+	−	C^{w}de/cdE	0.00005
				−	+	−	C^{w}de/CdE	0.000001
+	−	−	−	+	+	+	cDe/cde	2.05
							cDe/cDe	0.073
+	+	−	−	+	+	+	CDe/cde	31.2
							CDe/cDe	2.2
							cDe/Cde	0.03
				−	+	−	CDe/CDe	16.8
							CDe/Cde	0.5
+	+	−	+	+	+	+	C^{w}De/cde	1.5
							C^{w}De/cDe	0.11
							cDe/C^{w}de	0.0003
				−	+	−	C^{w}De/CDe	1.6
							CDe/c^{w}de	0.004
							C^{w}De/Cde	0.02
							C^{w}De/C^{w}De	0.04
							C^{w}De/C^{w}de	0.0001
+	−	+	−	+	+	+	cDE/cde	11.4
							cDE/cDe	0.8
							cDe/cdE	0.027
				+	−	−	cDE/cDE	2.25
							cDE/cdE	0.15
+	+	+	−	+	+	−	CDe/cDE	12.3
							CDe/cdE	0.4
							cDE/Cde	0.2
				+	+	+	CDE/cde	0.15
							CDE/cDe	0.01
							cDe/CdE	0.0005
				−	+	−	CDE/CDe	0.16
							CDE/Cde	0.02
							CDe/CdE	0.008
				+	−	−	CDE/cDE	0.06
							CDE/cdE	0.002
							Cde/CdE	0.003
				−	−	−	CDE/CDE	0.0004
							CDE/CdE	0.0004
+	+	+	+	+	+	−	C^{w}De/cDE	0.6
							C^{w}De/cdE	0.02
							cDE/C^{w}de	0.0015
				−	+	−	C^{w}De/CDE	0.008
							C^{w}De/CdE	0.0004
							CDE/C^{w}de	0.0002

Table 11-25. Comparison of the Rosenfield, Rh-Hr, and C-D-E nomenclature of the more common Rh antigens. The complete table including Rh1 to Rh40 is given by Issitt (1979)

Rosenfield	Rh-Hr	C-D-E
Rh1	Rh_0	D
Rh2	rh'	C
Rh3	rh"	E
Rh4	hr'	c
Rh5	hr"	e
Rh6	hr	f

Table 11-26. Four patterns of secretion of water-soluble A-B-H and Lewis antigens

Type	Secretion of		
	A-B-H	**Le^a**	**Le^b**
1 Sec Les	+ + + +	+	+ +
2 nS Les	−	+ + + +	−
3 Sec nL	+ + + +	−	−
4 nS nL	−	−	−

term "Rh_{null} disease" has been applied to the syndrome. In addition, Rh_{null} erythrocytes are not agglutinated by anti-**U** serum, are agglutinated by anti-**S** serum, and by both anti-**I** and anti-**i** sera (Schmidt and Vos, 1967).

Rh antibodies

If immunization takes place, either through pregnancy or blood transfusion, the antibodies formed may be of two types. The first are called saline agglutinins *(IgM antibodies)* since they agglutinate the corresponding erythrocytes in a saline medium. These appear in the early stages of sensitization or as the result of relatively mild antigenic stimulation. Intense immunization produces agglutinins that clump erythrocytes only in a medium high in protein or containing macromolecular substances such as PVP. These antibodies are albumin agglutinins *(IgG antibodies),* and their presence is generally indicative of a high degree of sensitization. In most severe cases both saline and albumin agglutinins are produced, but in a few only albumin agglutinins can be detected.

A third type of antibody reaction may be seen in highly sensitized persons. An antibody may be produced that unites with the respective erythrocyte without causing agglutination and renders it inagglutinable by saline antibodies. Such an antibody is called a *blocking antibody*. It is usually associated with albumin agglutinins but never with saline agglutinins. Blocking antibodies have also been called *incomplete antibodies* or crypt-agglutinoids. Whether or not they make up a third and distinct type of antibody (the effect may reflect only another property of IgG antibodies), their presence indicates severe sensitization. Their "blocking" action may confuse in vitro reactions, for when the titer of blocking antibodies is high, typing is unreliable if carried out in a saline medium. Blocking antibodies apparently pass quite readily through the placenta and may be found in the infant's blood, not only bound to the erythrocytes but also free in the serum. Such antibodies may be detected by the antiglobulin test (Coombs' test), the direct test for erythrocytes coated with blocking antibody, and the indirect test for *free antibody* in the serum (Chapter 13).

Lewis blood group system

Following the description of anti-**Le^a** (Mourant, 1946) and anti-**Le^b** (Andresen, 1948), the Lewis system seemed simple, involving two genes, *Le^a* and *Le^b*, dictating the agglutinogens Le^a and Le^b and phenotypes Lewis positive (20.5% of persons) and Lewis negative (79.5% of persons).

It was not long before it was realized that the Lewis system is not only extremely complicated but unique in many ways.

Peculiarities of the system are the following: (1) the antibodies usually are saline agglutinins reacting at room or lower temperature, although some samples of anti-Le^a are of the incomplete type and react at 37° C by the indirect antiglobulin reaction, (2) the Lewis antigens of erythrocytes are apparently acquired by adsorption from the plasma, (3) anti-Le^a reacts with an antigen seemingly inherited as a mendelian recessive (other erythrocyte antigens are codominant)—thus it has been found that when the parents are both Le(a−), the children may be either Le(a−) or Le(a+), (4) the red cell factors become manifest slowly and irregularly after birth—at birth, most bloods type as Le(a−b−), and it is not until about 2 years of age that repeat typings show the adult frequency of Le(a+) cells, (5) there is a striking difference in the frequency of Lewis-positive and Lewis-negative individuals in various races, and (6) anti-Le^b sera give many more positive reactions with group O and group A_2 cells than with cells of group B and A_1.

One characteristic feature of the Lewis system is its relationship to secretion of **A-B-H** substances in saliva (Table 11-26). In accordance with modern theory, it is postulated that the **A-B-H** and **Lewis** a and b substances found in the saliva of a secretor are the products of four independent gene systems. These are *Lele, Hh, Sese,* and *A-B-O* and act in sequence to form the **Le^a** substance, the **H** substance, the **A** and **B** substances, and determine the secretion of **A-B-H** substances in saliva and other body fluids. Persons who secrete **A-B-H** are phenotype Sec and those who do not are nS. Genes *Se* and *se* segregate independently from the A-B-O and Lewis genes and determine only the presence or absence of **A-B-H** substances in body fluids. The serologic specificity is determined by the A-B-O and Lewis gene products.

The Lewis system determines the presence or absence in saliva, plasma, and other body fluids of the water-soluble **Lewis** substance. Gene *Le* determines production of **Le** substance; gene *le* is an amorph and has no product. Secretors of **Lewis** substance therefore have the genotype *LeLe* or *Lele,* while nonsecretors have the genotype *lele.* Note that A-B-H secretors or nonsecretors are phenotypes Sec and nS, respectively, while Lewis secretors or nonsecretors are phenotypes Les and nL. Note also that the **Lewis** substance is adsorbed on the erythrocytes from the serum and is therefore not a primary characteristic of erythrocytes.

Since the **A-B-H** and **Lewis** substances are produced by competition for the same basic blood group substance, Lew-

Table 11-27. Lewis types*

	Saliva						Blood				
	Frequencies		Group-specific substances present in saliva§			Designations		Reactions of red cells with‖			
Designations	Whitest (%)	Blacks‡ (%)	Le	H	Le^H	Recommended	Commonly used	Anti-Le (anti-Le^x)	Anti-Le$_1$ (anti-Le^a)	Anti-Le^H (anti-Le^b)	
Les nS	23.1	18.6	+	−	−	Le$_1$	Le(a + b −)	+	+	−	
Les Sec	73.5	58.5	+	+	+	Le$_2$	Le(a − b +)	+	−	+	
nL Sec	2.8	17.0	−	+	− }	le	Le(a − b −)	−	−	−	
nL nS	0.6	5.9	−	−	− }						

*Slightly modified from Wiener, 1965.
†England.
‡Charleston, W. Va.
§Plus signs indicate the presence of the respective substance, as shown by inhibition of the corresponding antiserum; minus signs indicate that the substance is absent, i.e. inhibition does not occur in the tests.
‖Plus signs indicate agglutination; minus signs, absence of agglutination.

is secretors who are A-B-H nonsecretors (phenotype Les nS) will have more **Lewis** substance in saliva and other body fluids than those who are A-B-H secretors (phenotype Les Sec). Persons with phenotype Les nS will have erythrocytes strongly coated with **Lewis** substance and therefore highly reactive with anti-**Lewis** serum (Table 11-27). The Lewis system is defined therefore by the avidity of erythrocytes for **Lewis** substances in the plasma and their subsequent agglutination by anti-**Lewis** serum. The first antiserum described was anti-**Le^a**, followed about 2 years later by the discovery of anti-**Le^b**. Antisera have been described that react with both Le^a and Le^b cells; these have been called anti-**Le^x**. In the nomenclature recommended by Wiener (1965, Table 11-27), anti-**Le^x** is called anti-**Le**, and anti-**Le^a** is called anti-**Le$_1$**, while anti-**Le^b** is called anti-**Le^H** because of the similarity of reactions of anti-**H** and anti-**Le^H** with erythrocytes of group O and subgroup A$_2$. The designation of the Lewis factors as **Le^a** and **Le^b** implies that they are the result of allelic genes, which is not the case, but is still widely believed.

There are important racial and age differences in the Lewis system. The frequencies in Table 11-27 show that blacks are more likely to be Le^a negative. Also, the Lewis phenotype varies with age. Most newborns are Lewis type le (Le [a−b−]) when tested using saline technics; if the antiglobulin technic is used, about half of the newborns are Le(a+). During the first few months of life almost all infants adsorb the Le^a antigen on their erythrocytes and become Le(a+). By the age of 2 years, only about 20% are Le(a+), the adult frequency. Agglutination of Le(a+) cells is weakened during pregnancy. It should be noted that saliva should be used for Lewis phenotyping, using the inhibition technic.

Lewis antibodies usually are naturally occurring and, according to Wiener, are heteroimmune in origin. Since blacks more commonly have genotype *lele*, they are more likely to have Lewis antibodies. Naturally occurring Lewis antibodies are usually saline agglutinins reacting best at 16° C; they react best with type Le$_1$ cells. Immune antibodies from transfusion reactions due to Lewis sensitization are often hemolytic toward Le$_1$ cells and usually react also with type Le$_2$ cells after these are treated with ficin. Destruction

Table 11-28. Lutheran blood group system

Phenotype	Genotype	Frequency (%)	Reaction with	
			Anti-Lu^a	Anti-Lu^b
Lu(a+b−)	*Lu^{a}Lu^a*	0.1	+	0
Lu(a+b+)	*Lu^{a}Lu^b*	7.5	+	+
Lu(a−b+)	*Lu^{b}Lu^b*	92.4	0	+
Lu(a−b−)	?	Extremely rare	0	0

of complement by heating converts hemolytic to agglutinating antisera. Agglutination in saline media often shows a characteristic ''stringy'' appearance. Lewis antibodies may be responsible for severe hemolytic transfusion reactions. Hemolytic disease of the newborn due to anti-**Lewis** has not been described.

Erskine and Socha (1978) recommend that tests for Lewis antibodies be carried out with a panel of Le$_1$, Le$_2$, and le cells from group O individuals. The cells are ficinated. Each cell suspension is reacted with the serum being tested at 37° C. Immune antibodies will usually hemolyze Le$_1$ cells, Le$_2$ cells are partially hemolyzed or agglutinated, while le cells are not affected. In the rare instance of sensitization of **Le^H**, only the Le$_2$ cells will be hemolyzed. If the serum being tested is heated to destroy complement, agglutination rather than hemolysis will take place, either without further manipulation or after washing and adding antihuman globulin serum.

Lutheran blood group system

The Lutheran system (Table 11-28) depends on a pair of allelomorphic genes, *Lu^a* and *Lu^b*. About 8% of English white persons are Lutheran positive (genotypes *Lu^{a}Lu^a* and *Lu^{a}Lu^b*) and 92% are Lutheran negative (*Lu^{b}Lu^b*). The incidence of Lutheran-positive persons is higher in the United States (19.1%). Both **Lu^a** and **Lu^b** are antigenically active and both anti-**Lu^a** and anti-**Lu^b** have been responsible for hemolytic transfusion reactions and hemolytic disease of the

Table 11-29. Racial distribution of Kell types*

Population	Kell−	Kell+	% Gene frequency	
			k	K
Whites	91.6	8.4	95.7	4.3
Blacks	99.0	1.0	99.5	0.5
Chinese	99.5	0.5	99.7	0.3

*New York City, modified from Wiener, 1969.

Table 11-30. The Kell blood group system

Phenotype	Genotype	Frequency* (%)	Reactions with antisera	
			Anti-K	Anti-k
Kell+	KK	0.2	+	−
	Kk	8.2	+	+
Kell−	kk	91.6	−	+

*Approximate, for whites.

Table 11-31. Duffy blood group system

Phenotype	Genotype	Reaction with		Frequency (%)	
		Anti-Fy^a	Anti-Fy^b	White	Black
Fy(a+b−)	Fy^aFy^a and Fy^afy	+	0	17.2	9
Fy(a+b+)	Fy^aFy^b	+	+	48.5	2
Fy(a−b+)	Fy^bFy^b and Fy^bfy	0	+	34.3	22
Fy(a−b−)	fyfy	0	0	0	68

newborn. Darnborough et al (1963) describe an anti-Lutheran antibody having the double specificity of anti-Lu^a and anti-Lu^b. The phenotype Lu(a−b−) has been described by Crawford et al (1961) by Darnborough et al (1963), but is rare (incidence about 0.15%).

Kell blood group system

The Kell factor (**K**) was described by Coombs et al (1946) and identified by the antiglobulin technic. Three years later the antithetic factor **k** was described by Levine et al (1949), who named it Cellano after the name of the patient. It was then thought that the system was simple, Kell-positive individuals (approximately 8.8% of persons in the United States and 10.17% of persons in England) being of genotype KK or Kk, while the remainder are Kell negative and of genotype kk. There is a significant difference of the incidence of Kell-positive and Kell-negative persons among racial groups (Table 11-29).

Since then, the system has been extended by the discovery of antigens Penny (**Kp^a**), Rautenberg (**Kp^b**), K^0 (not an antigen but a type lacking all other Kell antigens), Peltz (**Ku**), and **McLeod.** Two additional factors are now included in the Kell system: **Js^a** (Giblett and Chase, 1959; the **Sutter** factor) and **Js^b** (Walker et al, 1963). **Js^a** is found only in blacks (about 19% positive). Anti-Js^a reacts best at 37° C using the antiglobulin technic. Usually only anti-**K** and anti-**k** antisera are used, and the reactions are given in Table 11-30. The rare type, K$_0$, is characterized by failure to agglutinate with both anti-**K** and anti-**k**. It should be noted that the Kell factor is absent from the erythrocytes in infants and young children who would then be typed as Kell negative regardless of their Kell type when tested later.

The Kell factors have been implicated in hemolytic transfusion reactions and hemolytic disease of the newborn. Since most persons are Kell negative, anti-**K** ranks third in the order of frequency of the antibodies implicated in hemolytic disease of the newborn and transfusion reaction (anti-

Rh$_0$ and anti-hr′ being more frequent). Anti-**k** is also a powerful antibody. In general, the Kell antigens are highly antigenic and are important. Kell antibodies react well with antiglobulin serum of antigamma specificity, but some also react with broad spectrum antiglobulin serum. They do not react well either in high-albumin media or with enzyme-treated cells. If the antiglobulin cross-matching technic is not used, there is real danger of missing highly potent antibodies. Freshly drawn red cells must be used for testing, for the reactivity diminishes on standing or storage.

Duffy blood group system

Antibodies in the Duffy system have been responsible for both hemolytic transfusion reactions and hemolytic disease of the newborn. In whites the system seems dependent on two alleles, Fy^a and Fy^b, and whites are of phenotype Fy(a+b−), Fy(a+b+), and Fy(a−b+) (Table 11-31). In blacks, however, about 68% fail to react with either anti-**Fy^a** or anti-**Fy^b** (phenotype Fy[a−b−] not found in whites); it has been postulated that this phenomenon is the product of a third gene, fy, probably inherited in the double-dose fyfy. Duffy-negative blacks are resistant to infection with Falciparum vivax (Miller et al, 1976).

Anti-**Fy^a** acts as an incomplete antibody, reacting best at 37° C by the indirect antiglobulin test. Most samples react with both antigamma and broad spectrum antiglobulin sera. Some samples of anti-**Fy^a** serum require complement. The strength of the agglutination reactions obtained depends in part on the reactivity of the test cells. Obviously, tests for the Duffy types are invalidated if the subject's red cells are coated by antibody, i.e., as in autoimmune antiglobulin positive hemolytic anemia. The same precaution applies to other blood groups detected by the antiglobulin reaction (Kidd, p. 513). The antibody is eluted very easily from the red cells, and the indirect antiglobulin tests, to detect Duffy reactions, must avoid excessive washing of the cells and careful control of incubation time. Anti-**Fy^a** may agglutinate

Table 11-32. Kidd blood group system

Phenotype	Genotype	Reaction with		Frequency (%)	
		Anti-Jk^a	Anti-Jk^b	White	Black
Jk(a+b−)	Jk^aJk^a and Jk^ajk	+	0	25	57
Jk(a+b+)	Jk^aJk^b	+	+	50	34
Jk(a−b+)	Jk^bJk^b and Jk^bjk	0	+	25	9
Jk(a−b−)	$jkjk$	0	0	Very rare	Very rare

enzyme-treated cells, but the antiglobulin technic is best. Anti-**Fy^b** shows essentially the same properties as anti-**Fy^a**.

Kidd blood group system

The antibodies in this system have been responsible for isolated hemolytic transfusion reactions and for hemolytic disease of the newborn. Both anti-**Jk^a** and anti-**Jk^b** have been implicated in hemolytic disease of the newborn. In general, the cases reported are characteristically not severe, although severe hemolytic disease has been found with either antibody. They are best detected by the indirect antiglobulin test using enzyme-treated cells and antiglobulin serum of broad specificity; complement must be present, and it is recommended that fresh serum be added to ensure this. Anti-**Kidd** sera tend to be unstable even when frozen. Most workers recommend adding fresh serum to the anti-**Kidd** sera before they are used.

This system consists of three alleles, very much like the Duffy system. The alleles are Jk^a, Jk^b, and jk. The reactions of the system are shown in Table 11-32.

I-i blood group system

In 1956 Wiener et al described a serum from a patient of blood group A$_1$B with hemolytic anemia of the cold-antibody type that reacted with all but 5 of 22,000 New Yorkers' blood. It was at first thought to identify another of the high-frequency factors and was called **I**. However, Jenkins et al (1960) described a patient who had naturally occurring anti-**I** in the serum; this was thought to represent an instance of blood factor **i**. Variants so far described are I$_1$, I$_2$, I$_3$ (some authors use the symbol I$_1$ and I$_{int}$ for the graded reactivity of I), i$_1$, i$_2$, and i$_{cord}$; the latter is the **i** factor present in cord erythrocytes, which supposedly develops into **I** in the adult. According to Moor-Jankowski et al (1964), the **I** antigen is also found in certain anthropoid apes and in rabbits. Most normal adults have the **I** antigen; the **i** antigens are found very rarely and i$_1$, rarer than i$_2$, has been found only in whites. Superficially, the genetic control would seem to depend on two genes, I and i, but it is probable that these are in fact modifying genes that affect the conversion of cord **i** to adult **I**.

Anti-**I** is the important antibody in the system. It can occur as an autoantibody in persons of phenotype I, as a natural antibody in persons of phenotype i$_1$ or i$_2$, or as an autoantibody in acquired hemolytic anemia of the "cold-antibody" type. It is reported (Jenkins et al, 1965) that 8%

Table 11-33. Frequency of Diego factor in various ethnic groups

Ethnic group	Frequency (%)
Whites	0
Blacks, North American	0
Blacks, African	0
Eskimos, Canadian Arctic	0
Norwegian Lapps	0
Swedish Lapps	0
South American Indians (Caribe)	35.5
South American Indians (Brasilid)	36-46
Mexican Indians	20
North American Indians (Chippewa)	10
Chinese	5
Japanese	8-12

of persons with infectious mononucleosis have anti-**i**. Agglutination of red blood cells by anti-**i** is a feature of congenital dyserythropoietic anemia, type II (HEMPAS) (Berrebi and Efrati, 1974). Acanthocytes have the same reactivity as cord red blood cells (Berrebi and Levene, 1976).

Diego blood group system

Levine et al (1956) discovered a previously undescribed antibody in a case of hemolytic disease of the newborn. The patient was a native of Venezuela, and when the antibody failed to react with the erythrocytes of hundreds of American whites, it was concluded that the factor belonged in the "family" or "private" group (see following discussion). However, subsequent studies have shown that its incidence in Mongolians is high and that it is almost never found in whites or blacks (Table 11-33). The factor was called **Di^a**. Anti-**Di^a** antibodies are of the incomplete type, best detected by the indirect antiglobulin test at 37° C. Factor **Di^b** was described some years later by Thompson et al (1967). Hemolytic disease of the newborn can occur when the mother is phenotype Di (a+b−), the child is phenotype Di (a+b+), and the mother's serum contains anti-**Di^b** antibody (Ishimori et al, 1976).

Sex-linked blood group system Xg

The genes of all blood groups are localized on autosomal chromosomes with the exception of the Xg^a characteristic, which is determined by gene Xg^a localized on the X chro-

Table 11-34. Some "private" and "public" blood factors

Factors	Comments
I. Private	
Wright (Wrᵃ)	Antibody may be naturally occurring; in hemolytic disease of the newborn the antibody is incomplete, detected only by indirect antiglobulin test; one example was described that reacted in saline media at 18° and 37° C but was nonreactive by the antiglobulin test
Levay	Reacts in saline media at 37° C
Graydon (Gr)	Reacts best in saline media at 18° C; probably identical with **Vw**
Jobbins	Reacts best in antiglobulin test
Becker	Reacts best in antiglobulin test
Ven	Reacts best in antiglobulin test
Berrens (Beᵃ)	Reacts in antiglobulin test, also in high-albumin medium and with enzyme-treated erythrocytes
Cavaliere (Ca)	Reacts best in antiglobulin test; probably identical with **Wrᵃ**
Romunda (Rm)	Reacts best in antiglobulin test
Batty (Byᵃ)	Reacts best in antiglobulin test
Swan (Swᵃ)	Reacts in all media; reaction weaker with enzyme-treated cells
Good	Reacts in all media but no reaction with enzyme-treated cells (papain)
Donna	Reacts in antiglobulin test with enzyme-treated cells (but not after bromelin treatment)
Buᵃ	Reacts in antiglobulin test
Nyberg (Nyᵃ)	Antibody agglutinates Ny(a+) cells in saline media, best at 4° and 28° C, and does not react with antiglobulin serum
Stones (Stᵃ)	Reacts with antiglobulin serum
Ridley (Riᵃ)	Reacts with antiglobulin serum
Gonzales (Goᵃ)	Reacts with antiglobulin serum
Schmidt (Sm)	Reacts with antiglobulin serum
II. Public	
Vel (Veᵃ)	Saline agglutinin at 18° C, hemolysin in the presence of complement, or in antiglobulin test at 37° C
Cartwright (Ytᵃ)	Reacts best in antiglobulin test, with enzyme-treated or untreated erythrocytes
I-i	Anti-**I** found as an autoantibody in individuals with acquired hemolytic anemia, cold-antibody type; reacts in saline media and with ficin-treated cells at 6° C
Gerbich (Ge)	Reacts best by antiglobulin reaction
Auberger (Au)	Reacts best by antiglobulin reaction with serum of antigamma specificity
Dombrach (Doᵃ)	Reacts best by antiglobulin reaction with papainized erythrocytes

mosome. This is the only sex-linked group. It is a useful system in medicolegal applications and of special interest to the geneticist as an additional genetic marker on the X chromosome.

"Private" (low-incidence) and "public" (high-incidence) blood factors

In the course of studying cases of hemolytic disease of the newborn, a variety of factors have been found that appear not to belong in any of the accepted blood group systems. Some of these are found only in the members of the family involved and so are called "private." Others can be detected in nearly all individuals studied and are therefore called "public" (Table 11-34).

SEROLOGIC TESTS IN DISPUTED PARENTAGE
Exclusion of paternity or maternity

More than 60 serologic and biochemical systems potentially useful in medicolegal cases involving disputed parentage were reviewed in a report by Miale et al (1976). While the application of all known systems would make exclusion of paternity of a falsely accused man almost certain, such extensive testing is neither feasible nor recommended. First, antisera for some serologic systems either are not available or are available only in one or very few laboratories. Second, in the case of "high frequency" factors the probability

of exclusion is very low (Table 11-35). Third, although the use of biochemical systems is sound, these procedures are technically difficult.

The Committee on Transfusion and Transplantation of the American Medical Association, working with representatives of the American Bar Association (Miale et al, 1976), officially recommended the use of six blood group systems and the HLA system for the exclusion of parentage. The probability of exclusion of nonfather for each system is given in Table 11-36. The cumulative probability for various sequences of test systems is given in Table 11-37. It is of interest that the cumulative probability of exclusion of nonfathers for these seven systems is nearly as high as that for the total list of more than 60 serologic and biochemical systems (excluding HLA). Other systems may be used as well: group specific component (Gc), haptoglobin, immunoglobulin haplotypes, red cell acid phosphatase phenotype, and red cell phosphoglucomutase phenotype. The joint AMA-ABA report recommends another change in current practice, the calculation of the *probability* of fatherhood. This is discussed in the following section.

This report has received criticism from various sources for various reasons. Sussman (1978) pointed out some typographical errors, for which the committee is grateful, but he also stated that "the erythrocyte enzyme, blood protein, and HLA systems have not been subject to the thorough study

Table 11-35. Mean probability of exclusion of nonfathers for potentially useful systems*†

System or test	Mean probability of exclusion of nonfathers			System or test	Mean probability of exclusion of nonfathers		
	Black	White	Japanese		Black	White	Japanese
ABO	.1774	.1342	.1917	Complement, third component	.0819	.1523	.0192
Auberger	.0105	.0186	—	Diaphorase	—	.0085	—
Cartwright (Yt)	.0069	.0395	—	Esterase D	—	.0913	—
Colton	0	.0266	—	Galactose-A-phosphate-uridyl-transferase	—	.0626	—
Cs	—	.0006	—	Glucose-6-phosphate dehydrogenase	.0932	0	0
Diego	.0030	0	.0304	Glutamic oxaloacetic transaminase (soluble)	0	0	.0113
Dombrock	.0661	.0518	—	Glutamic pyruvic transaminase (soluble)	.1285	.1875	.1826
Duffy	.0420	.1844	.1159				
Henshaw	.0151	0	—	Glutathione reductase	.2071	.2016	—
Hunter	.0170	.0026	—	Gm, serum groups	.2071	.2275	.1873
Kell	.0049	.0354	0	Group-specific component (Gc)	.0731	.1661	.1560
Kidd	.1545	.1869	.1573	Haptoglobin α	.1873	.1834	.1596
Lewis	.0262	.0024	.0193	Hemoglobin β	.0453	0	0
Lutheran	.0368	.0311	0	InV, serum group	.2366	.0601	.1664
M-N-S-s	.3206	.3095	.2531	Malic enzyme (NADP) soluble	.1258	.1681	—
P	.0026	.0266	.0809				
Penney	0	.0109	0	Parotid basic protein	.1163	.0050	0
Rh	.1859	.2746	.2050	Pepsinogen	.0126	.0126	0
Sd	—	.0052	—	Peptidase A	.0747	.1635	—
Secretor	.0305	.0296	.0238	Peptidase C	.0665	.0102	—
St	—	.0006	.0283	Peptidase D	.0459	.0108	—
Sutter	.0667	0	—	Phosphoglucomutase (locus 1)	.1344	.1457	.1476
U	.0001	0	—	Phosphoglucomutase (locus 3)	.1740	.1554	.1306
Vel	0	.0184	0				
Xg	.1615	.0965	.1344	Properdin factor B	—	.1443	—
Acetylcholinesterase	—	.1153	—	Pseudocholinesterase (locus 1)	.0052	.0158	0
Acid phosphatase	.1588	.2323	.1340	6-phosphogluconate dehydrogenase	.0335	.0229	.0586
Adenosine deaminase	.0283	.0452	.0291				
Adenylate kinase	.0059	.0428	0	Transferrin	.0410	.0064	.0079
Ag (x)	—	.0813	—	Xm, serum group	.1757	.1625	—
Alcohol dehydrogenase (locus 2)	—	.0452	—				
Alcohol dehydrogenase (locus 3)	—	.1824	—				
α-acid glycoprotein	.1834	.1773	.1583				
α₁-antitrypsin	.0180	.0806	.0170				
Amylase (urinary)	.0411	.0399	—				
Ceruloplasmin	.0504	.0059	.0214				

*From Miale et al, 1976.
†Dash = no data available.

Table 11-36. The seven test systems recommended for use in disputed parentage*

System	Mean probability of exclusion of nonfathers		
	Black	White	Japanese
A-B-O	.1174	.1342	.1917
Rh	.1859	.2746	.2050
M-N-S-s	.3206	.3095	.2531
Kell	.0049	.0354	0
Duffy	.0420	.1844	.1159
Kidd	.1545	.1869	.1573
HLA	.78-.80	.78-.80	.78-.80

*See Table 11-37 for cumulative probability of exclusion.

Table 11-37. Cumulative probability of exclusion of nonfathers

Systems*	Cumulative probability of exclusion (%)†		
	Black	White	Japanese
1	17.44	13.42	19.16
1 + 2	33.03	37.19	35.74
1 + 2 + 3	54.50	56.63	52.0
1 + 2 + 3 + 4	54.72	58.17	52.0
1 + 2 + 3 + 4 + 5	56.63	65.88	57.56
1 + 2 + 3 + 4 + 5 + 6	63.37	72.26	64.24
1 + 2 + 3 + 4 + 5 + 6 + 7	91.21	93.34	91.42

*1 = A-B-O, 2 = Rh, 3 = M-N-S-s, 4 = Kell, 5 = Duffy, 6 = Kidd, 7 = HLA.
†Cumulative probability is not the sum of individual probabilities, but is calculated using the formula: Probability = $1 - (1 - P_1)(1 - P_2) \ldots (1 - P_n)$ where P_1, P_2, and P_n are the probabilities of individual exclusions.

and research that the 100% acceptable systems have undergone.''

Specifically, he believes that the scarcity of monospecific HLA testing sera makes the application of this system impractical. However, Terasaki (1978) and Terasaki et al (1978) have published impressive data on the usefulness of HLA testing, not only in the exclusion of paternity but also in determining paternity. Sussman (1978) also does not agree that testing for the Duffy and Kidd groups should be done, but Polesky (1979) does include these systems. In his laboratory Polesky tests for blood group antigens first (A-B-O, Rh-Hr, M-N-S-s, K-k, Fy^a and Fy^b, Jk^a and Jk^b). The probability of exclusion of paternity using these six systems is 63.37% in blacks, 72.26% in whites, and 64.24% in Japanese. If more extensive testing is needed to reach an opinion, Polesky adds five serum proteins (Gm, haptoglobin, Gc protein, Bf [GBG], and Km) and five red cell enzymes (acid phosphatase, PGM_1, esterase D, adenylate kinase, and 6-PGD), which brings the cumulative probability of exclusion up to about 94%. In the joint AMA-ABA report (Miale et al, 1976) we recommended adding only the HLA system to the six blood groups studied, and these seven systems have cumulative probability of exclusion of 91.21% in blacks, 93.34% in whites, and 91.42% in Japanese.

At this time it is my recommendation that if a pathologist or immunohematologist gets involved in the question of disputed parentage, the first step would be testing for four to six blood group antigens. If a positive exclusion is then possible, there is no need for further testing. If exclusion is not possible, then further testing is indicated, with the systems chosen depending on the facilities and expertise available (Miale et al, 1976; Polesky and Krause, 1977; Terasaki, 1978; Poleski, 1979).

Types of exclusion

EXCLUSION OF NONFATHER. Five types of exclusion of a nonfather are possible.

1. The classic type in which the putative father is lacking a specificity that is present in the child and is absent in the mother so that the specificity found in the child must have been inherited from another man, i.e., child is K +, mother and putative father are K −.
2. Exclusion when the child lacks both specificities found in the putative father, i.e., child is group O, putative father is group AB.
3. The child is homozygous with respect to a specificity not present in both parents, i.e., child is *KK,* mother is *Kk* or *KK,* putative father is *kk.*
4. The child lacks a specificity for which the putative father is homozygous, i.e., child is *kk,* putative father is *KK.*
5. Indirect exclusion where the study of the parents of the mother and putative father or their other children seem to more clearly define their genetic makeup. For example, a person of phenotype (group) A_1 is either of genotype A^1A^1 or of genotype A^1O. The two genotypes cannot be distinguished by serologic studies on the given person. However, since the two genes are inherited one from each parent, parents of genotypes A^1A^1 and A^1A^1 cannot have a child of genotype A^1O.

Table 11-38. Verbal predicates, according to Hummel (1961) for different likelihoods of paternity (*W*), comparing the phenotype frequency of the putative father to that of a random man with the same blood group phenotype

W	Likelihood of paternity
99.80-99.90	Practically proved
99.1-99.75	Extremely likely
95-99	Very likely
90-95	Likely
80-90	Undecided
<80	Not useful

EXCLUSION OF NONMOTHER. As noted in the following sections, it is possible to exclude maternity in certain serologic patterns involving a given mother-child–putative father set. For example, a woman of group A_2 cannot be the mother of a child of group A_1B, regardless of the group of the father.

In the usual case of disputed paternity, the assumption is made that the woman is in fact the mother of the child of the mother-child–putative father set. This assumption is not always valid, in which case exclusion or nonexclusion of paternity is also not valid.

In addition to situations involving disputed paternity, the question of excluding maternity arises in cases of alleged child exchange, when the exclusion or probability of maternity is of primary importance.

IMPORTANCE OF GENETIC MUTATION. The possibility of mutation, which might invalidate the observed inheritance pattern, is very small, estimated to occur once in 40,000 persons. This is so infrequent that it can be ignored in the interpretation of the serologic findings.

The likelihood of paternity

For both medicolegal and socioeconomic reasons, it is desirable to estimate the likelihood of paternity in cases when the putative father is not excluded. This estimate is given to the court and is admissible evidence in many foreign countries. It should be noted that the estimate of likelihood of paternity is merely another piece of evidence to be adjudicated by the court.

In some special situations, as when there is genetic conformity between the child and putative father for an extremely rare specificity (not present in the mother), for example subgroup A_3 or the rare phenotype M^g, the likelihood of paternity is extremely high and obvious without resort to special calculations. Although such situations are not absolute proof of paternity the court can give this evidence due weight.

Usually the situation is not so simple. The serologist has to deal with various circumstances.

1. Calculation of likelihood of paternity in ''one-man'' cases, i.e., only one man has been named the putative father and he is not excluded. In this case the computation estimates the likelihood that the one man is in fact the father.
2. Calculation of likelihood of paternity in ''multiple men'' cases, where more than one man is known to be

The erythrocyte: abnormal forms and immunology   517

Table 11-39. Exclusion of paternity and maternity by the A_1A_2BO system*

Phenotype of mother	Phenotype of child					
	O	A_1	A_2	B	A_1B	A_2B
O	A_1B,A_2B	O,A_2,B,A_2B	O,B,A_1B	O,A_1,A_2	ME	ME
A_1	A_1B,A_2B	None	A_1B	O,A_1,A_2	O,A_1,A_2	O,A_1,A_2
A_2	A_1B,A_2B	O,A_2,B,A_2B	A_1B	O,A_1,A_2	ME	O,A_1,A_2
B	A_1B,A_2B	O,A_2,B,A_2B	O,B,A_1B	None	O,A_2,B,A_2B	O,B,A_1B
A_1B	ME	None	ME	None	O,A_2	O,B,A_1B
A_2B	ME	O,A_2,B,A_2B	A_1B	None	O,A_2,B,A_2B	O

*If the phenotype of the putative father appears in the box corresponding to the child-mother pair, the putative father is excluded. If ME appears in the box, there is maternal exclusion. Note the report of Perkins and Morel (1980) regarding the problem of subgroups of A in blacks.

involved and not excluded. In this case the computation estimates the likelihood of paternity for each of the involved men.

The great majority of situations fall under the first category.

In "one-man" cases, Hummel et al (1971, 1972) have proposed the application of the equation of Essen-Möller (1938). The plausibility of paternity, W. is calculated from:

$$W = \frac{1}{1 + \left(\dfrac{Y_1}{X_1} \times \dfrac{Y_2}{X_2} \times \dfrac{Y_3}{X_3} \cdots\right)}$$

where

Y = Frequency of various blood group phenotypes of men among the normal male population
X = Frequency of corresponding phenotypes of true fathers in the given mother-child combination

The calculation can be carried out from tables of genotype frequencies, but Hummel (1961) has prepared tables based on logarithms that facilitate the estimation of probability of paternity.

The calculated probability of paternity is not proof of paternity, even when it is close to 100%, but the greater the probability figure, the greater the likelihood of paternity (Walker, 1978). Langaney and Pison (1975) do not recommend calculating the probability of paternity. In any case, the calculation of W gives a "verbal predicate" of likelihood of paternity (Table 11-38). The information that an accused man is not excluded and the probability of paternity are reported to the court and represent evidence to be considered in arriving at a decision.

Use of individual systems
A-B-O (A₁-A₂-B-O) blood group system

Tests performed on subjects' red blood cells and serum with appropriate antisera, lectins, and cells of known blood group allow all subjects to be classified in one of the following categories: group O, group A_1, group A_2, group B, group A_1B, or group A_2B. The inheritance pattern is well established and allows a tabulation of phenotypes possible or not possible in children from a given mating (Table 11-39). It is possible to exclude maternity in some combinations of serologic factors determined from the mother-child-father combination (Table 11-39).

The following special features should be noted:

1. Subgroups of A are often incompletely developed at birth, and are usually fully developed by 1 year of age.

2. Subgroups of A give weak reactions with potent anti-A sera, stronger with group O serum, and may be missed entirely if the antiserum is weak.

3. There is an extremely rare genetic type called cis-AB (Reviron et al, 1968) or AB* (Salmon, 1971; p. 494) where the transmission of blood group AB appears to be by a single rather than two separate chromosomes, so that a cis-AB person can then be the parent of an O child and an O person can be the parent of a cis-AB child. Cis-AB also reacts weakly with anti-B, and more strongly with anti-B from A_2 blood than with anti-B from A_1 blood. In cis-AB individuals who are secretors, no B substance is demonstrable in their saliva, and the A substance may also be affected.

4. In the rare "Bombay" type the red cells contain no A,B, or H agglutinogens and may be typed as group O. However, the serum contains anti-A, anti-B, and anti-H.

5. In an occasional leukemic or preleukemic subject there is a change in the reactivity of the red cells, which simulates an actual change in blood group, i.e., red cells of a known group A or B person may simulate the reactions of group O cells. Acquired agammaglobulinemia in leukemia and other diseases may be characterized by the absence of isoagglutinins in the serum.

6. Change of red cell type has also been reported in subjects with colitis or carcinoma of the stomach, characterized by the red cells acquiring weak B characteristics, i.e., a person of group A_1 reacts as if the group were A_1B. This is called "acquired B." Acquired B should be suspected clinically, from the weak reaction with anti-B and from the presence of anti-B isoagglutinin in the serum.

7. Failure to demonstrate the expected isoagglutinins in the serum may be due to (1) acquired or congenital agammaglobulinemia, (2) a weak receptor, as in persons of subgroup A_4 or A_{el}, or (3) the rare blood chimera situation.

8. In the case of the rare weak subgroups of A, the presence of such a rare subgroup in the child and the putative father is strong likelihood of paternity.

The Rh blood group system

This system is more complicated than the ABO system, and knowledge has progressed from the first basic distinction between Rh+ and Rh− to the characterization of 40

Table 11-40. Exclusion of paternity or maternity by the Rh-Hr blood types*

Phenotype of putative mother	Phenotype of putative father				
	1 rh RH₀	2 rh' rh Rh₁ rh	3 rh' rh' Rh₁ Rh₁	4 rh" rh Rh₂ rh	5 rh" rh" Rh₂ Rh₂
1 rh Rh₀	2, 3, 4, 5, 6a, 6b, 7, 8, 9	3, 4, 5, 6a, 6b, 7, 8, 9	1, 3, 4, 5, 6a, 6b, 7, 8, 9	2, 3, 5, 6a, 6b, 7, 8, 9	1, 2, 3, 5, 6a, 6b, 7, 8, 9
2 rh' rh Rh₁ rh	3, 4, 5, 6a, 6b, 7, 8, 9	4, 5, 6a, 6b, 7, 8, 9	1, 4, 5, 6a, 6b, 7, 8, 9	3, 5, 6b, 7, 8, 9	1, 2, 3, 5, 6b, 7, 8, 9
3 rh' rh' Rh₁ Rh₁	1, 3, 4, 5, 6a, 6b, 7, 8, 9	1, 4, 5, 6a, 6b, 7, 8, 9	1, 2, 4, 5, 6a, 6b, 7, 8, 9	1, 3, 4, 5, 6b, 7, 8, 9	1, 2, 3, 4, 5, 6b, 7, 8, 9
4 rh" rh Rh₂ rh	2, 3, 5, 6a, 6b, 7, 8, 9	3, 5, 6b, 7, 8, 9	1, 3, 4, 5, 6b, 7, 8, 9	2, 3, 6a, 6b, 7, 8, 9	1, 2, 3, 6a, 6b, 7, 8, 9
5 rh" rh" Rh₂ Rh₂	1, 2, 3, 5, 6a, 6b, 7, 8, 9	1, 2, 3, 5, 6b, 7, 8, 9	1, 2, 3, 4, 5, 6b, 7, 8, 9	1, 2, 3, 6a, 6b, 7, 8, 9	1, 2, 3, 4, 6a, 6b, 7, 8, 9
6a rh' rh" Rh₁ Rh₂	1, 3, 5, 6a, 6b, 7, 8, 9	1, 5, 6b, 7, 8, 9	1, 2, 4, 5, 6b, 7, 8, 9	1, 3, 6b, 7, 8, 9	1, 2, 3, 4, 6b, 7, 8, 9
6b rhy rh Rhz rh	2, 3, 4, 5, 6a, 7, 8, 9	3, 4, 5, 6a, 8, 9	1, 3, 4, 5, 6a, 6b, 8, 9	2, 3, 5, 6a, 7, 9	1, 2, 3, 5, 6a, 6b, 7, 9
7 rhy rh' Rhz Rh₁	1, 3, 4, 5, 6a, 7, 8, 9	1, 4, 5, 6a, 8, 9	1, 2, 4, 5, 6a, 6b, 8, 9	1, 3, 4, 5, 7, 9	1, 2, 3, 4, 5, 6b, 7, 9
8 rhy rh" Rhz Rh₂	1, 2, 3, 5, 6a, 7, 8, 9	1, 2, 3, 5, 8, 9	1, 2, 3, 4, 5, 6b, 8, 9	1, 2, 3, 6a, 7, 9	1, 2, 3, 4, 6a, 6b, 7, 9
9 rhy rhy Rhz Rhz	1, 2, 3, 4, 5, 6a, 7, 8, 9	1, 2, 3, 4, 5, 6a, 8, 9	1, 2, 3, 4, 5, 6a, 6b, 8, 9	1, 2, 3, 4, 5, 6a, 7, 9	1, 2, 3, 4, 5, 6a, 6b, 7, 9

*From Wiener and Nieberg, 1963.

Instructions for use of table are as follows:

1. Determine the phenotypes of the blood of the mother, putative father, and the child or children using potent and specific antisera, including appropriate controls.
2. Assign the corresponding phenotype symbol and number to each individual tested.

phenotypes. By itself this system provides a 20% to 27% probability of excluding paternity of nonfathers.

Because of its complexity, the genetics and serologic principles of the system have come to be expressed by two quite dissimilar concepts, the CDE/cde nomenclature of Fisher and Race and the genetic and serologic principles expressed by the Rh-Hr nomenclature of Wiener. A review of the differences between the two is given elsewhere (p. 505). Experts in this field use both interchangeably, though some prefer one over the other. As applied to disputed parentage, both should lead to the same conclusion, but the lack of anti-d antiserum sometimes necessitates defining the "most probable" phenotype with the CDE/cde system.

When six antisera are used (anti-**Rh₀**, anti-**rh'**, anti-**rh"**, anti-**rhʷ**, anti-**hr'**, anti-**hr"**) plus anti-**hr** to distinguish between a few selected phenotypes, 28 phenotypes can be distinguished corresponding to 55 genotypes. Having determined the phenotype and genotype or possible genotypes (Table 11-23) of the mother-child–putative father situation, exclusion or nonexclusion of paternity or exclusion of maternity is decided by standard genetic diagrams.

> **Example:** Child's genotype: r'r'
> Mother's genotype: R¹r'
> Putative father's genotype: rr

Children of the given mother and putative father must have a genetic makeup that reflects the inheritance of one

	Phenotype of putative father			
6a rh' rh" Rh_1Rh_2	**6b** rh_y rh Rh_z rh	**7** rh_y rh' $Rh_z Rh_1$	**8** rh_y rh" $Rh_z Rh_2$	**9** rh_y rh_y $Rh_z Rh_z$
1, 3, 5, 6a, 6b, 7, 8, 9	2, 3, 4, 5, 6a, 7, 8, 9	1, 3, 4, 5, 6a, 7, 8, 9	1, 2, 3, 5, 6a, 7, 8, 9	1, 2, 3, 4, 5, 6a, 7, 8, 9
1, 5, 6b, 7, 8, 9	3, 4, 5, 6a, 8, 9	1, 4, 5, 6a, 8, 9	1, 2, 3, 5, 8, 9	1, 2, 3, 4, 5, 6a, 8, 9
1, 2, 4, 5, 6b, 7, 8, 9	1, 3, 4, 5, 6a, 6b, 8, 9	1, 2, 4, 5, 6a, 6b, 8, 9	1, 2, 3, 4, 5, 6b, 8, 9	1, 2, 3, 4, 5, 6a, 6b, 8, 9
1, 3, 6b, 7, 8, 9	2, 3, 5, 6a, 7, 9	1, 3, 4, 5, 7, 9	1, 2, 3, 6a, 7, 9	1, 2, 3, 4, 5, 6a, 7, 9
1, 2, 3, 4, 6b, 7, 8, 9	1, 2, 3, 5, 6a, 6b, 7, 9	1, 2, 3, 4, 5, 6b, 7, 9	1, 2, 3, 4, 6a, 6b, 7, 9	1, 2, 3, 4, 5, 6a, 6b, 7, 9
1, 2, 4, 6b, 7, 8, 9	1, 3, 5, 6a, 6b, 9	1, 2, 4, 5, 6b, 9	1, 2, 3, 4, 6b, 9	1, 2, 3, 4, 5, 6a, 6b, 9
1, 3, 5, 6a, 6b, 9	2, 3, 4, 5, 6a, 7, 8	1, 3, 4, 5, 6a, 8	1, 2, 3, 5, 6a, 7	1, 2, 3, 4, 5, 6a, 7, 8
1, 2, 4, 5, 6b, 9	1, 3, 4, 5, 6a, 8	1, 2, 4, 5, 6a, 6b, 8	1, 2, 3, 4, 5, 6b	1, 2, 3, 4, 5, 6a, 6b, 8
1, 2, 3, 4, 6b, 9	1, 2, 3, 5, 6a, 7	1, 2, 3, 4, 5, 6b	1, 2, 3, 4, 6a, 6b, 7	1, 2, 3, 4, 5, 6a, 6b, 7
1, 2, 3, 4, 5, 6a, 6b, 9	1, 2, 3, 4, 5, 6a, 7, 8	1, 2, 3, 4, 5, 6a, 6b, 8	1, 2, 3, 4, 5, 6a, 6b, 7	1, 2, 3, 4, 5, 6a, 6b, 7, 8

3. Find the assigned number of the mother and father in the side and top columns of the table and locate the box at which both intersect.

4. The child or children are not possible from this mating if their assigned numbers appear in this box.

5. Underlined phenotype numbers represent children for whom maternity is excluded.

6. This table is to be applied only to matings in which at least one of the parents is Rh_0 positive. Where both parents are Rh_0 negative, necessarily all Rh_0-positive children are excluded.

gene from each parent. Accordingly, the only children possible from this mating must have one of the following genotypes: R^1r or $r'r$. Since the child in this example is of genotype $r'r'$ the putative father is excluded.

Tables of exclusion have been constructed based on the more common genotypes of the mother-child–putative father combination (Table 11-40) but should not be used to the exclusion of the application of standard genetic diagrams as in the example above. The exclusion of maternity is based on the same principles:

The following special features should be noted:

1. Many commercial antisera labeled anti-**rh'** contain both anti-**rh'** and anti-**rh_i** and may in fact contain a preponderance of anti-**rh_i**. Anti-**rh_i** differs from anti-**rh'** in its inability to agglutinate cells having the rare agglutinogens rh_y and Rh_z (very rare in whites, less rare in Mongols). In the rare genotype Rh_zrh, the cells react with anti-**rh'** but not with anti-**rh_i**.

2. Many rare specificities exist in the system. These define extremely rare genotypes but do not affect the basic pattern.

The M-N-S-s blood group system

This system is superficially simple, based on two pairs of codominant allelic genes (*M* and *N*) and three phenotypes (M, MN, and N) associated with a second pair of codominant allelic genes (*S* and *s*) determining phenotypes S, Ss, and s. Transmission is by gene couplets *MS*, *Ms*, *NS*, and

Table 11-41. Exclusion of paternity by the M-N-S-s system when three antisera are used (anti-**M,** anti-**N,** and anti-**S**)

Mating	Children possible	Mating	Children possible
MS ×MS	MS, M	MNS ×MNS	MS, M, NS, N, MNS, MN
MS ×M	MS, M	MNS ×MN	MS, M, NS, N, MNS, MN
M ×M	M	MN ×MN	M, N, MN
MS ×MNS	MS, MNS, M, MN	MNS ×NS	MNS, MN, NS, N
MS ×MN	MS, MNS, M, MN	MNS ×N	MNS, MN, NS, N
M ×MNS	MS, MNS, M, MN	MN ×NS	MNS, MN, NS, N
M ×MN	M, MN	MN ×N	MN, N
MS ×NS	MNS, MN	NS ×NS	NS, N
MS ×N	MNS, MN	NS ×N	NS, N
M ×NS	MNS, MN	N ×N	N
M ×N	MN		

Ns. In addition, the agglutinogen U, present in all whites but absent in some blacks, is associated with both S and s. Four antisera (anti-**M,** anti-**N,** anti-**S,** and anti-**s**) determine nine phenotypes.

The combinations of phenotypes in the mother-child-putative father combination leading to exclusion of paternity or maternity are shown in Table 11-41. The chance of exclusion is about 24%. The possibilities of establishing maternal exclusion are limited to two situations: an MS woman cannot be the mother of an NS child, and an NS woman cannot be the mother of an MS child.

The following special features should be noted:

1. An exception to the rules that M parents cannot have an N child, or that N parents cannot have an M child, occurs in the rare instances (about 1:40,000, not to be confused with the rate of spontaneous mutation) where one of the pair of genes is M^g. Gene M^g determines an agglutinogen lacking M specificity, so the apparent exclusion in case of a putative father who is N with a child who is M might not hold if the father were M^gN and the child MM^g. Anti-M^g serum is not always available, but where exclusion is based only on the MN system all efforts should be made to test for M^g. In fact, the presence of gene M^g in both the father and the child would be a very strong likelihood of paternity.
2. The rare allele M^k inhibits the expression of the MN as well as the Ss locus.
3. In blacks, the He (Henshaw) factor should be taken into account. It is present in about 3% of blacks and absent in whites. Anti-**He** may be present in anti-**M** serum so that an N+ and He+ individual might mistakenly be typed as MN.
4. Commercial anti-N antisera should be rigidly controlled for overactivity or underactivity. Exclusion based on the MN blood group should use anti-N lectins to check the results.
5. Agglutinogen U should also be considered in blacks. It is present in all whites but absent in a small percentage of blacks. Blacks who are U negative also lack both S and s. Testing with anti-U serum can be helpful in interracial mother-child–putative father combinations, but only when one is U-negative.

The Kell blood group system

There are many specificities in this system, but only two are useful in disputed parentage, K and k. The use of two antisera, anti-**K** and anti-**k** defines three phenotypes, K, k, and Kk, corresponding to genotypes *KK, kk,* and *Kk.* This makes a simple system that needs no further elaboration, exclusion being along classic lines.

The following special features should be noted:

1. Use of both anti-**K** and anti-**k** when testing whites provides a chance of exclusion of about 3.5%. Since very few people are type K (Kell positive), testing with only anti-**K** reduces the chance of exclusion by only a few tenths of one percent.
2. The incidence of agglutinogen K is extremely small in blacks and is virtually zero in Chinese and Japanese. In these racial groups no exclusion may be expected on the basis of this blood group system. On the other hand, in an interracial situation the detection of K positivity could provide strong likelihood of paternity.

The Duffy blood group system

The antisera, anti-**Fy**^{a} and anti-**Fy**^{b}, define four phenotypes, Fy(a+b−), Fy(a+b+), Fy(a−b+), and Fy(a−b−), determined by allelic genes *Fy*^{a}, *Fy*^{b}, and *fy*. Gene *fy* has a high incidence in blacks (about 78%) but has not been identified in whites, so that in whites only the first three phenotypes are possible. Exclusion is along classic lines.

The following special feature should be noted.

If a person fails to react with either anti-**Fy**^{a} or anti-**Fy**^{b} (assuming no technical errors), this would be strong evidence that he or she is of black origin.

The Kidd blood group system

Two antisera, anti-**Jk**^{a} and anti-**Jk**^{b} define three phenotypes Jk(a+b−), Jk(a+b+), and Jk(a−b+), determined by the pair of genes *Jk*^{a} and *Jk*^{b}. Exclusion is along classic lines.

The following special feature should be noted.

A third gene has been postulated, *jk,* detemining a fourth phenotype, Jk(a-b-). This phenotype has been found in only one family of European whites, and only in single instances in a Filipino woman, a Chinese, and a Hawaiian-Chinese.

The HLA system

It has been known for some time that there exists in human beings a major histocompatibility system (HLA) of great complexity, composed of a series of many closely linked genes. Originally the serologically defined specificities of the HLA system were assigned to two linked loci, each with multiple alleles. These two loci are now designated HLA-A and HLA-B. More recently a third locus, HLA-C, was identified although its individual specificities are not easily identified in typing laboratories in the United States. A fourth locus, HLA-D, has also been identified by mixed lymphocyte culture reactions but is not yet readily detected by serologic means. The specificities (or the antigens) that are controlled by genes at each of these four loci are now identified by numbers. When the specificity is first recognized, this is indicated by placing a W in front of the number. Later, when general consensus is reached and the specificity firmly established by the World Health Organization Nomenclature Committee, the W is dropped and the number retained (Amos, 1975).

A "blank" in a genotype might indicate either homozygocity for a single specificity at a locus or, alternatively, it might indicate an inability to identify an antigen. This is usually clarified by family studies. The segregant series are now designated as HLA-A, HLA-B, HLA-C, HLA-D, and HLA-DR (Albert et al, 1978).An excellent review of the principles and methodology of this system is given in the monograph by Svejgaard et al (1979).

The HLA system is one of genetic dominance. Therefore, two antigens or specificities are possible for each segregating locus. At present, as many as eight tissue antigens can be identified in each individual. More practical limitations of tissue typing today, however, include only the specificites of HLA-A and HLA-B. A total of 53 specificities are now recognized within these two loci. Currently available tissue typing trays (for transplantation only) provided by the National Institutes of Health to each of over 200 typing laboratories in the United States allow for ready identification of 32 of the genotypic specificities. As time goes on, more and more reliable monospecific HLA antisera will become available to expert investigators. Using these trays, more than 255 haplotypes can be recognized with as many as 65,025 genotypes. The large number of antigens in the system makes it apparent that of all the individual systems, HLA typing offers the highest single-system probability of exclusion.

As in other genetic systems, HLA sometimes shows an unusually high association between antigens that constitute a single haplotype. This is referred to as genetic dysequilibrium. Often such associations are very selective for certain ethnic groups or subpopulations within various geographic regions of the world. There is a considerable amount of data available on haplotype frequencies (Jeannet et al, 1972; Mayr, 1971; Dausset et al, 1970). However, even larger numbers of special groups must be typed to provide the statistical basis for analysis of their HLA inheritance. Even when all haplotype frequencies are known, the HLA typing laboratory will still require a determination of racial and geographic origin to calculate the likelihood of exclusion of identification of paternity.

EXCLUSION OF PATERNITY. The calculation of probabilities for either exclusion or identification of a putative father is complicated by our inability to assign a haplotype designation to the father, even when we have identified all four HLA (A and B) antigens. If a putative father is shown to have both HLA antigens that constitute the paternal haplotype inherited by the child, he still could be excluded if studies of his father and mother revealed that he had inherited the antigens singly; i.e., one from each parent.

Using gene frequencies, it is possible to ascribe a general probability of exclusion by using the formula $(1-P)^4P$ (Soulier et al, 1974). The sum of these "probabilities of exclusion" then will give the total probability of exclusion.

LIKELIHOOD OF PATERNITY. The ability to establish a statistical likelihood that an accused man is the real father is an even more complicated problem. Here we must calculate the possibility that a man who has both antigens of the suspected paternal haplotype of a child may have inherited these antigens independently, one from each parent (a *trans* configuration). If they indeed have been inherited together as a true haplotype, they are said to be *cis* in nature and could have been inherited by the child. If the exact haplotype of the child that has been inherited from the father can be determined, then only those men who have both antigens could possibly be the father. If they have both antigens, the probability that they are in cis position is $2P-P^2$ (Speiser, 1975). The probability of trans configuration of the antigens can also be calculated.

These calculations are made knowing that the two antigens in question have been detected in a putative father. However, they ignore the possibility that the other two antigens have also been identified. If all four HLA antigens are known, then a more precise calculation of cis or trans possibilities can be made using haplotype frequency tables. Unfortunately, haplotype frequencies are now known only for the common haplotypes. Until all haplotype frequencies have been identified, we probably must be satisfied with simple calculation of serotype frequencies of antigens to determine the likelihood of paternity. Fortunately, the current data commonly allow for the ready identification of antigen frequencies after serologic identification using lymphocytotoxicity tests. Using antigen frequencies, it is possible to determine the likelihood that a man in the random population would possess both antigens that have been identified as paternal HLA antigens of the child in question. In the case of the rare antigens, this likelihood can be minimized (often less than 1%). However, with some common haplotypes, such as HLA-A3–HLA-B7, the general population demonstrates almost a 7.6% frequency. Family studies, of course, would be helpful in confirming that the putative father did indeed inherit the antigens in a cis configuration and therefore would be the most likely to be the father. However, it is difficult to see how the cooperation of family members could be obtained to allow family testing that would result in identification of paternity as opposed to exclusion.

As for some of the very rare blood group subgroups, there are very rare HLA specificities, i.e., HLA-AW35 or HLA-B14 that, if present in both the child and putative father but absent in the mother, would indicate a very high probability of paternity. Lee (1980) has calculated the paternity index (PI) for various mother-child-putative father trios.

Procedures and forms relating to the introduction of evidence

To satisfy the requirements of the law of evidence and to facilitate the introduction of evidence into the courts, it is recommended that standard procedures, including forms, be adopted. Procedures and forms document the full series of events relating to the testing procedures, beginning with the court's order (or other request) that samples be taken and tests made and ending with the expert's report to the court.

All parties should appreciate the confidential value of the test results. It is recommended that only requests from the court, an officer of the court, or an attorney be honored. Test results should be given only to the requesting agency or party unless there is written authorization for other distribution.

While it might seem desirable to encourage universal adoption of standard forms that satisfy all the requirements, it is probably sufficient to agree on a standard content of the forms.

The initial request

The initial order that blood and other samples be obtained and tested should identify the court or other requesting party, the case, the parties involved in the case and the purpose of the tests, i.e., exclusion of paternity, exclusion of maternity, etc. The request should direct the named parties to present themselves on the agreed upon date to the expert or to a laboratory at a designated place and time. Each person to be tested should receive a copy of the request. If the testing is to be done elsewhere than in the laboratory where the samples are obtained, the request should state the name and address of the expert to whom the samples should be shipped. Finally, the initial request should indicate the party or parties to whom the results of the tests and the opinion of the expert should be sent.

Identification of parties

It is essential that the persons to be tested in a case of disputed parentage be identified and the identification documented in such a way that there can be no question of identification in court. This can be achieved in various ways, but the following procedure is used by most experts.

1. All the persons to be tested should be present at the same time if at all possible. If one of the parties cannot be present at the designated time, he or she should be identified by his or her attorney and so recorded, in which case the attorney assumes the responsibility of acting as an officer of the court.
2. The following identification and documentation of identification should be made on an appropriate form or forms:
   a. Date blood samples are drawn.
   b. Name, address, social security number (if any), driver's license number (if any), and signature of each party, indicating which is the mother, which the child (or children), and which the putative father (or fathers).
   c. Permission of each person to be tested for blood and other samples to be obtained, including a state-

Table 11-42. Suggested binary code for A-B-O system*

| Blood group | Reactions with antiserum | | | Code |
	Anti-A	Anti-B	Anti-A₁	
O	−	−	−	000
A₁	+	−	+	101
A₂	+	−	−	100
B	−	+	−	010
A₁B	+	+	+	111
A₂B	+	+	−	110

*After Wiener, 1968c.

ment that he or she understands the purpose of the tests and an acknowledgment that he or she is aware of the penalties for misrepresentation of any fact relevant to the tests. The mother executes these requirements for children or minors.
   d. Right thumbprint of each party.* If the baby is less than 1 year of age, a footprint or palm print is probably better than a thumbprint.†
   e. Separate Polaroid photographs of each party, dated and signed on the back and countersigned by a witness, are recommended by some experts. The baby's photograph is signed by the mother.
   f. If blood samples are drawn elsewhere the above procedures should still be followed if at all possible, as the responsibility for identifying the parties involved rests with the person who obtains the blood samples. The specimens should be shipped by registered mail to establish the "chain of custody."

Identification of specimens

1. Anticoagulated (sodium citrate or ACD solution) and clotted venous blood is obtained from each party. Five to 10 ml of each should be obtained from adults and older children. In infants and small babies, capillary blood collected with micropipettes can be used. Heparinized blood is needed for HLA typing.
2. Each tube should be capped, labeled with the name of the donor and his or her relationship to the others (mother, baby, putative father), and initialed by the venipuncturist and the physician responsible for the testing.
3. Samples drawn elsewhere should be identified in the same way, then countersigned by the person receiving them and the physician responsible for the testing.
4. If saliva is collected, the above rules of identification also apply.

Guidelines for the expert

It is assumed that no specific technical instructions are necessary for an investigator who is qualified as an expert. The following guidelines are designed to ensure procedural uniformity.

---

*The Sirchie Fingerprint Laboratories, P.O. Box 30576, Raleigh, N.C. 27612.
†The Hollister Disposable Footprinter (Hollister, Inc., Libertyville, Ill. 60048) is convenient.

Table 11-43. Suggested binary code for Rh-Hr system*

Phenotype	Code†	Phenotype	Code	Phenotype	Code
rh	0000111	$rh_y rh''$	0110100	$Rh_2 Rh_2$	1010100
rh'rh	0100111	$rh_y rh_y$	0110000	$Rh_1 Rh_2$	1110110
rh'rh'	0100010	$rh'^w rh''$	0111110	$Rh_z rh$	1110111
$rh'^w rh$	0101111	$rh_y^w rh'$	0111010	$Rh_z Rh_1$	1110010
$rh'^w rh'$	0101010	Rh_0	1000111	$Rh_z Rh_2$	1110100
rh''rh	0010111	$Rh_1 rh$	1100111	$Rh_z Rh_z$	1110000
rh''rh''	0010100	$Rh_1 Rh_1$	1100010	$Rh_1^w Rh_2$	1111110
rh'rh''	0110110	$Rh_1^w rh$	1101111	$Rh_z^w Rh_1$	1111010
$rh_y rh$	0110111	$Rh_1^w Rh_1$	1101010		
$rh_y rh'$	0110010	$Rh_2 rh$	1010111		

*Modified from Wiener, 1968c.
†The code is based on agglutination reactions with antisera in the following order: anti-**Rh₀**, anti-**rh′**, anti-**rh″**, anti-**rh^w**, anti-**hr′**, anti-**hr″**, and anti-**hr**.

1. Tests should be performed in duplicate, using a different source of reagents for each, and each read independently by two observers.
2. An appropriate working form should be used to record the test results and appropriate controls. The form should show the date the tests were performed and the names of the technologists or physicians who performed the tests or read the results.

Report of the expert

Based on the test data, the expert sends a written report of the findings and conclusions to the attorneys representing the parties if testing is done in preparation for trial or to the court if the testing was ordered by the court. The report should be sufficiently detailed as to the findings and the expert's opinion based on the findings so as to minimize questions. If paternity is not excluded then, as recommended, a statement of the likelihood of paternity should be included in the final opinion. In that case, the report should state the method used for calculating likelihood of paternity.

It goes without saying that the data and report are confidential. All original data and documentation remain in the expert's files.

CODING OF PHENOTYPES

The use of computers for handling laboratory data is not an unqualified blessing. At times one wonders, between man and machine, who is master and who is servant. With regard to blood group genotypes, the problem is that input and output of phenotype and genotype data in the original form is, to the computer expert, an absurdity. Wiener has suggested a binary system that is logical and useful. Binary codes for the A-B-O and Rh-Hr systems are given in Tables 11-42 and 11-43. Note that the code is evolved by representing the agglutination reactions with antisera by "1" if there is agglutination and "0" if there is not.

12

"The best blood will at some time get into a fool or a mosquito."

Austin O'Malley

Transfusion of blood, blood products, and blood substitutes

HISTORY
  The National Blood Policy
INDICATIONS AND CONTRAINDICATIONS
  Anemia
    Anemia due to hemorrhage
    Aregenerative anemia
    Chronic hemolytic anemia
    Acute hemolytic anemia
    Megaloblastic anemia
    Anemia of chronic disease
  Leukemia
  Agranulocytosis
  Thrombocytopenia
  Hemorrhagic disorders
  Shock
  Hypoproteinemia
  General supportive therapy
CHOICE OF TRANSFUSION MATERIAL
  Stored blood
    Erythrocytes
    Leukocytes
    Platelets
    Coagulation factors
      Prothrombin (factor II)
      Factors V and VII
      Fibrinogen
      Factor VIII (antihemophilic globulin)
      Factor IX
      Factor X
      Factor XI
      Factor XII
      Factor XIII
  Fresh whole blood
  Plasma
  Packed red blood cells
  Platelet suspension
  Plasma fractions
    Albumin
    Fibrinogen
    Gamma (γ) globulin
    Factor VIII concentrate
    Factors II, VII, IX, and X concentrates
    Other fractions
  Plasma extenders and substitutes
  Cadaver (fibrinolytic) blood

Autologous (predonated) transfusion
  Plasmapheresis
FREQUENCY OF TRANSFUSION
  Transfusion for coagulation disorders
  Single-unit transfusion
ROUTES OF ADMINISTRATION
EXCHANGE TRANSFUSION
HAZARDS OF TRANSFUSION
  Transmission of disease
    Viral hepatitis
      Hepatitis A
      Non-A, non-B hepatitis
      Hepatitis B surface antigen and antibody
      Hepatitis B core antigen and antibody
      Hepatitis Be antigen and antibody
      Epidemiology of viral hepatitis
    Malaria
    Syphilis
    "Posttransfusion mononucleosis"
    Other infectious agents
  Transfusion reactions
    Hemolytic reactions
      Etiology
      Clinicopathologic correlation
      Investigation of a reaction
    Hypersensitivity reactions
      Allergic reactions
      Immediate dermal reactions
      Febrile reactions
      Serum sickness
      Anaphylactoid reactions
      Acute pulmonary edema
    Hemorrhagic reactions
      "Wash-out" effect on platelets
      Disseminated intravascular coagulation
      Posttransfusion thrombocytopenic purpura
    "Citric acid intoxication"
    Ammonia intoxication
    Circulatory overload

HISTORY

In an era when blood transfusions are given freely (3 units/100 population/year) (Myhre, 1974), if not with abandon, it is difficult to appreciate the long period of trial and error, the many frustrations preceding today's way of taking safety for granted. A brief review of the history of blood transfusion will not only serve to place the present in proper perspective, but also in the telling we reexperience 600 years or more of medical progress. As we pace off some of the memorable milestones, we find the story sometimes humorous, sometimes frightening, and always exciting.

Blood has always been respected as essential for the maintenance of life. The ancients undoubtedly had the experience of seeing life literally flow out of the body from battle or hunting wounds. At the height of the Roman Empire it became fashionable for patricians to commit suicide by exsanguination, thus dying gracefully and with decorum while surrounded by friends. In later centuries physicians reasoned that if a way could be devised to transfuse fresh blood, the procedure could be lifesaving. Medical treatment at that time leaned heavily on "bloodletting" as a means of ridding the body of "bad blood" and noxious humors. It seemed equally logical that the administration of "good blood" would benefit both the chronic and the acutely ill.

We must note that not until 1628 was it appreciated that blood flows in a closed system of arteries and veins. Lacking this knowledge, the obvious way to utilize it was to drink it or bathe in it. Although the Bible specifically forbids the Jews to ingest blood ("Ye shall not eat any thing with the blood," Lev. 19:26; "Ye shall eat no manner of blood," Lev. 7:26; "Be strong and avoid the temptation of eating blood," Deut. 12:23, etc.), no such admonitions kept the Romans from rushing into the arena to drink the blood of dying gladiators. In Egypt the pharaohs and princes bathed in human blood as a general restorative measure and, according to Pliny (Nat. Hist. 26:1), as a specific cure for leprosy.

The earliest administration of blood into the vein of a human is recorded by Villani as having taken place in 1492. This report has been the object of much controversy, and there are several versions of it, including one saying that the blood was drunk rather than transfused. According to Villani, Pope Innocent VIII had suffered a stroke and

. . . had for some time fallen into a kind of somnolency, which was sometimes so profound that the whole court believed him to be dead. All means to awaken the exhausted vitality had been resorted to in vain, when a Jewish doctor proposed to do so, *by a new instrument* [italics mine] of the blood of a young person, an experiment which hitherto had only been made on animals. Accordingly the blood of the decrepit old Pontiff was passed into the veins of a youth, whose blood was transfused into the veins of the old man. The experiment was tried three times and at the cost of the lives of three boys, probably from air getting into their veins, but without any effect to save that of the Pope.

The name of the physician is not recorded, nor is his fate, but it is safe to assume that no honors were showered on him.

More than a century passed before transfusion of blood is seriously mentioned again. In 1615 Andreas Livabius, a chemist practicing in the German city of Halle, wrote as follows:

Let there be a young man, robust, full of spirituous blood, and also an old man, thin, emaciated, his strength exhausted, hardly able to retain his own soul. Let the performer of the operation have two silver tubes fitting into each other. Let him open the artery of the young man and put into it one of the tubes, fastening it in. Let him immediately after open the artery of the old man, and put the female tube into it, and then the two tubes being joined together, the hot and spirituous blood of the young man will pour into the old one, as if it were from a fountain of life, and all of his weakness will be dispelled.

Discounting the therapeutic claims, this account is remarkable for the description of the technic of transfusing blood directly from donor to recipient.

Other investigators in Germany, France, and Italy were active in this field in the early 1600s, but the next significant advance was the description of the circulatory system by William Harvey in 1628. Prior to Harvey it was held that blood was generated in the liver and that it then moved back and forth in the blood vessels until it was used up. It is difficult to see how the early transfusionists, supposedly believing this, predicted such extravagant benefits from the injection of blood from donor's arm to recipient's.

William Harvey was born in Folkestone, England, on April 1, 1578. After graduation from Cambridge he studied in Padua under the famous anatomist Hieronymus Fabricius. It is noteworthy that Fabricius was at that time engaged in the study of the valves of veins, and indeed years later Harvey told Robert Boyle that Fabricius' work on the structure of veins first gave him the idea of "motion of blood in a circle." Harvey returned to London in 1602, became a Fellow of the College of Physicians in 1607, and in 1615 was named Lumllian lecturer of the College. In a lecture given on April 17, 1616, he clearly stated his concept of the circulation of the blood:

It is plain from the structure of the heart that the blood is passed continuously through the lungs to the aorta as by two clacks of a water bellows to raise water. It is shown by application of a ligature that the passage of blood is from the arteries into the veins. Whence it follows that the movement of the blood is constantly in a circle, and is brought about by the beat of the heart.

His book *Exercitatio anatomica de motu cordis et sanguinis in animalibus* was published 12 years later, in 1628, and may well be the most important medical treatise ever published. It not only provided a rational basis for transfusion but also dealt the final blow to the Galenic concept of blood and air that had ruled scientific thinking for fifteen centuries. According to Galen the liver was the organ that formed the blood, which flowed back and forth from the liver in two separate systems, arterial and venous. Harvey's thesis was in fact unacceptable to many physicians for many years (Brodin, 1978; Fishbein, 1978). He was not only subjected to criticism, but was caught on the Royalist side in the war between King Charles I and Oliver Cromwell. He stoutly defended his discovery for a few years and then devoted the rest of his life to a study of embryology.

Nevertheless, Harvey's discovery stimulated new approaches to blood transfusion in Europe, and there have been some nationalistic claims for priority. Francesco Folli of Florence is supposed to have performed a transfusion of blood into a human on August 13, 1654. The French claim that the Benedictine Monk Robert des Gabets performed a successful transfusion in 1658. In England, beginning in 1656, Sir Christopher Wren began to experiment with the injection of various solutions intravenously in dogs. His use of quills for cannulating a blood vessel provided his contemporaries with a useful, even though primitive, apparatus.

The credit for the first well-authenticated animal-to-animal transfusion goes to Richard Lower. He was a member of the Royal Society, and somewhat of a character, endowed with strong opinions, a caustic tongue, and many enemies. In 1665 and 1666 Lower, with the help of Dr. E. King, performed transfusions of blood from the carotid artery of one dog into another, and we find a reference to one of these demonstrations in the *Diary of Samuel Pepys* (November 14, 1666):

Here Dr. Croone told me, that, at the meeting at Gresham College to-night, which, it seems, they now have every Wednesday again, there was a pretty experiment of one dog let out, till he died, into the body of another on one side, while all his own run out on the other side. The first died upon the place, and the other very well, and likely to do well. This did give occasion to many pretty wishes, as of the blood of a Quaker to be let into an Archbishop, and such like; but, as Dr. Croone says, may, if it takes, be of mighty use to man's health, for the amending of bad blood by borrowing from a better body.

In November, 1667, Lower's colleague, Dr. King, transfused blood from a lamb into a Mr. Coga (Pepys' Diary, November 21, 1667):

Among the rest they discourse of a man who is a little frantic . . . , that is poor and a debauched man, that the College have hired for 20 *s.* to have some of the blood of a sheep let into his body; and it is to be done on Saturday next. They propose to let in about twelve ounces; which, they compute is what will be let in in a minute's time by a watch. They differ in the opinion they have of the effects of it; some think it may have a good effect upon him as a frantic man by cooling his blood, others that it will not have any effect at all. But the man is a healthy man, and by this means will be able to give an account what alteration, if any, he do find in himself, and so may be useful.

The transfusion was, surprisingly, uneventful, and again Pepys writes (November 30, 1966):

But here, above all, I was pleased to see the person who had his blood taken out. He speaks well, and did this day give the Society a relation thereof in Latin, saying that he finds himself much better since, and as a new man, but he is cracked a little in his head, though he speaks very reasonably, and very well. He had but 20 *s.* for his suffering of it, and is to have the same again tried on him: the first sound man that ever had it tried on him in England, and but one that we hear of in France, which was a porter hired by the virtuosos.

There is no further reference to Mr. Coga, and it must be assumed that, fortunately, the second transfusion was not carried out as planned.

At about the same time (June, 1667) Jean Baptiste Denis, court physician to Louis XIV, transfused 9 ounces of blood from the carotid artery of a lamb into a 16-year-old boy who, because of an obscure fever, had been treated by repeated venesection to the point of being moribund. The boy made a remarkable recovery, and Denis had a second success using a paid recipient. These successes did, however, give rise to a good deal of opposition and jealousy, and the situation was ripe for the disaster soon to come. The subject was an insane man and the first transfusion of sheep's blood was uneventful; the second caused, as we might expect, a reaction, described by Denis as follows: ". . . his arm became hot, the pulse rose, sweat burst out over his forehead, he complained of pain in the kidneys, and was sick at the stomach. The next day the urine was very dark, in fact black. . . ." In spite of this, Denis was urged by the man's wife to give a third transfusion, which he did, during which the recipient died. Denis' enemies could have no better weapon and prevailed on the widow to bring a charge of murder against Denis. He was eventually found not guilty, but the court prohibited further transfusions unless approved by the Faculty of Medicine of Paris. Since this august body had been critical of Denis' work from the first, the decision was tantamount to outlawing further experiments. In fact, 10 years later the French Parliament specifically prohibited blood transfusions in France, and when the Royal Society in England and the Magistrates in Italy followed suit, blood transfusion was effectively stopped for the next 150 years.

The revival of blood transfusion in the early 1800s is attributed to the work of an English obstetrician, James Blundell. Helpless in the face of fatal postpartum hemorrhage, Blundell (1818, 1828) directed his attention to the possibility of transfusing blood as a lifesaving measure. His approach was admirably scientific and systematic, so that he first perfected his apparatus and technic on animals. He devised the prototype of the modern syringe and several receptacles for transferring blood from the donor to the recipient. When he was satisfied with the results in animals, he felt justified in attempting transfusions in human beings. His first four attempts, in 1818, were on moribund patients and did not save them, but in subsequent cases he was able to save the lives of several women who would otherwise have died of hemorrhage. We must admire his work not only because of his careful reinvestigation of transfusion apparatus, but also because he was guided by a very specific and sound indication for transfusing blood.

Publication of Blundell's work stimulated worldwide interest, and for the first time serious reference to blood transfusion is found in American writings. Several American physicians claimed to have carried out successful transfusions, but it is difficult to single out one as the chief proponent of transfusion therapy. In the *Medical and Surgical History of the War of the Rebellion (1861-1865)*, reference is found to two successful transfusions in military hospitals. It seems unlikely that the number of transfusions would be so small had the practice been well established in American medicine.

In fact, Blundell's reports made a greater impact on the European than the American transfusionists. One interesting chapter in the history of transfusion is the use of milk by Canadian physicians during the middle 1800s (Oberman, 1969). The Canadian physician, Bovell (1855), used transfusion of cow's milk during the cholera epidemic of July, 1854. It is not clear how much milk was transfused, Bovell estimating 12 ounces and his colleague, Hodder, somewhat more. The rationale was the opinion of Donné that the "minute oily and fatty particles found in milk were convertible into the white corpuscles of the blood." It is not clear whether the transfusions were effective. The survival of some of the recipients caused Bovell and Hodder to apply to the City of Toronto far "a good cow and a few articles indispensable for the comfort and well-being of the patient." According to Hodder, "these were refused, and we thereupon sent in our resignation."

In the late 1800s transfusion of milk was tried by several American physicians. After some preliminary enthusiasm, all were forced to conclude that the practice was useless and dangerous. The introduction of isotonic saline solution as a transfusion material by Bull (1884) marked the end of milk as a potential blood substitute.

The year 1901 marks the beginning of the modern era of blood transfusion. It was in that year that Karl Landsteiner (1901) published his classic studies on the three blood types in human beings (A, B, and O), to which his associates De Castello and Sturli added the fourth (AB) in 1902. Landsteiner recognized that serologic incompatibility between donor and recipient could account for a transfusion reaction, but it was not until 7 years later that Ottenberg (1908) performed pretransfusion tests in vitro to determine compatibility. The discovery of the Rh factor by Landsteiner and Wiener (1940) and the many advances in immunohematology that followed provided the immunologic understanding required for modern, safe transfusion of blood.

In spite of these advances, modern transfusion practices would not have been possible without parallel advances in the technics of drawing, storage, and administration of blood. Most of the important advances occurred in the United States, and Rosenfield (1974, 1975) gives comprehensive reviews of the chronology of events and anecdotes about the investigators. Crile (1907) perfected the technic of direct anastomosis of donor's artery to recipient's vein, but this method had the disadvantages of sacrificing an artery in the donor and the inability to measure the amount of blood transfused. In 1914, Hustin in Belgium and Agote in Buenos Aires independently described the use of sodium citrate as an anticoagulant. In America, Lewisohn (1915) and Weil (1915) adopted and advocated the use of citrate. Rous and Turner (1916) showed that glucose added to the citrate improved the preservation of citrated blood, and this observation made possible the practice of indirect transfusion of stored blood. Loutit and Mollison (1943) described an improved acid-citrate-dextrose anticoagulant and preservative solution tht made possible the storage of whole blood up to 21 days.

The use of plasma for the emergency treatment of shock was advocated in the early 1900s, and in 1927 Strumia (Strumia and McGraw, 1941) pioneered the collection and storage of plasma. Elliott et al (1940) organized a similar operation in 1936, and stored plasma was used extensively in treating battle casualties during World War II. Wartime needs stimulated the development of blood procurement programs, research on plasma fractionation, preservation of blood and blood products, and the search for safe and effective blood substitutes. A method for freeze-drying plasma was perfected in 1942 by Flossdorf and Mudd. In 1941 Cohn et al (1944) began a series of brilliant studies on the fractionation of plasma by ethanol precipitation, initiating a new era in protein chemistry and making protein fractions available for use in therapy and research.

Looking ahead to the future, it seems likely that the next major step will be the routine use of frozen blood and, possibly, cadaver blood. It is not too improbable to anticipate the development of blood substitutes that will in great part eliminate the need for human donors. This would be a fitting climax to the story of Libavius, Wren, Lower, Blundell, and the adventuresome company of past and present transfusionists.

The National Blood Policy

Although the purpose of this chapter is to discuss the indications and contraindications for transfusion therapy and the proper utilization of blood and blood components, none of us can ignore the potential impact of the proposed National Blood Policy on the practice of transfusion therapy. The first portion of this section is factual. The remainder is my view of the genesis of the present situation, colored strongly by my feelings about the role of governmental agencies in regulating the practice of medicine.

Ignoring the long-standing conflict between the American Red Cross and the American Association of Blood Banks (AABB) (Surgenor, 1974), the story begins with the publication of two official reports on blood service and utilization in the United States.

The first was a study by the National Heart and Lung Institute published in 1972 (United States Department of Health, Education and Welfare, 1972). This was the result of a study on blood resources and utilization, and one of the important findings was that out of more than 9.3 million units of blood drawn in 1971, 2.7 million units were never used as whole blood because of outdating on storage.

An earlier report was derived from a study by a Committee of the National Research Council (National Academy of Sciences, National Research Council, 1970). This report also pointed to the poor utilization of blood and blood products and emphasized the high cost to patients who needed repeated transfusions, as in those with hemophilia.

To these justifiably alarming data was added the increasing awareness of the supposedly high incidence of transfusion hepatitis, widely publicized by a book written for the lay public (Titmuss, 1971). The concern of the public and physicians with this question became the focus of all discontent with blood banking, particularly when it was shown that *paid donors* were three times as likely as *volunteer donors* to carry the hepatitis virus in their blood.

The stage was set for two official acts that have had a major impact on transfusion practice. The first was the Blood Labeling Act in Illinois, passed in August, 1972, which stipulated that each unit of blood shall be labelled "purchased" or "donated." This was followed by a second bill (July, 1973) that stipulated that all blood requirements be met by volunteer donations. Purchased units of blood may be used only on written order of the physician, who also signs an affidavit that no other blood is available.

The second development was the publication of the

National Blood Policy (1974) in which the executive branch of the Federal government, through the Department of Health, Education and Welfare, sets forth a 10-point policy of blood procurement and utilization, specifically "to bring into being an all-voluntary blood donation system and to eliminate commercialism." It also identifies ". . . the Secretary of the Department of Health, Education and Welfare, or his designee, as responsible for the implementation of the policies enunciated above." Implementation of the national blood policy is assigned to the American Blood Commission, a special body representing professional, scientific, financial, consumer, and governmental sectors.

The American Blood Commission came into being in 1975. It is composed of representatives of 40 professional and lay organizations concerned directly or peripherally with blood transfusion. The goals of the commission are (1) an all-voluntary blood donation system; (2) an adequate, high-quality supply of blood sufficient to meet diagnostic and therapeutic requirements; (3) accessibility to the blood supply for all those who need blood products; and (4) efficiency and economy in providing blood services (Henry and Hubbell, 1980).

On the surface these aims are praiseworthy. In spite of this, there are reasons for concern.

It is obvious that the formulation and enforcement of the National Blood Policy is yet another attempt to establish governmental control over the conditions under which medicine may be practiced. The approach in this instance is familiar: first the existing system is judged to be bad by exaggerating its faults and ignoring its strengths, and then changes are legislated—supposedly for the public good. A second refinement has been added to this historically successful gambit: the affected people or organizations are threatened with punitive legislation unless they themselves carry out the restructuring changes.

The formation of the American Blood Commission is yet another example of the effectiveness of the government's approach. By the acceptance of its creation, there is an implied admission that the blood banking system is so bad as to need major restructuring. In addition, one has a right to be apprehensive when supporters of the American Blood Commission write: "Beyond carrying out the National Blood Policy, the American Blood Commission has been described by the Carter administration as a model, or prototype, of voluntary action. As an organizational prototype within a major subsystem in the American system of health care delivery, the Commission's significance therefore extends well beyond the realm of accelerating the development of an effective blood program; it demonstrates the viability and vitality of the American sector" (Henry and Hubbell, 1980).

Just how deficient is the system that must be restructured? Let us consider the four goals of the American Blood Commission.

The first goal is an all-voluntary blood donation system. It is badly worded, because the opposite of voluntary is involuntary; even the skid row bum who sells his blood in order to buy wine is a voluntary, even eager donor. The issue is in fact *paid* versus *nonpaid* donors. However, there are two classes of paid donors: the one who is admittedly danger-ous—the chronic alcoholic or the narcotic addict—and the paid, repeatedly screened professional donor, admittedly the safest of all donors because he has been proved most safe by the most reliable method, the transfusion of his blood into recipients. To lump both classes into the category of "undesirable" is obviously illogical. Furthermore, since we are concerned with an adequate supply of blood, the elimination of paid professional donors can, to some extent, have a negative impact on blood supplies. I believe that the American Blood Commission should consider this question and modify the first of the four goals. I would make the same recommendation to the Food and Drug Administration which, by regulation, requires that blood and blood components must be labeled as to type of donor, that is, whether paid or volunteer.

It is interesting also to put the question of paid versus nonpaid donor in proper quantitative perspective. In 1975, before any governmental regulations became effective, 92% of the units of blood collected by AABB members came from voluntary donors (a 26% increase over 1974), whereas 87% of all blood received by blood banks and transfusion services came from voluntary donors (Hemphill, 1975). By 1978, 95% to 97% of blood was collected from voluntary donors (Henry and Hubbell, 1980). It would seem that the problem is now small indeed.

The second goal of the Blood Commission, to ensure an adequate, high-quality supply of blood, can be met by either or both of two approaches: (1) increase the number of units drawn or (2) make better use of the available blood. How many more units can be drawn from voluntary donors remains to be seen. Much more likely is better utilization by the use of blood components whenever possible. This was initiated by blood bank professionals and actively instituted long before the government regulations (Smith and Elliott, 1951; Pool et al, 1964; Chaplin, 1969; Westphal, 1972; Buchholz, 1974; Valeri, 1975; Blajchman et al, 1979). The available data (American Red Cross Blood Services Operation Report, 1979) show that from 1973 to 1978 the reduction in the use of whole blood was accompanied by a fivefold increase in packed RBC use and fivefold increase in fresh-frozen plasma.

Physicians have been aware of the problem of transmitting disease, such as hepatitis, by the transfusion of blood from undesirable donors. Long before the Blood Commission was formed, blood banks have been active in developing reliable screening programs to detect the hepatitis B antigen. These programs have been effective in reducing the transmission of this type of hepatitis and should be credited to the bloodbanking professionals and not to government regulations. Most cases of viral hepatitis are non-A, non-B (p. 541), and unfortunately there is no routine test to identify the carrier of virus type A.

The third and fourth goals of the Blood Commission—accessibility to the blood supply and economy in providing blood services—depend to a great degree on achieving the first two goals. There are pros and cons for the concept of regional blood collecting and distributing centers, and it remains to be seen whether these will result in the hoped-for greater economy.

It should be noted in passing that whatever measures are

taken, blood will always be a finite resource. I have been interested in developing artificial blood substitutes that are better than the fluorocarbon emulsions developed in Japan, but research support for innovative approaches has been unavailable. There is no doubt in my mind that some day such artificial substitutes will be developed and that they will ease the blood supply problem to a great extent.

INDICATIONS AND CONTRAINDICATIONS

There is no doubt that transfusion of blood and blood products represents one of the major advances in medicine. The relative safety of transfusion therapy, however, should not obscure the fact that in spite of all preventive efforts, a small but significant number of untoward reactions can be expected. It is essential that the decision to administer blood be based on firm indications.

Sound transfusion therapy is guided by three principles: (1) the most important contraindication is the absence of a specific indication, (2) the anticipated therapeutic benefits should outweight the possibility of a bad reaction, and (3) maximum benefits will be obtained only if the transfusion material chosen is that which best supplies the patient's need. Not only is the use of blood components rather than whole blood more effective in some situations, but it makes possible maximum utilization of donor blood.

The indications and material of choice are listed in Table

Table 12-1. Indications for transfusion of blood or blood products and recommended transfusion material for each[a]

Indication	Recommended transfusion material
Anemia	
Aregenerative anemia[b]	Erythrocyte suspension
Anemia due to acute hemorrhage	Whole blood; erythrocyte suspension
Anemia refractory to treatment	Erythrocyte suspension
Hemolytic anemia[b]	Erythrocyte suspension
Hemolytic disease of newborn	Whole blood transfusion or exchange transfusion
Anemia of chronic hemorrhage	Erythrocyte suspension
Anemia of chronic renal disease	Erythrocyte suspension
Any severe anemia, as a lifesaving measure	Erythrocyte suspension
Correction of anemia before surgery	Erythrocyte suspension or whole blood
Leukemia	
Acute[c]	Whole blood; platelet suspension
Chronic	Whole blood
Agranulocytosis[d]	Leukocyte suspension
Hemorrhagic disease[e]	
Hemophilia (factor VIII deficiency)[f]	Fresh frozen type-specific plasma or factor VIII concentrate
Hypoprothrombinemia[f,g]	Plasma[h]
Factor V deficiency[f]	Fresh-frozen plasma
Factor VII deficiency[f]	Plasma[b]
Factor IX deficiency[f]	Factor IX concentrate
Factor X deficiency[f]	Factor X concentrate
Factor XI deficiency[f]	Plasma
Factor XII deficiency[f]	Plasma
Factor XIII deficiency	Plasma
Anticoagulant overdose (bishydroxycoumarin, heparin, etc.)[f]	Plasma
Hypofibrinogenemia[f]	Cryoprecipitate
Thrombocytopenic purpura[i]	Fresh whole blood or platelet transfusions
Von Willebrand's disease	Cryoprecipitate
Therapy of shock	Whole blood or plasma
Hypoproteinemia[j]	Plasma or albumin (Cohn's fraction V), salt-free as indicated
Hypogammaglobulinemia	Fresh plasma (commercial γ-globulin contains only IgG, not suitable for correcting IgA or IgM deficiency)

[a]Blood components rather than whole blood should be used whenever possible.
[b]See discussion in text for possible contraindications.
[c]Acute leukemias usually present a problem of anemia plus thrombocytopenia, the latter often being of greater importance.
[d]Limited value; beneficial effects are of short duration.
[e]For details of nomenclature see Chapter 17.
[f]If accompanied by severe hemorrhage or shock, supplementary and simultaneous transfusions with whole blood should be given.
[g]The term "hypoprothrombinemia" is used in the sense of a reduction of prothrombin only.
[h]The results of transfusion therapy alone are often disappointing.
[i]Nonthrombocytopenic purpura is not an indication for transfusion therapy unless there is marked blood loss.
[j]Limited value.

12-1. The books by Mollison, (1979), Huestis et al (1976), and Greenwalt et al (1977) are excellent general references for all aspects of transfusion practice.

Anemia

The first major indication is for the correction of anemia. The pathogenesis and etiology of anemia vary, and the benefits derived from transfusion are not the same in each case. In every case, however, the patient's deficiency in erythrocytes requires the transfusion of whole blood or preferably erythrocyte suspensions.

Anemia due to hemorrhage

In acute bleeding the combined loss in blood volume and the hypoxia from the loss of erythrocytes makes transfusion therapy essential if the amount of blood lost approaches 1,000 ml, or $\frac{1}{5}$ of the blood volume in children. The physician should exercise good clinical judgment if unnecessary transfusions are to be avoided. An otherwise healthy adult patient who loses 1,000 ml from a bleeding peptic ulcer needs no blood if the physicial activity is minimal and will regenerate red cells. A patient who loses 1,000 ml from a carcinoma eroding a large vessel may need a transfusion because the regenerative capacity is impaired. Duncalf and Underwood (1970) discuss the clinical circumstances that should be considered, summarized as follows:

1. The extent of blood loss and the degree of anemia (I have seen two patients with polycythemia vera who bled acutely from gastric ulcers but who required no therapy because their red blood cell count had dropped only to normal levels.)
2. Is the bleeding acute or chronic? (In chronic bleeding, there is time for cardiovascular compensation and the patient may be asymptomatic.)
3. Does the underlying disease (if the hemorrhage is not caused by trauma) or the status of the patient (postsurgical, acidotic, cardiac failure, pulmonary dysfunction) require immediate improvement in oxygenation?
4. Most important, can the patient be expected to do well without transfusion therapy, even if recovery from the loss of blood takes a little longer?

Whole blood or packed red blood cells are agents of choice. If bleeding is massive, the danger of depleting platelets and coagulation factors must be reckoned with.

In chronic bleeding the patient is usually relatively asymptomatic. Transfusion is seldom indicated. When needed, packed erythrocytes should be used.

Aregenerative anemia

In the aregenerative anemias there is a chronic deficiency in erythrocyte production. In the absence of an effective method of stimulating erythropoiesis, there is no choice but to transfuse packed red blood cells to make up the deficiency. The interval between transfusions is determined by the need to maintain the erythrocyte count at an adequate level. In some cases it is necessary to supply erythrocytes only during the critical period. In others the aregenerative phase extends over months or years, and numerous transfusions are required.

The physician should avoid treating the blood count rather than the patient. If the anemia is mild and the patient is asymptomatic, it is probably best not to administer blood. There is good evidence that blood transfusions can have a suppressive effect on bone marrow activity; e.g., DeMarsh and Alt (1948) have described anemia that followed the transfusion of blood in a patient with thrombocytopenia. Birkhill et al (1951) have shown that if blood is given to the point of producing polycythemia, a marked depression of bone marrow erythropoiesis occurs. Experimentally, Elmlinger et al (1952) have demonstrated a reduction of radioactive iron turnover following blood transfusion. These observations justify conservatism in the use of blood transfusions in general and in the presence of deficient bone marrow activity in particular. If the anemia is severe, however, the need for blood transfusion is of course greater than the possible danger of a supressive effect. The amount of blood given should not be directed toward restoring the erythrocyte count to normal levels, but rather toward keeping the patient asymptomatic at his or her usual or normal level of activity. In most cases, peripheral blood values of about 11 Gm/dl of hemoglobin, or 3.5 million erythrocytes/mm³ (3.5×10^{12}/l) are adequate.

Chronic hemolytic anemia

The same considerations apply to transfusion therapy in chronic hemolytic anemias. It is a common observation that many patients with chronic hemolytic anemia make a completely successful physiologic adjustment to their anemia and are asymptomatic. It is doubtful whether blood transfusion can be justified in these cases. We also find that such patients quickly return to pretransfusion levels after the blood transfusion, that transfused erythrocytes are often destroyed more rapidly than normal, and that the administration of large amounts of blood may overload the bile pigment and iron excretion mechanism.

There are many reports showing that a transfused patient who has a hemolytic anemia temporarily stops producing red blood cells. For example, Smith et al (1955) studied the suppressive effect of transfusions on erythropoiesis and hemoglobin synthesis that was most marked for about 2 weeks after the transfusion and persisted until most of the transfused red blood cells had been destroyed.

Acute hemolytic anemia

Blood transfusions may be necessary in acute hemolytic anemia as a lifesaving measure. A rapid drop in the number of circulating erythrocytes may be found, and the patient is often acutely ill. It should be remembered, however, that transfused red blood cells survive only a short time if the hemolytic anemia is being caused by antibodies in the patient's plasma. The patient's antibodies also make crossmatching very difficult, if not impossible. If hemolytic jaundice is already present, it may be aggravated by the added hemolysis of the transfused cells.

Megaloblastic anemia

While the peripheral blood count may be extremely low in pernicious and other megaloblastic anemias, the patient seldom has severe symptoms of anemia. In a rare case, blood transfusion is a lifesaving measure made necessary by impending cardiac failure.

It is extremely important to initiate complete peripheral blood and bone marrow studies before a transfusion is given. While there is some difference of opinion regarding the effect of blood transfusions on the megaloblastic morphology of bone marrow cells, there is no doubt that in some patients with pernicious anemia the transfusion of large amounts of blood produces a partial, or even complete, reversion of a megaloblastic to a normoblastic morphology. It is probable that patients respond in different degrees and that the amount of blood given is also important. Nevertheless, one cannot justify failure to perform a bone marrow aspiration while the blood transfusion is being prepared. A complete study of the peripheral blood is also important and obviously should be carried out before normal blood is administered.

Anemia of chronic disease

Blood transfusions are indicated in chronic anemias refractory to other treatment. In some the etiology is obscure, whereas in others, such as anemia that accompanies chronic renal insufficiency, the cause is known but cannot be corrected. There is then little choice but to administer blood periodically to maintain the peripheral blood count at a satisfactory level.

Leukemia

Blood transfusions are fundamental in the treatment of acute leukemia. In spite of advances in chemotherapy, they remain an important therapeutic weapon. The value of blood transfusions is of course not as an antileukemia specific but as supportive therapy, by means of which erythrocytes and platelets are supplied. Some claim longer survival when acute leukemia is treated with blood transfusions, but this is undoubtedly a result of correction of the anemia, thrombocytopenia, and hemorrhagic tendencies. Temporary benefits have been described when exchange transfusions are employed, but this is of greater theoretical interest than practical importance. Chemotherapy sometimes produces marked depression of bone marrow activity, making transfusions mandatory. Transfusions often keep the patient alive until chemotherapy can take effect. Platelet transfusions are indicated for the severely thrombocytopenic patient. In patients in whom chemotherapy is effective, the need for blood transfusions is often decreased or eliminated.

In chronic leukemia, transfusions are used to combat anemia or bleeding. The latter may be caused by thrombocytopenia, by the development of deficiencies of coagulation factors, or by circulating anticoagulants.

Agranulocytosis

Transfusions of whole blood or leukocyte suspensions are probably of little value in agranulocytosis. The survival time of transfused leukocytes in fresh whole blood is very short and in leukocyte suspensions even shorter, and there is no evidence to indicate that administration of concentrated leukocyte suspensions stimulates leukopoiesis. Granulocytes have HLA antigens that may lead to alloimmunization and subsequent transfusion reactions (Goldstein et al, 1971; see also p. 535).

Thrombocytopenia

Platelet transfusion is indicated in (1) thrombocytopenia caused by poor platelet production as in aplasia of the bone marrow, (2) thrombasthenia or thrombocytopathy, (3) thrombocytopenia of leukemia, and (4) thrombocytopenia caused by sequestration of platelets (in the spleen or extracorporeal pump). Except for platelet functional disorders (thrombasthenia or thrombocytopathy), it should be remembered that there is little danger of spontaneous hemorrhage caused by thrombocytopenia unless the platelet count is below 80,000/mm^3 (0.08×10^{12}/l) (Gardner, 1974). According to Harker and Slichter (1972) the bleeding time is prolonged when the platelet count is below 75,000/mm^3 (0.075×10^{12}/l). The probability of hemorrhage due to thrombocytopenia is greatest when the count is below 20,000/mm^3 (20×10^9/l) (Schiffer, 1978). Absolute criteria cannot be given, and the presence of clinical bleeding must modify the given general rule. Likewise, a patient with severe thrombocytopenia, but without clinical bleeding, should receive platelet transfusions prior to surgery. When the platelet count is normal, but the platelets are functionally abnormal, platelet transfusion is indicated prior to surgery, when bleeding is caused by trauma, or if there is severe bleeding in the absence of trauma.

A patient with an immunologic thrombocytopenic purpura should not receive platelet transfusions unless there is severe hemorrhage or if there is active bleeding prior to splenectomy. Chronic immunologic thrombocytopenic purpura (ITP) should not be treated with platelet transfusions. Platelet antibodies rapidly destroy transfused platelets, whether matched or not. The risk of developing platelet antibodies when platelet transfusion is indicated may be prevented in part by giving HLA-matching platelets (p. 538).

When it is probable that multiple platelet transfusions must be given, the platelets should be obtained from donors of the same ABO (Freireich et al, 1963) and HLA type as the patient. Sometimes it is necessary to take into account other intrinsic platelet antigens (p. 538). Since a significant number of red cells can be found in platelet concentrates, it is advisable to type the donor and recipient with respect to the Rh system to prevent sensitization of the recipient to some of the Rh antigens.

Hemorrhagic disorders

Transfusion of blood in hemorrhagic disease is a specific in the same sense that insulin is a specific in diabetes. Both replace the substance in which the body is deficient. Obviously, the kind of blood, plasma, or plasma fraction chosen is of great importance. Possible choices are discussed in the next section. Duration of the benefits must also be considered as a guide to the number and frequency of the transfusions.

Shock

When a patient is in shock, transfusions of whole blood or plasma are usually essential. The treatment of shock is always an individualized problem, the etiology and pathologic physiology varying from patient to patient. It is not always a simple problem of restoring blood volume. However, it is true that in most cases the immediate need is to increase blood volume. For this, whole blood is ideal, being in all respects superior to plasma. Not only does it immediately increase the oxygen-carrying capacity of the patient's blood, but it also provides an immediate and lasting expansion of blood volume by means of the transfused erythrocytes that are unable to escape from the vascular system.

Hypoproteinemia

Either plasma or albumin solutions can be used to correct hypoproteinemia, but actually they are of limited value. If the hypoproteinemia is reversible, plasma or albumin will supply needed protein during the critical period. However, most hypoproteinemias are caused by irreversible lesions such as occur in severe hepatic or renal disease, and the deficiency is only temporarily remedied by the administration of a fluid high in protein. When hypoproteinemia is associated with edema, transfusions of plasma or albumin help reduce the edema by increasing the osmotic pressure of the blood. Protein digests have been tried as substitutes for plasma, but clinical trials of the solutions presently available have not been as successful as animal experiments led us to expect.

General supportive therapy

The administration of blood to patients lacking the specific indications just mentioned is seldom justified and can be dangerous. Although it has often been claimed that blood helps the patient who is not doing well and speeds recovery, these benefits probably derive from the correction of an unrecognized condition for which blood transfusion is specific. The risk of a transfusion reaction is not justified in the absence of a specific indication.

CHOICE OF TRANSFUSION MATERIAL

The benefits derived from transfusion therapy are in direct proportion to the discrimination used in choosing the transfusion material. The aim in each case is to determine what is needed and then to choose, from the variety of agents available, the one that best supplies the deficit.

Stored blood

The development of blood banking has made stored whole blood readily available. Its usefulness is limited only by the changes that occur in storage.

Erythrocytes

When blood is drawn into acid-citrate-dextrose (ACD) solution and stored at 4° C, 90% of the transfused erythrocytes survive at the end of 14 days' storage. After 24 days of storage, only 70% of the erythrocytes survive. Most blood banks set a limit of 21 days' storage, after which the blood is considered unsuitable for transfusion. Blood drawn into citrate-phosphate-dextrose (CPD) solution is considered suitable for up to 28 days (Orlina and Josephson, 1969). The advantage of CPD solution is that the higher pH maintains glycolysis longer and the phosphate ions retard loss of red cell ATP and 2,3-DPG (Duhm and Gerlach, 1974).

Extensive studies in England and the United States during World War II led to the use of ACD for the preservation of blood. This mixture, although superior to simple citrate, does not prevent the eventual deterioration of erythrocytes. The deterioration consists of increased fragility and decreased utilization of glucose, with loss of potassium and organic phosphate (Fig. 12-1). Damaged erythrocytes disappear rapidly from the recipient's circulation (Fig. 12-2). Not only are nonviable cells useless to the recipient, but the danger of iron overload when frequent transfusions are necessary must be kept in mind. After blood is stored for 21 days in ACD solution at 4° C, about 80% of the erythrocytes will survive for at least 24 hours after the blood is transfused (Fig. 12-3). Stored sickle cell trait erythrocytes have the same survival as normal ones (Ray et al, 1959; Levin and Truax, 1960); blood from a donor with sickle cell trait provides no additional risk of hemolysis.

Improved methods for preserving blood continue to be a major civilian and military concern. Two lines of investigation show much promise.

The first deals with the reduction of erythrocyte metabolism by storage at temperatures below the standard 4° C. Erythrocyte metabolism virtually ceases at $-70°$ to $-140°$ C. It has been shown that erythrocytes suspended in glycerin and maintained at these low temperatures remain viable for years and can be warmed to body temperature without being injured (Huggins, 1964; Huggins and Grove-Rasmussen, 1965; Morrison et al, 1968). Addition of PVP (polyvinylpyrrolidone) or glycerol allows rapid freezing in liquid nitrogen and subsequent thawing with minimum hemolysis (Doebbler et al, 1966). Other cryoprotective agents are dimethylsulfoxide (Huggins, 1963) hydroxyethyl starch (Weatherbee et al, 1974), and hydroxyethylated amylopectin (Mischler and Parry, 1979).

The second approach deals with the addition of metabolites that maintain glucose metabolism in stored erythrocytes (Crouch and Bishop, 1963). The chief metabolic failure during storage is a progressive loss of ability to utilize glucose. Diminished anaerobic glycolysis is caused by the depletion of adenosine triphosphate. It has been found that by adding purine nucleosides such as inosine (Dawson, 1977), adenosine, and guanosine to the blood, the survival of erythrocytes is increased (Fig. 12-4). The improved survival is caused first by the splitting of the nucleoside into ribose, which enters into the pathway of aerobic glycolysis and then, as ribose-phosphate, generating adenosine triphosphate, which replenishes the run-down anaerobic cycle. It has been proposed recently that purine nucleosides be added routinely to ACD solution to prolong the useful storage time to 28 days or longer.

The oxygen dissociation curve (Fig. 12-5) expresses the ability of the erythrocyte to deliver oxygen to the tissues. It was once thought to be primarily dependent on temperature and pH, but now we appreciate that an additional shift to the right or left is dependent on the 2,3-diphosphoglyceric acid (2,3-DPG) within the erythrocyte. This has two important implications: (1) in anemia there is an increase in 2,3-DPG, shifting the curve to the right and resulting in an increase of the percentage of oxygen delivered and (2) on storage there is a decrease in 2,3-DPG, shifting the curve to the left and resulting in a decrease of the percentage of oxygen delivered (Chanutin and Curnish, 1967). The role of 2,3-DPG has been reviewed by Harkness (1971). His article gives a complete bibliography.

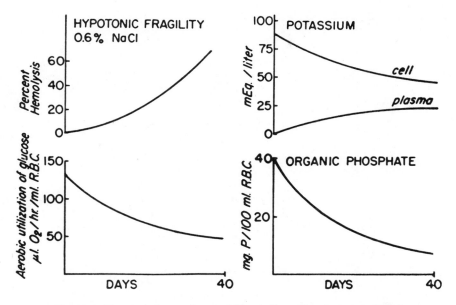

Fig. 12-1. Chemical changes in stored blood. (From Donohue et al, 1956.)

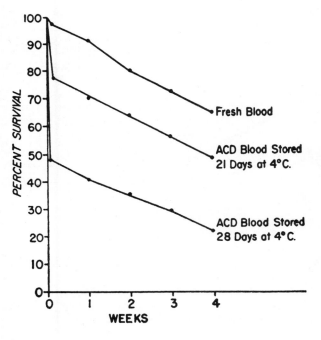

Fig. 12-2. Survival of stored erythrocytes (whole blood) after transfusion. (From Donohue et al, 1956.)

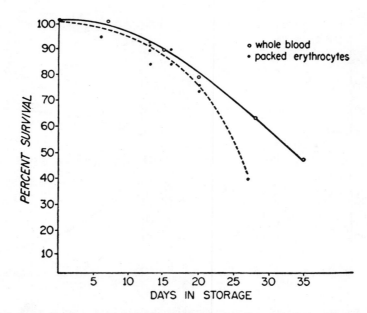

Fig. 12-3. Survival of stored erythrocytes (whole blood and packed erythrocytes) after transfusion. (From Donohue et al, 1956.)

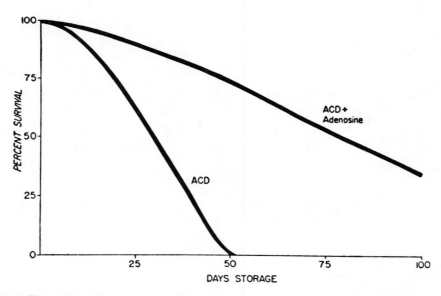

Fig. 12-4. Effect of adenosine on the survival of erythrocytes in stored blood. (From Donohue et al, 1956.)

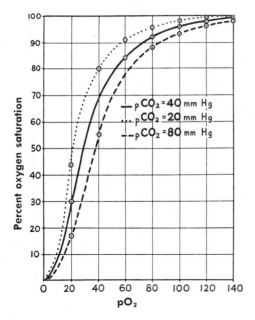

Fig. 12-5. Oxygen dissociation curves for human hemoglobin at various P_{CO_2}'s (at 37° C).

It has been known for many years that the erythrocyte is rich in 2,3-DPG, but not until 1967 was it found that 2,3-DPG causes a shift to the right of the oxygen dissociation curve. It is known that the configuration of the hemoglobin molecule changes with oxygenation and deoxygenation, the β-chains moving apart with deoxygenation (the molecule "breathes," so to speak) and the 2,3-DPG binding to the core of the molecule when the β-chains separate (Chapter 14).

The increase in 2,3-DPG in anemia improves the oxygenation of the tissues and, together with increased cardiac output, helps to compensate for the hypoxia secondary to a low concentration of hemoglobin. For example, it has been calculated that at a hemoglobin concentration of 5 Gm/dl, the shift to the right of the curve enables delivery of oxygen to the tissues comparable to a hemoglobin concentration of 10 Gm/dl. The same kind of 2,3-DPG-mediated right shift occurs in the adaptive response to the hypoxia occurring at high altitudes. An increase in 2,3-DPG and oxygen release occurs also in congenital cyanotic heart disease, obstructive lung disease, low-output cardiac failure, and vigorous exercise.

Blood stored in standard ACD or CPD shows a decrease in 2,3-DPG concentration, increasing oxygen affinity and reducing the ability to release oxygen. The concentration of 2,3-DPG drops rapidly and at the end of 1 week's storage is sufficiently low to shift the oxygen dissociation curve significantly to the left (Sugerman et al, 1970). The implications in transfusion therapy are obvious, for it is theoretically possible to transfuse a patient with blood that is near the storage expiration date and bring the hemoglobin concentration up to a respectable level but still have hypoxia at the tissue level.

There is no denying that the oxygen-releasing capacity of stored blood is impaired, but this becomes a factor in only a few clinical situations, as in massive exchange transfusions (Delivoria-Papadopoulus et al, 1971), and should not lead to an unreasonable increase in the use of fresh blood (Chaplin et al, 1974). For one thing, the concentration of 2,3-DPG increases rapidly, within hours, when depleted blood is transfused (Beutler et al, 1969; Dickerman et al, 1973). Also, there are only a few clinical situations in which a shift of the oxygen dissociation to the left would have significant clinical implications. In general, fresh, rather than stored, blood should be used only when an immediate restoration of tissue oxygenation is indicated, rather than in a few hours. Treatment of the respiratory syndrome in infants may be the chief, if not the only, situation where this applies.

In addition, it is feasible to prevent the loss of 2,3-PDG in stored blood. One approach is to add nucleosides to the blood (Chanutin, 1967; Strumia et al, 1970; Ness and Pennington, 1974). Adenine alone maintains levels of ATP but does not preserve 2,3-DPG. The combination of inosine and adenine, or inosine-adenine-guanine, prevents much of the loss of 2,3-DPG, particularly if the preservative is CPD rather than ACD (Sasakawa et al, 1978). Some have advocated the addition of pyruvate, which, converted to lactate by LDH, oxidizes reduced pyridine nucleotide back to nicotinamide adenine dinucleotide (NAD) and increases synthesis of 2,3-DPG. Mishler et al (1978, 1979) recommend the use of CPD solution containing one-half the standard amount of trisodium citrate. The newly licensed preservative designated CPDA-1, containing supplementary adenine and an increased amount of glucose, may be the best (Beutler and West, 1979). Finally, it should be noted that there is no loss of 2,3-DPG in red blood cells preserved by freezing.

Leukocytes

It is generally agreed that, even under optimum storage conditions, many leukocytes in whole blood disintegrate within 36 hours. Crosbie and Scarborough (1940) showed that 11% of the leukocytes are lost during the first day, 17% during the second day, 22% during the third to fifth days, and 24% during the sixth day. After 6 days of storage, only 25% of the leukocytes remains, and although they can be counted, they appear to have undergone degeneration. Even more important than the number of cells surviving is the observation that the remaining leukocytes have very little bactericidal activity by the end of the fourth day (McCullough et al, 1974). It is apparent, therefore, that little benefit is derived in leukopenia or agranulocytosis when the blood has been stored more than 1 day.

Leukocytes from normal donors can be harvested by continuous flow filtration leukapheresis (Djerassi et al, 1972) and other technics (McCullough, 1978) and have been used in the treatment of neutropenic patients (Schiffer et al, 1975). Lane and Windle (1979) have shown that after 24 hours of storage half of the granulocytes show abnormal random migration and chemotaxis, whereas after 48 hours the respiratory burst was decreased by 42%.

In most instances the indication for transfusing leukocytes is infection, established or threatened, in a neutropenic patient (Graw and Appelbaum, 1977; Vogler and Winton,

1977; Clift et al, 1978; Ruthe et al, 1978; Workman et al, 1978). Simultaneous treatment of the underlying disease is important. Schiffer et al (1979) emphasize the frequent occurrence of alloimmunization following granulocyte transfusions. Cohen et al (1979) review the occurrence of both fatal and nonfatal graft-versus-host reactions. Studies on leukocyte transfusions with cells collected from donors with chronic myelocytic leukemia (Morse et al, 1966a) have shown that most disappear quickly from the recipient's blood (half-life about 24 hours). Leukopheresis has been found of some value in removing white blood cells from patients with chronic myelocytic leukemia (Morse et al, 1966), chronic lymphocytic leukemia (Curtis et al, 1972), and reticuloendotheliosis (Fay et al, 1979).

Platelets

Platelets in whole blood disintegrate rapidly unless special precautions are taken in drawing blood. When drawn into ACD solution in standard vacuum glass bottles, the platelet count at the end of 24 hours is about $100,000/mm^3$ $(0.1 \times 10^{12}/l)$ and is $40,000/mm^3$ $(0.04 \times 10^{12}/l)$ at the end of the third day of storage. Platelet survival can be increased by drawing the blood into plastic containers or siliconized glass bottles and by using specially treated needles and tubing. Even so, when the patient needs platelets it is best to administer the blood within 24 hours after it is drawn. It should be emphasized that, when large amounts of stored blood are given, as in severe hemorrhage, there is a danger of producing thrombocytopenia because of the poor platelet content of stored blood. When treatment is indicated, thrombocytopenia is usually treated by the transfusion of platelet concentrates (p. 537). Plateletpheresis has also been used to lower the platelet count in thrombocythemia (Panlilio and Reiss, 1979).

Coagulation factors

The effect of storage on the coagulation factors was once the subject of bitter debate. It is now generally agreed that the survival of coagulation factors in stored blood depends on three things: (1) the method of blood collection, (2) the anticoagulant used, and (3) the inherent lability or stability of each factor. The desired hemostatic level for each coagulation factor is given on p. 540.

Optimum survival of the coagulation factors is obtained when blood is collected by gravity, rather than by suction, directly into chilled ACD solution. Prompt and complete mixing of the blood with the anticoagulant is essential. Two of the coagulation factors, V and VIII, are naturally labile even under optimum conditions but are even more labile when oxalate is used as the anticoagulant.

The literature contains contradictory conclusions as to the stability of various coagulation factors in blood and plasma. While it is agreed in general that some are labile and some are respectably stable, data from various investigators clearly indicate that the actual factor content of the blood or blood product is dependent less on a constant and predictable lability of the coagulation factor than on the following: (1) the factor content of the blood, since it can vary significantly within the range of normal, (2) the method of collection, (3) the storage temperature, (4) the speed with which fresh plasma is harvested and frozen, (5) the actual temperature of the deepfreeze cabinet, (6) the manner of thawing and administering frozen plasma, and (7) some unknown influences that can make 1 unit of frozen plasma markedly different from another processed in exactly the same way. These same considerations explain the variability of cryoprecipitate factor VIII concentrate.

PROTHROMBIN (FACTOR II). The one-stage prothrombin time of blood or plasma stored at 4° C becomes progressively longer. This is caused by reduced factor V activity rather than by loss of prothrombin. Prothrombin itself is fairly stable in ACD solution. A rapid drop to about 80% of normal takes place within 24 hours, after which deterioration is slow. About 70% of the prothrombin remains after 1 week of storage and about 60% remains after 3 weeks.

The treatment of choice for hypoprothrombinemia (in the sense of deficiency of vitamin K–dependent coagulation factors) is plasma, or whole blood if there is anemia secondary to acute hemorrhage, and simultaneous administration of vitamin K or one of the analogues. Vitamin K therapy is useless if the hypoprothrombinemia is the result of severe liver damage. Congenital deficiency of factor II does not respond to vitamin K and should be treated with plasma.

FACTORS V AND VII. Factor V is probably the most labile of the coagulation factors. In oxalate solutions 50% of factor V activity is lost after 24 hours and 85% after 1 week. It is more stable in ACD solution, the loss of activity amounting to about 30% in 24 hours and 50% after 1 week. In the treatment of factor V deficiency fresh plasma should be used. If there is anemia secondary to hemorrhage, fresh whole blood can be used. Vitamin K is of no value.

Factor VII, on the other hand, is stable, 70% to 90% remaining in blood after storing for 3 weeks. Factor VII deficiency should be treated by transfusing plasma and simultaneously giving vitamin K or one of the analogues.

FIBRINOGEN. Fibrinogen is thought to be relatively stable in blood stored at 4° C. After 1 or 2 weeks of storage it tends to precipitate spontaneously, often producing a gelatinous coating on the filter when the blood is administered. The *amount* of fibrinogen measurable in stored blood is not as important as the reactivity or *coagulability* of the fibrinogen. Fibrinogen in solution undergoes spontaneous deterioration, as evidenced by a progressive lengthening of the coagulation time when thrombin is added. Altered reactivity of the fibrinogen in stored blood probably takes place after a short period of storage. Heparin is the indicated therapeutic agent in the hypofibrinogenemia of acute disseminated intravascular coagulation (p. 843), but it is sometimes necessary to replace erythrocytes lost by hemorrhage. At times, supplemental fibrinogen is indicated, as when heparin therapy does not produce a rapid return to normal of the plasma fibrinogen concentration.

The effectiveness of lyophilized human fibrinogen may be due in part to protein impurities. The commercial product is by no means pure fibrinogen since it consists of 66% fibrinogen, 7% α-globulin, 13% β-globulin, 8% γ-globulin, and 6% albumin. This preparation has, in some patients, produced hemostasis out of proportion to the amount of fibrinogen it contained. Most preparations of fibrinogen (Cohn's fraction I) are rich in factor VIII.

Administration of fibrinogen is not without danger. The incidence of viral hepatitis is high, as high as 13% in one series, since the product cannot be sterilized. There is also evidence that administration of large amounts of fibrinogen can induce thrombosis.

FACTOR VIII (ANTIHEMOPHILIC GLOBULIN). Factor VIII disappears rapidly from stored blood, about half being lost after storage for 24 hours and two-thirds after 1 week. If a deficiency of this factor exists, treatment should consist of fresh whole blood (within 6 hours after it is drawn), freshly separated plasma, fresh frozen plasma, or one of the factor VIII concentrates (p. 538).

FACTOR IX. This factor is stable in stored whole blood.

FACTOR X. This factor is also stable. Frozen plasma shows negligible deterioration of this factor.

FACTOR XI. On the basis of transfusion experiments, Rosenthal and Sloan (1966) found this factor to be stable in both lyophilized and fresh frozen plasma.

FACTOR XII. Factors XI and XII are difficult to assay in vitro because of surface activation phenomena. On the basis of clinical experience it seems that fresh frozen plasma is effective in the treatment of the Hageman abnormality (factor XII deficiency).

FACTOR XIII. Factor XIII is stable, and either fresh or stored plasma is suitable for correcting a deficiency state. The half-life of factor XIII is 3 to 4 days, and the corrective effect of blood transfusion lasts for about 10 days. ·

Fresh whole blood

From the foregoing discussion it should be apparent that freshly drawn whole blood is in all cases superior to stored blood. However, there are practical considerations that make it desirable to use stored blood and blood components whenever possible. Fresh whole blood must be used when the recipient needs red blood cells in addition to platelets, leukocytes, or the labile coagulation factors.

Plasma

Plasma should be used when the patient does not require any of the formed elements. When transfusion therapy is used for the coagulation disorders, the choice between whole blood and plasma should be based on whether there is an associated deficiency of erythrocytes. Hemostasis is achieved more quickly if plasma is given since the entire volume of plasma actively transmits the coagulation factors, whereas the same volume of whole blood has half the effect.

Stored plasma is most useful in the treatment of shock and hypoproteinemia. Fresh plasma is the material of choice when dealing with a potentially labile component. Freshly separated and frozen plasma is ideal for supplying factors V and VIII.

Stored plasma usually represents a pool from a number of donors, the object being to reduce the concentration of each red blood cell agglutinin. It is usual to pool bloods in the ratio of 3 units of group O blood to 2 units of group A and 1 unit of group B. The anti-A and anti-B titers of the pooled plasma should be below 1:32. Because of this low agglutinin titer, plasma can usually be given without regard to the recipient's blood group. There is one important exception. When the recipient is a hemophiliac, almost certainly requiring repeated plasma transfusions over a period of years, it is recommended that only *type-specific* plasma be given, i.e., plasma prepared from blood of the same group as the patient. Frozen plasma retains factor VIII activity for many months, but must be used directly after thawing. The problem of pooled plasma as the vector of hepatitis virus is discussed on p. 541.

Packed red blood cells

Whenever a transfusion is given to supply erythrocytes, serious consideration should be given to the use of erythrocyte suspensions. There are a number of important advantages: (1) there is a greater economy of blood, which can be used for the preparation of both plasma and erythrocyte suspensions, (2) increased erythrocyte mass can be achieved with the least increase in blood volume, (3) there is a reduced incidence of transfusion reactions, and (4) the fact that erythrocyte suspensions have a low concentration of chloride, most of which remains in the separated plasma, may be important in patients with cardiac decompensation. It has been estimated that 80% or more of transfusions can be given as packed red cells (Chaplin, 1969).

Platelet suspension

As discussed previously, collecting blood without special precautions results in a striking decrease in platelet concentration. Blood drawn with special precautions into plastic containers is an excellent source of platelets, being particularly useful when the patient needs both platelets and erythrocytes. Within recent years a number of investigators have used concentrated platelet suspensions in the treatment of thrombocytopenia. It is possible in this way to administer a large quantity of platelets in a small volume. Bacterial contamination is a problem (Buchholz et al, 1971, 1973), but Cordle et al (1980) detected bacterial contamination in only 4 of 126 platelet concentrates prepared by a discontinuous flow centrifugal technic.

The biochemical changes that platelets undergo on storage are detailed by Baldini et al (1976). An optimum technic for preparing and storing platelet suspensions is outlined by Slichter and Harker (1976). Platelet survival data are in fact not necessarily indicative of platelet function. For example, platelets stored at room temperature do not correct aspirin-induced prolongation of the bleeding time even though they seem to survive normally (Handin and Valeri, 1971; Valeri, 1974b; Aster et al, 1976). Platelets stored at 4° C, on the other hand, have a short life span but better hemostatic effectiveness (Kahn and Meryman, 1976). Furthermore, there is evidence that antiplatelet antibodies are formed after the administration of platelet suspensions. There seems to be no danger when only a few units are given, but the risk is great when 10 units or more are transfused. In such situations, platelets given either in suspension or in fresh blood are destroyed almost immediately. Yankee et al (1973) and Lohrmann et al (1974) have shown that in such cases platelets from HLA compatible donors may be effective when unselected platelets are not. Mittal et al (1976) have shown that HLA-compatible platelets survive longer than mismatched platelets, and it is now generally accepted that only HLA-matched platelets should be used (Graw et al, 1977; Schiffer et al, 1978). Daly et al (1980) believe that empirical use of HLA-matched platelets is expensive and wasteful and suggest that a platelet count at 1 hour after the platelet transfusion can serve as an indication of the presence of HLA antibodies and the need for HLA matching for subsequent platelet transfusions. Also, Macpherson and Westphal (1979) have shown that non-HLA antibodies may play a significant role in determining the responses to platelet transfusions in multitransfused patients. There is no justification for using a platelet donor who has taken aspirin during the previous week, since these platelets will be functionally abnormal (Chapter 17). Even though platelet suspensions are usually pooled from several donors, a fraction of that pool will not benefit the recipient. The relation of specific platelet antigens Pl^{A1} and Pl^{B1} and corresponding antibodies to posttransfusion thrombocytopenic purpura is discussed on p. 548. A patient whose blood has platelet antibody should not receive platelets, either in fresh blood or in platelet-rich plasma or platelet concentrates.

Platelet suspensions should be used only when an acute bleeding episode in thrombocytopenia calls for the most rapid control of bleeding. At the present time platelet suspensions are not a routine method of treating thrombocytopenia. They are useful and effective in the supportive therapy of leukemia (Roy et al, 1973; Higby et al, 1974) when they are obtained by plateletpheresis (Koepke et al, 1975). A specific indication is nonimmunologic thrombocytopenia when the platelet count is 20,000/mm³ (0.02×10^{12}/l) or less (Gardner, 1974). Platelet transfusions may also be useful in the treatment of acute bleeding caused by platelet functional abnormalities or for preparing a patient with this type of abnormality for surgery. Platelet transfusions should not be used in immunologic thrombocytopenic purpura except for immediate control of severe bleeding.

Plasma fractions

Much progress is being made toward obtaining pure preparations of plasma protein components. The problem is of major importance, not only from the standpoint of making pure products available for therapy but also for the ultimate resolution of many problems dealing with fundamental protein interactions and blood coagulation.

Plasma fractions containing various coagulation factors have been prepared and studied, but at the present time only five preparations from human plasma are commercially available: albumin (fraction V), fibrinogen (fraction I), γ-globulin, factor VIII concentrate, and concentrates of factors II, VII, IX, and X.

Albumin

Human albumin in the form of Cohn's fraction V is useful in the treatment of shock, hypoproteinemia, and, specifically, hypoalbuminemia (Davison et al, 1974). A salt-free product is available for use when additional salt is contraindicated. It has been claimed that the addition of salt-poor albumin to blood in exchange transfusions increases the rate at which bilirubin is washed out. Administration of albumin

can be accompanied by hypotension caused by Hageman factor fragments (Alving et al, 1978). Pyrogenic reactions are also reported (Steere et al, 1978).

Fibrinogen

Human fibrinogen for therapy was once commercially available as fraction I. This product contained 66% fibrinogen and was also an excellent source of antihemophilic globulin (factor VIII). The FDA has arbitrarily ruled that human fibrinogen may no longer be sold for use in therapy and recommends that cryoprecipitate be used to treat hypofibrinogenemia.

Gamma (γ) globulin

Gamma globulin from human blood has been available for some time. It has been used in the prophylaxis and treatment of infectious diseases and in the specific treatment of hypogammaglobulinemia and agammaglobulinemia. It should be noted that commercial γ-globulin contains IgG but not IgA or IgM. Specific immunoglobulins, such as anti-Rh_0 immunoglobulin (p. 601), can be prepared from plasma containing a high titer of the desired immunoglobulin. Gamma globulin given for specific prophylaxis, i.e., to one exposed to viral hepatitis, should contain an adequate titer of the specific antibody.

Factor VIII concentrate

Factor VIII concentrates for the treatment of classic hemophilia are now readily available. The two products available are cryoprecipitate and purified factor VIII concentrates. The use of cryoprecipitate is not ideal, because our assays show an extremely variable, and sometimes disappointingly low, content of factor VIII. Optimum titers of factor VIII in cryoprecipitates require careful attention to collection and storage conditions (Kasper et al, 1975). On the other hand, commercial and assayed products (Hyland Laboratories, Courtland Laboratories) are excellent and of reliable potency. Cryoprecipitate should be used to treat von Willebrand's disease, since purified factor VIII preparations lack the missing von Willebrand factor (Chapter 17).

Factors II, VII, IX, and X concentrates

Concentrates of the "prothrombin complex" factors II, VII, IX, and X are now commercially available (Konyne, Cutter Laboratories; Prothrombin Complex, Hyland Laboratories). Other preparations are available in England, France, and the Netherlands. They are especially useful in the treatment of the second most common hemophilioid state, factor IX deficiency. Note that, like classical hemophilia, factor IX deficiency may be accompanied by an acquired anticoagulant. The concentrates are also useful in the treatment of congenital deficiencies of factors II, VII, or X, assuming that treatment is indicated.

Concentrates of factors II, VII, IX, and X (prothrombin complex) have been used since 1964 (Soulier et al, 1964) to correct deficiencies of the contained factors, usually for the most common factor IX deficiency (Breen and Tullis, 1969). The unmodified concentrates have in some instances caused thrombotic complications (Kasper, 1975), less frequently when heparin is added (Ménaché and Roberts, 1975). The thrombotic complications have been attributed to the presence of various activated coagulation factors (Kingdon et al, 1975; White et al, 1977; Elödi and Váradi, 1978; Chandra and Wickerhauser, 1979; Hultin, 1979; Seligsohn et al, 1979).

Supposedly because prothrombin complex preparations sometimes shift the coagulation system in the direction of thrombosis, they have been used to control bleeding in hemophiliacs having high titers of anti-VIII anticoagulant (Abildgaard et al, 1976; Kelly and Penner, 1976; Yolken and Hilgartner, 1978). Some investigators have used preparations in which the clotting factors have been purposely activated (Kurczinski and Penner, 1974). Success in achieving hemostasis in some of these patients has been reported with both types of preparations, but the mechanism by which the inhibitor is overcome is not clear. In fact, a recent survey (Kasper and Hemophilia Study Group, 1979) has shown that whereas in some patients the inhibitor titer is reduced by the treatment, a significant number show a rise in the inhibitor level. Castaldi and Smith (1980) have shown that in vitro there is more neutralization of the inhibitor in platelet-rich plasma than in platelet-poor plasma, and it is noteworthy that Bloom and Hutton (1975) used transfusions of fresh platelets in hemophiliacs having factor VIII inhibitor. The recommendation at this time is to use prothrombin complex in these cases only when the inhibitor is present in high titer.

Other fractions

Pilot studies have shown that other plasma fractions contain important coagulation factors. Fraction III-2 contains prothrombin and factor VII, fraction III-3 contains profibrinolysin, fraction IV-1 contains antifibrinolysin, and fraction IV-2 contains factor IX (PTC).

Plasma extenders and substitutes

At the present time there are no satisfactory substitutes for plasma. Acacia, dextran, methylcellulose, gelatin, and various macromolecular substances have been tried, but each has disadvantages. The search for the ideal substitute continues. When found, it will be of tremendous value in both civilian and military practice.

Cadaver (fibrinolytic) blood

The use of blood from human cadavers (the Russians prefer the term "fibrinolytic blood") was pioneered in Russia by Shamov (1937). Since that time the use of fibrinolytic blood has been accepted in Soviet medicine. At the Sklifosovsky Institute (Moscow) over 4,000 transfusions of fibrinolytic blood are now given annually. In the United States transfusions of fibrinolytic blood are reported by Kevorkian and Marra (1964).

There seems little reason to doubt the scientific value of this source of badly needed blood, and yet there has been a reluctance to become involved in the potential problems, mostly social and emotional, of using fibrinolytic blood. The reader is referred to the paper of Swan and Schechter

(1962) for a comprehensive review. Kiel (1969) gives a more recent account of the Russian experience.

Autologous (predonated) transfusion

Autologous transfusion, returning to the patient his own blood, has been used infrequently for many years but is receiving increasing attention (Newman et al, 1971; Cove et al, 1976; Kaplan et al, 1977; Eckardt et al, 1978; Silvergleid, 1979). This procedure has many advantages: (1) it eliminates the need for massive transfusion of stored blood and the complications that may arise; (2) it provides the patient with blood to which he cannot have an adverse reaction; and (3) it eliminates all possibility of trasmitting disease. Blood is drawn from a patient just prior to elective surgery so that it will be available if needed. This provides the safest blood possible as well as reducing the need for homologous blood.

Plasmapheresis

Plasmapheresis is the technic of withdrawing blood from a donor, separating and retaining the plasma, and returning the erythrocytes to the donor. In addition to being a valuable means of obtaining large amounts of plasma, the technic is useful in therapy. It has been used to treat macroglobulinemia where the removal of plasma reduces the viscosity of the blood and allows the removal of large quantities of the unwanted immunoglobulin.

FREQUENCY OF TRANSFUSION

In most cases the number and frequency of transfusions is determined by the results obtained. Determination of the blood volume, erythrocyte count, and hemoglobin concentration serves as a guide for stopping or continuing transfusion therapy. In special cases, particularly hemorrhagic disorders, the effective life of the transfused factor must be taken into account.

Transfusion for coagulation disorders

Here it is important to distinguish between the "biologic half-life" and the "half-disappearance time." When a factor is transfused into a patient having a deficiency of that factor, the disappearance curve is usually of the double-exponential type (semilog plot). The first, rapidly sloping portion reflects redistribution equilibria, while the second slope is a measure of the rate of the utilization of a factor after equilibria have been satisfied. The biologic half-life, determined from the slope of the second portion, has less relationship to the maintenance of therapeutic levels than does the half-disappearance time. Thus the biologic half-life is not necessarily useful in predicting the frequency of transfusion. The half-disappearance time (Table 12-2), i.e., the half-life of the transfused factor, is a better guide for therapy. Different figures can be found in various reports, but the differences are caused largely by variable assay technics and variable interpretations of semilogarithmic survival curves.

These figures indicate the length of time these transfused substances survive in the blood but are not an absolute indication of how soon the transfusion should be repeated. It is

Table 12-2. Survival (half-disappearance time) of coagulation factors after transfusion into subjects deficient in that factor

Factor	Half-disappearance time
Fibrinogen (I)	3-5 days
Prothrombin (II)	1-2 days
Factor V	4-12 hours
Factor VII	3-4 hours
Factor VIII	8-12 hours
Factor IX	24-36 hours
Factor X	2 days
Factor XI	1-3 days
Factor XII	1-3 days
Factor XIII	5-10 days

sometimes forgotten that the goal is to arrest the bleeding, and while survival figures and desired hemostatic levels are useful as a guide, the clinical result should dictate the frequency of transfusion. It is also true that if the patient continues to bleed severely, survival figures are meaningless since a great deal of the transfused factor may be lost.

In general, clinical judgment is just as valuable as factor assays when dealing with the hemotherapy of coagulation disorders. Laboratory studies may be a guide to the effectiveness of treatment, but if the patient continues to bleed, it matters little what the laboratory tests show. It is therefore difficult to give precise rules for how much blood, plasma, or concentrate to give and how frequently.

In hemophilia, for example, the preparation of a patient for surgery must be much more intense than the treatment of a spontaneous hemorrhage. The hemophiliac about to undergo surgery should receive sufficient factor VIII concentrate to bring the assay up to over 50% of the normal. This level should be maintained until there is complete healing of the wound. A hemophiliac with a major bleeding episode (hemarthrosis, muscle hematoma, hematoma in a vital area) need not be treated until normal factor VIII levels are reached, 40% of the normal being adequate. It is sometimes unappreciated that shortly after factor VIII concentrate is given, a very high concentration of factor VIII is reached and there is a gradual reduction over the next 8 to 12 hours. The question then arises as to when blood should be drawn for an assay. The situation is similar to the control of heparin therapy. It is probably best to determine if approximately half the desired level has been achieved 4 hours after the factor VIII concentrate is given. Theoretically, optimum and constant levels could be achieved by continuous intravenous drip, but as far as I know this has not been tried.

The hemophiliac with acquired antifactor VIII anticoagulant, estimated to occur in about 7% of treated hemophiliacs (Brinkhous et al, 1972), presents a difficult problem, usually attacked by administering very large amounts of factor VIII concentrate (Rizza and Biggs, 1973). I suspect that the assay of factor VIII is unreliable during therapy and prior to therapy when there is a powerful anticoagulant. There are reports of the successful use of prothrombin complex concentrate (factors II, VII, IX, X) in the treatment of hemophiliacs with acquired anticoagulant (p. 832).

Single-unit transfusion

It is difficult to defend the practice of transfusing only 1 unit of blood to a patient, and indeed the "single-unit transfusion" has been condemned by many. Unfortunately, a blanket condemnation is unfair. We should distinguish between a single-unit transfusion so intended and other circumstances in which the need for multiple transfusions is predicted, does not materialize, and thus only 1 unit is given. Morton (1969) presents a classification of single-unit transfusions that is recommended to those interested in this subject. He classifies single-unit transfusions as *conservative* if more than 1 unit might have been employed, *reasonable* if given in anticipation of a major blood loss that did not occur, and *questionable* or *unnecessary* when no definite indication is present. Even with these criteria it would seem that roughly one-third to one-fourth of all single-unit transfusions fall into the questionable or unnecessary category (Reece and Beckett, 1966).

ROUTES OF ADMINISTRATION

Blood or plasma is usually given intravenously. In most patients a superficial vein is readily accessible; if not, one of the deeper veins can be cannulated. Routes other than the intravenous route have been championed, but the experience in treating the victims of the Coconut Grove fire in Boston in 1942 showed that, even if the body is badly burned, the femoral vein is readily accessible and easily entered without cutdown.

The other possible routes are by way of an artery or into the bone marrow. Intra-arterial transfusions have been used, but the serious complication of a gangrenous limb developing after arterial spasm makes this route inadvisable. Transfusion into the marrow cavity has also been advocated, particularly when the veins are not readily accessible. The Turkel needle used for bone marrow biopsy can also be used for this purpose. Blood infused slowly into a marrow cavity is readily absorbed, and the risk of complications is very small. However, cannulation of a deep vein is generally preferred over bone marrow infusion.

EXCHANGE TRANSFUSION

Exchange transfusions present special technical and immunologic problems. They are used principally in the treatment of hyperbilirubinemia, with or without isoimmune hemolysis, in infants. Exchange has also been used in cases of chemical poisoning, in the emergency treatment of acute hemolytic anemia (Brody et al, 1970), in hepatic coma (Trey et al, 1966), in neonatal isoimmune thrombocytopenic purpura (Pearson et al, 1964), and in disseminated intravascular coagulation (Gross and Melhorn, 1971). Plasma exchange transfusion has been advocated for immune complex diseases, acute hepatic failure, and hemophilia with high-titer anticoagulant (Flaum et al, 1979). When the patient's plasma is replaced with solutions poor in coagulation factors, there is a danger of producing a significant hemostatic abnormality (Keller et al, 1979). In infants with hyperbilirubinemia the primary goal is to wash out bilirubin to prevent the development of kernicterus. In isoimmune hemolytic anemia in infants, and in acquired hemolytic anemia in adults, a second objective is to reduce the titer of hemolytic antibody. The first objective can be achieved simply by the process of removing bilirubin-rich blood and introducing bilirubin-poor blood, provided that the exchange is not done with incompatible blood, which is itself subject to hemolysis. The second objective deserves special immunologic consideration. Hemolytic antibodies are most commonly the result of A-B-O or Rh incompatibility, and this discussion will therefore relate primarily to this type of isoimmune disease.

In instances of Rh immunization the donor erythrocytes must not react with the hemolysin in the baby's blood. Accordingly, when anti-**Rh₀** is present, Rh₀-negative erythrocytes must be transfused. The same prinicple applies in cases of sensitization to other Rh factors or to factors in other blood groups. In addition to being Rh negative, the donor blood should be group O or group specific with the mother's blood, and the cross matching done against the mother's serum. For repeat transfusions, the second unit of blood should be compatible with the first unit as well.

In A-B-O immunization it is recommended that the donor cells be group O in every instance, although group O blood having a high titer of anti-**A** or anti-**B** must be avoided. The addition of group-specific A and B substance does not help much, since it does not neutralize immune anti-**A** and anti-**B.** Some recommend using washed group O erythrocytes resuspended in compatible plasma, and although this involves extra manipulation, it is immunologically the soundest procedure.

The indication for exchange transfusion is usually stated to be a serum bilirubin concentration of 18 to 20 mg/dl. This criterion, however, is modified by other considerations. Regardless of the total concentration of bilirubin, it is agreed that it is the unconjugated fraction that is toxic, particularly the bilirubin not bound to albumin. The rate at which the serum bilirubin concentration is increasing is very important. Also regardless of the total bilirubin concentration, exchange transfusion should be done in a jaundiced infant showing possible early signs of kernicterus or in a severely anemic infant. Prematurity is another consideration, for kernicterus is more likely in premature than in full-term infants. This is related to increased permeability of the blood brain barrier. Another factor to be taken into account is the increased liability of damaging the ganglion cells when there is hypoxia, hypoglycemia, or infection. The presence of coexisting subgaleal hemorrhage or cephalhematoma may increase the serum bilirubin concentration from breakdown of a large extravascular accumulation of hemoglobin. Hypoproteinemia, particularly hypoalbuminemia, indicates a reduced binding capacity for bilirubin. The same situation results from the administration to the mother of drugs that bind to protein (sulfonamides and salicylates). The administration of vitamin K to the mother also aggravates the situation, because it is hemolytic in large doses. Other drugs such as novobiocin interfere with glucuronide conjugation of bilirubin and increase the unconjugated bilirubin fraction.

HAZARDS OF TRANSFUSION

The untoward effects of blood or plasma transfusion fall into two categories: (1) transmission of disease from donor to recipient (Greenwalt and Jamieson, 1975) and (2) various types of transfusion reactions.

Transmission of disease

Three major diseases can be transmitted by blood or blood products: (1) viral hepatitis, (2) malaria, and (3) syphilis.

Viral hepatitis

Viral hepatitis has been classified traditionally into two types. Hepatitis caused by hepatitis virus A (HVA) is commonly called infectious hepatitis, has a short incubation period of 2 to 6 weeks, and is clinically mild with a very low mortality rate. Hepatitis caused by hepatitis virus B (HVB) is commonly called serum hepatitis, has a long incubation period of 6 to 26 weeks and is clinically severe with a mortality rate of 2% to 3%. Transmission of infectious hepatitis is usually by the fecal-oral route, but it can also be transmitted by blood transfusion. Transmission of serum hepatitis is usually parenteral, from blood or blood product transfusion, by contamination of a cut with the virus, or by infection through contaminated needles and syringes. Mosquitos may be insect vectors of the serum hepatitis virus in areas of high incidence, and subhuman primates may serve as a reservoir (Blumberg and Hesser, 1975).

Blumberg et al (1964, 1965) reported that antibodies to low-density human lipoproteins developed in some persons who had received multiple transfusions. The antigen defining this system was found in the serum of an Australian aborigine and came to be known as the Australia antigen. Several reports established the relationship of Australia antigen to serum hepatitis (Blumberg et al, 1968; Prince, 1968; Gocke and Kavey, 1969). The morphology, biology, immunology, and epidemiology of viral hepatitis is reviewed in detail by Dmochowski (1976).

At first most of the attention was focused on hepatitis caused by what is now known as the hepatitis B antigen. However, some cases of hepatitis were soon found to be unrelated to the hepatitis B antigen. Some of them were found to be caused by transmission of hepatitis A antigen detectable by immune electron microscopy of feces obtained during the acute phase of the disease (Feinstone et al, 1973). Soon it became obvious that some cases of hepatitis could be ascribed to transmission of neither the B nor the A virus, and these are designated non-A, non-B hepatitis. In fact, it is now estimated that about 90% of the cases of transfusion-associated hepatitis are non-A, non-B (Alter et al, 1975; Tabor and Gerety, 1979). Non-A, non-B hepatitis is also viral, but the virus has not been categorized. Bradley et al (1979) have transmitted non-A, non-B hepatitis from some lots of commercial factor VIII concentrate to chimpanzees and have demonstrated virus particles in the liver by immune electron microscopy.

The state of the art at this time provides sensitive "third generation" tests for the hepatitis B virus components and antibodies (radioimmunoassay) or reverse passive hemagglutination (Poleski and Taswell, 1975; Barbara et al, 1977; Hopkins et al, 1980). It is not common practice to screen blood donors for hepatitis A antigen and antibody, and all that is known about non-A, non-B hepatitis is based on epidemiologic studies in humans and chimpanzees. Therefore identification of the B antigens and antibodies in donors screens out what appears to be only a small fraction of potentially dangerous donors.

Before a discussion of hepatitis B, about which a great deal is known, some general comments on hepatitis A and non-B, hepatitis are appropriate.

HEPATITIS A. The present status of our knowledge about hepatitis A is reviewed by Holmes et al (1975), Purcell et al (1975), and Czaja (1979). The available evidence suggests that the probability of transfusion-transmitted hepatitis A is very small. First, the virus is excreted in the feces for only a few days during the acute phase, and the presence of the virus in the blood is unpredictable even during the acute phase. Second, serologic tests show that a significant number of nontransfused persons have antibodies to hepatitis A antigen as the result of subclinical disease and are presumably protected against reinfection. Fortunately, the type A hepatitis virus has not been associated with the development of chronic liver disease (Rakela et al, 1978).

NON-A, NON-B HEPATITIS. Non-A, non-B hepatitis transmitted by transfusion of blood or blood products probably accounts for up to 90% of all cases of transfusion-related hepatitis. It can produce severe, progressive liver disease but is often so anicteric and mild (Berman et al, 1979) that the disease may be unrecognized in its initial stages (Knodell et al, 1977). It should be noted, however, that because of the lack of a reliable serologic test for the agent or agents of non-A, non-B hepatitis, only limited data are available at this time.

HEPATITIS B SURFACE ANTIGEN AND ANTIBODY. Hepatitis B (HB) is caused by a virus usually transmitted by blood transfusion, contaminated needles, or entrance into an open wound. The complete B virus (HBV) is usually considered synonymous with the Dane particle (Kaplan et al, 1973). Surface and core antigens and corresponding antibodies have been identified.

Hepatitis B *surface* antigen (HBsAg) replicates in the liver cell independently of the core of the virus. It can be found in serum as three morphologically different forms: the outer coat of the intact Dane particle, a spherical 22-nm particle, or an elongated tubular structure (Robinson and Lutwick, 1976). However, it is only the outer coat of the Dane particle that contains nucleic acid and is infectious. Antigenic subtypes of HBsAg are known: a, d, y, w, r, e, and l (LeBouvier, 1971; Bancroft et al, 1972; Magnius et al, 1975; Bastiaans et al, 1979). Combinations of subtypes have been described in different geographic, racial, and socioeconomic groups (Nielsen et al, 1973; Perry and Chaudhary, 1973; Hopkins and Das, 1974). Subtyping of HBsAg is of no practical importance but is useful in epidemiologic studies.

The appearance of HBsAg in blood is the first manifestation of infection. Depending on the route of infection and the size of the inoculum, HBsAg antigenemia may be detectable 27 to 41 days after inoculation and 7 to 46 days before liver dysfunction is manifest (Barker and Murray, 1971). Surface antigenemia usually disappears during the recovery phase but persists if the liver damage progresses to chronic hepatitis (Nielsen et al, 1971). The presence of HBsAg in blood identifies a subject infected with the B virus even before the onset of clinical illness; it also identifies a chronic carrier of HBV.

The development of antibody to surface antigen, anti-HBs, may not be detectable for some months after the antigenemia disappears (Krugman et al, 1979). During this "serologic gap" between the disappearance of antigenemia and the appearance of antibody serologic tests will not detect individuals in the recovery phase, but blood from such donors is infective if positive for core antibody (Hoofnagle et al, 1978). Anti-HBs persists for at least 18 months and may be present indefinitely. A subject with anti-HBs is partially protected against reinfection.

HEPATITIS B CORE ANTIGEN AND ANTIBODY. Hepatitis B *core* antigen (HBcAg) is thought to be the 27-nm inner core of the complete Dane particle. It represents the nucleocapsid core, and its presence in blood connotes active infection, virus replication, and potential infectiousness.

Antibody to core antigen, anti-HBc, usually appears during the period of surface antigenemia, can be detected 12 to 20 weeks after infection and 4 to 10 weeks after the appearance of HBsAg, and its appearance coincides with the onset of clinical illness. When anti-HBc is the only antibody present in serum, it can be assumed that the subject has been infected and is in the early stage of recovery. When both anti-HBs and anti-HBc are present, the subject is probably in the late stage of convalescence. When the serum contains anti-HBc and HBsAg, the subject is either in the acute phase of hepatitis or has chronic hepatitis. In active liver disease, including the very serious fulminant hepatitis, the serum contains HBsAg, anti-HBs, and anti-HBc. When anti-HBc is present in high titer, there is active virus replication, and blood that contains it is infectious (Hoofnagle et al, 1978); but more recent evidence (Krugman et al, 1979) indicates that low levels of anti-HBc that persist with anti-HBs after recovery from type B hepatitis indicate immunity rather than virus infections.

In summary, the usual patterns seen in hepatitis type B are as follows: The typical type B hepatitis patient shows an early but transient elevation of serum HBsAg, and anti-HBs appears with recovery and may persist for a long time. Anti-HBc appears after HBsAg disappears, and the titer falls if the patient recovers. If the patient progresses to the chronic hepatitis carrier state, anti-HBc persists for a long time and in high titer. Subjects who are positive for anti-HBs but negative for anti-HBc are usually resistant to reinfection.

HEPATITIS Be ANTIGEN AND ANTIBODY. The hepatitis Be antigen (HBeAg) is a component of the Dane particle, probably the DNA polymerase in the core (Nielsen et al, 1974). All patients with acute hepatitis B have HBe antigenemia (Aikawa et al, 1978). This antigen appears in the blood shortly after HBsAg can be detected and usually disappears before the surface antigen does. If HBsAg persists, so does HBeAg, indicating a chronic process and the carrier state. Okada et al (1978) have reported mothers whose blood contains HBeAg transmitting viral hepatitis to their neonates; thus the presence of this antigen indicates a high degree of infectivity. The antibody to this antigen, anti-HBe, may persist for many weeks after the disappearance of HBsAg.

EPIDEMIOLOGY OF VIRAL HEPATITIS. The transmission of the virus by other than transfusion is important from the standpoint of epidemiology and safety for laboratory and other medical personnel. Nonparenteral (oral) transmission in humans has been achieved (Krugman et al, 1967), but most of the evidence is indirect and in most cases the mode of transmission is unknown. HBsAg has been demonstrated in feces, urine, bile, saliva, tears, and semen (Ward et al, 1972; Kistler et al, 1973; Heathcote et al, 1974; Vittal et al, 1974). The higher-than-average incidence of antigen positivity or hepatitis in health workers (Alter, 1975) and hospital personnel (Lewis et al, 1973), in the staff of hemodialysis units (London et al, 1969), in surgeons (Rosenberg et al, 1973), and in dentists (Feldman and Schiff, 1975) as well as many reports of case-clustering, suggest nonparenteral transmission. Venereal (oral or genital) transmission is postulated by some (Fulford et al, 1973; Dietzman et al, 1977), but in another study no difference was found in the hepatitis infection rates of female prostitutes and nuns (Adam et al, 1974). Handling virus-contaminated blood and other body fluids in the clinical laboratory is a potential hazard (Lauer et al, 1979). One hepatitis outbreak in a clinical laboratory has implicated cuts sustained while handling computer cards (Pattison et al, 1974). A survey in our laboratory revealed a very high incidence of HBsAg–positive control sera and materials (Wetli et al, 1973). Transmission of hepatitis B virus from asymptomatic mothers to their babies is possible (Odada et al, 1976).

As part of the current emphasis on an all-voluntary blood donor program, the point has been made repeatedly (Alter et al, 1972; Barker et al, 1975) that "commercial" blood carries with it a significantly higher incidence of transfusion hepatitis than that from voluntary donors. This is undoubtedly true when "commercial blood" is obtained from skid row donors or narcotic addicts. It may not be true, however, if one extrapolates this to include under "commercial" the professional donors who, it is true, are paid for donating the blood. For one thing, these professional donors usually donate blood many times and have been tested by the strictest of all tests—noninfection of the recipients. Another consideration is that the majority of cases of transfusion-related hepatitis are of the non-A, non-B type for which there are no screening tests. Thus even if an all-voluntary donor program is achieved and coupled with sensitive tests for hepatitis B antigens and antibodies, only a small percentage of all voluntary donors will be eliminated, and the problem of transfusion-related hepatitis will remain until the agent or agents of non-A, non-B hepatitis are identified and suitable screening tests are developed.

Blood components and products used parenterally can also transmit viral hepatitis. The chief offenders are (1) pooled plasma, presenting the possibility of a pool contaminated by one unit containing the virus, (2) human fibrinogen, (3) human prothrombin complex concentrates, (4) human factor VIII concentrates (Anderson et al, 1966; Mainwaring and Breuckner, 1966; Kasper and Kipnis, 1972; Sandler et al, 1973; Bradley et al, 1979), and (5) frozen and washed red blood cells (Haugen, 1979). These products should be considered potentially dangerous and should not be used without indications that are stronger than the hazard.

Clinical screening of donors aims at rejecting any who

have had jaundice, even when the etiology appears to be other than viral. Other reasons for rejection are low hemoglobin or hematocrit, medication, allergies, hypertension, and travel to areas where malaria is endemic (Standards for Blood Banks and Transfusion Services, 1976; Farrales et al, 1977). However, even if the donor is and has been well, he may be either in the incubation stage of the disease or a carrier and extremely dangerous. The virus of B hepatitis has been shown to be present in the blood during the incubation period of 40 to 180 days before the disease becomes manifest.

In spite of several enthusiastic reports of the efficacy of liver function tests in screening out preclinical or postclinical cases of hepatitis, the data in other reports prove quite clearly that liver function tests are practically useless for this purpose. This applies not only to flocculation tests but also to the more sophisticated serum enzyme determinations such as glutamic-oxaloacetic transaminase, glutamic-pyruvic transaminase, and isocitrate dehydrogenase.

The problem of killing the virus in blood or blood products has not been solved. Ultraviolet rays are effective when a very thin and uniform layer of plasma is exposed to their action under carefully controlled conditions. This is feasible when dealing with commercial products of small volume but not for the prophylactic treatment of large volumes of plasma. It seems that the best viricidal method combines ultraviolet irradiation with the addition of propiolactone. Administration of specific immunoglobulin (hepatitis B immune globulin, HBIG) to subjects exposed to the virus achieves excellent protection (Courouce-Pauty et al, 1975; Seeff et al, 1978).

Careful cleaning and adequate sterilization of needles and glassware are essential. Good practice requires that all equipment used for venipuncture or for obtaining blood be properly sterilized, either by dry heat or effective autoclaving. This specifically includes reusable syringes (Dull, 1961), since there is some reflux from syringe to bloodstream when blood is being drawn.

Malaria

As with viral hepatitis, a careful attempt is made to eliminate as a donor anyone who has had malaria. The subject of transfusion malaria is reviewed by Miller (1975). The parasite has been known to remain in the body for years after the initial attack. If a specific diagnosis was not made at that time, the donor is potentially dangerous. It is estimated that about 1,500,000 men have recently served in the armed forces in malaria-endemic areas. Chojnacki et al (1968) report the transmission of falciparum malaria by an asymptomatic Vietnam veteran. Of special interest in this report is the absence of parasites in the donor's peripheral blood and the presence of parasites in a bone marrow aspirate. There is a well-documented case of falciparum malaria transmitted by the transfusion of platelet concentrate (Garfield et al, 1978). The parasite of benign tertian malaria, *Plasmodium vivax*, does not survive longer than 96 hours in blood stored at the usual 4° C, but *Plasmodium malariae* and *Plasmodium falciparum* survive indefinitely under the usual conditions of blood storage. All three types fail to survive 5 days of storage at room temperature. Blacks who are blood group Duffy-negative are resistant to infection with *P. vivax* (Miller et al, 1976).

Syphilis

The transmission of syphilis by transfusion is not as great a problem as the transmission of malaria or viral hepatitis. However, from the medicolegal standpoint, the liability is great. Most patients would be indignant over acquiring a "social" disease in such an innocent manner.

The low incidence of transfusion-induced syphilis is partly caused by the low incidence of syphilis among blood donors. It may become more of a problem if the incidence of syphilis continues to rise. It is also probable that, as a result of public education, persons who know they have syphilis do not offer themselves as blood donors.

Any donor giving a history of syphilis is usually rejected regardless of whether the serologic test for syphilis is negative, even though adequate treatment probably made the blood safe. Serologically positive blood is also rejected, even though serologically positive tertiary syphilis is not transmissible by blood. The chief contraindication for using serologically positive blood is the transfer of serologic positivity to the recipient. In such a case, however, the serologic positivity is of relatively short duration. It has been claimed that serologic testing for syphilis is a public health measure as well, but the high incidence of biologic false positive tests in some groups or disease states (narcotic addicts, in disseminated lupus erythematosus and other collagen diseases, and even unexplained in normal persons) calls for intensive investigation of any positive test. The real problem is identifying the dangerous donor who has been exposed to syphilis, is infected, but has not yet developed a chancre, secondary syphilitic lesions, or a positive serologic reaction (Chambers et al, 1969). A male donor with a chancre is easily eliminated by the most superficial physical examination, but the usual examination given to female donors is not such as to reveal a chancre. Extragenital chancres are rare but should not be overlooked. I well remember a patient who had a chancre at the end of his big toe. He had emphatically denied sexual exposure but fortunately tried to get free advice with regard to the sore on his foot.

It is fortunate that *Treponema pallidum* is killed when blood is stored at 4° C for 96 hours or when plasma is similarly stored or frozen (Block, 1941). This alone is thought to eliminate much of the danger from the use of serologically negative blood containing organisms.

"Posttransfusion mononucleosis"

Recipients of blood have developed "posttransfusion mononucleosis" as the result of the donor being viremic. This complication was also reported after open-heart surgery in six patients who, before operation, had cytomegalovirusfixing (CMV-CF) antibody in their serum. It is not improbable that the syndrome described by Foster and Jack (1969) as "posttransfusion mononucleosis" and by Seaman and Starr (1962) as "febrile postcardiotomy lymphocytic splenomegaly" both reflect a lymphocytic reaction, possibly to cytomegalic virus, accompanied by a "virocyte" response in the peripheral blood. The criteria for this complication representing classic infectious mononucleosis have not been met. In fact, the disease is heterophile negative (see review by Bayer and Tegtmeier, 1976).

Other infectious agents

Isolated instances of transmission of other microorganisms are reported: brucellosis, trypanosomiasis, visceral leishmaniasis, toxoplasmosis, and Rocky Mountain spotted fever (Siegel et al, 1971; Janitschke et al, 1974; Wolfe, 1975; Wells et al, 1978).

Transfusion reactions

A number of untoward reactions may be produced by the transfusion of blood or plasma. These "transfusion reactions" are of different types and of various degrees of severity. The exact incidence, nationwide or in a given hospital, is not easily determined. In some cases there is failure to recognize or report transfusion reactions; in others, a coincidental change in the patient's condition may be attributed to blood transfusion. It is thought that transfusion reactions occur in about 5% of all transfusions. This figure may serve as a rough guide, an incidence higher than 5% calling for a careful appraisal of procedures and methodology and one lower calling for more accurate reporting.

Hemolytic reactions

Hemolytic reactions, although less frequent than other types, are the most important because they are potentially the most dangerous. When a hemolytic reaction occurs, it calls for a careful review of each step taken, from preparation to administration.

ETIOLOGY. Hemolysis is caused by incompatibility between the donor's and the recipient's blood. Either the donor's or the recipient's erythrocytes may be hemolyzed, the first by antibodies in the recipient's serum and the second by antibodies in the donor's serum. Errors in typing and cross matching are now rare, and most transfusions of incompatible blood can be attributed to clerical errors such as typing and cross matching the wrong patient or giving blood intended for one patient to another (Pineda et al, 1978a).

Hemolysis of donor erythrocytes is the more common; e.g., administration of group B blood to a recipient who is group A will produce hemolysis of donor (group B) erythrocytes because of the natural isoagglutinin anti-B in the recipient's blood. Hemolysis of the recipient's cells is possible when group O blood having a high titer of anti-A or anti-B agglutinins is given to recipients who are of group A, B, or AB. Because group O blood usually has low anti-A and anti-B titers, a person of this group has been considered a "universal donor," but obviously becomes a "dangerous universal donor" if the agglutinin titers are high.

It is generally thought that, to be safely used as universal donor blood, group O blood should have anti-A and anti-B titers of 1:100 or less. Natural isoagglutinins anti-A and anti-B can be neutralized in vitro by adding type-specific A and B substances prepared according to Witebsky's method. Immune anti-A and anti-B antibodies are not neutralized by type-specific substances and may produce a serious hemolytic reaction, even though the natural isoagglutinins have been neutralized.

Because group AB blood contains no natural isoagglutinins, a person of this blood group has been considered a "universal recipient." This concept is no longer valid. For one thing, the recipient's group AB erythrocytes can be hemolyzed by donor blood having high titers of anti-**A** or anti-**B** agglutinins. For another, persons of group AB may have *irregular isoagglutinins*. These agglutinins are called irregular because they are not regularly found in the A-B-O system. They have a narrower thermal range of activity, reacting best at 15° to 18° C, whereas the thermal range of regular isoagglutinins is 0° to 50° C. Irregular agglutinins are not immune antibodies produced by sensitization, but they may appear after one or more blood transfusions. They are anti-**O**, found in persons of subgroup A_1B and capable of agglutinating erythrocytes of group O or A_2, and anti-**A₁**, found in persons of subgroup A_2B and capable of agglutinating erythrocytes of group A_1 or A_1B.

Incompatibility with regard to Rh antigens may also produce a hemolytic reaction. Antibodies in the Rh system are always acquired and of the immune type, being produced by sensitization in the course of previous transfusions or pregnancy. If antibodies are present, they may produce hemolysis of donor erythrocytes when these are of the corresponding type. Most reactions in the Rh system result from the presence of anti-**Rh₀**, but reactions caused by anti-**rh′**, anti-**rh″**, anti-**hr′**, and others (Chapter 11) have been reported.

Very occasionally hemolytic transfusion reactions are caused by antibodies other than those to A-B-O or Rh antigens, such as Lewis, Kell, Duffy, Lutheran, and many others. These antibodies are produced only by previous sensitization.

Immune hemolysis may be by antibody plus complement or by antibody alone. Immune hemolysis mediated by complement occurs in this sequence: (1) immunoglobulin (IgG or IgM) attaches to the surface of the red blood cell, (2) the immunoglobulin molecule binds the first component of complement (C_{1q}) (Rosse, 1973a), (3) The complement system is sequentially activated (p. 556), ending with fixation of C9 and immediate intravascular lysis of the red blood cell, and (4) C3 divides into C3a, which acts as an anaphylotoxin, and C3b, which attaches to the red blood cell and serves to ready the red blood cell for ingestion by macrophages. Immune hemolysis by antibody alone involves immunoglobulins IgG_1 and IgG_3. These bind to the red blood cell and, like C3b, make it susceptible to phagocytosis by macrophages.

The occurrence of apparent hemolysis, as evidenced by hemoglobinemia and hemoglobinuria, but with no detectable antibody involvement should suggest three other possibilities: (1) the recipient has paroxysmal nocturnal hemoglobinuria (PNH) (p. 563), and hemolysis is caused by complement-mediated hemolysis of the PNH red blood cells (Götze and Müller-Eberhard, 1972); (2) hemolyzed blood has been administered (Ross, 1945); or (3) the transfused blood is from a donor with hemoglobin SC disease (Murphy et al, 1980).

CLINICOPATHOLOGIC CORRELATION. The typical clinical picture of an immediate severe hemolytic reaction consists of pain in the lumbar region, rapid elevation of temperature and pulse rate, chills, flushing of the skin, nausea, vomiting, and precordial pain. The symptoms are not the same in all patients and vary in severity. Occasionally there may be only a drop in blood pressure and an increase in pulse rate. Davidsohn and Stern (1955) report a case in which severe hemolysis was accompanied only by a mild urticaria. It is apparent that, relying on clinical observations alone, there may be considerable question as to whether a reaction has occurred. The decision may depend on the results of laboratory investigation. Clinical recognition of a transfusion reaction is almost impossible if it occurs in a patient under anesthesia, except for the signs of shock. Giving blood during surgery should be avoided if at all possible.

Hemolytic reactions sometimes occur some days after the administration of apparently compatible blood. These are designated "delayed hemolytic reactions" (Croucher et al, 1967; Holland and Wallerstein, 1968). The recipient usually has no demonstrable antibodies when the transfusion is given, but later antibodies are formed, possibly as an anamnestic response, which hemolyze the transfused red cells within a few days. There is evidence of hemolysis in all cases, but some recipients never have antibodies (Pineda et al, 1978b). These reactions are characterized by the development of a positive antiglobulin test and may be mild or, less often, as severe as the immediate reactions.

The course of events in a fatal reaction is hemolysis followed by hemoglobinemia, hemoglobinuria, jaundice, acute renal failure, oliguria, anuria, azotemia, and death. This sequence is reversible unless the renal damage is so severe that recovery is impossible. The severity of the reaction and its complications are in part proportional to the degree of hemolysis, and it is essential that a transfusion be stopped at the first sign of a reaction. The outcome in patients with severe renal damage often depends on the quality of medical care given. Heroic measures such as peritoneal dialysis and use of the artificial kidney should be taken when necessary, although some feel the results of conservative therapy to be better. Close observation is also essential during the recovery phase. A voluminous diuresis is common at this time, accompanied by a huge loss of sodium ions. This produces an electrolyte imbalance known as "salt-loss nephritis" or "salt-loss syndrome," which may be fatal if not recognized and treated.

The pathogenesis of the renal lesion has been the subject of intensive investigation. Originally described as *lower nephron nephrosis*, the renal damage is characterized by extensive tubular degeneration with necrosis, interstitial edema, and inspissation of hemoglobin and hemoglobin pigments in the lumina of the damaged tubules. It was once thought that tubular necrosis was caused by precipitated hemoglobin. Ischemia and intravascular coagulation are now considered the primary factors in the production of the renal lesions. Yuile et al (1949) have shown in experimental animals that hemoglobinuria by itself caused no degenerative lesions in the kidney, but when hemoglobinuria and ischemia were produced at the same time, degenerative lesions and hemoglobin casts followed. It is also important to note that, from the work of Peskin et al (1969) hemoglobin that is free of erythrocyte stroma does not cause renal damage or intravascular hemolysis. The old concepts of the pathogenesis of the renal lesion have been replaced by an appreciation that the tubular necrosis is caused by ischemia, decreased blood flow in the vessels of the renal cortex, and decreased glomerular filtration (Carriere et al, 1966; Hollenberg et al, 1968). This is probably preceded by several of the phenomena that accompany DIC, i.e., liberation of vasoactive amines, activation of the blood coagulation system with obstruction of the microvasculature by fibrin, etc. (p. 843).

INVESTIGATION OF A REACTION. It is imperative that an orderly procedure be followed whenever a reaction occurs or is suspected. In order to have on hand the specimens needed, it is essential to save pretransfusion blood specimens for at least 10 days after the transfusion is given.

The investigation is designed to reveal, first, whether hemolysis has occurred and, second, the cause. The materials needed and the studies to be performed are listed in Table 12-3.

Hemoglobinemia in the blood specimen obtained immediately after the reaction establishes the presence of hemolysis. It is often sufficient to identify hemoglobinemia by the red color of the serum. Quantitatively, the normal serum hemoglobin concentration is usually below 5 mg/dl. A serum hemoglobin concentration of 20 mg/dl or higher indicates abnormal hemolysis. Values of 100 mg/dl are not uncommon in severe reactions. Care must be taken to avoid causing hemolysis when drawing the blood specimen or separating the serum.

A drop in the serum haptoglobin concentration is also a delicate index of hemolysis. As noted in Chapter 10 the haptoglobin-hemoglobin complex is quickly cleared from the blood, so that when hemoglobin is liberated by hemolysis there is a concomitant consumption of serum haptoglobin. When stored blood is given in large quantities, a drop in the serum haptoglobin concentration should be expected and does not indicate that a hemolytic reaction has taken place. This transient drop in serum haptoglobin is simply due to the transfusion of free hemoglobin in the partially hemolyzed blood or from the hemolysis of stored cells at the end of their period of viability. However, a drop in serum haptoglobin following the administration of part of 1 unit of blood is an excellent indication that severe hemolysis has taken place.

Hemoglobinuria can be detected within 1 to 2 hours after the reaction. It is usually of short duration since hemoglobin is cleared rapidly from the blood. The appearance of hemoglobin in the urine may be delayed if there is oliguria. The degree of hemoglobinuria is of little significance, particularly when the specimen obtained represents in part urine already present in the bladder at the time of the reaction.

The presence of *methemalbumin* in the serum indicates previous hemoglobinemia. Although it is often possible to detect this abnormal pigment in the serum within a few hours after the reaction, it may not appear until 1 or 2 days later.

Hyperbilirubinemia can be detected within 6 to 12 hours. Jaundice appears 1 or 2 days later, depending on the degree of hyperbilirubinemia. The rise in serum bilirubin is caused mainly by a rise in the indirect-reacting fraction, although a lesser rise in the direct-reacting fraction is often seen as well.

Bilirubin, if produced in large amounts, is excreted in the urine, as are degradation products such as urobilinogen. The amount of urobilinogen excreted in the urine can be used to estimate how much hemoglobin has been destroyed.

When renal damage is severe, the retention of nitrogenous products in the blood produces an elevation of nonprotein nitrogen *(azotemia)* and, if sufficiently severe, a clinical picture of coma and convulsions. Azotemia usually becomes noticeable by the fourth day, at which time the urine flow will already have become scanty *(oliguria)* or absent *(anuria)*. During the recovery phase, large volumes of urine are excreted, the urinary sediment at first containing flushed-out hyaline casts and casts containing hemosiderin.

The cause of hemolytic transfusion reaction is sought by means of carefully planned and performed serologic tests of both the donor's and the patient's blood. When the cross matching is rechecked, the most sensitive methods should be used to confirm compatibility. If the standard high-protein cross matching shows the bloods to be compatible, this must be confirmed with enzyme-treated erythrocytes. Sensitization is detected by the direct antiglobulin test and antibodies in the recipient's serum can be detected by the indirect antiglobulin test. Nonagglutinating antibodies are identified by the indirect antiglobulin cross match technic. Antibodies may be absent from the recipient's serum soon after the reaction but may appear some days later. If an antibody is present, it must be identified if possible, not only for theoretical reasons but also to avoid another reaction if subsequent transfusions are necessary.

Hypersensitivity reactions

Hypersensitivity reactions are more common than hemolytic reactions and range in severity from mild to potentially fatal. They can be subdivided into: (1) allergic reactions to food or drug allergens, (2) immediate hypersensitivity dermal reactions, (3) febrile transfusion reactions, (4) serum sickness, (5) anaphylactoid reactions, and (6) acute pulmonary edema. With the exception of reactions caused by food and drug allergens and febrile reactions caused by bacterial contamination of donor blood, most hypersensitivity reactions are thought to be secondary to immunization to foreign immunoglobulin or to the presence of antilymphocyte or antiplatelet antibodies (Grumet and Yankee, 1974).

ALLERGIC REACTIONS. Allergic reactions to food or drug allergens may be both dermal (urticaria) and systemic (bronchial asthma). Most of these reactions are produced by the presence in the donor blood of an allergen to which the recipient is sensitive. Most of these allergens are thought to be derived from foods, and for this reason it is best to draw blood from fasting donors. It is also postulated that passive transfer of allergic antibodies from donor to recipient is possible and donors who are in an active state of allergy or who give a strong history of allergy should be rejected. Hypersensitivity to drugs is more difficult to define, but in the simplest form the recipient allergic to penicillin reacts to penicillin in the blood of the donor who is receiving this drug. In this example the reaction may be mild or severe as in the anaphylaxis group.

IMMEDIATE DERMAL REACTIONS. These reactions are

Table 12-3. Scheme for investigating a hemolytic transfusion reaction

A. Materials needed
1. Recipient's pretransfusion blood specimen
    a. For serum and cells
    b. For plasma
2. Recipient's posttransfusion blood specimens; draw immediately after the reaction and at intervals thereafter
    a. For serum and cells
    b. For plasma
3. Pilot tube for each unit of blood given
4. Remainder of blood in donor unit
5. Urine specimens from recipient; obtain immediately after the reaction and at intervals thereafter; catheterize if necessary

B. Test to be performed
1. Repeat A-B-O grouping on recipient's pretransfusion and posttransfusion blood samples, donor pilot tube, and blood in donor bottle or bottles, including reverse grouping, confirmation of group O with group O serum, and, if indicated, determination of subgroups of A and B
2. Repeat Rh typing on recipient's pretransfusion and posttransfusion blood samples, donor pilot tube, and blood in donor bottle or bottles, including tests for Rh variants (D^u) if the blood is Rh$_0$ negative
3. Repeat cross match of recipient's pretransfusion blood sample against pilot tube blood and blood in donor set by standard method (tests at room temperature and 37° C by saline, high-protein, and antiglobulin technics); if there is no incompatibility, repeat cross match using enzyme-treated donor red cells

4. Test recipient's pretransfusion and posttransfusion serum and donor's serum against a panel of group O cells of known antigen composition using standard saline and antiglobulin technics
5. Perform direct antiglobulin (Coombs') test on recipient's pretransfusion and posttransfusion blood, including microscopic reading of tests
6. Determine serum or plasma hemoglobin on recipient's immediate posttransfusion specimen; repeat at intervals
7. Determine the concentration of serum haptoglobin on the recipient's posttransfusion specimen; repeat at intervals
8. Test for presence of methemalbumin in serum from recipient, 6 and 48 hours after reaction
9. Determine blood urea nitrogen or nonprotein nitrogen at intervals to detect developing azotemia
10. Serial urinalysis for hemoglobin, urobilinogen, bilirubin, coproporphyrin, and albumin
11. Perform special immunologic studies for rare antibodies as indicated
12. If indicated, culture the blood remaining in donor bottle (at 4°, 20°, and 37° C)

C. Additional information to be obtained
1. History of previous transfusions, transfusion reactions, or sensitization caused by pregnancy
2. Amount of blood administered and rate of administration
3. Duration of blood storage before administration
4. Details of method of administration, particularly as to simultaneous administration of glucose or other solutions through same set

characterized by urticaria (hives) occurring during the infusion of whole blood, plasma, or plasma fractions. Those not caused by food or drug allergens are caused by hypersensitivity to immunoglobulin in the donor material. Dermal reactions respond well to antihistaminic drugs. A recipient prone to these reactions can be pretreated with antihistaminic drugs if additional transfusions need to be given. Washed erythrocyte suspensions can be used since the offending immunoglobulin is in the donor plasma.

FEBRILE REACTIONS. Febrile transfusion reactions are characterized by chills, fever, malaise, myalgia, and headache—a flu-like syndrome. The reaction is of two types: (1) reaction to a pyrogen in the transfused material or (2) reaction to antileukocyte or antiplatelet antibodies.

Pyrogenic reactions are characterized by an increase in body temperature. In the pure form, they are not accompanied by hemolysis. The rise in temperature occurs very shortly after the transfusion is given and may be accompanied by a mild or severe chill. A pyrogenic reaction is usually of short duration, lasting only a few hours.

The fever is often produced by pyrogenic substances contaminating the blood, plasma, or intravenous fluid. Pyrogens are usually the product of bacterial contamination or an impurity in the distilled water used for preparing intravenous solutions or the result of improperly cleaned intravenous tubing. Much has been done to prevent these pyrogenic reactions. Contamination from improperly cleaned apparatus has been eliminated by the use of disposable transfusion and intravenous sets. Careful pretesting of intravenous fluid for pyrogens before it is released by the manufacturer has reduced the incidence of pyrogenic reactions.

Bacterial contamination of blood and platelet concentrates (Walker, 1975) remains a serious problem and is probably the cause of many pyrogenic reactions. A meticulous aseptic technic must be employed in drawing and processing the blood to prevent bacterial contamination. It is also possible for the offending organism to be present in the blood at the time it is drawn. Storage at refrigerator temperature does not inhibit the growth of some bacteria. Others grow best at refrigerator temperature. If a pyrogenic transfusion reaction occurs, it is necessary to set up several cultures of the blood remaining in the bottle, incubating some at standard incubator temperature, others at room temperature, and still others at refrigerator temperature.

When a pyrogenic reaction is produced by intravenous fluid, the fluid remaining in the bottle should be saved for bacterial cultures and tested for the presence of pyrogens. Pyrogens can be detected by injecting the fluid into rabbits intravenously and noting whether a rise in temperature is produced. It is obvious that some pyrogenic reactions will be avoided if the blood or plasma is carefully inspected before it is given and discarded if there is any turbidity or evidence of bacterial growth.

Some febrile reactions are secondary to antileukocyte or antiplatelet antibodies, and are encountered in multitransfused patients or in previously pregnant women. The reaction is usually immediate but may be delayed several hours. Recipients who have had such a reaction should receive only leukocyte-free packed red blood cells or HLA-matched platelets.

SERUM SICKNESS. Reactions resembling serum sickness (fever, malaise, myalgia, arthritis, pericarditis) occur 1 to 5 days after the transfusion of whole blood, plasma, or plasma fractions. They are attributed to antiimmunoglobulin in the recipient's blood and can be avoided by using washed red cells or washed platelets.

ANAPHYLACTOID REACTIONS. Anaphylactoid reactions are characterized by shock, with symptoms of wheezing, shortness of breath, fall in blood pressure, and flushing. They are immediate and extremely dangerous and must be treated immediately with steroids, epinephrine, and oxygen. These reactions are also secondary to antiimmunoglobulin antibodies, usually anti-IgA, in the recipient (Leikola et al, 1973). Multitransfused patients and previously pregnant women are potential anaphylactoid reactors (Vos et al, 1973) as are IgA-deficient persons (Sandler and Zlotnick, 1976).

ACUTE PULMONARY EDEMA. Acute pulmonary edema with pulmonary infiltrates is reported following transfusion of plasma (Kernoff et al, 1972). This complication is thought to be secondary to a reaction between antileukocyte antibodies in the recipient and donor leukocytes or between recipient leukocytes and antileukocyte antibodies in the donor.

Hemorrhagic reactions

Hemorrhagic reactions, i.e., posttransfusion purpura, hematuria, gastrointestinal hemorrhage, or bleeding from an operation site, are of varied pathogenesis: (1) "wash-out" effect on platelets, (2) disseminated intravascular coagulation associated with a hemolytic transfusion reaction, or (3) posttransfusion thrombocytopenic purpura.

"WASH-OUT" EFFECT ON PLATELETS. Massive transfusion of platelet-deficient stored blood into a patient who is actively bleeding can lead to severe thrombocytopenia. Unless corrected by using fresh whole blood, the thrombocytopenia can then lead to continued bleeding.

DISSEMINATED INTRAVASCULAR COAGULATION. Disseminated intravascular coagulation (DIC, p. 843) is one complication of hemolytic transfusion reactions.

POSTTRANSFUSION THROMBOCYTOPENIC PURPURA. Posttransfusion thrombocytopenic purpura is a rare complication of blood transfusion. Typically the onset is about 1 week after blood transfusion into a previously transfused or previously pregnant woman (Shulman et al, 1961; Morrison and Mollison, 1966; Cimo and Aster, 1972; Abramson et al, 1974). The immunologic destruction of the recipient's platelets is attributed to the formation of a complement-fixing antiplatelet isoantibody of Pl[A1] specificity (Gerstner et al, 1979). In most cases the recipient's platelets are Pl[A1] negative so that is is assumed that prior immunization by transfusion occurred following transfusion of Pl[A1]–positive platelets. However Ziegler et al (1975) report posttransfusion purpura in a Pl[A1]–positive man, and Vaughan-Neil et al (1975) report one case attributed to Pl[B1] antibody. In the latter exceptions destruction of the recipient's platelets is probably of the *innocent bystander* type, i.e., nonspecific immune destruction by immune complexes not related to platelet antigens or antibodies. The demonstration of aggregation of normal platelets by the patient's plasma (Deykin

and Hellerstein, 1972; Abramson et al, 1974) has been used to detect platelet antibodies, but we have had no success with this technic.

There should be no difficulty in distinguishing this syndrome from DIC. The platelet count is very low, to levels seldom seen in DIC, and there is no evidence of hypofibrinogenemia or prolonged coagulation tests. Abramson et al (1974) showed plasmapheresis to be an effective method of therapy. Others have successfully used steroid therapy (Vaughan-Neil et al, 1975; Ziegler et al, 1975).

"Citric acid intoxication"

The arguments advanced to support the thesis that excesses of citrate in stored blood are toxic are alarmingly unscientific. The observations are that extremely rapid transfusion of ACD blood or the use of ACD blood for extracorporeal bypass apparatus or in exchange transfusions can produce toxic effects such as circulatory collapse and cardiac arrest. The explanation of the toxic effect is something else.

It has been proposed that the elevation of citrate concentration produces hypocalcemia that in turn causes circulatory collapse, but the only support for this comes from the observation that calcium gluconate may be effective in preventing cardiovascular collapse. It has also been shown that the administration of sufficient sodium citrate in a normal man (7.4 mg/kg, achieving blood levels of 77 mg/dl) produces hypotension, a drop in ionized calcium without a drop in total serum calcium, and electrocardiographic evidence of hypocalcemia. This is equivalent to the transfusion of 500 ml of ACD blood every 3 or 4 minutes into a 70-kg man. Since citrate is quickly metabolized in the liver, toxic levels could be reached more easily when ACD blood is transfused into a patient with liver disease, but I can find no study of citrate intoxication in patients having liver disease.

Actually, it seems almost certain that the toxic effects of massive ACD blood transfusion are the results of a combination of effects. The first may be referable to the citrate. The second is caused by the high potassium content of stored blood, particularly when given to patients already hyperkalemic. Stored blood may have a high concentration of potassium in the plasma, as much as 30 mEq/l. When the serum potassium concentration in the recipient reaches about 8 mEq/l, signs of potassium toxicity develop. Serum potassium concentrations in this range have been reported in infants subjected to exchange transfusion with ACD blood. Finally, stored ACD blood shows a significant drop in pH, from 6.8 to 6.4, after storage for 21 days. It has been shown that massive transfusion of stored blood at this pH caused death in 13 out of 16 dogs, whereas when the pH is restored to pH 7.3 to 7.9 before transfusion, all animals survived. The pH of arterial blood in the dogs transfused with acid blood drops to 6.84 within 15 minutes. "Transfusion acidosis" may be the most important effect of massive transfusion of ACD blood and could well make the debilitated patient more subject to the toxic effects of hyperkalemia and hypocalcemia.

Ammonia intoxication

A significant increase in the concentration of ammonia occurs on storage of ACD blood, to levels as high as 1,000 µg/dl at the end of 21 days. Patients with liver disease can be affected adversely by the increased ammonia concentration, to which must be added those listed in the discussion of "citric acid intoxication" (see preceding discussion).

Circulatory overload

Some reactions are apparently caused by an overload of the circulation when blood or fluid is given either in too large a volume or at too rapid a rate. The volume to be transfused should be determined by the patient's blood volume and age. The usual advice as to rate is to begin the transfusion at a rate of 5 ml/min for the first 20 minutes, then increase it so that 1 pint is given in 1½ to 2 hours. If the patient's blood volume is reduced, it is necessary and safe to give the blood as rapidly as possible. In children, elderly patients, or persons suffering from heart disease, blood and other intravenous fluids must be given slowly, the rate not to exceed 5 ml/min. This rate should be even slower if there is reason to suspect impending cardiac decompensation. The symptoms of circulatory overload are those of cardiac failure—dyspnea, cough, and cyanosis. Immediate treatment is required.

13

Anemia due to decreased erythrocyte survival—congenital and acquired hemolytic anemias

INTRODUCTION
RED CELL SURVIVAL
  Definitions
  Interpretation of survival curves
  Interpretation of erythrocyte survival data
CLASSIFICATION OF HEMOLYTIC DISEASE
PATHOGENESIS OF HEMOLYTIC DISEASE
  Structure of the erythrocyte membrane
  Transport of sodium and potassium
  Colloid osmotic hemolysis
  Immune hemolysis
  Complement
    The convertase system
    The activator system (alternate pathway)
    Other interactions of complement
    Autoimmune hemolysis
    Isoimmune hemolysis
    Drug-related hemolysis
      Immunohemolysis of the hapten type
      Immunohemolysis of the innocent bystander type
      Immunohemolysis of the alpha-methyldopa type
      Positive antiglobulin test only
      Nonimmunologic hemolysis
    Special types of complement-dependent hemolysis
      Paroxysmal cold hemoglobinuria (PCH)
      Paroxysmal nocturnal hemoglobinuria (PNH)
    Deficiencies of complement
  Hemolysis caused by deficiency of erythrocytic enzymes
    The glutathione-dependent system
    Glucose-6-phosphate dehydrogenase (G-6-PD) deficiency
    Pyruvate kinase deficiency
    Other enzymatic deficiencies
  Hemolysis caused by hereditary abnormality of the red cell membrane
    Hereditary spherocytosis (HS)
    Hereditary elliptocytosis
    Abetalipoproteinemia
    Hereditary stomatocytosis
    Lecithin-cholesterol acyltransferase (LCAT) deficiency
    Zieve's syndrome
    Congenital dyserythropoietic anemia, HEMPAS type
    High phosphatidylcholine hemolytic anemia (HPCHA)

  Mechanical fragmentation
    From cardiac valves
    Microangiopathic hemolytic anemia
    Exertional (march) hemoglobinuria
  The spleen and liver in sequestration hemolysis
  Erythrophagocytosis
METABOLISM OF HEMOGLOBIN AND BILE PIGMENTS IN
HEMOLYTIC DISEASE
  Hemoglobinemia
  Methemalbumin
  Hemoglobinuria
  Hemosiderinuria
  Quantitative relationships
    Source of bile pigments
    Fluctuations in pigment excretion
    Pigment excretion related to total hemoglobin
    "Corrected" fecal urobilinogen excretion
    Hemolytic index
    Fecal urobilinogen
      Normal values
      Limitations
    Urinary urobilinogen
      Collection of urine specimens
      Determination by dilution of a random sample
      Twenty-four—hour urine specimen
      Two-hour urine specimen
    Specificity of Ehrlich's aldehyde reaction
    Bilirubin in serum
      Regulation of bilirubin concentration in serum
      Hyperbilirubinemia and jaundice
      Partition of bilirubin
LABORATORY DIAGNOSIS OF HEMOLYTIC DISEASE
  Clinical-pathologic approach to the patient
  Importance of the peripheral blood smear
  Erythrocyte count and hemoglobin concentration
  Leukocyte count
  Platelet count
  Reticulocyte count
  Erythrocyte indices
  Erythrocyte morphology
    Spherocytosis
    Polychromatophilia

Distorted or disrupted erythrocytes
Erythrophagocytes
Drepanocytes (sickle cells)
Normoblasts
Codocytes (target cells)
Elliptocytes
Stomatocytes
Acanthocytes
Giant platelets
Heinz bodies
Siderocytes
Parasites
Osmotic fragility
Significance of measurements
Interpretation of results
After incubation
Investigation of metabolic abnormalities
Introduction
Autohemolysis
Heinz body formation
Glutathione stability test
Ascorbate test
Tests for unstable hemoglobins
Fluorescence test for G-6-PD deficiency
Fluorescence test for pyruvate kinase deficiency
Fluorescence test for glutathione reductase deficiency
Fluorescence test for triosephosphate isomerase deficiency
Orthocresol red test for pyruvate kinase deficiency
Methemoglobin reduction test for G-6-PD deficiency
Summary
Serologic investigations
Direct antiglobulin (Coombs') test
Principle of the test
The nature of antiglobulin serum
Value and limitations
Results in hemolytic anemia
Indirect antiglobulin test
γ-Globulin neutralization test
Agglutination of enzyme-treated erythrocytes
Agglutination in albumin and serum-albumin media
The use of low–ionic strength suspending media
Complete (saline) agglutinating antibodies
Hemolytic antibodies
Serologic studies in isoimmune hemolytic disease
CHARACTERISTICS OF THE MAJOR HEMOLYTIC ANEMIAS
Hereditary spherocytosis
Etiology and pathogenesis
Clinical aspects
Laboratory findings
Treatment
Elliptocytic hemolytic anemia
Etiology and pathogenesis
Clinical aspects
Laboratory findings
Treatment
Abetalipoproteinemia
Etiology and pathogenesis
Clinical aspects
Laboratory findings
Treatment
Paroxysmal nocturnal hemoglobinuria (PNH)
Etiology and pathogenesis
Clinical aspects
Laboratory findings
Treatment

G-6-PD deficiency
Etiology and pathogenesis
Clinical aspects
Laboratory findings
Treatment
Other enzymatic defects
Autoimmune hemolytic anemia (AIHA)
Etiology and pathogenesis
Warm antibody type
Cold antibody type
Drug-induced type
Treatment
Paroxysmal cold hemoglobinuria (PCH)
Etiology and pathogenesis
Clinical aspects
Laboratory findings
Treatment
Unstable hemoglobin hemolytic disease
Isoimmune hemolytic disease
Etiology and pathogenesis
Clinical aspects
Laboratory findings
Prevention and treatment

INTRODUCTION

One of the biologic differences between humans and lower species is that in humans there evolved complex systems for regulating the internal environment, thereby enabling them to achieve a high degree of independence from the external environment. One major improvement over lower forms was the development of the modern kidney to regulate the pH and electrolyte balance of the internal environment. Another was the improvement of the oxygen-carrying and exchanging capacity of the blood by enclosing the respiratory pigment, hemoglobin, inside a highly specialized membrane to form the human red blood cell.

Given these undeniably wonderful evolutionary improvements, it must be noted that human beings sometimes pay a dear price for them. As a highly developed species, we have improved our chances for survival, but we also have devised exquisitely efficient ways of destroying ourselves and others. Because of a highly developed and efficiently oxygenated brain, humans are capable of rational thought, but they also are capable of unfathomable irrationality. The red blood cell owes its almost miraculous function to a highly complex membrane, enzymatic systems to maintain the integrity of the membrane, and the normal hemoglobin within the cell. When all three are structurally and functionally normal, the red blood cell assumes the most efficient surface-to-volume ratio, the biconcave disk, is deformable without being damaged, and has a life span of about 120 days, during which time it makes an estimated half million circuits of the bloodstream. However, if the membrane has congenital structural abnormalities, or if its integrity is jeopardized by deficient enzymatic systems, external trauma, immunologic damage, or even because the cell contains an abnormal hemoglobin, then its life span is much shorter than 120 days. The short life span results in an increased rate of red blood cell destruction, which is the basic definition of hemolytic disease.

Should the life span of erythrocytes be decreased, progressive anemia would result unless the prehemolytic rate of erythropoiesis was simultaneously increased. Fortunately, increased erythropoiesis usually does occur in such cases. Various degrees of compensation are possible, the response being roughly proportional to the need. If the increased need is slight, the mitotic activity of polychromatophilic normoblasts may be sufficient. If severe, increased mitosis of pronormoblasts and basophilic normoblasts is necessary. This multiplication of young forms produces a many-fold increase in the number of mature forms. The result is an increase in total active erythropoietic tissue and replacement of fatty marrow by active marrow as well as an increase in the number of reticulocytes. Reticulocytosis is one of the important indications of increased erythropoiesis and, indirectly, of diminished erythrocyte survival.

Likewise, erythroid hyperplasia of the bone marrow is indirect evidence that an increased erythropoietic need exists. In the adult, sites that usually show only fatty marrow may be found to contain cellular marrow. In infants and children, who normally have little fatty marrow, marked hyperplasia of the marrow must be accommodated by an actual increase in size of the marrow cavities. This can often be seen in roentgenograms of the skull and long bones.

As a result of these compensatory changes, the difference between the rate of erythrocyte destruction and erythrocyte production is gradually narrowed until an equilibrium is reached and the peripheral erythrocyte count remains constant. This can occur at any level of peripheral blood values, depending on the severity of the need and the efficiency of medullary compensation. It has been calculated that increased erythropoiesis can achieve at most a sixfold increase in erythrocyte production, so that if erythrocyte survival is less than one sixth of normal, other mechanisms must come into play if an equilibrium is to be reached.

The terms applicable to the results of decreased erythrocyte survival must be carefully defined. *Hemolytic disease* is present whenever erythrocyte survival is less than normal. Hemolytic disease may be *compensated* if compensatory hyperplasia of the marrow and increased erythrocyte production are sufficient to balance the increased rate of erythrocyte destruction. In some cases the equilibrium is reestablished at almost normal blood values, and the hemolytic disease is not accompanied by anemia. In more severe cases an equilibrium is achieved at an anemic level and is called *compensated hemolytic anemia*. If the anemia is progressive, then it may be called *decompensated hemolytic anemia*. Decompensation is the result of one or both of two situations: the bone marrow reacts maximally, but erythrocyte survival is so short that complete compensation is not possible, or the marrow is unable to compensate to the required degree. In the latter case the term "dyserythropoietic hemolytic anemia" has been used. Finally, increased erythrocyte destruction is accompanied by an increased amount of liberated bilirubin. If this is greater than can be cleared from the bloodstream, or if there is subnormal bilirubin clearance because of liver dysfunction, *hemolytic jaundice* occurs. The amount of bilirubin liberated is in proportion to the amount of hemoglobin broken down and only indirectly related to the degree of abnormal erythrocyte survival.

RED CELL SURVIVAL

Under *normal* conditions erythrocyte destruction is limited to those cells which have reached old age. *Average survival time* in this case is equal to *life span*. In hemolytic disease, however, erythrocyte destruction is not limited to those cells which have become senile and are the most abnormal. There is also a random destruction of cells of all ages. Under these circumstances the average survival time is not the same as the potential life span.

Definitions

Erythrocyte survival data can be expressed in terms of *end point of elimination (full life span), half-life,* and *mean cell life*. End point of elimination measures the time required for a given group of erythrocytes to be eliminated from the circulation. Half-life is the time at which 50% of a given number of erythrocytes have been destroyed. Mean cell life is the *average* survival time. It should be obvious that erythrocyte survival measurements are meaningless if the patient is losing erythrocytes by bleeding.

There are two practical methods for measuring erythrocyte life span. The first is *random labeling* with ^{51}Cr or labeled diisopropyl fluorophosphate (DFP). The second is *cohort labeling* with glycine ^{14}C, glycine ^{3}H, glycine ^{15}N, or ^{59}Fe. In this method the erythrocytes are labeled as they are produced, and the total life span can be determined by measuring radioactivity for a sufficiently long period. Because cohort labeling requires expensive isotopes and a long period of observation, it is not the method of choice. Of the two random labeling technics, the ^{51}Cr method is the one most widely used. Cline and Berlin (1963), however, favor the use of labeled DFP, claiming better correlation with glycine ^{14}C measurements. The review by Berlin and Berk (1975) presents a complete discussion of red cell life span and of the methods used to measure it.

Interpretation of survival curves

The type of destruction taking place may be inferred from the shape of the survival curves obtained when percent survival is plotted against time. In general, when cell survival is dependent only on the senescence of the erythrocytes, the relationship is linear. This is seen in normal persons but seldom in those with hemolytic disease. The curve obtained in the latter is usually a modified exponential one. Since a pure exponential curve would express the random destruction of erythrocytes of all ages, it is thought that the curves obtained in hemolytic disease express a combination of random destruction of cells of all ages plus destruction of senile erythrocytes. The element of random destruction is dominant when erythrocyte survival time is shortened by the action of extracorpuscular (extrinsic) mechanisms. This is thought to be the case in idiopathic acquired hemolytic anemias, in hemolytic anemias associated with lymphoma and other malignancies, and in paroxysmal nocturnal hemoglobinuria.

Interpretation of erythrocyte survival data

Erythrocyte survival time in various hemolytic diseases is given in Table 13-1. The normal erythrocyte half-life is 28

Table 13-1. Erythrocyte survival in various hemolytic diseases, determined by ^{51}Cr method

Disease	Survival, days (half-life, T½)	Reference
Normal	28 to 38	Various authors
Sickle cell disease*	1 to 19	Weinstein et al, 1954
	3 to 11	Sprague and Peterson, 1958
Sickle cell trait*	27 to 38	Weinstein et al, 1954
Hb C disease*	19	Weinstein et al, 1954
Hb C trait*	28 to 32	Weinstein et al, 1954
Thalassemia (major)*	1 to 22	Erlandson et al, 1958; Vullo and Tunioli, 1958
Hereditary spherocytosis*	3 to 19	Dacie, 1960; Baird et al, 1971
Pyruvate kinase deficiency	1 to 21	Tanaka and Paglia, 1971
Acquired autoimmune hemolytic anemia	2 to 25	Weinstein and LeRoy, 1953; Constantoulakis et al, 1963
Megaloblastic anemia of pregnancy*	17 to 25	Hollingsworth and Adams, 1955

*Patient's erythrocytes into normal recipients.

to 38 days by the ^{51}Cr method, and a half-life of less than 26 days is considered abnormal; the shorter the measured half-life, the more severe the hemolytic disease.

Erythrocyte survival data may be summarized as follows. All hemolytic anemias are characterized by moderate to severe reduction in erythrocyte survival. Hemoglobinopathies that have heterozygous traits usually show normal survival, but moderately decreased survivals occasionally have been reported. One of three experimental conditions may be used: (1) survival of the patient's erythrocytes in the patient's own blood, (2) survival of normal erythrocytes in the patient's blood, and (3) survival of the patient's erythrocytes in normal blood.

In the first instance decreased survival may be a result of a defect either of the erythrocytes or in the plasma. This method does not allow a distinction to be made, but it may be useful in determining if shortened survival exists. It is also applicable in patients having a double defect. In the second type of experiment the decreased survival of normal erythrocytes in the patient's blood indicates that the hemolytic mechanism is present in the patient's plasma. In the third type, decreased survival indicates an inherent abnormality of the patient's erythrocytes.

CLASSIFICATION OF HEMOLYTIC DISEASE

All hemolytic phenomena involve an alteration of the red blood cell membrane. All that can be accomplished by further classification is to group these alterations according to etiology. Two groups are readily distinguished, one listing those mechanisms which damage an otherwise normal membrane, i.e., *extrinsic*, or *extracorpuscular*, effects, and those which can be attributed to some intrinsic abnormality of the cell membrane or the interior of the cell, i.e., *intrin-*

sic, or *corpuscular*, defects. This classic approach to the classification of hemolytic disease is still valid and useful, even though not all instances of hemolytic disease fall neatly into one or the other category; there are some syndromes that are caused by extracorpuscular agents acting on an abnormal or particularly susceptible membrane.

The etiologic classification presented in Table 13-2 is more meaningful when there is understanding of the various pathogenetic mechanisms discussed in the section that follows.

PATHOGENESIS OF HEMOLYTIC DISEASE
Structure of the erythrocyte membrane

At one time the erythrocyte membrane was considered to be structureless and inert, serving only to enclose and preserve the respiratory pigment, hemoglobin. The pioneering work of Ponder (1948) established the basic concepts later elaborated to give us the modern concept of structure. Ponder proposed that the erythrocyte surface consists of a highly oriented hemoglobin-lipoprotein ultrastructure (Fig. 13-1), the outer surface being predominantly lipoprotein. Moving away from the surface into the interior, the lipoprotein concentration decreases, the hemoglobin concentration increases, and there is gradual loss of orientation of the hemoglobin molecules.

Subsequently, investigations using modern technics of electrophoresis, chemical analysis, immunologic reactions, and electron microscopy have produced a great amount of data on the biochemical composition of the membrane. From these data, plus the ultrastructural appearance of the membrane by electron microscopy, several models of the structure of the membrane have been proposed. Before describing these new findings and the proposed models, it must be noted that there are unavoidable technical limitations of both the biochemical and electron microscopic studies. Because the membrane is such a small component of the red blood cell, the major component being hemoglobin, biochemical analyses of the membrane are done on hemoglobin-free "ghosts." However, the composition of a red cell ghost is related to the method used to prepare it (Ponder, 1948; Rega et al, 1967), and there is no way to be certain that some membrane protein or other constituents are not lost along with the hemoglobin. Likewise, because of the high electron density of hemoglobin, conventional electron microscopy is carried out on hemoglobin-free ghosts, and in the course of osmium fixation a great deal of membrane protein is lost (McMillen and Luftig, 1973). In spite of these technical limitations a great deal of information is now available on the chemical composition, and several models of the structure of the membrane have been proposed. Detailed reviews are given by Weed (1975), Eaton et al (1979), Lorand et al (1979), Lux (1979), Marchesi (1979), and Palek and Liu (1979).

A working model of the red cell membrane was proposed by Singer and Nicolson (1972) and has been modified only in minor details. The model assumes several levels of organization. The external layer contains glycoproteins that come to the surface from deeper layers and are interspersed between lipid molecules. A major glycoprotein has been

Table 13-2. Etiologic classification of hemolytic disease

I. Caused by intrinsic (corpuscular) defects
  A. Defect of erythrocyte membrane
    1. Hereditary spherocytosis (HS)
    2. Elliptocytosis
    3. Abetalipoproteinemia
    4. Stomatocytosis
      a. Hereditary
      b. Rh_{null} syndrome
    5. Paroxysmal nocturnal hemoglobinuria (PNH)
    6. Lecithin-cholesterol acyltransferase (LCAT) deficiency
    7. Zieve's syndrome
    8. Hereditary erythroid multinuclearity, congenital dyserythropoietic anemia, type II (HEMPAS)
    9. High phosphatidylcholine hemolytic anemia (HPCHA)
    10. Hereditary pyropoikilocytosis
  B. Defect of hemoglobin or heme synthesis
    1. Hemoglobinopathies (Chapter 14)
    2. Congenital erythropoietic porphyria (Chapter 10)
  C. Defect of intracellular enzyme (hereditary nonspherocytic hemolytic anemia)
    1. G-6-PD deficiency
    2. Pyruvate kinase deficiency
    3. Others (see p. 567)
II. Caused by extrinsic (extracorpuscular) agents
  A. Acquired autoimmune hemolytic anemia
    1. Idiopathic (primary)
    2. Symptomatic (secondary), associated with
      a. Disseminated lupus erythematosus
      b. Acute and chronic leukemias
      c. Lymphomas
      d. Carcinoma and sarcoma
      e. Multiple myeloma
      f. Gaucher's disease
      g. Ovarian dermoids and teratomas
      h. Myeloproliferative syndromes
      i. Periarteritis nodosa
      j. Thrombocytopenic purpura and hemolytic anemia (Evans' syndrome)
      k. Thrombocytopenic purpura and Landry-Guillain-Barré syndrome
      l. Thrombotic thrombocytopenic purpura
      m. Uremia
      n. Viral infections
      o. Waldenström's macroglobulinemia
      p. Ulcerative colitis
    3. Drug induced, immunologic
  B. Acquired isoimmune hemolytic anemia
    1. Rh incompatibility
    2. A-B-O blood group incompatibility
    3. Other blood group incompatibility
  C. Paroxysmal cold hemoglobinuria (PCH)
  D. Drugs and chemicals in susceptible individuals, nonimmunologic, related to enzymatic deficiency or unstable hemoglobin
    1. Antimalarials
      a. Primaquine
      b. Pamaquine
      c. Pentaquine
      d. Plasmoquine
      e. Quinocide
    2. Sulfonamides
      a. Sulfanilamide
      b. Sulfapyridine
      c. Sulfisoxazole
      d. Salicylazosulfapyridine
      e. Sulfamethoxypyridazine
      f. Sulfacetamide
    3. Salicylates and analgesics
      a. Aspirin

      b. Acetanilid
      c. Acetophenetidin
      d. Antipyrine
      e. Aminopyrine
      f. Paraaminosalicylic acid
    4. Other drugs
      a. Nitrofurantoin
      b. Nitrofurazone
      c. Furazolidone
      d. Furaltadone
      e. Sulfoxone
      f. Probenecid
      g. Acetylphenylhydrazine
      h. Naphthalene
      i. Methylene blue
      j. Vitamin K analogues
      k. Chloramphenicol
      l. Thiazosulfone
      m. Diaminodiphenylsulfone
      n. Trinitrotoluene
      o. Quinidine
      p. Quinine
      q. Copper sulfate
      r. Nalidixic acid
      s. Dimercaprol
      t. Mestranal
    5. Special agent
      a. Fava bean
  E. Drugs and chemicals, dose related, nonimmunologic
    1. Benzene
    2. Nitrobenzene
    3. Dinitrobenzene
    4. Lead salts
    5. Colloidal silver
    6. Aniline
    7. Phenacetin
    8. Acetanilid
    9. Phenylhydrazine
    10. Methyl chloride
    11. Vitamin K analogues
    12. Arsine
    13. Sodium chlorate
  F. Caused by infectious agents
    1. *Plasmodium* organisms
    2. *Bartonella bacilliformis*
    3. *Clostridium perfringens*
    4. *Streptococcus hemolyticus*
    5. *Staphylococcus aureus*
    6. *Treponema pallidum*
    7. Viruses
  G. Caused by mechanical injury
    1. March hemoglobinuria
    2. Aortic stenosis
    3. Cardiac valve prosthesis
    4. Disseminated intravascular coagulation (DIC)
    5. Microangiopathic anemias
  H. Caused by physical agents
    1. Burns
    2. Ultraviolet radiation
  I. Caused by vegetable or animal agents
    1. Castor bean
    2. Snake venoms
    3. Spider bite (necrotic arachnidism)
  J. Metabolic disorders
    1. Hypophosphatemia
    2. Malignant hypertension
    3. Wilson's disease
    4. Liver disease
    5. Vitamin E deficiency

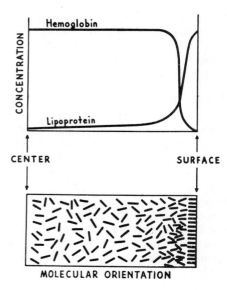

Fig. 13-1. Diagrammatic representation of surface structure of mammalian erythrocyte. (After Ponder, 1948.)

named glycophorin A and is a sialoglycopeptide. Glycophorin A and other sialoglycopeptides contain A-B-O, H, and Lewis antigens, and this outer layer is operationally designated the receptor domain. Beneath the glycoproteins there is a lipid bilayer containing dispersed globular proteins. According to the Singer-Nicolson model the lipid and protein zone is pictured as a fluid mosaic, i.e., various proteins are free to arrange themselves in a changing mosaic pattern because of the fluidity of the lipid bilayer. The other structure in the membrane is a protein that extends from the lipid bilayer into the interior of the cell, has adenosinetriphosphatase (ATPase) activity, and has been named *spectrin*. It is assumed that spectrin has contractile properties and that it is important in regulating the shape of the red blood cell. Erythrocyte deformability may be modulated by the rate of phosphorylation-dephosphorylation of spectrin (Smith and Moore, 1980).

Weed (1975) points out that the Singer-Nicolson fluid mosaic model probably is not sufficiently rigid to account for some of the conformational changes observed when red blood cells are subjected to various types of stress. The red blood cell is easily deformable by forces perpendicular to the surface but is resistant to stretching within the plane. Weed proposes that these properties are compatible with the concept that globular proteins are not moving at random within the lipid bilayer but instead are cross linked at the inner surface of the membrane. Marchesi (1979) suggests that the major structural protein, spectrin, interacts with other transmembrane proteins to form a relatively fixed support for the lipid bilayer. According to this concept the model of the membrane is assumed to be a fixed rather than a fluid matrix.

The lipids of the membrane are of three types: nonesterified cholesterol, phospholipids, and glycolipids. The cholesterol in the membrane of a mature erythrocyte is in equilibrium with plasma cholesterol. The greater portion of membrane lipids is composed of phospholipids: phosphatidyl-choline, phosphatidylethanolamine, sphingomyelin, phosphatidylserine, and traces of other phospholipids. The liberation of these thrombogenic phospholipids into the blood when there is massive hemolysis can give rise to the acute disseminated intravascular coagulation syndrome (DIC, Chapter 17). The glycolipid fraction is relatively small.

The proteins of the membrane have been separated by sodium dodecyl sulfate (SDS) gel electrophoresis into at least eight bands (Marschesi, 1979). They can be grouped into functional sets. Those exposed on the surface, such as glycophorin A, have contact or receptor functions, whereas those which penetrate to the inner surface of the membrane, such as spectrin, serve to stabilize the structure of the membrane. In addition to carrying some red blood cell antigens, glycophorin is rich in sialic acid, and this accounts for the negative charge on the red cell. It is also logical to assume that the glycoproteins on the surface of the red cell are responsible, wholly or in part, for the fact that macrophages do not ingest it unless the erythrocyte is at the end of its life span or the surface is abnormal.

Transport of sodium and potassium

The membrane is selectively semipermeable, allowing water and anions such as HCO_3^- and Cl^- to enter the cell and excluding *passive* passage of the cations Na^+ and K^+. This selective permeability is a result of the presence of pores between adjoining sets of plaque and phospholipid. These pores have a predominance of positive surface charges that gives them the unidirectional valve action. Transport of cations across the membrane requires energy, and for sodium and potassium the mechanism has been likened to a pump (Fig. 13-2). The energy is derived from high-energy phosphate (adenosinetriphosphate [ATP]) supplied by glycolysis. The pump mechanism is regulated by an enzymatic system (ATPase) in the cell membrane. Thus the structure and composition of the erythrocyte membrane allow both passive and active transport of small molecules, and active transport is dependent on the glycolytic system. The intact membrane is impermeable to large molecules such as hemoglobin.

Ionic equilibrium in the erythrocyte requires an exchange of intracellular Na for extracellular K. Although there is some exchange by simple diffusion, the major exchange is dependent on active transport. According to Hoffman (1966) there are two major cation pumps: pump I is ATP dependent and is inhibited by cardiac glycosides; pump II also requires energy but is not ATP dependent and is not inhibited by cardiac glycosides. Pump I accounts for about 70% of active cation transport.

Colloid osmotic hemolysis

Colloid osmotic hemolysis is the process whereby the erythrocyte undergoes hemolysis as the result of altered membrane permeability, failure of active cation transport, or both. To survive normally, the erythrocyte depends on an intact membrane functioning in conjunction with active cation transport. When these fail, water and ion equilibria are disturbed, the cell swells as the result of accumulating water and ions, and large molecules such as hemoglobin are lost through large defects in the continuity of the membrane.

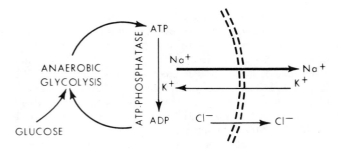

Fig. 13-2. Major cation pump system in the erythrocyte—pump I of Hoffman (1966). Three Na$^+$ cations are exchanged for two K$^+$ cations, and one Cl$^-$ anion leaves the cell by passive diffusion (the chloride shift).

Maintenance of the erythrocyte's normal shape is dependent in part on the integrity of the spectrin skeleton, on the composition of the lipid bilayer, and on control of its internal ionic milieu. The interior of the cell normally contains a preponderance of anions (hemoglobin, glycolytic intermediates, and glutathione) that are not permeable across an intact membrane. The membrane is normally permeable to water and to diffusion of Na$^+$ from a high extracellular to a low intracellular concentration. Without some protective mechanisms the imbibition of water would produce swelling and hemolysis. Normally this does not happen because the active cation transport pumps regulate the intracellular concentration of Na$^+$ and K$^+$, maintaining an intracellular-extracellular ratio of 1:12 for Na$^+$ and 25:1 for K$^+$. When this condition exists, the erythrocyte maintains its normal size and shape. In one case of congenital hemolytic anemia Wiley and Gill (1976) found increased influx of calcium ions.

Mild alterations in permeability result in slow influx of water and cations. The erythrocyte gradually becomes spheroidal, and the stretching of the surface membrane allows slow outward leakage of hemoglobin. This slow type of hemolysis is sometimes called *small hole* hemolysis to indicate a slow osmotic swelling and delayed hemolysis. In contrast, hemolysis mediated by complement is rapid and is not preceded by spheroidal transformation. The damage to the membrane is extensive, and hemolysis is acute, with rapid efflux of hemoglobin through large membrane defects. This type is appropriately called *large hole* hemolysis.

The energy for active transport of cations is derived from the metabolism of glucose. ATP is generated chiefly through anaerobic glycolysis. The enzymatic ATPase system is situated in the cell membrane. Even though ATP supplies the energy for the cation pumps, any process that accelerates cation exchange accelerates ATP use and glycolysis. Conversely, decreased glycolysis, as when the aging cell loses glycolytic enzymes, results in diminished formation of ATP, loss of cation and water homeostasis, and hemolysis.

Traditionally the major cation is thought to be sodium, but calcium also plays a part in the integrity of the red cell membrane. Associated with the ATPase activity of spectrin, there is an enzymatic control over the intracellular content of calcium ions. A rise in intracellular Ca^{++} is detrimental to

red cells, so the normal Ca^{++} concentration (5 to 10 μM/l RBC) must be maintained by a mechanism other than the sodium pump. The hypothetical calcium pump is based on either spectrin ATPase or, as suggested by Lorand et al (1979), by the activation of a special transamidase.

Immune hemolysis

Hemolysis (cytolysis of erythrocytes) may be caused by a variety of physical, chemical, or immunologic agents. In vivo this leads to diminished erythrocyte survival. Some of the agents active in vitro do not have physiologic counterparts, whereas others reflect damage of the erythrocyte membrane by other agents; e.g., decreased resistance to osmotic hemolysis is found in many situations where the membrane is altered. Immune hemolysis, on the other hand, represents a direct alteration of the membrane by immune complexes in the presence of complement. There is a third type of hemolysis, called nonimmune, that is dependent on complement but not on antigen-antibody complex.

In its simplest form immune hemolysis is dependent on the interaction of antigen receptors on the erythrocytic membrane with specific antibody in the presence of complement. Some hemolytic anemias of the autoimmune type do not have "specific" antierythrocytic antigen-antibody binding; the antigen-antibody complex may be entirely nonspecific with regard to the erythrocyte antigens but is bound to the surface of the erythrocyte and, with complement, produces hemolysis. The interaction of antigen, antibody, and complement alters the structure of the membrane. Defects or discontinuities in the membrane then are formed; as seen in electron photomicrographs, they may be as large as 80 to 100 Å (8 to 10 nm). As a result, the permeability of the membrane is altered, and as one of many possible consequences, hemoglobin escapes from the cell.

Complement

Complement is not a single substance but a complex of at least 11 interacting components. In 1896 Bordet found that serum contains a substance necessary for the lysis of erythrocytes and bacteria. The substance was not an antibody, since it was not increased by immunization. It was then found that lysis was dependent on two different substances, one heat stable (representing antibody) and the other heat labile. The latter was called *complement* because it complements the action of antibody. Subsequently complement was found to be a complex of components designated by the letter C' followed by successive numbers and symbols (Table 13-3). In recent publications the prime signs are omitted.

Complement components are all proteins and, with the exception of C1, are synthesized in macrophages (Ruddy et al, 1972). C1 is synthesized or assembled from subunits in the intestinal wall. Complement develops early in fetal tissues (Adinolfi, 1977).

Individual components and specific combinations of components interact in various immune reactions. C1a has an affinity for antigen-antibody complexes and aggregates of gamma globulin. The complex C4b,2a is involved in erythrophagocytosis. Fragments C3a and C5a are involved in the inflammatory reaction as anaphylatoxins. The complex C5,6,7 is involved in chemotaxis of leukocytes. The complex C8,9 mounts the final attack on the cell membrane.

The individual components of complement are found in blood in an inactive form. They are activated rapidly and in fixed sequence (Müller-Eberhard, 1975). Also, although the initial reactions involve single interactions, each subsequent product is capable of affecting many substrate molecules, so that the reaction sequence is progressively amplified. In the activated form the system is biologically active.

There are two mechanisms for the activation of the complement system: (1) the *convertase system,* and (2) the *activator system.* Of the two, the convertase system is the more important.

The convertase system

The convertase system of complement activation is involved in hemolysis and depends on esterase and convertase enzymatic reactions (Fig. 13-3).

In immune hemolysis the chain of events is set in motion by the binding of C1 to the antibody bound to the specific antigen on the cell membrane. C1 is a complex molecule composed of three subunits: C1q, C1r, and C1s. When these subunits complex with calcium ions and attach to the fixed immunoglobulin molecule through the C1q fragment, forming activated C1 (C1a), the C1s portion of the complex has esterase activity. Fixation of C1 requires that two IgG molecules or one IgM molecule has combined with the membrane antigen. Only IgG1, IgG2, IgG3, and IgM molecules are capable of fixing and activating complement. IgG4 is inactive in this complement reaction (Natvig and Kunkel, 1973).

C1s (esterase) cleaves C4 into fragment C4a and C4b, and C2 into C2a and C2b. The fragments C4a and C2b are small and float away free. Fragment C4b, however, binds to the cell membrane, while C2a attaches to C4b. This combination, requiring magnesium ions, produces the complex C4,2. This new complex has convertase activity, manifested by splitting C3 into a large C3b fragment and a small C3a fragment. C3a remains in the plasma and is an anaphylatoxin. C3b has a high affinity for all blood cell surfaces, and membrane-bound C3b is responsible for immune adherence of blood cells (Henson, 1969). C3b also attaches to the C4,2 complex to form complex C4,2,3, which cleaves C5 into C5a and C5b. C5b is bound to the cell membrane, and C6 and C7 then bind sequentially to it. The C5a fragment is, like C3a, an anaphylatoxin. The complex C5b,6,7 stimulates chemotaxis in leukocytes and is responsible for the first modification of the cell membrane, making it susceptible to attack by C8 and C9. Component C8 causes lysis, accelerated by C9.

Stereochemically, it must be assumed that all these reactions occur within a small area of the membrane. Müller-Eberhard (1975) proposes a three-site model of complement transfer to the target cell membrane. Site I is the location for the binding of C1 to antibody molecules. At site II the complex C4,2 is bound and then converted to C4,2,3. This complex then initiates the assembly of C5b,6,7,8,9 complex at site III, where the membrane lesion is produced. A fourth site is postulated at which fragment C3b binds independently to the cell membrane. In this configuration C3b is responsible for immune adherence reactions and for hemolysis of PNH erythrocytes.

Table 13-3. Properties of the components of complement*

Property	C1q	C1r	C1s	C2	C3	C4	C5	C6	C7	C8	C9
Synonym	11S component		C1 esterase		β1c globulin	β1e globulin	β1f globulin				
Sedimentation constant (S)	11.1	7.5	4.5	4.5	9.5	10.0	8.7	5.5	6.0	8.0	4.5
Electrophoretic mobility	γ2	β1	α	β1	β2	β1	β1	β2	β2	γ1	α
Molecular weight	400,000	190,000	85,000	115,000	180,000	206,000	180,000	128,000	121,000	154,000	80,000
Serum concentration (μg/ml)	180	100	80	25	1,500	450	75	60	60	80	150
Thermolability (56° C, 30 min)	+	+	+	+	0	0	+	0	0	+	+

*From Bruninga, 1971; Müller-Eberhard, 1975; Müller-Eberhard, 1976.

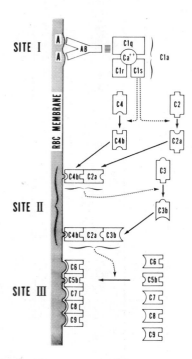

Fig. 13-3. Schematic representation of the sequence of activation of complement components and the relation of these to the red cell membrane. Sites I to III are probably in close proximity and not as shown in the figure. The arrangement of the complex C5b to C9 is not known, but is certainly not linear. (Modified from Bruninga, 1971; Müller-Eberhard, 1975.)

Antibodies that fix complement induce colloid osmotic hemolysis of the large hole type. Membrane permeability is altered by the large discontinuities (80 to 100 Å, 8 to 10 nm) in the membrane. Hemolysis is usually rapid, since the large pores in the membrane allow leakage of hemoglobin without swelling and spherocytosis. Some abnormal erythrocytes seem to be particularly susceptible to this type of damage; e.g., the erythrocytes in paroxysmal nocturnal hemoglobinuria (PNH, p. 596) are very susceptible to acid hemolysis. In this abnormality the membrane of the erythrocyte has a great avidity for C3b, and it is postulated that by binding many times the usual number of C3b fragments, the membrane develops an unusually large number of holes at an acid pH. The binding of C3b fragments to the membrane is in part caused by an amplified catalytic reaction of C4,2,3, one unit being able to catalyze the binding of multiple C3b fragments. Subpopulations having different degrees of avidity for C3b have been identified by various investigators (Packman et al, 1979). Treatment of PNH erythrocytes with neuraminidase enhances their susceptibility to hemolysis (Hause et al, 1978), and it has been suggested that the resulting increase in acid hemolysis and normalization of the sucrose test are caused by the loss of membrane sialic acid. Platelets and granulocytes from patients with PNH are also very susceptible to acid hemolysis, suggesting that the same type of membrane defect affects all three types of blood cells. Erythroid precursors also show increased sensitivity to complement-mediated hemolysis (Tumen et al, 1980).

After C3 fragments attach to the erythrocyte membrane, the PNH cells can be lysed by normal human serum. This is another type of complement-mediated hemolysis, since the binding of specific antibody to the surface antigen is not a prerequisite.

A third type of complement-mediated hemolysis requires neither a specific antigen-antibody combination at the surface nor an abnormal avidity of the cell membrane for C3. Antigen-antibody complexes are formed, but these are not related to the surface antigens of the erythrocyte. Pirofsky et al (1962) point out that the erythrocyte can simply offer a favorable surface environment for the interaction of nonspecific (with regard to erythrocyte antigens) antigen-antibody interaction. In other words, the erythrocyte acts as an involved but *innocent bystander*. They also point out that in this situation the antibody may appear to be directed toward the erythrocyte, i.e., an autoantibody, but that in fact the surface of the erythrocyte provides only the vehicle for the interaction. An example is the hemolytic anemia of hypersensitivity to penicillin, where the penicillin is bound to the erythrocyte surface and then reacts with penicillin antibody. The positive antiglobulin reaction that results is, in this sense, unrelated to any original erythrocyte antigen.

Immune complexes need not interact at the cell surface to induce immune hemolysis. Indeed, it is probable that the type of damage to various tissues produced by the properties of immune complexes is quantitatively more important than the specific attack by the antibody is to intrinsic cell antigens. The antibody, by itself, is not damaging until it combines with the antigen; the immune complex, however, is cytotoxic. It interacts with complement, activating C1 to the esterase, so that a complement-mediated membrane reaction takes place which is similar to that found when a specific antigen-antibody interaction occurs on the cell surface. Antigen-antibody complexes can produce a variety of other biologic effects such as stimulation of the fibrinolysis system, degranulation of mast cells, attachment to platelets and leukocytes, contraction of smooth muscle, increase in vascular permeability, and the production of fibrinoid degeneration in various tissues (Müller-Eberhard, 1976). Attachment of immune complexes to thrombocytes causes aggregation and thrombocytopenia, e.g., the thrombocytopenia secondary to quinine and quinidine. Attachment to the surface of the erythrocyte causes hemolytic anemia, e.g., the hemolytic anemia secondary to the drug stibophen and other drugs as well. In both instances the cellular damage is to innocent bystander cells to which neither the antigen nor the antibody is related. Regarding hemolytic anemia, the mechanism is immune but not autoimmune.

The activator system (alternate pathway)

The complement system can be activated by mechanisms other than esterase and convertase reactions (Götze and Müller-Eberhard, 1976). The chief alternate pathways involve activation by immunoglobulins, endotoxins, and cobra venom (Müller-Eberhard, 1976). There is also evidence that C5 can be activated by constituents of neutrophil granulocytes (Ward and Hill, 1970).

Some of the alternate pathways involve *properdin* (Pensky et al, 1968), a plasma glycoprotein described over 20 years ago as a protein in blood that has bactericidal properties in the presence of complement (Pillemer, 1958). Properdin activates a serum protein called *C3 proactivator* to an active enzyme that hydrolyzes C3 into C3a and C3b. As noted earlier, C3b can attach to the cell membrane independent of antigen-antibody interaction. However, attached C3b can combine with C5 and other sequential components.

Other interactions of complement

Activation of the complement system has other important biologic activities. Activation of the classic pathway by urate crystals induces the acute inflammatory reaction of gout (Giclas et al, 1979). Fragments C3a and C5a have phlogogenic (related to inflammation) activity and are called *anaphylatoxins*. They cause release of histamine from mast cells, stimulate chemotaxis of neutrophils, and cause contraction of smooth muscle. It has been shown that mast cells have specific membrane receptors for C3a (Laan et al, 1974) and that the uptake of radiolabeled C3a by mast cells correlates well with the amount of histamine released (Müller-Eberhard, 1975). Both C3a and C5a stimulate chemotaxis of neutrophils by activating a proesterase in the cell (Becker, 1972). The effect on smooth muscle is probably independent of histamine (Müller-Eberhard, 1975).

The interrelation between the complement, blood coagulation, and plasma kinin systems is shown in Fig. 13-4 and has been reviewed by Zimmerman (1976). Thrombin-induced platelet aggregation is enhanced by complement, and Polley and Nachman (1978) propose that the attachment of thrombin to the thrombin receptor on the platelet membrane generates a C3 convertase, which is different from the convertases of the classic or alternate pathways. A discussion of the coagulation and fibrinolytic systems is presented in Chapter 17.

Autoimmune hemolysis

In his book on the autoimmune hemolytic anemia Pirofsky (1969) classified the immunohemolytic anemias (hemolytic anemias having immunologic pathogenesis) into three groups: isoantibody immunohemolytic anemia, antiglobulin-positive immunohemolytic anemia, and autoimmune hemolytic anemia. This is in contrast with the usual classification consisting of isoantibody or isoimmune hemolytic anemia and autoimmune hemolytic anemia. Pirofsky's classification is based on the following definitions:

1. *Isoantibody immunohemolytic anemia* is hemolytic anemia resulting from an antibody produced in one individual attacking the erythrocytes of another, e.g., hemolytic disease of the newborn.

2. *Antiglobulin-positive immunohemolytic anemia* is hemolytic anemia resulting from an antibody produced by the affected person that attacks his own erythrocytes. This group is distinguished from the autoimmune group by these criteria: (1) the antibody either is not directed specifically against the erythrocyte or is directed against modified erythrocytes; (2) there is no evidence of true autoimmunization; and (3) the antiglobulin test, by definition, is always positive.

3. *Autoimmune hemolytic anemia* is hemolytic anemia caused by true autoantibody formation, the autoantibody attacking otherwise unmodified erythrocytes.

There is no disputing that at least three serologic mechanisms are involved in immunohemolytic disease: isoanti-

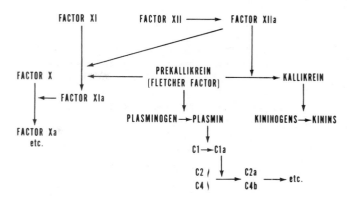

Fig. 13-4. Activation of complement by blood coagulation reactions. See also Chapter 17.

bodies, autoantibodies (in the strict sense), and antibodies mimicking autoantibodies but active because the erythrocyte is an innocent bystander in the interaction of antigen and antibody. However, it is misleading to categorize this group as characteristically antiglobulin-positive hemolytic anemias, since both the isoimmune and the autoimmune anemias are usually antiglobulin positive. If the immunohemolytic anemias of the autoimmune type call for classification into two subcategories, *true autoimmune* and *pseudoautoimmune* probably would be preferable. For the time being I prefer to use the traditional two-group classification, with the caution that an understanding of pathogenesis and serologic concepts is essential, as in any classification or definition.

The term "autoimmune" in this classification admittedly is not ideal. It encompasses the true autoimmune phenomenon, probably relatively rare, and the more common immune, but not strictly autoimmune, phenomena that affect the life span of erythrocytes.

As noted in Chapter 3, the term "autoimmunity" is not appropriate; "autoaggressiveness" would be better. The immune mechanism is based on "self-recognition," i.e., the body recognizing its own tissues and tissue products as being "self," or nonforeign. When the immune mechanism goes awry, there can be loss of self-recognition, and antibody formation results. Immune tolerance then no longer exists. There are at least eight ways in which this can happen. These mechanisms may not always operate in the development of true autoimmune hemolytic disease (antibodies directed specifically toward erythrocyte antigens) but may involve the erythrocyte in other ways.

1. Establishment of a foreign clone of cells. An immunocompetent and nonforeign cell undergoes a transformation (genetic, neoplastic, viral induced, etc.) and becomes modified so that it forms a clone which is now different from the normal clones. Such a clone could lose the ability to recognize host antigens as self and instead recognizes them as foreign. Antibodies against host tissues would be formed that would be autoaggressive. First, the new clone seems to be modified in its response to many autologous antigens. Since one clone is thought to produce only one antibody, it is more likely that not one but several foreign clones would be established. Second, the clone must persist and proliferate. Third, the antibody need not necessarily be directed

against erythrocyte antigens for hemolytic anemia to occur.

2. Emergence of forbidden clones. Burnet (1959) has postulated that during embryonic development clones of cells capable of responding to autologous antigens are inhibited or suppressed, whereas those clones which achieve self-recognition thrive. The suppressed clones are called *forbidden*, since their suppression is essential to the establishment of self-recognition. If a forbidden clone should emerge and become immunologically active, then autoimmunity can occur.

3. An immunodeficient state. The immunodeficient individual has a limited capacity for recognizing modified cells and antigens as self, so that a normal mechanism for maintaining immunologic homeostasis (i.e., the destruction of foreign cells) is deficient. This would allow the modified cells to become established and proliferate, analogous to the establishment of a forbidden clone. Again, it is probable that the result is not one but many forbidden clones.

4. Termination of the state of immune tolerance. This is defined as immunologic unresponsiveness to an antigen induced by exposure to the antigen during the neonatal period; e.g., if small amounts of serum albumin are injected into newborn animals, the adults become immunologically unresponsive to a challenging dose of albumin. When antigen is injected into an adult tolerant to it, the antigen is taken up by macrophages as usual but then is not transferred from macrophages to lymphocytes. The immunotolerant state is not always permanent, as was previously thought. When it is lost, the unresponsive cells are again capable of reacting to host cells and antigens. It is not obvious how this well-established concept applies to strictly autoimmune hemolytic anemia unless the erythrocyte antigens in the embryo or the newborn are suppressed and later elicit antibody response when tolerance is lost.

5. Removal of immunologic quarantine. Antigens stimulate antibody production only if they are available to macrophages and immunocompetent lymphocytes. In some anatomic situations (the nervous system, the cornea and lens of the eye, and the basement membrane of the seminiferous tubules of the testes), the tissues are either avascular or separated from the vascular system by impermeable barriers. Since lymphatic channels either do not exist or are scanty in these special locations, or since they may be avascular, as is the case in the cornea and lens of the eye, the tissues are effectively quarantined as far as the immunologic apparatus is concerned. There is no way for an antibody to be delivered to the receptor tissue. A third type of immunologic quarantine is the retention of intracellular constituents within the intact cell. One well-documented example of this is thyroglobulin, normally located only within the secretory cells of the thyroid gland. When thyroglobulin is injected into an animal, antithyroid antibodies are formed. A break in any of these types of quarantine can lead to the production of antibodies, since the released cells or cell products are foreign intruders to the immunologic system. Undoubtedly these mechanisms are responsible for a large variety of autoimmune reactions and affect many organs and tissues.

6. Modification of a self antigen. The immunologic system remains in a state of homeostasis as long as the antigens that it recognizes as self remain unchanged. Should such an antigen be modified by a change in specificity or some other characteristic by which it is recognized as self, it can become foreign to the immunocompetent cells, and a new type of antibody, a true autoantibody, can result. This concept has far-reaching implications and may be the most significant mechanism for autoimmunization.

7. Formation of haptens. Drugs and other chemicals can combine with protein to produce complex antigens that have the immunogenicity of the protein and the specificity of both the drug and the protein. In an antigenic complex the drug is called *hapten*. Although immunologic tolerance for the carrier protein cannot be broken by the protein-hapten complex, it is possible for the protein to become altered in the complex and to become foreign. Protein-hapten complexes are the most likely explanation for the drug-induced leukopenias, thrombocytopenias, and hemolytic anemias. This is not to say that the mechanism is necessarily, or even probably, truly autoimmune. If a new type of antibody were formed, it could damage cells through the mechanism of nonspecific antigen-antibody complexes discussed previously. Also, fixation of the offending drug on the surface of cells could direct the reaction to the cell surface, e.g., the erythrocyte, without the necessity of having a specific anti-erythrocytic antibody.

8. Nonexclusivity of mechanisms. Zuelzer et al (1966), for example, have made a convincing case for the combination of reactivation by infection with cytomegalovirus and impaired or altered immunologic reactivity.

The autoimmune hemolytic anemias can be classified on the basis of the serologic characteristics into two types: (1) the warm-antibody type, and (2) the cold-antibody type. This classification is descriptive of the behavior of the antibody, but it is more useful to classify the autoimmune hemolytic anemias on the basis of pathogenesis, as in Table 13-2, as (1) idiopathic (primary), and (2) symptomatic (secondary).

Isoimmune hemolysis

Whereas the autoimmune hemolytic anemias are related to antibodies of antierythrocytic specificity without blood group specificity (except in rare instances), isoimmune hemolysis is characterized by both antierythrocytic and blood group specificity.

Isoantibodies can be classified, with regard to thermal range, as either *cold acting* or *warm acting*. In 1904 Donath and Landsteiner showed that in paroxysmal cold hemoglobinuria (PCH) there was fixation of a hemolytic autoantibody in the patient's serum to the erythrocytes at a cold temperature, followed by complement-mediated hemolysis of the sensitized cells when warmed. Warm-acting antibodies were first described by Widal and by Chauffard and Troisier a few years later. The antiglobulin test described by Coombs et al (1945) documented the fixation of antibody to the erythrocytes. It was not long before it was found that such fixation, resulting in a positive antiglobulin (Coombs') test, occurred in many "idiopathic" hemolytic anemias.

Wiener (1944b) showed that anti-**Rh** antibodies existed as both warm-acting and cold-acting antibodies. Whereas the cold-acting antibodies agglutinated erythrocytes suspended in saline medium, the warm-acting antibodies became fixed to the erythrocytic membrane, saturating the antigenic site and thus blocking agglutination by cold-acting antibodies. The term "blocking antibodies" suggested by Wiener is descriptive and appropriate. Table 13-4 lists other terms used to describe the two types of antibodies. Cold-acting antibodies have been called *complete* because they cause direct agglutination, *saline* because they act in a saline medium, and *bivalent* because it was once believed that, in contrast, warm antibodies are univalent. Cold-acting antibodies are usually IgM immunoglobulins and are usually found to be naturally occurring. Warm-acting antibodies cause agglutination in albumin or serum media, are usually of the IgG type, and are usually found as the result of immunization. A clear distinction of properties is not always possible; e.g., it is not uncommon to find that immunization increases the titer of cold-acting antibody as well as producing immune warm-acting antibody. Several investigators have demonstrated that an antiserum containing what seems to be a single type of antibody is, in fact, heterogeneous

Table 13-4. Terms used to describe cold-acting and warm-acting erythrocytic antibodies

Cold acting	Warm acting
Complete	Incomplete
Agglutinating	Blocking or coating
Saline	Albuminoid or serum
Bivalent	Univalent
19S type	7S type
IgM type	IgG type*
Natural	Immune
Do not traverse placenta	Traverse placenta

(Yokoyama and Fudenberg, 1966). Also, it is now known that the cold-acting antibody of PCH is of the IgG rather than the expected IgM type. The thermal characteristics of autoantibodies and isoantibodies are given in Table 13-5.

The isoantibodies include the naturally occurring blood group antibodies such as anti-**A** and anti-**B** as well as immune antibodies produced by immunization to any of the blood groups, A-B-O, Rh, M-N-S, Kell, Duffy, Kidd, Lewis, and others (Chapter 11). Immune isoantibodies result from immunization in blood transfusion and pregnancy. They produce hemolytic disease in the form of hemolytic transfusion reactions or hemolytic disease of the newborn.

Transfusion immunization is the result of the administration of serologically incompatible erythrocytes. The recipient then produces antibodies to the antigens of the foreign cells. Some antigens can stimulate powerful antibody production, whereas others cannot. If powerful immune isoantibodies are produced, hemolytic disease will result when incompatible blood is given the second time.

Natural isoantibodies may also produce hemolytic disease if erythrocytes are given that are agglutinated or lysed by the corresponding natural isoantibody. In this case hemolytic disease does not depend on previous immunization. The reverse situation, administration of incompatible plasma, produces hemolysis of the recipient's erythrocytes.

Hemolytic disease of the newborn is caused by the development in the mother of isoantibodies to antigens present in the erythrocytes of the fetus. In the serologic sense, incompatibility exists between the fetus and the mother, e.g., when the mother is Rh_0 negative and the fetus Rh_0 positive, leakage of Rh_0-positive erythrocytes into the mother's circulation often causes immune anti-**Rh_0** antibodies to be formed (Schröder, 1975). Transmission of these antibodies through the placenta and into the circulation of the fetus then causes hemolysis of the baby's Rh_0-positive erythrocytes.

Table 13-5. Properties of antibodies responsible for hemolytic disease

Antibody	Thermal range	Optimum temperature	Comments
Autoantibodies			React with patient's own erythrocytes and heterologous erythrocytes of same
Autoagglutinins			blood group; may react less strongly with erythrocytes of different group and
Cold			may react weakly with erythrocytes of another species (chimpanzee and rhe-
Complete (natural)	0° to 5° C	0° to 5° C	sus monkey); warm antibodies usually agglutinate normal enzyme-treated
Incomplete (immune)	0° to 25° C	0° to 5° C	erythrocytes in saline-diluted patient's serum, but at times agglutinate better if
Warm			patient's serum is diluted with normal serum rather than with saline; warm
Incomplete (immune)	0° to 40° C	37° C	hemolysins rare; cold hemolysins require optimum pH of 6.5 to 6.8; inactive
Autohemolysins			below pH of 6; normal erythrocytes treated with trypsin as well as erythrocytes
Complete			from PNH very susceptible to action of cold autohemolysins; warm aggluti-
Cold	0° to 25° C	20° C	nins have blood group specificity (anti-**rh**″ and anti-**LW** among others); cold
Warm	37° C	37° C	agglutinins have anti-**il** specificity
Acid	0° and 37° C	0° or 37° C	
Isoantibodies (anti-**A-B-O,** anti-**Rh,** etc.)			When antibodies are γ-globulins, agglutination of sensitized cells by antiglobulin serum readily inhibited by small amounts of γ-globulin; isoantibodies do
Isoagglutinins			not react with patient's own erythrocytes or with heterologous erythrocytes of
Complete (natural)	0° to 40° C	20° C	same blood group; immune isohemolysin activity lost if complement de-
Incomplete (immune)	37° C	37° C	stroyed by heating serum at 56° C for 30 min
Isohemolysins			
Incomplete (immune)	37° C	37° C	

The same mechanism applies to other Rh antigens as well as to other blood groups.

Although the original description of hemolytic disease of the newborn involved incompatibility in the Rh blood group, subsequent experience has shown that roughly two thirds of the cases are caused by A-B-O incompatibility (usually in group A or B children of group O mothers). Of the remaining one third, most are caused by Rh incompatibility, with 2% or 3% caused by various other factors.

Massive destruction of the fetus' erythrocytes accounts for the pathogenesis of the disease. Breakdown of hemoglobin leads to rapidly developing hyperbilirubinemia. Because the glucuronide conjugating mechanism is deficient in the newborn, there is accumulation of unconjugated bilirubin, which in turn has an affinity for the basal ganglia of the brain (kernicterus) with resultant neurologic symptoms. The edema is probably the result of antigen-antibody reaction but may be caused in part by cardiac failure.

Drug-related hemolysis

Drug-related or drug-induced reactions sometimes result in hemolytic disease, sometimes in hemolytic anemia, and sometimes in a positive antiglobulin test with or without hemolytic disease. The immune reactions are reviewed by Worlledge (1969a, 1973) and by Miescher and Miescher (1978). Drug-related hemolysis is uncommon, but study of the varied mechanisms has expanded our understanding of the mechanisms of hemolysis.

Drug-related hemolysis falls into at least six categories: (1) hemolytic anemia, antiglobulin negative, caused by a deficiency of erythrocytic enzyme, (2) hemolytic anemia, antiglobulin positive, of the *hapten type,* in which the drug acts as an antigen, (3) hemolytic anemia, antiglobulin positive, of the *innocent bystander type,* in which the erythrocyte acts merely as the medium for expressing the immune reaction, (4) hemolytic anemia, antiglobulin positive, of the *alpha-methyldopa type,* (5) positive antiglobulin test without hemolysis or drug-induced antibodies, and (6) direct lytic effect on the erythrocyte, nonimmunologic and antiglobulin negative, caused by hemolysins of plant or animal sources or by lytic drugs.

IMMUNOHEMOLYSIS OF THE HAPTEN TYPE. The classic example of hemolytic anemia of the *hapten type* is that of penicillin sensitivity. Usually following high-dose intake, antipenicillin antibodies may develop in some persons. The penicillin is not by itself antigenic, but it acts as a hapten by coupling with an immunogenic carrier protein. The antibody to the complexed molecule has antipenicillin specificity. Antipenicillin antibody cannot by itself lyse red blood cells. However, if penicillin is administered subsequently, it binds to the surface of the red blood cells, serves as an acceptor of antibody, and the antigen-antibody complex then causes hemolysis. With few exceptions (Kerr et al, 1972) there is no fixation of complement, and the reaction is not complement mediated. The antiglobulin test (anti-γ) is usually strongly positive during active hemolysis. Getaz et al (1980) report a penicillin-like reaction in two patients receiving chemotherapy with Cisplatin (cis-diammine-dichloroplatinum).

There are some interesting features of penicillin sensitivity. According to Levine et al (1966) the benzylpenicilloyl group of benzylpenicillin is the major hapten. When penicillin sensitization occurs, and fortunately it is uncommon, it develops only after high-dose therapy. Sensitization usually follows intramuscular administration of penicillin and is rarely secondary to intravenous administration only. The antibody is usually of the IgG type but rarely may be IgA or IgM (Levine and Redmond, 1967). Although penicillin binds very firmly to the red cell membrane, bound antipenicillin antibody can be eluted and shown to be specific for penicillin derivatives.

IMMUNOHEMOLYSIS OF THE INNOCENT BYSTANDER TYPE. Whereas in hemolytic anemia of the hapten type the offending drug acts as a hapten and also fixes firmly onto the red cell membrane, in hemolytic anemia of the innocent bystander type the drug acts as hapten only and binds very loosely or not at all to the cell membrane. After antibodies to the drug are formed, they combine with free drug in the blood, and the antigen-antibody complex then attaches to whatever cells it encounters. When it attaches to red cells and causes them to lyse, it can truly be said that they are innocent bystanders, since they do not invite the attack by bearing the drug on the surface. However, innocence is probably not complete, since the red cell membrane does have receptors for the antigen-antibody complex, even if not immunologically specific. The antigen-antibody complex binds complement, and the hemolysis is complement mediated.

The classic example of acquired immunohemolytic anemia of the innocent bystander type is that secondary to intake of the drug stibophen (Shulman, 1964), which is used in the treatment of schistosomiasis. The antibody formed is IgG or IgM. Characteristically, the immune complex activates complement at the cell surface and then promptly breaks away, so that the antigamma antiglobulin test is usually negative, whereas the anticomplement antiglobulin test is usually positive (Croft et al, 1968). Furthermore the liberation of the immune complex leaves it free to attach to new cells and perpetuate the hemolytic process. Occasionally hemolysis may induce disseminated intravascular coagulation (Weiss et al, 1972).

The immune complex binds to platelet and leukocyte membranes as well, so that the triad of hemolytic anemia, leukopenia, and thrombocytopenia is not uncommon. In fact, adverse immune reactions of this type ascribed to other drugs often show thrombocytopenia or leukopenia as the major effect, e.g., quinidine and quinine sensitization cause severe thrombocytopenia, and only occasionally is there hemolysis of red cells (Freedman et al, 1956). Other drugs are implicated in adverse immune reactions of the innocent bystander type, responsible for various combinations of hemolytic anemia, leukopenia, and thrombocytopenia (Worlledge, 1973; Pisciotta, 1973; Miescher, 1973). The most important are phenacetin, paraaminosalicylic acid, sulfonamides, chlorpromazine, insulin, and isoniazid. Miescher (1973) gives an extensive list of drugs that should be considered, and drug-induced hemolytic anemias are reviewed by Garratty and Petz (1975). It should be noted that two problems are commonly encountered. First, the guilty drug is sometimes difficult to identify when the patient has been on a multidrug regimen. Second, it is not always possible to determine if the cell destruction is immunologic or caused by a direct toxic effect of the drug. It may be helpful to remember that immunologic cell destruction usually occurs very shortly after the drug intake, whereas toxic reactions are usually delayed.

IMMUNOHEMOLYSIS OF THE ALPHA-METHYLDOPA TYPE. Alpha-methyldopa (Aldomet) is a drug commonly used in the treatment of hypertension. About one fourth of the patients receiving this drug develop a positive antiglobulin (anti-γ) test, but only 1% to 5% of all subjects develop hemolytic anemia. In countries where enzymatic deficiencies of red blood cells are uncommon, methyldopa is said to be the most common cause of drug-induced hemolysis (Böttiger and Westerholm, 1973). The closely related drug, L-dopa, may also induce a positive antiglobulin test but not hemolysis (Goldberg and Bluestone, 1973).

This type of drug-induced immune reaction differs from the others in several respects. Neither the hapten nor the innocent bystander mechanism seems to be involved. In fact, it is not known how methyldopa induces the production of antibodies. Sensitization develops slowly, usually after some months of drug ingestion, and is dose related. Characteristically, the antiglobulin test reverts to negative when the drug is discontinued, usually within a few weeks or months, but sometimes persists for up to 2 years (Worlledge, 1969b). The antibody is heterogeneous, showing not only drug specificity but also Rh specificity, usually with rh' or rh" but sometimes with other Rh factors (Bakemeier and Leddy, 1968). The failure to react with Rh_{null} red blood cells, which lack all Rh antigens, suggests a specificity for Rh precursor substance. Patten et al (1977) report the occurrence of autoimmune hemolytic anemia with anti-Jk^a specificity in a patient taking methyldopa. Also characteristic of the immune reaction to methyldopa is the frequent occurrence of antibodies of nonerythrocytic specificity: antinuclear antibodies, rheumatoid factor, and antibodies against gastric mucosal cells. In the series reported by Perry et al (1971) antinuclear factor developed in 53% of the cases, rheumatoid factor in 18%, and positive lupus erythematosus (LE) cell preparations in 4%. Kirtland et al (1980) propose that methyldopa inhibits suppressor T-cells, leading to unregulated production of autoantibody by B-cells.

POSITIVE ANTIGLOBULIN TEST ONLY. About half to three-fourths of persons taking the antibiotic cephalothin (or cephaloridine) develop a positive antiglobulin test without evidence of red cell hemolysis (Gralnick et al, 1967; Molthan et al, 1967). Antiglobulin test positivity develops within a few days after inception of drug therapy, and no drug-specific antibodies can be demonstrated. This phenomenon is unexplained and seems to be unrelated to those cases which develop immunohemolysis during cephalothin therapy (Gralnick et al, 1971; Forbes et al, 1972).

NONIMMUNOLOGIC HEMOLYSIS. Hemolysins from animal sources (e.g., snake venoms), from microorganisms that produce hemolysins, and from physical agents such as hypotonic or hypertonic solutions attack the erythrocyte membrane directly and cause lysis. Some drugs (Table 13-2) also act directly on the erythrocyte membrane, the effect is dose related, and there is no individual susceptibility.

Although not absolutely excluded, this type of reaction is not of the hapten type, nor is it dependent on an enzymatic deficiency.

Some of the drugs that cause direct hemolysis are phenylhydrazine (Beutler et al, 1955), phenacetin (Shahidi and Hemaidan, 1969), vitamin K analogues in newborn and premature infants (Meyer and Angus, 1956), sodium chlorate (Lee et al, 1970), and industrial chemicals such as aniline or nitrobenzene derivatives (Lubash et al, 1964), arsine (Jenkins, G.C., et al, 1965), and lead (Dagg et al, 1965).

Special types of complement-dependent hemolysis

PAROXYSMAL COLD HEMOGLOBINURIA (PCH). Hemolysis of red cells in PCH is caused by a special hemolysin described by Donath and Landsteiner (1904) and called the Donath-Landsteiner (D-L) hemolysin or, better, D-L antibody. The hemolysis is complement dependent. Characteristically the reaction occurs in two phases: binding of D-L antibody at low temperature followed by hemolysis at body temperature.

Optimum fixation of antibody at cold temperature occurs in the presence of complement (Hinz et al, 1961) even though no hemolysis occurs at this time. The complement component that fixes to the cell membrane in the cold phase is C1q (Hinz and Mollner, 1964). In the warm phase the other components fix and interact sequentially in the classic convertase system.

The D-L antibody is an IgG immunoglobulin. The direct antiglobulin test using a serum of anti-γ specificity will be positive if performed in the cold, the temperature at which antibody is fixed to the cell surface. The direct antiglobulin test will be negative with anti-γ specific antiserum if the cells are washed at 37° C but will be positive with a broad-spectrum or anticomplement antiglobulin serum at any temperature. Typically, positive direct antiglobulin tests are obtained during an acute hemolytic attack and become negative after the attack. Indirect antiglobulin tests are then often positive. The antibody has anti-**P** specificity (Worlledge and Rousso, 1965) in contrast to the Ii specificity of other types of cold-acting antibodies.

It is interesting to note that the concentration of complement in the blood may be reduced markedly after one or more acute hemolytic episodes. It is recommended, therefore, that complement be added to one of the control tubes when testing for D-L antibody, in case the patient's serum is complement depleted.

PAROXYSMAL NOCTURNAL HEMOGLOBINURIA (PNH). Hemolysis in PNH is complement dependent, but, unlike PCH, no specific antibody is present. Hemolysis is caused entirely by a defect of the red cell membrane that renders the cell extremely susceptible to lysis by complement. There is fixation of C3 fragments to the erythrocytic membrane, enhanced at an acid pH, followed by hemolysis. After C3 fragments attach to the membrane, the erythrocytes can be lysed by normal, as well as PNH, serum. They also become more susceptible to antibody-mediated hemolysis, also because of increased susceptibility to complement hemolysis (Rosse and Dacie, 1966).

The nature of the membrane defect is not known, but there has been much speculation. The observation that the membrane defect is shared also by PNH granulocytes and platelets (Gardner and Murphy, 1972) and the frequent association with aplastic anemia (Dacie and Lewis, 1972) have led to the suggestion that the structural defect is the product of an abnormal clone of primitive stem cells (Oni et al, 1970; Lewis and Sirchia, 1972). It is difficult, however, to reconcile this concept with the observation that in different patients there are heterogeneous red cell populations with respect to sensitivity to hemolysis (Rosse, 1972, 1973b; Sirchia and Lewis, 1975; Packman et al, 1979).

It is almost certain that the complement component required to lyse PNH cells is C3 and that in vivo this is activated by the alternate or activator system involving properdin (Logue et al, 1973; Rosse et al, 1974). Hemolysis of PNH red blood cells in media of low ionic strength (sugar-water test) may involve the classic pathway of activating complement as well.

PNH erythrocytes lyse very quickly in acidified serum at a low ionic concentration. This is the basis for the *acid serum* test. The *sugar-water* test is probably effective because of the greater attachment of complement to the red cell membrane in a medium of low ionic strength.

Various explanations have been proposed for the membrane defect, but it is impossible to decide if the observed abnormalities reflect cause or effect: craters and pits on the membrane by electron microscopy (Lewis et al, 1971), a decrease in membrane acetylcholinesterase activity (Metz et al, 1960), increased sensitivity to peroxidation (Mengel et al, 1967), and altered membrane lipids (Mengel et al, 1972). The most impressive explanation is that membrane protein is deficient in thiol groups. Compounds capable of reducing the available thiol groups (L-cysteine, penicillamine, glutathione) can alter normal red cells so that they behave like PNH cells in all respects (Sirchia and Dacie, 1967; Mengel et al, 1972; Lewis et al, 1971; Goldstein, 1974).

Deficiencies of complement

Complement may be deficient when it is consumed in the course of complement-mediated reactions (disseminated LE, acute and chronic glomerulonephritis, serum sickness, subacute bacterial endocarditis) or when there is deficient synthesis (progressive glomerulonephritis, liver disease) (Schur, 1977). Hereditary deficiencies of various components (C1q, C1r, C1s, C2, C3, C4, C5, C6, C7, C8, C1 esterase inhibitor, and C3b inactivator) have been reported but are rare (Müller-Eberhard, 1976; Rosenfeld et al, 1976;

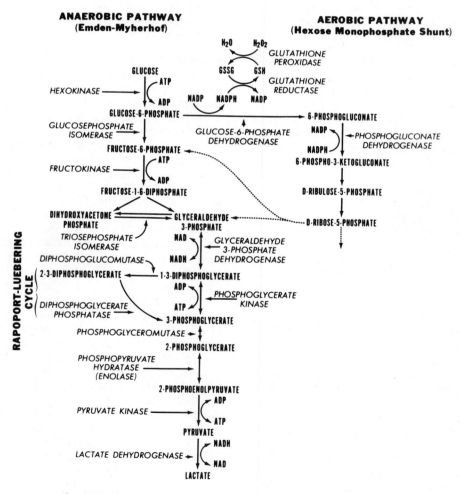

Fig. 13-5. Major pathways of glucose metabolism in the red blood cell.

Delâge et al, 1977; Glass et al, 1978; Hoppe et al, 1978; Snyderman et al, 1979; Inae et al, 1979).

Hemolysis caused by deficiency of erythrocytic enzymes

The energy and intermediates required by the erythrocyte for membrane function and cellular integrity are derived entirely from the anaerobic and aerobic metabolism of glucose (Rapoport, 1968). The metabolic pathways are shown in Fig. 13-5. The chief pathway, accounting for about 90% of the glucose used, is the anaerobic, or Embden-Meyerhof, pathway. About 10% of the glucose undergoes aerobic glycolysis in the hexose monophosphate shunt. The intermediate steps in the metabolism of glucose to lactate are regulated by enzymes, each of which is operative in one of the sequential steps. These enzymes may be deficient in at least two circumstances. The first is the natural process of red cell aging, characterized by a gradual loss of these enzymes. The other is the deficiency of an enzyme as an inherited deficiency.

A normal enzyme system in the erythrocyte is necessary for the maintenance of normal membrane structure and function, for the normal oxygenation of hemoglobin, and for the protection of hemoglobin against peroxidation. The deleterious effects of the enzymatic deficiencies can be attributed to impairment in the regeneration of ATP and other organic phosphates that supply the energy for the sequential metabolic steps. Traditionally, the hemolytic anemias secondary to enzymatic defects are called *nonspherocytic* to distinguish them from the classic hereditary spherocytosis.

When the role of an enzyme deficiency, such as that of pyruvate kinase in glucose metabolism, and the production of hemolytic anemia were defined, it seemed logical to investigate the possibility that other enzyme deficiencies also could cause hemolytic disease. In fact, there are isolated reports linking other enzymatic deficiencies and hemolysis, but, as recently reviewed by Beutler (1978a, 1979), some deficiencies are very rare or are not the cause of hemolytic disease. Table 13-6 lists the frequency of enzymatic defects found by Beutler (1979) in 350 cases studied. It is

obvious that enzymatic defects not listed are either extremely rare or possibly not even related to hemolytic disease.

The most common deficiencies are of G-6-PD and of pyruvate kinase.

The glutathione-dependent system

The protection of hemoglobin and enzymes is dependent on a system involving glutathione and glutathione-related enzymes, NADPH and G-6-PD. The reactions are shown in Fig. 13-6. It is essential to maintain a normal level of GSH if oxidation of hemoglobin and enzymes is to be kept under control, and this is a function of glutathione reductase. The control of peroxide is the function of glutathione peroxidase. If red cells are exposed to an oxidant drug, GSH is restored by the action of glutathione peroxidase and glutathione reductase.

Congenital primary deficiencies of the glutathione system have been reported (Beutler, 1979), but may not be acceptable. A deficiency of glutathione peroxidase may lead to a drug-related hemolytic anemia (Necheles et al, 1970a) on the basis of deficient protection against peroxidation. The same is true of glutathione reductase deficiency (Blume et al, 1968b) and a deficiency of glutathione caused by a deficiency of glutathione synthetase (Mohler et al, 1970). The integrity of the glutathione system is also dependent on the activity of G-6-PD (see the following section).

Glucose-6-phosphate dehydrogenase (G-6-PD) deficiency

G-6-PD deficiency is rare in North European whites and in American Indians but is common in American blacks and in many areas throughout the world (Burka et al, 1966; Saldanha et al, 1969; Stamatoyannopoulos et al, 1966a, 1970; Chan and Todd, 1972). Carson and Frischer (1966) estimate that about 100 million persons carry the trait.

A deficiency of G-6-PD makes the affected individual exceptionally susceptible to the development of drug-induced hemolytic anemia (Dern et al, 1954a, 1954b). The disease is not caused by an immunologic insult but by a biochemical defect. The occurrence of hemolytic anemia in black soldiers receiving the antimalarial drug primaquine led to the discovery that this type of hemolytic anemia is

Table 13-6. Frequency of significant enzymatic defects found by Beutler in 350 cases of suspected enzyme-deficient hemolytic anemia*

Enzymatic defect	Number of cases	Frequency (%)
G-6-PD	49	13.9
Pyruvate kinase	37	9.9
Glucosephosphate isomerase	6	1.7
Pyrimidine 5'-nucleotidase	5	1.4
Triosephosphate isomerase	3	0.9
Hexokinase	1	0.3
Aldolase	1	0.3
Diphosphoglycerate mutase phosphatase	1	0.3
All others	0	0

*Data from Beutler (1979).

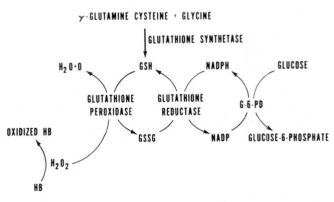

Fig. 13-6. Glutathione-dependent system.

caused by a deficiency of G-6-PD in erythrocytes. When deficient red blood cells are challenged by any one of several drugs, there is depletion of glutathione, formation of Heinz bodies, and inhibition of glucose use. All three factors favor membrane damage and phagocytosis by RE cells (see the review by Beutler, 1978b).

G-6-PD deficiency is sex linked (Desforges, 1976) so that the fully expressed defect is found in males and, like classic hemophilia, is transmitted from a heterozygous mother to the son. In heterozygous women the expression of the defect varies, and this has been attributed to random X-inactivation (Beutler et al, 1962). This mosaicism produces two populations of red blood cells in an affected female, one with normal enzyme activity and the other with deficient activity. On the average, then, the concentration of G-6-PD in heterozygous women is half the normal.

As in the case of variant hemoglobins (Chapter 14), over 80 molecular variants of G-6-PD are known (Beutler, 1978b). Although there is no clinical indication for identifying the variant in a given case, there is good evidence that the clinical severity is determined by the variant. The normal enzyme is designated B, and persons may be either B+ (normal enzymatic activity) or B− (deficient enzymatic activity). Enzyme A is found most commonly in blacks, those who are A+ being normal, and those who are A− being G-6-PD deficient and candidates for drug-induced hemolysis. All other variants are given geographic or proper names.

Except in rare instances, G-6-PD–deficient persons do not have hemolytic anemia unless challenged by drugs (Table 13-2), viral or bacterial infections, or metabolic disorders such as acidosis. There are some differences in response among different racial or geographic groups. Hemolysis is sometimes more severe in persons with G-6-PD deficiency of the Mediterranean type, whereas hemolysis secondary to ingestion of the fava bean (explained later) does not occur in A− blacks. Quinine, quinidine, and chloramphenicol are hemolytic in whites but not in blacks (Beutler, 1959b). Occasional cases of hemolytic disease of the newborn, nonimmunologic, associated with G-6-PD deficiency have been reported among Mediterranean and Oriental populations (Weatherall, 1960) but are even rarer in black newborns (Zinkham, 1963). Rarely, persons with G-6-PD deficiency have a mild congenital nonspherocytic hemolytic anemia in the absence of drug administration (Cloutier and Burgert, 1966).

Clinically, evidence of hemolysis appears 2 or 3 days after a susceptible subject takes the offending drug. There is back pain, hemoglobinuria, a rapid reduction of the red blood cell count and hemoglobin concentration, reticulocytosis, and icterus. The erythrocytes contain many Heinz bodies, except when hemolysis is caused by furadantin ingestion (Szeinberg et al, 1962). The antiglobulin test is negative. Recovery occurs within 1 week even if drug therapy is continued.

The hemolytic process tends to be more severe in subjects with G-6-PD deficiency of the Mediterranean type. In addition, these persons are susceptible to hemolysis following ingestion of the fava bean. This is called *favism* (Kattamis et al, 1969). In susceptible individuals an extremely severe,

sometimes fatal, hemolytic anemia follows ingestion of fava beans or even inhalation of pollen from the plant. The onset is almost immediate. In addition to the predisposing enzymatic deficiency, there are other unknown predisposing factors, since not all enzyme-deficient individuals are susceptible. An additional, but undetermined, genetic defect is postulated (Stamatoyannopoulos et al, 1966b). Subjects with a deficiency of the Canton variant of G-6-PD are also candidates for favism.

The severity of hemolysis in G-6-PD deficiency depends on the dose of the inducing drug, on the toxicity of the drug, and on the G-6-PD variant lacking in the subject (Carson and Frischer, 1966). Infection or metabolic disorders can induce hemolysis or accentuate drug-induced hemolysis. Renal damage reduces the elimination of an offending drug and can account for severe hemolysis when only a small dose of an oxidant drug is given. Although the most common is the black variant, the most severe hemolysis is seen in persons who have the Mediterranean variant.

The damage to the red cell that results from the administration of an oxidant drug is attributed to the failure to generate NADPH from NADP, a step dependent on G-6-PD. The oxidant drug causes the oxidation of GSH to GSSG, and, with the loss of GSH, the system responsible for controlling the oxidation of hemoglobin breaks down. As a result, a series of reactions occur that terminate in the formation of degradation products of hemoglobin, which then polymerize to form Heinz bodies (Allen and Jandl, 1961).

Pyruvate kinase deficiency

Pyruvate kinase (PK) deficiency is the second most common enzymatic deficiency associated with hereditary nonspherocytic hemolytic anemia (Valentine and Tanaka, 1978).

PK catalyzes the formation of pyruvate from phosphoenolpyruvate (Fig. 13-5), and this is accompanied by the transformation of ADP to ATP. It is probable that the decreased life span is secondary to the deficiency of ATP, since ATP is one of the major requirements for the maintenance of normal membrane function. The abnormality of the membrane is evident not only in the decreased life span of the red cells and increased destruction in the spleen and liver (Nathan et al, 1968b) but also in the shape abnormalities (discussed later) and loss of cell potassium (Keitt, 1966).

PK deficiency is inherited as an autosomal recessive trait, and only homozygous individuals have hemolytic anemia. Although most of the cases have been described in persons of North European origin, the defect has been described in diverse geographic and racial groups.

Hemolytic disease in PK deficiency is remarkably variable in severity. It ranges from hemolytic disease of the newborn, nonimmunologic but requiring exchange transfusions (Fung et al, 1969), to chronic hemolytic anemia that may be very mild in some cases and severe in others. It has been noted that adults with chronic hemolytic anemia caused by PK deficiency often give a history of anemia or jaundice in infancy or childhood. Aplastic crises have been encountered (Jacobasch and Boese, 1969). The spleen is enlarged only moderately, and although splenectomy has been beneficial in young children with severe anemia (Jacobasch and Boese, 1969), in most patients the results of splenectomy are disappointing. This is due in part to unabated destruction of red cells in the liver.

As expected, the degree of anemia and hyperbilirubinemia is variable. Reticulocytosis is a constant feature except in the rare occurrence of an aplastic crisis. Very high reticulocyte counts are seen after splenectomy, supposedly reflecting the increased susceptibility to hemolysis of the reticulocytes in the spleen (Nathan et al, 1968b). The blood smear shows the macrocytosis and polychromatophilia expected to accompany the reticulocytosis. Microspherocytes are not present. There may be occasional normoblasts when hemolysis is severe. Although not a constant feature, abnormalities of red cell shape may be encountered—tailed erythrocytes, irregularly distorted erythrocytes, or acanthocytes (Oski etal, 1964; Nathan et al, 1966). Leblond et al (1978a, 1978b) describe various bizarre red blood cell shapes in patients after splenectomy. The standard osmotic fragility of the red cells is normal, but there is increased autohemolysis after incubation for 48 hours, usually corrected by ATP but not glucose (Grimes et al, 1968), with enough exceptions (Tanaka and Paglia, 1971) to diminish the value of this test. The specific diagnosis of PK deficiency is based on the demonstration of the enzymatic deficiency in the erythrocytes. The deficiency is usually unequivocal in homozygotes, whereas heterozygotes show about half the normal enzymatic activity. However, in some cases there is marked disparity between the severity of the anemia and the degree of PK deficiency, and variant enzymes have been postulated (Paglia et al, 1968; Zuelzer et al, 1968). The antiglobulin test is of course negative. Goebel et al (1975) report the transformation of PK deficiency into acute leukemia.

Other enzymatic deficiencies

In addition to the deficiencies of G-6-PD or PK, a deficiency of other enzymes involved in the glycolytic pathways can result in hemolytic disease. These are rare. A summary of their features and pertinent references is given by Beutler (1978a).

Hemolysis caused by hereditary abnormality of the red cell membrane

Hereditary spherocytosis (HS)

Students who have been steeped in the complex marvels of modern medicine, such as electron microscopy, sometimes fail to take advantage of simple hematologic examinations, particularly the study of the blood smear. The diagnosis of hereditary spherocytosis is a case in point, since in most cases the blood smear will suggest the correct diagnosis.

Hereditary spherocytosis (congenital hemolytic anemia, familial spherocytosis, congenital hemolytic icterus, acholuric jaundice, hemolytic anemia of the Chauffard-Minkowski syndrome) is the oldest known hemolytic disease. Vaulair and Masius were the first to describe the characteristic spherocytosis in 1871. Chauffard, in 1907, and Minkowski, in 1910, described the disease in greater detail, and the cred-

it for describing the characteristic reticulocytosis and the increased osmotic fragility of the erythrocytes belongs to Chauffard. Excellent reviews are presented by Jandl (1968) and by Jandl and Cooper (1978).

The hemolytic state has a double component: there is decreased survival of erythrocytes that are intrinsically abnormal, and there is increased destruction of the abnormal erythrocytes in the spleen. Thus (1) normal erythrocytes transfused into a person having hereditary spherocytosis survive for a normal period, (2) erythrocytes from a person with hereditary spherocytosis transfused into a normal person show decreased survival, and (3) erythrocytes from a person with hereditary spherocytosis transfused into a person previously subjected to splenectomy show normal survival.

Increased osmotic fragility of the erythrocytes reflects the intrinsic defect but does not of itself explain the shortened survival, since survival in vivo is not dependent on the osmotic environment. Destruction of the abnormal erythrocytes occurs in the spleen, and somehow the spleen recognizes these abnormal erythrocytes, entraps them, and destroys them. It has been suggested that entrapment is a function of the spheroid shape of the abnormal erythrocytes, but this is not true, because even though the erythrocytes tend to be less spherical as a result of being made iron deficient, they are still trapped and destroyed in the spleen (Crosby and Conrad, 1960). In any case, splenectomy provides immediate and lasting improvement of the hemolytic disease, even though the bone marrow continues to produce intrinsically abnormal and spheroid erythrocytes. Only in rare cases do spherocytes disappear after splenectomy.

One demonstrable membrane lesion is excessive leakiness for sodium influx. This biochemical lesion sets up a chain of events: stimulation of the sodium pump to increase the elimination of intracellular sodium and, concomitantly, increased use of ATP and anaerobic glycolysis. When there is an ample supply of glucose, as when the cell is circulating freely in the blood, the pump can function well enough to regulate intracellular sodium. However, when the cells enter the spleen, their passage is delayed sufficiently to deplete the supply of glucose. The pump wheezes to a stop, and enough sodium enters the cell to cause colloid osmotic hemolysis. These sequences can be simulated in vitro, since the spherocytes are more susceptible to osmotic hemolysis after they have been incubated, and the increased osmotic hemolysis can be largely inhibited by supplying glucose. Schrier et al (1974) have shown that HS red cells have impaired drug-induced, endocytic vacuole formation, but the relationship of this phenomenon to decreased survival is not clear.

A second membrane lesion may explain both the cause of the membrane leakiness and the osmotic hyperhemolysis. It is postulated that there is an abnormality of membrane proteins that causes defective microfilament formation (Gomperts et al, 1972; Jacob et al, 1972). Since normal red cells exposed to a sulfhydryl group inhibitor behave like those of hereditary spherocytosis (Jacob and Jandl, 1962), there may be a relationship, still not clear, between the protein abnormality and the function of sulfhydryl groups.

An animal counterpart of the human disease has been

described in the deer mouse *(Peromyscus maniculatus)* (Anderson et al, 1960).

Hereditary elliptocytosis

Elliptocytosis is inherited as an autosomal dominant trait. The red cells assume the elliptical shape after leaving the bone marrow, since the normoblasts in the bone marrow are normal, as are reticulocytes in the blood. The newborn with hereditary elliptocytosis may show only a few elliptocytes. Not until the third or fourth month of age is the defect fully expressed. Zarkowsky (1979) finds that the elliptocytes in the newborn are unusually sensitive to heat, the fragmentation at 45° C resembling that seen in congenital pyropoikilocytosis (Zarkowsky et al, 1975). Once formed, the elliptocyte shows a membrane defect the opposite of that of hereditary spherocytosis, being abnormally permeable to sodium efflux. During the incubation of elliptocytes there is loss of intracellular sodium and a reduction of red cell ATP and 2,3-DPG activity (Peters et al, 1966). In addition, the elliptocyte has been shown to have two structural lesions. Murphy (1965) has shown that elliptocytes have a concentration of cholesterol at each end, and Rebuck and Van Slyck (1968) have shown that hemoglobin has the same unusual distribution.

Neither the biochemical nor the structural lesion explain why only 10% to 15% of patients with hereditary elliptocytosis have decreased red cell survival and hemolytic anemia (Geerdink et al, 1966). There is no reason to assume that asymptomatic elliptocytosis represents the heterozygous state, whereas elliptocytic hemolytic anemia represents the homozygous defect, although severe anemia has been seen in several persons believed to be homozygous (Pryor and Pitney, 1967). There is no correlation between the number of elliptocytes and decreased survival. Nor does the unusual shape have any relation to hemolysis. It is noteworthy that the erythrocytes of the llama are also elliptical but show no increased osmotic fragility; in fact, they do not lyse even in distilled water.

As in the case of hereditary spherocytosis, the elliptocytes that have a decreased life span are destroyed in the spleen, and as expected, there is enlargement of the spleen in these subjects. Elliptocytes do not disappear after splenectomy (Lipton, 1955). Elliptocytosis can occur in combination with hereditary spherocytosis and other red cell abnormalities (Aksoy et al, 1974a).

Abetalipoproteinemia

Because lipoproteins are a major component of the red cell membrane, and because the lipid composition of the membrane is dependent to a great extent on the lipid composition of the plasma, some abnormalities of lipid metabolism affect the red cell. Abnormalities of this type are seen in abetalipoproteinemia, hereditary stomatocytosis, lecithin-cholesterol acyltransferase (LCAT) deficiency, and Zieve's syndrome.

The liproproteins of plasma are of four types: (1) chylomicrons, (2) very low-density lipoproteins (VLDL) or pre-β-lipoproteins, (3) low-density lipoproteins (LDL) or β-lipoproteins, and (4) high-density lipoproteins (HDL) or α-lipoproteins. The lipoproteins are macromolecular complexes of lipids and proteins, and each type has a characteristic composition (Frederickson et al, 1978).

The absence of β-lipoprotein, *abetalipoproteinemia*, produces a rare but serious syndrome having the following features: acanthocytosis of the red cells, malabsorption of fat, retinitis pigmentosa, and neurologic damage. Because of the characteristic distortion of the shape of the red cells, the syndrome is sometimes called acanthocytosis. Although this is not incorrect, the preferred term is "abetalipoproteinemia."

The first report on abetalipoproteinemia (Bassen and Kornzweig, 1950) documented a new syndrome consisting of malformation of the erythrocytes and retinitis pigmentosa. The malformation of the red cells was named *acanthrocytosis* 2 years later (Singer et al, 1952), after the Greek stem *akantha* for thorn, and the superfluous letter *r* eventually was eliminated by later writers. The characteristic absence of β-lipoprotein from the blood was reported independently the same year by three investigators (Lamy et al, 1960; Mabry et al, 1960; Salt et al, 1960).

A review of the probable pathogenesis of the syndrome is presented by Fredrickson et al (1978). The evidence favors the concept that there is a complete lack of apoLDL (apoLP-ser) from abetalipoproteinemic plasma, caused by a genetic block in the synthesis of apoLDL. It is still uncertain if the relationship of abetalipoproteinemia and the acanthic malformation of the red cells is one of cause and effect. In favor of a direct relationship is the feature that acanthocytes are not found in the bone marrow and form only in the circulating blood. There are other red cell malformations that are related to abnormalities in plasma lipids, e.g., leptocytes in cirrhosis of the liver, and it is assumed that interaction between erythrocytes and plasma lipids produces abnormalities of the cell membrane. Experimentally, acanthocytosis can be produced in rats that are made abetalipoproteinemic (McBride and Jacob, 1968). On the other hand, acanthocytosis and hemolytic anemia have been found in situations where there is a normal plasma concentration of LDL, in alcoholic cirrhosis (Smith et al, 1964), and in pyruvate kinase deficiency (Oski et al, 1964; Baughan et al, 1968). Lipid analyses of acanthocytes have shown no constant abnormality. Generally, they contain relatively less phosphatidylcholine and more sphingomyelin and cholesterol than normal cells. The activity of the cholesterol-esterifying enzyme, LCAT, is reduced but not totally absent.

It is not certain that the hemolytic disease which sometimes accompanies abetalipoproteinemia has the same etiology in all the reported cases (Fredrickson et al, 1978).

Hereditary stomatocytosis

Stomatocytes (Fig. 13-15) are sometimes found in the blood in acute alcoholism (Douglass and Twomey, 1970) and are a feature of Rh$_{null}$ disease (p. 508). The hereditary type, accompanied by mild to severe hemolytic anemia, consists of several variants of uncertain kinship. The family studied by Lock et al (1961) was found to have stomatocytosis, moderately severe hemolytic anemia, severely increased osmotic fragility, and no improvement after splenectomy. The case reported by Miller et al (1965) showed striking hemolysis at a low temperature. The affected members of the family studied by Oski et al (1969) had mild hemolytic anemia. The red cells showed increased osmotic fragility and contained a high concentration of sodium and a low concentration of potassium, secondary to an unusually high permeability to sodium ions. Increased cation pump activity associated with low 2, 3-DPG and increased oxygen affinity are reported by Wiley et al (1979). Autohemolysis is increased if the test is performed at 37° C and is corrected by both glucose and ATP. Splenectomy is beneficial. Other variants have been described: stomatocytosis, mild hemolytic anemia, and normal osmotic fragility (Jackson and Knight, 1969); stomatocytosis, mild hemolytic anemia, and decreased osmotic fragility (Miller, D.R., et al, 1971); and stomatocytosis with increased cation permeability but no anemia or hemolytic disease (Honig et al, 1971).

Lecithin-cholesterol acyltransferase (LCAT) deficiency

A partial deficiency of LCAT is found in abetalipoproteinemia, but the absence of plasma LCAT is characteristic of a rare familial syndrome whose features are corneal opacities, proteinuria, codocytes (target cells), and low levels of plasma cholesteryl esters and lysolecithin (Norum et al, 1972). LCAT catalyzes the formation of cholesteryl esters from cholesterol by the transfer of an unsaturated fatty acid radical from lecithin. The high concentration of nonesterified cholesterol in the plasma probably is responsible for the formation of codocytes, as in obstructive jaundice with increased plasma unesterified cholesterol and lecithin (Cooper and Jandl, 1968). Patients with familial LCAT deficiency have moderately severe anemia caused in part by decreased red cell survival and in part by decreased erythropoiesis.

Zieve's syndrome

An unusual combination of hemolytic anemia, hyperglyceridemia, fatty infiltration of the liver, and jaundice in alcoholics has been described by Zieve (1958) and by Zieve and Hill (1961). The syndrome is interesting in that hyperglyceridemia by itself, as in the familial (type I) form, is not accompanied by hemolytic anemia. I have seen only one example of this type of hemolytic anemia, and the hemolysis was severe.

Congenital dyserythropoietic anemia, HEMPAS type

Hereditary erythroblastic multinuclearity with positive acidified serum test (HEMPAS) is one of three types of *congenital dyserythropoietic anemia (CDA)*, called dyserythropoietic because the marrow normoblasts show multinuclearity and bizarre malformations. CDA usually is classified into three categories (Heimpel and Wendt, 1968). Type I shows a mild macrocytic anemia with marked anisocytosis and poikilocytosis and suggestive megaloblastic dyspoiesis in addition to the characteristic dyserythropoietic changes in the bone marrow (Maeda et al, 1980). Type II is the HEMPAS variety (Enquist et al, 1972; Verwilghen et al, 1973) defined by normoblastic multinuclearity, bizarre morphology, anisocytosis, poikilocytosis, hemolytic anemia, and, most characteristic, red cells that are abnormally susceptible to acid hemolysis by about 60% of human sera. As noted (p. 596), HEMPAS cells are distinguished from PNH cells by

their failure to hemolyze in the sugar-water test. HEMPAS red cells are also hemolyzed by anti-**i** and anti-**I** antibodies. HEMPAS red blood cells have enhanced i and depressed H antigens so that they react strongly with anti-**i** and weakly with anti-**H** lectins (Bird and Wingham, 1976). Inheritance of type II CDA is autosomal recessive. Type III is probably inherited as an autosomal dominant and is the most heterogeneous, with multinuclearity of the normoblasts as the main common feature (Goudsmit et al, 1972). A possible fourth type (type IV) has been described by Benjamin et al (1975).

Hemolysis of HEMPAS cells is thought to be caused by an alloantibody (anti-HEMPAS) detectable only on the cells of HEMPAS patients. HEMPAS cells are more sensitive than normal cells to lysis by anti-**I** and complement (Rosse et al, 1974).

High phosphatidylcholine hemolytic anemia (HPCHA)

HPCHA represents another familial lipid disorder characterized by a faulty transfer of esterified fatty acid from phosphatidylcholine to phosphatidylethanolamine, with increased cation permeability (Shohet et al, 1973).

Mechanical fragmentation

Disruption of erythrocytes by mechanical trauma is seen in three clinically important situations: (1) in valvular cardiac disease and after cardiac surgery with insertion of prosthetic valves, (2) in microangiopathic hemolytic anemia, and (3) in exertional (march) hemoglobinuria.

From cardiac valves

The fragmentation of erythrocytes by extreme turbulence of the flowing blood is now well authenticated. It has been shown that mechanical hemolysis follows insertion of the Hufnagel aortic ball-valve or the Starr-Edwards aortic valve, and it has been suggested that improper approximation of the valve to the endocardial ring leaves a narrow space through which red cells pass at high velocity so that they are mechanically damaged. However, mechanical fragmentation also occurs in severe aortic stenosis prior to any surgical intervention. Shortened erythrocyte survival and the presence of large numbers of malformed red cells in the peripheral blood are evidence for mechanical hemolysis. In addition to turbulence trauma, there is evidence of unexplained immunologic reactions. Pirofsky et al (1965) found positive antiglobulin tests in six out of seven patients who had cardiac surgery. In some cases autoantibodies of anti-**hr″** specificity have been found. In another study Polesky et al (1969) found positive antiglobulin tests in about one third of 250 patients undergoing cardiac surgery. It is unlikely, however, that immunohemolysis plays an important role. There is no doubt that the chief mechanism is mechanical. There is no relationship between fragmentation and the materials used for prosthetic valves.

Microangiopathic hemolytic anemia

The term "microangiopathic hemolytic anemia" was suggested by Brain (1970) as a unifying concept for the hemolytic anemia found in association with thrombotic thrombocytopenic purpura, hemolytic-uremic syndrome in children, renal cortical necrosis, and some cases of malignant hypertension. The common denominator in these diseases is small-vessel disease. The peripheral blood smear shows typically fragmented or disrupted erythrocytes (schizocytes). It is postulated that at least some of the damage to the erythrocytes results from "clothesline-like" trauma to the cell as it is carried against strands of fibrin (Bull and Kuhn, 1970). The hemolytic-uremic syndrome has all the features of microangiopathic hemolytic anemia. The term is commonly used when the disease affects infants or young children, but it is not a different entity. The disease called thrombotic thrombocytopenic purpura is another that belongs in the group of microangiopathic hemolytic anemias. All these diseases or syndromes have in common the intravascular deposition of fibrin (Chapter 7).

Exertional (march) hemoglobinuria

Exertional, or march, hemoglobinuria was first described in 1881 in a soldier after a strenuous march. Many cases have been studied since then, and for many years the condition's pathogenesis defied an explanation. Davidson (1969) showed convincingly that the hemoglobinuria results from mechanical injury to blood in the feet during strenuous running on a hard surface. Bernard et al (1975) describe the association of march hemoglobinuria with transient deficiency of glutathione reductase and glutathione peroxidase.

The spleen and liver in sequestration hemolysis

Erythrocytes whose surface membrane has been damaged or altered hemolyze either in the bloodstream or after sequestration in the spleen and liver (Bowdler, 1975). Hemolysis in the bloodstream without sequestration is usually explosive and accompanied by shock, chills, abdominal pain, fever, hemoglobinemia, and hemoglobinuria, the classic syndrome of a hemolytic transfusion reaction. Hemolysis that follows sequestration is usually slow, and none of the signs and symptoms of acute hemolysis are found. Because hemolysis is gradual, there is rarely hemoglobinuria, the hemoglobin being removed by binding to haptoglobin.

A number of investigators have shown that, as a general rule, the sequestration of sensitized cells is greater in the liver than in the spleen, particularly when the sensitizing antibody is potent and of high titer. The spleen is generally responsible for sequestration and hemolysis of cells sensitized by weaker antibodies. In fact, both the liver and spleen contain major components of the RES. For clinical purposes there is no reason to separate hepatic from splenic sequestration, except that the spleen is surgically expendable. In hemolytic disease both are involved in the hemolysis of damaged cells. In some cases, such as in autoimmune hemolytic anemia of the warm-acting antibody type, splenectomy is followed by enlargement of the liver, since this organ assumes the major role in sequestration hemolysis.

We do not know how the cells of the RES recognize a cell that is to be destroyed. Sequestration hemolysis in the spleen may be, in part, only an exaggeration of the normal mechanism for disposing of senescent erythrocytes. Erythrocytes that are already damaged then would be merely more susceptible to lysis. Stasis undoubtedly plays a major role,

regardless of what type of damage the erythrocytes have suffered (Jandl and Cooper, 1972). With stasis there is reduced accessibility to glucose, a reduction in glycolysis, damage to the surface membrane, and loss of the normal shape and plasticity. Some postulate that a damaged membrane makes erythrocytes stick to reticuloendothelial cells, and there is evidence that erythrocytes damaged by diverse means such as antibodies, heat, inhibitors of sulfhydryl groups, protamine, or hexadimethrine bromide (Polybrene) are sequestered in the spleeen. Since reticuloendothelial cells cannot recognize, as far as we know, molecular differences in the hemoglobin inside the cell or distinguish normal from abnormal shapes, it follows that ultimately the recognition phenomenon is dependent on a damaged erythrocytic membrane.

Erythrophagocytosis

In addition to direct lysis or agglutination followed by delayed lysis, there is a third method by which sensitized erythrocytes may be destroyed—erythrophagocytosis. This is the ingestion of sensitized erythrocytes by polymorphonuclear leukocytes (Fig. 13-7), monocytes, and eosinophils. It is an occurrence not uncommon in hemolytic anemia, having been observed in the peripheral blood in a variety of hemolytic states. It can be produced in vitro by incubating sensitized erythrocytes with leukocytes.

Erythrophagocytosis by splenic macrophages is characteristic of the histopathology of the spleen in hemolytic anemias. There is little correlation between the degree of splenic erythrophagocytosis and the severity of the hemolytic state. Furthermore splenic erythrophagocytosis is sometimes seen when there is no evidence of hemolytic disease. It is difficult to assign a major role to splenic erythrophagocytosis if one takes the histopathologic evidence at face value. There is another very interesting possibility. Flanagan (1955), working in our laboratory, has shown that leukocytes which have ingested erythrocytes in vitro are markedly susceptible to mechanical trauma. If this is also true in vivo, then two interesting possibilities are presented. First, erythrophagocytosis may be an important method of erythrocyte destruction, and our failure to see this phenomenon more often may be because of the short survival or erythrophagocytes. Second, it may account for a simultaneous reduction in leukocytes, since these would be destroyed in considerable numbers. This is a possibility worth considering, since there is no completely satisfactory explanation of the leukopenia that occasionally accompanies immunologic disorders.

Erythrophagocytosis is at times very prominent in preparations made to demonstrate LE cells. It can be found in both the presence and the absence of LE and LE-like cells. We do not know if erythrophagocytosis in these cases can be assumed to indicate occult hemolytic disease or some other immune phenomenon, but we find it to be common not only in disseminated LE but also in rheumatoid arthritis and rheumatic fever.

METABOLISM OF HEMOGLOBIN AND BILE PIGMENTS IN HEMOLYTIC DISEASE

The basic aspects of hemoglobin metabolism are discussed in Chapter 10. At this time we are concerned with

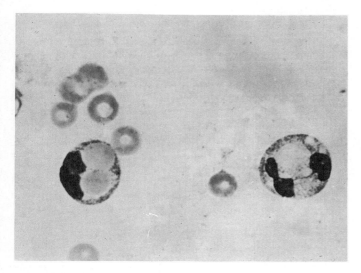

Fig. 13-7. Erythrophagocytosis of antibody-coated red blood cells by neutrophils, peripheral blood. (Wright's stain; ×950.)

some quantitative aspects referring specifically to hemolytic disease. These are basic to an appreciation of the value and limitations of laboratory tests concerned with any phase of hemoglobin metabolism.

Hemoglobinemia

When moderately accelerated erythrocyte destruction occurs, the rate of hemoglobin liberation is accelerated, and increased amounts of bile pigments must then be excreted. The pathways of hemoglobin breakdown are the same as under physiologic conditions, but the quantities involved are greater. If hemolysis is acute and massive, the rate of hemoglobin liberation is so high that large amounts of free hemoglobin are spilled into the blood. This is called hemoglobinemia. Plasma normally contains up to about 5 mg/dl (0.05 Gm/l) hemoglobin, but following acute intravascular hemolysis the plasma hemoglobin concentration may be many times this amount.

Free hemoglobin in plasma is quickly bound to haptoglobin to form a stable complex. Uncombined hemoglobin is found only after the haptoglobin is used up, in which case it is cleared by the kidneys and is found as free hemoglobin in the urine (hemoglobinuria). Hemoglobin-haptoglobin complex is cleared from the blood principally by the liver and bone marrow.

Methemalbumin

The fate of free hemoglobin depends, in part, on the level of concentration reached in the blood. At levels above about 135 mg/dl (1.35 Gm/l), hemoglobin is partially degraded in the bloodstream, forming a pigment that unites with plasma albumin to form methemalbumin (Fairley's pigment). It is probable that methemoglobin is a precursor of methemalbumin. Methemoglobin dissociates into heme and globin, and heme is bound either to hemopexin, forming a hemopexin-heme complex that is picked up by parenchymal liver cells (Müller-Eberhard, 1970), or to albumin to form methemalbumin (Sears, 1970). Methemoglobin in plasma shows an absorption band at 632 mμ. If the plasma contains methemalbumin, it can be identified by treating the plasma with

ammonium sulfide and ether, following which an ammonium chromogen is formed that has an intense absorption band at 558 mμ. This procedure is known as Schumm's test (Rosen et al, 1969).

The presence of methemalbumin in the blood is an indication that significant amounts of free hemoglobin were present at one time. Therefore methemalbumin is commonly found following severe intravascular hemolysis. Methemalbumin is not cleared from the blood in spite of occasionally reaching high concentrations. Its fate seems to be similar to that of the hemoglobin degraded by reticuloendothelial cells in that it is eventually broken down to bilirubin and other normal end products.

Hemoglobinuria

If the plasma hemoglobin concentration is greater than about 135 mg/dl (1.35 Gm/l), a second mechanism of elimination comes into effect. Renal clearance from the blood and excretion of free hemoglobin in the urine produce hemoglobinuria (see discussion on haptoglobin, p. 464).

Hemosiderinuria

In the course of excretion some hemoglobin is taken up by the tubular cells in the kidneys and broken down to hemosiderin. Following massive intravascular hemolysis sections of kidney show hemosiderin deposits in the tubular cells as well as hemoglobin casts in the tubules. Later the tubular cells that contain hemosiderin may be desquamated and are then found in the urinary sediment. Disintegration of the hemosiderin-containing tubular cells may liberate the hemosiderin granules, which can then be identified in the urinary sediment, to which they impart a rusty color. The hemosiderin-containing sediment gives a positive reaction for iron. The term "hemosiderinuria" is used when hemosiderin is present in the urine.

Quantitative relationships

The predictable way in which hemoglobin is broken down has led to intensive studies directed at establishing a quantitative relationship between the amount of hemoglobin destroyed and the amount of bile pigment excreted. If a constant and reliable relationship existed, it would be possible to determine accurately the amount of hemoglobin destroyed by measuring the end products. Unfortunately the relationship is only roughly quantitative.

Source of bile pigments

It is probable that some of the bile pigments excreted are derived from substances other than hemoglobin. One gram of hemoglobin theoretically yields 35 mg of bilirubin, a proportion that has been found to hold true in dogs with biliary fistulas. Assuming that a normal person destroys 6.25 Gm of hemoglobin each day (1/120 of the total hemoglobin), 220 mg of bilirubin should be formed daily and excreted as bilirubin and other end products. This is roughly equivalent to 35 mg of urobilinogen per day per 100 Gm of hemoglobin, or approximately 250 mg of urobilinogen per day. This amount can seldom be recovered, the daily excretion varying from 10 to 20 mg/day/100 Gm of hemoglobin. The major part of the difference is probably caused by the further degradation of urobilinogen into dipyrrole compounds that takes place in the bowel. The dipyrroles do not give a color reaction with Ehrlich's aldehyde reagent.

Studies with radioactive tracers have revealed another discrepancy. When glycine containing ^{15}N is fed to experimental animals, some of the isotopic nitrogen is used in the synthesis of hemoglobin. When this hemoglobin is broken down, ^{15}N-containing urobilinogen can be recovered in the feces. About 10% to 20% of the ^{15}N urobilinogen cannot be accounted for on the basis of being derived from hemoglobin. This urobilinogen is excreted before there is time for hemoglobin to be broken down and is therefore called *early-appearing urobilinogen*. Even larger amounts of nonhemoglobin are excreted in abnormal states; e.g., about 40% of the total excretion in pernicious anemia is nonhemoglobin urobilinogen. Its source is not known, and suggestions that it is derived from imperfect hemoglobin synthesis, excess protoporphyrin, early destruction of hemoglobin, or nonhemoglobin-derived bilirubin are all equally likely.

Fluctuations in pigment excretion

A third difficulty is introduced by the unpredictable daily fluctuations in urinary and fecal urobilinogen excretion. This is seen in normal persons and has no satisfactory explanation. In addition, there are abnormal situations that interfere with quantitative bile pigment degradation or excretion. Biirubin is cleared from the blood by the liver, so that abnormal liver function may markedly reduce the amount of bilirubin reaching the intestine and thus reduce the amount of fecal urobilinogen. At the same time, 35% to 70% of the urobilinogen formed in the intestine is normally reabsorbed and excreted in part in the urine, and the remainder is taken up by the liver. In the presence of liver disease reabsorbed urobilinogen is not cleared from the blood by the liver, and relatively large amounts are excreted in the urine. Degradation of bilirubin to urobilinogen depends chiefly on bacterial action. Fecal urobilinogen excretion will be decreased, therefore, if the intestinal flora is altered by antibiotics. Variations in intestinal motility affect the time available for bacterial action in the bowel, so that diarrhea and constipation account for other possible variables.

Pigment excretion related to total hemoglobin

Because of the variables discussed, the measurement of pigment excretion in absolute units is of limited value. It is also obvious that the amount of bile pigment excreted is proportional not only to the rate of hemoglobin breakdown but also to the amount of hemoglobin available; e.g., a child with hemolytic disease will excrete less fecal urobilinogen than an adult with hemolytic anemia of the same severity, since the child has less total circulating hemoglobin.

"Corrected" fecal urobilinogen excretion

An approximate correction can be made by relating fecal urobilinogen to body weight and blood hemoglobin level (Table 13-7) as follows:

"Corrected" daily fecal urobilinogen =

$$\text{Measured daily fecal urobilinogen} \times$$

$$\frac{\text{Normal Hb}}{\text{Patient's Hb}} \times \frac{\text{Normal weight}}{\text{Patient's weight}}$$

or

"Corrected" daily fecal urobilinogen (mg/24 hr) =

$$\frac{\text{Measured fecal urobilinogen} \times (\text{mg/24 hr})}{\dfrac{15 \text{ Gm/dl}}{\text{Patient's Hb (Gm/dl)}} \times \dfrac{70 \text{ kg}}{\text{Patient's weight (kg)}}}$$

Hemolytic index

Fecal urobilinogen can be more simply related to total circulating hemoglobin, the ratio being the hemolytic index, as follows:

$$\text{Hemolytic index} = \frac{\text{Fecal urobilinogen (mg/day)} \times 100}{\text{Total circulating hemoglobin (Gm)}}$$

The normal hemolytic index is 10 to 20. The usefulness of this ratio is illustrated in Table 13-7. Note that the severity of the disease is the same in these cases, as judged from the hemolytic index, but that the observed fecal urobilinogen values alone vary with the body weight and hemoglobin concentration. The decreased values for fecal urobilinogen can be, by themselves, misleading. Only when the hemolytic index is calculated does the true picture become apparent.

Fecal urobilinogen

The amount of fecal urobilinogen excreted is a rough, but useful measure of the amount of hemoglobin broken down. When more hemoglobin is destroyed, more bilirubin will be formed, and subsequent degradation of bilirubin will yield higher fecal urobilinogen levels. As discussed previously, it is not possible to express the relationship of hemoglobin to urobilinogen in an exact quantitative fashion. Nevertheless a rough proportionality exists when fecal urobilinogen values are interpreted on the basis of the patient's hemoglobin and body weight or total circulating hemoglobin. The higher the ratio of fecal urobilinogen to circulating hemoglobin, the higher the rate of hemoglobin destruction.

NORMAL VALUES. The amount of urobilinogen excreted in the feces by normal persons varies from day to day. Control data from our laboratory give us a normal average of 140 mg of fecal urobilinogen per 24 hours, with a standard

Table 13-7. Examples of application of "corrected" urobilinogen excretion and hemolytic index in hemolytic anemia

Patient weight (kg)*	Hemoglobin (Gm/dl)	Total circulating hemoglobin (Gm)	Fecal urobilinogen (mg/24 hr)		Hemolytic index
			Observed	Corrected	
Normal 70	15	735	150	150	20.4
No. 1 70	10	490	350	525	71.4
No. 2 40	10	280	200	525	71.4
No. 3 40	5	140	100	525	71.4
No. 4 20	10	140	100	525	71.4
No. 5 20	5	70	50	525	71.4

*Patients 1 through 5 have hemolytic disease, but not all have an abnormally high uncorrected fecal urobilinogen.

deviation of 47 mg, so that 95% of our normals fall in the range of 46 to 234 mg/24 hours. Normal values reported by others are 40 to 280 mg/day (Watson and Hawkinson, 1947). Determinations of fecal urobilinogen in single-stool specimens show such a wide range of normal values that they are practically useless—76.4 to 520 mg/100 Gm of feces.

LIMITATIONS. It is probable that much of the normal variation is accounted for by changes in intestinal motility and bacterial action. Hypermotility and diarrhea reduce the time for bacterial fermentation and therefore the amount of urobilinogen formed from the bilirubin. Constipation allows time for further breakdown of urobilinogen to dipyrrole and monopyrrole compounds that do not give a color reaction with Ehrlich's aldehyde reagent. Some variations may also be caused by variable rates of intestinal absorption of urobilinogen, although it is probable that under normal conditions urobilinogen is eventually returned to the intestinal excretory cycle.

Daily fluctuations may be avoided by pooling the feces obtained over a period of several days, as suggested by Watson and Hawkinson (1947). They recommend that fecal urobilinogen be determined on a thoroughly mixed 4–day stool specimen. There is no denying that this recommendation is sound, but the range of normals for 4-day collections is not much smaller than for 1-day specimens. The difficulties encountered in collecting and storing a 4-day specimen, plus the technical problem of thoroughly mixing the specimen before sampling, make us reluctant to adopt this method for routine studies. We feel that the information to be gained from the determination of fecal urobilinogen is generally available from serial determinations on 24-hour specimens.

Urinary urobilinogen

About 50% (35% to 70%) of the urobilinogen formed in the intestine is absorbed and returned to the liver. Normally it is partly reexcreted by the liver cells into the bowel and partly cleared from the blood and excreted in the urine. Therefore the measurable urobilinogen in the urine represents the portion reabsorbed from the bowel plus that cleared from the blood by the kidneys. The more urobilinogen absorbed from the bowel, the higher the output of urinary urobilinogen. The situation in hemolytic disease may be thought of as an exaggeration of the normal process, leading to increased amounts of bilirubin in the bowel, increased urobilinogen formed and excreted in the feces, and increased urobilinogen reabsorbed and excreted in the urine.

The amount of urobilinogen excreted in the urine depends not only on the amount present in the intestine but also on the rate of absorption and the efficiency with which it is cleared from the blood by the liver and kidneys. The daily and hourly fluctuations are even more striking than those in fecal urobilinogen excretion. Urinary urobilinogen probably depends to a greater extent on the efficiency of liver function than on the amount of urobilinogen formed in the bowel. Even in the presence of normal liver function, unexplained differences between fecal and urinary urobilinogen have been described. We have noted several cases of frank hemolytic disease in which striking increases in fecal urobilinogen were accompanied by normal urinary urobilinogen excretion. On the other hand, increases in urinary urobilinogen are the rule in the presence of parenchymatous liver disease, whether or not there is accelerated hemolysis.

COLLECTION OF URINE SPECIMENS. Three types of urine specimens are used for determining urobilinogen: (1) a random, or first morning, specimen, (2) a 24-hour specimen, and (3) a specimen representing the total urine output between the hours of 2 and 4 P.M. Determinations may be semiquantitative or quantitative.

DETERMINATION BY DILUTION OF A RANDOM SAMPLE. The addition of Ehrlich's reagent to urine containing urobilinogen produces a cherry-red color. This reaction is not specific for urobilinogen (p. 471). If the urine specimen is serially diluted, a point will be reached at which the color reaction can no longer be obtained. In a normal random specimen this is reached at a urine dilution of 1:10 or 1:20. Obviously, if dilution is carried further and the color reaction still occurs, the original specimen contained a larger than normal amount of urobilinogen. Thus a semiquantitative method for estimating urinary urobilinogen concentration is provided, the urine dilution being an expression of urobilinogen concentration. An increase above 1:20 is considered abnormal.

Although this method is simple, it is not recommended. Not only does the concentration of urobilinogen vary because of the factors previously discussed, but also the specific gravity of the urine affects it. A concentrated morning specimen therefore contains a higher concentration of urobilinogen than a later dilute specimen, depending on the ability of the kidneys to concentrate and dilute the urine. These variables markedly limit the significance of determinations on random specimens.

TWENTY-FOUR–HOUR URINE SPECIMEN. Fluctuation in urine concentration may be avoided by determining urinary urobilinogen in a 24-hour specimen. Normally 2 to 4 mg (3.4 to 68 μM/24 hr) of urobilinogen is excreted in the urine in 24 hours. In our laboratory we have found the average normal value to be 2.5 mg/24 hr (4.23 μM/24 hr) and the SD 0.5 mg (0.09 μM).

TWO-HOUR URINE SPECIMEN. In most cases maximum urinary urobilinogen excretion is between 2 and 4 P.M. For this reason a standard 2-hour collection is used instead of the 24-hour collection. It has been widely adopted, but it must be appreciated that in some cases the 2-hour excretion does not parallel the 24-hour one. It does have the advantage of simplifying the method of collection and reducing the volume of urine to easily handled amounts. Our normal for the standard 2-hour test is a mean of 1.5 mg (2.5 μM) and the SD 0.35 mg (0.6 μM).

Specificity of Ehrlich's aldehyde reaction

One criticism of all quantitative methods for determining urobilinogen, fecal as well as urinary, is the lack of specificity of the reaction with Ehrlich's aldehyde. The color is produced not only by urobilinogen but also by porphobilinogen and by tetrapyrrole degradation products of bilirubin such as mesobilirubinogen, *d*-urobilin, *d*-urobilinogen, and mesobilene-*B* (see Table 10-11, p. 471). The reaction measures all these chromogens, not urobilinogen alone. Therefore it has been proposed that the results be reported in terms of Ehrlich units rather than in milligrams of urobilinogen. In general, I am opposed to the use of arbitrary units, which in other situations have been responsible for unnecessary confusion. I prefer to report the results as milligrams of urobilinogen, with the understanding that what is being measured is *urobilinogen equivalents*.

Bilirubin in serum

When the rate of hemoglobin breakdown is normal, the total serum bilirubin is 0.3 to 0.8 mg/dl (5.1 to 13.7 μM/l) and is seldom higher than 1.5 mg/dl (25.7 μM/l). Of this, 0.1 to 0.2 mg/dl (1.7 to 3.4 μM/l) is of the direct-reacting type, the remainder being indirect reacting. Bilirubin, formed in reticuloendothelial cells, is liberated into the bloodstream and subsequently cleared from the blood by the liver (Chapter 10). It is probable that clearance requires several trips through the liver, the average survival time for bilirubin in the blood being about 1½ hours.

REGULATION OF BILIRUBIN CONCENTRATION IN SERUM. The bilirubin concentration of the serum is determined by three factors: (1) the amount of hemoglobin broken down, (2) the clearing efficiency of the liver, and (3) the presence or absence of bile duct obstruction.

As in the case of other bile pigments, the amount of bilirubin formed is proportional to the amount of hemoglobin that is degraded as well as to the rate of hemolysis; e.g., a normal person with a total circulating hemoglobin of about 750 Gm produces about 250 mg of bilirubin each day. This is cleared from the blood at a rate which results in a normal serum bilirubin concentration of about 0.5 mg/dl (8.6 μM/l). This represents the normal situation, 1/120 of the total hemoglobin, or about 6.25 Gm, producing 250 mg of bili-

rubin. If erythrocyte survival is shortened, the factor determining the amount of bilirubin produced is the amount of hemoglobin destroyed and not the rate of destruction per se. Twice as much bilirubin will be formed if survival is half the normal and the total circulating hemoglobin is approximately normal. On the other hand, half the normal survival and half the normal total circulating hemoglobin will produce a normal amount of bilirubin each day. It can be seen that hemolytic disease is not necessarily accompanied by an increased serum bilirubin concentration. When more bilirubin is produced, more is cleared from the blood by the liver and excreted into the intestine. In spite of this, the rate of clearance cannot always be increased to such an extent as to maintain the serum bilirubin concentration at a normal value. When the bilirubin concentration in the serum increases above 2 mg/dl (34 μM/l), *hyperbilirubinemia* results. An increase in serum bilirubin can also result from inability of the liver to clear bilirubin from the blood, either because of intrinsic hepatic damage or because of blockage of the bile ducts.

HYPERBILIRUBINEMIA AND JAUNDICE. Hyperbilirubinemia of moderate degree, below 3 to 4 mg/dl (51 to 68 μM/l), is not accompanied by the clinical sign of jaundice. Since the serum bilirubin in most chronic hemolytic anemias seldom exceeds concentrations of 4 to 5 mg/dl (68 to 86 μM/l), jaundice is not a common sign of chronic hemolytic disease. Bilirubin concentrations of 5 to 10 mg/dl (86 to 171 μM/l) are not uncommon in acute hemolytic episodes, but levels above 10 mg/dl (171 μM/l) are seldom encountered, except in the hemolytic disease of the newborn or in massive intravascular hemolysis following the transfusion of incompatible blood. Jaundice usually follows 1 or 2 days after the rise in serum bilirubin concentration, since time is required for diffusion of bilirubin into the tissues.

PARTITION OF BILIRUBIN. Partition of total serum bilirubin into *direct reacting* (1 minute) and *indirect reacting* (total minus 1 minute) may be helpful in distinguishing the jaundice of hemolytic disease from that of simple bile duct obstruction. When hyperbilirubinemia is caused by hemolytic disease, it might be expected that larger amounts of indirect-reacting bilirubin would be present in the blood. However, the increase in total serum bilirubin is almost never caused by a rise in the indirect-reacting bilirubin complex alone. An increase in the direct-reacting fraction will also be found, reflecting active conversion by the liver of the increased amounts of indirect-reacting bilirubin present in the blood. It is true, however, that in most uncomplicated cases of hemolytic disease the indirect fraction is greater than the direct, in contrast to the situation in obstructive jaundice in which the increase is chiefly, although not exclusively, in the direct-reacting bilirubin.

LABORATORY DIAGNOSIS OF HEMOLYTIC DISEASE
Clinical-pathologic approach to the patient

The complexities of pathogenesis, discussed in an earlier section, have resulted in a large number of tests useful in the study of hemolytic disease. Without a logical and pertinent approach the many tests available may be confusing rather than helpful. When they are used indiscriminately, one flounders around in a mass of data impossible to interpret. Before discussing the tests and the findings in individual diseases, we should consider how one decides which tests are indicated in various situations. The approach to the patient can be divided into two steps. First, it should be established, or suspected, that hemolytic disease is present. Second, the proper laboratory tests should be done to establish an exact pathogenetic diagnosis.

The suspicion that hemolytic anemia exists is based on four types of clinical and laboratory data (Table 13-8).

The presenting feature of hemolytic anemia is commonly anemia for which there is no obvious explanation. The suspicion that the process is hemolytic is strengthened by the presence of reticulocytosis (reticulocyte count and polychromatophilia of erythrocytes on smear) or hyperbilirubinemia. These findings suggest that the anemia is caused by excessive destruction of erythrocytes and that there is no failure of erythropoiesis, as evidenced by the reticulocytosis.

The history can be helpful not only in establishing the possibility of hemolytic anemia but also as a general guide to possible pathogenesis. A history of familial anemia is strongly suggestive. The age of the patient should be taken into account, since in a young person one might suspect a congenital or hereditary type of hemolytic anemia, whereas in an older person there is a greater possibility that the anemia is of the acquired type. One should determine whether the anemia is acute or chronic. The history of blood transfusion is important not only from the standpoint of possible isoimmunization but also as an indication of the chronicity of the anemia and, from the amounts of blood transfused, its severity. Since hemolysis is sometimes precipitated by the

Table 13-8. Clinical and laboratory data that suggest possibility of hemolytic disease

> **I.** General laboratory information
>   **A.** Anemia, etiology not obvious
>   **B.** Reticulocytosis
>   **C.** Hyperbilirubinemia
> **II.** History
>   **A.** Familial anemia
>   **B.** History of jaundice
>   **C.** History of red or brown urine
>   **D.** Acute or chronic anemia
>   **E.** History of blood transfusion
>   **F.** Intake of potentially hemolytic drug
>   **G.** Status after cardiac surgery
> **III.** Physical findings
>   **A.** Jaundice
>   **B.** Splenomegaly
>   **C.** Hepatomegaly
>   **D.** Lymphadenopathy
>   **E.** Valvular heart disease
>   **F.** Race and national derivation of patient
> **IV.** Concurrent disease
>   **A.** Viral infection
>   **B.** Bacterial infection
>   **C.** Lymphoma
>   **D.** Leukemia
>   **E.** Collagen disease
>   **F.** Liver disease

intake of drugs, it is essential to obtain a thorough history of drug intake. A history of red urine suggests hemoglobinuria and, if found, should be related to exposure to cold, strenuous exercise, and sleep pattern.

The physical findings alone are not especially characteristic in hemolytic anemia. However, as one progresses from the history through the physical examination, certain signs begin to assume significance when combined with the preliminary laboratory data and the historical findings. Splenomegaly and hepatomegaly are found commonly in various hemolytic anemias. Sometimes there is lymphadenopathy. Jaundice is the physical manifestation of hyperbilirubinemia; it may be absent if the serum bilirubin concentration is elevated only moderately. The race and national derivation of the patient are pertinent, since the most common hemolytic anemias in blacks are Hb-S hemoglobinopathy and G-6-PD deficiency. On the other hand, favism has never been reported in blacks. Orientals have a higher incidence of certain other hemoglobinopathies, such as Hb E and Hb H. People of Mediterranean origin have the highest incidence of thalassemia.

Finally, hemolytic anemia may be associated with intercurrent disease such as viral infections, bacterial infections, lymphomas, and leukemias. This type of symptomatic (secondary) hemolytic anemia is sometimes the first manifestation of one of these diseases. The presence of predisposing disease often suggests that the accompanying anemia is of the hemolytic type.

Importance of the peripheral blood smear

Good hematologic diagnosis and practice begin with a careful examination of the peripheral blood smear. The laboratory approach to the hemolytic anemias provides an excellent opportunity to put this into practice. Although other approaches are possible, the findings on the blood smear can be used to establish probable diagnoses and the direction for further investigation (Table 13-9). In many instances the abnormalities noted on the smear provide the first suspicion that hemolytic disease is present.

Erythrocyte count and hemoglobin concentration

Hemolytic disease and shortened erythrocyte survival are not necessarily accompanied by anemia. There can be, in some of the chronic hemolytic states, only a mild anemia if the compensatory erythroid hyperplasia in the marrow is sufficient to balance the increased rate of erythrocyte destruction. By definition, a hemolytic anemia is always accompanied by a significantly low erythrocyte count and hemoglobin concentration.

Anemia ranges from moderate to severe, depending on the nature of the disease process and the degree of compensatory hyperplasia in the marrow. Fluctuations are not uncommon in autoimmune hemolytic anemias, and the course of the disease is characterized by spontaneous remissions, during which evidence of gross hemolysis is absent.

A rapid drop in the erythrocyte count from a previously mild anemic level is indicative of a *hemolytic crisis*. The so-called aplastic type of crisis is extremely rare and is characterized by a low reticulocyte count, whereas a crisis with

Table 13-9. Findings on peripheral blood smears as an index of most probable diagnosis and guide to further investigation

Type I: Hemolytic disease present; erythrocytes generally normocytic and normochromic; some elliptocytes may be present
  A. Probability: Nonspherocytic hemolytic anemia
    1. Etiology: Enzyme deficiency
      a. Laboratory investigation
        (1) Autohemolysis test
        (2) Heinz body test
        (3) GSH stability test
        (4) Ascorbate test
        (5) Fluorescence test for G-6-PD deficiency
        (6) Methemoglobin reduction test for G-6-PD deficiency
        (7) Fluorescence tests for other enzymatic deficiencies
        (8) Quantitative enzyme assays
    2. Etiology: Unstable hemoglobin
      a. Laboratory investigation
        (1) Autohemolysis test
        (2) Measurement of methemoglobin
        (3) Heinz body test
        (4) Heat-stability test
    3. Etiology: Autoimmune hemolytic anemia
      a. Laboratory investigation
        (1) Autohemolysis test
        (2) Direct antiglobulin test
        (3) Indirect antiglobulin test
        (4) Special serologic procedures
    4. Etiology: PNH, PCH, or HEMPAS
      a. Laboratory investigation
        (1) Acid serum test
        (2) Sugar-water test
        (3) Bone marrow biopsy
Type II: Hemolytic disease present; microspherocytes present
  A. Probability: Hereditary spherocytosis
    1. Laboratory investigation
      a. Autohemolysis test with ATP and glucose added
      b. Osmotic fragility—fresh, incubated, and with added glucose
  B. Probability: Isoimmune hemolytic disease

    1. Laboratory investigation
      a. Blood grouping
      b. Direct antiglobulin test
      c. Indirect antiglobulin test
      d. Special serologic investigations
  C. Probability: Autoimmune hemolytic disease
    1. Laboratory investigation
      a. Autohemolysis test
      b. Direct antiglobulin test
      c. Indirect antiglobulin test
      d. Special serologic investigations
Type III: Hemolytic anemia present; numerous target cells present; hypochromia and microcytosis
  A. Probability: Hemoglobinopathy
    1. Laboratory investigation
      a. Test for erythrocyte sickling
      b. Measurement of Hb F
      c. Measurement of Hb A_2
      d. Hemoglobin electrophoresis
Type IV: Hemolytic disease present; many disrupted or distorted erythrocytes present
  A. Probability: Microangiopathic hemolytic anemia
    1. Laboratory investigation
      a. Autohemolysis test
      b. Quantitative fibrinogen
      c. Other coagulation studies for DIC syndrome
      d. Direct antiglobulin test
Type V: Hemolytic disease present; erythrocytes show acanthocytosis
  A. Probability: Acanthocytosis
    1. Laboratory investigation
      a. Lipoprotein electrophoresis
Type VI: Hemolytic disease present; half or more of the erythrocytes show elliptocytosis
  A. Probability: Elliptocytic hemolytic anemia
Type VII: Hemolytic disease present; erythrocytes show stomatocytic malformation
  A. Probability: Hereditary stomatocytosis

---

sudden hemolysis is followed by reticulocytosis. Severe crises are accompanied by dramatic clinical findings such as elevated temperature, nausea, vomiting, abdominal pain, tachycardia, and shock. According to some authors (Leikin, 1957) the aplastic type of crisis is characterized by an acute erythroid hypoplasia of the marrow and a maturation arrest of the granulocytic and thrombocytic elements, but in most cases hypoplasia of the marrow cannot be demonstrated. In some of the chronic hemolytic anemias one occasionally encounters a change from anemia to erythrocytosis. Although the concurrence of true polycythemia vera and hemolytic disease cannot be ruled out, it does seem that in some cases the erythroid proliferation gets out of control to produce a situation in which polycythemic red cell counts are encountered.

Leukocyte count

The leukocyte count usually contributes little to the diagnosis of chronic hemolytic disease. When the leukocyte count is abnormal, it usually reflects the disease underlying autoimmune hemolytic anemia, i.e., leukocytosis in leukemia or leukopenia in systemic LE. Chronic hemolytic anemias are usually characterized by normal or moderately elevated leukocyte counts. Striking elevations of the leukocyte count, with neutrophilia and a shift to the left, usually accompany more severe degrees of hemolysis. In an acute hemolytic crisis or following acute hemolysis from any cause, the leukocyte count may be strikingly elevated and at times reaches leukemoid levels. The very high leukocyte count plus the presence of myelocytes in the peripheral blood sometimes suggest the diagnosis of leukemia. An elevated leukocyte count is a reflection of increased medullary or extramedullary leukopoietic activity.

Leukopenia is occasionally encountered. It is sometimes seen in PNH and in idiopathic acquired hemolytic anemia. The combination of anemia with leukopenia suggests hypoplasia of the bone marrow, but in these cases the marrow is usually found to be normal to hypercellular.

Platelet count

The platelet count, like the leukocyte count, is usually normal or elevated. When the platelet count is elevated, it is again a reflection of hyperactivity of the bone marrow. Thrombocytopenia is common in PNH. Evans et al (1965) called attention to the coexistence of acute hemolytic anemia and thrombocytopenic purpura, each presumably caused by antibodies (Evans' syndrome, Fig. 13-25). Thrombocytopenia may also reflect underlying disease in secondary autoimmune hemolytic anemia, as in disseminated LE.

Reticulocyte count

The reticulocyte count, as measured, is expressed as the percent of red cells that contain stainable reticulum. Normally enough reticulocytes leave the bone marrow to maintain the number of circulating erythrocytes at a constant level. The normal reticulocyte count is 1% to 1.5%, with 3% as the upper limit of normal. (Deiss and Kurth, 1970, give the following normal values: 0.8% to 2.5% in men and 0.8% to 4.1% in women.)

The expression of reticulocytes as a percentile can be misleading when the red cell count is abnormal. A more accurate expression is in terms of the absolute number of reticulocytes (% reticulocytes $\times$ RBC count/mm^3 or/l). The absolute count ranges normally between 50,000 and 150,000/mm^3 (5×10^{10}/l and 15×10^{10}/l). Reticulocytosis is present when the upper limit is exceeded.

Reticulocytosis is one of the most important features of hemolytic anemia. The degree of reticulocytosis varies in the different types of hemolytic anemia and also is related to the course of the disease. In the more chronic types of hemolytic anemia, such as hereditary spherocytosis and sickle cell anemia, reticulocytosis is the rule. When the reticulocyte count is high, reticulocytes of the younger types are found. After acute hemolysis sufficient time must elapse to allow the bone marrow to become hyperplastic before reticulocytosis can be expected. Occasionally a chronic hemolytic anemia characterized by reticulocytosis will show an acute exacerbation of the anemia and a reduction of the reticulocyte count. In such cases it must be supposed that a maturation arrest has occurred in the bone marrow or that the reticulocytes are not being liberated. In most cases the acute crisis is followed by striking reticulocytosis.

Reticulocytosis reflects the erythropoietic activity of the marrow and the rate of delivery of reticulocytes into the peripheral blood. Because of this, reticulocytosis is not, per se, evidence for hemolysis. In the anemia of chronic hemorrhage, reticulocytosis is the result of compensatory erythroid hyperplasia in the marrow. The reticulocytosis that follows the administration of vitamin B$_{12}$ in pernicious anemia is the result of sudden release from a marrow already packed with reticulocytes. Note also that the newborn normally shows reticulocytosis of up to 6%.

Erythrocyte indices

There is usually little to be learned from a study of the erythrocyte indices in hemolytic disease. Since the indices are average figures for a varied population of erythrocytes, it is even possible that at times minor degrees of microsphe-

rocytosis or macrocytosis will be overshadowed by the large number of normal cells. On the other hand, cells that are either abnormally small or large may be seen by a careful study of the peripheral blood smear. A low MCV is usually seen in severe hereditary spherocytosis. In other types of chronic hemolytic anemia the MCV may be less than normal as a result of iron deficiency. In other cases the presence of macrocytes in the peripheral blood, as well as the large number of reticulocytes, may give moderately high MCV figures. The MCHC is usually low or normal, but slightly increased MCHC values have been reported in hereditary spherocytosis.

Erythrocyte morphology

A careful examination of the peripheral blood smear often gives much information to the careful and experienced observer. Some features are diagnostic, whereas others are merely suggestive of hemolytic disease.

Spherocytosis

Spherocytosis is readily recognized and indicates some degree of damage to the erythrocytes. In a stained smear these cells are small and lack the normal central pallor of the disk-shaped erythrocyte (Fig. 13-8). They appear darker than normal, not because of a greater hemoglobin content, but because the cell is spherical. Spherocytes do not form rouleaux.

Spherocytic erythrocytes do not always indicate congenital spherocytic anemia. A normal erythrocyte undergoes a disk-to-sphere transformation when its environment is altered, as when the pH is changed or the electrolyte concentration is altered. There are many agents that can produce this disk-to-sphere transformation in vitro, some, such as saponin, being hemolytic. A regular sequence of shape changes has been demonstrated, from a *disk* to a *crenated disk* to a *crenated sphere* to a *sphere*. If the concentration of lysin is sufficiently high, the sphere becomes a *prolytic sphere* and finally a *ghost,* the latter usually visible only by the phase microscopy. The disk-to-sphere transformation may be produced in the absence of lytic agents by placing a drop of saline-suspended normal erythrocytes between a glass slide and a coverslip. Significantly, this type of in vitro transformation is reversible, whereas congenital spherocytosis is not.

When spherocytic erythrocytes are seen in a blood smear, they may be either the *true spherocytes* of congenital spherocytosis and other hemolytic anemias or spherical forms of normal erythrocytes, i.e., *acquired spherocytes.* True spherocytes represent an irreversible shape change, not preceded by crenation, resulting in increased osmotic fragility. Acquired spherocytes may be produced in vitro as a result of altered pH, by the effect of the anticoagulant, by ionic shifts, or by metabolic exhaustion. Spherocytic forms increase in proportion to the length of time blood is stored, even at refrigerator temperature. Many spherocytic forms will be present after 3 weeks of storage. If this blood is used for transfusion, the patient's peripheral blood smear may reveal spherocytic forms derived from the donor blood. These cells are near the end of their life span and survive for only a short time.

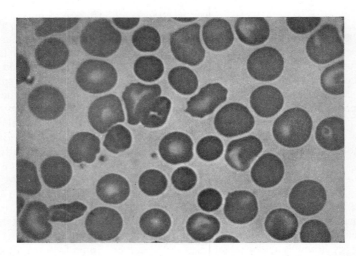

Fig. 13-8. Microspherocytes. Isoimmune hemolytic disease caused by A-B-O incompatibility. (Wright's stain; ×950.)

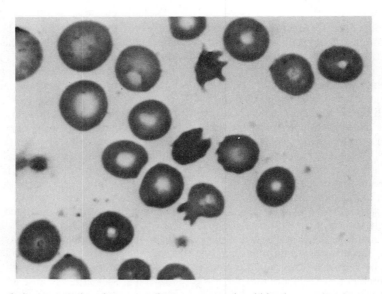

Fig. 13-9. Irregularly contracted erythrocytes (schizocytes), peripheral blood. Note that the spicules are shorter and more regular than in acanthocytes (see Fig. 13-23). (Wright's stain; ×1,250.)

True spherocytes are seen in *hereditary spherocytosis* or are produced in vivo by autoimmune and isoimmune reactions, by chemical agents, or by a physical agent such as high temperature. The hereditary spherocyte is probably delivered from the bone marrow as a normal disk-shaped erythrocyte. Reticulocytes and earlier precursors of the spherocyte are normal. The change to spherocytes takes place in the bloodstream, a change accompanied by decreased cell survival and hemolytic disease.

Careful examination of otherwise normal blood smears sometimes reveals the presence of a few spherocytic forms for which there is no obvious explanation. We have noticed a frequent coincidence in which there is slight spherocytosis with a splenomegaly that results from causes other than hemolytic disease. A few spherocytes are not uncommon in the leukemias, particularly in chronic myelocytic leukemia, and in the myeloproliferative syndromes.

Polychromatophilia

Polychromatophilia of the erythrocytes as seen in a Wright-stained peripheral blood smear is an indication of the presence of reticulocytes. Polychromatophilic cells are usually larger than normal and account for some of the macrocytic forms seen in the peripheral blood smear. In chronic hemolytic anemia macrocytes that are not polychromatophilic are occasionally seen.

Distorted or disrupted erythrocytes

Damage to the erythrocyte membrane may also produce irregularly contracted erythrocytes *(keratocytes, schizocytes)* that at first glance may be mistaken for crenated erythrocytes. However, a careful examination will reveal that the irregularities in the cell outline are spinelike (Fig. 13-9), not equally spaced as in a crenated cell, and quite distorted.

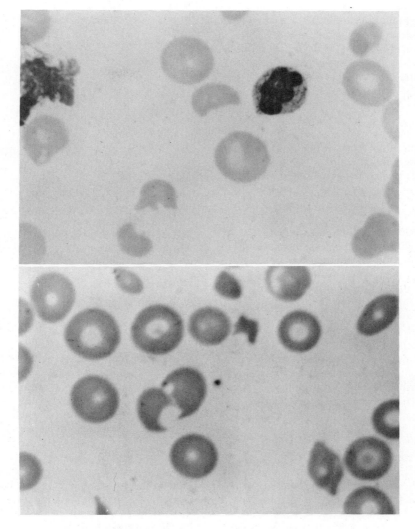

Fig. 13-10. Schizocytes, peripheral blood. (Wright's stain; ×1,250.)

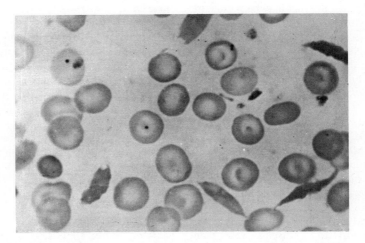

Fig. 13-11. Drepanocytes, routine blood smear. Note the Howell-Jolly bodies. (Wright's stain; ×950.)

In some of the severe hemolytic anemias the erythrocytes may show actual disruption (schizocytes), large numbers of broken cells being recognizable in the peripheral blood smear (Fig. 13-10). When these cells are hemispherical, they sometimes are referred to as *helmet cells*. At times they appear as though a wedge-shaped piece has been cut out of the cell.

Erythrophagocytes

The presence of erythrophagocytes (Fig. 13-7) has been reported in cases of hemolytic anemia. Such a finding strongly suggests the existence of immunohemolytic disease.

Drepanocytes (sickle cells)

In some cases of sickle cell anemia, sickle cells may be seen in routinely prepared peripheral blood smears (Fig. 13-11). Sickle cells are usually demonstrated by special technics directed at reducing the oxygen available to the erythrocytes. Sickling is not the exclusive property of cells containing Hb S (p. 624).

Normoblasts

Normoblasts are present in the peripheral blood in severe chronic hemolytic anemia, in acute hemolytic anemia, and in the hemolytic crisis of sickle cell anemia (Fig. 13-12). Normoblasts in the peripheral blood reflect the erythroid hyperplasia in the bone marrow and the accelerated release of erythroid cells.

Codocytes (target cells)

Target cells are not caused by hypoxia and can be seen in routine smears (Fig. 13-13). They are seen most commonly in the hemoglobinopathies (Chapter 14). When the peripheral blood smear reveals target cells, the presence of a hemoglobinopathy should be suspected. Target cells are sometimes seen in smears of normal blood as artifacts. They can be produced as artifacts when the blood smear is air dried in a very humid environment or by blowing on it and can be avoided by quick dehydration and fixation in absolute methyl alcohol.

Elliptocytes

One other erythrocyte abnormality that may be seen in the peripheral blood is elliptocytosis. This is an inherited abnormality of the erythrocyte and is not always indicative of hemolytic anemia, since elliptocytosis without abnormal hemolysis is more common than elliptocytic hemolytic anemia. The cells may be nearly normal in shape, oval, or rodlike (Fig. 13-14).

Stomatocytes

Hemolytic anemias have been described (Lock et al, 1961; Miller et al, 1965; Zarkowsky et al, 1968; Oski et al, 1969) that have some features of hereditary spherocytosis (mode of inheritance and osmotic fragility) but that do not show spherocytosis of the peripheral blood smear. The peripheral smear shows instead malformed erythrocytes with slitlike areas of central pallor (Fig. 13-15). Stomatocytes are also a feature of Rh_{null} disease (Sturgeon, 1970).

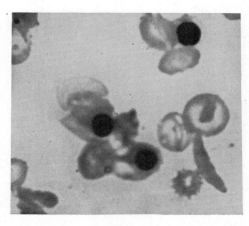

Fig. 13-12. Normoblasts, drepanocyte, and codocyte. Peripheral blood sickle cell anemia in crisis. (Wright's stain; ×1,160.)

Acanthocytes

Acanthocytosis (abetalipoproteinemia) (Fig. 13-23) is discussed on p. 568.

Giant platelets

Another finding in the peripheral blood smear that should lead one to think of hemolytic anemia or some other abnormality of hemopoiesis is the presence of giant platelets. These may be seen in either thrombocytopenia or thrombocytosis and may be present when hemolytic anemia is complicated by thrombocytopenia.

Heinz bodies

When hemolytic disease is suspected, it is at times important to perform special preparations. Heinz bodies are not seen in routinely prepared stained blood smears and must be looked for in wet preparations. They are an important diagnostic feature of hemolytic anemia caused by chemical compounds when the erythrocytes are deficient in G-6-PD or other enzymes or when an unstable hemoglobin is present. In an unstained preparation they appear as refractile round bodies ranging in size from a minute dot to about 3 μ in diameter (Fig. 13-24). Several Heinz bodies are usually present in the same cell. Heinz bodies can also be easily seen in supravitally stained preparations, in which they appear a lighter blue than the reticulum of reticulocytes.

Most patients having an unstable hemoglobin show Heinz bodies only after splenectomy or after being challenged with an oxidant drug. Heinz bodies are also seen in the α-thalassemia syndromes, Hb H being classified as an unstable hemoglobin. Erythrocytes from the newborn also show occasional Heinz bodies, supposedly the result of enzymatic immaturity.

Red blood cells from subjects having G-6-PD deficiency will show many Heinz bodies in each cell when exposed to acetylphenylhydrazine (Beutler et al, 1955). Normal red blood cells usually form only one Heinz body.

Siderocytes

Siderocytes are erythrocytes that contain granules visible when an iron stain is done. The granules appear as blue dots after Perls' Prussian blue stain and so are thought to contain

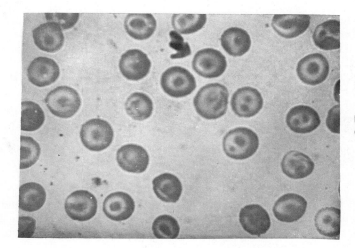

Fig. 13-13. Codocytes (target cells), peripheral blood smear. (Wright's stain; ×950.)

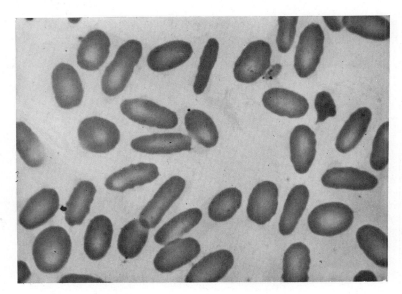

Fig. 13-14. Elliptocytosis.

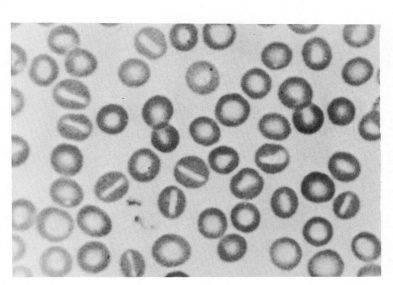

Fig. 13-15. Stomatocytes. (From Oski et al, 1969.)

ionized ferric iron. The relationship between the siderocytes described by Case (1945) and the inclusions described by Pappenheimer et al (1945) (Pappenheimer bodies) is not clear. Pappenheimer bodies stain purple with Wright's stain and also give a positive Prussian blue reaction. The siderocytes seen in hemolytic anemia have the same reaction, and the two are probably identical (Dacie and Doniach, 1947). The presence of siderotic granules in erythrocytes and precursors may give valuable data in the laboratory study of hemolytic disease. Normally, siderotic granules are common in orthochromic normoblasts, occasionally present in reticulocytes, and very scarce in erythrocytes. Siderocytes appear in the blood of a hematologically normal person after splenectomy. In the hemolytic anemias siderocytes are often found in moderate numbers; splenectomy also produces an increase (Table 13-10). It is thought that the spleen changes a siderocyte into a normal erythrocyte by "pitting" out the siderotic granule. If hemoglobin synthesis is normal, siderotic granules will be found in some of the normoblasts but in almost none of the erythrocytes. In some hemolytic anemias, 20% or more of the erythrocytes may be siderocytes, increasing to 80% or more after splenectomy. When hemoglobin synthesis is deficient because of a lack of available iron, siderotic granules are scarce both in normoblasts and in erythrocytes. (See also the discussion of sideroblastic anemias in Chapter 8.)

Parasites

Plasmodium and *Bartonella* organisms (Fig. 13-16) are readily identified in routine blood smears.

Osmotic fragility

The semipermeable characteristics of the surface membrane of an erythrocyte make each cell an osmometer that changes in volume with changes in the osmotic pressure of the external environment. A normal disk-shaped erythrocyte preserves its shape when suspended in serum or in an artificial salt solution of the same ionic concentration because

Table 13-10. Incidence of siderotic granules in normoblasts and erythrocytes in normal persons and in persons with hemolytic anemia*

Case	Siderocytes in peripheral blood (%)		Normoblasts containing siderotic granules (%)	
	Range	Average	Range	Average
Normal	0	0	24-81	49
Normal after splenectomy	0-14	4	11-54	26
Hereditary spherocytosis	0-2	0-2	12-87	43
Hereditary spherocytosis after splenectomy	2-45	10	12-72	42
Acquired hemolytic anemia	0-21	2.3	4-78	37
Acquired hemolytic anemia after splenectomy	1-67	20	30-51	41
Mediterranean anemia	0	0	21-55	41
Sickle cell anemia	0.2	0.2	44	44
Hemolytic disease of newborn infant	0-35	3.7	—	—

*After Douglas and Dacie, 1953.

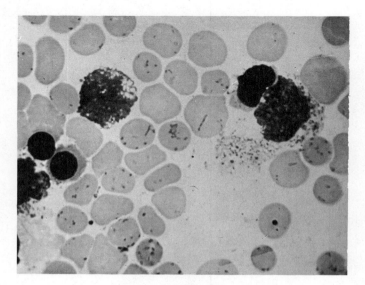

Fig. 13-16. Hemolytic anemia caused by *Bartonella bacilliformis,* bone marrow smear. Note the organisms within the erythrocytes. (Wright's stain; ×950.)

of the balanced ionic exchanges between cell and fluid. There being no shift of water into or out of the erythrocyte, the volume and shape remain essentially unchanged. The same cell suspended in distilled water will quickly undergo a disk-to-sphere transformation and will lyse.

It is disappointing that the mechanism of hypotonic lysis is not understood. It is true that lysis occurs when sufficient water enters the cell to stretch the membrane to the point where hemoglobin leaks out. The intermediate steps are in question. We can postulate that at first there is influx of cations and anions. Based on what we know now about the structure and function of the membrane, we must assume that the second step is an alteration of the membrane, either by stretching and enlargement of the pores or by activation of the cation pumps in an attempt to maintain internal osmolarity. The latter would soon exhaust ATP, and the membrane would become increasingly permeable to water. When a volume of 160% of normal is reached, the pores of the membrane core are sufficiently large to allow hemoglobin to leak out. The cell does not burst, and the ghost returns to the normal biconcave shape.

When the membrane is abnormal from the start, increased sensitivity to osmotic lysis is a function of the membrane abnormality. In hereditary spherocytosis, the erythrocytes are susceptible to sodium influx, whereas potassium efflux remains normal. The cation pumps are stimulated, increasing the utilization of ATP and glucose, but when these are exhausted, the influx of water is unimpeded. The same or similar mechanisms operate in erythrocytes having other types of membrane defects.

If it is assumed that a salt concentration of 0.85% is isotonic for the erythrocyte and that distilled water is the most abnormal ionic environment, then erythrocytes exposed to intermediate salt concentrations will undergo lysis, depending on the salt concentration and on the length of time that the erythrocyte has been exposed to the abnormal ionic environment.

Significance of measurements

Increased osmotic fragility, or decreased resistance to hemolysis, is a feature of spherocytes of all types and may therefore indicate congenital spherocytosis, idiopathic acquired hemolytic anemia, isoimmune hemolytic disease of the newborn infant (more common in A-B-O incompatibility than in Rh sensitization), and other hemolytic anemias. *Normal* osmotic fragility is found in symptomatic hemolytic anemia and in PNH. *Decreased* osmotic fragility is seen in sickle cell anemia and in hemolytic anemias characterized by abnormally flat target cells, as occurs in some of the hemoglobinopathies.

Interpretation of results

Procedures for determining osmotic fragility must take into account the importance of the relative volume of blood and saline mixture, the temperature at which the test is done, and the pH of the blood and saline mixture. Methods of reading the results vary. It is usually sufficient to add a measured amount of blood to a measured amount of saline solution of graded salt concentration and to record the saline concentration at which hemolysis can first be seen and the concentration at which all erythrocytes are hemolyzed (Fig. 13-17). If care is taken to perform this test exactly the same way for the patient and for the control, and if the same technic is used each time, the results are adequate to identify abnormal fragility. By this method, hemolysis normally begins at a salt concentration of 0.42% to 0.44% and is complete at 0.32%. Abnormal results are summarized in Table 13-11. A more accurate determination of osmotic fragility is that of Dacie and Lewis (1975a) (Fig. 13-18) in which the volumes of blood and saline mixture are carefully measured, and hemolysis is read in a photoelectric colorimeter. When the results are plotted, an osmotic fragility curve is obtained (Figs. 13-19 and 13-20). The curve is sigmoid, reflecting a heterogeneous erythrocyte population, the

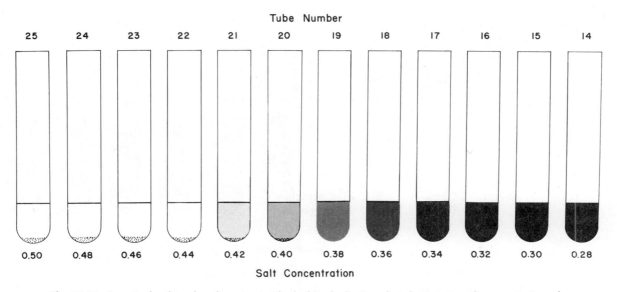

Fig. 13-17. Osmotic fragility of erythrocytes (method of Sanford). Hemolysis begins at a salt concentration of 0.44% and is complete at 0.32%.

Table 13-11. Osmotic fragility of erythrocytes in various diseases

Disease	Initial hemolysis (% saline ± 1 SD)	Complete hemolysis (% saline ± 1 SD)	Remarks
Normal	0.44 ± 0.02	0.32 ± 0.02	
Hereditary spherocytosis	0.68 ± 0.14	0.46 ± 0.10	Abnormal in all cases; initial hemolysis may occur in 0.85% saline solution
Acquired hemolytic anemia	0.52 ± 0.04	0.42 ± 0.04	Abnormal in most cases; degree varies with severity
Hemolytic disease caused by A-B-O incompatibility	0.50 ± 0.02	0.40 ± 0.02	Abnormal in many cases; degree varies with severity
Hemolytic disease caused by Rh incompatibility	0.60 ± 0.06	0.40 ± 0.04	Abnormal in many cases; degree varies with severity
Hemolytic anemia caused by drugs	0.50 ± 0.04	0.40 ± 0.04	Abnormal in most cases during onset; may be normal in later stages
Hemolytic anemia caused by burns	0.50 ± 0.04	0.40 ± 0.04	Abnormal in about 50% of cases during first few days; usually normal after a few days
Pernicious anemia	0.48 ± 0.04	0.36 ± 0.02	Occasionally very abnormal; normal in most cases
Congenital nonspherocytic hemolytic anemia	0.44 ± 0.02	0.32 ± 0.02	Fragility may be increased after blood is incubated
Elliptocytosis, asymptomatic	0.44	0.32	
Elliptocytosis with hemolytic anemia	0.50	0.32	
Thalassemia	0.38 ± 0.04	0.20 ± 0.06	Complete hemolysis may not be achieved until salt concentration of 0.1% is reached
Sickle cell anemia	0.36 ± 0.02	0.20 ± 0.04	Abnormal in all cases
Sickle cell trait (S/A)	0.44 ± 0.04	0.32 ± 0.04	Always normal
Hb C disease	0.34	0.22	Abnormal in almost all cases
Erythremia	0.40 ± 0.02	0.28 ± 0.02	Not a constant finding
Iron-deficiency anemia	0.38 ± 0.02	0.28 ± 0.02	Typical in severe anemia; not common otherwise
Obstructive jaundice (severe)	0.36 ± 0.02	0.28 ± 0.04	Decreased fragility usually noted in severely jaundiced patients

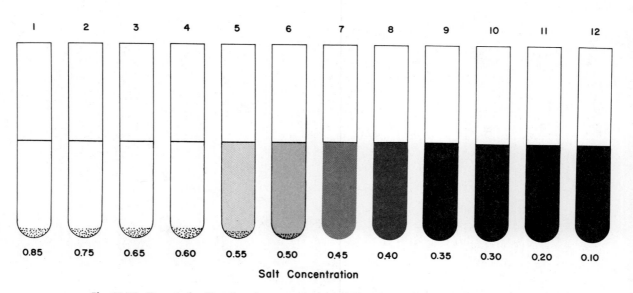

Fig. 13-18. Osmotic fragility of erythrocytes (method of Dacie). See plotted data in Fig. 13-19.

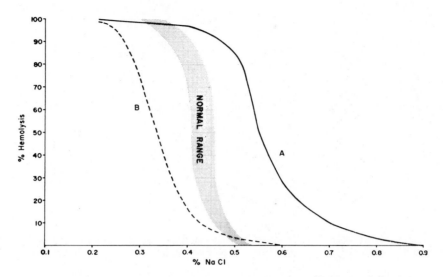

Fig. 13-19. Normal and abnormal osmotic fragility curves, plotted from photoelectric data obtained by Dacie's method. **A,** Increased osmotic fragility. **B,** Decreased osmotic fragility.

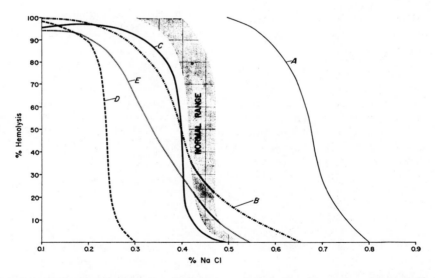

Fig. 13-20. Osmotic fragility of erythrocytes by Dacie's method. **A,** Hereditary spherocytosis. **B,** Thalassemia major. **C,** Thalassemia minor. **D,** Hb E disease. **E,** Hb E–thalassemia.

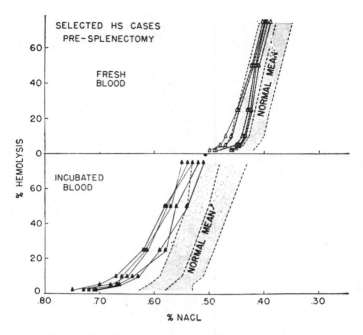

Fig. 13-21. Osmotic fragility in selected cases of congenital spherocytosis (HS). Note that in these cases the osmotic fragility is abnormal only after the blood is incubated at 37° C for 24 hours. (From Young, 1955.)

"tails" representing a small number of cells with osmotic fragility either higher or lower than the majority.

After incubation

Preincubation of blood at 37° C for 24 hours accentuates increased osmotic fragility, if present, and may reveal abnormal osmotic fragility not detectable with the standard test in which fresh whole blood is used (Fig. 13-21).

Investigation of metabolic abnormalities
Introduction

When hemolytic anemia has no characteristic red cell malformation and is of the nonspherocytic type, we assume that there is some metabolic abnormality which causes the accelerated hemolysis. From the many metabolic abnormalities discussed in the preceding section on pathogenesis, it is obvious that the identification of the specific metabolic defect calls for a variety of laboratory procedures. Some of these are specific, complex, and time consuming; others are nonspecific but still helpful; and still others are acceptably specific but qualitative or semiquantitative rather than ideally quantitative. Fairbanks and Fernandez (1969) have published an evaluation of tests for metabolic abnormalities with regard to their specificity, their sensitivity, and the relative ease with which they can be performed.

A step-by-step investigation of the glycolytic and energy pathways seems to be a rational approach but is in fact a Homeric odyssey fraught with complexities, problems of execution, and endangered by the whims of enzymatic analysis. Fortunately most instances of nonspherocytic anemia prove to be G-6-PD deficiency, pyruvate kinase deficiency, or caused by the presence of an unstable hemoglobin. These can be diagnosed with relative ease. The other abnormalities are rare.

Table 13-12. Tests useful in diagnosis and differential diagnosis of congenital nonspherocytic hemolytic anemia

Group I. Nonspecific tests
 A. Autohemolysis
 B. Heinz body formation
 C. GSH stability
 D. Ascorbate test
Group II. Screening tests that are specific but semiquantitative
 A. Fluorescence test for G-6-PD deficiency
 B. Fluorescense test for pyruvate kinase deficiency
 C. Fluorescence test for glutathione reductase deficiency
 D. Fluorescence test for triosephosphate isomerase deficiency
 E. Orthocresol red test for pyruvate kinase deficiency
 F. Methemoglobin reduction test for G-6-PD deficiency
Group III. Specific assays
 A. Assay of RBC G-6-PD
 B. Assay of RBC pyruvate kinase
 C. Heat denaturation test for unstable hemoglobins

The tests indicated in nonspherocytic hemolytic anemia fall into three categories (Table 13-12). The first includes simple nonspecific tests useful in establishing whether nonspherocytic hemolytic anemia exists and allowing some differentiation of types. The second category includes screening tests that are specific but only qualitative. The third are quantitative spectrophotometric tests (Beutler, 1975) that are specific but complex and time consuming.

Autohemolysis

When sterile defibrinated blood is incubated at 37° C, various degrees of autohemolysis take place. Normal eryth-

Table 13-13. Patterns of autohemolysis with and without added glucose or ATP

Disease	Unmodified	Glucose added	ATP added*
Hereditary spherocytosis	++ to ++++	±	±
Triosephosphate isomerase deficiency	++	±	±
G-6-PD deficiency	++	+	+
Unstable hemoglobinopathy	++	+	+
Hexokinase deficiency	++	+	+
Pyruvate kinase deficiency	++	++	0
Glutathione reductase deficiency	++	++	0
2,3-Diphosphoglycerate mutase deficiency	++	++	0
Isoimmune hemolytic disease	0	0	0
Acanthocytosis†	++	±	±
Thalassemia	0	0	0
Paroxysmal nocturnal hemoglobinuria (PNH)	++	++	?
Paroxysmal cold hemoglobinuria (PCH)	++‡	++	++
Stomatocytosis	++§	±	±
Elliptocytosis (hemolytic)	++	±	±

*Of doubtful value (Beutler, 1978c) because of acid pH.
†Autohemolysis inhibited by normal serum.
‡After sensitization of erythrocytes at refrigerator temperature.
§At 37°C; no hemolysis at 4°C.

rocytes show 0% to 0.5% hemolysis after 24 hours and 0.4% to 3.5% after 48 hours. Autohemolysis is increased in congenital spherocytosis, in all enzyme-deficient nonspherocytic hemolytic anemias, and in PCH (paroxysmal cold hemoglobinuria). Very rarely there is increased autohemolysis in autoimmune hemolytic anemia of the warm-antibody type. The test was once used extensively in the investigation of nonspherocytic hemolytic anemias, but its usefulness is limited, and semiquantitative assays of red cell enzymes give more specific information. Note that in hereditary spherocytosis there is striking autohemolysis corrected by added glucose. This may be found when there is normal osmotic fragility after incubation (Fukagawa et al, 1979).

If osmotic fragility tests are performed on blood incubated for 24 hours, it is usually found that those specimens showing increased autohemolysis will demonstrate increased osmotic fragility as well. Some persons with nonspherocytic hemolytic anemia show normal osmotic fragility with fresh blood but increased osmotic fragility after the blood is incubated.

Autohemolysis is a membrane phenomenon, and it is thought that incubation causes a loss of membrane lipids. Because of the membrane alteration, there is increased utilization of glucose and eventual depletion of ATP. As expected, glucose or ATP added to the blood sometimes protects against autohemolysis partially or completely, and the patterns of correction observed in various hemolytic anemias are sometimes useful in the differential diagnosis (Table 13-13).

Heinz body formation

Heinz bodies are formed when erythrocytes are exposed to reducing substances such as acetylphenylhydrazine or hydroxylamine. In normal blood the erythrocytes form single, large, marginal Heinz bodies (Fig. 13-24, *B*), and not all erythrocytes are affected. In those cases in which the

erythrocytes are sensitive to oxidant drugs such as primaquine each cell contains many Heinz bodies. Heinz body formation is found in G-6-PD deficiency, 6-PGD deficiency, glutathione reductase (GSSG-R) deficiency, GSH synthetase deficiency, glutathione peroxidase deficiency (GSH-Px), and triosephosphate isomerase deficiency. In hemolytic anemia caused by an unstable hemoglobin Heinz bodies are formed only after incubation of the blood for 48 hours at 37° C or, typically, after splenectomy. Note that Heinz body formation is negative in the second most common enzymatic deficiency—pyruvate kinase.

Glutathione stability test

Glutathione stability is abnormal in G-6-PD deficiency and, theoretically, in 6-PGD deficiency, GSH synthetase deficiency, glutathione peroxidase deficiency, and glutathione reductase deficiency. The test may be equivocal in the case of an unstable hemoglobin. It is normal in hereditary spherocytosis, pyruvate kinase deficiency, triosephosphate isomerase deficiency, and hexokinase deficiency.

Ascorbate test

The ascorbate test measures peroxidative denaturation of hemoglobin and was originally devised as a screening test for G-6-PD deficiency. It is simple, easy to perform, and sensitive. It gives a different pattern of results with various enzymatic defects than is seen with the test for Heinz bodies and with the autohemolysis and glutathione-stability tests. The ascorbate test is strongly positive in G-6-PD deficiency and the unstable hemoglobinopathies Köln, Santa Ana, and H. It is moderately positive in pyruvate kinase deficiency. It is normal in hereditary spherocytosis and in the unstable hemoglobinopathy Zürich.

Tests for unstable hemoglobins

The unstable hemoglobins are detected by the heat denaturation and isopropanol precipitation tests (Chapter 14).

Fluorescence test for G-6-PD deficiency

The fluorescence test for G-6-PD deficiency depends on the reaction:

$$\text{Glucose-6-phosphate} + \text{NADP} \xrightarrow{\text{G-6-PD}} \text{6-Phosphogluconate} + \text{NADPH}$$

In the presence of normal amounts of G-6-PD, fluorescence develops. When G-6-PD is absent (homozygotes), there is no fluorescence. This screening test is of limited value in the detection of heterozygotes.

Fluorescence test for pyruvate kinase deficiency

The fluorescence test for pyruvate kinase deficiency depends on the reactions:

$$\text{Phosphoenol pyruvate} + \text{ADP} \xrightarrow{\text{PK}} \text{Pyruvate} + \text{ATP}$$

$$\text{Pyruvate} + \text{NADH} \xrightarrow{\text{LDH}} \text{Lactate} + \text{NAD}$$

In the presence of normal amounts of pyruvate kinase there is decreased fluorescence. When pyruvate kinase is deficient, fluorescence persists.

Fluorescence test for glutathione reductase deficiency

The fluorescence test for glutathione reductase deficiency depends on the reaction:

$$\text{Oxidized glutathione} + 2\text{NADPH} \xrightarrow{\text{GSSG-R}} 2\text{GSH} + 2\text{NADP}$$

When glutathione reductase is normal, fluorescence decreases. When there is a deficiency of the enzyme, fluorescence persists.

Fluorescence test for triosephosphate isomerase deficiency

The fluorescence test for triosephosphate isomerase deficiency depends on the reactions:

$$\text{Glyceraldehyde-3-phosphate} \xrightarrow{\text{TPI}} \text{Dihydroxyacetone phosphate}$$

$$\text{Dihydroxyacetone phosphate} \xrightarrow{\substack{\text{Glycerophosphate} \\ \text{dehydrogenase}}} \text{Glycerophosphate} + \text{NAD}$$

When triosephosphate isomerase is normal, fluorescence decreases. When the enzyme is deficient, fluorescence persists.

Orthocresol red test for pyruvate kinase deficiency

The orthocresol red test has been proposed as specific for pyruvate kinase deficiency, but it probably is nonspecific. When the glycolytic degradation in the Embden-Myerhof pathway is normal, lactic acid is produced, lowering the pH. Orthocresol red is used as an indicator of the change in pH, since it changes from red to yellow at an acid pH. Since any enzymatic defect in the Embden-Myerhof pathway could result in failure to form lactate, it is doubtful whether this test is specific for pyruvate kinase deficiency. It may in fact be useful as a nonspecific screening test for the presence of an enzymatic defect.

Methemoglobin reduction test for G-6-PD deficiency

The methemoglobin reduction test devised by Brewer et al (1962) has the same sensitivity as the fluorescence screening test. It has the advantage of having been evaluated for heterozygous deficiency of G-6-PD (p. 565).

Summary

Which laboratory tests are done to detect a metabolic disturbance depends on the laboratory facilities available. The nonspecific tests listed in Table 13-12 can only indicate, at best, that a metabolic abnormality is present. The screening tests that are specific but semiquantitative are more difficult to perform and may not be as specific as originally proposed. On the other hand, kits are now available for specific assays of G-6-PD, pyruvate kinase, and rarer enzymes; if possible, specific enzymatic assays should be done along with the heat denaturation test for unstable hemoglobins.

Serologic investigations

Many of the laboratory examinations applicable to the study of hemolytic disease merely indicate the presence of the disease and give no information about the etiology; e.g., it is not unusual to encounter patients having refractory or progressive anemia with laboratory findings such as reticulocytosis, normoblastic hyperplasia of the bone marrow, and hyperbilirubinemia. A tentative diagnosis of hemolytic anemia may be entertained, to be confirmed if possible by erythrocyte survival studies selected to determine if survival is decreased and if the defect is intrinsic or extrinsic. Even if the diagnosis of hemolytic disease is confirmed, it is essential to determine, as exactly as possible, what abnormal mechanism is responsible for the diminished erythrocyte survival. Because of the frequency with which immunologic mechanisms are responsible for hemolytic disease, serologic investigations, carefully performed and interpreted, have become one of the major investigative tools for detecting the presence of hemolytic disease and determining its pathogenesis.

Some serologic studies, e.g., the direct and indirect antiglobulin (Coombs') test, detect the presence of antibodies in general. Others are designed to demonstrate the type and nature of these antibodies. It is important therefore to appreciate both the value and the limitations of the various tests to plan a logical and rewarding laboratory approach to diagnosis.

As discussed previously, hemolytic disease may be caused by either corpuscular or extracorpuscular defects. In the case of corpuscular defects the abnormality may be caused by several mechanisms, such as abnormal hemoglobin molecules, deficient enzyme systems, or defects of the erythrocytic membrane. These abnormalities are detected by means other than serologic tests. In extracorpuscular defects, however, abnormal erythrocyte survival is the result of the damage done to normal erythrocytes by some extracellular substance. Since most hemolytic disease caused by extracorpuscular defects is caused by either isoantibodies or autoantibodies, serologic methods are particularly important in the laboratory investigation of this type of hemolytic disease.

Hemolytic disease caused by isoantibodies is the result of either incompatibility of maternal and fetal blood groups during pregnancy or transfusion of incompatible blood. Serologic investigation of blood groups and isoantibodies is useful therefore in hemolytic disease of the newborn or infant and in patients of any age who develop hemolytic disease following the administration of blood.

Direct antiglobulin (Coombs') test

PRINCIPLE OF THE TEST. The direct antiglobulin test usually detects the presence of incomplete antibodies that become fixed to the surface of erythrocytes and that, by themselves, are not capable of producing agglutination (Fig. 13-22). Other mechanisms for a positive antiglobulin test are discussed on p. 563.

In 1908 Moreschi showed that erythrocytes sensitized (i.e., coated) with a heterologous protein are agglutinated by antibodies formed against that protein. Coombs et al (1945) revived and refined this concept, applying it directly to problems of immunohematology. They showed that erythrocytes exposed to antibodies, as in Rh hemolytic disease, would be agglutinated by an antiserum produced by immunizing a rabbit against human globulin or whole serum. In the *direct* test, sensitized erythrocytes are exposed directly to the action of antiglobulin serum. In the *indirect* test, suitable normal erythrocytes are first exposed to serum supposedly containing a coating antibody and then exposed to antiglobulin serum. Thus the direct test detects antibodies fixed to erythrocytes in vivo, whereas the indirect test is used to detect antibodies in serum.

THE NATURE OF ANTIGLOBULIN SERUM. The original concept of the reaction was that the red cells are coated with antibodies of the γ-globulin (IgG) type, and that agglutination is produced by the anti-IgG contained in the antiglobulin (Coombs') serum. Part of the evidence for this was that agglutination of sensitized erythrocytes can be inhibited by saturating the receptor sites with IgG before adding the antiglobulin serum.

We now appreciate that the antibodies responsible for hemolytic disease are not always of the IgG type. For this reason there occurred a change in the commercial antiglobulin reagents, from the classic monospecific anti-IgG type to one that also contains the most important non-γ component, anticomplement (anti-C3d). The new type of antiglobulin serum is called *broad spectrum* or, better, *polyspecific*.

A polyspecific antiserum containing anti-IgG and anti-C3d is used in the direct Coombs' test for the detection of immunohemolytic anemias: autoimmune hemolytic anemia, isoimmune hemolytic anemia, and hemolytic disease of the newborn. The direct test is positive in almost all cases of immunohemolytic anemia when a polyspecific antiserum is used (Petz and Garratty, 1975, 1978), whereas about one third give a false negative direct test if the antiserum used contains only anti-IgG. It is interesting that only an occasional case will give a positive test with anti-C3d alone. Stratton (1975) describes such a case, the sensitization being caused by anti-Jk^a. Facer et al (1979) found a high incidence of positive direct antiglobulin tests in children having malaria *(Plasmodium falciparum),* and the most frequent form of erythrocyte sensitization was with C3d. For practical reasons polyspecific antisera may contain antibodies other than anti-IgG and anti-C3d, e.g., some anti-IgM, anti-IgA, anti-C3c, or anti-C4, but these should not necessarily be considered "contaminants" (Worlledge and Blajchman, 1972). However, monospecific antisera should be used when the direct antiglobulin test using polyspecific antiserum is positive to determine the type of hemolytic anemia. The monospecific antisera available are anti-IgG, anti-C3d,

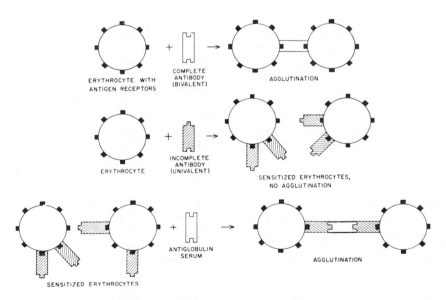

Fig. 13-22. Reactions between erythrocytes and antibodies. Agglutination by complete antibody, above; sensitization of erythrocytes by incomplete antibody, center; and agglutination of sensitized erythrocytes by a special complete antibody such as antiglobulin serum, bottom.

anti-**M**, and anti-**A**. Monospecific anti-**M** and anti-**A** antisera are not yet licensed but may be useful when there is evidence of *immune hemolytic anemia* but the direct test is negative with polyspecific (anti-IgG and anti-C3d) antiserum.

The use of polyspecific antiserum in the indirect test is recommended (Stratton, 1975; Wright and Issitt, 1979), but both the advantage and potential drawback should be noted. The advantage of an antiserum containing both anti-IgG and anti-C3d is that the reaction with certain antibodies (anti-**Jkª**, anti-**Leª**, anti-**Kell**, anti-**Duffy**, anti-**Kidd**) is weak or negative if monospecific anti-IgG is used, whereas it is positive with polyspecific antisera. The one potential disadvantage is that when a polyspecific antiserum is used for compatibility testing at room temperature, complement is fixed to the red cells, and when cold agglutinins are present, undesirable false positive reactions may occur. According to Giblett (1977), alloantibodies that do not react at 37° C are never responsible for in vivo hemolysis, and it is recommended that compatibility testing be carried out at 37° C only. Storage of blood samples at refrigerator temperatures is not a problem because the concentration of anticomplement antibodies in commercial Coombs' sera is insufficient to cause agglutination of red cells stored in autologous plasma or serum (Garratty and Petz, 1976; Issitt and Smith, 1976).

VALUE AND LIMITATIONS. The direct antiglobulin test is a sensitive index of the presence of incomplete antibodies. However, technical errors may give false positive or false negative results. Positive reactions may be obtained in some normal persons, but this may be caused by incompletely absorbed antiglobulin sera that contain anti-**T** or anti-**Tn** (Beck et al, 1976).

A false positive may result if the test is done on erythrocytes obtained from a clotted blood specimen that has been maintained at refrigerator temperature. This reaction is a result of the incomplete cold antibodies normally present in serum. The difficulty can be avoided by allowing the blood specimen to warm to room temperature before the erythrocytes are obtained. It also can be eliminated to a large degree by using oxalated or heparinized blood, since these anticoagulants inhibit the fixation of cold antibodies on erythrocytes. If the patient has cold antibodies in high titer, stricter precautions must be taken to avoid adsorption of the antibody on the erythrocytes. In this case it is recommended that blood be collected directly into saline solution warmed to 37° C.

Excluding false positive antiglobulin tests caused by incomplete cold antibodies, a positive test also will be shown by some patients in the absence of manifest hemolytic disease (Table 13-14). Most of these can be explained on the basis of hyperglobulinemia, which occurs in diseases such as rheumatoid arthritis, sarcoidosis, leukemia, lymphoma, and disseminated LE. However, other conditions characterized by hyperglobulinemia such as multiple myeloma and cirrhosis of the liver do not show positive antiglobulin tests. In the diseases mentioned, thought to give false positive tests, mild hemolytic anemia is sometimes present. In these cases the positive antiglobulin test may be significant. A false positive antiglobulin test is common in ulcer-

Table 13-14. Causes of false positive antiglobulin tests (i.e., a positive test not caused by the presence of specific antierythrocytic antibodies)

I. Technical
   A. Blood refrigerated and cells washed with cold saline solution
   B. Contamination with vapor from lipid solvents (acetone, toluene)
   C. Contamination with chromic or ferric salts
   D. Bacterial contamination of blood
   E. Prozone phenomenon caused by excess antibody (antiglobulin)
II. Nontechnical
   A. Reticulocytosis
   B. Valvular prosthesis
   C. Ulcerative colitis
   D. Pernicious anemia
   E. Methyldopa (Aldomet)
   F. Trypan blue
   G. Azo dyes
   H. Sodium cephalothin
   I. Penicillin
   J. Phenylhydrazine
   K. Quinine
   L. Acetophenetidin
   M. Normal person (rare)

ative colitis. Dacie (1953) emphasizes that false positive reactions are usually weak, are strongest in high concentrations of potent antiglobulin serum, and are not affected by the addition of a small amount of human γ-globulin (see following discussion of γ-globulin neutralization test).

False negative reactions are usually caused by technical shortcomings. One cause is incomplete washing of the erythrocytes. It is important to wash the test cells completely free of plasma or serum, since minute amounts of serum will inhibit the agglutination of sensitized erythrocytes by antiglobulin serum. Other false negative reactions are caused by weak antiglobulin sera, by the use of potent sera in inappropriate dilution, or by the use of too much antiglobulin serum (prozone phenomenon), contaminated antiglobulin serum, or dirty glassware. The technic used should be that recommended by the manufacturer.

RESULTS IN HEMOLYTIC ANEMIA. The direct antiglobulin test may be either positive or negative in hemolytic disease (Table 13-15). In general, it is positive in isoimmune hemolytic anemia caused by A-B-O, Rh, and other blood group incompatibilities. It is usually positive in "symptomatic" acquired autoimmune hemolytic anemia and negative in hemolytic disease caused by intracorpuscular defects. It must be concluded that the direct antiglobulin test, when positive, may be helpful in determining the presence of hemolytic anemia but that a negative result does not exclude that diagnosis.

Indirect antiglobulin test

In principle the indirect test is the same as the direct test, i.e., sensitized erythrocytes are agglutinated by antiglobulin serum. In the indirect test, however, normal erythrocytes of

Table 13-15. Direct antiglobulin (Coombs') test in various hemolytic anemias

Disease	Direct antiglobulin test	Remarks
Hereditary spherocytosis	Usually negative	May be positive during "crisis"; occasionally positive in absence of crisis
Congenital nonspherocytic hemolytic anemia	Negative	
Paroxysmal nocturnal hemoglobinuria (PNH)	Usually negative but sometimes positive	
Paroxysmal cold hemoglobinuria (PCH)	Positive or negative	Positive during acute attack, negative later; indirect test more often positive
March hemoglobinuria	Negative	
Porphyria erythropoietica	Negative	
Pernicious anemia	Negative but sometimes positive	
Erythrocytes sensitive to primaquine	Negative	Occasionally positive in acute malaria treated with quinine
Sickle cell anemia and other hemoglobinopathies	Negative	
"Idiopathic" acquired autoimmune hemolytic anemia	Positive	
"Symptomatic" acquired autoimmune anemia associated with:		
Disseminated lupus erythematosus	Usually positive	
Leukemia	Usually positive	
Lymphoma	Usually positive	
Carcinoma	Usually negative	
Ovarian dermoid, teratoma, and cyst	Positive or negative	
Periarteritis nodosa	Usually positive	
Thrombocytopenic purpura (Evans' syndrome)	Usually positive	
Thrombohemolytic (thrombotic) thrombocytopenic purpura	Usually negative	
Isoimmune hemolytic anemia		Acute hemolytic anemias caused by transfusion reactions usually show a negative Coombs' test; high degree of sensitization may later show positive reaction
A-B-O blood group incompatibility	Positive	
Rh incompatability	Positive	
Other blood group incompatibilities	Positive	
Hemolytic anemias caused by bacterial agents and protozoal parasites	Usually negative	
Hemolytic anemias caused by chemical agents	Positive or negative	
Hemolytic anemia of favism	Usually positive	Weaker reaction in children and mild cases; serum often contains incomplete warm antibodies
Hemolytic anemia associated with acute liver disease	Usually positive	Negative in mild anemia
Hemolytic anemia associated with uremia	Negative	

known phenotype first are exposed to the serum suspected of containing antibodies and then treated with antiglobulin serum. If the serum contains an antibody that, under the conditions of the test, is fixed on the erythroctyes, these will be agglutinated by the antiglobulin serum.

The indirect test is used to identify antibodies either in the patient's serum or in the eluate from sensitized erythrocytes. It may be used to determine if antibodies remain in the serum after the patient's own cells are saturated and to distinguish between two antibodies, one of which is fixed to the patient's cells. If both antibodies are free in the serum, each in turn can be absorbed by different cells having an affinity for the specific antibody.

By varying the conditions of the test, one can obtain much information as to the nature of the antibody; e.g., the test may be set up at various temperatures to determine the optimum temperature at which a reaction takes place, and thus the antibody can be identified as cold or warm. Acidification of the unknown serum does not affect the reaction of warm antibodies but does intensify the sensitizing ability of cold antibodies.

γ-Globulin neutralization test

Adding graded quantities of human γ-globulin to the antiglobulin serum permits separation of antiglobulin reactions into three types: (1) those inhibited by small amounts of γ-globulin, (2) those inhibited only by large amounts of γ-globulin, and (3) those which are intermediate between types 1 and 2. Reactions inhibited by small amounts of γ-globulin are the most common. They are referred to as the *γ-globulin type*. A typical reaction of this type is the inhibition of the agglutination of erythrocytes sensitized by anti-**Rh₀** when antiglobulin serum containing a very small amount of γ-globulin is added. Reactions inhibited by large amounts of γ-globulin only are referred to as *cold-antibody–type* reactions because this reaction is characteristic of erythrocytes sensitized by cold antibodies.

It should be noted that the γ-globulin neutralization test

assumes that the antibody coating the erythrocytes is of the γ type. The test does not apply when the antibody is of the non-γ type. However, it can be useful in demonstrating the presence of non-γ antibodies.

Agglutination of enzyme-treated erythrocytes

When normal erythrocytes are treated with a proteolytic enzyme, they are made agglutinable by a serum containing an incomplete antibody (i.e., the antibody does not cause agglutination of untreated cells). In practice the use of enzyme-treated erythrocytes is analogous to the use of the indirect antiglobulin test, since both are useful in the identification of incomplete antibodies.

The enzymes most commonly used are trypsin, papain, and ficin. Trypsin is expensive, and the trypsinization procedure is time consuming. Trypsinized erythrocytes are susceptible to agglutination by a normal serum panagglutinin. Papain and ficin have largely replaced trypsin. Papain is inexpensive and easy to use, and papainized erythrocytes detect incomplete autoantibodies better than the indirect antiglobulin test. Ficin gives the same results as papain, but the dry powder is irritating and should be handled with care. Pirofsky and Mangum (1959) have used another proteolytic enzyme, bromelin; in contrast to the other enzymes, bromelin detects incomplete antibodies fixed to the erythrocyte and is analogous to the direct antiglobulin test (Pirofsky et al, 1961).

A combination of mechanisms probably explains best how enzymes produce these effects. One is digestion of the surface to expose more antigenic sites. A second mechanism is a modification of the surface with release of N-acetylneuraminic acid and a reduction in surface electric ζ-potential so that the cells can come together and the shorter distance can be bridged by immunoglobulin molecules.

Detection of incomplete antibodies by means of enzyme-treated erythrocytes is not a substitute for the standard antiglobulin test. The two methods are complementary. Most comparative studies show that testing with enzyme-treated erythrocytes detects incomplete antibodies more often than does the antiglobulin test. Occasionally antibodies detectable with the antiglobulin test cannot be detected with enzyme-treated erythrocytes, i.e., anti-**K** and anti-**Fy^a**. Enzyme treatment also destroys M and N surface antigens. It is agreed that no single system suffices to detect all incomplete antibodies and that a combination of the antiglobulin test, enzyme-treated erythrocyte test, and agglutination in albumin media is recommended.

Agglutination in albumin and serum-albumin media

A third method of detecting incomplete antibodies depends on the agglutination of sensitized erythrocytes suspended in undiluted normal serum or in 20% albumin. This reaction is intense with highly sensitized cells. The degree of agglutination is roughly proportional to the degree of sensitization.

The use of low–ionic strength suspending media

The use of low–ionic strength suspending media in hemagglutination test systems has been shown to enhance red blood cell sensitization, to reduce the reaction time, and to reduce the incidence of false positive results (Moore and Mollison, 1976; Fitzsimmons and Morel, 1979).

Complete (saline) agglutinating antibodies

Complete agglutinating antibodies are capable of agglutinating normal group O erythrocytes in a saline medium. In acquired hemolytic anemia, if complete agglutinating antibodies are present, they are usually of the cold type.

In hemolytic anemia caused by cold antibodies the cold agglutinin titer is higher than 1:64 and sometimes as high as 1:64,000 or more. Group O cells, unmodified or enzyme treated, are tested against serial dilutions of the patient's serum at 2° C. Normal erythrocytes vary greatly in their ability to be agglutinated by cold antibodies. It is recommended therefore that cells from the same normal donor be used for all cold-agglutinin titrations. Some recommend using the patient's own erythrocytes, regardless of blood group.

Hemolytic antibodies

Warm hemolysins are rarely seen in acquired hemolytic anemia. Dacie and Cutbush (1954) studied one patient whose serum contained a warm hemolysin active against normal erythrocytes after acidification of the serum. In others they demonstrated the presence of warm antibodies that were hemolytic to enzyme-treated erythrocytes and erythrocytes from patients with PNH.

Cold hemolysins are capable of hemolyzing untreated normal erythrocytes in acidified serum. Although cold hemolysins are generally thought to be nonspecific with regard to the antigenic structure of the hemolyzed erythrocyte, they are most active against group O cells. The activity of cold hemolysins can also be demonstrated by using either enzyme-treated or PNH erythrocytes. In the latter case the serum must not be acidified.

Serologic studies in isoimmune hemolytic disease

Isoimmune hemolytic disease occurs in the newborn infant as a result of the serologic incompatibility of mother and fetus or at any age as a result of immunization by transfusion of incompatible blood. In either case it can be caused by immunization by many of the antigens of the erythrocyte. Acute hemolytic disease may also result from the transfusion of incompatible plasma. Acute hemolytic disease caused by incompatible blood transfusions may occur in patients without previous sensitization.

The diagnosis of isoimmune hemolytic disease seldom presents much difficulty. The circumstances usually lead one to strongly suspect its presence, as with hemolytic disease of the newborn.

Serologic diagnosis is standard and depends on (1) serologic characterization of the patient's and the mother's or donor's cells, (2) the direct antiglobulin test, (3) indirect antiglobulin tests using a panel of normal erythrocytes of known group and genotype, (4) serologic tests using enzyme-treated normal erythrocytes of known group and genotype, (5) titration of antibodies, and (6) selected special procedures.

Identification of the group and genotype of erythrocytes is covered in Chapter 11. This is the first step in determining whether serologic incompatibility is a possibility. In pregnancy recognition of the possibility that immunization exists leads to periodic serologic studies which detect the onset of immunization and dictate life-saving measures at the time of the infant's birth. In recent years we have seen a successful attack on the prevention of Rh-isoimmune disease of the newborn by the use of Rh immune globulin.

The direct antiglobulin test is useful in detecting isoimmune hemolytic disease. A positive test indicates that antibodies are present, but it does not otherwise identify or characterize the antibody present.

The indirect antiglobulin test, on the other hand, is extremely valuable in the detection and identification of isoimmune antibodies. Normal group O erythrocytes representing a "panel" of various Rh genotypes first are exposed to the unknown serum and then are tested with antiglobulin serum to determine if they have been sensitized. The antibody can be identified by noting to which type of erythrocyte it becomes fixed. By using panels of red blood cells having various antigens, it is possible to identify both the common and the uncommon antibodies as well as to detect the presence of more than one antibody. Some immune antibodies, e.g., anti-**K,** can only be detected by this test.

Enzyme-treated cells in saline suspension are agglutinable by sera containing the specific antibodies. This method is as useful as the indirect antiglobulin test and gives the same information.

Rh antibodies can be titrated in one of three ways: (1) normal erythrocytes plus serial dilutions of the patient's serum in saline solution, (2) enzyme-treated erythrocytes plus serial dilutions of the patient's serum in saline solution, and (3) normal erythrocytes suspended in 20% albumin plus serial dilutions of the patient's serum in serum from group AB blood.

In cases of hemolytic disease of the newborn suspected of being caused by A-B-O incompatibility it is necessary to determine the presence and titer of immune anti-**A** or anti-**B.**

CHARACTERISTICS OF THE MAJOR HEMOLYTIC ANEMIAS
Hereditary spherocytosis
Etiology and pathogenesis
Etiology and pathogenesis are discussed on p. 567.

Clinical aspects
Hereditary spherocytosis is familial, expressed in heterozygotes, and transmitted as a mendelian dominant, so that usually one of the parents of an affected person also manifests the disease (Young et al, 1951). However, there are reports of well-documented cases in which both parents are hematologically normal (Race, 1942). Hereditary spherocytosis is to be found in all races, although it is most common in whites. There is no sex predilection. It may become manifest at any age, from birth (Trucco and Brown, 1967) to as late as 77 years (Race, 1942), but roughly half the cases are first detected in children and the other half in adolescents and young adults (Young et al, 1951; Young, 1955).

Although typically more severe in the young age group, the disease varies greatly in its clinical features. It may be so mild as to be recognized with difficulty or may show only mild anemia. Godal and Refsum (1979) report on three athletes in whom the development of mild anemia during intensive training revealed the presence of unsuspected hereditary spherocytosis. In other cases a significant anemia and jaundice point to hemolytic disease, and in a young child the triad of anemia, jaundice, and splenomegaly suggests the diagnosis of hereditary spherocytosis. A given patient may show periods of remission and exacerbation, the latter often following acute infectious disease. Two types of "crises" occur. The more common is an acute episode, probably hemolytic, characterized by fever, abdominal pain, vomiting, lassitude, and sometimes coma. Rarer is the crisis called *aplastic* by Owren (1948). This may have a similar clinical picture, but it is accompanied by an arrest of erythropoiesis in the bone marrow, absence of reticulocytes in the peripheral blood, leukopenia, and thrombocytopenia. Gallstones of the pigment type, caused by chronic hemolysis, are increasingly more common as the patient grows older and may give rise to obstructive jaundice (Young et al, 1951).

Physical examination usually reveals moderate to extreme splenomegaly without hepatomegaly. The spleen may not be palpable in subclinical cases. Chronic ulcers or hyperpigmentation of the skin about the ankles is reported to occur in 5% to 10% of the cases. In severe cases there may be obvious jaundice, but it is seldom extreme unless there is obstructive jaundice as well.

Laboratory findings
Anemia may be absent, mild, or severe, depending on the severity of the disease. Most commonly the anemia is mild unless the patient is seen during an episode of acute exacerbation. The red cell indices are usually not helpful and in fact may be misleading. Since the spherocytes are approximately of normal volume, because they are thicker, the MCV is usually not decreased significantly unless the other cells are microcytic because of iron deficiency. When the disease is severe, the increased reticulocytes, usually between 5% and 20% but sometimes much greater, tend to increase the MCV, and when half or more of the red cells are reticulocytes, the MCV is high, in the range of macrocytic anemia. It is not uncommmon for a folate deficiency to develop in a long-standing hemolytic anemia (Delamore et al, 1961) so that not only are macrocytic red cells found in the blood, but also the bone marrow may show megaloblastic dyspoiesis. The MCH is normal or moderately decreased, again depending on whether the nonspherocytic cells are hypochromic. The MCHC is usually normal but may be slightly increased.

The blood smear is characteristic, showing a triple population of red cells, one microspherocytic, one either normal or variably hypochromic, and one consisting of large polychromatophilic reticulocytes. As previously noted, the relative proportion of these cells determines whether the MCV is low, normal, or high. Spherocytes are usually numerous, but in mild cases they are few. Although anisocytosis is sometimes striking because of the mixture of microspherocytes and large reticulocytes, there is little, if any, poikilocytosis. Normoblasts are uncommon but they may be seen in children with severe disease. Although these features of the blood smear usually are strongly suggestive of hereditary spherocytosis, the number of spherocytes is sometimes small. Even then the spherocytes are all about the same size. This is not true in other situations in which some spherocytes are found in the blood: following the transfusion of stored blood, in isoimmune hemolytic disease, in many of the other hemolytic anemias, and in splenic hyperactivity.

After splenectomy the microspherocytes of hereditary spherocytosis persist because the spleen must be present to effect hemolysis of these cells. However, the reticulocytosis disappears, since abnormal hemolysis is not taking place. Reticulocytopenia is a feature of the acute aplastic crisis, an acute episode of more severe anemia, leukopenia, thrombocytopenia, and aplasia of the erythroid population of the bone marrow (Owren, 1948).

Characteristically, the osmotic fragility of the erythrocytes is increased, both with fresh blood and with blood incubated for 24 hours at 37° C. The osmotic fragility of incubated cells may be definitely abnormal when standard osmotic fragility tests give normal or equivocal results. The abnormal osmotic fragility is corrected by glucose. If osmotic fragility is plotted, as in Fig. 13-20, the curve is normal in shape but shifted to the left. Note that when in a mild case there is only a small number of spherocytes, an abnormality of osmotic fragility may not be detectable.

Autohemolysis after incubation of sterile blood at 37° C for 24 hours is increased in both mild and severe cases and will be even more striking if the blood is incubated for 48 hours (Young et al, 1956). Langley and Felderhof (1968) report some cases with an atypical autohemolysis pattern. Normal blood seldom shows autohemolysis of more than 2% of the red cells, whereas in hereditary spherocytosis there is usually hemolysis of 5% to 25% of the red cells (50% or more after 48 hours of incubation). Autohemolysis of spherocytes is normal if glucose, sucrose, or ATP is added. Increased autohemolysis is not diagnostic of hereditary spherocytosis but is a valuable adjunct to the laboratory diagnosis, especially when the effect of added glucose or ATP is determined. Slight or moderate autohemolysis not affected by glucose or ATP (originally called autohemolysis type I) is seen in G-6-PD deficiency, unstable hemoglobin disease, and hereditary elliptocytosis. Moderate to severe autohemolysis corrected by ATP, but not by glucose (originally called autohemolysis type II), is seen in both PK and HK deficiency. Autohemolysis not corrected by either glucose or ATP is characteristic of immunohemolytic anemia. Many of the other hemolytic anemias show moderate autohemolysis that falls into no definite category.

The total serum bilirubin concentration is seldom greater than 6 mg/dl (103 μM/l) and is usually between 2 and 3 mg/dl (34 and 51 μM/l). In uncomplicated hereditary spherocytosis there is an increase in the 1-minute (unconjugated) fraction. When there is superimposed obstructive jaundice, the total bilirubin concentration may be very high, with a high conjugated fraction. The fecal excretion of urobilinogen is very high.

Other findings, not diagnostic, are erythroid hyperplasia of the bone marrow, a negative antiglobulin test (a positive reaction may be found when there is severe reticulocytosis,

but this is nonspecific), leukocytosis after an episode of acute lysis, extramedullary hemopoiesis in the spleen and sometimes along the vertebral column, and enlargement of the marrow cavity in the skull and long bones. Siderosis of the liver and spleen may be present.

Treatment

Splenectomy should be performed whenever the diagnosis of hereditary spherocytosis is established, even if the patient is asymptomatic and only moderately anemic. The only exception is when the diagnosis is made during the first year of life, at which time splenectomy carries an increased risk of postoperative infection.

After splenectomy the hemolytic anemia is completely eliminated even though spherocytes persist in the blood. If hemolytic anemia persists, either the cause has been misdiagnosed or the surgeon has failed to find and excise accessory spleens (MacKenzie et al, 1962). Leukocytosis and thrombocytosis occur postoperatively but should not cause concern.

Elliptocytic hemolytic anemia
Etiology and pathogenesis

Etiology and pathogenesis are discussed on p. 568.

Clinical aspects

The incidence of hereditary elliptocytosis is 0.02% to 0.05% of the general population (Bannerman and Renwick, 1962). Hemolytic anemia occurs in 10% to 15% of persons with hereditary elliptocytosis (Geerdink et al, 1966). In elliptocytosis without hyperhemolysis the subject is hematologically normal. When hemolytic anemia is present, there may be jaundice, splenomegaly, and leg ulcers (Wilson and Long, 1955; McCurdy, 1962). A hemolytic episode may be precipitated by an infection. Hemolysis and hyperbilirubinemia in the newborn with hereditary elliptocytosis may be confused with other types of neonatal hyperbilirubinemia (Austin and Desforges, 1969).

Laboratory findings

In a typical case of hereditary elliptocytosis one fourth to three fourths of the red cells are elliptical. These vary from obvious cells that are two to three times as long as they are wide to some that are not so elongated. Lipton (1955) found the average ratio of width to length to be 0.78:1, but this is smaller in the majority of cases. There should be no difficulty in distinguishing hereditary elliptocytosis from other conditions in which some red cells are oval (iron-deficiency anemia, thalassemia, megaloblastic anemias, and various hemolytic anemias), since these oval cells are never as elongated or as numerous as in hereditary elliptocytosis. Austin and Desforges (1969) described pyknotic red cells in neonatal elliptocytic hemolytic anemia. As noted, the newborn with hereditary spherocytosis may show only a few elliptocytes.

During an acute hemolytic episode the blood smear shows a few spherocytes, elliptocytes, and many polychromatophilic red cells, the latter reflecting a reticulocytosis. The reticulocyte count is usually between 10% and 20%. The anemia is usually mild, as is the hyperbilirubinemia. The haptoglobin concentration is decreased, as in all hemolytic processes. The antiglobulin test is negative. Autohemolysis is abnormal, but there should be no need to perform this test.

Treatment

Most cases of elliptocytosis are not complicated by hemolytic anemia and require no treatment. When there is hemolytic anemia, splenectomy should be performed. As in hereditary spherocytosis, the abnormally shaped cells persist in the blood after splenectomy, and according to Weiss (1963) there may be irregular and bizarre forms.

Abetalipoproteinemia

Etiology and pathogenesis

Etiology and pathogenesis are discussed on p. 568.

Clinical aspects

The clinical picture is typical. Affected children probably are homozygous for the defect and are usually born to normal parents, consanguineous in about half the cases reported. The child is normal at birth, but by about 1 year of age steatorrhea and abdominal distention develop, progressing in later childhood to ataxia, muscular weakness, and visual disturbances caused by pigmentary retinal degeneration. Anemia is not a major component of the disease, but the acanthocytes are a valuable diagnostic finding.

Laboratory findings

The spiny erythrocytes (acanthocytes, Fig. 13-23, B) and the absence of β-lipoprotein make a distinctive combination. The acanthocyte has long, spiny projections that are longer and more regularly spaced than the projections of irregularly contracted or burr erythrocytes. One half or more of the red cells show the characteristic shape, whereas other malformations (burr cells, spur cells) affect a minority of the red cells and may be accompanied by other evidence of red cell fragmentation (keratocytes or schizocytes). Spicule-bearing red cells resembling acanthocytes can be found in cirrhosis, in pyruvate kinase deficiency, and after splenectomy, but none of these conditions is accompanied by abetalipoproteinemia. The abnormal shape of acanthocytes can be partially or completely corrected by suspending the cells in 5% albumin or in an isotonic buffer at pH 5.8 or by adding small amounts of cationic detergents. The shape abnormality occurs after the cells are released from the bone marrow. Moderate autohemolysis is a constant feature; it can be corrected by the addition of small amounts of glucose, heparin, or normal serum. Osmotic fragility is normal or moderately decreased. There is intermittent increased hemolysis in vivo, as evidenced by moderately severe anemia, reticulocytosis, and decreased concentration of serum haptoglobin (Salt et al, 1960). Occasionally the anemia is severe (Fredrickson et al, 1978).

Serum lipids are markedly decreased. The serum choles-

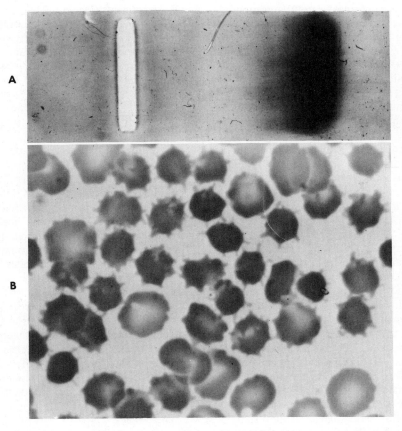

Fig. 13-23. Acanthocytosis and abetalipoproteinemia. **A,** Lipoprotein electrophoresis showing only α-lipoprotein. **B,** Acanthocytes, peripheral blood. (Wright's stain; ×950.)

terol is usually less than 60 mg/dl (1.6 mM/l), phospholipids less than 60 mg/dl (0.75 mM/l), and triglycerides less than 15 mg/dl (1.6 mM/l). No β-lipoprotein can be found on electrophoresis of the serum (Fig. 13-23, *A*). Specimens of small intestinal mucosa obtained by peroral biopsy show the villi to be normal in configuration, but the mucosal cells are engorged with lipid droplets (Fredrickson et al, 1978).

Treatment

There is no treatment that reverses the abetalipoprotein-emia. Some success is reported, with respect to the neurologic lesions, with administration of large doses of vitamins A and E (Fredrickson et al, 1978).

Paroxysmal nocturnal hemoglobinuria (PNH)
Etiology and pathogenesis

Etiology and pathogenesis are discussed on p. 563.

Clinical aspects

PNH occurs most frequently in middle-aged patients but also may be seen in children and in the elderly. There is no sex preference. The onset is insidious. Hemoglobinuria is present in the night or early morning urine specimens in the classic case, but often there are anemia and jaundice without hemoglobinuria. In others there is a pancytopenia that masks the diagnosis of PNH (Lewis and Dacie, 1967; Dacie and Lewis, 1972). Some cases of PNH terminate in acute leukemia (Kaufmann et al, 1969; Zittoun et al, 1975). When the hemoglobinuria is not nocturnal, careful questioning will reveal that it is still associated with sleep. Jaundice may be present in severe cases. Moderate splenomegaly is seen in about half the cases. Venous thromboses are not uncommon (Peytremann et al, 1972), and thrombosis of hepatic veins is a serious complication (Hartmann et al, 1980). Some or all of the features of DIC may accompany the thrombotic episodes. Nocturnal hemoglobinuria is paroxysmal rather than constant and may be precipitated by infections, blood transfusions, operations, menstruation, and a variety of drugs. In mild cases there may be anemia without hemoglobinuria. Occasionally an episode of hemoglobinuria follows the administration of heparin (Fritzsche and Martin, 1957), and heparin therapy probably is contraindicated in the treatment of thrombosis complicating PNH.

Laboratory findings

The peripheral blood usually shows no typical cellular abnormalities, but Pavlic and Bouroncle (1965) describe the presence of schizocytes during an acute attack. It is helpful to remember that spherocytosis is almost never seen in PNH. Anemia may be mild but is usually severe. During an aplastic episode there is anemia, leukopenia, and thrombocytopenia. Blood smears usually show a tendency toward macrocytosis of the erythrocytes. There is little or no anisocytosis or poikilocytosis. Reticulocytosis is common. Thrombocytopenia has been reported, as has leukopenia, but both are inconstant and show marked fluctuation. The bone marrow usually shows normoblastic hyperplasia, but there may be subtle megaloblastic change. It may show a reduction of all cell types if PNH follows or accompanies aplastic anemia. The two diseases frequently coexist, or

PNH may be followed by aplastic anemia or evolve into erythroleukemia (Cowall et al, 1979). The acid serum test (Ham test) is usually positive but may be negative, and it also may be positive in aplastic anemia, leukemia, and myloproliferative syndromes (Conrad and Barton, 1979). Hemolysis at an acid pH is also seen in hereditary spherocytosis and in 60% of the cases of hereditary dyserythropoietic anemia, HEMPAS (p. 569). The spherocytes of hereditary spherocytosis do not require complement, so that the control tubes with inactivated serum show no hemolysis in PNH and hemolysis with HS. These controls do not differentiate between PNH and HEMPAS. In PNH the sugar-water test of Hartmann and Jenkins (1966) is positive, but it is negative in HEMPAS. Hemoglobinuria in night or morning specimens is typical of the severe case but may be absent in mild cases. Hemoglobinemia, methemalbuminemia, and hyperbilirubinemia are present only when severe hemolysis occurs. Serum haptoglobin is decreased. Occasionally the antiglobulin (Coombs') test has been found to be positive, but it is usually negative. Intense siderosis of the kidneys and siderinuria are common.

Treatment

There is no treatment that alters the abnormality of the erythrocytes. The uncomplicated mild case should receive no treatment (Crosby, 1953). Treatment is directed toward the complications of infection, anemia, and thrombosis. A severe anemia can be rectified by transfusing *washed* red cell suspensions (Dacie, 1948), but the improvement is only temporary. The treatment of thrombosis, localized or generalized DIC, is usually ineffective (Peytremann et al, 1972) and may be dangerous if heparin is used (Fritzsche and Martin, 1957). A discussion of the problems to be considered in the treatment of PNH is given by Hartmann and Kolhouse (1972).

G-6-PD deficiency
Etiology and pathogenesis

Etiology and pathogenesis are discussed on p. 565.

Clinical aspects

G-6-PD activity is regulated by a gene on the X chromosome. In addition to being sex linked, the defect is incompletely dominant. The locus is closely linked to that for color blindness and hemophilia but not to that for Xg^a. The defect is fully expressed in homozygous males and variable in degree in heterozygous females. None of the other enzymatic defects are sex linked.

The hematologic effects of G-6-PD deficiency are varied, depending not only on the degree of expression of the defect but also on the enzymatic variant and on the race of the affected person. In some instances there is no hemolytic disease; in others there is mild chronic hemolysis not related to drug intake; and in still others the hemolytic disease is related to ingestion of one of the drugs listed in Table 13-2. Nevertheless it is possible to identify several major clinical variants.

The "black" type of G-6-PD deficiency was the first to be described. It was found that some black soldiers given antimalarial drugs developed mild to severe hemolytic anemia. Hemolysis tended to affect primarily older erythrocytes, so that in mild cases there was spontaneous improvement even when drug intake was continued. The susceptibility of erythrocytes to hemolysis was shown to be caused by a deficiency of G-6-PD. In the black male the deficiency is usually expressed as a sensitivity to an oxidant drug. About 10% (6% to 15%) of American black men have G-6-PD deficiency.

It was later found that G-6-PD deficiency has a widespread racial and geographic distribution. In whites and Orientals (''nonblack'' type of G-6-PD deficiency) there is greater susceptibility to the offending drugs, and the hemolytic episodes tend to be more acute and severe; e.g., nonblack–type deficient individuals are more susceptible to hemolysis following ingestion of chloramphenicol, quinine, and quinidine. They are also susceptible to hemolysis following ingestion of fava beans, whereas susceptible blacks are not.

Deficiency of G-6-PD seems to confer to the heterozygous female considerable resistance against falciparum malaria. Luzzatto et al (1969) suggest that the erythrocyte mosaicism which occurs in the heterozygous females accounts for the protective effect. Whatever the reason, it seems well established that the parasite prefers normal erythrocytes over those which are G-6-PD deficient.

A third clinical variant is seen in infants who are homozygous or heterozygous for G-6-PD deficiency. They have a high incidence of neonatal jaundice not related to any drug intake. It has been found that many of the adults who are shown to be G-6-PD deficient have had neonatal jaundice. One contributing factor may be that many infants normally have reduced glutathione peroxidase activity.

In addition to drug-induced hemolysis, susceptible individuals may develop acute hemolysis following viral infections or severe acidosis.

Laboratory findings

As expected, the peripheral blood findings range from completely normal to those of acute nonspherocytic hemolytic anemia. When there is mild compensated hemolytic disease, the anemia is mild or absent, and there is only moderate reticulocytosis and hyperbilirubinemia. In the acute hemolytic episodes the anemia is severe; there is marked hyperbilirubinemia and occasionally hemoglobinuria. The erythrocytes show no spherocytosis, may be entirely normal in appearance, or may be hypochromic in chronic hemolytic disease. During a severe acute episode there is leukocytosis, sometimes severe enough to be called a leukemoid reaction, and thrombocytosis.

The diagnosis of G-6-PD deficiency depends on both nonspecific and specific tests. Nonspecific tests are (1) a *positive autohemolysis test,* (2) a *positive Heinz body test* when blood is incubated with acetylphenylhydrazine (Fig. 13-24), (3) normal *osmotic fragility,* (4) *abnormal glutathione stability,* and (5) an *abnormal ascorbate test.* Specific identification of the enzymatic defect as a deficiency of G-6-PD is based on the specific quantitative assay of G-6-PD (Beutler, 1978a, 1978b).

The laboratory diagnosis of G-6-PD deficiency during an acute hemolytic episode is complicated by two features of

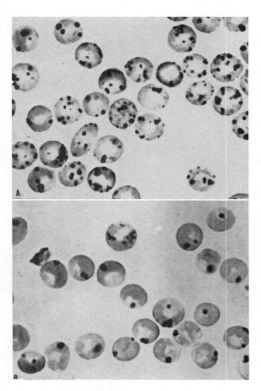

Fig. 13-24. Heinz body formation in sensitive, **A,** and nonsensitive, **B,** erythrocytes after incubation with acetylphenylhydrazine. (From Beutler et al, 1955.)

the acute hemolytic state: (1) hemolysis principally affects the older cells with the least enzymatic activity, leaving a disproportionate number of young erythrocytes with high enzyme activity; and (2) there is an increase in reticulocytes that are relatively rich in the enzyme.

Treatment

Severe acute hemolysis, especially in favism, should be treated by transfusing red cell suspensions to correct the anemia. Subjects with drug-sensitive hemolytic anemias should avoid drugs known to induce hemolysis (Table 13-2).

Other enzymatic defects

The second most common enzymatic defect associated with nonspherocytic hemolytic anemia is that of pyruvate kinase (Glader and Nathan, 1975; Valentine and Tanaka, 1978). The defect is inherited as an autosomal recessive characteristic. Mild to severe anemias have been described. The defect is identified by the specific fluorescence test.

The other enzymatic defects are very rare, and those interested are referred to Beutler (1978a, 1978b) and Valentine and Tanaka (1978).

Autoimmune hemolytic anemia (AIHA)
Etiology and pathogenesis

Etiologically, autoimmune hemolytic anemia is classified as idiopathic (primary, cause unknown) or symptomatic (secondary to various diseases, Table 13-2). Depending on

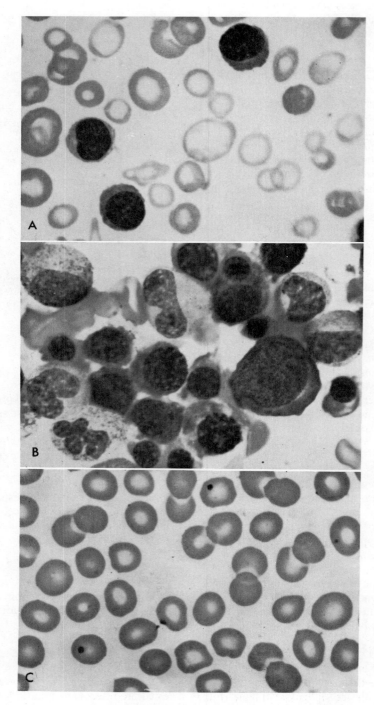

Fig. 13-25. Evans' syndrome. **A,** Peripheral blood smear. There are scattered normoblasts. **B,** Bone marrow. Note the erythroid hyperplasia. **C,** Peripheral blood, postsplenectomy. Note the Howell-Jolly bodies.

the serologic characteristics and the pathogenesis, it is also customary to classify these anemias as (1) the warm antibody type, (2) the cold antibody type, or (3) the drug-induced type (Issitt, 1977).

Warm antibody type

The anemia varies in severity and duration, and the onset is insidious. Hepatosplenomegaly is common, and lymphadenopathy is rare.

The blood smear shows some macrocytes, polychromatophilia, moderate anisocytosis, and some microspherocytes. Spherocytosis is striking in acute cases, and there may be normoblasts as well. Siderocytes are present in increased number. Erythrophagocytosis is found in many cases. There is variable reticulocytosis, sometimes as high as 50% or more. The leukocyte count may be elevated during an acute phase and may reach leukemoid levels (Porter and Lyle, 1974). The platelet count is usually normal, but there may be thrombocytopenia and purpura in combination with hemolytic anemia (Evans' syndrome, Fig. 13-25). The serum bilirubin concentration is elevated, typically the unconjugated fraction. The activity of serum lactate dehydrogenase is usually increased (Pirofsky, 1976). The bone marrow shows variable erythroid hyperplasia, depending on the severity and duration of the hemolytic anemia. The spleen is the site of erythrocyte destruction.

The osmotic fragility of the red blood cells is usually normal during a remission and increased in the acute phase. Autohemolysis is increased. The direct antiglobulin test is usually positive with polyspecific antisera but may be negative if there is low-grade sensitization of the red cells (Gilliland et al, 1971). If monospecific antisera are used, about 30% of the cases react with anti-IgG, about 50% with anti-IgG plus anticomplement, and about 20% with anticomplement (Issitt, 1974). Only rare cases show anti-IgA or anti-IgM specificity (Dacie and Worlledge, 1969). Antiglobulin−negative autoimmune hemolytic anemia has been reported in two subjects having IgA deficiency (Ghosh and Harris-Jones, 1974). On the other hand, a positive antiglobulin test not associated with hemolytic anemia is found in some narcotic addicts (Cushman and Maniatis, 1975) and in some normal individuals.

Warm antibodies commonly have anti−blood group specificity, usually for Rh antigens. When the specificity is for common factors, such as **rh″**, finding compatible blood for transfusion becomes a problem (Wiener et al, 1957). Usually the specificity is for several antigens. Dube et al (1975) have described a case having anti-N specificity.

Cold antibody type

Autoimmune hemolytic anemia of the cold antibody type is caused by antibodies maximally reactive at 0° to 10°C (Issitt, 1977) with occasional cases having a wide thermal range (Seldon et al, 1980). Typically a low titer is obtained if the test mixture is warmed to 37°C. The two most common cold agglutinins are anti-**I** and anti-**i**. Anti-**I** cold agglutinins are maximally reactive against red blood cells and are encountered as (1) pathologic autoantibodies in primary cold hemagglutination disease; (2) pathologic autoantibod-

ies in symptomatic cold hemagglutination disease secondary to leukemia, lymphoma, or pneumonia caused by *Mycoplasma pneumoniae* (in adults) or viral pneumonia (in children), usually in low titer; (3) low-titer autoantibodies in normal persons; or (4) alloantibodies in the rare adult having red blood cells of type i. Anti-**i** cold agglutinins are maximally reactive against cord red blood cells and are usually found (1) in patients with infectious mononucleosis caused by Epstein-Barr virus (EBV) and (2) rarely in other lymphoproliferative disorders and normal individuals (Rosenfield et al, 1965; Horwitz et al, 1977a).

When a polyspecific antiglobulin serum is used, the direct test is usually positive, and monospecific anticomplement antisera demonstrate only complement on the sensitized red blood cells. Complement is fixed in vivo at low temperatures, as on exposure to cold, leading to autoagglutination in peripheral blood vessels and acrocyanosis (Raynaud's disease). Autoagglutination in vitro can be avoided by placing drawn blood directly into a tube warmed to body temperature. It may be necessary to warm the glass slide before making a blood smear. If an erythrocyte count is performed manually, the diluting fluid must be warm. Erythrocyte counts with electronic particle-counting instruments can be completely erroneous because of autoagglutination.

High-titer cold antibodies are sometimes lytic. Acidified serum containing cold antibodies will lyse normal red cells at room temperature. Nonacidified serum containing cold antibodies will lyse trypsinized normal and PNH erythrocytes.

Drug-induced type

The pathogenesis of drug-induced immunologic injury to red blood cells is discussed on p. 562. Drug sensitization is often accompanied by a positive direct antiglobulin test, but hemolytic anemia is rare. In the case of sensitization of the hapten type (penicillin) and the innocent bystander type (such as stibophen) the indirect antiglobulin test will be positive when normal red blood cells are treated with the offending drug. A polyspecific antiserum should be used.

Treatment

The various therapeutic measures to be considered are reviewed by Pirofsky (1975). Severe anemia may indicate the need for blood transfusion, but this should be used only in life-threatening hypoxia or cardiac failure and with the realization that it may not be possible to find completely compatible donor blood. Steroid therapy is effective in about three fourths of the idiopathic type and about half the symptomatic type. If steroid therapy is ineffective or effective only in high doses over several weeks, then alternate approaches are indicated. Immunosuppressive therapy (azathioprine, chlorambucil, cyclophosphamide, amethopterin) is effective in about half the cases. Splenectomy should be considered if there is failure of steroid or immunosuppressive therapy plus evidence of major splenic red cell sequestration and destruction. Splenectomy is of no value in the cold-antibody type of autoimmune hemolytic anemia, because the liver is the major sequestering organ in this variant.

Paroxysmal cold hemoglobinuria (PCH)
Etiology and pathogenesis
Etiology and pathogenesis are discussed on p. 563.

Clinical aspects
Attacks of hemoglobinuria are precipitated by cold, but the duration of exposure and the degree of cold necessary to induce an attack vary from patient to patient. This corresponds to variations in thermal requirements in vitro. Hemolysis may occur immediately after exposure or some hours later. Pain in the legs, abdominal pain, and fever usually accompany an acute hemolytic episode. Constitutional symptoms or hemoglobinuria may occur separately. It was once thought that PCH is associated only with syphilis, but it is associated with a viral infection (Bird et al, 1976) or no obvious disease in about two thirds of the cases (Worlledge and Rousso, 1965).

Laboratory findings
The peripheral blood findings during a remission are not characteristic. During a paroxysm there may be an acute reduction in the concentration of erythrocytes and hemoglobin, followed by reticulocytosis. Hemoglobinemia accompanies acute hemolysis. If the plasma hemoglobin concentration rises above about 135 mg/dl (0.02 mM/l) of plasma, hemoglobinuria is found. The concentration of serum haptoglobin is reduced. Methemoglobin may be identified in the plasma after the paroxysm subsides. Leukopenia occurs during and immediately after a paroxysm, followed by leukocytosis. Erythrophagocytosis has been observed on blood smears made during an acute attack and apparently coincides with the leukopenic phase. The D-L reaction (p. 563) is positive at all stages of the disease, although during remission hemolysin activity may be minimal. Direct and indirect antiglobulin reactions are usually *positive* during a paroxysm and *negative* at other times. The positive antiglobulin reaction is complement and temperature dependent. The antibody can be assayed by the plaque-forming cell (PFC) method (Miyagawa et al, 1978). Scanning electron microscopy in one case (Djaldetti et al, 1975) has shown the red blood cells to have a wrinkled surface, a membrane alteration called *ropalocytosis* by Ghadially and Skinnider (1971). The significance of this ultrastructural finding is uncertain.

Treatment
PCH secondary to syphilis usually is improved by specific treatment for syphilis. PCH secondary to a viral infection usually disappears after the infection is over. Chronic and idiopathic cases of PCH usually require no therapy other than avoidance of cold. Transfusion should be avoided, but if necessary, the patient should be kept warm and should receive P-positive blood of homologous A-B-O and Rh groups kept at body temperature (Bird, 1977).

Unstable hemoglobin hemolytic disease
The unstable hemoglobins are discussed in Chapter 14.

Isoimmune hemolytic disease
Etiology and pathogenesis
Etiology and pathogenesis are discussed on p. 560.

Clinical aspects
Hemolytic transfusion reactions are discussed in Chapter 12. Hemolytic disease of the newborn may affect the fetus in utero or the infant at birth. Because the peripheral blood contains an abnormal number of normoblasts, the term "erythroblastosis fetalis" was once used. The presence of severe edema accounts for still another term no longer in favor, "hydrops fetalis." Normoblastosis and edema are absent in mild cases, but both are striking in the severely affected infant. Although some infants are only anemic at birth, the serum bilirubin concentration increases very rapidly, within 2 or 3 hours, and unless treated, there will be evidence of neurologic damage by the second day after birth. Splenomegaly and hepatomegaly are usually present, the degree of enlargement being proportional to the severity of the hemolytic syndrome. Petechial hemorrhages are not uncommon. The onset of neurologic damage may be marked by no more than irritability, but kernicterus soon produces tremors, a hyperactive Moro reflex, convulsions, and respiratory distress. Edema is striking in severely affected infants and is accompanied by hydrothorax and ascites.

Laboratory findings
The abnormalities found in the infant's blood are proportional to the severity of the disease. Anemia may be mild or severe. A hemoglobin concentration of 15 Gm/dl (2.3 mM/l) in cord blood is considered borderline normal and one of 13 Gm/dl (2.0 mM/l) definitely in the anemia range. The serum bilirubin of cord blood is elevated above 3 mg/dl (51.3 μM/l). If hyperbilirubinemia is not present at birth, it may develop during the next 24 hours. Indirect-reacting (unconjugated) bilirubin accounts for most of the increase and is responsible for the neurologic damage (Brodersen, 1977). The peripheral blood shows normoblastosis of various degrees, depending on the severity of the disease. More than 10 normoblasts per 100 leukocytes in the blood of a full-term infant may be considered suggestive of hemolytic disease. In premature infants as many as 40 normoblasts per 100 leukocytes can normally be found. Normoblastosis per se in an infant is not always indicative of isoimmune hemolytic disease, since it is also found in congenital syphilis, septicemia, inclusion disease, congenital heart disease, and the PJK syndrome (prematurity-jaundice-kernicterus).

The blood smear may show spherocytosis. This is usually slight in Rh incompatibility and striking in A-B-O incompatibility. Leukocytosis and thrombocytopenia are present if the disease is severe. Reticulocytosis is common.

Serologic studies of the infant's and mother's blood are necessary to determine the etiology. The blood group and genotype of the mother and the fetus are determined. The presence of an immune antibody is detected by direct and indirect antiglobulin tests. The direct antiglobulin test on cord blood is usually positive when a potent polyspecific antiglobulin serum is used. Some feel that the addition of bromelin increases the incidence of positive antiglobulin tests. A positive indirect antiglobulin test on cord blood demonstrates the presence of "free" immune antibody and when performed with a carefully selected panel of erythrocytes may specifically identify the antibody. If there is a possibility that hemolytic disease is caused by A-B-O incompatibility, the presence and titer of *immune* anti-**A** and anti-**B** antibodies in the mother's serum must be determined. An unsensitized mother will have no immune antibodies. In A-B-O hemolytic disease a mother with group O blood usually forms immune anti-**A** (A_1) antibodies, rarely anti-**B**. Isosensitization to antigens other than A-B-O or Rh_0 is rare (Wiener et al, 1964; Hanzlick and Senhauser, 1979).

Prevention and treatment

It is encouraging to end this chapter with the discussion of the one hemolytic anemia that can often be prevented (Walker, 1975; Bowman, 1978; Bowman et al, 1978). Human anti-**Rh_0** immune globulin has been used very successfully in women who are likely to develop anti-**Rh_0** antibodies and are then candidates for having a baby with isoimmune hemolytic disease. Candidates for the immune globulin are: (1) Rh_0-negative women undergoing abortion, (2) Rh_0-negative women with ectopic pregnancy, (3) postpartum Rh_0-negative mothers of an Rh_0-positive or D^u-positive infant, and (4) Rh_0-negative women of childbearing age who have inadvertently received a transfusion of Rh_0-positive blood (Abelson, 1974). The immune globulin should be given within 72 hours after abortion, delivery, or termination of an ectopic pregnancy. When the recipients are chosen carefully and the antiserum administered in proper dosage, the failure rate is judged to be as low as 2% (Woodrow, 1970). A count of the number of fetal cells in the mother's blood immediately postpartum estimates the amount of fetal-maternal hemorrhage (Clayton et al, 1973). Abelson (1974) gives a complete discussion of the indications, contraindications, and method of administering Rh immune globulin. Diamond (1974) reviews the development of modern prevention and treatment.

It goes without saying that Rh immune globulin will not prevent isoimmune hemolytic disease caused by incompatibility of other Rh factors or of the A-B-O and other blood groups (Finney et al, 1973; Spielmann et al, 1974; Weinstein and Taylor, 1975).

Another important measure is periodic antenatal monitoring of Rh_0-negative mothers to determine if sensitization is occurring. The genotype of the father may indicate the probability of sensitization, since the fetal cells must carry some of the paternal factors. Examination of the amniotic fluid to determine if it contains an excess of bilirubin (Bowman and Pollock, 1965) provides the pediatrician with important prognostic information.

Prompt treatment of an affected newborn by exchange transfusion serves to correct the anemia, reduce the hyperbilirubinemia, and eliminate antibody-coated cells (Mollison, 1979). Blood for exchange transfusion should be group O, Rh_0-negative, and freshly drawn to guarantee an adequate concentration of 2,3-DPG. The cross match is of donor cells against the mother's serum by the antiglobulin technic.

14

"... the rhymes are well
enough but not the reason,
and so it hath neither
rhyme nor reason."

Thomas Mann: *Joseph the Provider*

Anemia due to decreased erythrocyte survival—the hemoglobinopathies

INTRODUCTION
HISTORY
STRUCTURE OF HEMOGLOBIN
   Primary structure
   Secondary structure
   Tertiary structure
   Quaternary structure: the assembled molecule
NORMAL HEMOGLOBINS
   Hb A_1 ($\alpha_2\beta_2$)
   Hb A_2 ($\alpha_2\delta_2$)
   Hb F ($\alpha_2\gamma_2$)
   Hb A_{1c} (glycohemoglobin)
VARIANT HEMOGLOBINS
   Nomenclature
   Classification: structural
GENETIC CONTROL OF HEMOGLOBIN SYNTHESIS
   Inheritance patterns
   Synthesis of polypeptide chains
   Switch from fetal to adult hemoglobin
LABORATORY DIAGNOSIS IN THE HEMOGLOBINOPATHIES
   Introduction
   Tests for erythrocyte sickling
   Hb F: by alkali denaturation
   Hb F: erythrocyte distribution by acid elution
   Quantification of Hb A_2
   Ferrohemoglobin solubility
   Zone electrophoresis
   Ion-exchange chromatography
   Fingerprint technic
   Tests for unstable hemoglobin
   Hybridization technic
   Precautions in the laboratory diagnosis of the
     hemoglobinopathies
THE HEMOGLOBINOPATHIES
   Classification
   Geographic distribution
   Sickle cell anemia
     Hemoglobin synthesis
     Pathogenesis
     Clinical features
     Laboratory findings
   Sickle cell trait
   Screening for Hb S
   Hemoglobin C disease and trait
   Hemoglobin D disease and trait

Hemoglobin E disease and trait
Interaction between two structurally abnormal hemoglobins
   Sickle cell–Hb C disease
   Sickle cell–Hb D disease
   Other interactions
Unstable hemoglobin disease
Hemoglobinopathy associated with abnormal oxygen transport
   Increased oxygen affinity with erythrocytosis
   Decreased oxygen affinity with cyanosis
   Congenital methemoglobinemias
The thalassemia syndromes
   Geographic distribution
   Classification
   Genetics
   β-Thalassemia
     Homozygous
     Heterozygous
     Heterozygous β-thalassemia with another hemoglobinopathy
       Sickle cell–β-thalassemia
       Hb C–β-thalassemia
       Hb E–β-thalassemia
   $\delta\beta$-Thalassemia
     Homozygous
     Heterozygous
     Heterozygous $\delta\beta$-thalassemia with another hemoglobinopathy
   $\gamma\beta$-Thalassemia
   α-Thalassemia
     Homozygous
     Heterozygous
     Heterozygous α-thalassemia with another hemoglobinopathy
   δ-Thalassemia
   Hereditary persistence of fetal hemoglobin (HPFH)
     Heterozygous HPFH with another hemoglobinopathy
   The hemoglobin Lepore syndromes

INTRODUCTION

In the preceding chapter we considered some anemias caused by decreased erythrocyte survival where the abnormality, congenital or acquired, consisted of either an intrinsic biochemical and enzymatic defect or the mischance of normal erythrocytes in a hostile environment. In this chapter we will consider an especially interesting type of intrinsic erythrocytic abnormality, one in which there is a molecular lesion in hemoglobin synthesis leading either to the synthesis of "abnormal" hemoglobin molecules, the hemoglobin "variants," or to deficient synthesis of normal hemoglobin, as in the thalassemias. Whether the abnormality is in the structure of the polypeptide chains of the globin moiety of hemoglobin, whether the abnormality is in the *rate* of synthesis of one or more of the polypeptide chains, or whether there is a failure of the normal switch from fetal to adult hemoglobin production (Table 14-1), a *hemoglobinopathy* exists.

In about one-fourth of the hemoglobinopathies there is diminished erythrocyte survival leading to hemolytic disease and, when severe, to hemolytic anemia. The cause of the shortened erythrocyte survival is not always apparent, as discussed later (p. 638), but it must be assumed that in some situations a given hemoglobinopathy affects the membrane of the erythrocyte in such a way as to make it appear abnormal to the phagocytic cells of the RE system. Of equal interest is the question of why there is no decreased erythrocyte survival in other hemoglobinopathies.

HISTORY

In addition to clarifying the nature of once obscure anemias, the intensive research on the hemoglobinopathies has produced a massive body of data on the structure and function of hemoglobin and on the genetic controls over the synthesis of polypeptide chains. In recent years, this in turn has led to some success in the treatment of the most common hemoglobinopathy, sickle cell anemia, and to the promise that, given adequate basic information, other advances are possible in the treatment of disease at the molecular level.

Many investigators have contributed to the current knowledge. As far back as 1866, Körber discovered that two types of hemoglobin exist in human cord blood, one (Hb F for "fetal" hemoglobin) more resistant to denaturation by alkali than the other (Hb A for "adult" hemoglobin). The sickling phenomenon was observed by Herrick (1910) in the blood of a black suffering from severe anemia. Herrick was the first to use the term "sickle" when he described his findings as a "tendency of the erythrocytes to assume a slender sickle-like shape." Emmel (1917) not only observed the production of sickle cells in vitro but also recorded that sickling occurs not only in severly anemic but also in some nonanemic patients. Hahn and Gillespie (1927) showed that sickling occurred when the solution was oxygen deficient and that the shape change was reversible when the solution was oxygenated.

Table 14-1. General classification of the hemoglobinopathies

   I. Due to abnormal structure of one or more of the polypeptide chains of globin
  II. Due to abnormal rate of synthesis of one or more of the polypeptide chains of globin
 III. Hemoglobinopathies doubly heterozygous for two structural variants or a structural variant and thalassemia
  IV. The Lepore syndromes

After 1925 this line of investigation was paralleled by apparently unrelated studies on thalassemia, and soon these two streams merged into a mighty river of discovery. Prior to 1925 severe anemia in childhood was generally referred to as anemia of the von Jaksch type, "anemia infantum pseudoleukemica." Cooley and Lee (1925) described five children with severe anemia, splenomegaly, and bone changes and proposed that these findings made up a syndrome different from other types of anemia in infants and children (Cooley et al, 1927). The term "thalassemia" was introduced by Whipple and Bradford (1936), suggested by the Mediterranean background of affected children. During the same years (1925 to 1940) Italian hematologists reported the occurrence of anemia associated with hemolytic jaundice and decreased osmotic fragility of erythrocytes (Rietti, 1925; Greppi, 1928; Micheli et al, 1935). This syndrome, as defined by the Italian investigators, came to be known as anemia of the Rietti-Greppi-Micheli type, but its identity with the anemia described by Cooley was not considered, partly because the Italian cases were generally milder. It was not until Wintrobe et al (1940) described a mild hemolytic anemia in 14 members of three Italian families in Baltimore and in both parents of a child with typical severe thalassemia that it became obvious that the cases described by Rietti and the other Italian hematologists and the cases described by Wintrobe and his colleagues represented the mild heterozygous state of thalassemia (minor and minima), while the severe anemia, thalassemia major, represented the homozygous state (Chini and Valeri, 1949).

Pauling et al (1949) showed that the hemoglobin in sickle cell anemia (Hb S) migrated differently from normal hemoglobin (Hb A) when subjected to electrophoresis, a difference shown to be caused by an amino acid substitution in the globin polypeptide chain (Ingram, 1956, 1958). The new investigative technics, electrophoresis, "fingerprinting" of subunits of polypeptide chains, and amino acid analysis, were soon applied to the detection and characterization of many abnormal hemoglobins. Quite naturally the hemoglobins present in thalassemia were subjected to intensive study, and it was disappointing to find no evidence of structural abnormality in classic thalassemia. It seemed that some other defect in the genetic control was operative at the molecular level, and indeed some of the most interesting aspects of thalassemia involve studies of the genetic control of hemoglobin synthesis. Finally, the x-ray crystallographic studies of Perutz and his associates (Perutz, 1963, 1965; Perutz et al, 1965, 1968a, 1968b) provided the three-dimensional model of the hemoglobin molecule to which the various amino acid substitutions can be related.

The final story cannot yet be told, for we are on the threshold of important discoveries concerning the function of normal and abnormal hemoglobins, the genetic control over their synthesis, and the application of present and extended knowledge to the treatment of the hemoglobinopathies.

STRUCTURE OF HEMOGLOBIN

Human hemoglobin is composed of two pairs of polypeptide chains. Within each chain is nestled the heme prosthetic group. Since hemoglobin is a protein, it can be defined, first, in terms of its *primary* structure—the amino acid sequences and the covalent structure of the peptide chain. The *secondary structure* defines the arrangement in space of the helical structures making up the polypeptide chain. The *tertiary structure* is the arrangement in space of the secondary structures, the coiled shape of the polypeptide chain. The *quaternary structure* is the relationship of polypeptide chains to each other in the composition of the complete molecule.

Primary structure

The normal human hemoglobins are Hb A_1 (preferable to Hb A since there is an Hb A_2), which is the major component, Hb A_2, and Hb F.

Hb A_1 is composed of a pair of polypeptide chains designated α and a pair designated β, the molecular formula being $\alpha_2\beta_2$. The α-chain is defined by the sequence of 141 amino acids (Fig. 14-1), the β-chain by 146 amino acids (Fig. 14-2). Normal adult erythrocytes contain a very small fraction, designated Hb A_3, that increases as the hemolysate ages. It probably differs from Hb A_1 only in having a glutathione molecule attached to the β-chain (Muller, 1961). Other minor components, of no obvious importance, have been identified (Holmquist and Schroeder, 1966).

Hb A_2 is composed of a pair of α-chains and a pair designated δ, the molecular formula being $\alpha_2\delta_2$. The δ-chain is defined by the sequence of 146 amino acids (Fig. 14-3).

Hb F is composed of a pair of α-chains and a pair designated γ, the molecular formula being $\alpha_2\gamma_2$. The γ-chain is defined by the sequence of 146 amino acids (Fig. 14-4). Hb F in normal cord blood is a mixture of two types, one having ALA at position 136 and the other GLY (Schroeder et al, 1968). The two can be designated $\alpha_2\gamma_2^{136\ ala}$ and $\alpha_2\gamma_2^{136\ gly}$.

Three other hemoglobins can be considered normal, even though they are found in special situations. Hemoglobin Gower 1 is a tetramer of still another type of polypeptide chain, ϵ, and has the molecular formula ϵ_4. Hemoglobin Gower 2 contains a pair of normal α-chains and a pair of ϵ-chains and has the molecular formula $\alpha_2\epsilon_2$. Both are found in early human embryos (Huehns et al, 1964). The amino acid sequence of the ϵ-chain is not known. Traces of hemoglobin Portland 1 are found in normal cord blood and contain a pair of polypeptide chains designated ζ and a pair of γ-chains (Capp et al, 1970). The amino acid sequence of this sixth type of chain has not been determined.

Secondary structure

The amino acids in the polypeptide chains are not strung out in a straight line but are twisted around an imaginary axis in a helical conformation. Depending on the degree of rotation and the number of amino acids per 360° turn, three types of helixes are formed, designated α, π, and 3_{10}. About 60% of the polypeptide chains are in the α-helical conformation (Murayama, 1971).

```
 1   2   3   4   5   6   7   8   9  10  11  12  13  14  15
VAL-LEU-SER-PRO-ALA-ASP-LYS-THR-ASN-VAL-LYS-ALA-ALA-TRY-GLY

16  17  18  19  20  21  22  23  24  25  26  27  28  29  30
LYS-VAL-GLY-ALA-HIS-ALA-GLY-GLU-TYR-GLY-ALA-GLU-ALA-LEU-GLU

31  32  33  34  35  36  37  38  39  40  41  42  43  44  45
ARG-MET-PHE-LEU-SER-PHE-PRO-THR-THR-LYS-THR-TYR-PHE-PRO-HIS

46  47  48  49  50  51  52  53  54  55  56  57  58  59  60
PHE-ASP-LEU-SER-HIS-GLY-SER-ALA-GLN-VAL-LYS-GLY-HIS-GLY-LYS

61  62  63  64  65  66  67  68  69  70  71  72  73  74  75
LYS-VAL-ALA-ASP-ALA-LEU-THR-ASN-ALA-VAL-ALA-HIS-VAL-ASP-ASP

76  77  78  79  80  81  82  83  84  85  86  87  88  89  90
MET-PRO-ASN-ALA-LEU-SER-ALA-LEU-SER-ASP-LEU-HIS-ALA-HIS-LYS

91  92  93  94  95  96  97  98  99 100 101 102 103 104 105
LEU-ARG-VAL-ASP-PRO-VAL-ASN-PHE-LYS-LEU-LEU-SER-HIS-CYS-LEU

106 107 108 109 110 111 112 113 114 115 116 117 118 119 120
LEU-VAL-THR-LEU-ALA-ALA-HIS-LEU-PRO-ALA-GLU-PHE-THR-PRO-ALA

121 122 123 124 125 126 127 128 129 130 131 132 133 134 135
VAL-HIS-ALA-SER-LEU-ASP-LYS-PHE-LEU-ALA-SER-VAL-SER-THR-VAL

136 137 138 139 140 141
LEU-THR-SER-LYS-TYR-ARG
```

Fig. 14-1. α-Chain of human hemoglobin, sequence of amino acids. ALA = alanine, ARG = arginine, ASP = aspartic acid, ASN = asparagine, CYS = cysteine, GLU = glutamic acid, GLN = glutamine, GLY = glycine, HIS = histidine, ILU = isoleucine, LEU = leucine, LYS = lysine, MET = methionine, PHE = phenylalanine, PRO = proline, SER = serine, THR = threonine, TRY = tryptophan, TYR = tyrosine, VAL = valine. (After Lehmann and Carrell, 1969.)

```
  1    2    3    4    5    6    7    8    9   10   11   12   13   14   15
VAL-HIS-LEU-THR-PRO-GLU-GLU-LYS-SER-ALA-VAL-THR-ALA-LEU-TRY

 16   17   18   19   20   21   22   23   24   25   26   27   28   29   30
GLY-LYS-VAL-ASN-VAL-ASP-GLU-VAL-GLY-GLY-GLU-ALA-LEU-GLY-ARG

 31   32   33   34   35   36   37   38   39   40   41   42   43   44   45
LEU-LEU-VAL-VAL-TYR-PRO-TRY-THR-GLN-ARG-PHE-PHE-GLU-SER-PHE

 46   47   48   49   50   51   52   53   54   55   56   57   58   59   60
GLY-ASP-LEU-SER-THR-PRO-ASP-ALA-VAL-MET-GLY-ASN-PRO-LYS-VAL

 61   62   63   64   65   66   67   68   69   70   71   72   73   74   75
LYS-ALA-HIS-GLY-LYS-LYS-VAL-LEU-GLY-ALA-PHE-SER-ASP-GLY-LEU

 76   77   78   79   80   81   82   83   84   85   86   87   88   89   90
ALA-HIS-LEU-ASP-ASN-LEU-LYS-GLY-THR-PHE-ALA-THR-LEU-SER-GLU

 91   92   93   94   95   96   97   98   99  100  101  102  103  104  105
LEU-HIS-CYS-ASP-LYS-LEU-HIS-VAL-ASP-PRO-GLU-ASN-PHE-ARG-LEU

106  107  108  109  110  111  112  113  114  115  116  117  118  119  120
LEU-GLY-ASN-VAL-LEU-VAL-CYS-VAL-LEU-ALA-HIS-HIS-PHE-GLY-LYS

121  122  123  124  125  126  127  128  129  130  131  132  133  134  135
GLU-PHE-THR-PRO-PRO-VAL-GLN-ALA-ALA-TYR-GLN-LYS-VAL-VAL-ALA

136  137  138  139  140  141  142  143  144  145  146
GLY-VAL-ALA-ASN-ALA-LEU-ALA-HIS-LYS-TYR-HIS
```

Fig. 14-2. β-Polypeptide chain, sequence of amino acids. See legend for Fig. 14-1.

```
  1    2    3    4    5    6    7    8    9   10   11   12   13   14   15
VAL-HIS-LEU-THR-PRO-GLU-GLU-LYS-THR-ALA-VAL-ASN-ALA-LEU-TRY

 16   17   18   19   20   21   22   23   24   25   26   27   28   29   30
GLY-LYS-VAL-ASN-VAL-ASP-ALA-VAL-GLY-GLY-GLU-ALA-LEU-GLY-ARG

 31   32   33   34   35   36   37   38   39   40   41   42   43   44   45
LEU-LEU-VAL-VAL-TYR-PRO-TRY-THR-GLN-ARG-PHE-PHE-GLU-SER-PHE

 46   47   48   49   50   51   52   53   54   55   56   57   58   59   60
GLY-ASP-LEU-SER-SER-PRO-ASP-ALA-VAL-MET-GLY-ASN-PRO-LYS-VAL

 61   62   63   64   65   66   67   68   69   70   71   72   73   74   75
LYS-ALA-HIS-GLY-LYS-LYS-VAL-LEU-GLY-ALA-PHE-SER-ASP-GLY-LEU

 76   77   78   79   80   81   82   83   84   85   86   87   88   89   90
ALA-HIS-LEU-ASP-ASN-LEU-LYS-GLY-THR-PHE-SER-GLN-LEU-SER-GLU

 91   92   93   94   95   96   97   98   99  100  101  102  103  104  105
LEU-HIS-CYS-ASP-LYS-LEU-HIS-VAL-ASP-PRO-GLU-ASN-PHE-ARG-LEU

106  107  108  109  110  111  112  113  114  115  116  117  118  119  120
LEU-GLY-ASN-VAL-LEU-VAL-CYS-VAL-LEU-ALA-ARG-ASN-PHE-GLY-LYS

121  122  123  124  125  126  127  128  129  130  131  132  133  134  135
GLU-PHE-THR-PRO-GLN-MET-GLN-ALA-ALA-TYR-GLN-LYS-VAL-VAL-ALA

136  137  138  139  140  141  142  143  144  145  146
GLY-VAL-ALA-ASN-ALA-LEU-ALA-HIS-LYS-TYR-HIS
```

Fig. 14-3. δ-Chain of human hemoglobin, sequence of amino acids. See legend for Fig. 14-1. (After Schroeder et al, 1968.)

```
 1    2    3    4    5    6    7    8    9   10   11   12   13   14   15
GLY-HIS-PHE-THR-GLU-GLU-ASP-LYS-ALA-THR-ILU-THR-SER-LEU-TRY

16   17   18   19   20   21   22   23   24   25   26   27   28   29   30
GLY-LYS-VAL-ASN-VAL-GLU-ASP-ALA-GLY-GLY-GLU-THR-LEU-GLY-ARG

31   32   33   34   35   36   37   38   39   40   41   42   43   44   45
LEU-LEU-VAL-VAL-TYR-PRO-TRY-THR-GLN-ARG-PHE-PHE-ASP-SER-PHE

46   47   48   49   50   51   52   53   54   55   56   57   58   59   60
GLY-ASN-LEU-SER-SER-ALA-SER-ALA-ILU-MET-GLY-ASN-PRO-LYS-VAL

61   62   63   64   65   66   67   68   69   70   71   72   73   74   75
LYS-ALA-HIS-GLY-LYS-LYS-VAL-LEU-THR-SER-LEU-GLY-ASP-ALA-ILU

76   77   78   79   80   81   82   83   84   85   86   87   88   89   90
LYS-HIS-LEU-ASP-ASP-LEU-LYS-GLY-THR-PHE-ALA-GLN-LEU-SER-GLU

91   92   93   94   95   96   97   98   99  100  101  102  103  104  105
LEU-HIS-CYS-ASP-LYS-LEU-HIS-VAL-ASP-PRO-GLU-ASN-PHE-LYS-LEU

106  107  108  109  110  111  112  113  114  115  116  117  118  119  120
LEU-GLY-ASN-VAL-LEU-VAL-THR-VAL-LEU-ALA-ILU-HIS-PHE-GLY-LYS

121  122  123  124  125  126  127  128  129  130  131  132  133  134  135
GLU-PHE-THR-PRO-GLU-VAL-GLN-ALA-SER-TRY-GLN-LYS-MET-VAL-THR

136  137  138  139  140  141  142  143  144  145  146
GLY-VAL-ALA-SER-ALA-LEU-SER-SER-ARG-TYR-HIS
```

Fig. 14-4. γ-Polypeptide chain, sequence of amino acids. See legend for Fig. 14-1. Position 136 can be occupied by either ALA or GLY. (After Schroeder et al, 1968.)

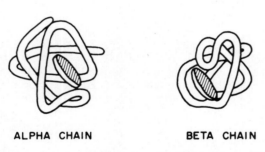

ALPHA CHAIN   **BETA CHAIN**

Fig. 14-5. The tertiary structure of the polypeptide chains of normal hemoglobin (Hb A₁). The heme group is shown as a disk, which in actual size is much smaller.

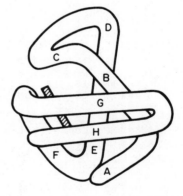

Fig. 14-6. β-Chain of human hemoglobin with the helices lettered **A** to **H.** (Modified from Schroeder and Jones, 1965.)

Tertiary structure

The conformation of the polypeptide chains is that of alternating helical and nonhelical segments coiled in what appears to be an irregular pretzel shape (Fig. 14-5). In fact, the coiling is such as to determine the orientation of polar groups (lysine and glutamic acid), dipolar groups (tyrosine and glutamine), and nonpolar groups (valine and leucine). In general, polar residues are excluded from the interior while large nonpolar residues usually lie either in the interior or in surface crevices.

The heme group in each polypeptide chain lies in a nonpolar pocket. One of the six coordination bonds of heme iron is linked with a histidine (87 HIS in the α-chain and 92 HIS in the β-chain), four are committed to the porphyrin ring, and the sixth is the site of combination with oxygen. The heme group contributes to the stability of the tertiary structure not only because of the histidine linkage but also through interaction with many nonpolar groups in the interior.

The helical portions of the polypeptide chains are designated by letters A to H (Fig. 14-6), beginning at the *N*-terminus. The nonhelical portions are designated by zones AB, BC, etc. The location of abnormalities in the polypeptide chains is defined by the number of the variant amino

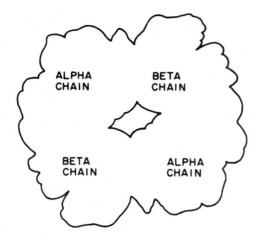

Fig. 14-7. Configuration of hemoglobin molecule, diagrammatic, as seen in horizontal cross section (see text).

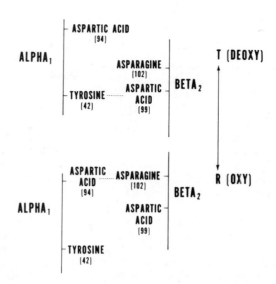

Fig. 14-8. Stereochemical changes occurring at the $\alpha_1\beta_2$ contact on oxygenation. The dotted line indicates a hydrogen bond. Note the shift in the hydrogen bond between tyrosine 42 and aspartic acid 99 to aspartic acid 94 and asparagine 102.

acid in the chain, also optionally by the helix in which the variation occurs. The latter convention will not be followed in this text.

Quaternary structure: the assembled molecule

The assembled molecule of hemoglobin consists of four interrelated subunits, each subunit consisting of a polypeptide chain and its heme moiety. In the case of normal human hemoglobin A_1, the molecule consists of two α and two β chains. The tetramer and the four hemes are so arranged as to enable the molecule to fulfill its role in the transport of oxygen from the lungs to the tissues and carbon dioxide from the tissues to the lungs. Detailed reviews of the stereochemistry of the hemoglobin molecule are given by Winslow and Anderson (1978), Perutz (1978), and Olsen (1979).

The tetramer forms a globular molecule having a central cavity (Fig. 14-7). The molecule is symmetric about the axis of the cavity and also in a plane perpendicular to this axis. The four subunits are held in this conformation by hydrophobic interactions at points of contact; about 60% of the contacts are between α_1 and β_1 chains ($\alpha_1\beta_1$ contacts), 33% are $\alpha_1\beta_2$ contacts, and the other 7% are $\alpha_1\alpha_2$ and $\beta_1\beta_2$ contacts. In each subunit the heme lies in a deep pocket of the globin chain, leaving only one edge of the heme exposed to receive the oxygen.

The structure of the normal hemoglobin molecule enables it to fulfill optimally the functions of delivering oxygen to the tissues and of eliminating carbon dioxide.

If the percent saturation of blood with oxygen is plotted against oxygen tensions (Po_2) from 0 to 100 mm Hg, the curve has the familiar sigmoid shape (Fig. 14-49). This is an expression of the characteristic oxygen pick-up and delivery system that provides for maximum saturation of hemoglobin with oxygen at the Po_2 existing in the lungs (100 mm Hg) and maximum release of oxygen at the Po_2 in the tissue (35 mm Hg). This is achieved by the combination of several interrelated physicochemical reactions.

According to Perutz (1978) the oxygen saturation and delivery system depends on the hemoglobin molecule

assuming either the R (relaxed) state or the T (tense) state. This is generally called the *allosteric* model (from the Greek *allos*, "other", and *stereos*, "solid"). The equilibrium between the R and T conformation is influenced by "allosteric effectors" such as protons or 2,3-DPG, which react with the hemoglobin molecule at nonheme sites. A second feature is the "heme-heme interaction," a sequential oxygenation of the four hemes in which the combination of oxygen with the first heme facilitates oxygenation with the second and subsequent ones. Deoxyhemoglobin is in the T conformation, and, as the first oxygen is added, salt bridges are successively broken or weakened and the molecule assumes the R conformation. When oxygen is released at the tissue level, the conformation returns to T. The simile used by Perutz (1978) is that "hemoglobin is not an oxygen tank but a molecular lung because it changes its structure every time it takes up oxygen or releases it."

The structural changes that take place are quite small, a matter of a few angströms. On oxygenation, the iron in the heme of the α-chain shifts 1 Å from a slight angle to the plane of the porphyrin ring into the plane of the ring. This is sufficient to change the distance between the heme-linked histidine and the plane of the porphyrin ring and to break salt bridges (a bond between N^+ and O^-) at the ends of the polypeptide chain as the molecule changes from the T to the R conformation. Another change that takes place is a switch in the hydrogen bonds (bonds between N and O through an intermediate H) between two subunits. Because the $\alpha_1\beta_1$ and $\alpha_2\beta_2$ subunits are held together by many hydrogen bonds, these dimers are inflexible. However, the contact between α_1 and β_1 is not so rigid, and the conformation changes when oxygen is introduced or released (Fig. 14-8).

The combination and release of oxygen with hemoglobin is affected by the concentration of H^+ (the Bohr effect), by the P_{CO_2}, and by the concentration of 2,3-DPG (p. 390). The carbon dioxide generated from cellular metabolism decreases the oxygen affinity of hemoglobin by lowering the pH and also by competitive binding for 2,3-DPG of N-terminal amino groups. The net effect is to shift the oxygen dissociation curve to the right.

The normal structure of the hemoglobin molecule is altered genetically in the "hemoglobinopathies." Some of the alterations lead to hemolytic disease or other clinical problems, whereas others are innocuous. The alterations of the hemoglobin molecule may be (1) point mutations having a single amino acid substitution, (2) mutations characterized by more than one amino acid substitution on the same chain, (3) deletions of amino acids, and (4) insertions and additions of amino acids. When the mutation causes significant clinical abnormalities, one or several of the following mechanisms are operative: (1) the substitution affects the heme pocket and the $\alpha_1\beta_1$ interface; (2) the substitution disrupts the α-helix conformation; (3) the substitution causes the deoxyhemoglobin molecules to form rigid fibers; (4) the mutation affects the oxygenation of heme iron; (5) the mutation affects the equilibrium between the T and R conformations.

NORMAL HEMOGLOBINS

Normal adult erythrocytes contain three hemoglobins, Hb A_1, Hb A_2, and Hb F. These can therefore be considered "normal" hemoglobins, even though in certain hemoglobinopathies the relative concentrations may be higher or lower than normal. On starch gel electrophoresis, one other distinct band, A_3, can be seen. This is of no significance, for it represents denatured hemoglobin plus nonhemoglobin stromal protein.

Hb A_1 ($\alpha_2\beta_2$)

Hb A_1 is the major component of normal adult blood and is responsible for oxygen transport. Minor components, designated Hb A_{1a} to Hb A_{1c}, have been found increased in diabetes mellitus (Tattersall et al, 1975). They migrate ahead of Hb A_1.

Hb A_2 ($\alpha_2\delta_2$)

Hb A_2 (Vella, 1977) is a minor component of normal adult blood. It can be separated from Hb A_1 by starch block (Fig. 14-23), cellulose acetate (Fig. 14-24), starch gel electrophoresis (Fig. 14-25), and chromatography. The values for the normal concentration of Hb A_2 depend on the method used (Appendix). Hb A_2 levels are low in both the normal and in sickle cell–$\beta+$ thalassemia and SS infants but are higher in sickle cell–$\beta+$ thalassemia than in SS or normal children by age 6 months to 1 year (Serjeant et al, 1978).

A variant of Hb A_2, designated A_2' (old designation Hb B_2), has been described by Horton and Huisman (1965). It is a genetically determined variant (Fig. 14-9) that may be found either alone or in combination with thalassemia. (Vella, 1977). Other variants of Hb A_2 are listed in Table 14-4.

Hb F ($\alpha_2\gamma_2$)

Fetal hemoglobin was discovered in 1866 by Körber, but Haurowitz, in 1929, was responsible for the first studies on the kinetics of the denaturation reaction. Hb F exhibits pro-found differences from Hb A_1. The two hemoglobins are immunologically different and show different oxygen dissociation properties. As oxyhemoglobin, Hb A_1 is readily denatured by alkali, whereas Hb F is not (Fig. 14-20).

Fetal hemoglobin can be demonstrated in blood smears by the method of Kleihauer et al (1957) or Neirhaus and Betke (1968). In hereditary persistence of fetal hemoglobin, all of the erythrocytes are found to contain some Hb F; when there is a mixed cell population, as in cord blood or other conditions accompanied by an elevated Hb F, there are scattered Hb F–containing erythrocytes among those that are normal (Fig. 14-10).

The elaboration of Hb F in fetal blood cells invites speculation, but little is actually known about how and why it happens. Hb F is characteristic of fetal blood (Cooper and Hoagland, 1972), but Hb A_1 is also elaborated throughout fetal life. There are wide variations in the relative amount of each hemoglobin at various fetal ages, but Hb A_1 has been detected as early as the thirteenth fetal week. In the newborn infant, half or more of the hemoglobin is of the fetal type. After birth, the concentration of Hb F falls rapidly if there is no hematologic disorder, and by the age of 1 to 2 years it has fallen to less than 1% (Fig. 14-11). In the D-trisomy syndrome, however, fetal hemoglobin is high at birth and remains high throughout infancy; there is often an unusually low concentration of Hb A_2.

Increased levels of Hb F are found in response to erythroid stimulation (Dover et al, 1979), in leukemia (Sheridan et al, 1976), in malignant osteopetrosis (Schilirò et al, 1978), in testicular malignancy (Dainiak and Hoffman, 1980), and in the secondary phase of aplastic anemia (Papayannopoulou et al, 1980).

Evidence exists that there is an association between Hb F and erythrocyte hexokinase type II. Hexokinase types I and III are present in adult erythrocytes, while type II is present only in the erythrocytes of newborn infants and of adults with hereditary persistence of fetal hemoglobin (Holmes et al, 1967).

At low oxygen tensions, Hb F is a more efficient carrier of oxygen than Hb A_1. It also releases carbon dioxide more readily. These properties are beneficial to the fetus. On the other hand, Hb F is more readily converted to methemoglobin than is Hb A_1, accounting for the greater susceptibility to methemoglobinemia shown by infants.

Hb A_{1c} (glycohemoglobin)

Normal blood contains a minor electrophoretically fast-moving fraction that has been shown to consist of four minor hemoglobins designated Hb A_{1a}, Hb A_{1a2}, Hb A_{1b}, and Hb A_{1c} (Bunn et al, 1978). The concentration of Hb A_{1c} is normally 3% to 6% of total hemoglobin. Hb A_{1c} differs from the Hb A_1 by the presence of one molecule of glucose bound to the N-terminal valine of every β-chain. It is formed in vivo from the combination of Hb A_1 with blood glucose, continuously and irreversibly, during the entire life span of erythrocytes (Bunn et al, 1976). Glycohemoglobin is also formed in vitro (Flückiger and Winterhalter, 1976). Sugars other than glucose bind to Hb A_1, and such combinations at sites other than β-chains produce the other minor components (Abdella et al, 1977; Bunn et al, 1979).

The concentration of Hb A_{1c} is increased two- to threefold in patients with diabetes mellitus (Rahbar, 1968; Rahbar et al, 1969b). The early hope was that this increase was a specific marker for diabetes (Paulsen, 1973), and this stimulated the development of clinically useful test systems (McDonald and Davis, 1979). However, the determination of Hb A_{1c} is not a specific test for diabetes. Variables that influence the quantitative results are the presence of Hb S, the hereditary persistance of fetal hemoglobin and other high-F syndromes, hyperlipemia, or the presence of a high proportion of young erythrocytes, as in hemolytic anemia or the anemia of chronic blood loss (Bernstein, 1980). Although glycosylation occurs progressively throughout the life span of the erythrocytes, Widness et al (1980) have shown that the level of Hb A_{1c} shows rapid fluctuations

related to acute changes in glucose concentration. Some of the rapidly formed glycohemoglobin may represent a loose complexing of glucose and Hb A_1, possibly at non-β loci (Bunn et al, 1979). At best, the measurement of Hb A_{1c} reflects the average blood glucose levels during the previous 2 to 4 weeks (Koenig et al, 1976a, 1976b; Gabbay et al, 1977; Gonen et al, 1977). Dix et al (1979) suggest that an elevation of Hb A_{1c} in the presence of a normal or "borderline abnormal" fasting blood glucose concentration is indicative of "latent diabetes," terms not easily definable. Dods and Bolmey (1979) found total glycosylated hemoglobin concentrations to correlate best with the 2-hour glucose tolerance test, but the criteria for a subject being diabetic or borderline on the basis of glucose tolerance are not so crit-

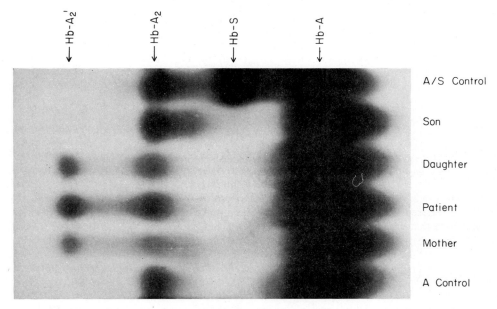

Fig. 14-9. Starch gel electrophoresis showing the separation of Hb A_2 and a family with Hb A_2'.

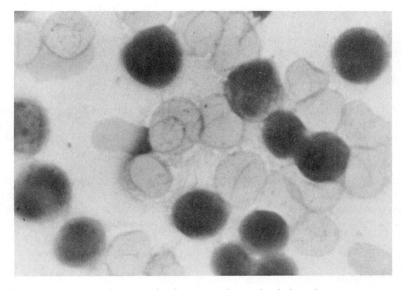

Fig. 14-10. Hb F demonstrated in RBCs by the stain technic. The dark erythrocytes contain Hb F.

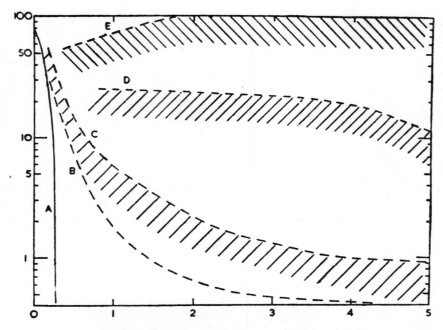

Fig. 14-11. Fetal hemoglobin levels after birth to 5 years of age. Ordinate: Hb F (%). Abscissa: Age (years). Curve **A,** Theoretical rate of disappearance of Hb F (80% at birth) assuming mean erythrocyte life span to be 100 days. Curve **B,** Rate of disappearance in normal children (slightly exaggerated since the Hb F concentration does not normally reach zero). Curve **C,** Maximal Hb F levels in thalassemia minor and sickle cell trait. Curve **D,** Maximal Hb F levels in sickle cell anemia in heterozygotes for two abnormal hemoglobins or thalassemia and an abnormal hemoglobin. Curve **E,** Upper level of Hb F in thalassemia major. (From White and Beaven, 1959.)

ical as to serve as the reference method. From the data available, it must be concluded that the value of quantifying glycohemoglobin for the diagnosis of diabetes or latent diabetes is limited.

VARIANT HEMOGLOBINS
Nomenclature

The first variant hemoglobins were designated by capital letters, but this nomenclature soon became impractical because of the numerous variants that had to be accomodated plus the confusion of several hemoglobins having the same assigned letter. This was usually based on electrophoretic mobility, but, since this is a function of the net charge on the molecule, two hemoglobins having identical mobility can in fact represent different substitutions resulting in identical net charges. The current convention is to assign a geographic name to a new hemoglobin, sometimes including a letter designation to indicate its electrophoretic mobility, i.e., Hb E Saskatoon indicates an electrophoretic mobility similar to other hemoglobins E. If the abnormal chain is known, the designation can be more precise, i.e., $\alpha_2\beta_2E$ Saskatoon. If the precise substitution is known, the definitive formula is self-explanatory, i.e., $\alpha_2\beta_2$22 GLU $\rightarrow$ LYS or $\alpha_2\beta_2^{22(B4)}$ GLU $\rightarrow$ LYS, the latter indicating that the abnormality is located on the B helix of the β-chain.

Classification: structural

Several hundred abnormal hemoglobins have been described. Most are characterized by the substitution of one amino acid only and can be classified according to the poly-peptide chain in which the substitution occurs: Table 14-2 (α-chain abnormalities), Table 14-3 (β-chain abnormalities), Table 14-4 (δ-chain abnormalities), and Table 14-5 (γ-chain abnormalities). Other variants representing tetramers, deletions, multiple substitutions, or additions are given in Tables 14-6 to 14-9. The unstable hemoglobins are listed in Table 14-12; the hemoglobins with altered oxygen affinity are listed in Tables 14-13 to 14-15. The fusion hemoglobins are listed in Table 14-18.

GENETIC CONTROL OF HEMOGLOBIN SYNTHESIS
Inheritance patterns

Some hemoglobinopathies show an autosomal dominant inheritance pattern, others an autosomal recessive. The autosomal dominant pattern is implied when, in the heterozygous individual, the hemoglobinopathy is accompanied by hematologic disease. In this case the term "disease" is used (e.g., *unstable hemoglobin disease*), even though the affected person is only heterozygous for the abnormality. The term "disease" is also applied when a person is homozygous for a defect. When a person is heterozygous for a defect and asymptomatic, the term "trait" is used. Most hemoglobinopathies are encountered in the heterozygous state, and most homozygous persons have severe disease. In some situations the homozygous state is not compatible with life, and a high number of stillbirths occurs.

Genetic counseling of persons having a hemoglobinopathy requires an understanding of inheritance patterns under certain conditions. The most frequently encountered situation, one parent heterozygous for Hb S (sickle cell trait) and

Text continued on p. 620.

Table 14-2. Variants of the α-chain*

Residue	Substitution	Name	Major abnormal property	Contacts	References
5(A3)	Ala → Asp	Hb J Toronto		External	Crookston et al (1965)
6(A4)	Asp → Ala	Hb Sawara	↑ O₂ affinity	External	Sumida et al (1973); Sasaki et al (1977)
	Asp → Asn	Hb Dunn			Jue et al (1979)
11(A9)	Lys → Glu	Hb Anantharj		External	Pootrakul et al (1975)
12(A10)	Ala → Asp	Hb J Paris I		External	Rosa et al (1965)
		J Aljezur			Trincao et al (1968)
15(A13)	Gly → Asp	Hb I Interlaken		External	Marti et al (1964)
		J Oxford			Liddell et al (1964)
		N Cosenza			Silvestroni et al (1967)
	Gly → Arg	Hb Ottawa			Vella et al (1974a)
		Siam			Pootrakul et al (1974)
16(A14)	Lys → Glu	Hb I		External	Beale and Lehmann (1965)
		I Philadelphia			Schneider et al (1966)
		I Texas			Bowman and Barnett (1967)
		I Burlington			O'Brien et al (1964)
		I Skamania			Baur (1968)
18(A16)	Gly → Arg	Hb Handsworth		External	Griffiths et al (1977)
19(AB1)	Ala → Asp	Hb J Kurosh		External	Rahbar et al (1976)
20(B1)	His → Tyr	Hb Necker Enfants-Malades		External	Wajcman et al (1980)
21(B2)	Ala → Asp	Hb J Nyanza		External	Kendall et al (1973a)
22(B3)	Gly → Asp	Hb Medellin		External	Gottlieb et al (1964)
23(B4)	Glu → Gln	Hb Memphis		External	Kraus et al (1965)
	Glu → Lys	Hb Chad			Boyer et al (1968)
	Glu → Val	Hb G Audhali			Marengo-Rowe et al (1968a)
27(B8)	Glu → Gly	Hb Ft. Worth		External	Schneider et al (1971)
	Glu → Val	Hb Spanish Town			Ahern et al (1976b)
30(B11)	Glu → Lys	Hb O Padova		α₁-β₁	Vettore et al (1974)
	Glu → Gln	Hb G Honolulu			Schneider and Jim (1961)
		G Singapore			Vella et al (1958)
		G Chinese			Swenson et al (1962)
		G Hong Kong			Swenson et al (1962)
31(B12)	Arg → Ser	Hb Prato	Slightly unstable	α₁-β₁	Marinucci et al (1979)
43(CE1)	Phe → Val	Hb Torino	Unstable; ↓ O₂ affinity	Heme	Beretta et al (1968)
	Phe → Leu	Hb Hirosaki	Unstable		Ohba et al (1975c)
44(CE2)	Pro → Leu	Hb Milledgeville	↑ O₂ affinity; n = 1.1 − 1.4	α₁-β₂	Honig et al (1980)
45(CE3)	His → Arg	Hb Fort de France	↑ O₂ affinity	Heme	Braconnier et al (1977)
	His → Gln	Hb Bari			Marinucci et al (1980)
47(CE5)	Asp → Gly	Hb Umi		External	Sumida (1975)
		Kokura			Sumida (1975)
		Michigan I			Shibata et al (1966)
		Michigan II			
		Yukuhashi II			Sumida (1975)
		L Gaslini			
		Tagawa II			Fujimura et al (1964)
		Beilinson			DeVries et al (1963)
		Mugino			Sumida (1975)
	Asp → His	Hb Hasharon	Unstable		Halbrecht et al (1967)
		Sinai			Ostertag and Smith (1968)
		Sealy			Schneider et al (1968)
		L Ferrara			Bianco et al (1963); Tentori (1977)
	Asp → Asn	Hb Arya	Slightly unstable		Rahbar et al (1975a)
48(CE6)	Leu → Arg	Hb Montgomery		Surface	Brimhall et al (1975)
49(CE7)	Ser → Arg	Hb Savaria		External	Szelényi et al (1980)
50(CE8)	His → Asp	Hb J Sardegna		External	Tangheroni et al (1968)
51(CE9)	Gly → Asp	Hb J Abidjan		External	Cabannes et al (1972)
	Gly → Arg	Hb Russ			Reynolds and Huisman (1966)
53(E2)	Ala → Asp	Hb J Rovigo	Unstable	External	Alberti et al (1974)

*Tables 14-2 to 14-9 courtesy Ruth N. Wrightstone, with additions.

Continued.

Table 14-2. Variants of the α-chain—cont'd

Residue	Substitution	Name	Major abnormal property	Contacts	References
54(E3)	Gln → Arg	Hb Shimonoseki		External	Miyaji et al (1963a)
		Hikoshima			Miyaji et al (1963a)
	Gln → Glu	Hb Mexico			Jones et al (1968a)
		J Paris II			Rosa et al (1966)
		Uppsala			Fessas et al (1969)
56(E5)	Lys → Glu	Hb Shaare Zedek		External	Abramov et al (1980)
	Lys → Thr	Hb Thailand			Pootrakul et al (1977)
57(E6)	Gly → Arg	Hb L Persian Gulf		External	Rahbar et al (1969a)
	Gly → Asp	Hb J Norfolk			Baglioni (1962b)
		Kagoshima			Imamura (1966)
		Nishik I, II, III			Yanase et al (1968)
58(E7)	His → Tyr	Hb M Boston	↓ O_2 affinity; $n = 1.2$	Heme: "distal"	Gerald and Efron (1961)
		M Osaka			Shimizu et al (1965)
		Gothenburg			Hansen et al (1960)
		M Kiskunhalas			Hollán et al (1967)
60(E9)	Lys → Asn	Hb Zambia		External	Barclay et al (1969)
61(E10)	Lys → Asn	Hb J Buda		External	Brimhall et al (1974)
63(E12)	Ala → Asp	Hb Pontoise		Surface	Thillet et al (1977)
64(E13)	Asp → Asn	Hb G Waimanalo		External	Blackwell et al (1973)
		Aida			Ramot et al (1972)
	Asp → His	Hb W India			Sukumaran et al (1972)
	Asp → Tyr	Hb Perspolis			Rahbar et al (1976)
68(E17)	Asn → Asp	Hb Ube 2		External	Miyaji et al (1967)
	Asn → Lys	Hb G Philadelphia			Baglioni and Ingram (1961)
		G Knoxville I			Chernoff and Pettit (1965)
		Stanleyville I			Bowman et al (1966)
		D Washington			Chernoff and Pettit (1965)
		D St. Louis			Minnich et al (1962)
		G Bristol			Dance et al (1964)
		G Azakuoli			Chernoff and Pettit (1965)
		D Baltimore			Chernoff and Pettit (1965)
71(E20)	Ala → Glu	Hb J Habana		External	Colombo et al (1974)
72(EF1)	His → Arg	Hb Daneskgah-Tehran		External	Rahbar et al (1973)
74(EF3)	Asp → His	Hb Mahidol		External	Pootrakul and Dixon (1970)
		G Taichung			Blackwell and Liu (1970)
		Q Thailand			Lorkin et al (1970b)
	Asp → Asn	Hb G Pest			Brimhall et al (1974)
	Asp → Gly	Hb Chapel Hill			Orringer et al (1976)
75(EF4)	Asp → His	Hb Q Iran		External	Lorkin et al (1970b)
	Asp → Tyr	Hb Winnipeg			Vella et al (1973)
	Asp → Asn	Hb Matsue-Oki			Ohba et al (1977b)
	Asp → Gly	Hb Mizushi			Iuchi et al (1980a)
78(EF7)	Asn → Lys	Hb Stanleyville II		External	Van Ros et al (1968)
80(F1)	Leu → Arg	Hb Ann Arbor	Unstable	Surface	Adams et al (1972)
81(F2)	Ser → Cys	Hb Nigeria		External	Honig et al (1978b)
82(F3)	Ala → Asp	Hb Garden State		External	Winter et al (1978)
84(F5)	Ser → Arg	Hb Etobicoke	↑ O_2 affinity; unstable	Internal	Crookston et al (1969)
85(F6)	Asp → Asn	Hb G Norfolk	(?) ↑ O_2 affinity; $n = 2.6$	External	Lorkin et al (1975b); Cohen-Solal et al (1975)
	Asp → Tyr	Hb Atago			Fujiwara et al (1971)
	Asp → Val	Hb Inkster			Reed et al (1974)

Table 14-2. Variants of the α-chain—cont'd

Residue	Substitution	Name	Major abnormal property	Contacts	References
86(F7)	Leu → Arg	Hb Moabit	Unstable; ↓O$_2$ affinity	Heme	Knuth et al (1979)
87(F8)	His → Tyr	Hb M Iwate M Kankakee M Oldenburg	Ferri-Hb; ↓O$_2$ affinity; $n = 1.0$	Heme; "proximal"	Miyaji et al (1963b) Heller et al (1962) Pik and Tönz (1966)
90(FG2)	Lys → Asn	Hb J Broussais Tagawa I		External	De Traverse et al (1966) Yanase et al (1968)
	Lys → Thr	Hb J Rajappen			Hyde et al (1971)
91(FG3)	Leu → Pro	Hb Port Phillip	Unstable	α$_1$-β$_2$	Brennan et al (1977b)
92(FG4)	Arg → Gln	Hb J Cape Town	↑O$_2$ affinity: $n = 2.2$	α$_1$-β$_2$	Botha et al (1966); Lines and McIntosh (1967)
	Arg → Leu	Hb Chesapeake	↑O$_2$ affinity; $n = 2.2$		Clegg et al (1966)
94(G1)	Asp → Tyr	Hb Setif	Unstable	α$_1$-β$_2$	Wajcman et al (1972)
	Asp → Asn	Hb Titusville	↓O$_2$ affinity; ↑ dissocia- tion; $n = 1.06$		Schneider et al (1975a)
	Asp → His	Hb Sunshine Seth			Schroeder et al (1979)
95(G2)	Pro → Leu	Hb G Georgia	↑ Dissociation	α$_1$-β$_2$	Huisman et al (1970)
	Pro → Ser	Hb Rampa	↑ Dissociation; ↑O$_2$ affinity		DeJong et al (1971); Smith et al (1972)
	Pro → Ala	Hb Denmark Hill	↑O$_2$ affinity; $n = 1.8 - 2.4$		Wiltshire et al (1972)
	Pro → Arg	Hb St. Lukes	↑ Dissociation		Bannister et al (1972)
102(G9)	Ser → Arg	Hb Manitoba	Slightly unstable	Central	Crookston et al (1970)
109(G16)	Leu → Arg	Hb Suan-Dok	Unstable	Internal	Sanguansermsri et al (1979)
112(G19)	His → Asp	Hb Hopkins II	Unstable; ↑O$_2$ affinity; $n = 2.2$	External	Charache and Ostertag (1970); Clegg and Charache (1978)
	His → Arg	Hb Strumica Serbia			Niazi et al (1975) Beksedic et al (1975)
114(GH2)	Pro → Arg	Hb Chipas		α$_1$-β$_1$	Jones et al (1968a)
115(GH3)	Ala → Asp	Hb J Tongariki		External	Gajdusek et al (1967)
116(GH4)	Glu → Lys	Hb O Indonesia Buginese X Oliviere		External	Baglioni and Lehmann (1962) Lie-Injo and Sadono (1958) Sansone et al (1970)
	Glu → Ala	Hb Ube 4			Ohba et al (1978)
120(H3)	Ala → Glu	Hb J Meerut J Birmingham		External	Blackwell et al (1974) Kamuzora et al (1974)
126(H9)	Asp → Asn	Hb Tarrant	↑O$_2$ affinity; $n = 1.8$	α$_1$-β$_1$	Moo-Penn et al (1977b)
127(H10)	Lys → Thr	Hb St. Claude		Central	Vella et al (1974b)
	Lys → Asn	Hb Jackson			Moo-Penn et al (1967c)
136(H19)	Leu → Pro	Hb Bibba	Unstable; ↑ dissociation	Heme	Kleihauer et al (1968)
141(HC3)	Arg → Pro	Hb Singapore		External, deoxy, salt bonds to H9, H10, NA1, other α-chain, oxy: mobile Bohr	Clegg et al (1969)
	Arg → His	Hb Suresnes	↑O$_2$ affinity; $n = 2.06$		Poyart et al (1976)
	Arg → Ser	Hb J Cubujuqui			Sáenz et al (1977)
	Arg → Leu	Hb Legnano	↑O$_2$ affinity		Mavilio et al (1978)
	Arg → Gly	Hb J Camaguey			Martinez et al (1978)

Table 14-3. Variants of the β-chain

Residue	Substitution	Name	Major abnormal property	Contacts	References
1(NA1)	Val → Ac-ala	Hb Raleigh	↓ O$_2$ affinity; ↓ dissociation	DPG binding	Moo-Penn et al (1977a)
2(NA2)	His → Arg	Hb Deer Lodge		DPG binding	Labossiere et al (1972)
6(A3)	Glu → Val	Hb S	Sickling	External	Ingram (1959)
	Glu → Lys	Hb C			Hunt and Ingram (1960)
	Glu → Ala	Hb G Makassar			Blackwell et al (1970a)
7(A4)	Glu → Gly	Hb G San José		External	Hill et al (1960)
	Glu → Lys	Hb Siriraj			Tuchinda et al (1965)
9(A6)	Ser → Cys	Hb Porto Alegre	Polymerization; ↑O$_2$ affinity; ↓ heme-heme	External	Bonaventura and Riggs (1967); Tondo et al (1974)
10(A7)	Ala → Asp	Hb Ankara		External	Arcasoy et al (1974)
14(A11)	Leu → Arg	Hb Sögn	Unstable	Surface	Monn et al (1968)
	Leu → Pro	Hb Saki	Unstable		Beuzard et al (1975); Milner et al (1976)
15(A12)	Trp → Arg	Hb Belfast	Unstable; ↑O$_2$ affinity; *n* diminished	Internal	Kennedy et al (1974); Gacon et al (1976)
16(A13)	Gly → Asp	Hb J Baltimore J Trinidad J Ireland N New Haven J Georgia		External	Baglioni and Weatherall (1963) Weatherall (1964) Weatherall (1964) Chernoff and Perillie (1964) Wong et al (1971)
	Gly → Arg	Hb D Bushman			Wade et al (1967)
17(A14)	Lys → Glu	Hb Nagasaki		External	Maekawa et al (1970)
	Lys → Asn	Hb J Amiens			Elion et al (1979)
19(B1)	Asn → Lys	Hb D Ouled Rabah		External	Elion et al (1973)
	Asn → Asp	Hb Alamo			Lam et al (1977)
20(B2)	Val → Met	Hb Olympia	↑O$_2$ affinity; *n* = 2.5-2.7	External	Stamatoyannopoulos et al (1973)
22(B4)	Glu → Lys	Hb E Saskatoon	Unstable	External	Vella et al (1967a)
	Glu → Gly	Hb G Taipei			Blackwell et al (1969b)
	Glu → Ala	Hb G Saskatoon Hsin Chu G Coushatta G Taegu			Vella et al (1967b) Blackwell et al (1968) Bowman et al (1967) Blackwell et al (1968)
	Glu → Gln	Hb D Iran			Rahbar (1973)
23(B5)	Val → Asp	Hb Strasbourg	Slightly unstable	Internal	Garel et al (1976b); Forget (1977)
24(B6)	Gly → Arg	Hb Riverdale-Bronx	Unstable	Internal	Ranney et al (1968)
	Gly → Val	Hb Savannah	Unstable		Huisman et al (1971)
	Gly → Asp	Hb Moscva	Unstable; ↓O$_2$ affinity; *n* near normal		Idelson et al (1974)
25(B7)	Gly → Arg	Hb G Taiwan Ami		External	Blackwell and Liu (1968)
26(B8)	Glu → Lys	Hb E		External	Hunt and Ingram (1961)
	Glu → Val	Hb Henri Mondor	Unstable (slight)		Blouquit et al (1976)
27(B9)	Ala → Asp	Hb Volga Drenthe	Unstable	Internal	Idelson et al (1975) Kuis-Reerink et al (1976)
28(B10)	Leu → Gln	Hb St. Louis	Unstable; ferri-Hb; ↑O$_2$ affinity; *n* = 2.2	Internal	Cohen-Solal et al (1973); Thillet et al (1976b)
	Leu → Pro	Hb Genova	Unstable; ↑O$_2$ affinity; *n* = 1.0		Sansone et al (1967)
29(B11)	Gly → Asp	Hb Lufkin		Internal	Schmidt et al (1977)
30(B12)	Arg → Ser	Hb Tacoma	Unstable; ↓ Bohr and heme-heme; normal O$_2$ affinity; *n* = 2.8	α$_1$-β$_1$	Brimhall et al (1969)
32(B14)	Leu → Pro	Hb Perth Abraham Lincoln	Unstable	Internal	Jackson et al (1973) Honig et al (1973)
	Leu → Arg	Hb Castilla	Unstable		Garel et al (1975)
35(C1)	Tyr → Phe	Hb Philly	Unstable; ↑O$_2$ affinity; *n* = 1.3	α$_1$-β$_1$	Rieder et al (1969)
37(C3)	Trp → Ser	Hb Hirose	↑O$_2$ affinity; *n* = 1.5	α$_1$-β$_1$	Yamaoka (1971)
	Trp → Arg	Hb Rothchild			Gacon et al (1977)
39(C5)	Gln → Lys	Hb Alabama		α$_1$-β$_2$	Brimhall et al (1975)
	Gln → Glu	Hb Vassa	Slightly unstable		Kendall et al (1977)

Table 14-3. Variants of the β-chain—cont'd

Residue	Substitution	Name	Major abnormal property	Contacts	References
40(C6)	Arg → Lys	Hb Athens-Ga Waco	↑ O_2 affinity; $n = 2.8$; unstable	α_1-β_2	Brown et al (1976) Moo-Penn et al (1977d)
	Arg → Ser	Hb Austin	↑ O_2 affinity; ↑ disso- ciation; n reduced		Moo-Penn et al (1977d)
41(C7)	Phe → Tyr	Hb Mequon		Heme	Burkett et al (1976)
42(CD1)	Phe → Ser	Hb Hammersmith Chiba	Unstable, ↓ O_2 affinity; $n = 2.25$	Heme	Dacie et al (1967) Ohba et al (1975b)
	Phe → Leu	Hb Louisville Bucuresti	Unstable; ↓ O_2 affinity; $n = 1.85$		Keeling et al (1971) Bratu et al (1971)
43(CD2)	Glu → Ala	Hb G Galveston G Port Arthur G Texas		External	Bowman et al (1964) Bowman et al (1964) Bowman et al (1964)
	Glu → Gln	Hb Hoshida			Iuchi et al (1978)
46(CD5)	Gly → Glu	Hb K Ibadan		External	Allan et al (1965)
47(CD6)	Asp → Asn	Hb G Copenhagen		External	Sick et al (1967)
	Asp → Gly	Hb Gavello			Marinucci et al (1977)
	Asp → Ala	Hb Avicenna			Rahbar et al (1979)
48(CD7)	Leu → Arg	Hb Okaloosa	Unstable; ↓ O_2 affinity; $n = 2.85$	Surface	Charache et al (1973)
50(D1)	Thr → Lys	Hb Edmonton		External	Labossiere et al (1971)
51(D2)	Pro → Arg	Hb Willamette	↑ O_2 affinity; unstable; $n = 2.9$	α_1-β_1	Jones et al (1976c)
52(D3)	Asp → Asn	Hb Osu Christiansborg		External	Konotey-Ahulu et al (1971)
	Asp → Ala	Hb Ocho Rios			Beresford et al (1972)
	Asp → His	Hb Summer Hill			Wilkinson et al (1980)
56(D7)	Gly → Asp	Hb J Bangkok J Meinung J Korat J Manado		External	Clegg et al (1966) Blackwell and Liu (1966) Blackwell and Liu (1966) Blackwell et al (1970b)
	Gly → Arg	Hb Hamadan			Rahbar et al (1975b)
57(E1)	Asn → Lys	Hb G Ferrara	Unstable	External	Giardina et al (1978)
58(E2)	Pro → Arg	Hb Yukuhashi Dhofar	Unstable	External	Yanase et al (1968) Marengo-Rowe et al (1968b)
59(E3)	Lys → Glu	Hg I High Wycombe		External	Boulton et al (1971)
	Lys → Thr	Hb J Kaohsiung J Honolulu			Blackwell et al (1971b) Blackwell et al (1972c)
	Lys → Asn	Hb J Lome			Wajcman et al (1977)
60(E4)	Val → Leu	Hb Yatsushiro		Internal	Kagimoto et al (1978)
61(E5)	Lys → Glu	Hb N Seattle		External	Jones et al (1968b)
	Lys → Asn	Hb Hikari			Shibata et al (1964)
62(E6)	Ala → Pro	Hb Duarte	Unstable; ↑ O_2 affinity; $n = 2.9$	External	Beutler et al (1974)
63(E7)	His → Arg	Hb Zürich	Unstable; ↑ O_2 affinity; $n = 1.8$	Heme; "distal"	Muller and Kingma (1961)
	His → Tyr	Hb M Saskatoon M Emory M Kurume M Radom M Arhus M Chicago Leipzig Hörlein-Weber Novi Sad M Erlangen	Ferri-Hb; ↑ O_2 affinity; $n = 2.1$-2.3		Gerald and Efron (1961) Gerald and Efron (1961) Shibata et al (1961) Murawski et al (1963) Hobolth (1965) Josephson et al (1962) Betke et al (1960) Hörlein and Weber (1948) Efremov et al (1974) Kohne et al (1975)
	His → Pro	Hb Bicêtre	Unstable; autoxidizing		Wajcman et al (1976)
64(E8)	Gly → Asp	Hb J Calabria J Bari J Cosenza	Unstable	Internal	Tentori (1974) Tentori (1974) Tentori (1974)
65(E9)	Lys → Asn	Hb J Sicilia		External	Ricco et al (1974)
	Lys → Gln	Hb J Cairo			Garel et al (1976a)
66(E10)	Lys → Glu	Hb I Toulouse	Unstable; Ferri-Hb	External; ?heme	Rosa et al (1969)

Continued.

Table 14-3. Variants of the β-chain—cont'd

Residue	Substitution	Name	Major abnormal property	Contacts	References
67(E11)	Val → Asp	Hb Bristol	Unstable	Heme	Steadman et al (1970)
	Val → Glu	Hb M Milwaukee I	Ferri-Hb; ↓O$_2$ affinity; $n = 1.2$		Gerald and Efron (1961)
	Val → Ala	Hb Sydney	Unstable		Carrell et al (1967)
68(E12)	Leu → Pro	Hb Mizuho	Unstable	Internal	Ohba et al (1977a)
69(E13)	Gly → Asp	Hb J Cambridge J Rambam		External	Sick et al (1967) Salomon et al (1965)
70(E14)	Ala → Asp	Hb Seattle	Unstable; ↓O$_2$ affinity; $n = 2.6$	Heme	Kurachi et al (1973)
71(E15)	Phe → Ser	Hb Christchurch	Unstable	Heme	Carrell and Owen (1971)
73(E17)	Asp → Tyr	Hb Vancouver	↓O$_2$ affinity; $n = 2.7$	External	Jones et al (1976b)
	Asp → Asn	Hb Korle Bu G Accra			Konotey-Ahulu et al (1968) Lehmann et al (1964)
	Asp → Val	Hb Mobile	↓O$_2$ affinity; $n = 2.7$		Schneider et al (1975b)
74(E18)	Gly → Val	Hb Bushwick	Unstable	External	Rieder et al (1975)
	Gly → Asp	Hb Shepherds Bush	Unstable; ↑O$_2$ affinity; $n = 2.2\text{-}2.4$		White et al (1970)
75(E19)	Leu → Pro	Hb Atlanta	Unstable	Internal	Hubbard et al (1975)
	Leu → Arg	Hb Pasadena	Unstable; ↑O$_2$ affinity		Johnson et al (1980)
76(E20)	Ala → Asp	Hb J Chicago		External	Romain et al (1975)
77(EF1)	His → asp	Hb J Iran		External	Rahbar et al (1967)
79(EF3)	Asp → Gly	Hb G Hsi-Tsou	↑O$_2$ affinity	External	Blackwell et al (1972b); Benesch et al (1975)
	Asp → Tyr	Hb Tampa			Johnson et al (1980)
80(EF4)	Asn → Lys	Hb G Szuhu Hb Gifu		External	Blackwell et al (1969c) Imai et al (1970)
81(EF5)	Leu → Arg	Hb Baylor	Unstable; ↑O$_2$ affinity; $n = 2.0$	Internal	Schneider et al (1976a)
82(EF6)	Lys → Asn → Asp	Hb Providence	↓O$_2$ affinity; $n = 2.5\text{-}2.7$	DPG binding	Moo-Penn et al (1976a); Bonaventura et al (1976)
	Lys → Thr	Hb Rahere	↑O$_2$ affinity; n normal		Lorkin et al (1975a)
	Lys → Met	Hb Helsinki	↑O$_2$ affinity; $n = 2.3$		Ikkala et al (1976)
83(EF7)	Gly → Cys	Hb Ta-li		External	Blackwell et al (1971a)
	Gly → Asp	Hb Pyrgos			Tatsis et al (1976)
85(F1)	Phe → Ser	Hb Bryn Mawr Buenos Aires	Unstable; ↑O$_2$ affinity	Internal	Bradley et al (1972) de Weinstein et al (1973)
87(F3)	Thr → Lys	Hb D Ibadan		External	Watson-Williams et al (1965)
88(F4)	Leu → Arg	Hb Böras	Unstable; ↑O$_2$ affinity	Heme	Hollender et al (1969)
	Leu → Pro	Hb Santa Ana	Unstable		Opfell et al (1968)
89(F5)	Ser → Asn	Hb Creteil	↑O$_2$ affinity; $n = 1.2$	Internal	Thillet et al (1976a)
	Ser → Arg	Hb Vanderbilt	↑O$_2$ affinity		Paniker et al (1978)
90(F6)	Glu → Lys	Hb Agenogi	↓O$_2$ affinity; n normal	External	Miyaji et al (1966)
91(F7)	Leu → Pro	Hb Sabine	Unstable	Heme	Schneider et al (1969a)
	Leu → Arg	Hb Caribbean	Unstable; ↓O$_2$ affinity		Ahern et al (1976a)
92(F8)	His → Tyr	Hb M Hyde Park M Akita	↑O$_2$ affinity; ferri-Hb	Heme; "proximal"	Heller et al (1966); Shih et al (1980) Shibata et al (1969)
	His → Gln	Hb St. Etienne Istanbul	Unstable; ↑O$_2$ affinity; ↑ dissociation; $n = 1.8$		Beuzard et al (1972) Aksoy et al (1972)
	His → Asp	Hb J Altgeld Gardens	Normal O$_2$ affinity		Adams et al (1975)
	His → Pro	Hb Newcastle			Finney et al (1975)
95(FG2)	Lys → Glu	Hb N Baltimore Hopkins I Jenkins N Memphis Kenwood		External	Clegg et al (1965) Gottlieb et al (1967) Dobbs et al (1966) Bayrakci et al (1964) Hamilton et al (1969)
	Lys → Asn	Hb Detroit			Moo-Penn et al (1978a)
97(FG4)	His → Gln	Hb Malmö	↑O$_2$ affinity; $n = 1.87$	α$_1$-β$_2$	Lorkin et al (1970a)
	His → Leu	Hb Wood	↑O$_2$ affinity; $n = 1.5$		Taketa et al (1975)

Table 14-3. Variants of the β-chain—cont'd

Residue	Substitution	Name	Major abnormal property	Contacts	References
98(FG5)	Val → Met	Hb Köln	Unstable	Heme; α_1-β_2	Carrell et al (1966)
		San Francisco (Pacific)	↑ O_2 affinity; $n = 1.46$		Woodson et al (1970)
		Ube I	Unstable		Ohba et al (1973)
	Val → Gly	Hb Nottingham	Unstable; ↑ O_2 affinity; n "impaired"		Gordon-Smith et al (1973)
	Val → Ala	Hb Djelfa	Unstable; ↑ O_2 affinity; $n = 1.0$-2.3		Gacon et al (1975b)
99(G1)	Asp → Asn	Hb Kempsey	↑ O_2 affinity; $n = 1.0$	α_1-β_2	Reed et al (1968)
	Asp → His	Hb Yakima	↑ O_2 affinity; $n = 1.1$		Jones et al (1967)
	Asp → Ala	Hb Radcliffe	↑ O_2 affinity; $n = 1.1$		Weatherall et al (1977)
	Asp → Tyr	Hb Ypsilanti	↑ O_2 affinity		Rucknagel et al (1967)
100(G2)	Pro → Leu	Hb Brigham	↑ O_2 affinity	α_1-β_2	Lokich et al (1973)
101(G3)	Glu → Lys	Hb British Columbia	↑ O_2 affinity; $n = 1.6$	α_1-β_2	Jones et al (1976a)
	Glu → Gln	Hb Rush	Unstable		Adams et al (1974)
	Glu → Gly	Hb Alberta	↑ O_2 affinity; $n = 1.0$		Mant et al (1976-77)
	Glu → Asp	Hb Potomac	↑ O_2 affinity		Charache et al (1978)
102(G4)	Asn → Lys	Hb Richmond	Asymmetric hybrids	Heme; α_1-β_2	Efremov et al (1969)
	Asn → Thr	Hb Kansas	↓ O_2 affinity; ↑ dissociation; $n = 1.3$		Bonaventura and Riggs (1968)
	Asn → Ser	Hb Beth Israel	↓ O_2 affinity; $n = 1.0$-1.8		Nagel et al (1976)
103(G5)	Phe → Leu	Hb Heathrow	↑ O_2 affinity; $n = 1.2$	Heme	White et al (1973)
104(G4)	Arg → Ser	Hb Camperdown	Slightly unstable	Central cavity	Wilkinson et al (1975)
	Arg → Thr	Hb Sherwood Forest			Ryrie et al (1977)
106(G8)	Leu → Pro	Hb Southampton Casper	↑ O_2 affinity; $n = 1.5$; unstable		Hyde et al (1972); Koler et al (1973)
	Leu → Gln	Hb Tübingen	Unstable; ↑ O_2 affinity; $n = 2.15$		Kleihauer et al (1971); Kohne et al (1976)
107(G9)	Gly → Arg	Hb Burke	Unstable; ↓ O_2 affinity; $n = 2.1$	Internal	Jones and Koler (1976)
108(G10)	Asn → Asp	Hb Yoshizuka	↓ O_2 affinity; $n = 2.3$-3.0	α_1-β_1	Imamura et al (1969)
	Asn → Lys	Hb Presbyterian	↓ O_2 affinity		Moo-Penn et al (1978)
109(G11)	Val → Met	Hb San Diego	↑ O_2 affinity; $n = 2.02$-2.24	Internal	Nute et al (1974)
111(G13)	Val → Phe	Hb Peterborough	Unstable; ↓ O_2 affinity; n near normal	Internal	King et al (1972)
112(G14)	Cys → Arg	Hb Indianapolis	Very unstable	α_1-β_1	Adams et al (1978)
113(G15)	Val → Glu	Hb New York		Internal	Ranney et al (1967)
115(G17)	Ala → Pro	Hb Madrid	Unstable	α_1-β_1	Outeirino et al (1974)
117(G19)	His → Arg	Hb P Galveston		External	Schneider et al (1969b)
119(GH2)	Gly → Val	Hb Bougardirey-Mali		α_1-β_1	Chen-Marotel et al (1979)
	Gly → Asp	Hb Fannin-Lubbock	Slightly unstable		Schneider et al (1976b); Moo-Penn et al (1976b)
120(GH3)	Lys → Glu	Hb Hijiyama		External	Miyaji et al (1968a)
	Lys → Asn	Hb Riyadh, Karatsu		External	El-Hazmi and Lehmann (1976); Miyaji et al (1977)
	Lys → Gln	Hb Takamatsu			Iuchi et al (1980b)
121(GH4)	Glu → Gln	D Los Angeles	↑ O_2 affinity	External	Baglioni (1962c)
		D Punjab			Ozsoylo (1970); Ramot et al (1969)
		D North Carolina			Smith and Conley (1959)
		D Portugal			Wasi et al (1968)
		Oak Ridge			Imamura and Riggs (1972)
		D Chicago			Bowman and Ingram (1961)
	Glu → Lys	Hb O Arab			Baglioni and Lehmann (1962)
		Egypt			Kamel et al (1970)
	Glu → Val	Hb Beograd			Efremov et al (1973)
124(H2)	Pro → Arg	Hb Khartoum	Unstable	α_1-β_1	Clegg et al (1969)
	Pro → Gln	Hb Ty Gard	↑ O_2 affinity		Bursaux et al (1978)

Continued.

Table 14-3. Variants of the β-chain—cont'd

Residue	Substitution	Name	Major abnormal property	Contacts	References
126(H4)	Val → Glu	Hb Hofu		Surface	Miyaji et al (1968b)
127(H5)	Gln → Glu	Hb Hacettepe		α_1-β_1	Altay et al (1976)
128(H6)	Ala → Asp	Hb J Guantanamo	Unstable	α_1-β_1	Martinez et al (1977)
129(H7)	Ala → Asp	Hb J Taichung		Surface	Blackwell et al (1969a)
	Ala → Glu or Asp	Hb K Cameroon			Allan et al (1965)
	Ala → Pro	Hb Crete	↑ O_2 affinity		Maniatis et al (1979)
130(H8)	Tyr → Asp	Hb Wien	Unstable	Internal	Lorkin et al (1974)
131(H9)	Gln → Glu	Hb Camden Tokuchi		α_1-β_1	Wade Cohen et al (1973) Ohba et al (1975a)
132(H10)	Lys → Gln	Hb K Woolwich		Surface	Allan et al (1965)
134(H12)	Val → Glu	Hb North Shore	Unstable	Internal	Arends et al (1977); Brennan et al (1977c)
135(H13)	Ala → Pro	Hb Altdorf	Unstable; ↑ O_2 affinity; $n = 1.0$	Central	Marti et al (1976)
136(H14)	Gly → Asp	Hb Hope	Unstable	Central	Minnich et al (1965)
138(H16)	Ala → Pro	Hb Brockton	Unstable	Central	Moo-Penn et al (1980a)
139(H17)	Asn → Lys	Hb G Manhasset	↓ O_2 affinity	Central	Nagel et al (1980)
141(H19)	Leu → Arg	Hb Olmsted	Unstable	Heme	Lorkin et al (1970a)
142(H20)	Ala → Pro	Hb Toyoake	Unstable; ↑ O_2 affinity	Central	Hirano et al (1980)
	Ala → Asp	Hb Ohio	↑ O_2 affinity		Moo-Penn et al (1980b)
143(H21)	His → Arg	Hb Abruzzo	↑ O_2 affinity; $n = 2.7$	DPG binding	Tentori et al (1972)
	His → Gln	Hb Little Rock	↑ O_2 affinity; $n = 2.5$-3.0		Bromberg et al (1973)
	His → Pro	Hb Syracuse	↑ O_2 affinity; $n = 1.1$		Jensen et al (1975)
144(HC1)	Lys → Asn	Hb Andrew Minneapolis	↑ O_2 affinity; $n = 2.4$	External	Zak et al (1974)
145(HC2)	Tyr → His	Hb Bethesda	↑ O_2 affinity; $n = 1.1$	Hydrogen bond to Val FG5; same β-chain in deoxy form	Hayashim et al (1971)
	Tyr → Cys	Hb Rainier	↑ O_2 affinity; alkali resistant; $n = 1.5$		Hayashim et al (1971)
	Tyr → Asp	Hb Ft. Gordon Osler Nancy	↑ O_2 affinity; $n = 1.0$		Kleckner et al (1975) Charache et al (1975) Gacon et al (1975a)
	Tyr → Term	Hb McKees Rocks	↑↑ O_2 affinity; $n = 1.0$		Winslow et al (1976)
146(HC3)	His → Asp	Hb Hiroshima	↑ O_2 affinity; $n = 2.4$	α_1-β_2	Perutz et al (1971)
	His → Pro	Hb York	↑ O_2 affinity; $n = 1.8$		Barem et al (1976)
	His → Arg	Hb Cochin–Port Royal	Normal oxygen affinity; $n = 3.0$		Wajcman et al (1975)

Table 14-4. Variants of the δ-chain

Residue	Substitution	Name	References
2(NA2)	His → Arg	Hb A_2 Sphakiá	Jones et al (1966b)
12(A9)	Asn → Lys	Hb A_2 NYU	Ranney et al (1969)
16(A13)	Gly → Arg	Hb A_2' (B_2)	Ball et al (1968)
20(B2)	Val → Glu	Hb A_2 Roosevelt	Rieder et al (1976)
22(B4)	Ala → Glu	Hb A_2 Flatbush	Jones and Brimhall (1967)
43(CD2)	Glu → Lys	Hb A_2 Melbourne	Sharma et al (1974)
51(D2)	Pro → Arg	Hb A_2 Adria	Alberti et al (1978)
69(E13)	Gly → Arg	Hb A_2 Indonesia	Lie-Injo et al (1971)
116(G18)	Arg → His	Hb A_2 Coburg	Sharma et al (1975)
136(H14)	Gly → Asp	Hb A_2 Babinga	De Jong and Bernini (1968)

Table 14-5. Variants of the γ-chain

Residue	Substitution	Name	References
1(NA1)	Gly → Cys (136 gly)	Hb F Malaysia	Lie-Injo et al (1974)
5(A2)	Glu → Lys (136 ala)	Hb F Texas I	Jenkins et al (1967); Ahern et al (1972)
6(A3)	Glu → Lys	Hb F Texas II	Larkin et al (1968)
7(A4)	Asp → Asn (136 gly)	Hb F Auckland	Carrell et al (1974)
12(A9)	Thr → Lys	Hb Alexandra	Loukopoulos et al (1969)
16(A13)	Gly → Arg (136 gly)	Hb F Melbourne	Brennan et al (1977a)
22(B4)	Asp → Gly (136 ala)	Hb F Kuala Lumpur	Lie-Injo et al (1973)
61(E5)	Lys → Glu (136 ala)	Hb F Jamaica	Ahern et al (1970)
75(E19)	Ilu → Thr	Hb F Sardinia	Grifoni et al (1975)
80(EF4)	Asp → Tyr (136 ala)	Hb F Victoria Jubilee	Ahern et al (1975)
97(FG4)	His → Arg (136 ala)	Hb F Dickinson	Schneider et al (1974)
108(G10)	Asn → Lys	Hb F Ube	Omura et al (1975)
117(G19)	His → Arg (136 gly)	Hb F Malta I	Cauchi et al (1969)
	His → Arg (136 ala)	Hb F Malta II	Huisman et al (1972b)
121(GH4)	Glu → Lys (136 ala)	Hb F Hull	Sacker et al (1967)
121(GH4)	Glu → Lys (136 gly)	Hb F Carlton	Brennan et al (1977a)
125(H3)	Glu → Ala (136 gly)	Hb F Port Royal	Brimhall et al (1973)
130(H8)	Try → Gly (136 gly)	Hb F Poole	Lee-Potter et al (1975)

Table 14-6. Hemoglobin variants, other abnormalities

Name	Structure	Location or nature of abnormality	References
Hb α^A	α_4	Four α-chains	Huehns et al (1961)
Hb Barts	γ_4	Four γ-chains	Hunt and Lehmann (1959)
Hb δ^{A_2}	δ_4	Four δ-chains	Dance and Huehns (1962)
Hb Gower I	ϵ_4	Four ε-chains	Huehns et al (1964)
Hb Gower II	$\alpha_2\epsilon_2$		Huehns et al (1964)
Hb H	β_4	Four β-chains	Jones et al (1959)
Hb Portland 1	$\gamma_2\zeta_2$	ζ-chains instead of β	Capp et al (1970)

Table 14-7. Hemoglobin variants with deleted residues

Residue	Deletion	Name	Major abnormal property	References
α141	ARG → O	Hb Koellicker		Marti et al (1967)
β6 or 7	Glu → O	Hb Leiden	Unstable; slightly ↑O_2 affinity	DeJong et al (1968)
β17-18	(Lys-Val) → O	Hb Lyon	↑O_2 affinity	Cohen-Solal et al (1974)
β23	Val → O	Hb Freiburg	↑O_2 affinity	Jones et al (1966a)
β42-44 or 43-45	(Phe-Glu-Ser) → O or (Glu-Ser-Phe) → O	Hb Niteroi	↓O_2 affinity; unstable	Praxedes and Lehmann (1972)
β56-59	(Gly-Asn-Pro-Lys) → O	Hb Tochigi	Unstable; O_2 affinity not known	Shibata et al (1970)
β74-75	(Gly-Leu) → O	Hb St. Antoine	Unstable; normal O_2 affinity	Wajcman et al (1973)
β75	Leu → O	Hb Vicksburg		Newman et al (1979)
β87	Thr → O	Hb Tours	↑O_2 affinity; unstable	Wajcman et al (1973)
β91-95, 92-96, or 93-97	(Leu-His-Cys-Asp-Lys) → O	Hb Gun Hill	Unstable; ↑O_2 affinity	Bradley et al (1967)
β131	Gln → O	Hb Leslie Deaconess	Unstable; normal O_2 affinity	Lutcher and Huisman (1975); Moo-Penn et al (1975); Lutcher et al (1976)
β141	Leu → O	Hb Coventry		Casey et al (1976)

Table 14-8. Hemoglobin variants with more than one point mutation in the same polypeptide chain

Residue	Substitution	Name	Major abnormal property	References
β6	Glu → Val ⎫	Hb C Harlem;	Normal O_2 affinity	Bookchin et al (1967)
β73	Asp → Asn ⎭	Hb C Georgetown		Lang et al (1972)
β6	Glu → Lys ⎫	Hb Arlington Park	Not done	Adams and Heller (1973)
β95	Lys → Glu ⎭			
α78	Asn → Asp ⎫	Hb J Singapore	Not done	Blackwell et al (1972a)
α79	Ala → Gly ⎭			
β6	Glu → Val ⎫	Hb C Ziguinchor		Goossens et al (1975)
β58	Pro → Arg ⎭			
β6	Glu → Val ⎫	Hb S Travis	↑ O_2 affinity	Moo-Penn et al (1977c)
β142	Ala → Val ⎭			

Table 14-9. Hemoglobin variants with extended chains

Location	Residue	Name	Major abnormal property	References
α141	31 additional residues: Tyr-Arg-Gln-Ala-Gly-Ala-Ser-Val-[140] Ala-Val-Pro-Pro-Ala-Arg-Trp-Ala-Ser-Gln-Arg-Ala-Leu-[150][160] Leu-Pro-Ser-Leu-His-Arg-Pro-Phe-Leu-Val-Phe-Glu[170]	Hb Constant Spring		Clegg et al (1971)
α141	31 additional residues: identical to Hb Constant Spring except for residue 142, which is lysine instead of glutamine	Hb Icaria		Clegg et al (1974)
α141	16 or 17 additional residues: Tyr-Arg (Ser,Ala,Gly,Ala,[140] Ser,Val,Ala,Val,Pro,Pro,Ala)-Arg(?,Ala,Ser,Gln)-Arg-[150] COOH	Hb Koya Dora		DeJong et al (1975)
β146	11 additional residues: Thr-Lys-Leu-Ala-Phe-Leu-Leu-Ser-[150] Asn-Phe-Tyr	Hb Tak	↑ O_2 affinity	Flatz et al (1971); Imai and Lehmann (1975); Lehmann et al (1975)
α139-141	Thr-Ser-Asn-Thr-Val-Lys-Leu-Glu-Pro-Arg (Frameshift)[140]	Hb Wayne		Seid-Akhaven et al (1972)
β145	Lys-Ser-Ile-Thr-Lys-Leu-Ala-Phe-Leu-Leu-Ser-Asn-Phe-Tyr-[144][150][155] COOH	Hb Cranston	Unstable	Bunn et al (1975)
α118-119	Ala-Glu-Phe-Thr-*Glu-Phe-Thr*-Pro (insertion)[115][116][117][118][119]	Hb Grady Dakar		Huisman et al (1974) Garel et al (1976c)

the other normal, produces half normal children and half heterozygous for Hb S. No homozygous (with respect to the hemoglobinopathy) children are possible. If one parent is homozygous (sickle cell disease) and the other is normal, all of the children will be heterozygous (sickle cell trait). If one parent is homozygous and the other is heterozygous, half of the children will be homozygous (disease) and half will be heterozygous (trait). In the rare situation in which one parent is doubly heterozygous for an abnormality on the same chain (Hb S trait and Hb C trait, for example) and the other is normal, the heterozygous children will inherit either one or the other, but not both, and none will be double heterozygous like the affected parent. Even rarer is the situation in which one parent is doubly heterozygous for two defects determined by diffent loci; the heterozygous children may

inherit either or both defects. Doubly heterozygous children can also result from mating of parents who are each heterozygous for a different defect.

Synthesis of polypeptide chains

The synthesis of the polypeptide chains of globin is controlled by separate *structural genes*. The information as to the product to be synthesized is carried from the structural gene to the *ribosomes* by *messenger RNA* (mRNA). Synthesis of polypeptide chains occurs at the ribosome level (Fig. 14-12). Six types of globin polypeptide chains are known: alpha (α), beta (β), delta (δ), gamma (γ), epsilon (ε), and zeta (ζ). The biosynthesis of hemoglobin is reviewed by Benz and Forget (1974) and Winslow and Anderson (1978).

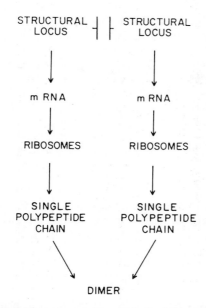

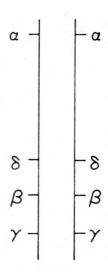

Fig. 14-12. Simplified scheme of the synthesis of the single polypeptide chains and formation of the dimer, under control of a pair of structural loci. Detailed definitions of the mechanisms of transcription (synthesis of mRNA from DNA) and translation (synthesis of protein by mRNA) are given by Nienhuis and Anderson (1974), Rabinovitz (1974), and Lodish (1976).

Fig. 14-13. A "working" diagram of the arrangements of four of the structural genes for hemoglobin synthesis. The α- and non-α-loci probably lie on different chromosomes, represented in the diagram by a distance between the two. The δ-, β-, and γ-loci are closely linked. The order may in fact be γ, δ, β (Kendall et al, 1973), but because of the close linkage the actual order is not very important. Both the α- and γ-loci may be multiple (see text). Not shown are loci for ϵ- and ζ-chains, since their position is not known.

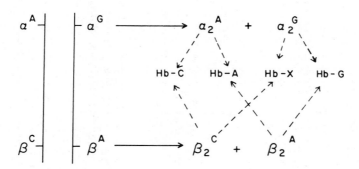

Fig. 14-14. Structural loci and the combination of dimer chains to form four different hemoglobins in one individual. It is assumed that the individal possesses four separate structural loci, α^A produces an α_2^A dimer, α^G produces an α_2^G dimer, β^C produces $\alpha\beta_2^C$ dimer, and β^A produces a β_2^A dimer. These combine to form the four hemoglobins. (After Baglioni and Ingram, 1961.)

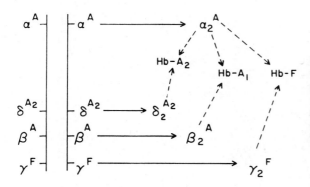

Fig. 14-15. Structural loci and combination of dimers to form the three normal hemoglobins. As in Fig. 14-14, α_2, β_2, γ_2, and δ_2 dimers are synthesized and recombined to form Hb A_1, Hb A_2, and Hb F. Since normal adult blood contains about 3.5% Hb A_2, 1% to 2% Hb F, and the remainder Hb A_1, the different chains must be produced in different quantities if, as is in fact true, few or no excess chains are normally found in normal normoblasts.

All evidence points to the arrangement of genes as shown in Fig. 14-13. The chromosomes that carry these genes have not been fully identified; there is evidence that some of the loci are on chromosome 2 and others on B group chromosome 4 or 5 (Price et al, 1972). The diagram reflects present opinion that the α- and β-chain loci are not closely linked and lie some distance apart, but that the β- and δ-loci are closely linked (Boyer et al, 1963) as are the γ- and β-loci (Gilman and Smithies, 1968; Kendall et al, 1973b). For example, α-chain synthesis is not influenced in β-thalassemia, whereas there is activation of δ-chain or γ-chain synthesis, or of both. The occurrence of simultaneous suppression of both δ- and β-chain synthesis in $\delta\beta$-thalassemia suggests that the loci for these chains are near each other.

There is at least one exception to the assumption that each type of polypeptide chain is determined by a single gene. Position 136 on the γ-chain can be occupied by either glycine or alanine (Schroeder et al, 1968; Cauchi et al, 1969). Thus at least two types of fetal hemoglobin can be synthesized, one containing the γ-136 gly chain and the other the γ-136 ala chain, designated Gγ and Aγ, respectively (Massa et al, 1980). This implies the presence of two allelic genes at the γ-locus, but a study of two variants of Hb F, Hb Malta I and Hb Malta II, has led to the conclusion that there are in fact four structural genes for Hb F and that these are nonallelic (Huisman et al, 1972).

The question of possible multiple loci for structural genes controlling the synthesis of other types of chains is raised by Lehmann and Carrell (1969), particularly regarding α-chain synthesis in some α-chain variants. Hollán et al (1972) have in fact studied one individual having two α-chain variants (Hb J Buda and Hb G Pest) in addition to normal α-chains, suggesting the presence of three structural genes at the α-locus ($\alpha^{G\ Pest}$, $\alpha^{J\ Buda}$, and α^A). Other examples indicating multiple α-chain loci have been reported (Ostertag et al,

1972; DeJong et al, 1975). Recent data show that the α-gene is duplicated, that the two loci are closely linked on each chromosome, and that they are located on chromosome 16 (Deisseroth et al, 1977). Deletion of one to four genes dictates the severity of α-thalassemia (Kan et al, 1979).

The evidence derived from the study of individuals having multiple hemoglobins as well as from dissociation and recombination experiments in vitro indicates that two single polypeptide chains of the same type combine to form dimers, and that dimers of different types then combine to form various tetramer combinations; e.g., the individual studied by Baglioni and Ingram (1961) was shown to have four hemoglobins: Hb A$_1$, Hb G Philadelphia, Hb C, and Hb X. According to the genetic hypothesis, the four structural loci and the recombination of dimers form the four different hemoglobins, as shown in Fig. 14-14. In the normal adult, dimers of α^A-, β^B-, and γ^F-chains are formed, though not in equal proportion. They then combine as shown in Fig. 14-15. Since there is no substantial evidence in favor of variable affinity for each other among the various dimers, it is assumed that the proportion of the various hemoglobins formed is related to the rate of synthesis of the different chains.

Switch from fetal to adult hemoglobin

The condition known as "hereditary persistence of fetal hemoglobin" is defined as the persistence of high levels of fetal hemoglobin into adult life, usually in the absence of severe hematologic disturbances. The latter feature distinguishes it from other hemoglobinopathies with hematologic signs and symptoms and higher than normal levels of fetal hemoglobin. It occurs mainly in blacks, but cases have been described in other races and in several countries. Only one person homozygous for this abnormality has been described. The others are heterozygous, sometimes in combi-

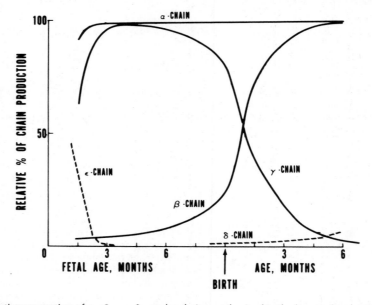

Fig. 14-16. Relative proportion of α-, β-, γ-, δ-, and ϵ-chains synthesized in the human fetus and neonate. (After Ingram, 1963; Kabat, 1972.) Synthesis of Hb A$_1$, is detectable in human embryos 35 mm in crown-rump length (55 gestational days) (Kazazian and Woodhead, 1973) even though it is not detectable in the blood by electrophoresis until the embryo is 80 gestational days of age (Pataryas and Stamatoyannopoulos, 1972).

nation with Hb S, Hb C, α-thalassemia, or δ-thalassemia.

To better understand the genetic basis for this syndrome, it is desirable to first discuss the "switch mechanism" from fetal to adult hemoglobin that, in normal individuals, begins in utero and is complete by the fifth or sixth month after birth (Fig. 14-16). The synthesis of α-chains remains constant throughout, but at about the sixth month of fetal life the synthesis of γ-chains begins to decrease, while synthesis of β-chains begins. By 6 months of age only a few γ-chains are synthesized in a normal person, enough to make only a little Hb F (less than 2%). By this time, β-chain synthesis is optimum and Hb A$_1$ is the major component of adult blood. The switch from Hb F to Hb A is related to the degree of biologic maturation of the fetus and not to the incident of birth (Bard, 1973).

This sequence requires a mechanism for "switching off" the synthesis of γ-chains and "switching on" the synthesis of β-chains. Since it must be assumed that both structural γ- and β-genes are present from the day of conception, it is necessary to assume a mechanism for regulating the activity of these genes. Several models have been proposed, but all of them are still speculative. Ingram (1963) falls back on Jacob and Monod's (1961) model for the regulation of protein synthesis and postulates *operator* genes that turn structural genes on and off and *regulator* genes that, in turn, control the activity of operator genes. Baglioni et al (1961) suggest that there is no hemoglobin synthesis in the early normoblast and that this cell has a built-in mechanism for repressing synthesis of hemoglobin of any type. Then, as the cell matures, the repressing system is lost and the structural genes are turned on. As a corollary, the repressing mechanism is lost earlier in rapidly proliferating early normoblasts, accounting for increased levels of fetal hemoglobin in hematologic disorders where there is increased proliferation of erythroid cells. It is difficult to see how this applies to

a variety of diseases, such as leukemia and aplastic anemia, which may show higher than normal levels of Hb F (Beaven et al, 1960; Jones, 1961; Miller, 1969; Nyman et al, 1970; Özsoylu and Balci, 1970).

Some light has been shed on this question by studies on the hemoglobin switching mechanism in sheep and goats (Huisman et al, 1969). In these animals there is a switch from Hb A$_1$ ($\alpha_2\beta_2^A$) to Hb C ($\alpha_2\beta_2^C$) in response to anemia, hypoxia, or erythropoietin administration. The evidence indicates that the synthesis of the new hemoglobin is not from a clone of new cells but rather by selective gene action on the same erythroid precursors, probably through a change in globin mRNA (Nienhuis and Anderson, 1972; Nienhuis and Bunn, 1974).

LABORATORY DIAGNOSIS IN THE HEMOGLOBINOPATHIES
Introduction

The hemoglobinopathies of clinical significance are characterized by mild to extremely severe anemia refractory to treatment. The peripheral blood smear shows several of the following features that, while not absolutely diagnostic, should suggest the possibility that a hemoglobinopathy is present: microcytosis, hypochromia, codocytes, normoblastosis, anisocytosis, poikilocytosis, deformed erythrocytes resembling drepanocytes, and intraerythrocytic crystal formation. When hemolysis is severe, as in the hemolytic crisis of sickle cell anemia, there is not only severe normoblastosis but also striking leukocytosis—the shift to the left suggesting an infectious disease. Since the anemia of a hemoglobinopathy is of the hemolytic type, there is usually reticulocytosis, with the blood smear showing polychromatophilia, diffuse basophilia, basophilic stippling, and scattered macrocytic erythrocytes. In the newborn the findings may be those of isoimmune hemolytic disease but without proof of

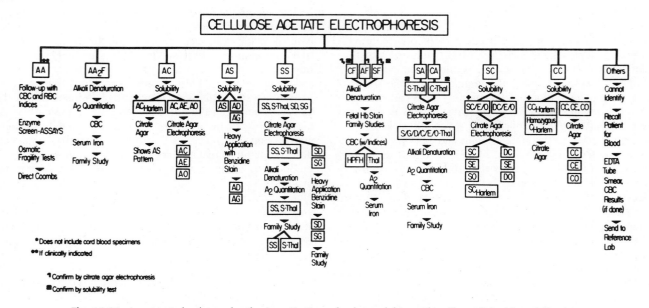

Fig. 14-17. A suggested scheme for the investigation of a hemoglobinopathy. (From Schmidt and Brosius, 1975.)

sensitization. Instead of anemia, erythrocytosis is characteristic of the hemoglobinopathies characterized by increased oxygen affinity (p. 646).

Clinically, the signs are proportional to the severity of the hemolytic process and are sometimes characteristic of special hemoglobinopathies. Chronic hemolytic anemia may be associated with pallor, tachycardia, and splenomegaly. Cyanosis should alert one to the possibility of congenital methemoglobinemia or of a hemoglobinopathy associated with a hemoglobin having decreased oxygen affinity (p. 649).

Family studies are extremely important, not only for the diagnosis in a given case but also for establishing carriers of a hemoglobinopathy. Without access to the members of the patient's family the nature of the hemoglobinopathy sometimes remains unproved.

Excellent descriptions of methods used in the study of the hemoglobinopathies are given by Schmidt (1975), Schmidt and Brosius (1975), and Schmidt et al (1974). It is recommended that an unknown specimen be studied first by cellulose acetate electrophoresis followed by appropriate differential studies (Fig. 14-17). Recommended methods are given in the Appendix.

Ultrastructural studies of normoblasts in some hemoglobinopathies (Hb Hammersmith and Hb Nottingham) have revealed many morphologic abnormalities (Frisch et al, 1974) in some of the normoblasts, presumably those synthesizing the abnormal hemoglobin. The abnormalities included binucleated and multinucleated normoblasts, abnormalities of the nuclear envelope, alteration in the structure and density of the chromatin, microtubules, many iron-laden mitochondria, and a variety of nuclear and cytoplasmic inclusions. Similar changes are seen in congenital dyserythropoietic anemia (Breton-Gorius et al, 1973) and in severe iron-deficiency anemia (Hill et al, 1972). It seems that the ultrastructural lesions are indicative of cellular injury of varied etiology.

Tests for erythrocyte sickling

When erythrocytes containing Hb S are exposed to a reduced oxygen tension, they become markedly distorted, assuming a sickle-like shape (Fig. 14-18) with irregular filamentous projections. The sickling phenomenon is a reflection of the "crystallization" of hemoglobin into the characteristic shape. A red blood cell containing Hb S can undergo reversible sickling if the reducing environment is not too severe, but after several episodes of reversible sickling the sickling becomes irreversible (Lessin and Jensen, 1974).

By electron microscopy (Fig. 14-19) one finds that drepanocytes have formed filaments that stack to form twisted rods. The rods are made up of 14 filaments formed by Hb S molecules, in a helical conformation (Dykes et al, 1978). According to Murayama (1966) these changes result from the formation of a hydrophobic bond between the valine in position 1 and the valine in position 6, allowing a cyclic structure to form between the histidine in position 2 and the threonine in position 4 (Fig. 14-20). This rigidly oriented portion of the β-chain then fits into a complementary portion of the adjoining α-chain to produce the linear stacking. More recently Murayama (Murayama and Nalbadian, 1973) has proposed that sickling occurs by the interaction of

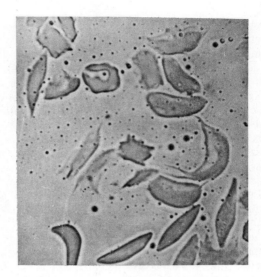

Fig. 14-18. Drepanocytes, metabisulfite preparation. (×950.)

hydrophobic bonds between tetramers of Hb S and proposes a test (Murayama test) said to be specific for Hb S. The formation of drepanocytes is strongly suggestive of the presence of Hb S, but it must be noted that erythrocytes containing other variants (Table 14-10) also have been found to sickle under appropriate reducing conditions. Erythrocytes of some animal species can also sickle: deer, sheep, mongoose, racoon, hamster, and squirrel (Kitchen et al, 1964, 1968; Hawkey and Jordan, 1967; Whitten, 1967). In the deer, sickling is induced by oxygenation, is not accompanied by increased cell destruction, and should be called "pseudosickling."

Various methods can be used to demonstrate sickling. Sickling of abnormal erythrocytes may be produced by placing a drop of blood on a slide, applying a coverslip, and sealing the preparation. As the preparation stands, the oxygen is consumed. Sickling will appear in a few hours in the case of sickle cell anemia and more slowly in sickle cell trait. It is claimed that in sickle cell trait not only does sickling develop more slowly but also fewer drepanocytes are produced and are of a less bizarre morphology than in sickle cell disease, but this is an unreliable differentiation of the heterozygous from the homozygous state. Sickling may be hastened by placing a rubber band tightly around the finger and leaving it in place for 5 minutes before making a wet-drop preparation of capillary blood. Maximum sickling is produced by adding a reducing agent, such as sodium metabisulfite ($Na_2S_2O_5$) or sodium dithionite ($Na_2S_2O_4$), to the blood. Less powerful sickling agents are cultures of *E. coli* and cell-free filtrates of the cultures. Phenothiazines inhibit sickling in vitro at concentrations higher than 128 μg/ml; they also reverse sickling induced by metabisulfite (McFadzean et al, 1969).

Erythrocytes sickle if they contain Hb A and Hb S or only Hb S. Erythrocytes may not sickle if the concentration of Hb S is lower than is required for sickling (25% or more) (Huntsman, 1974). A high concentration of Hb F apparently inhibits the sickling reaction, as evidenced by the

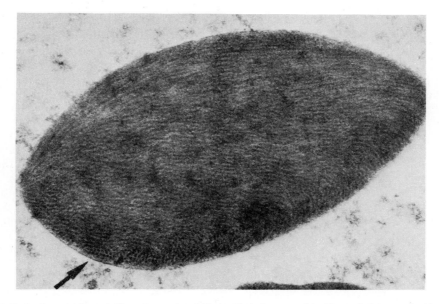

Fig. 14-19. Erythrocyte from sickle cell anemia, sickled with sodium metabisulfite and photographed by electron microscopy. Note the high degree of organization of the rods of Hb S. (From White, 1969.)

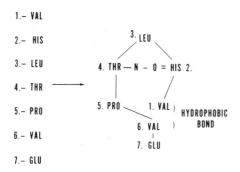

Fig. 14-20. Molecular rearrangement of the *N*-terminal portion of the β-chain of Hb S in the sickling reaction. (After Murayama, 1966.)

Table 14-10. Human hemoglobinopathies in which the erythrocytes can be made to sickle

Hemoglobinopathy	Reference
Hb S	Itano and Pauling, 1949
Hb I	Schwartz et al, 1957
Hb I—thalassemia	Atwater et al, 1960
Hb Bart's	Lie-Injo, 1961
Hb C Georgetown*	Pierce et al, 1963
Hb Alexandra	Thompson and Holloway, 1963
Hb C Harlem*	Bookchin et al, 1968
Hb Pôrto Alegre	Bonaventura and Riggs, 1967
Hb Memphis/S	Kraus et al, 1967
Hb C Ziguinchor	Goossens et al, 1975
Hb S Travis	Moo-Penn et al, 1977

*Hb C Georgetown and Hb C Harlem are identical (Table 14-8).

failure to produce sickling in the erythrocytes of newborns having sickle cell trait (Watson et al, 1948; Charache and Conley, 1964). Unreliable sickling reactions have been observed both when the blood hemoglobin concentration is very low (2 Gm/dl; 0.31 mM/l) or when there is polycythemia.

Hb F: by alkali denaturation

Quantification of Hb F by densitometry is not recommended (Schmidt et al, 1974). The recommended method is based on differential denaturation by alkali. The mechanism by which some hemoglobins are denatured by alkali while others are not is not well understood. Suffice it to say that Hb F is resistant to denaturation (under the conditions of the standard tests), whereas Hb A_1 is not. Hb Bart's, Hb J, and Hb Rainier (Hayashi et al, 1971) are reported to have greater resistance to alkali denaturation than Hb A_1. All other hemoglobin variants are, like Hb A_1, denatured by strong alkali.

It is important to appreciate that while the value of this method is unquestioned, denaturation is not an all-or-none reaction; it is a function of time, pH, and altered solubility (Fig. 14-21). When a solution of oxyhemoglobin is made highly alkaline, the hemoglobin molecule is denatured and thereby is made insoluble at a normal pH. Hb F has a slower rate of denaturation than Hb A_1. After Hb A_1 is completely denatured in a mixture, the semilogarithmic plot of the fraction of undenatured hemoglobin against time yields a straight line; extrapolated back to the starting time, the line intersects the ordinate at a point representing undenatured hemoglobin. This principle has been shown to be most accurate when the amount of undenatured hemoglobin is relatively great. At low concentrations of undenatured hemoglobin, some degree of inaccuracy is unavoidable. The filtrate

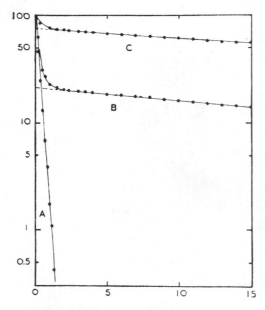

Fig. 14-21. Rate of denaturation of oxyhemoglobin by alkali. Ordinate: Residual hemoglobin (%). Abscissa: Time (minutes). **A,** Normal adult. **B,** Infant aged 4½ months with Hb S–Hb C and 21% Hb F. **C,** Cord blood, 76% Hb F. (From White and Beaven, 1959.)

is in fact a mixture of undenatured hemoglobin and dissolved denatured hemoglobin, whereas the precipitate contains a small amount of absorbed undenatured hemoglobin.

Normal values depend on the technic used (Appendix). The method recommended by White (1974) has a normal value of up to 2%.

Hb F: erythrocyte distribution by acid elution

The acid elution technic for determining the distribution of Hb F among red blood cells (Kleihauer et al, 1957; Nierhaus and Betke, 1968) is valuable in the study of blood containing a high concentration of Hb F. In hereditary persistence of fetal hemoglobin all the red blood cells contain Hb F, whereas in other hemoglobinopathies only some of the cells contain Hb F (Fig. 14-10).

Quantification of Hb A₂

Quantification of Hb A_2 by cellulose acetate electrophoresis followed by elution or scanning is much less accurate than by chromatography. According to Shibata et al (1975) the precision of Hb A_2 estimation by various technics is (1) cellulose acetate electrophoresis and densitometry, CV = 20%, (2) cellulose acetate electrophoresis followed by elution with Drabkin's solution, CV = 3.7%; column chromatography, CV = 2.6%. The range of normal persons using the electrophoresis method is 1.5% to 6%, whereas the range using DEAE-cellulose chromatography is 1.5% to 3% (Huisman, 1974). Reiss et al (1975) have published an improved method for quantifying Hb A_2 by cellulose acetate electrophoresis, with normal values of 2.55% ± 0.60 (2SD). The preferred method (chromatography) is given in the Appendix.

Ferrohemoglobin solubility

It has been noted that, when manually determining the blood hemoglobin concentration, erythrocytes containing Hb S hemolyze incompletely in the cyanide reagent. A cloudy, rather than clear, solution results, which should alert one to the presence of Hb S. This helpful observation is of course not possible when an automated method is used. A number of commercial kits are available for the detection of insoluble Hb S. Recommendations are being prepared for presentation to the Food and Drug Administration to allow regulation of these and other products (Schmidt, 1974). Solubility tests are easily and less expensively performed without recourse to kits (see Appendix).

Application of solubility measurements to hemoglobin solutions shows that, while oxyhemoglobin A_1 and S behave similarly, ferrohemoglobin S has a much lower solubility than any other ferrohemoglobin (Itano, 1953; Goldberg, 1958; Cook and Raper, 1971). This feature is useful in distinguishing Hb S and Hb D, since these have identical electrophoretic mobilities at pH 8.6. Likewise, ferrohemoglobin C has a higher solubility than ferrohemoglobin A. Solubility readings for the various hemoglobins found in homozygous hemoglobinopathies are $C > A_1 > G > S$. The solubility test is not specific for Hb S, since other hemoglobins have low solubility: Hb Kings County (Sathiapalan and Robinson, 1968), Hb Stanleyville II (Perutz and Lehmann, 1968), Hb C Harlem (Bookchin et al, 1967), and possibly other non-S hemoglobins that sickle as well as some unstable hemoglobins.

Zone electrophoresis

Electrophoresis on various media identifies those hemoglobins which, because of a change in electrical charge, have characteristic mobilities (Fig. 14-22). Many hemoglobin variants have the same charge and therefore the same electrophoretic mobility. Electrophoresis on filter paper is the original technic used but has been replaced by technics that give sharper separation of hemoglobin components. Regardless of the medium used, the principles are the same. The rate of migration is determined by the net charge on the molecule; this charge is stabilized by keeping the pH constant. Mobility is also influenced by the ionic strength of the buffer, decreasing as the ionic strength increases. Accordingly, a pH value is chosen that allows the different charges on various hemoglobin molecules to be reflected in different mobilities. Routine electrophoresis at pH 8.4 to 8.6 provides excellent resolution of hemoglobins A_1, F, S, and C (Figs. 14-23 and 14-25). Electrophoresis in citrate agar of pH 6 to 6.5 (Schneider, 1974b) gives a better separation of Hb F from Hb A_1. It is particularly useful in separating some hemoglobins having nearly the same mobility at pH 8.6 (Hb C from Hb E, Hb S from Hb D [Figs. 14-23 and 14-24], and Hb Little Rock from Hb A_1 [Bromberg et al, 1973]). Likewise, an ionic strength is chosen that is low enough to permit optimum migration but not so low as to interfere with current conductivity (see Appendix). Blood specimens should be freshly drawn and processed. Artifacts simulating "new" hemoglobin variants have been produced by prolonged storage of whole blood, particularly at warm temperatures (Pearson et al, 1961). If an unstable hemoglobin is

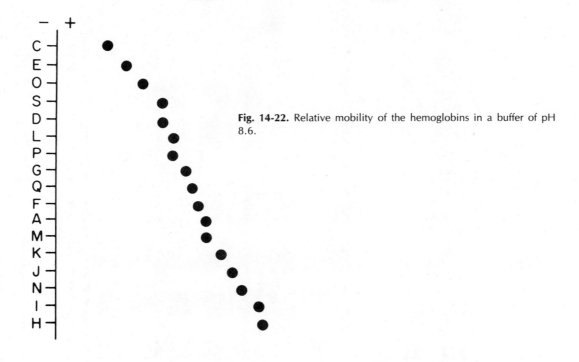

Fig. 14-22. Relative mobility of the hemoglobins in a buffer of pH 8.6.

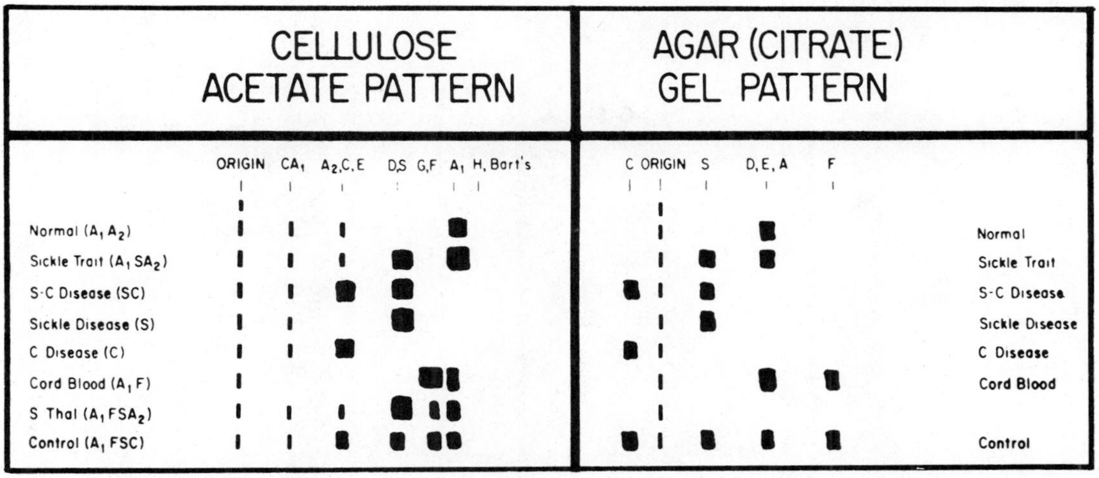

Fig. 14-23. Electrophoretic separation of hemoglobins. The diagram on the left is with cellulose acetate at a pH of 8.4. CA$_1$ is the weak band of carbonic anhydrase sometimes seen with both normal and abnormal hemolysates. The diagram on the right is with citrate agar at pH 6.0. (From Schmidt and Brosius, 1975.)

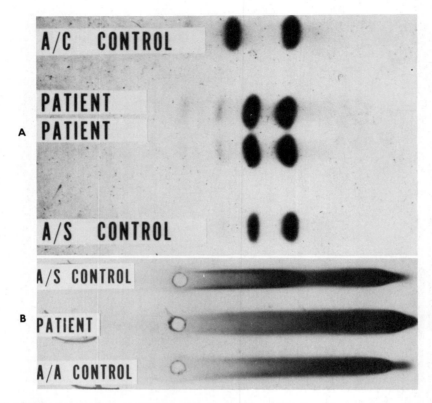

Fig. 14-24. Identification of Hb D on citrate agar electrophoresis at pH 6. Routine electrophoresis on cellulose acetate at pH 8.6 could be mistaken for an A/S pattern, **A,** but at pH 6 on citrate agar, **B,** the abnormal Hb D migrates differently from Hb S.

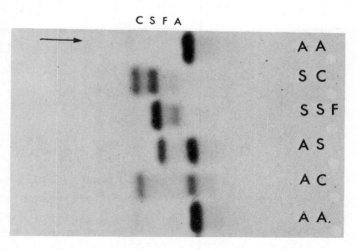

Fig. 14-25. Separation of various hemoglobins by electrophoresis on cellulose acetate, pH 8.6.

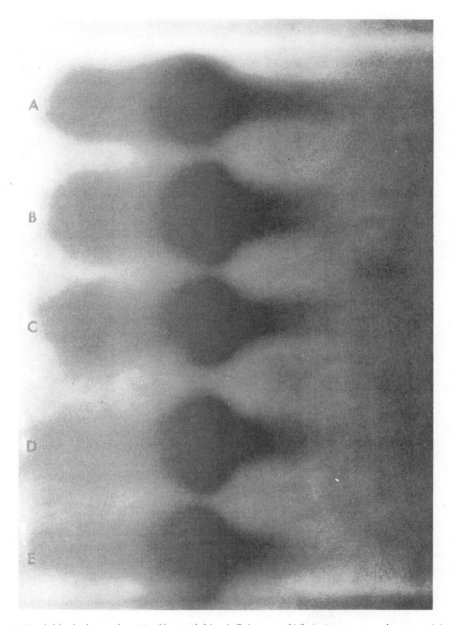

Fig. 14-26. Starch block electrophoresis of hemoglobin. **A-C,** increased Hb A_2 (component closer to origin at left) in thalassemia. **D,** and **E,** Normal amount of Hb A_2 in a normal person. The major component is Hb A_1.

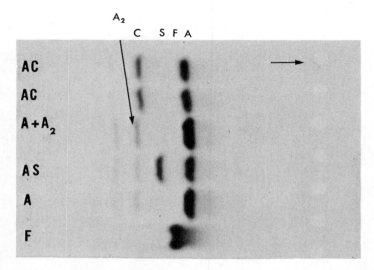

Fig. 14-27. Hemoglobin electrophoresis on cellulose acetate, pH 8.6, showing the relative mobility of Hb A_2.

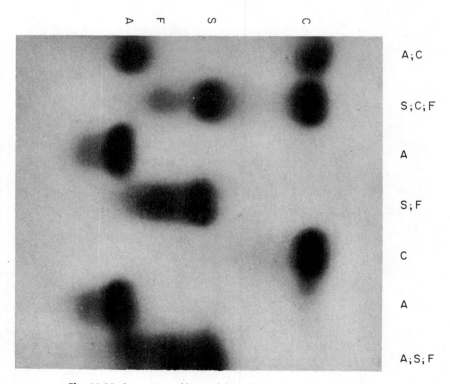

Fig. 14-28. Separation of hemoglobins by starch gel electrophoresis.

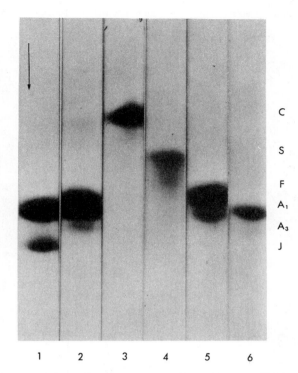

Fig. 14-29. Electrophoretic migration of hemoglobins in acrylamide gel. **1,** Hb A–Hb J; **2,** adult, mother of patient in **1;** 3, homozygous Hb C; **4,** homozygous Hb S; **5,** normal newborn; **6,** normal adult.

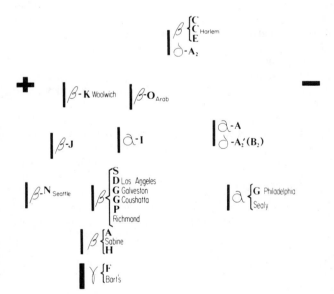

Fig. 14-30. Relative mobilities of globin chains, cellulose acetate, urea-barbital buffer, pH 8.7. (From Schmidt and Brosius, 1975.)

suspected, it is essential to avoid any delay between obtaining the sample and performing the test. For the stable hemoglobin variants, hemolysates in the deoxygenated form are stable for several months.

Electrophoresis on starch block was used by Kunkel and Wallenius to separate and quantify the minor Hb A_2 component. The technic gives excellent results (Fig. 14-26) but is laborious. The A_2 component is readily identified by celulose acetate electrophoresis (Fig. 14-27). Electrophoresis on starch gel (Fig. 14-28) is one of the two most sensitive methods for separating hemoglobin variants, the second being acrylamide gel electrophoresis (Fig. 14-29).

Electrophoresis of the globin chains of hemoglobin on cellulose acetate in both acidic and alkaline buffers containing urea or 2-mercaptoethanol is a promising method for characterizing hemoglobins (Schneider, 1974b; 1978). Hemolysate undergoes electrophoresis in the presence of mercaptoethanol to split the heme from the globin, after which each globin chain migrates at a characteristic rate, depending on pH and composition of the buffer (Fig. 14-30).

Ion-exchange chromatography

The most sensitive technics for separating and quantifying hemoglobin fractions are based on ion-exchange chromatography (Jonxis and Huisman, 1968; Huisman, 1972) (Appendix).

Fingerprint technic

The fingerprint technic, developed by Ingram (1958), is based on tryptic digestion of hemoglobin, followed by filter paper electrophoresis in one direction and chromatography at a right angle. Trypsin splits the polypeptide chain only at those points where the basic amino acids lysine and arginine occur. The resulting chromatogram (Fig. 14-31) is a two-dimensional map of the tryptic peptides, each peptide being located in a definite and characteristic position. The term "fingerprint" is indeed descriptive. Gross differences in hemoglobin polypeptides are detected by this technic; e.g., Ingram first identified a polypeptide difference between the fingerprints of Hb A_1 and Hb S, the difference being in the first tryptic peptide in the β-chain (βT_1).

When an abnormal tryptic peptide is identified, it can be isolated (by column chromatography) and its exact amino acid composition determined by appropriate methods.

Tests for unstable hemoglobin

Most unstable hemoglobins are not identifiable as such by electrophoretic methods. The instability is caused by unstable internal bonding, and the tests used to detect unstable hemoglobins depend on the effect on unstable bonds. Two tests are recommended. In the *heat stability test* (Dacie et al, 1964) a hemolysate of the patient's blood and a control normal are heated to 50° C, a temperature at which unstable hemoglobins precipitate within a short time (Appendix). The isopropanol precipitation test (Carrell and Kay, 1972)· depends on accelerated precipitation of unstable hemoglobin by isopropanol (Appendix). Carrell (1974) recommends that both tests be used in testing for unstable hemoglobins.

Red blood cells containing an unstable hemoglobin form

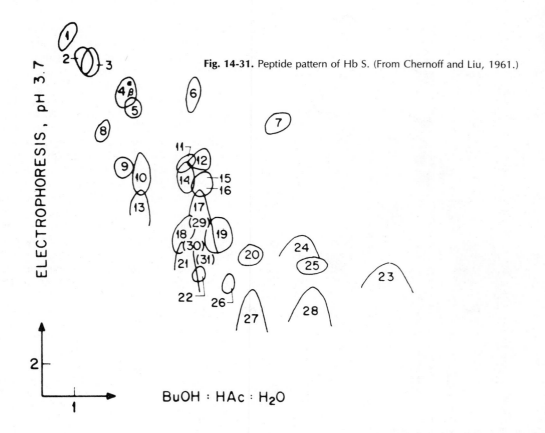

Fig. 14-31. Peptide pattern of Hb S. (From Chernoff and Liu, 1961.)

Heinz bodies when stained supravitally with brilliant cresyl blue (Appendix), but this test is less specific than the two just mentioned. Heinz bodies are also formed in G-6-PD deficiency (Chapter 13) and in some thalassemias. In unstable hemoglobin disease no Heinz bodies may be seen unless the patient is splenectomized (Papayannopoulou and Stamatoyannopoulos, 1974). The test may be useful in distinguishing between Hb H and Hb I (Rigas et al, 1956), for on prolonged exposure to crystal violet the inclusions of Hb H are very fine in contrast to the typical Heinz bodies of Hb I disease.

Hybridization technic

When a hemoglobin solution is made either acid (pH below 5.0) or alkaline (pH 11.0 to 11.6), the hemoglobin molecule dissociates into subunits half the size of the original molecule. Upon bringing the pH back to neutral the subunits recombine spontaneously.

Vinograd (1959) discusses the possible sequences of dissociation and recombination. It is probable that dissociation is from the whole molecule (e.g., $\alpha_2\beta_2$) to asymmetric half molecules (in this case $\alpha\beta$) to individual chains (α and β). The individual chains then can recombine to form new symmetric half molecules and, in turn, the original molecule. If these events occur in a mixture of subunits from two different hemoglobins, recombination can occur between subunits of one hemoglobin and those of the second as well as between subunits from the same source. Thus ''hybrid'' hemoglobin molecules can be formed, differing in physical properties (e.g., electrophoretic mobility and behavior on

chromatography) and therefore identifiable as being different from either of the two original hemoglobin molecules.

This technic has been used extensively to detect whether an abnormality of the hemoglobin molecule resides in the α- or the β-chain. It is also useful in proving the identity or difference between two hemoglobins; e.g., if the two hemoglobins so studied have identical α- and β-chains (or other chains), recombination will not form a hybrid different from the original molecules. If the chain composition is different, on the other hand, a new identifiable hybrid will be formed.

It has been found that canine hemoglobin is excellent for hybridization studies, since dissociation of the molecule of canine hemoglobin gives α- and β-subunits different from the α- and β-subunits of human hemoglobins. Therefore hybridization of human hemoglobin ($\alpha_2{}^A\beta_2{}^A$) with canine hemoglobin ($\alpha_2{}^{can}\beta_2{}^{can}$) will yield two new hybrid molecules ($\alpha_2{}^A\beta_2{}^{can}$ and $\alpha_2{}^{can}\beta_2{}^A$). The same principles apply to hybridization experiments using canine hemoglobin and an abnormal human hemoglobin; e.g., hybridization of canine hemoglobin with Hb Lepore ($\alpha_2[\delta\text{-}\beta]_2$) yields the hybrids $\alpha_2{}^{can}(\delta\text{-}\beta)_2$ and $\alpha_2{}^A\beta_2{}^{can}$, showing that Hb Lepore contains normal α-chains.

Precautions in the laboratory diagnosis of the hemoglobinopathies

It goes without saying that the laboratory diagnosis of a hemoglobinopathy requires meticulous technic to avoid erroneous and misleading data. Furthermore, a great deal of sophistication is required to interpret the data. One major

Table 14-11. Classification of the major hemoglobinopathies

I. Hemoglobinopathy caused by abnormal structure of one or more of the polypeptide chains of globin
  A. Associated with decreased red cell survival
    1. Altered molecular structure associated with abnormal red cell shape and membrane characteristics
      a. Hb S disease and trait
      b. Hb C disease and trait
      c. Hb D disease and trait
      d. Hb E disease and trait
    2. Interaction between two structurally abnormal hemoglobins
      a. Hb S–Hb C disease
      b. Hb S–Hb D disease
    3. Interaction between a structurally abnormal hemoglobin and thalassemia
      a. Hb S–β-thalassemia
      b. Hb S–$\delta\beta$-thalassemia
      c. Hb C–thalassemia
      d. Hb E–β-thalassemia
      e. Hb D–β-thalassemia
      f. Hb G–β-thalassemia
      g. Hb J–β-thalassemia
    4. Altered molecular stability associated with Heinz body formation: the unstable hemoglobins

  B. Associated with abnormal oxygen transport
    1. Increased oxygen affinity with erythrocytosis
    2. Decreased oxygen affinity with cyanosis
    3. Congenital methemoglobinemias
II. Hemoglobinopathy caused by abnormal rate of synthesis of one or more of the polypeptide chains of globin
  A. β-Thalassemia
  B. $\delta\beta$-Thalassemia
  C. α-Thalassemia
  D. δ-Thalassemia
  E. Hereditary persistence of fetal hemoglobin (HPFH)
III. Hemoglobinopathy doubly heterozygous for two structural variants or a structural variant and thalassemia
  A. Hb S–Hb C
  B. Hb S–thalassemia
IV. The Lepore syndromes
  A. The Lepore hemoglobinopathies
  B. The "anti-Lepore" hemoglobinopathies

---

pitfall is a superficial interpretation of routine electrophoretic patterns without appreciating that many structural variants have identical mobilities. One example that comes to mind is the thalassemic syndromes in which Hb A_1 is very low or absent, so that, superficially, the electrophoretic pattern is interpreted as a homozygous structural variant.

Clinical correlation is essential, especially when interpreting the significance of Hb F and Hb A_2 levels. Hb F levels are elevated in some cases of pernicious anemia (Beaven et al, 1960), aplastic anemia (Shahidi et al, 1962; Brabec et al, 1970), PNH (Weatherall and Clegg, 1972), refractory anemia with megaloblastic erythropoiesis (Rosa et al, 1971), sideroblastic anemia (Lie et al, 1968), pure red cell aplasia (Beaven et al, 1960), the second trimester of pregnancy (Pembrey and Weatherall, 1971), molar pregnancy (Bromberg et al, 1957), thyrotoxicosis (Lie-Injo et al, 1967), the juvenile form of chronic myelocytic leukemia, Philadelphia chromosome negative (Beaven et al, 1960; Maurer et al, 1972; Shapira et al, 1972), and other acute leukemias of childhood (Miller, 1969). Isolated cases are reported, too numerous to document, of elevated Hb F associated with a great variety of malignancies. Hb A_2 is elevated in megaloblastic anemias, whereas low Hb A_2 levels are found in untreated iron-deficiency anemia (Josephson et al, 1958). Thus normal levels of Hb A_2 may be found in β-thalassemia heterozygotes if they are in a phase of severe iron deficiency (Wasi et al, 1968). Low Hb A_2 levels may be seen in erythroleukemia (Aksoy and Erdem, 1967). Heller et al (1963) have noted unusually low levels of Hb S when sickle cell trait is combined with megaloblastic anemia. An elevation of Hb H has been found in leukemia (Beaven et al, 1963) and in erythroleukemia (Rosenzweig et al, 1968; Hamilton et al, 1971).

THE HEMOGLOBINOPATHIES
Classification

A working classification of the hemoglobinopathies is given in Table 14-11.

Geographic distribution

The occurrence of the major hemoglobinopathies in the United States is a reflection of migration from Europe, Asia, and Africa. The distribution of the major hemoglobinopathies in these lands is shown in Figs. 14-32 to 14-35.

While it is clear that the influx of immigrants and slaves into this country established the hemoglobinopathies in the New World, the geographic distribution in Europe, Africa, and Asia has intrigued many investigators (Lehmann, 1959a, 1959b; Gelpi, 1973). The distribution of the sickle cell gene has received the most attention.

The first assumption that might be made is that there were independent, spontaneous mutations in widely scattered areas, giving rise to separate foci of Hb S individuals. This seems unlikely, both because the mutation rate is low, 5×10^{-8} per gene pair per generation (Frota-Pessoa and Wajntal, 1963), and because the distribution of other hemoglobinopathies should be the same throughout the Old World.

It seems almost certain that the sickle cell gene was an isolated mutation in Central Africa (Sandler et al, 1978) and that its current distribution is the result of several factors: the slave trade between East Africa and Arabia, Iraq, and India; Arab conquest of the lands bordering the Mediterranean Sea and the Indian Ocean; the effect of endemic falciparum malaria, and interaction between sickle cell trait, thalassemia, and G-6-PD deficiency. It is not surprising that there are whites (nonblacks or non-Orientals) having Hb S in both

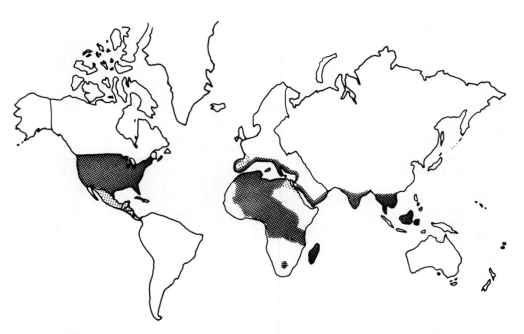

Fig. 14-32. Worldwide distribution of hemoglobinopathies (shaded areas). Nonshaded areas are not necessarily free of hemoglobinopathies but the incidence is either limited to sporadic cases or no data are available on frequency.

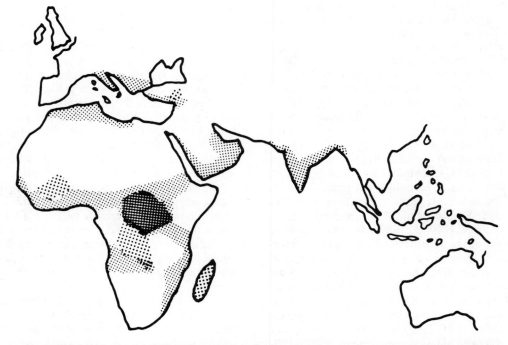

Fig. 14-33. Distribution of sickle cell gene (shaded area). Darker areas represent a greater frequency.

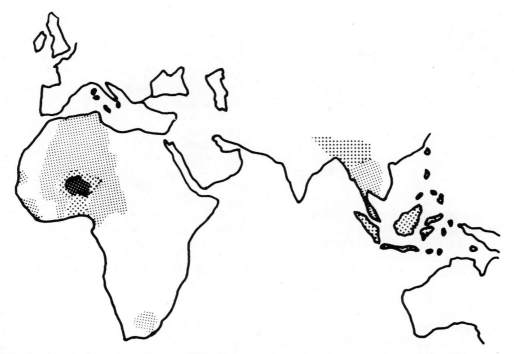

Fig. 14-34. Distribution of Hb C gene (in Africa) and Hb E gene (in Asia). Darker areas represent a greater frequency.

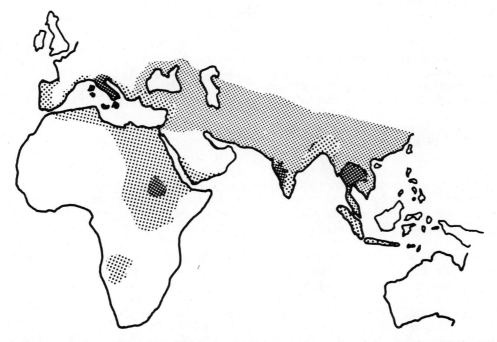

Fig. 14-35. Distribution of the several thalassemia genes (shaded areas). Darker areas represent a greater frequency. β-thalassemia is common in the Mediterranean area, whereas α-thalassemia is common in the Near East.

Europe and Asia—southern Italy and Sicily, the Lake Copais district and the Chalcidice peninsula of Greece, the Eti-Turks in southern Turkey (Altay et al, 1978), and some tribal groups in India (Gelpi and Perrine, 1973).

It seems probable that the Hb C mutation originated in West Central Africa, that for Hb D in India and the Near East, and that for Hb E in Southeast Asia. Thalassemia may have originated anywhere in the Mediterranean basin.

Sickle cell anemia
Hemoglobin synthesis

Hb S has the structural formula $\alpha_2\beta_2^{6\ val}$, indicating a substitution of valine for the glutamic acid at position 6 (Fig. 14-36).

In both sickle cell anemia and sickle cell trait the varieties of hemoglobin produced depend on the structural genes controlling hemoglobin synthesis. As shown in Fig. 14-37, B, the structural genes for β-chains in sickle cell anemia are of the β^s variety, so that only the characteristic β^s chains are synthesized. These combine with normal α-chains to form Hb S. No Hb A_1 is synthesized, since all of the β-chains are of the S variety. Synthesis of δ- and γ-chains proceeds at a normal rate, so that the amount of Hb A_2 and Hb F is usually normal but may be increased. In sickle cell trait (Fig. 14-37, A) both normal and abnormal chains are formed so that, in addition to Hb A_2 and Hb F, both Hb S and Hb A_1 are produced. Furthermore, since fewer abnormal chains are usually produced than normal ones (Bank, 1970), the amount of Hb A_1 usually exceeds that of Hb S. If the amount of Hb S is greater than Hb A_1, an interacting Hb S–thalassemia should be suspected. The same is true if Hb F is significantly increased.

Pathogenesis

The patient with sickle cell anemia not in crisis is relatively asymptomatic, depending on the severity of the anemia and the degree of compensation. The complications can be attributed to (1) hemolytic disease and (2) vascular occlusive disease (Fig. 14-38).

The hemolytic element is responsible for the anemia (McCurdy and Sherman, 1978). Increased pigment excretion increases the incidence of gallstones (Perrine, 1973). Compensatory hyperplasia of bone marrow with enlargement of marrow spaces accounts for the radiologic findings of thinning of the cortices and sometimes demineralization and osteoporosis. Siderotic pigmentation of the spleen and liver can be striking, particularly if many transfusions are given.

The vascular occlusive disease is the result of complex interactions (Finch, 1972; Rickles and O'Leary, 1974). Almost certainly the primary event is sickling of the erythrocytes with sluggish blood flow and sludging in venules and capillaries. Increased adherence of erythrocytes containing Hb S to cultured vascular endothelium (Hebbel et al, 1980) suggests that this may contribute in vivo to microvascular occlusion. The sludging favors the development of hypoxia and acidosis, accentuates the sickling malformation (Milner, 1974), and produces local hypoxia and, in various organs, ischemic necrosis. Local stasis, hypoxia, and acidosis provide the trigger for adhesion of platelets to the damaged endothelium and subendothelial tissue (Chapter 17), favoring local thrombus formation. There is also activation of coagulation factor XII (Hageman), possibly the release of tissue thromboplastin, combining with the action of aggregated platelets to further favor thrombosis. Since the development of microthrombi is widespread, a sort of disseminated intravascular coagulation (DIC) is established. Superimposed on this may be the classic type of DIC triggered by the release of thromboplastic lipids from the hemolyzing red blood cells. Leichtman and Brewer (1978) have documented the occurrence of DIC by demonstrating an elevation of fibrinopeptide A by radioimmunoassay. A significant increase in blood coagulation factor VIII has been found by Abildgaard et al (1967) in children with sickle cell anemia, but the importance of this elevation as a factor in thrombosis is difficult to assess. Because oral contraceptives often cause an increase in factor VIII levels and predispose to thrombosis, it has been recommended that women with sickle cell trait should not take oral contraceptives (Haynes and Dunn, 1967). The role of the fibrinolytic system is also difficult to evaluate. In classic DIC there is activation of the system, a probable protective function in dissolving microthrombi, but in sickle cell anemia in crisis several investigators have found decreased fibrinolytic activity (Mahmood, 1969). This also favors thrombosis by delaying resolution of thrombi.

The most dramatic and dangerous feature of sickle cell anemia is the occurrence of acute episodes of "crisis," characterized by pain in the extremities, chest, abdomen, or back, and low grade fever. Diggs (1965) classifies crises into two types, those based on vascular occlusion, the "painful crises," and those of a hematologic nature (hemolytic or aplastic). Data from the Colorado Sickle Cell Treatment and Research Center (Mahoney and Githens, 1979) show that 20% of patients with sickle cell anemia (Hb S/S) and 28.6% of patients with sickle cell–Hb C disease or sickle cell–thalassemia develop crises at altitudes above 2000 m. Approximately 20% of those having S/C or S/thalassemia hemoglobinopathy had crises when flying in pressurized commercial planes, whereas none of the S/S patients encountered any difficulties in flight.

Hemolytic crises may occur in children, but acute hemolysis is not a feature in the adult. The "aplastic" crisis is rare (MacIver and Parker-Williams, 1961). There is an apparent acute failure to release cells from the bone marrow, as evidenced by exacerbation of the anemia, absence of reticulocytes from the blood, and thrombocytopenia.

Crises are often precipitated by an acute infection, to which patients with sickle cell anemia are particularly susceptible. The most common are severe infection of lungs, urinary tract, or skeletal system (Barrett-Connor, 1971). There is a danger that an acute illness in a subject with sickle cell anemia is ascribed to a crisis while a severe infection is overlooked.

It might have been anticipated that the publicity given to sickle cell anemia by the screening programs would produce occasional instances of factitious or hysterical "pseudocrises," aptly named the "hemoglobin Munchausen syndrome" (Lindenbaum, 1974).

The anemia is caused mostly by decreased red blood cell

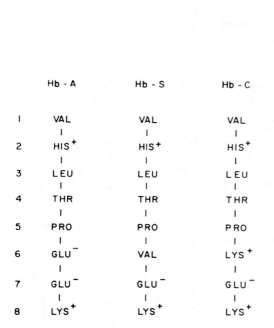

	Hb - A	Hb - S	Hb - C
1	VAL	VAL	VAL
2	HIS$^+$	HIS$^+$	HIS$^+$
3	LEU	LEU	LEU
4	THR	THR	THR
5	PRO	PRO	PRO
6	GLU$^-$	VAL	LYS$^+$
7	GLU$^-$	GLU$^-$	GLU$^-$
8	LYS$^+$	LYS$^+$	LYS$^+$

Fig. 14-36. Substitution for amino acid No. 6 in the β-chain of normal hemoglobin to form Hb S or Hb C (amino acids 1 to 8, tryptic peptide 1).

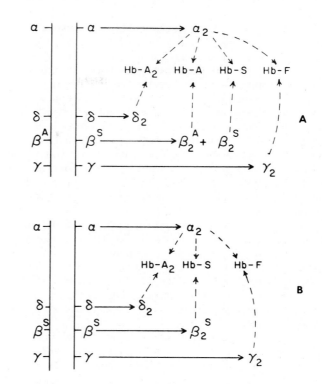

Fig. 14-37. The genetic control of the hemoglobins present in sickle cell anemia, **B,** and sickle cell trait, **A.**

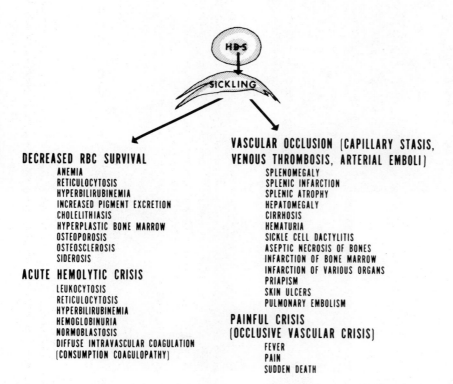

DECREASED RBC SURVIVAL
    ANEMIA
    RETICULOCYTOSIS
    HYPERBILIRUBINEMIA
    INCREASED PIGMENT EXCRETION
    CHOLELITHIASIS
    HYPERPLASTIC BONE MARROW
    OSTEOPOROSIS
    OSTEOSCLEROSIS
    SIDEROSIS

ACUTE HEMOLYTIC CRISIS
    LEUKOCYTOSIS
    RETICULOCYTOSIS
    HYPERBILIRUBINEMIA
    HEMOGLOBINURIA
    NORMOBLASTOSIS
    DIFFUSE INTRAVASCULAR COAGULATION
    (CONSUMPTION COAGULOPATHY)

VASCULAR OCCLUSION (CAPILLARY STASIS, VENOUS THROMBOSIS, ARTERIAL EMBOLI)
    SPLENOMEGALY
    SPLENIC INFARCTION
    SPLENIC ATROPHY
    HEPATOMEGALY
    CIRRHOSIS
    HEMATURIA
    SICKLE CELL DACTYLITIS
    ASEPTIC NECROSIS OF BONES
    INFARCTION OF BONE MARROW
    INFARCTION OF VARIOUS ORGANS
    PRIAPISM
    SKIN ULCERS
    PULMONARY EMBOLISM

**PAINFUL CRISIS
(OCCLUSIVE VASCULAR CRISIS)**
    FEVER
    PAIN
    SUDDEN DEATH

Fig. 14-38. Pathogenesis of the signs and symptoms found most commonly in sickle cell disease. Aplastic crises are rare and are omitted from the diagram because the pathogenesis is unknown.

survival, but there is also an element of ineffective erythropoiesis. The diminished red cell survival is explainable by a series of inferences. In vitro studies with sickling erythrocytes show, on deoxygenation, a series of morphologic changes terminating in the drepanocyte with long microfilaments (Jensen and Klug, 1973). Upon oxygenation the sickled cell reverts to the normal shape. If this reversible sickling is produced a number of times, the cell loses its ability to revert to the normal shape when oxygenated and irreversible sickling is established. The inability to revert to the normal shape is probably caused by progressive loss of microfilaments and damage to the cell membrane (Padilla et al, 1973), with resulting decreased survival of the cell (Bensinger and Gilette, 1974). The membrane may also be damaged by the precipitation of hemoglobin, forming small Heinz bodies (Lessin and Jensen, 1972). These changes lead to intravascular fragmentation, a minor mechanism (Naumann et al, 1971), and extravascular phagocytosis by RE cells (Bensinger and Gilette, 1974). Other features, such as reduced membrane lipids (Jensen and Klug, 1973), may be involved in the phagocytosis of these abnormal cells by RE phagocytic cells.

Diggs and Williams (1963) have reported good success in treating the occlusive crisis with papaverine (0.065 Gm intramuscularly, repeated every 2 to 4 hours for 24 hours).

In 24 out of 32 cases there was good, to dramatic, relief of pain. Of the various vasodilators that have been tried, this seems most promising. Based on the observation that erythrocytes containing Hb S sickle more readily in an acid than in an alkaline medium, sodium lactate intravenously and sodium citrate by mouth have been found to be effective in treating a crisis (Barreras and Diggs, 1964). Hyperbaric oxygenation reduces the number of circulating sickle cells but does not affect the painful crisis (Laszlo et al, 1969). The current status of antisickling therapy is discussed by Brewer (1976). Partial exchange transfusion has been used in the treatment of crises in adults (Brody et al, 1970) and during pregnancy (Ricks, 1968; Morrison and Wiser, 1976), as well as in children (Lanzkowsky et al, 1978). Orlina et al (1978) emphasize the frequency of alloimmunization in multiple-transfused patients with sickle cell disease.

Clinical features

Sickle cell anemia is usually discovered in childhood, and persons so affected seldom live beyond young adulthood. Although plagued by numerous complications, it is remarkable to note how well most of the patients adjust to the chronic anemia.

Sickle cell hemoglobinopathy occurs chiefly in blacks or in persons of black ancestry. The incidence of the sickle cell

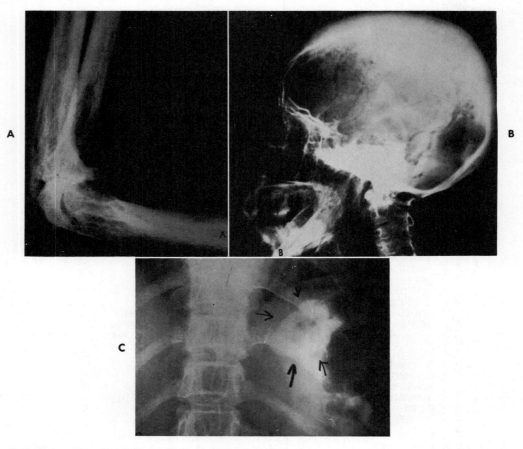

Fig. 14-39. Sickle cell anemia. **A,** Elbow showing coarsening of trabecular pattern. **B,** Skull, **C,** Small calcified spleen (autosplenectomy). (Courtesy Dr. R. E. Parks.)

abnormality in American blacks varies in different localities from 7% to 13%. The homozygous state occurs in about 2.5% to 3.5% of blacks having a positive test for sickling or about 160/100,000 population (Motulsky, 1973a). The incidence of both the heterozygous and the homozygous form is higher in some parts of Africa and India (Livingstone, 1967). An interesting account of sickle cell disease in Ghana is given by Konotey-Ahulu (1974), and the unusually high incidence and mild clinical course of sickle cell anemia in Saudi Arabia is discussed by Gelpi (1979). The disease is also more benign in Israeli Arabs (Roth et al, 1978).

The symptomatology is quite variable, as might be expected in a disease embracing the features of hemolysis, anemia, and vascular occlusion. From time to time, acute episodes occur, characterized by fever, abdominal or joint pain, leukocytosis, and jaundice. Sometimes pneumonia is either part of the crisis or precipitates one. Osteomyelitis, pneumococcal meningitis, and septicemia are frequent complications, probably because of deficient serum opsonizing

activity (Winkelstein and Drachman, 1968). Splenomegaly is found in childhood (Fig. 2-26, p. 68), but in later years the spleen decreases in size as the result of numerous infarcts and diffuse fibrosis. The spleen is sometimes completely atrophic and calcified (Figs. 14-39 and 2-25, p. 67). Cardiac enlargement secondary to the chronic anemia is common. The jaundice is chronic and may vary in severity. There may be superimposed obstructive jaundice, sometimes caused by gallstones (Fig. 14-40). Engorgement of the cavernous sinuses of the penis with sludged sickled erythrocytes occasionally produces painful and embarrassing priapism. Necrosis of the renal papillae produces hematuria (Allen, 1964). This is common, and sickle cell disease should be ruled out in a black with hematuria. Hematuria may be seen also in other hemoglobinopathies: homozygous Hb C (Thomas et al, 1955); β-thalassemia (Robertson, 1972); A/D hemoglobinopathy (Gunnells and Grim, 1967). Unexplained hematuria in whites may also be secondary to a hemoglobinopathy (Chiorazzi et al, 1974; Sperber and Tessler, 1974; Crane et al, 1977). The bone lesions reflect either the striking erythroid hyperplasia of the bone marrow

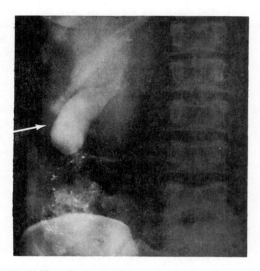

Fig. 14-40. Sickle cell anemia. Coarsening of trabecular pattern in vertebral bodies. Arrow points to radiotranslucent stone in the gallbladder, a common complication in chronic hemolytic disease. (Courtesy Dr. R. E. Parks.)

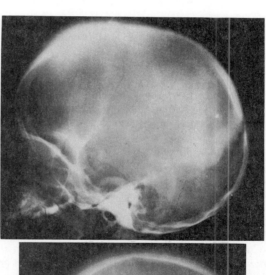

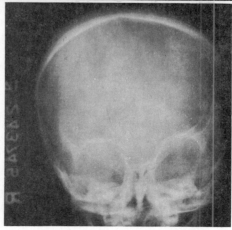

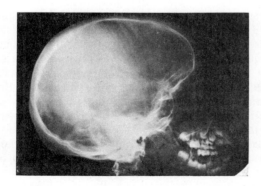

Fig. 14-41. Sickle cell anemia. Note the thickening of the skull caused by widening of the diploic space and thinning of the inner and outer tables, the most common manifestation in the skull of a patient with sickle cell anemia. (Courtesy Dr. R. E. Parks.)

Fig. 14-42. Sickle cell anemia. Skull of 20-month-old black girl. Note the hair-on-end appearance, occasionally seen in sickle cell anemia though supposedly characteristic of β-thalassemia. (Courtesy Dr. R. E. Parks.)

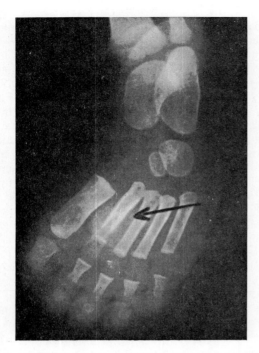

Fig. 14-43. Sickle cell anemia. Aseptic necrosis of metatarsal bone in a 15-month-old black boy. (Courtesy Dr. R. E. Parks.)

(enlargement of the marrow space, Figs. 14-41 and 14-42) or aseptic necrosis on the basis of ischemia (Fig. 14-43). Infarction of the bone marrow is common, particularly during stasis crisis. A complete review of the pathology of bone and joint lesions is given by Diggs (1967). Neurologic damage is not uncommon and can also be attributed to ischemia. The most common skin manifestation is ulcers of the ankles, but it should be noted that ulcers can also be found in other hemoglobinopathies.

Laboratory findings

The anemia is usually severe. Peripheral blood smears show moderate degrees of *anisocytosis, poikilocytosis,* and *hypochromia.* Codocytes are present. Drepanocytes (sickled erythrocytes) can sometimes be seen on stained smears. Barreras et al (1968) have described keratocytes (blister cells) and schizocytes (irregularly contracted or fragmented erythrocytes) in the blood smears from patients with sickle cell anemia and pulmonary emboli. These are probably formed, as in microangiopathic hemolytic anemia (Chapter 13) or acute DIC (Chapter 17), by the impingement of erythrocytes on strands of fibrin. There may be a few *normoblasts,* increased during an acute hemolytic episode. Even during quiescent periods there is a *reticulocytosis* (5% to 10%) and polychromatophilic normoblasts in the peripheral blood smear. During a hemolytic crisis there is *leukocytosis* with a shift to the left, but there is no increase in leukocyte alkaline phosphatase (Wajima and Kraus, 1968). Leukocytosis is also common when the patient is not in crisis. During an aplastic crisis, on the other hand, the reticulocyte count is very low, and there may be leukopenia and thrombocytopenia. In adults with splenic atrophy, the blood smear also shows features of asplenia, particularly many Howell-Jolly

bodies (Pearson et al, 1969). The *osmotic fragility* of the erythrocytes is decreased. Serum immunoglobulin concentration is normal or slightly increased, but there is a deficiency of serum opsonizing activity against pneumococci. Neely et al (1969) report that serum LDH activity is about twice the normal and that it is markedly elevated during a crisis.

The bone marrow usually shows striking normoblastic erythroid hyperplasia, but in an aplastic crisis there is maturation arrest of the erythrocyte precursors. As in all severe hemolytic anemias, the bone marrow sometimes contains intermediate megaloblasts.

Sickle cell preparations show the typical sickling. In most cases there may be a moderate elevation of Hb F (up to 8%), but in occasional instances fetal hemoglobin may be increased to as high as 20%. When the fetal hemoglobin is increased, family studies should be done to rule out interaction with thalassemia. There is one report, however, of sickle cell disease in two adult black siblings with 20% Hb F uniformly distributed in all red cells and in whom interaction with HPFH or thalassemia seems to have been ruled out (Makler et al, 1974). Electrophoresis at pH 8.6 shows only one component migrating as Hb S (Fig. 14-25). The hemoglobin can be further identified on the basis of ferrohemoglobin solubility and electrophoresis on citrate agar at pH 6 to 6.5.

The National Hemoglobinopathy Standardization Laboratory of the Centers for Disease Control has recommended that cellulose acetate electrophoresis be used as the primary procedure in all sickle cell screening programs in which counseling is being performed (Schmidt, 1973; Schmidt and Brosius, 1974). Since Hb S, Hb D, and Hb G Philadelphia migrate together at pH 8.6, additional identification of Hb S is needed, i.e., solubility study and citrate-agar electrophoresis at pH 6 to 6.5.

Sickle cell trait

The simple sickle cell trait, the heterozygous Hb S and Hb A_1 combination, affects about 8% of American blacks (Boggs, 1974b), is usually asymptomatic (Cooper and Toole, 1972), and is not accompanied by anemia. Rarely, however, aseptic necrosis of femoral heads does occur (Keeling et al, 1974), as in sickle cell anemia. The red blood cells contain both Hb S and Hb A_1 and, in spite of some contrary opinions, cannot be distinguished from homozygous Hb S red cells on the basis of sickling tests alone. Electrophoresis shows both Hb A_1 and Hb S, in equal proportion or with a preponderance of Hb A_1. The presence of Hb S in less than the expected amount should make one suspect a previous transfusion of blood containing Hb S, as illustrated by the interesting case reported by Gibaud et al (1974). When more Hb S than Hb A_1 is found, interaction with thalassemia should be suspected. Red cell life span is normal (Barbedo and McCurdy, 1974). Sickling can occur in vivo if the environment is sufficiently low in oxygen (Conn, 1954). Rupture of the infarcted spleen can occur therefore in sickle cell trait as well as in sickle cell anemia. Sudden death can occur, as reported by Jones et al (1970), when there is hypoxia and strenuous exercise. Sickling crises may occur in flight, even in pressurized aircraft (Green et al, 1971). Strenuous excercise with hemoglobinuria is reported to have precipitated a crisis (Zimmerman et al, 1974). However, well-conditioned football players with sickle cell trait usually do not have problems (Murphy, 1973), although there has been at least one death of a football player with sickle cell trait following a strenuous practice session (Horn, 1980). A comprehensive review of the effects of exercise and altitude on the morbidity of sickle cell trait is given by Sears (1978).

An interesting relationship has been noted between the incidence of falciparum malaria and sickle cell trait. The geographic distribution of both is remarkably similar, but, instead of being at greater risk because of two serious diseases, persons with sickle cell trait seem resistant to infection with malaria. In addition, the mortality from malaria in children with sickle cell trait is less than in those who are normal (Allison, 1954, 1964). To a lesser degree, persons having Hb C trait (Hb A$_1$ and Hb C) are also resistant to malaria. It is hypothesized that the higher mortality from sickle cell anemia is balanced by the increased survival of those with sickle cell trait (Motulsky, 1964). There is no good explanation why red cells containing Hb S are not to the liking of the parasite. Some suggestions are that the parasite cannot metabolize Hb S (Allison, 1954), or that sickling interrupts the life cycle (Mackey and Vivarelli, 1954) or passage to the tissue phase (Miller et al, 1956). Recently Miller et al (1975) have reported that Duffy blood group negative human erythrocytes are resistant to infection by *Plasmodium knowlesi,* an agent infectious for Duffy positive human erythrocytes. Duffy negativity is also related to resistance to vivax malaria (Mason et al, 1977). The suggestion that Duffy blood group determinants are receptors for *P. vivax* may point to as yet unappreciated blood group receptors for malaria on the surface of erythrocytes.

While the combination of Hb S and Hb A$_1$ is a benign situation, the combination of Hb S with a second hemoglobinopathy may lead to severe disease.

Screening for Hb S

Mass screening surveys are underway to identify previously undiagnosed persons with sickle cell trait with the goal of reducing the incidence of sickle cell disease. Screening newborn infants for sickle cell anemia is mandatory in four states: New York, Georgia, Kentucky, and Louisiana. While superficially praiseworthy, these programs present some problems that have concerned thoughtful physicians (Motulsky, 1973b; McCurdy et al, 1974; Hampton et al, 1974; Motulsky, 1974; Rucknagel, 1974; O'Brien, 1974; Rowley, 1978).

We are concerned here with the laboratory aspects of mass screening, and some comments are in order.

Our concern is with the choice of methods for screening, with the skill of the technologists using the methods, and with the degree of sophistication brought to the interpretation of test results.

As discussed in preceding sections, no one test is sufficient to specifically identify the presence of Hb S. Sickling tests are good to a point, owing their success to the fact that, in most instances, a hemoglobin that sickles is in fact Hb S, but there are others that also sickle. Solubility tests are useful but no more specific for Hb S because so many other variants also have low solubility. The commercial Sickledex

test (Ortho Foundation) is not specific for Hb S. Electrophoresis on cellulose acetate at pH 8.6 is good, but should be performed also at pH 6 to 6.5 on citrate agar to distinguish Hb S from Hb D, Hb C from Hb E, and others. None of the above tests will detect thalassemia as the primary disease or the interaction of a structural variant with thalassemia unless the peripheral blood smear and electrophoretic patterns are interpreted by a knowledgeable physician. Family studies are often necessary. When a hemoglobinopathy is discovered, the facilities for special studies, selected for the individual problem rather than by "routine," should be available. Obviously, programs dedicated only to identifying "sicklers" are scientifically inadequate and sociologically immoral (Rubin and Rowley, 1979).

There is another aspect that should be disturbing. It seems inevitable when mass public health programs are instituted that the technical simplicity of the procedures is emphasized and the work force that is needed is assigned to semiskilled workers. If this is the only way a program can be carried out I doubt whether it is worth doing, for the interpretation of laboratory data cannot be more accurate than the data.

Hemoglobin C disease and trait

In hemoglobin C synthesis a positively charged lysine is substituted for the glutamic acid in position 6 of the β-chain (Fig. 14-36). Hb C disease is rare, the incidence in the U.S. being about 22/100,000 blacks (Motulsky, 1973a). The disease is mild (Smith and Krevans, 1959) with intermittent episodes of abdominal discomfort, splenomegaly, and slight jaundice. Hb C trait (Hb C plus Hb A$_1$) affects about 3% of American blacks (Boggs, 1974b) and is asymptomatic, although cases of priapism have been reported.

The hematologic findings are more impressive than the clinical picture. The peripheral blood smear shows many codocytes and an occasional microspherocyte. Intraerythrocytic crystals of hemoglobin (Fig. 14-44), sometimes within rod-shaped red cells, can be found if searched for. Crystallization can be induced if washed red cells suspended in sodium citrate solution are allowed to stand for some hours in a wet coverslip preparation (Fig. 14-45).

Hemoglobin C in combination with another hemoglobinopathy can produce severe disease.

Hemoglobin D disease and trait

Both Hb D disease (homozygous Hb D) and Hb D trait (Hb D plus Hb A$_1$) are extremely rare (Chernoff, 1958), and both are asymptomatic. The peripheral blood smear shows a variable number of codocytes. On routine electrophoresis at pH 8.6, Hb D migrates like Hb S, so that Hb D trait might be misdiagnosed as sickle cell trait. Red cells containing Hb D do not sickle. As for some of the other hemoglobinopathies, Hb D in combination with Hb S or thalassemia leads to severe disease.

Hemoglobin E disease and trait

Hemoglobin E is rarely encountered in the United States but is one of the common abnormal hemoglobins in Asia (Chernoff et al, 1956; Aksoy, 1960). A very complete review of the distribution and population dynamics of Hb E is given by Flatz (1967). It has been estimated that Hb E occurs in about 20,000,000 persons, of which 80% live in

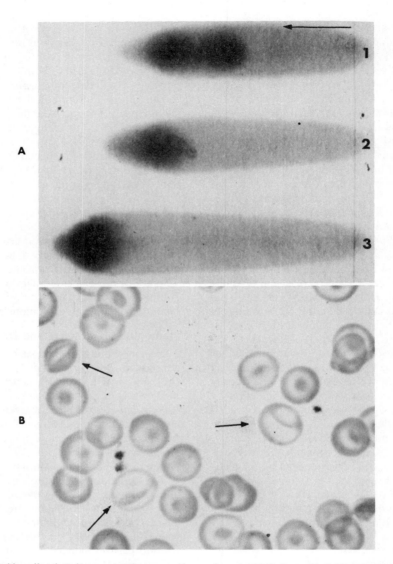

Fig. 14-44. Sickle cell–Hb C disease. **A,** Filter paper electrophoresis. **(1)** Patient with sickle cell–Hb C disease; **(2)** sickle cell anemia control; **(3)** normal control. **B,** Blood smear. Note the intraerythrocytic crystals (arrows) and many codocytes. (Wright's stain; ×950.)

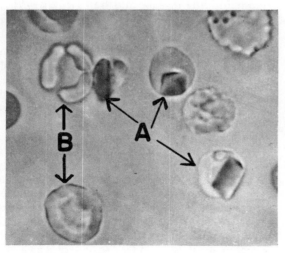

Fig. 14-45. Intraerythrocytic hemoglobin crystals in blood from a patient with sickle cell–Hb C disease. **A,** Intraerythrocytic crystals; **B,** aggregation of hemoglobin along cell margins. (Unstained, sealed, moist preparation.) (From Kraus and Diggs, 1956.)

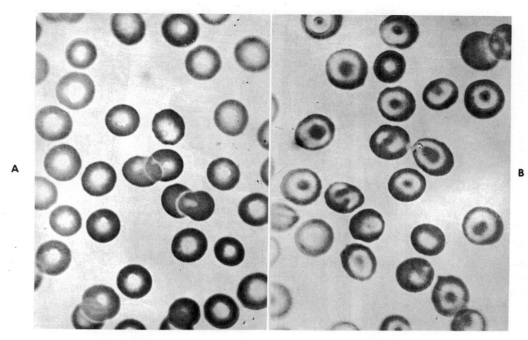

Fig. 14-46. Blood smears **A,** Hb E trait. **B,** Hb E disease. (From Chernoff et al, 1956.)

Southeast Asia. The homozygous state is characterized by mild hemolytic anemia and the peripheral blood smear shows many codocytes (Fig. 14-46, *B*). Fairbanks et al (1980) report a case of homozygous Hb E disease without anemia and mimicking β-thalassemia minor. The heterozygous (Hb E plus Hb A_1) state is asymptomatic, and the peripheral blood smear shows no codocytes (Fig. 14-46, *A*). According to Fairbanks et al (1979) the trait often shows a low MCV, but microcytosis caused by iron deficiency was not ruled out.

Interaction between two structurally abnormal hemoglobins

As noted in the preceding sections the heterozygous combination of a structurally abnormal hemoglobin with Hb A_1 is either asymptomatic or is accompanied by mild hemolytic anemia. However, the combination of two structurally abnormal hemoglobins often leads to severe disease only slightly less severe than the major homozygous hemoglobinopathies.

The most important interactions are the combination of Hb S and Hb C (sickle cell–Hb C disease), between Hb S and Hb D (sickle cell–Hb D disease), and between various structurally abnormal hemoglobins (Hb S, Hb C, Hb D, and Hb E) and thalassemia (Huisman, 1979). The thalassemia interactions are discussed following the discussion of the thalassemia syndromes.

Sickle cell–Hb C disease

The person with sickle cell–Hb C disease inherits one hemoglobinopathy from each parent. Since these are the two most common hemoglobinopathies, there is a fairly high incidence in blacks of the combination: 120 births out of 100,000 and 80 persons per 100,000 of all ages in the Unit-

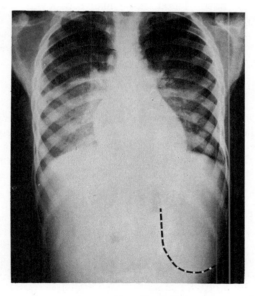

Fig. 14-47. Splenomegaly in sickle cell–Hb C disease. Note the bilateral basal pneumonia, a presenting sign that is not infrequent. (Courtesy Dr. R. E. Parks.)

ed States (Motulsky, 1973a) and as high as 25% of the population in some regions of Africa.

The symptoms of the disease vary from moderate to severe, the course being generally less severe than that of sickle cell disease. There may be hematuria, musculoskeletal pain, and abdominal pain (River et al, 1961). Splenomegaly is common (Fig. 14-47) in adults, in contrast to the low incidence in adults with sickle cell anemia. Aseptic necrosis of bone (Fig. 14-48) is also more common than in

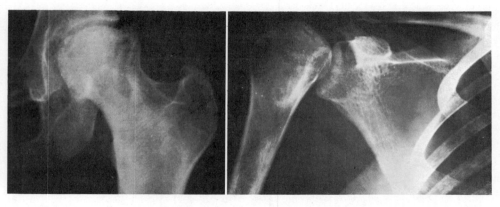

Fig. 14-48. Sickle cell–Hb C disease. Aseptic necrosis of femoral and humoral heads in a 27-year-old black female. (Courtesy Dr. R. E. Parks.)

sickle cell anemia. Pregnancy in women with sickle cell–Hb C disease is a potentially serious situation (Henderson et al, 1961), and we have seen several fatal complications. The cause of death is a crisis-like episode, resembling the vascular occlusive phenomena of sickle cell disease, and in our cases necropsy showed pulmonary and cerebral bone marrow and fat emboli as well (Ober et al, 1959). General anesthesia may precipitate a fatal crisis (Rockoff et al, 1978).

The peripheral blood shows many codocytes and some intraerythrocytic crystals (Figs. 14-44 and 14-45). Hemoglobin electrophoresis shows only Hb S and Hb C, and the red blood cells sickle. In the absence of complications there is only moderate anemia.

Sickle cell–Hb D disease

The interaction of Hb S and Hb D is uncommon (Smith and Conley, 1959; Cawein et al, 1966) as would be expected from the low frequency of Hb D. Of the various hemoglobins D (Tables 14-2 and 14-3), only the combination of Hb S–Hb D Punjab is characterized by moderate hemolytic anemia. Hb S–Hb D Ibadan is asymptomatic (Weatherall and Clegg, 1972).

Other interactions

A number of other interactions have been reported, all rare (Kumpati et al, 1978). Some of these are Hb S–Hb J Baltimore; Hb S–Hb K; Hb S–HPFH (hereditary persistence of fetal hemoglobin); Hb S–Hb E and Hb S–Hb G Philadelphia. Hb S in combination with Hb O Arab has been found in the United States (Javid, 1973) and can be mistaken for sickle cell–Hb C disease because of the identical electrophoretic mobility of Hb C and Hb O. This combination gives rise to a moderately severe form of sickle cell disease (Milner et al, 1970). Hb S–Hb J hemoglobinopathy is completely asymptomatic (Gellady and Schwartz, 1973).

Unstable hemoglobin disease

Many hemoglobinopathies have been described that are characterized by the presence of a hemoglobin variant less stable than normal hemoglobin. Some are asymptomatic while others are the cause of a severe hemolytic anemia with Heinz body formation. Inheritance is autosomal dominant, and the known cases are heterozygous. The homozygous state is probably incompatible with fetal survival. The unstable hemoglobins are listed in Table 14-12. The division into three clinical groups follows the classification of Winslow and Anderson (1978).

Those unstable hemoglobins associated with hemolytic anemia have a characteristic picture. Intermittent jaundice is precipitated by an acute infection (Zinkham et al, 1979b) with the passage of dark urine caused by excretion of dipyrrholes derived from the breakdown of heme. Splenomegaly is found in almost every case. There may be thrombocytopenia caused by platelet sequestration in the enlarged spleen. The red blood cells show moderate anisocytosis and poikilocytosis, reticulocytosis (some have questioned the reliability of distinguishing reticulocytes from Heinz bodies [Koler et al, 1973]), and some punctate basophilia. In nonsplenectomized patients Heinz bodies are present during an acute episode of jaundice. During a quiescent period Heinz bodies are scarce or absent but can be induced by allowing the blood to stand at room temperature for 24 to 48 hours (Dacie et al, 1964), or by adding sodium nitrate (Chernoff and Horton, 1969) or acetylphenylhydrazine (Beutler et al, 1955) to the blood. It is probable that Heinz bodies are in fact formed, but removed by the spleen because Heinz bodies can be found without the use of inducing agents in 50% to 100% of the red cells following splenectomy.

These hemoglobins are less stable than normal hemoglobin in the sense that relatively mild thermal or chemical trauma induces a precipitation of hemoglobin and the formation of Heinz bodies. The chief instability is caused by instability of heme binding so that the heme dissociates easily from the globin (Jacob, 1970; Rieder, 1974). This is followed by rapid precipitation of abnormal β-chains (the complex reactions preceding precipitation are outlined by Rachmilewitz, 1974), forming the Heinz bodies that become attached to the red cell membrane (Winterbourne and Carrell, 1974). This in turn produces increased permeability of the cell membrane and shortened survival of the red cells. The free heme molecules are broken down into the dipyrrholes that color the urine. The liberated α-chains remain free and are sometimes seen as a trailing protein on electrophoresis. There is evidence that in Hb Leiden there is in fact an excess of α-chain production (Rieder and James, 1974).

Table 14-12. Clinical classification of unstable hemoglobins*†

Hemoglobin	Substitution	Remarks‡
Group I: severe or moderately severe hemolytic anemia		
Hb Torino	α43 Phe → Val	AOA; DH
Hb Ann Arbor	α80 Leu → Arg	
Hb Bibba	α136 Leu → Pro	
Hb Savannah	β24 Gly → Val	
Hb Volga	β27 Ala → Asp	
Hb Genova	β28 Leu → Pro	
Hb Abraham Lincoln	β32 Leu → Pro	Same as Hb Perth
Hb Castilla	β32 Leu → Arg	
Hb Hammersmith	β42 Phe → Ser	Same as Chiba; AOA
Hb Dhofar	β58 Pro → Arg	Same as Yukuhashi
Hb Bicêtre	β63 His → Pro	
Hb Bristol	β67 Val → Asp	AOA
Hb Mizuho	β68 Leu → Pro	
Hb Christchurch	β71 Phe → Ser	
Hb Shepherd's Bush	β74 Gly → Asp	AOA; DH
Hb Santa Ana	β88 Leu → Pro	
Hb Borås	β88 Leu → Arg	AOA
Hb Sabine	β91 Leu → Pro	
Hb Istanbul	β92 His → Gln	Same as St. Etienne; AOA
Hb Newcastle	β92 His → Pro	
Hb Nottingham	β98 Val → Gly	AOA
Hb Köln	β98 Val → Met	Same as Ube I, San Francisco; AOA
Hb Casper	β106 Leu → Pro	Same as Southampton; AOA
Hb Burke	β107 His → Arg	AOA
Hb Wien	β130 Tyr → Asp	
Hb Olmsted	β141 Leu → Arg	
Hb H	β4	No heme-heme interaction and no Bohr effect; AOA
Hb F Poole	γ130 Try → Gly	
Group II: mild hemolytic anemia		
Hb Hirosaki	α43 Phe → Leu	
Hb L Ferrara	α47 Asp → His	See Table 14-2 for synonyms
Hb Strumica	α112 His → Arg	Same as Serbia
Hb Leiden	β6 or 7 Glu → O	AOA
Hb Belfast	β15 Try → Arg	AOA
Hb Freiburg	β23 Val → O	AOA; C
Hb Riverdale-Bronx	β24 Gly → Arg	
Hb Philly	β35 Tyr → Phe	
Hb Louisville	β42 Phe → Leu	Same as Bucuresti; AOA
Hb Tochigi	β56-59 → O	
Hb Zürich	β63 His → Arg	DH
Hb Duarte	β63 Ala → Pro	AOA
Hb I Toulouse	β66 Lys → Glu	
Hb Sydney	β67 Val → Ala	
Hb Seattle	β70 Ala → Asp	AOA; C
Hb Bushwick	β74 Gly → Val	
Hb Atlanta	β75 Leu → Pro	
Hb Pasadena	β75 Leu → Arg	
Hb Bryn Mawr	β85 Phe → Ser	Same as Buenos Aires; AOA
Hb J Altgeld Gardens	β92 His → Asp	
Hb Gun Hill	β92-96 → O; or 91-95 → O; or 93-97 → O	DH; β-chains lack heme; AOA
Hb St. Etienne	β92 His → Gln	β-chains lack heme
Hb Rush	β101 Glu → Gln	
Hb Tübingen	β106 Leu → Glu	AOA; C
Hb Peterborough	β111 Val → Phe	AOA; DH
Hb Madrid	β115 Ala → Pro	
Hb Altdorf	β135 Ala → Pro	AOA
Hb Hope	β136 Gly → Asp	AOA

*Modified from Winslow and Anderson (1978), with addition of recently reported variants.
†References given in Tables 14-2 to 14-9.
‡DH, Drug hypersensitivity; AOA, abnormal oxygen affinity; C, cyanosis.

Continued.

Table 14-12. Clinical classification of unstable hemoglobins—cont'd

Hemoglobin	Substitution	Remarks
Group III: no clinical anemia or unspecified severity		
Hb Prato	α31 Arg → Ser	
Hb Arya	α47 Asp → Asn	
Hb J Rovigo	α53 Ala → Asp	
Hb Etobicoke	α84 Ser → Arg	AOA
Hb Moabit	α86 Leu → Arg	
Hb Port Phillip	α91 Leu → Pro	
Hb Setif	α94 Asp → Tyr	
Hb Manitoba	α102 Ser → Arg	
Hb Suan Dok	α109 Leu → Arg	
Hb Hopkins 2	α112 His → Asp	AOA
Hb Dakar	α112 His → Gln	
Hb Sögn	β14 Leu → Arg	
Hb Saki	β14 Leu → Pro	
Hb Lyon	β17, 18 Lys, Val → O	
Hb E Saskatoon	β22 Glu → Lys	
Hb Strasbourg	β23 Val → Asp	
Hb Moscova	β24 Gly → Asp	
Hb E	β26 Glu → Lys	Oxidatively unstable
Hb Henri Mondor	β26 Glu → Val	
Hb Volga	β27 Ala → Asp	Same as Drenthe
Hb St. Louis	β28 Leu → Gln	
Hb Tacoma	β30 Arg → Ser	AOA
Hb Vaasa	β39 Gln → Glu	
Hb Athens-Georgia	β40 Arg → Lys	AOA
Hb Okaloosa	β48 Leu → Arg	AOA
Hb Willamette	β51 Pro → Arg	AOA
Hb G Ferrara	β57 Asn → Lys	
Hb J Bari	β64 Gly → Asp	Same as J Cosenza and J Calabria
Hb St. Antoine	β74, 75 Gly, Leu → O	
Hb Baylor	β81 Leu → Arg	AOA
Hb Tours	β87 Thr → O	AOA
Hb Caribbean	β91 Leu → Arg	
Hb Djelfa	β98 Val → Ala	AOA
Hb Camperdown	β104 Arg → Ser	
Hb Indianapolis	β112 Cys → Arg	
Hb Fannin-Lubbock	β119 Gly → Asp	
Hb Khartoum	β124 Pro → Arg	
Hb Guantanamo	β128 Ala → Asp	
Hb Leslie	β131 Gln → O	Same as Deaconess; AOA
Hb North Shore	β134 Val → Glu	
Hb Brockton	β138 Ala → Pro	AOA
Hb Toyoake	β142 Ala → Pro	AOA
Hb Cranston	Elongated β-chain	

While this seems to be the usual mechanism for instability, there are others. There may be weakening instead of the $\alpha_1\beta_1$ contact, as in Hb Philly and Hb Tacoma; a distortion of the entire molecule, as in Hb Freiburg, Hb Gun Hill, and Hb Leiden; or a distortion of a helical sequence, as in Hb Genova, Hb Santa Ana, Hb Sabine, and Hb Bibba.

The laboratory identification of unstable hemoglobins is discussed on p. 631. Electrophoresis under standard conditions is not helpful. Electrophoretic mobilities are summarized by White and Dacie (1971). Various degrees of trailing behind Hb A_1 may suggest the presence of α-chains and other degradation products. It may be helpful to note that hemolysates containing unstable hemoglobin precipitate spontaneously after a few days of storage. There is an increase in alkali-resistant hemoglobin that may not represent Hb F.

Some confusion in the classification of these hemoglobinopathies arises from the observation that some also have altered oxygen affinity (De Furia and Miller, 1972). However, not all the variants having altered oxygen affinity have unstable characteristics.

Hemoglobinopathy associated with abnormal oxygen transport

Increased oxygen affinity with erythrocytosis

Some hemoglobin variants have increased oxygen affinity that is sometimes sufficient to inhibit optimum release of oxygen. This causes hypoxia, stimulation of erythropoietin,

Table 14-13. Hemoglobins with increased oxygen affinity

Residue	Substitution	Name	Residue	Substitution	Name
α-Chain			87(F3)	Thr → O	Hb Tours
6(A4)	Asp → Ala	Hb Sawara	88(F4)	Leu → Arg	Hb Borås
44(CE2)	Pro → Leu	Hb Milledgeville	89(F5)	Ser → Asn	Hb Creteil
45(CE3)	His → Arg	Hb Fort de France		Ser → Arg	Hb Venderbilt
84(F5)	Ser → Arg	Hb Etobicoke	92(F8)	His → Gln	Hb St. Etienne, Istanbul
85(F6)	Asp → Asn	Hb G Norfolk	97(FG4)	His → Gln	Hb Malmö
92(FG4)	Arg → Gln	Hb J Cape Town		His → Leu	Hb Wood
	Arg → Leu	Hb Chesapeake	98(FG5)	Val → Met	Hb Köln, San Francisco (Pacific), Ube I
95(G2)	Pro → Ala	Hb Denmark Hill		Val → Gly	Hb Nottingham
	Pro → Ser	Hb Rampa		Val → Ala	Hb Djelfa
112(G19)	His → Asp	Hb Hopkins-II	99(G1)	Asp → Asn	Hb Kempsey
126(H9)	Asp → Asn	Hb Tarrant		Asp → His	Hb Yakima
141(HC3)	Arg → His	Hb Suresnes		Asp → Tyr	Hb Ypsilanti
	Arg → Leu	Hb Legnano		Asp → Ala	Hb Radcliffe
			100(G2)	Pro → Leu	Hb Brigham
β-Chain			101(G3)	Glu → Lys	Hb British Columbia, Hb Alberta, Hb Potomac
9(A6)	Ser → Cys	Hb Porto Alegre	103(G5)	Phe → Leu	Hb Heathrow
15(A12)	Try → Arg	Hb Belfast	106(G8)	Leu → Pro	Hb Southampton, Hb Casper
17-18(A14-15)	Lys, Val → O	Hb Lyon		Leu → Gln	Hb Tübingen
20(B2)	Val → Met	Hb Olympia	109(G11)	Val → Met	Hb San Diego
28(B10)	Leu → Gln	Hb St. Louis	121(GH4)	Glu → Gln	Hb D Los Angeles, D Chicago, D Punjab, D North Carolina, D Portugal, Oak Ridge
	Leu → Pro	Hb Genova			
35(C1)	Tyr → Phe	Hb Philly			
37(C3)	Try → Ser	Hb Hirose			
40(C6)	Arg → Lys	Hb Athens-Ga., Waco	124(H2)	Pro → Gln	Hb Ty Gard
	Arg → Ser	Hb Austin	129(H7)	Ala → Pro	Hb Crete
51(D2)	Pro → Arg	Hb Willamette	135(H13)	Ala → Pro	Hb Altdorf
62(E6)	Ala → Pro	Hb Duarte	142(H20)	Ala → Pro	Hb Toyoake
63(E7)	His → Arg	Hb Zürich		Ala → Asp	Hb Ohio
	His → Tyr	Hb M Saskatoon, M Emory, M Kurume, M Hida, M Radom, M Arhus, M Chicago, Leipzig, Hörlein-Weber, Novi Sad, M Erlangen	143(H21)	His → Arg	Hb Abruzzo
				His → Gln	Hb Little Rock
				His → Pro	Hb Syracuse
			144(HC1)	Lys → Asn	Hb Andrew-Minneapolis
75(E19)	Leu → Arg	Hb Pasadena	145(HC2)	Tyr → His	Hb Bethesda
78(E18)	Gly → Asp	Hb Shepherds Bush		Tyr → Cys	Hb Rainier
79(EF3)	Asp → Gly	Hb G Hsi-Tsou		Tyr → Asp	Hb Ft. Gordon, Osler, Nancy
81(EF5)	Leu → Arg	Hb Baylor			
82(EF6)	Lys → Thr	Hb Rahere		Tyr → Term	Hb McKees Rocks
	Lys → Met	Hb Helsinki	146(HC3)	His → Asp	Hb Hiroshima
85(F1)	Phe → Ser	Hb Bryn Mawr, Buenos Aires		His → Pro	Hb York
				Elongated	Hb Tak

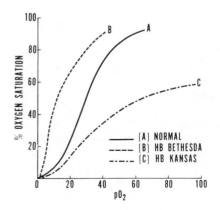

Fig. 14-49. Oxygen dissociation curves. **A,** For normal whole blood. **B,** For Hb Bethesda (increased oxygen affinity). **C,** For Hb Kansas (low oxygen affinity). (Data from Bunn et al, 1972; Bonaventura and Riggs, 1968.)

Table 14-14. Hemoglobins with increased oxygen affinity[*]

Hemoglobin	Substitution	Erythrocytosis
Hb Chesapeake	α92 Arg → Leu	Yes
Hb J Capetown	α92 Arg → Gln	No
Hb Yakima	β99 Asp → His	Yes
Hb Kempsey	β99 Asp → Asn	Yes
Hb Ypsilanti	β99 Asp → Tyr	Yes
Hb Rainier	β145 Tyr → Cys	Yes
Hb Hiroshima 1	β146 His → Asp	Yes
Hb Hirose	β37 Try → Ser	No
Hb Malmö	β97 His → Gln	Yes
Hb Bethesda	β145 Tyr → His	Yes
Hb Little Rock	β143 His → Gln	Yes
Hb Olympia	β20 Val → Met	Yes
Hb Heathrow	β103 Phe → Leu	Yes
Hb San Diego	β109 Val → Met	Yes
Hb Andrew–Minneapolis	β144 Lys → Asn	Yes
Hb Denmark–Hill	α95 Pro → Ala	No
Hb Rampa	α95 Pro → Ser	No
Hb Georgia	α95 Pro → Leu	No
Hb Brigham	β100 Pro → Leu	Yes
Hb Köln	β98 Val → Met	No
Hb Creteil	β89 Ser → Asn	Yes
Hb Lyon	β17 Lys ⎱ → 0 18 Val ⎰	No
Hb Leiden	β6 or 7 Glu → 0	No
Hb Bryn Mawr	β85 Phe → Ser	No
Hb Nottingham	β98 Val → Gly	No
Hb Belfast	β15 Try → Arg	No
Hb Hopkins 2	α112 His → Asp	No
Hb Syracuse	β143 His → Pro	Yes
Hb Abruzzo	β143 His → Arg	Yes
Hb Duarte	β62 Ala → Pro	No
Hb Wood	β97 His → Leu	Yes
Hb Nancy (Osler; Fort Gordon)	β145 Tyr → Asp	Yes
Hb Tak	Elongated β-chain	No
Hb Shepherd's Bush	β74 Gly → Asp	No
Hb McKees Rocks	β145 Tyr → term	Yes
Hb Willamette	β51 Pro → Arg	No
Hb Baylor	β81 Leu → Arg	No
Hb Altdorf	β135 Ala → Pro	No
Hb Ohio	β142 Ala → Asp	Yes
Hb Rahere	β82 Lys → Thr	Yes
Hb Vanderbilt	β89 Ser → Arg	Yes
Hb Radcliffe	β99 Asp → Ala	Yes
Hb Alberta	β101 Glu → Gly	Yes
Hb York	β146 His → Pro	Yes
Hb Suresnes	α141 Arg → His	Yes
Hb Tarrant	α126 Asp → Asn	No
Hb Austin	B40 Arg → Ser	No
Hb Helsinki	β82 Lys → Met	Yes
Hb British Columbia	β101 Glu → Lys	Yes
Hb Potomac	β100 Glu → Asp	Yes

[*]References in Tables 14-2 and 14-3.

Table 14-15. Hemoglobins with decreased oxygen affinity

Residue	Substitution	Name
α-Chain		
43(CE1)	Phe → Val	Hb Torino
58(E7)	His → Tyr	Hb M Boston, M Osaka, Gothenburg, M Kiskunhalas
86(F7)	Leu → Arg	Hb Moabit
87(F8)	His → Tyr	Hb M Iwate, M Kankakee, M Oldenburg
94(G1)	Asp → Asn	Hb Titusville
β-Chain		
1(NA)	Val → Ac-Ala	Hb Raleigh
24(B6)	Gly → Asp	Hb Moscva
42(CD1)	Phe → Ser	Hb Hammersmith, Chiba
	Phe → Leu	Hb Louisville, Bucuresti
48(CD7)	Leu → Arg	Hb Okaloosa
67(E11)	Val → Glu	Hb M Milwaukee-I
70(E14)	Ala → Asp	Hb Seattle
73(E17)	Asp → Tyr	Hb Vancouver
	Asp → Val	Hb Mobile
82(EF6)	Lys → Asn → Asp	Hb Providence
90(F6)	Glu → Lys	Hb Agenogi
91(F7)	Leu → Arg	Hb Caribbean
102(G4)	Asn → Thr	Hb Kansas
	Asn → Ser	Hb Beth Israel
107(G9)	Gly → Arg	Hb Burke
108(G10)	Asn → Asp	Hb Yoshizuka
	Asn → Lys	Hb Presbyterian
111(G13)	Val → Phe	Hb Peterborough
139(H17)	Asn → Lys	Hb G Manhasset

impaired release of oxygen to the tissues (Wagner, 1974). In the case of some hemoglobins with high oxygen affinity, the substitution interferes with the interface of $\alpha_1\beta_2$ contacts in such a way as to favor the oxy-structure (Perutz, 1970b). In other cases there is interference at the terminal carboxy of the β-chain. This complex stereochemical system is reviewed by Nagel and Bookchin (1974). In Hb Little Rock there is impaired binding of 2,3-DPG in deoxyhemoglobin. Some of the unstable hemoglobins also have abnormal oxygen affinity (Table 14-12), but those with high oxygen affinity are not associated with erythrocytosis.

The inheritance of these hemoglobinopathies is autosomal dominant (Berglund, 1972). The presenting sign is erythrocytosis, which may be mistakenly attributed to stress or other nonspecific causes, since these hemoglobinopathies are detected only by special methods (starch gel electrophoresis in TRIS-EDTA buffer pH 8.6, agar gel electrophoresis pH 6.2, or oxygen affinity determinations [Lichtman et al, 1976]). Because of the familial tendency, these hemoglobinopathies can be misdiagnosed as familial erythrocytosis. The specific diagnosis is made by measuring the oxygen affinity of the blood. In most instances the erythrocytosis is marked, but there is no leukocytosis or thrombocytosis. There are no other abnormal hematologic findings, and the erythrocytosis does not predispose to complications. Blood

and erythrocytosis (Stamatoyannopoulos et al, 1971; Stephens, 1977) (Tables 14-13 and 14-14).

In most of these variants the location of the substitution is such as to impair heme-heme interaction so that the oxygen dissociation curve becomes hyperbolic. The mutation also reduces the Bohr effect, so that the oxygen dissociation curve is shifted to the left (Fig. 14-49). This accounts for

Table 14-16. Classification of the thalassemias

I. β-Thalassemia
  A. Homozygous β^+-thalassemia: $\alpha_2\beta_2^{thal\,+}$
  B. Homozygous β^0-thalassemia: $\alpha_2\beta_2^{thal\,0}$
  C. Heterozygous β^+-thalassemia: $\alpha_2\beta\beta^{thal\,+}$
  D. Heterozygous β^0-thalassemia: $\alpha_2\beta\beta^{thal\,0}$
II. δβ-Thalassemia
  A. Homozygous δβ-thalassemia: $\alpha(\delta\beta)^{thal}\alpha(\delta\beta)^{thal}$
  B. Heterozygous δβ-thalassemia: $\alpha\beta\alpha(\delta\beta)^{thal}$
  C. Doubly heterozygous δβ-β-thalassemia: $\alpha\beta^{thal}(\delta\beta)^{thal}$
III. α-Thalassemia
  A. Homozygous α-thalassemia: $\alpha^{thal\,1}\beta\alpha^{thal\,1}\beta$
  B. Heterozygous α-thalassemia: $\alpha\beta\alpha^{thal\,1}\beta$
  C. Homozygous mild α-thalassemia (H disease): $\alpha^{thal\,1}\beta\alpha^{thal\,2}\beta$

  D. Heterozygous mild α-thalassemia: $\alpha\beta\alpha^{thal\,2}\beta$
  E. Heterozygous α-Q-Thalassemia: $\alpha^{thal\,1}\beta\alpha^Q\beta$
  F. Heterozygous α-Constant Spring thalassemia: $\alpha^{thal\,1}\beta\alpha^{Constant\,Spring}\beta$
IV. δ-Thalassemia
  A. Homozygous δ-thalassemia: $\alpha_2\beta_2(\delta_2^{thal})$
  B. Heterozygous δ-thalassemia: $\alpha_2\beta_2(\delta^{thal})$
V. The Lepore syndromes: $\alpha_2(\delta\beta)_2$
VI. Hereditary persistence of fetal hemoglobin (HPFH)
  A. Negro type
  B. Greek type
  C. Swiss type
VII. Double heterozygosity of above categories with each other or structural variants

erythropoietin levels are normal, thus ruling out some other types of erythrocytosis, but these subjects respond normally to blood loss anemia with an increase in erythropoietin excretion (Hayashi et al, 1971).

Decreased oxygen affinity with cyanosis

In most instances unstable hemoglobins (Table 14-15) have a high oxygen affinity. In a few there is decreased oxygen affinity causing cyanosis (Hb Seattle, Hb Freiburg, and Hb Tübingen). Hb Peterborough and Hb Hope have decreased oxygen affinity and are considered mildly unstable (Steinberg et al, 1976), but instability may be a matter of degree in some instances. Variants that have a low oxygen affinity and cause cyanosis, but are not considered unstable, are Hb Agenogi, Hb Yoshizuka, Hb Kansas, Hb Titusville, and Hb Beth Israel (Nagel, 1976). Most cases of congenital hemoglobinopathy-associated cyanosis are caused by the presence of hemoglobin M variants.

Congenital methemoglobinemias

Congenital (hereditary) methemoglobinemia includes (1) methemoglobinemia associated with deficient reducing systems, (2) methemoglobinemia associated with excessive oxidative activity, and (3) methemoglobinemia associated with the abnormal hemoglobins designated M.

To discuss methemoglobinemia without duplication, all three types are discussed in Chapter 10. We need only say here that the amino acid substitutions in the hemoglobins M are such that the hemoglobin iron remains in the ferric state, forming a stable bond with tyrosine rather than the usual histidine. In this conformation the molecule is stabilized and is a poor carrier of oxygen.

The thalassemia syndromes
Geographic distribution

As shown in Fig. 14-35, β-thalassemia is most prevalent in areas surrounding the Mediterranean Sea. Migration from this area has carried the gene to other parts of the world. The gene may also be found when the Mediterranean origin is obscured by the passage of several generations or by intermarriage. Thalassemia can and does occur in persons of other than Mediterranean or Oriental ancestry. For no obvious reason thalassemia is both rare and mild in American blacks (Braverman et al, 1973).

α-Thalassemia is also found in the Mediterranean area but is particularly prevalent in Southeast Asia, the Middle East, and the Orient.

Classification

The clinical classification of thalassemias into *thalassemia major, thalassemia intermedia, thalassemia minor,* and *thalassemia minima* is purely clinical and refers only to the clinical severity in a given person. A subject with thalassemia major has severe anemia usually beginning in infancy, one with thalassemia intermedia has less severe anemia, one with thalassemia minor may have little or no anemia but have abnormal morphology of the red cells, while one with thalassemia minima may be normal except that the presence of a thalassemia gene is inferred from family studies.

There is little correlation between the clinical classification and the genetic type of thalassemia. While it is true that thalassemia major is often the expression of homozygous β-thalassemia, a very severe disease can be found in other types as well as in doubly heterozygous states (thalassemia interacting with a structural variant such as Hb S). In addition, there is a wide spectrum of clinical severity for each of the genetic types. The most striking examples are in homozygous β-thalassemia that, while usually severe, is sometimes surprisingly mild (Gabuzda et al, 1963; Erlandson et al, 1964) especially in blacks (Went and MacIver, 1961). This probably represents two varieties of β-thalassemia: β^+-thalassemia (mild), and β^0-thalassemia (severe).

The classification and characterization of the thalassemias on a genetic basis is preferred even though there are still areas of uncertainty. The subject is well covered by Weatherall and Clegg (1972) and by Weatherall (1978).

A genetic classification of the thalassemia syndromes is given in Table 14-16.

Genetics

In contrast to the hemoglobinopathies associated with structural hemoglobin variants, the thalassemias are characterized by the presence of mutant genes that suppress the *rate of synthesis* of globin chains (Bank and Marks, 1966; Bank et al, 1968). Originally thought to result from the presence of either one or a pair of suppressor thalassemia genes at the normal loci (e.g., α^{thal} at the α-locus, β^{thal} at the β-locus), the situation has been found to be more complex, with a strong possibility that several suppressor genes are in fact operative, as for the γ-locus.

The mechanism that dictates the diminished rate of production of globin chains is still not entirely clear. With some important exceptions (Nienhuis et al, 1971; Clegg and Weatherall, 1972; Rieder, 1972), the best hypothesis is that there is faulty transcription leading to deficient amounts of chain-specific mRNA (Benz and Forget, 1971; Housman et al, 1973; Kacian et al, 1973; Benz et al, 1975). This in turn leads to a decreased rate of synthesis of globin chains. In some instances, as in α-thalassemia, there is evidence favoring deletion of α-loci (Ottolenghi et al, 1976). Whether chain-specific mRNA is deficient because of faulty transcription or because of gene deletion, the result is the same—diminished rate of production of globin chains.

Inheritance of thalassemia is autosomal, but it is difficult to classify further as to dominant or recessive because the heterozygous state is not always symptomatic.

β-*Thalassemia*

HOMOZYGOUS. In the homozygous state, β-thalassemia is almost always a serious disease. Synonyms are Cooley's anemia and thalassemia major. It manifests in infants, with failure to thrive, pallor, moderate icterus, and massive hepatosplenomegaly. As a consequence of chronic hemolysis and many blood transfusions there is siderosis of the spleen, liver, and other organs. The disease is usually fatal in childhood; infection or cardiac failure are common complications. Sometimes the disease is surprisingly mild and a few affected persons survive into adulthood. Kan et al (1975) report that a prenatal diagnosis can be made from aspirated placental blood.

β-Thalassemia is characterized by diminished (β^+-thalassemia) or absent (β^0-thalassemia) synthesis of the β-chains. In accord with current thinking, Benz et al (1975) found that β-chain–specific mRNA is absent in β^0-thalassemia. Some cases of β^0-thalassemia are caused by gene deletions (Ramirez et al, 1976), in some there is no gene deletion but β-specific mRNA can be detected (Tolstoshev et al, 1976), in some hybridizable mRNA is present but there is no β-chain synthesis (Kan et al, 1975), and in some cases from Ferrara, Italy, there is normal mRNA that cannot be translated (Conconi et al, 1975).

The laboratory findings are characteristic. A summary of the hematologic features of the thalassemia syndromes is given in Table 14-17. The blood picture is that of a hypochromic and microcytic anemia, with very low red blood cell count and hemoglobin, low MCV, MCH, and MCHC. The smear shows marked anisocytosis, poikilocytosis, hypochromia, codocytes, polychromatophilia, and a few, to very many, normoblasts. The reticulocyte count is usually in the range of 5% to 10%. The leukocyte count is moderately elevated with a moderate to sometimes striking shift to the left. The platelet count is usually normal, but sometimes pooling of platelets and leukocytes in the massively enlarged spleen results in thrombocytopenia and leukopenia.

The bone marrow is hyperplastic with a preponderance of normoblasts. Occasional intermediate megaloblasts may be present and, rarely, there is superimposed severe folate deficiency with frank megaloblastosis. Foamy histiocytes resembling Gaucher cells are not uncommon but are not numerous. There is an abundance of iron. Early normoblasts may contain inclusion bodies representing precipitated excess α-chains; the excess chains are sometimes seen as trailing in electrophoretic patterns.

The osmotic fragility of the erythrocytes is decreased, sometimes markedly. The serum bilirubin concentration is moderately increased. Serum iron concentration is high with almost complete transferrin saturation. Erythrocyte survival is diminished and this, combined with maturation arrests of polychromatophilic cells in the bone marrow (Yataganas et al, 1973), results in anemia. Ultrastructural studies of normoblasts in β-thalassemia major have shown nuclear and membrane abnormalities, intranuclear inclusions, and cytoplasmic inclusions (Polliack et al, 1974a), changes reflecting ineffective erythropoiesis.

The hemoglobins in blood vary in the two types of homozygous β-thalassemia. In the more common, the thal+ or high F type, Hb F is markedly elevated, Hb A_2 levels are variable, and Hb A_1 is decreased. In the thal^0 or high A_2 type, the Hb F level is low, the Hb A_2 level is high, and, because of complete absence of β-chain synthesis, no Hb A_1 is present. In the high F type, stains for Hb F in red cells shows it to be distributed heterogeneously, in contrast with the finding in HPFH. The diagram in Fig. 14-50 may be helpful in understanding the basis for the combination of hemoglobins found in the homozygous thalassemias.

The severe anemia is treated with blood transfusions, and eventually there is iron overload (Pearson and O'Brien, 1975). Some of the iron is derived from the transfused erythrocytes, some from increased intestinal absorption of iron (Heinrich et al, 1973). Iron-chelating agents (e.g., deferoxamine) are used to control tissue iron deposition (Graziano et al, 1978).

HETEROZYGOUS. Heterozygous β-thalassemia has no characteristic clinical picture, varying from a moderately severe anemia to a completely asymptomatic picture. It encompasses the clinical designation of thalassemia intermedia to thalassemia minor (thalassemia trait). Pallor and splenomegaly may be present in the more severe cases. Hyperbilirubinemia is rare and, when present, may be a sign of other concomitant disease such as Gilbert's syndrome (Cartei and Dini, 1975). Some cases of β-thalassemia trait with unusually severe clinical and hematologic findings may belong in the category of "inclusion-body β-thalassemia trait" described by Stamatoyannopolous et al (1974). An excess of α-chain production in those cases produces numerous inclusions in normoblasts. The mild cases have no signs or symptoms and are often detected only in the course of family studies.

In almost all cases the blood shows some degree of hypochromia and microcytosis, easily dismissed as mild iron-deficiency anemia. Failure to respond to iron therapy gives a clue as to its true nature. The combination of low MCV and elevated Hb A_2 identifies many but not all cases of heterozygous thalassemia (Zannis-Hadjopoulos et al, 1977). In the severe form the blood smear may appear typically thalassemic (as in the homozygous disease). Osmotic fragility is almost always decreased. Hb A_2 is elevated (Rowley, 1976;

Table 14-17. Hematologic features of the thalassemia syndromes

Syndrome	Blood morphology	Anemia	HB A₁	Hb A₂	Hb F	Other features
Homozygous β⁺-thalassemia	Thalassemic ++++	++++	↓+++	↑, N, ↓	↑+++	Free α-chains and inclusions; Hb F heterogeneously distributed
Homozygous β⁰-thalassemia	Thalassemic ++++	++ to ++++	0	N	↑++++	Free α-chains and inclusions; Hb F heterogeneously distributed
Heterozygous β-thalassemia	Thalassemic ++	0 or +	N or ↓+	↑++(3.5-7%)	N, ↑(0-7%)	Free α-chains
Homozygous δβ-thalassemia	Thalassemic +	+	0	0	↑++++	Hb F in all red blood cells
Heterozygous δβ-thalassemia	Thalassemic ±	0	N	N	↑++	Hb F heterogeneously distributed
Heterozygous δβ-thalassemia	Thalassemic + to ++	0 or +	0 to ↓+++	N	↑++++	Hb F heterogeneously distributed
Homozygous α-thalassemia	Thalassemic ++++	++++	0	0	0	Hydrops fetalis; Hb Bart's up to 100%; ± Hb H; ± Hb Portland; red blood cells sickle
Homozygous "mild" α-thalassemia	Thalassemic +++	++ to +++	↓+	↓+	N	Hb H and Hb Bart's present
Heterozygous α-thalassemia	Thalassemic ++	0 to +	N	N	N	Hb Bart's in newborn; ± Hb H
Homozygous δ-thalassemia	Normal	0	N	0	N	
Heterozygous δ-thalassemia	Normal	0	N	↓+	N	
Lepore, homozygous	Thalassemic +	0 to +	0	0	↑++++	Hb Lepore 10-25%; Hb F heterogeneously distributed
Lepore, heterozygous	Normal	0	N	N	↑++	Hb Lepore ± 10%
HPFH—Negro type Heterozygous	Normal	0	↓+	↓+	↑17-38%	Hb F homogeneously distributed
HPFH—Negro type Homozygous	Normal	0	0	↓+	↑ to 100%	Hb F homogeneously distributed
HPFH—Greek type	Normal	0	↓+	N	↑10-19%	Hb F homogeneously distributed
HPFH—Swiss type*	Normal	0	N	N	↑1-3%	Hb F heterogeneously distributed

*A doubtful entity.

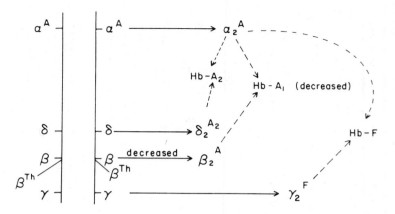

Fig. 14-50. Hemoglobin synthesis in homozygous β-thalassemia. The pattern is for the thal+ type, in which there is depressed synthesis of β-chains, normal synthesis of α- and δ-chains, and hyperactivity of the γ-locus. This results in decreased HB A$_1$, normal Hb A$_2$, and high Hb F. There are excess α-chains because of the unavailability of β-chains.

In the thal^0 type it is assumed that there is complete lack of β-chain synthesis with hyperactivity of the δ-chain locus. Accordingly Hb A$_2$ is increased, Hb A$_1$ is absent, Hb F is normal or slightly increased, and α-chains are again in excess.

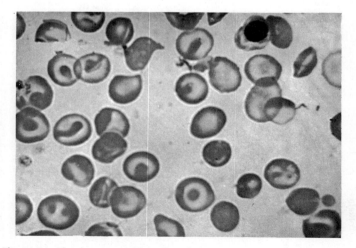

Fig. 14-51. Blood smear, sickle cell–β-thalassemia. (Wright's stain; ×950.)

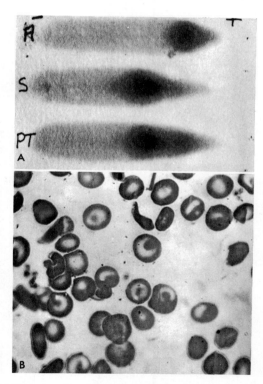

Fig. 14-52. Interacting sickle cell–β-thalassemia. **A,** Paper electrophoretic pattern showing the major component to be Hb S. **B,** Peripheral blood smear.

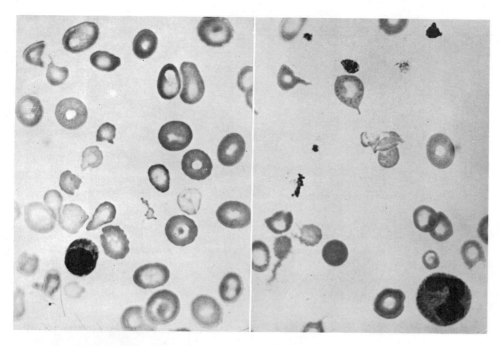

Fig. 14-53. Peripheral blood smears in Hb E–β-thalassemia. (From Chernoff et al, 1956.)

Dinçol et al, 1979), while Hb F is normal or slightly elevated. There may be some variation from this pattern depending on whether the heterozygosity is of the thal$^+$ or thal^0 type.

HETEROZYGOUS β-THALASSEMIA WITH ANOTHER HEMOGLOBINOPATHY. The association of rare variants with β-thalassemia warrants little discussion: Hb D–thalassemia (Lehmann, 1959a; Sukumaran et al, 1960), Hb G–thalassemia (Hill et al, 1962), Hb J–thalassemia (Wilkinson et al, 1967). A discussion of the more common combinations follows.

SICKLE CELL–β-THALASSEMIA. The interaction of Hb S and thalassemia produces two modalities of clinical severity: one is severe and resembles sickle cell anemia, while the other one is a benign variant that resembles sickle cell trait (Weatherall, 1964). Affected twins have been shown to have different degrees of clinical severity (Joishy et al, 1976).

The severe cases show moderately severe anemia, microcytosis, hypochromia, anisocytosis, and poikilocytosis (Fig. 14-51). The reticulocyte count is in the 10% to 20% range. Tests for sickling are positive. Hemoglobin electrophoresis shows Hb S always in excess of Hb A$_1$ (Fig. 14-52) and increased Hb A$_2$ and Hb F. In some cases there seems to be complete suppression of Hb A$_1$, probably an expression of the β$^{thal\ 0}$ gene with complete inhibition of β-chain synthesis. The absence of Hb A$_1$ can lead to an erroneous diagnosis of sickle cell anemia (s/s). Data for globin chain synthesis in Hb S–β^0-thalassemia are given by Felice et al (1979).

The mild cases have little or no anemia, but the blood smear is thalassemic. Reticulocytosis is less marked. The electrophoretic findings are the same as in the severe cases except that absence of Hb A$_1$ is unusual.

HB C–β-THALASSEMIA. Like sickle cell thalassemia, Hb C–thalassemia may be either severe or mild. In blacks the combination is usually benign (Weatherall, 1964), whereas the Italian, Turkish, and Algerian cases are severe (Portier et al, 1960). The blood picture is as in Hb C disease. Hemoglobin electrophoresis shows a marked preponderance of Hb C, up to 90%, with some Hb A$_1$ and moderately increased Hb F. Since there is no way to separate hemoglobin A$_2$ from Hb C, there is no information on Hb A$_2$ levels. It is assumed that in the cases with very low Hb A$_1$ levels the thalassemia gene is of the β$^{thal\ 0}$ variety.

HB E–β-THALASSEMIA. This has been found in Thailand, an area of high frequency for Hb E (Wasi et al, 1969). The picture is of a moderately severe anemia, hepatomegaly, splenomegaly, and growth retardation. The hemotologic findings are as in severe β-thalassemia (Fig. 14-53). Hemoglobin electrophoresis shows Hb E, large amounts of Hb F, and no Hb A$_1$.

δβ-*Thalassemia*

δβ-Thalassemia was originally called F-thalassemia, normal Hb A$_2$ thalassemia, or β-thalassemia type 2. It is thought to differ from β-thalassemia in that it represents defective synthesis of both δ- and β-chains (Zuelzer et al, 1961; Stamatoyannopoulos et al, 1969; Weatherall and Clegg, 1972). The basic defect is the deletion of the δ and β structural genes (Ottolenghi et al, 1976).

HOMOZYGOUS. Homozygous individuals are mildly anemic and show a moderately microcytic hypochromic blood picture, with codocytes, anisocytosis, and poikilocy-

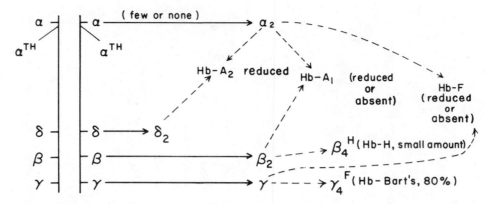

Fig. 14-54. Hemoglobin synthesis in homozygous α-thalassemia. The almost complete suppression of α-chain synthesis provides no α-chains for the synthesis of Hb A_1, Hb A_2, or Hb F. Instead the γ-chains are free to form Hb Bart's while some of the free β-chains form variable amounts of Hb H. A few of the γ-chains combine with embryonic ζ-chains to form Hb Portland.

tosis. Red cell osmotic fragility is decreased. The only hemoglobin present is Hb F, and no Hb A_1 or A_2 is detectable. Since there is only Hb F in the red cells, it is found homogeneously distributed in all the cells, and this alone might cause confusion with HPFH.

HETEROZYGOUS. The heterozygous state is asymptomatic, usually with no anemia or splenomegaly, but some cases show mild anemia (Pagnier et al, 1979). The MCH is usually less than normal. Hb F is increased in the range of 5% to 20% and heterogeneously distributed. Hb A_1 and A_2 are normal.

The doubly heterozygous state for δβ- and β-thalassemia presents a variable clinical picture, some resembling β-thalassemia homozygotes while others have mild anemia and some splenomegaly. The peripheral blood picture is moderately to severely thalassemic. Characteristically Hb F is markedly elevated, ranging from 60% to 95%, and is heterogeneously distributed. Hb A_2 is normal.

A heterozygous form of δβ-thalassemia and β-thalassemia has been described in which the β-thalassemia gene is thought to be inactive or "silent" (Schwartz, 1969). Characteristically the Hb F is only moderately high.

HETEROZYGOUS δβ-THALASSEMIA WITH ANOTHER HEMOGLOBINOPATHY. The combination of sickle cell–δβ-thalassemia is not common (Stamatoyannopoulos et al, 1967) but is interesting because it confirms the difference between β-thalassemia and δβ-thalassemia (Russo and Mollica, 1962). The picture is usually that of mild hemolytic anemia associated with splenomegaly. The peripheral blood picture is moderately thalassemic. Hemoglobin electrophoresis shows elevated Hb F, normal Hb A_2, and Hb S. There is complete absence of Hb A_1.

Only one family with the combination of Hb E–δβ-thalassemia is reported (Wasi et al, 1969).

γβ-*Thalassemia*

A form of γβ-thalassemia has been described (Kan et al, 1972) that is associated with hemolytic anemia in the newborn.

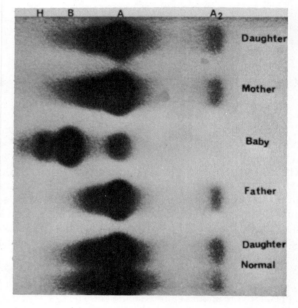

Fig. 14-55. Starch gel electrophoresis, pH 8.6, showing the presence of Hb H and Hb Bart's in a baby with hydrops fetalis caused by α-thalassemia. What seems to be an Hb A component is not, since the authors were able to show that it contained no α-chains. (From Kan et al, 1967.)

α-*Thalassemia*

HOMOZYGOUS. Homozygous α-thalassemia is encountered in two forms (Adams and Steinberg, 1977). The most severe represents homozygosity of two severe (symptomatic) $α^{thal_1}$ genes and is incompatible with life. Affected infants are stillborn, hydropic, and have marked hepatomegaly in the absence of isoimmune (ABO or Rh) hemolytic disease. The hemoglobin is almost entirely Bart's ($γ_4$), with some Hb H ($β_4$) and a small fraction of Hb Portland ($γ_2ζ_2$). Red cells containing large amounts of Hb Bart's sickle, and this is one of the non-S hemoglobinopathies characterized by sickling. The derivation of the hemoglobins found is shown in Fig. 14-54, and the starch gel electrophoretic pattern of a typical case of hydrops fetalis caused by homozygous α-thalassemia is shown in Fig. 14-55.

A less severe form of homozygous α-thalassemia (Hb H disease) results when one gene is a symptomatic α^{thal_1} and the other a "mild" α^{thal_2}, which is "silent" in carriers. Clinical manifestation varies from mild to severe. The blood picture is thalassemic and also shows extreme poikilocytosis and many small red cell fragments. The blood contains 4% to 30% Hb H, smaller amounts of Hb Bart's, and normal to low amounts of Hb A_2. In affected children the level of Hb Bart's is high at birth while that of Hb H is low, but the ratio shifts as they get older. Hb H is an unstable hemoglobin and also has a high oxygen affinity. On electrophoresis at alkaline pH, Hb H migrates more rapidly than Hb A and at the same rate as Hb I. It separates sharply from other hemoglobins at pH 6.5. Red cells containing Hb H produce many inclusions when incubated with brilliant cresyl blue. They are similar to Heinz bodies but consist of precipitated Hb H. Red cell survival is diminished because of damage to the red cell membrane by the precipitated hemoglobin and to poor handling of the inclusions by the pitting function of the spleen.

Instances of acquired Hb H disease are of great theoretical interest. Acquired Hb H disease has been reported in erythroleukemia (Rosenzweig et al, 1968; Beaven et al, 1978), acute granulocytic leukemia (Old et al, 1977), chronic granulocytic leukemia (Beaven et al, 1963), sideroblastic anemia (Boehme et al, 1978; Yoo et al, 1980), and in myeloproliferative syndromes (Hamilton et al, 1971; Veer et al, 1979).

HETEROZYGOUS. The clinical severity of heterozygous α-thalassemia depends on whether the single thalassemia gene is a^{thal_1} or α^{thal_2}. With the "mild" gene there may be little or no anemia, slight thalassemic red cell morphology, and moderately decreased osmotic fragility of the red cells. Hb Bart's is present at birth but is usually less than 2%. With the symptomatic gene there is mild anemia, definite thalassemic morphology of the red cells, decreased osmotic fragility of the red cells, and elevation of Hb Bart's at birth in the range of 4% to 14%. The presence of Hb Bart's is one of the diagnostic features. It may be present in small amounts in normal cord blood, not uncommonly in blacks, but it disappears by the age of 3 months. In heterozygous α-thalassemia, Hb Bart's persists, sometimes into adulthood. There are also traces of Hb H that produce inclusions in some of the red cells on exposure to brilliant cresyl blue.

HETEROZYGOUS α-THALASSEMIA WITH ANOTHER HEMOGLOBINOPATHY. α-Thalassemia has been found in association with Hb Q, Hb I, Hb Constant Spring, Hb S, Hb O, and Hb New York.

Hb Q–α-thalassemia is common in Orientals (Lie-Injo et al, 1966). The condition resembles Hb H disease, with moderate anemia and an intermediate thalassemic blood picture. Hb H inclusion bodies are present. Hemoglobin electrophoresis shows Hb H, Hb Bart's, Hb Q, and Hb Q_2 (variant Hb A_2 containing α^Q chains).

Hb I–α-thalassemia has been found in only one family (Atwater et al, 1960). Clinically mild, the subject's red cells sickled with sodium metabisulfite. Hemoglobin electrophoresis showed 70% Hb I with no increase in Hb F.

Hb Constant Spring has been found to have an additional 31 residues attached to the C-terminal end of the α-chain. Its combination with α-thalassemia sometimes results in typical Hb H disease (Milner et al, 1971; Kan et al, 1974). There is now strong genetic and biosynthetic evidence that in Hb Constant Spring there is a deficit of α-chains and that when it interacts with α-thalassemia it accounts for about half the cases of Hb H disease in southeast Asia (Fessas et al, 1972; Wasi et al, 1972).

Steinberg et al (1975) have investigated black adults with sickle cell trait who had lower than expected concentrations of Hb S and propose that some cases represent interaction of Hb S with mild α-thalassemia. Interaction of Hb S with α-thalassemia is reported by Aksoy (1963b).

A patient triply heterozygous for Hb S, Hb O Arab, and α-thalassemia is reported by Ballas et al (1977).

δ-Thalassemia

In homozygous δ-thalassemia there is complete suppression of δ-chains. Consequently, no Hb A_2 is formed (Ohta et al, 1970). In the heterozygous state Hb A_2 is present but in small quantity. Neither condition is accompanied by anemia, and this thalassemia is completely harmless.

Hereditary persistence of fetal hemoglobin (HPFH)

HPFH is a completely benign condition characterized by the persistence of large amounts of fetal hemoglobin into adult life. Three types have been described: the *Negro type,* the *Greek type,* and the *Swiss type.* HPFH is included in the thalassemic syndromes because there is suppression of β-chain synthesis with compensation by persistent γ-chain synthesis. The relation to the $\delta\beta$-loci is discussed by Bethlenfalvay et al (1975).

The Negro type (Conley et al, 1963) occurs in both the heterozygous and homozygous states. Heterozygotes have 17% to 38% Hb F homogeneously distributed among all the red cells, decreased Hb A_1, and slightly decreased Hb A_2. In the homozygous state (Wheeler and Krevans, 1961; Siegel et al, 1970; Ringelhann et al, 1977) all of the hemoglobin is Hb F. The blood shows many target cells with some anisocytosis and poikilocytosis. Inheritance is autosomal codominant. As noted (p. 622) there are two structural variants of normal fetal hemoglobin. Schroeder and Huismann (1970) studied 29 black families with HPFM with respect to the ratio of one type to the other and showed that the group studied was heterogeneous, some characterized by the predominance of one or the other type of chain while others had an equal ratio of the two.

The Greek type (Fessas and Stamatoyannopoulos, 1964) has been found only in the heterozygous state. The percentage of Hb F is lower than in the Negro type and Hb A_2 is normal. Inheritance is the same as in the Negro type.

The Swiss type (Pawlak and Kozlowska, 1970) shows a persistence of low levels of Hb F (1% to 3%) into adult life and the Hb F is *heterogeneously* distributed. These levels of Hb F are so close to the normal adult level of up to 2% as to make this a doubtful category.

Table 14-18. Fusion hemoglobins

Hemoglobin	Structure	Fusion site	References
Hb Lepore Hollandia	$\alpha_2(\delta\text{-}\beta)_2$	$\delta 22$ and $\beta 50$	Barnabas and Muller (1962)
Hb Lepore Baltimore	$\alpha_2(\delta\text{-}\beta)_2$	$\delta 50$ and $\beta 86$	Ostertag and Smith (1969)
Hb Lepore Washington	$\alpha^2(\delta\text{-}\beta)_2$	$\delta 87$ and $\beta 116$	Huisman et al (1963)
Lepore Augusta			Labie et al (1966)
Hb G			Jonxis and Huisman (1968)
Lepore Boston			Jonxis and Huisman (1968)
Lepore Bronx			Ranney and Jacobs (1964); Barkhan et al (1964)
Lepore Cyprus			Beaven et al (1964)
Hb Pylos			Jonxis (1968)
Hb Miyada	$\alpha_2(\beta\text{-}\delta)_2$	$\beta 12$ and $\delta 22$	Ohta et al (1971)
Hb P Nilotic (?Congo)	$\alpha_2(\beta\text{-}\delta)_2$	$\beta 22$ and $\delta 50$	Badr et al (1973); Efremov (1978)
Hb Lincoln Park	$\alpha_2(\beta\text{-}\delta)_2$	$\beta 22$ and $\delta 50$ plus deletion of Val 137	Honig et al (1978a)
Hb Coventry	$\alpha_2(\beta\text{-}\delta)_2$	$\beta 12$ and $\delta 22$ plus deletion of Leu 141	Casey et al (1976); Efremov (1978)
Hb Kenya	$\alpha_2(\gamma\text{-}\beta)_2$	$\gamma 81$ and $\beta 86$	Huisman et al (1972a); Kendall et al (1973b)

HETEROZYGOUS HPFH WITH ANOTHER HEMOGLO-BINOPATHY. HPFH in combination with a structural hemoglobin variant or thalassemia results in a benign combination with few hematologic abnormalities (Charache and Conley, 1969).

There is no anemia in HPFH–Hb S; the blood shows some anisocytosis and poikilocytosis and variable numbers of target cells. Tests for sickling are positive (Weatherall and Clegg, 1972). Electrophoresis shows only Hb F, Hb S, and Hb A_2, with complete absence of Hb A_1 caused by absence of normal β-chains. Hb F concentration varies from 15% to 35%, with homogeneous distribution. The latter is important in differentiating HPFH–Hb S from sickle cell anemia with high Hb F.

HPFH–Hb C is also asymptomatic. The blood smear shows many target cells and moderate anisocytosis and poikilocytosis. Electrophoresis shows only Hb C and Hb F. (Hb A_2 has the same mobility as Hb C and has not been measured.) There is no Hb A_1. Hb F levels vary from 28% to 37%.

HPFH–β-thalassemia resembles mild thalassemia minor, with minimal anemia and only rarely splenomegaly. The blood smear shows a typical thalassemic red cell morphology. Hb F levels range from 67% to 71%, uniformly distributed throughout the red cells. Hb A_2 is normal. Hb A_1 is completely absent if the combination is with β^0-thalassemia (Fogarty et al, 1974).

HPFH–α-thalassemia has been reported only one time (Fessas et al, 1962) and seems harmless.

The hemoglobin Lepore syndromes

After Hb Lepore was shown to be constructed from a normal complement of α-chains and two abnormal chains consisting of portions of both δ- and β-chains (Baglioni, 1962a), other similar hemoglobins, also called Lepore, were identified and given different geographic names (Table 14-18).

The structure of the fused chain is thought to result from fusion of a portion of the structural gene corresponding to the N-terminus of the δ-chain with a portion of the structural gene corresponding to the C-terminal end of the β-chain to form a fused $\delta\beta$ structural gene (Fig. 14-56). The "leftover" portions of the structural genes fuse to form an "anti-Lepore" structural gene, probably manifest in Hb Miyada, Hb P Congo, and Hb P Nilotic (Congo and Nilotic may be identical), Hb Coventry, and Hb Lincoln Park (Efremov, 1978).

The homozygous state resembles β-thalassemia, with severe anemia from childhood. The major hemoglobin is Hb F (up to 75%) with Hb Lepore making up the difference since there is no detectable Hb A_1 or Hb A_2. The heterozygous state is usually asymptomatic. The blood (Fig. 14-57) shows some microcytosis and hypochromia, target cells, low MCV, and decreased osmotic fragility of the red cells. There is seldom anemia. Hb A_1 and Hb A_2 are normal, there is a slight to moderate increase in Hb F, and about 10% Hb Lepore is present (Fig. 14-57). Hb Lepore is a slow-migrating hemoglobin with an electrophoresis mobility at pH 8.6 identical with that of Hb S and Hb D. Isoelectric focusing (IEF) (Basset et al, 1978) is an excellent way of identifying the Lepore variants.

Double heterozygosity for Hb Lepore and another hemoglobinopathy is recorded for β-thalassemia, $\delta\beta$-thalassemia, Hb S, Hb C, Hb Peterborough, and Hb J Oxford (Quattrin and Venturto, 1974).

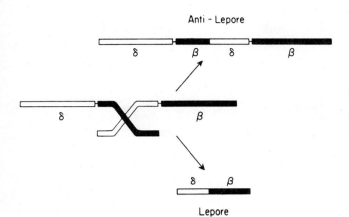

Anti - Lepore

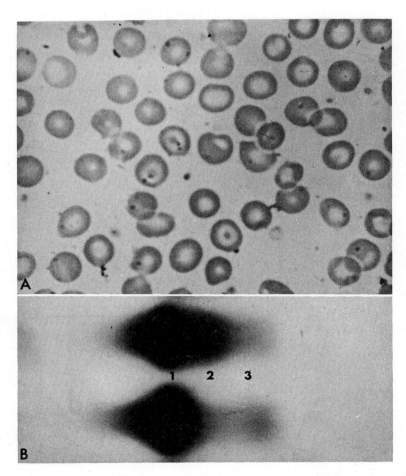

Fig. 14-56. Production of Lepore and anti-Lepore fusion genes during meiosis by the postulated mechanism of unequal, nonhomologous crossing over. (From Stamatoyannopoulos and Nute, 1974. By permission.)

Fig. 14-57. Lepore trait. **A,** Blood. (Wright's stain; ×950.) **B,** Starch block electrophoresis, Lepore trait above the normal control below; **1** is Hb A_1, **2** is Hb Lepore, and **3** is Hb A_2.

15

Leukocytes: leukocytosis, leukopenia, and functional abnormalities

NEUTROPHIL GRANULOCYTES: NORMAL AND ABNORMAL
  FUNCTION
  Introduction
  Granulopoiesis in inflammation
  Release of granulocytes
  Neutrophil migration
  Chemotaxis
  Defective chemotaxis and random motility
    Deficiencies of the complement system
    Abnormalities of the kinin-generating system
    Inhibition of chemotactic factors
    Decreased cell-derived products
  Abnormal adherence and membrane deformability
  Abnormal random migration
  Abnormal chemotaxis
  Phagocytosis and killing of bacteria
EOSINOPHIL LEUKOCYTES
  Chemotaxis
  Phagocytosis
  Killing of bacteria
BASOPHIL LEUKOCYTES
MONOCYTES
LEUKOCYTOSIS AND LEUKOPENIA
  The normal WBC count and differential
    The normal WBC count
    Effect of age
    Deviation from basal conditions
    Other influences
  The normal leukocyte differential count
    Relative versus absolute values
  Leukocytosis
    Definitions
    Significance of leukocytosis
    Neutrophilic leukocytosis
      Quantitative aspects
      Qualitative changes
    Eosinophilic leukocytosis
    Basophilic leukocytosis
    Lymphocytosis
      Infectious mononucleosis
        Clinical picture
        Laboratory findings
        Heterophil antibody
        Presumptive test
        Differential absorption test

    Monospot test
    Infectious lymphocytosis
  Monocytosis
Systemic lupus erythematosus
  Clinical picture
  LE cell phenomenon
    Formation of LE cells
    Morphology
    Tart cell (nucleophagocytosis)
    Associated laboratory findings
    Significance of LE cells
    Specificity of the LE phenomenon
    Antinuclear antibodies by fluorescence
Leukopenia
  Definitions
  Etiology
  Neutropenia
    Chronic neutropenia in childhood
    Neonatal neutropenia
    Cyclic neutropenia
    Familial neutropenia
    Other neutropenic syndromes
  Lymphopenia
  Eosinopenia

NEUTROPHIL GRANULOCYTES: NORMAL AND ABNORMAL FUNCTION
Introduction

Preceding chapters have dealt with the structure and function of erythrocytes. These specialized blood cells are released into the blood and normally remain in the vascular system throughout their life span. Their escape from the blood is accidental or incidental to morbid processes. Since the primary functions of the red blood cells are to effect gas exchange and maintain equilibria between the blood and extravascular space, they are of no use to the body unless they remain in the circulating blood.

Leukocytes, on the other hand, are found in the blood not because they perform essential functions there but because the blood is a useful carrier, serving only to convey them from the site of formation to the extravascular location where they function. Their sojourn in the blood is merely a matter of convenient transportion and probably of minor importance in their life cycle. Unlike the erythrocytes, leukocytes are of no value to the body until they escape from the blood and reach the extravascular space.

The leukocytic response to inflammation gives us the opportunity to obtain quantitative data for leukocytes in an accessible fluid, blood, since they use the blood to reach the site where they will go to work. Clinical and experimental data show that certain patterns of leukocytic response can be expected in different types of disease so that the white blood cell count and differential are helpful adjuncts to diagnosis.

In addition to quantitative data, there is now much data on leukocytic function and dysfunction. It is essential to understand the normal functional mechanisms by which leukocytes are attracted to the site of inflammation and how they function when they arrive there. In some cases the defense mechanism is deficient because there is a shortage of leukocytes. In others, the leukocytes are functionally abnormal and unable to participate in the defense of the host.

The participation of granulocytes in the inflammatory reaction involves a series of reactions. First, the bone marrow receives a directive that more granulocytes are needed. This is followed by the stimulation of the release reaction whereby granulocytes leave the bone marrow and enter the blood. Next, the leukocytes are specifically directed to invade the inflammatory site, where the granulocytes participate in their various functional reactions. Finally, resolution of the inflammatory reaction is accompanied by inhibition of further proliferation and release and also by a decrease in the stimulatory factors that initiated the sequence.

All of these reactions continue to be investigated, using both in vitro and in vivo methods. Some of the reactions are understood better than others.

Granulopoiesis in inflammation

An overview of granulopoiesis is given in Chapter 1. We are concerned here specifically with the granulocyte response to inflammation.

It is probable that during the time of increased need more granulocytes are made available by a combination of reactions: (1) increased activity in the stem cell compartment, (2) increased mitotic activity in the bone marrow, (3) shortened generation time, (4) accelerated transit time through the marrow, and (5) accelerated release from the bone marrow (Cronkite and Vincent, 1969; Robinson and Mangalik, 1975).

Stimulation of the stem cell compartment can be understood if studies of the colony-forming cell in vitro are transfered to the in vivo situation. The cell that generates granulocytic colonies is thought to be identical with the multipotential stem cell (Dicke et al, 1971). Although morphologically indistinguishable, the stem cell that gives rise to neutrophils, monocytes, and eosinophils in semisolid culture media has been designated CFU-C while the stem cell that forms spleen colonies consisting of granulocytes and erythrocytes has been designated CFU-S. CFU-S stem cells are considered to be pluripotential, whereas CFU-C stem cells are considered to be the immediate stem cell for the

neutrophil, monocyte, and eosinophil series. Colony formation in vitro from a CFU-C cell does not occur unless one of a family of substances called "colony-stimulating factors" is added to the medium. These are derived from various sources, but one of the best sources is from normal blood cells (Chervenick and Boggs, 1970). At first it was assumed that the granulocyte itself is the source of colony-stimulating factor; it is now thought that the source of the factor is the monocyte and the macrophage (Golde and Cline, 1974). Colony-stimulating factor has many of the biochemical properties of erythropoietin (Stanley and Metcalf, 1972). For now it may be assumed that colony-stimulating factor represents a true *granulopoietin* acting directly on stem cells. It is required both for stimulation of CFU-C stem cells and also for subsequent maturation (Paran and Sachs, 1968). Colony-stimulating activity in serum is increased following the administration of endotoxin (Quesenberry et al, 1973), following the induction of neutropenia by antineutrophil serum (Shadduck and Nagabhushanam, 1971), in response to stress (Weiner and Robinson, 1971), and during viral infections, particularly infectious mononucleosis (Metcalf and Wahren, 1968). These observations justify relating the initiation of the granulocyte response at the level of the stem cell compartment to colony-stimulating factor. As discussed in the following section, colony-stimulating factor also participates in the increased activity in the maturation compartment (progranulocytes and myelocytes).

It would be very tidy if a lack of colony-stimulating factor could be related to neutropenic states and an excess to myeloproliferative syndromes and leukemia. Unfortunately, such is not the case (Amato et al, 1976). Variable levels of colony-stimulating factor have been found in human cyclic neutropenia (Guerry et al, 1974), whereas in conditions of human leukemia and preleukemic states most investigators find a marked lack of endogenous production of colony-stimulating factor (Iscove et al, 1971; Senn and Pinkerton, 1972; McCulloch, 1975). However, increased production of colony-stimulating factor has been found in some cases of chronic myelocytic leukemia (Robinson and Pike, 1970b), whereas in the acute transformation from chronic to acute myelocytic leukemia, production of colony-stimulating factor is diminished (Goldman, 1974). There is at present no acceptable explanation for the contradictory reports.

Release of granulocytes

The total blood granulocyte pool (TBGP) consists of the marrow granulocyte pool (MGP), the circulating granulocyte pool (CGP), and the marginated granulocyte pool (MGP). While some agents, notably epinephrine or strenuous exercise, appear to mobilize leukocytes, this is accomplished by a shift from the marginated to the circulating pool and is of minor importance in the inflammatory response. Clearly, the major mobilization in the inflammatory response affects the very large marrow pool, by far the largest marrow pool of granulocytes. A number of "leukocytosis-releasing factors" have been described (Chapter 1), and it is postulated that they effect a leukocytosis by a direct effect on the marrow capillaries and sinusoids, making the endothelial lining and basement membrane more permeable to the younger cells (Stohlman et al, 1973). The administration of lithium carbonate increases the total granulocyte pool and can cause neutrophilic leukocytosis (Rothstein et al, 1978). The granulocytes leave the blood by penetrating between endothelial cells, as in the localized inflammatory exudation, but the releasing factors are not necessarily of inflammatory origin. In fact, releasing factors are quite different from those that stimulate granulopoiesis (Broxmeyer et al, 1974).

Neutrophil migration

A detailed review of tests of leukocyte function is given in Crowley et al (1980b).

Neutrophils must leave the blood and enter the perivascular space to perform their role in the defense mechanism. Migration through the endothelium and basement membrane is a functional characteristic of granulocytes (neutrophils and monocytes) not completely dissociated from chemotaxis, which is discussed in the following section.

All studies of granulocyte migration in vivo are based on the pioneer work of Rebuck and associates (Rebuck and Crowley, 1955) using the skin window coverslip technic. A refinement that provides somewhat better quantitative data is the plastic skin chamber technic (Senn and Jungi, 1975) or the rubber chamber used by Hellum and Solberg (1977). The cellular reaction is different in the two technics. In the Rebuck skin window, a sequence of morphologic transformations is seen, characterized by the appearance of macrophages after 6 to 8 hours. In the plastic skin window technics the cellular response is predominantly of neutrophils. It has been suggested that the Rebuck technic is a model of a foreign body reaction, whereas the plastic skin window studies reflect better the neutrophil migration in response to inflammation (Senn and Jungi, 1975). However, the Rebuck technic is probably a better indication of the total efficiency of the cellular system in response to inflammation.

In normal persons, three types of responses have been found: a "peak" response in which a peak response occurs within 6 to 12 hours and then declines, an "up-slope" response that is slower but sustained, and a "high-plateau" response characterized by a rapid rise maintained at a high level. These responses are characterized and reproducible for different individuals and may represent individuality in the response to infection.

Abnormalities in neutrophil migration are (1) a decrease in neutrophil migration after age 40, (2) a decrease in mobilization in acute alcoholism, (3) a decrease in acute leukemia (granulocytic and lymphocytic), (4) a decrease in chronic myelocytic leukemia, (5) a decrease in myeloproliferative syndromes, (6) a decrease in chronic lymphocytic leukemia, (7) normal migration in Hodgkin's disease, (8) decreased migration in multiple myeloma, and (9) decreased migration in cirrhosis of the liver. In most of these situations there is a well recognized increased susceptibility to infection.

Chemotaxis

Neutrophils and monocytes are actively motile, showing *random motility* (nondirected movement), sometimes erroneously called "mobility," and *chemotaxis* (directed movement). It is assumed that chemotaxis is an important factor in attracting the leukocyte to the inflammatory site, but in spite of numerous in vitro studies the relative importance of random motility and chemotaxis to the inflammatory response remains to be established (Gallin and Wolff, 1975; Keller et al, 1975; Miller, 1975a).

Chemotaxis is regulated by (1) *cytotaxins,* substances that induce chemotaxis, (2) *cytotaxigens,* substances that induce the formation of cytotaxins, (3) *cytotaxin inactivators,* and (4) *inhibitors* of chemotaxis.

Many exogenous and endogenous substances have been shown to have chemotactic activity. In plasma or serum, chemotactic activity is related to reactions in the complement-kallikrein-fibrinolysin system. Products of reactions within this system that have cytotactic activity are plasminogen activator; kallikrein; complement components C5a, C3a, and C567; and the fibrin degradation product, fibrinopeptide B. Plasminogen activator has chemotactic activity for neutrophils and monocytes, while kallikrein is chemotactic for neutrophils, monocytes, and basophils. Chemotaxis can also be stimulated by the peptide N-formyl-methionyl-leucyl-phenylolamine (Marasco et al, 1980). Newborns, infants, and young children show decreased monocytic and granulocytic chemotaxis (Klein et al, 1977).

Cell-derived products, from the breakdown of granulocytes and macrophages, participate in the chemotactic response by (1) having chemotactic activity, (2) acting as cytotaxigens, (3) inactivating chemotactic factors, and (4) immobilizing leukocytes in the area of inflammation. Products of bacterial growth and viral replication are chemotactic for neutrophils and monocytes.

Cytotaxin inhibitors and inactivators play an important role in "turning off" the cellular response to inflammation. The chief source of inhibitors and inactivators is serum, and these neutralize the chemotactic activity of complement components, plasminogen activator, and kallikrein. An inactivator of C5a is released from neutrophils after phagocytosis. Another product of neutrophils has been called the neutrophil immobilizing factor (NIF), and it is postulated that this is responsible for concentrating neutrophils at the site of inflammation by inhibiting their motility. Rabson et al (1978) have shown that prostaglandin A_1 inhibits both random migration and chemotaxis, and they postulate that during the inflammatory response the release of prostaglandin A_1 serves to increase neutrophil accumulation at the site.

Eosinophils, basophils, and lymphocytes also show chemotactic responses. Eosinophil chemotaxis is activated by histamine, C3a, and C5a, and a specific eosinophilic chemotactic factor called ECF-A, probably histamine, released during the anaphylactic reaction. Basophilic chemotactic factors are C3a, C5a, kallikrein, and lymphokines released by the interaction of lymphocytes with specific antigen. Lymphocytic chemotaxis is dependent on lymphokines.

There is some degree of specificity of the chemotactic agents for the different types of blood cells and this almost certainly plays a part in determining the nature of the cellular population in the area of inflammation.

Defective chemotaxis and random motility

Defective chemotaxis or random migration is now associated with clinical syndromes generally characterized by deficient resistance to infection and specifically by deficient

Table 15-1. Classification of abnormalities of chemotaxis and random migration*

I. Abnormalities of chemotactic factors
  A. Caused by substrate deficiencies
    1. Of complement components
    2. Of the kinin-generating system
      a. Hageman factor (XII) deficiency
      b. Fletcher factor (prekallikrein) deficiency
  B. Caused by inhibition of complement activation
    1. Systemic lupus erythematosus
    2. Cirrhosis of the liver
  C. Caused by inhibition of chemotactic factor, not complement related
    1. In Hodgkin's disease
    2. In children with severe recurrent infections
    3. In acute cutaneous anergy
  D. Caused by decreased cell-derived products
    1. In the Wiskott-Aldrich syndrome
    2. In the Sézary syndrome
II. Abnormalities of cell response
  A. Abnormal adherence
    1. Alcoholism
    2. Secondary to adrenocortical steroid therapy
  B. Abnormal membrane deformability
    1. In the Chediak-Higashi syndrome
    2. Neonatal granulocytes
  C. Abnormal random and directed (chemotactic) migration
    1. Lazy leukocyte syndrome
  D. Abnormal directed (chemotactic) migration
    1. Defective chemotaxis and hyperimmunoglobulinemia E
      a. Job's syndrome
      b. Mucocutaneous mycosis
      c. Atopic eczema
    2. Hypogammaglobulinemia
    3. Diabetes mellitus
    4. Rheumatoid arthritis
    5. Felty's syndrome
    6. Neoplasms

*Modified from Gallin and Wolff, 1975; Miller, 1975.

Table 15-2. Measurable abnormalities of granulocyte motility in some conditions

Condition	Absolute neutrophil count	Rebuck skin window response	Chemotaxis	Random motility
Chediak-Higashi	Low	Diminished	Diminished	Normal
Neonate	Normal	Moderately diminished	Diminished	Moderately diminished
Lazy leukocyte syndrome	Low	Diminished	Diminished	Diminished
Diabetes	Normal	Moderately diminished	Diminished	Normal
Familial chemotactic defect	Normal	Normal	Diminished	Normal
Defective chemotaxis and cell-mediated immunity	Normal	Moderately diminished	Diminished	Normal
Crohn's disease*	Normal	Diminished†	Normal	Normal

*Segal and Loewi (1976).
†Neutrophil migration.

cellular defenses. A classification of these abnormalities is given in Table 15-1.

The study of leukocytic function is not at present a routine laboratory procedure, but its importance is such that it will undoubtedly be used more widely in the future. The parameters that are usually measured are (1) the absolute neutrophil count, (2) the Rebuck skin window technic (Rebuck and Crowley, 1955), (3) chemotaxis by a Boyden-type assay (Boyden, 1962; Keller et al, 1975), and (4) random motility (Bryant et al, 1967; Miller, 1975a). Table 15-2 summarizes the abnormalities of these parameters in various disorders of granulocytic motility.

Deficiencies of the complement system

Abnormality of chemotactic activity has been described in deficiency of C1r (Day et al, 1972; Gallin, 1975), C2 (Gallin, 1975), C3 (Alper et al, 1970), C5 (Rosenfeld and Leddy, 1974); dysfunction of C5 (Miller and Nilsson, 1970); and abnormalities of the alternate pathway of complement activation in sickle cell anemia (Johnston et al,

1973). Abnormal chemotaxis related to inhibition of a normal complement system has been described in disseminated lupus erythematosus (Clark et al, 1974) and cirrhosis of the liver (DeMeo and Andersen, 1972).

Abnormalities of the kinin-generating system

The kinin-generating system has several components that have chemotactic activity. Gallin and Kaplan (quoted in Gallin and Wolff, 1975) found that human plasma deficient in Hageman factor (XII) exhibits deficient chemotactic activity after kaolin activation unless purified factor XII was added to the plasma. The same pattern has been described in serum deficient in Fletcher factor (prekallikrein) (Weiss et al, 1974). However, since the complement system is normal in these deficiency states, an increased susceptibility to infection is not found.

Inhibition of chemotactic factors

Inhibitors of chemotaxis are described that inhibit through mechanisms probably not complement related. Normal serum contains inhibitors of chemotaxis, but in some situations these inhibitors are present in high titer. This has been described in Hodgkin's disease (Ward and Berenberg, 1974), in a child with chronic granulomatous disease (Ward and Schlegel, 1969), in some children with severe recurrent bacterial or viral infections (Smith et al, 1972; Soriano et al, 1973), and in subjects with acute cutaneous anergy (Van Epps et al, 1974). At least one of the probably heterogeneous family of inhibitors is an α_2-macroglobulin (Gallin and Kaplan, 1974).

Decreased cell-derived products

Once arrived at the inflammatory site, granulocytes and monocytes liberate cellular constituents that take part in the inflammatory response in various ways: (1) of themselves they act as cytotaxins to attract additional leukocytes; (2) they act as cytotaxigens, interacting with complement to generate cytotactic components; (3) they inactivate chemotactic factors; and (4) they immobilize leukocytes, preventing them from leaving the field of battle. Since some of these actions are antagonistic to each other, the net result is dictated by which ones predominate at various times.

Normally, the active cell-derived products are the *lymphokines* (p. 85) and *transfer factor* (p. 85). Lymphocytes and monocytes release chemotactic lymphokines when exposed to specific antigen (Ward et al, 1970), and these affect all types of blood cells: neutrophils, monocytes, lymphocytes, basophils, and eosinophils (Ward et al, 1971; Kay and Austen, 1972; Altman et al, 1973; David, 1973). Antigen-stimulated leukocytes also release transfer factor, involved in the delayed hypersensitivity reaction (Lawrence, 1974).

A decreased production of cytotaxins from neutrophils during phagocytosis has been described (Gallin and Wolff, 1975) but is not associated with clinical abnormality. Abnormal lymphokine production, on the other hand, has been found to be a feature of the Wiskott-Aldrich syndrome (sex-linked thrombocytopenia, hemorrhagic dermatitis, and increased susceptibility to infection). Altman et al (1974) found excessive chemotactic lymphokine production in this syndrome, associated with decreased monocytic chemotaxis. It was postulated that the high level of lymphokines overwhelmed the monocytes and rendered them nonreactive to the chemotactic stimulus. Kirkpatrick and Gallin (1975) have found that the dialyzable chemotactic factor derived from the T-lymphocytes of the Sézary syndrome has weak activity, but its significance is unclear.

Abnormal adherence and membrane deformability

In order to leave the blood and enter the extravascular space, neutrophils must first adhere to the endothelium and then traverse the endothelial lining and subendothelial tissues. Both are poorly understood membrane phenomena, the first probably not unlike the adhesiveness of platelets, the second dependent on plasticity of the cell membrane. Adherence to vascular endothelium is a normal function of the neutrophil membrane, is responsible for the normal margination that makes up the normal marginated pool and, when excessive, may account for neutropenia (Fehr and Jacob, 1977). According to Crowley et al (1980a) normal

adhesiveness and anchoring requires a granulocytic protein having a molecular weight of 110,000 daltons.

Abnormal adherence accompanies adrenocortical steroid therapy and alcohol and aspirin ingestion (MacGregor et al, 1974). It is reflected in abnormal neutrophil accumulation in the Rebuck skin window (Dale et al, 1974) in subjects receiving prednisone. Abnormal adherence, usually combined with other cellular abnormalities, has been demonstrated in a few subjects with recurrent infections (Edelson et al, 1973). In vitro, this property of granulocytes is quantified by exposing them to glass beads or other artificial materials.

Deformability of the cell is necessary if it is to insinuate itself between endothelial cells. In the Chediak-Higashi syndrome the granulocytes appear to be abnormally rigid (Clark and Kimball, 1971), supposedly because the cytoplasm contains large inclusions, although Oliver et al (1975) suggest that the decreased deformability is related to the effect of cyclic GMP (but not cyclic AMP) on microtubule deformability. Neonatal granulocytes are also more rigid than normal (Miller, 1975b). Abnormal neutrophil motilization was found in alcoholics by Brayton et al (1970). This defect is classified under "abnormal adherence" in Table 15-1.

Abnormal random migration

After neutrophils reach the extravascular site of inflammation, their normal random motility is changed to directed motility (chemotaxis) when faced with a gradient of chemotactic activity. Abnormalities of migration fall into two general groups, combined abnormal random plus directed migration, and abnormal directed migration only.

The "lazy leukocyte syndrome" (Miller et al, 1971) is characterized by recurrent infections, neutropenia, normal granulocyte reserve in the bone marrow, abnormal Rebuck skin window response, abnormal random and directed migration of neutrophils, and diminished neutrophilic response to epinephrine, endotoxin, and etiocholanolone (Patrone et al, 1979). Similar cases reported by Edelson et al (1973) also showed impaired bactericidal activity and nitro-blue tetrazolium reduction. Boxer et al (1974) investigated a subject with this syndrome and, based on electron microscopy of the neutrophils, concluded that the cells are deficient in actin microfilaments. Pinkerton et al (1978) also believe the defect to be altered structure or function of the microfilamentous protein in the membrane.

Abnormal chemotaxis

Whereas both random and directed migration are abnormal in the lazy leukocyte syndrome, there are abnormalities, not infrequent if one considers all categories, in which the defect is in directed migration (chemotaxis) only.

I saw a middle-aged man many years ago whose body was covered with deep staphyloccocal abscesses and boils of many years' duration. In retrospect, he fits the syndrome now given the biblical name of "Job's syndrome" (Davis et al, 1966) (Job 2:7-8: "So went Satan forth from the presence of the Lord, and smote Job with sore boils from the sole of his foot unto his crown. . . ."). Other subjects have been studied by Clark et al (1973) and Hill et al (1974a). Characteristically, there is normal random migration but abnormal chemotaxis of granulocytes. Many of the cases have markedly elevated levels of immunoglobulin E, but there are other syndromes characterized by hyperimmunoglobulinemia E, defective chemotaxis, and recurrent nonstaphylococcal infections. Miller et al (1973) have described patients in whom the infection was caused by *Trichophyton rubrum,* while others had atopic eczema or chronic cutaneous candidiasis (Miller, 1975). It might be well to restrict the use of the term "Job's syndrome" to those cases characterized by staphylococcal abscesses.

Defective chemotaxis has also been found associated with hypogammaglobulinemia, usually of all immunoglobulin classes (Gallin, 1975). The patient described by Steerman et al (1971) had hypogammaglobulinemia, defective chemotaxis, and impaired phagocytosis, bactericidal activity, and nitroblue reduction. Defective chemotaxis and hyperimmunoglobulinemia E had been reported by Hill and Quie (1974), but Fontan et al (1976) found that this syndrome is reversible when an underlying allergy responded to an allergen-free diet.

Abnormal chemotaxis has been found in diabetes mellitus, both the adult and juvenile forms (Mowatt and Baum, 1971a; Hill et al, 1974b). The relative importance of defective chemotaxis as related to susceptibility to infection in such a complex disease is difficult to establish.

Deficient neutrophil chemotaxis is a feature of rheumatoid arthritis (Mowatt and Baum, 1971b) and Felty's sydrome (Zivkovic and Baum, 1972). Defective monocyte chemotaxis has been found in some patients with neoplasms (Snyderman and Stahl, 1975).

Phagocytosis and killing of bacteria

The sequences occurring during phagocytosis and killing of bacteria were described vividly by Metchnikoff (1887) about 80 years ago. He noted that leukocytes are first attracted to the microbe, engulf them (he said "englobe them"), are incorporated into clearly visible vacuoles, and are then destroyed. Many thousands of publications since then have, piece by piece, filled in the details of the complex biochemical and biophysical reactions that take place in the course of this easily observed phenomenon. These are reviewed by Stossel (1975), Baehner (1975), Klebanoff and Clark (1978), and Rosen and Klebanoff (1979).

Eosinophils can be phagocytic (see Plate 60), but the chief phagocytic cells are the polymorphonuclear neutrophil, the monocyte, and the monocyte-derived macrophages. Neutrophils are of primary importance because they are more numerous and are mobilized more promptly.

Phagocytosis and killing of bacteria require a sequence of reactions that can be outlined as (1) recognition by neutrophils that bacteria should be engulfed and killed, (2) phagocytosis of bacteria, (3) incorporation of bacteria into phagocytic vacuoles, and (4) bacterial killing.

It is uncertain whether neutrophils require a special directive to engulf bacteria to the exclusion of debris at the site of inflammation. Chemotactic substances liberated by bacterial growth may be involved in the creation of the gradient necessary to bring the neutrophil and the microorganism together. Then the microorganism is rendered susceptible to phagocytosis by the fixation onto the cell membrane of substances called *opsonins.* Two classes of substances play major roles in opsonization—complement components and immunoglobulins.

The complement components that act as opsonins are C3 (Alper et al, 1970) and C5 (Miller and Nilsson, 1970). C3 can be activated by either the classic or the properdin system. Experimental studies show that phagocytes in vitro bind and ingest antibody-coated particles 100 times more efficiently when the particles are also coated with activated complement components (Ehlenberger and Nussenzweig, 1977). By the same token, if the granulocyte's receptors for activated complement components should be saturated, as in massive intravascular activation of the complement system, the cell would no longer be able to respond to additional complement components and would be functionally "paralyzed" (Bowers et al, 1977; Jacob, 1978).

The immunoglobulins that act as opsonins are IgG, subclasses IgG_1 and IgG_3, and IgM, especially when they are microorganism specific and complement fixing (Abramson et al, 1970). The antibody molecule acts as a link between the microorganism and the phagocytic cell, the Fab portion attaching to the microorganism while the Fc portion attaches to specific receptor sites of the membrane of the phagocytic cell, polymorphonuclear neutrophils, and macrophages (Ishizaka et al, 1970).

Phagocytosis is accomplished through engulfing the organism by embracing it with two pseudopods and then internalizing it by reestablishing the continuity of the neutrophil membrane. The pseudopodia contain actin polymer microfilaments that act as contractile structures responsible for the extension and retraction of pseudopods (Pollard and Weihing, 1974). Boxer et al (1974) have described abnormal locomotion, ingestion, and degranulation in association with poorly polymerizable actin. Phagocytosis is accompanied by complex biochemical events, including the activation of lipases and increased conversion of lysolecithin to lecithin (Baehner, 1975). The neutrophil also exhibits a fivefold to tenfold increase in the activity of the hexose monophosphate shunt and increased oxygen consumption, the "respiratory burst" (Johnston, 1978). This leads to increased formation of hydrogen peroxide (Rosen and Klebanoff, 1979) and superoxide radicals (Simchowitz and Spilberg, 1979). The oxidative reactions are mediated by NADPH oxidase, NADP oxidase, and amino acid oxidase (Paul et al, 1970). Reduction of the redox dye nitroblue tetrazolium (NBT) is based on the transfer of hydrogen to the dye during the respiratory burst, the reaction occurring within the phagocytic vacuole. The NBT reduction test is therefore a valuable measure of the respiratory burst.

When the microorganism is ingested, it comes to lie within a phagocytic vacuole, the phagosome. Then another migration phenomenon takes place. The nonspecific azurophilic and the specific neutrophilic granules migrate toward the phagosome and discharge their contents into the phagosome, first the lysomal enzymes of the specific granules and shortly thereafter those of the primary granules. In so doing, the granules lose identity and the cell is said to undergo "degranulation." The specific granules supply alkaline phosphatase, aminopeptidase, lysozyme, lactoferrin, and collagenase, while the primary granules supply acid phosphatase, myeloperoxidase (commonly, peroxidase), some lysozyme, and several other enzymes. It is noteworthy that the cell cytoplasm undergoes a pH change from alkaline to acid, so that the liberation first of enzymes acting at an alkaline pH followed by enzymes acting at an acid pH corresponds to a favorable intracellular environment.

One bactericidal system involves the interaction of the hydrogen peroxide formed during the respiratory burst with a halide ion (iodide or chloride) and myeloperoxidase. One effect is the iodination of the microorganism, which is lethal, another is peroxidation of chloride, and a third is the reaction of hydrogen peroxide with myeloperoxidase leading to the formation of bactericidal aldehydes. It is also possible that some other products of the respiratory burst (superoxide anion and singlet oxygen) are themselves bactericidal (Goldstein et al, 1975).

The second bactericidal system is not peroxide dependent. This is based on the bactericidal activity of lysozyme and lactoferrin. Lysozyme acts best on bacteria already damaged by antibody and complement, and thus may be more important in the digestive process. Lactoferrin is an iron-binding protein that inhibits bacterial growth by chelating the iron required by certain bacteria. After the organism is killed, all that remains is for it to be digested by the action of lysozyme and of acid hydrolytic enzymes.

Bactericidal activity may be deficient at one of several points in the described sequence. There may be: (1) a disorder of opsonization, (2) a diminished phagocytosis, (3) a disorder of granule formation or function, or (4) an impaired intracellular microbicidal activity.

Congenital deficiencies of complement components C3 (Alper et al, 1970) and C5 (Miller and Nilsson, 1970) are accompanied by defective opsonization. Newborn infants have low levels of C3 and C5 in their serum (Adinolfi, 1970) and decreased opsonizing activity for some microorganisms (McCracken and Eichenwald, 1971). An abnormality of the alternate pathway of complement activation in sickle cell disease (Johnston et al, 1973) may explain in part a high susceptibility for pneumococcal or meningococcal infection. It must be noted that complement is also required for normal chemotaxis.

Diminished ingestion of bacteria may be a result of a shortage of neutrophils, as in the neutropenic syndromes or acute leukemia (Chilcote and Baehner, 1974). Plasma from patients with multiple myeloma inhibits phagocytosis. In viral infections the virus binds to the surface of leukocytes, which are then less phagocytic (Sawyer, 1969).

A congenital lack of myeloperoxidase (Salmon et al, 1970; Breton-Gorius et al, 1975) is responsible for diminished bacterial killing because myeloperoxidase is a cofactor in the iodination of the ingested microorganism. Acquired deficiency of myeloperoxidase in neutrophils has been identified in acute myelocytic and myelomonocytic leukemia (Davis et al, 1971). Delayed bacterial killing by leukocytes from patients with the Chediak-Higashi anomaly is attributed to delayed granulation and transfer of enzymes from the abnormal lysosomes into the phagosome (Stossel et al, 1972).

The most common bactericidal defect is seen in *chronic granulomatous disease* (CGD). This is a severe, inherited disorder of granulocytes, monocytes, and histiocytes causing a serious susceptibility to infection. The term "granulomatous" reflects the histopathologic finding of widespread granulomatous lesions associated with pigmented histiocytes. There is no defect in phagocytosis, but the ingested microorganisms are not killed. The biochemical lesion is reflected in the absence of the respiratory burst normally expected in phagocytic cells and lack of hydrogen peroxide formation. Defective microtubule assembly measured by the concentration of concavalin A on the surface of neutrophils ("capping") is also a feature of CGD (Oliver et al, 1977). Subjects with CGD are susceptible to infection with catalase-positive organisms (*Staphylococcus aureus, Staphylococcus albus, Klebsiella aerobacter,* all Enterobacteriaceae [*Escherichia, Proteus, Serratia,* etc.] except *Shigella dysenteriae* [A] type 1, *Pseudomonas, Yersinia, Brucella,* some *Neisseria* sp., *Candida albicans,* and *Aspergillus*) because these organisms do not generate hydrogen peroxide. Catalase-negative organisms (pneumococci, streptococci, *Haemophilus influenzae, Streptococcus fecalis, Clostridia* sp., *Lactobacilli*) generate sufficient hydrogen peroxide for the myeloperoxidase microbicidal system and are killed normally. A selective bactericidal dysfunction characterized by impaired killing of *Staphylococcus aureus* has been described (Davis et al, 1968). A defect in one of the oxidase systems is assumed to be responsible for the lack of peroxide generation (Baehner et al, 1970).

A valuable tool in the investigation of CGD has been the nitroblue tetrazolium (NBT) reduction test. Baehner and Nathan (1968) found that this redox dye is reduced to a purple formazan compound in normal, actively phagocytizing cells but not in cells from CGD. The color development is caused by the NBT acting as a hydrogen acceptor, and the reaction takes place within the phagosomes. The NBT reduction test can be made quantitative (Baehner and Nathan, 1968) by extracting the reduced dye and measuring the concentration spectrophotometrically, or semiquantitative by using a slide test (Windhorst et al, 1967). The test has been used to identify subjects with CGD and to investigate the mode of inheritance. The disease is transmitted either as a sex-linked or autosomal recessive trait (Chandra et al, 1969; Kontras and Bass, 1969; Windhorst et al, 1969.) The carrier state characteristically shows about half the normal dye reduction and a mixed population of neutrophils, half normal and half NBT negative. Normally, neutrophils, monocytes, eosinophils, and platelets are able to reduce NBT. In an affected individual, failure to reduce NBT is shown by neutrophils, histiocytes, and eosinophils.

With rare exceptions (Douwes, 1972) the NBT reduction test is a reliable adjunct to the diagnosis of CGD. It has a poor reputation, however, when it is applied to the differentiation between bacterial and other infections. Lace et al (1975) discuss the variation in methodology and the high degree of unreliability when applied to clinical states other than CGD, listing 43 nonbacterial infections and other clinical states associated with false-positive NBT tests and the many reports of bacterial infections accompanied by false-negative results. The "stimulated" NBT reduction test using latex incubation (Jedrzejczak et al, 1975) or endotoxin

(Merzbach and Obedeanu, 1975) is more sensitive than the standard test in detecting leukocytic dysfunction in patients with neoplastic disease (Haim et al, 1977), but the results may be age related, since NBT reduction declines with advancing age. Repine at al (1979) have modified the slide test (Ochs and Igo, 1973) by using phorbol myristate acetate instead of endotoxin.

A few cases are reported of microbicidal deficiency having metabolic abnormalities different from the classic CGD. These include a combined defect in chemotaxis, phagocytosis, and intracellular killing (Tan et al, 1974); glutathione peroxidase deficiency (Holmes et al, 1970); complete deficiency of leukocyte G-6-PD (Cooper et al, 1972); and lipochrome histiocytosis (Rodey et al, 1970).

EOSINOPHIL LEUKOCYTES
Chemotaxis

The complement components C3, C5, and C567 are chemotactic for eosinophils that respond in the same way as neutrophils (Ward, 1969). A specific eosinophil chemotactic factor has been extracted from sensitized guinea pig lung and named the eosinophil chemotactic factor of anaphylaxis (ECF$_A$) (Kay et al, 1971). A similar factor is formed by the interaction of IgE and antigen (Kay and Austen, 1971). Under special circumstances, histamine acts as an eosinophil chemotactic factor (Clark and Kaplan, 1975).

Phagocytosis

Eosinophils are actively phagocytic for microorganisms (Cline et al, 1968), antigen-antibody complexes, and debris, but phagocytosis of bacteria is less avid than by neutrophils (Mickenberg et al, 1972). The degranulation reaction after phagocytosis is similar to that in neutrophils (Cotran and Litt, 1969).

Killing of bacteria

Eosinophils are less bactericidal than neutrophils in spite of a more intense oxidative response to phagocytosis (Mickenberg et al, 1972). The difference may be caused by the eosinophil peroxidase being different from the myeloperoxidase of neutrophils (Archer et al, 1965; Bujak and Root, 1974; Migler et al, 1978). Eosinophils and neutrophils are equally effective in the killing of newborn larvae of *T. spiralis* (Bass and Szejda, 1979).

BASOPHIL LEUKOCYTES

Basophil leukocytes exhibit chemotaxis and phagocytic activity (Cline and Lehrer, 1968; Dvorak and Dvorak, 1975), but their physiologic role is played by the discharge of the contents of the specific granules to the exterior (Dvorak and Dvorak, 1979). It is probable that human basophils contain all the blood histamine and that this is localized in the basophilic granules. The basophil granules stain metachromatically with toluidine blue, indicating the presence of acid mucopolysaccharide, thought to be heparin or a heparin-like substance (Amman and Martin, 1961). A platelet aggregating factor (PAF) is released from sensitized human basophils by antigen or anti-IgE antibodies (Benveniste, 1974).

IgE plays a major role in the secretion of histamine from basophils (Ishizaka and Ishizaka, 1973). IgE binds to the surface of basophils and mast cells exclusively, and human basophils have 10,000 to 40,000 molecules of membrane-bound IgE (Stallman and Aalberse, 1977). The interaction between antigen and IgE at the surface initiates a sequence of reactions involving degranulation and release of histamine and other substances.

IgE-mediated basophil degranulation requires the bridging of two adjacent molecules of IgE by anti-IgE antibody or by specific antigen. Complement is not required. The first step, called the activation phase, follows antigen binding and is mediated by cyclic AMP (Lichtenstein and Henney, 1974). The release reaction requires calcium. According to Kelly and White (1974) lymphocytes and neutrophils participate in the histamine release reaction by supplying a histamine-releasing factor. This histamine-releasing factor generates an inhibitor of histamine release at 38° C, which may play an important role in limiting the duration and extent of the inflammatory reaction. Basophils participate in the skin reaction of allergic contact dermatitis (Aspegren et al, 1963; Fregert and Rorsman, 1964) and in the delayed hypersensitivity reaction by degranulation and release of histamine (Dvorak et al, 1974). This reaction is slow compared with the almost immediate release of histamine when the basophils of atopic patients are exposed to specific allergen (Chan, 1972).

MONOCYTES

The monocyte-macrophage system is discussed in Chapter 3.

LEUKOCYTOSIS AND LEUKOPENIA
The normal WBC count and differential
The normal WBC count

The normal WBC count can be defined for a given population after taking into account age, sex, and race. The range of normal values for a given population is made larger by deviations from the basal condition, a complication that, for practical reasons, is unavoidable. Because of the spread in normal ranges, the decision that a count is abnormally high or low should be made with caution. One other factor that comes into play is that the normal range represents in part the variation among subjects, all of whom are normal. There is no doubt that each person is his own reference for what is normal, provided that such data are available when he or she was not sick.

Significant differences in methodology have been introduced by the widespread adoption of instruments that count blood cells electronically and by instruments that use various methods to determine the leukocyte differential. Given the unavoidable methodologic errors in performing WBC counts manually in hemocytometer chambers and the demonstrably better reproducibility of electronic counts, it was hoped that new data obtained with automatic instruments would define better the range of normals. This was in fact one of the aims of a symposium sponsored by the College of American Pathologists in 1977 (Koepke, 1979). However, the symposium dealt almost exclusively with WBC differentials. I have not been able to find recent data that are as detailed as those from Albritton (1952) used in

Table 15-3. Normal leukocyte count in blood*

Age	Leukocyte count (cells/mm³)		Leukocyte count, SI units (cells × 10⁹/l)†	
	Average	95% range‡	Average	95% range
At birth	18,100	9,000-30,000	18.1	9.0-30.0
12 hr	22,800	13,000-38,000	22.8	13.0-38.0
24 hr	18,900	9,400-34,000	18.9	9.4-34.0
1 wk	12,200	5,000-21,000	12.2	5.0-21.0
2 wk	11,400	5,000-20,000	11.4	5.0-20.0
4 wk	10,800	5,000-19,500	10.8	5.0-19.5
2 mo	11,000	5,500-18,000	11.0	5.5-18.0
4 mo	11,500	6,000-17,500	11.5	6.0-17.5
6 mo	11,900	6,000-17,500	11.9	6.0-17.5
8 mo	12,200	6,000-17,500	12.2	6.0-17.5
10 mo	12,000	6,000-17,500	12.0	6.0-17.5
12 mo	11,400	6,000-17,500	11.4	6.0-17.5
2 yr	10,600	6,000-17,000	10.6	6.0-17.0
4 yr	9,100	5,500-15,500	9.1	5.5-15.5
6 yr	8,500	5,000-14,500	8.5	5.0-14.5
8 yr	8,300	4,500-13,500	8.3	4.5-13.5
10 yr	8,100	4,500-13,500	8.1	4.5-13.5
12 yr	8,000	4,500-13,500	8.0	4.5-13.5
14 yr	7,900	4,500-13,000	7.9	4.5-13.0
16 yr	7,800	4,500-13,000	7.8	4.5-13.0
18 yr	7,700	4,500-12,500	7.7	4.5-12.5
20 yr	7,500	4,500-11,500	7.5	4.5-11.5
21 yr	7,400	4,500-11,000	7.4	4.5-11.0

*Data from Albritton, 1952.
†To convert the WBC in traditional units (cells/mm³) to SI units (cells/l), the number in thousands is multiplied by 10⁹; e.g., 10,600/mm³ = 10.6 × 10⁹/l. To convert the WBC in SI units to traditional units, the number is expressed in thousands; e.g., 10.6 × 10⁹/l = 10.6 thousands/mm³.
‡Average value ±2 SD.

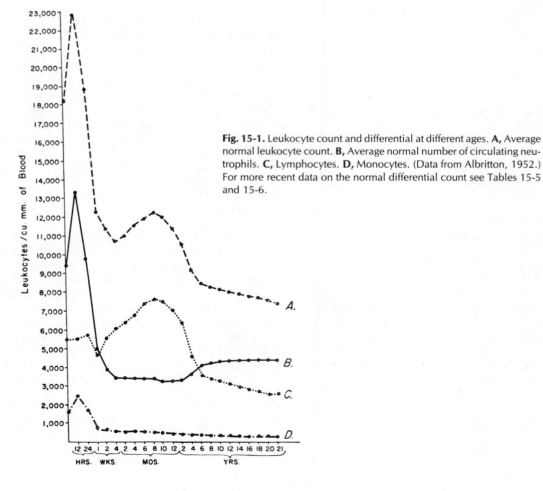

Fig. 15-1. Leukocyte count and differential at different ages. **A,** Average normal leukocyte count. **B,** Average normal number of circulating neutrophils. **C,** Lymphocytes. **D,** Monocytes. (Data from Albritton, 1952.) For more recent data on the normal differential count see Tables 15-5 and 15-6.

Table 15-3 and Fig. 15-1. The data given by Dacie and Lewis (1975a) for five age groups (adults, infants 1 day old, infants 1 year old, children 4 to 7 years, and children 8 to 12 years) are not significantly different. Altman and Dittmer (1961) also give data, for five broad groups, that are not significantly different from those of Albritton (1952).

Effect of age

The leukocyte count is normally higher in the newborn infant than in the adult (Table 15-3; Fig. 15-1). It rises to an even higher level 12 hours after birth and then shows a gradual decline until the adult level is reached at about 21 years of age. There is no significant change after this point. The values for total WBCs and total neutrophil cells in neonates are given by Manroe et al (1979). It should be noted that blood for this study was obtained from either warmed or unwarmed heelstick, occasionally by venipuncture, and that the values are not significantly different from those given in Albritton (1952) (Fig. 15-1).

Deviation from basal conditions

Under basal conditions, when an adult is in a state of complete physical and mental relaxation, the total leukocyte count is seldom higher than 7,000 cells/mm³ (7 × 10⁹/l), most counts falling in the range of 4,500 to 7,000 cells/mm³ (4.5 to 7.0 × 10⁹/l). With moderate activity, such as is usual daily activity, the leukocyte count is higher than under basal conditions but seldom higher than 11,000/mm³ (11.0 × 10⁹/l) (Albritton, 1952; Orfanakis et al, 1970). Strenuous exercise, on the other hand, produces a significant increase in the total number of leukocytes, the count often rising to 14,000/mm³ (14 × 10⁹/l) or 15,000/mm³ (15 × 10⁹/l) (Ahlborg and Ahlborg, 1970). The rise occurs promptly and disappears within an hour. Most of this increase can be accounted for by an increase in the circulating pool at the expense of the marginated pool. The leukocytosis that follows exercise is proportional to the intensity, rather than to the duration, of the exercise.

It should be noted that blood counts are seldom performed on subjects who are in a basal condition. This caveat is particularly important when one is interpreting the leukocyte count and differential of newborns. Christensen and Rothstein (1979) have shown that counts from vigorously crying babies show a significant leukocytosis and shift to the left when compared with counts obtained when the baby is quiet.

Leukocytosis is also produced by emotional stress. Some inconstant differences exist between the response produced by epinephrine and that produced by ACTH. After administration of epinephrine, there is a sharp increase in neutrophils, lymphocytes, and eosinophils, followed by a second phase during which there is a further rise in neutrophils and a drop in lymphocytes and eosinophils. When ACTH is given instead, the response is about the same, without the initial rise in eosinophils. When ACTH is given to a person with impaired adrenal function, only the neutrophilic response takes place.

Other influences

Many of the "physiologic" variations in the leukocyte count are probably reflections of physical or emotional stress. Some examples are the leukocytosis that follows convulsive seizures (epileptic or induced), anesthesia, and paroxysmal tachycardia. Marked leukocytosis has been reported in severe electric shock. There is some difference of opinion as to whether a significant leukocytosis follows food intake. This "digestive leukocytosis" is certainly not striking. Other "physiologic" variations have been described, such as in pregnancy or as a result of high altitude or other meteorologic factors, but these do not stand the scrutiny of statistical analysis. Cyclic variation in the number of neutrophils in blood of healthy men probably represents the effect of normal biorhythm (Morley, 1966). Statland et al (1978) have shown sometimes striking diurnal and week-to-week variations. Several studies comparing leukocyte counts in healthy whites and blacks have shown that, in both children and adults, the leukocyte count in blacks is significantly lower and attributable to lower values for neutrophils (Karayalcin et al, 1972; Caramihai et al, 1975; van Assendelft et al, 1979).

The normal leukocyte differential count

The leukocyte differential count also varies at different ages (Table 15-4). This procedure is subject to considerable variation, since the distribution of leukocytes may vary from smear to smear and from area to area in the same smear, a distribution error of 15% or more being possible. The range of normal values is wide.

The traditional method for preparing a WBC differential count is by direct microscopic inspection by a physician or technologist of a Wright's-stained blood smear, tabulating the relative percent of each cell type when 100 or more leukocytes are seen and identified. It has been estimated by market surveys that over 1 million WBC differential counts are done each day in the United States. Putting aside for the moment the question of whether this many differentials are necessary adjuncts to patient care, it can be assumed that in a routine hematology laboratory differential counts are the most time-consuming of the procedures.

The development of automated differential counters would seem a logical step toward avoiding many of the problems inherent in manual differential counting: (1) the time and fatigue load on the technologist, (2) the statistical variance from the true value when the usual 100 cells are identified, and (3) individual observer variances in the criteria used for cell identification. However, instrumentation has created a new set of problems. Most of these were discussed at the Symposium on Differential Leukocyte Counting held in Aspen in 1977, and the proceedings of this symposium should be read by anyone who performs differential cell counts, by any technic.

The five automated differential counters available as of this writing fall into two categories: those which are digital image processing systems (the Corning LARC, the Coulter diff3, the Abbott ADC 500, and the Geometric Data Hematrak) and one that is a cytochemical flow-through system (Technicon Hemalog-D). The characteristics of each are summarized by Triplett (1979). Evaluations of individual systems are given by Trobaugh and Bacus (1979), Gilmer (1979), and Pierre (1979). Dutcher et al (1979) give a comparative evaluation of the Hematrak, LARC, and Hemalog-D.

Table 15-4. Normal leukocyte differential count in blood*

Age	Segmented neutrophils		Band neutrophils†		Eosinophils		Basophils		Lymphocytes		Monocytes	
	%	No./mm³‡	%	No./mm³‡	%	No./mm³‡	%	No./mm³‡	%	No./mm³‡	%	No./mm³‡
At birth	47 ± 15	8,400	14.1 ± 4	2,540	2.2	400	0.6	100	31 ± 5	5,500	5.8	1,050
12 hr	53	12,100	15.2	3,460	2.0	450	0.4	100	24	5,500	5.3	1,200
24 hr	47	8,870	14.2	2,680	2.4	450	0.5	100	31	5,800	5.8	1,100
1 wk	34	4,100	11.8	1,420	4.1	500	0.4	50	41	5,000	9.1	1,100
2 wk	29	3,320	10.5	1,200	3.1	350	0.4	50	48	5,500	8.8	1,000
4 wk	25 ± 10	2,750	9.5 ± 3	1,150	2.8	300	0.5	50	56 ± 15	6,000	6.5	700
2 mo	25	2,750	8.4	1,100	2.7	300	0.5	50	57	6,300	5.9	650
4 mo	24	2,730	8.9	1,000	2.6	300	0.4	50	59	6,800	5.2	600
6 mo	23	2,710	8.8	1,000	2.5	300	0.4	50	61	7,300	4.8	580
8 mo	22	2,680	8.3	1,000	2.5	300	0.4	50	62	7,600	4.7	580
10 mo	22	2,600	8.3	1,000	2.5	300	0.4	50	63	7,500	4.6	550
12 mo	23	2,680	8.1	990	2.6	300	0.4	50	61	7,000	4.8	550
2 yr	25	2,660	8.0	850	2.6	280	0.5	50	59	6,300	5.0	530
4 yr	34 ± 11	3,040	8.0 ± 3	710	2.8	250	0.6	50	50 ± 15	4,500	5.0	450
6 yr	43	3,600	8.0	670	2.7	230	0.6	50	42	3,500	4.7	400
8 yr	45	3,700	8.0	660	2.4	200	0.6	50	39	3,300	4.2	350
10 yr	46 ± 15	3,700	8.0 ± 3	645	2.4	200	0.5	40	38 ± 10	3,100	4.3	350
12 yr	47	3,700	8.0	640	2.5	200	0.5	40	38	3,000	4.4	350
14 yr	48	3,700	8.0	640	2.5	200	0.5	40	37	2,900	4.7	380
16 yr	49 ± 15	3,800	8.0 ± 3	620	2.6	200	0.5	40	35 ± 10	2,800	5.1	400
18 yr	49	3,800	8.0	620	2.6	200	0.5	40	35	2,700	5.2	400
20 yr	51	3,800	8.0	620	2.7	200	0.5	40	33	2,500	5.0	380
21 yr	51 ± 15	3,800	8.0 ± 3	620	2.7	200	0.5	40	34 ± 10	2,500	4.0	300

*Average values based on the average normal leukocyte counts in Table 15-3, modified to conform with data from my own laboratory.
†Note that these values are higher than those found in other references. They have been obtained by using strict criteria in differentiating segmented from band forms. We do not classify a neutrophil as a segmented form unless a typical threadlike filament is visible.
‡To convert the number of cells in traditional units (cells/mm³) to SI units (cells/l), the number in thousands is multiplied by 10^9; e.g., 8,400/mm³ = 8.4×10^9/l.

These instruments are without a doubt marvels of biochemical engineering. Insofar as they can relieve the time and fatigue factors of manual differential counts, they can fulfill this purpose. By having the ability to count, at a relatively small increment in instrument time, more leukocytes than the usual 100, they can increase precision. Because it was soon apparent that the performance of the digital image processing system can be affected by the quality of the smear and of the staining process, they have forced the design of attachments that make standardized smears from venous blood and for standardized staining procedures (Marshall, 1977). These advantages have also resulted in studies that have defined the range of normal differential counts. In one study (van Assendelft et al, 1979) differential counts on 5,800 persons were performed manually (100 cells) by five technologists at the Center for Disease Control (Atlanta) (Table 15-5). This study did not utilize an automated differential counter and, except for a significantly lower stab count possibly reflecting different criteria for this cell, the figures are not significantly different from those of Albritton (1952). Klee and O'Sullivan (1979) compared 200-cell manual differential counts with those obtained from 10,000 cell counts using the Hemalog-D (Table 15-6). The Hemalog-D system uses cytochemical reactions to identify leukocytes and is not able to differentiate stabs from segmental neutrophils. I consider this a major criticism of this system.

One of the supposedly major advantages of automated differential counters is the facilty with which more than the usual 100 leukocytes can be identified. This is carried to an extreme in the Hemalog-D, the system designed to classify 10,000 leukocytes/sample. While it is accepted that the more cells counted, the greater the precision, two questions arise: (1) If the precision is in fact greater, is it clinically useful? and (2) If the precision is in fact greater, is it statistically significant?

With regard to the first question, it is still to be proved that the greater precision is clinically useful. There are sug-

Table 15-5. Estimated mean percentage leukocyte distribution for U.S. population, by group, race, and sex*

Age/group Race-sex	Cell type						Sample size
	Segmented neutrophils	Band neutrophils	Lymphocytes	Monocytes	Eosinophils	Basophils	
25-34 yr							
White							
Male	57.0	0.3	37.3	3.1	2.2	0.1	499
Females	59.2	0.4	35.8	2.6	1.9	0.1	643
Black							
Males	54.8	0.0	39.3	3.2	2.6	0.1	62
Females	52.9	0.1	41.6	2.8	2.4	0.2	91
35-44 yr							
White							
Males	58.0	0.3	36.2	3.2	2.2	0.1	381
Females	60.9	0.3	34.6	2.3	1.8	0.1	480
Black							
Males	55.4	0.1	39.5	2.8	2.1	0.1	49
Females	53.7	0.1	41.5	3.1	1.5	0.1	88
45-54 yr							
White							
Males	59.0	0.3	35.4	3.1	2.1	0.1	534
Females	59.4	0.2	35.6	2.9	1.8	0.1	647
Black							
Males	54.5	0.2	40.2	2.8	2.1	0.2	88
Females	53.5	0.1	42.0	2.6	1.7	0.1	94
55-64 yr							
White							
Males	60.0	0.2	34.7	2.9	2.1	0.1	440
Females	57.6	0.2	37.4	2.9	1.8	0.1	491
Black							
Males	54.4	0.0	40.8	2.9	1.9	0.0	61
Females	53.8	0.1	41.2	3.2	1.6	0.1	70
65-74 yr							
White							
Males	59.8	0.3	34.2	3.2	2.4	0.1	417
Females	58.6	0.2	36.3	2.9	1.9	0.1	447
Black							
Males	54.4	0.2	40.0	3.0	2.3	0.1	83
Females	52.9	0.1	42.0	2.9	2.0	0.1	78

*Reproduced, with permission, from van Assendelft, O.W., et al. In Koepke, J.A., editor: Differential leukocyte counting, Skokie, Ill., 1979, College of American Pathologists. Absolute counts are not given because the WBC counts are not available.

Table 15-6. Reference values (2.5 to 97.5 percentiles) for leukocyte differential counts, comparing 200-cell manual differentials with 10,000-cell Hemalog-D differentials*

	200-cell differential		Hemalog-D differential	
	Percentage counts	Absolute counts	Percentage counts	Absolute counts
Adults				
Neutrophils	43.5-79.5	2,266-7,676	47.5-76.8	2,000-7,150
Lymphocytes	13.0-43.0	832-3,140	16.2-43.0	1,100-3,000
Monocytes	2.0-11.0	123-804	1.0-10.3	60-750
Eosinophils	0-7.5	0-492	0.4-5.9	25-380
Basophils	0-2.0	0-156	0.2-1.3	10-100
Male children (age 5-16 yr)				
Neutrophils	32.5-70.0	1,420-5,200	38.5-71.5	1,700-5,200
Lymphocytes	21.0-55.0	1,200-3,600	19.4-51.4	875-3,300
Monocytes	2.5-12.5	120-886	1.1-11.6	28-825
Eosinophils	2.0-12.0	39-686	0.9-8.1	41-460
Basophils	0.0-2.5	20-118	0.2-1.3	16-80
Female children (age 5-16 yr)				
Neutrophils	36.0-73.5	1,550-6,500	41.9-76.5	1,700-7,500
Lymphocytes	18.0-53.0	1,290-3,600	16.3-46.7	1,078-3,000
Monocytes	2.0-13.0	112-850	0.9-9.9	45-750
Eosinophils	2.0-11.5	29-750	0.8-8.3	40-650
Basophils	0.0-3.0	20-130	0.3-1.4	7-140
Children (age 0-4 yr)				
Neutrophils	16.0-60.0	1,000-12,000	Total leukocyte count 3,800 to 10,900/mm^3 for	
Lymphocytes	20.0-70.0	1,500-8,500	adults, and 4,000 to 9,000 for children ages 5-16	
Monocytes	0-7.0	0-450	years	
Eosinophils	0-8.0	0-600		
Basophils	0-1.0	0-400		

*Reproduced, with permission, from van Assendelft, O.W., et al. In Koepke, J.A., editor: Differential leukocyte counting, Skokie, Ill., 1979, College of American Pathologists.

gestions that the greater precision in classifying eosinophils and basophils may have clinical usefulness (Klee and O'Sullivan, 1979), but the same data (Table 15-6) show that the improved precision in counting eosinophils and basophils when 10,000 leukocytes are classified with the Hemalog-D rather than counting 200 cells manually is probably not significant.

Rümke (1976, 1979) discusses the second question, the significance of the numerical results when the number of leukocytes classified is increased. These data apply only to digital image processing systems utilizing a stained blood smear. Table 15-7 is based on a statistical analysis, and although it does prove improved precision when the number of leukocytes identified is larger than 100, the question of whether these degrees of improved precision are clinically useful remains unanswered.

One other question must be faced, and that is whether 1 million differential counts per day are all contributing significantly to patient care. In my opinion the number of differential counts (and other laboratory procedures) could be significantly reduced if they would be requested only when clinically useful information is sought. The differential count is useful in detecting and following the course of infectious diseases and myeloproliferative or lymphoproliferative disorders. It has little value as a screening test for chronic nonhematologic diseases. Inspection of the smear for abnormalities of red blood cells and platelets may be more valuable than the differential leukocyte count. Perhaps

the need to automate the differential leukocyte count would not be so pressing if, as an estimate, two thirds to three fourths could be eliminated without affecting patient care.

Relative versus absolute values

The leukocyte differential count expresses in percent the relative number of the various types of leukocytes present in the peripheral blood. Because each is a relative value, the differential count alone has limited value; e.g., if the percentage of one type of cells is increased, it can be said that cells of that type are relatively more numerous than normal, but we still do not know whether this reflects a decrease in cells of another type or an actual increase in the number of the cells that are relatively increased. Relative values can obviously be misleading.

On the other hand, if the relative percentile values are known from the differential count and if the total leukocyte count is also known, it is possible to calculate *absolute* values that are not subject to misinterpretation. The absolute value for each type of leukocyte is obtained by multiplying the percentile value by the total leukocyte count, as follows:

Absolute value (leukocytes/mm^3) =

$$\frac{\text{Relative value}}{(\%)} \times \frac{\text{Total leukocyte count}}{(\text{cells/mm}^3)}$$

For example, if the total leukocyte count is 10,000/mm^3 (10 × 10^9/l) and the differential count shows 50% seg-

Table 15-7. The 95% confidence limits for various percentages of leukocytes of a given type as determined by differential counts on stained blood smears*†

a	n = 100	n = 200	n = 500	n = 1,000
0	0-4	0-2	0-1	0-1
1	0-6	0-4	0-3	0-2
2	0-8	0-6	0-4	1-4
3	0-9	1-7	1-5	2-5
4	1-10	1-8	2-7	2-6
5	1-12	2-10	3-8	3-7
6	2-13	3-11	4-9	4-8
7	2-14	3-12	4-10	5-9
8	3-16	4-13	5-11	6-10
9	4-17	5-14	6-12	7-11
10	4-18	6-16	7-13	8-13
15	8-24	10-21	11-19	12-18
20	12-30	14-27	16-24	17-23
25	16-35	19-32	21-30	22-28
30	21-40	23-37	26-35	27-33
35	25-46	28-43	30-40	32-39
40	30-51	33-48	35-45	36-44
45	35-56	37-53	40-50	41-49
50	39-61	42-58	45-55	46-54
55	44-65	47-63	50-60	51-59
60	49-70	52-67	55-65	56-64
65	54-75	57-72	60-70	61-68
70	60-79	63-77	65-74	67-73
75	65-84	68-81	70-79	72-78
80	70-88	73-86	76-84	77-83
85	76-92	79-90	81-89	82-88
90	82-96	84-94	87-93	87-92
91	83-96	86-95	88-94	89-93
92	84-97	87-96	89-95	90-94
93	86-98	88-97	90-96	91-95
94	87-98	89-97	91-96	92-96
95	88-99	90-98	92-97	93-97
96	90-99	92-99	93-98	94-98
97	91-100	93-99	95-99	95-98
98	92-100	94-100	96-100	96-99
99	94-100	96-100	97-100	98-100
100	96-100	98-100	99-100	99-100

*Reproduced, with permission, from Rümke, C.L. In Koepke, J.A., editor: Differential leukocyte counting, Skokie, Ill., 1979, College of American Pathologists.

†n is the total number of cells counted; **a** the observed percentage of cells of the given type. 0 and 100 confidence limits are to be interpreted as nearly 0 and nearly 100.

mented neutrophils, the absolute number of neutrophils is 50% of 10,000, or 5,000 neutrophils/mm³ of blood (5 × 10⁹/1). Average normal values are given in Table 15-4. The examples on pp. 672 and 673 will serve to demonstrate the usefulness of absolute values.

Leukocytosis
Definitions

Leukocytosis is defined as an increase above normal in the number of leukocytes in the peripheral blood. In considering what is normal, constantly keep in mind the data in Tables 15-3 and 15-4. The ranges given represent the 95% range, 5% of normal persons falling outside of this range.

It is customary to distinguish between *physiologic leuko-*

Table 15-8. Causes of physiologic leukocytosis

Newborn infant and older infant
Exercise
Emotional disturbance (fever, excitement, pain, etc.)
Menstruation
Exposure to cold
Anesthesia
Obstetric labor
Paroxysmal tachycardia
Sunlight
Ultraviolet irradiation
Artificially induced fever
Convulsive seizures

cytosis (Table 15-8) and *pathologic leukocytosis*. The former is caused by physiologic conditions, such as exercise. The latter is caused by disease. The importance of making this distinction is to remind ourselves to eliminate physiologic factors before assuming leukocytosis to be pathologic.

An increase in circulating leukocytes is only rarely caused by a proportional increase in leukocytes of all types. When it occurs, it is usually caused by acute hemoconcentration and may be called *balanced leukocytosis*. More commonly, the increase in the leukocyte count is produced by an increase in one cell type only, making the terms "neutrophilic leukocytosis" (neutrophilia), "lymphocytic leukocytosis" (lymphocytosis), "monocytosis," "eosinophilia," and "basophilic leukocytosis" applicable to each type. A relative increase may have various interpretations, as discussed previously, depending on whether the leukocyte count is low, normal, or high. Pathologic leukocytosis is always accompanied by an *absolute* increase in one or another type of leukocyte. Necheles (1980) gives complete summaries of quantitative disorders of leukocytes.

Significance of leukocytosis

Changes in the number, type, and morphology of the leukocytes in the peripheral blood are extremely valuable indicators of the presence and cause of some disease states. There is a wealth of laboratory and clinical data showing that certain diseases are accompanied by a specific type of leukocytosis that is roughly proportional to their clinical severity.

Occasionally leukocytosis is found in which there is no evidence of clinical disease. Such a finding suggests the presence of occult disease and should stimulate an intensive search for the cause. There is an occasional person in whom a deviation from the normal leukocyte picture defies all attempts at explanation. This is an important point and a matter of common experience. It is equally important not to substitute extensive hematologic studies for clinical thoroughness and acumen. I have seen one medical service completely frustrated by an elderly patient with senile dementia who had an apparently unexplainable leukocyte count of 55,000/mm³ (55 × 10⁹/1) and a neutrophilic leukocytosis. The cause eventually came to light when the resident performed a pelvic examination and found a decomposing potato in the patient's vagina.

EXAMPLE 1: Adult, WBC, 9,000/mm³ (9 × 10⁹/l)

	Differential count (%)	Absolute values (cells/mm³)	Absolute values (cell × 10⁹/l)
Segmented neutrophils	51.0	4,600	4.6
Band neutrophils	8.0	720	0.72
Lymphocytes	34.0	3,060	3.06
Eosinophils	2.0	180	0.18
Basophils	1.0	90	0.09
Monocytes	4.0	360	0.36

Conclusion—The relative distribution and absolute values for each type of leukocyte are within normal limits.

EXAMPLE 2: Adult, WBC 9,000/mm³ (9 × 10⁹/l)

	Differential count (%)	Absolute values (cells/mm³)	Absolute values (cells × 10⁹/l)
Segmented neutrophils	60.0	5,400	5.4
Band neutrophils	20.0	1,800	1.8
Lymphocytes	10.0	900	0.9
Eosinophils	3.0	270	0.27
Basophils	1.0	90	0.09
Monocytes	6.0	540	0.54

Conclusion—There is a relative and absolute increase in neutrophils and a relative and absolute decrease in lymphocytes.

EXAMPLE 3: Adult, WBC 30,000/mm³ (30 × 10⁹/l)

	Differential count (%)	Absolute values (cells/mm³)	Absolute values (cells × 10⁹/l)
Segmented neutrophils	60.0	18,000	18.0
Band neutrophils	20.0	6,000	6.0
Lymphocytes	16.0	4,800	4.8
Eosinophils	2.0	600	0.6
Basophils	0.5	150	0.15
Monocytes	1.5	450	0.45

Conclusion—Although the differential count is essentially the same as that in example 2, in this case there is a relative and absolute increase in neutrophils and only a relative decrease in lymphocytes. Note also that there is an increase in circulating eosinophils.

EXAMPLE 4: Adult, WBC 9,000/mm³ (9 × 10⁹/l)

	Differential count (%)	Absolute values (cells/mm³)	Absolute values (cells × 10⁹/l)
Segmented neutrophils	20.0	1,800	1.8
Band neutrophils	1.0	90	0.09
Lymphocytes	72.0	6,500	6.5
Eosinophils	2.0	180	0.18
Basophils	1.0	90	0.09
Monocytes	4.0	360	0.36

Conclusion—There is a relative and absolute decrease in neutrophils and a relative and absolute increase in lymphocytes.

EXAMPLE 5: Adult, WBC 20,000/mm³ (20 × 10⁹/l)

	Differential count (%)	Absolute values (cells/mm³)	Absolute values (cells × 10⁹/l)
Segmented neutrophils	20.0	4,000	4.0
Band neutrophils	1.0	200	0.2
Lymphocytes	72.0	14,400	14.4
Eosinophils	2.0	400	0.4
Basophils	1.0	100	0.1
Monocytes	4.0	800	0.8

Conclusion—There is a relative decrease in neutrophils, but the actual number of neutrophils is not decreased. There is a relative and an absolute increase in lymphocytes. The high white cell count is caused by an increase in lymphocytes.

EXAMPLE 6: Adult, WBC 2,500/mm³ (2.5 × 10⁹/l)

	Differential count (%)	Absolute values (cells/mm³)	Absolute values (cells × 10⁹/l)
Segmented neutrophils	18.0	450	0.45
Band neutrophils	0.0	0	0.0
Lymphocytes	75.0	1,870	1.87
Eosinophils	1.0	25	0.025
Basophils	1.0	25	0.025
Monocytes	5.0	125	0.125

Conclusion—There is a relative increase in lymphocytes, but there is no increase in the absolute number of lymphocytes. There is a relative and absolute decrease in neutrophils. The low total leukocyte count is caused by a decrease in neutrophils. Note that in examples 5 and 6 the differential counts are essentially the same but have a totally different significance.

False elevation of the white blood cell count can occur when the cell count is performed with an electronic particle counter if the blood contains cryoglobulins (Emori et al, 1973) or cryoglobulin crystals (Shah et al, 1978). False high counts can also result from incomplete lysis of red blood cells or when there are numerous normoblasts.

Neutrophilic leukocytosis

Neutrophilic leukocytosis is usually caused by one of three types of stimuli: infection by bacteria, metabolic or drug intoxication, and necrosis of tissue. A list of the specific causes of neutrophilic leukocytosis is given in Table 15-9.

QUANTITATIVE ASPECTS. Neutrophilic leukocytosis refers to an increase of neutrophilic leukocytes above 6,500/mm³ (6.5 × 10⁹/l) of blood. It has been described in individuals who are otherwise normal (Ward and Rheinhard, 1971).

Whether the neutrophilic leukocytosis is moderate or severe depends on the (1) cause of the neutrophilia, (2) virulence of the invading organism, (3) hematologic reactivity of the patient, (4) localization of the inflammatory process, and (5) modification by therapy.

The neutrophilia caused by other than bacterial agents is usually mild to moderate. Invasion with certain bacteria, such as *Staphylococcus aureus, Diplococcus pneumoniae,* and *Streptococcus hemolyticus,* is usually accompanied by marked neutrophilia, whereas organisms such as *Salmonella typhosa* and *Mycobacterium tuberculosis* produce little or no neutrophilia. Other bacteria are intermediate in their ability to produce neutrophilia. Neutrophilia is also seen in certain fungal *(Actinomyces),* viral (rabies, poliomyelitis, and herpes zoster), and spirochetal *(Leptospira icterohaemorrhagiae)* infections.

The virulence of the organism may modify the considerations mentioned, highly virulent organisms producing a more marked neutrophilia than those of low virulence. The virulence of the invading organism cannot, however, be invariably separated from the resistance of the host. The latter depends on immunity and other factors.

The hematologic reactivity of different patients can vary, the same stimulus causing different degrees of leukocytosis in different persons. Children respond to infection with a greater degree of neutrophilic leukocytosis than adults, whereas some elderly patients respond weakly or not at all, even when the infection is severe. Neonates with sepsis

more often present with neutropenia rather than neutrophilia (Manroe, et al, 1979). Persons of any age who are weak and debilitated may fail to respond with a significant neutrophilic leukocytosis. When an infection becomes overwhelming and the patient's resistance is exhausted, it will be found that, as death approaches, the number of neutrophilic leukocytes in the blood decreases and may even reach a leukopenic level.

A localized inflammatory process such as an abscess produces a greater neutrophilic leukocytosis than one that is generalized, such as bacteremia. In general, the degree of neutrophilia is proportional to the amount of tissue involved in the inflammation, since the leukocytosis-promoting substances are probably derived from necrotic cells. A large abscess would therefore stimulate a more severe neutrophilia than simple invasion of the bloodstream by bacteria.

Steroid therapy modifies the leukocytic response and may cause serious diagnostic errors. Although ACTH given to a normal person produces neutrophilia, tissue resistance is weakened when ACTH is given to a person suffering from a severe infection, and the infection can spread rapidly without producing the expected leukocytosis. What would normally be an important sign is thus obscured, and the physician can be badly misled.

A significant rise in serum potassium (spurious hyperkalemia) has been recorded when blood having a very high white cell count is allowed to stand after clotting occurs. In addition to release of platelet potassium when the platelet count is high (Hartmann et al, 1958) and from granulocytes (Bronson et al, 1966), spurious hyperkalemia has also been found in chronic lymphocytic leukemia (Froment et al, 1965; Bellevue et al, 1975).

QUALITATIVE CHANGES. Any stimulus that produces neutrophilic leukocytosis also causes immature neutrophilic leukocytes to be released into the blood. Neutrophilia is therefore usually accompanied by a *shift to the left* in the differential count, the degree of shift being roughly proportional to the magnitude of the neutrophilia. If the neutrophilia is moderate, there may be only an increased number of band neutrophils, but if it is severe, metamyelocytes and myelocytes can be found.

The presence of immature neutrophils is sometimes the only indication that infection is present. In elderly persons, for example, or if the infection is overwhelming, there can be a shift to the left even when there is little or no leukocy-

Table 15-9. Causes of neutrophilic leukocytosis

I. Acute infections by pyogenic bacteria and other organisms (Nettleship, 1938; Wintrobe, 1939; Hill and Duncan, 1941; Hilts and Shaw, 1953; Holland and Mauer, 1963; Dubos and Hirsch, 1965; Horsfall and Tamm, 1965)
   A. Localized or limited such as
      1. Abscesses
      2. Osteomyelitis
      3. Otitis media
      4. Acute pyelonephritis
      5. Acute appendicitis
      6. Pneumonia
      7. Salpingitis
      8. Meningitis (pyogenic or tuberculous)
      9. Tonsillitis
      10. Acute cholecystitis
      11. Thrombophlebitis, etc.
   B. Generalized such as
      1. Acute rheumatic fever
      2. Scarlet fever
      3. Septicemia
      4. Peritonitis
      5. Empyema
      6. Anthrax
      7. Cholera
      8. Plague, etc.
II. Reactive to metabolic, chemical, or physical stimuli (Wintrobe, 1939; Hill and Duncan, 1941; Tullis, 1947; Jensson, 1958; Colman and Shein, 1962; Biörck et al, 1964; Rey and Wolf, 1968)
   A. Metabolic
      1. Uremia
      2. Acidosis (diabetic and other)
      3. Eclampsia
      4. Gout (acute)
      5. Cushing's syndrome
   B. Chemical
      1. Epinephrine
      2. ACTH
      3. Lead
      4. Digitalis
      5. Mercury
      6. Camphor
      7. Arsenic
      8. Kerosene
   C. Insect venom
      1. Black widow spider
   D. Reaction to parenterally given foreign protein
   E. Reaction to parenterally given bacterial vaccines
   F. Electric shock
III. Tissue necrosis from any cause (Wintrobe, 1939; Meyer and Rotter, 1942; Hilts and Shaw, 1953; Chen and Walz, 1958; Harrison, 1966)
   A. Myocardial infarction
   B. Gangrene
   C. Extensive burns
   D. Secondary to bacterial invasion
   E. Necrosis in rapidly growing malignant neoplasms
   F. Degeneration in benign neoplasms
IV. Acute hemorrhage
   A. Internal
   B. External
V. Acute hemolysis (Chapter 13)
   A. Hemolytic transfusion reactions
   B. Acute hemolytic anemia
   C. Crisis in chronic hemolytic anemia
VI. Myeloproliferative disorders (Chapter 16)
VII. Myelocytic leukemia (Chapter 16)
VIII. Chronic idiopathic neutrophilia (Ward and Rheinhard, 1971)
IX. Familial (Bousser and Neydé, 1947; Bjure et al, 1962; Cutting and Lang, 1964)
X. Cyclic (Coventry, 1953)

tosis. On the other hand, absence of a shift to the left in the presence of severe infection indicates a poor prognosis.

An opposite *shift to the right* is characterized by the presence of adult segmented neutrophils only. It is common in pernicious anemia. We have also noted this shift to the right in cases of chronic morphine addiction.

A severe infection or toxic state sometimes makes the granules of the neutrophils coarse and dark staining. It has been suggested that the more *toxic granulation* present in the neutrophils, the more severe the infection. A "degenerative index" has been proposed. This index gives the ratio between neutrophils showing toxic granulation and the total number of neutrophils. We do not find it particularly useful, recommending instead a careful survey of the blood smear. The smear must be thin and well stained, since poor staining causes basophilic staining of neutrophilic granules as an artifact.

Döhle bodies are small (1 to 2μ), round or oval, gray-blue bodies found in the cytoplasm of neutrophilic leukocytes in severe infections, burns, and some cases of thrombocytopenic purpura. They are common in scarlet fever but, contrary to early beliefs, are not specific for this disease (Chapter 4). They are said not to be present in rubella.

Eosinophilic leukocytosis

Eosinophilic leukocytosis is an increase above 400 eosinophils/mm³ (0.4 × 10⁹/1) of blood. Because eosinophilia having no obvious significance is a frequent finding in hospitalized infants (Burrell, 1953; Lawrence et al, 1980), the upper limit of normal for this group of patients should be at least 500/mm³ (Table 15-3). The causes of eosinophilia are listed in Table 15-10.

In general, the eosinophilic response is produced by allergies, foreign proteins, and protein breakdown products (Hardy and Anderson, 1968). Eosinophilia is striking in some allergic disorders, particularly if they are acute. In acute bronchial asthma, eosinophils in the blood may number up to 5,000/mm³ (5 × 10⁹/1) and are also found in the sputum. Connel (1968) reports that one third to one fourth of the eosinophils in the eosinophilia of allergic rhinitis and symptomatic asthma contain vacuoles not seen in nonallergic individuals. Eosinophilic hyperplasia of the bone marrow and eosinophilic infiltration of the myocardium have been reported in asthmatic patients. Chronic skin diseases, some allergic in type, are often accompanied by eosinophilia. Both parasitic *infestation* (skin involvement) and *infection* (systemic) are usually accompanied by eosino-

Table 15-10. Causes of eosinophilic leukocytosis

I. Allergic disorders (Cape, 1954; Jacob et al, 1964; Donohugh, 1966; Fiegenberg et al, 1967; Girard et al, 1967; Connell, 1968; Lecks and Kravis, 1969)
   A. Bronchial asthma
   B. Hay fever
   C. Urticaria
   D. Angioneurotic edema
   E. Erythema multiforme
   F. Löffler's syndrome
   G. Allergic eczema
   H. Dermatitis venenata
   I. Gastrointestinal (food) allergy
   J. Dermatitis herpetiformis
   K. Tropical (parasitic) eosinophilia (see III)
   L. Periarteritis nodosa
   M. Erythema neonatorum
   N. Hypersensitivity to potassium iodide, penicillin, and other drugs
II. Chronic (nonallergic) skin diseases (Kiang and Choa, 1949; Donohugh, 1966; Lecks and Kravis, 1969)
   A. Pemphigus
   B. Exfoliative dermatitis
   C. Psoriasis
   D. Ichthyosis
   E. Pruritus caused by jaundice
   F. Leprosy
III. Parasitic infection or infestation (Cartwright, 1949; Beaver and Danaraj, 1958; Conrad, 1971)
   A. Trichinosis (Trichinella spiralis)
   B. Echinococcosis (Echinococcus granulosus)
   C. Cysticercosis (Cysticercus cellulosae)
   D. Toxoplasmosis (Toxoplasma gondii)
   E. Schistosomiasis (Schistosoma, 3 species)
   F. Clonorchiasis (Clonorchis sinensis)
   G. Filariasis (Wuchereria bancrofti)
   H. Necatoriasis (Necator americanus)
   I. Strongyloidiasis (Strongyloides stercoralis)
   J. Ascariasis (Ascaris lumbricoides)
   K. Ancylostomiasis (Ancylostoma duodenale)
   L. Scabies (Sarcoptes scabiei)
   M. Gnathostomiasis (Gnathostoma spinigerum)
   N. Visceral larva migrans (Toxicara canis)

IV. Hemopoietic disorders (Hardy and Anderson, 1968; Benvenisti and Ultman, 1969)
   A. Hodgkin's disease
   B. Sarcoidosis
   C. Pernicious anemia
   D. Sickle cell anemia
   E. Postsplenectomy
   F. Chronic myelocytic leukemia (eosinophilic leukemia)
   G. Eosinophilic leukemoid reactions
   H. Polycythemia vera
V. Miscellaneous (Berger, 1921; Friedman, 1935; Isaacson and Rapoport, 1946; Riisager, 1959; Hungerford and Karson, 1960; Naiman et al, 1964; Buka, 1965; Ranke, 1965; Heddle et al, 1969)
   A. Fibroplastic parietal endocarditis (Löffler's)
   B. Diffuse and circumscribed eosinophilic gastroenteritis
   C. Eosinophilic peritonitis
   D. Scarlet fever
   E. Chorea
   F. Following x-irradiation
   G. Ulcerative colitis
   H. Tumors of ovary
   I. Tumors of uterus (adenocarcinoma, carcinoma of cervix, uterine leiomyoma)
   J. Primary carcinoma of the liver
   K. Tumors of serous surfaces
   L. Tumors of bone
   M. Caseous tuberculosis of lymph nodes
   N. Poisoning with pilocarpine
   O. Poisoning with copper sulfate
   P. Poisoning with camphor
   Q. Poisoning with phosphorus
   R. Bite of black widow spider (Latrodectus mactans)
   S. Familial (hereditary)
   T. Idiopathic
   U. Sulfonamide administration
   V. Magnesium deficiency
   W. Eosinophilic fasciitis (Abeles et al, 1979)
   X. Eosinophilic gastroenteritis (McNabb et al, 1979)

philia, usually moderate in intestinal parasitism and severe when there is systemic involvement. Systemic involvement has given rise to some of the highest recorded eosinophilias. Superficial infestation usually shows only moderate eosinophilia. Active invasion of tissue with the larval forms accounts for infiltration of the local tissue with eosinophils as well as for the eosinophils in the blood. The cause of eosinophilia in many other conditions is obscure. It may be familial in some (Naiman et al, 1964), while others have a nonfamilial, persistent eosinophilia whose etiology cannot be found. An interesting group of hypereosinophilic syndromes is presented in Chapter 5 (Figs. 5-39 to 5-42). It should be noted that eosinophilia can be masked by concomitant administration of steroids. I have heard of one case of infection with *Strongyloides intercoralis* in which the eosinophilia was masked by steroid therapy, and the infection was fatal.

Hypereosinophilia (50% to 90%; 20,000 to 70,000/mm³)

in acutely ill patients has been called the "hypereosinophilic syndrome" (Chusid et al, 1975; Parillo et al, 1978; Van Slyck and Adamson, 1979). The pathogenesis is varied, some cases being chronic granulocytic leukemias, others having various causes. It is obviously important to identify those cases which represent granulocytic leukemia, by examination of bone marrow and blood and by chromosome studies (Bitran et al, 1977). There is one report (Gittman et al, 1978) of hypercalcemia associated with hypereosinophilia of unknown etiology.

Basophilic leukocytosis

An increase in basophils in the peripheral blood is found most commonly in chronic myelocytic leukemia and in the myeloproliferative disorders (particularly polycythemia vera). Basophilic leukocytosis has also been noted in erythroderma, urticaria with severe eosinophilia, urticaria pigmentosa, and ulcerative colitis. Basophilic infiltration (here the question of basophils versus tissue mast cells comes up) into the tissues and exudates of various skin lesions has recently received a good deal of attention; e.g., infiltration of lesions with basophilic leukocytes has been noted in scabies, eczema, miliaria, erythema multiforme, herpes zoster, herpes simplex, contact dermatitis, positive reactions in various skin tests, and drug eruptions (Aspegren et al, 1963). When the lesions are characterized by vesicles, the fluid in the vesicles contains basophils. Diffuse infiltration into various organs is found in *systematic mast cell disease* (Sagher and Even-Paz, 1967) characterized by hepatosplenomegaly, bone lesions, fever, and signs and symptoms referable to the release of histamine from basophils (flushing, diarrhea, nausea, and vomiting). Mast cells may be found in the peripheral blood in the mast cell leukemia variant (Plate 52).

Shelley (1963) described the "indirect basophil degranulation test" for detecting sensitivity to drugs or allergic reactions to drugs. The test is based on the theory that basophil granules release histamine when there is an antigen-antibody reaction. As a result, visible changes occur in the granules. This test has been applied to penicillin-sensitive persons (Katz et al, 1964) and, while the correlation is not perfect, it has yielded a higher percentage of correlation than others that have been tried. It is recommended that the test be done some weeks after a penicillin reaction, for the test may be negative immediately after. Positive results have been obtained in persons sensitive to drugs other than penicillin, notably aspirin. The literature on the basophil degranulation test is reviewed by Kirshbaum et al (1967).

Lymphocytosis

Lymphocytosis is an increase in the number of lymphocytes above 9,000/mm^3 (9 × 10^9/1) in infants and young children, 7,000/mm^3 (7 × 10^9/1) in older children, and 4,000/mm^3 (4 × 10^9/1) in adults. Conditions causing lymphocytosis are listed in Table 15-11. In general, lymphocytosis accompanies viral infections, exanthems, some chronic infections, and lymphocytic leukemia. Two diseases, infectious mononucleosis and infectious lymphocytosis, are particularly important.

INFECTIOUS MONONUCLEOSIS. This is an acute infectious disease of viral origin that presents a protean clinical picture and is characterized by atypical lymphocytes in the peripheral blood *and* a positive differential absorption test for heterophil antibody. Atypical lymphocytes alone are not enough to satisfy the diagnostic criteria since similar cells are seen in a variety of viral diseases (see subsequent discussion). The serologic test for heterophil antibodies of the infectious mononucleosis type must be positive. Heterophil antibody-negative mononucleosis may be due to other than the Epstein-Barr virus (EBV) (see further), for example, cytomegalovirus (Jordan et al, 1973), toxoplasmosis (Evans, 1972), or unknown agents (Horwitz et al, 1977a,b; Evans, 1978). By definition, this section deals with the most common, that caused by infection with EBV.

As time goes on, there is more evidence for the suspected viral etiology, almost certainly EBV (Schleupner and Overall, 1979). Peters (1967) has demonstrated specific heterophil-reactive antigen in the kidney during the acute phase of infectious mononucleosis. Gerber et al (1969) have shown

Table 15-11. Causes of pathologic lymphocytosis

I. Acute viral infections
  A. Infectious mononucleosis
  B. Infectious lymphocytosis
  C. Mumps
  D. Chicken pox
  E. German measles
  F. Viral hepatitis
II. Chronic infections
  A. Syphilis, secondary stage
  B. Syphilis, congenital
  C. Tuberculosis
  D. Brucellosis
  E. Pertussis
III. Hemopoietic disorders
  A. Lymphocytic leukemia
  B. Leukosarcoma
  C. Non-Hodgkin's lymphomas
IV. Miscellaneous
  A. Carcinoma of the breast

that complement-fixing antibodies to a herpes-like virus (HLV) developed in each of 21 patients with documented infectious mononucleosis. In the course of the disease, antibodies develop to the herpes-like virus (EBV) associated with a cell line derived from a Burkitt lymphoma (Gerber et al, 1968). Moses et al (1968) have described a herpes-like virus in the nucleus and cytoplasm of cultured lymphocytes from infectious mononucleosis. In infectious mononucleosis there is a parallel rise in the heterophil titer and in the titer of anti-EBV antibodies (Henle et al, 1968; Hewetson et al, 1973). The EBV has been implicated as the agent responsible for the development of lymphocytic leukemia after infectious mononucleosis (Levine et al, 1972). The evidence for transmission from person to person by saliva and respiratory droplets is not conclusive (Hoagland, 1967), even though Niederman et al (1976) have found EBV in a significant number of oropharyngeal specimens from patients with infectious mononucleosis. This suspected mode of transmission has given infectious mononucleosis the designation "the kissing disease." The different incidence among students at the University of California (1,212 cases/100,000 students/academic year) and the University of Hawaii (37 cases/100,000 students/academic year) is subject to several explanations (Chang et al, 1979.)

CLINICAL PICTURE. Infectious mononucleosis can mimic many other diseases and varies from a mild syndrome recognized with difficulty to a severe incapacitating disease. It may be epidemic or sporadic. Typically, it affects young persons and is extremely rare after 40 years of age (Shapiro and Horowitz, 1959; Carter et al, 1978). Sporadic cases usually show a more characteristic course. The incubation period is usually about 11 days but may be longer. The prodromal period lasts for 4 or 5 days and shows no characteristic clinical features and no hematologic or serologic changes. The fully developed disease lasts from 7 to 21 days. There are three common clinical types: (1) the pharyngeal type, with sore throat as the chief complaint, (2) the typhoidal type, with severe constitutional symptoms, and

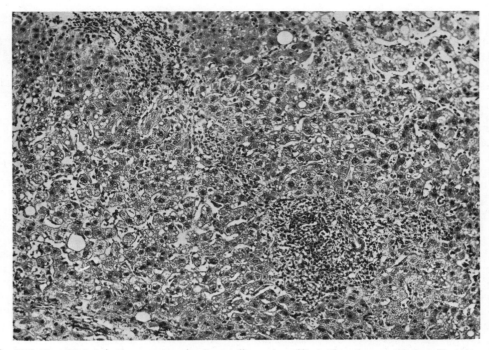

Fig. 15-2. Hepatitis in infectious mononucleosis, paraffin section of liver. There is accumulation of lymphocytes, both small and reactive, in the portal areas, with no necrosis of parenchymal cells. (Hematoxylin-eosin stain; ×95.)

(3) the glandular type, with striking cervical lymphadenopathy. Any given patient may show a mixed symptomatology (Finch, 1969). Fever is usually present and may be as high as 106° F. Splenomegaly is found in about half the patients and hepatomegaly in about one tenth. Rupture of the spleen, spontaneous or following trauma, is a rare complication (Rutkow, 1978). A macular or maculopapular rash occurs in about one fifth of the patients. It may be confused with the eruption of typhus, typhoid, or scarlet fever. Petechiae on the hard palate are common. Other hemorrhagic phenomena (petechiae and ecchymoses of skin, nasopharyngeal bleeding, hematuria, and gastrointestinal bleeding) may be encountered but are rare. The period of convalescence is usually short but can last for months or years. The more severe complications are (1) hepatitis (incidence: 50% to 90% based on hyperbilirubinemia, elevated SGOT, and other serum enzyme activity) (Fig. 15-2), (2) laryngeal edema (incidence: rare), and (3) Guillain-Barré syndrome (incidence: very rare).

Two aspects of the clinical features deserve special emphasis. The first is the question of whether infectious mononucleosis can occur a second time, as a relapse or recurrence. Almost certainly the answer is "no." I have not been able to find a single report in which all three criteria essential for diagnosis (clinical picture, atypical lymphocytes in the peripheral blood, and a high heterophil antibody titer exhibiting the characteristic absorption pattern) have been met for both the original bout and the alleged recurrence. Joncas et al (1974) have shown that an elevated heterophil antibody titer may persist for as long as 23 months. Most reports are based on an anamnestic rise in the hetero-

phil titer (Hoagland, 1963) or on the clinical diagnosis of a systemic disease having the features of infectious mononucleosis. Occasionally the disease runs a chronic course with temporary improvement, and such a case might appear to represent a recurrence (Sumaya, 1977).

The second feature is the high incidence of parenchymal liver disease, ranging from mild to severe. Death resulting from massive liver necrosis is reported by Chang and Campbell (1975). Clinically, this is manifested as lassitude for some weeks after the blood and serologic abnormalities return to normal. On the basis of hyperbilirubinemia and serum enzyme abnormalities, hepatitis of various degrees is a feature in 50% to 90% of the proved cases of infectious mononucleosis (Horwitz et al, 1980).

LABORATORY FINDINGS. Anemia is rare. However, a few cases of acquired hemolytic anemia have been described (Keyloun and Grace, 1966; Deaton et al, 1967).

The *leukocyte count* is elevated in about half the cases and normal or less than normal in the others. When elevated, it is seldom above 20,000/mm^3 (20 × 10^9/l), although in children counts as high as 63,000/mm^3 (63 × 10^9/l) are recorded. Leukopenia is not unusual early in the course of the disease, leukocyte counts as low as 1,500/mm^3 (1.5 × 10^9/l) having been reported.

The *leukocyte differential count* shows 50% to 97% lymphocytes that are atypical (Plate 58). Downey divided them into three types. Type I cells show an oval, slightly lobulated nucleus containing coarse strands and masses and poorly demarcated parachromatin. The cytoplasm is pale blue, vacuolated, and foamy. Type II cells are usually larger; their nucleus shows a finer chromatin pattern and sharper parachromatin, and the cytoplasm is usually less foamy. Type III cells show a round to oval nucleus and a deeply basophilic cytoplasm. Type III cells sometimes closely resemble plasma cells. Another type of cell sometimes encountered in significant numbers is one that has the normal structure of a large lymphocyte, except for many azurophilic granules. The distinction between the three chief cell types has no practical significance. The characteristic cells are of the T type (Sheldon et al, 1973) or both T and B (Enberg et al, 1974; Giuliano et al, 1974); they appear atypical because they are in fat lymphocytes undergoing blastoid transformation. These reactive lymphocytes usually appear by the fourth or fifth day but sometimes not until the fourteenth day of the illness. They usually persist for about 1 month, but in exceptional cases are present for 3 months or more. The morphology of these cells by electron microscopy is described in detail by Schumacher et al (1969).

Cells having an appearance identical to those in infectious mononucleosis are not uncommon in other viral infections. These are illustrated in Chapter 4. In our experience the infectious mononucleosis cell is indistinguishable from the "virocytes" seen in viral hepatitis and viral respiratory and systemic diseases. During the winter of 1956 we studied a large number of apparently epidemic cases that clinically resembled mild infectious mononucleosis. Many reactive lymphocytes were present in the peripheral blood smear, which in all cases appeared typical of infectious mononucleosis. However, only four out of the 58 patients studied had a positive test for heterophil antibodies of the infectious mononucleosis type. These patients may well fit into the group called "cytomegalovirus mononucleosis" described by Klemola et al (1969).

With the exception of the heterophil test, other laboratory findings are not diagnostic of infectious mononucleosis. The *platelet count* is usually normal. It is rarely low, with purpura as the chief sign. Severe thrombocytopenia led to massive cerebral damage and death in one of our cases, and this very rare but lethal complication is also reported by Goldstein and Porter (1969). *Albuminuria* and *hematuria* may be present, but there is no other evidence of abnormal renal function. Cowdrey (1966) reports an increased concentration of uric acid in the serum of 22 patients with the disease. When hepatitis is a complication, there may be *icterus* of the plasma, an elevated *serum bilirubin,* increased amounts of *urinary urobilinogen,* and abnormal *liver function tests*. Since there is usually an increase in immunoglobulins, flocculation or turbidity tests of liver function are unreliable; elevation of SGOT, LDH, and alkaline phosphatase activity in serum occurs in almost all patients having hepatitis. Residual liver damage is common. In all cases there is a rise in the serum concentration of immunoglobulins, predominantly IgM (Fig. 3-19), which probably represents heterophil antibody (Yoshida and Nahmias, 1967). In some cases the *spinal fluid* contains up to 1,000 lymphocytes/mm³ (1 × 10^9/l) and increased amounts of protein. *Serologic tests for syphilis* may be positive, but whereas it was once thought that the incidence of biologic false-positive tests for syphilis was about 10%, the data from more recent series show the incidence to be less than 1% (Cabrera and Carlson, 1968).

Table 15-12. Absorption patterns for various heterophil antibodies*

Condition	Absorbed by	
	Forssman antigen†	Beef erythrocytes
Normal	Yes	No or partial
Infectious mononucleosis	No or slight	Yes
Serum sickness or sensitization	Yes	Yes

*If absorption is "yes," there will be no agglutination, and if it is "no," there will be agglutination when the absorbed serum is added to sheep erythrocytes.
†Guinea pig or horse kidney.

There may be hemolytic anemia (Deaton et al, 1967), sometimes caused by cold agglutinins of anti-i specificity (Capra et al, 1969) and sometimes caused by aggravation of concomitant hemolytic disease such as hereditary spherocytosis (Godal and Skaga, 1969). Most instances of hemolytic anemia are of the antiglobulin-positive autoimmune type (Worledge and Dacie, 1969), but some are antiglobulin negative, while others are caused by cold agglutinins (Dickerman et al, 1980).

HETEROPHIL ANTIBODY. The definitive diagnosis of infectious mononucleosis depends on demonstration in the blood of a heterophil antibody that is only partially, or not at all, absorbed by tissue containing the *Forssman antigen*. In 1911 Forssman described an apparently serologically nonspecific (i.e., heterophil) antigen in the tissues of a variety of animals. Injection into rabbits of tissues containing this antigen produced antibodies (heterophil antibodies) against sheep's erythrocytes. Forssman antigen is present in tissue from the guinea pig, horse, dog, cat, mouse, and tortoise and is absent in tissue from humans, ox, sheep, rat, goose, pigeon, eel, and frog. In general, when the tissue contains Forssman antigen, the erythrocytes in the animal do not.

Paul and Bunnell (1932) found that the serum of patients with infectious mononucleosis would agglutinate sheep erythrocytes. Although normal persons often have antibodies that agglutinate sheep erythrocytes, the titer in infectious mononucleosis is much higher. The titer in normal persons is usually no higher than 1:56, whereas in infectious mononucleosis it may be as high as several thousand. The titration of agglutinating antibodies is sometimes called the Paul-Bunnell test.

It was once thought that the agglutinating antibodies present in the serum of patients with infectious mononucleosis were heterophil antibodies of the Forssman type. It is certain, however, that a different type of heterophil antibody is produced in infectious mononucleosis. Heterophil antibodies, not of the infectious mononucleosis type, are found normally in serum (in low titer), are produced by a variety of infectious agents, and are the result of immunization. Chiefly as the result of the studies of Davidsohn et al (1955) and Davidsohn and Lee (1962, 1964), the Forssman antibody present in the serum of normal persons has been shown to be wholly absorbed by tissues containing Forssman antigen (such as guinea pig or horse kidney) and only partially absorbed by beef erythrocytes. On the other hand, the heterophil antibody in infectious mononucleosis is not signifi-

Table 15-13. Typical serologic findings in infectious mononucleosis

Example	Presumptive test	Differential test after absorption with		Interpretation
		Forssman antigen	Beef erythrocytes	
1	1:448	0	1:224	Negative for infectious mononucleosis
2	1:448	1:224	1:224	Negative for infectious mononucleosis
3	1:448	1:224	0	Positive for infectious mononucleosis
4	1:448	1:112	0	Positive for infectious mononucleosis
5	1:448	1:56	0	Positive for infectious mononucleosis
6	1:224	1:28	0	Positive for infectious mononucleosis
7	1:56	1:28	0	Positive for infectious mononucleosis
8	1:56	1:14	0	Positive for infectious mononucleosis
9	1:28	1:28	0	Positive for infectious mononucleosis
10	1:28	1:14	0	Positive for infectious mononucleosis
11	1:28	1:7	0	Positive for infectious mononucleosis

cantly absorbed by Forssman antigen and is absorbed by beef erythrocytes. Heterophil antibody in a titer of 1:112 or higher is also found in serum sickness but can be differentiated from the other two in that it is absorbed by both Forssman antigen and beef erythrocytes (Table 15-12).

PRESUMPTIVE TEST. The presumptive test measures the titer of heterophil antibodies in the serum but does not differentiate between types. It is generally agreed that about 98% of normal persons have a heterophil antibody titer of 1:56 or less. It is almost never higher than 1:112 as a result of infections other than infectious mononucleosis or in cases in which there has been sensitization to horse serum. The heterophil antibody titer is usually 1:224 or higher in infectious mononucleosis. In the absence of sensitization and if the clinical and hematologic findings are typical, a titer of 1:224 is presumed to indicate infectious mononucleosis.

DIFFERENTIAL ABSORPTION TEST. The differential absorption test of Davidsohn et al (1955) is specific. Infectious mononucleosis is present when there is no absorption of heterophil antibody with Forssman antigen, or slight absorption only, and complete absorption of the antibody with beef erythrocytes. A positive result for infectious mononucleosis depends less on the titer obtained after absorption than on the fact that a measurable quantity of non-Forssman antibody remains after absorption with Forssman antigen (Table 15-13). Note that in examples 9, 10, and 11 the presumptive test gives a titer in the normal range, while the differential test is diagnostic of infectious mononucleosis. Although this combination is not common, it is seen often enough to pose a serious objection to using the presumptive test only.

MONOSPOT TEST. The value of the differential absorption test has been proved by many years' experience. Recently, however, a rapid, simple, and equally specific test, the Monospot test (Ortho Pharmaceutical Corp.), has been made available commercially. We are using it exclusively in our laboratory. Myhre and Nakayama (1976) report that the Mono-chek test (Hyland Laboratories) equals the Monospot test in accuracy.

The test is based on the observation (Lee et al, 1968) that the agglutinin titer for heterophil antibodies is about three times higher when horse erythrocytes are used than it is with the traditional sheep erythrocytes. They also found that fresh horse erythrocytes preserved in citrate were more sensitive and specific than formalin-treated erythrocytes. Furthermore, differential absorption can be performed and the heterophil titer determined with horse erythrocytes. A slide test was then developed that includes differential absorption. The system provides for both a presumptive test and a quantitative titration. Because the amount of serum needed is small, it is possible to collect capillary blood when venipuncture is difficult or otherwise undesirable. Because the test system is more sensitive than one using sheep erythrocytes, positive results are obtained with lower titers of heterophil antibodies and persist for a longer time. The test is performed on a slide and is read at 1 minute after the reagents are mixed. The method is given in the Appendix.

The specificity of the Monospot test is excellent and as good as that of the standard differential absorption test. Lee et al (1968) encountered one false-positive test in a child with acute leukemia (the standard test was negative). Evans et al (1969) reported two false-positive results with the Monospot test in 501 sera tested. Wahren (1969) found the Monospot test positive in all cases of verified infectious mononucleosis and no false negative reactions. Wolf et al (1970) reported a positive Monospot test in two patients with lymphoma (one with Hodgkin's disease and the other with lymphocytic lymphoma, poorly differentiated). Merrill and Barrett (1976) reported the occurrence of a positive Monospot test in a patient with histiocytic medullary reticulosis. False-positive results are also found in malaria (Reed, 1974). Horwitz et al (1979b) report the persistence of false-positive Monospot tests for up to 6 years.

INFECTIOUS LYMPHOCYTOSIS. Acute infectious lymphocytosis is a benign infectious and contagious disease occurring in children (Putnam et al, 1968). The etiologic agent is not known but is presumed to be a virus, either Coxsackie A (Horwitz and Moore, 1968) or adenovirus (Olson et al, 1964). In an epidemic studied by Horwitz and Moore (1968) an enterovirus of the Coxsackie type was isolated in 21% of the patients' stool specimens, and neutral-

Table 15-14. Causes of monocytosis, nonleukemic*

I. Infectious diseases
    A. Subacute bacterial endocarditis
    B. Pulmonary tuberculosis
    C. Brucellosis
    D. Typhoid fever
    E. Rickettsial infections
    F. Kala-azar
    G. Trypanosomiasis
    H. Leishmaniasis
II. Other diseases
    A. Ulcerative colitis
    B. Regional enteritis
    C. Sarcoidosis
    D. Collagen diseases
    E. Hodgkin's disease
    F. Non-Hodgkin's lymphomas
    G. Gaucher's disease

*Modified from Maldonado and Hanlon, 1965; Golde, 1975.

izing antibodies to that virus increased in titer in many of the affected children. The symptomatology is not unlike that of infectious mononucleosis, but there is no lymphadenopathy or splenomegaly. There is nether anemia nor thrombocytopenia. The blood findings are characteristic. The leukocyte count is usually elevated, up to 100,000/mm³ (100 × 10⁹/l), and the differential count shows a preponderance (60% to 92%) of small, mature lymphocytes that appear entirely normal. Characteristically, there are no smudged cells as in chronic lymphocytic leukemia. Tests for heterophil antibodies are negative.

Monocytosis

Monocytosis is an increase in the number of monocytes above 750/mm³ (0.75 × 10⁹/l) in children and 440/mm³ (0.44 × 10⁹/l) in adults. Monocytosis is a feature of monocytic leukemia (Chapter 16), and this must be distinguished from the benign reactive states discussed here. By itself it is not as diagnostic of disease as other types of leukocytosis. Monocytosis (Table 15-14) is sometimes seen in subacute bacterial endocarditis, brucellosis, typhoid, rickettsial infections, kala-azar, chronic ulcerative colitis, regional enteritis, collagen diseases, trypanosomiasis, Hodgkin's disease, and Gaucher's disease (Maldonado and Hanlon, 1965), but not consistently enough to rely on in diagnosis. In pulmonary tuberculosis, on the other hand, monocytosis frequently accompanies acute and active infection. It subsides during the healing or inactive phase, at which time a lymphocytosis may occur. The ratio of the absolute number of monocytes to lymphocytes (M:L ratio) is high when the disease is acute and low during recovery.

Rosenthal, in 1936 described cases of monocytosis and agranulocytosis that he named ''leukopenic infectious monocytosis.'' Stone and Redmond (1963) have described another case. Both would be considered instances of a benign neutropenia were it not for the striking monocytosis that marked the onset of the disease. The disease is an acute febrile illness mimicking infectious mononucleosis (but without the characteristic serologic reaction) or acute leuke-

mia. Complete and spontaneous recovery occurs within a few weeks. However, Cassileth (1967) reports an interesting case in which the patient first had agranulocytosis induced by chlorpromazine, then marked monocytosis, and acute leukemia 18 months later. Pretlow (1969) reports an interesting case in which the patient had monocytosis for 11 years that culminated in acute monocytic leukemia.

Systemic lupus erythematosus
Clinical picture

The clinical aspects of this disease are discussed by Maddock (1965), Dubois (1974), Kaslow and Masi (1978), and Masi and Kaslow, (1978).

LE cell phenomenon

The LE (lupus erythematosus) cell is a neutrophilic leukocyte that has ingested a homogeneous globular mass of altered nuclear material. With few exceptions, formation of this cell is seen only when the preparation is made from the blood of a person having systemic lupus erythematosus. LE cell formation does not occur in every case of disseminated lupus erythematosus, the incidence of positive tests being at best about 80%. In cases of proved lupus erythematosus the characteristec LE cell usually disappears during spontaneous or steroid-induced remissions. In the group of 20% that do not show LE cells, many show extracellular globular material (see next section), but of course this is not diagnostic.

LE cells in aspirated bone marrow were first described by Hargraves et al (1948) and later developments were reviewed by Hargraves (1969). It was later shown that these cells do not exist in the bone marrow in vivo but can be found when aspirated bone marrow is allowed to stand in vitro. The phenomenon can be reproduced with peripheral blood. Various technics using peripheral blood have largely replaced the one using bone marrow.

FORMATION OF LE CELLS. Formation of LE cells depends on a plasma factor, the *LE plasma factor,* found in the blood and other body fluids obtained from patients with lupus erythematosus. Specifically, the factor is a γ-globulin and is one of the five antibodies found in the serum in lupus erythematosus: (1) antinuclear antibody, (2) antinucleoprotein antibody, (3) anti-DNA antibody, (4) antihistone antibody, and (5) antinucleolar antibody. It is stable in serum stored at refrigerator temperature and in the frozen state and is not destroyed by heat unless the serum is heated to 65° C. When leukocytes from the same patient, from normal persons, and even from other species are suspended in serum containing the LE plasma factor (antinucleoprotein antibody, IgG type) and the mixture is incubated, the LE plasma factor produces a depolymerization of DNA in the nucleus of some cells. Depolymerization is accompanied by liberation of nuclear material that appears as free homogeneous globular masses. When these masses are ingested by neutrophilic leukocytes, the typical LE cells are formed. Phagocytosis is complement dependent (Blondin and McDuffie, 1970). Occasionally the mass is ingested by cells other than neutrophils (Plate 60). It is not known whether the LE plasma factor attacks some of the living leukocytes to produce the free globular bodies or whether it attacks only

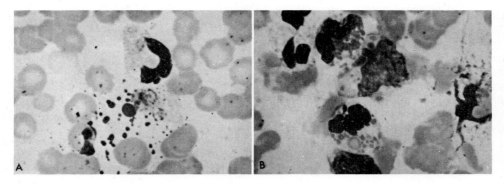

Fig. 15-3. Extracellular globular material, **A,** and early LE cell formation, **B,** in a preparation also showing many typical LE cells.

dead or damaged leukocytes. There is strong evidence that the intensity of LE cell formation is proportional to the number of platelets present, and this suggests that liberated platelet substances are somehow involved in the reaction.

MORPHOLOGY. The LE cell has a typical appearance when the preparation is stained with Wright's stain (Plate 60). It is a neutrophilic leukocyte distended by an intracytoplasmic homogeneous red-purple body. The nucleus is compressed to one side, its appearance is distorted, and the phagocytic cell, pregnant with the large inclusion, appears larger than normal. The inclusion in the LE cell is homogeneous and redder than the usual color of unaltered chromatin. The criterion of almost complete homogeneity of structure must be rigidly followed.

TART CELL (NUCLEOPHAGOCYTOSIS). A similar cell, called the "tart cell" because it was first described in a patient named Tart, is produced by phagocytosis of a nucleus, usually by a monocyte (Plate 60). Nucleophagocytosis does not indicate disseminated lupus erythematosus, and it is important therefore to distinguish between the tart cell and the LE cell (Heller and Zimmerman, 1956). In a tart cell the ingested nucleus retains some characteristic nuclear structure such as recognizable chromatin clumps, nucleoli, or nuclear membrane. Sometimes the inclusion is fairly homogeneous, but it is never as "smooth" as in the LE cell and usually has a darker-staining rim. Tart cells may be seen in drug sensitivity and have been produced experimentally by mixing leukocytes with antileukocyte serum (Zimmerman et al, 1953).

ASSOCIATED LABORATORY FINDINGS. Preparations that contain LE cells may show two other characteristic phenomena: the presence of extracellular globular material (Fig. 15-3) (Arterberry et al, 1964; Golden and McDuffie, 1967) and the formation of "rosettes." It is probable that these phenomena represent stages intermediate to the formation of the LE cell. When the globular material is extracellular, it has the same homogeneous appearance and staining as the intracellular inclusion. Both are Feulgen positive. Free masses may be small or large. Rosettes are formed when neutrophilic leukocytes surround one of these bodies. The body is eventually ingested by one cell, although it is occasionally possible to see two cells sharing the meal.

While the finding of LE cells is most helpful in the diagnosis of disseminated lupus erythematosus, the percentage

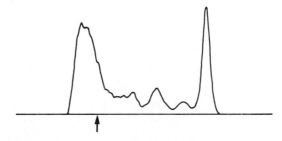

Fig. 15-4. Electrophoresis of serum proteins in disseminated lupus erythematosus.

of false-negative preparations (not inconsiderable, about 20%) makes accessory laboratory findings worthy of consideration. The peripheral blood usually shows lymphopenia (Rivero et al, 1978) and thrombocytopenia. As a matter of fact, thrombocytopenia should always suggest the possibility of disseminated lupus. Mild anemia is usually present, but severe hemolytic anemia can occur. The serum proteins show striking alterations (Barton, 1959). On electrophoresis (Fig. 15-4) there is a decrease in albumin, α_2-globulin, and β-globulin, with an increase in α_1-globulin and usually a striking increase in γ-globulin. It has been noted that the protein pattern is influenced by the degree of proteinuria, and the γ-globulin fraction in serum can be lower than normal when proteinuria is severe. The technic of immunoelectrophoresis allows a more sensitive separation of serum protein fractions and shows a decrease in albumin, normal α_2-globulin, increased haptoglobin, decreased β_1A-globulin, increased β_2A- and β_2M-globulin, and increased γ-globulin. The pattern in systemic lupus with hepatitis is essentially the same (Fischer, 1962) with the exception of decreased haptoglobin. The increase in the γ-globulin fraction is probably the most characteristic feature of this autoimmune disease. It is not unusual to find antithyroid and antiglomerular antibody as well. Serum complement activity is low, with low concentrations of C2 and C3. Levels of β_1c- and β_1a-globulin are low in patients with active lupus nephritis. Serologic tests for syphilis are positive in about 20% of the cases.

Purpura caused by thrombocytopenia, sometimes amegakaryocytic (Griner and Hoyer, 1970), is not uncommon (Clark et al, 1978) but occasionally there is severe bleeding not attributable to thrombocytopenia. Investigation reveals a prolonged venous clotting time, prolonged prothrombin time, and prolonged partial thromboplastin time. The coagulation abnormality is related to the development of a circulating anticoagulant that, in general, behaves as an inhibitor of intrinsic thromboplastin (Chapter 17) (Exner et al, 1978). The lupus anticoagulant is usually of the IgG type and inhibits prothrombin activator either directly or by interfering with the formation of Xa-V-phospholipid complex.

SIGNIFICANCE OF LE CELLS. In most cases the finding of LE cells indicates the presence of disseminated lupus erythematosus. However, not all patients with this disease show the LE phenomenon, nor is there always a correlation between the presence of LE cells and the clinical severity of the disease. The administration of corticosteroids usually, but not always, abolishes LE cell formation (Rothfield and Pace, 1962). It should be noted that there is no LE formation in discoid lupus erythematosus without systemic involvement.

SPECIFICITY OF THE LE PHENOMENON. The specificity of the LE phenomenon is still being argued. Supposedly, typical LE cells have been found in rheumatoid arthritis,

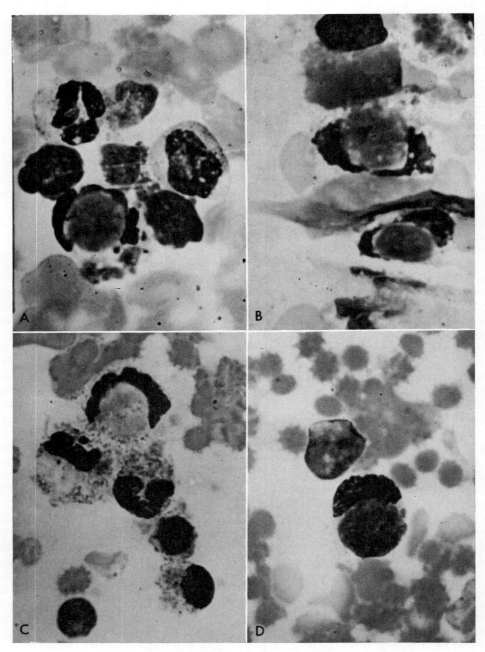

Fig. 15-5. LE cell phenomenon as a result of hydralazine intake.

hemolytic anemia, glomerulonephritis, drug reaction (particularly penicillin reactions), and serum sickness. Some of these reports must be discounted, first, because the cells illustrated are not convincing, and second, because many of the diseases listed may be part of the lupus erythematosus syndrome or precede the development of the typical syndrome. There remain, however, some cases in which apparently typical LE cells have been found in the absence of lupus erythematosus. These are few and do not invalidate the many observations that point to a high degree of correlation between lupus erythematosus and LE cell formation.

Of special interest are the drug-induced lupus syndromes (Alarcón-Segovia, 1969; Dubois, 1975). The first drug implicated was hydralazine hydrochloride, which is used in the treatment of hypertension. About 10% of persons receiving the drug developed a syndrome that was clinically, serologically, and pathologically indistinguishable from lupus erythematosus. The LE cells found are typical (Fig. 15-5). Later, it was found that other drugs have lupus-inducing or lupus-activating potential (Table 15-15). Some of the drugs deserve special mention. The drugs most commonly implicated are hydralazine (Hildreth et al, 1960; Alarcón-Segovia et al, 1967; Condemi et al, 1967), the anticonvulsant drugs (Benton et al, 1962), and procainamide hydrochloride (Colman and Sturgill, 1965; Fakhro et al, 1967; McDevitt and Glasgow, 1967; Lappat and Cawein, 1968). These drugs are thought to produce the reaction through unknown, but not allergic, mechanisms. The other drugs listed probably elicit allergic reactions that, in turn, bring about the LE syndrome (Lee et al, 1966). Of special interest is the drug methyldopa, known to cause a positive antiglobulin test and apparently also capable of inducing the LE phenomenon (Sherman et al, 1967).

Table 15-15. Drugs implicated in production of LE syndrome

I. Drugs producing the effect by unknown alterations of nucleoprotein
  A. Hydralazine hydrochloride (Apresoline)
  B. Anticonvulsant drugs
    1. Dilantin
    2. Mesantoin
    3. Tridione
    4. Primidone
    5. Ethosuximide
  C. Procainamide hydrochloride
  D. Phenelzine sulfate (Nardil)
II. Drugs producing the effect through allergic reactions
  A. Sulfonamides
  B. Penicillin
  C. Methyldopa
  D. Oral contraceptives
  E. Isoniazid
  F. Tetracycline
  G. Streptomycin
  H. Griseofulvin
  I. Phenylbutazone
  J. Methylthiouracil
  K. Propylthiouracil
  L. Reserpine

ANTINUCLEAR ANTIBODIES BY FLUORESCENCE. Antinuclear antibodies can be demonstrated by immunofluorescence. The indirect fluorescent antibody (IFA) or antinuclear antibody (ANA) test is based on the development of nuclear fluorescence when antinuclear antibody is fixed to nuclear material and then reacts with fluorescein-conjugated antihuman γ globulin (Friou, 1967; Beck, 1969; Ritchie, 1970).

The LE antibody is usually of the IgG type but may be of the IgM or IgA type. It has been shown to be an antibody to DNA-histone nucleoprotein. It reacts with the nuclei of a variety of cells: normal human leukocytes, cells from chronic myelocytic leukemia, leukocytes from various mammalian species, spermatozoal nuclei, and tissue cell nuclei. Normal rat liver is the most commonly used substrate for immunofluorescence studies. The reaction of fluorescein-conjugated antihuman γ-globulins is both quantitative and qualitative.

Quantitatively, the titer of antibodies can be determined by carrying out the test with serially diluted serum (Ritchie, 1967). The highest dilution of serum giving a positive fluorescence is reported as the titer of antibody. Normal serum gives fluorescence in the range of 1:1 to 1:20, most normal sera showing a titer of 1:5 or less. Normal serum from elderly subjects has a higher titer of antinuclear antibody than in the young or middle-aged. In disseminated lupus erythematosus, titers of 1:20 to 1:40,960 have been found, most sera showing a titer of 1:40 or greater, with the highest titers in the acute phase of the disease. Similar high titers are found in rheumatoid arthritis (1:1 to 1:40,960, with most instances in the range of 1:1 to 1:320) and in scleroderma (1:1 to 1:40,960, with most instances between 1:40 and 1:1,280).

Qualitatively, several patterns of fluorescence are seen (Fig. 15-6) (Bickel, 1968). In the *diffuse* pattern, commonly found in disseminated lupus erythematosus, the whole nucleus shows diffuse fluorescence. In the *peripheral* pattern, also seen in the acute phase of lupus erythematosus, the periphery of the nucleus fluoresces more intensely than the center. In the *speckled* pattern, most common in scleroderma, the nucleus shows minute points of fluorescence tending to concentrate at the center. In the *nucleolar* pattern, seen in collagen diseases other than disseminated lupus erythematosus, the nucleoli show intense fluorescence, while other nuclear material does not. Pure patterns falling into these categories are uncommon; usually mixed patterns are seen, although one feature may be predominant (Bonomo et al, 1965). It has also been noted that the pattern may vary at different serum dilutions.

Neither the titer of antibody nor the fluorescent pattern alone is an absolute diagnostic or differential criterion. The present status of the art may be summarized as follows:

1. Whereas the LE phenomenon is positive in only about 80% of the cases of disseminated lupus erythematosus, the indirect fluorescence test is positive in almost 100% of the cases.

2. A negative fluorescence test usually rules out lupus erythematosus, but there are exceptions.

3. Whereas the LE test can become negative in the course of steroid therapy, the titer of antinuclear antibody is not

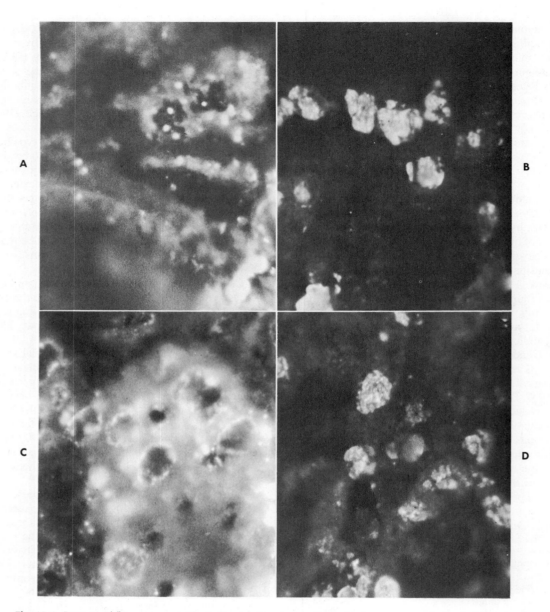

Fig. 15-6. Patterns of fluorescence in the indirect antinuclear antibody fluorescence test. **A,** Nucleolar pattern. **B,** Homogeneous pattern. **C,** Peripheral pattern. **D,** Speckled pattern.

affected by steroids. A dropping titer indicates true clinical remission rather than a steroid effect.

4. The titer of antibody is not diagnostic of the various collagen diseases, but in combination with other laboratory and clinical data, some generalizations are possible. First, a titer of less than 1:20 in a patient suspected of having lupus erythematosus practically excludes the diagnosis. Second, a high titer, together with a peripheral fluorescence pattern, is strong evidence of lupus erythematosus. Third, a high titer with a diffuse, nucleolar, or speckled pattern is not diagnostic and is seen in lupus erythematosus, scleroderma, rheumatoid arthritis, and Sjögren's syndrome. The diffuse pattern is more common in mild, than in acute, lupus erythematosus.

5. The indirect fluorescent antibody test is always positive in drug-induced LE-like syndromes. The LE test may be positive or negative. The fluorescence test may be positive before the full expression of the drug-induced state and is useful in predicting the complication.

6. In addition to anti-DNA antibodies (native DNA), there may be antibodies to a ribonuclease-insensitive acidic nuclear protein, designated anti-Sm, and immune deposits in the dermis (the lupus band test. [LBT]) (Moses and Barland, 1979).

7. Antinucleolar antibodies in high titer favor the diagnosis of systemic sclerosis over other diseases in the collagen group.

Leukopenia
Definitions

Leukopenia is a reduction in the number of leukocytes in blood below the normal for the patient's age, sex, race, etc.

In adults, leukopenia can be defined as the reduction in the number of leukocytes in the peripheral blood below 4,000/mm^3 (4 × 10^9/l). In some instances the leukopenia is caused by a reduction in all types of leukocytes and may be called *balanced leukopenia*. Usually, however, the leukopenia is caused by a reduction of only one type of leukocyte, in which case it can be more exactly defined as neutropenia (granulocytopenia, agranulocytosis), lymphopenia, eosinopenia, etc. *Neutropenia* is a reduction in neutrophilic leukocytes below 1,500/mm^3 (1.5 × 10^9/l) in children and below 1,800/mm^3 (1.8 × 10^9/l) in adults. *Lymphopenia* is a reduction in lymphocytes below 1,400/mm^3 (1.4 × 10^9/l) in children and below 1,000/mm^3 (1 × 10^9/l) in adults. *Eosinopenia* is a reduction in eosinophils below 200/mm^3 (0.2 × 10^9/l) in either children or adults. Basophils occur in such small numbers that a reduction is difficult to determine. A reduction in the number of monocytes is significant only in regard to the lymphocyte/monocyte ratio in pulmonary tuberculosis. Neutropenia has the greatest clinical significance.

Etiology

Some of the conditions listed in Table 15-16 will always produce leukopenia if the dose or exposure is sufficiently high. Among these are various types of ionizing radiation, whether externally or parenterally administered in the form of radioactive isotopes. The hematologic depressant drugs used in the chemotherapy of leukemia and lymphomas are equally toxic. Leukopenia is characteristic of some of the infections listed, such as typhoid and paratyphoid fever, tularemia, and some of the viral infections, whereas in others it is a variable occurrence. Leukopenia caused by drugs is uncommon, and some of the drugs listed have produced leukopenia only in rare instances. Most leukopenias caused by drugs are neutropenias.

It is thought that drugs cause neutropenia either because of hypersensitivity or because of their direct toxic effect on leukocytes and leukocyte precursors. Drugs that produce neutropenia in only a small number of cases probably do so because of the person's hypersensitivity. The drug may act as a hapten that combines with one of the protein constituents of the leukocytes to form a complex antigen. When for reasons that are not yet clear the patient develops antibodies to such an antigen, the antibody is cytotoxic and produces either lysis of the leukocytes or agglutination with subsequent removal by the lung and destruction. Some drugs are directly cytotoxic. This type of reaction usually develops slowly and is chronic, whereas the acute leukopenias are usually caused by hypersensitivity. It has been pointed out that many of the drugs capable of producing leukopenia contain the benzene ring or other ring structures.

It is sometimes necessary to take into account a given person's normal baseline value. One of my senior technologists has, over a period of 20 years, had a WBC count ranging between 3,500 and 4,200/mm^3, all types of leukocytes being equally reduced. He has not been subject to infections or had any other difficulties.

Neutropenia

Severe neutropenia causes the body to be markedly susceptible to overwhelming bacterial invasion. The acute clinical condition resulting from neutropenia may be called *acute agranulocytosis, agranulocytic angina,* or *malignant leukopenia*. There is an acute onset of prostration, chills, and fever. The gangrenous ulceration of the mucous membranes, particularly of the mouth and throat, gives rise to the term ''angina.'' The leukocyte count is low, sometimes well below 1,000/mm^3 (1 × 10^9/l). There is no leukocytic response to infection, and the mortality rate is 20% to 50% even with adequate antibiotic treatment. The differential count shows an almost complete absence of neutrophilic leukocytes. The few that may be present are segmented forms showing degenerative changes in the nucleus and cytoplasm. There is usually no anemia or thrombocytopenia when the reaction is caused by hypersensitivity. The bone marrow may be hypoplastic, normal, or hyperplastic. When hypoplastic, it may show only myeloblasts, progranulocytes, and myelocytes, the more mature granulocytes being absent.

Chronic neutropenia is not too severe a disease, and the patient may be asymptomatic. The leukocyte count is seldom below 3,000/mm^3 (3 × 10^9/l). The neutrophils are reduced but seldom absent. Chronic neutropenia may be caused by myelotoxic agents also responsible for producing anemia and thrombocytopenia. The bone marrow may then show many of the variants discussed in the chapter on myeloproliferative disorders.

Some chronic neutropenias cannot be attributed to any of the agents listed in Table 15-16. Some authors feel that as many as 20% to 30% fall in this group. It may well be that a significant number of these are caused by antineutrophil antibodies (Boxer et al, 1975; Lalezari et al, 1975). Among them are some syndromes that are clinically characteristic.

CHRONIC NEUTROPENIA IN CHILDHOOD. Chronic granulocytopenia in childhood is an interesting entity occurring in early life (Zuelzer and Bajoghli, 1964). The leukocyte count is as low as 2,000/mm^3 (2 × 10^9/l), with neutrophils markedly reduced both in relative and absolute numbers. The clinical course is benign, with no striking increase in susceptibility to infection, for it has been shown that in these cases there is an adequate granulocytic response to infection or, experimentally, to bacterial toxin. The bone marrow shows a depletion of adult granulocytes. It has been proposed that the granulocytopenia is caused by increased destruction or sequestration of leukocytes rather than by a maturation arrest. There is no evidence to indicate that leukoagglutinins are present.

Less than 20 acceptable cases of this syndrome have been reported. The syndrome is distinguished from aplastic anemia by the absence of anemia and thrombocytopenia and from leukemia by the absence of splenomegaly, lymphadenopathy, and immature cells in the peripheral blood. It is distinguished from neonatal neutropenia (see next section) in that the neutropenia in that syndrome is transient, occurs in the newborn, and is caused by transplacental leaking of maternal leukoagglutinins. It is distinguished from infantile genetic agranulocytosis by the familial incidence and high mortality of the latter syndrome. Cyclic neutropenia is, as the name implies, cyclic, whereas chronic granulocytopenia in childhood is not.

NEONATAL NEUTROPENIA. Neonatal neutropenia

Table 15-16. Causes of neutropenia

I. Infections (Castaneda and Guerrero, 1946; Horsfall and Tamm, 1965)
  A. Typhoid fever
  B. Paratyphoid fever
  C. Tularemia
  D. Brucellosis
  E. Influenza
  F. Measles
  G. Infectious hepatitis
  H. Psittacosis
  I. Infectious mononucleosis
  J. Rubella
  K. Scrub typhus
  L. Sandfly fever
  M. Dengue
  N. Malaria
  O. Relapsing fever
  P. Kala-azar
  Q. Miliary tuberculosis
  R. Septicemia
  S. Overwhelming bacterial infections
II. Cachexia and inanition
III. Hemopoietic disorders (Amorosi, 1965; Collier and Brush, 1966)
  A. Pernicious anemia
  B. Aleukemic leukemia
  C. Aplastic anemia
  D. Hypersplenism
  E. Gaucher's disease
  F. Felty's syndrome
IV. Anaphylactoid shock
V. Chemical agents (Finch, 1972; Wintrobe et al, 1974)
  A. Sulfonamides
    1. Prontosil
    2. Neoprontosil
    3. Sulfanilamide
    4. Sulfapyridine
    5. Sulfathiazole
    6. Gantrisin
    7. Sulfaguanidine
    8. Sulfamerazine
    9. Succinylsulfathiazole
  B. Antibiotics
    1. Chloramphenicol
    2. Penicillin
    3. Streptomycin
  C. Antihistaminics
    1. Pyribenzamine
    2. Antergan
    3. Methaphenilene (Diatrin)
  D. Analgesics
    1. Antipyrine
    2. Aminopyrine
    3. Phenylbutazone
    4. Phenacetin
  E. Anticonvulsants
    1. Dilantin
    2. Mesantoin
    3. Trimethadione (Tridione)
    4. Phenurone

F. Antithyroid drugs
    1. Thiouracil
    2. Propylthiouracil
    3. Methylthiouracil
    4. Methylmazole
    5. Carbimazole
    6. Tapazole
  G. Hemopoietic depressants
    1. Urethane
    2. Nitrogen mustard
    3. Triethylenemelamine
    4. Diaprim
    5. Aminopterin
    6. Methotrexate
    7. 6-Mercaptopurine
    8. Phenylhydrazine
    9. Myleran
    10. Demecolcine
  H. Organic arsenicals
    1. Acetarsone
    2. Arsphenamine
    3. Mapharsen
    4. Neoarsphenamine
    5. Sulfarsphenamine
  I. Miscellaneous
    1. Quinine
    2. Cinchophen
    3. Vioform
    4. Aniline
    5. Dinitrophenol
    6. Salts of heavy metals
    7. Chlorpromazine
    8. Pronestyl
    9. Tibione
    10. Atabrine
    11. DDT
    12. Diparcol
    13. Presidon
    14. Barbiturates
    15. Plasmoquin
    16. Funagillin
    17. Diamox
    18. Colchicine
VI. Neonatal immunoneutropenia (Lalezari et al, 1960; Halvorsen, 1965)
VII. Physical agents
  A. Ionizing radiation (Chapter 16)
VIII. Etiology obscure
  A. Disseminated lupus erythematosus (Copeland et al, 1958)
  B. Cyclic neutropenia (Morley et al, 1967)
  C. Chronic granulocytopenia in childhood (Zuelzer and Bajoghli, 1964)
  D. Familial neutropenia (Gänsslen, 1941; Bjure et al, 1962; Cutting and Lang, 1964)

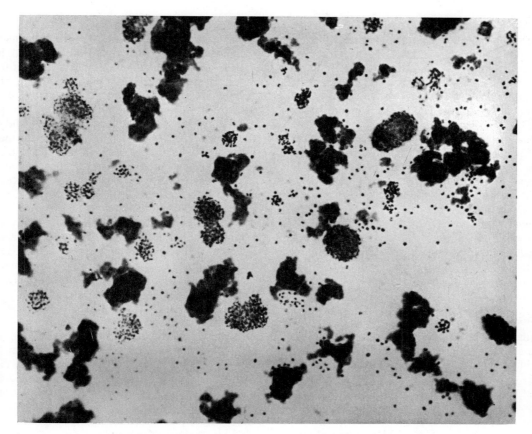

Fig. 15-7. Positive leukocyte agglutination test in isoimmune neonatal neutropenia. (From Lalezari et al, 1960.)

(isoimmune neonatal neutropenia) presents typical clinical and laboratory findings. There is severe neutropenia, which is transient if death does not occur from overwhelming infection. The mother's serum contains a potent leukoagglutinin (Fig. 15-7) that is active against the child's leukocytes but not against the mother's own leukocytes (Lalezari et al, 1960; Halvorsen, 1965). The bone marrow shows an absence of mature neutrophils. The pathogenesis of this disease is thought to be the same as that for isoimmune hemolytic disease of the newborn, i.e., the mother produces antibodies against the baby's leukocytes and the antibodies cross the placenta into the baby's blood and there destroy the granulocytes. It must be noted, however, that leukoagglutinins are demonstrable in many (19% to 24%) parous women (Payne, 1962), so that the rarity of isoimmune neutropenia is surprising.

CYCLIC NEUTROPENIA. Cyclic neutropenia is also rare. It is marked by severe neutropenia occurring cyclically, usually every 21 days (Page and Good, 1957; Videbaek, 1962). It is sometimes familial (Morley et al, 1967) and is probably inherited as an autosomal dominant trait of high penetrance and variable expressivity. The bone marrow shows hypoplasia of the granulocytic series during the neutropenic attack, reverting to normal as the attack passes. Leukoagglutinins have not been demonstrated. The disease is chronic. Clinically, the neutropenic phase is often complicated by various infections, often affecting the mucosa of the mouth and pharynx.

FAMILIAL NEUTROPENIA. The term "familial neutropenia" (Cutting and Lang, 1964) refers to a heterogeneous group of syndromes, having as the common denominator the inheritance of the disease as a dominant, nonsex-linked trait. Included in this group are *familial benign chronic neutropenia* (Gänsslen, 1941; Bousser and Neydé, 1947) and *chronic familial neutropenia* (Levine, 1959). The disease is mild or asymptomatic and characteristically affects several members of the family. The leukocyte count is moderately depressed (3,000 to 5,000/mm^3, 3 to 5 × 10^9/l), with a relative and absolute decrease in neutrophils. There is no splenomegaly.

OTHER NEUTROPENIC SYNDROMES. Splenomegaly is characteristic of two other neutropenic syndromes: *chronic hypoplastic neutropenia* (Lipton, 1969) and *primary splenic neutropenia* (Wiseman and Doan, 1939). In the former, splenectomy is of no value, while in the latter it is curative. Whether or not this is sufficient to distinguish each as a separate entity is doubtful, although chronic hypoplastic neutropenia is characterized by a hypoplastic bone marrow, whereas in primary splenic neutropenia the bone marrow is normal or hyperplastic and the benefit derived from splenectomy indicates that hypersplenism could account for the leukopenia.

Still another neutropenic syndrome can be defined. *Infantile genetic agranulocytosis* (Kostmann, 1956) is a severe disease with onset in early infancy, severe infections, and early death. It is familial but the inheritance is as a nonsexlinked recessive trait, a pattern that also separates this disease from the more benign familial neutropenias discussed in the previous sections. Cases of a disease similar to that described by Kostmann have been reported under another name, *congenital neutropenia*, (MacGillivray et al, 1964). Two cases terminating as acute leukemia are recorded (Gilman et al, 1970; Rosen and Kang, 1979).

As would be expected, there are instances of neutropenia that do not fit even these general categories and have been called *chronic idiopathic granulocytopenia* (Krill et al, 1964; Kyle and Linman, 1968; Caligaris-Cappio et al, 1979). Of great interest is the syndrome called *reticular dysgenesia* by De Vaal and Seynhaeve (1959). It is characterized by both neutropenia and lymphopenia in the peripheral blood. It is reasonable to suppose that the difficulty in classifying the neutropenia reflects the lack of knowledge of basic mechanisms, the situation being similar to that encountered in classifying the myeloproliferative syndromes.

Lymphopenia

Lymphopenia in infants and children (alymphocytosis) is related to thymic hypoplasia and is accompanied by congenital agammaglobulinemia (Chapter 3). Because of the thymic hypoplasia, the syndrome is called *thymic alymphoplasia* (Gitlin and Craig, 1963; Gitlin et al, 1964). The syndrome described by De Vaal and Seynhaeve (1959), *reticular dysgenesia,* may be the same, although in the two patients they described the peripheral blood showed complete absence of both lymphocytes and granulocytes, whereas most infants in whom a diagnosis of thymic alym-

phoplasia has been made show leukopenia (200 to 600/ mm^3, 0.2 to 0.6 × 10^9/l), with a striking reduction, but not complete absence, of lymphocytes and granulocytes. The thymus and other lymphoid tissues show almost no lymphocytes. Hassall's corpuscles are absent, indicating that the thymic aplasia is well established before they normally appear by the tenth week of fetal life. The bone marrow shows absence of granulocyte precursors, and the cause of the double defect is unknown. It bears on the question of the origin and development of blood cells in that the defect does not involve the other cell series. There is also a lack of mature plasma cells, accounting for the hypogammaglobulinemia (Hitzig and Willi, 1961).

Lymphopenia in the adult is not uncommon in disseminated lupus erythematosus, Hodgkin's disease, and lymphosarcoma. It is one of the early signs of the acute radiation syndrome. It is also seen in terminal renal failure and in cardiac failure. Lymphopenia is a normal response to stress (Hurdle et al, 1966; Cronkite, 1967a; Zacharski and Linman, 1971).

Eosinopenia

Eosinopenia can be produced by the administration of ACTH when adrenocortical function is normal. Eosinopenia in stress situations and in Cushing's disease reflects increased adrenocortical activity (Beeson and Bass, 1977). The eosinopenia is produced by temporary retention of eosinophils in the bone marrow. Eosinopenia in acute infection is not dependent on endocrine mechanisms but is mediated by products of the inflammatory reaction (Bass et al, 1980).

16

"This is the very Reason why that which I plainly perceive to be Mambrino's Helmet, seems to thee to be only a Barber's Bason, and perhaps another Man may take it to be something else."

Cervantes: *Don Quixote*

Aplastic anemia, myeloproliferative disorders, leukemia, and lymphoma

APLASTIC ANEMIA
  Definition
  Pathogenesis
  Acquired aplastic anemia
    Ionizing radiation
      Types of ionizing radiation
      Cellular effects of ionizing radiation
      Sensitivity of various tissues
      Hemopoietic effects of radiation injury
      Chronic exposure to X-radiation
      Chronic exposure to thorium radiation
      Radiation injury from isotopes
      Acute radiation syndrome
    Chemical agents
    Laboratory findings
  Familial aplastic anemia
  Aplastic anemia and viral hepatitis
  Idiopathic aplastic anemia
  Relationship with other blood disorders
PURE RED CELL APLASIA
  Red cell aplasia, Diamond-Blackfan type
  Chronic red cell hypoplasia in adults
    Idiopathic hypoplasia
    Red cell aplasia associated with thymoma
    Metabolic inhibition of erythropoiesis
    Erythroid hypoplasia in hemolytic anemia
MYELOPROLIFERATIVE DISORDERS
  Introduction
  Pathogenesis
  General clinical and laboratory features
  Polycythemia vera (erythremia)
    Definitions
    Clinical picture
    Laboratory findings
      Blood as a whole
      Erythrocyte count
      Hemoglobin concentration
      Leukocyte count
      Platelet count
      Peripheral blood smear
      Other findings
      Bone marrow
      Iron metabolism and erythrocyte survival
      Blood coagulation and hemostasis

Secondary polycythemia (erythrocytosis)
    Etiology
      Polycythemia at high altitudes
      Pulmonary disease
      Hypoventilation hypoxia
      Congenital heart disease
      Chronic acquired heart disease
      Abnormal hemoglobin pigments
      Hemoglobinopathies
      Tumors and miscellaneous conditions
      Erythrocytosis in the newborn
      Benign familial erythrocytosis
      Relative erythrocytosis
  Differential diagnosis of polycythemias
  Myelofibrosis and agnogenic myeloid metaplasia
  Osteopetrosis
  Leukoerythroblastosis
  Familial myeloproliferative disease
  Thrombocytosis and thrombocythemia
  Leukemoid reactions
  Di Guglielmo's syndrome
LEUKEMIA
  Historical background
  Definition
  Incidence
  Etiology
    Epidemiology of leukemia
    Leukemogenic effect of ionizing radiation
    Role of viruses
    Leukemogenic chemicals
    Chromosomal abnormalities
    Summary
  Classification
    The traditional classification
    The acute leukemias
      French-American-British (FAB) classification of acute leukemia
      Immunologic cell markers
      Cytochemistry
      Electron microscopy
      Stem cell leukemia
      Acute lymphocytic leukemia (L1, L2, L3)
      Acute myelocytic leukemia
        Acute granulocytic leukemia (M1, M2)
        Hypergranular progranulocytic leukemia (M3)

Acute monocytic (Histiocytic) leukemia (M5)
Acute myelomonocytic leukemia (M4)
Acute erythroleukemia (M6)
Acute megakaryoblastic leukemia
Plasma cell leukemia
  Blood and bone marrow
Mast cell leukemia
  Blood and bone marrow
Leukemic reticuloendotheliosis ("hairy cell" leukemia)
  Blood and bone marrow
Leukosarcoma
The chronic leukemias
  Chronic lymphocytic leukemia
    Blood and bone marrow
    Other findings
  Chronic granulocytic (myelocytic) leukemia
    Blood and bone marrow
    Other findings
  Chronic erythremic myelosis
    Blood and bone marrow
  Dysmyelopoietic syndromes
MULTIPLE MYELOMA, PRIMARY MACROGLOBULINEMIA, AND OTHER IMMUNOGLOBULINOPATHIES
  Introduction
  Multiple myeloma
    Definition
    Blood
    Bone marrow
    Protein abnormalities
    Other findings
  Primary macroglobulinemia (Waldenström)
  γ-Heavy-chain disease
  α-Heavy-chain disease
  μ-Heavy-chain disease
  Monoclonal immunoglobulinopathy without neoplasm
  Monoclonal immunoglobulinopathy associated with neoplasm
  Cryoglobulinemia and pyroglobulinemia
MALIGNANT LYMPHOMA
  Introduction
  Classification
  Non-Hodgkin's lymphoma
    Nodular lymphoma
    Diffuse lymphoma
    Burkitt's lymphoma
    Clinical correlations
    Other features of non-Hodgkin's lymphomas
  Hodgkin's disease
    Classification
    Lymphocytic predominance type
    Nodular sclerosis type
    Mixed cellularity type
    Lymphocyte depletion type
    Clinical presentation and staging
    Staging laparotomy
    Criteria for diagnosis
    Clinical correlations
PSEUDOLYMPHOMA

APLASTIC ANEMIA
Definition

Although a case of severe anemia, leukopenia, and hemorrhagic manifestations was described by Ehrlich in 1888, the term "aplastic anemia" *(anemie pernicieuse aplastique)* was first used by Chauffard in 1904. Since that time the term has been applied rather loosely to syndromes marked by anemia, leukopenia, and thrombocytopenia, presumably on the basis of depressed marrow function. As more and more studies of the bone marrow in pancytopenia were made, it was noted that, while the marrow was hypoplastic or aplastic ("aregenerative") in some cases, as would be expected, in others the marrow was normal or even hyperplastic (Vilter et al, 1960; Frisch and Lewis, 1974). In the latter instances the term "aplastic" could be applied only when modified by such phrases as *atypical aplastic anemia, pseudoaplastic anemia,* and *refractory anemia with hyperplastic bone marrow.* The term "refractory" reflects the unresponsiveness to therapy that is common in pancytopenias regardless of the state of the bone marrow. Though commonly used, "refractory" is not a good term. There are many examples of once "refractory" diseases for which successful therapy was later discovered. A refractory anemia is simply one that does not respond to any known agent. A distinction can also be made between a *familial* form of aplastic anemia (the Fanconi type) and the more common *acquired* type. All things considered, while none of the suggested names is entirely satisfactory unless further modified, the term "aplastic anemia" has the advantage of common usage. This section deals with what might be called "classic" aplastic anemia, in which pancytopenia is the result of an aplastic marrow, excluding infiltrative marrow disease.

Pathogenesis

Studies spanning many years have gradually accumulated evidence for some specific physical or chemical agents as the cause for bone marrow damage (Table 16-1). Ionizing radiation and chemicals are examples of accepted etiologic agents. However, when these and other possible etiologic factors are ruled out, there have always remained many cases of unknown etiology, lumped together as "idiopathic." In these cases, particularly, therapy has been empiric or merely supportive.

Within the last few years new methods have been used to study aplastic anemia, so that we see the beginning of a sounder classification based on pathogenesis. It is now apparent that at least three defects may produce aplastic anemia: (1) absent or defective hemopoietic stem cells, (2) an intrinsic defect in the hemopoietic microenvironment, and (3) suppression of hemopoiesis by immunologic or other suppressive mechanisms (Boggs and Boggs, 1978; Fitchen and Cline, 1978; Karp et al, 1978; Kagan et al, 1979).

Most cases of aplastic anemia are the result of absent or defective hemopoietic stem cells. Agar cultures of the bone marrow show that only a few hemopoietic colonies form, indicating a reduced number of stem cells (CFU-C) in the patient's bone marrow (Kurnick et al, 1971; Kagan et al, 1979). It is probable that the degree of injury dictates future events in the stem cell compartment, so that in a sense the effect is dose related, as in radiation injury or drug toxicity. Most of the etiologic factors in Table 16-1 affect the stem cell compartment. As would be predicted, bone marrow transplantation is indicated when the number of hemopoietic colonies in agar cultures of bone marrow cells is small, indicating diminished or defective CFUs.

The possibility of a second mechanism in aplastic ane-

Table 16-1. Classification of aplastic anemia, excluding aplastic anemia accompanied by infiltrative marrow disease

I. Bone marrow injury caused by physical or chemical agent	30. Pyrimethamine
A. Ionizing radiation	31. Quinidine
B. Chemical agents (see Table 16-5)	32. Ristocetin
1. Aminopyrine	33. Sulfonamides
2. Arsenicals, organic	34. Streptomycin
3. Atabrine (quinacrine)	35. Stoddard's solvent
4. Benzene hydrochloride (Lindane)	36. Thiouracils
5. Benzol	37. Triflupromazine
6. Bismuth salts	38. Trimethadione
7. Chloramphenicol	39. Trinitrotoluene
8. Chlordane	40. Tripelennamine hydrochloride
9. Chlorophenothane (DDT)	**II.** Congenital aplastic anemia (Diamond-Blackfan type)
10. Chlorpromazine	**III.** Familial aplastic anemia
11. Colchicine	**A.** Associated with developmental anomalies (Fanconi type)
12. Dinitrophenol	**B.** Without developmental anomalies (Estren and Dameshek type)
13. Phenytoin sodium	
14. Folic acid antagonists	**IV.** Chronic erythrocytic hypoplasia in adults
15. Gold salts	**V.** Aplastic anemia associated with thymoma
16. Lithium carbonate	**VI.** Metabolic inhibition of bone marrow
17. Mepazine	**A.** Malignancy
18. Mercury salts	**B.** Infection
19. Methimazole	**C.** Renal failure
20. Methylethylphenylhydantoin	**D.** Endocrinopathies
21. Naphthalene	**E.** Chronic liver disease
22. Nitrogen mustard and derivatives	**F.** Viral hepatitis
23. Paraphenylenediamine (hair dyes)	**G.** Allergy
24. Perphenazine	**H.** Pancreatic insufficiency
25. Phenindione	**VII.** Erythroid hypoplasia of bone marrow in hemolytic disease
26. Phenylbutazone	**VIII.** Idiopathic aplastic anemia
27. Prochlorperazine	
28. Promazine	
29. Promethazine	

mia, an abnormal microenvironment, has been supported by finding that in some cases a normal number of hemopoietic colonies are formed on agar culture of bone marrow cells. This implies that the marrow contains a normal number of CFUs but that their environment is not conducive to differentiation (Metcalf and Moore, 1971). Boggs and Boggs (1976) have suggested that depletion of the stem cell compartment may be followed by replication and differentiation of stem cells, i.e., recovery, or replication without differentiation, i.e., no recovery. When stem cells are able to produce hemopoietic colonies in vitro but not in vivo, it can be assumed that the microenvironment in the bone marrow is somehow abnormal or inhibitory to differentiation. In this probably rare situation the transplantation of bone marrow may be ineffective unless the microenvironment is altered or preconditioned. It is probable that the effect of androgens is to alter the microenvironment.

The third pathogenetic mechanism in aplastic anemia is inhibition of stem cells by immunologic or other suppressive activities (Cline and Golde, 1978). Suppression may be of at least two types: one inhibits differentiation by altering the microenvironment, and the other inhibits proliferation. It is not always possible to identify the exact suppressive mechanism, but some interesting studies have been published. Ascensao et al (1976) described a patient whose marrow culture produced few agar colonies, but after treatment of

bone marrow cells with antithymocyte globulin and complement, they were able to form many hemopoietic colonies. Kagan et al (1976), Haak et al (1977b), and Hoffman et al (1977) have shown that the blood of some patients with aplastic anemia contains lymphocytes (T-lymphocytes) (Amare et al, 1978) that suppress the development of hemopoietic colonies by normal bone marrow. There are also reports of ineffective androgen therapy unless antilymphocyte globulin is administered, (Speck et al, 1978). The rare instance of an unsuccessful bone marrow graft between identical twins can be ascribed to the presence of inhibitory factors. It is significant that hemopoietic recovery in some patients treated with immunosuppressive agents has been by proliferation of an autologous rather than an infused donor bone marrow (Territo, 1977). It is also noteworthy that cases of aplastic anemia treated with antilymphocyte globulin do not reject mismatched bone marrow (Speck et al, 1978).

These studies are important in that they may provide a rational basis for deciding on the most effective therapeutic regimen for a patient with aplastic anemia. At this time the following guidelines seem justified. If agar cultures show a lack of CFU-C and no evidence of immunologic inhibition, then bone marrow transplantation (Storb et al, 1978) has a reasonable chance of success. If there is evidence of immunologic suppression, then immunosuppressive therapy should be used, either alone or in combination with bone marrow transplantation or androgen therapy (Freedman et al, 1979). Fitchen et al (1979) describe successful therapy by exchange plasmapheresis in a patient having an IgG inhibitor in her plasma.

Acquired aplastic anemia
Ionizing radiation

Joliet and Curie discovered radioactivity about 85 years ago. For better or worse, the atomic age had begun. Although Roentgen's discovery of X-rays preceded the discovery of radioactivity, it was not until Joliet and Curie's discovery had been applied in both war and peace that we appreciated the effects of ionizing radiation. The effect of chronic exposure to X-rays is minor when compared with the severity of acute radiation injuries from a nuclear explosion.

Three factors determine the effect of ionizing radiation on hemopoietic tissue: (1) the type of ionizing radiation, (2) the tissue's sensitivity to ionizing radiation, and (3) the susceptibility of different species to ionizing radiation.

TYPES OF IONIZING RADIATION. The α- and β-rays have little penetrating power. External irradiation with these rays has no effect on hemopoietic tissue since it is well beyond the reach of α- and β-rays. Both α- and β-rays can be damaging, however, when radioactive substances, ingested or given parenterally, are deposited in the bones and bone marrow.

The γ-rays, X-rays, and neutrons penetrate easily and pass through the thickness of the body. In so doing they are capable of damaging deep-lying hemopoietic organs. Dangerous exposure to γ-rays may occur through improper or prolonged handling of radioactive materials. X-rays are used in roentgenology for diagnosis and treatment. The dosage is usually controlled, and the danger of overexposure is carefully avoided. Large doses are sometimes given purposely in the treatment of carcinomas and other neoplasms. Atomic bomb explosions produce a very intense emission of γ-rays and neutrons. The radiation released in Hiroshima was 25% neutrons and 75% γ-rays, whereas the radiation in Nagasaki was almost purely γ-rays. The greater severity of radiation effects in Hiroshima is related to the high neutron exposure (Finch, 1979).

Radiation *exposure* is measured in *roentgens;* a roentgen is a unit representing the amount of radiation that will produce a certain amount of ionization in a unit volume of air. The *absorbed dose* is measured in *rads,* which are units of absorbed energy. One rad is 100 ergs/gram of tissue. In the case of X-rays, 1 roentgen (R) of exposure is roughly equivalent to 1 rad of absorbed dose. Other types of ionizing radiation do not necessarily have the same absorption effect as X-rays; their biologic effectiveness therefore varies. The biologic effects can be compared with each other in terms of the *rem unit*. This is defined as a quantity of ionizing radiation such that its biologic effectiveness is the same as that of 1 rad of intermediate voltage X-rays. One rem is also roughly equal to 1 rad in the case of β- and γ-rays from radioactive isotopes.

CELLULAR EFFECTS OF IONIZING RADIATION. Cellular damage is not produced by rays passing through a cell,

but rather by the part of the ray that is absorbed. Mechanisms of cellular damage are reviewed by Montgomery et al (1964) and by Little (1968). After absorption, ionization and secondary emission cause profound changes in cellular metabolism. One effect is the inhibition or disruption of cellular enzyme systems, particularly those involving enzymes containing sulfhydryl groups. A marked inhibition of DNA synthesis is also produced in the nucleus of the cell, as a result of which mitosis is no longer possible. It has been suggested that the damaging effect of ionizing radiation may be due to the liberation of oxygen, and it has been demonstrated that animals placed in an atmosphere of low oxygen tension are less liable to radiation injury.

In addition to local effects at the site of irradiation, there is evidence to show that some effect is produced at distant points; e.g., leukopenia may occur as a result of intense localized X-irradiation even though the bone marrow is not in the path of radiation (Bond and Cronkite, 1957). It has also been observed that irradiation at one site causes a shrinking in the size of lymphomatous lymph nodes at another, even when the nodes are shielded. The manner in which these distant effects are produced is unknown.

SENSITIVITY OF VARIOUS TISSUES. Different body tissues and cells show various degrees of sensitivity to radiation injury (Table 16-2). In the bone marrow, radiosensitivity of the cells in order of decreasing sensitivity are lymphocytes, normoblasts, granulocytes, and megakaryocytes (Cronkite, 1967b).

HEMOPOIETIC EFFECTS OF RADIATION INJURY. Lymphocytes are the most susceptible blood cells. Within a few hours after a lymph node is exposed to gamma irradiation, disintegration of the nuclei of the lymphocytes occurs. This is followed by the breakup of these cells and ingestion of the fragments by phagocytic cells; 24 to 36 hours after the injury, only fixed and phagocytic reticulum cells remain. When the spleen is irradiated, the lymphoid cells of the white pulp also show these changes. Atypical binucleated lymphocytes are sometimes found in the peripheral blood of persons exposed to ionizing radiation (Dickie and Hempelmann, 1947; Roy-Taranger et al, 1965).

About 3 days after high-dose, whole-body irradiation, marked lymphopenia is seen in the peripheral blood. Transient neutrophilic leukocytosis usually occurs at the same time. By the sixth day there is neutropenia as well as lymphopenia (Brown and Abbatt, 1955). Anemia develops much later, even though normoblasts are very susceptible to radiation injury. This is explained by the long life span of erythrocytes and by the fact that adult erythrocytes are not easily damaged by ionizing radiation. On the seventh or eighth day, few or no megakaryocytes can be found in the bone marrow, and the peripheral blood shows severe thrombocytopenia. No obvious relationship exists between irradiation and the number of circulating eosinophils. Either eosinopenia or eosinophilia may occur after massive irradiation, the latter to a sometimes striking degree. In the recovery phase following severe radiation injury, the peripheral blood findings are determined by the rate of regeneration from the various parent cells.

There is no longer any doubt that the incidence of leukemia is increased in proportion to the exposure to ionizing

Table 16-2. Susceptibility of various cells to radiation injury in order of decreasing sensitivity*

Lymphocytes	Basal cells of epidermis
Normoblasts	Connective tissue cells
Germinal epithelium of testis	Bone cells
	Liver cells
Myeloblasts	Pancreatic cells
Monocytes	Renal cells
Megakaryocytes	Nerve cells
Epithelium of intestinal mucosa	Muscle cells
	Reticulum cells
Germinal cells of ovary	

*Data from Cronkite and Bond, 1960.

Table 16-3. Sources of exposure to ionizing radiation

A. Natural sources
1. Cosmic rays
2. From naturally occurring radioactive materials

B. Artificial sources
1. Medical
   a. Diagnostic X-ray procedures
   b. Radiotherapy
   c. Radioisotopes
2. Occupational
3. Radioactive contamination
   a. Nuclear bombs
   b. Disposal of radioactive wastes
   c. Accidental

Table 16-4. Biologic effects of radiation*

Dose rate (R/wk)	Total dose (rem)	Description	Effect
0.001		Cosmic rays at sea level	None detectable
0.002-0.005		Natural background	None detectable
0.001		Fallout from bomb tests	None detectable
0.01		Entire population—whole body	Maximum permissible for general population
0.1		Whole body after age 18	Maximum permissible for radiation workers
0.02	50	Entire population—whole body	Statistical life span shortening
0.04	60	Entire population—gonadal—to age 30	Estimated doubling of mutation rate
0.3		Whole body	None detectable
1.5		Hands	None detectable
5.0	5,000	Radium in bone (0.5 μc); 20 yr	Marginal bone tumor induction
7.0		Whole body—long term	Leukopenia
50.0		Whole body—long term	Carcinogenesis
	0.02-0.2	Chest examination—local	None detectable
	10-30	Gasrointestinal series—local	None detectable
	1.5-100	Teeth—local	None detectable
	5-250	Fluoroscopy—local	None detectable
	2-4	Whole body—in utero	Doubling of childhood cancer
	200	Single dose—to thyroid gland—in children	Marginal cancer induction
	300	Single dose—skin	Hair loss
	300-1,000	Single dose—skin	Erythema
	1,500	Single dose—eyes	Cataracts
	2,000	Single dose—skin	Marginal cancer induction
	6,000	Single dose—tumor	Lethal to tumor
	25	Single dose—whole body	Blood cell changes
	50	Single dose—whole body	Marginal radiation sickness
	150	Single dose—whole body	Recoverable radiation sickness
	200	Single dose—whole body	Marginal radiation death
	450	Single dose—whole body	LD_{50} in humans
	900	Single dose—whole body	LD_{100} in humans
	300	Single dose—ovaries	Sterility
	500	Single dose—testes	Sterility
	10^3 to 10^4	Single dose	Lethal to insects
	10^4 to 5×10^6	Single dose	Lethal to bacteria
	10^6 to 5×10^7	Single dose	Lethal to viruses
	2×10^8	Single dose	Radiation polymerization of plastics

*Data from Aronow et al, 1962. See also Pasternack and Heller, 1968; Penfil and Brown, 1968.

radiation. In both Hiroshima and Nagasaki the incidence of leukemia in survivors rose two to five times as high as the baseline, the peak occurring 7 years after the exposure (Moloney, 1955). Most radiation-induced leukemias are of the granulocytic type. A higher incidence of malignant lymphoma and multiple myeloma has also been found (Nishiyama et al, 1973). While exposure to ionizing radiation from explosion of fission and thermonuclear bombs is the most fearsome threat, other sources of radiation are equally dangerous (Tables 16-3 and 16-4).

CHRONIC EXPOSURE TO X-RADIATION. Early experimenters, who did not appreciate the danger of chronic exposure to X-radiation, suffered such complications as hyperkeratosis and squamous cell carcinoma of the skin. Modern radiologists are more conscious of the danger of overexposure; yet before better safety measures were adopted, the incidence of leukemia was nine times higher in this group than for doctors in general (March, 1950, 1961). Chronic exposure can produce mild leukopenia characterized by relative and absolute granulocytopenia and relative lymphocytosis. There may be mild anemia, with some macrocytosis. Leukocytosis, polycythemia, and leukemoid reactions have been described. The platelet count may drop; if it is below $100,000/mm^3$ ($0.1 \times 10^{12}/l$), there is strong evidence of overexposure.

The hematologic effects of radiation injury also depend on the manner of exposure. Martland (1929) described radium poisoning in workers engaged in painting watch dials with a luminous paint containing radium. The radium was ingested as a result of wetting the paintbrush between their lips. The patients showed profound anemia and necrosis of the bones of the jaws, and some died of sepsis. At necropsy the bone marrow was found to be hyperplastic, no fatty marrow remaining in the long bones. The radium had been deposited in the bones and was thus in close proximity to the bone marrow.

Following Martland's reports, others were found and the syndrome was further defined. Hematologically, the findings are an excellent example of the multiple manifestations of abnormal myeloproliferation. Early in the disease, typical aplastic anemia with pancytopenia and hypocellular bone marrow is seen. Later the marrow becomes hyperplastic, and the peripheral blood shows macrocytic erythrocytes, immature leukocytes, and sometimes striking leukocytosis with leukemoid reaction. Neoplasms of the bone and nearby tissues are also found in some cases (Woodard and Higinbotham, 1962).

CHRONIC EXPOSURE TO THORIUM RADIATION. Thorium dioxide in the form of a colloidal suspension (Thorotrast) was once used for contrast radiography, but because of its potential danger to hemopoietic tissues, it has been replaced by other types of contrast media. Thorium has a half-life of 1.4×10^{10} years. The α-particles are emitted primarily, but β- and γ-radiation is also emitted. Thorium gradually breaks down to mesothorium, thorium X, and thorium A, B, and C derivatives that also strongly emit α-particles. After intravascular injection, thorium localizes in the liver, spleen, and bone marrow. In the spleen, progressive fibrosis is produced. Instances of aplastic anemia as a result of marrow damage have been described, as have leukemia and malignant tumors at the site of injection. These deleterious results may become apparent many years after administration of thorium (Duane, 1957).

RADIATION INJURY FROM ISOTOPES. The use of isotopes in research and treatment is now widespread. Careful control of material and the observation of rigid technics by handlers minimize the danger. The dosage needed to determine erythrocyte survival rate, blood volume, and thyroid function is small and not dangerous to the patient. On the other hand, when large doses are used in therapy, as with radioactive gold for peritoneal carcinomatosis, radioactive iodine for carcinoma of the thyroid, and radioactive phos-

phorus for leukemia or polycythemia, the danger of radiation injury is greater. There is evidence that the incidence of leukemia has increased among patients with polycythemia who were treated with radioactive phosphorus (Modan and Lilienfeld, 1965), but this may be due in part to the longer survival of the treated patients (Lawrence et al, 1969). Current use of radioactive isotopes makes it necessary to handle radioactive bodies with particular precautions. A recommended guide for pathologists in the morgue, embalmers, and undertakers is published by the National Bureau of Standards (1958).

ACUTE RADIATION SYNDROME. On August 6, 1945, an atomic bomb was detonated 2,000 feet above the city of Hiroshima. Three days later another was detonated above Nagasaki. At the point of explosion, a temperature of several million degrees developed, causing instantaneous vaporization of fissionable material and fission products—a blinding mass of radioactive gases that formed a fireball. Rising quickly into the troposphere, it dispersed and the effects became negligible. The area under the blast was subjected to grim devastation from the shock wave and the fiery heat. In Hiroshima about 80,000 persons died and an equal number were injured. Those who survived the blast and fire were exposed to γ-radiation and neutron radiation, the dose received depending on the victim's distance from the hypocenter and on the degree of shielding provided by the more substantial buildings (Arakawa, 1960).

It has been concluded that radiation damage was minor compared to the effect of the shock wave and fire (Hachiya, 1955; Gerstner, 1958). One estimate cites radiation damage as the dominant feature in about 10% of the casualties. Understandably, these figures are only estimates. In Hiroshima, 72 out of the 190 doctors perished, and most hospitals were destroyed. The medical care available during the first few days was no more than improvised first aid. Most of those not killed instantly, but seriously injured by a combination of mechanical, thermal, and radiation injury, died during these few days. About one-seventh of the casualties were affected by radiation alone. Their case histories provide grim definition of the acute radiation syndrome.

Clinically, these casualties sought medical aid in two waves. The first group, later found to include those survivors nearest the explosion, complained of anorexia, vomiting, diarrhea, and extreme weakness. The symptoms began a few days after the explosion. Many died a few hours or days after the first symptoms appeared. Death was the result of circulatory collapse and electrolyte imbalance; the chief pathologic lesion was a denudation of gastrointestinal mucosa (Liebow et al, 1949). Those surviving into the second week developed leukopenia, high fever, purpura, bloody diarrhea, bleeding from the gums, epistaxis, and hemoptysis. By the end of the second week almost all were dead.

The second wave of casualties affected by radiation did not appear until 3 or 4 weeks after the explosion. It was later determined that these persons were farther from the hypocenter than those in the first wave or were in heavy concrete buildings near the hypocenter. They too had noted some malaise, but this soon passed and was followed by a 3-week interval during which they were not ill. The first ominous sign was loss of scalp hair. This was soon followed by malaise, fever, ulceration of the mouth, leukopenia, thrombocytopenia, and purpura. Leukopenia and thrombocytopenia were most pronounced during the third to fifth week after exposure, and about half of those so affected died during this period. Death was caused by severe bleeding and overwhelming respiratory or enteric infection. In the survivors, the purpura and fever diminished during the fifth or sixth week, and there was improvement accompanied by the gradual return of normal leukocyte and platelet counts. Anemia was a late manifestation, noticeable by the fourth week and becoming most severe in the tenth to twelfth week. Examination of the bone marrow showed atrophy beginning during the third week and becoming maximal during the fifth week, with gradual recovery over the next month or two.

What has been described are the two typical forms of the acute radiation syndrome: the *gastrointestinal,* affecting persons receiving large doses of radiation, and the *hemopoietic,* affecting persons receiving smaller doses. Variations in both and transitional forms between the two were encountered, as would be expected. Follow-up studies of survivors emphasized the relationship between exposure to ionizing radiation and the development of leukemia. Lange et al (1954, 1955) have made a detailed report of 75 cases of leukemia occurring in the survivors. They show the incidence of leukemia to be highest in the group subjected to the greatest exposure. Of the 75 persons, 51 had granulocytic leukemia, the majority of those affected being adults. Only one had lymphocytic leukemia. The largest number of cases occurred in 1950, 5 years after exposure. In a second report, Moloney and Lange (1954) described the hematologic sequence in ten victims who had undergone careful serial studies before leukemia developed. Seven had acute or subacute leukemia; three had chronic myelocytic leukemia. One person was hematologically normal only 10 weeks before the onset of acute leukemia. Those with chronic granulocytic leukemia had evidence of hematologic abnormality long before leukemia could be recognized. They showed mild anemia, chronic thrombocytopenia, and leukocytosis, with immature leukocytes and many basophilic leukocytes in the peripheral blood. This is the best documentation, from the viewpoint of etiology, of a dysmyelopoietic syndrome (p. 729) preceding the development of acute leukemia.

Radiation injuries from the air bursts over Hiroshima and Nagasaki did not tell the whole story. The number of radiation casualties was small compared to the number of blast and burn injuries. The bombs used then are now considered small in comparison to the hydrogen bomb. It remained for another incident to emphasize the danger of fallout when a nuclear weapon is exploded at ground level.

In the early morning of March 1, 1954, a thermonuclear bomb was exploded at ground level on the atoll of Bikini. Upon touching the ground, the resultant fireball instantaneously vaporized thousands of tons of soil that, bombarded by intense neutron radiation, formed a cloud of highly radioactive material. As the fireball rose, a partial vacuum was formed at the base, and very strong surface winds swept many additional tons of surface material and debris into the radioactive holocaust. As a result, a huge cloud of radioactive dust rose to a great height and was blown great distances by airstreams at high altitude. The radioactive dust then settled on regions below in the form of a fallout that emitted highly penetrating radiation.

Though the explosion was a test shot and its effects had supposedly been thoroughly anticipated, 28 Americans and 239 natives on the Marshall Islands of Utirik, Ailinginae, Rongerik, and Rongelap Atoll were seriously affected by the fallout. One child, 1 year old, was ill but recovered; acute granulocytic leukemia developed 18 years later (Conard, 1975).

Twenty-three Japanese fishermen were also affected, and their story is typical of the effects of fallout. On the morning of the explosion their boat lay about 100 miles off Bikini. While laying out their nets, they saw a red glow on the horizon to the west. Some minutes later they heard two sharp explosions. Three hours later a white ash began to fall on their boat and continued falling for about 5 hours. Within a few hours the crew was stricken with drowsiness, fatigue, and gastrointestinal symptoms. By the fourth day, however, the men had completely recovered and were well except for minor skin lesions on the return voyage to Japan, which lasted 13 days. By the time they reached port, only two men had skin lesions serious enough to require hospitalization. However, within 2 weeks evidence of progressive marrow failure appeared in all members of the crew. Most had progressive leukopenia and thrombocytopenia; a few had abnormal bleeding. They remained in serious condition, but 8 weeks after exposure there was evidence of improvement, slower in some cases than in others. Recovery would probably have been complete in all cases had not 17 of the men contracted acute hepatitis, from which one died.

It will be noted that the effects of fallout were identical to those produced in persons heavily exposed to the air bursts. It has been estimated that each group was exposed to about the same air dose of penetrating radiation, 200 to 400 R. With doses in this range, regardless of the source of penetrating radiation, the effect is primarily hemopoietic. With higher doses, bone marrow damage is severe, but the acute involvement of the gastrointestinal tract overshadows the hematologic changes; death may occur before the hematologic effects are well developed. Massive doses in the range of 2,000 R or more usually cause death within 2 days, convulsions, tremors, and ataxia indicating lethal damage to the central nervous system. Of practical importance is the conclusion that the effects of a certain dose of penetrating radiation are the same whether the exposure takes place all at once or over a few days' time. In the event of a thermonuclear attack in wartime it is most unlikely that even reasonably accurate measurements of the radiation dose would be available. The management of casualties by those persons who are left would necessarily be guided by the clinical picture and laboratory findings.

Chemical agents

Many different chemical agents have been thought responsible for producing anemia, agranulocytosis, thrombocytopenia, pancytopenia, hypoplasia or aplasia of the bone marrow, and atypical myeloproliferative syndromes. In most cases a direct causal relationship is difficult to prove. Some agents, such as benzol and benzol derivatives, are almost certainly myelotoxic; many clinical and experimental observations support this belief. The supposed toxicity of other agents rests on less reliable evidence. Because it is important to identify the toxic agent, one is inclined to persist in questioning the patient until a history of exposure to a potentially toxic chemical is obtained. In the absence of in vitro methods for confirming the clinical impression, it is not always possible to be certain that a given drug is indeed the offending agent. This is particularly true in dealing with drugs in common use, such as the antibiotics. It is important to note also that there have been, and will continue to be, cases of "idiopathic" aplastic anemia for which it is impossible to blame any drug. There is a wide variation in individual susceptibility, some persons being very resistant to drugs known to be toxic, and others being liable to a severe reaction from a drug considered innocuous. At one time the Subcommittee on Blood Dyscrasias (Committee on Research, Council on Drugs) of the American Medical Association published a semiannual summary of reports of blood dyscrasias caused by drugs. The Committee did not assume the responsibility of evaluating the reports it received. Table 16-5 lists some of the drugs that have been implicated, without definite proof in most cases, in production of bone marrow depression.

Benzol (C_6H_6) is an important myelotoxic drug widely used in industrial processes and as a base for many other chemicals and drugs. Benzol itself is a common industrial solvent and is used extensively in the rubber, paint, and lacquer industries. It is volatile, and the toxic reaction follows inhalation of the fumes. In recent years the practice of glue sniffing provides an additional, nonindustrial source of exposure to benzene and other volatile hydocarbons. Several cases of aplastic anemia, one fatal, have been attributed to habitual glue sniffing (Powars, 1965). The most common effects of exposure to benzol are mild macrocytic anemia, thrombocytopenia, and leukopenia. Severe anemia is found only when the marrow is severely damaged. Thrombocytopenia and macrocytosis may be the first signs of toxicity. Leukopenia is usually a late manifestation. The bone marrow may be hypoplastic or hyperplastic. Either leukemoid reactions or leukemia can develop. It is noteworthy that Rawson et al (1941) found that in six cases of "agnogenic myeloid metaplasia" there was a history of exposure to either benzol or carbon tetrachloride. This affirms the close relationship between one myeloproliferative syndrome and another.

Gold salts, usually gold thiosulfate, can produce aplastic anemia, but they are no longer used as frequently as they once were in the treatment of arthritis. *Organic arsenicals* such as arsphenamine, neoarsphenamine, acetarsone (Stovarsol), sulfarsphenamine, bismuth arsphenamine sulfonate (Bismarsen), and oxophenarsine hydrochloride (Mapharsen) are used in treating syphilis and trypanosomiasis. About 1 in 90,000 persons receiving organic arsenicals develops various degrees of bone marrow depression (Freeman, 1944; Kyle and Pease, 1965). Another compound, tryparsamide, is nontoxic.

Aplastic anemia has followed exposure to *mustard gas*

Table 16-5. Some drugs implicated in hemopoietic suppression*

Acetophenetidin (1, 3)	Cycloheximide (3)	Para-aminosalicylic acid (3, 4)
Acetylsalicylic acid (aspirin) (1, 2, 3)	Dextromethorphan HBr (2)	Penicillin (1, 2, 3, 4)
Acetyl sulfisoxazole (3)	Diethylstilbestrol (2)	Phenobarbital (1, 2, 3, 4)
Aminosalicylic acid (3, 4)	Phenytoin (Dilantin) (4)	Phenylbutazone (Butazolidin) (1, 2, 3)
Ammonium thioglycolate (3)	Dipyrrone (3)	Primidone (1)
Amodiaquin HCl (3)	Ethinamate (2)	Prochlorperazine (Compazine) (2, 3)
Arsenicals (1, 2, 3, 4)	Fumagillin (3)	Pyrimethamine (Daraprim) (1, 2, 3)
Arsphenamine (1, 2)	γ-Benzene hexachloride (1, 3)	Quinidine (2)
Atabrine (1, 2)	Hair lacquer (3)	Quinine (2, 3)
β-Naphthoxyacetic acid (2)	Imipramine HCl (3)	Reserpine (2)
Benzene (1, 2, 3, 4)	Iproniazid (1)	Stibophen (2)
Bishydroxycoumarin (3, 4)	Isoniazid (1, 3, 4)	Streptomycin (1, 2, 3)
Carbamide (2)	Lead (1)	Sulfamethoxypyridazine (Kynex) (2, 3, 4)
Carbon tetrachloride (1)	Lithium carbonate (1)	Tetracycline (3)
Carbutamide (Orabetic) (2)	Mephenytoin (Mesantoin) (1, 2)	Thenalidine tartrate (3)
Chloramphenicol (1, 2, 3, 4)	Meprobamate (1, 2, 3)	Thioridazine HCl (3)
Chlordane (1)	Methaminodiazepoxide (Librium) (3)	Tolazoline HCl (1, 2
Chlorophenothane (DDT) (1, 2)	Methapyrilene HCl (4)	Tolbutamide (1, 2, 3)
Chlorothiazide (3)	Methylpromazine (3)	Tolbutamide (Orinase) (2)
Chlorpheniramine maleate (3)	Mezapine (2)	Trifluoperazine (1, 3)
Chlopromazine (Thorazine) (3)	Nitrofurantoin (4)	Trifluoperazine (Stelazine) (3)
Chlorpropamide (2)	Novobiocin (4)	Trimethadione (Tridione) (1, 2)
Chlortetracycline (1, 3)	Nystatin (2)	
Cinophen (3)	Oxyphenabutazone (2)	
Coldricine (2, 3)		

*More than 500 are listed in the last report of the American Medical Association Subcommittee on Blood Dyscrasias. The drugs listed in this table are those which when given alone have been implicated in the production of dyscrasias. Most reports are of isolated cases with no firm evidence other than clinical experience. 1 = pancytopenia; 2 = thrombocytopenia; 3 = leukopenia; 4 = anemia.

and the administration of *nitrogen mustard* compounds in the treatment of leukemia and lymphoma. The effect of mustard compounds is very much like that of ionizing radiation. Some of the *antibiotics,* such as the sulfonamides, streptomycin, and chloramphenicol, have been blamed for producing marrow depression, the latter supposedly because of the toxic effect of the benzene ring it contains. An instance of chloramphenicol-induced aplastic anemia is detailed in Case 9, Fig. 5-35, p. 250. There is no doubt that chloramphenicol is an extremely dangerous drug (Yunis and Bloomberg, 1964; Best, 1967). From the hematologist's viewpoint, it should be outlawed. In none of the instances we have seen of aplastic anemia induced by chloramphenicol could the use of the drug be justified. Reversible erythropoietic depression occurs in about half of all patients who are given the drug. The incidence of irreversible marrow depression is low (about 1 in 100,000 persons), but the mortality rate is high in this group. Characteristic of chloramphenicol toxicity is vacuolization of the normoblasts in the bone marrow and an increase in the serum iron concentration and iron-binding capacity. It is thought that chloramphenicol attacks stem cells at the level of mitochondrial protein synthesis (Yunis, 1973). Aplastic anemia caused by chloramphenicol may transform into acute leukemia (Gadner et al, 1973).

Drugs used in the treatment of epilepsy, particularly trimethadione (Tridione) and mephenytoin (Mesantoin), occasionally produce aplastic anemia (Huijgens et al, 1978). According to Yunis et al (1967) the toxic effect of phenytoin (Dilantin) is the inhibition of DNA synthesis in erythroid cells, probably at the step of deoxyribotide synthesis. During World War II, quinacrine hydrochloride (Atabrine), an antimalaria drug, was found to sometimes produce aplastic anemia. According to Custer (1946) the incidence of this complication was about 1 out of every 35,000 soldiers who took the drug.

The mechanism by which a drug produces pancytopenia is not always a simple matter of a primary depression of hemopoiesis. It is true that ionizing radiation, folic acid antagonists, and nitrogen mustards apparently have a direct cytotoxic effect. Other agents seem to depend to a large extent on individual susceptibility. The sensitivity may be immunologic. It has been postulated that in some cases the drug acts as a hapten that combines with a protein constituent of the cell to form a complex antigen. Immune bodies formed in response to such an antigen would be capable of cytotoxic action. Such action can be exerted against immature cells in the bone marrow as well as against cells in the peripheral blood, the two effects combining to produce peripheral cytopenia. In almost all cases of aplastic anemia, whether congenital or acquired, there is an increase in the level of fetal hemoglobin (Hb F), up to 15% of total pigment (Shahidi et al, 1962). This interesting finding may indicate that the injury to early erythroid cells produces not only maturation arrest but also a reversion to the fetal system of hemoglobin synthesis (Chapter 14). It has been suggested that those patients with higher levels of Hb F are more likely to undergo remission of the aplastic anemia (Bloom and Diamond, 1968).

The hemolytic anemias caused by immune bodies and the immune thrombocytopenias are examples of peripheral cytotoxic effects. In isoimmune hemolytic anemia there may be a myelotoxic effect as well. Cannemeyer et al (1955) have found that sensitivity to para-aminosalicylic acid may produce lymphadenopathy, splenomegaly, and hepatomegaly. Abnormal lymphocytes, indistinguishable from infectious mononucleosis cells, are found in the peripheral blood. They suggest that these findings reflect hyperactivity of reticuloendothelial cells that have been stimulated to form antibodies. It is noteworthy that aplastic anemia is a rare complication of infectious mononucleosis (Van Doornik et al, 1978).

The prognosis in drug-induced aplastic anemia is not easily assessed. While the disease should be considered serious, the course in a given case may be mild or severe. When a possible etiologic agent is discovered, it is imperative that administration of that drug, and of all other potentially dangerous drugs, be discontinued immediately. If this is followed by improvement, it may support the supposed causal relationship, but a spontaneous remission may also have taken place. For the same reason, it is not always possible to evaluate the effectiveness of therapy.

Therapy is based on keeping the patient alive with transfusions of fresh blood while trying to stimulate hemopoiesis by other means. Corticosteroids and androgens are sometimes effective. Some investigators feel that splenectomy is beneficial though seldom curative. Even with optimum care about half of the persons showing severe pancytopenia die within 3 to 24 months. Those who survive past this time sometimes have a spontaneous remission that cannot be credited to the therapeutic regimen.

Laboratory findings

The laboratory findings in a classic type of complete marrow aplasia are a pancytopenia, with extremely low leukocyte, erythrocyte, hemoglobin, and platelet counts. The erythrocytes in the peripheral blood smear are normocytic and hypochromic; there is a lack of reticulocytes, and the leukocyte differential shows an almost complete absence of neutrophils and a predominance of lymphocytes. As noted, Hb F may be elevated, and erythropoietin levels are usually increased.

This classic picture may not be found when there is partial damage to the bone marrow or, as is not infrequent, when one cell type is depressed more than the others. For example, neutropenia and thrombocytopenia may be severe while the anemia is mild, a not uncommon reaction to drugs responsible for marrow depression. As discussed in the following section, aplasia of the marrow in other myeloproliferative syndromes may have a leukoerythroblastic peripheral blood picture.

In the classic type of aplastic anemia (by definition, pancytopenia and aplastic bone marrow), biopsied marrow tissue shows little or no hemopoietic tissue. However, a biopsy, even at multiple sites, does not necessarily represent all the marrow space. In fact, a more complete examination at necropsy usually shows some islands of hemopoietic tissue, often hyperplastic (Fig. 5-2, p. 213) (Frisch and Lewis, 1974). Frisch et al (1975) have studied the ultrastructural features of the erythroid cells in these isolated islands of regeneration and found megaloblastic changes as well as other evidence of "dyserythropoiesis," i.e., binucleated and multinucleated cells, intercellular bridges containing microtubules, cytoplasmic cisternal structures, intranuclear inclusions, and anomalies of the nuclear membrane. Whether these erythroid anomalies are a primary component of the disease, as these authors imply, is intriguing but questionable. The wonders revealed by the electron microscope sometimes remind me of how Leeuwenhoek looked at spermatozoa for the first time with his primitive microscope and saw a tiny man (homunculus) within them.

Familial aplastic anemia

The syndromes included in this category are characterized by pancytopenia in children, and this distinguishes them from pure red cell aplasia of the Diamond-Blackfan type. There is usually a familial tendency, another distinguishing feature. Two types of familial aplastic anemia have been described.

The type described by Fanconi in 1927 (Schmid, 1967) (*anemia perniciosiforme constituzionale infantile*) has the following features. Affected children show numerous somatic and metabolic abnormalities; growth failure, skeletal anomalies, micocephaly, mental retardation, hypogonadism, hypogenitalism, nephrosis, glycosuria, aminoaciduria, and pigmentation of the skin. The hematologic feature is aplasia of the bone marrow, often accompanied by fibrosis, anemia, leukopenia, and thrombocytopenia. The spleen is very small in most patients. It should be noted that before the syndrome is fully established, the bone marrow may be normocellular or even hypercellular.

The second type, described by Estren and Dameshek (1947) (familial hypoplastic anemia of childhood), shows the same hematologic features but without the anomalies of the Fanconi type. Out of eight patients reported, seven died by the age of 10 years; one had a splenectomy and survived beyond this age.

Aplastic anemia and viral hepatitis

A severe form of aplastic anemia may follow the onset of viral hepatitis. Ajlouni and Doeblin (1974) summarize 88 cases in the literature and describe two additional cases. The age and sex distribution parallel that of viral hepatitis, and an 88% mortality rate is reported. It is not known why some subjects develop aplastic anemia when the majority do not. There may be an individual susceptibility to cellular damage by the virus, and it is perhaps pertinent to note that Worledge and Dacie (1969) reported a case of fatal aplastic anemia following infectious mononucleosis.

Idiopathic aplastic anemia

When careful clinical and laboratory investigations reveal no apparent cause for an aplastic anemia, there remains only the classification "idiopathic" (Movitt et al, 1963). Half or more of all cases of aplastic anemia fall into this category (Corrigan, 1974). Although one should always be reluctant to fall back on any term that includes the word "idiopathic," it is equally undesirable to implicate an etiologic agent when the proof is unreasonably remote. In aplastic anemia, particularly, the more searching the history, the more likely it is to uncover exposure to a drug or agent that conceivably may have had a toxic action on the bone marrow. This is a very difficult problem, and in the absence of an in vitro test it becomes a matter of probability, elimination, and, at times, rejection of a ready-made but untrue explanation.

Relationship with other blood disorders

It has been suggested that during or after aplastic anemia a clone of abnormal erythroid and stem cells arises that proliferates and gives rise to sideroblastic anemia (Geary et al, 1974), leukemia (Delamore and Geary, 1971), or paroxysmal nocturnal hemoglobinuria (Lewis and Dacie, 1967). Conversely, sideroblastic anemia may convert to aplastic anemia (Brittin et al, 1968).

PURE RED CELL APLASIA

The syndromes described under this category have in common a suppression of erythropoiesis with little or no abnormality of leukocyte or platelet production. The literature contains many reports of pure red cell aplasia in which the term "aplastic anemia" is used, but since they represent selective aplasia of the erythroid series, the term "aplastic anemia" should be avoided.

Red cell aplasia, Diamond-Blackfan type

The Diamond-Blackfan type of pure red cell aplasia was first mentioned by Josephs in 1936 and defined later by Diamond and Blackfan (1938) and Diamond et al (1961). Diamond et al (1976) and Alter and Nathan (1979) present comprehensive reviews. It is an anemia that is usually not present at birth but becomes manifest at 2 to 3 months of age. It is slowly progressive and usually refractory to treatment. While anemia becomes severe, there is only mild leukopenia, and the platelet count is normal. The bone marrow shows either a hypoplasia of the erythroid series or a maturation arrest at the basophilic normoblast stage. The basophilic normoblasts are sometimes atypical and large, with large, irregular nucleoli. Failure of erythropoiesis is reflected by the very few or absent reticulocytes in the peripheral blood. Rarely, the disease terminates in acute leukemia (D'Oelsnitz et al, 1975; Krishnan et al, 1978). Hammond et al (1968) report an elevation of erythropoietin titer.

The etiology is unknown (Freedman et al, 1976). There is no evidence of decreased erythrocyte survival. However, the demonstration of an inhibitor in the sera of patients with this type of red cell aplasia suggests an immunologic suppression (Ortega et al, 1975; Nathan et al, 1978a, 1978b; Steinberg et al, 1979). Corticosteroid therapy is effective in most cases (Diamond, 1978), as in the thymoma cases. Since the chief defect is anemia, transfusion with whole blood or packed red cells is indicated.

Chronic red cell hypoplasia in adults

Erythrocytic hypoplasia in adults is of two types: (1) that associated with thymoma and (2) the idiopathic type.

Idiopathic hypoplasia

According to Seaman and Koler (1953) the idiopathic type is defined by (1) chronic normocytic or macrocytic anemia, (2) decreased or absent reticulocytes, (3) marked erythroid hypoplasia in an otherwise normocellular bone marrow, (4) normal leukocyte and platelet counts, and (5) no evidence of extramedullary hemopoiesis.

Although this syndrome is uncommon, it would appear to have a varied etiology (Tsai and Levin, 1957). A few of the reports concern persons also exposed to such drugs as the sulfonamides, benzol, bismuth, and neoarsphenamine (Bithell and Wintrobe, 1967). In the series reported by Schmid (1963) about 10% of the cases terminated as leukemia. Goldstein and Pechet (1965) described the occurrence of erythrocytic hypoplasia 30 years after the onset of pernicious anemia.

Some cases of anemia, usually mild, still remain that show erythroid hypoplasia of the bone marrow and none of the features that would place them in any other category. In our experience, erythrocytic hypoplasia may be secondary to malignancy, infection, or renal failure.

Red cell aplasia associated with thymoma

About half of all cases of red cell aplasia in adults are associated with the presence of a thymic neoplasm (thymoma). Several observations indicate that the thymic tumor is responsible for the red cell aplasia. For example, surgical removal of the tumor is beneficial in about half the cases (Hirst and Robertson, 1967). Specific immunologic suppression of normoblasts and erythroid precursors is the probable pathogenesis, since antibodies to erythroid cells and stem cells have been demonstrated in some cases (Krantz and Kao, 1967; Field et al, 1968; Krantz, 1973; Krantz et al, 1973). Some patients have had an excellent response to steroid therapy (Krantz, 1973) or immunosuppressive drugs (Krantz and Kao, 1969). The occurrence of red cell aplasia in association with various immune phenomena, such as in systemic lupus erythematosus (LE) (Cassileth and Myers, 1973) and isoimmune hemolytic disease (Giblett et al, 1956), lends independent support to the possibility of immunologic suppression of erythropoiesis (Robins-Browne et al, 1977). The thymic tumor is most commonly of the spindle cell type or spindle cell–lymphocytic type (Roland, 1964; Min et al, 1978). River (1966) reports an interesting case in which erythroid aplasia and a positive LE test developed 3 months after thymectomy. There was no anemia before surgery. This patient also had an elevated level of plasma eythropoietin.

There is moderate to severe anemia. The erythrocytes are normocytic and normochromic. There is an absence of reticulocytes in the blood. The leukocytes and platelets are normal. The serum iron concentration is greater than normal, with almost complete saturation of iron-binding capacity, reflecting the lack of hemoglobin synthesis. The bone marrow shows a marked reduction of maturing erythroid cells. In contrast, granulopoiesis and thrombopoiesis are normal.

Metabolic inhibition of erythropoiesis

"Metabolic inhibition of erythropoiesis" is not a good term, but it will do to describe mild normochromic anemia accompanied by erythroid hypoplasia of the bone marrow in patients having malignancy (Banerjee and Narang, 1967;

Napoli and Wallach, 1976), infection, renal failure, endocrinopathies, chronic liver disease, pancreatic insufficiency, and occasionally allergy. In many of these states, anemia is attributable to detectable factors such as decreased erythrocyte survival, but often a thorough investigation serves only to eliminate all such mechanisms, leaving only the anemia (refractory to treatment), the hypoplasia of the bone marrow, and one of the conditions listed. There would be little justification for this category were it not for the observation that an anemia, otherwise refractory to all therapy, frequently improves when the underlying condition is remedied (Napoli and Wallach, 1976). The transient pure red cell aplasia seen in some cases of viral hepatitis may be caused by cell-mediated immunologic suppression (Wilson et al, 1980).

Erythroid hypoplasia in hemolytic anemia

Temporary or prolonged hypoplasia of the erythroid elements in the bone marrow (the so-called *aplastic crisis*) is occasionally seen in congenital spherocytic anemia, in sickle cell anemia, and in paroxysmal nocturnal hemoglobinuria (PNH) (Bauman and Swisher, 1967). The pathogenesis of the hypoplasia in these conditions is not known. Of particular interest with respect to pathogenesis are reports of erythroid hypoplasia in idiopathic immune hemolytic anemia in which it may be supposed that a circulating antibody, whose presence is confirmed by a positive antiglobulin test, affects erythroid precursors as well as adult erythrocytes.

MYELOPROLIFERATIVE DISORDERS
Introduction

The iron-deficiency, megaloblastic, and hemolytic anemias are readily classified according to pathogenesis and morphology. The clinical syndromes are sharply defined, and the diagnostic criteria are commonly accepted. Thus in most cases therapy is based on sound physiologic principles. In contrast, the hematologic disorders discussed here have long puzzled both the clinician and the pathologist. Indeed, each in his own way has contributed to the confusion, though each has long been concerned with the problems presented and with the search for understanding.

The concept to be developed is that of a group of related but sometimes inconstant syndromes having as a common denominator the proliferation of hemopoietic elements, proliferation that may be either benign or malignant, medullary or extramedullary. These diseases are called the myeloproliferative disorders. The term was introduced by Dameshek (1951) in an editorial speculating on the possibility of a common etiologic agent for myelocytic leukemia, polycythemia vera, agnogenic myeloid metaplasia, thrombocythemia, megakaryocytic leukemia, and erythroleukemia. Dameshek's suggestion was well received, and the term he proposed was promptly adopted; he seemed to have voiced the half-formed thoughts of many investigators. While his suggestion that there may be a common myeloproliferative stimulus, hormonal or steroid in nature, remains only a speculation, the concept that apparently dissimilar diseases are related insofar as each is a manifestation of abnormal hemopoietic stimulation has deepened our understanding of the clinical and hematologic findings. Note that although *granulocytes* is a more exact term for cells containing gran-

Table 16-6. Myeloproliferative disorders

Polycythemia vera (erythremia)	Leukoerythroblastosis
	Thrombocytosis
Myelofibrosis	Leukemoid reactions
Myelosclerosis	Di Guglielmo's syndrome
Agnogenic myeloid metaplasia	Leukemia (nonlymphocytic)

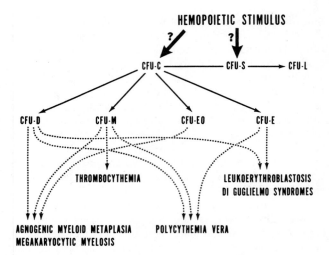

Fig. 16-1. Derivation of the myeloproliferative syndromes, excluding leukemia. Stem cell nomenclature as in Table 1-1, p. 4.

ules, their origin from bone marrow, as distinct from lymph nodes, gave rise to the term *myeloid*. In general the two terms are synonymous and are considered so in this text.

Previously, pathologists and hematologists had directed their efforts toward establishing criteria to distinguish among and identify diseases showing in various combinations features such as (1) leukocytosis or leukopenia with immature cells (myeloid or erythroid) in the peripheral blood, (2) bone marrow that might be aplastic, sclerotic, hyperplastic, infiltrated with tumor cells, or normal, (3) various degrees of splenomegaly and hepatomegaly, (4) anemia, and (5) polycythemia. The question of leukemia versus a benign process overshadowed all others.

In the previous edition of this book the polymorphous features of the myeloproliferative syndromes were tabulated according to the chief presentation of the syndrome. Most of the terms are now of only historical interest. The most commonly used terms are given in Table 16-6.

Pathogenesis

Current thinking is that myeloproliferative syndromes represent clonal proliferation of hemopoietic stem cells (Adamson and Fialkow, 1978; Jacobson et al, 1978) (Fig. 16-1). The evidence for this is strong, at least for some of the common syndromes. For example, the patient with agnogenic myeloid metaplasia studied by Jacobson et al (1978) was heterozygous at the X-linked G-6-PD locus; thus both type A and type B isoenzymes were found in nonhematopoietic cells. In contrast, only one type of G-6-PD isoenzyme (type A) was found in granulocytes, red blood cells, and platelets. The same isoenzyme distribution was found in polycythemia vera (Adamson et al, 1976) and in primary myelofibrosis (Kahn et al, 1975). A second line of evidence for the clonal origin is derived from chromosome studies. The evidence that chronic granulocytic leukemia is clonal is strong because of the characteristic Ph[1] (Philadelphia) chromosome in all types of blood cells. Characteristic chromosome patterns in other myeloproliferative disorders are less convincing. Nevertheless, it must be accepted that the myeloproliferative syndromes are the result of monoclonal proliferation at the stem cell level. Less convincing is the concept that since the fibrosis in the bone marrow is reactive, the fibroblasts are not derived from the same clone (Laszlo, 1975).

Many of the myeloproliferative syndromes carry a significantly high risk of terminating as leukemia (Rosenthal and Moloney, 1977), and in this sense some consider them to be "preleukemic." This is discussed on p. 729. There are reports, too numerous to list, of transformations from one disease pattern to another, e.g., from polycythemia vera to

myelofibrosis (Van Den Berghe et al, 1979b; Pettit et al, 1978), or from multiple myeloma to myelofibrosis (Coughlin et al, 1978). The protean nature of the myeloproliferative syndromes is exemplified in the report of Dao et al (1977), in which 33 patients had various abnormalities: 2 had a monoclonal gammopathy, 5 had a positive antiglobulin test, 19 had the i antigen on the erythrocytes, and 3 had a positive heterophil test.

General clinical and laboratory features

The clinical or laboratory findings that call attention to the existence of myeloproliferative disease can be quite varied, as would be expected. In general, however, one or more of the following might be the presenting sign or symptom: (1) anemia, (2) polycythemia, (3) leukocytosis, (4) presence of teardrop erythrocytes (Fig. 16-2), macrocytes, and nucleated erythroid precursors in the peripheral blood smear, (5) thrombocytosis, (6) thrombocytopenia, (7) purpura or other hemorrhagic manifestations, (8) splenomegaly, (9) hepatomegaly, (10) fibrotic, sclerotic, aplastic, or hyperplastic bone marrow, and (11) portal hypertension.

The occurrence of anemia in the myeloproliferative disorders deserves special mention. It is a variable finding and, when present, may be mild to moderately severe. In most instances, anemia is due to ineffective erythropoiesis or shortened erythrocyte survival secondary to splenomegaly. In some instances the marrow is found to be megaloblastic and the anemia of the macrocytic type. Occasionally the anemia is hemolytic, associated with a positive antiglobulin test, and of the autoimmune type.

Polycythemia vera (erythremia)
Definitions

Polycythemia refers to an increase in the concentration of erythrocytes in the peripheral blood to above normal. As discussed in Chapter 7, the upper limit of normal in the erythrocyte count depends partly on statistical considerations. In statistical language it is "almost certain" that an

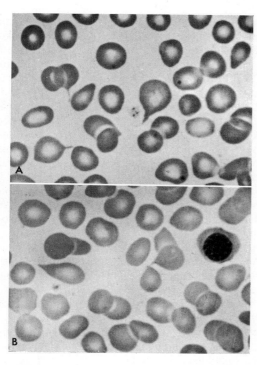

Fig. 16-2. Teardrop erythrocytes in myeloproliferative disorder, peripheral blood. (Wright's stain; ×950.)

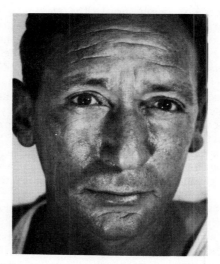

Fig. 16-3. Polycythemia vera. Note ruddy cyanosis and typical suffusion of the eyes.

erythrocyte count of more than 5.7 million/mm^3 (5.7 × 10^{12}/l) in women and 6.4 million/mm^3 (6.4 × 10^{12}/l) in men represents a polycythemic level. Even so, there are some "normal" individuals in whom these values are exceeded (Fessel, 1965).

Polycythemia may be *primary* or *secondary*. Primary polycythemia is usually called *polycythemia vera.* Its etiology is unknown, but it is essentially a myeloproliferative disorder. Secondary polycythemia, sometimes called *erythrocytosis,* accompanies a variety of conditions to which it is probably secondary. It is customary to separately classify a third group, *relative polycythemia,* or *relative erythrocytosis,* caused by decreased plasma volume, but we consider this to fall into the secondary group.

Clinical picture

The disease was first described by Vaquez in 1892 and defined by Osler in 1903 and 1904. It is usually called polycythemia vera, but synonymous terms are "Vaquez' disease," "Osler's disease," "Vaquez-Osler disease," "erythremia," "polycythemia rubra," "myelopathic polycythemia," "erythrocytosis megalosplenica," and "cryptogenic polycythemia."

Lawrence (1955) presents a summary of the clinical and laboratory findings in 303 persons with polycythemia. Of this group, 231 had polycythemia vera and 72 had either secondary or relative polycythemia.

Of the patients with polycythemia vera, 7% have a family history of polycythemia, leukemia, or pernicious anemia. The most common signs and symptoms are (1) ruddy cyanosis (62%) (Fig. 16-3), (2) headache (45%), (3) dyspnea or orthopnea (34%), (4) dizziness or vertigo (28%), (5) eye complaints (27%), and (6) epigastric discomfort (26%). The incidence of thrombotic phenomena is high, affecting about one-third of the patients (13% have thrombophlebitis of the leg or arm, 10% have cerebral thrombosis, 4% have coronary thrombosis, and 4% have thromboses other than cerebral or coronary).

The first symptoms usually occur between 30 and 40 years of age; the disease is most common between 50 and 60 years of age (Osgood, 1965). There is a slight preponderance of men affected (1.3:1) (Modan, 1965). Splenomegaly is common when the disease is in relapse or untreated, some authors reporting an enlarged spleen in as many as 90% of the patients (Wasserman, 1976). The spleen may be enlarged to the brim of the pelvis; hepatomegaly is seen in about one-third of the patients (Tinney et al, 1943).

The etiology of polycythemia vera is unknown. It is not caused by hypoxia, since the incidence of primary polycythemia is low among people living at high altitudes. It has been suggested that polycythemia vera is the result of local hypoxia of the bone marrow caused by capillary thickening and subintimal fibrosis of the arterioles and arteries, but most investigators do not agree with this concept (Hecht and Samuels, 1952). The titer of erythropoietin in plasma is usually normal (Erslev et al, 1979), in contrast to elevated titers in secondary polycythemia; an exception is the case reported by Dainiak et al (1979). In tissue culture, erythroid cells from patients with polycythemia vera respond normally to erythropoietin (Golde and Cline, 1975). Various chromosomal abnormalities have been found (Shabtai et al, 1978). A high degree of unsaturated vitamin B$_{12}$ binding capacity resulting from an increase in transcobalamin III helps to differentiate polycythemia vera from secondary polycythemias (Rachmilewitz et al, 1977).

Polycythemia vera is basically a myeloproliferative disorder characterized by abnormal proliferation of erythroid, leukocytic, and megakaryocytic elements. Each is responsible for certain complications. The elevated erythrocyte count and increased total erythrocyte mass produce a high viscosity of the blood (Dintenfass, 1966) and thus predispose to thrombosis. Proliferation of leukocytic elements often oversteps the boundary of benign proliferation and terminates as a true leukemia (Tubiana et al, 1968). Proliferation of megakaryocytic elements produces an increase in blood platelets in the peripheral blood. Thrombocytosis may have opposite effects: (1) it often seems to favor the development of thrombosis (Chievitz and Thiede, 1962) and (2) it sometimes produces abnormal bleeding, the hemorrhagic state being caused by an inhibitory effect on plasma thromboplastin generation or by abnormal platelet function (Chapter 17).

The incidence of leukemia is high, varying between 14% and 20% in different groups of patients with polycythemia (Tubiana et al, 1968; Lawrence et al, 1969; Weinfeld et al, 1977). The incidence is higher in patients surviving for a long period without treatment but is low among those receiving adequate treatment. All gradations are seen, from leukocytosis, through leukemoid reactions, to leukemia. Almost all leukemias are of the chronic granulocytic type, but the terminal episode may be acute. The splenomegaly is primarily congestive, but many show prominent extra-medullary hemopoietic foci. Some patients also show myelofibrosis.

Laboratory findings

BLOOD AS A WHOLE. The blood is dark and thick. Its increased viscosity is proportional to the increased erythrocyte concentration and may be more than twice the normal. Arterial oxygen saturation is normal (Bader et al, 1963).

The blood volume is usually increased because of an increase in the total erythrocyte mass (Berlin et al, 1950). The plasma volume may be normal or even decreased. It is almost never increased. Because of the variation in plasma volume, the hematocrit does not always parallel the total erythrocyte mass. It is, however, always increased, the highest recorded hematocrit being 92% in a patient with an erythrocyte count of 10.37 millon/mm^3 (10.37 $\times$ 10^{12}/l) (Zadek, 1927).

The sedimentation rate is slow. The MCV may be normal or low; Wintrobe et al (1974) report one patient with an MCV of 61 fl. The MCH is usually normal, but it may be low in patients who have had repeated hemorrhages or venesections. The MCHC is also either normal or low.

ERYTHROCYTE COUNT. The erythrocyte count in untreated patients is usually between 7 and 10 million/mm^3 (7 to 10 $\times$ 10^{12}/l). Unusually high erythrocyte counts are usually accompanied by low MCV values. Lower than normal counts are seen after severe hemorrhage and in terminal leukemia.

HEMOGLOBIN CONCENTRATION. The hemoglobin concentration is usually between 18 and 24 Gm/dl (2.79 to 3.72 mM/l) of blood. It may be proportionately lower than the erythrocyte count when the erythrocytes are hypochromic. Low hemoglobin values are seen following severe hemorrhage and in terminal leukemia.

LEUKOCYTE COUNT. Untreated patients usually show an elevated leukocyte count above 15,000/mm^3 (15 $\times$ 10^9/l). It may be 50,000/mm^3 (50 $\times$ 10^9/l) or more when there is a leukemoid reaction or leukemia. The degree of leukocytosis is approximately in proportion to the increase in erythrocyte count. Most large series of patients studied include some who do not have an elevation of the leukocyte and platelet count, and these cases can present a problem in differentiating polycythemia vera from erythrocytosis. The leukocytes show an elevated alkaline phosphatase score.

PLATELET COUNT. The platelet count is usually increased, sometimes to several million per cubic millimeter. It may be normal or low following therapy that suppresses hemopoiesis and sometimes in acute terminal leukemia. Hyperkalemia caused by increased release of potassium from the excessive number of platelets is called "spurious hyperkalemia" (Hartmann et al, 1958; Myerson and Frumin, 1960).

PERIPHERAL BLOOD SMEAR. The blood smear in the untreated patient is usually characteristic. There is a shift to the left of the neutrophilic leukocytes; immature forms such as myelocytes and even myeloblasts can be seen. Normoblasts are also found in many cases—sometimes as many as 88/100 leukocytes, but usually fewer. Large masses of platelets can be seen when the platelet count is high, and giant platelets are common. Fragments of megakaryocytes are seen sometimes. It may be difficult to prepare satisfactory blood smears because of the high viscosity of the blood.

OTHER FINDINGS. There may be a high concentration of uric acid in the blood. Gout is described in 13 out of 231 patients in one series and in 11 out of 125 patients in another. Hyperuricemia occurs, in general, in about 10% of patients having various myeloproliferative disorders (Yü, 1965). The oxygen saturation of arterial blood is usually normal. The concentration of Hb F is elevated in about 10% of patients (Hoffman et al, 1979).

BONE MARROW. The bone marrow is hypercellular. There is little fatty marrow, even in the shafts of the long bones. It is sometimes aspirated with difficulty, making trephine biopsy necessary. Smears show a large number of cells of all types, with a sometimes striking increase in megakaryocytes. The percentile values are usually normal since there is hyperplasia of all cell types. Sometimes there is a relatively greater increase in the granulocyte series. Basophils are numerous, both in the bone marrow and in the peripheral blood, and they account for the elevated histamine concentration in the blood (Gilbert et al, 1966). With the onset of leukemia, the differential count shows a preponderance of granulocytes, with many immature forms. In acute leukemia there is a preponderance of myeloblasts. Occasionally the bone marrow is found to be acellular or fibrotic (Fig. 16-4).

IRON METABOLISM AND ERYTHROCYTE SURVIVAL. The data available on the life span of erythrocytes in polycythemia vera are contradictory (Pollycove et al, 1966). Some investigators have found the life span to be normal. However, determinations with ^{14}C-labeled glycine suggest that the erythrocyte population in polycythemia vera consists of some cells with decreased survival and some with a normal life span. The rate of turnover of radioactive iron is high (Brodsky et al, 1968a). This may be caused by an increased overall production of erythrocytes plus a rapid rate of iron turnover in erythrocytes having a short survival.

BLOOD COAGULATION AND HEMOSTASIS. The bleeding time and venous coagulation time are normal. Clot retraction is sometimes increased when there is thrombocytosis, and the clot becomes friable. Patients with polycythe-

mia are prone to both thrombosis and hemorrhage. Both may be related in part to the thrombocytosis. Blood from polycythemia vera is more coagulable than normal in the sense that larger amounts of heparin or citrate are required to keep it fluid. On the other hand, we have shown that as the concentration of platelets increases, there is a progressive

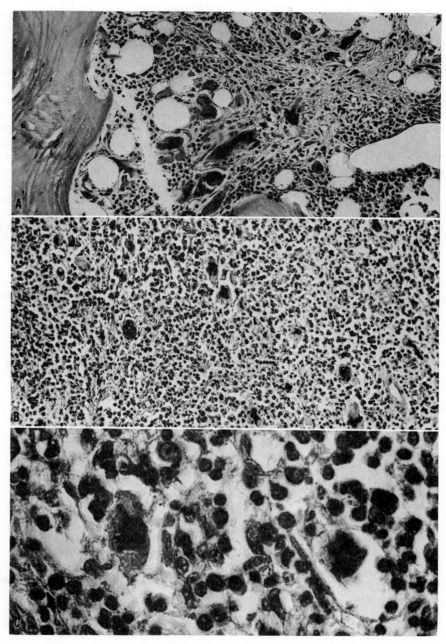

Fig. 16-4. Polycythemia vera followed by myelofibrosis and megakaryocytic myelosis in a 77-year-old white man. Diagnosis of polycythemia vera was established 7 years before death, and the patient was treated with [32]P. Five years later the WBC count rose to 45,000 mm³ (45 × 10⁹/l), and the peripheral blood picture was leukemoid. One year later the peripheral blood picture changed again to a leukoerythroblastic form with many immature leukocytes and 17% normoblasts. During his last year of life the patient developed progressive anemia characterized by markedly decreased ^{51}Cr-erythrocyte survival. Splenectomy was performed. Death occurred postoperatively. **A,** Postmortem bone marrow. (Hematoxylin-eosin stain; ×130.) **B,** Spleen. (Hematoxylin-eosin stain; ×130.) **C,** Spleen. (Hematoxylin-eosin stain; ×585.)

inhibition of intrinsic thromboplastin generation (Fig. 17-12, p. 796). This may account for the hemorrhagic phenomena, but it is not clear why only some of the patients with thrombocytosis bleed abnormally. Some patients are extremely sensitive to bishydroxycoumarin (Dicumarol); this may be an indication of liver damage caused by circulatory congestion and anoxia.

Secondary polycythemia (erythrocytosis)
Etiology

Secondary polycythemia is usually caused by hypoxia arising from decreased atmospheric pressure, impaired pulmonary ventilation (Fig. 16-5), congenital heart disease, arteriovenous aneurysm, chronic acquired heart disease, or the presence of abnormal hemoglobin pigments such as methemoglobin or a hemoglobin variant with increased oxygen affinity (p. 646). The oxygen saturation of arterial blood is low in each of these conditions, in contrast to the normal saturation in polycythemia vera. In a small number of cases the polycythemia is secondary to a tumor or hormonal disorder. In general, secondary polycythemia is associated with high levels of erythropoietin, whereas in polycythemia vera the erythropoietin level in urine or blood is usually lower than normal. This is very helpful in distinguishing between polycythemia vera and erythrocytosis.

POLYCYTHEMIA AT HIGH ALTITUDES. Most of the definitive studies on the polycythemia seen at high altitudes have been carried out in Peru, a country of high mountain peaks, where an estimated 165,000 persons live at altitudes between 14,000 and 16,400 feet above sea level. People living at these altitudes have an increased erythrocyte count and an increased hemoglobin concentration. The blood volume may be normal or increased. There is no leukocytosis, thrombocytosis, or splenomegaly.

Those who live at sea level and ascend rapidly to high altitudes usually develop symptoms of hypoxia such as dizziness, fatigue, nausea, and prostration. This is usually called "acute mountain sickness." A reticulocytosis occurs and is followed by a gradual increase in the erythrocyte count and hemoglobin concentration. At first there is a decrease in blood volume, chiefly because of a decreased plasma volume, which accounts in part for the rapid increase in the erythrocyte count. Later there is stimulation of erythropoietin production and an absolute increase in red cell mass (Whitcomb et al, 1970). When a person returns to sea level, the hematologic values gradually revert to normal. It is interesting to note that persons living at high altitudes have a high rate of plasma iron turnover, but when they descend to sea level, hemoglobin synthesis slows down markedly, and the rate of plasma iron turnover becomes a tenth of what it was at high altitude. Some persons who remain at a high altitude have "chronic mountain sickness" or "Monge's disease" (Hecht, 1971), usually accompanied by an increase in red cell 2,3-DPG (Eaton et al, 1969). Treatment with progestational agents (Lyons, 1976) has been found to increase ventilation and to reduce the hematocrit (Kryger et al, 1978).

PULMONARY DISEASE. Any interference with pulmonary ventilation can produce chronic hypoxia and secondary polycythemia. Some etiologic factors are emphysema, sili-

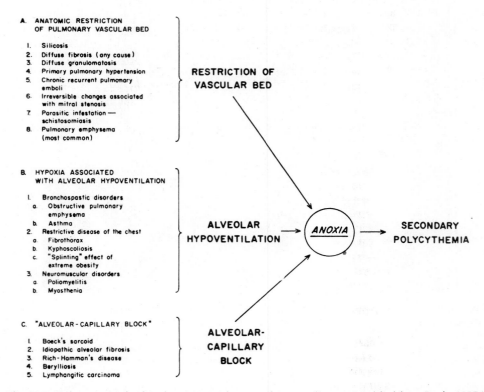

Fig. 16-5. Pathogenesis of polycythemia secondary to pulmonary disease. (Modified from Dack, 1957.)

cosis, cavernous hemangiomas, and pulmonary vascular fibrosis (Ayerza's syndrome) (Porto, 1948).

Several authors have pointed out that chronic hypoxia does not always lead to erythrocytosis. In these cases the hypoxia does stimulate erythropoietin production, but for unknown reasons there is no erythropoietic response.

HYPOVENTILATION HYPOXIA. Hypoxia from hypoventilation not secondary to pulmonary disease can lead to increased erythropoietin production and erythrocytosis. This is seen in the "Pickwickian syndrome" (extreme obesity and hypoventilation) (Burwell et al, 1956) and in "Ondine's curse" (somnolence and hypoventilation of central nervous system origin) (Mellins et al, 1970).

CONGENITAL HEART DISEASE. Polycythemia is secondary to congenital heart disease when the lesion is such as to allow the mixing of arterial and venous blood, thus causing a reduced oxygen saturation in the blood. Polycythemia can be expected in pulmonary stenosis with a septal defect, in patent ductus arteriosus, in persistent truncus arteriosus, in tetralogy of Fallot, and in simple septal defects (Bing et al, 1948).

CHRONIC ACQUIRED HEART DISEASE. Polycythemia is not common in chronic acquired heart disease but is sometimes seen in chronic rheumatic valvulitis and in congestive failure (Hedlund, 1953). There is one report (Levinson and Kincaid, 1961) of erythrocytosis associated with myxoma of the right atrium.

ABNORMAL HEMOGLOBIN PIGMENTS. Chemicals such an aniline, aniline derivatives, coal tar derivatives, gum shellac, phosphorus, and the nitrites produce methemoglobinemia or sulfhemoglobinemia, thereby reducing the oxygen-carrying capacity of the blood. Hypoxia of long standing may then bring about secondary polycythemia (Jaffe, 1966). Heavy smoking may cause erythrocytosis by increasing the concentration of carboxyhemoglobin (Sagone and Balcerzak, 1973; Smith and Landaw, 1978).

HEMOGLOBINOPATHIES. Erythrocytosis secondary to the presence of hemoglobin with increased oxygen affinity is discussed on p. 646.

TUMORS AND MISCELLANEOUS CONDITIONS. Erythrocytosis may be found in association with obesity (the Pickwickian syndrome), fibromyomas of the uterus, hypernephroma of the kidney, hydronephrosis, polycystic kidney disease, bilateral renal cysts, carcinoma of the kidney, the nephrotic syndrome, Cushing's syndrome, hyperaldosteronism, pheochromocytoma, masculinizing ovarian tumor, brain tumor, and carcinoma or hepatoma of the liver (Tso and Hua, 1974; Okazaki et al, 1979). Erythrocytosis is found in some cases of Lindau's disease (cerebellar hemangioblastoma and cysts of the kidney). This type of erythrocytosis is attributed to inappropriate secretion of erythropoietin, as discussed on p. 21. I have seen several cases of erythrocytosis secondary to the administration of large doses of testosterone, an association described also by Kennedy (1962).

ERYTHROCYTOSIS IN THE NEWBORN. Erythrocytosis in the newborn may be the result of congenital adrenal hyperplasia (Gold and Michael, 1959), maternal-fetal transfusion (Michael and Mauer, 1961), or fetal-to-fetal transfusion in uniovular, monochorionic twins (Hodapp, 1962). In the last situation, polycythemia is the result of a shunt of erythrocytes from one twin, who becomes anemic, to the other. The hematocrit is very high (83% in one case), so that the polycythemia would seem to be a result of a relative increase in erythrocyte mass.

BENIGN FAMILIAL ERYTHROCYTOSIS. Familial erythrocytosis has been described in a few families (Yonemitsu et al, 1973; Adamson et al, 1973; Howarth et al, 1979). It differs from polycythemia vera in that it is a benign condition not accompanied by leukocytosis, thrombocytosis, or other features of polycythemia vera. There is an absolute increase in total red cell mass, and the condition is not secondary to any disease known to produce secondary polycythemia.

RELATIVE ERYTHROCYTOSIS. Relative erythrocytosis is not secondary to hypoxia. It is caused by a decrease in total plasma volume resulting from acute dehydration or from "stress." Some persons develop relative polycythemia in response to nervous stress or strain. This is sometimes called "Gaisböck's disease" (Hall, 1965) or Gaisböck's syndrome (Stefanini et al, 1978). The oxygen saturation of the blood remains normal. The erythrocytosis is usually mild in degree, and there is no leukocytosis, thrombocytosis, or splenomegaly. Relative erythrocytosis may be secondary to hypertension (Emery et al, 1974).

Differential diagnosis of polycythemias

Differentiation of the three types is usually not difficult. *Polycythemia vera* is characterized by polycythemia, leukocytosis, thrombocytosis, and such features of a myeloproliferative disorder as splenomegaly and immature cells in the peripheral blood. In some cases the leukocytosis and thrombocytosis are only moderate, but the bone marrow is usually hyperplastic. The arterial blood shows a normal oxygen saturation. There is no elevation of erythropoietin levels. *Secondary polycythemia* shows polycythemia alone, without the other characteristics of polycythemia vera. The oxygen saturation of the blood is reduced, and a possible etiologic factor can usually be found. The erythropoietin level is usually elevated. *Relative polycythemia (relative erythrocytosis)* shows a normal oxygen saturation and none of the features of polycythemia vera. The total plasma volume is decreased.

Determination of blood and plasma volumes may be helpful in distinguishing polycythemia vera from secondary polycythemia but is seldom diagnostic in itself. In polycythemia vera the total blood volume and total erythrocyte mass are increased. Plasma volume is normal or decreased. The blood volume is also increased in secondary polycythemia, although in some cases the increase is slight. The blood volume in relative polycythemia is normal, but the plasma volume is decreased.

Myelofibrosis and agnogenic myeloid metaplasia

"Myelofibrosis" and "agnogenic myeloid metaplasia" are terms used to describe the characteristics of a myeloproliferative syndrome characterized by fibrosis and granulocytic hyperplasia in the bone marrow and by proliferation of granulocytes in the spleen and liver (Feldman, 1974). Extramedullary hemopoiesis may occur at other sites and can take

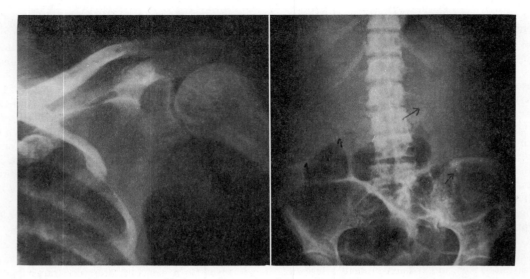

Fig. 16-6. Myeloproliferative disorder, generalized myelosclerosis with splenomegaly and hepatomegaly. Leukemoid reaction in peripheral blood. (Courtesy Dr. R.E. Parks.)

the form of pseudotumors (Waitz et al, 1978). It is a monoclonal proliferation, and it is believed by most that the fibrosis is reactive to the proliferative disease. The terms "myeloid metaplasia" and "agnogenic myeloid metaplasia" are so traditional that they will probably survive forever, but the proliferation of blood cells is not a metaplastic process, since this implies the transformation from one type of tissue to another.

Myelofibrosis is a disease of middle or advanced age, but occasionally it is seen in childhood (Rosenberg and Taylor, 1958), sometimes associated with Down's syndrome (Evans, 1975). The chief symptoms of the chronic disease are progressive anemia, splenomegaly, and hepatomegaly (Figs. 16-6 and 16-7). The anemia is usually normochromic. The blood smear usually shows the characteristic "teardrop" cells, and their number is reduced after splenectomy (DiBella et al, 1977). As the disease progresses, there may be increasing neutrophilic leukocytosis with the appearance of some immature granulocytes and sometimes a frankly leukemoid picture. In the later stages the fibrosis in the bone marrow may be so severe that the term "osteosclerosis" is justified. Biopsy of bone marrow by aspiration yields either a dry tap or hypercellular marrow, depending on the degree of fibrosis or the sampling by chance of a hyperplastic area. Core biopsy is usually indicated and confirms the fibrosis and the cellular hyperplasia. At times, megakaryocytes are numerous, and in that case the term "megakaryocytic myelosis" has been used (Fig. 16-8). Sometimes a leukoerythroblastic picture (increased leukocytes and normoblasts [Plate 64]) is seen. About 20% of the cases terminate as acute granulocytic leukemia (Silverstein and Linman, 1969; Ward and Block, 1971). There is some evidence indicating that myelofibrosis is an immunologic reaction (Lewis and Pegrum, 1978) and that the fibrosis can be reversed by cytostatic therapy (Kelemen et al, 1977). Occasional patients have antiglobulin-positive hemolytic anemia (Khumbanonda et al, 1969). In rapidly developing

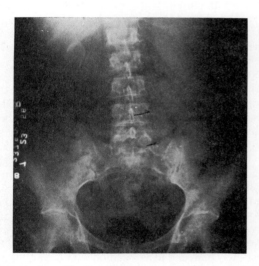

Fig. 16-7. Myeloproliferative disorder, myelofibrosis and splenomegaly. Arrows outline the enlarged spleen.

anemia the bone marrow may also contain megaloblasts (Fig. 16-9).

The proliferating granulocytes in the spleen and liver are probably functional. In a study by Cabot et al (1978) it was shown that splenectomy carries a poor risk if the hemopoietic activity in the bone marrow, as measured by the ^{59}Fe sacral uptake, is insufficient. The liver involvement may cause portal hypertension, development of esophageal varices, and ascites (Ligumski et al, 1978).

Most cases of myelofibrosis run a chronic course, and when leukemia is the terminal event, it occurs some years after the initial diagnosis. In contrast, there are now many reports of an acute form of the syndrome called "acute myelofibrosis," "acute megakaryocytic myelofibrosis," "acute (malignant) myelosclerosis," or "malignant myelo-

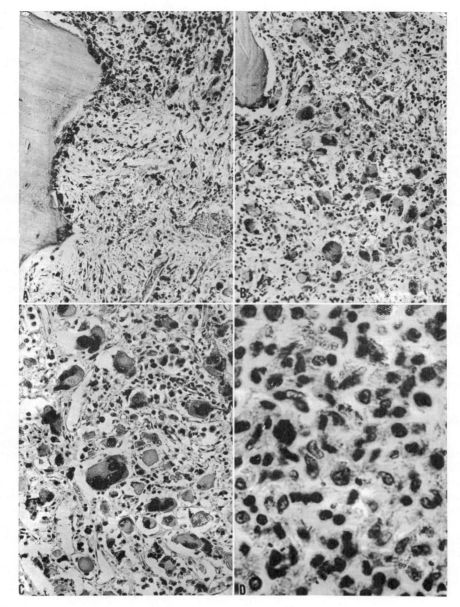

Fig. 16-8. Myelofibrosis with megakaryocytic myelosis of the spleen in a 61-year-old white man. Onset occurred 6 months before death, with pancytopenia, fatigue, and weight loss. There was progressive pancytopenia, and death resulted from thrombocytopenia and hemorrhage. The bone marrow was fibrotic, with striking megakaryocytic proliferation. The spleen was small, weighing 60 Gm, but showed striking megakaryocytic myelosis. **A** and **B,** Bone marrow. (Hematoxylin-eosin stain; ×130.) **C,** Bone marrow. (Hematoxylin-eosin stain; ×350.) **D,** Spleen. (Hematoxylin-eosin stain; ×585.)

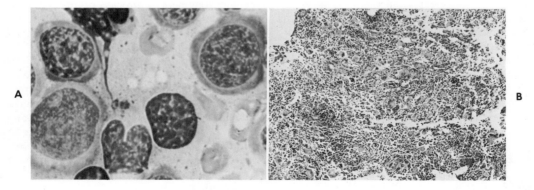

Fig. 16-9. Megakaryocytic myelosis with megaloblastic dyspoiesis in the bone marrow in a middle-aged white man. The patient had been granulocytopenic for 5 years; there was an acute onset of anemia with splenomegaly. **A,** Bone marrow smear. (Wright's stain; ×1,425.) **B,** Paraffin section of bone marrow. (Hematoxylin-eosin stain; ×90.) (Courtesy Dr. Leo P. Cawley.)

sclerosis'' (Estevez et al, 1974; Lubin et al, 1976; Spector and Miller, 1978; Ali and Janes, 1979; Bearman et al, 1979; Weisenburger, 1980). The acute syndrome is characterized by pancytopenia, rare or absent teardrop red blood cells, hyperplastic bone marrow showing a marked increase in reticulin, no significant splenomegaly, and a rapidly progressive clinical course (Bearman et al, 1979). Because the clinical course and cellular pictures are not unlike those of acute granulocytic leukemia, it would seem that one criterion for the diagnosis of acute myelofibrosis would be the absence of the Ph[1] chromosome. Yet I have found only one report in which this is mentioned (Van Slyck et al, 1970), and in that report the chromosomal marker was present. In fact, the existence of acute myelofibrosis as an entity, distinct from leukemia, has been questioned (Bird and Proctor, 1977).

Osteopetrosis

Osteopetrosis (malignant infantile osteopetrosis, Albers-Schönberg disease) is a rare disease in children characterized by densely radiopaque bones, anemia, thrombocytopenia, and leukoerythroblastosis (Yu et al, 1971; Lehman et al, 1977). The course is variable, but often the disease is rapidly fatal. Therapy with prednisone is beneficial (Reeves et al, 1979).

Leukoerythroblastosis

The term ''leukoerythroblastosis'' is applied to any situation in which the manifestation in the blood of a myeloproliferative disorder is the presence of immature granulocytes and normoblasts. Traditionally this picture has been associated with replacement of normal marrow cells by foreign cells, myelophthisis, and usually metastatic tumor (Leland and Macpherson, 1979; Delsol et al, 1979). Weick et al (1974) reviewed 215 instances of leukoerythroblastosis and found marrow infiltration with primary hematologic malignancy in 63%, whereas a surprisingly high percentage (37%) had a variety of other diseases. It must be concluded that leukoerythroblastosis does not necessarily have an ominous connotation.

Familial myeloproliferative disease

Randall et al (1965) have described a familial form of myeloproliferative disease affecting nine children who are first or second cousins living in a rural area within a radius of several hundred miles in the southeastern corner of Colorado. The disease is characterized by onset during childhood, splenomegaly, hepatomegaly, anemia, thrombocytopenia, and leukocytosis. Quite remarkable and characteristic is the finding that while the leukocytosis is sometimes striking (up to 128,000/mm^3, 128 × 10^9/1), the leukocytes show a very low alkaline phosphatase ''score.'' This usually points to granulocytic leukemia rather than to a myeloproliferative disorder, and indeed the first diagnosis made in some of these children was that of granulocytic leukemia. However, neither the morphologic features of the peripheral blood, bone marrow, liver, and spleen nor the clinical course in surviving children supports the diagnosis of leukemia. Furthermore, in no cases was the Ph[1] chromosome found.

Six additional families having familial myeloproliferative disease have been reported by Kaufman et al (1978). Luddy et al (1978) have described a familial myeloproliferative syndrome involving three siblings who also had either thrombocytopenia or abnormal platelet aggregation with collagen, adenosine diphosphate (ADP), and epinephrine. The terminal event in all three was leukemia (granulocytic or monocytic). The mother and five other siblings had a variety of hematologic abnormalities.

The low alkaline phosphatase activity in the leukocytes sets these cases apart from all other nonleukemic myeloproliferative disorders. Because of this, the report of this variant is extremely interesting.

Thrombocytosis and thrombocythemia

When the platelet count (normal 258,800, SD 57,000) is higher than 500,000/mm^3 (0.5 × 10^{12}/1) of blood, there is thrombocytosis. Thrombocytosis is common in chronic granulocytic leukemia and a constant feature of classic polycythemia vera. In these states the proliferation of megakaryocytes in the bone marrow and the thrombocytosis in the peripheral blood reflect the underlying proliferative disorder that affects other cell types as well. Thrombocytosis in these and other myeloproliferative disorders is, in a sense, secondary and not unexpected.

Occasionally the proliferation of megakaryocytes in the bone marrow and thrombocytosis in the peripheral blood occur as a ''primary'' disease in the sense that there is little or no evidence of proliferation, medullary or extramedullary, of erythroid cells and leukocytes. The primary disease has been called ''haemorrhagic thrombocythaemia'' (Schechter et al, 1962). Actually, thrombocytosis is a myeloproliferative disorder whether or not it is seen first as a proliferation of megakaryocytes alone.

Clinically, thrombocytosis or thrombocythemia frequently causes either severe bleeding or thrombosis. With a platelet concentration of 1 million/mm^3 (1 × 10^{12}/1) or more, a defect in thromboplastin generation is demonstrable (p. 796). The defect is most severe when the platelet concentration is highest. When, with treatment, the platelet count is reduced, there is also an improvement in the hemorrhagic disease. Instead of abnormal bleeding, however, some patients show a striking tendency to form thrombi. While this is perhaps most common in the thrombocytosis that follows splenectomy, it is puzzling that one cannot predict in advance which patients with a high platelet count will have abnormal bleeding and which will form thrombi.

Of all the myeloproliferative disorders, this is one in which treatment is directed primarily toward returning the cell count to normal. This has been accomplished with a number of agents used in cancer chemotherapy (Robertson, 1970; Bensinger et al, 1970).

The term ''spurious hyperkalemia'' (Hartmann et al, 1958) has been suggested for the elevated potassium concentration in the serum of patients with thrombocytosis. The potassium concentration is in proportion to the platelet count, and when the count is about 2 million/mm^3 (2 × 10^{12}/1), the potassium concentration is about 8 mEq/l (8 mM/l). The increased potassium is released from the platelets during the release reaction. When the platelet count is reduced by chemotherapy, the serum potassium concentration falls in proportion.

Leukemoid reactions

A leukemoid reaction is one in which the peripheral blood findings resemble those found in leukemia, with the important difference that while leukemia is a neoplastic proliferation and is malignant in nature, leukemoid reactions are benign proliferations.

It is difficult to define leukemoid reaction more precisely.

There is no absolute criterion for the leukemoid blood picture, either in the leukocyte count or in the differential count. Leukemoid reactions mimic leukemia and may show the same quantitative and qualitative changes. In fact, the undesirable term "pseudoleukemia" is sometimes used (Sanal et al, 1979). Nor is there an absolute dividing line between marked leukocytosis and leukemoid reactions,

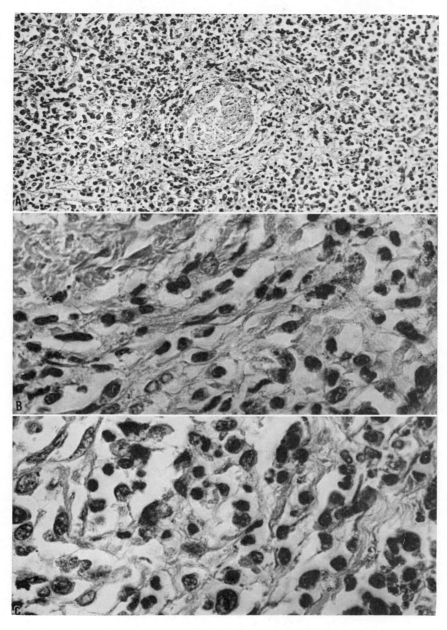

Fig. 16-10. Leukemoid reaction or granulocytic leukemia in a 38-year-old white man. There was a history of leukocytosis for 11 years before a gastrectomy for peptic ulcer. At operation the spleen was found to be moderately enlarged but was not removed. WBC count at that time was 49,700 (49.7 × 10⁹/l); the differential count showed 2% blasts, 24.5% myelocytes, 13% metamyelocytes, 40% segmented neutrophils, and 2% normoblasts. One year before death (4 years postgastrectomy) the patient was treated with cobalt irradiation, following which he developed pancytopenia. Simultaneously there was sudden enlargement of the spleen. Although leukopenic, the differential count on peripheral blood showed 20% blasts. ^{51}Cr-erythrocyte survival was very short (half-life of 7 days). Splenectomy was performed. Death occurred from staphylococcus septicemia. The spleen weighed 3,300 Gm. Necropsy did not reveal typical histopathologic lesions of leukemia. **A,** Spleen. (Hematoxylin-eosin stain; ×130.) **B** and **C,** Spleen. (Hematoxylin-eosin stain; ×585.) Note the siderosis in **B** and **C.**

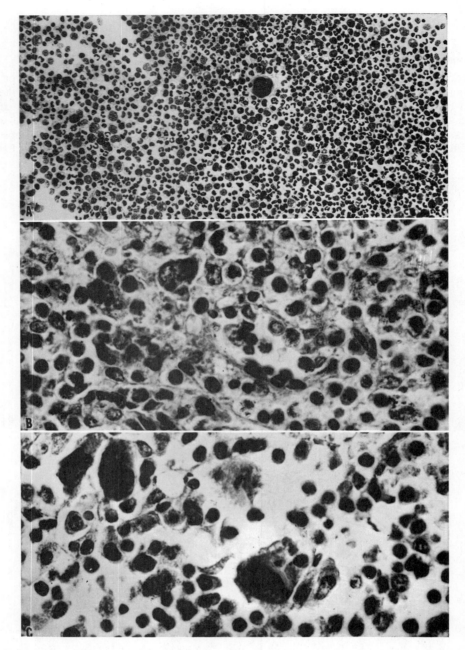

Fig. 16-11. Leukemoid reaction with hepatosplenomegaly and megakaryocytic myelosis, with minimal fibrosis, of the spleen in a 71-year-old white man. The patient was admitted to the hospital because of mental confusion and leukocytosis 1 year before death. Leukocyte count at admission was 74,000 mm^3 (74 × 10^9/l), and there was a shift to the left, with immature granulocytes. The bone marrow during life was hyperplastic. There was striking splenomegaly. Necropsy revealed glioblastoma multiforme of the right frontal lobe, splenomegaly (960 Gm spleen), and cardiac failure. **A,** Antemortem bone marrow aspiration. (Wright's stain; ×130.) **B,** Paraffin section of spleen. (Hematoxylin-eosin stain; ×450.) **C,** Paraffin section of spleen. (Hematoxylin-eosin stain; ×585.)

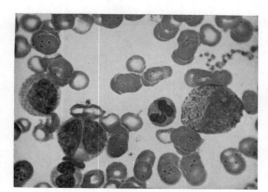

Fig. 16-12. Leukemoid reaction, peripheral blood. (Wright's stain; ×950.)

Table 16-7. Conditions that may cause a leukemoid reaction

I. Infections
  A. Granulocytic (myelocytic) reactions
    1. Pneumonia
    2. Empyema
    3. Endocarditis
    4. Meningitis
    5. Diphtheria
    6. Bubonic plague
    7. Septicemia
    8. Tuberculosis
    9. Leptospirosis
  B. Lymphocytic reactions
    1. Whooping cough
    2. Chickenpox
    3. Mumps
    4. Infectious mononucleosis
    5. Infectious lymphocytosis
    6. Congenital syphilis
    7. Tuberculosis
  C. Monocytic reactions
    1. Tuberculosis
II. Intoxications
  A. Eclampsia (myelocytic)
  B. Burns (myelocytic)
  C. Mustard gas (myelocytic)
  D. Mercury poisoning (myelocytic)

III. Tumors
  A. Embryonal cell carcinoma of kidney (myelocytic)
  B. Carcinoma of breast (lymphocytic)
  C. Carcinoma of colon (myelocytic)
  D. Carcinoma of stomach (lymphocytic)
  E. Hodgkin's disease (myelocytic)
IV. Myeloproliferative disorders (Table 16-6)
V. Miscellaneous
  A. Acute hemolysis (myelocytic)
  B. Acute hemorrhage (myelocytic)
  C. Pernicious anemia following liver therapy (myelocytic)
  D. Megaloblastic anemia of pregnancy following folic acid therapy (myelocytic)
  E. Recovery from agranulocytosis (myelocytic)
  F. After parenteral iron-dextran complex (myelocytic)
  G. Chronic exposure to ionizing radiation
  H. Acute rheumatoid arthritis (myelocytic)

although in the latter the leukocyte count is usually above 50,000/mm³ ($50 \times 10^9/1$). Qualitatively, there are more immature cells in leukemoid reactions than in the usual leukocytosis (Figs. 16-10 to 16-12). It is the presence of immature cells as much as the high leukocyte count that gives the leukemoid blood picture the appearance of leukemia.

In some instances the differentiation between leukemoid reactions and leukemia is extremely difficult if not impossible. Both hematologic and clinical findings may be compatible with leukemia. Splenic puncture sometimes helps to distinguish one from the other, particularly in the case of granulocytic proliferations. In granulocytic leukemoid reactions the splenogram shows some immature myeloid cells and a high percentage of normal splenic lymphocytes, whereas in granulocytic leukemia the predominant cells are myeloid. The bone marrow in a myelocytic leukemoid reaction usually shows a larger proportion of mature cells than in myelocytic leukemia, but the marrow differential count may be much the same in both conditions. As a rule, leukemoid reactions are not accompanied by the anemia or thrombocytopenia so common in leukemia. When any one of the possible causes of leukemoid reaction is present, the likelihood of leukemoid reaction rather than leukemia is increased. The alkaline phosphatase score is invariably high in leukemoid reactions, usually low in frank granulocytic leukemia, and intermediate when the disease is in transition from a myeloproliferative disorder to granulocytic leukemia. The presence of the Ph¹ chromosome is evidence for granulocytic leukemia rather than a leukemoid reaction, but its absence is inconclusive.

When a differential diagnosis between the two cannot be made, it is necessary to follow the patient carefully to determine the course of the disease. Whereas leukemia is usually progressive, leukemoid reactions are usually transient, and with the subsidence of infection or other stimulus, the blood picture returns to normal. Leukemoid reactions may, however, persist for a long time. I have seen cases in which not even the necropsy findings were definitive.

Table 16-7 lists the conditions known to cause or accompany a leukemoid reaction.

Di Guglielmo's syndrome

The excellence of the concept of the "myeloproliferative disorders" is proved by considering how it has clarified Di Guglielmo's syndrome. In 1912 Copelli reported a case of "erythromatosis" characterized by normochromic anemia, splenomegaly, extramedullary erythropoiesis in the liver and spleen, and abnormal erythropoiesis in these organs and the marrow. Although he did not call them so, his description of the abnormal erythroid cells suggests megaloblasts. In 1917 Di Guglielmo reported the case of a patient with erythroleukemia showing mixed erythroblastic, leukocytic, and megakaryocytic proliferation. From this he derived the concept of leukemic erythroblastic proliferation analogous to the leukemic proliferation of other cell types. Actually, the first recognized case of "pure" erythroblastic proliferation was reported by Di Guglielmo himself in 1923. He described two more in 1926. There followed a few reports of cases that resembled those of Di Guglielmo, but a tendency was noted in most instances for mixed erythroblastic-leukocytic proliferation even when the erythroblastic element was dominant. Hence the term "erythremic myelosis" was introduced. It was noted also that sometimes the terminal event was acute granulocytic leukemia; this leukemic element accounts for the term "erythroleukemia." The spectrum of variants that make up the Di Guglielmo syndrome presents an excellent example of transitions from benign to malignant proliferation.

Cases of pure erythroblastic proliferation, the situation originally envisaged by Di Guglielmo, are extremely rare. Moeschlin (1940) reviewed the cases reported and concluded that only five were acceptable. Two of those were reported by Di Guglielmo. Investigators such as Dameshek and

Baldini (1958), who have studied patients with this disease who survived for some years, point out that it is characteristic for this disease to begin as a predominantly erythroblastic proliferation, progress to a mixed erythroblastic-myeloblastic phase, and terminate as an acute myeloblastic leukemia. Di Guglielmo (1946) himself later expanded his original concept of pure erythroblastic proliferation to include these transitional forms, the "polyphasic" group, and even included proliferative processes that affect other cell types

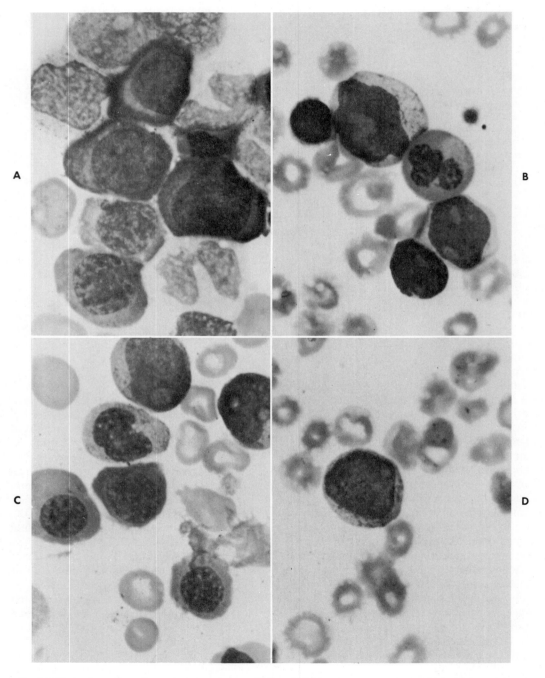

Fig. 16-13. Acute erythremic myelosis in a 4-year-old boy. **A-C,** Bone marrow aspiration biopsy. **D,** Peripheral blood. (Wright's stain; ×1,150.)

almost exclusively. Thus it becomes apparent that although the proliferative process is primarily erythroblastic in rare instances (Di Guglielmo's "acute erythremic disease" or "genuine erythroblastosis"), most patients show the polyphasic pattern common to all myeloproliferative disorders. Dameshek and Baldini (1958) call these cases "Di Guglielmo's syndrome." The term "Di Guglielmo's disease" should be reserved for the rare cases in which the proliferation is primarily erythroid.

Two features are characteristic of Di Guglielmo's syndrome. One is the megaloblastic nature of the proliferating red cell precursors (Figs. 16-13 and 16-14), and the other is atypical bilirubin metabolism.

The nucleated red blood cells in the bone marrow have been described as "atypical," "bizarre," "megaloblastoid," "paramegaloblastic," and occasionally frankly megaloblastic. There is no doubt, however, that the features described are those of intermediate or fully developed megaloblasts. The failure to call them megaloblasts comes not from the lack of megaloblastic characteristics but from a reluctance to use this term in diseases other than those that respond in a characteristic fashion to folic acid or vitamin B_{12}. Yet cells having characteristics intermediate between megaloblasts and normoblasts are encountered in such dissimilar diseases as hemolytic anemia, leukemia, and lymphoma. There is no response to vitamin B_{12} in Di Guglielmo's syndrome.

The extreme erythroblastic proliferation in the bone mar-

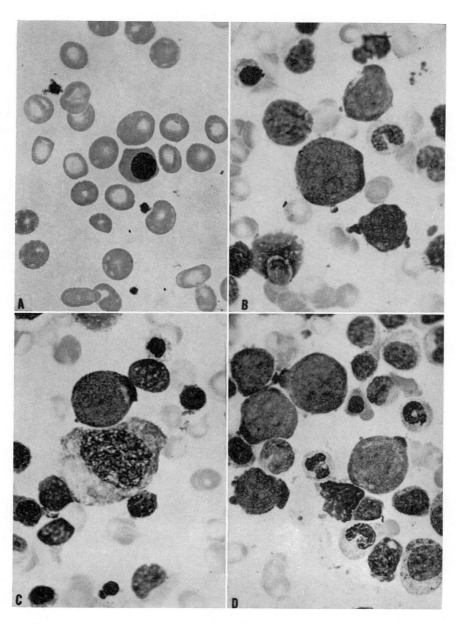

Fig. 16-14. Chronic erythremic myelosis. **A,** Peripheral blood. **B-D,** Bone marrow smear. (Wright's stain; ×950.)

row suggests that usually seen in acute hemolytic anemia. Indeed, there is usually hyperbilirubinemia and increased excretion of urobilinogen. There is not, however, reticulocytosis or significantly decreased erythrocyte survival (^{51}Cr, Dameshek and Baldini, 1958). In addition, the antiglobulin test is usually negative. Dameshek and Baldini (1958) postulate a "heme diversion" situation, similar to that in pernicious anemia, whereby a significant amount of bilirubin is derived from sources other than erythrocyte hemoglobin. As in pernicious anemia, the reticulocytopenia points to ineffective erythropoiesis.

LEUKEMIA
Historical background

It is interesting to note that, historically, leukemia is a relatively new disease. It is new not only in the sense that the first description dates back only 140 years but also because nowhere in biblical or Graeco-Roman writings is there any reference to a disease that might, in retrospect, be considered to be leukemia. This is, in a way, surprising, for the gross appearance of the blood that led Virchow to coin the name *Weisses Blut,* or leukemia, and the sometimes striking splenomegaly and hepatomegaly should have come to the attention of physicians of ancient times. Can this mean that leukemia did not exist before the early 1820s? Or is it merely fortuitous or attributable to lack of gross and, particularly, microscopic criteria? It is impossible to tell, and yet the possibility of a "new" disease is at least as likely as that of an old disease undescribed. As a matter of fact, if one takes Shimkin's (1955) data for gross mortality caused by leukemia during the years 1921 to 1951 and extrapolates back to the baseline (Fig. 16-15), the intersection is at about the year 1850. Admittedly, such an exercise is open to many criticisms, but the conclusion that perhaps leukemia did not exist prior to the early 1800s does have some support from other sources. According to medical historians, the serious study

of human anatomy dates back at least four centuries, and yet no reference to splenomegaly, at least, can be found in the early treatises.

In any case, within a period of about 10 years (1838 to 1847) definitive reports appeared on the occurrence and significance of splenomegaly and the first descriptions of leukemia. Richard Bright's paper in 1838 entitled *Observations on Abdominal Tumors and Intumescence; Illustrated by Cases of Diseases of the Spleen* was soon followed by several descriptions of leukemia as studied both postmortem and during life. In France, in 1839, a 44-year-old woman with splenomegaly died after being admitted to the Hôtel Dieu in Paris under the care of Barth. At necropsy, Donné examined the blood microscopically and found that "a considerable proportion of the cells had all the characteristics of pus cells." Donné (1844) reported this and other cases in 1844. In Scotland, Craigie (1845) and Bennett (1845) both reported cases characterized by splenomegaly, hepatomegaly, lymphadenopathy, and many globules of "purulent matter" or "pus corpuscles" in the blood.

Up to this point the disease had not been named, and, since Donné, Craigie, and Bennett each thought they were dealing with "suppuration of the blood" as evidenced by the large number of "pus corpuscles" in the blood, it can be said fairly that they described but did not further define the disease.

It remained for Virchow (1845) to point out that the disease was not "pyemic," for careful necropsy studies failed to disclose a primary infection that might have spread to the blood. Because the blood in his case was grossly "yellowish white," he referred to the condition as *Weisses Blut.* Two years later he proposed the name "leukemia" and in subsequent years amplified and further defined the disease (Virchow, 1865), pointing out that in addition to the increase in white blood cells there is a decrease in red blood cells. He also distinguished between (chronic) granulocytic leukemia

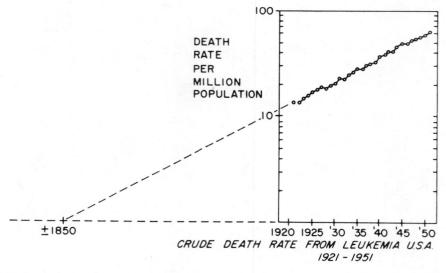

Fig. 16-15. Extrapolation of gross mortality data for leukemia, 1921-1951, back to the baseline. If the extrapolation is warranted, it suggests a very low incidence before 1850. (Data for the years 1920-1950 from Shimkin, 1955.)

("splenic leukemia") and (chronic) lymphocytic leukemia (enlargement of the lymph nodes and presence in the blood of lymphocytes).

It is not possible to estimate the effect of these studies on the developments in morphologic hematology soon to come, but there is a recurring pattern to medical discovery whereby events that must happen do indeed take place. Clearly, it was necessary to concentrate on the morphology and origin of blood cells before the disease could be better understood. From 1877 on, Paul Ehrlich (1891) developed differential staining methods and classified granulocytes as neutrophilic, eosinophilic, and basophilic. Naegeli (1900) (Fig. 16-16) introduced the term "myeloblast" for the primitive cell found in the marrow and in the blood in some leukemias, and there followed a period of years when the concern was directed toward the origin and development of blood cells.

By 1930 the morphologic variants of acute and chronic leukemia were well established, and nothing has been added since then except in details. There have been two major milestones within recent years. The first is the therapeutic attack on the disease by use of corticosteroids and chemotherapy. The second is the relatively recent work on cytogenetics, cell markers, cytochemistry, and immunochemistry.

Definition

Leukemia is a neoplastic disease characterized by the abnormal proliferation of hemopoietic cells in the bone marrow and other organs. By definition, these cells can be expected to appear in the peripheral blood.

Several points made in this definition warrant some discussion. There should be little argument against including the term "neoplastic" in defining a disease that is invariably fatal; yet the preceding discussion on the many facets of proliferative disease should emphasize the difficulty of drawing a sharp line between the benign and the malignant forms. It will be remembered that at one time pernicious anemia was considered an anemia universally fatal and therefore "pernicious." The megaloblast of pernicious anemia is no less "malignant" in appearance than the myeloblast or the lymphoblast of acute leukemia. Both diseases can be thought of as malignant until treated—clinically malignant because of the fatal outcome and pathologically malignant because of abnormal morphologic features.

We no longer think of pernicious anemia as a neoplastic proliferation, of course, having learned that the proliferation, producing morphologically abnormal cells but at the same time ineffective for making erythrocytes, is a reflection of an underlying enzymatic defect we can correct. Leukemia today is as much an enigma as pernicious anemia was

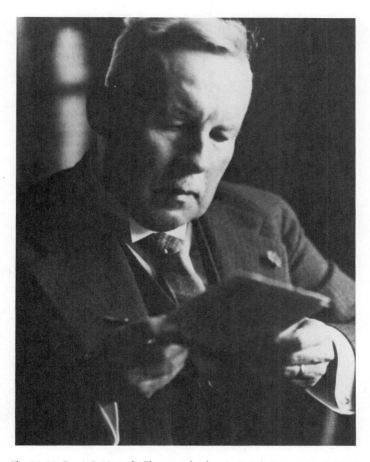

Fig. 16-16. Dr. A.E. Naegeli. Photograph taken in Zurich, Switzerland, 1933.

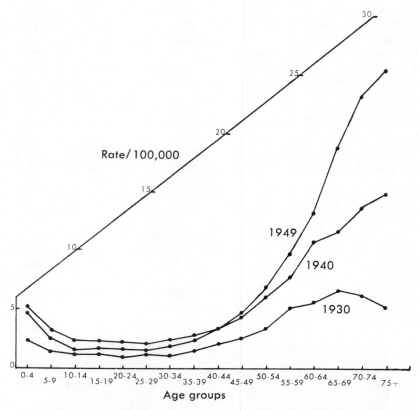

Fig. 16-17. Incidence of leukemia deaths by age in 1930, 1940, and 1949. (From Cooke, 1954.)

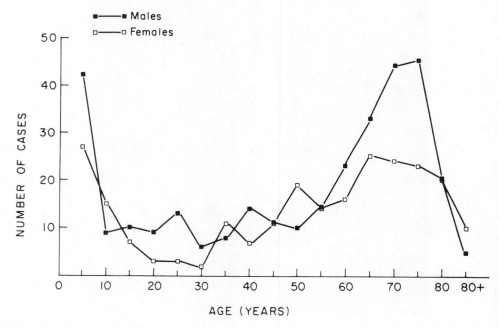

Fig. 16-18. Age and sex distribution of 553 cases of leukemia. (Drawn from data of Gunz and Hough, 1956.)

in the preceding century. One important difference is that whereas the problem of pernicious anemia was solved by basic research and happy coincidence by finding the missing factor so that maturation was redirected toward normal erythropoiesis, leukemia is being approached as the problem of finding a ''magic bullet'' that will kill the leukemic cells with the least damage to the host. The analogy is intriguing.

In the sense that the proliferation of hemopoietic cells seems without purpose and is detrimental to the host, leukemia is a malignant proliferation. We now realize that proliferation can begin anywhere, though typically it occurs first in the organs that react in ''benign'' proliferation—the bone marrow, the spleen, the lymph glands, and the liver. Do the leukemic cells found in other organs and tissues originate there, or do they represent colonization at distant sites in the sense of classic metastases? It is not unlikely that, at least in part, leukemic cells originate in various tissues. If, as we believe, undifferentiated stem cells are widely distributed in the body, there is no reason to suppose that the stimulus for proliferation would affect only those in the bone marrow. On the other hand, the presence of leukemic cells in the peripheral blood can precede sequestration into various organs, a process characteristic of the life cycle of normal leukocytes. In either case, the infiltration of normal tissue by leukemic cells causes abnormal function of that tissue and is responsible for most of the symptoms. The presence of large numbers of leukemic cells in the peripheral blood is not, by itself, harmful.

Incidence

It is agreed in all reports that the incidence of leukemia has shown a steady increase during the past 40 years. The most complete data are based on mortality figures. Admittedly the incidence of a disease and the mortality are usually significantly different, but mortality data are more complete. In the United States the mortality from leukemia in 1940 was about 3.9/100,000; in 1954 it was about 6.5/100,000 (Court-Brown and Doll, 1957); and in 1964 it was about 8/100,000 (Segi and Kurihara, 1964). An upward trend is found in other countries as well. For the same years the mortality in Canada rose from 3 to 5.1 to 7/100,000; in Denmark, from 4.8 to 7.1 to 7.6/100,000; in Scotland, from 3.8 to 4.8 to 5.6/100,000; and in England and Wales, from 2.6 to 4.9 to 6/100,000. Perhaps a small portion of the increase can be ascribed to better diagnosis, but even when allowance is made for this and similar factors, there remains what appears to be a true increase in incidence. Recently Fraumeni and Miller (1967) and Devesa and Silverman (1978) reported a decline, the first observed in leukemia mortality in the United States. The cause of the downturn remains speculative.

It is interesting to note that although this increased incidence appears in all age groups, there has been a proportionately greater increase in the incidence of leukemia in older persons (Fig. 16-17). If the incidence is plotted according to age (Fig. 16-18), two peaks are noted, one between 3 and 4 years of age and one between 70 and 80 years of age. In the older age group there is a significantly greater increased incidence in men. Almost all of this is attributable to the higher incidence of chronic lymphocytic leukemia in men. Fig. 16-19 shows that the incidence of childhood leukemia is greater in whites than it is in nonwhites, and also greater in males than in females. The relative frequency of the various types of leukemia in childhood is approximately as follows: out of 258 cases (Meighan, 1964), there were 225 acute (and subacute) lymphocytic leukemias, 13 acute granulocytic, 13 acute monocytic, 4 acute (type unspecified), and 3 chronic granulocytic.

Statistics on the relation of age to type of leukemia show that, although any type of leukemia can occur at any age, there is a consistent pattern in most series. Acute leukemia is more common than chronic leukemia at all ages and is most frequent in children and the elderly. Chronic granulocytic leukemia is rare in childhood, becoming increasingly more frequent in older age groups. Chronic lymphocytic leukemia is rare before 35 years of age but is the most common form of chronic leukemia in older persons.

Data on the relative frequency of each cytologic type of leukemia vary somewhat in different series (Gunz and Baikie, 1974), but in general the distribution in the United States is as follows: chronic lymphocytic leukemia, 25%; chronic granulocytic leukemia, 22%; chronic myelomonocytic leukemia, 3%; and acute leukemia, 50% (not always classifiable as to cell type, but roughly 20% lymphoblastic, 20% myeloblastic, and 10% myelomonoblastic). Chronic lymphocytic leukemia is rare in China, Japan, and India.

Etiology

The etiology of leukemia is not known. There are four partially overlapping approaches to an investigation of etiology. The first is the epidemiologic, the second concerns the leukemogenic effect of ionizing radiation, the third deals with the role of viruses, and the last deals with genetic (chromosomal) determinants.

Epidemiology of leukemia

In a sense the four approaches just mentioned all require a consideration of epidemiologic factors, but in this section we are concerned primarily with the question of whether leukemia, regardless of the fundamental etiologic factor concerned, exhibits features suggesting that it affects certain populations with greater frequency than others.

There are a number of observations, so far not explained, that describe a high localized incidence (clustering) of leukemia (Bartsch et al, 1975) and indicate that some groups are more susceptible than others (Fraumeni, 1969). As examples, the peak incidence in white children in the range of 3 to 4 years of age (Fig. 16-19) is not found in nonwhite children. There is a greater frequency in males than in females. There is a predilection for persons from the upper socioeconomic group, and as far as leukemia in children is concerned, almost all the affected children I have seen have been unusually handsome and endearing. There is no clear-cut or highly significant difference in the incidence of leukemia in various regions of the United States, and indeed the incidence in various countries varies but little. The exceptions are Japan and China (Wells and Lau, 1960), with an incidence about half that found in the United States and Europe. The lower incidence in Japan can be accounted for

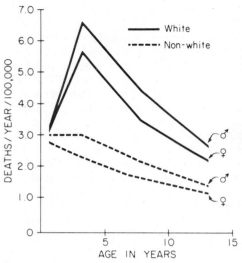

Fig. 16-19. Mortality from acute leukemia in white and black children, 1950-1959. (Data from Ederer et al, 1965.)

Table 16-8. Familial incidence of various types of leukemia*†

	Chronic lymphocytic	Acute lymphocytic	Chronic granulocytic	Acute granulocytic	Stem cell	Monocytic
Chronic lymphocytic	13	—	—	—	—	—
Acute lymphocytic	0	1	—	—	—	—
Chronic granulocytic	9	1	4	—	—	—
Acute granulocytic	3	0	3	4	—	—
Stem cell	2	2	2	1	0	—
Monocytic	0	0	0	1	0	0

*Data from Videbaek, 1947.

†The table shows the frequency with which one type of leukemia (left) is associated with the same or other types (across) within the same families.

by the lower incidence in middle-aged Japanese and by the rarity of chronic lymphocytic leukemia in the older age group. The rarity of chronic lymphocytic leukemia in the Japanese is an example of a true epidemiologic difference, and it is interesting to note that chronic lymphocytic leukemia has not developed in anyone in the group exposed to ionizing radiation at Hiroshima and Nagasaki (Finch et al, 1969). One other racial group shows a significant difference in incidence: African children have the lowest incidence of leukemia among children of all groups, even though they seem particularly prone to a characteristic type of lymphoma (Burkitt's tumor). Where reliable data are available (accurate reporting plus adequate medical diagnostic facilities), they show the incidence of leukemia to be rising at a fairly constant rate. As of now, no one has been tempted to relate the rising incidence of leukemia to the increasing consumption of cigarettes. I do not see how those who can prove anything by statistics can resist the temptation to do so.

The occasional occurrence of familial leukemia is always striking, but there is some question as to how much weight to give it. The most often quoted study (Videbaek, 1966), plus other reports, indicates there are about 100 occurrences of familial leukemia. The data from Videbaek's study are shown in Table 16-8. The data from Guasch (1954) are basically the same. In general the most common familial leukemia is the chronic lymphocytic type (Blattner et al, 1976);

the next most frequent association is between chronic lymphocytic and chronic granulocytic leukemia. Gunz et al (1978) report on 13 cases of leukemia, 12 of them acute, in three generations of a family.

While there is no doubt that familial leukemia does occur, the question is whether its frequency is greater than might be expected. Some investigators (e.g. Videbaek, 1966) think it is, while others (Morganti and Cresseri, 1954) show that it is not. There are many pitfalls in collecting this type of information, the chief one being that when familial incidence is being studied, the starting point is an individual with the disease, a good example of "Berkson's fallacy" in statistical analysis (Berkson, 1959). All in all, the evidence for a familial predisposition for leukemia is questionable, even though leukemia and other neoplasms do sometimes affect several persons in the same family. Ly et al (1978) report on the onset of acute leukemia within the same week in a husband and wife. One had acute granulocytic and the other acute myelomonocytic. Based on the frequency of acute leukemia in adults in Norway, the probability for simultaneous leukemia in a couple is 1:400 million.

The incidence of leukemia in identical twins is also subject to differing interpretations. While 15 pairs of identical twins having leukemia are recorded, the true incidence of leukemia in one identical twin only is unknown. There is an interesting report (Goh and Swisher, 1965) of chronic granulocytic leukemia in one identical twin while the other was normal. The leukemic twin had the Ph[1] chromosome, but the normal one did not. Five other pairs of twins have been reported, and only in one pair was the Ph[1] chromosome present in both twins (Tokuhata et al, 1968). However, Chaganti et al (1979) found identical cytogenetic abnormalities in twins who developed acute lymphocytic leukemia.

Leukemogenic effect of ionizing radiation

There is no longer doubt that ionizing radiation is a leukemogenic factor. The atomic bomb detonations over Hiroshima and Nagasaki have provided irrefutable evidence for it. In survivors in Hiroshima, the first cases of leukemia appeared about 18 months after exposure, with a peak incidence between 1950 and 1956 (the explosions occurred in 1945). Although there is some disagreement about the threshold of exposure as related to the incidence of leukemia, it is generally agreed that the highest incidence occurred in exposed individuals who were caught within a radius of 1,500 meters from the hypocenter, and that, in general, the incidence is higher in those who received large doses of ionizing radiation. According to some (Lawrence, 1964), it is expected that between 1 and 6 out of a million exposed to 1 rad/year would be expected to develop leukemia. This amount of ionizing radiation seems small, but it should be noted that a little over 0.1 rem is absorbed every year from natural cosmic and terrestrial radiation. To this is added exposure from diagnostic X-ray films (about 0.02 rem/roentgenogram for examination of the chest, 0.15 rem for gallbladder studies, and 0.2 rem for upper or lower gastrointestinal study using a barium meal or enema). These figures do not take into account overexposure when the operator is careless. It should be noted, also, that the exposure from fluoroscopy is about 4 rems/minute.

X-irradiation for therapeutic purposes can account for massive exposure, particularly when directed to the spine and pelvis (containing about 65% of the bone marrow). Court-Brown and Doll (1957) have reported 33 cases of leukemia in 13,352 patients who received irradiation to the spine and pelvis for ankylosing spondylitis. Radiotherapy for Hodgkin's lymphoma has also been implicated as the stimulus for development of acute leukemia (O'Donnell et al, 1979).

Other types of exposure to ionizing radiation should be mentioned briefly. The incidence of leukemia was once greater in radiologists than in other physicians or in the unselected population (Seltser and Sartwell, 1965) but has decreased sharply since 1940 (Warren, 1970). Children whose mothers have had roentgenographic pelvimetry while pregnant have a higher incidence of leukemia than nonexposed children (MacMahon, 1962). The incidence of leukemia is also greater among children who are treated with X-irradiation for thymic enlargement (Hempelmann et al, 1975). Unexplained is the observation that ionizing radiation does not induce chronic lymphocytic leukemia (Finch et al, 1969).

How does ionizing radiation sometimes induce leukemia? We do not know. Ionizing radiation induces chromosomal aberrations, chiefly aneuploidy (chromosome number deviating from the normal complement of 46), but also structural abnormalities such as fragmentation, dicentric chromosomes, and ring chromosomes. However, there is no evidence that these radiation-induced chromosomal changes are related in any way to the leukemogenic effect. In fact, it is likely that a concordance of several etiologic factors must occur, of which radiation is one, before leukemogenesis occurs.

Role of viruses

If any of the theories of the etiology of leukemia can be said to be more "likely" than the others, then that implicating viruses is certainly the one, not because there is much evidence to implicate viruses in human leukemia, but because viruses are so definitely implicated in leukemia of lower animals. But even here, leukemogenesis is more likely when the virus interacts with genetic predisposition and other leukemogenic agents.

That leukemia can be induced (leukosis) in fowls by cell-free filtrates of tissues from an affected fowl has been known since 1908 and has since been studied extensively. The viruses have been isolated and characterized, and virus clusters have been seen by electron microscopy in fowl leukemia cells. In mammals the transmission of mouse leukemia was accomplished when Gross (1951) showed that leukemia could be transmitted from a high-leukemia strain of mouse (AK) to another strain (C_3H) provided that the recipient animals were newborn. The original transmission experiments, using intact cells, were no more than grafts into susceptible animals, but later studies showed that the agent was truly ultrafilterable and specific, and that it could be sedimented by ultracentrifugation and inactivated by heating to 50° C for 30 minutes. A summary of current knowledge of tumor viruses is given in Table 16-9, and the role of viruses in leukemogenesis in animals and man is reviewed by Gunz and Baikie (1974) and by Rapp and Buss (1974).

The extensive experimentation that followed Gross's work has really contributed little to the question of the role of viruses in human leukemogenesis. It has been shown that leukemogenic viruses induce a malignant transformation of human cells in tissue culture, induce chromosomal aberrations, etc. However, the most direct attacks on transmission of human leukemia, i.e., the injection of leukemic human blood into normal human recipients, have met with uniform failure. It has been suggested, with much justification, that there are factors interacting with the virus agent, such as genetic predisposition, the effect of ionizing radiation, and latency of the virus until activated by one or more intrinsic or extrinsic factors (Lindenmann, 1974).

One possible explanation of how a virus acts as a leukemogen is that viral RNA is converted to cellular DNA by "reverse transcription" mediated by the enzyme "reverse transcriptase" (Temin, 1964, 1971; Sarin et al, 1976; Viola et al, 1976). By this mechanism, the virus makes a DNA copy of itself, which then serves as the template for virus RNA synthesis (Gillespie and Gallo, 1975). Sarin and Gallo (1974), Gallo et al (1970), and Baltimore (1976) have shown that cells from some patients with acute leukemia contain a reverse transcriptase that differs from polymerases isolated from normal cells or PHA-stimulated lymphocytes.

Table 16-9. Representative tumor viruses*

Group-name	Virus	Natural host	Species for in vivo tumors	Species for in vitro transformation	Pathologic classification of tumors†
Myxovirus-like (RNA)	Rous sarcoma				
	Bryan strain	Chicken	Chicken, turkey	Chicken	M
	Schmidt-Ruppin strain	Chicken	Chicken, rat, monkey, mouse, hamster, guinea pig	Chicken, human (?)	M
	Avian leukosis complex	Chicken	Chicken	Chicken	M
	Fujinami	Duck	Duck	Duck, chicken	M
	Gross virus	Mouse	Mouse, rat	—	M
Poxvirus (DNA)	Yaba	Monkey	Monkey	—	B
	Milkers' nodules	Cow	Human	—	B
	Fibroma	Rabbit	Rabbit	Rabbit (?)	B
	Molluscum contagiosum	Human	Human	—	B
Polyoma (DNA)	Polyoma	Mouse	Mouse, hamster, guinea pig, rabbit, rat	Mouse, hamster, rat	M
	SV40	Rhesus monkey	Hamster	Hamster, mouse, human	M
	Human wart	Human	Human	—	B
	Shope papilloma	Rabbit	Rabbit	—	B → M
	Bovine papilloma	Cow	Cow, hamster, mouse	Cow (?), mouse	M (?)
	Canine papilloma	Dog	Dog	—	B
Adenovirus (DNA)	Adenovirus type 3	Human	Hamster	—	M
	Adenovirus type 7	Human	Hamster	—	M
	Adenovirus type 12	Human	Hamster, mouse, rat	Hamster (?)	M
	Adenovirus type 18	Human	Hamster	—	M
	Adenovirus type 31	Human	Hamster	—	M

*From Goodheart, 1965.
†M = malignant; B = benign.

Reverse transcriptase is also found in cell cultures of other human neoplasms (Bowen et al, 1973; Hehlmann et al, 1973). These studies have served to strengthen the leukemogenic role played by viruses and may indicate a measurable enzymatic difference between normal and neoplastic cells.

Leukemogenic chemicals

Chemical carcinogens have been known for many years, but only one chemical, benzene, is strongly implicated in leukemogenesis (Vigliani and Saita, 1964; Aksoy et al, 1974b; Infante et al, 1977; Aksoy and Erdem, 1978). Of current importance is the strong evidence that chemotherapy for other diseases (Hodgkin's lymphoma, non-Hodgkin's lymphoma, multiple myeloma, carcinoma) can induce leukemia (Clément, 1979; Foucar et al, 1979; Kapadia et al, 1980). The role of potentially carcinogenic chemicals is discussed by Miller (1978).

Chromosomal abnormalities

The association of a variety of chromosomal abnormalities with leukemia is well established. These are probably not related directly to the etiology of leukemia but serve as markers of a damaged or altered cell (Nowell and Finan, 1977; Verma and Dosik, 1977; Golomb et al, 1978a; Ben-

edict et al, 1979; Sessarego et al, 1979; Shiloh et al, 1979; Testa et al, 1979; Trujillo et al, 1979).

It was once thought that the abnormal chromosome marker found in the majority of cases of *chronic* granulocytic leukemia, the Ph^1 (Philadelphia) chromosome, represented an abnormality of chromosome 21. This seemed to explain the high incidence of leukemia in children with mongolian idiocy (Down's syndrome), a genetic defect with an abnormality of chromosome 21 (trisomy 21) (Sutow and Welsh, 1958; Jackson et al, 1968). Unhappily for that idea, the Ph^1 chromosome is now thought to involve chromosome 22 instead (9:22 translocation), so that most of what has been written about the role of chromosome 21 in chronic granulocytic leukemia must be discarded. In fact, attempts to relate leukemia to chromosome changes have been disastrous, with the exception of the Ph^1 chromosome. *Acute* leukemias usually show abnormalities of chromosomes 8 and 21 rather than chromosome 22 (Yamada and Furusawa, 1976), but a significant number of adult acute lymphocytic leukemias are Ph^1-positive (Bloomfield et al, 1977). The Ph^1 chromosome has also been found in multiple myeloma (Van Den Berghe et al, 1979a). An additional example is the birth and death of the Ch^1 (Christchurch) chromosome in chronic lymphocytic leukemia (Fitzgerald and Hamer, 1969; Sandberg and Hossfeld, 1970).

Table 16-10. Traditional classification of leukemia

I. Stem cell (undifferentiated cell) leukemia	**V.** Myelomonocytic
II. Lymphocytic	**A.** Acute myelomonocytic (Naegeli type)
A. Acute lymphocytic leukemia	**B.** Chronic myelomonocytic (Naegeli type)
B. Chronic lymphocytic leukemia	**VI.** Erythremic myelosis (Di Guglielmo's syndrome)
III. Granulocytic	**A.** Acute erythremic myelosis
A. Acute granulocytic (myelocytic) leukemia	**B.** Chronic erythremic myelosis
B. Chronic granulocytic (myelocytic) leukemia	**VII.** Megakaryocytic leukemia
C. Acute progranulocytic (promyelocytic) leukemia	**VIII.** Leukemic phase of lymphoma and myeloma
D. Chronic neutrophilic leukemia	**A.** Plasma cell leukemia
IV. Monocytic (histiocytic, Schilling type)	**B.** Mast cell leukemia
A. Acute monocytic (histiocytic) leukemia	**C.** Leukemic reticuloendotheliosis ("hairy cell" leukemia)
	D. Leukosarcoma, etc.

Fialkow (1967) has proposed the intriguing concept that immunologic damage can lead to chromosomal damage and then to neoplastic transformation.

Summary

While each of the factors discussed plays a role in the etiology of leukemia, the best guess at this time is that the induction of leukemia is a multiphasic process involving both genetic and extrinsic mutations. What has been observed so far is the puzzle in parts. What is hoped for is the discovery of how the various leukemogenic stimuli act in sequence or in collusion.

Classification

The traditional classification

Traditionally leukemia has been classified on the basis of (1) duration of the disease, (2) predominant cell type in the blood and bone marrow, and (3) leukocyte count in the peripheral blood. Recently a new classification of acute leukemia has been proposed by a joint French-American-British (FAB) cooperative group. There is some justification in remarking that progressively more sophisticated classification schemes are often mistaken for increased knowledge and understanding.

On the basis of duration, persons with *acute* leukemia have a short life expectancy (6 months or less), and those with *chronic* leukemia have a long life expectancy (12 months or more). Some use the term "subacute" to indicate a duration intermediate between acute and chronic, i.e., 6 to 12 months. Others use subacute to refer to the transitional stage between chronic leukemia and the acute terminal variant. In practice, there is no way of predicting survival except in the most general terms, and classification according to duration is accurate only in retrospect. Furthermore, the use of improved supportive therapy, chemotherapy, and steroids to induce remissions makes accurate classification on the basis of duration impossible. Accordingly, the term "subacute" will not be used to refer to the duration of the disease.

On the basis of the cells found in the blood and bone marrow, leukemia can be classified, first, as to cell type and, second, as to cellular maturity. In most cases, classification as to cell type makes it possible to distinguish between lymphocytic, granulocytic, and other leukemias.

Classification according to cellular maturity often parallels the classification as to duration. Thus acute leukemias usually show a large number of immature cells, and chronic leukemias usually show a significant number of well-differentiated cells. Morphologically, subacute leukemias are intermediate between acute and chronic, but here also the distinction between a "subacute" population and the "acute" or "chronic" is difficult to define. With the exception of an apparent transition from chronic lymphocytic to acute lymphocytic leukemia (Fig. 5-66, p. 313), the term "subacute" will not be used.

On the basis of the leukocyte count in the peripheral blood, leukemia can be classified as *leukemic, subleukemic,* and *aleukemic.* In leukemic leukemia the leukocyte count is higher than normal (the normal value depends on the age but is usually much higher than 15,000/mm³ [15×10^9/l]). In subleukemic leukemia the leukocyte count is less than normal, but there are sufficient abnormal cells to suggest the diagnosis of leukemia. In aleukemic leukemia the leukocyte count is less than normal, and the blood supposedly contains no abnormal cells. Obviously the distinction between subleukemic and aleukemic leukemia depends mostly on the diligence with which one searches for abnormal cells. In our experience, abnormal cells can usually be found if a smear of the buffy coat is examined. A given patient may show leukemic and subleukemic phases.

The traditional classification of leukemia is given in Table 16-10. The new FAB classification of acute leukemia and the new data on which it is based are discussed in the following section.

The acute leukemias

FRENCH-AMERICAN-BRITISH (FAB) CLASSIFICATION OF ACUTE LEUKEMIA. The FAB classification of acute leukemia (Bennett et al, 1976) assumes two broad categories of acute leukemia: lymphoblastic and myeloblastic. It then subclassifies each on the basis of (1) the morphology on Romanovsky-stained smears of blood and bone marrow and (2) certain cytochemical reactions (myeloperoxidase, naphthol AS or ASD acetate with fluoride inhibition). Since that report, new technics have been used to characterize the categories in the FAB classification. These include conventional markers for T and B cells, activity of terminal DNA nucleotidyltransferase, serum lysozyme, surface markers,

Table 16-11. FAB classification of acute lymphocytic leukemia and the characteristics of each type

Type	Synonym	Characteristics
L1	Acute lymphocytic leukemia in childhood	Predominant cell is small (< 12 μm) and varies little in size. Nucleus round, seldom clefted; chromatin homogeneous; nucleoli inconspicuous. Cytoplasm moderately basophilic, variably vacuolated. Not phagocytic. Many cells positive with anti-null acute lymphocytic leukemia serum. About one-fourth have T-cell markers. High terminal transferase activity. Cytochemical reactions as in Table 16-13.
L2	Acute lymphocytic leukemia in adulthood	Predominant cell is larger than in L1, and cells vary in size. Nuclear outline irregular, often clefted; nuclear chromatin pattern variable; one or more nucleoli present. Cytoplasm moderately abundant, variably basophilic, variably vacuolated. Not phagocytic. About half of the cells are positive with anti-null acute lymphocytic leukemia serum. About one-fourth have T-cell markers. High terminal transferase activity. A few cases have the Ph[1] chromosome. Cytochemical reactions as in Table 16-13.
L3	Burkitt-type	Predominant cell is large and varies little in size. Nucleus round to oval with smooth outline; one or more prominent nucleoli. Cytoplasm moderately abundant, deeply basophilic; vacuolization often prominent. Frequently phagocytic. Negative with anti-null acute lymphocytic leukemia serum. All have B-cell markers. Cytochemical reactions as in Table 16-13.

Table 16-12. FAB classification of acute myeloblastic leukemia and the characteristics of each type

Type	Synonym	Characteristics
M1	Myeloblastic leukemia without maturation	Predominant cell is a nongranular blast. Nuclear chromatin pattern delicate; one or more nucleoli. Cytoplasm scanty, rarely contains a few granules, rare Auer rods. Cytochemical reactions as in Table 16-13.
M2	Myeloblastic leukemia with maturation	Cells show maturation beyond the progranulocyte stage, with about 50% blasts and progranulocytes. Cells older than blasts have abundant cytoplasm, contain azurophilic granules and often Auer rods. Myelocytes, metamyelocytes, and mature granulocytes may be agranular. In rare cases the cells are predominantly eosinophilic. Cases showing also erythroid hyperplasia but with less than 50% normoblasts and no megaloblasts are included in this group rather than in M6. Cytochemical reactions as in Table 16-13.
M3	Hypergranular progranulocytic leukemia	Majority of cells have heavily granulated cytoplasm; granules stain variably pink, red, or purple; Auer bodies common and often multiple. Cytochemical reactions as in Table 16-13. A variant type is characterized by minimal or no granulation in the cytoplasm and a bilobed, multilobed, or reniform nucleus.
M4	Myelomonocytic leukemia	Cells characteristically have a monocytoid nucleus and granulocytic cytoplasm. The monocytoid nucleus distinguishes this type from M2. Promonocytes and monocytes with azure granules are present in both blood and bone marrow. Cytochemical reactions as in Table 16-13.
M5	Monocytic (histiocytic) leukemia	Cells predominantly monoblasts (M5a). Nucleus has lacy chromatin structure, one or more nucleoli. Cytoplasm abundant, with rare fine pink granules. The more differentiated form (M5b) shows monoblasts, promonocytes, and monocytes, the more mature cells having many dustlike pink granules. Cytochemistry as in Table 16-13.
M6	Erythroleukemia (Di Guglielmo's syndrome)	Of the cells in the bone marrow, 50% or more are normoblasts or megaloblasts, sometimes having bizarre nuclei. Nucleated erythroid cells in blood also atypical. There is an increase in myeloblasts and progranulocytes. Auer bodies may be present. Megakaryocytes often atypical. Frequently converts to M1, M2, or M4. Cytochemical reactions as in Table 16-13.

E-rosette formation, membrane immunoglobulin, anti-null acute lymphocytic leukemia antiserum, and Fc and C3 receptors (Gralnick et al, 1977). Table 16-11 gives the extended FAB classification and features of acute lymphocytic leukemia and Table 16-12 of acute myeloblastic leukemia.

Two characteristics of acute leukemia have been generally accepted: (1) the extreme variability of morphology as seen in Romanovsky-stained smears and (2) the variable and usually unpredictable response to therapy. The purpose of the FAB classification is to sort out the various morphologic variants into types and, more recently, to add to morphologic studies the cytochemical and immunochemical features of each type. It is hoped that in turn this will allow better discrimination in therapy and prognosis. Unless applicable to therapy, mere classification is only an intellectual exercise.

There are at this time very few data that prove the worth of the FAB classification. From the very beginning it has been recognized that the best response to chemotherapy is seen in the acute lymphocytic leukemia of childhood (Zuelzer, 1978). In fact, it was fortuitous that the first chemotherapeutic attack on acute leukemia involved childhood leukemia (Farber et al, 1948), the type now called L1. As an

Table 16-13. Cytochemical reactions in the acute leukemias

Reaction[a]	M1	M2	M3	M4	M5	M6	L1,2,3[b]
Peroxidase	+	+++	+++	+++	+	+ to ++[c]	Neg.[d]
Sudan black B	+	+++	+++	+++	+	+ to ++[c]	Neg.
NASDA[e]	+	+++	+++	+++	+++	+ to ++[c]	Neg.
Fluoride inhibition	No	No	No	Variable	Yes	No	—
PAS[f]	+	+	+	++	++	+	++ to +++
Lysozyme[g]	Neg.	Low	Low	Intermediate	High	Low	Neg.

[a] + = positive in a few cells; + + = more than 25% of cells are positive; + + + = 50% or more of cells are positive.
[b] T-cell acute lymphocytic leukemias often show acid phosphatase positivity in the Golgi region (Stein et al, 1976). Diffuse acid phosphatase reactivity is characteristic of myeloblasts.
[c] Depending on the number of granulocytes.
[d] Arbitrarily, when more than 3% of the blasts are peroxidase positive, the disease is classified as other than acute lymphocytic leukemia.
[e] Naphthol ASD chloroacetate.
[f] Periodic acid–Schiff reaction.
[g] In serum or urine.

aside, Farber's trial of the antifolate aminopterin was based on the misconception that folic acid accelerated the malignant process. The characteristics of other types of leukemia are also well known, i.e., the association of disseminated intravascular coagulation with hypergranular promyelocytic leukemia (Gralnick and Sultan, 1975), now designated M3. It remains for prospective studies to demonstrate the value of the new classification. It should be noted that the FAB classification is applicable only to overt, untreated acute leukemia. It does not apply to chronic leukemias. The lower limit suggested for an unequivocal diagnosis of acute myelocytic leukemia is a combined percentage of myeloblasts and progranulocytes greater than 50%.

IMMUNOLOGIC CELL MARKERS. New markers are being used (Catovsky, in Gralnick et al, 1977), in addition to the conventional T- and B-cell markers for lymphocytes (Brouet et al, 1976). Presumably, lymphoid cells can be classified, first, on the basis of their being T, B, or null cells, by means of conventional technics. Approximately three-fourths of acute leukemias in children and one-half in adults lack B- or T-cell markers and are classified as ''null acute lymphocytic leukemia'' (Catovsky, 1977). This category of acute lymphocytic leukemia can be identified more specifically by the use of an anti-null acute lymphocytic leukemia serum (Greaves et al, 1975). However, Davey et al (1979) have shown that the ''null'' lymphoblast from most cases of acute lymphocytic leukemia is a B cell in an early stage of development.

The enzyme terminal DNA nucleotidyltransferase is present in high concentration in thymocytes and is absent in normal T- or B-lymphocytes. It is being applied to characterize further the null acute lymphocytic leukemias (Coleman et al, 1976). High activity has been found in the majority of patients with L1 and L2 leukemia, both in null acute and T-cell acute (E-rosette–positive) lymphocytic leukemia (Mertelsmann et al, 1978). Transferase activity in myeloblasts is very low (Hutton and Coleman, 1976). Blasts having either or both high transferase activity and strong activity with anti-null acute lymphocytic leukemia serum have been found in patients with Ph[1]-positive chronic granulocytic leukemia in blast transformation (Janossy et al, 1976;

Oken et al, 1978). This suggests that terminal transferase and the null acute lymphocytic leukemia antigen are markers for a common stem cell, CFU-S. However, some corollary assumptions may be required, one being that there exist several repressor mechanisms, so that when a pluripotent stem cell is the target for the leukemogenic stimulus, some committed stem cells are affected but not others (Fialkow et al, 1979).

Surface marker immunoglobulins are characteristic of B cells. Since they are uncommon in acute lymphocytic leukemia, Catovsky, in Gralnick et al (1977), suggests that B-cell acute lymphocytic leukemia represents the leukemic phase of poorly differentiated lymphomas, either Burkitt's (L3) or lymphosarcoma (Mann et al, 1976). Monoblasts and monocytes may have receptors for the Fc portion of IgG and for C3b (Abramson et al, 1976). The selective release of lysozyme from monoblasts and promonocytes distinguishes these cells from myeloblasts and lymphoblasts. High concentrations of lysozyme in urine or serum are found in almost all cases of acute monocytic (M5), acute myelomonocytic (M4), and chronic myelomonocytic leukemia.

CYTOCHEMISTRY. Cytochemical reactions provide additional parameters for classifying the acute leukemias (Table 16-13).

ELECTRON MICROSCOPY. Electron microscopy is yet another parameter for classifying acute leukemia (Glick, 1976). Glick et al (1980) studied 100 cases of acute leukemia in adults by a combination of traditional morphology, cytochemistry, and electron microscopy. These cases were classified as follows: 1 M1, 8 M2, 4 M3, 32 M4, 12 M5 undifferentiated (M5a), 26 M5 differentiated (M5b), and 17 unclassifiable consisting of primitive stem cells showing negative cytochemical reactions.

STEM CELL LEUKEMIA. The application of cytochemical, immunochemical, and immunologic methods to the investigation of acute leukemia has succeeded in most cases in identifying the cell type. There remain a few cases that cannot be characterized except that the predominant cell is an undifferentiated stem cell. If the patient survives for a reasonable time, an acute leukemia previously classified as stem cell leukemia may show an identifiable cell population. This category should not be used unless all methods have failed to identify the cell type.

ACUTE LYMPHOCYTIC LEUKEMIA (L1, L2, L3). Childhood acute lymphocytic leukemia (L1) is the most common malignancy in children, with an incidence of about 34/million children under the age of 15 years. The onset may have various symptoms: low-grade fever, malaise, pallor, bruising, lymphadenopathy, bone pain, or various combinations of symptoms.

The blood usually shows anemia, thrombocytopenia, and lymphocytosis with a variable number of lymphoblasts. When the leukocyte count is high, the number of blasts will also be high.

Bone marrow aspiration sometimes yields a dry tap because the marrow is markedly hypercellular. Bone marrow obtained by either aspiration or core biopsy shows it to consist almost entirely of lymphoblasts having a characteristic morphology and other features (Table 16-11). Occasionally the morphology will be as in L2, and rarely (about 1%) as in L3. There is general agreement that children having the L1 variant have the best response to therapy (Miller et al, 1979). Acute lymphocytic leukemia (type L1) lymphoblasts are heterogeneous as to immunologic markers and other features, so that type L1 is essentially a morphologically homogeneous subtype. Various trials have attempted to correlate immunologic characteristics with prognosis, but such correlations are so far not conclusive (Chessells et al, 1977; Smithson et al, 1979).

Conversion of acute lymphocytic leukemia after chemotherapy to acute myelocytic and chronic myelocytic leukemia is reported by Hutter et al (1979). The conversion after therapy of acute lymphocytic leukemia to malignant histiocytosis (histiocytic medullary reticulosis of Scott and Robb-Smith) is discussed by Karcher et al, (1978).

Acute lymphocytic leukemia in adults is usually of the L2 type. Both the response to therapy and the prognosis are poorer than in type L1. Type L3 is a morphologic variant resembling the cells in Burkitt's lymphoma but, in contrast to types L1 and L2, is probably homogeneously of B-cell origin.

ACUTE MYELOCYTIC LEUKEMIA. Acute myelocytic leukemia (Plate 41) is classified by the "lumpers" as acute nonlymphocytic leukemia and by the "splitters" into six subtypes (M1 to M6, FAB classification, Table 16-12). There is something to be said for both approaches to classification, but the first is not relevant to either morphology or clinical course. The clinical presentation of acute myelocytic leukemia is essentially the same as in all acute leukemias. Lymphadenopathy is uncommon, whereas splenomegaly and hepatomegaly are common. Thrombocytopenia is not as common as in acute lymphocytic leukemia (Boggs et al, 1962).

ACUTE GRANULOCYTIC LEUKEMIA (M1, M2). Type M1 is acute myeloblastic leukemia without maturation; i.e., the predominant blast is a nongranular myeloblast. Type M2 is acute myelocytic leukemia with maturation; 50% of the cells are myeloblasts and progranulocytes, the remainder being myelocytes and more mature cells. Auer bodies (Plates 43 and 44) are found in 5% to 20% of cases, but all cases are characterized by the presence of "ϕ-bodies." These are not

seen by the usual peroxidase reaction but are hydroperoxidase positive (Hanker et al, 1978; Hanker et al, 1979). The ϕ-bodies disappear during a remission. They are not found in the blast crisis of chronic lymphocytic leukemia. Concurrent folate or vitamin B_{12} deficiency (Chanarin, 1969) can occur in all types of acute leukemia and accounts for the presence at times of megaloblasts in the bone marrow and hypersegmented neutrophils in the blood. Tumors composed of myeloblasts or of myeloblasts and progranulocytes have been called "myeloblastomas," "chloromas," and more recently, "granulocytic sarcomas" (Rappaport, 1966; Muss and Moloney, 1973).

HYPERGRANULAR PROGRANULOCYTIC LEUKEMIA (M3). The rare variant M3, hypergranular progranulocytic leukemia, is characterized by the presence in blood and bone marrow of many atypical progranulocytes. These contain large clublike or rod-shaped azurophilic or azure-blue granules (Bernard et al, 1963). The granules may be basophilic (Liso et al, 1974). A variant shows minimal or no granulation in the cytoplasm and a bilobed, multilobed, or reniform nucleus.

Progranulocytic leukemia is often accompanied by a hemorrhagic diathesis (Rand et al, 1969; Polliack, 1971; Gralnick and Sultan, 1975). It is thought that the cells release a thromboplastic substance that triggers the development of disseminated intravascular coagulation (DIC, p. 843), but the thromboplastic substance is probably not of granular origin, since DIC may be a complication of other acute leukemias (Baker, WG et al, 1964; Leavey et al, 1970; Rosner et al, 1970; Pitney, 1971).

ACUTE MONOCYTIC (HISTIOCYTIC) LEUKEMIA (M5). Acute monocytic leukemia (M5) is rare, and many of the cases in the old literature should have been classified as the more common myelomonocytic (M4) type.

Leukocytosis is usually moderate and never as marked as in acute lymphocytic or granulocytic leukemia. Anemia and thrombocytopenia are common. The differential count shows a preponderance of monoblasts, an occasional promonocyte, few or many monocytes, and some reduction in neutrophils. The bone marrow is more difficult to interpret because, in addition to the numerous monoblasts, there may be a normal or even increased number of progranulocytes and myelocytes.

The monoblast of acute monocytic leukemia has a very delicate convoluted, or folded, nucleus, variable amounts of cytoplasm, and no cytoplasmic granules. In contrast, the nucleus of the blast cell in acute myelomonocytic leukemia resembles that of a myeloblast. It has been said that Auer rods are not seen in monoblasts, but I have found them in one typical case. It is helpful to find later cells of the monocytic series, with the characteristic fine pink granulation, but sometimes the granulation is absent. In contrast, the cytoplasm of more mature cells of the myelomonocytic series contains the typical granulation seen in the granulocytic series.

The cytochemical features are given in Table 16-13. An increase in serum and urine muramidase is characteristic of both acute monocytic and acute and chronic myelomonocytic leukemia. It is helpful in distinguishing these from other leukemias but offers little in the more difficult problem of distinguishing between the monocytic and myelomonocytic types (Berg and Brandt, 1970; Zucker et al, 1970). The increased excretion of muramidase can cause renal tubular dysfunction (Muggia et al, 1969). IgG monoclonal immunoglobulinopathy was associated with this leukemia in the cases reported by Meuret et al (1974) and by Law et al (1976). Allen et al (1973) reported a case associated with macroglobulinemia and Bence Jones proteinuria.

ACUTE MYELOMONOCYTIC LEUKEMIA (M4). Acute myelomonocytic leukemia (M4) is more common than type M5. The myelomonocytic series is characterized by cells having a monocytoid nucleus and a granulated cytoplasm. In the acute leukemia the earliest blast cells have few characteristic morphologic features, although the nucleus is often indented or folded. Early in the maturation series the monocytoid nucleus is still obvious, but the cytoplasm has large granules similar to those seen in the granulocytic series. Both the blood and bone marrow will show variable proportions of myelomonoblasts and promyelomonocytes. The chronic form of this leukemia, chronic myelomonocytic leukemia, is now considered to be a dysmyelopoiesis that may progress to acute leukemia. In practice, the dividing line between the acute and the chronic disease is somewhat subjective, depending on the number and immaturity of the cells and on the number of adult monocytes in the blood.

The cytochemical features are given in Table 16-13. Cannat and Seligmann (1973) describe immunologic abnormalities in juvenile acute myelomonocytic leukemia. Kjellström et al (1979) report the occurrence of familial "acute monocytic leukemia," but in at least one of their cases the features are those of myelomonocytic leukemia.

ACUTE ERYTHROLEUKEMIA (M6). Acute erythroleukemia (M6) probably represents the acute variant of Di Guglielmo's syndrome. The leukocyte count is moderately elevated, and the differential count shows normoblasts and megaloblasts. The bone marrow morphology is more diagnostic, the predominant cells being bizarre megaloblasts, with many immature granulocytes (Scott et al, 1964) (Fig. 16-13). Polycythemia vera may precede the development of acute erythroleukemia (Van den Bogaert and Van Hove, 1971). There is sometimes an increase in Hb F (Chernoff, 1955). In some cases Hb H has been found, but it is not clear if this is reported for the acute or the chronic cases of Di Guglielmo's syndrome. Kass and Schnitzer (1975) consider acute erythroleukemia to be a transitory stage in the evolution of acute myeloblastic leukemia.

ACUTE MEGAKARYOBLASTIC LEUKEMIA. Proliferation of megakaryocytes is a common feature of many myeloproliferative syndromes, especially those which are acute. Very few cases meet the strict criteria for the classification of acute megakaryocytic leukemia. Breton-Gorius et al (1978a) have convincingly demonstrated that megakaryocytic cells have a characteristic peroxidase, "platelet peroxidase," that can serve as an enzymatic marker for the identification of megakaryoblasts. Cells more mature than the megakaryoblast should show PAS positivity (Efrati et al, 1979).

PLASMA CELL LEUKEMIA
BLOOD AND BONE MARROW (Plate 53). Plasma cell leukemia that is not the terminal acute phase of multiple myelo-

ma (p. 732) is rare (Pruzanski et al, 1969). Most of the cases are part of multiple myeloma (Fishkin et al, 1972; Zawadzki et al, 1978). Although a few plasma cells are usually seen in the blood in multiple myeloma, the leukemic phase may show 80% to 90% of the cells to be plasma cells. Polliack et al (1974b) report a case that showed an unusual immunoglobulinopathy with K and L light-chains and γ-heavy-chains in the urine.

MAST CELL LEUKEMIA
BLOOD AND BONE MARROW (Plate 52). A few cases of acute leukemia have been reported in which the predominant cell is the tissue mast cell (Efrati et al, 1957; Waters and Lacson, 1957; Friedman et al, 1958). It should be differentiated from chronic granulocytic leukemia with many basophils. Mast cells and basophils both stain metachromatically with toluidine blue, so this does not distinguish one from the other, but Gustafson and Pihl (1967) claim that ruthenium red reacts specifically with mast cell granules. Mast cell leukemia is closely related to systemic mastocytosis (Sagher and Even-Paz, 1967).

LEUKEMIC RETICULOENDOTHELIOSIS ("HAIRY CELL" LEUKEMIA)
BLOOD AND BONE MARROW (Plate 55). Leukemic reticuloendotheliosis was described by Ewald (1923) as a disease characterized by splenomegaly and mononuclear cells with cytoplasmic projections in the blood. Recently, this disease has received a great deal of attention, out of proportion to the low incidence, because of the vivid description of the flagellated cells as "hairy cells" and because of the excellent response to splenectomy (Schrek and Donelly, 1966; Yam et al, 1968; Trubowitz et al, 1971; Flandrin et al, 1973; Catovsky et al, 1974b; Katayama and Finkel, 1974). However, Jansen et al (1978) found no significant difference after 2 years between groups of persons who had undergone splenectomy and those who had not. Golomb et al (1978b) reached the same conclusion. The histopathology of the spleen (Burke et al, 1974) and bone marrow (Burke, 1978) is characteristic. Some investigators believe that the cells are of histiocytic origin (Daniel and Flandrin, 1974; Jaffe et al, 1974), but most studies indicate that they are leukemic B-lymphocytes (Ghadially and Skinnider, 1972; Burns et al, 1973; Stein and Kaiserling, 1974; Stuart and Dewar, 1979). They are thought by some to synthesize IgG and are not phagocytic (Schrek and Donnelly, 1966), but Palutke and Tabaczka (1979) have shown that the immunoglobulin on the surface of the cells is adsorbed from the serum. Saxon et al (1978) describe a case of hairy cell leukemia with T-lymphocyte characteristics. The hairy projections can be seen with some difficulty in routine Wright-Giemsa–stained smears and easily by phase contrast and electron microscopy (Schnitzer and Kass, 1974; Golomb et al, 1975; Quan et al, 1980), and not all cells show them. The cells otherwise look like young lymphocytes. The cells are strongly acid phosphatase positive, and the acid phosphatase, with some exceptions (Schaefer et al, 1975), is not degraded by tartrate. Positivity for α-naphthyl butyrate esterase was found in all 14 cases studied by Higgy et al (1978). It should be noted that more than the presence of hairy cells is needed to make the diagnosis of leukemic reticuloendotheliosis (see Plate 12).

LEUKOSARCOMA. The term "leukosarcoma" was introduced by Sternberg in 1904. It is nonspecific in that many of the non-Hodgkin's lymphomas may, at one time or another, invade the blood (Schnitzer and Kass, 1973) (Fig. 16-55).

The chronic leukemias

The chronic leukemias are (1) chronic lymphocytic leukemia and (2) chronic granulocytic leukemia. Other nonacute leukemias are difficult to classify. These are (1) chronic neutrophilic leukemia, (2) chronic myelomonocytic leukemia, and (3) chronic erythremic myelosis. Chronic granulocytic leukemia is arbitrarily separated from the acute leukemias on the basis of having less than 50% blasts and progranulocytes in the bone marrow (FAB recommendation). There is no doubt that when the bone marrow contains over 50% blasts, the leukemia should be classified as acute, but I doubt whether a patient showing anemia, thrombocytopenia, and 30% blasts and progranulocytes should be classified as having the chronic disease. In the case of acute lymphocytic leukemias the classification is "nonacute lymphocytic leukemia" when more than 3% of the blasts are peroxidase positive (Bennett in Gralnick et al, 1977). This terminology is bound to cause some confusion, since the alternatives to "nonacute" are "subacute" or "chronic," neither of which is applicable.

CHRONIC LYMPHOCYTIC LEUKEMIA

BLOOD AND BONE MARROW (Plate 51). There is usually no anemia, or a very mild one, in the absence of a complicating acquired autoimmune hemolytic anemia. Occasionally a normochromic normocytic anemia develops in a patient whose disease spans many years, usually with an extremely high and rising leukocyte count. Antiglobulin-positive acquired hemolytic anemia develops in 10% to 20% of patients (Chapter 13). Thrombocytopenia is seldom present but may develop as part of the autoimmune reaction (Boggs et al, 1966). The leukocyte count is usually high, most frequently in the range of 50,000/mm³ (50 × 10⁹/l) to 150,000/mm³ (150 × 10⁹/l), but in an occasional case it may be only slightly elevated. Leukocyte counts performed with electronic cell counters are notoriously inaccurate in chronic lymphocytic leukemia and should be checked by manual counts. The differential count of blood leukocytes shows an almost pure population of small lymphocytes, with a reduction in neutrophils. The lymphocytes are small but may appear larger in very thin smears (Fig. 4-13, p. 137). They may show more irregularity of the nuclear shape, in the form of a cleft or indentation (the "buttock cell"), than is usually seen in normal lymphocytes (Schrek et al, 1970). They match the clinical picture in appearing suprisingly nonneoplastic. They are usually of B-cell origin (Belpomme et al, 1974), but Sagone and Murphy (1975) present evidence for a mixed population, with a small percentage being of T-cell origin (Marks et al, 1978) and others neither B nor T in origin (Branda et al, 1978b; Kirov et al, 1980). Foon et al (1980) have reported that in some cases the lymphocytes have both B- and T-cell characteristics. Extremely characteristic is the finding of smudge forms. The number varies from a few to very many, and the ratio of smudged to intact lymphocytes may be five or more to one. The smudging is caused by an abnormally high mechanical fragility and is produced when the smear is prepared. The smudged lymphocytes usually show a central clear area that probably represents the nucleolus. I have in the past called the smudged cells "Gumprecht ghosts," but I note that Bessis (1973b) also applies this term to smudged cells in other leukemias. An atypical finding sometimes seen in the lymphocytes of chronic lymphocytic leukemia is the presence in the cytoplasm of pale rod-shaped inclusions (de Man and Meiners, 1962) that can be mistaken as Auer rods but that do not have the expected cytochemical reactions and probably represent immunoglobulin crystallization (Clark et al, 1973). In one case (McCann et al, 1978) the inclusions consisted of λ light chains. The cytoplasm sometimes contains PAS-positive inclusions and sometimes PAS-negative inclusions.

The bone marrow usually contributes little to the diagnosis so obvious from the blood smear. The predominant cell is a small lymphocyte similar to those in the blood, but in thin portions these may appear larger, and one might be tempted to call them prolymphocytes. In fact, only a rare lymphoblast and prolymphocyte are to be found. Paraffin sections of marrow particles confirm the hypercellularity and the diffuse infiltration with small lymphocytes. Massive infiltration may produce a pancytopenia.

OTHER FINDINGS. When autoimmune hemolytic anemia complicates the disease, it is of the antiglobulin-positive type. There may be other evidence of inappropriate formation of immunoglobulins: monoclonal gammopathy (Azar et al, 1957), agammaglobulinemia (Prasad, 1958), cryoglobulinemia (Rawnsley and Shelley, 1968), and cryofibrinogenemia (Jager, 1962). Some cases of chronic lymphocytic leukemia have a terminal complication called Richter's syndrome (Long and Aisenberg, 1975), the features of which are a terminal phase in which there are weight loss, lymphadenopathy, lymphocytopenia, immunoglobulinopathy, and the histologic picture of a pleomorphic malignant lymphoma. Another variant picture has been called "chronic lymphosarcoma cell leukemia," characterized by the presence in blood of lymphocytes that are large, that have abundant cytoplasm, and whose nucleus has a reticular pattern with a single nucleolus (Zacharski and Linman, 1969).

Apparently, typical chronic lymphocytic leukemia can undergo various transformations: to acute granulocytic leukemia (Lawlor et al, 1979), to malignant histiocytosis (Wick et al, 1980), or to multiple myeloma (Kough and Makary, 1978; Pedersen-Bjergaard et al, 1978). The coexistence of chronic lymphocytic leukemia and diffuse histiocytic lymphoma is sometimes called Richter's syndrome (Armitage et al, 1978). Transformation to prolymphocytic leukemia seems to be of two types. In the first there is a gradual change from the typical small lymphocyte to prolymphocytes (Brouet et al, 1973b; Enno et al, 1979) that retain the original B-cell markers. This disease is progressive and refractory to treatment and could easily be classified as acute or subacute. The second type is considered by some to be a variant of chronic lymphocytic leukemia (Galton et al, 1974; Bearman et al, 1974a; Kjeldsberg et al, 1980). It is characterized by massive splenomegaly, no lymphadenopathy, and many prolymphocytes in the peripheral blood, bone marrow, and spleen (Bearman et al, 1978a). Cytochemically the prolymphocytes are rarely PAS positive and in some cases are acid-phosphatase positive (paranuclear or diffuse), β-glucuronidase positive, and α-naphthyl-acetate positive. All cases in the series of Bearman et al (1978a) were naphthol ASD acetate positive, with little inhibition by fluoride, and in one case the cells were acid-phosphatase positive, suggestive of T-cell origin. Some cases have round or oval nuclei; in others the nucleus is clefted. It is likely that prolymphocytic leukemia is not a homogeneous type, since there is much variability in morphology, cytochemical reactions, and surface markers in the reported cases (Bearman et al, 1978a; Pallesen et al, 1979; Woessner et al, 1978). However, Katayama et al (1980) believe that β-lineage prolymphocytic leukemia is a distinct clinicopathologic entity.

CHRONIC GRANULOCYTIC (MYELOCYTIC) LEUKEMIA

BLOOD AND BONE MARROW (Plate 46). Some degree of anemia is present, and the red cells are normochromic and normocytic. The leukocyte count is usually elevated, in the range of 50,000 to 300,000/mm³ (50 to 300 × 10⁹/l) or more, although sometimes a subleukemic count is encountered. The blood smear is so cellular as to appear to be aspirated marrow. The leukocyte differential shows a few myeloblasts, usually less than 10%, a few progranulocytes, and many myelocytes, metamyelocytes, and band and polymorphonuclear neutrophils. Basophils are increased and sometimes eosinophils are also. Chronic granulocytic leukemia with marked eosinophil proliferation has been called "eosinophilic leukemia" (Benvenisti and Ultman, 1969), but this is only a variant, and the term has no clinical or pathologic significance. The same applies to "basophilic leukemia" (Mitrakul et al, 1969), and Rebuck (1978) proposes the term "basophilic leukemic conversion of chronic granulocytic leukemia". The platelet count is increased in over half the patients, and at times the platelet count is 1,000,000/mm³ (1 × 10¹²/l) or higher. The combination of granulocytic predominance, increased basophils, and thrombocythemia makes the diagnosis of an uncomplicated case an easy matter.

Characteristically, the adult neutrophils present in chronic granulocytic leukemia have very little alkaline phosphatase activity, so that the score is very low (Hayhoe et al, 1964). This is helpful in differentiating chronic granulocytic leukemia from polycythemia vera (high alkaline phosphatase), from leukemoid reactions (high alkaline phosphatase), and from the majority of cases of myeloproliferative syndrome (high alkaline phosphatase). Because of exceptions, one must not place undue emphasis on this particular laboratory finding. For example, alkaline phosphatase may be normal or high in chronic granulocytic leukemia in remission (Xefteris et al, 1961) or with superimposed infection (Perillie, 1967) and in some cases of myelosclerosis (Merker and Heilmeyer, 1960). Low alkaline phosphatase scores are found in PNH and pernicious anemia (Merker and Heilmeyer, 1960; Tanaka et al, 1960), but these diseases are not likely to enter into the differential diagnosis of chronic granulocytic leukemia. Judging from studies on Japanese survivors of the atomic bombing, a gradual diminution of alkaline phosphatase activity indicates transition into a leukemic phase (Moloney and Lange, 1954).

Aspirated bone marrow shows approximately the same distribution of granulocyte forms as in the blood smear. Basophils are increased, and they often appear partially disrupted and may be ignored by the inexperienced morphologist. There is some reduction of normoblasts. Megakaryocytes are usually more numerous than normal, especially in samples from patients with a high platelet count. Lipid-filled histiocytes resembling Gaucher cells are sometimes present (Lee and Ellis, 1971). Occasional patients with granulocytic leukemia show the acquired type of Pelger-Huët anomaly (Plate 39). Paraffin sections show extreme cellularity.

OTHER FINDINGS. The description of the Ph¹ (Philadelphia) chromosome (Fig. 16-20) in chronic granulocytic leukemia has provided an important diagnostic and prognostic aid.

The Ph¹ chromosome is a chromosome formed by a translocation between the long arm of chromosome 22 and the long arm of chromosome 9 (O'Riordan et al, 1971; Rowley, 1973). Translocation to the short area of chromosome 6, as well as to other chromosomes, is reported by Mammon et al (1976). Note that it was originally thought to be derived from chromosome 21. It has been found to be present in 90% of the patients with chronic granulocytic leukemia (typical) and absent in 10% (atypical chronic granulocytic leukemia) (Mitelman et al, 1976). Ph¹-negative chronic granulocytic leukemia is seen primarily in very young children (Hardisty et al, 1964), but it may occur in adults (Tjio, 1966; Kardinal et al, 1976) and in older children (8 to 9 years of age) (Whang-Peng et al, 1968). It is an acquired, rather than inherited, abnormality, and all the evidence points to its clonal origin; i.e., the hemopoietic cells that have it are derived from the same clone of Ph¹-positive stem cells (Fialkow et al, 1967; Fitzgerald et al, 1971). In active or relapsing Ph¹-positive chronic granulocytic leukemia, the Ph¹ chromosome is found in granulocytes, normoblasts, and megakaryocytes (Rastrick et al, 1968). It is not found in any other cell type with the possible exception of type L2 acute lymphocytic leukemia (Table 16-11). There are two important implications.

First, it should be expected that in chronic granulocytic leukemia there will be a proliferation of granulocytes, normoblasts, and megakaryocytes. There is no denying the proliferation of granulocytes and megakaryocytes, but erythroid proliferation is rare. Perhaps the only indication of abnormal erythroid proliferation is seen in chronic granulocytic leukemia in childhood, in which a significant elevation of the level of fetal hemoglobin (Hb F) in blood is common (Bloom et al, 1966; Weatherall et al, 1968).

Second, since the disease is clonal, the presence of the Ph¹ chromosome in granulocytes, megakaryocytes, and normoblasts and its absence in lymphocytes, plasma cells, and megaloblasts suggest either that only CFU-Cs are stimulated or, if the precursor CFU-Ss are stimulated, that there must be suppression of proliferation of CFU-Ls.

It is generally agreed that Ph¹-negative chronic granulocytic leukemia differs from the typical Ph¹-positive leukemia in adults in that the course is more rapidly progressive and response to chemotherapy is poor (Whang-Peng et al, 1968; Canellos et al, 1976). Ph¹-positive chronic granulo-

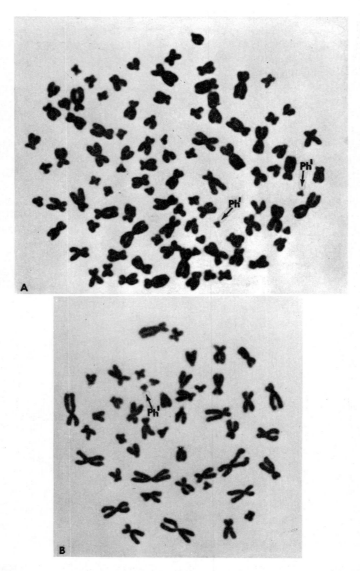

Fig. 16-20. Philadelphia chromosome (Ph¹) in myelocytic leukemia. **A,** Metaphase of a tetraploid marrow cell from a chronic granulocytic leukemia patient with two Ph¹ chromosomes. **B,** Metaphase of a diploid marrow cell from a chronic granulocytic leukemia patient with one Ph¹ chromosome. (Courtesy J. Whang and J.H. Tjio.)

cytic leukemia in children is "typical" in that the course and prognosis is like that in the adult (Ph¹-positive) form. There are still unresolved questions about Ph¹-negative chronic granulocytic leukemia in adults. Gunz and Baikie (1974) state categorically that the disease is not chronic granulocytic leukemia if the Ph¹ chromosome is absent. This is difficult to accept, in view of two studies (Whang-Peng et al, 1968; Ezdinli et al, 1970) showing that the survival of Ph¹-positive adults with typical chronic myelocytic leukemia was 4 to 5 times longer than that of Ph¹-negative adults. Warburton and Bluming (1973) describe a Philadelphia-like short Y chromosome that, in males, can be mistaken for the true Ph¹ chromosome.

When the leukocyte count is high, there is rapid consumption of glucose in drawn blood, and false low glucose levels will be obtained (Hanrahan et al, 1963). The serum potas-

sium concentration may be high (spurious hyperkalemia) as a result of the release of potassium from the large number of platelets. Hypercalcemia and hyperphosphatemia, presumably secondary to bone destruction, have been reported; most authors reporting these findings fail to mention if there was an increase in the serum protein concentration (Jordan, 1966; Ballard and Marcus, 1970). The serum vitamin B_{12} level is high, as the result of an increase in transcobalamin I (Herbert, 1968), but this elevation is sometimes seen in other chronic myeloproliferative disorders.

Chronic granulocytic leukemia often converts to a terminal acute leukemia called the "blast crisis" (Barton and Conrad, 1978). Two morphologic types are found (Gralnick and Bennett, 1970). Some cases are typically myeloblastic, while others are thought to be lymphoblastic (Rosenthal et al, 1977). The myeloblastic variant often shows the Ph¹ chromosome, which the lymphoblastic cases do not. The lymphoblast variant is characterized by high terminal transferase activity (Sarin et al, 1976) and by immunologic markers (Bacigalupo et al, 1978). Rarely in juvenile chronic granulocytic leukemia the blast crisis is characterized by erythroid blast cells (Smith and Johnson, 1974; Hoffman and Zanjani, 1978), anemia, and a high concentration of fetal hemoglobin. Breton-Gorius et al (1978b) report a case of blast crisis in which the cells were morphologically and cytochemically characteristic of megakaryoblasts.

CHRONIC ERYTHREMIC MYELOSIS

BLOOD AND BONE MARROW. In the chronic form of Di Guglielmo's syndrome—chronic erythremic myelosis—the blood and bone marrow show immature granulocytes as well as evidence of megaloblastic dyspoiesis (Dameshek and Baldini, 1958). I find a curious reluctance to call the abnormal erythroid cells megaloblasts, many authors preferring to call them "atypical" or "bizarre." In fact, recognition of the megaloblastic dyspoiesis is important in the definition of the syndrome and for differentiation from other anemias such as sideroblastic anemia and other myeloproliferative syndromes. The megaloblastosis of chronic erythremic myelosis does not respond to therapy with vitamin B_{12}, and there is no reduction in the level of serum vitamin B_{12}. Characteristically, many of the erythroid cells contain PAS-positive inclusions (Hayhoe et al, 1964). Kass (1977c) reviews some of the other biochemical and enzymatic changes that may be found in the abnormal erythroid cells. Perinuclear iron deposits (ringed sideroblasts) may be present (Bessis, 1973b) in this disease but are not diagnostic, since they are found in the sideroblastic anemias as well. The conversion of polycythemia vera to chronic erythremic myelosis is described (Eastman et al, 1968).

Dysmyelopoietic syndromes

The term "dysmyelopoietic" refers to cases in which the bone marrow shows qualitative and quantitative changes suggestive of acute leukemia but having a chronic course that does not necessarily terminate as acute leukemia (Sultan, in Gralnick et al, 1977). The unfortunate term "preleukemia" should not be used (Salomon and Tatarsky, 1969; Fisher et al, 1973; Kass, 1979). The term "smoldering acute leukemia" is at least descriptive of the natural history of some cases (Knospe and Gregory, 1971). Since, however, most patients live for years without developing an acute leukemia (Dreyfus, 1976), no term that includes the word "leukemia" should be used. This would be a "crepe hanging" situation (Siegler, 1975).

It is well known that many hematologic disorders carry the risk, usually low, of transforming into acute leukemia (Table 16-14). It is probably unjustified to refer to all these disorders as dysmyelopoietic diseases. The current recommendation is to apply the term to only three diseases: (1) refractory anemia with excess blasts, (2) chronic myelomonocytic leukemia, and (3) idiopathic sideroblastic anemia.

Refractory anemia with excess blasts (RAEB) is probably the most common dysmyelopoietic syndrome (Dreyfus, 1976; Streuli et al, 1980). The patients are middle aged or older, with insidious onset of anemia and weakness. The

Table 16-14. Some disorders with high risk of developing into leukemia

Refractory anemia with excess blasts (RAEB) (see text)
Chronic myelomonocytic leukemia (see text)
Polycythemia vera (Lawrence et al, 1969)
Myelofibrosis (Silverstein and Linman, 1969)
Sideroblastic anemia (Catovsky et al, 1971a)
Aplastic anemia (Pierre, 1974)
Paroxysmal nocturnal hemoglobinuria (PNH) (Kaufmann et al, 1969)
Trisomy 21 (Down's syndrome) (Jackson et al, 1968)
Ataxia-telangiectasia (Lampert, 1969)
Congenital hypoplastic anemia (Fanconi's syndrome) (Crossen et al, 1972)
Bloom's syndrome (Sawitsky et al, 1966)
Congenital agranulocytosis (Kostmann's disease) (Gilman et al, 1970)
Pure red cell aplasia (Schmid, 1963)
Monocytosis (Hurdle et al, 1972)

anemia is normochromic and normocytic. There may be any combination of leukopenia, anemia, and thrombocytopenia. The platelets are ultrastructurally abnormal and functionally abnormal, producing a thrombocytopathy with abnormal hemostasis (Sultan and Caen, 1972; Maldonado, 1976). There is no monocytosis. The bone marrow is hypercellular, containing atypical normoblasts and up to 30% myeloblasts and progranulocytes. Auer rods are not present, and these are considered characteristic of the frankly leukemic state. Serum and urine lysozyme levels are normal. The course is chronic with little change clinically or morphologically, but in one-fourth of the cases there is eventual evolution of acute myelocytic or acute myelomonocytic leukemia. Chemotherapy in the quiescent stage is not only useless but invariably dangerous (Dreyfus, 1976).

Chronic myelomonocytic leukemia is now classified as a dysmyeloplastic syndrome (Geary et al, 1975; Zittoun, 1976). It resembles the RAEB syndrome clinically and hematologically, except that the blood shows an increase in promonocytes and monocytes, up to 2,000/mm³ (2×10^9/l), and there is an increase in serum and urine lysozyme levels. The likelihood of developing acute (myelomonocytic) leukemia is fairly high.

Idiopathic sideroblastic anemia (p. 413) is a chronic syndrome that terminates in acute leukemia in about 10% of the cases. Dyserythropoiesis is more marked than in the other two dysmyeloplastic syndromes, with many ringed sideroblasts and increased deposits of iron in macrophages. There is no monocytosis in the blood, and the serum and urine lysozyme levels are normal.

MULTIPLE MYELOMA, PRIMARY MACROGLOBULINEMIA, AND OTHER IMMUNOGLOBULINOPATHIES
Introduction

In some diseases and in some nondisease situations, the serum or both urine contain increased amounts of immunoglobulin or immunoglobulin fragments. The increased serum or urine fraction is found as a monoclonal, or rarely biclonal, peak by electrophoresis, and the nature of the

Table 16-15. Conditions in which increased amounts of immunoglobulin or immunoglobulin fragments are found in serum or urine or both

Condition	Remarks
I. Multiple myeloma	
A. Type: IgG in serum only	Incidence: About 40% of all myelomas
B. Type: IgG in serum plus Bence Jones protein in urine	Incidence: About 20% of all myelomas
C. Type: IgA in serum only	Incidence: About 13% of all myelomas
D. Type: IgA in serum plus Bence Jones protein in urine	Incidence: About 5% of all myelomas
E. Type: Bence Jones protein only in urine and/or serum (light-chain disease)	Incidence: About 20% of all myelomas
F. Type: Mixed IgG and IgA in serum	Incidence: Rare
G. Type: Mixed IgG and IgM in serum	Incidence: Rare
H. Type: IgD in serum	Incidence: Rare
I. Type: IgE in serum	Incidence: Rare
J. Type: β_2-lipoprotein myeloma	Incidence: Rare, associated with xanthomatosis (Neufeld et al, 1964)
K. Type: No protein abnormality	Incidence: About 1% of all myelomas
II. Primary macroglobulinemia (Waldenström)	
III. γ-Heavy-chain disease (Franklin)	Anomalous protein is heavy-chain fragment of IgG or IgA
IV. α-Heavy-chain disease	
V. μ-Heavy-chain disease	Anomalous protein is heavy-chain fragment of IgM
VI. Monoclonal immunoglobulinopathy without neoplasm	
VII. Monoclonal immunoglobulinopathy associated with neoplasm	
VIII. Cryoglobulinemia	
IX. Pyroglobulinemia	
X. Para-amyloidosis	

Table 16-16. Structures of immunoglobulins in multiple myeloma and other immunoglobulin abnormalities*

Disease	L-chains	H-chains
Multiple myeloma		
IgG myeloma	κ or λ	γ
IgA myeloma	κ or λ	α
IgD myeloma	κ or λ	δ
IgE myeloma	κ or λ	ε
Bence Jones protein	κ or λ	None
γ-Heavy-chain disease	None	γ
α-Heavy-chain disease	None	α-A₁ subclass
μ-Heavy-chain disease	None	μ
Macroglobulinemia (IgM)	κ or λ	μ

*See Chapter 3 for structure of the immunoglobulins.

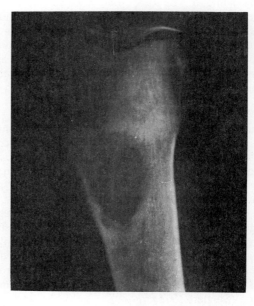

Fig. 16-21. Multiple myeloma. First manifestation was soft swelling of the leg, with solitary cystic lesion of the femur ("solitary" myeloma). The patient later developed generalized disease. (Courtesy Dr. R.E. Parks.)

abnormal component is identified by immunoelectrophoresis. The structure of the immunoglobulins is discussed in Chapter 3. Table 16-15 lists the conditions discussed in this section. The composition of the immunoglobulins found in these diseases is given in Table 16-16.

Multiple myeloma
Definition

Multiple myeloma (plasma cell myeloma) is a neoplasm of proliferating plasma cells of B-lymphocyte origin. Multiple myeloma and the lymphomas are considered lymphoproliferative disorders, in contrast to the myeloproliferative disorders. Overt clinical disease may be preceded by many years by monoclonal gammopathy (Kyle and Bayrd, 1965; Norgaard, 1971). The disease may present as a solitary tumor involving a bone (Fig. 16-21), *solitary myeloma,* or as diffuse osseous and organ involvement, *multiple myeloma.* Solitary myeloma may remain localized or may change into multiple myeloma. The features of the fully developed disease are related to the bone destruction, the replacement of normal bone marrow by plasma cells, and the hyperproteinemia and hyperglobulinemia (Kyle, 1975).

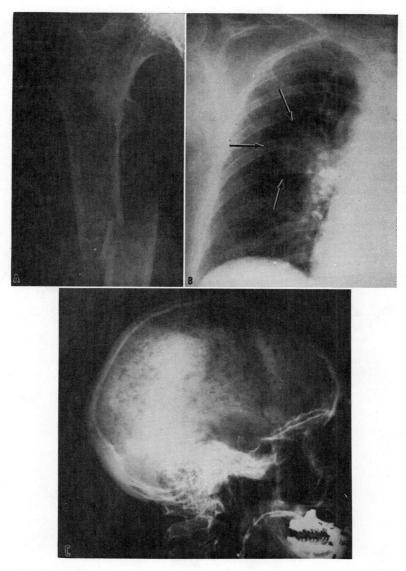

Fig. 16-22. Multiple myeloma. **A,** Pathologic fracture of the femur. **B,** Myelomatous infiltration of the lung. **C,** Involvement of the skull. (Courtesy Dr. R.E. Parks.)

The incidence of multiple myeloma is about 3/100,000, with a significantly higher incidence in black persons (McPhedran et al, 1972). The disease is rare in persons less than 30 years of age (Porter, 1963; Maeda et al, 1973), and the incidence increases with increasing age, with a peak incidence in the 60s or 70s (Carbone et al, 1967; McPhedran et al, 1972). There is no sex difference. Myeloma-like lesions have been found in skeletons of prehistoric American Indians (Morse et al, 1974).

Symptoms resulting from bone involvement are localized and consist of rheumatoid pain, swelling, deformity, or pathologic fracture (Fig. 16-22). The ribs, sternum, vertebral bodies, and skull are involved most frequently, but any bone containing marrow can be involved. There is a severe susceptibility to infection (Fahey et al, 1963) secondary to decreased concentrations of functional immunoglobulins.

The immunoglobulin deficiency is due in part to defective synthesis (Harris et al, 1971) and in part to increased catabolism (Solomon et al, 1963). There may be infiltration with plasma cells into almost any organ or tissue (Pasmantier and Azar, 1969). Other complications are renal failure secondary to the excretion of large amounts of protein, calcium, and uric acid (Schubert et al, 1972); a "hyperviscosity syndrome" caused by the hyperglobulinemia, particularly in the IgM type (Kopp et al, 1967; Tuddenham et al, 1974a); hypersensitivity to cold related to the presence of cryoglobulins (Osserman, 1959); abnormal bleeding caused by thrombocytopenia, interaction of myeloma globulins with coagulation factors, and abnormal platelet function (Niléhn and Nilsson, 1966; Cohen et al, 1970; Lackner et al, 1970); amyloidosis, especially in IgD myeloma (Friman et al, 1970; Glenner et al, 1973; Kyle and Bayrd, 1975); various neurologic symptoms (Osserman, 1959); and hypercalcemia (Cohen and Rundles, 1975).

In spite of these ominous complications the prognosis has improved as the result of appropriate chemotherapy (Alexanian et al, 1968).

Blood

The blood findings are those of a mild to severe myeloproliferative disorder. A mild, though sometimes severe, anemia is usually present. Polycythemia has been reported (Franzén et al, 1966) but is probably coincidental. The leukocyte count is usually normal or low but may be elevated. The blood smear may show normal erythrocytes with a few macrocytes, a few normoblasts, and, when the leukocyte count is high, immature myeloid cells. The smear usually shows extensive rouleau formation caused by the hyperglobulinemia. The presence of cold hemagglutinins often makes enumeration of the erythrocytes somewhat difficult unless the diluting fluid is warmed. The sedimentation rate is rapid as a result of rouleau formation.

If blood smears are examined with sufficient care, plasma cells will usually be found even in the supposedly nonleukemic phase. Plasma cells will be found almost invariably if the buffy coat is examined. When the peripheral blood contains many plasma cells, one is justified in making the diagnosis of plasma cell leukemia. Plasma cell leukemia occurs in about 2% of myeloma patients (Pruzanski et al, 1969). Polliack et al (1977) report B-cell acute lymphocytic leuke-

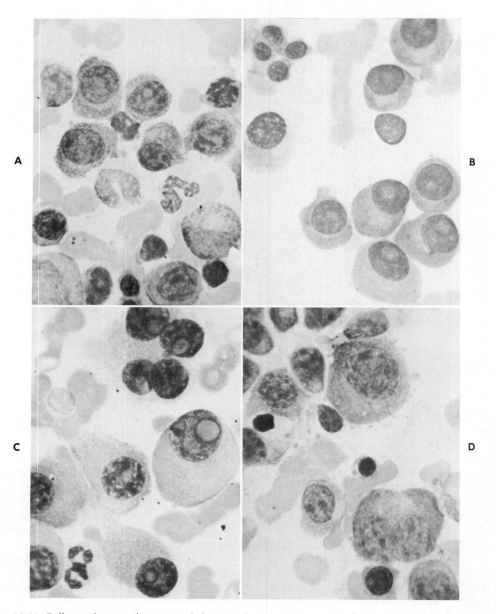

Fig. 16-23. Different degrees of maturity of plasma cells in multiple myeloma, bone marrow smears. **A,** Most mature. **D,** Least mature. (Wright's stain; ×950.)

mia as the terminal event. Terminal acute myelocytic leukemia (Tursz et al, 1974) and acute myelomonocytic leukemia (Parker, 1973) have also been reported.

Bone marrow

Typical bone marrow findings are illustrated in Plate 56. One of the two types of plasma cells is usually predominant. The first is a mature plasma cell indistinguishable from that normally found in the bone marrow (Fig. 16-23, *A*). The other is large, has a high nucleus-to-cytoplasm ratio and a fine nuclear structure, and may show one or more giant nucleoli (Fig.· 16-23, *B-D*). These atypical cells are sometimes called myeloma cells but are better classified as plasmablasts and proplasmacytes. They may show eosinophilic globular inclusions (Russell bodies) or Auer rods. Normal plasma cells are moderately acid-phosphatase positive, but the cells in multiple myeloma are almost uniformly strongly positive (Bataille et al, 1980). They may be phagocytic (Fitchen and Lee, 1979). Pseudo-Gaucher cells are sometimes found (Scullin et al, 1979). Many investigators have attempted to correlate the morphology of the plasma cells with the type of immunoglobulin synthesized, the aggressiveness of the disease, and the response to therapy. In general, there is little correlation. Waldenström (1961) and other investigators find that the "flaming plasma cell," or "thesaurocyte," usually is found in myeloma of the IgA type. Megaloblastic changes are sometimes seen (Hoffbrand et al, 1967).

Multiple myeloma in which the adult type of plasma cell is found tends to be less severe than that in which the cells are more primitive. While early cases may not show a striking increase, plasma cells usually account for more than 10% of the cells in the bone marrow, in contrast with benign plasmacytosis (in immunization, liver disease, etc.) in which plasma cells number less than 10%. Even so, it may be somewhat difficult to distinguish multiple myeloma and plasmacytosis from other causes unless there are characteristic roentgenologic, clinical, or laboratory findings.

Whether sparse or numerous, the plasma cells are often found in clumps.

Protein abnormalities

Abnormal protein metabolism is a characteristic feature of multiple myeloma. The types of immunoglobulin abnormality found in multiple myeloma are classified in Tables 16-15 and 16-16 and are illustrated in Figs. 16-24 to 16-35. The high concentration of immunoglobulin produces hyperviscosity and impaired blood flow and vascular insufficieny (McGrath and Penny, 1976). The separation of myeloma immunoglobulins on starch gel is shown in Fig. 16-36. Rarely, serum proteins are normal (Effert et al, 1960).

The laboratory evidence of protein abnormalities consists of one or more of the following: (1) hyperproteinemia caused by hyperglobulinemia, (2) electrophoretic evidence of an abnormal globulin component in the serum, (3) Bence Jones protein in the urine, (4) electrophoretic evidence of an abnormal globulin component in the urine with or without Bence Jones protein, (5) cryoglobulinemia, (6) macroglobulinemia, (7) pyroglobulinemia, and (8) identification and classification of the abnormal protein component (serum or urine) by immunoelectrophoresis.

Hyperproteinemia is seen in about 75% of the cases, ranging from 7.5 Gm to as high as 23.3 Gm/dl (750 to 2,330 Gm/l) of serum. The hyperproteinemia is caused by an increase in the globulin components so that the A/G ratio is reversed. Myeloma without serum or urine protein abnormalities has been called "hyposecretory myeloma" (Cabanel et al, 1973). Less than two dozen examples have been described. Equally rare are myelomas secreting two types of immunoglobulin (Rudders et al, 1973).

Bence Jones protein in the urine is found in approximately half the cases. Some claim that it can be found in a larger percentage of cases if at least six urine specimens are examined chemically at intervals. The technic used for detecting Bence Jones protein is critical (Naumann, 1966). It is identified by its characteristic solubility reactions on heating and

Text continued on p. 746.

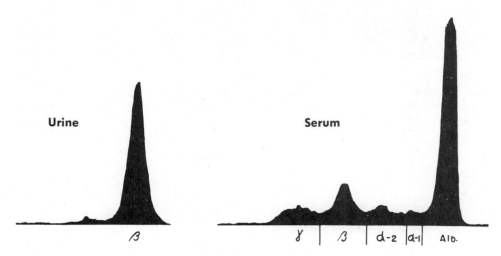

Fig. 16-24. Serum and urine electrophoresis patterns in a patient with multiple myeloma. The serum pattern is normal in this case, but the urine pattern shows an abnormal β-globulin constituent.

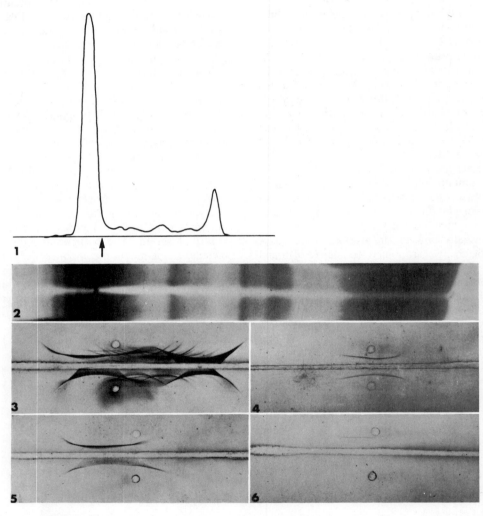

Fig. 16-25. Multiple myeloma. **1,** Electrophoresis showing abnormal peak in the γ area. **2,** Starch gel electrophoresis showing abnormal γ bands. **3-6,** Immunoelectrophoresis, normal control at top, patient at bottom: **3,** polyvalent antiserum; **4,** anti-IgA serum; **5,** anti-IgG serum showing abnormal γ component; **6,** anti-IgM serum showing decrease of IgM.

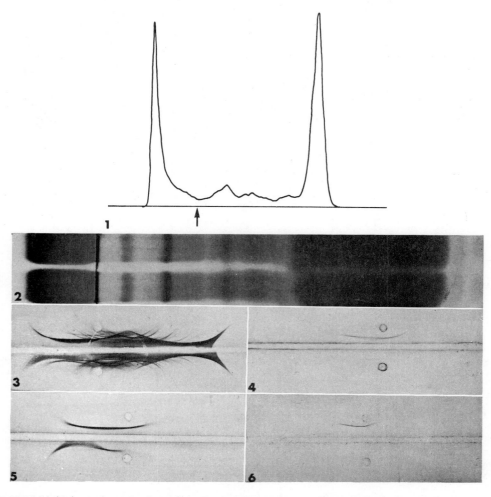

Fig. 16-26. Multiple myeloma. **1,** Electrophoretic pattern showing abnormal γ peak. **2,** Starch gel electrophoresis showing abnormal γ band. **3-6,** Immunoelectrophoresis, normal control at top, patient at bottom: **3,** polyvalent antiserum showing abnormal γ components; **4,** anti-IgA serum showing reduction of IgA; **5,** anti-IgG serum showing abnormal and increased IgG component; **6,** anti-IgM serum showing decreased IgM.

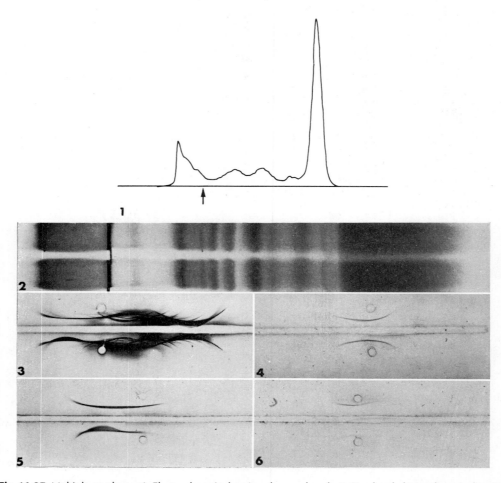

Fig. 16-27. Multiple myeloma. **1,** Electrophoresis showing abnormal peak. **2,** Starch gel electrophoresis showing abnormal γ component. **3-6,** Immunoelectrophoresis, normal control at top, patient at bottom: **3,** polyvalent antiserum; **4,** anti-IgA; **5,** anti-IgG showing increased IgG; **6,** anti-IgM showing decreased IgM.

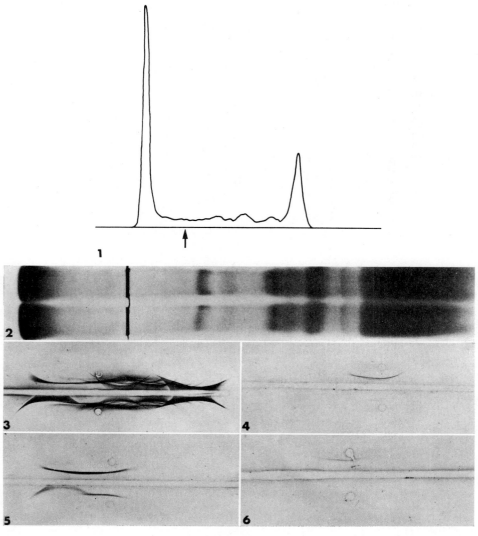

Fig. 16-28. Multiple myeloma. **1,** Electrophoresis showing abnormal γ peak. **2,** Starch gel electrophoresis showing homogeneous γ component. **3-6,** Immunoelectrophoresis, normal control at top, patient at bottom: **3,** polyvalent antiserum; **4,** anti-IgA showing decreased IgA; **5,** anti-IgG showing two IgG components; **6,** anti-IgM showing decreased IgM.

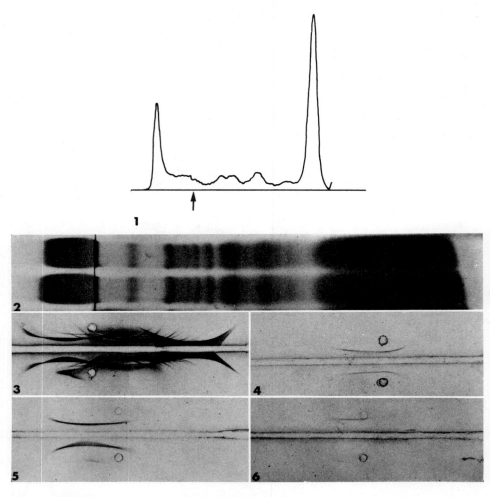

Fig. 16-29. Multiple myeloma. **1,** Electrophoresis showing abnormal γ peak. **2,** Starch gel electrophoresis showing abnormal γ component. **3-6,** Immunoelectrophoresis, normal control at top, patient at bottom: **3,** polyvalent antiserum; **4,** anti-IgA showing normal IgA; **5,** anti-IgG showing decreased IgG; **6,** anti-IgM showing decreased IgM.

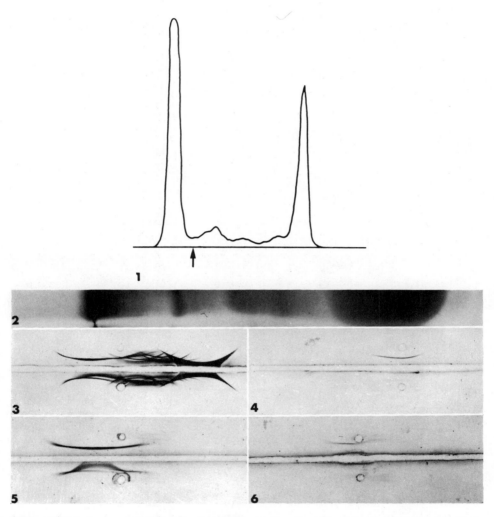

Fig. 16-30. Multiple myeloma. **1,** Electrophoresis showing abnormal γ peak. **2,** Starch gel electrophoresis show-ing abnormal component migrating partially in the γ and partially in the β area. **3-6,** Immunoelectrophoresis, normal control at top, patient at bottom: **3,** polyvalent antiserum showing two γ components; **4,** anti-IgA showing reduced IgA; **5,** anti-IgG showing several components; **6,** anti-IgM showing a reduction of IgM.

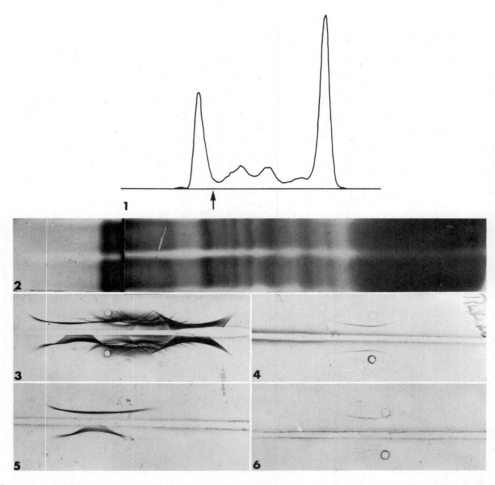

Fig. 16-31. Multiple myeloma. **1,** Electrophoresis showing abnormal γ peak. **2,** Starch gel electrophoresis show-ing multiple abnormal bands in the γ and β areas. **3-6,** Immunoelectrophoresis, normal control at top, patient at bottom: **3,** polyvalent antiserum; **4,** anti-IgA; **5,** anti-IgG; **6,** anti-IgM.

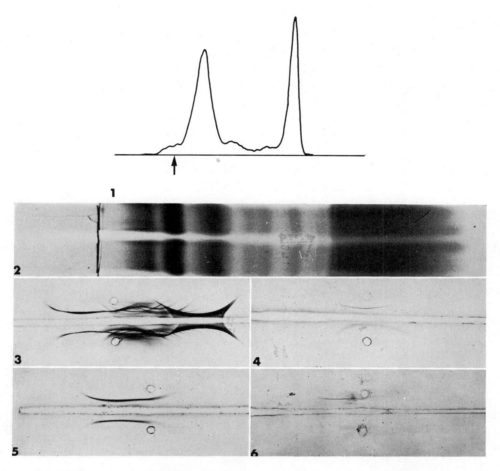

Fig. 16-32. Multiple myeloma. **1,** Electrophoresis showing abnormal β peak. **2,** Starch gel electrophoresis showing abnormal β components. **3-6,** Immunoelectrophoresis, normal control at top, patient at bottom: **3,** polyvalent antiserum; **4,** anti-IgA showing increased IgA; **5,** anti-IgG; **6,** anti-IgM.

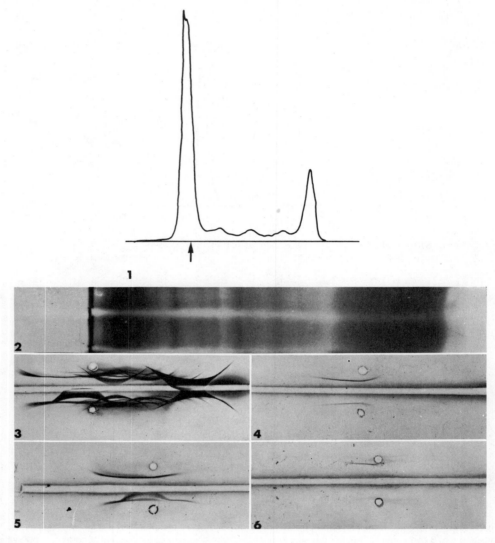

Fig. 16-33. Multiple myeloma. **1,** Electrophoresis showing abnormal peak in the γ and β areas. **2,** Starch gel electrophoresis showing abnormal component in the β area. **3-6,** Immunoelectrophoresis, normal control at top, patient at bottom: **3,** polyvalent antiserum; **4,** anti-IgA; **5,** anti-IgG showing several abnormal components; **6,** anti-IgM.

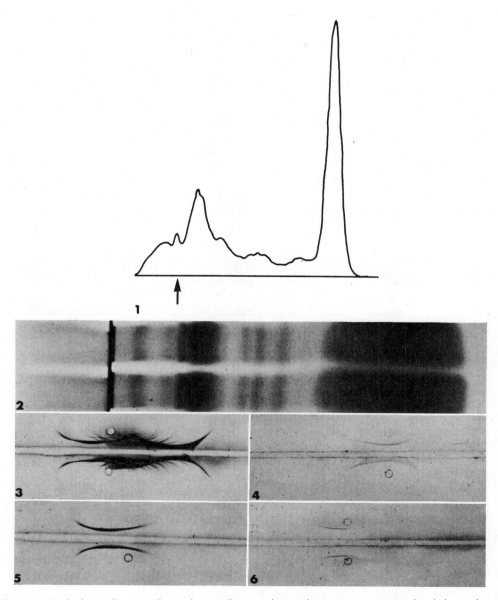

Fig. 16-34. Multiple myeloma. **1,** Electrophoresis showing abnormal β component. **2,** Starch gel electrophoresis showing an abnormal β component. **3-6,** Immunoelectrophoresis, normal control at top, patient at bottom: **3,** polyvalent antiserum; **4,** anti-IgA showing increased IgA; **5,** anti-IgG; **6,** anti-IgM.

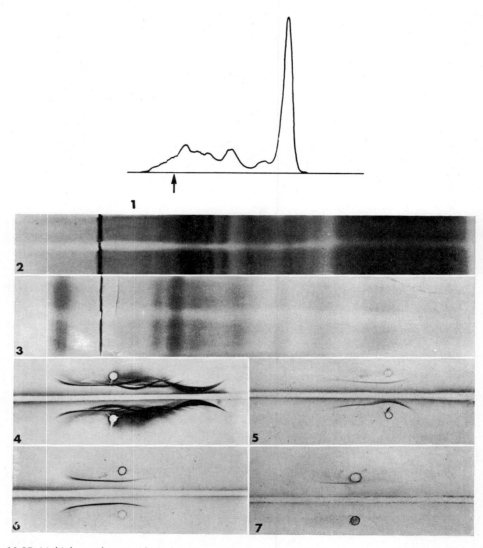

Fig. 16-35. Multiple myeloma in clinical remission after therapy. **1,** Electrophoretic pattern showing no striking abnormality. **2,** Starch gel electrophoresis of serum showing questionable bands in the β area. **3,** Starch gel electrophoresis of urine showing a Bence Jones component (to the left of the origin) and abnormal β component (to the right of the origin). **4-7,** Immunoelectrophoresis of serum, normal control at top, patient at bottom: **4,** polyvalent antiserum; **5,** anti-IgA showing an increased IgA; **6,** anti-IgG; **7,** anti-IgM.

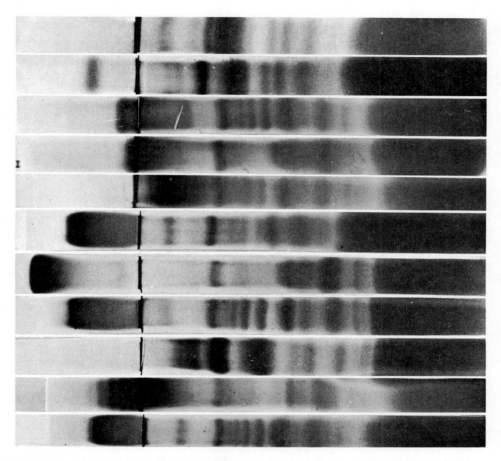

Fig. 16-36. Various patterns of serum protein abnormalities in multiple myeloma. Note that these 11 cases appear to be quite heterogeneous on starch gel. Compare with the multiple myelomas illustrated in Figs. 16-24 to 16-35. Starch gel electrophoresis, Amidoschwarz stain.

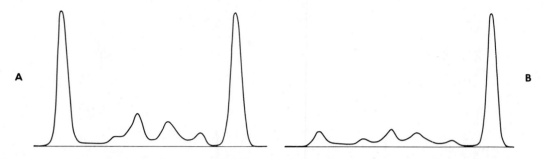

Fig. 16-37. Normalization of serum protein pattern in myeloma in remission. **A,** Initial cellulose acetate pattern (November 1969). **B,** Pattern in April 1976 following continuous intermittent treatment with melphalan and prednisone.

Table 16-17. Immunoglobulin changes in disease*†

	IgG	IgA	IgM		IgG	IgA	IgM
Immunoglobulin dis- orders				Infection			
Lymphoid aplasia	− − −	− − −	− − −	Pulmonary tuberculosis	+	N	N
Agammaglobulinemia	− − −	− − −	− − −	Trypanosomiasis	N(+)	N(+)	+ + +
Selective IgG, IgA deficiency	− − −	− − −	N or + +	Lupus erythematosus	+ +	+	+
				Rheumatoid arthritis	+	+	+
Selective IgA, IgM deficiency	N	− − −	− − −	Hepatic disease			
				Laennec's cirrhosis	+ +	+ + +	N
An-IgA- globulinemia	N	− − −	N	Biliary cirrhosis	N	N	+ +
				Acute hepatitis	+	+	+
Ataxia-telangiectasia	N	− − −	N	Hepatoma	N	N	−
Multiple myeloma, macroglobulinemia				Leukemia, lymphoma, etc.			
G (γ) myeloma	+ + +	− −	− −	Acute lymphoblastic leukemia	N	−	N
A (β₂A) myeloma	− −	+ + +	− −	Chronic lymphocytic leukemia	−	− −	− − −
M macroglobulinemia (Waldenström)	−	−	+ + +	Acute myeloblastic leukemia	N	N	N
Bence Jones proteinuria	−	−	−	Chronic myelocytic leukemia	N	−	N
Gastrointestinal protein loss	− −	− −	− −				
Nephrotic syndrome	− −	−	N	Hodgkin's disease	N	N	N

*From Fahey, 1965.
†N signifies normal; −, − −, and − − − signify progressively more severe reduction below normal; +, + +, and + + + signify progressively greater increases above normal.

cooling. Urine containing this protein shows a white, cloudy precipitate when heated to 60° C. The precipitate dissolves when the temperature is increased to boiling and reappears when the urine is cooled. It should be noted that Bence Jones protein is occasionally found in the urine when there is no hyperglobulinemia and that it may be absent in the presence of striking hyperglobulinemia. The finding of Bence Jones protein is not absolutely diagnostic of multiple myeloma since it is occasionally found in leukemia and in other benign and malignant bone marrow involvement.

Electrophoretic analysis of urine containing Bence Jones protein shows it to have a mobility between α_2-globulin and γ-globulin. Electrophoretic analysis of urine specimens giving a negative Bence Jones reaction occasionally reveals that an abnormal globulin is nevertheless present (Fig. 16-24). An appreciation of this finding indicates the desirability of performing electrophoretic analysis of urine spec-

imens in suspected cases, whether or not a Bence Jones reaction is obtained. Since the advent of immunoelectrophoretic methods, we believe that the demonstration of light chains in urine by these technics should replace the classic Bence Jones reaction. Some believe that subtyping of the light chains into κ or λ types is of value since several investigators have proposed that response to chemotherapy (melphalan) is good when light chains of the κ type are excreted and poor when excreted chains are of the λ type.

Other findings

Hypercalcemia is present in about half the cases. The mechanism by which hypercalcemia is produced is probably a combination of bone resorption and calcium retention caused by hyperplasia of the parathyroid glands and secondary to severe renal damage. The concentration of phosphorus and alkaline phosphatase in the blood is often normal.

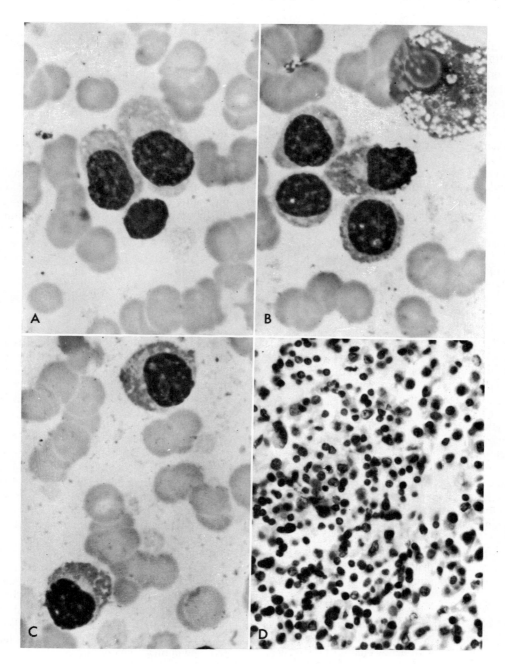

Fig. 16-38. Bone marrow, Waldenström's macroglobulinemia.

Renal damage is common, is sometimes severe (McIntyre, 1979), and is confirmed by high values for blood nonprotein nitrogen, urea nitrogen, creatinine, and uric acid. Albuminuria, cylindruria, and defective renal function tests are seen. Transcobalamin II levels are very high (Carmel and Hollander, 1978). Splenic puncture usually yields material that is diagnostic of myeloma. Tests of the coagulation system usually show many abnormalities (abnormal clot retraction, prolonged plasma prothrombin time, and defective thromboplastin generation) resulting from the interference by the high concentration of immunoglobulin rather than from deficiency of the coagulation factors. Fig. 16-37 illustrates the progressive improvement in the serum protein pattern during the course of melphalan therapy.

Primary macroglobulinemia (Waldenström)

Macroglobulins (immunoglobulin IgM) may be found in a variety of conditions (Table 16-17), but primary macroglobulinemia is a distinct syndrome closely related to multiple myeloma. It is also of B-cell origin. It was described by Waldenström in 1944, and the syndrome commonly bears his name (Argani and Kipkie, 1965; Bayrd et al, 1965).

The bone marrow shows a typical proliferation of "lymphoreticular" or "lymphoplasmacytoid" cells (Fig. 16-38), and it is thought that these cells are responsible for the synthesis of the macroglobulin in the blood (Fig. 16-39). While the cellular proliferation is responsible for the hepatomegaly (about 50% of the cases), splenomegaly (about 50% of the cases), and lymphadenopathy (about 30% of the cases), most of the symptomatology of the disease (and most of the laboratory findings) can be attributed to the effects of the macroglobulin. Thus an increase in the sedimentation rate, autohemagglutination, rouleau formation, hemorrhagic manifestations caused by the thrombocytopenia and interference with coagulation systems by the macroglobulin, and peripheral vascular occlusion (hyperglobulinemic purpura) are found. An accompanying deficiency in synthesis of normal IgG immunoglobulins accounts for the increased susceptibility to infection.

Macroglobulinemia is sometimes secondary to other diseases (Table 16-17). The cases illustrated in Figs. 16-40 and 16-41 are examples of macroglobulinemia secondary to disseminated lupus erythematosus and rheumatoid arthritis.

γ-Heavy-chain disease

Franklin et al (1964) reported the first instance of a gammopathy characterized by an excess of free heavy chains (H-chains). Osserman and Takatsuki (1964) reported an additional three cases. Frangione and Franklin (1973) and Franklin et al (1978) present a review of all the known cases.

The features of the syndrome are (1) proliferation of cells of the plasmacytic and lymphocytic series associated with the clinical pattern of malignant lymphoma (lymphadenopathy, hepatosplenomegaly), (2) excessive production of H-chains, γ type, and (3) decrease in the synthesis of normal immunoglobulins. The H-chain component is found in both serum and urine. Except in one case, there is no Bence Jones proteinuria. Feremans et al (1979) report a case of this disease characterized by λ–Bence Jones proteinuria and macroglobulinemia.

The H-chains in this disease are of several types (Frangione and Franklin, 1973), depending on where the molecular break takes place (Franklin et al, 1978).

α-Heavy-chain disease

Seligmann et al (1968b) and Seligmann and Rambaud (1969) described another type of heavy-chain disease characterized by the accumulation of heavy chains of the α type. There is infiltration of the lamina propria of the intestinal wall with lymphocytes, plasma cells, and histiocytes, accompanied by a malabsorption syndrome (Rambaud and Matuchansky, 1973). This disease has also been called "Mediterranean abdominal lymphoma" because the first cases studied occurred in persons living in countries bordering the Mediterranean (Brandtzaeg and Baklien, 1974), and most cases reported subsequently have come from the Mediterranean area. However, Cohen et al (1978) report α-H-chain disease associated with North American polyploid gastrointestinal lymphoma. Recent reviews by Seligmann (1975) and Selzer et al (1979) are recommended.

μ-Heavy-chain disease

A rare variant of the heavy-chain diseases, μ-heavy-chain disease, was described by Ballard et al (1970). Only a few additional cases have been discovered (Dammacco et al, 1974; Brouet et al, 1979). Most of the subjects had lymphoma or chronic lymphocytic leukemia (Josephson et al, 1973). The bone marrow shows lymphocytosis and vacuolated plasma cells.

Monoclonal immunoglobulinopathy without neoplasm

A heterogeneous and, as of now, poorly understood group of disorders is characterized by a monoclonal immunoglobulinopathy and no other detectable abnormality. Some cases are reported in which monoclonal immunoglobulinopathy precedes by years the development of multiple myeloma or primary macroglobulinemia. In the series reported by Osserman and Takatsuki (1963) this group makes up 10% of 400 cases of gammopathy. Of the 40 cases, 32 are of the IgG type, 7 of the IgA type, and 1 of the IgM type.

Monoclonal immunoglobulinopathy associated with neoplasm

Roughly half of the cases of monoclonal immunoglobulinopathy are associated with lymphomas and are of the IgG type. The others are associated with a variety of neoplasms, the most common being carcinoma of the rectosigmoid, carcinoma of the breast, carcinoma of the prostate, and tumors of the oropharynx (Migliore and Alexanian, 1968; Solomon, 1977).

Cryoglobulinemia and pyroglobulinemia

Cryoglobulins are globulins that precipitate out of *serum* at temperatures below 37° C. Most precipitate when serum is cooled to refrigerator temperature (4° C) (Figs. 16-42 and 16-43), but some show a gelatinous form even at room temperature. They redissolve at 37° C. Cryoglobulins may have immunologic characteristics of IgA, IgG, or IgM globulins, with corresponding molecular weights. Cryoglobulins are common in plasma cell myeloma (Rice, 1956; Costanzi et al, 1965) but are also found in association with other neoplasms (lymphosarcoma, chronic lymphocytic leukemia, and carcinomatosis), in infectious diseases (kala-azar, Sjögren's syndrome, subacute bacterial endocarditis, and malaria), in various systemic diseases (rheumatoid arthritis, periarteritis nodosa, and disseminated lupus erythematosus), and in miscellaneous disorders (myeloproliferative disorders and portal cirrhosis) (Goldberg and Barnett, 1970). In one case of cold cryopathy the protein has been found to be IgG (Grossman et al, 1972).

Cryofibrinogen is a cold-insoluble form of fibrinogen, precipitating out of *plasma* at refrigerator temperature (Ritzmann et al, 1963; Glueck and Herrmann, 1964). Cryofibrinogen precipitate characteristically dissolves in saline solution, but not in distilled water, at 37° C, and the solution is clottable by thrombin. Cryofibrinogenemia is found most commonly in multiple myeloma but may be associated with the same diseases that exhibit cryoglobulins. Cryofibrinogenemia is not uncommon in toxemia of pregnancy (McKay and Corey, 1964). An "essential" form has been described that is not associated with a disease state but is often associated with purpura and gangrene of the extremities secondary to peripheral vascular occlusion. It is commonly found

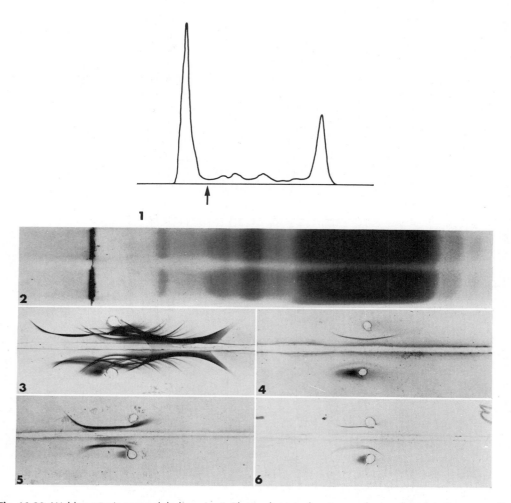

Fig. 16-39. Waldenström's macroglobulinemia. **1,** Electrophoresis showing an abnormal peak in the γ area. **2,** Starch gel electrophoresis showing that the abnormal protein component does not migrate in either direction from the origin. **3-6,** Immunoelectrophoresis, normal control at top, patient at bottom: **3,** polyvalent antiserum; **4,** anti-IgA; **5,** anti-IgG; **6,** anti-IgM showing increased IgM. Note failure of the protein to diffuse out of the wells.

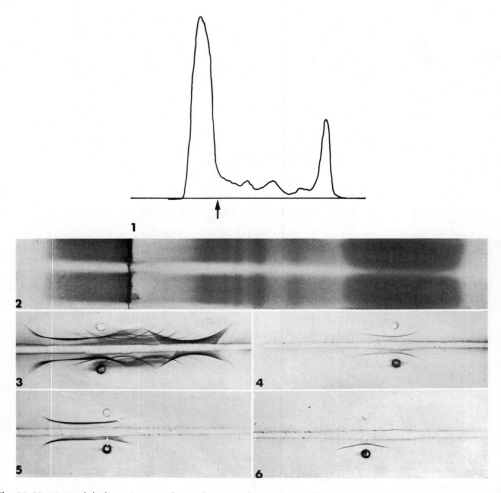

Fig. 16-40. Macroglobulinemia secondary to lupus erythematosus. **1,** Electrophoresis showing abnormal γ peak. **2,** Starch gel electrophoresis showing some migration into the γ area. **3-6,** Immunoelectrophoresis, normal control at top, patient at bottom: **3,** polyvalent antiserum; **4,** anti-IgA; **5,** anti-IgG; **6,** anti-IgM showing increased IgM.

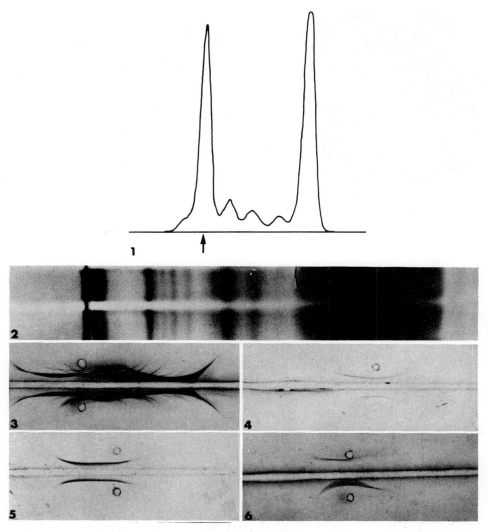

Fig. 16-41. Macroglobulinemia secondary to rheumatoid arthritis. **1,** Electrophoresis showing abnormal peak at origin. **2,** Starch gel electrophoresis showing very slight migration into the β area. **3-6,** Immunoelectrophoresis, normal control at top, patient at bottom: **3,** polyvalent antiserum; **4,** anti-IgA; **5,** anti-IgG; **6,** anti-IgM showing increased IgM.

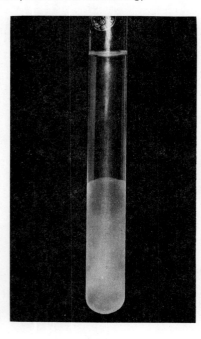

Fig. 16-42. Cryoglobulin. About half of the serum volume is made up of cryoglobulin precipitated at refrigerator temperature. See Fig. 16-43 for electrophoretic studies.

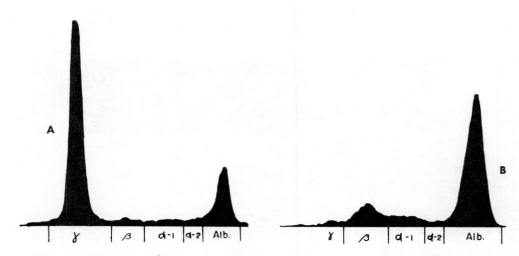

Fig. 16-43. Serum electrophoretic patterns of specimen shown in Fig. 16-42. **A,** Whole serum at 37° C (cryoglobulin in solution). **B,** Supernatant serum after cryoglobulin was removed by cold precipitation and centrifugation.

during the acute phase of familial Mediterranean fever (Shamir et al, 1974).

Pyroglobulins are heat precipitable from serum at 56° C and redissolve when the serum is cooled. They are not found as commonly as cryoglobulins, but in most instances they are associated with multiple myeloma (Brachfeld and Myerson, 1956; Fisher et al, 1963). They may be discovered accidentally when serum is inactivated by heat for various serologic tests. In a few cases, pyroglobulins have been found in an apparently normal person.

MALIGNANT LYMPHOMA
Introduction

Lymphomas are extramedullary proliferations of lymphoreticular cells. They are usually thought to be neoplasms, but they vary greatly in degree of malignancy and in response to therapy. Lymphomas, like lymphocytic leukemia, can properly be considered as "lymphoproliferative diseases" paralleling the concept of "myeloproliferative disorders," considered earlier in this chapter. When they are clonal, as they usually are, it can be assumed that the proliferating cell is the CFU-L or its derivatives (Fig. 1-5, p. 6). As pointed out earlier, the distinction between lymphoma and leukemia is sometimes arbitrary, and it is not unusual to find that the distinction becomes progressively more arbitrary as the disease progresses.

Classification

It is generally agreed that the classification of Rappaport (1966) (Table 16-18) as modified by Byrne (1977) (Table

Table 16-18. Classification of lymphomas according to Rappaport (1966)

I. Nodular lymphomas
  A. Lymphocytic lymphoma
    1. Poorly differentiated
    2. Moderately differentiated
    3. Well differentiated
  B. Lymphoma, mixed cell type
  C. Reticulum cell sarcoma (histiocytic lymphoma) (Gall, 1958)
  D. Hodgkin's disease (see Table 16-21)
II. Diffuse lymphomas
  A. Lymphocytic lymphoma
    1. Poorly differentiated
    2. Moderately differentiated
    3. Well differentiated
  B. Lymphoma, mixed cell type
  C. Reticulum cell sarcoma (histiocytic lymphoma) (Gall, 1958)
  D. Hodgkin's disease (see Table 16-21)

Table 16-19. Modified Rappaport classification of non-Hodgkin's lymphomas (Byrne, 1977)

I. Nodular lymphomas
  A. Lymphocytic, poorly differentiated
  B. Mixed cell, lymphocytic and histiocytic
  C. Histiocytic
II. Diffuse lymphomas
  A. Lymphocytic, well differentiated
  B. Lymphocytic, poorly differentiated
  C. Mixed cell, lymphocytic and histiocytic
  D. Histiocytic
  E. Lymphoblastic
  F. Undifferentiated, Burkitt type
  G. Undifferentiated, non-Burkitt type

Table 16-20. Modified classification of lymphomas (Lukes and Collins, 1974, 1975)

I. Modified type (U cell)
II. T-cell types
  A. Mycosis fungoides and Sézary's syndrome
  B. Convoluted lymphocyte
  C. ? Immunoblastic sarcoma
  D. ? Hodgkin's disease
III. B-cell types
  A. Small lymphocyte (chronic lymphocytic leukemia)
  B. Plasmacytoid lymphocyte
  C. Follicular-center cell types (follicular, diffuse, follicular and diffuse, and sclerotic)
    1. Small cleaved cell
    2. Large cleaved cell
    3. Small noncleaved cell
    4. Large noncleaved cell
  D. Immunoblastic sarcoma
IV. Histiocytic type
V. Unclassifiable

16-19) is the most useful (Jackson, 1979). The Rappaport classification is based exclusively on the histopathology of the lymphoma, and there are numerous data correlating the histopathology of the lesion with the patient's survival and response to therapy. The availability of immunologic and enzymatic cell markers has suggested the possibility that alternate classifications based on cell markers might be clinically more useful (Jaffe et al, 1977; Berard et al, 1978; Brubaker and Whiteside, 1979; Brubaker et al, 1979; Frizzera et al, 1979; Pinkus and Said, 1979). Such a classification was proposed by Lukes and Collins (1974, 1975) (Table 16-20). There is some correlation between the Rappaport and the Lukes-Collins classifications (Bloomfield et al, 1979), but whether the latter is more applicable to the patient's management remains to be seen (Nathwani et al, 1978).

Non-Hodgkin's lymphoma
Nodular lymphoma

The non-Hodgkin's lymphomas are defined as malignant lymphomas arising from, or differentiating toward, germinal center cells. As a rule they exhibit a follicular or nodular growth pattern. This nodular pattern may be associated with a diffuse pattern. Occasionally only a diffuse pattern is seen, but a reticulin stain may still reveal remnants of a nodular pattern.

Lymphomas with a nodular pattern have to be distinguished from reactive follicular hyperplasia. The criteria for separating these two entities are well summarized by Rappaport et al (1956). They are based on architectural and cytologic features. In nodular lymphomas the architecture is partially or completely effaced. This is true of all malignant lymphomas and is best appreciated by a study of the subcapsular area, which is normally occupied by the peripheral sinus. Obliteration of the subcapsular sinus is particularly well seen with reticulin stains. Neoplastic nodules vary moderately in size and shape and are evenly distributed throughout cortex and medulla. Reactive follicles are especially prominent in the cortical portion of the lymph node and vary considerably in size and shape. Reaction centers are more sharply demarcated than neoplastic follicles.

Reticulin fibers may be condensed at the periphery of neoplastic nodules, while they are slightly altered around reactive follicles (MacKenzie, 1959). Cytologically, reactive follicles show debris-containing macrophages and frequent mitotic figures. In neoplastic nodules, macrophages are inconspicuous and mitotic figures are scarce.

Examples of some nodular types of lymphomas are shown in Figs. 16-44 and 16-45.

Diffuse lymphoma

Lymphomas are classified as diffuse when, because of a diffuse growth pattern, the architecture of the lymph node is effaced. Examples of some diffuse lymphomas are given in Figs. 16-46 to 16-48.

Burkitt's lymphoma

Burkitt's tumor (lymphoma, undifferentiated, Burkitt type) is a diffuse, lymphoma with characteristic clinical and histologic features. Burkitt's tumor was first reported as a jaw sarcoma of East African children (Burkitt, 1958). It was identified as a malignant lymphoma by O'Conor and Davies (1960). In American patients, abdominal and pelvic

Text continued on p. 759.

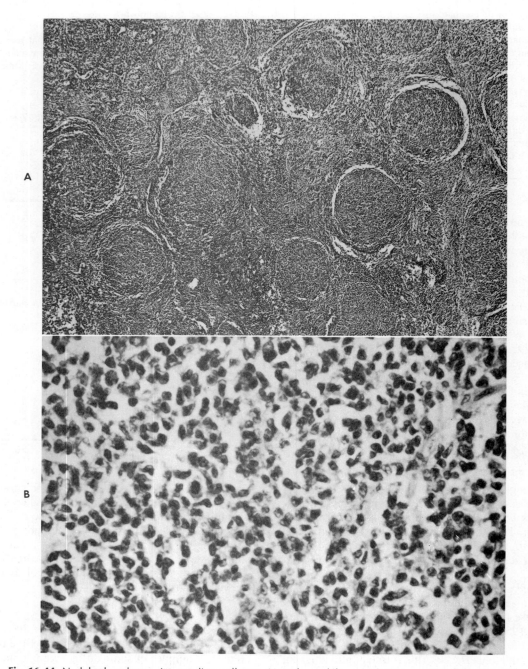

Fig. 16-44. Nodular lymphoma, intermediate cell type. Note the nodular growth pattern, **A,** and the distorted irregular nuclear membranes, **B.** (Hematoxylin-eosin stain: **A,** ×100; **B,** ×850.)

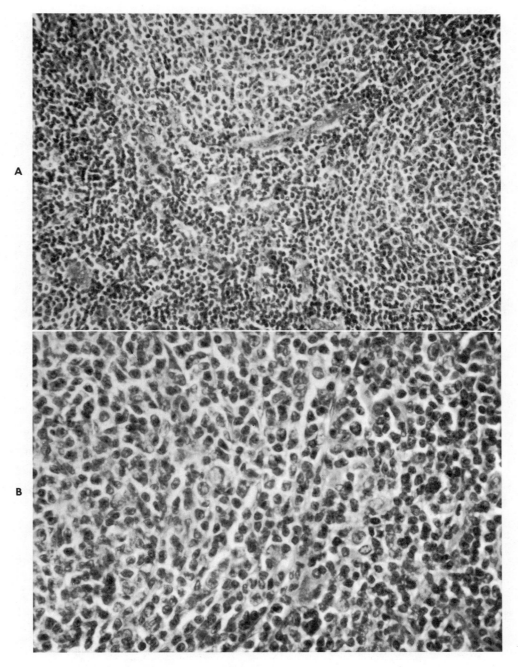

Fig. 16-45. Nodular lymphoma, mixed cell type. (Hematoxylin-eosin stain; **A,** ×350; **B,** ×850.)

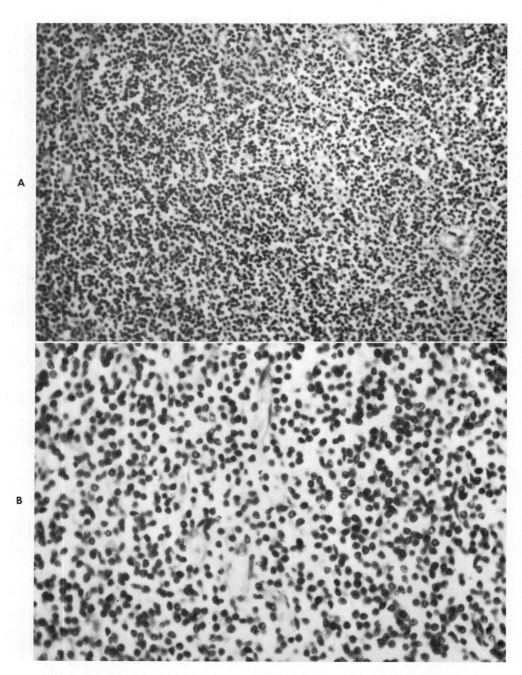

Fig. 16-46. Diffuse lymphoma, small cell type. (Hematoxylin-eosin stain; **A,** ×350; **B,** ×850.)

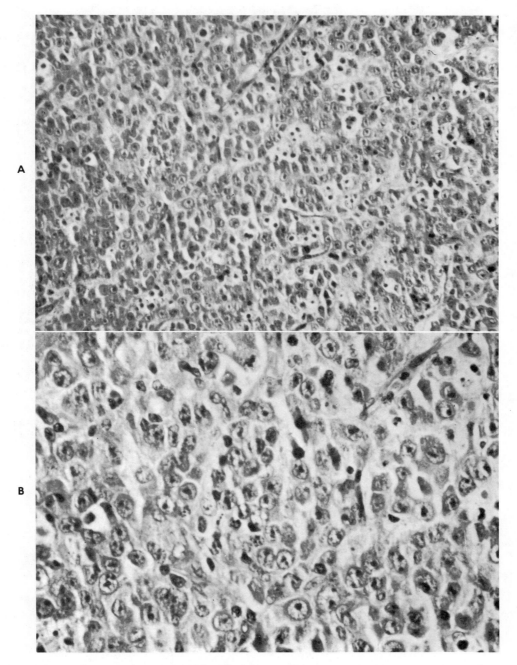

Fig. 16-47. Diffuse lymphoma, poorly differentiated (? lymphoblastic). (Hematoxylin-eosin stain; **A,** ×350; **B,** ×850.)

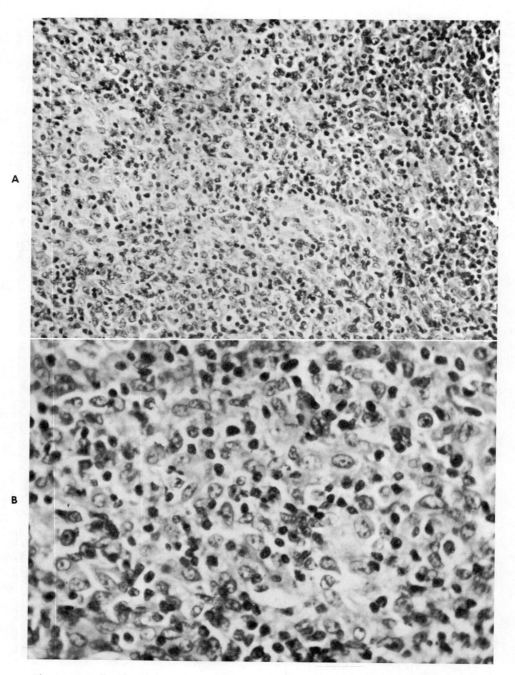

Fig. 16-48. Diffuse lymphoma, mixed cell type. (Hematoxylin-eosin stain; **A,** ×350; **B,** ×850.)

involvement is far more frequent than jaw involvement. Bone marrow involvement is also more frequent in American patients. In a series of 30 American patients 23 had an abdominal tumor (Arseneau et al, 1975; Banks et al, 1975). Four of these showed ovarian involvement. Lymphadenopathy was the sole presenting physical finding in only 3 cases. Facial bones were involved in 5 cases and were the presenting sites of tumor in 3 cases. Involvement of the bone marrow was documented in 5 of the 26 patients whose bone marrows were available. Good correlation between lactic dehydrogenase values and stage of Burkitt's tumor has been reported. Complete remissions were obtained in 13 of the 30 patients treated with chemotherapy. Metabolic complications related to therapy included azotemia, hyperkalemia, hyperuricemia, hyperphosphatemia, and hypocalcemia. Of the 13 patients who had a complete remission, 9 were free of disease for 37 to 80 months.

Histologically, Burkitt's tumor is composed of "blasts" with pyroninophilic and Giemsa-positive cytoplasmic rims. Nucleoli are prominent. Characteristic of this neoplasm is a "starry sky" appearance caused by the presence of benign-appearing phagocytic cells containing debris. Some PAS-positive material can be identified in these macrophages. The histologic features of Burkitt's tumor have been defined by the World Health Organization (Berard et al, 1969) and are reviewed by Wright (1971).

In 17 autopsied cases of Burkitt's tumor the most consistent feature was widespread organ involvement, predominantly in the extralymphatic sites (Banks et al, 1975). All had tumor in two or more gastrointestinal organs. Twelve had hepatic involvement and 16 had tumor in kidneys. Involvement of lungs was present in 11 cases and of the central nervous system in 9. Cardiovascular organs and the musculoskeletal system were infiltrated with tumor in 6 patients. Diffuse peripheral lymph node involvement was seen in only 1 patient. The spleen was involved in 10 and the bone marrow in 12 of the 17 autopsied cases. Chemotherapeutic agents appeared to alter the cytologic appearance of the tumor. The cells exhibited marked pleomorphism resembling malignant histiocytes. Reed-Sternberg–like cells were seen occasionally.

Clinical correlations

There is less information available on clinicopathologic correlations for the "non-Hodgkin's" lymphomas than for Hodgkin's disease. In a large series of cases (Jones et al, 1973), nodular lymphomas were found in 44% of the group and diffuse lymphomas in 56%. Patients under 35 years of age and those over 60 years of age tended to have diffuse lymphomas. When they were first diagnosed, 39% of the patients had stage IV disease. Systemic symptoms did not adversely affect survival. They were present in 24% of patients with diffuse and 18% of patients with nodular lymphomas. Patients with nodular lymphomas survived significantly longer than patients with diffuse lymphomas. Malignant lymphomas, whether nodular or diffuse, have a better prognosis if they exhibit a tendency to sclerosis (Millett et al, 1969). The small cell lymphomas fare better than the large cell lymphomas.

Other features of non-Hodgkin's lymphomas

Monoclonal immunoglobulinopathy is not uncommon (Krauss and Sokal, 1966; Alami et al, 1969). Acquired autoimmune hemolytic anemia and antiglobulin-positive and idiopathic thrombocytopenic purpura are complications (Jones, 1973). Salmon (1974) calls the complications encountered in non-Hodgkin's lymphomas "paraneoplastic syndromes" and discusses their pathogenesis. Biopsied bone marrow tissue should be examined carefully in view of the high incidence of bone marrow involvement (Vinciguerra and Silver, 1974). Bone marrow involvement may lead to megaloblastic dysplasia and macrocytic anemia (Fig. 16-49). The leukemic phase of lymphoma is characterized by the presence of immature lymphoid (lymphosarcoma) cells in blood (Figs. 16-50 and 16-51).

Hodgkin's disease
Classification

In contrast with lymphocytic and histiocytic lymphomas, there is fairly good agreement as to the histologic classification of Hodgkin's disease. The current classification (Rye classification) is a simplification of the one proposed by Lukes et al (1966) (Table 16-21) and was established at a conference on Hodgkin's disease held in Rye, New York, in 1965.

According to the Rye classification, which has been almost universally adopted, Hodgkin's disease is subdivided into four types: (1) lymphocyte predominance, (2) nodular sclerosis, (3) mixed cellularity, and (4) lymphocyte depletion (Lukes, 1971). In general, the more mature lymphocytes there are, the better the prognosis. The various histologic types of Hodgkin's disease should not be thought of as fixed and rigid categories. Thus, a patient who initially presents with lymphocytic predominance type, in time may change to the mixed and finally to the lymphocyte depletion type. However, the nodular sclerosis type of Hodgkin's disease remains so, even though, during its cellular phase, it may have the diverse histologic appearance of the other types of Hodgkin's disease in addition to the nodular structure, the bands of collagen, and the Reed-Sternberg cells.

A histologic diagnosis of Hodgkin's disease requires the demonstration of Reed-Sternberg cells (Fig. 16-52). The classic or diagnostic type of Reed-Sternberg cell is a large cell with an abundant acidophilic to amphophilic cytoplasm, which is pyroninophilic. It may contain two or more nuclei or a lobated nucleus with prominent, large, acidophilic, round, inclusion-like nucleoli, which are surrounded with perinucleolar halos. In addition to this diagnostic type of Reed-Sternberg cell there are three variants: (1) the lacunar type of Reed-Sternberg cell, characteristic of the nodular sclerosis type of Hodgkin's disease, (2) a polyploid type of Reed-Sternberg cell seen in the lymphocyte predominance type, and (3) the pleomorphic, sarcomatous variant seen in the lymphocyte depletion type (Lukes, 1971). In general the number of Reed-Sternberg cells found is inversely proportional to the number of lymphocytes present. It should be remembered that Reed-Sternberg cells by themselves are not sufficient for a diagnosis of Hodgkin's disease, since morphologically identical cells can be seen in other diseases

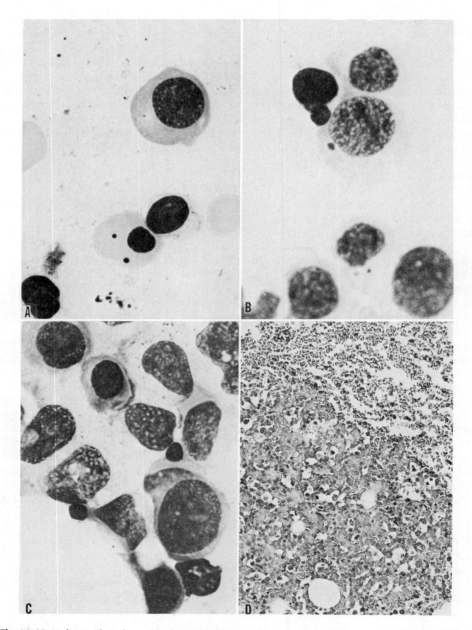

Fig. 16-49. Malignant lymphoma involving the spleen and bone marrow with associated megaloblastic dyspoiesis in the bone marrow in a 71-year-old white man. There was refractory macrocytic anemia with weakness and difficulty in swallowing. Bone marrow aspiration biopsy revealed intermediate megaloblasts and many naked nuclei. Paraffin section of marrow revealed solid areas of lymphosarcoma. **A-C,** Bone marrow smears. (Wright's stain; ×1,000.) **D,** Paraffin section of bone marrow. (Hematoxylin-eosin stain; ×144.) (Courtesy Dr. Dan Seckinger.)

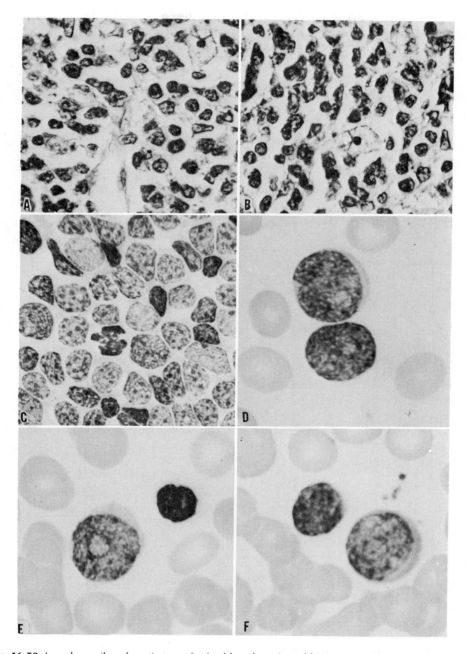

Fig. 16-50. Lymphoma (lymphocytic type, ? mixed lymphocytic and histiocytic) with terminal leukemic phase (leukosarcoma) in a 50-year-old white man. Onset of adenopathy and splenomegaly occurred 1 year before death. Biopsy of lymph nodes revealed lymphoma. One year later there was an acute change in the peripheral blood: WBC count 21,600/mm³ (21.6 × 10⁹/l) with 65% atypical lymphocytes. Splenic puncture revealed the same type of cell population. **A** and **B,** Lymph nodes. (Hematoxylin-eosin stain; ×585.) **C,** Splenic puncture. (Wright's stain; ×585.) **D-F,** Peripheral blood. (Wright's stain; ×1,425.)

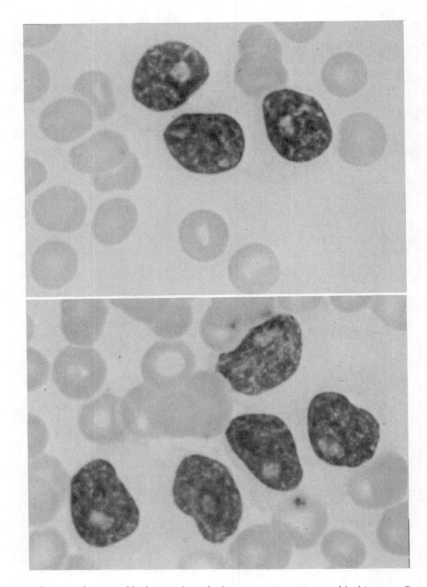

Fig. 16-51. Lymphoma with terminal leukemic phase (leukosarcoma) in a 67-year-old white man. Onset occurred 1 year before death and was marked by splenomegaly and weight loss. In spite of chemotherapy, there was little improvement. The terminal picture was that of the leukosarcoma phase; WBC count was 35,200/mm³ (35.2 × 10⁹/l)—92% of the cells as illustrated. Peripheral blood. (Wright's stain; ×1,425.)

Table 16-21. Histologic types of Hodgkin's disease, with comparison of old nomenclature, that proposed by Lukes et al (1966), and modified Lukes classification*†

Old terminology	Lukes (1966)	Modified Lukes‡
	I. Lymphocytic and histiocytic	**I.** Hodgkin's disease, lymphocytic predominance
Hodgkin's paragranuloma	**A.** Diffuse (lymphocytes predominant)	
Lymphoreticular medullary reticulosis		
Benign Hodgkin's disease		
Reticular lymphoma		
Follicular lymphoma, Hodgkin's type	**B.** Nodular (lymphocytes predominant)	
Hodgkin's granuloma	**C.** Nodular or diffuse (histiocytes predominant)	
Lymphocytic Hodgkin's disease		
Hodgkin's granuloma	**II.** Mixed	**II.** Hodgkin's disease, mixed type
Fibromyeloid medullary reticulosis		
Hodgkin's granuloma with sclerosis	**III.** Nodular sclerosis	**III.** Hodgkin's disease, nodular sclerosis type
	IV. Diffuse sclerosis	**IV.** Hodgkin's disease, lymphocytic depletion type
	V. Reticular	
Hodgkin's granuloma	**A.** With nonpleomorphic Reed-Sternberg cells	
Reticulo-Hodgkin's disease		
Hodgkin's sarcoma	**B.** With pleomorphic Reed-Sternberg cells	

*Modified from Lukes et al, 1966.
†I believe that the classification proposed by Lukes is more descriptive and useful than the modified nomenclature in column 3, but the modified nomenclature is widely used.
‡Modified Lukes classification recommended at Conference on Hodgkin's Disease, Rye, New York, September, 1965.

such as infectious mononucleosis. They have to be found in association with other characteristic histologic features before a diagnosis of Hodgkin's disease can be established.

Lymphocytic predominance type

The proliferation of small lymphocytes with a varying number of mature histiocytes may involve the lymph node diffusely or focally (Fig. 16-53). When the node is involved diffusely, it resembles a malignant lymphoma of the small (well differentiated) lymphocytic type or chronic lymphocytic leukemia. The diagnosis of Hodgkin's disease is made when classic Reed-Sternberg cells are found (Fig. 16-52). These are rare, and many sections may have to be examined before one is found. The scarcity of diagnostic Reed-Sternberg cells is as important for the diagnosis of the lymphocyte predominance type of Hodgkin's disease as is the abundance of lymphocytes. In addition to the rare diagnostic Reed-Sternberg cell, a rather characteristic variant is more frequently found in the lymphocytic predominance type of Hodgkin's disease. It consists of a large, polyploid, twisted nucleus with fine nuclear chromatin and only small nucleoli.

Nodular sclerosis type

Two criteria are essential for the diagnosis of the nodular sclerosis type: bands of collagen and the lacunar type of Reed-Sternberg cell (Fig. 16-54). The most distinctive feature of the lacunar Reed-Sternberg cell is a pericellular halo that is seen in formalin-fixed tissue and is caused by the retraction of the cytoplasm leaving only a small amount of perinuclear, acidophilic cytoplasm. The nuclei of the lacunar cells are hyperlobated and vary in size. Prominent nucleoli are always present. With Zenker's fixation the pericellular halo is not present, and these cells may be overlooked.

In addition to these two criteria, nodular sclerosis exhibits diverse histologic appearances resembling the other histologic types of Hodgkin's disease. Occasionally the entire node may be replaced by dense, hyalinized collagen.

Nodular sclerosis is the most common histologic type of Hodgkin's disease. It is seen somewhat more frequently in women and predominantly affects mediastinal, supraclavicular, and cervical lymph nodes.

Mixed cellularity type

In the mixed cellularity type the architecture of the lymph node is obliterated by proliferating lymphocytes, histiocytes, eosinophils, polymorphonuclear leukocytes, and plasma cells (Fig. 16-55). Focal necrosis may be present. There is usually some fibrosis, which varies in degree in different portions of the node. Diagnostic Reed-Sternberg cells are frequent. Mixed cellularity also serves as an unclassified type and includes all cases that lack the typical features for the remaining types.

Lymphocyte depletion type

The lymphocyte depletion type is a group that contains the diffuse fibrosis and reticular types of the classification of Lukes et al. "Diffuse fibrosis" is an inaccurate term for the histologic alteration observed. The lymph nodes are depleted of lymphocytes and exhibit a deposit of a homogenous, nonfibrillary, nonbirefringent eosinophilic material, best described as hyaline (Fig. 16-56). Stains for amyloid are negative. This process is often associated with the reticular type of Hodgkin's disease, which shows proliferation, focal

Text continued on p. 770.

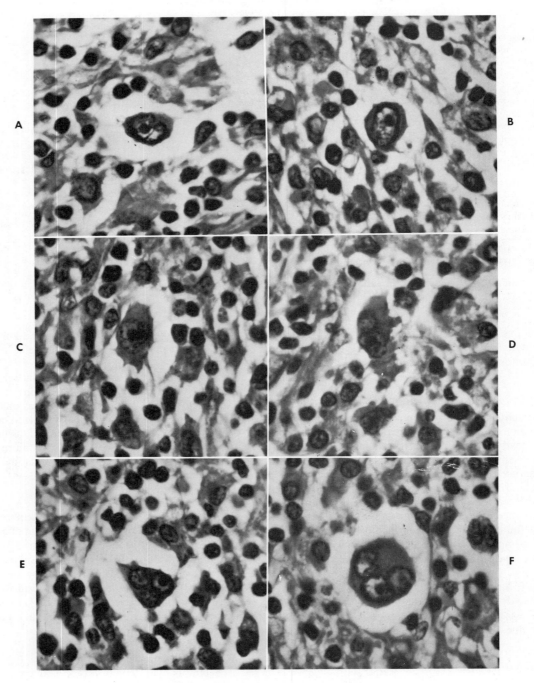

Fig. 16-52. Reed-Sternberg cells, Hodgkin's disease.

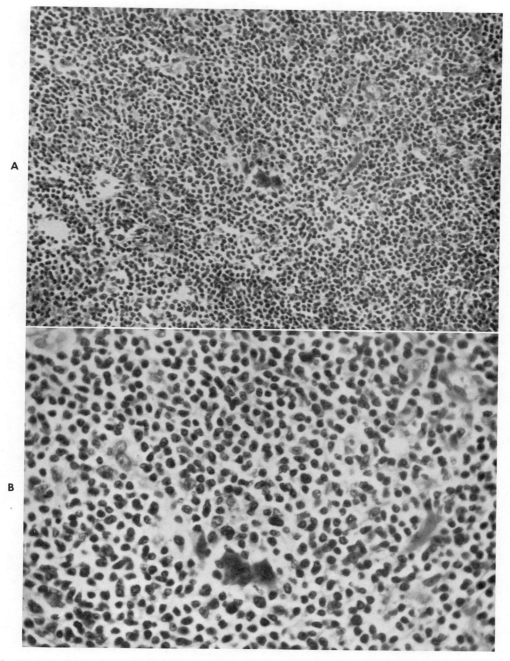

Fig. 16-53. Hodgkin's disease, lymphocytic predominance. Note the polyploid Reed-Sternberg cell, characteristic of this type. (Hematoxylin-eosin stain; **A,** ×350; **B,** ×850.)

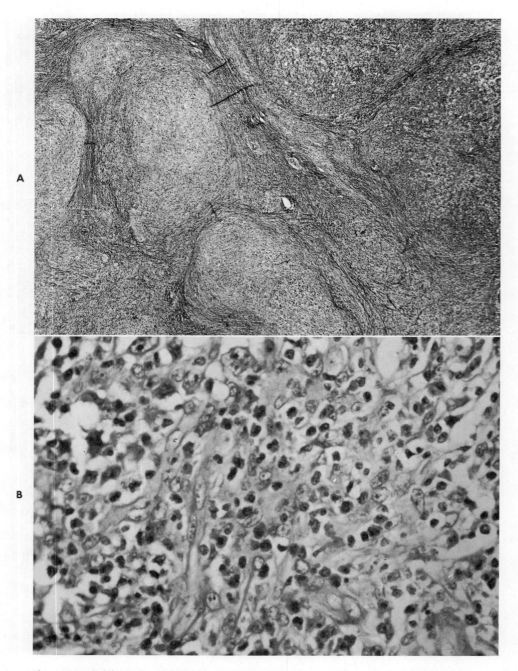

Fig. 16-54. Hodgkin's disease, sclerosing, nodular. (Hematoxylin-eosin stain; **A,** ×90; **B,** ×850.)

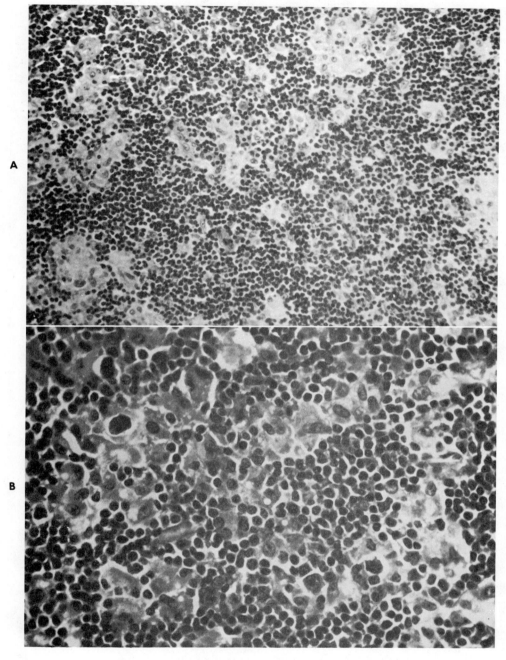

Fig. 16-55. Hodgkin's disease, mixed cellularity type. (Hematoxylin-eosin stain; **A,** ×350; **B,** ×850.)

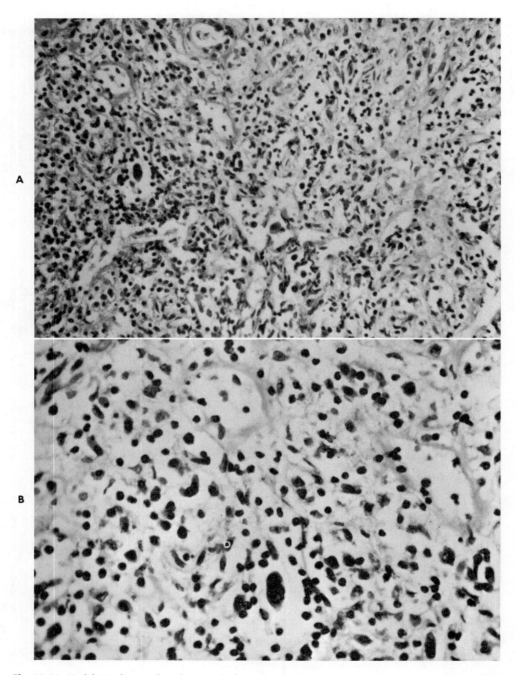

Fig. 16-56. Hodgkin's disease, lymphocytic depletion type. (Hematoxylin-eosin stain; **A,** ×350; **B,** ×850.)

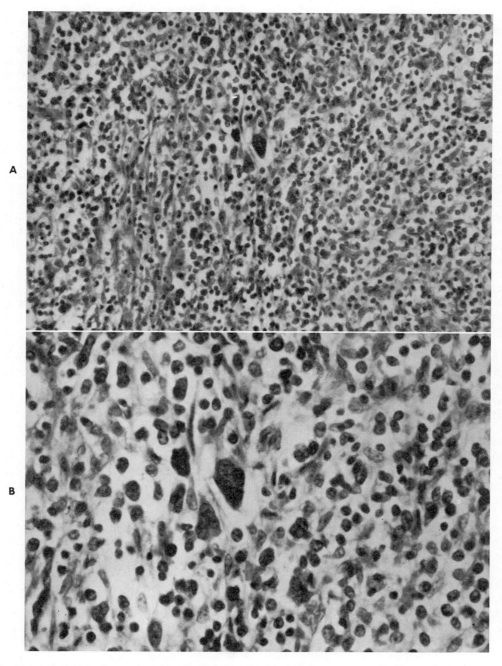

Fig. 16-57. Hodgkin's disease, lymphocytic depletion type (Hodgkin's sarcoma), with pleomorphic Reed-Sternberg cells. (Hematoxylin-eosin stain; **A,** ×350; **B,** ×850.)

or diffuse, of highly atypical reticulum cells with varying numbers of diagnostic Reed-Sternberg cells (Fig. 16-57). In addition, there may be numerous pleomorphic Reed-Sternberg cells with bizarre nuclei and absent or giant eosinophilic nuclei.

The lymphocytic depletion type of Hodgkin's disease often is seen clinically as a rapidly progressive disease with fever, pancytopenia, and lymphocytopenia, and frequently without peripheral lymphadenopathy (Neiman et al, 1973; Bearman et al, 1978b). The distribution of the lesions is predominantly subdiaphragmatic, with extensive involvement of liver, spleen, retroperitoneal lymph nodes, and bone marrow.

Clinical presentation and staging

The most common clinical presentation of malignant lymphoma is painless lymphadenopathy. The "lump" feels rubbery firm, and the diagnosis is established by biopsy and histologic examination. The lymph node or nodes involved may be in any of the lymph node–bearing areas of the body. If internal lymph nodes are involved, the presenting symptoms may be caused by pressure by the nodes on important structures, such as pressure by hilar nodes on bronchi, causing cough. If the disease is widespread, the patient may have systemic symptoms such as fever and weight loss. Mycosis fungoides is a special type of malignant lymphoma in which cutaneous plaques and tumors are present. Burkitt's tumor or lymphoma is predominantly a tumor of childhood that is seen as a rapidly growing tumor usually extranodal in location.

A detailed scheme for the clinical staging of Hodgkin's disease has been worked out (Carbone et al, 1971). It correlates well with prognosis and helps in deciding whether radiotherapy or chemotherapy should be used. The same clinical staging is also applicable to the non-Hodgkin's lymphomas, though less experience is available with staging in these entities. It must be emphasized that clinical and pathologic staging classifications apply only to the patient at the time of disease presentation and before definitive therapy. The lymphatic structures are defined as the lymph nodes, spleen, thymus, Waldeyer's ring, appendix, and Peyer's patches. Stage I is involvement of a single lymph node region or of a single extralymphatic organ or site (I_E). Stage II is involvement of two or more lymph node regions on the same side of the diaphragm or localized involvement of an extralymphatic organ or site in addition to one or more lymph node regions on the same side of the diaphragm (II_E). Stage III is involvement of lymphatic structures on both sides of the diaphragm that may be associated with localized involvement of an extralymphatic organ or site (III_E), involvement of the spleen (III_S), or both (III_{SE}). Stage IV is diffuse or disseminated involvement of one or more extralymphatic organs or tissue with or without associated lymph node involvement. Each stage is further subdivided into A or B categories, B for those with defined general symptoms and A for those without. General symptoms include (1) unexplained weight loss of more than 10% of the body weight in the 6 months before examination, (2) unexplained fever with temperatures about 38° C, and (3) night sweats.

Staging laparotomy

Staging laparotomy with splenectomy and biopsy of liver, retroperitoneal nodes, and bone marrow is performed to determine the extent of the disease, as well as the extent of radiotherapy or chemotherapy or both. This procedure is performed most often to confirm the extent of the disease in patients who clinically appear to have stage I or II disease. Approximately 25% of spleens, clinically unsuspected, are involved with Hodgkin's disease when studied by the pathologist (Rosenberg, 1971). On the other hand, about 50% of clinically enlarged spleens will not exhibit Hodgkin's disease on detailed pathologic examination. It is unusual for the liver to be involved in the absence of splenic Hodgkin's disease. The overall demonstration of liver involvement by laparotomy is about 5%. The bone marrow must be examined histologically to establish a diagnosis of Hodgkin's disease, although at times the appearance of neoplastic reticulum cells in smears of aspirated bone marrow is equally diagnostic (Fig. 5-77, p. 337). Marrow for histologic examination may be obtained by aspiration (Rywlin et al, 1970), by trephine, or by an open surgical technique. The yield of positive bone marrow biopsies is 9% in untreated patients whose disease is beyond stage II (Rosenberg et al, 1971).

Criteria for diagnosis

Staging laparotomies resulting in the submission to the pathologist of relatively small biopsies of liver and bone marrow have raised the question as to minimum criteria necessary for the diagnosis of Hodgkin's disease (Rappaport et al, 1971). The criteria are not as stringent as for the initial diagnosis of Hodgkin's disease, and diagnostic Reed-Sternberg cells with eosinophilic, inclusion-like nucleoli are not required. Mononuclear cells, with nuclear features of Reed-Sternberg cells (Hodgkin cells) in one of the characteristic cellular environments of Hodgkin's disease, should be regarded as indicative of liver or bone marrow involvement. The presence of atypical lymphoreticular cells that fall short of these criteria should be reported as "suggestive of Hodgkin's disease." The presence of nonspecific lymphoreticular infiltrates or sarcoidlike granulomas should not be considered as evidence of Hodgkin's disease (Kadin et al, 1970). Focal fibrosis of the bone marrow, associated with lymphoreticular cells in the absence of mononuclear or multinuclear cells with nuclear features of Reed-Sternberg cells, should be regarded as strongly suggestive of Hodgkin's disease in an untreated patient with histologically proven Hodgkin's disease.

Hodgkin's disease of the spleen primarily involves the white pulp and varies from microscopic foci to grossly visible nodules. In treated patients, features of any of the histologic types of Hodgkin's disease may be identified, with the possible exception of lymphocyte predominance (Lukes, 1971). In the lymphocyte depletion type, the malpighian corpuscles are hyalinized and Reed-Sternberg cells are scarce. In the reticular variant of lymphocyte depletion, bizzare, pleomorphic Reed-Sternberg cells are frequent and are associated with varying numbers of diagnostic Reed-Sternberg cells.

When vascular invasion is observed in sections of lymph nodes or spleen, there is a greater prevalence of disseminated and extranodal Hodgkin's disease (Strum et al, 1971).

Clinical correlations

In a study of 176 previously untreated cases of Hodgkin's disease (Keller et al, 1968), it was found that after 6 years the highest number of survivors were in the lymphocyte predominance group. The largest histologic group, comprising half the cases, was in the nodular sclerosis group. The second largest group was mixed cellularity. The lymphocyte predominance and lymphocyte depletion groups were about equal in frequency and constituted together approximately 10% of the patients. Patients with lymphocyte predominance were almost entirely in clinical stages I and II, while lymphocyte depletion cases were largely in stages III and IV. The data from Keller et al (1968) show that survival is related to the stage of the disease. Survival rate after 4½ years was 90% for stage I, 65% for stage II, 40% for stage III, and 20% for stage IV. According to histologic type, 90% survival was found for patients with the lymphocytic predominance type, 70% survival for the nodular sclerosis type, and slightly less than 40% survival for the lymphocytic depletion and mixed cellularity types. There was also a high degree of correlation between extensive disease and systemic symptoms. Thus nearly four-fifths of stage IV cases had systemic symptoms, while three-fourths of stage II cases had none.

The vast majority of patients with active Hodgkin's disease display a defect in cell-mediated immunity. This defect contributes to the variety of bacterial, viral, mycotic, and protozoal infections to which these patients are prone (Aisenberg, 1972).

PSEUDOLYMPHOMA

Lymph nodes can undergo reactive changes that are usually benign in nature but in which the histopathology mimics one of the lymphomas. Typically, such changes are found in lymph nodes after immunization. An excellent review of these lesions can be found in the monograph by Jackson (1979).

17

"Upon this gifted age, in its dark hour,
Falls from the sky a meteoric shower
Of facts . . . they lie unquestioned, uncombined.

Wisdom enough to leech us of our ill
Is daily spun; but there exists no loom
To weave it into fabric";

Edna St. Vincent Millay: *Collected Sonnets*

Hemostasis and blood coagulation

INTRODUCTION: COAGULATION PAST,
    PRESENT, AND FUTURE
    Coagulation past
    Coagulation present
    Coagulation future
HEMOSTASIS
    Mechanisms of hemostasis
BLOOD COAGULATION
    The classic theory
    The "modern" theory
    The blood coagulation sequence
    The coagulation factors
        Fibrinogen
        Prothrombin
        Thromboplastin
        Thrombin
        Factor V
        Factor VII
        Factor VIII
        Factor IX
        Factor X
        Factor XI
        Factor XII
        Factor XIII
        The Fletcher factor
        The Fitzgerald factor
        Other coagulation factors
    Nonhemostatic functions of the coagulation system
    Hemostasis in the newborn
PHASE I
    Platelets and hemostasis
        Introduction
        Platelet morphology
        The platelet membrane
        Organelles
        Energy metabolism
        Interaction of platelets with subendothelial tissues
    Platelet function
        Shape change
        Platelet adhesion
        Platelet aggregation
        Platelet release reactions
    Role of platelet factor 3
    Role of factors XI and XII

Laboratory studies in phase I abnormalities
    Platelet morphology
    Bleeding time
    Tourniquet test
    Clot retraction
    Platelet factor 3 release
    Platelet factor 4 release
    Release of serotonin
    Platelet adhesiveness (retention)
    Platelet aggregation
    Deficiency of contact factors
Classification of platelet disorders
Thrombocytopenic states
    Caused by excessive destruction or sequestration
        Due to immunologic mechanisms
            Idiopathic thrombocytopenic purpura (ITP)
            Symptomatic thrombocytopenic purpura
        Due to splenomegaly and sequestration in the spleen
        Due to sequestration not in the spleen
        Due to mechanical destruction
        Due to miscellaneous factors
    Caused by deficient production
        Due to bone marrow suppression
        Deficient thrombocytopoiesis, mechanism unknown
        Congenital, neonatal, or familial thrombocytopenic
            syndromes
Functional platelet abnormalities
    Thrombasthenia
    Storage pool disease
    Bernard-Soulier syndrome
    Thrombopathic thrombocytopenia
    Von Willebrand's disease and variants
    Congenital afibrinogenemia
    Thrombocytopathy associated with established congenital
        diseases or syndromes
    Absent collagen-induced aggregation
    Acquired thrombocytopathy caused by drugs
    Congenital enzymatic deficiencies
    Acquired thrombocytopathy secondary to other diseases
Thrombocytosis and thrombocythemia
PHASE II: THROMBOPLASTINOGENESIS
    Factors involved
    Interaction of factors
    Naturally occurring inhibitors
    Pathologic inhibitors

Hemorrhagic disorders in phase II
Laboratory investigation of phase II abnormalities
  Bleeding time
  Coagulation time of venous blood
  Prothrombin time
  Partial thromboplastin time
  Recalcification time of plasma
  Prothrombin consumption test
  Thromboplastin generation test
  Identification of the factor deficiency by differential
    APTT studies
  Assays of coagulation factors
Hemophilia (factor VIII deficiency)
  History
  Genetics
    Inheritance
    Factor VIII synthesis
  Incidence
  Severity
  Clinical findings
  Multiple factor deficiencies
  Laboratory diagnosis
Factor IX deficiency
  Genetics
  Laboratory diagnosis
Factor X deficiency
Factor XI deficiency
Factor XII deficiency
Summary
Therapy of phase II abnormalities
  General considerations
  Hemophilia
  Factor IX deficiency
  Factor X deficiency
  Deficiency of factor XI or XII
PHASE III: THROMBINOGENESIS
  Reactions
  Role of vitamin K
  Hemorrhagic disorders in phase III
    Congenital deficiencies
      Deficiency of factor II
      Deficiency of factor V
      Deficiency of factor VII
    Acquired deficiencies
      Vitamin K deficiency in adults
      Hemorrhagic disease of the newborn
      The "lupus anticoagulant"
      Oral anticoagulants
        Drug interaction with coumarin drugs
        Standardization of therapeutic range based on standard
          reference plasmas
PHASE IV: FIBRIN FORMATION AND FIBRINOLYSIS
  Mechanism of the reaction
    Action of thrombin
    Physiologic fibrin
    Fibrinolysis
      Activation by bacterial filtrates
      Activation by tissue activator
      Activation by urokinase
      Inhibitors of fibrinolysis
  Hemorrhagic disorders caused by abnormalities in phase IV
    Dysfibrinogenemia
    Afibrinogenemia and hypofibrinogenemia
      Congenital afibrinogenemia
      Acquired hypofibrinogenemia
    Diffuse intravascular coagulation (DIC)

    Definition
    Synonyms
    Etiology
    Pathogenesis
      Induction by endotoxin
      Role of inflammation
      Role of immune reactions
      Activation of the extrinsic coagulation system
    Classification
    Laboratory diagnosis
  Increased fibrinolytic activity
  Summary: differentiation of DIC from hyperfibrinolysis
  Immunoglobulinopathies
  Deficiency of factor XIII
  Summary
HEMORRHAGIC DISORDERS CAUSED BY VASCULAR DEFECTS
  Scurvy
  Hereditary hemorrhagic telangiectasia
  Thrombotic thrombocytopenic purpura
  Allergic purpura
  Connective tissue disorders
  Autoerythrocyte sensitization
  The prethrombotic ("hypercoagulable") state
    Platelets
      Platelet count
      Platelet adhesiveness
      Platelet aggregation
      Platelet survival and turnover
      Components of the release reaction
    Coagulation factors
    Products of fibrinogen to fibrin conversion or fibrinolysis
    Reduced fibrinolytic activity
    Serum lipoproteins
    Conclusion
LABORATORY DIAGNOSIS OF HEMORRHAGIC DISORDERS
  Preoperative tests
  Laboratory control of anticoagulant therapy
    Control of oral anticoagulant therapy
    Control of heparin therapy
  Investigation of a hemorrhagic disorder

INTRODUCTION: COAGULATION PAST, PRESENT, AND FUTURE
Coagulation past

It might be rewarding to consider what stimulated the early interest in blood coagulation. We can profitably begin with the mid-1800s, at which time most investigators were concerned with coagulation as it related to the problems of phlebitis, arterial thrombosis, and embolism. Jean Cruveilhier, elected to the first Chair of Pathologic Anatomy in Paris, had stated in 1837 that inflammation of the veins (phlebitis) was the basic pathologic process in disease. In Vienna, in 1842, Rokitansky expounded the theory that all diseases are a manifestation of a chemical imbalance in blood whereby it becomes coagulated in capillary vessels, the coagulant stimulus being products of inflamed tissues. In 1843 Rudolph Virchow, generally considered the father of cellular pathology, began a series of fundamental chemical studies on blood and concluded that *fibrin* was formed in the course of coagulation from a precursor in blood that he named *fibrinogen*. He then turned his attention to intravascular thrombosis and in 1845 described the process of embolism, previously unappreciated. Virchow's combined chemical and anatomic approach to the problem of thrombosis is perhaps the first great milestone. Note that it seemed then that the coagulation of blood was important in its relation to thrombosis rather than abnormal bleeding. We will come back to this point later.

Shortly after this, in 1860, Alexander Schmidt began his studies on the chemistry of blood coagulation. He showed a remarkable facility for first proposing and then abandoning one theory after another. He was, so to speak, the first "flexible" coagulationist. Nevertheless, he and his contemporary, Hammarsten, contributed the following fundamental concepts: (1) the conversion of fibrinogen to fibrin is enzymatic; (2) the enzyme (*fibrin-ferment*) is *thrombin* and is a component of the washed blood clot; (3) thrombin is derived from an inactive precursor called *prothrombin;* (4) activation of prothrombin to thrombin is effected by constituents of leukocytes and tissues called *zymoplastic* agents; and (5) calcium salts are essential for the process of coagulation. The last point was reinforced by the observation of Arthus and Pages that oxalate and citrate could inhibit coagulation.

The basic expression of the classic coagulation theory was presented by Paul Morawitz in 1905. He stated that prothrombin, fibrinogen, and calcium are present in circulating blood and that prothrombin activation is accomplished by *thrombokinase* (from disintegrating leukocytes and platelets or, in intravascular thrombosis, from diseased tissues). He assumed the presence of *antithrombins* in circulating blood that keep the reaction in check if thrombokinase is present in low concentration.

Thus the classic reactions are two:

I. Prothrombin $\xrightarrow{\text{Thrombokinase Ca}^{++}}$ Thrombin

II. Fibrinogen $\xrightarrow{\text{Thrombin}}$ Fibrin

Now it must be noted that this was a most important contribution, since these basic steps have been modified only by the addition of complex intermediate reactions. It dominated the following 40 years of research in the field. Again, it continued to relate the mechanisms of blood coagulation to the problem of intravascular thrombosis.

Before going into the "modern" era, we should emphasize the relative disinterest during the 1800s in what we now call the *hemorrhagic* diseases. Purpura was then, as now, a clinical sign and, because it affects the skin, was of interest only to the dermatologist. It was described by Werlhof in 1735, and Haberdeen first described the anaphylactoid type in 1735 even though it now bears the names of Schönlein (1837) and Henoch (1868). The relationship of purpura to some abnormality in the blood was first pointed out by both Andrew Duncan and George Johnston in 1822. They both described the absence of clot retraction in purpura, but as yet no explanation was available. The prolonged bleeding time (or "flowing time") was noted the following year (1823) by William Stoker, but it was not until 1910 that Duke published his method for determining the bleeding time and emphasized the very fundamental difference between the coagulation time and the bleeding time.

The relationship of platelets to purpura did not become apparent for many years. Platelets were first recognized as cellular entities in 1842 by Donné, but it was not until 1895 that Hayem reported the association of thrombocytopenia and purpura. Interestingly, Hayem, up to the time he died in 1933, and most authorities in the mid-1800s, considered platelets to be breakdown products of leukocytes or the source of erythrocytes. The first clear statement that platelets are an important part of the blood coagulation mechanism was given by Bizzozero in 1882.

The only other hemorrhagic diathesis recognized during this period was hemophilia. Though the "bleeding disease" was known to the ancients, the term "hemophilia" was coined by Hopff in 1828. Schönlein, in 1837, referred to it as hemorrhaphilia—undoubtedly better derived but destined to never being adopted. It was recognized that blood clotted slowly in this disease, and the sex-linked inheritance pattern was appreciated. It was also known that the clotting time of whole blood could be corrected by normal plasma but not by serum. However, the early coagulationists blamed a lack of calcium and, later, every new blood clotting factor as it was described. It was not until 1937 that Patek and Taylor established that hemophilia was a deficiency state of a substance normally present in blood—antihemophilic globulin.

There are two particularly interesting chapters in the history of hemophilia. The first took place in 1840. At that time, Samuel Lane operated on an 11-year-old boy for squint and encountered severe postoperative bleeding. He learned then that the boy was a known bleeder, and when the bleeding continued, he felt obliged to resort to the procedure of blood transfusion being advocated by Blundell (Chapter 12). Accordingly, about 170 ml of fresh whole blood from a normal female donor was transfused using Blundell's method and equipment. Bleeding stopped almost immediately. This is undoubtedly the first blood tranfusion used in the treatment of hemophilia, but this observation made little impact.

The second interesting note refers to Addis' observation in 1911 that both normal plasma and the globulin fraction from normal plasma corrected the prolonged clotting time of hemophilic whole blood. Since it was known that the globulin fraction contained prothrombin, by then firmly established as an important coagulation factor, Addis concluded that hemophilic blood was deficient in prothrombin. Because of his stature as an eminent physician, Addis' concept prevailed until the 1930s when it was finally refuted by Quick (one-stage prothrombin time) and by Warner et al (two-stage prothrombin assay). Later coagulationists have often shown an atavistic kinship with Addis, because he showed, without meaning to, the fundamental difference between an observation and the validity of the conclusions drawn from it.

Coagulation present

What we consider to be the modern era is perhaps arbitrary and might vary with the writer. In view of the coagulation renaissance in the 1930s, we think of the year 1930 as the dividing line between past and present. However, because of developments, from the 1930s to the present, in the physiology and role of platelets in normal and abnormal hemostasis and the evidence that coagulation factors have two properties, procoagulants and immunologically detectable proteins, an even more modern era can be identified. The following is an historical overview.

Just as a major river comes into being by the contribution of diverse tributaries, so is today's knowledge the result of several lines of investigation that at one time seemed to be unrelated and sometimes even contradictory. For our purpose here, we will consider seven major contributions: (1) the work of Dam, Schönheyder, McFarlane, Almquist, Stokstad, Tage-Hausen, and Doisy on vitamin K; (2) the work of Roderick, Quick, and Link et al on toxic sweet clover disease; (3) the development of Quick et al of the "one-stage prothrombin time" test; (4) the development of the "two-stage" assay for prothrombin by Warner et al; (5) the discovery of factor V deficiency by Owren; (6) the discovery of molecular variants of antihemophilic factor by Shanberge, Denson, Biggs, and Ratnoff, followed by the discovery of molecular variants of other coagulation factors; and (7) the contributions of many investigators to the present understanding of platelet physiology, abnormal function, and thrombosis.

First, the story of vitamin K. In 1929 Dam observed that chicks fed a synthetic diet developed a hemorrhagic state that could not be prevented or cured by citrus juice. This hemorrhagic state in chicks was described by others, but there are recurring references to the cause being a deficiency of vitamin C in the face of undeniable evidence that vitamin C had nothing to do with it. The observation of McFarlane in 1931 that the blood failed to clot was universally ignored until 1935, at which time Schönheyder rediscovered it. In the same year, Dam coined the term "Koagulation-vitamin," vitamin K, for the substance missing from the chicks' diet and responsible for the bleeding abnormality.

The nature of the bleeding defect could not be clarified until the technics for studying it became available. In this area as well as in many others Quick's one-stage test was a bell, however imperfect, in the dense fog of coagulation theory. Basing his approach on the classic theory of Morawitz, Quick measured the clotting time of plasma when an optimum amount of calcium ions and thromboplastin was added. If Morawitz's theory was correct, the clotting time in such a test system should be a function of the only unknown (other than fibrinogen) in the mixture, i.e., prothrombin. This Quick believed and fought for during the early years. When he applied his test to the blood of the bleeding chicks in 1937, he found the prothrombin time to be prolonged and concluded that the prothrombin decreased in chicks when they were put on a vitamin K–free diet.

Meanwhile (1936) Warner et al had developed another system for assaying prothrombin, the so-called two-stage test. This was also based on the classic theory, but the reaction was made to happen in two steps; in the first, thrombin was generated from prothrombin, and in the second, thrombin was measured. We now appreciate that the two-stage method is more closely a measure of prothrombin than the Quick method, more by chance than design, for both are based on the classic two-step theory and both were devised before the other factors affecting the conversion of prothrombin were discovered. In any case, when these two tests

were applied to various bleeding disorders, serious discrepancies were found. The discrepancies led to intense and sometimes bitter controversy.

It took some years to unravel the difference, but there is no doubt that the development of the one-stage and two-stage tests, plus the stimulating battles between the two camps, initiated the modern era of blood coagulation. The positive accomplishments that can be attributed mostly to Quick's test were these: (1) the major reactions in the classic theory of Morawitz were confirmed; (2) it showed that hemophilia is not caused by a prothrombin deficiency; (3) it pinpointed the cause of bleeding in hemorrhagic disease of the newborn, in obstructive jaundice, and in Dam's chicks as being in the prothrombin conversion phase; (4) it provided Link et al with the assay method needed for the identification of the toxic agent in spoiled sweet clover; (5) it provided the basic technic for the laboratory control of oral anticoagulant therapy; and last, but not least, (6) it provided the means by which deficiency of factors V, VII, or X were discovered.

Owren's description of the hemorrhagic diathesis caused by lack of factor V illustrates not only how Quick's test was essential for further discoveries but also how the brilliant simplicity of some experiments is indeed the mark of genius. In 1943 in Norway, Owren attended a 29-year-old woman who had been admitted to the hospital because of severe bleeding. Although the coagulation time of whole blood was prolonged, the other tests were normal (platelet count, fibrinogen concentration, and serum calcium concentration). The possibility of a prothrombin deficiency occurred to Owren, but to test for it by Quick's method he needed brain thromboplastin reagent. A commercial reagent was not available, and rabbits had become almost extinct since they were a nonrationed item during the German occupation. Owren was forced to hunt down the rabbits and prepare his own brain extract. He did indeed find the "prothrombin time" to be prolonged, but he also showed that it could be restored to normal by $BaSO_4$-adsorbed normal plasma, a reagent known to be free of prothrombin. Thus the defect could not be in prothrombin, but in a new factor that he called V because the classic theory already named four factors (fibrinogen, prothrombin, thromboplastin, and calcium).

The isolation of bishydroxycoumarin (dicumarol) by Link et al as the toxic agent in spoiled sweet clover was followed a year later (it is said to have been completed on April Fool's Day, 1940) by its synthesis by Huebner. This and other coumarin compounds have been applied to the problems of exterminating rats and of preventing thromboembolism in humans. There is no doubt as to their efficacy as rodenticides; in the prevention of thromboembolism, some still hold reservations, and these are in part related to the laboratory control. Bishydroxycoumarin was first used in humans in 1941 by Butt et al and by Bingham et al. The laboratory control of oral anticoagulant therapy will be covered in a later section. We might point out here, however, that the coumarin drugs effect a reduction of four coagulation factors (prothrombin, VII, IX, and X), and their mode of action could not be clarified until the other factors besides prothrombin were identified.

Although spoiled sweet clover disease of cattle was a major economic problem, the discovery of its cause seemed to have little reference to human problems. Indeed, once it was shown to be caused by improperly cured hay, all that was required to prevent the disease was to be more careful about storing hay. What is important is that by a happy occurrence of events the physician was given a new tool with which to attack the problem of thromboembolic disease. Actually, this was a fortunate development, for the coagulationists had become so concerned with the biochemistry of coagulation and with the hemorrhagic diseases caused by a lack of old and new factors that the really important problems in hemostasis—why blood normally remains fluid in the vascular system and why thrombosis sometimes occurs—threatened to be overshadowed by the relatively few hemorrhagic diatheses. This is not to say that clinical bleeding is a minor and undramatic problem, but for every case of hemophilia there are hundreds of cases of coronary artery thrombosis and thromboembolic disease. Furthermore, it will be pointed out that only a remote relationship exists between coagulation of the blood and the clinical sign of abnormal bleeding. This will be discussed later.

We should mention here the studies of Seegers and colleagues over the past many years. Seegers begins with "purified" bovine prothrombin (it does not fulfill all requirements for 100% purity) and shows that, by varying conditions in vitro, it is possible to identify a number of "prothrombin derivatives," each having characteristic features and each substituting for one or the other of the "standard" coagulation factors. Thus he sees prothrombin as the fundamental molecule in blood coagulation, proposing that under various conditions (in vitro) it yields products that, in addition to thrombin (several varieties), include autoprothrombin C (active factor X?), autoprothrombin I (several varieties described, Ip and Ic, the first equivalent to factor VII and the second to factor X?), autoprothrombin II (equivalent to factor IX?), autoprothrombin III (derivative of prothrombin when Ca ions, Ac globulin, and autoprothrombin C are added), and platelet cofactor I (equivalent to factor VIII).

Seeger's in vitro experiments are admirable in many ways. The prothrombin derivatives he described have been isolated in fairly pure form, and, in microgram amounts, have been shown to correct the clotting defect in vitro of corresponding hemorrhagic disorders. This is, without doubt, the most misleading experiment in blood coagulation. Still, his concept of what can happen in vitro, and the extension of this to in vivo phenomena, is so basically different from the accepted theory that one does know what to do with it. We leave it for history to settle.

Whatever the chemical truth, it does not for now invalidate the laboratory procedures used to sort out the hemorrhagic disorders. When a test is done, though our supposition as to what happens may eventually be shown to be sheer nonsense, it can still be valid if it detects an entity, distinguishes it from others, and correlates well with other tests and with the clinical picture. Everyone would like to use "pure" test systems instead of crude blood fractions, and someday this may be feasible. For the present we must do the best we can with the methods available.

The discovery of molecular abnormalities of the factor VIII molecule, and later of other coagulation factors, has opened a new vista of the coagulation process. Just as Pauling's demonstration of an electrophoretic difference between Hb S and Hb A initiated an era of molecular biology in the hemoglobinopathies and in biochemical constituents such as proteins and enzymes, so has the demonstration of molecular abnormalities in many of the coagulation factors initiated an era in which we think of the coagulation factors in terms of molecular biology and pathology.

The last advances to mark the modern era involve platelets and platelet function and, in fact, may be the most important contribution to the solution of the enigma of normal and abnormal hemostasis. It should be obvious that the coagulation abnormalities, while dramatic, are of minor importance as compared with one of the most common and most serious diseases afflicting modern human beings—thrombosis and thromboembolic disease. It is in this area that the platelet has come to occupy a deservedly prominent place. The role of platelets has also seemed to place blood coagulation in proper perspective as one, probably minor, contributor to the hemostatic process.

Finally, I have never been able to completely ignore the suspicion that coagulation as we now know it is an unlikely physiologic system. Unlike most other biologic situations, we postulate a complex system of reactants and reactions that breaks down completely when any one step is abnormal or any one factor deficient. There is no compensation for a deficiency; there are no classic feedback mechanisms that we know of. The complexity of the system seems unnecessary, for in the classic theory the two basic reactions are all that is needed for the formation of fibrin. There is no denying that the various hemorrhagic diseases are distinct entities, but it seems unlikely that nature created so many coagulation factors just to produce a variety of diseases. It is more probable, if we may speculate, that what we have are molecular variants of a small number of coagulation proteins, something in between the modern schemes and Seeger's concept. One possible alternate scheme is presented by Mann (1970).

Also speculative is the relation of the cyclic nature of some bleeding disorders to environmental factors. We have found that patients having von Willebrand's disease show striking cyclic remissions and exacerbations not only of the severity of bruising but also in objective measurements such as the bleeding time and tourniquet test. Andrews (1960) presents evidence for a significantly higher incidence of posttonsillectomy bleeding at the time of a full moon than at any other time. Similar observations have been made on the relation of bleeding from peptic ulcers to the phase of the moon. The relationship of disease to weather is the subject of a classic multivolume work by Petersen (1934-1938), but there are few controlled studies on the periodicity of bleeding. Perhaps more coagulationists would benefit by leaving the laboratory and seeing patients as clinical problems; just as certainly many clinicians would benefit from visiting the laboratories now and then.

Coagulation future

Tocantins made the pertinent comment that "we have been looking too long at the problem of hemostasis through the keyhole of blood coagulation."

the future. In the more formal portion of this chapter we will be concerned with the general problem of hemostasis. As a matter of fact, as time goes on it becomes increasingly obvious that the coagulation of blood becomes less and less important as the primary factor in hemostasis. We need only mention a few examples to support this. No blood is less coagulable than that congenitally lacking in fibrinogen, and yet congenital hypofibrinogenemia is seldom accompanied by spontaneous hemorrhage. In fact, even menstruation may be normal. Another example is the Hageman deficiency, which in vitro behaves as the most severe of the thromboplastin generation abnormalities but which is clinically asymptomatic in almost all cases. Our most severe case of Hagemen deficiency is that of a retired boxer who certainly was subjected to more than average trauma. And yet he was not considered a "bleeder."

Indeed, it is impossible to relate the coagulation of blood to the *onset* of spontaneous bleeding, admitting that abnormal coagulation can account for *continuing* bleeding as the result of trauma. Trauma is itself an interesting variable. Even in hemophilia the *onset* of intra-articular bleeding commonly follows only a slightly more strenuous exertion than usual, such as throwing a baseball or a sudden twisting motion. How this can be related to abnormal thromboplastin generation has escaped me for many years.

The other side of the coin, thrombosis, also defies a relationship to the coagulability of the blood as a whole. Here the abnormality is almost certainly a local phenomenon at a point where the conditions for keeping blood fluid no longer exist. The probable effectiveness of anticoagulants in preventing the extension of a thrombus, or possibly a recurrence of thrombosis, cannot in good faith be ascribed to the prolonged prothrombin time or prolonged coagulation time. Nor in our experience can one implicate a prothrombin time below the arbitrary "therapeutic level" as a cause of the hematuria sometimes seen as a complication of anticoagulant therapy. I do not see how erythrocytes leak through the capillary walls of the glomerulus just because the prothrombin time is prolonged. Obviously there is more to it.

The point is that we are coming around in full circle, placing coagulation in proper perspective as far as hemostasis is concerned. The early investigators became interested in coagulation because they considered thrombosis the basic pathologic process in disease. In the modern era, coagulationists had to go through the in vitro phase to work out basic reactions. These are still not completely clarified, and these investigations must continue. In recent years we have seen some early rewards from the application of the coagulation mechanisms to the phenomena of localized and generalized thrombosis. There is no doubt that we are more interested than ever in the reactions that occur at the endothelial surface and that result in thrombosis. Clarification of these reactions will hopefully lead to eliminating one of the major causes of human disease.

Finally, coagulationists and all other scientists should periodically look at Macfarlane's (1966) Platoesque illustration (Fig. 17-1) of the difference between shadow and substance. Almost everything we examine in physiology and pathology is a shadow of the real thing that is being studied. The illustration shows beautifully that dissimilar, yet familiar, shadows can be cast by an object of totally unfamiliar form, outside normal experience. To quote Macfarlane, ". . . a reconstruction of this real shape could be obtained by combining the evidence of different shadows, even though they appear to be giving conflicting information."

HEMOSTASIS

Hemostasis is the physiologic process by which spontaneous or induced hemorrhage is stopped. The term has several applications. Bleeding from a large severed vessel may be stopped by mechanical hemostasis and from a smaller vessel by spontaneous hemostasis involving physiologic mechanisms. Mechanical hemostasis is a surgical or first aid problem. The hemorrhagic disorders arising from deficient physiologic hemostasis, however, are initially a laboratory

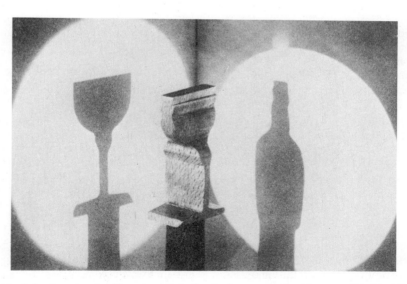

Fig. 17-1. Macfarlane's example of how two dissimilar shadows are derived from a solid object that resembles neither. (From Macfarlane, 1966.)

concern. The correction of such hemorrhagic disorders calls for the intelligent application of laboratory data and an effective liaison between pathologist and clinician.

Thromboembolic disease is an expression of pathologic hemostasis, caused by the hemostatic process occurring at the wrong place and certainly at the wrong time. As we will see, the "hypercoagulable state," in the sense of a set of measurable conditions in the blood that make it likely to form thrombi, is still difficult, if not impossible, to define and predict. In another sense, the occurrence of pathologic hemostasis, as in thrombus formation, is certainly a localized hypercoagulable state beginning in the lumen of blood vessels.

Mechanisms of hemostasis

Hemostasis results from the interaction of several mechanisms at the site of injury. The primary mechanism is the reaction of platelets with endothelium and subendothelial tissues. As the result of platelet properties of adhesiveness, aggregation, and the release of cell components, two major effects are produced. The first, significantly effective at the small vessel level, is vasoconstriction caused by serotonin released from platelets. The second is the activation of the blood coagulation mechanism in the microenvironment of the platelet aggregate, resulting in the deposition of fibrin on the "white thrombus" formed by the aggregated platelets and thus the "hemostatic plug" (Sixma and Wester, 1977). In fact, platelets have on them or in them most of the reactants necessary to effect local hemostasis, including key factors such as fibrinogen and prothrombin, so that they are a microcosm of hemostatic function. A later effect is activation of the fibrinolytic system, serving to dissolve the formed fibrin and thus restore, partially or completely, the patency of the blood vessel.

If, as is generally believed, normal hemostasis is effected by normally functioning platelets and their interaction with the endothelial cells lining the vascular system, we can justifiably consider this as the first phase of hemostasis. We will also see that platelet phospholipid (platelet factor 3, PF3) is required in some of the reactions involving the blood coagulation factors.

The traditional distinction between "intrinsic" and "extrinsic" pathways may not be as sharp as it was once thought. When cells are damaged, various phospholipids are released from the cell membrane. Those phospholipids released from damaged tissue cells do seem to have the special property of activating factor X by complexing with factor VII in the presence of calcium ions, bypassing XII, XI, and IX, but this is probably more important physiologically, and in some pathologic states, than it is biochemically. Activation of factor IX by the factor VII–tissue thromboplastin complex is another convergence of the classic extrinsic and intrinsic pathways (Østerud and Rapaport, 1980).

BLOOD COAGULATION
The classic theory

The classic theory of blood coagulation (Rossi, 1972) proposed by Morawitz (1905) assumes the interaction of four plasma components: (1) prothrombin, (2) thromboplas-

tin, (3) thrombin, and (4) fibrinogen. Ionized calcium is required for the basic reactions, which may be outlined:

I. Prothrombin + Ca^{++} + Thromboplastin → Thrombin
II. Fibrinogen + Thrombin → Fibrin

During the last 30 years, many investigators have considered the problems of blood coagulation, perhaps in part because of the peculiar fascination this subject has for biochemist and physician alike. The undoubted progress has been a mixed blessing, since with it came much confusion of terms.

The "modern" theory

The "modern" theory began to form with the discovery that the conversion of prothrombin to thrombin also involves factors V and VII. At about the same time it was found that hemophilia was caused by the deficiency of a substance in the blood called factor VIII and that a reduction of this factor would cause an incomplete conversion of prothrombin to thrombin. The classic theory had to be modified to include the newly discovered factors, the number of which increased rapidly for a time.

The numerical system for identifying accepted coagulation factors proposed by Koller and adopted in the first edition of this book has since been recommended for universal use by the International Committee on Nomenclature of Blood Clotting Factors (Table 17-1). Numbers are easily handled and are useful for grouping the probable synonyms. It avoids the problem of precedence, since some terms were proposed on the basis of preliminary observations or inconclusive experiments and were later redefined. It also avoids the use of terms that imply a greater knowledge of the mode of action or nature of the factor than is justified by the data. New factors retain the name proposed by the discoverer until they are accepted and given a number.

Almost all studies on blood coagulation have been done with crude or impure fractions. This does not mean the results are worthless—merely that they should be interpreted cautiously. Another important source of error is the failure to distinguish between a fraction *containing* a certain factor and *being* that factor or, worse, the failure to distinguish between *observed activity* and the *factor* postulated from it.

The blood coagulation sequence

There are several ways in which the sequence of events that terminate with the polymerization of fibrinogen can be presented. The scheme shown in Fig. 17-2 has a number of advantages.

First, the sequence is presented in four phases, or sets of reactions, representing major clinical categories of hemostatic abnormalities. Phase I, the "initiator," "trigger," or "contact" phase, clearly separates the role of platelets in hemostasis from subsequent reactions. When I first used this scheme, there was not as much known about the role of platelets in hemostasis and abnormalities of platelet function. In the intervening years this has been shown to be a most important hemostatic step. Furthermore, as we consider hemostatic abnormalities we can readily classify quanti-

Table 17-1. Blood coagulation factors—standard nomenclature and synonyms

Factor	Probable synonyms
Factor I	Fibrinogen
Factor II	Prothrombin (Schmidt) Thrombogen Serozyme (Bordet and Delange) Plasmozyme
Factor III	Thromboplastin Thrombokinase (Morawitz) Cytozyme (Bordet)
Factor IV	Calcium
Factor V	Proaccelerin (Owren) Prothrombin accelerator (Fantl and Nance) Labile factor (Quick) Plasma Ac globulin (Ware and Seegers) Thrombogen (Nolf)
Factor VI (obsolete)*	Accelerin (Owren) Serum Ac globulin (Ware and Seegers)
Factor VII	Serum prothrombin conversion accelerator (SPCA) (Alexander) Stable prothrombin conversion factor (Owren) Co-thromboplastin (Mann and Hurn) Proconvertin-convertin (Owren) Serum accelerator (Jacox) Autoprothrombin I (Seegers)
Factor VIII	Antihemophilic globulin (AHG) Antihemophilic factor (AHF) Thromboplastinogen (Quick) Platelet cofactor I (Seegers)
Factor IX	Plasma thromboplastin component (PTC) (Aggeler) Christmas factor (Biggs) Plasma factor X (Schulman and Smith) Platelet cofactor II (Seegers) Autoprothrombin II (Seegers)
Factor X	Stuart factor (Hougie et al) Autoprothrombin III (Seegers)
Factor XI	Plasma thromboplastin antecedent (PTA) (Rosenthal et al)
Factor XII	Hageman factor (Ratnoff and Colopy)
Factor XIII	Fibrin-stabilizing factor (Laki and Lorand; Lorand)

*Recently Murano and Bick (1980) have tried to revive it by making the incredible suggestion that it is "probably responsible for all 'false positive' results in the clinical laboratory."

tative and qualitative platelet abnormalities as phase I defects and direct the tests to be performed in the orderly approach to the laboratory diagnosis. Characteristically, patients whose hemostatic problem falls into phase I have a prolonged bleeding time and a history of purpura, ecchymoses, and other abnormal bleeding. The "contact" factors, XI and XII, probably play their major role in phase II, but we now know that they also provide one of the stimuli for initiating the reactions of platelet adhesiveness and aggregation.

Second, just as it is useful to identify the reactions that occur in phase I and the hemostatic abnormalities that can be

attributed to a malfunction at that phase, the identification of three subsequent phases provides a ready scheme for describing these reactions and for classifying the hemorrhagic states that are caused by abnormalities at various points of the sequence. Phase II, "thromboplastinogenesis," represents that portion of the intrinsic coagulation system that leads to the generation of plasma thromboplastic activity. Hemophilia and the hemophilioid states are abnormalities of this phase. Given a prolonged partial thromboplastin time, it can be assumed that there is a defect in this phase. In phase III, "thrombinogenesis," prothrombin is converted to thrombin. Other factors involved in this conversion can be conveniently placed here as can differential studies utilized in identifying the specific defect. Abnormalities in phase III are characterized by a prolonged plasma prothrombin time. In phase IV, thrombin brings about the polymerization of fibrinogen to fibrin, and the abnormalities in this phase include quantitative and qualitative alterations in fibrinogen, a deficiency of fibrin-stabilizing factor (XIII), increased fibrinolytic activity, or some interference with fibrinogen polymerization. The detailed discussion of how this scheme can be helpful in the diagnostic approach to a patient is given in a later section.

This schematic presentation shows two other features not presented by other schemes. The first is the recognition that thrombin is a catalyst for reactions in phases I, II, and III. The second is the inclusion of physiologic inhibitors for each phase.

The catalytic action of thrombin in phases I and II and its actions as an autocatalyst in phase III (Therriault et al, 1957) provides a biochemical amplifier not unlike the progressively accelerating reactions of a thermonuclear explosion. In any in vitro test system that leads to the formation of a clot, there is a lag phase during which nothing seems to be happening when observed visually. This is followed by an acute phase during which there is very rapid fibrin formation. The catalytic and autocatalytic action of thrombin provides one explanation for what is observed. Beginning activation of phase I provides a small amount of platelet phospholipid, which in turn is utilized to generate a small amount of plasma thromboplastin followed by a small amount of thrombin. This amount of thrombin is not sufficient to convert fibrinogen to fibrin, but as it accelerates the reactions in phases I and II and even the rate of thrombin formation in phase III, the rate of production of the end products of the reactions is progressively amplified. When a critical concentration of thrombin is reached, the conversion of fibrinogen to fibrin occurs very rapidly. This beautifully simple reaction is almost anticlimactic, following, as it does, a series of complex and poorly understood events.

Such an autocatalytic process would be disastrous unless mechanisms exist for controlling it. Such inhibitory mechanisms are present at each phase. In phase I, it is normal endothelium that prevents the platelet and contact factors from triggering the coagulation sequence. At the second phase, naturally occuring antithromboplastins can inhibit the reactions, and in phase III antithrombins are inhibitory. In phase IV there are no known physiologic inhibitors of fibrin formation, but the reaction is stopped by fibrinopep-

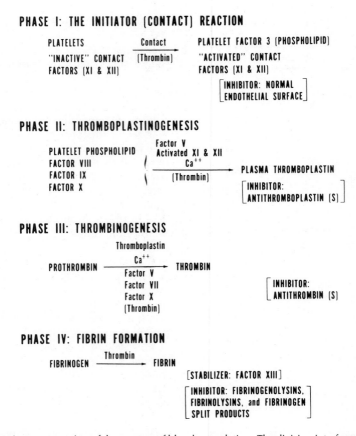

PHASE I: THE INITIATOR (CONTACT) REACTION

PLATELETS   Contact   PLATELET FACTOR 3 (PHOSPHOLIPID)

"INACTIVE" CONTACT   (Thrombin)   "ACTIVATED" CONTACT
FACTORS (XI & XII)   FACTORS (XI & XII)

$$\left[\text{INHIBITOR: NORMAL ENDOTHELIAL SURFACE}\right]$$

PHASE II: THROMBOPLASTINOGENESIS

Factor V
PLATELET PHOSPHOLIPID   Activated XI & XII
FACTOR VIII Ca^{++}
FACTOR IX   (Thrombin)   PLASMA THROMBOPLASTIN
FACTOR X

$$\left[\text{INHIBITOR: ANTITHROMBOPLASTIN (S)}\right]$$

PHASE III: THROMBINOGENESIS

          Thromboplastin
          Ca^{++}
PROTHROMBIN —————— THROMBIN
          Factor V
          Factor VII
          Factor X
          (Thrombin)

$$\left[\text{INHIBITOR: ANTITHROMBIN (S)}\right]$$

PHASE IV: FIBRIN FORMATION

        Thrombin
FIBRINOGEN —————— FIBRIN

$$[\text{STABILIZER: FACTOR XIII}]$$

$$\left[\text{INHIBITOR: FIBRINOGENOLYSINS, FIBRINOLYSINS, and FIBRINOGEN SPLIT PRODUCTS}\right]$$

Fig. 17-2. Schematic representation of the process of blood coagulation. The division into four phases is arbitrary and is used only as a convenient scheme for classifying the hemorrhagic disorders and the tests used to study them. Thrombin in parentheses in phases I, II, and III indicates that it acts as a catalyst rather than a reactant.

tides and by the adsorption of excess thrombin into the fibrin clot. The fibrinolytic system is not inhibitory but it does provide a way to dissolve fibrin, often reestablishing the patency of a vessel occluded by thrombus. One other inhibitory mechanism, the clearance of activated factors, especially Xa (Deykin et al, 1968) and macromolecular substances such as fibrinogen polymers and possibly plasma thromboplastin (Spaet et al, 1961), may be physiologic as well as of importance in the genesis of DIC.

Although these physiologic inhibitory systems are important for hemostatic homeostasis, when pathologically hyperactive they can have a deleterious effect. For example, pathologic levels of inhibitors (circulating anticoagulants or excessive fibrinolytic activity) can cause bleeding either by inhibiting the end product or by dissolving fibrin as soon as it is formed.

The third feature of the scheme shown in Fig. 17-2 is that it makes no assumptions beyond what can be proved experimentally. It has become popular to consider the coagulation process as a "waterfall" sequence (Davie and Ratnoff, 1964) or a "cascade" sequence (Macfarlane, 1964) (Fig. 17-3). These are conceived as enzymatic cascades in which there is a sequential proenzyme-to-enzyme transformation, the "activated" coagulation factor at each step acting in turn as the enzyme that activates the proenzyme in the next step,

the activated factor being identified by the lowercase letter "a." It is probably true that at least some of the coagulation factors are converted from a nonactivated to an activated form (serine proteases), but there is no evidence that this applies to all of them. In fact, Macfarlane (1966) modified the cascade sequence, making factor V a "cofactor" rather than a proenzyme, admitting also that other portions of the cascade sequence are based either on indirect or circumstantial evidence. It is true that indirect evidence must suffice until such a time as pure factors can be reacted in controlled systems, but this does not mean that a hypothesis should be accepted uncritically.

The concept of proenzyme-to-enzyme transformation is based on in vitro studies which show that some of the coagulation factors yield products that have enzymatic activity. These factors are II, VII, IX, X, XI, and XII. There is no evidence that factors V and VII have corresponding activated forms (Hemker, 1975).

It is obvious that many of the reactions involved in coagulation are not well defined and remain hypothetical. It might be well to be more cautious, and for now a compromise might be to outline the reactions as in Fig. 17-4, with the reservation that the proof of some of these is also in the future. Even if these reactions or the cascade hypothesis is eventually found to be correct, there is no way by which

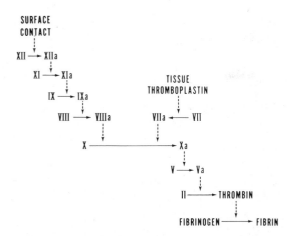

Fig. 17-3. The "cascade" hypothesis of Macfarlane (1964). The "waterfall" hypothesis of Davie and Ratnoff (1964) is identical, substituting curved for straight arrows.

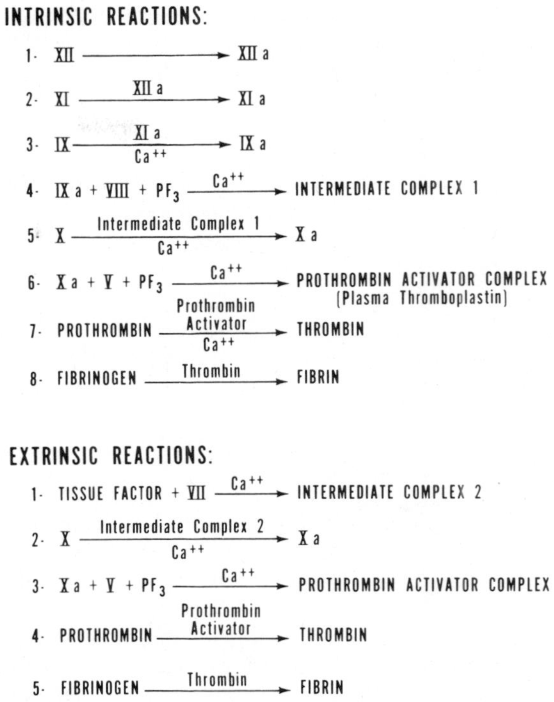

INTRINSIC REACTIONS:

1. $XII \longrightarrow XII\,a$

2. $XI \xrightarrow{XII\,a} XI\,a$

3. $IX \xrightarrow[Ca^{++}]{XI\,a} IX\,a$

4. $IX\,a + VIII + PF_3 \xrightarrow{Ca^{++}}$ INTERMEDIATE COMPLEX 1

5. $X \xrightarrow[Ca^{++}]{Intermediate\ Complex\ 1} X\,a$

6. $X\,a + V + PF_3 \xrightarrow{Ca^{++}}$ PROTHROMBIN ACTIVATOR COMPLEX (Plasma Thromboplastin)

7. PROTHROMBIN $\xrightarrow[Ca^{++}]{Prothrombin\ Activator}$ THROMBIN

8. FIBRINOGEN $\xrightarrow{Thrombin}$ FIBRIN

EXTRINSIC REACTIONS:

1. TISSUE FACTOR + VII $\xrightarrow{Ca^{++}}$ INTERMEDIATE COMPLEX 2

2. $X \xrightarrow[Ca^{++}]{Intermediate\ Complex\ 2} X\,a$

3. $X\,a + V + PF_3 \xrightarrow{Ca^{++}}$ PROTHROMBIN ACTIVATOR COMPLEX

4. PROTHROMBIN $\xrightarrow{Prothrombin\ Activator}$ THROMBIN

5. FIBRINOGEN $\xrightarrow{Thrombin}$ FIBRIN

Fig. 17-4. Intrinsic and extrinsic reactions in the coagulation sequence.

intermediate reactions can now be applied to the laboratory approach to a patient who has a hemostatic abnormality. Here is where the four-phase scheme, admittedly an oversimplification, is most useful. To quote Macfarlane (1966), "It is important to distinguish between academic interest and physiological relevance."

The coagulation factors

All the coagulation factors, with some interesting exceptions, are synthesized in the liver. Of the three portions of the factor VIII molecule (p. 809), only the procoagulant portion is synthesized in the liver, the antigenic portion and the von Willebrand factor being synthesized by endothelial cells. Plasma factor XIII is probably synthesized in the liver, whereas platelet factor XIII is synthesized in megakaryocytes. Four of the coagulation factors synthesized in the liver are vitamin K dependent (II, VII, IX, and X); the others are not.

Most of the coagulation factors have been isolated and purified from animal or human plasma. In many instances the factor purified from animal blood (usually bovine) appears to be biochemically and functionally identical to products prepared from human blood, but at times there are significant differences in reactivity and species specificity.

Fibrinogen

Fibrinogen is the glycoprotein clotted by thrombin. It is present in normal plasma in a concentration of 250 to 400 mg/dl. It is a fibrillar protein of the keratin-myosin family and has a molecular weight of about 340,000. The molecule is elongated, measuring 450 to 500 Å (45 to 50 nm), at pH 9.5 (Tooney and Cohen, 1972). The molecule appears to be made up of three globular portions (Fowler and Erickson, 1979), the outer two about 60 Å (6 nm) in diameter and the middle one about 50 Å 5 nm) in diameter, connected by strands 15 Å (1.5 nm) in width and 140 to 165 Å (14 to 16.5 nm) in length. The molecule is probably composed of a dimer of three nonidentical pairs of polypeptide chains (α, β, and γ) held together by 29 disulfide bonds. Three of the disulfide bonds bind the dimeric halves of the molecule to each other (Blombäck and Blombäck, 1972). The structure and amino acid composition of the native chains and of the fibrinopeptides are given by Doolittle (1980). Its isoelectric point is at pH 5.5. It is precipitated from plasma at 56° C, at which temperature it is partially denatured. It is partially adsorbed from plasma by prothrombin adsorbents, being least adsorbed by tricalcium phosphate and most adsorbed by aluminum and magnesium hydroxide.

The clotting of fibrinogen is a sol-gel change involving complex molecular arrangements. The clotting of fibrinogen by thrombin involves the splitting away of terminal fibrinopeptides, two fibrinopeptides A and two fibrinopeptides B, from α- and β-chains (Laki, 1968). Thrombin splits the arginylglycine peptide bonds, the release of fibrinopeptide A being faster than that of fibrinopeptide B. Snake venom (Reptilase) releases only fibrinopeptide A (Blombäck et al, 1957). The remaining portion of the fibrinogen molecule is now a fibrin monomer. Fibrin polymers of high molecular weight are formed by end-to-end and side-to-side polymerization. In the absence of calcium and factor XIII these polymers are soluble in dilute acid or concentrated solutions of urea. Factor XIII stabilizes the polymer by introducing γ-glutamyl-ε-lysine peptide links, forming linkages between dimers of γ-chains and also between dimers of α-chains (McKee et al, 1970; Chen and Doolittle, 1971). As in the hemoglobin variants, abnormal fibrinogens have been discovered that have altered polymerization characteristics and amino acid substitutions in polypeptide chains. Because there is a rapid rate of fibrinogen turnover in the blood, it has been suggested that polymerization and depolymerization of fibrinogen occur normally and continuously in the bloodstream and possibly at the endothelial surface of the blood vessels.

Whereas fibrinogen is cleaved by thrombin to form polypeptides A and B, the proteolytic action of other enzymes yields different fibrinogen degradation products (Mihalyi, 1980).

Prothrombin

Assuming that the clotting of fibrinogen is produced by thrombin, it is necessary to postulate an inactive precursor (prothrombin) in the circulating blood. It follows that no clot (in vitro) or thrombus (in vivo) can form unless prothrombin is converted to thrombin.

Prothrombin is synthesized in the liver and found in plasma at a concentration of about 10 mg/dl. It is the most abundant of the coagulation factors. Human prothrombin has a molecular weight of about 71,600 (Mann and Elion, 1980).

The conversion of prothrombin to thrombin is brought about by a "prothrombin activator complex" consisting of activated factor X (Xa) acting as the proteolytic enzyme, of factor V acting as a "cofactor" of phospholipid, and of calcium ions. The complex of Xa, V, and phospholipid is bound to the prothrombin molecule by calcium bridges. Calcium bridges require that the prothrombin molecule have calcium-binding sites. These are provided by a postribosomal modification of the prothrombin molecule synthesized in the liver cell, the carboxylation of the glutamic acid residues to form γ-carboxy glutamic acids. This carboxylation is vitamin K dependent. In the absence of vitamin K or the presence of vitamin K antagonists (oral anticoagulants) the carboxylation does not occur, and the prothrombin molecule is incomplete and unable to be converted to thrombin by the Xa-V-phospholipid complex. The incomplete prothrombin molecule has been called PIVKA II (protein induced by vitamin K antagonists). The incomplete molecule is biologically inactive (Stenflo, 1970) and binds only one ion of calcium per mole instead of four bound by the carboxylated molecule (Stenflo and Ganrot, 1973).

The proteolytic action of Xa is effected at two sites, cleaving the prothrombin molecule into polypeptide fragments and thrombin. Cleavage of one site results in the formation of prothrombin fragment $1 \cdot 2$ (F$1 \cdot 2$) and prothrombin 2 (P2), the single-chain precursor of thrombin. Cleavage of P2 results in the formation of active thrombin consisting of two chains connected by a disulfide bridge (Mann and Elion, 1980).

One prothrombin unit has been defined as the amount of prothrombin capable of forming one unit of thrombin. Normal plasma contains about 350 units of prothrombin per milliliter.

Normal prothrombin, in common with some of the other factors, is adsorbed from oxalated plasma by $Mg(OH)_2$, $BaSO_4$, and $Ca_3(PO_4)_2$, from citrated plasma by $Al(OH)_3$, and by Seitz filter asbestos pads. Adsorbed prothrombin may be eluted from the adsorbent by various methods, but since other globulins are also adsorbed by these substances, the eluates are by no means pure.

For some years the measurement of prothrombin in plasma was the subject of bitter and confusing debate. It is now obvious that the Quick one-stage method measures the sum total of the prothrombin conversion phase and therefore measures prothrombin and factors V, VII, and X. The two-stage results are a closer approximation of prothrombin as such, but since both results are modified by the presence of antithrombin and antithromboplastin as well as by a reduction in fibrinogen in the one-stage test, an abnormal result calls for further investigation. Nevertheless, both methods are valuable and will be discussed at greater length.

Thromboplastin

A concept found in most blood coagulation hypotheses assumes the need for a substance that, in the presence of calcium ions, brings about the conversion of prothrombin to thrombin. This substance is called thromboplastin.

The concept of thromboplastic activity is based on the observation that tissue extracts contain a substance that is able to accelerate the coagulation of unmodified whole blood or of recalcified plasma. Since tissue extracts cannot clot pure fibrinogen, it was assumed that the action took place in an earlier stage. Having postulated a substance such as thromboplastin, it is obvious that it cannot exist in the blood in an active state; therefore most theories include a mechanism for thromboplastin formation from inactive precursors.

It is not entirely justified to apply the action of tissue extracts on blood to the mechanisms of spontaneous blood clotting. Yet the concept of thromboplastic activity in blood coagulation was, until recently, based almost entirely on in vitro reactions between plasma and tissue extracts. The concept now is that tissue extracts contain "tissue thromboplastin" and—more or less by analogy—that a "plasma thromboplastin" exists that has a similar action. This distinction must be constantly maintained. In the scheme outlined in Fig. 17-4, thromboplastic activity is synonymous with "prothrombin activation." The prothrombin activator in the intrinsic system is synonymous with plasma thromboplastin. In the extrinsic system, the thromboplastin from tissues that is required to initiate the reactions is active because a prothrombin activator is formed. It is not known whether intrinsic and extrinsic prothrombin activators are the same or different substances.

The active principles in tissue thromboplastin have not been categorized. The whole tissue extracts convert prothrombin to thrombin in the presence of calcium ions, whereas the lipid-solvent extractable portion (partial thromboplastin) reacts with the hemophilioid factors but not with prothrombin. Partial thromboplastin consists chiefly of cephalin and is analogous to platelet phospholipid. Thromboplastic activity is present in all animal tissues as well as in plant cells, microorganisms, saliva, milk, amniotic fluid, and Russell's viper and other venoms. However, preparations made from different tissues or by different extraction methods behave somewhat differently, and data obtained with one are not necessarily applicable to the others.

The popularity of Quick's "one-stage prothrombin"

determination in the control of therapy with bishydroxycoumarin and similar anticoagulants led to the development of commercial preparations of thromboplastin. They vary as to source, method of preparation, use of stabilizer, etc. They are standardized against normal and abnormal plasma (p. 385). It should be emphasized, however, that the fact that two substances give the same clotting time does not indicate that they are the same or interchangeable. The picture is further complicated by the fact that tissue extracts contain variable quantities of the lipid inhibitors.

Plasma thromboplastin is the theoretical counterpart of the thromboplastic activity in tissue juice. Blood contains all the ingredients necessary for coagulation, making it independent of tissue thromboplastin. Blood therefore contains substances capable of interacting in such a way as to form a plasma thromboplastin analogous to tissue thromboplastin. The evolution of plasma thromboplastic activity can be measured by means of the thromboplastin generation test, but the characterization of plasma thromboplastin as a definite substance has not been achieved. The reactions thought to occur in the generation of plasma thromboplastin will be discussed in a later section.

Quick and Hickey (1960) showed that hemolysates of erythrocytes contain a substance that participates in the generation of intrinsic thromboplastin. They have named this substance "erythrocytin." Erythrocytin is formed in the plasma from the interaction of platelet factor 3 and active contact product (phase I of the scheme shown in Fig. 17-2) and then adsorbed either into or onto the erythrocytes. The erythrocytin in the erythrocytes is not normally available for participation in the intrinsic reactions but can be an important trigger of diffuse intravascular coagulation when there is extensive intravascular hemolysis. Likewise, hemolyzed blood is not suitable for coagulation studies.

Thrombin

With all the supposed complexity of the various stages and reactions that terminate in the formation of thrombin, the relative simplicity of this substance and its straightforward action are somewhat of an anticlimax. Thrombin is defined as being the active agent that clots fibrinogen. Crude preparations having powerful thrombic activity are easily prepared and commercially available. The purest thrombin product is prepared from purified prothrombin (Thompson and Davie, 1971). The molecular weight of human thrombin is about 32,000. Its isoelectric point is between pH 5.6 and 5.75. The molecule consists of two polypeptide chains, one heavy and one light chain, held together by disulfide bonds. The amino acid sequences have been determined by Magnusson (1972). Thrombin is inhibited by difluorophosphate (DFP) (Magnusson, 1972) and has esterase activity toward arginine esters such as TAME (tosyl arginine methyl ester) (Weinstein and Doolittle, 1972). Thrombin is inhibited by antithrombin III, and the rate of inhibition is accelerated by heparin (Rosenberg and Damus, 1973).

The action of thrombin is so powerful that it can clot several hundred times its weight of fibrinogen. It is probable that it acts as an enzyme, splitting arginyl-glycyl bonds at the N-terminal of the α- and β-chains of the fibrinogen molecule (Workman and Lundblad, 1980). When fibrin is formed, it adsorbs thrombin and in so doing acts as antithrombin and as an important brake to the reaction.

Given a fibrinogen solution or plasma with identical reactivity, thrombin can be measured in units, according to the speed with which it produces clotting. Various units of measurements have been proposed, all equally satisfactory for comparing thrombin solutions. However, the conditions for using a given unit system should be carefully noted. The most careful standardization procedure defines 1 unit of thrombin as the amount that clots 1% fibrinogen in 15 seconds at 37° C, pH 7.3, and sodium chloride concentration of 0.154M.

Factor V

The conversion of prothrombin to thrombin in the presence of calcium ions and tissue thromboplastin only is a relatively slow process. It can be speeded up by various substances once called "accelerators," but it will be seen from Fig. 17-4 that "accelerators" actually are involved in intermediate reactions, and factor V is more properly considered a "cofactor" by complexing with Xa and phospholipid to convert prothrombin to thrombin. The presence of factor V increases the activity of Xa more than threefold. Thrombin itself acts as a prothrombin conversion accelerator but is not usually considered one of the accelerators in spite of its considerable activity in this respect. Nevertheless, it is probably the most important accelerator of prothrombin conversion in vivo.

The accelerators present in plasma received the earliest and most thorough attention. Nolf (1908) was the first to find that the residual plasma from which prothrombin had been prepared contained a factor, "thrombogen," which speeded up the conversion of prothrombin to thrombin. Quick (1943) described a gradual lengthening of the one-stage prothrombin time when oxalated plasma was stored. Since this could be corrected by fresh plasma, he suggested that the "prothrombin complex" consisted in part of a *labile factor*. Similar accelerators were described by Fantl and Nance (1946) (prothrombin accelerator), by Owren (1947) (factor V), and by Ware and Seegers (1948) (Ac globulin). It is supposed that all these terms are synonyms for the same factor, although this is not certain. In our scheme this is called factor V.

Factor V occurs in the plasma of all normal persons. It is synthesized in the liver. The factor deteriorates in oxalated plasma (more slowly in citrated plasma). It is apparently labile when the pH is increased to 10.5, with a maximum stability at a pH range of 5 to 9. Factor V is used up when human plasma is clotted, but considerable factor V activity remains in bovine serum. Factor V is not adsorbed from plasma by Seitz filtration, $BaCO_3$, $BaSO_4$, $Ca_3(PO_4)_2$, or $Al(OH)_3$.

The theory that factor V (proaccelerin) is the precursor of factor VI (accelerin) is derived chiefly from the observation that more activator is found in bovine blood after clotting than before. Factor V was therefore thought to be a precursor that becomes a more active accelerator through the action of thrombin (plasma Ac globulin is the precursor and serum Ac globulin the active accelerator) (Ware and Seegers, 1948). The designation "factor VI" has been discarded (see footnote to Table 17-1). Most of the biochemical data on factor V are derived from studies with the bovine factor (Colman, 1980).

Factor VII

Factor VII in plasma is stable, in contrast to the lability of factor V, and is undiminished in serum stored for 4 days at 25° to 37° C. Stored serum is a useful source of factor VII. Factor VII (as well as factors II, IX, and X) is adsorbed from oxalated plasma or serum by $BaSO_4$, $BaCO_3$, and $Ca_3(PO_4)_2$ or from citrated plasma by $Al(OH)_3$ and can then be eluted from adsorbent by a sodium citrate solution. It may then be further purified by various technics. Factor VII can also be removed from plasma by Seitz filtration. Factor VII (as well as factors II, IX, and X) is decreased during therapy with bishydroxycoumarin and related vitamin K– inhibiting drugs.

Purified factor VII has been prepared by several workers (Gladhaug and Prydz, 1970; Jesty and Nemerson, 1974; Jesty, 1980). Factor VII purified from plasma has a molecular weight of about 63,000 (Prydz, 1965), whereas that purified from serum (factor VIIa) has a molecular weight of 44,700 (Gladhaug and Prydz, 1970). Factor VII is converted to "active" VIIa by tissue thromboplastin, and VIIa in turn activates factor X. An alternate mode of activation of factor VII is by kallikrein (Gjønnaess, 1972; Saito and Ratnoff, 1975), but this is slow and of doubtful physiologic importance. This alternate activation probably comes into play when plasma is stored at refrigerator temperature (Laake and Østerud, 1974). Normal plasmas usually do not show significant cold activation, but marked activation is found in plasma from pregnant women or women taking oral contraceptives (Gjønnaess and Fagerhol, 1974). Factor XIIa is a potent activator of VII (Kisiel et al, 1977). Traditionally, the coagulation pathway involving tissue thromboplastin and factor VII has been called "extrinsic," and it seemed to be distinct and separate from the pathway called "intrinsic." The observations that factor VII can be activated by kallikrein or XIIa has, to a great measure, eliminated the supposed individuality of each pathway.

A point that students sometimes find confusing needs clarification. All of the coagulation factors are present in normal plasma. Some, factors V and VIII, are consumed when blood clots and are therefore absent in serum. Others, factors VII, IX, and X, are activated when blood clots and the excess remaining can be found in serum in a more active form than that in plasma.

Factor VIII

The numerical designation of VIII was assigned to the blood coagulation factor deficient in classic hemophilia. Since that time it has become apparent that what we now call the factor VIII molecule exhibits several activities in addition to providing the antihemophilic factor. Those various activities will be described in the section on von Willebrand's disease and in the section on hemophilia. It should be noted that the older studies of factor VIII considered only its procoagulant and antihemophilic activity (Cooper, 1980). In this section some of the classic studies are reviewed.

In 1906 Weil observed that the addition of normal blood to hemophilic blood corrected the prolonged coagulation time. In 1911 Addis showed that the remedial factor was present in the globulin fraction prepared from normal plasma. Patek and Taylor (1937) showed that normal plasma contains a substance, later called factor VIII, that corrects the long coagulation time of hemophilic blood. The period from 1937 to 1951 saw the most intensive studies on the antihemophilic factor. Confirmation of the presence of antihemophilic activity in the globulin fraction of normal plasma and of the effectiveness of this fraction in vivo was followed by the demonstration that the antihemophilic activity of normal plasma is found chiefly (but not entirely) in Cohn's fraction I and III, whereas the same fractions prepared from hemophilic blood showed no activity.

The isolation and purification of factor VIII are difficult and were not achieved to any significant degree until recent years Hershgold et al (1966; 1971) have achieved a 10,000-fold concentration of human factor VIII; their concentrate is chemically, physically, and immunologically homogeneous. This material was injected into rabbits, and the anti-factor VIII antiserum was used to study the immunologic reactivity of factor VIII in normal plasma, hemophilic plasma, and plasma from patients with von Willebrand's disease. Using the hemagglutination inhibition technic, Stites et al (1971) showed that material either antigenically similar or identical to factor VIII is present in similar amounts in both normal and hemophilic plasma and serum.

The biosynthesis of factor VIII is discussed in detail by Webster et al (1975). All the evidence points to the liver as the primary site of synthesis, although there is also evidence that the liver may synthesize an inactive precursor of factor VIII and that the spleen converts the precursor to the biologically active molecule. For now the role of extrahepatic tissues in the assembly of the molecule of factor VIII remains unclear, particularly that of the spleen. For example, there is no deficiency of factor VIII in splenectomized persons, and Rizza and Eipe (1971) found that the rise in factor VIII procoagulant activity that normally occurs after strenuous exercise is found in both normal and asplenic subjects.

Purified factor VIII is a glycoprotein with a molecular weight of 1.1 million (Hershgold et al 1971; Legaz et al, 1973).

Factor VIII is considered labile in blood drawn into ACD solution, but estimates of the rate of decay vary from 24 hours to several days. In fact, a 50% decay of factor VIII in stored blood has been shown to occur very quickly, the remainder decaying at a rate of about 2% per day (Bowie et al, 1964). Potent concentrates have been prepared as cryoglobulin precipitate (Pool and Shannon, 1965) and by glycine precipitation of normal plasma (commercially available from Hyland Laboratories and from Courtland Laboratories). Plasma can be heated to 56° C for 5 minutes to remove fibrinogen without any loss of antihemophilic activity; yet there is a rapid loss of activity when frozen plasma is thawed slowly. The antihemophilic activity of fresh plasma is not impaired by Seitz filtration or by adsorption with $Ca_3(PO_4)_2$, $BaSO_4$, $BaCO_3$, or $Al(OH)_3$. Factor VIII levels are increased above the normal in multiple myeloma, particularly of the IgG type. Reports of increased factor VIII levels in some conditions (e.g., malignancy, trauma, and hyperthyroidism) are of doubtful significance in view of the methodologic error in assay procedures.

It is generally agreed that factor VIII is required for adequate evolution of plasma thromboplastin. It seems that (1) factor VIII is normally present in excess, for normal thromboplastin generation occurs even at 40% of normal factor VIII concentration and is not significantly reduced until factor VIII is reduced to 10% to 20% of normal and (2) in the course of the reaction, factor VIII seems to be almost completely utilized. Until at least four other factors necessary for thromboplastin generation were described (factors IX, X, XI, and XII), it was assumed that factor VIII was the one antecedent of thromboplastin (hence the suggested terminology of "thromboplastinogen"). However, a deficiency of factors IX, X, XI, or XII also gives rise to deficient thromboplastin generation. The relationship of these thromboplastic factors in the formation of intrinsic prothrombin activator is shown in Fig. 17-4 and will be discussed in detail in subsequent sections.

Factor IX

Following scattered observations on the occasional phenomenon of one "hemophilic" blood having a corrective effect on another "hemophilic" blood, it was shown by Aggeler et al (1952) that in a case clinically resembling hemophilia the defect was not in factor VIII. They called the defective factor "plasma thromboplastin component" (PTC), since it was necessary for the formation of thromboplastin. In the same year a similar case was described by Schulman and Smith (1952). Again, the deficiency was shown to be not of factor VIII but of a different and distinct "plasma factor." Also in the same year Biggs et al (1952) reported seven cases that resembled hemophilia, but the patients were not deficient in factor VIII. The new clotting factor was called the "Christmas factor," from the name of the first patient they studied in detail. According to the standard international nomenclature this factor is IX.

Factor IX is present in plasma in the nonactivated form and in serum as activated IXa. It is present in the 40% to 50% $(NH_4)_2SO_4$ plasma fraction and in Cohn's fractions III and IV-1, but is absent from Cohn's fraction I. It is completely adsorbed from oxalated plasma by Seitz filtration and by the usual prothrombin adsorbents, from which it may be eluted by 0.2M sodium citrate solution. It is very stable when stored at refrigerator temperature and is moderately heat stable. Factor IX is reduced following administration of bishydroxycoumarin. Molecular variants of factor IX have been described.

Purified factor IX has been prepared by several workers (reviewed by Davie et al, 1975; Kingdon and Lundblad, 1975; Chung et al, 1980), and the amino acid sequence of bovine factor IX has been determined by Fujikawa et al (1974a). Bovine factor IX has a molecular weight of about 55,400 and, like many of the other coagulation factors, is a glycoprotein. Purified human factor IX is said to have a molecular weight of 72,000 (Andersson et al, 1975). Factor IXa is said to have a molecular weight of 46,500 (Fujikawa et al, 1974b). Factor IXa has esterase activity toward ben-

zoyl arginyl ethyl ester and other synthetic substrates and activates factor X to Xa (see later) by cleaving an arginyl-isoleucine peptide bond (Fujikawa et al, 1974c).

Factor X

The designation "factor X" has been assigned to the Stuart (or Stuart-Prower) factor described by Hougie et al (1957). It was originally called Stuart after the family name of the patient.

The deficiency is unusual in that it seems to affect both phases II and III of our scheme and is involved in both intrinsic and extrinsic reactions. It will be noted (Fig. 17-4) that the reason for this is that factor X takes part in intermediate reactions in both systems. The one-stage plasma prothrombin time is long, as is the Stypven time. There is also defective plasma thromboplastin generation, as evidenced by an abnormally short serum prothrombin time, long partial thromboplastin time, and abnormal thromboplastin generation test in the serum-substituted run.

Human factor X is a glycoprotein having a molecular weight of about 58,900 (Jackson, 1980). Several workers have prepared purified and highly concentrated preparations (Bajaj and Mann, 1973; Esnouf et al, 1973). It is made up of a light and a heavy chain held together by disulfide bonds, and the amino acid sequence of the light chain of bovine factor X has been determined by Enfield et al (1975) and DiScipio et al (1977). Factor X is converted to Xa by factors IXa and VIII in the presence of phospholipid and calcium, as well as by trypsin and Russell's viper venom (Bajaj and Mann, 1973). Activation of X to Xa by trypsin involves the cleavage of a small peptide from the heavy chain, whereas activation by tissue thromboplastin and factor VII may involve more extensive liberation of peptides (Jesty and Nemerson, 1974). Factor Xa is a serine protease and has esterase activity against tosyl arginine methyl ester (Adams and Elmore, 1971) and other synthetic substrates. It is inhibited by the complex heparin-antithrombin III (Yin et al, 1971b). Molecular variants have been described.

Factor XI

Factor XI is a glycoprotein with a molecular weight of about 160,000 (Schiffman and Lee, 1974; Bouma and Griffin, 1977; Griffin and Bouma, 1980). It is converted to XIa by XIIa, and XIa has endopeptidase activity toward factor IX (Fujikawa et al, 1974b) and esterase activity toward benzoyl arginine ethyl ester (Kingdon et al, 1964) and other synthetic substrates. Studies with human factor XI (Schiffman and Lee, 1974) showed surprisingly that it can be activated by trypsin but not by XIIa alone. These authors suggest that activation of factor XI by factor XIIa requires an additional substance that is not prekallikrein. The activation of XI is, however, dependent on the interaction of several substances. A deficiency of high–molecular weight (HMW) kininogen (Fitzgerald trait, Williams trait, Flaujeac trait) is accompanied by severely defective contact-activation reactions. Optimal activation of factor XII requires prekallikrein and HMW kininogen (Griffin and Cochrane, 1976). It is now thought that factor XII is bound to a foreign surface and is activated to XIIa. XIIa in the presence of HMW kininogen is a potent activator of factor XI to XIa and prekallikrein to kallikrein (Meier et al, 1976). During contact activation, HMW kininogen links both factor XI and prekallikrein to the foreign surface where they can be activated by surface-bound XIIa. Once formed, XIa remains bound to the surface, whereas kallikrein is freed (Thompson et al, 1977). Platelets may (Walsh, 1972c) or may not (Schiffman et al, 1977) participate in the activation of factor XI.

Factor XI can be adsorbed selectively by celite under carefully controlled conditions. It is adsorbed only slightly by BaSO₄.

Factor XII

Preparations of human factor XII show it to have a molecular weight of 110,000 to 120,000 (Cochrane and Wuepper, 1971). A summary of the properties of factor XII is given by Schiffman (1980). Most preparations are from bovine plasma (Komiya et al, 1972) and have a molecular weight of about 95,000. Factor XII is activated to XIIa by collagen and other subendothelial connective tissue, celite, kaolin, charcoal, micronized silica, and elagic acid (Ratnoff and Crum, 1964). Factor XIIa activates XI to XIa and prekallikrein to kallikrein. Factor XII is adsorbed by celite but only at such a celite concentration that factor XI is adsorbed also. There is little or no adsorption by BaSO₄.

Factor XIII

Factor XIII, the fibrin stabilizing factor, is a plasma glycoprotein having a molecular weight of 320,000 and made up of dissimilar pairs of α- and β-chains (Folk and Chung, 1973). Factor XIII has also been isolated from disrupted platelets, but this is not the same as the plasma factor, since it has a molecular weight of 146,000 to 165,000 and is composed of only a pair of α-chains (Bohn, 1972). The site of biosynthesis of plasma factor XIII is the liver, whereas platelet factor XIII is synthesized in megakaryocytes. It is not clear why the two forms are different, but both are active, since the enzymatic activity resides in the α-chains (McDonagh and McDonagh, 1980). Platelet factor XIII is a nongranular component (Lopaciuk et al, 1976) and is not released during the platelet release reaction (Joist and Niewiarowski, 1973).

Factor XIII is converted to XIIIa by the action of thrombin in the presence of calcium ions. The activation involves two steps. The first reaction is dependent only on thrombin and consists of splitting away two small peptides from the α-chains. The second is calcium dependent and results in the dissociation of the tetramer into an α₂ dimer, the active factor, and a β₂ dimer that is inactive. Factor XIIIa has a molecular weight of about 140,000 (Chung et al, 1974).

Factor XIIIa acts as a transglutaminase. It stabilizes the fibrin clot by forming intermolecular cross linkages between glutamine and lysine residues (Pisano et al, 1971) of adjacent fibrin monomers. Peptide bonds are formed between two γ-chains of fibrin to form γ dimers and among multiple α-chains to form α polymers (McDonagh et al, 1971). The stabilized clot is resistant to lysis by acid or urea. Solubility of fibrin clots by acid or urea is not involved in human hemostasis but the absence of factor XIII in vivo may be accompanied by abnormal bleeding. Plasma from factor XIII–deficient individuals fails to support fibroblastic proliferation in tissue culture.

The Fletcher factor

A deficiency of a new coagulation factor, named Fletcher after the name of the family with the defect, has been reported by Hathaway et al (1965) and by Hattersley and Hayse (1970). The new factor seemed to behave as a contact factor but was found to be distinct from factors XI and XII (Hathaway and Alsever, 1970). It is now considered synonymous with plasma prekallikrein (Wueper, 1973; Mandle and Kaplan, 1980; Schachter, 1980). The deficiency state is characterized by a prolonged activated partial thromboplastin time that becomes shorter only on prolonged contact activation (Abildgaard and Harrison, 1974). The APTT is not prolonged if the activator is elagic acid (Hathaway and Alsever, 1970). The interrelations of prekallikrein, factors XI and XII, the kinin system, and the complement system are discussed on p. 795. In addition to providing a link between coagulation, fibrinolysis, and kininogen activation, there is evidence that the Fletcher factor functions as an activator of factor VII in vitro (Gjønnaess, 1972; Saito and Ratnoff, 1975). This may be another possible link between the intrinsic and extrinsic pathways if it is shown to be operative in vivo.

The Fitzgerald factor

This factor was found to be deficient in an asymptomatic 71-year-old man (Saito et al, 1975; Waldman et al, 1975). The deficiency state resembles deficiencies of factor XII or Fletcher factor, because of a diminished activation as measured by the activated partial thromboplastin time, but was shown to be a new deficiency. The Fitzgerald, Flaujeac, Williams, and Reid factors are now considered to be (HMW) kininogens (Donaldson, 1980). However, Schiffman et al (1975) claim that the Fitzgerald factor is identical with their contact activation cofactor (CAC).

Other coagulation factors

The "Nishimine" factor deficiency was described by Yoshida et al (1961a). The deficiency affected a child born of consanguineous parents. The clinical findings resembled those of von Willebrand's disease.

The "Tatsumi" factor was also described by Yoshida et al (1961b). The deficiency affected several individuals, sons and daughters of consanguineous parents.

Pechet et al (1966, 1967) have described the "Dynia defect" in one subject with multiple bleeding episodes and in four asymptomatic relatives. It has been proposed that the factor is involved either in the reaction between IXa and VIII or in the activity of Xa. Hougie et al (1975, 1978) have described a mild hemorrhagic diathesis transmitted as an autosomal dominant caused by a deficiency of a new factor named "Passovoy."

Nonhemostatic functions of the coagulation system

Several reactions in the coagulation sequence have other important physiologic roles (Koller, 1966; McKay, 1972).

The deposition of fibrin is characteristic of the inflammatory reaction and probably serves to entrap and localize the infectious organisms. Deposition of fibrin in lymphatic vessels also tends to prevent dissemination of bacteria and bacterial products. The protective action of fibrin in bacterial infection is an important feature of infection with coagulase-positive *Staphylococcus aureus,* the staphylococcal coagulase being an active participant in the fibrin deposition. On the other hand, streptococci produce streptokinase; this fibrinolytic agent tends to break down the fibrin barriers, and streptococcal infections are characteristically spreading in nature.

It is well known that the fibrin network is important in the process of wound healing. Fibroblasts have been shown to migrate along the fibrin strands, eventually forming the fibrous scar. Beck et al (1961) have shown that there is delayed wound healing in cases of afibrinogenemia or of factor XIII deficiency. Here the fibrin network is loose and seems to offer insufficient support for fibroblastic proliferation. It is reported that small wounds in these deficiency states form large unsightly scars.

Fibrin is also essential for the implantation of metastatic tumor cells and possibly for the proliferation of tumor tissue (Laki,1974). It is probable that dissemination of tumor cells by way of the bloodstream is a common occurrence, but the tumor cells do not implant at distant sites unless provided with an adhesive fibrinous surface or mass (Ogura, 1967). There is some evidence, although not conclusive, that anticoagulants and fibrinolytic agents do indeed reduce the incidence of tumor metastases. Implantation may be aided by liberation from tumor cells of clot-promoting thromboplastic substances.

The role of activated factor XII (XIIa) in the activation of the kinin system is discussed on p. 795. Factor XIIa has been shown to increase vascular permeability (Ratnoff and Miles, 1964) and leukocyte migration (Graham et al, 1965b). Kellermeyer (1967) showed that factor XII is implicated in the development of gouty arthritis: urate crystals activate factor XII, which produces both increased vascular permeability by itself and by activation of prekallikrein, and increased leukocyte migration by activation of the complement system. Hageman factor–dependent pathways in disease states are reviewed by Colman and Wong (1977).

Hemostasis in the newborn

The blood of the normal newborn at, or shortly after, birth shows a mild deficiency of factors II, VII, X, and XI (Aballi and De Lamerens, 1962; Bleyer et al, 1971; Buchanan, 1978). Factors V and VIII levels are normal. The deficiency is due in part to immaturity of synthetic systems and in part to failure of the deficient factors to cross the placenta from mother to fetus. The deficiency is more marked in premature infants. Characteristically, the plasma prothrombin time and partial thromboplastin time in the newborn at term are slightly prolonged, being about 10% to 15% longer than the normal adult values. Both tests become even more prolonged by the third or fourth day after delivery and then gradually approach the normal adult values, reached at 6 to 12 months of age. Comparison of the results of the one-stage

prothrombin time and the two-stage assay for prothrombin shows that prothrombin (factor II) is the most depressed. In the premature infant the prothrombin time and partial thromboplastin time are usually prolonged (about 20% to 25% longer than the normal adult values), and any further decrease after birth or other complications may cause a severe bleeding diathesis (Barnard et al, 1979). When the prothrombin time and partial thromboplastin time are used for presurgery screening in the newborn, the results should be interpreted in the light of this expected relative physiologic deficiency. The newborn also exhibits defective platelet aggregation reactions (Pandolfi et al, 1972) and slightly abnormal release reaction (Corby and Zuck, 1976; Whaun et al, 1980).

PHASE I
Platelets and hemostasis
Introduction

Hemostasis, the physiologic reaction responsible for the arrest of bleeding, is normally one of the defense mechanisms of the body. As noted earlier, it depends on the proper functioning of the coagulation sequence and, more importantly, on normal activity of platelets and factors XI and XII. In a vascular system lined by normal endothelium, blood remains fluid because neither the platelets nor the contact factors have occasion to come into play. In other words, the normal vascular endothelium is nonthrombogenic. However if a vessel is cut, it will be noted that there is almost immediate adhesion of platelets to the edges of the cut vessel (Hovig et al, 1968; Wester et al, 1979). This is the "trigger" reaction that initiates a sequence of events leading to the formation of the "hemostatic plug." Failure of the sequence, because of malfunction of the trigger reaction or because of subsequent reactions, leads to abnormal bleeding.

The pathologic counterpart of physiologic hemostasis is thrombosis—the formation of an intravascular coagulum that partially or completely occludes the lumen of a blood vessel. The tissue or organ receiving its blood supply from that vessel, in the case of an occluded artery, undergoes ischemic necrosis (ischemic—lacking a blood supply), and in organs such as the heart or the brain the effect can be fatal. If the thrombus occludes a vein, the venous return of blood is impeded and portions of the thrombus can become dislodged and carried to other sites, a process called embolism.

The adhesion of platelets to the damaged blood vessel lining serves as the trigger for both physiologic and pathologic hemostasis. The reactions are basically the same, differing only in minor details, and will be discussed in subsequent sections.

Platelet morphology

Platelets are formed in the Golgi region of the cytoplasm of megakaryocytes and are released into the blood by fragmentation of the cytoplasm. Thrombocytopoiesis is controlled by thrombopoietin. Most of the platelets are produced by megakaryocytes in the bone marrow (Thiëry and Bessis, 1956), but a few may be derived from pulmonary

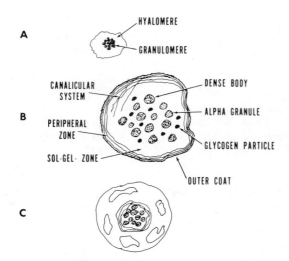

Fig. 17-5. Morphology of platelets by light and electron microscopy. **A,** Morphology by light microscope. **B,** Ultrastructure of a normal platelet. **C,** Ultrastructure of platelet during the release reaction.

megakaryocytes (Kaufman et al, 1965). After acute platelet depletion, 4 to 5 days are required to restore the platelet count to normal (Krevans and Jackson, 1955), but when platelet life span is estimated by isotopic labeling, the life span is 9 to 12 days (Bithell et al, 1967). The discrepancy is not explained and it is likely that the true life span falls somewhere between the two figures; repopulation after acute depletion may be at a rate faster than normal, and isotopic labels are notorious for leaching out of the primary target and labeling other cells.

After release, two thirds of the platelets are in circulating blood and one third is sequestered in the spleen (Penny et al, 1966). The normal pooling of platelets in the spleen is related to the sluggish blood flow through that organ and not to an active sequestration process. Most instances of thrombocytopenia accompanying splenomegaly can be attributed to increased pooling in the enlarged organ rather than to hyperfunction of sequestration by the spleen, "hypersplenism." However, it is probable that platelets at the end of their life span are sequestered and destroyed chiefly by the spleen (Aster, 1969). After splenectomy the liver becomes the chief site of platelet destruction. It is not likely that a significant number of platelets is consumed in the course of normal hemostasis. However, in disseminated intravascular coagulation half or more are aggregated and entrapped in fibrin thrombi.

When seen in a routine blood smear, platelets are 2 to 3 μ (2 to 3 μm) in diameter and two zones can be distinguished, the central granular "granulomere" and the clear "hyalomere" (Fig. 17-5, A). In normal blood a few platelets may be found that are about 4 μ (4 μm) in diameter, and these are young, newly released cells. When there is increased platelet production many of the larger platelets will be found (Karpatkin, 1972), probably in proportion to the number of active megakaryocytes (Garg et al, 1971).

Electron microscopy has provided not only details of platelet ultrastructure but also the means for correlating

structure and function (Zucker-Franklin, 1970; White, 1971; Holmsen, 1972; White, 1972a, 1972b; Zucker-Franklin and Grusky, 1972; Hovig, 1974; White and Gerrard, 1976).

The platelet membrane

The ultrastructure of a normal platelet is shown in a simplified diagram in Fig. 17-5, B. The outermost portion of the cell membrane is a shaggy coat called the "exterior coat", in which are found various glycoproteins. In the course of adhesion, aggregation, and the release reaction (p. 794) the outer coat retains its structure. Below the outer coat lies the "unit membrane." It appears to be trilaminar, but this may be the result of a fixation artifact. The cell membrane is pierced by a tortuous canalicular system that is probably utilized for the release of internal metabolites and possibly for some of the adsorptive reactions.

Although the cell membrane is made up of the outer coat and the trilaminar membrane, no clear definition is available yet as to what constituents are located in one or the other. The characteristics of the cell membrane are more important than the location of specific compounds. The one special feature assigned to the outer coat is that it comes into play in the adhesion and aggregation reactions. Otherwise, it is convenient to consider the constituents and reactions of the membrane as a functional unit without reference to the two morphologic structures. Also, the biochemical compounds that are in or on the membrane, and in the interior of the cell for that matter, are legion and only those pertinent to the hemostatic function will be considered.

A number of enzymes are associated with the membrane. Important ones are ATPase, ADPase, nucleoside diphosphokinase, and glucosyl transferases. ATPase, ADPase, and nucleoside diphosphokinase are probably involved in ADP-induced platelet aggregation (Salzman et al, 1966; Guccione et al, 1971). Glucosyl transferases (galactosyltransferase and collagen: glucosyltransferase) react with the galactosyl residues of collagen in the adhesion reaction (Jamieson, 1974) and possibly with glycoprotein residues on the surface of other platelets in the aggregation reaction (Roseman, 1970). There is evidence that the collagen receptor is fibronectin (Bensusan et al, 1978; Arneson et al, 1980). The platelet membrane carries a net negative charge due mostly to sialic acid residues. The negatively charged residues are not distributed evenly but in groups so that in the aggregation reaction in vitro constant stirring is needed to bring the negatively charged groups into contact with the positively charged gaps.

In addition to the collagen receptors, the platelet membrane has receptors for ADP, serotonin, epinephrine, thrombin, and the von Willebrand factor. These are probably different and specific; for example, a small amount of ADP, either added or from hemolyzed red blood cells, will make the platelets refractory to additional ADP but not to other aggregating agents such as collagen or epinephrine. The ADP receptors are binding sites for extracellular ADP in the primary wave of platelet aggregation. Serotonin receptors are responsible for the transport of serotonin from the plasma into the dense bodies in the interior of the platelet. Epinephrine (α-receptors) and thrombin receptors are binding sites for extracellular epinephrine and thrombin in the primary wave of aggregation. The receptors for the von Willebrand factor are selective for that factor (p. 808), and platelets are not aggregated by ristocetin unless the von Willebrand factor is present. It is assumed that each of the receptors is specific as far as the primary wave of aggregation is concerned.

The submembrane area contains *microfilaments* and thicker *microtubules.* The close proximity of the microfilaments to the unit membrane (Sixma and Molenaar, 1966) suggests that they are involved in maintaining the normal disk shape and retraction of pseudopods. Microfilaments isolated from disrupted platelets have been found to contain the contractile proteins *actin* and *myosin,* the latter similar to myosin filaments in muscle (Behnke et al, 1971). The terms "actomyosin" and "thrombosthenin" refer to platelet contractile proteins (Lüscher and Bettex-Galland, 1972). Booyse and Rafelson (1969) postulate that thrombin produces an increase in ATP that effects a dissociation of thrombosthenin to F-actin and actomyosin. Actomyosin has high ATPase activity, and the conversion of ATP to ADP results in the reassociation of the two fragments into the whole molecule of thrombosthenin. Thrombosthenin has contractile properties and causes retraction of the clot in which the platelets are trapped. This hypothesis is based in part on known properties of other contractile proteins. Thrombosthenin requires calcium ions for contractile activity (Nachman et al, 1967) and causes clot retraction by migrating into pseudopods formed during the shape change and then acting as a retractile protein to bring about clot retraction (Booyse and Rafelson, 1969). Clot retraction, then, is dependent on a normal number of platelets. Between zero and $100,000/mm^3$ ($0.1 \times 10^{12}/l$), the degree of clot retraction is directly proportional to the platelet count. Absent or very poor clot retraction is also seen in thrombasthenia (p. 804) but not in other abnormalities of platelet function. The force of clot retraction (about 10^4 dyne/cm^2) (Rubinstein, 1962) is probably sufficient to participate in hemostasis in vivo.

The microtubules form a complex canalicular system, some lying beneath the cell membrane and some penetrating the matrix of the platelet. There are two systems of microtubules. One is thought not to open to the exterior, contains electron-dense material, and is called the "dense tubular system." These microtubules probably are involved in calcium sequestration (White, 1972c). The other tubular system opens to the exterior. The most interesting feature of the open microtubular system is that it connects the interior of the platelet with the outside where some microtubules pass through the cell membrane. In the interior, microtubules come in close approximation to the granules and dense bodies, and at least some of the materials released from the granules in the course of release reactions find their way to the exterior through the system of microtubules. In addition, the open microtubules provide a communication between the plasma and the platelet interior. This is responsible for the platelet acting as a "sponge," adsorbing many plasma constituents, notably serotonin and coagulation factors, which then appear to be primary platelet constituents when platelet lysates are analyzed. Tubules that do not communi-

cate with the exterior (dense tubules) are sometimes seen in relation to a Golgi body, but only about 10% of the platelets contain a Golgi apparatus and its role is probably of minor importance.

Organelles

The interior of the platelet, the sol-gel zone, contains two types of granules, the α-*granules* and the *dense bodies*, a few *mitochondria,* and some *glycogen* deposits.

The α-granules are more numerous and less electron dense than the dense bodies. There is also a functional distinction, although this is partly speculative. α-Granules are enclosed by a unit membrane and contain hydrolytic enzymes (acid-phosphatase, β-glucuronidase, cathepsin) (Marcus et al, 1966) and are not unlike lysosomes. The dense bodies are rich in serotonin and according to White (1968) are derived from α-granules. They also contain nonmetabolic ATP and ADP, platelet factor 4, and catecholamines (Holmsen et al, 1969b). Serotonin is complexed with ATP (Maynert and Isaac, 1968). Analyses of the "granule fraction" of disrupted platelets do not always distinguish between α-granules and dense bodies. In addition to the constituents named above, many others have been identified in the granule fraction, and even more in disrupted whole platelets. There is no way of knowing at this time how many of these are truly platelet constituents rather than substances adsorbed from the plasma. It is almost certain that all the protein coagulation factors except factor XIII are adsorbed from the plasma (p. 794) and that platelet phospholipid (platelet factor 3) is derived from the platelet membrane (Marcus et al, 1971). Adenine nucleotides are primary constituents and are important in the energy metabolism of the platelet as well as in the aggregation reactions.

Energy metabolism

Platelets have an active energy metabolism that provides energy for the maintenance of normal structural integrity and for the aggregation and release reactions. Energy is supplied by ATP regenerated from the metabolism of glucose by the glycolytic and tricarboxylic acid cycles (Doery et al, 1970). Glucose is adsorbed from the plasma. The content of nucleotides (ATP/ADP) is not plasma dependent, and it is probable that platelets receive their complement of nucleotides in the megakaryocyte cytoplasm without any significant de novo synthesis after platelets are released (Holmsen, 1972). Adenine nucleotides are distributed in two pools, the *metabolic pool* involved in energy-supplying reactions, and the *storage pool,* available for the release reaction (Holmsen et al, 1969a). Because nucleotides from the storage pool and serotonin are normally released together during the release reaction, it is assumed that they both reside in the dense bodies.

Cyclic AMP (cAMP, adenosine 3'-5' cyclic monophosphate) is an important regulator of nucleotide metabolism and therefore of platelet reactions (Salzman et al, 1972; Schneider, 1974). As shown in Fig. 17-6, platelet cAMP is derived from ATP by the action of adenyl cyclase. cAMP is transformed to 5' AMP by cyclic phosphodiesterase, and this reaction reduces the cAMP concentration. cAMP activates phosphokinase, which, in the course of phosphorylat-

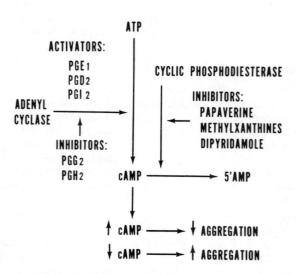

Fig. 17-6. Role of cAMP in platelet aggregation.

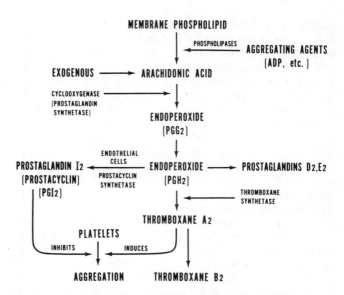

Fig. 17-7. Metabolism of arachidonic acid in platelets and the role of thromboxane in platelet aggregation.

ing other enzymes, forms ADP from ATP. The amount of intracellular ATP is also a limiting factor, and Schneider (1974) suggests that phosphorylase kinase activated by Ca^{++} and proteolytic enzymes generates ATP by direct mobilization of glycogen.

In general, increased cAMP causes inhibition of platelet reactions. Thus agents that activate adenyl cyclase (prostaglandin E_1 or PGE_1, PGD_2 and PGI_2) and agents that inhibit cyclic phosphodiesterase (papaverine, dipyridamole [Persantin], and methylxanthines) increase cAMP and are effective inhibitors of platelet function (Mills and Smith, 1972). Whether the opposite situation holds, that agents that cause increased platelet reactivity do so by reducing cAMP, is still controversial. Some may be inhibitors of adenyl cyclase: epinephrine, prostaglandin E_2 (PGE_2), collagen, thrombin (Mills and Smith, 1972; Salzman et al, 1972), and ADP (Mellwig and Jakobs, 1980). According to Kloeze (1969) the activating effect of PGE_1 and the inhibiting effect of PGE_2 can be expressed by the formula:

$$\% \; max.\Delta A = -494 - 99 \log [PGE_1] + 26 \log [PGE_2]$$

where % max.ΔA = Maximum decrease in light absorbance in the aggregation reaction
$[PGE_1]$ and $[PGE_2]$ = Molar concentrations

Prostaglandin D_2 (PGD_2) also stimulates formation of cAMP (Mills and MacFarlane, 1974), probably through a different receptor than the one for PGE_1.

As shown in Fig. 17-7, the prostaglandins are derived from arachidonic acid. In platelet metabolism, arachidonic acid adsorbed from the plasma (Russell and Deykin, 1976) is converted to prostaglandin endoperoxidases by the enzyme cyclooxygenase, which is derived from the platelet membrane (Hamberg and Samuelsson, 1974). It is believed that the primary effect of aspirin and indomethacin is the inhibition of cyclooxygenase leading to decreased production of thromboxane A_2. The prostaglandins are precursors of thromboxane A_2, which induces platelet aggregation

(Malmsten et al, 1975; Smith et al, 1976). Thromboxane A_2 also induces contraction of smooth muscle in the arterial wall (Ellis et al, 1976). Prostaglandin endoperoxidases are transformed by arterial microsomes to prostaglandin I_2 (PGI_2; prostacyclin), an unstable compound that is about 30 times more potent than PGE_1 as an inhibitor of platelet aggregation (Moncada et al, 1976). These findings suggest that the initiation of thrombus formation depends not only on platelet adhesiveness but also on a biochemical balance between generated substances that favor aggregation of platelets and contraction of smooth muscle, e.g., thromboxane A_2, and substances that inhibit platelet aggregation and relax smooth muscle, e.g., PGI_2 (Needleman et al, 1977). It is also possible that atheromatous plaques favor platelet adhesiveness and aggregation by allowing thromboxane A_2 synthesis to take place in the vessel wall (Ally et al, 1980) as well as by impeding the passage of platelet prostaglandins into the arterial wall and thus eliminating the formation of PGI_2 (Table 17-2).

Inhibition of cyclooxygenase has at least three effects. Inhibition of platelet cyclooxygenase by aspirin in small doses leads to decreased synthesis of thromboxane A_2 and a decrease in platelet aggregation. However, large doses of aspirin also inhibit cyclooxygenase in the vessel wall and thus diminish formation of PGI_2, removing the inhibitor to aggregation. The effect of aspirin as a platelet-inhibitory drug is therefore very dose dependent, particularly since at low doses only platelet cyclooxygenase is inhibited (Amezcua et al, 1979). Patrono et al (1980) have shown that a 200-mg dose every 72 hours is adequate to inhibit synthesis of thromboxane A_2. A complete review of the clinical pharmacology and of the results of clinical trials with antiplatelet drugs is given by Gallus (1979). The drugs that have been most extensively tried in various thromboembolic diseases are aspirin, sulphinpyrazone, and dipyridamole, alone or in combination and sometimes in combination with heparin or oral anticoagulants. Last, the metabolism of prostaglandins

Table 17-2. Conversion of prostaglandin peroxide (PGH$_2$) to prostacyclin (PGI$_2$) by different layers of the arterial wall*

Layer	Conversion (%)
Intima	31.8 ± 2.5
Internal elastic	4.3 ± 0.1
Media	3.9 ± 0.9
Adventitia	2.7 ± 0.9

*Data from Moncada et al (1977).

and cAMP is interrelated, in that PGE$_1$ favors the formation of cAMP and inhibits aggregation, whereas PGE$_2$ inhibits formation of cAMP, decreases the concentration of cAMP, and favors aggregation.

Interaction of platelets with subendothelial tissues

The normal intact lining of blood vessels, the *endothelium*, is a truly nonthrombogenic surface because it is nonadhesive for platelets. The sequence of platelet reactions in vivo is initiated when the subendothelial tissue, to which platelets adhere strongly, is exposed. This occurs when a vessel is transected or when endothelial cells are lost (Fig. 17-8).

Immediately beneath the endothelium in capillaries, small veins, and heart valves lies a special type of connective tissue called the *basement membrane*. This consists of a network of fine fibrils varying from 50 to 100 Å (5 to 10 nm) in thickness. Deeper still lie fibers of *collagen*. The subendothelial area of large arteries is significantly different. It consists of irregular particles of *basement membrane* fibrils, electron-dense *microfibrils,* and electron-lucent *elastin* (Stemerman, 1973). The basement membrane does not form a continuous layer, and the elastin is in relation to the internal elastin lamina. Little or no collagen is found subintimally in large arteries but is abundant in deeper portions of the vessel wall.

It follows that platelets are exposed to different types of connective tissue depending on the type of blood vessel involved and the type of injury. Transection of vessels exposes platelets to deep-lying collagen and other fibrils, but simple loss of endothelium exposes basement membrane fibrils in capillaries, veins, and cardiac valves and to electron-dense microfibrils in arteries. The demonstration that collagen suspension in vitro induced release of ADP (Hovig, 1963) and activated factor XII (Wilner et al, 1968) pointed to collagen fibrils at first as the interacting subendothelial tissue. The interaction with collagen apparently plays an important role in forming the hemostatic plug when a small vessel is cut. Selective removal of the endothelium of an artery results in adhesion of platelets in a monolayer to microfibrils with little morphologic change in the platelets, whereas adhesion to collagen causes marked alteration of platelet structure (Stemerman, 1973).

Adhesion of platelets to denuded subendothelial tissue is accompanied by a polymorphonuclear and mononuclear reaction and later by restoration of the endothelial lining (Stemerman and Ross, 1972) over a less well organized subendothelial zone. Removal of the regenerated endotheli-

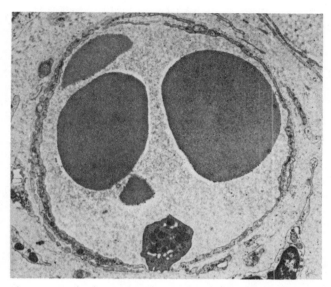

Fig. 17-8. A platelet entering the gap between endothelial cells produced by distending the vessel. (From Zucker: Sci Am **242:**86, 1980; print courtesy Dr. H.R. Baumgartner.)

um results in a heightened thrombogenic response characterized by fibrin deposition at the surface and in the subendothelium and by migration of platelets into the subendothelial tissue (Stemerman, 1973). This accentuated thrombogenic reaction may involve the liberation of tissue products from the altered vessel wall. During the healing phase the subintimal tissue is markedly thickened. A very similar intimal thickening is considered a precursor of atherosclerosis in human beings (Movat et al, 1958).

The manifestations of inadequate hemostasis are a prolonged bleeding time and clinical hemorrhagic manifestations. The bleeding time measures how long it takes for effective hemostasis to be established and, since this is primarily dependent on normal platelet function, the test is one of the measurable parameters of platelet function. The clinical manifestations of abnormal hemostasis are discussed in a later section (p. 804). We can note here that purpura, the formation of pinpoint subcutaneous hemorrhages (petechiae), is related primarily to abnormal platelet function. Whether spontaneous or induced by the tourniquet test, it is the result of red blood cells leaking out through gaps between the endothelial cells. When such gaps are formed, either spontaneously or as the result of increased intraluminal pressure and dilatation of the vessel, they are normally occluded by platelets (Tranzer and Baumgartner, 1967; Gimbrone et al, 1969; Wojcik et al, 1969). When platelets are deficient in number or function this does not happen, and red blood cells can escape. Not uncommonly, platelet abnormalities cause enough subcutaneous bleeding to produce bruises after minimal trauma.

Platelet function

The platelet performs its hemostatic function by responding to a variety of stimuli by undergoing a predictable sequence of reactions (Fig. 17-9): (1) shape change (2) adhesiveness, (3) primary aggregation, (4) secondary aggregation, and (5) release reactions. The sequence is completed

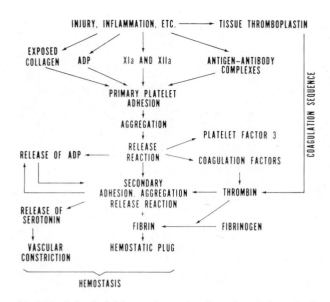

Fig. 17-9. Role of platelets and associated reactions in hemostasis.

if the stimulus (inducer) is sufficiently strong and no inhibitors are operative. If the stimulus is weak or inhibitors sufficiently strong, then the sequence can stop, and even reverse, before it is completed. The nature of the inducer also controls whether the entire sequence is followed. The fully developed hemostatic process also involves activation of the blood coagulation sequence.

Shape change

All inducers of platelet adhesion and aggregation cause the platelet shape to change from a disk to a spiny sphere (Mustard and Packham, 1970). The shape change is not calcium dependent, since it is not inhibited by EDTA, a powerful inhibitor of adhesion and aggregation. The shape change does not change the cell volume (Born, 1970). Since the shape change precedes the adhesion reaction at optimum concentrations of strong inducers, it is assumed that the spiny processes promote adhesion to foreign surfaces as well as cell-to-cell adhesion (aggregation). The shape change is reversible if it is brought about by a very low concentration of the inducer, for example, by a low concentration of thrombin. The change from disk to spiny sphere sometimes decreases the light transmission of platelet-rich plasma, which is reflected in an almost immediate small dip in the baseline tracing in an aggregometer. Born (1972) suggests that the shape change produced by various agents is the result of platelet ADP interacting with contractile protein at or near the cell surface. Ultrastructural studies have shown that the shape change is accompanied by a shift toward the interior of the circumferential microtubules and of organelles. Everything points to the shape change being a preparatory step for more violent release reactions.

Platelet adhesion

Platelet adhesion refers to the process whereby platelets adhere to something other than platelets, i.e., basement membrane, microfibrils, collagen, glass, other "foreign surfaces." The platelets can be thought to have a "sticky" surface, but the conditions for adhesion vary with different substrates. Platelet adhesion to glass requires the presence of calcium ions, whereas adhesion to basement membrane or collagen does not. Adhesion to collagen is dependent on the formation of an enzyme-acceptor complex between the collagen glucosyltransferase of the platelet membrane and the galactosyl residues of collagen (Jamieson, 1974). Adhesion to microfibrils differs from the interaction with collagen in that it requires calcium ions (Baumgartner et al, 1971). Adhesiveness to collagen can be measured specifically by the method of Legrand et al (1979). Platelet adhesion is an essential step in the hemostatic reaction, and decreased adhesion is found in the functional platelet abnormalities. Concentrated factor VIII corrects the abnormal adhesion found in von Willebrand's disease (Bouma et al, 1972) and rabbit antihuman factor VIII inhibits this correction, but the inhibition probably affects the von Willebrand portion of the normal factor VIII molecule (Weiss et al, 1973b). Platelet adhesion is not affected by aspirin (Bick et al, 1976) despite its prolonging the bleeding time (Mielke et al, 1969).

Platelet aggregation

Platelet aggregation is the adhesion of platelets to other platelets. Aggregation in vivo is induced by a variety of stimuli (Fig. 17-9), and the reaction can be studied in vitro by adding various inducers of aggregation to platelet-rich plasma and measuring the change in light transmission in an aggregometer instrument. Platelet aggregation is accompanied by the release reaction. Clinical situations associated with abnormal aggregation are discussed on pp. 804-819.

The aggregation reactions seen in vitro are dependent on pH, temperature, mechanical stirring, calcium ion concentration, number of platelets in the platelet-rich plasma, elapsed time between the performance of the aggregation tests and the preparation of platelet-rich plasma, "plasmatic atmosphere," and type and concentration of the aggregation-inducing agent.

Optimum aggregation requires that the pH of the platelet-rich plasma be between 6.8 and 8.5. At a pH a few tenths less than 6.8 no aggregation can be induced. Correction of a low pH to 7.4 restores normal aggregation. Aggregation is also very temperature dependent. The optimum temperature is 37° C. Below 32° C no aggregation takes place. Mechanical stirring with a magnetic bar at a constant optimum speed is essential. Stirring is necessary to bring platelets within aggregating distance of each other. In vivo this is a by-product of blood flow (Rozenberg and Dintenfass, 1964).

Aggregation has an absolute requirement for calcium ions. It is inhibited by removing all calcium ions with EDTA. When sodium citrate is used as an anticoagulant, enough ionized calcium is free to supply the calcium requirement. However, if the sodium citrate concentration is too high, insufficient calcium ions remain in solution (Ts'ao et al, 1976). We use 3.2% sodium citrate (0.109M), 1 part to 9 parts of venous blood for all coagulation studies, and find that this concentration is better than higher ones for aggregation studies.

Everyone working with aggregation is aware that difficulties will be encountered if the platelet count in platelet-rich plasma is too low. Levine (1976) reports that ADP and collagen produce normal aggregation with platelet counts (of the platelet-rich plasma) as low as 50,000/mm^3 (0.05 × 10^{12}/l), while epinephrine produces normal aggregation when the platelet count is as low as 75,000/mm^3 (0.075 × 10^{12}/l). The same report shows, however, that this conclusion holds when a high final concentration of ADP is used (1 × 10^{-5}/M) but not at a final concentration of 1 × 10^{-6}/M. I feel that the concentration of platelets is important, but the degree of aggregation and the distinction of primary and secondary phases depends equally as much on the final concentration of the aggregating agent and on the sensitivity of the instrument used to detect and record aggregation.

It is important to note that the time between the preparation of the platelet-rich plasma and the performance of aggregation studies is another technical variable. Confusing results are obtained if the interval is either too short or too long. During centrifugation the platelets become partially unreactive, a condition commonly called "platelet shock," the nature of which is unknown. Aggregation by epinephrine, we find, is particularly poor and usually monophasic if this aggregation is performed as soon as the platelet-rich plasma is obtained. To avoid this, plasma is allowed to stand at room temperature for about 30 minutes before beginning the aggregation studies, and epinephrine is one of the last aggregating agents used. After citrated plasma stands for 2 to 3 hours, the platelets begin to show spontaneous aggregation and become partially refractory to aggregating agents. Holmsen (1972) states that platelet reactivity is stable for up to 8 hours if ACD anticoagulant is used in place of citrate.

The role of plasma constituents, the "plasmatic cofactors" in the "plasmatic atmosphere," has been investigated extensively. The concept that a plasmatic atmosphere of proteins is a requirement for normal platelet function was proposed many years ago (Roskam, 1923). Deutsch et al (1955) and Bounameaux (1957) first attempted to identify the plasma components.

Fibrinogen was identified as a plasmatic cofactor for normal platelet function from observations that in clinical cases of congenital afibrinogenemia there is diminished ADP-induced platelet aggregation (Gugler and Lüscher, 1963; Inceman et al, 1966; Rodman et al, 1966; Weiss and Rogers, 1971). Only minute amounts of fibrinogen are required, and it has been pointed out that so-called afibrinogenemic plasma sometimes does contain small amounts of fibrinogen (Rodman et al, 1966). A second known cofactor is the von Willebrand factor, the von Willebrand portion of the factor VIII molecule (Zimmerman et al, 1971a), which is a requirement for platelet aggregation by ristocetin (Howard et al, 1973; Weiss et al, 1973c). A possible third cofactor is factor XII (Okonkwo et al, 1970; Bang et al, 1972).

The assignment of cofactor activity to some of the coagulation proteins led to investigations of the role of other coagulation factors. Attempts to identify these as cofactors by the use of plasmas having specific deficiencies of coagulation factors have not been rewarding (Bang et al, 1972), although we have recently studied a child with congenital deficiency of factor XI who also had very abnormal platelet aggregation. Edgin et al (1980) report a case of acquired

deficiency of factor X with a long bleeding time, abnormal aggregation with epinephrine and collagen, but normal aggregation with ADP or ristocetin. We have recently used immunologic neutralization to show that some or all of the factors in the "prothrombin complex" (factors, II, VII, IX, and X) are required for normal platelet aggregation (Miale and Kent, 1975). We have suggested that these, and possibly all, coagulation factors are adsorbed onto or into the platelet from the plasma and that they are involved in the platelet aggregation reaction. The concept of the platelet as a "sponge" is not new (Adelson et al, 1961). In addition to serotonin (Mills et al, 1968), immunoglobulins (Nachman, 1965), plasminogen (Nachman, 1965), myxovirus (Terada et al, 1966), and Australia antigen (Furukawa et al, 1975), platelets adsorb coagulation factors V (Hjort et al, 1955; Walsh, 1972a), VIII (Karpatkin and Karpatkin, 1960), IX (Biggs et al, 1968), XI and XII (Horowitz and Fujimoto, 1965; Walsh, 1972b), and contain XIII. It can be postulated that all of the coagulation proteins are adsorbed onto platelets from the plasma and react, together with phospholipid in the membrane, in the formation of the fibrin deposited on and in aggregates of platelets. It is not improbable that the reactions of the platelet membrane replicate the entire coagulation sequence in a microcosmic setting. The generation of thrombin at the platelet membrane is obviously related to the aggregation reaction (Johnson et al, 1965). How the participation of coagulation factors relates to the release of ADP remains a mystery.

A number of inducers can bring about platelet aggregation. It is believed by most that maximum aggregation is caused by ADP released during the release reaction (Mills et al, 1968). The strongest evidence for this is from the observation that the addition of ADP-inactivating enzymes to the system inhibits most of the aggregation response and, more recently, that failure of ADP release during the release reaction results in poor aggregation. However, some observations are difficult to reconcile with the hypothesis that ADP is the chief effector of aggregation. For example, platelets can be made unresponsive to ADP (Packham et al, 1969) but will aggregate if epinephrine is added (O'Brien, 1966). It has been suggested that because epinephrine decreases platelet cAMP it is this that increases the responsiveness of the unresponsive platelets, but this is speculative. It now appears that the aggregation reactions are related in part to the activation of prostaglandin synthesis, but this probably does not apply to aggregation by ristocetin.

Whatever the nature of the reactions may be, it is found that different aggregating agents produce different aggregation responses. The response is also dependent on the concentration of aggregation inducer in the platelet-rich plasma. Suboptimal amounts of any of the aggregating agents produce a weak first wave reaction soon followed by deaggregation. Ideal amounts of collagen give a characteristic single wave response after a lag period of about 1 minute. Ideal amounts of ADP produce a primary wave of aggregation followed by a secondary wave in about 70% to 80% of subjects (McMillan, 1966). In our laboratory, the percent of supposedly normal individuals that show a biphasic aggregation is somewhat lower. There is no explanation for the failure of some normal persons to have biphasic responses. Epinephrine causes a double wave aggregation in almost all normal individuals, although we occasionally obtain only a primary wave response. Ideal amounts of thrombin produce a double wave response, but it is difficult to achieve this ideal and most responses are monophasic. Ristocetin is a strong aggregating agent that gives single wave aggregation, but occasionally a secondary wave is obtained. Primary wave aggregation is reversible when suboptimum concentrations of aggregating agents are used. The secondary wave, however, is irreversible. These reactions are illustrated and discussed further on p. 799.

Platelet release reactions

The "release reaction" (Holmsen et al, 1969a) refers to the release of platelet substances into the surrounding medium. As shown in Fig. 17-9, the primary sequence of adhesion-aggregation-release reaction is accompanied by the release of ADP (and other substances, as discussed later), which produces a second sequence of adhesion-aggregation-release reaction that results in a second release of platelet materials. The second release reaction that is produced when ADP or epinephrine is the aggregation-inducing agent accounts for the secondary wave of aggregation seen in the aggregometer tracings. Collagen produces a single wave of aggregation because it probably causes a maximum release reaction by itself. This outline must be modified a little, however, by the probability that the release reactions are not so distinct from each other, and various degrees of release probably occur continuously, beginning with the first platelet reaction, building up to maximum release with collagen or thrombin or during the secondary wave of aggregation with ADP or epinephrine.

The release reaction is secretory and is energy dependent (Karpatkin, 1967; Muenzer et al, 1975). It is not the result of platelet disruption, and the platelet membrane remains unbroken. However, the structure of the platelet is altered markedly. Swollen pseudopods containing microtubules encircle the cell. Granules and organelles are compacted in the center of the cell and are surrounded by tubules and filaments (Fig. 17-5, *C*) (Hovig, 1968). The granules gradually become indistinct and the dense bodies disappear as their contents are released through the canalicular system (White, 1968). A few platelets do undergo lysis throughout the aggregation and release sequences (Holmsen, 1972), and this may be one of the mechanisms for making available membrane-associated platelet factor 3 and coagulation factors.

A number of substances are released during the release reaction (Hirsh and Doery, 1971). Some are incidental insofar as they play no obvious role. For example, several enzymes are released that have no known function related to hemostasis, among them acid phosphatase, resulting in increased enzymatic activities in plasma. Potassium is also released, and, if enough platelets are involved, a high serum concentration of potassium results in "spurious hyperkalemia." Other released materials do contribute to the hemostatic process: serotonin, ATP, ADP, calcium, platelet factor 3, and platelet factor 4. Platelet factor 4 (PF$_4$) has a high antiheparin activity (Levine and Wohl, 1976). Other antiheparin platelet proteins (low-affinity PF$_4$, β-thromboglobulin (Moore and Pepper, 1976), and platelet basic pro-

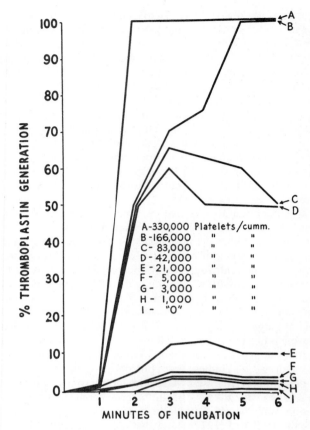

Fig. 17-10. Effect of platelet concentration on generation of plasma thromboplastin. The concentrations shown are for platelets per cubic millimeter of final incubation mixture.

tein (PBP) (Guzzo et al, 1980) have low antiheparin affinity. β-Thromboglobulin (BTG) is increased when platelet life span is decreased (Ludlam, 1979) and in thrombocytopenic patients with acute leukemia (Kutti et al, 1980). Serotonin is a powerful vasoconstrictor; ADP produces the explosive secondary wave of aggregation; calcium ions are necessary in the coagulation sequence responsible for fibrin formation; platelet factor 3 is also involved in fibrin formation; and platelet factor 4 may favor fibrin deposition.

When the early investigators were attempting to unravel the mysteries of the platelet, much of the work consisted of analyzing disrupted platelets. Over the years a number of substances present in platelet lysates were glorified by being called "platelet factors," and the list includes ten numbered 1 to 10 in Arabic numerals to distinguish them from the Roman numerals assigned to coagulation factors. The first one to be discredited was factor 1, which was shown to be adsorbed factor V (Hjort et al, 1955). Vicic et al (1980) have shown that factor V is released during the release reaction and that it is probably derived from α-granules. Platelet factor 5 is supposedly intrinsic platelet fibrinogen, which has since been found to be identical with plasma fibrinogen and is undoubtedly also adsorbed from plasma (Ganguly, 1969). Factor 10 is adsorbed serotonin. In fact, only two platelet

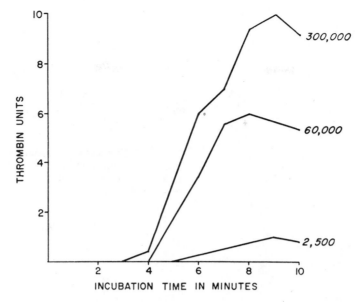

Fig. 17-11. Relationship between platelet concentration and thrombin formation. The concentration shown is the number of platelets per cubic millimeter of plasma used to generate thrombin.

constituents can be said to be platelet factors, platelet factor 3 and platelet factor 4. The role of platelet factor 3 is discussed in the following section. Platelet factor 4 has heparin-neutralizing activity (Harada and Zucker, 1971; Walsh et al, 1974) by blocking the action of antithrombin III (Yin et al, 1971b).

Role of platelet factor 3

Two basic reactions must take place in the intrinsic system before fibrinogen can be polymerized to fibrin; plasma thromboplastin must be generated from precursors, and prothrombin must be converted to thrombin. In the absence of platelets, resulting in deficiency of platelet factor 3, there is deficient generation of plasma thromboplastin (Fig. 17-10), deficient conversion of prothrombin to thrombin (Fig. 17-11), and incomplete prothrombin consumption (Table 17-3). It is interesting to note that, in vitro at least, increasing the number of platelets does not cause hypercoagulability and in fact a very high platelet count is accompanied by deficient thromboplastin generation (Fig. 17-12).

Platelet factor 3 is a phospholipid, commonly called cephalin, but the activity of crude cephalin preparations, such as the lipid fraction of tissue extracts, probably owes its activity to the presence of phosphatidyl ethanolamine and phosphatidyl serine (Slotta, 1960) (Fig. 17-13).

Role of factors XI and XII

As shown in Fig. 17-9, activated factors XI and XII are two of the inducers involved in platelet reactions. These factors are also involved in the early steps of the coagulation sequence (Fig. 17-2). In addition, they are involved in the activation of the fibrinolytic system, discussed on p. 840, in the activation of the kinin system in the inflammatory reaction, and in the activation of the complement system (Fig. 17-14). The activation of XII to XIIa on contact with suben-

Table 17-3. Relationship between platelet concentration and prothrombin consumption*

Patient number	Platelets/mm³ of blood†	Serum prothrombin time‡
1	2,500,000	14 sec
2	1,750,000	15 sec
3	640,000	20 sec
4	310,000	27 sec
5	225,000	35 sec
6	110,000	21 sec
7	77,000	15 sec
8	50,000	13 sec
9	24,000	12 sec
10	20,000	12 sec
11	14,000	12 sec
12	8,000	12 sec
13	6,000	12 sec
14	750	10 sec

*Fourteen different patients having normal plasma prothrombin times (one stage). Patient no. 14 had acute leukemia; patients nos. 8 to 13 had thrombocytopenic purpura; patient no. 1 had polycythemia vera; and patient no. 2 had chronic myelocytic leukemia.
†Direct counts by phase microscopy.
‡Method is given in Appendix. Normal value > 21 seconds.

dothelial tissues in vivo, with glass and other foreign surfaces, or with particulate substances in vitro results in the activation of XI to XIa and X to Xa, etc. in the coagulation sequence. Factor XIIa also converts prekallikrein (Fletcher factor) to active kallikrein, which activates plasma kininogens to bioactive kinins (Melmon and Cline, 1967). According to Özge-Anwar et al (1972), factor XIIa activates prekallikrein through a derivative that they call "factor XIIf." Schiffman and Lee (1974) claim that the interaction of fac-

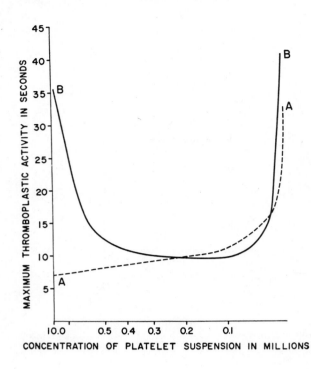

Fig. 17-12. Effects of varying platelet concentration on the generation of plasma thromboplastin. **A** represents the standard system. **B** is the dilute system in which alumina plasma is diluted 1:20 and serum is diluted 1:40. (From Miale and Garrett, 1957.)

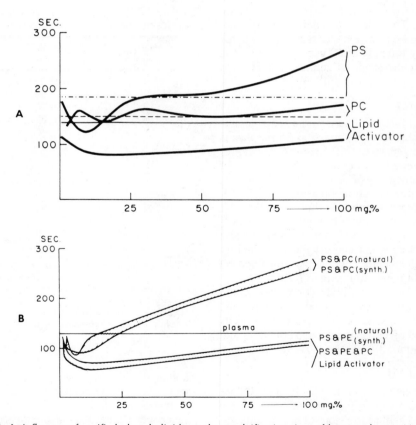

Fig. 17-13. A, Influence of purified phospholipids on the recalcification time of human plasma. Note that PS promotes clotting at a low concentration and inhibits it at a high concentration. PC has no significant effect. **B,** Influence of mixtures of phospholipids on the recalcification time of human plasma. Note that PS + PC and PS + PE + PC have the same activity as lipid activator. PS + PC are active at low concentration; at higher concentration the inhibitory activity of PS predominates. **PS** = phosphatidyl serine; **PC** = phosphatidyl choline; **PE** = phosphatidyl ethanolamine. *Lipid activator* is from acetone-dried human brain by extraction with petroleum ether at room temperature. (Courtesy Dr. Karl H. Slotta.)

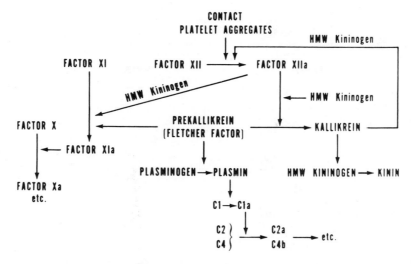

Fig. 17-14. Interactions of hemostatic and nonhemostatic reactions. The role of high molecular weight (HMW) kininogen is according to Mandle et al (1976).

tors XI and XII requires a ''contact activation cofactor'' (CAC), which may be identical with the Fitzgerald factor. Fletcher factor also has factor XI–activating activity (Hathaway and Alsever, 1970). Fletcher factor deficiency is asymptomatic, but the partial thromboplastin time is prolonged.

Laboratory studies in phase I abnormalities
Platelet morphology

In most abnormalities involving platelets the morphology of the platelets on stained blood smears is unremarkable. A wide variation in size with many large platelets usually accompanies severe thrombocytopenic states. Platelets that are larger than normal are young (Karpatkin, 1972). Large platelets are common in the myeloproliferative disorders and postsplenectomy. Characteristically large platelets are seen in the Bernard-Soulier syndrome (Fig. 17-22) and in thrombopathic thrombocytopenia. Large platelets are a feature of the May-Hegglin syndrome. In Greece and other Mediterranean countries multisystem congenital abnormalities have been described in which abnormally large platelets (hereditary macrothrombocytopathia) are found (Epstein et al, 1972). In healthy persons from Mediterranean countries, macrothrombocytopenia is a benign variable (Von Behrens, 1975). The platelets are described as smaller than normal in the Wiskott-Aldrich syndrome. Recently, we have observed by phase microscopy that patients with chronic liver disease have many very small platelets along with those of normal size.

Bleeding time

The bleeding time is an in vivo measurement of hemostatic efficiency. It should be performed according to the Ivy technic as modified by Mielke et al (1969) or with the bleeding time device Simplate (General Diagnostics). In platelet functional disorders the bleeding time is prolonged, and in thrombocytopenic states it is inversely proportional to the platelet count when this is below $60,000/\text{mm}^3$ ($0.06 \times 10^{12}/l$). The bleeding time is also prolonged in von Wille-

brand's disease. The bleeding time is determined primarily by the interaction of platelets with subendothelial tissues and not by the integrity of the coagulation mechanisms, so that it is usually normal in coagulation disorders. It is reported to be prolonged occasionally in intensely transfused hemophiliacs (Hathaway et al, 1973), but a platelet dysfunction has also been demonstrated in such cases. We have found the bleeding time to be prolonged only rarely in congenital coagulation disorders. Patients on long-term oral anticoagulant therapy, on the other hand, usually have a moderately prolonged bleeding time. Aspirin prolongs the bleeding time by 2 to 3 minutes, occasionally more, in most normal persons (Quick, 1966; Mielke et al, 1969) and usually markedly in subjects with von Willebrand's disease (Stuart et al, 1979).

Tourniquet test

It is assumed that increasing the intravascular pressure in the arm by inflating a blood pressure cuff to midway between systolic and diastolic blood pressure causes gaps to form between endothelial cells and that these gaps normally are occluded by platelets (Fig. 17-8), so that there is no extravasation of red blood cells (Tranzer and Baumgartner, 1967; Gimbrone et al, 1969; Wojcik et al, 1969). This is how normal ''vascular integrity'' is maintained. The tourniquet test is usually positive in severe thrombocytopenic states and in von Willebrand's disease. Aspirin intensifies the positivity in von Willebrand's disease. The test is inconsistently positive in other platelet functional abnormalities.

Clot retraction

It was once thought that all platelet functional abnormalities are characterized by abnormal clot retraction, but we appreciate now that decreased or absent clot retraction is found only in thrombasthenia. Papayannis and Israëls (1970) found decreased or absent clot retraction in clinically normal family members of subjects with thrombasthenia. Clot retraction is normal when the platelet count is 100,000/

Table 17-4. Abnormal platelet factor 3 release in congenital thrombocytopathy as revealed by the thromboplastin generation test (TGT)*†

Incubation mixture			Clotting time, seconds at minutes						Remarks
Ads. plasma 1:5	Serum 1:10	Platelet susp.	1	2	3	4	5	6	
N	N	N	32	20	9	8	8	8	Normal baseline
PT	N	N	29	19	9	8	8	9	Patient's plasma is normal
N	PT	N	34	21	9	8	8	8	Patient's serum is normal
N	N	PT	39	26	26	26	27	28	Patient's platelets are abnormal

Other findings:
1. Platelet count 295,000/mm³
2. Clot retraction; normal
3. Prothrombin consumption: serum prothrombin time, 14.5 sec.

*In this and in subsequent tables N = reagent from normal control, PT = reagent from patient being studied.
†The patient's platelets are deficient in the generation of intrinsic thromboplastin.

Table 17-5. Conditions in which there is decreased platelet adhesiveness (decreased retention)

Thrombasthenia
Thrombocytopathies
von Willebrand's disease
Hypofibrinogenemia
Thrombocytosis
Uremia
Scurvy
Immunoglobulinopathies
During adequate heparin therapy
During adequate oral anticoagulant therapy

mm³ $(0.1 \times 10^{12}/l)$ or higher, but between 0 and 100,000/mm³ $(0$ and $0.1 \times 10^{12}/l)$ the degree of retraction is directly proportional to the platelet count. Clot retraction may appear to be decreased in hyperfibrinogenemic states. In hypofibrinogenemic states only a small clot forms, and this may mimic increased retraction or lysis of the clot. Clot retraction is normal in siliconized glass tubes but not in tubes coated with collodion.

Platelet factor 3 release

Platelet factor 3 becomes available during the platelet release reaction. Since factor 3 release from the platelet membrane is secondary to aggregation, it is an indirect measurement of this reaction and a direct measurement of the release reaction. No conclusion can be drawn regarding the entire release reaction from factor 3 measurements because under some conditions serotonin release does not parallel factor 3 release (Sixma and Nijessen, 1970). Furthermore, platelet factor 3 is a membrane constituent whereas serotonin is granule bound. Platelet factor 3 can be measured indirectly by the prothrombin consumption test (Table 17-3), the thromboplastin generation test (Table 17-4), or by the celite test. These measure the contribution of platelet factor 3 in the generation of intrinsic thromboplastic activity and subsequently the conversion of prothrombin to thrombin. When used for this purpose it is assumed that the platelet count is normal and that there is no deficiency of coagulation factors.

Platelet factor 3 release (or availability) is abnormal in acquired and congenital platelet defects. In severe thrombocytopenia there can be only a small amount of platelet factor 3 released, which mimics abnormal release.

Platelet factor 4 release

Platelet factor 4 is probably granule bound and its release parallels the release of serotonin. It is not a commonly measured parameter of platelet function. Methods are given by Poplawski and Niewiarowski (1965) and by Fuster et al (1973).

Release of serotonin

The measurement of serotonin released during the aggregation reaction is probably the most direct and reliable estimate of the release reaction, but this procedure is used only in specialized laboratories. The best technic is based on the measurement of isotopically labeled serotonin.

Platelet adhesiveness (retention)

Platelet adhesiveness is determined in vitro by measuring the retention of platelets by a column of glass beads, admittedly a nonphysiologic model. In the original Salzman technique blood was pulled through the column by the vacuum of a Vacutainer tube, but this technique has been replaced by one that pushes the blood through the column at a constant rate using an infusion pump.

Adhesiveness to glass beads is a complex phenomenon depending not only on the adhesive property of platelets but also on the amount of ADP released from red blood cells, the concentration of plasma fibrinogen, the viscosity of the blood, the rate of flow through the column, the number and size of the glass beads, the length of the column, and the type of plastic used to construct the column (Bowie and Owen, 1971). Some investigators (Bowie et al, 1969) make their own columns and believe that they give meaningful results. Our experience with several types of commercial columns has been generally unsatisfactory. Normal values have shown such a broad range (9.9% to 79.6% retention in our latest study) that a distinction between normals and abnormals has not been possible.

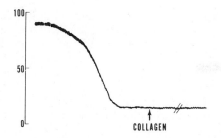

Fig. 17-15. Aggregation of normal platelets by collagen.

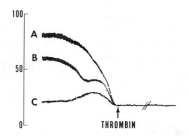

Fig. 17-16. Aggregation of normal platelets by varying concentrations of thrombin. **A** and **B**, Optimum concentrations; **C**, too weak.

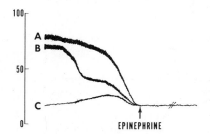

Fig. 17-17. Aggregation of normal platelets by varying concentrations of epinephrine. **A**, Excessive; **B**, optimum; **C**, suboptimum.

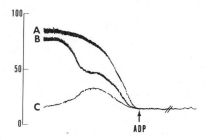

Fig. 17-18. Aggregation of normal platelets by varying concentrations of ADP. **A**, Excessive; **B**, optimum; **C**, suboptimum.

For the past few years we have depended on the in vivo method of Borchgrevink (1960a). In almost all cases the results of the in vivo method have correlated with the clinical picture and other laboratory findings, whereas the glass bead retention is unpredictable. Fig. 17-31 shows an instance of serious discrepancy in a von Willebrand variant. I believe that the in vivo method gives us the greater degree of correlation with the clinical picture and other laboratory findings. Theoretically, it is a physiologic measurement of the role of platelets in hemostasis, for the serial platelet counts made from the incision reflect the degree of platelet adhesiveness to subendothelial tissues. It is important to note that the incision for the in vivo method must be carefully standardized, using either the Mielke template or the Simplate. Our range of retention for normal subjects is 56% to 95%. In 19 patients having a prolonged bleeding time and other abnormalities the range of in vivo adhesiveness was 0% to 39%.

Abnormal adhesiveness (decreased retention) is encountered in a variety of conditions (Bowie and Owen, 1973) (Table 17-5) and is an additional parameter of platelet function in a patient being investigated for a bleeding problem. There are also many reports of *increased* retention (in neoplasia, after surgery, after trauma, in pregnancy, during oral contraceptive intake, in cirrhosis of the liver, in ischemic heart disease, in homocystinuria, during cardiopulmonary bypass, and in diabetes mellitus), but I would discount the importance of these observations. Under the most rigidly controlled conditions, the retention test using glass bead columns is disappointingly nonreproducible.

Platelet aggregation

The aggregation reaction that occurs in vivo is reproduced in vitro by adding an aggregating agent to platelet-rich plasma. The aggregation reactions can be measured and plotted using one of several instruments that measure and record the change in optical density that occurs as the evenly dispersed platelets form large clumps.

Four aggregating agents are used: (1) a suspension of collagen, (2) adenosine diphosphate (ADP), (3) epinephrine, and (4) thrombin. Ristocetin is used when von Willebrand's disease, thrombasthenia, or Bernard-Soulier syndrome is suspected, but we use it routinely.

The in vitro aggregation response is markedly dependent on the final concentration of aggregating agent in the test system. With all agents, suboptimum concentrations cause weak aggregation and may be followed by deaggregation. On the other hand, an excessive concentration may overcome an aggregation defect and will mask the secondary wave expected with some aggregating agents. Although we can begin with concentrations that usually produce normal aggregation, it is often necessary to try stronger or weaker concentrations.

Aggregation by collagen at any but very low concentrations gives a single wave response (Fig. 17-15). Characteristically this is preceded by a lag period of 1 to 2 minutes, not seen with any of the other aggregating agents.

With thrombin a suboptimum concentration produces slight aggregation followed by deaggregation (Fig. 17-16, *C*). With an optimum concentration there is good aggregation, usually monophasic (Fig. 17-16, *A*), but occasionally a biphasic response is obtained (Fig. 17-16, *B*). An excess of thrombin will clot the plasma and invalidate the test.

When epinephrine is used as the aggregating agent, a biphasic curve is usually obtained with an optimum concentration (Fig. 17-17, *B*). If the concentration is too high the biphasic response is lost (Fig. 17-17, *A*), while with subop-timum concentrations poor aggregation is followed by deag-gregation (Fig. 17-17, *C*). On a few occasions a biphasic response cannot be obtained in normal individuals.

Aggregation by ADP shows patterns similar to those obtained with epinephrine (Fig. 17-18). In about 30% to 40% of supposedly normal persons a biphasic ADP response cannot be obtained at any concentration of ADP.

Spontaneous aggregation in platelet-rich plasma without added aggregating agents may accompany a thrombotic epi-sode (Yon et al, 1976).

Deficiency of contact factors

In addition to the interaction between contact factors and platelets already discussed, the contact factors (XI, XII, Fletcher, and Fitzgerald) are required for proper generation

---

Table 17-6. Classification of platelet disorders

I. Thrombocytopenia (insufficient platelets) (Table 17-7)
II. Thrombasthenia and thrombocytopathy (functionally abnormal platelets) (Table 17-8)
III. Thrombocytosis and thrombocythemia (excessive platelets) (Table 17-10)

Table 17-7. Classification of thrombocytopenia

I. Caused by excessive destruction or sequestration
  A. Due to immunologic mechanisms
    1. Idiopathic thrombocytopenic purpura (ITP)
    2. Symptomatic thrombocytopenic purpura
      a. Apronalide (Sedormid) purpura
      b. Quinidine purpura
      c. Quinine purpura
      d. Digitoxin
      e. Chlorothiazide derivatives
      f. Chlorpropamide
      g. Meprobamate
      h. Phenylbutazone
      i. Sulfonamides
      j. Antihistaminics
      k. Other drugs (Shulman, 1972)
      l. Neonatal immunologic thrombocytopenic purpura
      m. Isoimmune neonatal thrombocytopenic purpura
      n. Systemic lupus erythematosus
      o. Evans' syndrome
      p. Infectious mononucleosis
      q. Other viral diseases (chicken pox, smallpox, rubella, measles, measles vaccination, Thai hemorrhagic fever)
      r. After blood transfusion
      s. During heparin therapy
  B. Due to splenomegaly and sequestration in the spleen
    1. Gaucher's disease
    2. Felty's syndrome
    3. Congestive splenomegaly
    4. Lymphomas with predominantly splenic involvement
    5. Miliary tuberculosis of spleen
    6. Sarcoidosis
    7. Myeloproliferative disorders with splenomegaly
    8. Septicemia with splenomegaly
  C. Due to sequestration not in the spleen
    1. Cavernous hemangiomas (Kasabach-Merritt syndrome)
    2. Multiple hemangiomas
    3. Diffuse intravascular coagulation, thrombotic thrombocyto-penic purpura, microangiopathic hemolytic anemia, etc.
  D. Due to mechanical destruction
    1. Extracorporeal circulation
    2. Cardiac valve prostheses
  E. Due to miscellaneous factors
    1. Massive hemorrhage
    2. Massive transfusion of platelet-poor (bank) blood
    3. Chronic alcoholism
II. Caused by deficient production
  A. Bone marrow suppression of thrombocytopoiesis
    1. Potentially myelotoxic drugs (partial list)
      a. Antifolates
      b. Nitrogen mustard
      c. Chloramphenicol
      d. Gold salts
      e. Dinitrophenol
      f. Streptomycin
      g. Penicillin
      h. DDT
      i. Benzol
      j. Organic chemicals
    2. Physical and animal agents
      a. Ionizing radiation
      b. Artificial fever
      c. Heat stroke
      d. Burns
      e. Insect bites
    3. Bone marrow replacement (metastatic tumor, miliary tuber-culosis, lymphomas, myelofibrosis, etc.)
    4. Deficient thrombocytopoiesis, mechanism unknown
      a. Pernicious anemia
      b. Paroxysmal nocturnal hemoglobinuria
      c. Prematurity
      d. Uremia
      e. Cyanotic congenital heart disease
      f. Platelet tidal dysgenesis
    5. Congenital, neonatal, or familial thrombocytopenic syn-dromes
      a. Wiskott-Aldrich syndrome
      b. May-Hegglin anomaly
      c. Chediak-Higashi syndrome
      d. Bilateral aplasia of radius
      e. Hyperglycinemia
      f. Tyrosinosis
      g. Congenital deficiency of thrombopoietin
      h. Hereditary sex-linked thrombocytopenia
      i. Hereditary nonsex-linked thrombocytopenia

of intrinsic thromboplastin. These reactions will be discussed in the section on phase II (p. 819).

Classification of platelet disorders

Classification of platelet disorders is shown in Table 17-6.

Thrombocytopenic states

Direct platelet counts by phase microscopy show a normal range of about 200,000 to 400,000/mm³ (0.2 to 0.4 × 10¹²/l). Brecher and Cronkite (1950) and Brecher et al (1953) give the mean as 250,000/mm³ (0.25 × 10¹²/l) and the 95% range as 140,000 to 400,000/mm³ (0.14 to 0.4 × 10¹²/l). In our laboratory the normal values derived from 180 normal subjects are a mean of 259,000/mm³ (0.259 × 10¹²/l), 95% range 145,000 to 375,000/mm³ (0.145 to 0.375 × 10¹²/l), highest normal 380,000/mm³ (0.38 × 10¹²/l), lowest normal 130,000/mm³ (0.13 × 10¹²/l). Since platelet counting by phase microscopy is the reference method, electronic cell counts should show the same normal values and distribution. False low counts (spurious thrombocytopenia) are occasionally caused by platelet satellism (Greipp and Gralnick, 1976) (Plate 64) or cold agglutinins (Kjeldsberg et al, 1974). Comparison of the count with the estimated number of platelets on the blood smear will usually serve to detect gross discrepancies. A progressive drop in the platelet count, sometimes to thrombocytopenic levels, is found during normal pregnancy (Sejeny et al, 1975).

Thrombocytopenia may be severe (10,000 to 20,000/mm³, 0.01 to 0.02 × 10¹²/l) or mild (60,000 to 100,000/mm³, 0.06 to 0.1 × 10¹²/l). No dysfunction or clinical bleeding is expected with platelet counts higher than about 60,000/mm³ (0.06 × 10¹²/l).

Caused by excessive destruction or sequestration

DUE TO IMMUNOLOGIC MECHANISMS. Thrombocytopenia resulting from platelet destruction by immunologic mechanisms is called "idiopathic" (idiopathic thrombocytopenic purpura, ITP) when no cause can be found for the development of platelet-destroying antibodies or antigen-antibody complexes. Immunologic thrombocytopenic purpura secondary to drug hypersensitivity or other agents is called "symptomatic" thrombocytopenic purpura. Although there is good evidence that the thrombocytopenic states listed under the heading *Due to immunologic mechanisms* in Table 17-7 are caused by antibodies acting against platelets, the methods for detecting antiplatelet antibodies are sufficiently unreliable (Dixon and Ross, 1975) that we cannot be confident that other thrombocytopenic states do not have an immunologic component.

In immunologic thrombocytopenias the damaged platelets are not lysed in the circulation but are sequestered by the spleen and liver (Shulman et al, 1965; Aster and Keene, 1969; Harker, 1970). Although the spleen may be the site of synthesis for platelet antibodies (Karpatkin et al, 1972a), the beneficial effect of splenectomy is caused primarily by the elimination of a sequestering organ. The effect of corticosteroids is probably also splenic. Immunosuppressive therapy is useful when neither steroid therapy nor splenectomy is effective (Finch et al, 1974).

IDIOPATHIC THROMBOCYTOPENIC PURPURA (ITP). Idiopathic thrombocytopenic purpura (ITP) presents as two clinically different syndromes: the acute type and the chronic type (Gardner, 1965; Baldini, 1972a; Wintrobe et al, 1974).

Acute ITP is more common in children (Choi and McClure, 1967). There is often a history of respiratory infection, rubella, or other exanthems. The onset is sudden, with two types of symptoms and signs: (1) purpura and ecchymoses of the skin and of the mucous membranes and (2) symptoms resulting from bleeding from the gastrointestinal or urinary tract, or intracranial or vaginal bleeding. The spleen is not enlarged and there is no lymphadenopathy. The course is usually benign, most children responding to steroid therapy within a few weeks or months. About 10% of the cases, however, progress to the chronic form.

Chronic ITP may follow acute ITP. In adults it is characterized by an insidious onset—usually a long history of easy bruising or abnormal bleeding. The clinical course is long, usually characterized by remissions and relapses, modified, of course, by therapy with steroids or by splenectomy. As in the acute form, the spleen is usually not palpable but, when enlarged, may be three to four times the normal weight.

The most striking laboratory finding is the *thrombocytopenia*. In the acute form the platelet count may be extremely low, to levels of only a few thousand per cubic millimeter of blood. In blood smears, platelets may seem to be scarce or completely absent. Giant platelets as well as small platelets are common (Khan et al, 1975). In the chronic form there is also thrombocytopenia, but it is often less severe than in the acute form. The bleeding time is almost always prolonged, and the tourniquet test is positive. All blood coagulation tests are normal except for prothrombin consumption and clot retraction; these are found to be abnormal in proportion to the number of platelets. There is no anemia or leukocytosis unless there has been extensive internal or external bleeding. The release of potassium from a large number of platelets results in a high serum potassium concentration (spurious hyperkalemia) (Hartmann et al, 1958; Ingram and Seki, 1962).

The *bone marrow* is not diagnostic. Megakaryocytes are plentiful (in contrast to thrombocytopenias caused by marrow depression), and although there may be an increase in young megakaryocytes and in forms having little granulation of the cytoplasm, these changes are not of themselves diagnostic. The changes that are found do not explain the thrombocytopenia, which is caused by decreased platelet survival, but rather the altered morphology either is caused by the same antibody that affects circulating platelets (McKenna and Pisciotta, 1962) or is a reflection of accelerated thrombopoiesis. The morphologic changes in the megakaryocytes can be said to be compatible with the diagnosis of ITP, but the diagnosis depends on the sum total of other findings. Nevertheless, the bone marrow should be studied to rule out diseases to which thrombocytopenia can be secondary, i.e., leukemia. Foamy histiocytes are present in some cases of ITP (Table 2-3, p. 47) and should not be mistaken for Gaucher cells.

The pioneer studies of Harrington et al (1951, 1953) provided strong evidence that in ITP the blood contains a substance, presumably an antibody, that causes damage to platelets and decreased platelet survival by sequestration in the spleen. Animal experiments as well as human studies have reinforced the concept that ITP is an immunologic disorder. However, while various immunologic studies (demonstration of platelet agglutinins, platelet lysins, positive platelet antiglobulin test, etc.) are invariably abnormal in experimental thrombocytopenia, the results in humans are inconstant, and different investigators have obtained conflicting results (Harrington et al, 1956; Shulman et al, 1965; Karpatkin and Siskind, 1969; Karpatkin et al, 1972b). More recently a solid-phase radioimmunoassay method has been shown to be a major improvement over the other methods (Hymes et al, 1979). The antibody is probably an IgG immunoglobulin. Hymes et al (1980) have found that the antibody in serum is of the IgG3 subclass, whereas antibody bound to platelets is poly-γ specific.

There is evidence that antiplatelet antibodies cross-react with endothelial cells (Morrison and Baldini, 1969). Whether this is a factor contributing to the formation of petechiae and ecchymoses is uncertain.

SYMPTOMATIC THROMBOCYTOPENIC PURPURA. One group of symptomatic thrombocytopenic purpuras is related to *hypersensitivity to certain drugs* (Gynn et al, 1972; Shulman, 1972). The classic ones are apronalide (Sedormid, a sedative no longer in use), quinine, and quinidine. Other purpuras related to drug intake very probably fall into this group when the drug effect is not a direct suppression of bone marrow thrombopoiesis.

Although apronalide is no longer used, it was Ackroyd's classic studies many years ago which showed that purpura caused by a drug could have an immunologic basis. He showed that in susceptible individuals (1) the intake of this drug can cause a clinical disease indistinguishable from ITP, (2) the drug plus the patient's serum (complement present) causes lysis of platelets, and (3) in the absence of complement, the drug plus the patient's serum causes only agglutination.

Of the other drugs listed in Table 17-7, the most commonly implicated are quinidine (Bolton and Dameshek, 1956; Bolton, 1956) and quinine (Helmly et al, 1967). Belkin (1967) reports an instance of quinine purpura that followed ingestion of quinine in the form of the common "tonic" mix. His designation of this purpura as "cocktail purpura" is most appropriate.

The mechanism of platelet damage is undoubtedly immunologic. The evidence indicates that the antibody causes an alteration of the platelet membrane by fixation of complement, that it is specifically antidrug (rather than antiplatelet), and that the platelets are "innocent bystanders" (Chapter 13), the drug and antibody complex fixing onto the platelet surface.

Evans' syndrome (hemolytic anemia plus thrombocytopenic purpura) may be an instance in which both erythrocytes and platelets are innocent bystanders in nonspecific (with regard to these cells) antigen-antibody reactions.

Thrombocytopenic purpura may precede or accompany the fully developed autoimmune diseases, particularly *disseminated lupus erythematosus* (Eversole, 1955) and the thrombocytopenia may precede the other manifestations of this disease by many years (Rabinowitz and Dameshek, 1960). Thrombocytopenic purpura is sometimes seen in *chronic lymphocytic leukemia* (Ebbe et al, 1962), the *lymphomas,* and the storage diseases (Green et al, 1971). It has been suggested that in these diseases some clones of immunocytes lose the capacity to distinguish between "self" and "not self" and thus produce antibodies to autologous platelets. Sequestration in an enlarged spleen may be equally important.

Symptomatic thrombocytopenic purpura may accompany infectious mononucleosis and other viral infections (Ackroyd, 1949; Angle and Alt, 1950; Billo and Wolff, 1960; Clarke and Davies, 1964; Morse et al, 1966b). We have seen one fatality in infectious mononucleosis caused by thrombocytopenia and cerebral hemorrhage. Terada et al (1966) have shown that myxoviruses are adsorbed onto, and can be eluted from, platelets; these reactions are accompanied by damage to the platelet membrane. Viruses can also be adsorbed by megakaryocytes (Dmochowski, 1960). Whether platelets are active as viral carriers during various viremic states is speculative. For the present we may be justified in assuming that they are and include in this category other viral diseases (chicken pox, smallpox, rubella, measles, and measles vaccination). Especially interesting is the thrombocytopenia that is sometimes seen in infants born to mothers who have had rubella (Bayer et al, 1965; Saidi et al, 1969).

In a few cases, severe thrombocytopenic purpura follows the transfusion of compatible blood (Morse, 1967; Mueller-Eckhardt et al, 1980). This has been shown to be caused by the development of a powerful antiplatelet antibody designated anti-Pl^{A1} (anti-Zw^a). Most of the patients reported with this unusual complication have been multiparous women.

Thrombocytopenia has been found to occur during intermittent intravenous heparin therapy (Babcock et al, 1976). Transient thrombocytopenia is not clinically important, but in some cases the thrombocytopenia is severe and persistent and is thought by most to have an immune etiology (Ansell and Deykin, 1980).

Neonatal immunologic thrombocytopenic purpura is sometimes seen in infants born of mothers who have, or have had, ITP. In some cases the mother is normal, and *isoimmune neonatal thrombocytopenic purpura* is a result of maternal fetal incompatibility with respect to platelet or platelet–leukocyte antigens (Pearson et al, 1964; Grenet et al, 1967; Colombani et al, 1968). In this connection it should be noted that when there is an anti-Pl^{A1} antibody, transfusion of compatible Pl^{A1}-negative platelets should be used (Adner et al, 1969).

DUE TO SPLENOMEGALY AND SEQUESTRATION IN THE SPLEEN. We have already noted that platelets damaged by antigen-antibody complexes are sequestered and destroyed by the normal spleen. The conditions discussed in this section produce thrombocytopenia by sequestering normal and undamaged platelets, and it is assumed that no immunologic mechanism is necessary.

As noted in Chapter 2, an enlarged spleen serves as a reservoir to shunt blood cells out of the circulation. While damaged cells such as immunologically damaged erythrocytes and platelets are destroyed in large number after being trapped in the spleen, it is also true that when there is massive splenomegaly many normal cells are trapped (Aster, 1965; Rowley and Jacobs, 1972). There may be accelerated destruction as well, but this is caused by normal lytic splenic mechanisms acting for a long period of time on cells that are sequestered. We assume that this is the chief mechanism for thrombocytopenia in *Gaucher's disease, Felty's syndrome, congestive splenomegaly, lymphosarcoma with predominantly splenic involvement, miliary tuberculosis of the spleen, sarcoidosis, myeloproliferative disorders with splenomegaly,* and *septicemia with splenomegaly.* When the bone marrow is involved or when there may be associated immunologic abnormalities, the pathogenesis of the thrombocytopenia may involve several mechanisms.

DUE TO SEQUESTRATION NOT IN THE SPLEEN. Infants having *cavernous hemangiomas* or *multiple large hemangiomas* (Atkins et al, 1963; Brizel and Raccuglia, 1965) are sometimes thrombocytopenic (the Kasabach-Merritt syndrome) (Hoak et al, 1971; Rodriguez-Erdmann et al, 1971). Sequestration of platelets in the tumors has been demonstrated by radioactive tagging, and the thrombocytopenia disappears when the tumor is excised or shrunk by irradiation. Occasionally, multiple hemangiomas are associated with splenomegaly, so that there is then a second mechanism for platelet sequestration.

Trapping of platelets in the fibrin network, which is deposited throughout the vascular system in the syndromes characterized by diffuse intravascular coagulopathy, accounts in part for the thrombocytopenia that is such a common sign in the syndrome (p. 846).

DUE TO MECHANICAL DESTRUCTION. Extracorporeal circulation of blood produces moderate destruction of platelets. The cause is primarily mechanical (trauma, adhesion to tubing, etc.), but the use of stored blood for priming is a contributing factor to the thrombocytopenia. In experimental animals, the addition of PGI_2 to blood prevents thrombocytopenia during cardiopulmonary bypass (Plachetka et al, 1980). Adhesion to artificial cardiac valves has been reported to cause moderate thrombocytopenia (Lander et al, 1965).

Behrendt et al (1968) report nonthrombocytopenic postperfusion purpura as a new syndrome. Most of their patients also had atypical lymphocytes in the peripheral blood.

DUE TO MISCELLANEOUS FACTORS. Thrombocytopenia can result from massive hemorrhage, usually from the gastrointestinal tract, by simple loss. If such a patient is given massive replacement therapy with stored blood, the thrombocytopenia is accentuated by the administration of platelet-poor blood. The combination of continuing hemorrhage and blood replacement with stored blood can result in severe thrombocytopenia.

Thrombocytopenia is reported in chronic alcoholism (Lindenbaum and Hargrove, 1968; Ryback and Desforges, 1970) as well as following intravenous infusion of ethyl alcohol (Post and Desforges, 1968). The mechanism is unknown; both a peripheral effect on platelets and sequestration have been postulated. Thrombocytopenia is one of the features of acute disseminated intravascular coagulation. Congenital thrombocytopenia is described in aplasia of the radius (Nilsson and Lundholm, 1960). Thrombocytopenia is reported in association with the Köln hemoglobinopathy (Hutchinson et al, 1964). Flury et al (1975) reported thrombocytopenia in Waldenström's macroglobulinemia in which IgM protein acted as an antibody against platelets.

Caused by deficient production

DUE TO BONE MARROW SUPPRESSION. The pathogenesis of thrombocytopenia caused by bone marrow damage is usually self-evident. The myelotoxic drugs produce hypoplasia or aplasia of the cellular elements. Megakaryocytes are reduced along with other cell lines. Occasionally a drug will produce only thrombocytopenia, but such cases are unusual. Ionizing radiation is the classic example of damage to the bone marrow by a physical agent, and the effects of intensive doses are devastating to all marrow elements. When there is infiltration of the bone marrow by tumor, miliary tuberculosis, lymphomas, or fibrous tissue, one factor in the production of thrombocytopenia is the replacement of normal marrow, but since there are usually other complications (splenomegaly, extramedullary hemopoiesis, etc.) in these conditions, it is not always possible to accept a simple "crowding out" phenomenon as the explanation for the thrombocytopenia. In fact, some of the myeloproliferative syndromes show extensive megakaryocytic hyperplasia of the bone marrow and megakaryocytic proliferation in the spleen as well. Some of these patients show thrombocytopenia while others show thrombocytosis. In these cases there is seldom good correlation between the number of megakaryocytes and the platelet count in the peripheral blood. It is probable that in some cases the proliferating megakaryocytes do not produce platelets. In addition, there are a few reports implicating a platelet functional abnormality in the myeloproliferative disorders.

DEFICIENT THROMBOCYTOPOIESIS, MECHANISM UNKNOWN. Deficient thrombocytopoiesis is seen in miscellaneous metabolic disorders such as pernicious anemia, paroxysmal nocturnal hemoglobinuria, and prematurity. For lack of knowledge, it is assumed that there is some metabolic interference with thrombocytopoiesis, but undoubtedly research in the years to come will further refine the classification. For example, the strong immunologic factor in pernicious anemia and paroxysmal nocturnal hemoglobinuria may also operate in the production of thrombocytopenia.

CONGENITAL, NEONATAL, OR FAMILIAL THROMBOCYTOPENIC SYNDROMES. The *Wiskott-Aldrich syndrome* consists of thrombocytopenia, eczema, and predisposition to infection (Cassimos et al, 1960; Krivit et al, 1966). There is also a platelet functional defect. The inheritance pattern is that of a sex-linked recessive disorder. Thrombocytopenic bleeding and overwhelming viral or bacterial infections are characteristic. The susceptibility to infection is probably related to defective cellular resistance. Most patients are reported to have low or absent hemagglutinin titers, with essentially normal serum immunoglobulins.

A few cases of *hereditary, sex-linked, recessive thrombocytopenia* not associated with eczema and infection have been reported. These are probably mild or incomplete variants of the Wiscott-Aldrich syndrome.

Defective thrombocytopoiesis is reported in the *May-Hegglin anomaly* (Davis and Wilson, 1966). The same mechanism is presumed to account for the thrombocytopenia associated with *Chediak-Higashi anomaly, bilateral aplasia of the radius, hyperglycinemia,* and *tyrosinosis.* In *congenital deficiency of thrombopoietin* (Schulman et al, 1960), the thrombocytopenia is related to defective production.

Hereditary nonsex-linked thrombocytopenia has been reported as *hereditary thrombocytopenia* (Myllylä et al, 1967). The defect is manifested either as an autosomal dominant or an autosomal recessive. Similar cases are reported by other authors. It is difficult at present to decide on a satisfactory classification of these familial disorders.

Functional platelet abnormalities

The classification of the various ways in which platelets fail to function normally is probably the most important advance in the area of normal and abnormal hemostasis. In spite of intensive research there are still many observations to be reconciled, and a definitive classification has not been achieved as yet. The classification I find useful (Table 17-8) is compatible with the data available from various investigators as well as from our own cases, but is subject to change as more information becomes available.

Thrombasthenia

In 1918 Glanzmann reported a hemorrhagic disorder characterized by poor clot retraction. He proposed that the defect was related to poor platelet function and called the syndrome "thrombasthenia." Just as Glanzmann's cases do not make up a homogenous group (some were probably thrombocytopenic states), so the terms "Glanzmann's thrombasthenia" and "thrombasthenia, Glanzmann type" were applied to cases of platelet dysfunction prior to the classification of the various types of dysfunction.

In our classification we restrict the term thrombasthenia for cases showing the following: (1) normal platelet count, (2) prolonged bleeding time, (3) absent or poor clot retraction, (4) abnormal platelet retention, and (5) weak or absent aggregation with collagen, ADP, epinephrine, thrombin, or ristocetin (Figs. 17-19 and 17-20). This is the only platelet function disorder in which poor or absent clot retraction is expected (Reichert et al, 1975).

The disorder is transmitted as an autosomal recessive trait (Pittman and Graham, 1964; Caen et al, 1966) and is usually severe. It is a puzzling platelet abnormality, for the platelets normally undergo the shape change when exposed to ADP (Zucker, et al, 1966), and the release reaction is also normal in spite of the absence of aggregation (Caen et al, 1966; Weiss and Kochwa, 1968). Clot retraction is usually poor or absent (Caen, 1972), a feature seen only in thrombasthenia.

The major abnormality is the lack of glycoprotein (glycoprotein II) from the platelet surface (Nurden and Caen, 1974). Some studies have shown that the platelets in this disorder have a diminished amount of thrombasthenin (Booyse et al, 1972). It is possible that this accounts for the poor clot retraction and poor or absent response to normally released constituents.

Table 17-8. Classification of functional platelet disorders

I. Thrombasthenia
II. Thrombocytopathy
  A. Storage pool disease
    1. Decreased release of nucleotides
    2. Decreased content of nucleotides
    3. Decreased PF_3 release
  B. Bernard-Soulier syndrome
  C. Thrombopathic thrombocytopenia
  D. Abnormal prostaglandin synthesis
    1. Congenital cyclooxygenase deficiency
    2. Congenital thromboxane synthetase deficiency
    3. Congenital phospholipase deficiency
  E. Deficient plasmatic cofactors
    1. Congenital afibrinogenemia
    2. von Willebrand's disease and variants
    3. Congenital absence of other plasma factors
    4. Absence of ionized calcium
  F. Defective nucleotide metabolism
  G. Drug induced
    1. Inhibitors of prostaglandin metabolism
    2. Stimulators of cAMP system
  H. Pathogenesis not defined

At one time thrombasthenia promised to be a homogeneous disease with predictable features, but it is now apparent that there are variants. In our cases (Figs. 17-19 and 17-20) there is absent aggregation with ristocetin, but others claim that aggregation by ristocetin is normal (Weiss, 1975). Another possible variant has been called *essential athrombia* (Inceman et al, 1962; Inceman and Tangun, 1975). It differs from classic thrombasthenia in that clot retraction is normal or only slightly abnormal. Aggregation is not seen with collagen, epinephrine, thrombin, or ADP, but ristocetin-induced aggregation is normal.

Storage pool disease

This is the first of many congenital or acquired platelet functional abnormalities called thrombocytopathy and distinguished from thrombasthenia on the basis that thrombasthenia shows diminished or absent clot retraction and the platelets are not aggregated by any of the usual agents, including ristocetin.

The release of intrinsic (nonmetabolic) ADP from the dense granules is thought to be a prerequisite of the aggregation reactions, especially of the secondary wave of aggregation produced by ADP or epinephrine. In the same year there appeared three independent reports of a platelet functional abnormality characterized by impaired release of ADP (Hardisty and Hutton, 1967; O'Brien, 1967; Weiss, 1967). It was assumed that intrinsic ADP was not released because the platelets were not aggregated by collagen or epinephrine, whereas added ADP produced only a primary wave response.

Recent data indicate that thrombocytopathies characterized by an abnormal release reaction are a heterogeneous group. The term "storage pool disease" is reserved for those cases having a deficiency of dense granule-associated

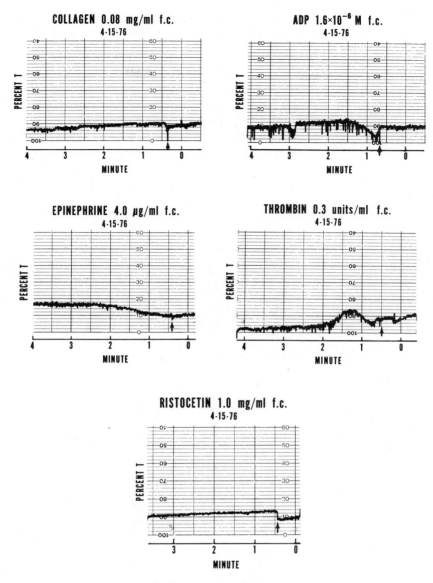

Fig. 17-19. Abnormal aggregation patterns in thrombasthenia. The patient is a 33-year-old woman with a history of lifelong abnormal bleeding. Hysterectomy was performed 5 years ago because of uncontrollable menorrhagia. There is defective aggregation with all agents; defective platelet retention (P. J., Table 17-4); 3+ tourniquet test; bleeding time, 6'20"; factor VIII:C assay, 74%; factor VIII:Ag, 137%; and clot retraction decreased (f.c. = final concentration of aggregating agent).

ADP (Holmsen and Weiss, 1972; Weiss and Ames, 1973). In variants having a normal amount of ADP in the dense granules there is a failure of the release mechanism (Weiss, 1972). The term "aspirin-like" defect is sometimes applied to these cases.

In storage pool disease, electron microscopy shows only a rare dense body and a normal number of α-granules (White et al, 1971). The dense bodies normally contain both ATP and ADP, with a high ADP/ATP ratio. In storage pool disease the reduction of ADP results in a low ADP/ATP ratio (Holmsen, 1972). This type of platelet abnormality has also been found in rats (Tschopp and Zucker, 1972). In those animals it has been found that the young platelets being released from megakaryocytes have very few dense bodies,

suggesting that there is abnormal thrombopoiesis with poor incorporation of ADP into platelets at the time of production.

Recent data show that the distinction between deficient storage pool and deficient release of ADP may not be entirely valid. Holmsen et al (1975) have shown that platelets from storage pool disease have defective release of granule-associated constituents, from both dense and α-granules. Even more interesting is the report that platelets from storage pool disese can convert arachidonic acid to prostaglandin intermediates but cannot respond to the aggregation-inducing stimulus (White and Witkop, 1972). In contrast, aspirin-treated platelets do not form prostaglandin intermediates.

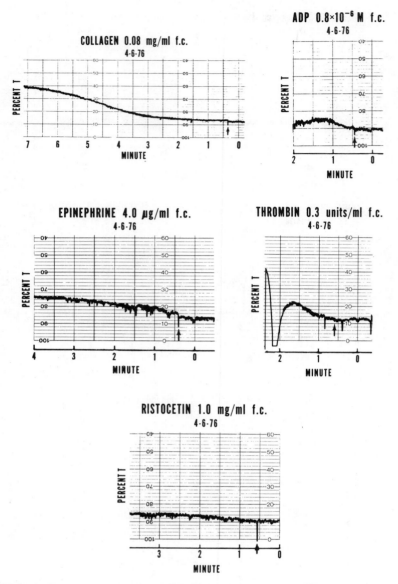

Fig. 17-20. Abnormal aggregation patterns in thrombasthenia. The patient is a 56-year-old woman with a strongly positive history of abnormal menstrual periods, nosebleeds, and bleeding after tooth extractions. Platelet aggregation studies as shown. Other findings included 1+ tourniquet test; normal clot retraction; bleeding time, 6′; factor VIII assay greater than 100%; factor VIII–related antigen, 120%; and platelet retention abnormal. This patient was diagnosed as having thrombasthenia in spite of the normal clot retraction.

A deficiency of nonmetabolic ADP in platelets has been reported in a variety of diseases: (1) Hermansky-Pudlak syndrome (Hardisty et al, 1972); (2) Wiskott-Aldrich syndrome (Baldini, 1972b); (3) thrombocytopenia with absent radii syndrome (tar baby syndrome) (Day and Holmsen, 1972a); and (4) Chediak-Higashi syndrome (Bell et al, 1976).

Deficiencies of enzymes involved in prostaglandin metabolism can mimic an abnormal release reaction. Congenital deficiency of cyclooxygenase (Malmsten et al, 1975) resembles the aspirin effect except that there is decreased platelet retention, not seen in the aspirin effect. A deficiency

of thromboxane synthetase (Weiss and Lages, 1977) can also mimic the aspirin effect by blocking the conversion of prostaglandin G_2 to thromboxane A_2.

Another type of abnormal release involves platelet factor 3 (PF_3). Isolated cases are reported in which a hemorrhagic tendency is accompanied by diminished PF_3 release, other tests of platelet function being normal (Sultan et al, 1976). Schwartz et al (1974) report the association of PF_3 deficiency and glucose-6-phosphate dehydrogenase deficiency.

In storage pool disease (deficient granule–associated ADP) there is a normal platelet count, a variably prolonged

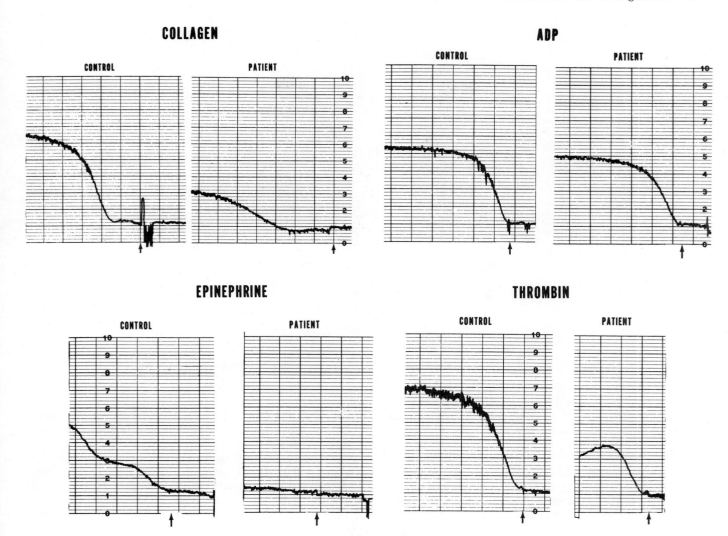

Fig. 17-21. Aggregation patterns in congenital thrombocytopathy (abnormal release reaction). Patient is a 30-year-old woman with a history of easy bruising, profuse menstrual periods, and severe bleeding after rhinoplasty. Bleeding time 9′ and 12′+, tourniquet test 2+.

bleeding time, and deficient platelet aggregation with collagen, epinephrine, and thrombin. Addition of ADP produces only a small primary wave. Sometimes there is decreased PF_3 availability. If the ADP content is normal but there is failure of the release reaction, there is deficient platelet aggregation with collagen, epinephrine, and thrombin and a fairly normal response to added ADP (Fig. 17-21). In both types platelet adhesiveness is usually decreased.

Bernard-Soulier syndrome

Bernard and Soulier (1948) described a syndrome characterized by a prolonged bleeding time, abnormal prothrombin consumption, and giant platelets. Since then a few additional cases have been studied and some of the features of the platelet abnormality defined (Bithell et al, 1972). The defect is inherited as an autosomal recessive, and consanguinity is common.

There is mild to moderate thrombocytopenia, the bleeding time is abnormally long, and clot retraction is normal. PF_3 availability is poor when measured by the prothrombin consumption test but normal by the kaolin method (Cullum et al, 1967). Platelet adhesiveness is decreased. The blood smear shows many, but not all, platelets to be very large (Fig. 17-22), approaching the size of lymphocytes, and the dense central granulation produces a pseudonucleated appearance. Platelets are aggregated normally by ADP, epinephrine, collagen, and thrombin, but not by ristocetin or crude bovine fibrinogen (Caen et al, 1973). The abnormal ristocetin aggregation is not corrected by normal plasma, suggesting that the platelets in this syndrome lack the receptor for von Willebrand factor (Weiss et al, 1974).

The platelet lesion is a lack of membrane glycoprotein other than the one lacking in thrombasthenia (Nurden and Caen, 1075). It is noteworthy that the platelets in thrombasthenia are also not aggregated by ristocetin. Walsh et al (1975) found that these abnormal platelets do not bind coag-

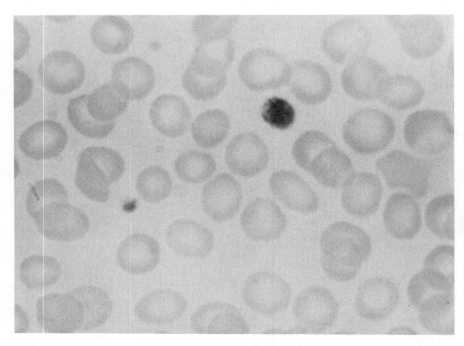

Fig. 17-22. Giant, morphologically abnormal platelet in the Bernard-Soulier syndrome. (Courtesy Dr. H. James Day.)

ulation factors V and XI. This probably accounts for the abnormal prothrombin consumption test.

Thrombopathic thrombocytopenia

The defect called "thrombopathic thrombocytopenia" (Quick and Hussey, 1963; Kurstjens et al, 1968) resembles the Bernard-Soulier syndrome in that it is also characterized by thrombocytopenia and the presence of giant platelets. It differs in the inheritance pattern, which in this disease is autosomal dominant. It is rare, and the abnormality has not been studied extensively. Baadenhuijsen et al (1971) have shown deficient aggregation by collagen and poor platelet factor 3 availability. Ultrastructural studies by Vossen et al (1968) and Libánská et al (1975) revealed a reduction of platelet granules. Quick (1965) reported the coexistence of thrombopathic thrombocytopenia and von Willebrand's disease in one family. The case reported by Beck (1980) as "idiopathic thrombocytopenia with giant platelets" showed a prolonged bleeding time, impaired aggregation by collagen, ADP, and adrenaline, but normal aggregation with ristocetin.

The relationship of this thrombocytopathy to the "Mediterranean giant platelet syndrome" or "hereditary macrothrombocytopathia" seen in the Mediterranean countries is not clear. The Mediterranean form is sometimes associated with other congenital anomalies, such as deafness, nephritis, and immunoglobulinopathies (Epstein et al, 1972). The Alport syndrome (Eckstein et al, 1975) includes congenital renal dysfunction, thrombocytopenia, and giant platelets.

von Willebrand's disease and variants

The bleeding disorder variously called von Willebrand's disease or von Willebrand's syndrome was discovered by von Willebrand in 1926 among inhabitants of the Åland islands. The original description is of a mild to moderately severe bleeding tendency with the clinical features of epistaxis, easy bruising, and profuse menstrual bleeding in affected females. Characteristically, the platelet count was normal and the bleeding time prolonged. Nilsson et al (1957a, 1959) reinvestigated the families studied by von Willebrand and concluded that 16 out of 17 cases had decreased levels of factor VIII, and that in all cases the platelets were qualitatively and quantitatively normal. However, a few years later Salzman (1963) showed that there was defective platelet retention on glass bead columns, and Borchgrevink (1960a) demonstrated abnormal retention in vivo, indicating that this parameter of platelet function is abnormal. More attention was focused on the platelets in this disease when it was shown that sometimes they are not aggregated normally by ristocetin (Howard and Firkin, 1971). Ristocetin is an antibiotic that was shown to produce thrombocytopenia (Gangarosa et al, 1960) and is now used only for in vitro studies. Ristocetin is a mixture of two components, A and B; the A component acts in platelet aggregation (Jenkins et al, 1975).

The reports that the abnormal platelet retention and bleeding time are corrected by transfusing normal plasma (Nilsson et al, 1957b) or cryoprecipitate (Weiss and Rogers, 1972) and that, in vitro, the addition of factor VIII concentrates also corrects the defective aggregation of platelets by ristocetin (Bouma et al, 1972; Weiss et al, 1973a) led to the conclusion that the hemostatic defect in von Willebrand's disease is the lack of a normal blood factor, the von Willebrand factor (vWF), necessary for proper platelet function. The vWF is not identical with antihemophilic factor, since hemophiliac plasma corrects the von Willebrand defects

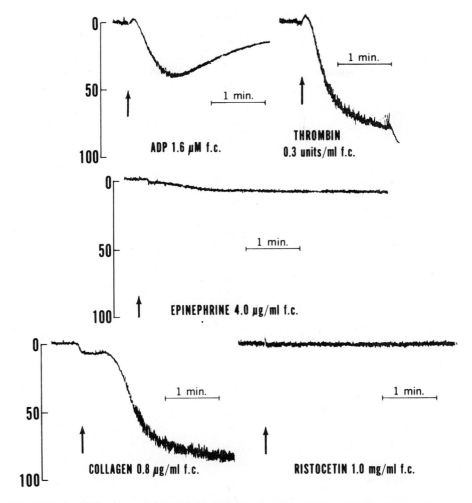

Fig. 17-23. Patterns of platelet aggregation in severe von Willebrand's disease. Note the absence of aggregation of platelet-rich plasma by ristocetin. The poor aggregation with epinephrine and ADP is atypical. This patient was a 28-year-old girl who at age 7 had trauma to the jaw with severe bleeding. She has had two episodes of minor bleeding into her left knee joint. Severe bleeding after tooth extraction required 43 units of cryoprecipitate to stop the bleeding. We suspected that she had developed an antibody to VIII:vWF but have been unable to confirm it. Other studies showed VIII:C of 7%, VIII:Ag of 0% (Fig. 17-25), VII:vWF of 0%. She is probably the homozygous daughter of heterozygous parents (mother has 42% VIII:Ag, 130% VIII:C, 90% VIII:vWF, and weak aggregation with ristocetin, 42%; father has 52% VIII:Ag, 108% VIII:C, 12.5% VIII:vWF, and weak aggregation with ristocetin, 28%).

(Weiss et al, 1973a), including the defective ristocetin-induced platelet aggregation (Weiss et al, 1973b).

Up to that time the term "factor VIII" was used as a specific designation of the antihemophilic factor. It soon became apparent that the "factor VIII" molecule is composed of more than that portion deficient in classic hemophilia. The demonstration that the factor VIII molecule consists of a procoagulant portion that is active in coagulation and an immunologic portion not involved in coagulation (Zimmerman et al, 1971a) was important also in confirming the existence of a vWF, since in classic von Willebrand's disease there is a reduction of both the antihemophilic factor and the immunologically detectable portion of the factor VIII molecule. Finally, transfusion of normal or hemophiliac plasma into a patient with von Willebrand's disease produces a sustained elevation of the factor VIII–related

antigen and of the antihemophilic factor, in contrast with the short survival of transfused antihemophilic factor in classic hemophilia (Veltkamp and Van Tilburg, 1973). More recently it has been shown that the transfusion of normal plasma, hemophiliac plasma, or normal cryoprecipitate produces high levels of antihemophilic factor, factor VIII–related antigen, and of the von Willebrand factor (Chediak et al, 1977). The pathogenesis of the hyperresponse to transfusion is unknown.

It is no longer possible to use the general term "factor VIII." A convention has been adopted that refers to the various activities of the factor VIII macromolecule: *VIII:C* refers to the antihemophilic activity, the procoagulant activity; *VIII:Ag* is the antigenic activity that can be quantified by various immunologic methods; *VIII:vW* is the activity lacking in severe classic von Willebrand's disease and responsi-

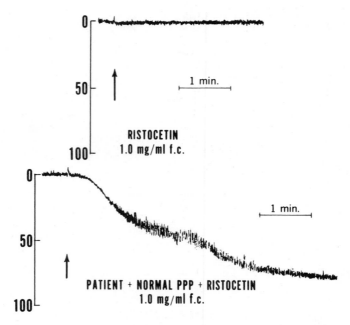

Fig. 17-24. Severe von Willebrand's disease (same patient as in Fig. 17-23) showing correction of deficient ristocetin aggregation by normal platelet-poor plasma.

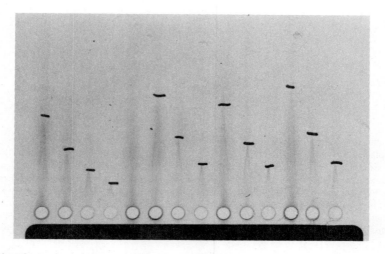

Fig. 17-25. Rocket electrophoresis for quantifying VIII:Ag. The height of the rocket is directly proportional to the amount of VIII:Ag. Wells from left to right: (1) normal, undiluted; (2) normal, 1:2; (3) normal, 1:4; (4) normal, 1:8; (5) vWD disease (patient in Fig. 17-23); (6) hemophilia carrier undiluted; (7) hemophilia carrier, 1:2; (8) hemophilia carrier, 1:4; (9) classic hemophilia (factor VIII deficiency) undiluted; (10) classic hemophilia, 1:2; (11) classic hemophilia, 1:4; (12) hemophilia carrier undiluted; (13) hemophilia carrier, 1:2; and (14) hemophilia carrier, 1:4. Note the lack of VIII:Ag in von Willebrand's disease, the normal amount in classic hemophilia, and the higher than normal amount in the hemophilia carriers.

ble for mediating the aggregation of platelets by ristocetin and adhesiveness of platelets to subendothelium. VIII:vW is also an acute phase reactant and is increased in myocardial infarction and postoperative states (Cucuianu et al, 1980).

The classic case of von Willebrand's disease should have the following features: (1) prolonged bleeding time, (2) defective platelet adhesiveness, (3) normal aggregation of platelets by collagen, ADP, epinephrine, or thrombin but abnormal aggregation by ristocetin, (4) very low levels of VIII:C, VIII:Ag, and VIII:vW, and (5) hyperresponse following infusion of normal cryoprecipitate. The procoagulant activity is measured by the traditional clotting assay for "factor VIII." The VIII:Ag is usually measured by the Laurell rocket technique, but other techniques have been used (Stites et al, 1971; Hoyer, 1972). Crossed immunoelectrophoresis has been used to detect variant VIII:vW molecules

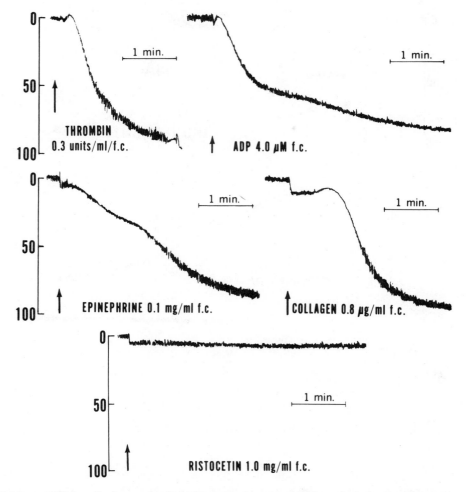

Fig. 17-26. von Willebrand's disease, familial. This patient is a 7-year-old boy who had severe bleeding at age 1 from a torn frenulum. He has had easy bruising and frequent nosebleeds. Bleeding time 9'45"; in vivo adhesiveness 29%; 48% VIII:C; 30% VIII:Ag; 0% VIII:vW. The data for the mother are shown in Fig. 17-27.

in a kindred with autosomal dominant von Willebrand disease and in asymptomatic heterozygotes (Green and Philip, 1980). It should be noted that animal antihuman VIII antisera have anti-VIII:Ag and anti-VIII:vW activity, whereas human anti-VIII antibodies developing in hemophiliacs have only anti-VIII:C activity. VIII:vW is quantified by using washed fixed platelets (Brinkhous et al, 1975; Olson et al, 1975). The method used in my laboratory is given in the Appendix.

Examples of classic von Willebrand's disease are shown in Figs. 17-23 to 17-27.

The lesion in the classic von Willebrand's disease is a defective interaction between the platelets and the subendothelial tissues. Experimentally, a segment of rabbit aorta can be denuded of endothelial cells by a balloon catheter, and the adhesion of platelets to subendothelial tissues can be determined following various perfusion procedures (Baumgartner, 1973). Tschopp et al (1974) used this model to show that in von Willebrand's disease adhesion of platelets to subendothelial tissues is deficient and that normal adhesiveness could be restored by normal plasma or factor VIII

concentrate. The plasma factor required for normal adhesion is the von Willebrand factor, VIII:vW. Because patients with severe von Willebrand's disease have very little or no VIII:Ag in their plasma, some have assumed that VIII:Ag and VIII:vW are one and the same (Jaffe and Nachman, 1975). However, there is also strong evidence that they are not identical. First, the hyperresponses to cryoprecipitate transfusion in von Willebrand's disease show that VIII:Ag levels are higher and persist longer than VIII:vW levels (Chediak et al, 1977). Second, variants of von Willebrand's disease (see further) sometimes show discordant levels of VIII:Ag and VIII:vW. Endothelial cells synthesize VIII:Ag but not VIII:C. Normal platelets are rich in VIII:Ag (Fig. 17-28), probably absorbed from the plasma.

Purified "factor VIII" is a glycoprotein having a molecular weight of over 1 million and exhibits three distinct properties that by suitable methods can be shown to reside in subunits: (1) a procoagulant activity involved in the intrinsic coagulation pathway; (2) an antigenic portion that has no other activity; and (3) a portion, the von Willebrand factor necessary for platelet aggregation by ristocetin. These func-

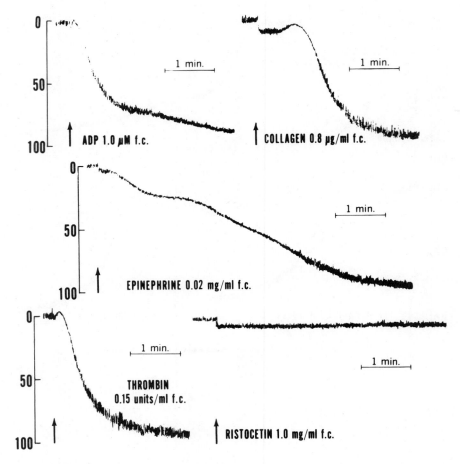

Fig. 17-27. von Willebrand's disease, familial. This patient is a 28-year-old woman, the mother of the 7-year-old boy shown in Fig. 17-26. Bleeding time 15'; 36% VIII:C; 25% VIII:Ag; 0% VIII:vW; platelet adhesiveness (in vivo) 32%. This woman had frequent nosebleeds, most severe between ages 3 and 11; bled 2 days and 3 weeks after hysterectomy, requiring several transfusions. This patient's mother had frequent nosebleeds all her life.

tional units are not necessarily identical with subunits of low molecular weight obtained by various procedures.

A diagram showing a tentative scheme for the relationship of the three functional properties to the whole molecule is shown in Fig. 17-29. It is possible to fit most of the observations into this concept. The three subunits are under separate genetic control, as judged from the corresponding deficiency states. The synthesis of the procoagulant portion is regulated by a recessive gene on the X chromosome; the antigen portion by a non-X autosomal gene, since it is normal in hemophilia; the von Willebrand factor is under a third controlling mechanism, since in von Willebrand's disease antigenic and procoagulant activities are of different degrees and the trait is transmitted as an autosomal dominant. The complex factor VIII molecule assembled from the three functional units has all the expected activities. Whether a ''super'' genetic system regulates the rate of synthesis of the functional units is speculative, although such a control would account for the combination of various proportions of subunits. I believe that this scheme is not very far from the true situation (Firkin and Howard, 1976; Over et al, 1980). This is not incompatible with the report that the antigen-

procoagulant complex in von Willebrand's disease is deficient in carbohydrate (Gralnick et al, 1976), for the carbohydrate moiety is believed to be associated with the VIII:vW. Rick and Hoyer (1975) have found that the factor VIII procoagulant moiety is of low molecular weight. VIII:vW is probably the larger portion of the compound molecule (Over et al, 1980).

Of particular importance is the antigenic portion of the molecule. Quantification using an immunologic technic (Fig. 17-25) reveals some interesting differences in various factor VIII–related disorders. In hemophilia the amount of VIII:Ag is normal and often greater than normal, in the hemophiliac carrier it is normal or, usually, greater than normal, and in von Willebrand's disease it is very low or undetectable. Since VIII:Ag and VIII:vW are probably not identical, the measurement of VIII:Ag alone is not sufficient to sort out the von Willebrand syndromes (Barrow et al, 1979).

Cultured human endothelial cells synthesize VIII:Ag, which is adsorbed by platelets (Nachman and Jaffee, 1976). VIII:Ag has also been found in vascular subendothelium (Rand et al, 1980). Tuddenham et al (1974b) were able to

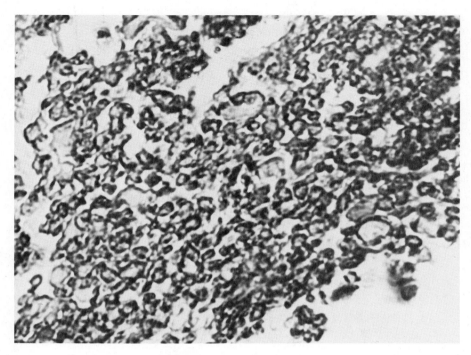

Fig. 17-28. The surface of normal washed (×4) platelets is rich in VIII:Ag, as shown the immunoperoxidase technique (×450). These washed platelets were, however, not aggregated by ristocetin.

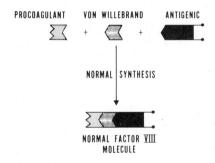

Fig. 17-29. Schematic representation of the three functional units of the factor VIII molecule.

demonstrate factor VIII–related antigen in endothelial cells of human fetuses at a gestational age of 8 to 20 weeks.

The aggregation of normal platelets by ristocetin assumes that they have a surface receptor for the VIII:vW factor, which in turn is a receptor for the molecule of ristocetin. In the absence of VIII:vW, as in severe von Willebrand's disease, platelets lack this receptor, and aggregation by ristocetin does not take place. There is no ready explanation of why platelets in thrombasthenia and Bernard-Soulier syndrome are not aggregated by ristocetin, unless we assume that the platelets in these diseases also lack the VIII:vW receptor (Weiss et al, 1974). Abnormal ristocetin aggregation is occasionally seen in acute leukemia, infectious mononucleosis, and immunologic thrombocytopenic purpura.

Cases of classic severe von Willebrand's disease are rel-

atively rare. More commonly seen are subjects who have a strong history of abnormal bleeding (easy bruising, nosebleeds, bleeding after surgery or delivery, bleeding after tooth extraction, excessive menstrual bleeding), sometimes with a strong family history implying autosomal inheritance. These patients are usually classified as "variants" of von Willebrand's disease, although it is possible that they represent the heterozygous state of a mild von Willebrand disease (Veltkamp and Van Tilburg, 1973). Various combinations of laboratory findings may be found (Bowie et al, 1976). Most common in our experience is the combination of prolonged bleeding time and diminished adhesiveness. Sometimes intermediate levels of VIII:Ag, VIII:vW, and VIII:C are seen; sometimes one or all are normal. The aspirin tolerance test is useful in doubtful cases (Stuart et al, 1979). Before giving the aspirin, a bleeding time is performed and blood is drawn for platelet aggregation studies. Then 10 to 15 grains of aspirin are given to the patient and the bleeding time repeated 2 hours later. A marked prolongation of the bleeding time favors the diagnosis of a von Willebrand variant. Examples of von Willebrand variants are shown in Figs. 17-30 to 17-36.

There are even more puzzling reports of genetic variants of von Willebrand's disease, one of which does not show the hyperresponse to infused factor VIII (Holmberg and Nilsson, 1973), as well as other differences (Firkin et al, 1973; Alexandre et al, 1975; Ekert and Firkin, 1975; Bowie et al, 1976), including a qualitatively abnormal VIII:Ag (Kernoff et al, 1974; Thomson et al, 1974; Gralnick et al, 1975).

An acquired von Willebrand syndrome has been reported in association with disseminated lupus erythematosus (Si-

Text continued on p. 818.

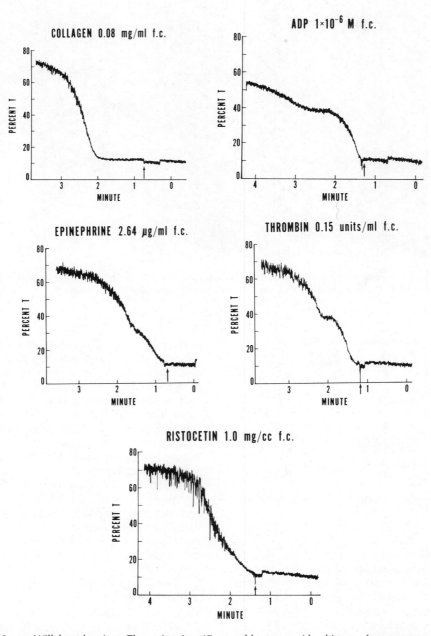

Fig. 17-30. von Willebrand variant. The patient is a 47-year-old woman with a history of recurrent nosebleeds, profuse menstrual bleeding, and postoperative bleeding. The only abnormalities were prolonged bleeding time (over 10′) and abnormal platelet retention (Fig. 17-31). Normal aggregation with all agents as shown. Levels of VIII:C and VIII:Ag are normal.

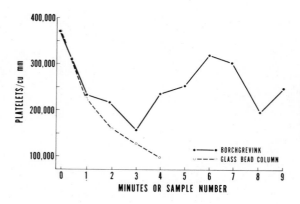

Fig. 17-31. Abnormal platelet adhesiveness by the in vivo method, von Willebrand variant, patient in Fig. 17-30. Note that the glass bead retention is normal. We find the early reduction followed by a secondary rise to be common when adhesiveness is abnormal and the bleeding time prolonged.

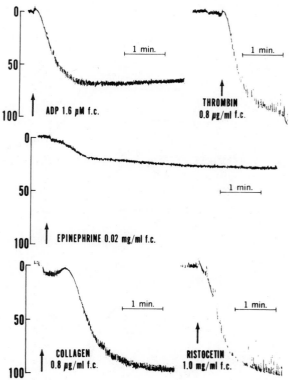

Fig. 17-32. von Willebrand variant. Patient is a 24-year-old woman with easy bruising and severe postoperative bleeding after extraction of wisdom teeth. Bleeding time 9'; 100% VIII:C; 49% VIII:Ag; 28% VIII:vW; platelet adhesiveness (in vivo) 10% (Fig. 17-33). The poor response to epinephrine is unexpected, but we have seen it in a number of patients with a von Willebrand variant. Abnormal aggregations with collagen and ADP, corrected by cryoprecipitate, are reported in a variant by Sheridan and Pinkerton (1980).

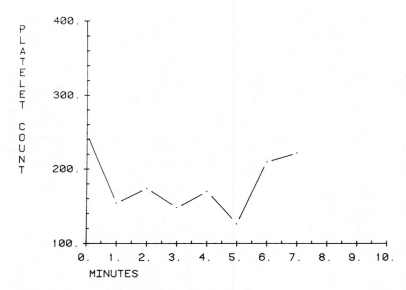

Fig. 17-33. In vivo (Borchgrevink) adhesiveness in the patient shown in Fig. 17-32. (Graph by Prophet Computer System, Division of Research Resources, N.I.H.)

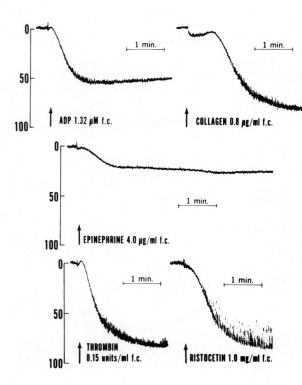

Fig. 17-34. von Willebrand variant. Patient is a 29-year-old woman with severe menorrhagic and postpartum hemorrhage on two occasions. There is a strong family history indicating autosomal inheritance. Her grandfather bled severely after prostatectomy, an uncle had delayed bleeding after surgery, and the mother had menorrhagia requiring hysterectomy. Bleeding time 10'45"; 58% VIII:C; 63% VIII:Ag; 50% VIII:vW; platelet adhesiveness (in vivo) 32%.

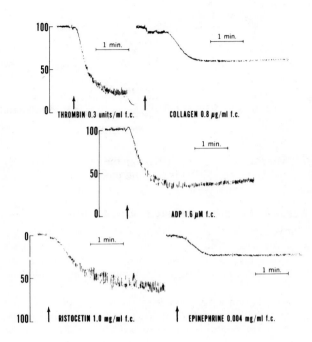

Fig. 17-35. von Willebrand variant. Patient is a 23-year-old woman. She has had frequent nosebleeds, severe menorrhagia, bleeding after dental extraction, and postpartum bleeding. Her mother required hysterectomy for menorrhagia. Bleeding time 11'50"; 60% VIII:C; 28% VIII:Ag; 70% VIII:vW; 0% platelet adhesiveness (in vivo) (Fig. 17-36).

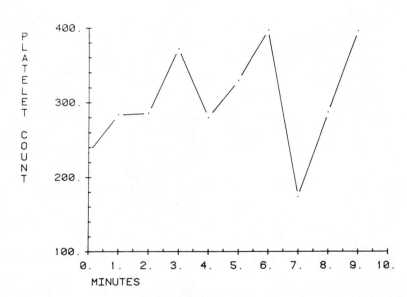

Fig. 17-36. In vivo (Borchgrevink) adhesiveness in the patient shown in Fig. 17-35. (Graph by Prophet Computer System, Division of Research Resources, N.I.H.)

Table 17-9. A partial list of drugs that inhibit platelet function

Aspirin
Phenylbutazone (Butazolidin)
Ibuprofen (Motrin)
Indomethacin (Indocin)
Dipyridamole (Persantine)
Propranolol (Inderal)
Antihistamines
Theophylline
Clofibrate (Atromid)
Phenothiazines
Tricyclic antidepressants (Elavil)
Colchicine
Furosemide (Lasix)
Nitrofurantoin (Furadantin)
Penicillins
Gentamycin
Corticosteroids
Hydrazinophthalazine (hydralazine)
Lithium

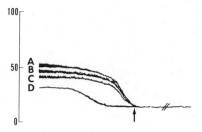

Fig. 17-37. Effect of aspirin ingestion on platelet aggregation. **A,** With epinephrine; **B,** with ADP; **C,** with thrombin; and **D,** with collagen. Compare with Figs. 17-15 to 17-18.

mone et al, 1968) and various other diseases (Ingram et al, 1973; Mant et al, 1973; Handin et al, 1976; Wautier et al, 1976; Cass et al, 1980). Cramer et al (1976) found a reduction of factor XII in 9 of 39 patients with von Willebrand's disease.

The ideal treatment for von Willebrand's disease is plasma or cryoprecipitate. Some purified factor VIII concentrates, effective in treating hemophilia, supply little vWF (Green and Potter, 1976).

Congenital afibrinogenemia

Congenital afibrinogenemia is responsible for two hemostatic defects, one caused by lack of fibrin formation and the other by abnormal platelet function. Fibrinogen is necessary for ADP-induced aggregation and normal retention. It is suggested that membrane-bound fibrinogen, probably the carboxyterminal part of the α-chain, is required for normal aggregation with ADP, collagen, and thrombin (Niewiarowski and Stewart, 1978). The aggregation defect can be demonstrated in vitro if the fibrinogen concentration is less than 15 mg/dl and if a low concentration of ADP is used (Inceman et al, 1966; Hellem, 1968; Mustard and Packham, 1970; Weiss and Rogers, 1971).

Thrombocytopathy associated with established congenital diseases or syndromes

Mild to severe platelet dysfunction has been reported in the May-Hegglin anomaly (Lusher et al, 1968a), in the Wiskott-Aldrich syndrome (Kuramoto et al, 1970), in the Ehlers-Danlos syndrome and other connective tissue disorders (Estes, 1968), in albinism (Hardisty et al, 1972), in thrombocytopenia with absent radii (Day and Holmsen, 1972a), and in glycogen storage disease I (Czapek et al, 1973; Kao et al, 1980).

Absent collagen-induced aggregation

Three instances of absent collagen-induced aggregation have been reported (Hirsh et al, 1967; Papayannis et al,

1971; Mielke and Rodvien, 1976). In the cases described by Caen and Legrand (1972) it was the patients' collagen that reacted abnormally with otherwise normal platelets.

Acquired thrombocytopathy caused by drugs

Many drugs are known to affect platelet function. Only a few of the most commonly used ones are listed in Table 17-9. Complete lists and discussions of drug effects are given by Mustard and Packham (1970) and Packham and Mustard (1974).

The most commonly used drug, aspirin, deserves special mention. After an oral dose of 300 to 600 mg, aspirin inhibits platelet aggregation to a significant degree (Fig. 17-37). There is diminished aggregation with collagen and thrombin and absence of the secondary wave with ADP or epinephrine. It has been shown that the effect of aspirin is caused by defective release of nonmetabolic platelet ADP and of serotonin (Evans et al, 1968), as well as platelet factors 3 and 4 (Zucker and Peterson, 1968). Aspirin intake causes a prolongation of the bleeding time but does not affect glass-bead retention (Bick et al, 1976). Aspirin interferes with prostaglandin metabolism, and the effect is dose related. The inhibitory effect of aspirin lasts for the life span of the platelets and is measurable for as long as several days after aspirin is ingested. It should be noted that there are dozens of proprietary drugs that contain aspirin (Leist and Banwell, 1974). During investigation of a patient with a possible platelet defect a history of drug intake is essential but is sometimes unreliable. We have adopted the policy of asking the patient to refrain from taking *any* medication for 1 week prior to being investigated.

The possibility that a complete understanding of platelet function and its alteration by drugs will lead to a pharmacologic approach to the prevention of thrombosis is an exciting prospect (Genton et al, 1975). Aspirin may well prove to be the most effective inhibitor of platelet aggregation.

Congenital enzymatic deficiencies

Aside from acquired enzymatic deficiencies caused by drugs, there are a few reports of congenital deficiencies of enzymes active in prostaglandin metabolism. Malmsten et al (1975) and Lagarde et al (1978) have identified a deficiency of platelet cyclooxygenase as the cause of an abnormal release reaction. Weiss and Lages (1977) report a possible congenital defect in platelet thromboxane synthetase. If enzymatic defects should prove to be the cause of congenital abnormalities in cases showing an abnormal release reaction, a major reclassification of thrombocytopathies will be necessary.

Acquired thrombocytopathy secondary to other diseases

Uremia is accompanied by multiple hemostatic defects, two of which, thrombocytopenia and thrombocytopathy, are of primary importance (Eknoyan et al, 1969; Rabiner and Molinas, 1970). Thrombocytopathy is reported in various myeloproliferative disorders (chronic myelocytic leukemia, myelofibrosis, polycythemia vera, and thrombocythemia) (Caen et al, 1969; Spaet et al, 1969). Defective platelet function has been reported in cirrhosis of the liver (Thomas et al, 1967), disseminated lupus erythematosus (Weiss and Eichelberger, 1963), pernicious anemia (Stefanini and Karaca, 1966), scurvy (Wilson et al, 1967), and immunoglobulinopathies (Vigliano and Horowitz, 1967; Perkins et al, 1970). Most of these abnormalities should be reinvestigated with more modern technics.

Thrombocytosis and thrombocythemia

The terms "thrombocytosis" and "thrombocythemia" are applied to abnormally high platelet counts. By definition and common usage, "thrombocytosis" is used when the elevated platelet count is secondary to another disease, whereas "thrombocythemia" is used when the elevated platelet count reflects a primary megakaryocytic proliferation. A classification is given in Table 17-10.

The platelet count is greater than 500,000/mm^3 (0.5 × 10^{12}/l) and may be in the millions/mm^3. The increased number of platelets can produce either abnormal bleeding (Boyle, 1962) or thrombosis (Gunz, 1960; Frick, 1969). Abnormal bleeding results from a combination of thrombocytopathy and interference with thromboplastin generation. The role of a high platelet count in the production of thrombosis is discussed by Zucker and Mielke (1972). It is not known what predisposes some subjects to hemorrhage and others to thrombosis. The liberation of large amounts of acid phosphatase and potassium (Davey and Lander, 1965) from the large platelet mass causes serum concentrations of these substances to be elevated.

Elevation of the platelet count in reactive thrombocytosis is usually not as great as in thrombocythemia. Because it is usually transient there are fewer hemorrhagic and thrombotic complications.

Thrombocytosis is reported in acute rheumatic fever and rheumatoid arthritis (Marchasin et al, 1964), in chronic inflammatory bowel diseases (Morowitz et al, 1968), and in cirrhosis of the liver (Marchasin et al, 1964). Thrombocytosis secondary to hematologic diseases has been noted after severe hemorrhage (Desforges et al, 1954), in iron-deficiency anemia (Schloesser et al, 1965), in hemolytic anemia (Marchasin et al, 1964), and in the recovery stage after thrombocytopenia (Ogston and Dawson, 1969).

Thrombocytosis may be found in association with manifest or occult neoplasms (Davis and Mendez Ross, 1973). Moderate thrombocytosis is sometimes seen after major surgery (Breslow et al, 1968). Thrombocytosis after splenectomy is the rule (Hirsh and Dacie, 1966), usually maximum

Table 17-10. Classification of thrombocytosis and thrombocythemia

I. Thrombocytosis
 A. Secondary to inflammatory reactions
  1. Acute rheumatic fever
  2. Rheumatoid arthritis
  3. Ulcerative colitis
  4. Regional enteritis
  5. Tuberculosis
  6. Cirrhosis of the liver
  7. Osteomyelitis
 B. Secondary to blood disorders
  1. Polycythemia vera
  2. Chronic granulocytic leukemia
  3. Myelofibrosis
  4. Acute hemorrhage
  5. Iron-deficiency anemia
  6. Hemolytic anemias
  7. Rebound thrombocytosis
 C. Secondary to malignancy
  1. Carcinoma
  2. Hodgkin's disease
  3. Non-Hodgkin's lymphomas
 D. Postoperative
 E. Postsplenectomy
 F. Response to Vincristine administration
 G. Tidal platelet dysgenesis
II. Thrombocythemia

during the second or third week. Administration of Vincristine produces thrombocytosis by accelerating platelet production (Robertson et al, 1972). In "platelet tidal dysgenesis" there are regular fluctuations in the platelet count between thrombocytopenic and thrombocytotic levels (Engström et al, 1966).

The term "thrombocythemia" refers to myeloproliferative syndromes having as the chief component the proliferation of megakaryocytes and a high blood platelet count, and the term "essential thrombocythemia" is used (Harker and Finch, 1969). However, the proliferation is never limited to megakaryocytes, usually involving leukocytes as well, so that there is no sharp dividing line between essential thrombocythemia and the thrombocythemia that is part of the myeloproliferative syndrome. A few cases of essential thrombocythemia in children have been reported (Barnhart et al, 1980). Several authors have reported defective aggregation responses (Kaywin et al, 1978; Barnhart et al, 1980).

PHASE II: THROMBOPLASTINOGENESIS
Factors involved

As shown in Fig. 17-2, phase II of the coagulation sequence involves reactions that lead to the formation of plasma (intrinsic) thromboplastic activity. The development of this intrinsic thromboplastic activity involves the interaction of several coagulation factors: (1) platelet phospholipid (platelet factor 3) made available during platelet reactions in phase I, (2) factor VIII, (3) factor IX, (4) factor X, (5) factor XI, (6) factor XII, and (7) factor V. When any one is reduced below certain critical limits, there is less plasma thromboplastin formed and the subsequent reaction, the conversion of prothrombin to thrombin, is deficient.

Interaction of factors

The sequence in which the factors involved in phase II interact has been known for some time (Fig. 17-4), although there are still unanswered questions as to the kinetics of the reactions.

The sequence is initiated in vitro by the activation of factor XII through contact with a foreign surface, glass, kaolin, celite, or other materials and with collagen and other subendothelial connective tissues in vivo. In vivo there is also the interaction of platelets with subendothelial tissue (p. 791), with the liberation of tissue thromboplastin which brings factor VII into play, bypassing the contact reactions. Factor XIIa activates factor XI to XIa. The details of this reaction are still unclear. The reactions are probably not calcium dependent. Some believe that the reaction between XIIa and XI is that of enzyme to substrate (Ratnoff, 1972). Others believe that the interaction of XIIa and XI results in the formation of an "activation product" complex (Macfarlane, 1966) that acts as an enzyme for the next step in the sequence, the activation of factor IX to IXa in the presence of calcium ions and its inhibition both by anticoagulants that complex calcium and by heparin.

It is generally agreed that the key reaction in thromboplastin generation involves the activation of factor X to Xa. It is probable that IXa, VIII, and platelet factor 3 form a lipid-protein complex in the presence of calcium ions that activates factor X to Xa (Hemker and Kahn, 1967). Factor X is activated to Xa also by Russell's viper venom (Esnouf and Williams, 1962) and the reaction product formed in the extrinsic system.

The next step, the formation of a "prothrombin activator" (plasma thromboplastin) involves the formation of a complex between factor Xa, factor V, and platelet factor 3 in the presence of calcium ions (Jobin and Esnouf, 1967; Chuang et al, 1972). There is no activation of factor V to Va as proposed in the original "cascade" or "waterfall" hypothesis. Intrinsic plasma thromboplastin or prothrombin activator is sometimes called "prothrombinase."

Thrombin acts as a catalyst at several points. It accelerates availability of platelet factor 3, accelerates the formation of intermediate complex 1, accelerates the formation of prothrombin activator, and acts as an autocatalyst in the conversion of prothrombin to thrombin.

I do not know where the thromboplastin-like material in red blood cells fits into the coagulation scheme. Quick and Hickey (1960) reported that red blood cell hemolysate brings about good prothrombin consumption when added to platelet-poor plasma, even if clotting is carried out in a silicone-coated test tube. They call the active material in the hemolysate "erthyrocytin" and propose that this substance is first formed by the interaction of "plasma contact factor" and platelet factor 3 and is then taken into the erythrocytes. One implication of this observation is that hemolysis must be carefully avoided when delicate coagulation tests are performed. Another implication is that intravascular hemolysis may initiate serious intravascular coagulation reactions.

Bentley and Krivit (1960) have used the erythrocytin reaction to study the carrier state in hemophilia. They base their study on the observation that erythrocytin does not correct the abnormal consumption of platelet-poor hemophilic plasma, supposedly because erythrocytin reacts with factor VIII (and IX). If, then, minute amounts of normal plasma are added to a system of erythrocytin and hemophilic plasma, the prothrombin consumption is in direct proportion to the amount of factor VIII added. This technic was found sensitive to a difference of between 0.0005 and 0.0008 ml of normal plasma. Using this technic to assay the amount of factor VIII in the plasma of carrier females, they found that the carriers did indeed have low levels of factor VIII, intermediate between normal persons and persons with hemophilia. This is an interesting application of the observations on erythrocytin.

Naturally occurring inhibitors

There are several mechanisms that inhibit various stages of the coagulation sequence. These are called "naturally occurring" to distinguish them from pathologic inhibitors such as antifactor VIII (p. 826). One is the removal of excess thrombin by the fibrin clot (Klein and Seegers, 1950). This was inappropriately called antithrombin I. A second is the inhibitory activity of fibrin degradation products (Larrieu et al, 1972). The most important is antithrombin III, which has been shown to act at several points of the sequence. Its most important activity is the neutralization of factor Xa (Yin et al, 1971b). Antithrombin III probably inactivates thrombin and plasmin (Egeberg, 1965a) and is identical with heparin cofactor (Yin et al, 1971b). A reduction in antithrombin III activity, whether congenital (Egeberg, 1965b) or as the result of oral contraceptive intake (Miale and Kent, 1974), predisposes to thrombosis, and antithrombin III may become the key to some of the thrombotic diseases (see p. 854).

Pathologic inhibitors

A variety of pathologic inhibitors to coagulation factors have been described (Shapiro and Hultin, 1975). All are antibodies to individual coagulation factors and are discussed in the sections on deficiencies of coagulation factors. One inhibitor, the "lupus anticoagulant," inhibits the prothrombin activator complex Xa-V-phospholipid-Ca and is discussed on p. 836.

Hemorrhagic disorders in phase II

Assuming that sufficient platelet factor 3 is made available from phase I, the disorders in phase II are caused by a deficiency (as defined later) of the factors involved in the generation of plasma thromboplastin (Table 17-11) or the development of pathologic antithromboplastic activity. The deficiency of factor VIII causes hemophilia. Deficiency of factors IX, X, XI, or XII cause the respective hemorrhagic states, and this group is sometimes called the "hemophilioid" diseases. A severe deficiency of factor V also leads to defective generation of plasma thromboplastin, but since the commonly used partial thromboplastin time test is relatively insensitive to the level of factor V, whereas the reaction with tissue extract is very sensitive, a deficiency of factor V is

Table 17-11. Terminology of phase II defects

Deficiency	Corresponding terminology
Factor VIII	Classic hemophilia, hemophilia A
	PTF-A deficiency
	Hemophilia I
Factor IX	Christmas disease
	PTC deficiency
	Hemophilia B
	PTF-B deficiency
	Hemophilia II
	Hemophilioid state C*
	Deuterohemophilia
Factor X	Stuart clotting defect
	Factor X deficiency
	Stuart-Prower defect†
Factor XI	PTA deficiency
	PTF-C deficiency
	Hemophilioid state D*
Factor XII	Hageman deficiency

*Hemophilioid state A = factor V deficiency; hemophilioid state B = factor VII deficiency.
†The "Prower" defect may or may not be identical with the Stuart defect.

best studied as a phase III abnormality. Note that after the Xa-V-phospholipid-Ca complex is formed, the remainder of the coagulation sequence follows a common pathway.

Laboratory investigation of phase II abnormalities

It is obvious that normal function is phase II is dependent not only on factors involved in this phase but also on an adequate amount of platelet factor 3 made available from platelets during phase I reactions. This needs to be taken into account when interpreting some of the tests used to detect an abnormality in phase II. A summary of the features of phase II abnormalities is given in Table 17-12.

Bleeding time

The bleeding time is usually normal in all phase II abnormalities, but on rare occasions it may be prolonged (Bounameaux, 1963), especially in intensively transfused hemophiliacs, in which case the prolonged bleeding time may be caused by altered platelet function (Hathaway et al, 1973). The bleeding time is very rarely prolonged in factor IX deficiency (Blackburn et al, 1962). In practice the bleeding time is not usually performed if the history clearly implicates a phase II abnormality. It is an important test, however, in the differential diagnosis of von Willebrand's disease from mild hemophilia.

Coagulation time of venous blood

The coagulation time of venous blood in untreated glass test tubes is typically most prolonged in hemophilia and least prolonged in factor X deficiency. Carefully performing the venipuncture using the two-syringe technic, we have not encountered any case of mild hemophilia with a normal coagulation time. The coagulation time is surprisingly long in the mildest of phase II abnormalities—factor XII defi-

ciency. With the advent of more sensitive tests this is no longer an important test in a screening study. We are again doing it almost routinely to detect the abnormal clot retraction in thrombasthenia (p. 804). The test is also useful in the gross detection of hypofibrinogenemia and hyperfibrinolysis.

Prothrombin time

The one-stage prothrombin time of plasma using tissue thromboplastin is normal in uncomplicated deficiency of factors VIII, XI, or XII. It is usually normal in factor IX deficiency except for the Bm variant (p. 830), in which case it is normal with the usual thromboplastin but prolonged when bovine thromboplastin is used. A prolonged prothrombin time with either tissue thromboplastin or Russell's viper venom and a prolonged partial thromboplastin time are characteristic of factor X deficiency, but caution is advisable in diagnosing factor X deficiency only because of this pattern. A similar pattern is seen in factor V deficiency, different only in that the prothrombin time is much more abnormal than the partial thromboplastin time. Note also that both the prothrombin time and partial thromboplastin time tests are prolonged in afibrinogenemia and in the presence of pathologic or administered anticoagulants and inhibitors.

Partial thromboplastin time

The partial thromboplastin time (PTT) of plasma is the coagulation time when a "partial thromboplastin" is used. A partial thromboplastin is the lipid portion of tissue extracts and differs from the complete tissue extract in its reactivity with various coagulation factors (Fig. 17-38). It reacts like platelet factor 3, for which it can be substituted. It is most sensitive to the levels of factors VIII, IX, X, XI, or XII, although the PTT is also prolonged in severe deficiency of factor V. The PTT is prolonged in prothrombin deficiency only when this factor is almost completely absent. The PTT is most useful, therefore, as a screening test to detect a deficiency of factors VIII, IX, X, XI, or XII. The addition of an activating agent (kaolin, celite, elagic acid, or micronized silica) to the partial thromboplastin reagent provides maximum activation of factors XI and XII and clotting times shorter than with the unmodified reagent. It is customary to refer to the test performed with the unmodified reagent as the PTT and to the one with activating agent as the activated PTT or APTT. The latter is now used in most laboratories. As in other tests that depend on the formation of fibrin as the end point, the PTT and APTT will be prolonged in afibrinogenemia. The tests are also abnormal in the presence of an anticoagulant (acquired anticoagulant, heparin). The PTT and APTT are prolonged in intensive oral anticoagulant therapy because of a reduction in factors IX and X. Because partial thromboplastin is a substitute for platelet factor 3, the PTT and APTT are normal in quantitative and qualitative platelet defects. The tests will be abnormal in von Willebrand's disease if the level of factor VIII is very low.

Recalcification time of plasma

The recalcification time of plasma parallels the results obtained with the venous coagulation time. It is more accu-

Table 17-12. Summary of clinical and laboratory findings in deficiency of factors VIII, IX, X XI and XII

Characteristics	Factor VIII deficiency (hemophilia)	Factor IX deficiency (Christmas disease)	Factor X deficiency (Stuart defect)	Factor XI deficiency (PTA)	Factor XII deficiency (Hageman)
Sex	Males predominant; females possible but rare	Males predominant; females possible but rare	Both sexes	Both sexes	Both sexes
Hereditary pattern	Sex-linked recessive; carried by female; transmitted to male	Sex-linked recessive; carried by female; transmitted to male	Not sex linked; carriers heterozygous; bleeders homozygous; trait highly penetrant; autosomal recessive	Not sex linked; autosomal dominant or co-dominant	Not sex linked; autosomal recessive
Severity of hemorrhage	Severe	Moderately severe	Moderately severe	Mild to moderately severe	Usually none or very mild
Clinical manifestations of bleeding	Follows minimal trauma; joints frequently involved	Follows minimal trauma; joints sometimes involved	Follows trauma; spontaneous nasal and gingival bleeding; joints rarely involved	Spontaneous bleeding rare; joints rarely involved	Usually none or very mild
Coagulation time	Prolonged, to many hours	Prolonged, to 1 hour	Slightly prolonged	Usually normal	Markedly prolonged
Bleeding time	Normal; very rarely prolonged	Normal; very rarely prolonged	Normal	Usually normal; very rarely prolonged	Usually normal
Prothrombin, factors V and VII, platelets, fibrinogen	All normal	All normal	All normal	All normal	All normal
Prothrombin time	Normal	Normal	Prothrombin time prolonged with tissue thromboplastin and snake venom	Normal	Normal
Partial thromboplastin time	Prolonged	Prolonged	Prolonged	Prolonged	Prolonged
Recalcification time	Prolonged	Prolonged	Prolonged	Slightly prolonged	Prolonged
Prothrombin utilization	Deficient	Deficient	Deficient	Moderately deficient	Deficient
Deficient thromboplastin generation when	Al(OH)$_3$ plasma substituted	Serum substituted	Serum substituted	Patient's serum plus patient's plasma substituted	Patient's serum plus patient's plasma more abnormal than serum only
Defect corrected by (see also Table 17-21):					
1. Fresh normal blood or plasma	Yes	Yes	Yes	Yes	Yes
2. Stored normal blood or plasma	No	Yes	Yes	Yes	Yes
3. Normal serum, stored	No	Yes	Yes	Yes	Yes
4. Factor VIII–deficient plasma	No	Yes	Yes	Yes	Yes
5. Factor IX–deficient plasma	Yes	No	Yes	Yes	Yes
6. Factor X–deficient plasma	Yes	Yes	No	No	Yes
7. Factor XI–deficient plasma	Yes	Yes	Yes	No	Yes
8. Factor XII–deficient plasma	Yes	Yes	Yes	Yes	No

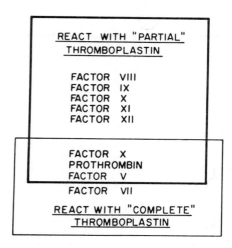

Fig. 17-38. Reaction of "complete" and "partial" thromboplastin with the various coagulation factors. The sensitivity of partial thromboplastin to the level of factor II and factor V is slight, and a deficiency of factor X is the one that gives significantly prolonged clotting times with both a complete and a partial thromboplastin.

rate because it can be performed under controlled laboratory conditions. We use it as a check of the APTT, for the control of heparin therapy (p. 857), and for the detection of naturally occurring circulating anticoagulants. The test should always be performed on platelet-rich plasma. In very severe thrombocytopenia the recalcification time will be moderately prolonged.

Prothrombin consumption test

The one-stage prothrombin time of serum obtained under controlled conditions is a measure of how much prothrombin (and other associated factors) remains after the blood clots, and thus it is an indirect reflection of the efficiency of phase I in providing platelet factor 3 and of the reactions in phase II. If either of these phases is abnormal, little prothrombin will be consumed and the serum prothrombin time will be short. If there is no quantitative or qualitative platelet abnormality and no abnormality of phase III the test measures the efficiency of plasma thromboplastin generation in phase II. The test will be abnormal in deficiency of factors VIII, IX, X, XI, or XII. Note that it is also abnormal in factor V deficiency, but this should not enter into the interpretation, since this test is not performed if the prothrombin time of plasma is prolonged.

Thromboplastin generation test

The preceding tests are useful in the detection of a phase II defect. The thromboplastin generation test (TGT) is more sensitive and specific. First, it will distinguish between a defect in the plasma (deficiency of factors V and VIII) and one in the serum (deficiency of factors IX, X, XI, or XII). Second, it can be used to measure platelet factor 3 availability if the patient's platelets are used in the system. Third, it provides a sensitive test for the presence of anticoagulants. Fourth, with specific correction mixtures, it will establish which one of the various factors is deficient. Note that both factor V and factor X deficiency give a prolonged PT and

PTT in the screening study, and this should be taken into account in interpreting the results of the TGT test. The TGT is now seldom used, but we find it much more sensitive in identifying a defect in phase II than the differential APTT studies.

Identification of the factor deficiency by differential APTT studies

If it is concluded from a prolonged APTT that the deficiency is of factors VIII, IX, X, XI, or XII, the APTT can be used in conjunction with easily prepared normal blood fractions (Table 17-13) to identify the specific abnormality (Table 17-14). Many laboratories find this a more convenient system than the TGT, but the correction reactions are difficult to interpret when the patient's APTT is only moderately prolonged. The same system can be made even more specific by using plasmas having a known deficiency to determine if there is correction of the patient's plasma by the plasma of known deficiency. No correction will occur if the two deficiencies are of the same factor.

Assays of coagulation factors

If a factor deficiency has been identified by a differential correction study (APTT or TGT system), a final proof is provided by an assay of the deficient factor. Assays are used by some to follow the effect of therapy, but I believe that this is seldom necessary, since normalization of the APTT almost always indicates that a hemostatically effective level of the deficient factor has been achieved. Assays give the appearance of being accurate, since the end point is measured in seconds and tenths of seconds, but in fact a reproducibility of less than 5% (CV) is difficult to achieve. Furthermore, assays require substrates having known deficiencies. These are expensive if lyophilized substrates are purchased or if patient's plasma is stored frozen to be used as a substrate, it may have limited stability.

Hemophilia (factor VIII deficiency)
History

Hemophilia is one of the oldest diseases of humanity. The earliest reference to the disease is found in the fifth century Talmud (Rosner, 1969), in which a familial bleeding disorder is described that led to the Rabbinic decree that the sibling of two brothers who died of bleeding after circumcision should not be circumcised. The early writers recognized that the disease was transmitted through the mother, for they made the point that it mattered not whether the boys were by the same or different fathers. Later, in the sixteenth century, Rabbi Joseph Karo pointed out that hemophilia could also be transmitted through the male; he prohibited circumcision of the third son of a man whose earlier sons, born of different mothers, died of bleeding after circumcision. Modern Rabbinic authority forbids circumcision in any child in whom the diagnosis of hemophilia can be established.

McKusick (1962) calls attention to what may be the earliest record of hemophilia in America. An obituary in the *Salem* (Mass.) *Gazette* dated March 22, 1791, tells of the death of Isaac Zoll, 19 years of age, in Frederick County (Va.) as the result of a slight cut of the foot. The account then reads as follows: ''From the time of his receiving the

Table 17-13. Factor content of various blood fractions and products

	I	II	V	VII	VIII	IX	X	XI	XII
Fresh normal plasma	Yes	Yes	Yes	Yes	Yes	Yes	Yes	Yes	Yes
Aged normal plasma	Yes*	Yes	No	Yes	No	Yes	Yes	Yes	Yes
Serum	No	Yes†	No	Yes	No	Yes	Yes	Yes	Yes
Al(OH)₃-adsorbed citrated plasma	Yes‡	No	Yes	No	Yes	No	No	Yes (reduced)	Yes
BaSO₄-adsorbed oxalated plasma	Yes‡	No	Yes	No	Yes	No	No	Yes (reduced)	Yes
Seitz-filtered plasma	Yes	No	Yes	No	Yes	No	No	Yes (reduced)	Reduced
Plasma from intensive bishydroxycoumarin-treated patient	Yes	Reduced	Yes	Reduced	Yes	Reduced	Reduced	Yes	Yes

*But reduced and of diminished reactivity on prolonged storage.
†Significant amounts remain just after clotting, gradually diminishing as serum ages.
‡Prolonged or intensive adsorption removes significant amounts of fibrinogen and other factors.

Table 17-14. Differential correction studies for phase II abnormalities, deficiency of factors VIII to XII, based on APTT

Deficiency	APTT corrected by			
	Normal plasma*	Aged normal serum†	BaSO₄-adsorbed plasma‡	Celite-adsorbed plasma§
Factor VIII	Yes	No	Yes	Yes
Factor IX	Yes	Yes	No	Yes
Factor X‖	Yes	Yes	No	Yes
Factor XI	Yes	Yes	Yes	No
Factor XII	Yes	Yes	Yes	Yes

*Normal plasma contains factors VIII, IX, X, XI, and XII (as well as all other factors).
†Aged normal serum does not contain factor VIII but contains "activated" IX, X, XI, and XII. It is aged to eliminate residual prothrombin and thrombin.
‡BaSO₄-adsorbed (oxalated) plasma is deficient in IX and X, but contains VIII, XI, and XII.
§Normal plasma adsorbed with celite, as specified on p. 925, is deficient only in factor XI.
‖Plasma deficient in factor X will show both a prolonged PT and prolonged PTT.

wound, till he expired, no method could be devised to stop the bleeding; if the wound was bound up, the blood gushed out at his mouth or nostrils. Five brothers to the above person have bled to death, at different periods, from (various) accidents. The father of the above persons has had two wives, and by each several children; those who died in this singular manner all of the first wife.''

Brinkhous (1975) reviews the history of hemophilia from the early reports to modern times. The first case of hemophilia recorded in the medical literature was published in 1793, but it was the report of Otto, in 1803, that attracted wide attention and led to other specific reports in the world literature. The term ''hemophilia'' was introduced by Hopff, a student of Schönlein, in 1828. It was not until 1893, when Wright published his study on the determination of the clotting time, that the abnormal coagulation in hemophilia could be measured.

The relationship between hemophilia and hemarthrosis was established in a classic paper by König in 1892. He described the clinical and pathologic picture of hemophilic hemarthrosis and warned against surgical intervention based on erroneous diagnosis of tuberculous and other arthropathies. Handicapped by the lack of specific therapy, he made the pertinent point that ''the question as to what to do for

bleeders' joint is completely secondary to the question of what *not* to do.''

The demonstration that the clotting of blood could be abnormal stimulated speculation and research. In 1904 Morawitz proposed the classic coagulation scheme (p. 774), and it was postulated that thrombokinase (tissue thromboplastin) or calcium was deficient in hemophilia. In 1911 Addis showed that the deficiency was not of calcium and proposed instead a deficiency of a plasma globulin, which, based on what was known at that time, he believed to be prothrombin. Platelets were also implicated by some as being defective in the release of thromboplastin, but this explanation was also refuted by other investigators.

In 1936 and in subsequent years Patek and Taylor published definitive evidence that the defect in hemophilia was the lack of a ''globulin substance,'' later named ''antihemophilic globulin.'' The work of Quick (one-stage prothrombin time) and Brinkhous et al (two-stage prothrombin assay) had conclusively shown that prothrombin was normal in hemophilia. The same investigators then showed in 1947 that the conversion of prothrombin to thrombin was dependent on the interaction of platelets and antihemophilic globulin. Thus the classic clotting theory, already modified by the addition of the new factors V and VII, was further

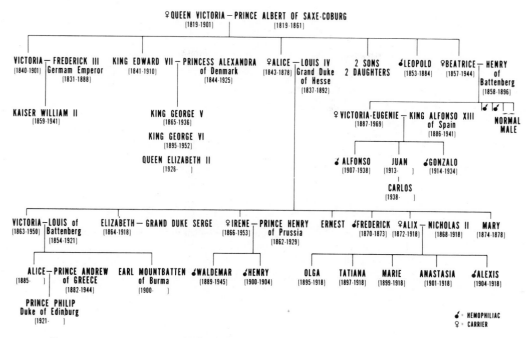

Fig. 17-39. Transmission of hemophilia in the Royal House of Stuart and other royal lineages.

expanded to include the role of antihemophilic globulin (factor VIII). Finally, with the definition of the defect in classic hemophilia, it became possible to identify hemophilia-like diseases caused by a deficiency of new coagulation factors IX, X, XI, or XII.

Hemophilia, like porphyria (p. 445), afflicted some of the royal houses of Europe (Fig. 17-39). Queen Victoria (1819-1901) was a hemophiliac carrier responsible for hemophiliacs in four subsequent generations. Her second and fifth daughters were carriers and her son Leopold was a hemophiliac. Through these people, various royal lineages in Europe and Russia became involved in later generations.

Genetics

The genetics of hemophilia must be discussed from two different aspects, the inheritance of the disease and the genetic control of factor VIII biosynthesis (Graham, 1975).

INHERITANCE. Hemophilia is inherited as a sex-linked recessive trait (Kerr, 1965). The expected inheritance patterns are shown in Fig. 17-40 and have been confirmed in studies with hemophiliac dogs (Brinkhous and Graham, 1950). The most common matings are of a hemophiliac male with a normal female or of a normal male with a carrier female. Except in the rarer matings, the disease is transmitted by a carrier female to affected male children. A careful family history should be obtained to establish the inheritance pattern, remembering however that a negative family history is not uncommon either because of unavailable data for at least four generations or because the disease arises from a new mutation. A close linkage between the X chromosome loci of hemophilia and a variant of G-6-PD (Boyer

and Graham, 1965) and between hemophilia and color blindness (Whittaker et al, 1962) has been reported.

Hemophiliac females are not as rare as once thought. More than 60 cases have been documented (Kerr, 1965; Morita et al, 1971). Graham et al (1975) report a very interesting kindred in which hemophilia was inherited as a dominant characteristic affecting three generations of women. Graham (1975) points out that in addition to the mating of a hemophiliac male to an unrelated carrier female, genetic homozygosity in a female can be caused by consanguinity in a hemophilia kindred, incestuous illegitimacy, mutation in the germ line of a person marrying into a hemophilia kindred, postzygotic somatic mutation, genetic abnormality in a phenotypic female with one X chromosome bearing the hemophilia gene (testicular feminization, Turner's syndrome, etc.), extreme lyonization in a heterozygote, or various anomalies affecting the X chromosome. All other possible causes of a low factor VIII level in a female should be ruled out, especially von Willebrand's disease. A case of spontaneous hemophilia in a genotypically normal 11-year-old girl is reported by Afifi (1974).

The detection of the carrier female is of great importance in genetic counseling. The early approach to this was to base the diagnosis of the carrier state on a reduced level of factor VIII procoagulant (VIII: C). Theoretically, the carrier female should have about half the normal concentration of factor VIII, based on the Lyon hypothesis. The Lyon hypothesis (Lyon, 1968) is that early in embryonic development one X chromosome in the somatic cell of the female is inactivated in a random fashion. Thus, is some of the cells of a carrier, the paternal (hemophiliac) X chromosome is active, while in others it is the maternal X chromosome that is active. The amount of factor VIII synthesized would

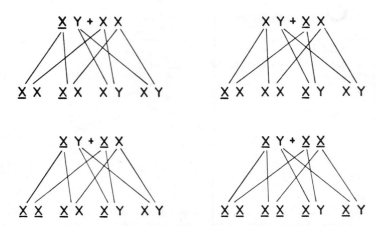

Fig. 17-40. Inheritance pattern in hemophilia. These are the theoretical distributions that can result from the matings shown. In practice, it is sometimes difficult to predict the distribution if the children are few. X̲, Hemophilia chromosome. X̲Y, Hemophiliac male. XY, Normal male. XX, Normal female. X̲X, Carrier female. X̲X̲, Hemophiliac female.

depend on the proportion of cells having an active X chromosome. It would be expected that when the percentage of maternal and paternal X chromosomes inactivated is about equal, the level of factor VIII should be approximately half the normal. However, chance inactivation need not affect an equal number of maternal and paternal chromosomes. In fact, when a large number of obligatory carrier females (i.e., one who has given birth to a hemophiliac) is studied, the mean value for factor VIII is about half the normal but the range is broad, from very low to normal (Veltkamp et al, 1968). There is much overlap with the normal range (45% to 163% of "normal" in our laboratory) and elevation of the factor VIII level is a feature of oral contraceptive therapy and pregnancy (Crowell et al, 1971).

Recent evidence that factor VIII is in fact a complex molecule (see further) has provided a much more reliable method for the detection of the carrier state (Bennett and Huehns, 1970; Zimmerman et al, 1971b; Bouma et al, 1975; Meyer et al, 1975; Veltkamp, 1975a; Ratnoff and Jones, 1976). It can be shown that in the female carrier there is an increase in factor VIII–related antigen (Fig. 17-25), so that the ratio of antigen to procoagulant is greater than 1 and, as it exceeds 2 (or is less than 0.5 if the ratio is procoagulant to antigen), the probability of the carrier state approaches 95% in some series but not in others (Bouma et al, 1975; Meyer et al, 1975). Usually hemophilia carriers have normal or high levels of VIII:Ag, but we have studied a family in which the mother of two mild hemophiliac sons, therefore an obligatory carrier, had 57% VIII:Ag and 39% VIII:C.

FACTOR VIII SYNTHESIS. The molecular structure of factor VIII is still unsettled. We propose a three-piece molecule (p. 809), the VIII:C portion having a sex-linked control, whereas the VIII:Ag and VIII:vW portions are under autosomal control. Reviews of this complex subject with many references can be found in Wagner and Cooper (1975), Van Mourik et al (1975), Denson (1975), and Bennett and Bloom (1975).

Incidence

Hemophilia is usually seen in white individuals, with an occasional case reported in Chinese or black persons (Bullock et al, 1957). It is estimated to affect 3 or 4 out of every 100,000 persons. It is the most common defect in phase II of our scheme (about 85% of the abnormalities are factor VIII deficiencies, about 14% are factor IX deficiencies, and the other three hemophilioid diseases make up the rest). In the *familial* form it follows the predicted patterns of inheritance. In the *sporadic* form the disease apparently occurs as the result of spontaneous mutation. Since the gene is recessive, hemophilia would soon disappear if new cases did not arise by spontaneous mutation. However, before a case is considered to be of the sporadic type, other possibilities should be considered: (1) illegitimacy, (2) mild and unrecognized familial incidence, (3) chance factors in the progeny producing only unrecognized female carriers for several generations, or (4) falsification of the history by the patient or family.

Severity

Hemophilia may be clinically mild (Kitchens, 1980) or severe. A fairly close correlation exists between the severity of the disease and the degree of reduction in the amount of procoagulant factor VIII in the blood. Within families, the severity of the disease tends to be the same (Roberts, 1971). The disease is clinically more severe, and more difficult to treat, when a hemophiliac develops a factor VIII inhibitor. The incidence varies but is about 10% (5% to 20%, Weiss, 1975). Inhibitor development is more common in intensely treated, severe, young hemophiliacs. The titer of inhibitor falls gradually in the absence of replacement therapy but rises very quickly when cryoprecipitate or other replacement therapy is used.

Acquired inhibitors of factor VIII have been found in nontransfused children without underlying coagulation abnormality (Shapiro and Hultin, 1975). The children studied by

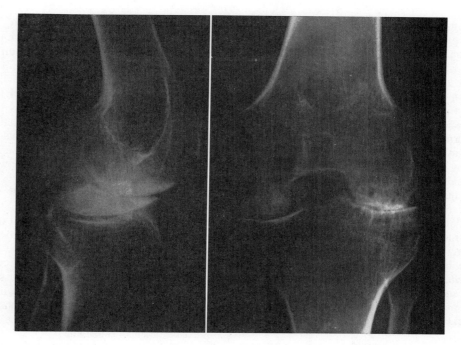

Fig. 17-41. Hemophiliac arthropathy of the knee. Note the atrophy, destruction of cartilages, and deepening of intracondylar space. (Courtesy Dr. R.E. Parks.)

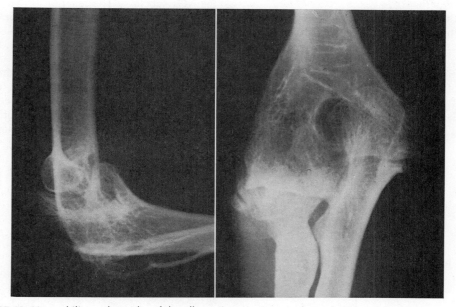

Fig. 17-42. Hemophiliac arthropathy of the elbow. Same patient as shown in Fig. 17-41. (Courtesy Dr. R.E. Parks.)

Brodeur et al (1980) had various acquired anticoagulants (anti-VIII, anti-IX, lupus-type anticoagulant).

Clinical findings

The clinical picture and treatment are discussed comprehensively in Brinkhous and Hemker (1975). Bleeding may occur during infancy or may manifest itself later in life.

Bleeding from the ligated umbilical cord is most unusual, but bleeding following circumcision in an unsuspected case can be profuse. Britten (1966) reports an instance of hemophilic bleeding on the first day of life from the site of intramuscular injection of vitamin K. In later life, subcutaneous and intramuscular hemorrhages may follow trivial injury. Although painful and incapacitating, these hemorrhages are seldom fatal unless they occur in an area where compression of vital structures presents a serious problem (Veltkamp, 1975b). Hemorrhage from the nose, mouth, and lips may be severe, but the most incapacitating feature of the severe form of the disease is bleeding into joints, a feature more characteristic of hemophilia than of any other hemorrhagic diathesis. Any joint may be involved, but repeated hemorrhage into the knees, ankles, and elbows produces the greatest restriction of normal activity. Joint hemorrhage is usually recurrent and may appear following no obvious trauma except that normally accompanying joint motion. Although one hemorrhage seldom produces advanced joint changes, each subsequent injury causes progressive erosion of the joint surface (Figs. 17-41 and 17-42), marked limitation of motion caused by both pain and ankylosis, and disuse inevitably followed by muscular atrophy and contractions. Gastrointestinal bleeding is common and, although at times the bleeding site cannot be identified, the most common cause is duodenal ulcer. Hematuria is common, and indeed bleeding may be seen from, and into, almost any organ or tissue. One of the rarer syndromes is severe low abdominal pain caused by either intramural bowel hemorrhages or hemorrhage into the iliopsoas muscle.

Hemophiliacs are not completely immune to thrombosis, and there are a few reports of myocardial infarction in hemophiliacs (Borchgrevink, 1959; Meili et al, 1968).

Multiple factor deficiencies

The coexistence of two factor deficiencies is so rare that it excites only the geneticist. Some of the reports are based on questionable evidence. Some that are acceptable are (1) coexistence of factor V and factor VIII deficiency (Seligsohn and Ramot, 1969), (2) coexistence of factor VIII and factor IX deficiency (Robertson and Trueman, 1964,) and (3) coexistence of factor VII and factor VIII deficiency (Gobbi, 1966; Girolami et al, 1976; Machin and Miller, 1980).

Laboratory diagnosis

The bleeding time is usually normal, as is the plasma prothrombin time. Prothrombin consumption, venous coagulation time, plasma recalcification time, and partial thromboplastin time (PTT and APTT) are all abnormal (Fig. 17-43). Fig. 17-44, *A*, shows that the PTT does not become abnormal if the factor VIII assay is greater than 40% of normal. Fig. 17-44, *B*, shows the relationship between factor VIII assay and the PTT in normal subjects. Assays of factor VIII procoagulant parallel the clinical severity of the disease, with mild hemophiliacs showing assay values of 5% to 25% and severe ones 0% to 5%. Typical differential studies are shown in Table 17-15.

The detection of an acquired inhibitor to factor VIII is important because, in the presence of the inhibitor, the disease is aggravated and therapy becomes a problem (Penner and Kelly, 1975; Shapiro and Hultin, 1975). Weiss (1975) reviews the various methods for detecting and titrating the inhibitor. We have relied on the cross-recalcification time test almost exclusively (Table 17-16), although inhibition of the APTT works equally well. Whichever method is used, the time and temperature dependence of the anticoagulant must be taken into account.

The inhibitor found in hemophiliacs has been shown to be an antibody (Roberts et al, 1975) against VIII:C. The antibody has been shown to be of the IgG class ($\gamma_2\kappa_2$) by Lusher et al (1968b). Andersen and Terry (1968) found it to be of the γG_4 subclass. The reaction between antigen and antibody is unusual in that it is both time and temperature dependent. The inhibitor is best demonstrated at 37° C and reacts very slowly at room temperature. High titer inhibitors neutralize VIII:C almost immediately, but when the inhibitor is of low titer the test mixture, regardless of the method used, should be incubated for at least 60 minutes to allow maximum manifestation of inhibitor activity. The inhibitor is specific for VIII:C (Yang and Kuzur, 1977).

An inhibitor against VIII:C is occasionally found in post-

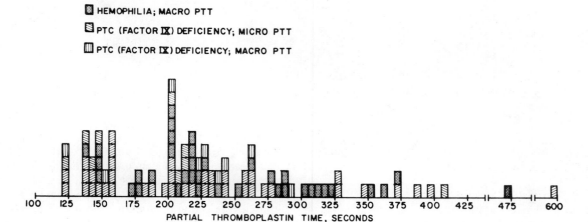

Fig. 17-43. Nonactivated partial thromboplastin time test in factor VIII and factor IX deficiencies.

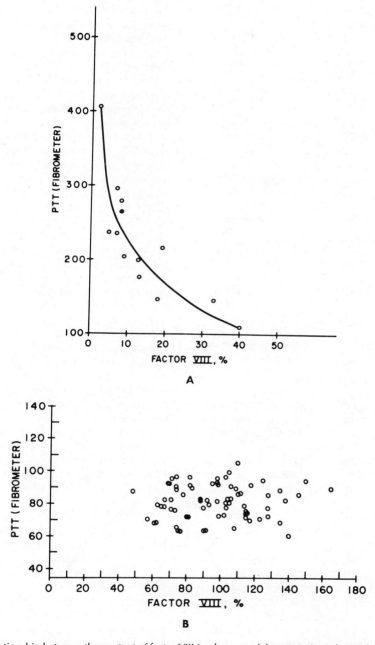

Fig. 17-44. Relationship between the content of factor VIII in plasma and the nonactivated partial thromboplastin time. **A,** Factor VIII assay versus PTT in 13 proved hemophiliacs. **B,** Factor VIII assay versus PTT in 72 normal subjects.

Table 17-15. Differential APTT studies
in factor VIII deficiency

Test material	Partial thromboplastin time*
Patient's plasma	164 sec
80% patient plasma + 20% normal plasma	60 sec
80% patient plasma + 20% aged serum	172 sec
80% patient plasma + 20% BaSO$_4$–adsorbed plasma	65 sec
80% patient plasma + celite-adsorbed plasma	66 sec
80% patient plasma + 20% VIII–deficient plasma	168 sec
20% patient plasma + 80% VIII–deficient plasma	158 sec

*Automated APTT, General Diagnostics, Morris Plains, N.J.

Table 17-16. Detection of an acquired anticoagulant
in hemophilia using the cross-recalcification
time test*

Test material	Time
100% patient plasma	590 sec
75% patient plasma + 25% normal plasma	343 sec
50% patient plasma + 50% normal plasma	283 sec
25% patient plasma + 75% normal plasma	210 sec
100% normal plasma	95 sec

*Recalcification time tests, mixtures incubated at 37° C for 60 min before testing. The patient was a 28-year-old hemophiliac who had received many transfusions of blood or plasma with a gradual development of refractoriness to transfusion therapy.

partum normal females (Voke and Letsky, 1977; Michiels et al, 1978) and elderly normal subjects and in diseases other than hemophilia (Roberts et al, 1975; Soulier and Boffa, 1980): rheumatoid arthritis, disseminated lupus erythematosus, temporal arteritis, ulcerative colitis, pemphigus vulgaris, dermatitis herpetiformis, macroglobulinemia, neoplasms, penicillin reactions, and abscess formation (Shapiro and Hultin, 1975).

Factor IX deficiency
Genetics

Factor IX deficiency was distinguished from hemophilia in 1952. Biggs et al (1952) called it "Christmas disease" after the family name of their patient. Aggeler et al (1952) called it "plasma thromboplastin component deficiency" (PTC deficiency). The pattern of inheritance is the same as in hemophilia, one of the reasons that some prefer the designation "hemophilia B." Handley and Lawrence (1967) report an acquired deficiency of factor IX in the nephrotic syndrome.

The disease is inherited as a sex-linked recessive trait. Although, on the average, the bleeding abnormality is less severe than in factor VIII deficiency, it can be clinically indistinguishable from it. Like hemophilia, the severity of factor IX deficiency tends to be the same for affected members of a family. The occurrence of myocardial infarction in

factor IX deficiency is reported by Brody and Beizer (1965).

Immunologic studies have shown that this hemorrhagic disorder is caused by a number of abnormal factor IX molecules (Roberts and Cederbaum, 1975). Patients with factor IX deficiency can be divided into three categories, based on the neutralization of factor IX in the patient's blood by anti-factor IX antibody, i.e., cross-reactivity as in the studies with hemophiliacs. One group is designated CRM$^+$, characterized by full antigenic, but variably diminished procoagulant, activity of factor IX. The second group is designated CRM$^-$, characterized by absence of both antigenic and procoagulant activity. The third group is designated CRM^R, showing equally reduced, but present, antigenic and procoagulant activity.

A variant (Hougie and Twomey, 1967) is called hemophilia Bm, distinguished from normal factor IX by a prolonged plasma prothrombin time when bovine brain thromboplastin is used. This variant is also heterogeneous, some bloods being CRM$^+$ and others CRM$^-$ when tested with human anti-IX (Meyer et al, 1971). Another variant was described by Veltkamp et al (1970) that differs from the usual factor IX deficiency in that the concentration of factor IX increases and the bleeding tendency improves as the patients get older. This variant has been named hemophilia B Leyden. The variant named hemophilia B Chapel Hill (Roberts and Cedarbaum, 1975) differs from the others because, unlike the usual factor IX, the molecule does not undergo a reduction in molecular weight on activation. Finally, in vitamin K deficiency or administration of oral anticoagulants, a variant factor IX molecule is synthesized that has normal immunologic, but reduced procoagulant, activity (Natelson and Coltman, 1972). It is apparent that factor IX deficiency shows a great degree of molecular heterogeneity. Bithell et al (1970) have described a factor IX variant in a female with Turner's syndrome. Antibodies to factor IX develop with about the same frequency as in hemophilia (Weiss, 1975). Like antibody to factor VIII, anti-IX is an immunoglobulin of γG_4 subclass (Pike et al, 1972). Goodnight et al (1979) present evidence that the antibody circulates as the IX antigen-antibody complex.

Laboratory diagnosis

Screening tests do not distinguish this deficiency from hemophilia. It is identified by correction studies (Table 17-17) and by specific assay.

Factor X deficiency

The Stuart family was first reported as having factor VII deficiency. Studies of Hougie et al (1957) not only showed this family to have a defect different from those previously described, but they also clearly showed that the cases previously called factor VII deficiency formed a heterogeneous group.

Blood deficient in the Stuart factor shows defective activity in both phases II and III. The venous clotting time is slightly prolonged; the one-stage prothrombin time with tissue thromboplastin is markedly prolonged; the Stypven time is also prolonged (it is normal in true factor VII deficiency); the partial thromboplastin time is prolonged; prothrombin

Table 17-17. Differential APTT studies in factor IX deficiency

Test material	Partial thromboplastin time*
Patient's plasma	120 sec
80% patient plasma + 20% normal plasma	67 sec
80% patient plasma + 20% aged serum	51 sec
80% patient plasma + 20% BaSO₄– adsorbed plasma	125 sec
80% patient plasma + 20% celite– adsorbed plasma	74 sec
80% patient plasma + 20% IX–deficient plasma	124 sec
20% patient plasma + 80% IX–deficient plasma	126 sec

*Automated APTT, General Diagnostics, Morris Plains, N.J.

Table 17-18. Differential APTT studies in factor X deficiency*

Test material	Partial thromboplastin time†
Patient's plasma	131 sec
80% patient plasma + 20% normal plasma	76 sec
80% patient plasma + 20% aged serum	44 sec
80% patient plasma + 20% BaSO₄– adsorbed plasma	128 sec
80% patient plasma + 20% celite– adsorbed plasma	77 sec
80% patient plasma + 20% X–deficient plasma	133 sec
20% patient plasma + 80% X–deficient plasma	129 sec

*Plasma prothrombin time also prolonged (41 sec, control 12 sec).
†Automated APTT, General Diagnostics, Morris Plains, N.J.

Table 17-19. Differential APTT studies in factor XI deficiency

Test material	Partial thromboplastin time*
Patient's plasma	110 sec
80% patient plasma + 20% normal plasma	54 sec
80% patient plasma + 20% aged serum	39 sec
80% patient plasma + 20% BaSO₄– adsorbed plasma	63 sec
80% patient plasma + 20% celite– adsorbed plasma	113 sec
80% patient plasma + 20% XI–deficient plasma	109 sec
20% patient plasma + 80% XI–deficient plasma	114 sec
80% patient plasma + 20% XII–deficient plasma	60 sec

*Automated APTT, General Diagnostics, Morris Plains, N.J.

consumption is impaired; and thromboplastin generation is abnormal when the patient's serum is substituted. Differential APTT studies (Table 17-18) and specific assay are used to identify the deficiency. There may be associated defects in platelet aggregation (Edgin et al, 1980). Occasionally, in severe deficiencies, the bleeding time is prolonged (Bounameaux, 1963).

The defect has been described in both males and females and varies from severe to mild. It is inherited as an autosomal recessive characteristic. Graham et al (1957) believe that the hemorrhagic diathesis is manifest when the patient is homozygous for the defect. Reduced levels of factor X in some of the children of bleeders indicate a heterozygous state.

An acquired form of factor X deficiency has been described in several cases of amyloidosis (Korsan-Bengtsen et al, 1962; Howell, 1963; Krause, 1977) following exposure to fungicides and in association with renal and adrenal cortical malignancies. Acquired deficiency of factor X in amyloidosis is caused by the binding of factor X to amyloid fibrils (Triplett et al, 1977). Haupt (1965) reports decreased factor X levels in children having various types of thrombocytopenia. In one case (Bayer et al, 1969) a 12-year-old boy developed a severe deficiency of factor X without apparent cause and improved spontaneously. Factor X deficiency in a neonate is reported by Machin et al (1980).

A variant factor X deficiency has been described by Girolami et al (1970, 1971, 1975). They propose the term "factor X Friuli" after the name of the area in northern Italy in which the disease was found. The variant is distinguished from the classic defect by a normal (or slightly prolonged) Stypven time as well as by an anomalous result when assayed by the Bachmann technic (Stypven-cephalin).

Factor XI deficiency

The deficiency state affects both males and females and is inherited as an autosomal dominant with incomplete penetrance (Rosenthal and Sanders, 1954; Rosenthal, 1954). The homozygous state shows low levels of factor XI and may exhibit moderately severe bleeding, whereas the heterozygote has intermediate to almost normal levels of factor XI

and is usually asymptomatic (Ingram and Rizza, 1976). Since most persons with this deficiency are heterozygous, they are either asymptomatic or have very minimal signs of abnormal bleeding. Hemarthroses are rare. Abnormal bleeding may occur only after trauma or surgery.

The incidence of factor XI deficiency is low. Most cases are found in Jewish persons and predominantly in the New York and Los Angeles areas. Reports of very high incidence are certainly based on unreliable methodology. For example, Conrad et al (1965) diagnosed 65 out of 85 abnormalities as factor XI deficiency! The diagnosis was based on a thromboplastin generation test system in kit form; the results obtained with these kits are easily misinterpreted. Typical differential studies are shown in Table 17-19.

Factor XII deficiency

Factor XII deficiency is inherited as a recessive trait affecting both males and females (Ratnoff and Steinberg, 1962). It is customary to refer to it as the Hageman trait, but the term "trait" is poorly chosen, for there are both homozygous- and heterozygous-deficient persons. Interestingly, even the homozygous patient is usually asymptomatic. Only a few instances of abnormal bleeding are reported. In contrast, the laboratory studies are markedly abnormal (Table 17-20). All of our patients have been asymptomatic, and detection has been made by screening coagulation tests. The first deficiency of factor XII discovered in our coagulation laboratory was in an 81-year-old former boxer with no history of being a "bleeder" in the ring.

As a historical note, Ratnoff et al (1968) report that Mr. John Hageman, the patient after whom the deficiency was named, died in 1968. The cause of death was massive pulmonary embolism 12 days after sustaining multiple fractures.

Summary

The differential studies useful in phase II abnormalities are summarized in Table 17-21.

Therapy of phase II abnormalities
General considerations

In none of the phases do the coagulation abnormalities require that substitution therapy achieve a blood assay of 100% of the deficient factor. Each deficiency has a "hemostatic level" at which the abnormal bleeding ceases (Table 17-22). These numbers do not substitute for clinical observation, for if the patient continues to bleed, a hemostatic effect has not been achieved regardless of the assay value.

Hemophilia

The treatment of hemophilia is discussed by Owen and Bowie (1975) and by Roberts and McMillan (1975). In the absence of trauma a hemophiliac will not have bleeding episodes if the factor VIII level is about 25%. During a bleeding episode the hemostatic level to be achieved is about 30% of normal. Normalization of the APTT occurs at a factor VIII level of about 40%, and we recommend this test to follow the effectiveness of therapy rather than the more difficult and expensive assay of factor VIII. We have found the factor VIII assays of cryoprecipitates so variable that we recommend instead one of the commercially available factor VIII concentrates. The treatment of a hemophiliac who has a factor VIII antibody consists of using massive infusions of potent concentrate. The presence of anti-**A** or anti-**B** in concentrates may cause a hemolytic anemia (Ashenhurst et al, 1976; Orringer et al, 1976).

Buchanan and Kevy (1978), among others, have used prothrombin complex concentrates to treat hemophiliacs with inhibitors. Most reports are favorable but failures are reported (Parry and Bloom, 1978). There is no evidence that treatment with prothrombin complex concentrates is less expensive than the use of VIII concentrates or that there is less risk of hepatitis (Allain and Krieger, 1975; Blatt et al, 1977). There is a risk that prothrombin complex concentrates are thrombogenic (Cederbaum et al, 1976; Campbell et al, 1978), although there is one report (Prager et al, 1979) of 3 million units being given without complications. It is also reported that some recipients of these concentrates develop an anamnestic rise in antibody titer (Palascak and Shapiro, 1977). In the multicenter therapeutic trial reported

Table 17-20. Differential APTT studies in factor XII deficiency

Test material	Partial thromboplastin time*
Patient's plasma	302 sec
80% patient plasma + 20% normal plasma	54 sec
80% patient plasma + 20% aged serum	54 sec
80% patient plasma + 20% BaSO$_4$– adsorbed plasma	65 sec
80% patient plasma + 20% celite– adsorbed plasma	51 sec
80% patient plasma + 20% XII–deficient plasma	280 sec
20% patient plasma + 80% XII–deficient plasma	330 sec

*Automated APTT, General Diagnostics, Morris Plains, N.J.

by Lusher et al (1980) the effect of prothrombin complex concentrates was compared with that of a placebo (albumin) and, not surprisingly, the concentrates were more effective than the placebo in the treatment of hemarthroses complicated by an anticoagulant. The most interesting finding in this study was that 25% of the patients receiving the placebo reported the treatment to be effective.

Prophylactic treatment has been adopted by many physicians treating hemophiliacs (Aronstam et al, 1976). However, since factor VIII antibodies in hemophilia develop only in multiply transfused hemophiliacs, with rare exceptions, the physician should balance this problem against the beneficial effects of prophylaxis.

Factor IX deficiency

The treatment of factor IX deficiency is discussed by Owen and Bowie (1975) and by Soulier and Steinbuch (1975). In treating an acute bleeding episode or when preparing a patient for major surgery, one should attempt to achieve and maintain the factor IX level at about 15% to 25% of normal. Concentrates of factors II, VII, IX, and X should be used. Large amounts may be needed if the patient has developed a factor IX antibody. Many concentrates are unfortunately thrombogenic (Kingdon et al, 1975; Cederbaum et al, 1976). This should be taken into account when deciding whether to use one for therapy.

Factor X deficiency

Mild bleeding episodes can be treated with fresh or frozen plasma, but more severe problems should be treated with factors II, VII, IX, and X concentrate (Dike et al, 1972). The hemostatic level is 10% to 20% of normal.

Deficiency of factor XI or XII

Bleeding occurs only rarely, and fresh or frozen plasma is effective.

PHASE III: THROMBINOGENESIS
Reactions

As shown in Fig. 17-4, the conversion of prothrombin to thrombin is preceded by the prothrombin activator complex of factor Xa, factor V, and platelet factor 3. Prothrombin activator complex converts prothrombin to thrombin in the

Table 17-21. Differential diagnosis of defects in phase II, including contact factors

Test	Factor VIII deficiency	Factor IX deficiency	Factor X deficiency	Factor XI deficiency	Factor XII deficiency	Inhibitor present
Coagulation time	Prolonged	Prolonged	Prolonged	Prolonged	Prolonged	Prolonged
Prothrombin time	Normal	Normal	Prolonged	Normal	Normal	Slightly to moderately prolonged*
Prothrombin consumption	Impaired	Impaired	Impaired	Impaired	Impaired	Impaired
Partial thromboplastin time	Prolonged	Prolonged	Prolonged	Prolonged	Prolonged	Prolonged
Corrected by:						
Normal plasma	Yes	Yes	Yes	Yes	Yes	No
Aged serum	No	Yes	Yes	Yes	Yes	No
BaSO₄–adsorbed plasma	Yes	No	No	Yes	Yes	No
Celite-adsorbed plasma†	Yes	Yes	Yes	No	Yes	No
Thromboplastin generation						
Platelets	Normal	Normal	Normal	Normal	Normal	Normal
Plasma	Deficient	Normal	Normal	Normal or deficient‡	Normal or deficient‡	Normal or deficient
Serum	Normal	Deficient	Deficient	Normal or deficient‡	Normal or deficient‡	Normal or deficient
Corrected by:						
Normal plasma	Yes	Yes	Yes	Yes	Yes	No
Aged or normal serum	No	Yes	Yes	Yes	Yes	No
Celite-adsorbed plasma†	Yes	Yes	Yes	No	Yes	No

*Not corrected by fresh, normal BaSO₄-adsorbed plasma or stored serum.
†15 mg celite/ml of plasma.
‡Reported variously to be (1) abnormal only when both patient's plasma and serum are used, (2) abnormal when only serum is substituted, and (3) abnormal when only plasma is substituted. Should be confirmed by cross-correction using known deficient substrates.

Table 17-22. Hemostatic levels to be achieved in the treatment of coagulation factor deficiencies

Deficiency	Hemostatic level (% of normal)
Factor VIII	25-30
Factor IX	15-25
Factor X	10-20
Factor XI	10-20
Factor XII	3-5
Factor XIII	3-5

Table 17-23. Prothrombin time with tissue extract and Russell's viper venom (Stypven) in phase III abnormalities

Deficiency	Prothrombine time	
	With tissue extract	With venom
Prothrombin	Prolonged	Prolonged
Factor V	Prolonged	Prolonged
Factor VII	Prolonged	Normal
Factor X	Prolonged	Prolonged

presence of calcium ions. Prothrombin activator complex is common to both the intrinsic and the extrinsic pathways, but the extrinsic pathway involves the interaction of tissue factor with factor VII.

For convenience, phase III reactions are those which depend on extrinsic activation by tissue factor or Russell's viper venom. The two activators have different activities, tissue factor being dependent on factor VII, whereas Russell's viper venom activates factor X to Xa in the presence of phospholipid independently of factor VII (Table 17-23). Whereas abnormalities in phase II are detected conveniently with the PTT, abnormalities in phase III (congenital or caused by oral anticoagulants) are detected with the one-stage prothrombin time (PT). Note, however, that a prolonged prothrombin time can result from other factors:

fibrinogen concentration below 60 mg/dl (1.74 μm/1); pathologic circulating anticoagulants against thrombin, factor X, or factor V; or the administration of heparin.

Role of vitamin K

One additional feature that sets this phase apart from the others is that some of the factors involved in the PT test depend on vitamin K for adequate synthesis. These are known as the vitamin K–dependent factors: prothrombin and factors VII, IX, and X. Factor IX does not participate in the reaction with tissue factor and, in factor IX deficiency, the PT test is normal. Factor V is not a vitamin K–dependent factor. Synthesis of the vitamin K–dependent factors is inhibited by oral anticoagulants, and the PT test is used principally for the control of oral anticoagulant therapy.

Table 17-24. Differential diagnosis of defects in phase III

Test	Prothrombin deficiency	Factor V deficiency	Factor VII deficiency	Anticoagulant present
Prothrombin time, one-stage, tissue thromboplastin	Prolonged	Prolonged	Prolonged	Prolonged
Corrected by:				
Normal stored serum	No	No	Yes	No
Fresh BaSO₄ plasma	No	Yes	No	No
Stored oxalate plasma	Yes	No	Yes	No
Prothrombin assay, two-stage	Reduced	Normal	Normal or reduced	Reduced*
Factor V assay	Normal	Reduced	Normal	Normal*
Factor VII assay	Normal	Normal	Reduced	Normal*
Antithrombin titer	Normal	Normal	Normal	Increased
Prothrombin time, using Russell's viper venom	Prolonged	Prolonged	Normal	Prolonged

*Assays for prothrombin and other factors not reliable when an anticoagulant is present in high titer.

Table 17-25. Detection of congenital, pure prothrombin deficiency*

Test material	Prothrombin time
Patient's plasma	20 sec
Patient's plasma 80% + N plasma 20%	14.6 sec
Patient's plasma 80% + BaSO₄-adsorbed plasma 20%	21 sec
Patient's plasma 80% + N serum 20%	20.5 sec
Patient's plasma 80% + N stored plasma 20%	15 sec

Conclusion: Correction of prothrombin time by normal plasma and normal stored plasma indicates a deficiency of prothrombin. Stypven time was prolonged, the nonactivated partial thromboplastin time was 86 sec (normal). Two-stage prothrombin assay showed 2.4% of normal prothrombin concentration.
*Patient was a 14-year-old girl with profuse menstrual bleeding.

Table 17-26. Detection of factor V deficiency, in this case a congenital deficiency of this factor alone

Test material	Prothrombin time
Patient's plasma	28 sec
Patient's plasma 80% + N plasma 20%	14 sec
Patient's plasma 80% + BaSO₄-adsorbed plasma 20%	14 sec
Patient's plasma 80% + N serum 20%	27 sec
Patient's plasma 80% + N stored plasma 20%	26 sec

Conclusion: Correction of prothrombin time by normal plasma and BaSO₄-adsorbed normal plasma indicates a deficiency in factor V. Confirmed by a factor V assay of 13% of normal.

The role of vitamin K in the synthesis of factors II, VII, IX, and X is reviewed by Gallop et al (1980). The vitamin K cycle consists of oxidation of vitamin K to vitamin K-2,3-epoxide in the presence of carbon dioxide. This compound is responsible for the carboxylation of a glutamic acid residue in the protein moiety, catalyzed by a carboxylase enzyme. Vitamin K is regenerated from vitamin K-2,3-epoxide by vitamin K epoxide reductase. Carboxylation of the protein is necessary for calcium binding; for example, normal (carboxylated) factor II binds 10 to 12 moles of calcium per mole of protein in contrast with less than 1 mole of 351cium for the acarboxyprothrombin.

Vitamin K deficiency or the administration of coumarin drugs results in the synthesis of variant molecules of factors II, VII, IX, and X (Stenflo, 1975) that are antigenically identical with the normal factors but that are inactive in coagulation and do not bind calcium. This is interpreted as indicating that vitamin K acts late in the synthetic sequence, being required only for the attachment of γ-carboxyglutamic acid residues as a calcium-binding site. The demonstration of antigenically identical, but inactive, molecules of prothrombin may clarify in part the question of abnormal proteins formed during oral anticoagulant therapy. These were called PIVKA (protein induced by vitamin K antagonists) by Hemker et al (1963) and later PIVKA II for the abnormal

prothrombin molecule, PIVKA IX for the abnormal factor IX molecule, and PIVKA X for the abnormal factor X molecule (Lindhout and Kop-Klaassen, 1975). The noncarboxylated prothrombin molecule is not converted to thrombin by tissue thromboplastin, but it is converted by *Echis carinatus* venom (Corrigan and Earnest, 1980). There is no good evidence that the PIVKA variants exert an anticoagulant effect (Girolami et al, 1977).

Hemorrhagic disorders in phase III

It should be noted that no deficiency of tissue factor has been found. The deficiencies classified as phase III abnormalities are characterized by a prolonged plasma PT with tissue extracts. Factor X–deficient plasma also has a prolonged prothrombin time, but this deficiency has been discussed as a phase II abnormality. The differential diagnosis of phase III abnormalities is given in Table 17-24.

Congenital deficiencies

Congenital deficiency of factors II, V, or VII are rare.

DEFICIENCY OF FACTOR II. Of the reported cases of congenital deficiency of prothrombin (factor II) only a few have been investigated adequately (DeBastos et al, 1964; Seeler, 1972a). Both men and women are affected, but the cases are too few to establish the mode of inheritance. The

Table 17-27. Detection of factor VII deficiency, congenital

Test material	Prothrombin time
Patient's plasma	32 sec
Patient's plasma 80% + N plasma 20%	15 sec
Patient's plasma 80% + BaSO$_4$-adsorbed plasma 20%	17 sec
Patient's plasma 80% + N serum 20%	17 sec
Patient's plasma 80% + N stored plasma 20%	31 sec

Conclusion: Correction of prothrombin time by normal plasma and serum indicates a deficiency of factor VII. The Stypven time was normal, and the factor VII assay was 2% of normal.

Table 17-28. Combined prothrombin and factor VII deficiency in patient receiving bishydroxycoumarin (Dicumarol)

Test material	Prothrombin time
Patient's plasma	33 sec
Patient's plasma 80% + N plasma 20%	14 sec
Patient's plasma 80% + BaSO$_4$-adsorbed plasma 20%	34 sec
Patient's plasma 80% + N serum 20%	15 sec
Patient's plasma 80% + N stored plasma 20%	16 sec

Conclusion: Correction of prothrombin time by normal plasma, normal serum, and normal stored plasma indicates a double defect factor VII and prothrombin. The pattern is typical of bishydroxycoumarin effect. Reduction of factors IX and X was also demonstrated by specific assays.

Table 17-29. Prolongation of prothrombin time by an anticoagulant, in this case intensive therapy with heparin

Test material	Prothrombin time
Patient's plasma	60 sec
Patient's plasma 80% + N plasma 20%	58 sec
Patient's plasma 80% + BaSO$_4$-adsorbed plasma 20%	59 sec
Patient's plasma 80% + N serum 20%	57 sec
Patient's plasma 80% + N stored plasma 20%	56 sec
Patient's plasma 20% + N plasma 80%	35 sec

Conclusion: Failure to correct prothrombin time with any of the reagents, including normal plasma, indicates an anticoagulant effect rather than a deficiency of a factor. Note that the patient's plasma prolongs the prothrombin time of normal plasma.

bleeding tendency can be severe, with easy bruising, epistaxis, and bleeding after surgery. I have seen only one case of this defect (Table 17-25). The PT is prolonged and is corrected by normal and stored plasma, and the two-stage assay shows low values of factor II.

Variant molecules of factor II have been discovered: prothrombin Barcelona (Josso et al, 1975; Rabiet et al, 1978), prothrombin San Juan (Shapiro, 1975), prothrombin Padua (Girolami, 1975), prothrombin Brussels (Kahn, 1975), prothrombin Cardeza (Shapiro et al, 1969), and prothrombin Quick (Owen et al, 1978). All have moderately depressed biologic activity but a normal amount of immunologically reactive protein.

DEFICIENCY OF FACTOR V. Congenital deficiency of factor V is rare. Owren's (1947) studies of a woman with a hemorrhagic disease dating back to her childhood led to his description of a new clotting factor that he called "factor V." He called the disease "parahemophilia." Only about 60 congenital cases have been reported (Mellinger and Duckert, 1971; Seeler, 1972a), and in some instances the disease has been familial. Transmission follows an autosomal recessive or partially dominant pattern. The identification by differential studies and assay is shown in Table 17-26.

DEFICIENCY OF FACTOR VII. Congenital factor VII deficiency has been described by a number of investigators. Alexander et al (1951) recognized that the deficiency was caused by the lack of a serum prothrombin conversion accelerator (SPCA). The coagulation studies in a case we have studied are shown in Table 17-27. Seegers and Alkjaersig (1955) studied the blood from one of Alexander's patients and concluded that the deficiency was in the conversion of prothrombin to autoprothrombin I. It is interesting to note that in most cases of acquired factor VII deficiency, there is an accompanying deficiency in prothrombin. Newcomb et al (1956) reported a congenital deficiency of both prothrombin and factor VII. Nour-Eldin and Wilkinson (1959), Verstraete et al (1962), and Hall et al (1975) reported a combined deficiency of factors VII and IX. However, the possibility of oral anticoagulant drug intake or heparin administration should always be considered when multiple defects of the prothrombin complex are encountered (Tables 17-28

and 17-29). A probable factor VII inhibitor in a patient with bronchogenic carcinoma is reported by Campbell et al (1980).

Acquired deficiencies

VITAMIN K DEFICIENCY IN ADULTS. Vitamin K is a fat-soluble vitamin necessary for the synthesis of prothrombin and factors VII, IX, and X (the "vitamin K–dependent" coagulation factors). It is postulated that vitamin K acts at the ribosomal level in the liver cell to convert a precursor to the four active clotting factors. There is evidence that vitamin K acts on the synthesis of factors in the prothrombin complex after the translational stage.

Vitamin K (Menadione, Hykinone, Synkayvite) has little activity in humans in the treatment of coumarin-induced or acquired vitamin K deficiency. On the other hand, the analogue vitamin K$_1$ (Phytonadione, Mephyton, Aquamephyton, Konakion) is active and is the drug of choice. All of the vitamin K preparations are suitable for prophylaxis.

Vitamin K is available from two sources: from foods (as vitamin K$_1$) and as a product of bacterial action in the gastrointestinal tract (as vitamin K$_2$). It is absorbed from the bowel when bile salts are present and can be traced to the liver, where prothrombin synthesis takes place. Thus there are four possible reasons for the development of vitamin K deficiency: (1) deficient nutritional intake, (2) defective synthesis in the bowel, (3) poor absorption from the bowel, and (4) lack of utilization by a diseased liver.

A pure nutritional deficiency in adults is so rare, if it occurs at all, as to need no discussion. In infants, however, it has been shown that vitamin K deficiency can be accentuated by a diet of some infant formulas low in vitamin K (Moss, 1969). Defective synthesis, on the other hand, can result from any long-standing gastrointestinal disorder. Particularly in steatorrhea, deficient synthesis is complicated by defective absorption because of increased bowel motility and decreased fat absorption. Long-term antibiotic therapy can sufficiently reduce the bacterial flora to produce a vitamin K deficiency. In hemorrhagic disease of the newborn it is thought that the vitamin K deficiency is produced by deficient synthesis in a bowel not yet supplied with normal bacterial flora, combined with the absence of bile salts. Defective absorption is seen in obstructive jaundice, where the bile does not enter the bowel. After normal absorption, vitamin K activity is dependent on normal liver function for the synthesis of functional prothrombin and associated factors.

Treatment of acquired prothrombin and factor VII deficiency with vitamin K must take into account the pathogenesis of the deficiency. Vitamin K by mouth is not effective in obstructive jaundice unless bile salts are given at the same time. The defective absorptive mechanism can be bypassed by giving vitamin K parenterally. If the hemorrhagic diathesis is secondary to hepatocellular disease, vitamin K will not be effective, regardless of the route of administration. In this event it will be necessary to depend on blood transfusion to supply the deficient coagulation factors.

Vitamin K_1 is most effective in deficiencies associated with obstructive jaundice, following bishydroxycoumarin administration, and in hemorrhagic disease of the newborn. It has no significant effect in the congenital deficiencies or in acquired factor V deficiency. It is best to recognize these limitations and to avoid giving large doses in an effort to achieve the impossible. Vitamin K toxicity (hemolytic anemia, hyperbilirubinemia, and even kernicterus) is a recognized complication of overdosage in infants.

HEMORRHAGIC DISEASE OF THE NEWBORN. Hemorrhagic disease of the newborn is defined as bleeding during the first few days of life related to vitamin K deficiency. It can be prevented in most instances by giving vitamin K_1 to the mother before delivery or to the infant at birth. The deficiency is manifested by bleeding from the cord and other sites, and coagulation studies show a prolonged prothrombin time and a deficiency of the vitamin K–dependent factors. Severe neonatal bleeding can occur if the mother has been taking anticonvulsant drugs (hydantoins) and barbiturates (Bleyer and Skinner, 1976). The hemorrhagic disease is worsened by several potentially additive circumstances. There is, first, a physiologic deficiency of coagulation factors in the newborn. Second, there is immaturity of liver synthetic processes, particularly in the premature infant. Third, there is little synthesis of vitamin K in the bowel until the bacterial flora is well established. Finally, any concurrent disease such as sepsis, respiratory distress, or thrombocytopenia may precipitate serious hemorrhage. When an

infant has atresia of the bile ducts, no bile enters the gastrointestinal tract and vitamin K cannot be absorbed even though it is being synthesized in adequate quantities.

Vitamin K deficiency may develop during the first few months of life as a result of a vitamin K–deficient diet (breast feeding without supplements or infant formulas low in vitamin K).

THE "LUPUS ANTICOAGULANT." The occurrence of a coagulation inhibitor in approximately 5% of systemic lupus erythematosus cases was first described by Conley and Hartman (1952). Because of its unusual properties it has been called the "lupus anticoagulant," even though it can occur in other autoimmune disorders (Boxer et al, 1976), after the administration of drugs that induce the LE syndrome (Davis et al, 1978), after psychotropic drug therapy (Zucker et al, 1978; Zarrabi et al, 1979), and after viral infection (Beck et al, 1979) and various other diseases (Gandalfo et al, 1977).

Characteristically, the lupus anticoagulant produces a moderately long prothrombin time and a prolonged activated partial thromboplastin time not corrected by normal plasma. It is identified by its property of inhibiting highly diluted tissue thromboplastin (Boxer et al, 1976; Schleider et al, 1976). Yin and Gaston (1965) proposed that the anticoagulant was directed against the phospholipid portion of the prothrombin activator complex (Xa-V-phospholipid-calcium), and this is supported by recent studies (Clyne et al, 1980). The lupus anticoagulant has been shown to be an immunoglobulin of the IgG or IgM type (Yin and Gaston, 1965; Thiagarajan et al, 1980). Thiagarajan et al (1980) also showed that the antibody inhibits phosphatidylserine and phosphatidic acid and that the anticoagulant effect can be corrected by normal platelets. The dilute thromboplastin test for the lupus anticoagulant is not abnormal in patients with acquired anti-VIII:C antibodies.

Patients with the lupus anticoagulant usually have no hemorrhagic symptoms unless there is a concomitant thrombocytopenia or platelet functional abnormality (Feinstein and Rapaport, 1972, Lechner, 1974). Surprisingly, however, the occurrence of thrombosis is not unusual (Bowie et al, 1963; Åberg and Nilsson, 1972; Angles-Cano et al, 1979; Mueh et al, 1980). The pathogenesis of this thrombotic tendency is not known. In those who have autoimmune disease one can postulate that immunologic vasculitis or the presence of circulating immune complexes may predispose to thrombosis, but this mechanism cannot be invoked on all cases.

There are some reports of the simultaneous occurrence of the lupus anticoagulant and coagulation factor deficiencies, but the apparent deficiencies are artifactual, because of the inhibitory effect of the anticoagulant. The factor X inhibitor found in two cases of leprosy by Ness et al (1980) is such an example.

ORAL ANTICOAGULANTS. Bishydroxycoumarin (Dicumarol) and related compounds are being used extensively in the treatment of acute and chronic thrombotic disease. Their use is based on their ability to lengthen the one-stage prothrombin time and thus supposedly reduce the possibility of spontaneous thrombosis or the extension of an existing thrombosis.

As noted, administration of coumarin drugs results in the

formation of variant (nonactive) coagulation factors. There is evidence that the system required for the production of the vitamin K antagonist varies in activity among persons because some have been described that are abnormally resistant to coumarin drugs, presumably on the basis of a deficient enzyme system (O'Reilly, 1970). The common observation that, among individuals, there is a wide variation in the dose required to maintain the same intensity of anticoagulant therapy also suggests an enzyme system of variable activity. Such a system would also explain the influence of various drugs (e.g., the barbiturates) in decreasing the effectiveness of oral anticoagulants by competing for the same enzyme system. Other drugs, however, such as phenylbutazone, potentiate the effect of coumarin drugs.

Intake of coumarin drugs for suicidal or pseudosuicidal purposes seems to be increasing in frequency. Bowie et al (1965) have reviewed the subject of the "anticoagulant malingerers" or "Dicumarol eaters." We also have in our file one instance in which bishydroxycoumarin was used in an attempted homicide.

Therapy with any of the anticoagulant drugs is usually controlled by prothrombin time determinations (Miale, 1962). Any of the commercially available tissue thromboplastins may be used, but shifting from one thromboplastin preparation to another in the middle of therapy is not recommended, since the results obtained with one thromboplastin are not always comparable to those obtained with another. The standard test using undiluted plasma is reliable. The unknown factors introduced when plasma is diluted make the diluted test (12.5% plasma) of doubtful value. It is now our practice to report results only in seconds.

Oral anticoagulants are of two types: *coumarin derivatives* such as bishydroxycoumarin (Dicumarol), ethyl biscoumacetate (Tromexan), acenocoumarol (Sintrom), phenprocoumon (Liquamar, Marcumar), and warfarin sodium (Coumadin, Panwarfin, Athrombin-K), and the *derivatives of indandione* such as phenindione (Hedulin, Danilone, Indon), diphenadione (Dipaxin, Didandin), and anisindione (Miradon).

Each preparation has advantages and disadvantages. Bishydroxycoumarin is absorbed incompletely from the upper gastrointestinal tract, requires about 72 hours to develop the maximum effect, and the effect persists for 4 to 7 days after the drug is discontinued. Ethyl biscoumacetate is rapidly and completely absorbed, requires 18 to 24 hours to reach maximum effectiveness, and the effect persists for 1 to 2 days. Acenocoumarol is rapidly and completely absorbed, requires 24 to 36 hours to reach maximum effectiveness, and the effect persists for 3 to 4 days. Phenprocoumon is slowly but completely absorbed, requires 2 to 3 days to reach maximum effectiveness, and the effect persists for 5 to 7 days. Warfarin sodium requires 1 to 2 days to reach maximum effectiveness and the effect persists for 3 to 5 days. The indandione derivatives, on the other hand, act quickly and without a cumulative effect; within 24 hours after the drug is discontinued the prothrombin time returns to normal. Because of toxic reactions such as leukopenia, dermatitis, and renal damage, they are not widely used in this country.

After absorption, the coumarins are strongly bound to serum albumin, although there is some evidence that they are also bound to liver tissue and, in the case of bishydroxycoumarin, to serum globulins. Only a small fraction, 3% to 10%, of the total plasma concentration represents drug not bound to protein, and it is this free fraction, in equilibrium with bound drug, that is pharmacologically active.

Coumarins are metabolized in hepatic microsomes, and a number of degradation products have been identified in plasma, urine, bile, and feces. Coumarin metabolites have little or no hypoprothrombinopenic effect. There is little excretion of the unmodified drugs in the urine because their binding with albumin prevents glomerular filtration.

There have been arguments over the years as to the best laboratory technic for monitoring the effect of anticoagulant therapy. We have followed a large number of patients on long-term oral anticoagulant therapy, and the results of various measurements are shown in Fig. 17-45. It is quite apparent from this example that there is no parameter that is "out of step" with the prothrombin time or with other tests.

The optimal dose of the coumarin-indandione drugs is that which combines maximum protection against thromboembolism with the lowest incidence of induced bleeding, but data on dosage as related to effectiveness are disappointingly scarce. Wright et al (1954) showed that oral anticoagulant therapy maintained at 2 to 2½ times the control prothrombin time have good therapeutic results with minimal complications. Borchgrevink (1960b) reported a significantly higher mortality rate for inadequately treated patients. It follows that the prothrombin time must be in the range of 2 to 2½ times the normal for anticoagulant therapy to be effective. In fact, there is evidence that small doses of oral anticoagulants increase platelet adhesiveness whereas adequate doses inhibit.

DRUG INTERACTION WITH COUMARIN DRUGS. In addition to the coagulation factors known to be involved in the prothrombin time test, there are other situations that may cause unexplained fluctuations in the prothrombin time. These include drugs, febrile illness, dehydration, and alcoholic weekends. Not to be forgotten are the drug-enhancing effect of liver dysfunction and the drug-neutralizing effect of increased intake of vitamin K. We have seen one instance where food intake seemed to interfere with the therapeutic level. A patient who had been completely stable on a warfarin sodium dosage of 30 mg/week for 2 years developed a craving for grapes and ate about 2 pounds each day. Within a week she was out of control (prothrombin time: 12 seconds). In the absence of other causes, we suspected that the grapes were the culprit. When she stopped eating them, she returned to her previous steady state.

Not only does diet affect oral anticoagulant therapy, but there are also many drugs that can potentially interact with oral anticoagulants and potentiate their effect (Table 17-30). In some cases the combined intake of an oral anticoagulant and another drug results in a different interaction, the oral anticoagulant potentiating the effect of the other drug. Several mechanisms are involved in these interactions: (1) inhibition of microsomal enzyme activity in the liver cell, (2) activation of microsomal enzyme activity, (3) displacement of the oral anticoagulant from binding sites on plasma proteins, (4) an antivitamin K effect, either by decreasing the absorption of vitamin K from the gastrointestinal tract or by

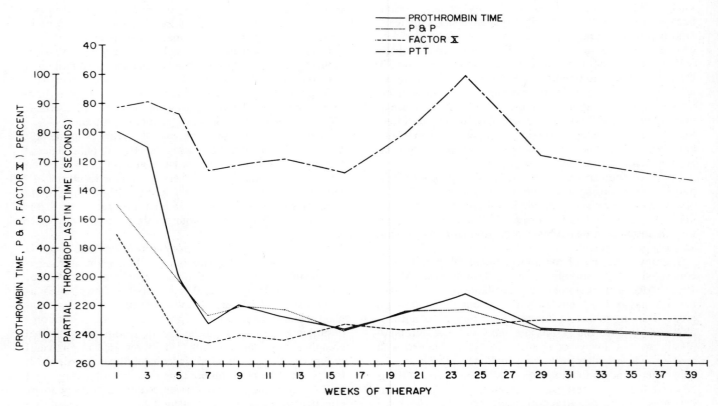

Fig. 17-45. Laboratory control of long-term anticoagulant therapy. Patient received warfarin (Coumadin), and good control was maintained. Note that all four tests run roughly parallel. Note also that in spite of fairly intensive anticoagulant therapy, the effect on the intrinsic system, as measured by the nonactivated partial thromboplastin time, is relatively slight. The method used for the assay of factor X is specific for factor X only if the concentration of prothrombin is normal.

Table 17-30. Potential interaction of various drugs with coumarin oral anticoagulants

I. Drugs sometimes influencing anticoagulant effect
  A. Accentuated anticoagulant effect
    1. Alcohol
    2. Aspirin
    3. Acetaminophen (Tylenol)
    4. Chloramphenicol
    5. Clofibrate (Atromide S)
    6. Ethchlorvynol (Placidyl)
    7. Glucagon
    8. Methylphenidate (Ritalin)
    9. Phenylbutazone (Butazolidin)
    10. Phenyramidol (Analexin)
    11. Quinidine
    12. Quinine
    13. Methandrostenolone (Dianabol)
    14. Thyroid preparations (dextrothyroxine)
    15. Tolbutamide (Orinase)
    16. Neomycin

    17. Metronidazole (Flagyl)
    18. Sulfisoxazole (Gantrisin)
  B. Decreased anticoagulant effect
    1. Barbiturates
    2. Chloral hydrate
    3. Glutethimide (Doriden)
    4. Griseofulvin
    5. Oral contraceptives
    6. Ethchlorvynol (Placidyl)
    7. Diphenylhydantoin (Dilantin)
    8. Adrenocortical steroids
    9. Cholestyramine
II. Coumarin drug influencing effect of other drugs
  A. Barbiturates: increased serum barbiturate concentration
  B. Chlorpropamide (Diabinese): hypoglycemia
  C. Phenytoin (Dilantin): increased serum concentration
  D. Tolbutamide (Orinase): hypoglycemia

affecting its transport or metabolism, and (5) effect on hemostatic factors other than the vitamin K–dependent ones, such as on platelet adhesiveness. The subject of drug interactions is reviewed by Koch-Weser and Sellers (1971), Udall (1970), Robinson and Sylwester (1970), and Robinson et al (1971).

Since one cannot but be impressed by the list of drugs taken by the average patient, both in and outside the hospital, drug interactions are increasingly important. In our experience, when an irate physician blames the laboratory performance of the prothrombin time test when his patient's condition seems to be difficult to control or goes out of control for no obvious reason, it is found that the patient is receiving several of the drugs listed. Individuality of response accounts for the fact that, fortunately, not all patients are affected by these drug interactions. The finding that some persons are constitutionally resistant to coumarin drugs, while others exhibit moderate degrees of resistance, as compared to the average, indicates that individual factors operate in both drug effects and drug interactions. Sometimes patients who are receiving oral anticoagulants take it on themselves to vary the prescribed dose, usually because they relate the dosage to well-being or to a feeling of weakness.

STANDARDIZATION OF THERAPEUTIC RANGE BASED ON STANDARD REFERENCE PLASMAS. For some years there has been much effort expended to arrive at a national and international "standardization" of the prothrombin time test. Details of the controversy are given by Miale and Kent (1972). In fact, the true goal has not been to standardize the test procedure but rather to achieve some uniformity in the use of oral anticoagulants and in the intensity of therapy.

Our approach in the United States has been to use artificially prepared reference plasmas, with assayed values for the vitamin K–dependent factors, as a common reference material against which the various thromboplastins are measured (Miale and LaFond, 1969a). This proposal was accepted by the Standards Committee of the College of American Pathologists (Miale and LaFond, 1969b). Kahan and Norén (1975) have used lyophilized normal and abnormal plasmas to calibrate three different thromboplastins. When measured against the same reference plasmas, the various thromboplastins give different prothrombin time values, and these cannot be made to correspond by the use of curves that give percentile activity. We have recommended that the use of such curves be discontinued and the prothrombin time results given only in seconds.

If the prothrombin time of the standard reference plasmas is determined by using various commercial thromboplastins and the prothrombin time is plotted against the reciprocal of the factor VII level in the standard reference plasmas, divergent lines having different slopes will be obtained (Fig. 17-46). Since factor VII is the chief reactant with tissue factor and is the one most predictably depressed by oral anticoagulants, the therapeutic range is equivalent to a factor VII level of 10% to 20% (Miale, 1980). The suggested therapeutic level for each thromboplastin is given in Table 17-31.

This schedule guarantees the same intensity of anticoagulant therapy when a patient is tested in laboratories using

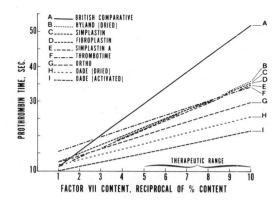

Fig. 17-46. Plot of the prothrombin time against the reciprocal of the factor VII assay of standard reference plasmas. The therapeutic range is equivalent to a factor VII level of 10% to 20% of normal.

Table 17-31. Therapeutic levels for various commercial thromboplastins, representing a reduction of the factor VII level to 10% to 20% of normal

Thromboplastin	Therapeutic range (sec)
British comparative	30-53
Hyland (dried)	22-36
Simplastin	22-36
Fibroplastin	22-30
Simplastin A	21-30
Thrombotime	24-30
Ortho	15-30
Dade (dried)	17-26
Dade (activated)	15-21

different thromboplastins. Aside from the obvious advantage to the patient who travels from one area to another, it can be hoped that standardization of therapy will help to solve some of the problems that arise when evaluating the benefit of oral anticoagulant therapy as practiced in various centers and countries.

We should also remember that the accuracy and precision of the prothrombin time test depend on care in the technic used (see Appendix). As in all laboratory studies, a system of quality control must be followed. The daily use of commercial normal and abnormal plasmas, such as Verify Normal, I, and II (General Diagnostics), is highly recommended.

PHASE IV: FIBRIN FORMATION AND FIBRINOLYSIS
Mechanism of the reaction

After the complexity of the reactions leading up to it, phase IV is a miracle of simplicity and directness. The interactions of the various precursors have one goal, the formation of a substance, thrombin, which alone can produce the desired sol-gel change of fibrinogen to fibrin.

Action of thrombin

Thrombin acts as a hydrolytic enzyme (Laki, 1968) causing a breakdown of the fibrinogen molecule into fibrin

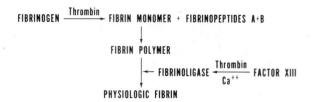

Fig. 17-47. Reactions in phase IV. Fibrin formation. Fibrinoligase is activated factor XIII (XIIIa).

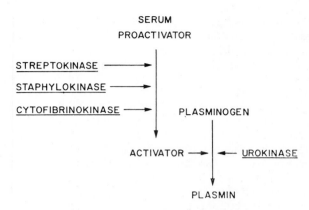

Fig. 17-48. Fibrinolytic system of blood. Not shown are the inhibitors, one of which (antifibrinolysin) inhibits plasmin, whereas others (anti-streptokinase, etc.) inhibit bacterial activators. Chloroform extraction of plasma probably destroys or removes antifibrinolysin.

monomer and polypeptides A and B, Fig. 17-47. Molecules of fibrin monomer then form larger and larger molecules of fibrin polymer by successive steps (Brass et al, 1976), in which first the single molecules and then the polymer molecules come together in an end-to-end and side-to-side fashion. The final fibrin polymer forms a gel that we recognize as the clot (Murano, 1974).

Thrombin acts as an enzyme, in that minute amounts will clot a very large amount of fibrinogen. It would seem that thrombin merely initiates the reaction, after which polymerization takes place independently of the thrombin. The properties of the fibrin clot depend on the pH and ionic concentration of the medium. If these conditions are not favorable, ultimate polymerization may not occur, and the intermediate polymer molecules will remain in solution without forming a gel. The presence of macroglobulins in the blood or an abnormal amount of globulin, as in multiple myeloma, causes a gelatinous clot to form that shows no retraction. If the environment is favorable, the gel consists of large fibrin aggregates that have a molecular weight of about 4.5 million.

Physiologic fibrin

These reactions have been studied in vitro, and there is little doubt that they are basically the same in vivo. There are some important differences in the end product. The clot formed in the blood, physiologic fibrin, is not soluble in a solution of urea, whereas fibrin formed in vitro from pure fibrinogen is readily soluble in urea. The greater stability of physiologic fibrin is due to the action of two agents, calcium, and a fibrin-stabilizing factor (factor XIII). It is thought that in the presence of factor XIII a strong stable linkage (probably S—S bonds) is formed between fibrin monomers, whereas in the absence of factor XIII the linkage is weak (probably H—bonds only), so that the clot is less stable, its solubility in urea being a measurable property of the weaker linkage. The fibrin-stabilizing system involves the change of factor XIII to an active transpeptidase (called "fibrinoligase" by Lorand [1972] and "plasma transamidase" by Loewy [1972]). Transpeptidation involves the reaction between ε-amino-lysine and γ-glutamyl-carbonyl groups of adjacent fibrin molecules, and it is this bridge that stabilizes physiologic fibrin so that it can no longer be dissolved by 1% monochloroacetic acid or 5M urea (Finlayson, 1974).

The formation in vitro of fibrin polymer molecules of intermediate size suggests that there exists in vivo a dynamic equilibrium between fibrinogen and fibrin, an equilibrium characterized by the formation of intermediates of varying molecular weight (Mosesson, 1974). This in effect means that fibrinogen does not exist in the blood in the pure monomolecular form only, but that it is being constantly polymerized and depolymerized. The rapid rate of fibrinogen turnover in the blood lends support to this idea.

Fibrinolysis

Both normal and pathologic depolymerization of fibrin depend on the activity of a fibrinolytic system in the blood. This system can be considered the last of several hemostatic mechanisms that either prevent or correct what might otherwise become catastrophic situations (McNicol and Davies, 1973). We have already noted that the autocatalytic reactions concerned with blood clotting are kept under control by natural inhibitors that restrict intravascular clotting and prevent whole-body thrombosis. When a thrombus does form, its natural history is dissolution; in most instances the patency of the blood vessel is restored. Dissolution of the thrombus is a function of the in vivo fibrinolytic system of *plasminogen* and *plasmin*. Much of our knowledge of this system is derived from in vitro studies of various fibrinolytic systems.

Observations regarding proteolytic activity in the blood are among the oldest in the history of blood coagulation. The enzymatic theory of blood coagulation made much of the observation of Delezenne and Pozerski, in 1903, that plasma shaken with chloroform developed proteolytic (fibrinolytic) activity. Morawitz, in 1906, observed that the incoagulable blood in cases of sudden death was itself fibrinolytic. Opie and Barker, in 1907, determined that the fibrinolytic activity of serum is found in the globulin fraction.

Interestingly, further progress was the result of Tillett and Garner's studies, reported in 1933, with extracts of β hemolytic streptococci. They found that when cell-free extracts of streptococcal cultures were added to clotted plasma, the clot dissolved. They assumed that the lytic substance was an enzyme elaborated by streptococci, and they called the enzyme fibrinolysin. However, Milstone, in 1941, found that streptococcal extracts had no effect on purified fibrinogen unless a small amount of serum, or of the globulin fraction, was added. By 1948 Kaplan et al and MacLeod had defined the reaction with streptococcal enzyme. It was shown that the streptococcal enzyme (streptokinase) was an activator of a profibrinolysin *(plasminogen)* in human blood or serum; this was activated to a fibrinolytic substance *(plasmin)*.

The fibrinolytic system of blood is shown in Fig. 17-48. It will be noted that tissue activator (cytofibrinokinase) is the only one that may be active in vivo. It is derived primarily from endothelial cells (Ali, 1967). The rest of the activators cannot be involved under natural conditions, but urokinase and streptokinase are being used as thrombolytic agents (Prentice and Davidson, 1973).

ACTIVATION BY BACTERIAL FILTRATES. Streptokinase is a product of actively growing hemolytic streptococci (Lancefield group A, human C and G). Most preparations of streptokinase are mixtures of streptokinase and streptodornase. The latter is a deoxyribonuclease. Staphylococci produce a kinase, staphylokinase, that behaves like streptokinase, though more slowly.

ACTIVATION BY TISSUE ACTIVATOR. Tissue fragments and extracts have the ability to activate plasminogen. The active substance is bound firmly to tissue proteins but can be extracted with potassium thiocyanate.

ACTIVATION BY UROKINASE. The presence of a proteolytic enzyme in urine has been known for many years. It is now agreed that the fibrinolytic activity of urine is caused by an enzyme, urokinase, capable of activating plasminogen (Lesuk et al, 1976). It is a proteolytic enzyme, capable of hydrolyzing tosyl arginine methyl ester (TAME) and lysine ethyl ester. Milk, tears, and saliva contain a similar, but not identical, enzyme. It should be noted that trypsin is also an activator of plasminogen.

INHIBITORS OF FIBRINOLYSIS. Blood contains one or more inhibitors of fibrinolysis. The chief antifibrinolysin has been found to migrate with the α_2-globulins. However, human albumin (fraction V) has considerable antifibrinolytic activity. Within the last few years it has been shown that ϵ-aminocaproic acid, an analogue of lysine, blocks plasminogen activation and also neutralizes plasmin (Bennett and Ogston, 1973). This substance has already been tested in vivo in fibrinolytic states and the results are encouraging. Note, however, that it is indicated only when a "primary" fibrinolytic syndrome is present and absolutely contraindicated when the fibrinolysis is secondary to diffuse intravascular coagulation.

Hemorrhagic disorders caused by abnormalities in phase IV

The hemorrhagic diseases caused by deficient function in this phase fall into four categories: (1) those caused by afibrinogenemia, hypofibrinogenemia, or dysfibrinogenemia, (2) those caused by excessive fibrinolytic activity, (3) those associated with dysproteinemia in which there is an interference with the formation of fibrin, and (4) those caused by deficiency of factor XIII (fibrin-stabilizing factor). Disorders of phase IV are listed in Table 17-32.

Dysfibrinogenemia

A number of instances have been recorded in which fibrinogen is quantitatively normal but functionally abnormal (Table 17-33). Characteristically there is a prolongation

of clotting tests, particularly the thrombin time test, simulating the presence of an anticoagulant, a low or normal plasma concentration of fibrinogen when estimated from a clot, normal amounts by immunologic technics and precipitation methods, and normal assays for all other coagulation factors. In some cases there is a hemorrhagic diathesis, in others wound dehiscence, and in others no clinical abnormality. It is thought that in most dysfibrinogenemias the abnormal fibrinogen fails to polymerize. Various anomalies have been demonstrated (Ratnoff and Bennett, 1973). Fibrinogen Detroit has an amino acid substitution (arginine → serine, residue 19) in the α-chain (Kudryk et al, 1976). Fibrinogen Baltimore and some others show delayed release of fibrinopeptides when acted upon by thrombin (Beck et al, 1971). Fibrinogen Zurich I and II and Paris I show poor polymerization (Funk and Straub, 1970; Finlayson et al, 1980). Fibrinogen Zurich I shows also poor release of fibrinopeptide A (Hofmann et al, 1979). Fibrinogen Oklahoma shows deficient cross-linking of fibrin monomers (Hampton, 1968). The recently described fibrinogen Lille has a structural defect at the NH_2 terminal region of the molecule (Denninger et al, 1978). In some of the other variants, combinations of abnormalities have been noted (Ratnoff and Bennett, 1973; Mammen, 1974). Von Felten et al (1969b) and Gralnick et al (1978) report cases of dysfibrinogenemia associated with hepatoma and suggest that the hepatoma was responsible for the synthesis of an abnormal, possibly fetal, fibrinogen. Qualitative abnormalities of fibrinogen are reported in cirrhosis of the liver and hepatitis (Aiach et al, 1973).

Congenital dysfibrinogenemias are usually either asymptomatic or accompanied by mild hemorrhagic disease. However, in some cases there has been thromboembolic disease: in fibrinogens Paris II, New York, Oslo, Copenhagen, Baltimore, and Marburg. D'Souza et al (1979) report the occurrence of thromboembolic disease in a patient with a high concentration of an abnormal fibrinogen thought to be acquired rather than congenital because the abnormality was not present in three children of the patient.

Afibrinogenemia and hypofibrinogenemia

The term "afibrinogenemia" implies a complete lack of fibrinogen in the blood. Although it is sometimes impossible to demonstrate any fibrinogen by chemical tests, some is usually detectable by immunologic tests. It is probably more accurate to refer to "hypofibrinogenemia" in all cases. By common usage, afibrinogenemia refers to the absence of fibrinogen by chemical tests, and hypofibrinogenemia refers to the reduction in fibrinogen concentration below 100 mg/dl of plasma. The concentration must fall below 60 to 100 mg/dl to be clinically significant.

CONGENITAL AFIBRINOGENEMIA. Congenital afibrinogenemia is rare, only a few dozen cases having been reported (Jackson et al, 1965). Most patients with this disorder have shown a tendency to bleed severely after trauma. Only a few have shown spontaneous hemorrhages, even though the blood was completely incoagulable. Studies on patients with this condition have not revealed the cause of the disease, but the data obtained have been extremely valuable. Fibrinogenopenic blood permits the study of the reac-

Table 17-32. Defects of hemostasis due to abnormalities in phase IV

I. Dysfibrinogenemia
II. Afibrinogenemia and hypofibrinogenemia
   A. Congenital
   B. Simple acquired (without increased fibrinolysis)
      1. Liver disease
      2. Congenital syphilis
      3. Diseases involving bone marrow, spleen, and RES
   C. Diffuse intravascular coagulation (DIC)—consumption coagulopathy
      1. In infectious disease
         a. Sepsis (various organisms)
         b. Gram-negative shock
         c. Viral or rickettsial infections
            (1) Varicella (hemorrhagic, purpura fulminans)
            (2) Generalized vaccinia
            (3) Smallpox
            (4) Rubella (hemorrhagic)
            (5) Rubeola (hemorrhagic black measles)
            (6) Generalized herpes zoster
            (7) Hemorrhagic fevers (Thailand, Bolivian, Argentinian, Philippine, Kyasanur Forest disease)
            (8) Rocky Mountain spotted fever
            (9) Scrub typhus
            (10) Viral hepatitis
      2. In obstetric complications
         a. Premature separation of placenta
         b. Retained dead fetus or placental tissue
         c. Septic abortion
         d. Amniotic fluid embolism
         e. Hydatidiform mole
         f. Placenta previa
         g. Placenta accreta
         h. Eclampsia
         i. Ruptured uterus
         j. Cesarean section
      3. In intravascular hemolysis
         a. Hemolytic transfusion reaction
         b. Acute hemolytic anemias (except PNH)
         c. Venomous snake bite
         d. Hypotonic hemolysis (intravenous hypotonic solution, transurethral prostatectomy)
      4. In neoplasms
         a. Acute leukemia (acute progranulocytic)
         b. Lymphomas
         c. Carcinoma (pancreas, prostate, ovary, breast, bladder, stomach)
         d. Neuroblastoma, metastatic
         e. Rhabdomyosarcoma, metastatic
         f. Kasabach-Merritt syndrome
         g. Hemangiomatous transformation of the spleen or liver
      5. In autoimmune disease and hypersensitivity reactions
         a. Drug reactions
         b. Lupus erythematosus
         c. Acute glomerulonephritis
         d. Renal homograft rejection
         e. Other autoimmune reactions
      6. Postoperative
         a. Pulmonary surgery
         b. Shock
      7. In benign tumor (giant cavernous hemangioma of liver, Kasabach-Merritt syndrome)
      8. Miscellaneous
         a. Heat stroke
         b. Extensive burns
         c. Cyanotic congenital heart disease
         d. Sarcoidosis
         e. Hyaline membrane disease
         f. Asphyxia (newborn)
         g. Combat casualties
         h. Hypobaric erythrocytosis (experimental)
         i. Fat embolism
         j. Dissecting aneurism of aorta
         k. Amyloidosis
III. Increased fibrinolytic activity (primary)
   A. Cirrhosis of liver
   B. Acute hemorrhage
   C. Severe burns
   D. Shock
   E. Heat stroke
   F. Barbiturate poisoning
   G. Methyl alcohol intoxication
   H. Stress (fear, convulsive shock, emotional)
   I. Congenital heart disease
   J. Therapeutic administration of fibrinolytic agents
IV. Interference with fibrin polymerization
   A. Multiple myeloma
   B. Macroglobulinemia
   C. Cryoglobulinemia
V. Deficiency of factor XIII (fibrin-stabilizing factor)

tions by which thrombin is formed, without the complication of fibrin clots being formed (Alexander et al, 1954).

When fibrinogen is given intravenously to a patient with afibrinogenemia, there is first a rapid shift of fibrinogen from the blood to the extravascular pool. Within 48 hours, only half of the administered fibrinogen can be found in the blood. After this time the fibrinogen concentration in the blood drops logarithmically. The half-life of radioactive-tagged (^{35}S-labeled *dl*-methionine) fibrinogen is 5.6 days. Tagged fibrinogen given to normal subjects has a half-life of about 110 hours and a mean disappearance rate of about 15% per day. Decreased synthesis of fibrinogen, with resulting hypofibrinogenemia, has been found in patients receiving L-asparaginase (Bettigole et al, 1970).

ACQUIRED HYPOFIBRINOGENEMIA. Acquired hypofibrinogenemia is of two general types: simple acquired hypofibrinogenemia caused by deficient synthesis of fibrinogen and hypofibrinogenemia caused by excessive consumption (diffuse intravascular coagulation). Sometimes hypofibrinogenemia is found in conjunction with increased fibrinolytic activity, but this is usually not a true hypofibrinogenemia; the fibrinolysin alters the fibrinogen molecule so that it is unclottable and therefore not measurable by technics based on chemical analysis of the clot.

Fibrinogen is synthesized in the parenchymal cells of the liver, and most instances of chronic acquired hypofibrinogenemia can be attributed to liver disease. In some instances, low plasma fibrinogen concentrations are found

Table 17-33. Molecular variants of fibrinogen

Fibrinogen variant	Reference	Fibrinogen variant	Reference
Amsterdam	Janssen and Vreeken, 1971	Montreal	Lacombe et al, 1973
Baltimore	Beck et al, 1971	Nancy	Streiff et al, 1971
Bethesda I	Gralnick et al, 1971	New York	Al-Mondhiry et al, 1975
Bethesda II	Gralnick et al, 1973	Oklahoma	Hampton, 1968
Buenos Aires II	Amsellem et al, 1978	Oslo	Egeberg, 1967
Cleveland I	Forman et al, 1968	Paris I	Mosesson et al, 1976
Cleveland II	Crum et al, 1974	Paris II	Samama et al, 1969
Copenhagen	Hansen et al, 1980	Paris IV	Amsellem et al, 1978
Detroit	Kudryk et al, 1976	Parma	di Imperato and Dettori, 1958
Giessen I	Krause et al, 1973	Philadelphia	Martinez et al, 1974
Giessen II	Krause et al, 1975	St. Louis	Gaston et al, 1971
Giessen III	Matthias et al, 1977	Troyes	Soria et al, 1972a
Iowa City	Jacobsen and Hoak, 1973	Valencia	Aznar et al, 1974
Lille	Denninger et al, 1978	Vancouver	Jackson and Beck, 1970
London	Lane et al, 1980	Vienna	Mammen, 1974
Los Angeles	Zietz and Scott, 1970	Wiesbaden	Winckelmann, 1973
Louvain	Verhaeghe et al, 1974	Zürich I	von Felten et al, 1969a
Marburg	Fuchs et al, 1977	Zürich II	Funk and Straub, 1970
Metz	Soria et al, 1972b		

in association with bone marrow or splenic involvement by tumor or granuloma. This had led to the supposition that fibrinogen is also synthesized by reticuloendothelial tissue, but studies with antifibrinogen fluorescent antibody show that fibrinogen is present only in liver cells.

Hypofibrinogenemia has been described in congenital syphilis; it may be supposed that here it also reflects involvement of the liver and the RES.

Diffuse intravascular coagulation (DIC)

DEFINITION. The diffuse intravascular coagulation (DIC) syndrome is defined as the sum total of the reactions and consequences related to diffuse intravascular deposition of fibrin. At one time there was confusion in the classification of conditions characterized by various combinations of hypofibrinogenemia, evidence of intravascular coagulation, and increased fibrinolysis. It is now possible to sort out that heterogeneous group into two general groups. One, extremely rare, is characterized by the primary development of a potent fibrinolysin; the other, more common, is the syndrome characterized by DIC (McKay, 1973). In the latter there may be a secondary increase in fibrinolytic activity.

SYNONYMS. Disorders included under the classification DIC are some previously called *acquired afibrinogenemia and hypofibrinogenemia*. Synonyms for DIC are *disseminated fibrin thromboembolism, defibrination syndrome, fibrinolytic thromboembolism, thrombosis-fibrinolysis-thrombocytopenia syndrome*, and *consumption coagulopathy*. In addition to these, *thrombotic thrombocytopenic purpura*, the *microangiopathic hemolytic anemia syndromes*, and the hemorrhagic diathesis associated with *acute progranulocytic leukemia* (p. 724) can be included in this category.

ETIOLOGY. The etiology of the DIC syndrome is varied and the conditions that may be associated with it are listed in Table 17-32.

PATHOGENESIS. In simplest form, DIC is produced when any of several mechanisms activate the coagulation sequence intravascularly. Either the intrinsic or extrinsic system or both are activated. The activation may be localized or generalized. Activation results in the deposition of fibrin within the blood vessels and a diminution of those coagulation factors that are consumed in the course of the clotting reaction. Microthrombi are most frequent in the kidneys, followed by the lungs, spleen, adrenals, heart, brain, and liver, in descending order of frequency (Watanabe et al, 1979).

The reactions that occur in the syndrome are complex. Most are interdependent and interreactive, but for convenience they can be discussed under four headings.

INDUCTION BY ENDOTOXIN. An experimental model for DIC is the effect of injecting endotoxin intravenously into rabbits. If two injections of endotoxin are given 24 hours apart, the second injection produces the Shwartzman reaction. The effects of the first and second injection of endotoxin are diagramed in Fig. 17-49. The first injection serves primarily to produce blockage of the RES; platelet aggregates and some fibrin deposition can be seen in the small vessels of various organs. The second injection produces full-scale intravascular deposition of fibrin, the most characteristic lesion being thrombosis of renal glomerular capillaries. If the RES is blockaded by Thorotrast, only one injection of endotoxin is necessary to produce the Shwartzman reaction.

As shown in Fig. 17-49, endotoxin also activates factor XII, which, in turn, contributes to the formation of thrombin by the intrinsic system and then of thrombi.

The Shwartzman reaction is implicated in the development of DIC in gram-negative septicemia and acute meningococcemia. An example of DIC in gram-negative sepsis is shown in Fig. 17-50. Thrombotic thrombocytopenic purpura may be another example of the Shwartzman reaction in humans (p. 802).

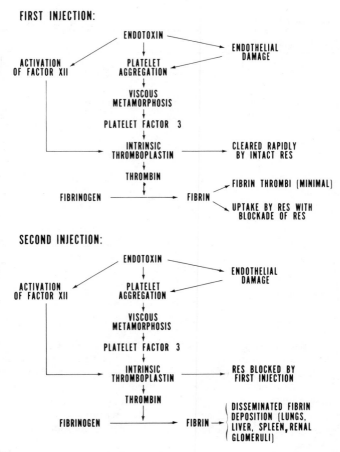

Fig. 17-49. Effect of the first and second injection of endotoxin in production of the Shwartzman reaction. (Based on data from Spaet et al, 1961; McKay, 1965.)

ROLE OF INFLAMMATION. Inflammatory reactions other than those accompanied by endotoxin release can cause DIC by their effect on platelets, by the activation of the intrinsic and extrinsic coagulation process, and by the release of serotonin and the activation of the plasma kinin system.

The response of platelets to various aggregating agents is discussed on p. 799. Products of inflammation such as serotonin and ADP can produce platelet aggregation and activation of the intrinsic system. Other aggregating agents that may be involved in the inflammatory reaction are histamine, immune complexes, and adrenaline.

The plasma kinin system (Fig. 17-14) is related to the intrinsic coagulation system through the shared action of activated factor XII. The kinins have many pharmacologic activities, but in the context of DIC it is the capillary permeability effect that is most important. It is probable that through this effect the products of inflammation diffuse more readily into the blood and then activate the extrinsic coagulation system. The activation of factor XII can be produced by a variety of mechanisms: (1) by endotoxin, as just noted, and (2) by collagen exposed after the endothelial lining of vessels is denuded by endotoxin, other products of inflammation, serotonin, or hypoxia.

ROLE OF IMMUNE REACTIONS. Both specific and nonspecific immune reactions can be involved in DIC. Specific antiplatelet antibodies produce breakdown of platelets, liberation of platelet factor 3, and activation of the intrinsic coagulation system. Immunologic lysis of erythrocytes by antibodies specific for red cell antigens also activates the intrinsic coagulation mechanism through the release of erythrocin and possibly other active phospholipids. The classic example of this is the massive intravascular hemolysis that results from the transfusion of incompatible blood. Note, however, that the most severe expression of DIC secondary to hemolysis occurs when there is the added element of shock. In some instances where there is intravascular hemolysis without shock, as in paroxysmal nocturnal hemoglobinuria, there is no significant DIC. Reactions caused by antiplatelet or antierythrocyte antibodies are not complement dependent.

The immunologic trigger need not be specific in the form of antiplatelet or antierythrocyte antibodies. Immune complexes of various types can attach to and lyse platelets and erythrocytes that act as "innocent bystanders" (Chapter 13). These lytic reactions are complement dependent.

ACTIVATION OF THE EXTRINSIC COAGULATION SYSTEM. Although it is likely that both the intrinsic and the

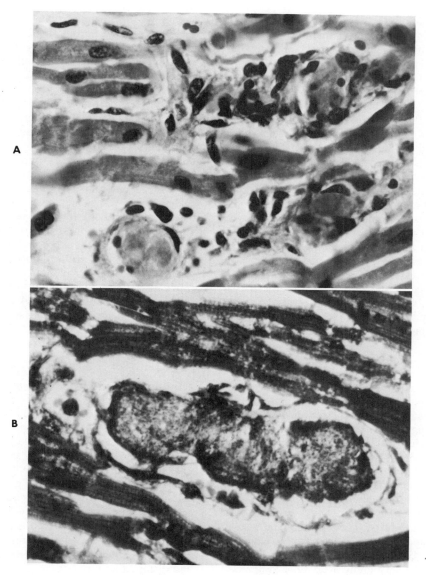

Fig. 17-50. DIC lesions of myocardium in a 2½-week-old infant who died of gram-negative sepsis and DIC. Platelet count 5,000/mm³ (5 × 10⁹/l), fibrinogen not detectable, no end point in prothrombin time and partial thromboplastin time test. (**A,** Hematoxylin-eosin stain; ×450; **B,** phosphotungstic acid–hematoxylin stain; ×450.)

extrinsic coagulation systems are activated in DIC secondary to the inflammatory reaction, there are some situations where the extrinsic system is primarily involved. In such instances, tissue thromboplastin enters the bloodstream, resulting in widely disseminated thrombosis. This mechanism is involved in DIC secondary to obstetric complications (premature separation of the placenta, retained dead fetus or placental tissue, amniotic fluid embolism, etc., Table 17-32). In septic abortion the pathogenesis is related to the endotoxin and inflammation mechanism. Carcinomas, particularly when they are large and have central necrosis, can be accompanied by DIC resulting from the products of tumor necrosis seeping into the blood to act as activators of the extrinsic system.

CLASSIFICATION. In addition to the etiologic classification given in Table 17-32, the DIC syndromes can be classified as *acute* or *chronic* and as *generalized* or *localized*.

Most DIC syndromes are acute, but there may be a chronic course in carcinomatosis. Also, DIC is usually generalized, but there are some important examples of predominantly localized mirothrombosis. Lupus nephritis, glomerulonephritis, and the glomerular thrombosis in the experimental Shwartzman reaction are examples of the localized reaction. With the advent of organ transplants, we have come to appreciate that the transplant rejection reaction is an example of the localized syndrome, triggered in this case by the immunologic mechanism.

LABORATORY DIAGNOSIS. The laboratory findings in the *acute* DIC syndrome are characteristic of a profound hemostatic defect that involves abnormalities in all four phases of blood coagulation. Given an understanding of the pathogenesis of the syndrome, the findings are easily explained. It need not be said that single tests ordered without understanding are certain to be misleading.

As would be expected, acute intravascular coagulation results in a reduction of the involved factors (hence "consumption coagulopathy") and abnormality of tests dependent on these factors. Plasma fibrinogen is reduced, sometimes to extremely low levels; the blood may seem not to form a clot, the formed clot may retract to a small mass, or the fibrinogen screening test will show a reduced concentration of fibrinogen, confirmed by the chemical determination. Factors II, V, and VIII are reduced; in conjunction with the low concentration of fibrinogen, the plasma prothrombin time and partial thromboplastin time tests will give a long clotting time or may show no end point at all. It is important to remember that in some disease states (cancer) and in pregnancy the predisease level of fibrinogen may be twice or more than the usual. The reduction in coagulation factors can be confirmed by specific assays, but this is usually unnecessary. Other coagulation factors may also be diminished, but less predictably. However, factor XIII is always diminished in proportion to the reduction of fibrinogen.

The platelet count is almost always reduced, sometimes to extremely low levels and sometimes out of proportion to the reduction in other factors. This is the result of the platelet aggregation that occupies such a central position in DIC, but in addition, there is increased sequestration of aggregated platelets and trapping of platelets and platelet aggregates in the fibrin network. Here also it is important to remember that some diseases (chronic granulocytic leukemia, myeloproliferative syndromes, cancer) are accompanied by high platelet counts so that there may be a reduction of platelets because of DIC but no thrombocytopenia.

The clotting of fibrinogen is accompanied by the release of fibrinopeptide split products. Their physiologic role is considerable; their diagnostic importance has been exaggerated. They contribute to the pathogenesis of DIC by their action as inhibitors of fibrinogen polymerization. Split products also interfere with platelet aggregation, but this would not seem to be an adverse effect in this situation. The addition of thrombin (diluted to give a normal clotting time of 15 to 18 seconds) to the patient's plasma (thrombin time) will result in a clotting time that is longer than normal because of the inhibitory effect of split products and also because of the reduced concentration of fibrinogen. The usefulness of this test is limited when the concentration of fibrinogen is sufficiently low to account for a long thrombin time regardless of whether inhibitory split products are present. In this case one should perform a thrombin time on a mixture of the patient's plasma and normal plasma to determine if the patient's plasma is inhibitory. The standard cross-recalcification time test for anticoagulant activity is also applicable. Split products can be identified and also measured by using antihuman antiserum (gel diffusion, immunoelectrophoresis, radioimmunoassay, and hemagglutination inhibition). Split products also induce rapid clumping of staphylococci, the so-called staphylococcus clumping test. Other tests that may be useful are the ethanol gelation test and the plasma

protamine paracoagulation test. The ethanol gelation test measures soluble fibrin complexes that the staphylococcus clumping test does not. The protamine paracoagulation test measures fibrin monomers and fibrin fragment X (Fung and Woodson, 1976).

At best, the presence of fibrin split products confirms that there has been cleavage of fibrin. It does not distinguish between the two major syndromes of DIC and primary fibrinolysis. Very powerful fibrinolysins will also cause the release of fibrin split products, although there is some evidence that there may be a difference in the ratio of low– to high–molecular weight products in the two conditions. Furthermore, split products may be present in the serum of normal pregnant women and in various types of renal failure not associated with DIC. It should be apparent that the demonstration of split products does not by itself indicate DIC. It so happens that there are probably 99 cases of DIC for every case of pure primary fibrinolysis; this incidence accounts for the high correlation between the presence of split products and the diagnosis of DIC. Fibrin split products remain in the circulation for 24 to 72 hours after they are released, so their presence does not necessarily indicate that the process of DIC is continuing or that it correlates with the return to normal of fibrinogen, platelets, and coagulation factors.

After DIC is well established, there is usually a secondary activation of the fibrinolytic system. This serves a protective and restorative function and should not be inhibited. Antifibrinolytic therapy (e.g., Amicar) is obviously contraindicated in DIC. In our experience this secondary fibrinolytic activity is not as powerful as that found in the primary fibrinolytic syndromes, and usually the euglobulin lysis time is only moderately prolonged.

Changes in red cell morphology are occasionally helpful. The presence of irregularly contracted erythrocytes and of schizocytes indicates some type of intravascular damage. The damage is mechanical when erythrocytes are pushed through a fibrin network. In microangiopathic hemolytic anemia and the hemolytic-uremic syndrome, fragmented and distorted erythrocytes are usually present. Schizocytes are found in about 10% of other DIC syndromes. The presence of cold-precipitable fibrinogen (cryofibrinogen) is not uncommon in DIC and may be a helpful diagnostic index.

The *acute* syndrome of DIC usually presents little problem in diagnosis. A few problems deserve mention. Based on an understanding of pathogenesis, it should be expected that the abnormality of various laboratory findings will vary depending on the acuteness and severity of the syndrome, the interval between the onset and the laboratory tests, and different rates of return to normal. For example, early in the syndrome, thrombocytopenia and afibrinogenemia may be the most abnormal of the findings. During recovery, assuming that the initial cause of DIC has been removed, the abnormalities may return to normal at different rates, so that the findings might be confusing. Sometimes the platelet count becomes higher than normal during the recovery phase, and such a finding might be confusing. Some reports stress the development of accelerated clotting during the recovery phase.

In the *chronic* DIC syndrome the process of intravascular coagulation and consumption of coagulation factors is low grade, and the laboratory tests may not be as strikingly abnormal as in the acute syndrome. The chronic form of DIC is usually seen in disseminated lupus erythematosus, preeclampsia, thrombotic thrombocytopenic purpura, and the hemolytic-uremic syndrome. Serial activation of the coagulation system may show an "overshoot" of fibrinogen between attacks.

Finally, the therapeutic benefit from anticoagulant therapy with heparin is most remarkable when the triggering stimulus for DIC is no longer operative and there are no other complications. The newborn, for example, is so labile with respect to acid-base balance and oxygen requirements that these must be well regulated if therapy for DIC is to be completely effective. The same applies to treatment of any other underlying disease responsible for DIC. Some of the so-called therapeutic failures are attributable to the false hope that heparin alone will work miracles (Green et al, 1972).

Increased fibrinolytic activity

Increased fibrinolytic activity (primary, not part of the DIC syndrome) is seen in shock, acute hemorrhage, cirrhosis of the liver, barbiturate poisoning, methyl alcohol intoxication, and severe anxiety states such as occur during air raids and examinations. Rarely, acute leukemia and carcinomatosis are accompanied by extremely strong fibrinolytic activity without evidence of DIC. Not uncommonly, excessive fibrinolytic activity is seen in normal persons for no apparent reason.

When there is very powerful fibrinolytic activity, the fibrinolysin has both a fibrinolytic and fibrinogenolytic effect. Hyperfibrinolysis reduces the levels of factors I, II, and V. As a result, there is hypofibrinogenemia and prolongation of the plasma prothrombin time and partial thromboplastin time, and fibrin split products can be demonstrated. It will be noted that the pattern is similar to that in DIC, but some differences are usually helpful.

The clotting tests are seldom as prolonged in hyperfibrinolysis as they are in DIC, for the reduction in factors II and V is not as great as when they are used up in intravascular coagulation. Factor VIII levels are normal in hyperfibrinolysis but decreased in DIC. The presence of fibrin split products does not distinguish one condition from the other. There is evidence, however, that the split products produced by thrombin action and those produced by fibrinolysin are qualitatively different. When fibrinolysin (plasmin) attacks fibrinogen, a series of fragments are formed. Fragment X is a large fibrinogen derivative that is subsequently cleaved into a high molecular fragment Y and a low molecular fragment D. Fragment Y is further split into additional D fragments and low–molecular weight E fragments. Fragment X is clottable by thrombin, but fragments D and E are not. On the other hand, the action of thrombin on fibrinogen results in the formation of fibrinopeptides A and B.

As noted earlier (Fig. 17-49), DIC is usually accompanied by moderate to severe thrombocytopenia. In hyperfibrinolysis syndromes the platelet count is usually normal but there is an important exception. Fibrinogen split products

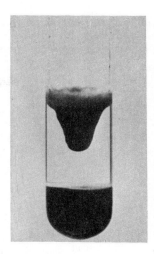

Fig. 17-51. Increased fibrinolysis; 24-hour incubation at 37° C.

can cause platelet aggregation, and it is possible to have thrombocytopenia when the fibrinolytic process is so severe that there is a high concentration of fibrinogen split products. The thrombocytopenia, however, is fortunately less common than in DIC.

Probably the most helpful tests are those which measure the fibrinolytic system. If clotted blood is incubated at 37° C, it is sometimes possible to establish the presence of a powerful fibrinolysin by observing that the clot gradually lyses (Fig. 17-51). The euglobulin lysis test measures plasminogen activators and plasmin; in primary hyperfibrinolysis the test gives rapid lysis, while in secondary fibrinolysis in the late stage of DIC it is only moderately abnormal. It is also helpful to remember that a secondary increase in fibrinolysin in DIC occurs after the syndrome is well established, so that clinical correlation should play an important role in interpreting the laboratory results.

It may be helpful to remember that, while changes in erythrocyte morphology and the presence of cryofibrinogen may be found in DIC, they are not a feature of the hyperfibrinolytic state.

ε-Aminocaproic acid (EACA) is being used as an inhibitor of fibrinolysis (Bennett and Ogston, 1973). It is a synthetic amino acid similar to lysine but lacking the α-amino group. Since activators of plasminogen act by splitting lysine bonds in the plasminogen molecule, it is thought that EACA and lysine act as competitive inhibitors. It is effective but it must be used only when the increased fibrinolytic activity is primary and not associated with DIC (Prentice, 1975).

Summary: differentiation of DIC from hyperfibrinolysis

It is not always easy to distinguish between the two syndromes, but fortunately certain patterns are predictable (Table 17-34). I would emphasize that the diagnosis begins at the bedside and it is there that the suspicion is aroused that one or the other situation is likely. Evidence of abnormal

Table 17-34. Differentiation of acute DIC and hyperfibrinolysis

Test	DIC	Hyperfibrinolysis
Prothrombin time	Prolonged	Prolonged
Partial thrombo-plastin time	Prolonged	Prolonged
Fibrinogen concentration	Low	Low
Thrombin time	Prolonged	Prolonged
Platelet count	Usually low	Usually normal
Fibrinogen split products	Present	Present
Euglobulin lysis time	Usually normal	Prolonged
Cryofibrinogen	Present	Absent
Erythrocyte morphology	Sometimes abnormal	Normal

bleeding plus thrombosis or thromboembolism indicates DIC. The existence of a disease known to predispose to DIC is another helpful criterion. Not too much reliance should be placed on the presence of fibrinogen degradation products only in making a diagnosis of DIC. Finally, it should be noted that primary hyperfibrinolysis is extremely rare and that antifibrinolytic therapy should be used only when there is no evidence of DIC.

Immunoglobulinopathies

Some persons with multiple myeloma, cryoglobulinemia, or macroglobulinemia show hemorrhagic tendencies related in part to interference with the thrombin-fibrinogen reaction. Purpura may be caused by increased vascular fragility or thrombocytopenia, but there is also interference with spontaneous blood coagulation.

When an abnormal concentration of immunoglobulin is present (Chapter 16), there is interference with the conversion of fibrinogen to fibrin. The clot that forms spontaneously in vitro is gelatinous, fails to retract, and histologically does not show the normal fibrin strands. Absence of clot retraction is seen even when the platelet count is normal. When thrombin is added to plasma containing abnormal globulin, the clotting time is much longer than normal; when the plasma is diluted, the thrombin time is restored to normal. Mixtures of normal and abnormal plasma confirm the clot-retarding effect of abnormal globulins.

In our experience the results of other coagulation studies are often confusing; e.g., the one-stage prothrombin time can be prolonged, not because of a defect in phase III but because the abnormal globulin acts like an antithrombin. The determination of prothrombin consumption is often difficult because the gelatinous nature of the blood clot makes it difficult to obtain serum.

Deficiency of factor XIII

About 65 families with congenital deficiency of factor XIII have been described (McDonagh et al, 1974). Factor XIII is required for the cross-linking of fibrin. The deficiency is congenital, shows no sex preference, and has caused (1) bleeding from the umbilical cord, (2) hematomas, (3) bleeding after trauma (abnormal wound healing with severe scarring has been reported in some patients [Amris and Ranek, 1965]), and (4) prepartal and postpartum bleeding. All of the laboratory tests are normal except for the specific assays for factor XIII (Fig. 17-52). An instance of bleeding caused by an inhibitor of factor XIII is reported by Godal (1970) and McDevitt et al (1972). Factor XIII is moderately reduced in sepsis, multiple fractures, and DIC when quantified by the specific dansyl cadaverine method (Hedner et al, 1975). The defect is readily corrected by transfusing fresh or frozen plasma.

Summary

The differential diagnosis of phase IV abnormalities is given in Table 17-35.

HEMORRHAGIC DISORDERS CAUSED BY VASCULAR DEFECTS

As our knowledge of hemostasis increases, the number of hemorrhagic disorders thought to be caused by primary vascular damage decreases. Granting that there are some persons who have easy bruising or purpura without any demonstrable abnormalities ("purpura simplex," etc.), some can be better categorized when platelet function and other studies are done. The disorders discussed here are those in which we can believe vascular integrity to be at fault.

Scurvy

The integrity of the capillary wall depends in part on the presence of a "cement substance" between individual endothelial cells and in part on the juxtacapillary "ground substance" (Chambers and Zeveifack, 1947). Both contain hyaluronic acid. Experimentally, a local application of hyaluronidase has been shown to produce hemorrhage at the metarteriole of the exposed mesoappendix of the rat. Vitamin C (ascorbic acid) is one of the substances required for the synthesis of hyaluronic acid; the purpura associated with scurvy (ascorbic acid deficiency) (Fig. 17-53) can be explained on the basis of defective cement and ground substances (Frederici et al, 1966) or defective collagen synthesis (Bevelaqua et al, 1976) and will respond to the administration of vitamin C. While this explains the bleeding in scurvy, in other syndromes there is no demonstrable deficiency of vitamin C, and administration of this vitamin has no effect.

Hereditary hemorrhagic telangiectasia

Hereditary hemorrhagic telangiectasia (Rendu-Osler-Weber disease) is clearly distinguishable from other vascular defects. It is inherited as an autosomal dominant of high penetrance (Bird and Jaques, 1959), though a few cases are recorded in which the family was normal. The disease is characterized by nodular or spider-like telangiectasias that may be found on the skin and mucosal surfaces (Fig. 17-54). The lesions can be found in internal organs, most often the gastrointestinal tract and lungs (Ecker et al, 1960), but also in other organs. Bleeding from an abnormal area is com-

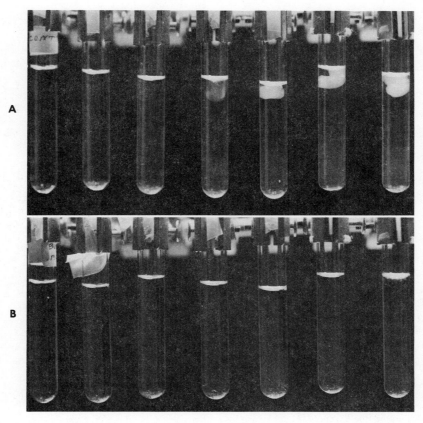

Fig. 17-52. Clot-solubility test for factor XIII (see method in Appendix). **A,** Normal test. **B,** Patient deficient in factor XIII.

Table 17-35. Differential diagnosis of defects in phase IV*

Test	Hypofibrinogenemia	Afibrinogenemia	Increased fibrinolysin	Deficiency of factor XIII†
Bleeding time	Normal	Normal or prolonged	Normal or prolonged	Normal
Coagulation time	Prolonged	Blood does not clot	Normal or prolonged	Normal
Clot retraction	Small clot; may be confused with lysis	No clot	Clot lysis	Normal
Prothrombin time	Prolonged	No end point	Normal‡	Normal
Assays for prothrombin, factor V, and factor VII	Normal	Normal	Normal‡	Normal
Plasma + thrombin	Small clot; time prolonged	No clot forms	Normal§	Normal
Fibrinogen (chemical determination)	Reduced below 60 to 100 mg/100 ml	Absent	Normal or reduced	Normal
Fibrinolysin titer	Normal	Normal	Increased	Normal

*See Table 17-34 for differentiation of DIC from hyperfibrinolysis.
†Only abnormality present (solubility of clot in urea or monochloroacetic acid) must be specifically tested.
‡Abnormal if fibrinolysin is sufficiently powerful to destroy fibrinogen and other factors.
§Abnormal if fibrinolysin is sufficiently powerful to produce a high concentration of split products or reduced fibrinogen concentration.

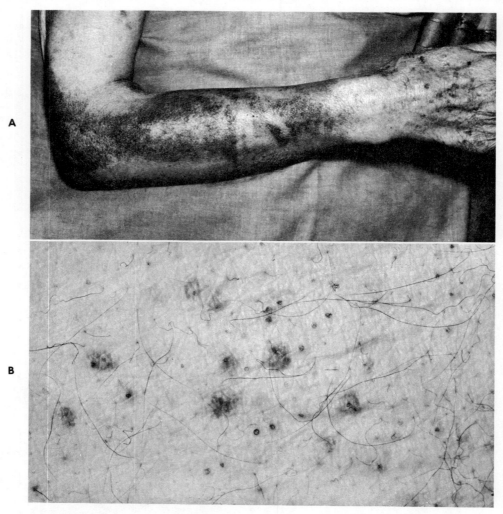

Fig. 17-53. Purpura due to scurvy. **A,** Subcutaneous ecchymoses and purpura. **B,** Close-up showing the typical perifollicular hemorrhages.

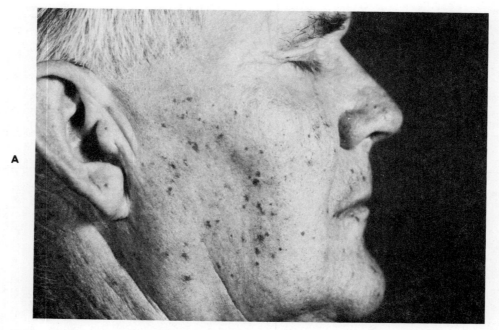

Fig. 17-54. Hereditary hemorrhagic telangiectasia. **A,** Face; **B,** close-up of skin lesions; **C,** tongue; and **D,** lip.

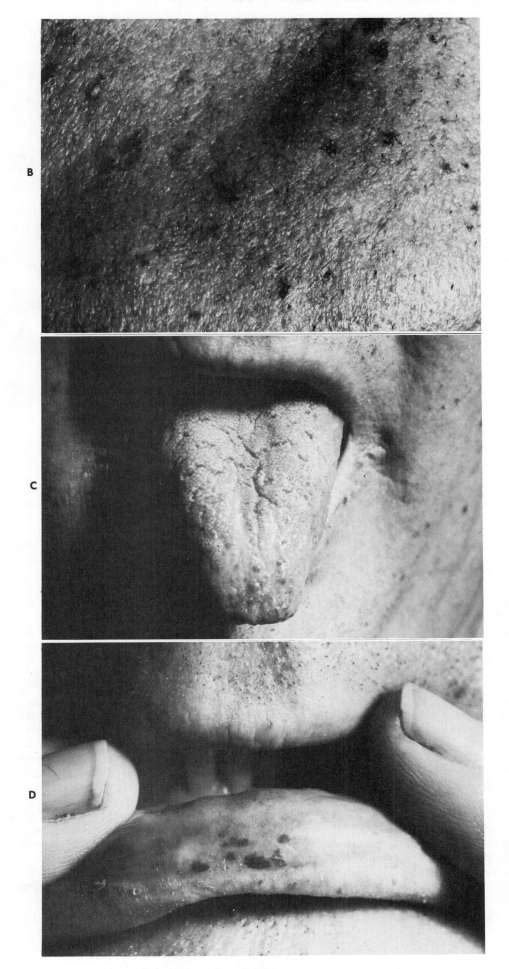

Fig. 17-54, cont'd. For legend see opposite page.

mon. When accessible it can be controlled by pressure; internal bleeding, when severe, becomes a surgical problem.

Thrombotic thrombocytopenic purpura

Thrombotic thrombocytopenic purpura (TTP), or "Moschkovitz syndrome," is classified here as a vascular abnormality on the basis of intimal and subintimal changes that are thought to be the primary lesion (Feldman et al, 1966). Because thrombocytopenia is an almost constant finding, it is sometimes classified as a thrombocytopenic purpura. Because there is intravascular aggregation of platelets and disposition of fibrin, it also has some of the features of DIC. The thrombocytopenia is assumed to have an immunologic basis (Mant et al, 1972; Weisenburger et al, 1976; Heyns et al, 1979). Biopsy of gingival tissue shows the typical histopathologic features in about half the cases (Goodman et al, 1978).

TTP differs from other similar disorders in several ways. The anatomic lesions seem to be characteristic, consisting of proliferation of endothelial cells, aggregation of platelets, occlusion of small vessels by hyalin-like material consisting in part of fibrin, and the deposition of similar material in the subendothelium. Based on these findings it is logical to hypothesize that the vascular lesions are primary, that they lead to platelet aggregation, thrombocytopenia, and the production of a DIC-like syndrome.

Clinically, the disease is almost always rapidly fatal, shows variable response to heparin therapy, and probably responds best to the combination of splenectomy plus steroids (Amorosi and Ultmann, 1966) or, more recently, to transfusion of plasma, exchange transfusion, and antiplatelet drugs (Eckel et al, 1977; Pisciotta et al, 1977; Peterson et al, 1979). Almost all patients show a syndrome of fever, thrombocytopenia, hemolytic anemia (antiglobulin negative), renal disease, and neurologic signs. At necropsy, microvascular occlusion is found in almost all organs. The etiology of TTP is unknown. In view of its rarity, the occurrence of the disease in siblings (Paz et al, 1969) and in a husband and wife (Watson and Cooper, 1971) as coincidence is unlikely. In one case there was coexistence of giant lymph node hyperplasia and thrombotic thrombocytopenic purpura (Couch, 1980).

Allergic purpura

The term "allergic purpura" (anaphylactoid purpura, Henoch-Schönlein purpura) is applied to a syndrome consisting of purpura and systemic manifestation such as abdominal or joint pain (Ruhrmann, 1963). It frequently follows infectious diseases. The platelet count and coagulation studies are normal. Many cases placed in this group are caused by drug hypersensitivity (Ackroyd, 1953).

Connective tissue disorders

The dermatologist recognizes a group of skin diseases called "pigmented purpuric eruptions" (Shamberg's progressive pigmentary dermatitis, angioma serpiginosum, Majocchi's disease, pigmented purpuric lichenoid dermatitis) (Herzberg, 1968). In the Ehlers-Danlos syndrome (Fig. 17-55), subcutaneous and other types of hemorrhages are

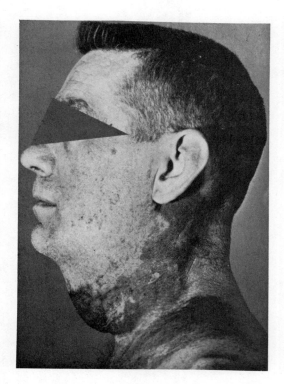

Fig. 17-55. Ehlers-Danlos syndrome. (Courtesy Dr. August Miale, Jr.)

caused by a combination of increased vascular fragility plus various coagulation abnormalities (Goodman et al, 1962; Robitaille, 1964; Mason and Rigby, 1965).

Autoerythrocyte sensitization

This unusual disorder is difficult to categorize. It is usually encountered in middle-aged women, and ecchymoses, supposedly not resulting from trauma, are preceded by a stinging or painful sensation (Ratnoff and Agle, 1968). The ecchymoses can be reproduced by intradermal injection of the patient's own red blood cells or hemolysate. The only patient I have studied who showed all these features was a neurotic lady whose ecchymoses were strikingly symmetric and suggested self-induced lesions.

The prethrombotic ("hypercoagulable") state

The study of detectable changes in the blood in thromboembolic disease involves two very different situations, abnormalities in established thrombosis and abnormalities when a subject is at risk from thrombosis. Because there are measurable abnormalities in some cases of established thrombosis, it is sometimes assumed that the same changes in blood have predictive value in the subject who will develop thrombosis (Collins et al, 1976). In fact, the literature is replete with reviews of the so-called hypercoagulation state that do not distinguish between the two situations and as a consequence often use the term "hypothetical hypercoagulation state." Since there is nothing hypothetical about established thrombosis, it is obvious that the problem is the identification of the subject at risk from thrombosis, the *prethrombotic* state.

Subjects at risk from thrombosis fall into two categories: (1) those who have an underlying disease that predisposes to thrombosis, and (2) those who are clinically healthy but who will develop thrombosis.

The two most common situations predisposing to thrombosis are malignancies and surgical procedures. Over 100 years ago, Trousseau pointed out that "phlebitis" should suggest the possibility of occult cancer. The association of malignancy and thrombosis has been reported many times since (Pochedly et al, 1973; Brodsky, 1974; Reagan and Okazaki, 1974; Sun et al, 1974; Lipinska et al, 1976), especially in carcinoma of the pancreas, where the incidence of venous thrombosis may be as high as 50% (Sproul, 1938). Cancers of the lung (Fisher et al, 1951), ovary (Henderson, 1955), or stomach (Fisch et al, 1951) also have a high incidence of venous thrombosis. The high incidence of thrombosis in mucin-producing carcinomas is attributed to the activation of factor X by mucin (Pineo et al, 1974; Rohner et al, 1967). Tumor extracts other than mucin also activate factor X directly (Gordon et al, 1975).

Thrombosis is one of the complications of the postoperative state (Madden and Hume, 1976). The incidence in orthopedic procedures varies from 35% to 57% and is about 25% in major abdominal or thoracic surgery. Predisposing factors are previous venous thrombosis, varicose veins, obesity, malignancy, and age older than 61 (Kakkar, 1972).

Some of the abnormalities found in established thrombosis, especially when it is extensive or disseminated, as in DIC, are the result of thrombus formation and not the cause. For example, the presence of degradation products of fibrinogen or fibrin indicate that thrombosis has already taken place. Likewise, fibrinogen, factor V, or factor VIII may be nonspecific reactants, so that elevation of their concentration in blood may be reactive rather than causal.

There are also important quantitative considerations. Whereas extensive disseminated thrombosis is usually accompanied by measurable changes in the blood, such is usually not the case when a small thrombus is formed, possibly because the changes are too small to be quantified by currently available techniques. Likewise, the prethrombotic state may well be accompanied by some alterations too subtle to measure.

Keeping these reservations in mind, we can look at various points in the hemostatic system and consider whether any of the described abnormalities apply to the identification of the prethrombotic state.

Platelets

PLATELET COUNT. In a normal person the total platelet pool is about 750 billion platelets. Even with a portion of the pool sequestered in the spleen and other sites, the number of platelets in circulating blood is in the billions. Widespread acute intravascular coagulation is accompanied by a significant reduction in the platelet count, but the formation of a localized thrombus does not involve enough platelets to reduce the count. By the same token, thrombocytopenia is not an indication of the prethrombotic state.

On the other hand, thrombocytosis in the myeloproliferative syndrome or following splenectomy is often associated with thrombosis (Hirsh and Dacie, 1966; Virmani et al,

1979). In polycythemia vera there is also an increase in the red cell mass, hematocrit, and blood viscosity (Dintenfass, 1966), and a subject with both thrombocytosis and a high hematocrit with increased viscosity must be considered a candidate for thrombosis (Dormandy, 1980). I believe it is fair to say that thrombocytosis is an indication of the prethrombotic state and may in fact be the only platelet abnormality unequivocally related to thrombosis.

PLATELET ADHESIVENESS. Platelet adhesiveness as measured with glass bead columns is admittedly difficult to standardize and reproduce (Bowie and Owen, 1971), although some investigators have confidence in this method (Bowie and Owen, 1973). In my laboratory, we have replaced this method with the in vivo technique described by Borchgrevink (1960a) because we find it to be more sensitive and specific for measuring decreased adhesiveness in a variety of thrombocytopathies. Neither test has proved to have value in either established thrombosis or in the prethrombotic state.

PLATELET AGGREGATION. Enhanced platelet aggregation using standard amounts of various aggregating agents has been reported in some patients having a variety of diseases: in diabetes with vascular complications (Kwaan et al, 1972; Sagel et al, 1975), in type II hyperbetalipoproteinemia (Carvalho et al, 1974a; Carvalho et al, 1974b), in angina pectoris (Salky and Dugdale, 1973), and in survivors of myocardial infarction (Frishman et al, 1974). It is unwarranted to attach great significance to these reports, given the striking variability in response found in even normal subjects to the same concentrations of aggregating agents. Some of the observed responses in disease states may be attributed to failure to adjust the citrate concentration according to the hematocrit when the patient is anemic (Kelton et al, 1980).

Some investigators have attempted to detect "hyperaggregability" by using low concentrations of aggregating agents (Collins et al, 1976; Colman, 1978), but there are no standard criteria for establishing the effective low concentrations of aggregating agents (Salky and Dugdale, 1973; Frishman et al, 1974; O'Malley et al, 1975; Lake et al, 1977). In my laboratory, all attempts to detect hyperaggregability by low concentrations of ADP or epinephrine have failed.

Perhaps more significant is the detection of autoaggregation, i.e., in the absence of added aggregating agents. Normally, untreated platelet-rich plasma in an aggregometer shows less than 10% aggregation after 10 to 15 minutes. Increased autoaggregation has been found in some cases of thrombocythemia (Preston et al, 1974) and thrombocytosis (Vreeken and vanAken, 1971), in about one-third of diabetic patients (O'Malley et al, 1975), and in patients with arterial insufficiency (Wu and Hoak, 1976). While there is no evidence that autoaggregation precedes the thrombotic state, I believe that this test should be done whenever platelet aggregation studies are performed.

It has been suggested that spontaneous platelet aggregation occurs in vivo in various vascular disorders (Wu and Hoak, 1974; Fleischman et al, 1975; Kalendovsky et al, 1975; Wu and Hoak, 1975; Wu et al, 1976). Since platelet aggregates can only be detected after the blood is drawn, it may not be warranted to extrapolate in vitro findings to the in vivo status, particularly when dealing with platelets. Even so, the presence of platelet aggregation is not a constant finding in vascular disease, and there is no evidence that it has predictive value.

PLATELET SURVIVAL AND TURNOVER. Some investigators have found that in various vascular diseases there is in some cases decreased platelet survival measured by injection of ^{51}Cr-labeled autologous platelets (Harker and Slichter, 1970, 1972b, 1974; Steele et al, 1973) or by measuring the time required for platelets to return to normal after aspirin ingestion (Schwartz, 1974; Stuart et al, 1975). There is no evidence that decreased survival or increased turnover is an indicator of the prethrombotic state.

COMPONENTS OF THE RELEASE REACTION. Two components of the release reaction have been studied in thromboembolic disease, platelet factor 4 (PF$_4$) and β-thromboglobulin.

Elevated levels of PF$_4$, measured usually as antiheparin activity, have been found in a variety of vascular disorders (Okuno and Crockatt, 1977). There is no doubt that a significant number of platelets must release their various components before antiheparin activity is measurable. For example, PF$_4$ levels are elevated in immunologic thrombocytopenia (Dana et al, 1976). The specific platelet protein, β-thromboglobulin, is elevated in deep vein thrombosis and pulmonary embolism (Ludlam et al, 1975), but, like PF$_4$, it reflects the breakdown of many platelets and its predictive value is doubtful.

Coagulation factors

It might seem logical to assume that, since a deficiency of coagulation factors leads to hemorrhagic diatheses, an excess of factors or accelerated activation of the factors might lead to thrombosis. However, in spite of some reports that increased levels of factors I, II, V, VII, or VIII are associated with thrombosis (Poller, 1957; Gaston, 1966; Penick et al, 1966; Kropatkin and Izak, 1968; Gjønnaess and Fagerhol, 1974), it is fair to say that no consistent relationship has been found between increased levels of those factors and either established as impending thrombosis. It must be noted that fibrinogen, factor V, and factor VIII levels are elevated nonspecifically in inflammation. Furthermore, given normal ranges of 50% to 150% for most of the coagulation factors, it is difficult to assign great significance to values between 100% and 150%.

However, one coagulation factor, X, is pertinent in thrombotic disease, not because increased levels are associated with thrombosis, but because of the interaction of the activated form, Xa, with the natural serine protease antithrombin, antithrombin III (AT III), also called Xa inhibitor (XaI).

The naturally occurring antithrombins are AT III, α-1 antitrypsin, and C1 inactivator, but the last two are of minor importance (Harpel and Rosenberg, 1976). AT III is responsible for about 75% of the antithrombin activity in plasma (Abildgaard, 1967). It inhibits all of the activated factors (IXa, Xa, XIa, XIIa) as well as thrombin, and the inhibition is increased markedly in the presence of heparin (Wessler and Yin, 1974; Rosenberg, 1975). Since Xa is required for

the conversion of prothrombin to thrombin, a reduction of AT III, its natural inhibitor, should favor thrombosis. In fact, familial AT III deficiency, inherited as an autosomal dominant trait, has been found to be associated with thrombosis (Egeberg, 1965; van der Meer et al, 1973; Marciniak et al, 1974; Gruenberg et al, 1975. This association is so striking that assays of AT III may be of value in detecting the prethrombotic state (Sagar et al, 1976a). At first it was difficult to explain how a 50% reduction in AT III could cause thrombosis, but Reeve (1980) has shown that during factor X activation Xa rises as the simple reciprocal of AT III while thrombin rises as the reciprocal of the square of AT III. Thus the thrombin level doubles at an AT III level of 70% and quadruples at an AT III level of 50%.

The interaction of Xa and AT III deserves some additional comments. It was once thought that the major action of AT III was an inhibitor of Xa rather than of thrombin directly, but it has been shown that purified human AT III inactivates thrombin at a higher rate than it inactivates Xa (Odegard and Lie, 1978). Also, molecular variants of AT III, such as AT III Budapest (Sas et al, 1975) and others (Sørensen et al, 1980) are characterized by a normal level of immunologically detectable protein and decreased antithrombic activity. Another variant has shown a normal amount of AT III but a decreased rate of interaction with Xa (Gitel et al, 1978).

The value of another coagulation test, the activated partial thromboplastin time (APTT) seems well documented. It has been shown that an APTT of less than 28 seconds (with a reagent giving a mean normal of 37 seconds) in postoperative patients is a good indication that there is a risk of thrombosis (McKenna et al, 1977).

Products of fibrinogen to fibrin conversion or fibrinolysis

Thrombin cleaves fibrinogen into fibrin monomers and fibrinopeptides A and B. Digestion of fibrin by plasmin produces different cleavage products, X, Y, D, and E, having progressively smaller molecular weights. Fibrinopeptide A is elevated in cellulitis, various infectious processes, and LE (Nossel, 1976). Fibrin monomers copolymerize with intermediate fibrin polymers, fibrinogen, and fibrin degradation products and are probably best identified by gel exclusion chromatography (Fletcher and Alkjaersig, 1972). In any case, there must be a significant amount of fibrinogenolysis by thrombin before fibrinopeptide A or fibrin monomers are present in abnormal amounts, and there is no evidence that such elevations are of predictive value. The same is true of fibrin degradation products produced by the action of plasmin, with the possible reservation that increased levels of soluble complexes are reported in women taking oral contraceptives (Alkjaersig et al, 1975) and in patients with coronary artery disease (Anayo-Galindo et al, 1976).

The common screening tests for split products and fibrin degradation products (staphylococcus clumping, protamine sulfate paracoagulation, and ethanol gelation) are positive only when there is extensive thrombosis. Radioimmunoassays of fibrinopeptide A and fragment E are more sensitive but not so sensitive as to be positive when there is only a small thrombus. The same is true of gel exclusion chromatography, but the technique is more difficult and not yet recommended for other than research purposes. There is no evidence that any of these tests will detect a prethrombotic state (Johnston et al, 1980).

Reduced fibrinolytic activity

Activation of the fibrinolytic system is one of the natural mechanisms for minimizing thrombosis or for dissolving thrombi. Most probably, there is normally a balanced equilibrium between fibrinogen, fibrin, and fibrin monomers, shifted toward fibrin monomers at sites of incipient fibrin deposition by the release of plasminogen from neighboring endothelial cells.

Reduced fibrinolytic activity, then, favors thrombus deposition. Reduced fibrinolytic activity may be caused by an increase in inhibitors of plasmin: α-2-macroglobulin, AT III, α-1-antitrypsin and C1 inactivator.

There is good evidence that reduced fibrinolytic activity may precede thrombosis and so may be useful in detecting a prethrombotic state. Decreased fibrinolytic activity has been found in women taking oral contraceptives (Åstedt et al, 1973), in pregnancy (Åstedt, 1972), in postoperative patients (Ygge, 1970), and in obesity (Almer and Janzon, 1975). In one study it was found that the risk of thrombosis was greater in patients having high α-1 antitrypsin levels (Gallus et al, 1973a). In two other series the patients at risk had prolonged euglobulin lysis times (Mansfield, 1972; Gordon-Smith et al, 1974). It is noteworthy that fibrinolytic activity is less in leg veins than in arm veins (Robertson et al, 1972), and this parallels the rarity of venous thrombosis in arm veins.

Serum lipoproteins

In type II familial hyperbetalipoproteinemia there is a high incidence of vascular disease (Jensen et al, 1967; Slack, 1969), especially stroke (deGennes et al, 1968; Colman, 1978). It is advisable to investigate the family, since homozygotes are more subject to thrombotic disease than are heterozygotes.

Hyperaggregability of platelets has been reported (Carvalho et al, 1974a), possibly because the platelet membrane adsorbs a great deal of β-lipoprotein from the plasma (Shattil et al, 1977).

Conclusion

It is clear at this time that no single test can be counted on to detect the prethrombotic state. The following six determinations as a group are recommended:
1. Platelet count
2. Hematocrit
3. Activated partial thromboplastin time
4. Antithrombin III
5. Plasma fibrinolytic activity
6. Lipoprotein fractionation

These tests are indicated particularly in clinical situations known to have a high incidence of thrombosis. I believe, also, that it will be important to study a group of individuals serially over a period of years, since a shift of the test values from an individual's baseline may be more informative than one-time testing.

LABORATORY DIAGNOSIS OF HEMORRHAGIC DISORDERS

In spite of the many uncertainties of the basic mechanisms of hemostasis, a fairly rational and systematic approach to the laboratory diagnosis can be made.

Problems of hemostasis are presented to the clinical pathologist for various reasons. A patient may be actively bleeding or have a history of abnormal bleeding, sometimes familial. In some instances, tests for hemostatic integrity are routinely ordered prior to surgery to determine beforehand if the patient has an abnormal tendency to bleed. In other cases, one or more laboratory tests indicate that there may be a problem of abnormal hemostasis, and it is then necessary to determine, first, if such is the case and, second, what disease the patient has. Last, there is the common problem of laboratory control of anticoagulant therapy.

Experience has led us to group these problems in three categories: (1) preoperative tests of hemostatic function, (2) laboratory control of anticoagulant therapy, and (3) investigation of patients having a manifest or suspected hemorrhagic disorder.

Preoperative tests

Until a few years ago it was considered good medical practice to perform bleeding time and clotting time tests on patients scheduled for surgery. I am not sure when these tests were first advocated as a "routine" preoperative procedure, but I am sure that this routine was adopted because some patients had suffered severe or fatal postoperative bleeding.

It has been interesting to observe the illogical sequence of events that has culminated in the recommendation that routine tests should be abandoned. First, we find the methods modified to the point of unreliability; witness the relaxation of technic in doing a proper bleeding time, the adoption of worthless "short-cut" methods of determining what can only be facetiously called the "coagulation time"—capillary tube methods, puddle-the-blood-on-the-slide methods and even "refinements" of these. As a result, whatever value the basic tests may have had was destroyed. The next step, that preoperative tests are unreliable and unnecessary, is obviously illogical. Preoperative screening for hemorrhagic disease is as desirable and necessary now as it was some years ago.

Granted, the short-cut methods were adopted, in part, because of the difficulty of obtaining venous blood from infants and children. What was needed were reliable methods that utilized blood obtained by skin puncture. Such methods have been developed in our laboratory and in our opinion provide a reliable routine for preoperative screening.

The most valuable of these is the *micro-partial thromboplastin* test (Appendix). After the technic was worked out, the test was performed routinely on 681 patients admitted to our hospital for surgery. The results are shown in Fig. 17-56. Six hundred seventy-nine fell within the distribution curve for 387 normal persons. Two fell outside the normal range and, on complete investigation, were proved to have classic hemophilia. One of the two was an infant scheduled for circumcision, and it is interesting to note that a normal

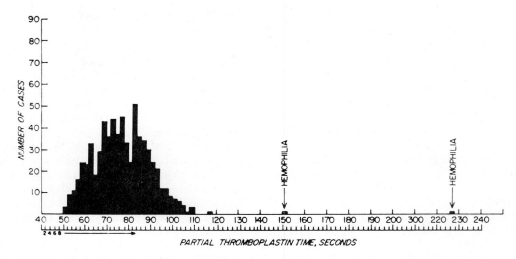

Fig. 17-56. Distribution of micro-partial thromboplastin time (PTT, nonactivated) in 681 presurgery patients. The two patients with prolonged times were later proved to have classic hemophilia.

result had been obtained when a capillary clotting time test was done.

The other microtechnic developed in our laboratory is the *micro-prothrombin time* (Appendix). This technic is a reliable and completely comparable substitute for the standarad one-stage prothrombin time performed on venous blood.

Our experience with these tests leads us to propose an approach to the problem of presurgery screening tests:

1. *History and physical examination:* This is most important but does not obviate the need for laboratory tests. The infant just referred to did not have a family history of hemophilia, and many of the hemophiliacs studied in our laboratory have been sporadic cases. When a positive family history is obtained, or when there is a personal history of abnormal bleeding, (purpura, easy bruising, nosebleeds, menstrual difficulty, bleeding after minimal trauma or after surgery, etc.), nothing less than a complete investigation will do. If the family and personal history are negative, the routine that follows should be sufficient.

2. *Auxiliary laboratory studies:* A complete blood count with an estimation of the number of platelets from a properly prepared smear should be performed.

3. *Prothrombin time:* Use the microtechnic in infants and young children.

4. *Partial thromboplastin time:* Use the microtechnic in infants and young children.

5. *Bleeding time:* This is optional but desirable if there is a history of easy bruising. Two of the most severe instances of postoperative bleeding I have seen were in two patients with von Willebrand's disease. One had undergone rhinoplasty and the other a "face-lifting" procedure. In retrospect, each had a history of easy bruising and other abnormalities, but the significance of the history was not appreciated.

Laboratory control of anticoagulant therapy

Two types of anticoagulants are in common clinical use: (1) drugs that lengthen the coagulation time—heparin and synthetic heparin-like drugs and (2) drugs that lengthen the prothrombin time—bishydroxycoumarin and related compounds and the indandione derivatives.

Control of oral anticoagulant therapy

This is discussed on p. 837.

Control of heparin therapy

Heparin acts as an anticoagulant at several points of the coagulation sequence (Yin et al, 1971b). It reacts with antithrombin III as a cofactor to inhibit factor Xa and the other activated factors (IXa, XIa, and XIIa). It also inhibits the formation or the activity of the Xa-V-PF$_3$ complex. These reactions can be said to be antithromboplastic. It also has a direct antithrombic effect (Briginshaw and Shanberge, 1974; Machovich, 1975), and it inhibits the platelet release reaction. In vitro it affects all the coagulation tests. It is generally agreed that the most important effect of heparin is to enhance the effect of antithrombin III, and several mechanisms have been proposed (Rosenberg and Damus, 1973; Machovich, 1975). It is most likely that heparin acts by displacing Xa from the phospholipid complex (Walker and Esmon, 1979).

There are many unresolved questions regarding heparin. In one study (Abbott et al, 1977) in animals it was found that the incidence of hemorrhage was higher following administration of heparin of intestinal mucosal origin compared with that of lung origin. In human subjects, there is a discrepancy between the two types of heparin when the anticoagulant activity is measured by the APTT or the Xa assay (Barrowcliffe et al, 1977), mucosal heparin producing higher blood concentrations than lung heparin when the Xa assay was used. No difference was noted in assays based on the APTT. The implication is that the APTT underestimates the anticoagulant effect if it is assumed that heparin binds to AT III at a 1:1 molecular ratio (Einarsson and Andersson, 1977). However, the clinical importance of which type of heparin is "better" is still unknown.

Because the molecular weight of heparin varies widely

(Jaques, 1979, 1980), crude heparin has been fractionated into fractions of low and high molecular weight, in an attempt to arrive at a uniform product with predictable anticoagulant properties. So far the data are contradictory. Barrowcliffe et al (1977) found that anti-Xa activity increased with low–molecular weight fractions while the APTT activity decreased. Antithrombin III binding of low–and high–molecular weight fractions is the same (Barrowcliffe, 1980). Shanberge et al (1978) found that the high–molecular weight fraction produced a higher and longer-lasting anticoagulant effect. Barrowcliffe et al (1979) found that the low–molecular weight and the high–molecular weight fractions had similar anti-Xa activity but that in the APTT assay the high–molecular weight fraction was about twice as potent. It should be noted that various fractionation technics have been used and the discrepancies may well be related to how the fractions are prepared. There is a considerable variation in the potency of various commercial preparations (Jaques et al, 1973).

In spite of some enthusiasts, we do not use the APTT to control heparin therapy, since we and others (Bern, 1975; Teien and Abildgaard, 1976) have found it to be erratic. More attention should be paid to the difference in heparin sensitivity of various commercial APTT reagents (Sibley et al, 1973). Reagents using elagic acid are notably insensitive, and, in any case, for any series investigating the results of heparin therapy the reagent used should be recorded. In the series reported by Salzman et al (1975), the incidence of bleeding was no less when heparin therapy was monitored with the APTT than when it was not monitored at all. We prefer to monitor heparin therapy with the recalcification time of platelet-rich plasma. It is extremely important to use platelet-rich plasma because the platelets contain antiheparin (factor 4), and platelet-deficient plasma does not reflect the in vivo effect. For the same reason, if the platelet count of the plasma varies from time to time, the recalcification time may appear to be erratic. Gulliani et al (1976) recommend the whole blood recalcification time for monitoring heparin therapy.

Perhaps more important than the test used is an appreciation of the sequence of inhibition with respect to time. If the heparin is given as an intravenous bolus, a maximum anticoagulant effect is reached about 1 hour later, and the effect decays over the next 3 to 4 hours. In this method of heparin therapy, it is obviously important to know when the blood sample is drawn with respect to the time the heparin was infused. Since there is some difference among recipients as to the intensity and the duration of the anticoagulant effect, the first heparin dose should be monitored at 2 and 5 hours and before the next dose for subsequent periods.

More even therapeutic levels are achieved by continuous intravenous drip or infusion (Salzman et al, 1975), which is recommended not only because it is better for the patient but also because it avoids the distrust of the laboratory test, which may seem to be erratic because the blood samples are drawn at random times.

The value of low-dose (mini-dose) heparin therapy is still being debated. Regimens have varied from 2,000 units to 10,000 units of heparin given subcutaneously 1 to 9 hours preoperatively followed by 2,500 to 5,000 units hourly, 6,

8, or 12 hours postoperatively. One other variable is the use of calcium heparin in Europe, whereas in the United States sodium heparin is used (Thomas et al, 1976). In most series the incidence of postoperative thromboembolic disease has been reduced (Kakkar et al, 1972; Gallus et al, 1973b; Sagar et al, 1976b), with some exceptions (Hampson et al, 1974). One of the supposed advantages of low-dose regimens is that laboratory monitoring is not necessary; but, since patients receiving heparin fall into one of three categories (hyporesponders, normoresponders, and hyperresponders) (Brozovic et al, 1975; Gurewich et al, 1978), it is recommended that the response should be monitored, at least at the beginning of the treatment period. There is no agreement as to what test to use. Gurewich et al (1978) use an unspecified APTT reagent supposedly sensitive to as little as 0.05 units of heparin/ml of plasma.

Heparin is neutralized by protamine sulfate. In vitro 1 mg of protamine sulfate neutralizes about 100 USP units of heparin, but this is only a rough guide for the neutralizing dose in vivo (Jaques, 1975). An excess of protamine will result in prolonged PT and APTT tests, but the thrombin time is normalized.

When anticoagulant therapy is begun with heparin and then changed to an oral anticoagulant, the heparin effect should be allowed to end, usually 6 hours after the last dose, before the PT can be used to monitor the oral anticoagulant therapy.

Investigation of a hemorrhagic disorder

The challenge of investigating a hemorrhagic disorder can usually be met without difficulty, provided several considerations are kept in mind: (1) a careful personal and family history should be obtained and a thorough physical examination should be performed; (2) the technics of the blood coagulation tests are performed with the highest degree of accuracy and care; (3) investigations should be done before therapy is given; and (4) a planned outline and sequence of tests should be followed.

Although laboratory diagnosis gives the final answer, the importance of a careful history and physical examination cannot be overemphasized. Bleeding per se does not indicate a hemorrhagic disorder caused by defective hemostasis, nor does the absence of current bleeding rule out an existing disorder. It is essential to know the nature of present or past episodes, the possible inciting causes, the intake of drugs, what therapy was given, and when it was given. A careful family history should be obtained, keeping in mind the inheritance patterns of the hereditary disorders. The physical examination should include a careful inspection of the skin surface and mucous membranes. Physical evidence of blood dyscrasias such as lymphadenopathy, hepatomegaly, and splenomegaly should be looked for. It is our practice to follow a set routine of laboratory studies as indicated by the history, and to collect such blood at one time as will provide the specimens needed for the necessary tests. The advantages of following a given routine are several. We like to repeat basic tests such as the blood count because it would be foolish to do elaborate tests without first doing the simple ones that give information as to the presence of anemia or leukemia. In addition, the preliminary data often suggest the

Table 17-36. Recurrent patterns in typical hemorrhagic disorders

Test	Defect in phase I	Defect in phase II	Defect in phase III	Defect in phase IV
Bleeding time	Prolonged[a]	Normal or prolonged	Normal[b]	Normal[b]
Coagulation time	Normal	Prolonged	Normal[b]	Prolonged[c]
Clot retraction	Poor	Normal	Normal	Increased[d]
Tourniquet test	Positive[e]	Negative[f]	Negative[f]	Negative
Platelet count	<100,000[g]	Normal	Normal	Normal
Prothrombin time	Normal	Normal	Prolonged	Prolonged[c]
Prothrombin consumption	Impaired	Impaired	Normal[h]	Normal[h]
Partial thromboplastin time	Normal	Prolonged	Normal[i]	Prolonged
Thromboplastin generation test	Normal[k]	Abnormal	Normal[i]	Normal

[a]May be normal at some times in von Willebrand's syndrome.
[b]May be prolonged in very severe deficiencies.
[c]No clot may form.
[d]May lyse (excessive fibrinolysin).
[e]May be negative.
[f]May be positive.
[g]May be normal (thrombocytopathia or thrombasthenia) or increased (thrombocythemic bleeding).
[h]Of no value; may be difficult to determine.
[i]Prolonged in severe deficiency of factor V.
[k]Normal in thrombocytopenia if platelet concentration is adjusted to normal; abnormal in platelet dysfunction states (see also Table 17-7).

pattern to be followed in outlining the tests to be performed. Last, the attending physician may want to give transfusions or other therapy before the laboratory studies are completed, or the patient's condition may require immediate therapy. It is well, therefore, to obtain sufficient blood when the patient is first seen and before therapy is begun.

In the majority of instances, diagnosis is made simple by the fact that certain patterns characterize a disease or a group of closely related diseases (Table 17-36). It is also fortunate that the presence of more than one defect is extremely rare. A second defect will be recognized if the complete diagnostic scheme is followed.

There was gear there'd make a beggarman as rich as Lima Town,
Copper charms and silver trinkets from the chests of Spanish crews.
Gold doubloons and double moydores, louis d'ors and portagues.
Masefield: *Spanish Waters*

Appendix—methods

THE BLOOD SPECIMEN
  Obtaining venous blood
    Routine venipuncture, p. 860
    External jugular puncture, p. 861
    Femoral puncture, p. 861
    Internal jugular puncture, p. 861
    Longitudinal sinus puncture, p. 861
  Obtaining capillary blood, p. 861
  Use of anticoagulants
    Sodium citrate, p. 862
    EDTA salts, p. 862
**CELL COUNTING AND WHOLE BLOOD
MEASUREMENTS**
  The hemocytometer, p. 862
  Erythrocyte count (hemocytometer), p. 863
  Leukocyte count (hemocytometer), p. 864
  Platelet count (phase contrast), p. 864
  Reticulocyte count, p. 865
  Circulating eosinophil count, p. 866
  Absolute basophil count, p. 866
  Microhematocrit, p. 867
  Erythrocyte indices, p. 867
  Sedimentation rate
    Westergren method, p. 867
    Landau-Adams method, p. 867
SMEARS, DIFFERENTIAL COUNTS, AND SPECIAL STAINS
  Preparation of blood smears, p. 867
  Wright-Giemsa stain, p. 868
  May-Grünwald-Giemsa stain, p. 869
  Giemsa stain (original azure blend type), p. 869
  Differential leukocyte count, p. 869
  Peroxidase reaction (Graham-Knoll), p. 869
  Peroxidase stain (substitute reagent for benzidine), p. 870
  Sudan black B stain for lipids, p. 870
  Alkaline phosphatase stain (Kaplow), p. 871
  Acid phosphatase with tartrate resistance, p. 871
  Periodic acid–Schiff reaction (PAS), p. 872
  Naphthol ASD acetate, plain and with fluoride inhibition, p. 872
  Deoxyribonuclease digestion for identification of DNA, p. 873
  Ribonuclease reaction for identification of RNA, p. 873
  The Feulgen reaction, p. 873
  Demonstration of siderocytes, p. 874
  Nonhemoglobin storage iron in bone marrow smears, p. 874
  Nitro blue tetrazolium (NBT) test, qualitative, p. 874
HEMOGLOBIN AND HEMOGLOBIN DERIVATIVES
  Hemoglobinometry, p. 875
  Cyanmethemoglobin method, p. 875
  Abnormal hemoglobin compounds

Spectroscopy, p. 876
Identification of abnormal compounds, p. 876
Urinary porphyrins, p. 877
Porphobilinogen (qualitative), p. 877
Porphyrins (qualitative), p. 877
Porphyrins: quantitative assay of urinary coproporphyrin,
  uroporphyrin, δ-aminolevulinic acid, and porphobilinogen,
  p. 877
  Coproporphyrin and uroporphyrin, p. 878
  δ-Aminolevulinic acid and porphobilinogen, p. 879
  Porphobilinogen, p. 880
  δ-Aminolevulinic acid, p. 880
Porphobilinogen (semiquantitative method), p. 880
Quantitative methemoglobin in blood, p. 881
Assay of serum iron concentration, p. 882
TESTS FOR HEMOLYTIC DISEASE
  Osmotic fragility of erythrocytes
    Method of Sanford, p. 883
    Method of Dacie, p. 883
    Osmotic fragility after incubation, p. 883
  Acid serum test for paroxysmal nocturnal hemoglobinuria, p. 884
  Sugar-water test for paroxysmal nocturnal hemoglobinuria,
    p. 884
  Demonstration of Donath-Landsteiner (D-L) hemolysin, p. 884
  Autohemolysis, p. 884
  Alkali denaturation test for fetal hemoglobin, p. 885
  **Demonstration of fetal hemoglobin in red blood cells: acid
    elution technic,** p. 885
  Susceptibility to Heinz body formation, p. 886
  Tests for unstable hemoglobins
    Inclusion bodies (Heinz bodies), p. 886
    Hemoglobin H inclusion bodies, p. 886
    Heat denaturation test, p. 886
    Isopropanol precipitation test, p. 887
  Demonstration of sickle cells
    Sodium bisulfite method, p. 887
  Solubility test for Hb S, p. 887
    Centrifugation test to differentiate sickle cell trait from sickle
    cell anemia, p. 888
  Hemoglobin electrophoresis
    Preparation of hemolysate, p. 888
    Hemoglobin electrophoresis (cellulose acetate: alkaline pH),
      p. 889
    Hemoglobin electrophoresis (agar gel, acid pH), p. 890
    Differential electrophoresis for hemoglobin H, p. 890
    Globin chain separation
      At alkaline pH, p. 891
      At acid pH, p. 891

Quantification of Hb A_2 and Hb S by microchromatography, p. 892

Quantification of serum haptoglobin (cellulose acetate), p. 893

Quantitative hemoglobin in plasma and urine, p. 894

PROTEIN ELECTROPHORESIS AND IMMUNOELECTROPHORESIS

Separation of serum proteins using cellulose acetate, p. 894

Separation of serum lipoproteins using Agarose gel, p. 896

Immunoelectrophoresis, polyvalent and monovalent, p. 897

Quantification of immunoglobulins, p. 899

Quantification of ceruloplasmin, p. 900

Fetoglobin (fetuin, α-fetoprotein, α-fetoglobulin), p. 900

Concentration and protein electrophoresis of urine, p. 901

Urine immunoelectrophoresis for κ and λ light chains, p. 901

Cold-precipitable protein study, p. 902

SEROLOGY AND IMMUNOLOGY

General laboratory technic

Cell washing, p. 903

Reading and grading test tube agglutination, p. 903

Preparation of red cell suspensions

Cells for A-B-O reverse grouping, p. 903

Cells for antibody identification, p. 903

Cells for antibody identification using freshly drawn blood, p. 903

A-B-O blood grouping technics

Cell grouping (adults): slide method, p. 904

Cell grouping: test tube method, p. 904

Serum or reverse grouping: test tube method, p. 904

Cell grouping (cord blood): slide method, p. 904

Subgroups of A or AB blood

Use of anti-A_1 serum (absorbed anti-A or anti-A lectin), p. 904

Use of group O serum, p. 905

Rh typing

Slide test, p. 905

Modified or rapid tube test, p. 905

Tube test, p. 905

Method for Rh_0 variant (D^u), p. 906

Direct antiglobulin (Coombs') test, p. 906

Screening for irregular antibodies, p. 906

Antibody identification, p. 907

Antibody elution technics

Heat elution method, p. 907

Rubin ether method, p. 908

Testing the heat eluate in A-B-O hemolytic disease, p. 908

Testing the eluate for antibody of unknown specificity, p. 908

Absorption of nonspecific cold agglutinins, p. 908

Investigation of a positive direct antiglobulin test, p. 909

Prenatal serologic studies, p. 909

Titration of irregular antibodies in maternal serum

Saline titration, p. 909

Albumin-antiglobulin titration, p. 909

Titration of anti-A and anti-B isoagglutinins

Screening for naturally occurring anti-A and anti-B antibodies, p. 910

Neutralization of naturally occurring anti-A and anti-B antibodies, p. 910

Serologic studies on newborn infants, p. 910

Demonstration of free homologous antibody in cord serum, p. 911

Cold agglutinins, p. 911

Demonstration of leukoagglutinins, p. 912

Heterophil antibody: Monospot test, p. 912

Demonstration of LE cells, p. 912

Clotted blood method, p. 913

Rotary bead method, p. 913

Fluorescent antinuclear antibody test: qualitative method, p. 913

Fluorescent antinuclear antibody test: quantitative method, p. 915

COAGULATION TESTS

Venous coagulation time: glass technic, p. 915

Clot retraction, p. 915

Ivy bleeding time using Simplate, p. 915

Tourniquet test, p. 916

Platelet adhesiveness: in vivo method, p. 917

Platelet aggregation, p. 918

Platelet factor 3 availability (Celite method), p. 919

Plasma recalcification time, p. 919

Cross-recalcification times for screening circulating anticoagulants, p. 920

Detection of the lupus anticoagulant, p. 920

One-stage prothrombin time (Quick), p. 920

One-stage prothrombin time: microtechnic, p. 921

Evaluation of a prolonged one-stage prothrombin time, p. 922

Factor II assay, p. 923

Factor V assay, p. 923

Factor VII assay, p. 923

"Stypven" time, p. 923

Prothrombin consumption, p. 924

Partial thromboplastin time

Macromethod, nonactivated, p. 924

Macromethod, activated, p. 925

Micromethod, nonactivated or activated, p. 925

Evaluation of a prolonged partial thromboplastin time, p. 925

Thromboplastin generation test, p. 926

Factor VIII (VIII: C) assay, p. 929

Factor VIII–related antigen (VIII: Ag) by electroimmunoassay (EIA), p. 929

Ristocetin co-factor (VIII: vW) assay by aggregometry, p. 931

Factor IX assay, p. 932

Factor X assay, p. 932

Factor XI assay, p. 932

Factor XII assay, p. 932

Semiquantitative assay of fibrin-stabilizing factor (factor XIII), p. 933

Detection of Fletcher factor deficiency, p. 933

Antithrombin III

By thrombin neutralization, p. 934

By rocket electroimmunoassay, p. 934

By radial immunodiffusion, p. 935

Assays utilizing chromogenic or fluorogenic substrates, p. 935

Thrombin time, p. 936

Protamine paracoagulation test, p. 936

Ethanol gelation test, p. 936

Fibrinolysis (screening), p. 936

Euglobulin lysis time (fibrinolysin activity), p. 937

Heparin assay, p. 938

THE BLOOD SPECIMEN
Obtaining venous blood
Routine venipuncture

All equipment used for venipuncture should be dry and sterile. When a tourniquet is used, it should be just tight enough to occlude the venous return. The tourniquet should be released as soon as the vein is entered.

A two-syringe technic should be used whenever blood is obtained for coagulation studies. After the vein is entered, about 1 ml of blood is withdrawn into the first syringe. This syringe is disconnected from the needle that is left in place in the vein, and a second syringe is attached. Silicone-coated or plastic syringes and needles should be used to obtain venous blood for coagulation studies.

After the required amount of blood is obtained, the needle is withdrawn, pressure is applied with a sterile gauze square, and the arm is elevated to assist in collapsing the punctured vein.

Blood is distributed from the syringe by removing the needle and gently expressing the blood into the test tube. The blood is made to run down the side of the tube. Avoid using the last milliliter of blood in the syringe, particularly if it is frothy.

If the vacuum tube technic is used, the tube is fixed to its adapter-held needle so that the innermost shaft of the needle holds the stoppered tube in place but does not completely penetrate the stopper so as to lose the vacuum. The patient's arm is prepared and the vein entered in the usual way. After the vein is entered, the adapter is held firmly and the vacuum tube is forced onto the needle shaft so that the rubber stopper is penetrated. If the vein has been properly entered, blood will gush into the tube. The tube should be allowed to fill to its capacity. Discomfort will be experienced by the patient if vacuum remains in the tube as the needle is removed from the vein. Also, if an improper volume of blood is mixed with the premeasured quantity of anticoagulant, gross errors in hematocrit and other values can result.

If only one tube of blood is required, the tourniquet is released and the needle and tube are removed as with a syringe. If more than one tube of blood is required, after the first tube has filled, place a finger of the left hand on the skin over the vein where the tip of the needle lies, apply pressure to stop the flow of blood, pull the filled tube from the needle shaft, and quickly replace with another vacuum tube. Release the finger pressure and the tube will fill. This may be repeated as often as necessary for the quantity of blood required.

If an anticoagulant is in the tube, the tube should be inverted several times right after it has been removed from the holder in order to mix thoroughly.

Some vacuum tubes are stored inverted, and the anticoagulant collects around the rim of the tube and the bottom of the stopper. If not previously tapped down, the anticoagulant will cake when wet with blood and no amount of agitation or mixing seems to dissolve it.

The vacuum-tube type used presently is the B-D Vacutainer* that has a three-piece outfit: needle, adapter or holder, and tube. The holder of the B-D unit is not disposable, although the needle and tubes are.

External jugular puncture

In very small infants, blood is usually obtained from the internal jugular vein, the external jugular vein (preferred for coagulation studies), or the longitudinal sinus. An external jugular or a femoral puncture is used in larger infants (over 18 months of age) or in small children. After the age of 3 years, the median basilic vein over the antecubital fossa is the usual site for venipuncture.

Procedure

1. Wrap infant in a mummified manner.
2. Turn his head to one side and let it hang over the side of a table.
3. Sterilize area.
4. Provoke the child to cry to distend the external jugular vein.
5. Pull the skin tight over the puncture site, insert the needle directly over the vein, and then enter the vein cleanly.
6. When the needle is withdrawn, apply pressure and hold the child upright for a few minutes.

Femoral puncture

Procedure

1. An assistant is needed to hold the child securely.
2. The assistant stands behind the infant, leans over his head and trunk, and holds his leg in a semifrog position. The arms

*Becton-Dickinson & Co., Rutherford, N.J.

of the infant are held down by the assistant's upper arms and elbows.

3. The operator, after locating the femoral pulse just below the inguinal ligament, inserts the needle, aiming slightly medial to the pulse beat.
4. The needle is inserted until the bone is barely touched.
5. While suction is exerted, the needle is *slowly* withdrawn until a small amount of blood enters the syringe.
6. If the flow ceases, the needle is pushed deeper and is slowly withdrawn as before. It is important to remember that both the syringe and the legs must be held stationary to ensure drawing the maximum amount of blood.
7. After the needle is withdrawn, pressure is maintained over the area for a few minutes.

Internal jugular puncture
Procedure

1. Wrap infant securely in a sheet.
2. Place him on a table and adjust the position so that his head falls over the side. With neck extended, his head is turned slightly to one side. This makes the posterior margin of the sternocleidomastoid muscle on the opposite side stand out.
3. Sterilize area.
4. The needle is inserted just deep to and behind the posterior margin of the sternocleidomastoid muscle, approximately halfway between its origin and insertion. The needle is then advanced under the muscle, parallel to the skin surface and in the direction of the suprasternal notch, for a distance of 1½ to 2 inches.
5. The needle is then slowly withdrawn while a negative pressure is kept on the syringe until a point is reached at which blood enters the syringe.
6. After blood is obtained, hold the child upright and apply pressure over the area for a few minutes.

Longitudinal sinus puncture

This method of venipuncture can be used on infants when the anterior fontanelle is open. The fontanelle is diamond shaped, and the superior sagittal sinus runs just under the scalp from the anterior to the posterior angle of the fontanelle. The puncture is best made at the posterior angle where the sinus is largest. Care must be exercised not to enter the subarachnoid space.

Procedure

1. Wrap child securely in a sheet.
2. Outline the bony margins of the fontanelle with Mercurochrome.
3. Sterilize area.
4. Insert needle at about a 30- to 90-degree angle, not more than ⅛ inch deep.

Obtaining capillary blood

Capillary blood is obtained by puncturing the skin with a sharp blade. In adults and children the finger is preferred. In infants the puncture should be done at the heel.

Heel punctures should be done on the lateral portion of the heel pad and should be no deeper than 2.4 mm in order not to enter the calcaneus bone. The posterior of the heel should not be used, since the depth from skin to bone is about half that of the lateral aspect of the heel. Sites of previous punctures should be avoided.

A sterile dry blade should be used. Sterile disposable blades are now available. We prefer a scalpel blade, discarding it after use. Wiping blades or needles with alcohol or other disinfectants will not prevent transmission of the virus of hepatitis.

Squeezing or milking should be avoided, although it is permissible to massage the area lightly before the puncture is performed.

The first drop of blood should be wiped away with a dry sponge.

References

Blumenfeld et al, 1979
Hammond, 1980

Use of anticoagulants
Sodium citrate

Soluble citrates act as anticoagulants by combining with calcium to form an insoluble calcium salt.

A 3.2% (0.109M) solution of trisodium citrate is used to collect blood for the thromboplastin generation test, the prothrombin time test, and other coagulation tests—1 part citrate solution to 9 parts blood.

ACD solution (trisodium citrate 1.32 Gm, citric acid 0.48 Gm, dextrose 1.47 Gm, and distilled water to 100 ml) is used by some to collect and store erythrocytes in the investigation of hemolytic anemia—0.25 ml of ACD solution per milliliter of blood.

EDTA salts

Sodium and potassium salts of ethylenediamine tetra-acetic acid (EDTA) act as anticoagulants by forming insoluble calcium salts. Either the disodium or the dipotassium salt can be used. It preserves cellular elements better than sodium citrate and is suitable for routine hematologic and blood typing procedures. Blood anticoagulated with EDTA cannot be used for coagulation or platelet function studies. Dipotassium EDTA is available as dipotassium Versenate. It is used in a concentration of 1 mg of dry powder/ml of blood. When dry EDTA is used, the blood sample should be inverted gently a number of times to effect complete solution of the EDTA in blood. A solution of EDTA may be used, 0.1 ml of 1% EDTA/ml of blood.

Reference

Hadley and Weiss, 1955

CELL COUNTING AND WHOLE BLOOD MEASUREMENTS
The hemocytometer

The hemocytometer, or counting chamber, is used for direct cell counts. Admittedly, cell counts in most laboratories are now automated. Nonetheless, it is possible that at some time all the sophisticated cell counting instruments will strike for better working conditions and technologists will then have to relearn how to count cells manually. Also, the hemocytometer has other applications (cell counts in spinal fluid, cast counts in urine sediments, etc.).

The standard hemocytometer is constructed so that the distance between the bottom of the cover glass and the surface of the chamber is 0.1 mm. The surface of the chamber contains two specially ruled areas. Each ruled area consists of a square, 3 mm on each side, divided into nine "large" squares, each side of these being 1 mm, and the area being 1 mm^2 (Fig. A-1). The four large corner squares (1, 2, 3, and 4), each 1 mm^2 in area, are subdivided into 16 smaller squares to facilitate cell counting. These four corner squares are used for counting leukocytes. The center square, also 1 mm^2 in area, is subdivided into 25 smaller squares, each $\frac{1}{5}$ mm on each side and $\frac{1}{25}$ mm^2 in area. Each of the 25 small squares is further subdivided into 16 smaller squares for convenience when erythrocytes are counted. Squares A, B, C, D, and E in Fig. A-1 are used for erythrocyte counts.

Hemocytometer chambers and cover glasses should meet the specifications of the National Bureau of Standards, NBS Form 80, Aug. 1, 1941. Chambers and coverslips meeting these specifications are so marked by the manufacturer. To meet specifications, the depth of the standard chamber must not vary more than ±2% (±0.002 mm), the length of any side of the 1 mm squares must not

exceed ±1% (±0.01 mm), and cover glasses must be plane on both sides within 0.002 mm.

The boundary lines of the central 1 mm^2 are double, sometimes triple. When double, the boundary of the square is the outer line. When triple, the boundary is the middle of the three lines.

The calculation of the cell count should *not* be reduced to a set formula of counting certain squares and multiplying by a factor. The method is inflexible if a factor is used; if the routine is varied, the factor no longer applies and serious errors will be made. Instead, if cells in 1 mm^2 are counted in a chamber having a depth of 0.1 mm, calculate the count according to the following general formula:

$$\text{Count (cells/mm}^3) = \text{Cells/mm}^2 \times 10 \times \text{Dilution}$$

In every case, cells are counted in a certain number of squares, and the count for an area of 1 mm^2 is calculated by a simple proportion, as follows:

$$\frac{\text{Cells counted}}{\text{Area counted (mm}^2)} = \frac{\text{Cells/mm}^2}{1}$$

The calculated number of cells per square millimeter is then multiplied by 10 (the depth of the chamber is 0.1 mm; therefore the cells counted in 1 mm^2 multiplied by 10 gives the cells in 1 mm^3 of the diluted specimen) and then by the dilution to give cells per cubic millimeter of undiluted specimen. The count per cubic millimeter is further multiplied by 10^6 to give cells/l.

If the chamber has a depth of 0.2 mm (see Circulating eosinophil count), a different factor is used for the depth of the chamber.

The statistical error of cell counting is discussed in Chapter 7. Technical errors are potentially greater. The following points must be kept in mind:

1. A freely flowing drop of capillary blood must be used.
2. When anticoagulated blood is used, the specimen must be carefully mixed by inverting the tube of blood at least 20 times before sampling. Do not shake, as this introduces air bubbles or foam, which make accurate pipetting impossible. Tilt the well-mixed tube to a 45-degree angle or slightly more, and pipet from the lip of the tube, following this same procedure as for capillary blood.
3. The blood-diluting pipets must be clean and dry.
4. The pipet must be filled quickly, and the blood must be drawn accurately, using an aspirating tube attached to the pipet, up to the desired line. If the line is overshot slightly, it is permissible (but not desirable) to expel the excess blood by touching the tip of the pipet against some nonporous material. If the line is overshot by a good distance, it is necessary to use a fresh pipet.
5. No air bubbles should be present in the blood column.
6. The tip of the pipet must be wiped free of blood before it is introduced into the diluting fluid.
7. The diluting fluid must be drawn into the pipet with steady suction, avoiding loss of blood from the pipet.
8. The fluid must be drawn up accurately to the line above the bulb, holding the pipet as nearly vertical as possible to avoid trapping air in the pipet. Quickly place the index finger of your free hand over the tip of the pipet and remove the aspirating tube.
9. The pipet must be shaken for at least 3 minutes, preferably in a mechanical shaker, or by hand. Care should be exercised not to shake the pipet endwise, but in a figure-eight pattern or by rotating vigorously between the fingers. The chamber is filled immediately after the pipet is shaken.
10. At least one third of the contents of the pipet is discarded before filling the chamber.
11. The chamber is filled by capillary attraction, regulating the flow of fluid from the pipet in such a way that the chamber fills quickly and smoothly. The chamber must be filled

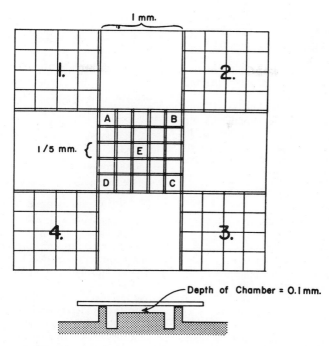

Fig. A-1. Hemocytometer. Squares **1, 2, 3,** and **4** are used for counting leukocytes; squares **A, B, C, D,** and **E** are used for counting erythrocytes.

completely, but fluid must not spill over into the moats. Allow the cells to settle in the counting area for approximately 2 minutes; then proceed with the counting.

12. The hemocytometer chamber and cover glass must be clean and dry before use. Grave errors are introduced by fingerprints or an oily film.

13. Pipets should have a maximum error of ±1%. Inferior grades should not be used.

Interpretation

The theoretical error of hemocytometer counts is discussed in Chapter 7.

Erythrocyte count (hemocytometer)
Principle

Blood is diluted with a fluid that is isotonic with the erythrocytes. The diluted specimen is introduced into the hemocytometer chamber, and the erythrocytes are counted. Diluting fluids used for erythrocyte counts do not destroy the leukocytes. These are normally so few that they do not interfere with enumerations of the erythrocytes. When there are many, they are easily identified and are not counted.

Diluting fluid (Gower's)

Sodium sulfate, anhydrous (CP)	12.5 Gm
Glacial acetic acid	33.3 ml
Distilled water to	200.0 ml

In our laboratory, Isoton* is used as the diluent for hemocytometer counts.

Method

1. Fill an erythrocyte diluting pipet with blood to the 0.5 line.
2. Dilute with diluting fluid to the 101 line above the bulb.

*Coulter Diagnostics, Hialeah, Fla.

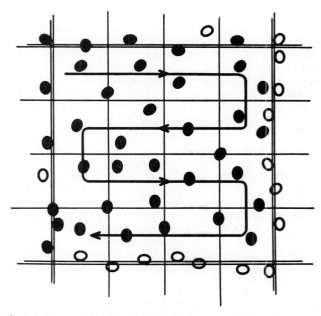

Fig. A-2. Manner of counting erythrocytes in one of the small squares. Dark cells are counted and light cells are omitted. The diagram shows 36 erythrocytes in an area of $\frac{1}{25}$ mm^2.

3. Under these conditions the blood is diluted 1:200.
4. Fill both sides of the hemocytometer chamber.
5. Count (45× objective) the cells in 5 of the 25 small squares in the central area (A, B, C, D, and in E in Fig. A-1) of each chamber. This represents an area of $\frac{1}{25} \times 5$ mm^2 or $\frac{1}{5}$ mm^2 for each chamber. The difference between the highest number of cells and the lowest among the 10 squares should be no larger than 25.
6. In counting cells, compensate for the random distribution at

the margin of each of the five small squares by counting those cells that touch the left and upper *outer* line (in chambers with double lines) and disregarding those that touch the right and lower *inner* line (Fig. A-2).

7. Calculate the number of erythrocytes per cubic millimeter of undiluted blood by taking into account the area counted, the depth of the chamber, and the dilution.

8. In extremely anemic persons, decrease the dilution of blood to 1:100 by filling the pipet to the 1 line instead of the 0.5 line or to 1:20 by using a leukocyte-diluting pipet instead. In severe polycythemia, increase the dilution by filling with blood to the 0.2 or 0.3 line of the erythrocyte diluting pipet (dilutions are then 1:500 and 1:333, respectively).

Normal values

See discussion in Chapter 7.

All adults: Average 5.1 million/mm³, 95% range 4.1 to 6.1 million (5.1×10^{12}/l; 95% range 4.1 to 6.1×10^{12}/l).

Adult males: Average 5.4 million/mm³, 95% range 4.4 to 6.4 million (5.4×10^{12}/l; 95% range 4.4 to 6.4×10^{12}/l).

Adult females: Average 4.8 million/mm³, 95% range 3.8 to 5.8 million (4.8×10^{12}/l; 95% range 3.8 to 5.8×10^{12}/l).

Children: See Chapter 7.

Remarks

In case of autoagglutination of the red cells, use 0.85% saline solution instead of the usual diluent. Warming the pipet by rotating vigorously in the palms of the hands usually disperses persistent clumps. It may be necessary to also warm the hemocytometer.

Leukocyte count (hemocytometer)
Principle

Blood is diluted with a fluid that lyses the nonnucleated erythrocytes but not the leukocytes or the nucleated erythrocyte precursors. Lysis is produced by any acid solution. Türk's solution contains a dye that stains the nuclei, but the real value of the dye is to help in distinguishing the leukocyte-diluting fluid from others.

It must be emphasized that the cells counted are not necessarily all leukocytes. When the blood smear shows nucleated erythrocytes, the cell count must be corrected to the true leukocyte count.

Diluting fluid (Türk's)

Glacial acetic acid	1 ml
Gentian violet, 1% aqueous	1 ml
Distilled water to	100 ml

Filter before using.

Method

1. Fill a leukocyte-diluting pipet with blood to the 0.5 line.
2. Dilute with Türk's fluid to the 11 line above the bulb (1:20 dilution).
3. Shake, fill the hemocytometer chamber, and count (10× objective) the cells in each of the four large corner squares (1 mm² each) on both sides of the chamber. The rule for including or excluding cells is the same as for the erythrocyte count. The difference between the highest and the lowest number of cells among the eight squares should be no larger than 15.
4. Calculate the leukocyte count on the basis of cells counted, area counted, and the dilution.
5. If the count is above 50,000 cells/mm³ (50×10^9/l) of blood, it is best to repeat it using a higher dilution. For very high leukocyte counts, dilute in an erythrocyte pipet.
6. If nucleated erythrocytes are present, the leukocyte count can be corrected according to the following formula:

$$\text{Corrected count} = \text{Observed count} \times \frac{100}{100 + \% \text{ Nucleated erythrocytes}}$$

For example, if the observed leukocyte count is 20,000/mm³ (20×10^9/l) and 50 nucleated erythrocytes are counted per 100 leukocytes, the corrected leukocyte count is as follows:

$$20,000 \times \frac{100}{150} = 13,333 \text{ leukocytes/mm}^3 \ (13.3 \times 10^9/l)$$

Interpretation

See discussion of leukocytes in Chapter 15.

Platelet count (phase contrast)

The readiness with which platelets agglutinate and adhere to a foreign surface necessitates special precautions during the collection of a blood specimen and immediate dilution in an anticoagulant solution. Their small size makes direct counting in a hemocytometer chamber more difficult than other cell counts.

A number of methods for platelet counting have been proposed. We feel that the least reliable methods are those in which platelets are estimated indirectly from supravital preparations; the most reliable is that of Brecher and Cronkite, in which platelets are counted in a special counting chamber using phase microscopy. No other manual method is recommended at this time. Laboratories that are required to perform many platelet counts have used a specially adapted Coulter electronic counter. We have evaluated the Technicon Autocounter for platelets and found that counts with this instrument correlate very well with phase counts.

Equipment and reagents

1. Flat bottom, thin counting chamber (special thin chamber for phase microscopy)*
2. No. 1 coverslips, best grade
3. Phase microscope equipped with long working distance phase condenser, 43× annulus, and 43× phase objective
4. Erythrocyte-diluting pipets, certified ±1% error
5. Siliconized serologic test tubes, to be used for counts from venous blood
6. Diluting fluid: 1% ammonium oxalate in distilled water
   a. Store in refrigerator and always filter just before using.
   b. It is best to make it up in small amounts.

Method

1. Make a deep clean puncture with a sharp Bard-Parker blade. Wipe away first drop of blood.
2. Fill to 0.5 line from the second drop, dilute to the 101 line with the diluting fluid, and immediately shake in a mechanical shaker for 3 minutes.
3. For platelet counts from venous blood, the preferred anticoagulant is EDTA (1 mg/ml of blood or 0.1 ml of a 1% EDTA solution/ml of blood).
4. Fill the special chamber in the usual way. Note that a thin No. 1 coverslip is used to cover the chamber. The chamber must be scrupulously clean.
5. Place chamber in a Petri dish containing a wet pledget of cotton. Let stand for at least 20 minutes.
6. Using medium-dark phase contrast, count the platelets in the 25 small squares (1 mm²) of the erythrocyte counting area on both sides of the chamber (total area counted is 2 mm²).

---

*American Optical Corp., Buffalo, N.Y.

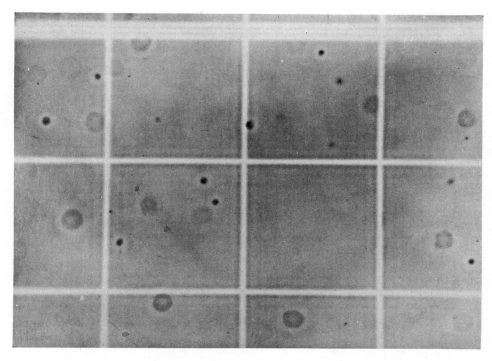

Fig. A-3. Appearance of platelets (the small, darker structures) by phase microscopy. (×430.)

7. Calculate the number of platelets per cubic millimeter of blood according to the area counted, the depth of the chamber (0.1 mm), and the dilution (1:200).

Remarks

Platelets are seen as round or oval purple bodies (Fig. A-3) that sometimes show dendritic processes. Structures such as dirt particles are refractile; platelets are not.

If there is clumping of platelets, the count must be discarded, and a fresh specimen must be obtained. Uniform shaking for 3 minutes is essential. Shaking by hand is not satisfactory. When the platelet count is low, count 9 mm^2 on each side.

Normal values

According to Brecher and Cronkite, the mean normal platelet count is about 250,000/mm^3, 95% range (± 2 SD) 140,000 to 440,000/mm^3 (0.25×10^{12}/l; 95% range 0.14 to 0.44 $\times 10^{12}$/l).

In our laboratory the mean normal platelet count (180 normal subjects) was found to be 258,800, SD 57,038 (0.258×10^{12}/l; SD 0.05×10^{12}/l). In round figures our mean normal is 259,000 platelets/mm^3, 95% range 145,000 to 375,000 platelets/mm^3 (0.259×10^{12}/l; 95% range 0.145 to 0.375 $\times 10^{12}$/l). The highest normal found was 380,000/mm^3 (0.38×10^{12}/l) and the lowest normal 130,000/mm^3 (0.13×10^{12}/l).

The error of the method expressed as the coefficient of variation (CV) is about 8% in our laboratory. This was determined by duplicate counts on the same patients.

References

Brecher and Cronkite, 1950
Brecher et al, 1953

Reticulocyte count

Reticulocytes are immature nonnucleated erythrocytes that still retain some basophilic substance (Chapter 11). Under certain conditions the basophilic substance appears as a reticulum when these cells are exposed to vital stains. Several dyes are suitable, but we prefer New Methylene Blue (CI 52030).*

Reagent

1. New Methylene Blue solution
   a. Dissolve 0.5 Gm of new methylene blue and 1.6 Gm potassium oxalate in distilled water and make up to 100 ml.
   b. Filter before use.

Method

1. Draw capillary blood or freshly drawn venous blood up to the 0.5 line in a leukocyte-diluting pipet, and then draw in an equal volume of New Methylene Blue solution by filling until the blood column reaches the 1 mark. A small air bubble may be let in before the dye solution.
2. Draw blood and dye into the bulb, mix well, and let stand about 15 minutes.
3. Expel a small drop of the mixture on a slide and smear in the usual fashion. Do not counterstain.
4. Count the reticulocytes encountered while 1,000 erythrocytes are examined under oil immersion. The number of reticulocytes counted divided by 10 equals the percent of reticulocytes present.

Remarks

This technic can be used for the demonstration of Heinz bodies. They will appear as homogeneous light-blue bodies in nonreticulated erythrocytes.

Reference

Brecher, 1949

---

*Hartman-Leddon Co., Philadelphia, Pa.

Circulating eosinophil count

The number of eosinophils per cubic millimeter of blood can be estimated from the differential leukocyte count and the total leukocyte count, but this method is not sufficiently accurate. By the use of special diluting fluids that hemolyze the erythrocytes and stain the eosinophils, eosinophils can be counted directly in a counting chamber.

Diluting fluids are of two types. One type contains an acid dye (eosin or phloxine) to stain the eosinophils, distilled water to lyse the erythrocytes, acetone to prevent lysis of the eosinophils, and sodium carbonate to accelerate staining of the eosinophils. The second type contains an acid dye (eosin or phloxine), propylene glycol to lyse the erythrocytes, and sodium carbonate to accelerate staining. Either diluent is satisfactory, but we prefer the type containing propylene glycol.

Diluting fluid

Propylene glycol	50 ml
Distilled water	40 ml
Phloxine, 1% aqueous	10 ml
Sodium carbonate, 10% aqueous	1 ml

Filter and store at room temperature. Discard after 1 month.

Method

1. Draw capillary or venous blood to the 1 line in a leukocyte-diluting pipet. Routinely, two pipets are filled.
2. Fill to the 11 line with diluting fluid.
3. Shake very briefly and let stand for 15 minutes.
4. Shake for 30 seconds in a mechanical shaker.
5. Fill the Speirs-Levy counting chamber. It consists of four chambers per slide, each with ten 1×1 mm squares that are subdivided into 16 smaller areas. The depth of each chamber is 0.2 mm.
6. Fill chambers 1 and 3 from one pipet and 2 and 4 from the other pipet.
7. Allow to stand for 15 to 20 minutes in a Petri dish containing a wet pledget of cotton.
8. Count all four chambers and calculate the total eosinophil count as follows:

$$\text{Eosinophils/mm}^3 = \frac{\text{No. of eos. counted} \times \text{Dilution} \times \text{Depth}}{\text{No. of square millimeters counted}}$$

$$\text{Eosinophils/mm}^3 = \frac{X \times 10 \times 5}{40}$$

Normal value

50 to 250 eosinophils/mm³ of blood (0.05 to 0.25×10^9/l).

Remark

Direct eosinophil counts are used to determine the degree of eosinopenia or the eosinopenic response to ACTH.

Interpretation

Eosinopenia

1. In hyperadrenalism (Cushing's disease), counts of 0 to 30/mm³ (0 to 0.03×10^9/l) are characteristic.
2. Response to stress in the presence of normal adrenal function (postoperative).
3. Decrease of at least 50% from baseline value 4 hours after the intramuscular injection of 25 mg of ACTH indicates normal adrenocortical function.
4. Absence of eosinopenic response indicates hypoadrenalism (Addison's disease).

Absolute basophil count

Principle

Based on neutral red staining, saponin hemolysis, and formaldehyde fixation. Neutral red is a supravital as well as a pH indicator dye. Being a pH indicator dye, it emphasizes the acidic nature of the basophil granules that contain an acid mucopolysaccharide, most probably heparin. The basophil granules stain a bright, brick-red color, while the other leukocytes remain colorless to light pink. Occasionally an eosinophil is seen, but its granules stain yellow to orange. Erythrocytes are hemolyzed by the saponin solution.

Stock solutions

1. Buffer solution, 1%, pH 5.4*
2. Neutral red stain solution, 0.012%
   a. Dissolve 6 mg of pure neutral red dye in 50 ml of pH 5.4 buffer solution
   b. Prepare each week.
3. Saponin* hemolyzing solution, 4%
   a. Dissolve 40 mg saponin in 0.1 ml of pH 5.4 buffer solution.
   b. Make fresh daily.
4. Formalin (40% formaldehyde)

Working solutions

1. Neutral red, saponin solution
   a. Add 0.25 ml saponin hemolyzing solution to 1 ml of freshly filtered neutral red stain solution.
2. Formaldehyde fixative solution
   a. Dilute 0.5 ml of formalin in 3.5 ml of pH 5.4 buffer solution.

Method

1. Add 0.05 ml blood (fresh, venous, heparinized) to polyethylene microcentrifuge tube. (Blood drawn in plastic or siliconized glass syringes minimizes the surface adherence of basophils.)
2. Add 0.4 ml neutral red hemolyzing solution. Cork and mix.
3. Add 0.05 ml formaldehyde fixative solution. Mix.
4. Load four chambers of a Spiers-Levy eosinophil counting chamber.
5. Allow chamber to sit 10 minutes on a piece of moistened filter paper in covered Petri dish.
6. Read under high dry power ($\times 430$) using bright light, plus a CS 160 didymium filter.
7. For capillary blood, use 20 mm³ pipet for blood and formaldehyde measurement. In this instance only 0.16 ml of neutral red hemolyzing solution is used.

Calculation

One and one-fourth times the total number of basophils in all ten 1×1 mm squares in each of the four chambers equals the absolute number of basophilic leukocytes in each cubic millimeter of blood.

Formula: Number of cells $\times$ dilution, divided by the volume (8 mm³).

Normal values

Adults and children are considered as the same: 20 to 50/mm³ (0.02 to 0.05×10^9/l). An absolute basophil count of over 50 (0.05×10^9/l) is referred to as basophilia and a count under 20 (0.02×10^9/l) as basopenia.

---

*Hartman-Leddon Co., Philadelphia, Pa.

Reference

Shelley and Parnes, 1965

Microhematocrit
Principle

See discussion of hematocrit in Chapter 6.

The advantage of using a known and constant relative centrifugal force makes the microhematocrit less subject to technical variations than the macromethod of Wintrobe.

The microhematocrit method may be used with either venous or capillary blood. Special centrifuges and computers are offered by several manufacturers.

Method

1. Use heparinized capillary tubes for capillary blood and plain tubes for EDTA blood.
2. Fill capillary tube about two-thirds full and seal the empty end by heating carefully in a small flame. While sealing, hold the capillary tube at a right angle to the flame.
3. Centrifuge for 2 minutes (or as recommended by manufacturer).
4. Read the hematocrit in the microhematocrit reader.

Normal values

Normal hematocrit values vary with the age of the patient (see Table 6-3, p. 361).

We find this method to have a 1.5% error (32 determinations on the same specimen of blood, average hematocrit 41%, SD ±0.6%).

Reference

Strumia et al, 1954

Erythrocyte indices

Mean corpuscular volume (MCV)

$$MCV = \frac{\text{Hematocrit} \times 10}{\text{Erythrocyte count (millions/mm}^3)}$$

Mean corpuscular hemoglobin (MCH)

$$MCH = \frac{\text{Hb (Gm/dl} \times 10)}{\text{Erythrocyte count (millions/mm}^3)}$$

Mean corpuscular hemoglobin concentration (MCHC)

$$MCHC = \frac{\text{Hb (Gm/dl} \times 100)}{\text{Hematocrit}}$$

Normal values

MCV: Mean 90, SD 5, 95% range 80 to 100 (fl)
MCH: Mean 30, SD 2, 95% range 26 to 34 (pg, or 0.40 to 0.53 fmol)
MCHC: Mean 34, SD 1.5, 95% range 31 to 37 (%)

Sedimentation rate

The factors affecting the sedimentation rate of erythrocytes are discussed in Chapter 6. We find two of the methods most useful: the Westergren method when only the sedimentation rate is determined and the micromethod of Landau-Adams when only a small amount of blood is available. Normal values are given in Chapter 6.

Westergren method
Method

1. Use venous blood containing dry potassium or sodium EDTA anticoagulant.

2. Draw blood into the Westergren tube up to the zero mark. Place tube in special rack.
3. Read the depth of fall of the erythrocyte column at the end of 60 minutes. Readings may be taken every 15 minutes if desired.

Remarks

The sedimentation rate obtained by this method is not corrected for anemia.

In 1973 the International Committee for Standardization in Hematology proposed adoption of a "standard" method using the Westergren tube, but specified that blood be drawn into liquid sodium citrate anticoagulant. Adoption of this method requires a blood sample that can be used only for estimating the sedimentation rate. We prefer the method given above.

Landau-Adams method
Method

1. Fix the special suction attachment on a dry Landau microsedimentation pipet* and draw 5% sodium citrate solution up to the first line.
2. From a capillary puncture, draw blood into the pipet until the fluid column reaches the upper mark.
3. Wipe the end of the pipet. Draw the blood into the bulb, leaving a few millimeters in the stem to avoid air bubbles.
4. Mix contents of pipet; slowly transfer the blood back into the stem; then draw back into the bulb and mix again. Repeat, mixing three times in all, finishing with the blood in the stem. The blood column may be at any point in the stem, but must not be in the tip. No bubbles should be present in the column.
5. Close off the tip of the pipet with the thumb, remove the suction attachment, place pipet in special sedimentation rack, and read at the end of 60 minutes.

Reference

Landau, 1933

SMEARS, DIFFERENTIAL COUNTS, AND SPECIAL STAINS
Preparation of blood smears

The pros and cons of the coverslip versus the slide method can be summarized as follows: (1) "perfect" coverslip smears are better than "perfect" slide smears because the leukocytes are more evenly distributed; (2) it is difficult to make consistently "perfect" coverslip smears; (3) anyone can learn to make "perfect" slide smears; and (4) the average quality of slide smears is better than that of average coverslip smears.

Materials

Obtain new clean slides, either precleaned by the manufacturer or washed with soap and water. They may be stored in 95% alcohol and wiped with a lint-free cloth before using.

Method

1. Make a capillary puncture and wipe away the first drop of blood.
2. Touch the slide to the second drop, transferring a *small* drop of blood to the side about ½ inch from one end.
3. Lay the slide on a flat surface. Place the end of a second slide, balanced on the fingertips at an angle no greater than 30 degrees, in front of the drop of blood.

---

*Curtin Scientific Co., Houston, Texas.

4. Pull the spreader slide back into the drop of blood. When the blood has spread along two thirds of the width, push the spreader slide forward with a steady even motion. The weight of the slide is the only pressure applied.
5. Allow the smear to air dry. Do not blow on it.

Remarks

1. The entire smear should cover no more than half the area of the slide.
2. No portion of the smear should extend to the edges of the slide.
3. There should be no ridges, lines, or holes.
4. There should be 10 or more low-power fields in which the erythrocytes barely touch but do not overlap.
5. Leukocytes should be evenly distributed.
6. Use of a spreader slide with cut-off corners does not prevent margination of leukocytes if the technic is poor. If the smear is made quickly and properly, unacceptable margination can be avoided.
7. A poor smear makes proper staining and identification of leukocytes difficult. For best results, stain within 1 hour. Unstained smears can be stored if they are fixed for 30 seconds in absolute methyl alcohol.
8. If venous blood only is available, a satisfactory smear (either coverslip or slide) may be made from a small drop of blood from the needle immediately after the blood has been drawn.
9. Smears made from fresh EDTA-treated blood are usually satisfactory, but should never be used in dyscrasias or if any abnormality of the red or white cells is suspected.
10. The errors to avoid are as follows:
    a. Use of too large a drop of blood
    b. Delay between transferring the drop of fresh blood to the slide and making the smear
    c. Use of a spreader slide having a chipped or unpolished end
11. Automated differential counting instruments use either "push" or "spun" smears. Spun smears are superior because the distribution of white blood cells is more even.

Wright-Giemsa stain
Reagents

1. Wright's stain

Wright's stain powder*	9 Gm
Giemsa stain powder†	1 Gm
Glycerin, U.S.P.	90 ml
Methanol‡	2,910 ml

   a. Mix reagents in a large brown bottle and tightly stopper.
   b. Shake bottle of stain for at least 5 minutes daily for a week and then set aside to age for at least a month before use.
   c. Small volumes of the stain are filtered into dropper bottles as needed. Whatman No. 2 filter paper is used.
   d. It is *imperative* that the *alcohol* used be of the *brand* specified, as this is the most critical of the reagents. The specified brand has consistently given excellent results.

---

*Wright's blood stain crystalline compound, certified, Hartman-Leddon Co., Philadelphia, Pa.
†Giemsa stain (original azure blend type), certified, Hartman-Leddon Co., Philadelphia, Pa.
‡Methyl alcohol, anhydrous (absolute) CH_3OH (methanol-acetone free), AR, Mallinckrodt Chemical Works, St. Louis, Mo.

2. Stock phosphate buffer
   a. 0.067M sodium phosphate, dibasic (Na_2-HPO_4, anhydrous, 9.47 Gm/l)
   b. 0.067M potassium phosphate, monobasic (KH_2PO_4 9.08 Gm/l)
3. Working buffer, pH 6.4

0.067M Na_2HPO_4	26.5 ml
0.067M KH_2PO_4	73.5 ml
	100.0 ml vol

   a. The stock solutions are made separately, stored in large, brown, stoppered bottles, and mixed to the desired pH, 6.4, as needed.

Method

1. The air-dried smears are fixed by a quick dip (approximately 15 seconds) in a Coplin jar containing absolute methanol. The jar is covered when not in use and the methanol is changed several times during the day as the alcohol takes on water. Absolute alcohol can be used for a long time if anhydrous $CuSO_4$ is added. Anhydrous $CuSO_4$ is white and takes up water from the alcohol, turning pale blue as it becomes hydrated. A quick dip is all that is required for fixation of peripheral smears, as Wright-Giemsa stain acts as an additional fixative. The fixed smears are allowed to air dry.
2. The smears are placed on a horizontal plane (a rack is used for slides, rubber corks for coverslips), blood side up, and flooded with Wright-Giemsa stain. Leave on for about 1 minute.
3. The smears are then once again flooded with an equal volume of buffer solution. Blow gently on the smear to mix. Let the smears stand for 8 to 10 minutes. (The optimum time is determined by trial and error.)
4. Rinse thoroughly with a stream of running tap or distilled water.
5. Wipe the back of the smears with a wet gauze and stand them on end to dry.

Remarks

A satisfactory stain should give the following results:
1. Red cells: Yellowish red
2. Neutrophils: Dark purple chromatin, pale pink cytoplasm, lilac granules
3. Eosinophils: Dark purple chromatin, pale blue cytoplasm, bright red granules
4. Basophils: Dark purple chromatin, dark blue granules
5. Lymphocytes: Dark purple chromatin, sky-blue cytoplasm
6. Monocytes: Medium blue chromatin, gray-blue cytoplasm, fine lilac granules
7. Platelets: Violet to purple granulomere, light blue hyalomere

When the stain is being washed off, the smear must be quickly flooded with water to avoid precipitation of the scum on the smear. If precipitation has formed on the smear, the smear may be salvaged by destaining with either absolute methanol or with Wright-Giemsa stain. The technic is to flood the smear with the alcohol or Wright-Giemsa stain and then very quickly rinse with running water. Repeat the procedure as many times as necessary. After the desired destaining, air dry the smear and restain. Precipitation is usually caused by allowing the Wright-Giemsa stain to dry on the smear before the buffer is added.

Insufficient washing will result in a bluish cast.

After washing is completed, the smear must *not* be placed flat on the table. Stand on end or edge in a slide tray and dry quickly. Smears may be gently blotted dry with soft cleansing tissue or lens paper.

After stained coverslip smears have dried, they are mounted, blood side down, on a clean glass slide, using a mounting agent such as Permount.*

When a film appears on the *back* side of smears, the smear may be cleaned by wiping with an alcohol-dampened tissue.

When bone marrow smears are to be stained with Wright-Giemsa stain, longer fixation times (30 seconds or more) and slightly longer staining times are used. These are determined by trial and error.

The main purpose of the absolute methanol fixation *before* staining is to minimize the chance of waterlogging caused by atmospheric humidity.

May-Grünwald-Giemsa stain
Reagents

1. May-Grünwald powder†
2. Giemsa powder, certified‡
3. Absolute methanol§
4. Glycerin
5. Phosphate buffer, pH 7.2
   a. Mix 71.5 ml 0.067M Na_2HPO_4 (9.47 Gm anhydrous salt/l of distilled water) plus 28.5 ml 0.067M KH_2PO_4 (9.08 Gm anhydrous salt/l of distilled water).
   b. Prepare fresh when needed.

Preparation of stains

1. May-Grünwald stain
   a. Grind 0.3 Gm of powder in 100 ml of methanol.
   b. Allow to stand at least 2 to 3 days.
   c. Before use, filter and dilute with equal volume of phosphate buffer.
2. Giemsa stain
   a. Dissolve 0.6 gm of Giemsa powder in 50 ml of absolute methanol and 25 ml of glycerin.
   b. Allow to stand 2 to 3 days.
   c. Before use, filter and dilute 1 vol of stain plus 9 vol of buffer.

Method

Air-dried blood or bone marrow smears are processed in Coplin jars as follows:
1. Fix in absolute methanol for 15 minutes.
2. Transfer without blotting to diluted May-Grünwald solution for 15 minutes.
3. Drain off stain on filter paper without blotting and transfer to diluted Giemsa solution for 30 minutes.
4. Transfer to phosphate buffer (pH 7.2) and agitate for 10 to 20 seconds.
5. Remove and blot dry.

Reference

Hayhoe et al, 1964

Giemsa stain (original azure blend type)
Reagent

1. Liquid Giemsa blood stain‖
   a. Dilute 1:20 with distilled water.

---

*Fisher Scientific Co., Pittsburgh, Pa.
†Edward Gurr, Ltd., London (Esbe Laboratory Supplies, Toronto, Can.).
‡Hartman-Leddon Co., Philadelphia, Pa.
§Mallinckrodt Chemical Works, St. Louis, Mo.
‖Hartman-Leddon Co., Philadelphia, Pa.

Method

1. Fix air-dried blood or bone marrow smears in absolute methanol (Mallinckrodt) for 30 seconds. Allow to air dry.
2. Either flood the slides with the diluted Giemsa stain on a staining rack or stain slides in a Coplin jar for 20 to 30 minutes.
3. Rinse well with running tap water and allow to air dry.

Remarks

As the Giemsa stain is water based, material to be stained must be fixed before staining—cellular material with methanol, bacterial material by heat or alcohol. Giemsa stain is widely used to stain thick blood smears for malarial parasites. In this instance the smear is *not* fixed prior to staining because the water in the stain will lake the red cells and the parasites will remain. Rack staining is preferred for this technic.

Differential leukocyte count

The purpose of a differential leukocyte count, whether on a smear of peripheral blood, bone marrow, splenic punctate, or lymph node puncture, is to establish the relative frequency of each type of cell. The differential leukocyte count on peripheral blood follows a definite routine, but on bone marrow and other smears, suitable thin fields are chosen at random.

Method (peripheral blood smears)

1. Inspect smear under low power. Observe the distribution of leukocytes and choose that portion of the smear, usually near the thin end, where there is no overlapping of erythrocytes. Shift to the oil immersion objective.
2. Move the slide from the extreme upper edge of the smear to the extreme lower edge, counting and classifying each leukocyte in the successive fields. Shift over one field and proceed to the upper edge, still classifying each leukocyte. Continue in this fashion until the required number of cells is counted.

Remarks

The number of cells counted depends on the leukocyte count and on the accuracy required. At least 100, preferably 200, cells should be classified when the leukocyte count is normal. Classify 300 leukocytes when the count is between 20,000 and 50,000/mm³ (20 to 50×10^9/l) of blood and 400 or 500 cells when the count is above 50,000/mm³ (50×10^9/l) of blood.

Always note and report on the morphology of the erythrocytes and on the morphology and number of platelets. When the platelet count is normal, an average of 3 to 5 platelets is seen per oil immersion field.

At least 500 cells should be classified for a bone marrow differential count and for differential counts on splenic and lymph node punctures.

Normal values

Normal values are given in the appropriate sections of the text.

Interpretation

The error of the differential count depends on the number of cells classified and on the frequency of each type (Table 15-7, p. 671).

Peroxidase reaction (Graham-Knoll)

The enzyme peroxidase is present in the granules of myeloid cells. It acts on hydrogen peroxide, liberating oxygen. The liberated oxygen oxidizes benzidine to a brown compound (Fig. A-4).

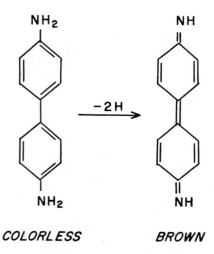

COLORLESS   BROWN

Fig. A-4. Color reaction in the peroxidase stain.

Therefore any structure containing peroxidase stains brown by this reaction.

Reagents

1. Alcoholic formalin, 10%
   a. Mix 10 ml of 40% ("full strength") formalin with 90 ml of 95% ethyl alcohol.
2. Peroxidase reagent
   a. Enough benzidine to cover the point of a knife (approximately 25 mg) is dissolved in 6 ml of 95% ethyl alcohol.
   b. Add 4 ml of distilled water and 0.02 ml of 3% hydrogen peroxide. The hydrogen peroxide must be fresh.
   c. The peroxidase reagent should be freshly prepared before using.

Method

1. Fix smears exactly 30 seconds in alcoholic formalin. Rinse with tap water and air dry.
2. Flood the slide with peroxidase reagent and leave on for 5 minutes. Rinse thoroughly with tap water and dry.
3. Counterstain with dilute Giemsa stain for 20 minutes.

Interpretation

Cells are either peroxidase positive or negative (see Table 4-8, p. 206).

Remarks

Best results are obtained by using fresh hydrogen peroxide and freshly prepared smears. The peroxidase reaction becomes gradually weaker when smears are more than 1 day old.

The amount of hydrogen peroxide added must be carefully measured. If too much hydrogen peroxide is used, the enzyme is destroyed before oxygen can be liberated. If not enough hydrogen peroxide is added or if the solution is old, the reaction will be weak or negative.

Peroxidase stain (substitute reagent for benzidine)
Reagents

1. Buffered formalin acetone, pH 6.6

Na_2HPO_4	20 mg
KH_2PO_4	100 mg
H_2O	30 ml
Acetone	45 ml
Formalin	25 ml

2. Stain, pH 5.5

3-amino-9-ethylcarbazole*	10 mg
Dimethylsulfoxide	6 ml
0.02M acetate buffer, pH 5.0 to 5.2	50 ml
0.3% hydrogen peroxide	0.4 ml

3. Mayer's hematoxylin

Method

1. Fix *thin* blood smears in buffered formalin acetone 15 seconds at room temperature. Wash gently.
2. Incubate slides for 2½ minutes in filtered stain at room temperature.
3. Wash gently in running tap water and counterstain with Mayer's hematoxylin for 8 minutes.
4. Wash, dry, and mount in glycerol-gelatin.

Interpretation

Peroxidase activity is represented by red-brown granular deposits. The distribution of dye is identical to that seen in benzidine stains.

Comment

This technic is suggested as an alternative to methods employing benzidine, since federal regulations now prohibit use of benzidine and its derivatives in concentrations above 0.1% unless rigorous safety precautions are taken. These supposedly carcinogenic compounds will likely become unavailable in the future.

Reference

Graham et al, 1965a

Sudan black B stain for lipids

Sudan black B stains a wide variety of lipids, including neutral fats, phospholipids, and sterols. Sudan black B is useful in distinguishing myeloid cells from other cells, since the granules of myeloid cells are sudanophilic. Sudan black B does not differentiate the various lipids. Phospholipids can be identified by Baker's acid hematin reaction.

Reagents

1. Sudan black B solution
   a. Add 0.3 Gm of Sudan black B to 100 ml of absolute ethyl alcohol.
   b. Shake frequently for 1 to 2 days or until all the dye is dissolved.
   c. Filter.
2. Buffer
   a. Mix a solution of 16 Gm of pure phenol in 30 ml of absolute ethyl alcohol with a solution of 0.3 Gm of disodium phosphate crystals ($Na_2HPO_4 \cdot 12H_2O$) in 100 ml of distilled water.
3. Sudan black B staining solution
   a. Mix 60 ml of the Sudan black B solution (1) with 40 ml of the buffer (2).
   b. Filter. The mixture should be neutral or slightly alkaline.
4. Dilute the Giemsa stain (1:20).
5. Fixative: 40% formalin (full strength)

Method

1. Fix air-dried smears in formalin vapor for 10 minutes by placing the slides to be fixed in a closed staining jar, the bottom of which is covered with 40% formalin.

---

*Aldrich Chemical Co., Milwaukee, Wis.

2. Immerse slides for 30 minutes in Sudan black B staining solution.
3. Wash thoroughly for several minutes in absolute ethyl alcohol.
4. Counterstain with dilute Giemsa's stain for 40 minutes.
5. Air dry.
6. Sudan black B staining is an excellent substitute for the peroxidase stain using benzidine. Granules that are peroxidase positive are also Sudan positive. Additional advantages are that lipids are more stable than peroxidases and smears need not be fresh for the Sudan black B stain.

Results

See Table 4-8, p. 206.

Alkaline phosphatase stain (Kaplow)
Reagents

1. Fixative solution

Formalin (40% formaldehyde)	10 ml
Absolute methanol	90 ml

   a. Between use, store in freezing unit of refrigerator.
2. Stock solution: 0.2M propanediol
   a. Dissolve 10.5 Gm of 2-amino-2 methyl-1,3-propanediol in 500 ml distilled water.
   b. Store in refrigerator.
3. Working solution: 0.05M propanediol buffer, pH 9.75
   a. To 25 ml of stock 0.2M propanediol solution, add 5 ml of 0.1N HCl.
   b. Dilute to 100 ml with distilled water.
   c. Store in refrigerator.
4. Substrate mixture, pH 9.5 to 9.6

Sodium α-naphthyl phosphate	35 mg
Fast blue RR (diazonium salt of 4-benzol-2:5 methoxy-aniline)	35 mg
Working 0.05M propanediol buffer, pH 9.75	35 ml

   a. Prepare immediately before use.
   b. Filter directly into Coplin jar and use at once.
5. Counterstain: Harris hematoxylin
   a. Use full strength; filter before using.

Method

1. Prepare blood films as usual.
2. Immerse slides in fixative for 30 seconds at ±5° C. Wash in running tap water for 10 seconds.
3. Incubate in substrate mixture for 15 minutes at room temperature. Wash in running tap water for 10 seconds.
4. Counterstain with Harris hematoxylin for 3 to 4 minutes. Wash in running tap water for 10 seconds and air dry.
5. A smear of normal peripheral blood is stained as a control. We recommend blood from a patient late in pregnancy or in the delivery room as a strongly positive control.

Remarks

Smears may be made from either capillary or venous blood, but capillary blood should be used whenever possible. Venous blood collected in oxalate or heparin can be used, but smears should be made as soon after collection as possible. Blood collected in EDTA is not suitable.

Staining should be done within 8 hours after the smears are made. If it is to be done later, the smear is fixed in the formalin-methanol. After fixation, smears can be saved for later staining for up to 8 weeks.

Stained smears should not be coverslipped, as mounting media produce variable loss of staining intensity.

The degree of positivity of each of 100 neutrophils is rated on the basis of a 0 to 4 scale, the score for a given smear being the sum of the ratings for 100 leukocytes.

0	Colorless
1	Diffuse but slight positivity, with occasional granules
2	Diffusely positive, with moderate number of granules
3	Strongly positive, with numerous granules
4	Very strongly positive, with very dark, confluent granules

In general, only myeloid cells show alkaline phosphatase activity and these but weakly when normal.

Increased phosphatase activity is noted in the leukocytosis caused by various infections, but not in chronic myelocytic leukemia (Chapters 4 and 16). (High: over 100; normal: 15 to 70; low: less than 20.)

References

Kaplow, 1955, 1963

Acid phosphatase with tartrate resistance
Principle

The cells in leukemic reticuloendotheliosis ("hairy cell" leukemia) contain an acid phosphatase isoenzyme that is resistant to tartrate inhibition. This is used to differentiate them from other cells in the peripheral blood.

Reagents

1. Fixative: 3% glutaraldehyde in 60% acetone
2. 0.2M acetate buffer, pH 5.2

0.2M acetic acid	40 ml
0.2M sodium acetate	160 ml

   Refrigerate.
3. 0.2M tartrate
   a. Dissolve 3.002 Gm L(+)Tartaric acid* in 50 ml distilled water. Add approximately 35 ml of 1N sodium hydroxide. Adjust to pH 4.9 by careful addition of more 1N sodium hydroxide. Add sufficient distilled water to make 100 ml of solution. *Refrigerate.*
4. Incubation mixture A: Prepare fresh. Naphthol AS-BI phosphoric acid, sodium salt* 15 mg. Add 1 to 2 drops of dimethyl formamide (DMF) to dissolve. To a beaker containing the above add:

0.2M acetate buffer pH 5.2	25 ml
Distilled water	25 ml
Fast Red Violet LB*	35 mg

   Filter through Whatman No. 1 filter paper into Coplin jar. Add 2 drops 10% $MnCl_2$.
5. Incubation mixture B: Prepare fresh.

Incubation mixture A	36 ml
0.2M tartrate	4 ml

Method

1. Fix two air-dried smears in glutaraldehyde-acetone for 1 to 2 minutes.
2. Place one smear in incubation mixture A and one in incubation mixture B.
3. Incubate for 1 to 2 hours at 37° C.
4. Wash in running water for 10 minutes.
5. Counterstain with Mayer's Hematoxylin* for 10 minutes.
6. "Blue" in ammonia water.
7. Wash and dry.

---

*Sigma Chemical Co., St. Louis, Mo.

Results

Nearly all nucleated cells and platelets will have varying degrees of red reaction product on the smear incubated in mixture A. All nucleated cells plus platelets will either be completely devoid of red reaction product or will contain only minute amounts on the smear from mixture B.

"Leukemic histiocytes" (hairy cells) will be richly positive on smears from either mixture A or B.

Remarks

The tartrate-resistant acid phosphatase does occur in some other conditions including atypical lymphocytes from infectious mononucleosis and rare cases of chronic lymphocytic leukemia and lymphosarcoma. However, the cells are very faintly positive as contrasted with the strongly positive "hairy cells."

Reference

Li et al, 1970. Modified by Dr. T.M. Dutcher; personal communication.

Periodic acid–Schiff reaction (PAS)
Principle

Polysaccharides, mucopolysaccharides, and mucoproteins are demonstrated by the PAS reaction. Periodic acid (HIO_4) is an oxidant that breaks the C—C bonds in various structures, where these are present as 1:2-glycol groups (CHOH—CHOH), converting them into dialdehydes (CHO · CHO). The equivalent amino or alkylamino derivatives of 1:2-glycol or its oxidation product (CHOH · CO) are also attacked and converted into dialdehydes. The particular property of periodic acid is that it does not further oxidize the resulting aldehydes and these can therefore be localized by combination with Schiff's reagent to give a substituted dye that is red in color. Carbonyl groups are said to be oxidized to carboxylic groups and are thereby prevented from subsequent reaction with Schiff's reagent. The red dyestuff formed by union of fuchsinsulfurous acid with dialdehyde is a new compound and not reoxidized fuchsin. The amount of color developed by the reaction is dependent on the amount of reactive glycol structure present.

Reagents

1. Periodic acid solution
   a. Dissolve 5 Gm of periodic acid crystals in 500 ml distilled water.
   b. Store in a dark bottle; keeps for 3 months.
2. Basic fuchsin
   a. Dissolve 5 Gm of basic fuchsin in 500 ml of hot distilled water. When cool, filter.
   b. Saturate with SO_2 gas* by bubbling for 1 hour.
   c. The solution, in a conical flask, is extracted with 2 Gm of activated charcoal for a few seconds in a hood, and immediately filtered through a Whatman No. 1 filter into a dark bottle.
   d. Fresh solution is prepared every 2 to 3 months.
3. SO_2 water
   a. Saturate distilled water with SO_2 by bubbling gas through it for a few minutes.
   b. Make up and use fresh.

Method

1. Fix air-dried smears for 10 minutes in solution of 10 ml 40% formalin and 90 ml absolute ethanol.
2. After brief washing with tap water, immerse the smears for 10 minutes in a Coplin jar containing periodic acid solution, wash again, and blot dry.
3. Immerse in Schiff's basic fuchsin in a Coplin jar for 30 minutes. Cover Coplin jar.
4. Rinse in several changes of SO_2 water for 2 to 3 minutes.
5. Wash in tap water for 5 to 10 minutes and counterstain with Harris hematoxylin for 10 to 15 minutes.

Results

PAS-positive cells show pink to red coloration. Negative cells show *no* pink color. A method for scoring PAS positivity based on the amount of pinkness and type of granules has been proposed by some investigators, but we do not consider scoring necessary.

Control smears are flooded with diastase solution (diastase of malt,* 0.5% [0.5 Gm diastase of malt in 100 ml distilled water; good for 1 week in refrigerator]) for 30 minutes before treatment with periodic acid. Wash for 2 minutes in running tap water.

References

Pearse, 1961
Hayhoe et al, 1964

Naphthol ASD acetate, plain and with fluoride inhibition
Principle

The particular esterase isoenzymes hydrolyze the substrate and liberate a napthhol or phenol, which couples with a diazonium salt and produces a colored insoluble product.

Reagents

1. Formalin (40%)
2. Phosphate buffer

0.1M Na_2HPO_4 (14.2 Gm/l)	60 ml
0.1M KH_2PO_4 (13.6 Gm/l)	40 ml

3. Naphthol ASD acetate

Naphthol ASD acetate	16 mg
Acetone	3 ml
Propylene glycol	2 ml

4. Fast blue BB salt
5. Sodium fluoride

Method

1. Fix smears in formalin vapor for 10 minutes, wash carefully and air dry.
2. Incubation mixture consists of 100 ml phosphate buffer, 5 ml naphthol ASD acetate solution, and 200 mg Fast Blue BB salt. Mix thoroughly in a magnetic stirrer for 3 to 4 minutes.
3. Filter 50 ml incubation mixture through Whatman No. 1 filter paper into a Coplin jar. Label *Plain*.
4. Immediately dissolve 75 mg sodium fluoride in remaining incubation mixture. Filter into a Coplin jar and label *Na F*.
5. Place one fixed smear in *Plain* Coplin jar and another in *Na F*. Incubate 70 minutes at room temperature.
6. Remove slides and wash in a Coplin jar of tap water, waving the slides back and forth very gently to avoid dislodging blood or bone marrow film.

---

*Available in 16-oz cans from commercial refrigeration companies; as "Can-O-Gas" from Virginia Chemicals & Smelting Co., West Norfolk, Va.

*Fisher Scientific Co., Pittsburgh, Pa.

7. Counterstain in Harris hematoxylin stain for 10 minutes. Wash gently as in previous step.
8. Air dry or blot dry and examine under oil immersion.

Interpretation

The reaction in the *Plain* mixture is manifested by the presence of blue granules in the nucleus and cytoplasm of both monocytes and granulocytes, but monocytes and monoblasts show the greatest degree of positivity. However, in the smears exposed to *Na F* the granulocytes remain positive, while in the monocytes the reaction is markedly or completely inhibited (Table 4-8, p. 206). It should be noted that many monocytes retain a small degree of activity.

References

Flandrin and Daniel, 1971
Yam et al, 1971

Deoxyribonuclease digestion for identification of DNA

DNA is basophilic; structures containing it stain blue with Giemsa stain. After digestion with deoxyribonuclease, which specifically destroys DNA, areas that are basophilic in a control smear stained with Giemsa stain are colorless in the enzyme-treated smear stained with Giemsa stain. RNA is not affected by this enzyme.

Reagents

1. Deoxyribonuclease solution
   a. Dissolve 1.4 Gm of sodium acetate in 10 ml of distilled water.
   b. Dissolve 2.46 Gm of magnesium sulfate in 10 ml of distilled water.
   c. Combine the two solutions and add 80 ml of distilled water.
   d. Dissolve 4.0 mg of deoxyribonuclease* in 50 ml of the above.
2. Dilute Giemsa stain
   a. Dilute 1 ml of stock Giemsa stain (dissolve 3.8 Gm of dry Giemsa stain powder in 200 ml of glycerin by holding at 60° C for 2 hours; then add 312 ml of absolute methyl alcohol) to 10 ml with distilled water.

Method

1. Choose two smears of equal thickness. Fix both in absolute methyl alcohol for 15 minutes.
2. Air dry both slides. One is the control slide; the other is treated with the enzyme solution.
3. Place one slide in deoxyribonuclease solution at 37° C for 30 to 60 minutes. Wash in water and air dry.
4. Stain the control (untreated) and the enzyme-treated slide in dilute Giemsa stain for 30 minutes. Air dry.

Results

When the control and the enzyme-treated slides are compared, it will be noted that DNA-containing chromatin is basophilic on the control slide and almost colorless on the enzyme-treated slide. Nucleoli are prominent on the enzyme-treated smear, since they are composed of basophilic RNA that is not affected by deoxyribonuclease. When present on the control smear, cytoplasmic basophilia, due to RNA, is unaffected by enzyme digestion. (See Table 4-8, p. 206.)

---

*Worthington Biochemical Corp., Freehold, N.J.

Ribonuclease reaction for identification of RNA

The principle is the same as that of deoxyribonuclease digestion of DNA. Here the enzyme ribonuclease is specific for RNA. DNA is not affected.

Reagents

1. Ribonuclease solution
   a. Dissolve 1.4 Gm of sodium acetate in 10 ml of distilled water.
   b. Dissolve 2.46 Gm of magnesium sulfate in 10 ml of distilled water.
   c. Combine the two solutions and add 80 ml of distilled water.
   d. Dissolve 4 mg of ribonuclease* in 50 ml of the preceding.
2. Dilute Giemsa stain (1:20)

Method

1. Choose two smears of about equal thickness. Fix both in absolute methyl alcohol for 15 minutes.
2. Air dry both slides. One is the control slide; the other is treated with the enzyme solution.
3. Place one slide in ribonuclease solution for 30 to 60 minutes at 37° C. Wash in water and air dry.
4. Stain the control (untreated) and the enzyme-treated slide in dilute Giemsa stain for 30 minutes. Dry.

Results

Areas normally basophilic because they contain RNA will be colorless on the enzyme-treated smear. (See Table 4-8, p. 206.)

The Feulgen reaction

The Feulgen reaction is specific for DNA. Acid hydrolysis frees the aldehyde groups of the deoxypentose sugar component of DNA. The aldehyde groups then react with the leukofuchsin in Schiff's reagent to produce a pink-purple color at the site where DNA is present.

Reagents

1. Fixative: Absolute methyl alcohol
2. 1N hydrochloric acid
   a. Dilute 36.4 ml concentrated HCl (sp gr 1.19) to 1,000 ml with distilled water.
3. Schiff's reagent
   a. Dissolve, by shaking, 1 Gm of basic fuchsin in 200 ml of boiling distilled water.
   b. Cool to about 50° C, filter into a clean flask, and add 20 ml of 1N HCl.
   c. Cool to room temperature and add 1 Gm of anhydrous sodium bisulfite.
   d. Let stand at room temperature at least 24 hours before using. Store in a dark bottle and use at room temperature. The reagent should be pale yellow. When it turns red, it should be discarded.
4. SO_2 water
   a. Dilute 10 ml of a 10% solution of anhydrous sodium bisulfite and 10 ml of 1N HCl to 200 ml with tap water. Keep tightly stoppered.

Method

1. Fix the air-dried smear (blood, bone marrow, etc.) in absolute methyl alcohol for 15 minutes.

---

*Worthington Biochemical Corp., Freehold, N.J.

2. Immerse in tap water for 5 minutes.
3. Place in 1N HCl at 60° C for 4 minutes.
4. Wash in cold 1N HCl and rinse with distilled water.
5. Immerse in Schiff's reagent for 1 to 1½ hours.
6. Wash for 2 minutes in each of three changes of SO_2 water.
7. Immerse in tap water for 5 to 10 minutes. Air dry.

Results

Nuclear chromatin and nuclear remnants stain red-pink to red-violet. The greater the concentration of DNA, the more intense the staining. Therefore the nuclear chromatin of immature cells is pale staining; that of mature cells stains intensely. (See Table 4-8, p. 206.)

Remark

DNA can be specifically identified by using the technic of deoxyribonuclease digestion.

Demonstration of siderocytes

Siderocytes are erythrocytes containing granules of iron that give a positive Prussian blue reaction. Only an occasional siderocyte is found in normal blood, but a large number are present in the hemoglobinopathies, in lead poisoning, and after splenectomy (Chapter 11).

Reagents

1. Potassium ferrocyanide solution
   a. Dissolve 2 Gm of potassium ferrocyanide in 100 ml of distilled water.
2. HCl, 1% (by volume)
3. Aqueous safranin, 0.1%

Method

1. Fix blood smear in absolute methyl alcohol for 10 minutes. Air dry.
2. Stain for 10 minutes in a *freshly mixed* solution of equal parts of potassium ferrocyanide solution and HCl.
3. Wash in distilled water. Counterstain for 1 minute with 0.1% safranin. Wash and air dry.
4. Examine under oil immersion. Determine what percent of the erythrocytes contains blue-green granules.

References

Kaplan et al, 1954
Mills and Lucia, 1949

Nonhemoglobin storage iron in bone marrow smears

Storage iron is estimated by noting the amount of hemosiderin in the bone marrow. Special stains for iron can be done either on paraffin-embedded sections or on smears.

Reagents

1. Absolute methyl alcohol
2. HCl, 5%
3. Potassium ferrocyanide, 2%

Method

1. Fix bone marrow smear in absolute methyl alcohol for about 3 minutes.
2. Prepare Prussian blue stain *just before using* (10 ml of 5% HCl plus 30 ml 2% ferrocyanide). Fill a Coplin jar.
3. Immerse smear in the *freshly prepared* reagent for about 30 minutes.
4. Wash with tap water until pink.
5. Dry and mount.

Result

Iron deposits stain blue.

Remarks

Smears previously stained with Wright's stain can be stained for iron by this method. Kaplan's method (Kaplan et al, 1954) is better for intracellular siderotic granules.

Reference

Sundberg and Broman, 1955

Nitro blue tetrazolium (NBT) test, qualitative

Principle

The NBT test is based on the observation that a metabolic change and an increased reduction of nitro blue tetrazolium (NBT) dye occur when leukocytes are involved in phagocytosis in vivo. The percentage and absolute number of polymorphonuclear leukocytes that reduce the colorless tetrazolium salts to water-insoluble black formazan deposits in the cytoplasm of neutrophils exposed to a solution of NBT are strikingly increased in persons with bacterial infections as compared with normal persons or persons with nonbacterial illnesses.

Materials and reagents

1. 0.2% NBT* in physiologic saline solution. (NBT is very light sensitive and must be stored in the dark. Under such conditions, it should be stable for months.)
2. 0.15M phosphate-buffered saline solution, pH 7.2. Add 4.97 Gm $NaH_2PO_4 \cdot H_2O$ and 16.18 Gm $NaHPO_4$ to a liter flask. Dissolve in sufficient amount of physiologic saline to make 1 liter. Check pH.
3. Siliconized concave microslides
   a. Acid-cleaned slides (use either potassium dichromate or 50% nitric acid).
   b. Rinse in clear water.
   c. Immerse slides for at least 5 seconds in a solution of 1 part Siliclad (Clay Adams) to 100 parts water.
   d. Rinse in water.
   e. Dry at 212° F for 10 minutes. Drying may also be accomplished at room temperature for 24 hours.

Method

1. Venous blood is collected in heparin or in capillary tubes from finger or heel sticks. Mix thoroughly by gentle shaking.
2. Approximately 0.1 ml of blood is transferred onto a clean, siliconized, concave microslide and mixed with an equal amount of NBT solution (a mixture of equal amounts of 0.2% NBT in physiologic saline solution and 0.15M phosphate buffered saline solution, pH 7.2).
3. Place the slide in a plastic container containing a wet paper towel to provide humidity. Incubate at 37° C for 25 minutes.
4. Mix well but gently with the tip of a disposable Pasteur pipet. Make regular smears (as for peripheral blood smears). Use special care to avoid damage to the cells and avoid extremely thin or thick smears.
5. Air dry slides and counterstain with Wright's stain.
6. Examine slides microscopically under oil immersion and count 100 neutrophils. Classify neutrophils as NBT negative or NBT positive (large black deposits). Count cells only positively identifed as neutrophils.
7. Report percent of positive NBT neutrophils.

---

*Sigma Chemical Co., St. Louis, Mo.

Normal values

0% to 10%.

Remarks

1. Modifications of the time and type of incubation (hot air, water bath, etc.) are noted in the literature. Variation in time of incubation does not appear to alter the results significantly; however, the type of incubation does affect the results and therefore should be followed to avoid misinterpretation.
2. Slides used for making the smears are cleaned with 95% ethyl alcohol.
3. In cases of leukopenia, buffy coat preparations can be made and used instead of whole blood for the incubation mixture. Similarly, after incubation the mixture can be placed in capillary tubes and spun to obtain smears of the buffy coat.
4. Interpretation and counting of smears
   a. Reduced NBT (formazan deposits) can be seen in neutrophils, monocytes, eosinophils, and clumps of platelets; thus it is important that only cells definitely identified as neutrophils be counted.
   b. The dye must reside within the cytoplasm of the cell.
   c. Any distorted or otherwise equivocal cell should not be counted. If in counting 100 neutrophils, the number of equivocal cells added to the number of definitely positive neutrophils raises the final count into a positive NBT response range, an additional 100 or more neutrophils should be counted to establish the NBT response unequivocally.
   d. Avoid the edges and extreme end of the feathered edge of the slide because, here, cells have a greater tendency to be clumped and distorted.
   e. When occasional clusters of neutrophils are encountered, only the individual neutrophils that can be clearly identified are counted.
5. Elevated NBT responses are characteristic of normal newborn infants, in chronic granulomatous disease, and in patients with untreated or ineffectively treated bacterial infections, tuberculosis, some viral infections, fungal infections, some parasitic infections, and lymphomas.

References

Charette and Komp, 1972
Matula and Paterson, 1971
Park, 1971
Park et al, 1968
Strukelj and Zemva, 1973

HEMOGLOBIN AND HEMOGLOBIN DERIVATIVES

Two aspects of hemoglobinometry are of particular importance to the clinical laboratory: measurement of blood hemoglobin concentration (hemoglobinometry) and identification and quantification of hemoglobin derivatives.

Hemoglobinometry

Only two methods are acceptable for clinical hemoglobinometry: *spectrophotometric* measurement as *oxyhemoglobin* and *spectrophotometric* measurement as *cyanmethemoglobin*.

The oxyhemoglobin method measures that hemoglobin capable of being converted into oxyhemoglobin; it will not measure carboxyhemoglobin and other abnormal hemoglobin compounds. The cyanmethemoglobin method measures all hemoglobin and hemoglobin derivatives, with the possible exception of sulfhemoglobin. There is something to be said for each method.

The measurement of oxyhemoglobin represents the oxygen-carrying capacity of the blood, ignoring hemoglobin compounds that are not physiologically active. Physiologically, the amount of hemoglobin capable of combining with oxygen is more important than total hemoglobin. On the other hand, compounds such as carboxyhemoglobin may, in heavy smokers and in persons engaged in certain industries, make up as much as 1 to 1.5 Gm of the total hemoglobin. Failure to measure these compounds results in lower hemoglobin values, may exaggerate the degree of anemia, and can yield false low values for MCH and MCHC. The cyanmethemoglobin method measures total hemoglobin, active or not in oxygen carrying, and gives truer data for the calculation of MCH and MCHC. It can be argued that the inclusion of a portion of physiologically inactive hemoglobin by the cyanmethemoglobin method is just as serious a drawback as the failure to measure total hemoglobin by the oxyhemoglobin method.

At this time we feel that the cyanmethemoglobin method is the method of choice for routine hemoglobinometry, but that every laboratory should be ready to perform the oxyhemoglobin method in special instances. This is easily done if the original calibration by the iron method is used to construct two curves, one for oxyhemoglobin and one for cyanmethemoglobin. It is then a simple matter to use the oxyhemoglobin method when desired. Use of the two methods together will give, by the difference, an indication of the amount of abnormal hemoglobin pigments. One particular advantage of the cyanmethemoglobin method is that a cyanmethemoglobin standard is available commercially, making it possible for smaller laboratories to have a simple method for calibrating spectrophotometers and periodically checking the results.

Cyanmethemoglobin method
Principle

Blood is laked, and the hemoglobin is converted to cyanmethemoglobin by the cyanide in the diluting fluid.

Reagents

1. Cyanide reagent

Sodium bicarbonate ($NaHCO_3$)	1 Gm
Potassium cyanide (KCN)	50 mg
Potassium ferricyanide ($K_3Fe[CN]_6$)	200 mg
Distilled water to	1,000 ml

2. Cyanmethemoglobin certified standard (Hycel)*

Method

1. Prepare tubes containing 5 ml of the cyanide reagent.
2. Add 0.02 ml of capillary or venous blood, rinsing the pipet at least three times.
3. Mix thoroughly and let stand for at least 10 minutes before reading.
4. Read in a spectrophotometer, wavelength 540 mμ. Read equivalent hemoglobin from the calibration curve or table.

Remarks

The dilution chosen for the oxyhemoglobin and cyanmethemoglobin methods is largely a matter of convenience. Dilution tubes containing 5 ml of diluent are conveniently and accurately prepared by using an automatic pipet that delivers the same amount of diluent each time.

The 0.02-ml pipets (Sahli type) should have a minimum certified calibration of $\pm 1\%$. For the most precise work, each pipet should be calibrated in one's own laboratory, but this is not necessary for clinical purposes if $\pm 1\%$ pipets are used.

The cyanide reagent for the cyanmethemoglobin method should be made fresh each week. It is best to make up only what will be

---

*Hycel Inc., Houston, Tex.

needed each day. When discarded, it should not be poured into a sink previously used to dispose of acid solutions. Acid reacts with cyanides to liberate deadly hydrocyanic acid. The concentration of cyanide in this reagent is low, and the reagent is not dangerous, the lethal dose being about 4 liters.

Calibration curves for transmittance (T) against concentration of the cyanmethemoglobin standard should be drawn on semilog graph paper according to the manufacturer's directions. Plain graph paper can be used if OD readings are used instead. T and OD readings are obviously not interchangeable.

Cyanmethemoglobin reagent* may be used in place of the cyanide reagent. This diluent, used as specified by the manufacturer, will not completely lyse erythrocytes containing HB S or Hb C or some erythrocytes from patients with advanced liver disease. While this is a useful screening method for these conditions, complete hemolysis can usually be achieved by diluting the commercial solution 1:1 with distilled water.

Normal values

The difference between oxyhemoglobin values and cyanmethemoglobin values in normal individuals depends on several factors:

1. Carboxyhemoglobin, included in the cyanmethemoglobin value but not in the oxyhemoglobin, is higher in heavy smokers than in nonsmokers.
2. Apparent differences may be caused by using different values for hemoglobin iron. This might apply if an instrument is calibrated for oxyhemoglobin by the iron method while the manufacturer's readings for the cyanmethemoglobin standard are accepted.

Abnormal hemoglobin compounds

The abnormal hemoglobin compounds can be identified spectroscopically and by simple chemical reactions. Some can be quantitated, but in general this is not necessary, and the usual quantitative methods are not very accurate.

Spectroscopy

We find the hand spectroscope manufactured by the Zeiss Co. to be excellent. It is relatively inexpensive, easy to use, and so constructed that the unknown solution can be simultaneously compared with one of known composition.

Use of the spectroscope

1. Either daylight or fluorescent light can be used. With daylight, the Fraunhofer D line is found at 590 mμ. With fluorescent light, two closely adjacent yellow lines are found at 577 and 579 mμ, a single green line at 546 mμ, and a single purple line at 436 mμ.
2. For optimum results the intensity of the light source and the concentration of the solution to be examined must be adjusted to give sharp and narrow absorption bands. This is usually a matter of trial and error until the characteristics of a particular spectroscope are learned.
3. The slit should be open just far enough to give a full spectrum and easily visible, sharp Fraunhofer lines.
4. Examination is facilitated if the instrument allows simultaneous comparison of a known and unknown solution or of a treated and untreated specimen.
5. Oxyhemoglobin is always present in blood, and the identification of an abnormal compound depends on how much interference is encountered by the oxyhemoglobin absorption bands (see Fig. 10-12, p. 462).

Collection of specimens

1. Blood is usually collected in dry oxalate.
2. Heparin is the anticoagulant of choice when methemoglobin is suspected.
3. Blood to be examined for carboxyhemoglobin is best collected in tightly stoppered tubes using dry sodium citrate as the anticoagulant.
4. Extreme care must be taken in all cases to prevent hemolysis.
5. Urine should be examined as soon as possible after it is voided.
6. Erythrocytes and plasma may be examined separately. This is essential when looking for methemalbumin.

Preparation of known solutions

Absorption bands may be identified by reference to a standard chart (Fig. 10-12, p. 462). For direct comparison, however, and for training purposes, solutions of known composition can be prepared as follows:

1. Oxyhemoglobin: Add 1 drop of blood to 15 ml of water; dilute until two bands are seen, at 578 and 540 mμ.
2. Carboxyhemoglobin: Dilute blood 1:50 with water; saturate with illuminating gas.
3. Reduced hemoglobin: Dilute blood 1:50, add a few milligrams of $Na_2S_2O_4$, and mix gently.
4. Sulfhemoglobin: Dilute blood 1:50. To 5 ml, add 0.9 ml of 0.1% phenylhydrazine hydrochloride and 0.1 ml of water saturated with H_2S gas. A convenient source of H_2S is marketed under the trade name Aitch-Tu-Ess.*
5. Methemoglobin (neutral): Dilute blood 1:50 with water; add a crystal of potassium ferricyanide.
6. Methemoglobin (alkaline): To 10 ml of neutral methemoglobin, add 1 or 2 drops of concentrated ammonium hydroxide.
7. Methemalbumin: Incubate at 40° C 1 vol of oxyhemoglobin solution and 4 vol of sterile plasma.
8. Acid porphyrin: Add slowly, with constant stirring, 0.1 ml of blood to 9.9 ml of concentrated sulfuric acid. Use concentrated sulfuric acid if further dilution is necessary.
9. Alkaline porphyrin: Add slowly 1 ml of blood to 10 ml of concentrated sulfuric acid. Pour cautiously into 350 ml of cold distilled water. Harvest the precipitate that forms; add to it a small amount of concentrated ammonium hydroxide and filter. Dilute as necessary with concentrated ammonium hydroxide.

Identification of abnormal compounds

If a recording spectrophotometer is available, curves characteristic of hemoglobin compounds and derivatives can be used for identification of unknown solutions (see Figs. 10-13 to 10-18, pp. 462-463). Characteristic absorption bands can also be detected by using a spectroscope.

Oxyhemoglobin

Two bands are present, one at 578 and the other at 540 mμ. Add a few milligrams of $Na_2S_2O_4$; the two bands are replaced by a single band of reduced hemoglobin at 556 mμ.

Carboxyhemoglobin

The suitably diluted solution shows one band at 535 and one at 572 mμ. These bands are similar to those of oxyhemoglobin, but are shifted slightly to the right (purple). Add a few milligrams of $Na_2S_2O_4$; if the bands persist, carboxyhemoglobin is present. A

---

*Hycel Inc., Houston, Tex.

*Hengar Co., Philadelphia, Pa.

wide band of reduced hemoglobin will also be present, extending from 540 to 570 mμ; if the specimen is sufficiently diluted, this band will be very faint and will not obscure the carboxyhemoglobin bands.

Methemoglobin

A band is present at 630 mμ; it disappears when either a few milligrams of KCN or of $Na_2S_2O_4$ are added. Atypical reactions may be seen in congenital methemoglobinemia.

Sulfhemoglobin

A band is present at 618 mμ, it persists when a few milligrams of KCN are added, but disappears on addition of either $Na_2S_2O_4$ plus saturation with CO, $Na_2S_2O_4$ plus 2 ml of 10% NaOH, or a few drops of 3% H_2O_2.

Methemalbumin

Examine *plasma* for a band at 624 mμ. The band disappears after addition of $Na_2S_2O_4$; it persists after addition of KCN. Confirm by Schumm's test as follows: layer ether over an aliquot of untreated plasma and add one tenth vol of saturated solution of yellow ammonium sulfide; mix and observe spectroscopically. If methemalbumin is present, an absorption band at 558 mμ is seen.

Myoglobin

Examine *urine* for bands at 582 and 542 mμ. These are too close to the bands of oxyhemoglobin to permit distinction when daylight is used but can be distinguished when fluorescent light is used because the position of the double Fraunhofer lines at 577 and 579 mμ makes comparison easier (Bowden et al, 1956).

Urinary porphyrins

Examine untreated urine for the following band:

Alkaline porphyrin: 612, 568, 538, and 504 mμ
Acid porphyrin: 602 and 557 mμ
Metallic porphyrin: 568 and 538 mμ

Porphobilinogen (qualitative)

Ehrlich's reagent reacts with the pyrrole group present in hemoglobin derivatives, producing a red color. Accordingly, a red color is produced in the presence of porphobilinogen, urobilinogen, indole, and other pyrrole compounds. The red aldehyde compound formed when *p*-dimethylaminobenzaldehyde reacts with porphobilinogen is insoluble in chloroform, whereas the aldehydes of other pyrroles are completely soluble in chloroform.

Reagents

1. Ehrlich's reagent
   a. Dissolve 0.7 Gm *p*-dimethylaminobenzaldehyde (analytical reagent*) in 150 ml of concentrated HCl and 100 ml of distilled water.
2. Saturated aqueous sodium acetate
   a. Add 150 Gm of sodium acetate to 100 ml of distilled water.
   b. Dissolve by heating gently. Cool.

Method

1. Acidify about 10 ml of urine with concentrated HCl to a pH of 3.5 to 5.
2. To about 2.5 ml of acidified urine in a large test tube, add 2.5 ml of Ehrlich's reagent. Mix quickly and then add 5 ml of the saturated solution of sodium acetate.

---

*Eastman Kodak Co., Rochester, N.Y.

3. If a red color develops, add a few milliliters of chloroform and mix thoroughly. Repeat the chloroform extraction until the chloroform is colorless.

Results

If porphobilinogen is present, the aqueous fraction remains red. If the color is caused by urobilinogen or indole, it will be taken up by the chloroform, and the aqueous fraction becomes colorless. (See Chapter 10 and Table 10-11, p. 471.)

Reference

Watson and Schwartz, 1941

Porphyrins (qualitative)

The porphyrins have a pink-to-red fluorescence when viewed by ultraviolet light at about 4,000 Å. Uroporphyrin can be separated from coproporphyrin because of different solubilities in acid solutions.

Reagents

1. HCl, 5%
   a. Add 50 ml of concentrated HCl slowly to 200 ml of distilled water.
   b. Dilute to 370 ml.

Method

1. Transfer 25 ml of urine to a separatory funnel and add 10 ml of glacial acetic acid.
2. Extract twice with 50-ml portions of ether, collecting and combining the ether extracts. The aqueous residue is saved for a subsequent step (5).
3. Wash the combined ether extracts in a separatory funnel with 10 ml of 5% HCl. Collect the HCl fraction and view by ultraviolet light (4,000 Å).
4. A strong red fluorescence indicates the presence of large amounts of coproporphyrin. Confirm spectroscopically.
5. View by ultraviolet light the aqueous portion saved from the ether extraction in step 3. Red fluorescence indicates the presence of uroporphyrin. Confirm spectroscopically and by the Waldenström method, as follows:
6. Using dilute (0.37%) HCl, adjust the aqueous residue to a pH of 3 to 3.2.
7. Extract twice with 50 ml portions of ethyl acetate. Save and combine the ethyl acetate extracts.
8. Extract the ethyl acetate three times with 2-ml portions of 9.2% HCl (25% by volume). Combine the acid extracts and view by ultraviolet light. Red fluorescence indicates uroporphyrin. Confirm spectroscopically.

Remarks

Small amounts of coproporphyrin are present in normal urine. Uroporphyrin is not normally present in the urine.

Ethyl acetate will not extract all the Waldenström uroporphyrin and little or none of the pure uroporphyrin type I found in congenital porphyria. However, ethyl acetate extraction will concentrate the more commonly occurring Waldenström uroporphyrin sufficiently to detect its presence.

Porphyrins: quantitative assay of urinary coproporphyrin, uroporphyrin, δ-aminolevulinic acid, and porphobilinogen

Principle

Urinary porphyrins are determined on urine collected over a 24-hour period. The urine is maintained at an alkaline pH and collected in a dark bottle. Contact with metal should be avoided.

For coproporphyrin and uroporphyrin an aliquot of urine is

placed in a separatory funnel, acidified, and coproporphyrin extracted by ethyl acetate and reextracted into 1.5N HCl. The aqueous portion of the first extractions contains uroporphyrin. It is passed through an aluminum hydroxide column to adsorb uroporphyrin, which is then released by 1.5N HCl. Both porphyrins are read in a fluorometer against coproporphyrin standards. A conversion factor is used to calculate uroporphyrin concentration.

For determining δ-aminolevulinic acid, the urine is passed through a Dowex-2 column that adsorbs porphobilinogen (PBG), while allowing aminolevulinic acid (ALA) to pass through. PBG is eluted with acetic acid and quantitated with Ehrlich's reagent. The ALA portion is passed through a Dowex-50 column that adsorbs it. ALA is eluted with sodium acetate, then condensed with acetylacetone to form a pyrrole that reacts with Ehrlich's reagent.

Collection of urine

Plastic-capped dark bottles containing 5 Gm anhydrous sodium carbonate are used for 24-hour collection, and the individual random specimens are added as soon as possible. Phosphate that may precipitate at this pH may adsorb porphyrins so that the specimen must be well mixed before measuring total volume and sampling. Refrigeration of urine is desirable, and analysis should be made within a week.

Coproporphyrin and uroporphyrin
Reagents

1. Anhydrous Na_2CO_3 for collection
2. Saturated sodium acetate
   a. Heat 100 ml distilled water to about 70° C.
   b. Add 125 Gm $NaC_2H_3O_2 \cdot 3H_2O$, mix, and transfer to screw-capped container.
   c. On cooling, crystals must form to indicate saturation.
3. Buffered acetic acid, 4 parts glacial acetic acid to 1 part saturated sodium acetate
4. Ethyl acetate, ACS
5. Sodium acetate, 3%
   a. Dissolve 30 Gm Na acetate ($3H_2O$) and make up to volume of 1 liter.
6. Alcoholic iodine solution, 1%
   a. Use 1 Gm iodine crystals/100 ml 95% alcohol.
   b. Keep in refrigerator in brown bottle.
7. 1.5N HCl
   a. Use 5 ml concentrated HCl made up to 37 ml with water.
8. Aluminum oxide
   a. Check new lots to see if adsorption of uroporphyrin is adequate.
   b. Use Alcoa chromatographic alumina F-20 or Baker and Adamson ignited powder aluminum oxide.
9. Acetone, ACS
10. Acetone, 50% in acetic acid, 1%
    a. Combine 250 ml acetone, 245 ml water, and 5 ml glacial acetic acid.
11. Acetic acid, 1%
    a. To 1 ml glacial acetic acid, add water to make up to 100 ml.
12. Coproporphyrin standard
    a. Stock standard: 50 μg in 100 ml of 1.5N HCl (Coproporphyrin-1*).
    b. Working standard: 5μg% or 0.05 μg/ml. Dilute 1 vol of stock standard with 9 vol of 1.5N HCl.
    c. To check instrument performance and curve, make the following secondary working standards. To 1 vol of

---

*Sigma Chemical Co., St. Louis, Mo.

stock standard, add 4 vol of 1.5N HCl; mix. To a series of 10 ml volumetric flasks, add 1, 2, 3, 4, and 5 ml of this standard, make to volume with 1.5N HCl, and mix. These dilutions are equivalent to 0.01, 0.02, 0.03, 0.04, and 0.05 μg/ml. Read in fluorometer against a 1.5N HCl blank after setting instrument on zero with dummy cuvette and with aperture for required sensitivity. If a higher value is needed, read also the undiluted secondary working standard (equivalent to 0.1 μg/ml).
    d. Working standard is stable (sealed) at room temperature for 1 year. Should be checked against a standard kept in the refrigerator (be sure to bring to room temperature).

Method

1. Check and record the pH of the urine. If less than 6.5 or over 9.5, the results of porphyrin analysis may be unreliable.
2. Pipet a 5-ml aliquot of urine into a 250-ml separatory funnel.
3. Add in order:

Distilled water	20.0 ml
Buffered acetic acid	5.0 ml
Ethyl acetate	100.0 ml
Alcoholic iodine, 1%	0.1 ml

4. Shake funnel 100 times, allowing gases to escape as needed. Let phases separate.
5. Drain aqueous portion (bottom layer) containing uroporphyrin into a 500-ml flask.
6. Wash ethyl acetate phase four times with 20 ml portions of 3% sodium acetate. Shake each ten times and allow to separate before adding aqueous phase to uroporphyrin flask (step 5). The two phases must separate completely. Read each wash in fluorometer against Na acetate blank. With each extraction the reading decreases, ideally to 0, but if too many extractions are done, the reading will again increase as a result of extraction of nonuroporphyrin compounds. Generally, no more than four washes are indicated.

Quantification of coproporphyrin

1. Extract the ethyl fraction with 5-ml portions of 1.5N HCl, shaking 100 times for each. Drain aqueous phase into graduated cylinder. Beginning with the third extraction, compare fluorometer reading to the 1.5N HCl blank. Continue to repeat extraction as long as pink fluorescence is present in the HCl extract. Pool all extracts and make up to convenient (measured) volume (usually 25 ml) with 1.5N HCl. Mix.
2. Blank Turner fluorometer with dummy cuvette, using as filters primary 405 and secondary 25 and high-sensitivity door. Use an appropriate range setting and fill the cuvettes to within ⅜ to ½ inch of the top. Record readings of the 1.5N HCl blank, the unknown, and the 0.05 μg working standard.
3. If the reading of the unknown is higher than that of the standard, make appropriate dilution of the unknown with 1.5N HCl. Mix.

Calculation

$$\frac{\text{Unknown blank}}{\text{Standard blank}} \times \frac{E}{U} \times D \times S \times V \times 0.925 =$$

$$\text{Coproporphyrin (μg/24 hr specimen)}$$

where
E = Volume of 1.5N HCl extract
U = Initial volume of urine used
D = Additional dilutions made
S = Concentration of standard (μg/ml)
V = 24 hr volume of urine
0.925 = Correction factor for ethyl acetate enhancement

Normal values

See Chapter 10.

Quantification of uroporphyrin

1. Prepare alumina column. Cover the holes in plate of 22 × 200 mm chromatograph tube with a thin layer of cotton. Dampen cotton with 50% acetone. Attach tube to 500-ml suction flask. Make column 5 to 7 cm high with slurry of Al_2O_3 and 50% acetone—1% acetic acid solution.
2. Slowly add aqueous portion from step 6 on p. 878 to column and let drip through or use only gentle suction so that uroporphyrin concentrates at upper portion of column. (Check with ultraviolet lamp.)
3. Wash column until free of blue-green fluorescence of urine by filling chromatograph tube with 1% acetic acid and using suction to remove. Repeat until fluorescence disappears (use ultraviolet lamp and check final washing with fluorometer). To avoid excessive dilution, draw off excess acetic acid and discard contents of flask.
4. With tube in suction flask, add 5 ml of 1.5N HCl and watch with ultraviolet lamp as pink fluorescence of uroporphyrin passes down column.
5. When uroporphyrin reaches bottom, place 16 × 150 mm test tube into flask and insert chromatograph tube into test tube. Allow 5 ml of 1.5N HCl to drip through column into test tube. Pour eluate into graduated cylinder.
6. Repeat step 5 until pink fluorescene is gone; check by fluorometer reading. Pool all eluates and make up to convenient volume with 1.5N HCl. Mix.
7. Using 12 × 75 mm cuvettes for 1.5N HCl blank, 0.05 μg/ml coproporphyrin standard, and uroporphyrin unknown, record readings derived for each using high-sensitivity door, primary filter 405, secondary filter 25, and fluorometer set at 0 with dummy cuvette. If unknown reads higher than standard, dilute appropriately with 1.5N HCl.

Calculation

$$\frac{\text{Unknown reading} - \text{blank}}{\text{Standard reading} - \text{blank}} \times$$

$$S \times 0.925 \times 0.75 \times \frac{E}{U} \times D \times V =$$

Uroporphyrin (μg in 24 hr specimen)

where   S = Concentrated standard (μg/ml)
    0.925 = Correction for ethyl acetate enhancement of 1.5N HCl
    0.75 = Correction of coproporphyrin to uroporphyrin equivalent
    E = Total volume of 1.5N HCl extract
    U = Volume of urine originally extracted
    D = Dilution of 1.5N HCl eluate to read below standard
    V = 24-hr volume urine

Normal values

See Chapter 10.

δ-Aminolevulinic acid and porphobilinogen
Reagents

1. Resins and chromatography columns
   a. Use a column 0.9 × 30 cm with ground glass connection and fritted filter. Place a plug of glass wool above filter and add sufficient resin slurry to make column 2 ± 0.1 cm in height. After the Dowex-2 X-8 column is so prepared for the PBG and prior to addition of sample, it is washed with 5 ml of distilled water, discarding the wash. The Dowex-50 X-8 column for the ALA is washed with 25 ml of distilled water, which is discarded.
   b. Dowex-2 X-8 resin (200-400 mesh) for PBG. Place about 200 Gm of this resin in a 1-liter beaker. Remove fine particles by repeated suspension and sedimentation in 400 to 600 ml of distilled water, decanting until the supernatant is clear. Convert to acetate with 3N sodium acetate until the eluate is free of chloride (check with silver nitrate or 5-diphenylcarbazone). Then wash until free of sodium acetate (check for sodium in flame spectrophotometer). Store the resin in a glass jar in two times its volume of distilled water.
   c. Dowex-50 X-8 resin (200-400 mesh) for ALA. About 200 Gm of this resin is washed initially the same way as the Dowex-2 X-8. Then it is converted to sodium form by letting it stand overnight in two times its volume of 2N NaOH. After this, wash with distilled water until neutral and convert to acid form by treating alternately with an equal volume of 4N HCl and 6 vol of 2N HCl. Store the resin in a glass jar in two times its volume of 1N HCl.
   d. The resins keep 3 or 4 months at room temperature.
2. 3N sodium acetate: 40.8 Gm sodium acetate trihydrate/100 ml
3. 0.5N sodium acetate: 6.8 Gm sodium acetate trihydrate/100 ml
4. Acetate buffer, pH 4.6
   a. Add 57.5 ml glacial acetic acid (1 mole) to 136 Gm of sodium acetate trihydrate (1 mole) and dilute to 1 liter with distilled water.
5. 2N NaOH: 80 Gm/l.
6. 4N HCl: 333 ml of concentrated acid/l.
7. 6N HCl: 500 ml of concentrated acid/l.
8. 2N HCl: 166 ml of concentrated acid/l.
9. 1N HCl: 83 ml of concentrated acid/l.
10. Acetylacetone (2,4-pentanedione)
11. Regular Ehrlich's reagent: 2% (w/v) *p*-dimethylaminobenzaldehyde in 6N HCl
12. Modified Ehrlich's reagent
    a. Dissolve 1 Gm of *p*-dimethylaminobenzaldehyde in about 30 ml of glacial acetic acid.
    b. Add 8 ml of perchloric acid (70%) and make to 50 ml with glacial acetic acid.
    c. This reagent is somewhat unstable. Prepare immediately before use.
13. 1M acetic acid: 57.5 ml concentrated acid/l.
14. 0.2M acetic acid: 11.5 ml concentrated acid/l.
15. Porphobilinogen standards*
    a. Stock standard: Use 10 mg of PBG (mol wt 226) per 100 ml of water.
    b. Make five dilutions with water to make standards containing 1.0, 0.8, 0.6, 0.4, and 0.2 mg% PBG. These are equivalent to PBG concentrations in urine of 10, 8, 6, 4, and 2 mg%.
    c. Add 2 ml of regular Ehrlich's reagent to 2 ml of each standard and to 2 ml of water for the blank.
    d. Mix immediately and read at exactly 5 minutes in 12-mm cuvettes at 555 mμ against the blank at 100% T. Plot standard curve.
16. δ-Aminolevulinic acid standards†
    a. Stock standard: Use 67 mg of ALA · HCl (mol wt 167.5)

---

*Obtained as PBG · H_2O (mol/wt 244) from Dew Laboratory, Tampa, Fla.; or Porphobilinogen, synthetic, pfs, Sigma Chemical Co., St. Louis, Mo.

†Obtained as ALA · HCl from Mann Research Laboratories, New York, N.Y.

dissolved and diluted to 1,000 ml with water. Stock standard and dilutions correspond to:
(1) Stock = 5.25 mg ALA/100 ml urine
(2) 16 ml stock + 4ml H_2O = 4.2 mg ALA/100 ml urine (sol b)
(3) 12 ml stock + 8 ml H_2O = 3.15 mg ALA/100 ml urine (sol c)
(4) 10 ml sol b + 10 ml H_2O = 2.1 mg ALA/100 ml urine (sol d)
(5) 10 ml sol d + 10 ml H_2O = 1.05 mg ALA/100 ml urine

b. Add 1 ml of H_2O to a 10-ml volumetric flask and to five others add 1 ml of a diluted standard, appropriately labeled.

c. Add 7.0 ml 0.5M sodium acetate and 0.2 ml acetylacetone to all and then make to volume with pH 4.6 acetate buffer.

d. Stopper, mix, and place in boiling water bath for 10 minutes.

e. Cool to room temperature, make to volume with buffer, mix, and to 2-ml aliquots, add 2 ml modified Ehrlich's reagent.

f. Read in 12-mm cuvettes after exactly 15 minutes at 553 mμ with blank set at 100%. Plot appropriately.

Porphobilinogen
Method

1. Check urine pH and adjust to pH 6.0 ± 1. Mix well and place 1 ml on Dowex-2 column. Allow to drip through.
2. Allow two separate 2-ml water aliquots to pass through column. Collect all from 1 and 2 and save for ALA (note a).
3. Transfer 2 ml 1M acetic acid to column. Collect in 10-ml volumetric flask.
4. Transfer 2 ml 0.2M acetic acid to column. Collect in same flask (note b).
5. Dilute to 10 ml volume with water. Mix.
6. The color determination is done on a 2-ml aliquot to which 2 ml regular Ehrlich's reagent is added. A blank of 2 ml water is treated the same way. Mix immediately. After mixing, read in exactly 5 minutes against reagent blank at 100% T at 555 mμ in 12-mm cuvettes. Read from chart.

Calculation

$$\text{Unknown mg\%} \times \frac{\text{24-hr vol}}{100} = \text{mg/24 hr}$$

Note a: If ALA is high, elute with two more aliquots of 2 ml water. Add to pool.
Note b: If PBG is high, elute two more times with 2 ml of 0.2M acetic acid. Add to pool from step 4.

Normal value
Up to 4 mg PBG/24 hour.

δ-Aminolevulinic acid
Method

1. Quantitatively transfer all of the eluate from step 2 above to Dowex-50 column.
2. Wash column free of adsorbed urea with 16 ml water, checking last part with Ehrlich's reagent to see if all yellow reaction with urea is gone.
3. Add 3 ml 0.5M sodium acetate. Allow to drain and discard (note a).

4. Elute ALA with 7 ml 0.5 sodium acetate, collecting in a 10-ml volumetric flask (note b).
5. Set up blank 10-ml flask containing 1 ml water and standard 10-ml flask containing 1 ml of standard equivalent to 3.15 mg%. To each add 7 ml 0.5M sodium acetate.
6. To all add 0.2 ml acetylacetone and dilute to mark with pH 4.6 acetate buffer. Mix.
7. Place stoppered flasks in boiling water bath for 10 minutes.
8. Cool to room temperature and if needed bring back to volume with pH 4.6 buffer. Mix.
9. To 2-ml aliquots of each, add 2 ml modified Ehrlich's reagent, mix, and transfer to 12-mm cuvettes.
10. After 15 minutes and before 30 minutes have elapsed, read at 553 mμ against blank.
11. Either calculate against standard or read in mg% from curve and correct for 24-hour volume.

Note a: Color of column should become lighter only part of the way down, not all the way.
Note b: If ALA is high, elute with second 7-ml portion of 0.5M sodium acetate into another 10-ml flask and carry through rest of procedure. Add the values obtained from the second to that of the first.

Calculation

$$\text{Unknown mg\%} \times \frac{\text{24-hr vol}}{100} = \text{mg/24 hr}$$

Normal value

Up to 4 mg of ALA/24 hours.

References

The methods outlined here are from the following references, with modifications by Dr. J.N. Patterson and Miss Doris Dede.
Mauzerall and Granick, 1956
Schwartz et al, 1951, 1960

Porphobilinogen (semiquantitative method)
Principle

Porphobilinogen reacts with Ehrlich's p-dimethylaminobenzaldehyde reagent to form a red compound called porphobilinogen aldehyde. Saturated sodium acetate is added to increase the urobilinogen color and to cause its complete extraction into the solvent (chloroform). If there is still red color in the aqueous layer, extract with butanol. Rule out drug interference by running a blank on the urine with HCl alone.

This method is useful as an adequate screening method and for estimating the approximate concentration.

Reagents

1. Ehrlich's reagent
   a. Mix 0.7 Gm p-dimethylaminobenzaldehyde and 150 ml concentrated HCl.
   b. Add 100 ml distilled water to make 250 ml.
   c. Final solution should be colorless or straw color.
2. Sodium acetate, ACS saturated aqueous
3. Congo red paper
4. N-Butyl alcohol, ACS
5. HCl, concentrated ACS
6. Chloroform, ACS
7. HCl, 60%
   a. Make 60 ml concentrated acid up to volume with 100 ml distilled water.

8. Stock standard: 10 mg% dye
   a. Use 5 mg of Pontacyl Carmine 2 B* and 95 mg of Pontacyl Violet 6 R* dissolved in and made up to 1,000 ml with 0.5% acetic acid.
9. Working standard
   a. Varying concentrations of the stock dye solution are made with 0.5% acetic acid and compared with known concentrations of urobilinogen aldehyde used for instrument calibration.
   b. Read in 19 × 15 mm cuvettes in a Coleman Jr. spectrophotometer against a 0.5% acetic acid blank set at 100% at 565 mμ. In plotting the values, or in calculating the value, PBG is arbitrarily assigned as 1 unit/1 mg of urobilinogen.

Pontacyl dye mixture (mg/100 ml)	Urobilinogen (mg/100 ml) = units of PBG
2.040	0.6
1.700	0.5
1.360	0.4
1.020	0.3
0.850	0.25
0.680	0.20
0.510	0.15
0.340	0.10
0.170	0.05
0.085	0.025

Method

1. Place 2.5 ml urine and 2.5 ml Ehrlich's reagent into a 19 × 150 mm cuvette and mix for 30 seconds. A red color develops if porphobilinogen is present.
2. Add 5 ml saturated sodium acetate and mix well. The red color, if present, may intensify (note a). The Congo red paper should remain red when the solution is checked here (note b). If no pink or red color, report PBG as negative.
3. If color is present, add 5 ml chloroform. Shake and allow to separate; chloroform carries urobilinogen and nonspecific Ehrlich reactors to the bottom of the tube. A negative result is indicated by no pink color in the aqueous phase.
4. If pink-red color is present in the aqueous layer, remove it, place in another tube, and add 5 ml of butyl alcohol. Shake vigorously, and allow the layers to separate (note c).
   a. A negative result is indicated by having no pink or red color in the lower aqueous layer.
   b. If there is an intense color in the butanol layer and a pink color still in the aqueous layer, remove the butanol layer into another tube and extract the aqueous layer again with butanol to be sure all the urobilinogen or other Ehrlich's reacting substances are removed (note d).
5. After the butanol extraction is completed, if the aqueous layer is still pink, red, or red-violet, prepare a blank in a 19 × 150 mm Coleman cuvette by placing 5 ml saturated sodium acetate, 2.5 ml Ehrlich's reagent, and mix. Then add 2.5 ml of urine (note a) with mixing, then 5 ml butanol with shaking, and allow to separate (note c).
6. Place the blank in the Coleman Jr. spectrophotometer and set at 100% T at a wavelength of 565 mμ.
7. Read and record the %T of the unknown and obtain the value from the prepared standard curve.

---

*DuPont de Nemours & Co., Inc., Wilmington, Del.

Calculation

$$P \times \frac{A}{U} \times \frac{V}{100} \times D = \text{Units of PBG/24 hr}$$

where P = Units of PBG in unknown read from calibration curve
  A = Total volume of diluted aqueous solution, usually 10 ml (2.5 ml urine, 2.5 ml Ehrlich's reagent, and 5 ml saturated sodium acetate)
  U = 2.5 ml urine (amount used in test)
  V = Total 24-hr volume of specimen in ml
  D = Dilution factor if urine was diluted with water prior to measuring 2:5 ml

Note a: If the color is very intense, start procedure again, using 2.5 ml of a quantitatively diluted urine. If this is necessary, the 2.5 ml or urine in the blank should be of this same dilution.
Note b: The Congo red paper is used to be sure all the HCl in the Ehrlich's reagent has been converted to acetic acid. A blue color would indicate the conversion had not taken place. Check the saturation of sodium acetate and the making of the Ehrlich's reagent. A known amount more of saturated acetate may have to be added to obtain a red color with the Congo red paper.
Note c: If the layers do not separate clearly, filter through moistened coarse filter paper.
Note d: Check for drug causing the red color in the aqueous portion by adding 2.5 ml 60% HCl to 2.5 ml of urine. If no red color develops, you can conclude that the color in the test is caused by PBG. Conclusive proof of PBG is to examine urine and Ehrlich's mixture of step 1 without delay with a hand spectroscope to see if there are two absorption bands, one at 560 to 570 mμ and a second weaker band at 515 to 530 mμ.
Note e: For other color reactions, see Table 10-11, p. 471.

References

Schwartz et al, 1944
Watson and Hawkinson, 1947
Watson and Schwartz, 1941

Quantitative methemoglobin in blood

Methemoglobin has a characteristic absorption peak at 630 mμ. Cyanide converts the methemoglobin to cyanmethemoglobin. The difference in absorption before and after the addition of the cyanide is a measure of the amount of methemoglobin present. Total hemoglobin is determined by converting all the hemoglobin into cyanmethemoglobin and reading at 540 mμ. The determination of F_M and F_T needs be done only once for a given instrument.

Reagents

1. Potassium ferricyanide, 20%
   a. Dissolve 20 Gm of potassium ferricyanide in distilled water. Heat gently.
   b. Cool and dilute to 100 ml. Dispense from a dropper bottle.
   c. To prepare a 5% solution, dilute 1 vol of the 20% solution with 3 vol of distilled water.
2. 0.067M phosphate buffer, pH 6.6
   a. Dissolve 9 Gm of $Na_2HPO_4 \cdot 12H_2O$ and 5.7 Gm of anhydrous KH_2PO_4 in distilled water and dilute to volume of 1 liter.
   b. To prepare 0.017M buffer (pH 6.6), dilute 1 vol of the 0.067M solution with 3 vol of distilled water.
3. Sodium cyanide, 10%
   a. Dissolve 5 Gm of sodium cyanide in 50 ml of distilled water. Dispense from a dropper bottle.
4. Neutralized sodium cyanide
   a. Add 1 vol of 12% acetic acid (12 ml of glacial made up to 100 ml with distilled water) to 1 vol of 10% sodium cyanide.

b. The reagent should be prepared in a hood, adding the acid to the cyanide. The solution should be used within an hour after preparation and dispensed from a dropper bottle.

Method for methemoglobin

1. Add 0.1 ml of capillary or oxalated venous blood collected under oil to 10 ml of 0.017M phosphate buffer.
2. Mix and let stand 5 minutes.
3. Read OD at 630 mμ, using distilled water as the blank. OD reading = D_1.
4. Add 1 drop of neutral sodium cyanide.
5. Mix and let stand 2 minutes.
6. Read at 630 mμ. OD reading = D_2.
7. $(D_1 - D_2) \times F_M$ = Gm of methemoglobin/dl of blood.

Method for total hemoglobin

1. Add 1 drop of concentrated NH_4OH to a 10 ml sample of buffer and blood described in step 1 under *methemoglobin*.
2. To a 2-ml aliquot, add 8 ml of 0.067M phosphate buffer.
3. Add 1 drop of 20% potassium ferricyanide, mix, and let stand 2 minutes for maximum conversion of hemoglobin to methemoglobin.
4. Add 1 drop of 10% sodium cyanide.
5. Mix and let stand 2 minutes to convert methemoglobin to cyanmethemoglobin.
6. Read at 540 mμ, using a blank of 10 ml 0.067M phosphate buffer and 1 drop of 20% potassium ferricyanide. OD reading = D_3.
7. $D_3 \times F_T$ = Gm of total hemoglobin per dl of blood.

Determination of F_M

1. No. 1 tube (unknown): 9.9 ml 0.017M phosphate buffer + 0.1 ml 5% potassium ferricyanide solution. No. 2 tube (blank): 10 ml 0.017M phosphate buffer + 0.1 ml 5% potassium ferricyanide solution.
2. Add 0.1 ml of blood to the unknown. The hemoglobin concentration of this blood should be determined by the standard method.
3. Mix and allow to stand 2 minutes.
4. Read D_1 at 630mμ, using distilled water as the blank.
5. After reading, add 1 drop of neutralized sodium cyanide to both unknown and blank.
6. Mix, let stand 2 minutes, and read again at 630 mμ, setting the OD at 0 with the blank. Reading = D_2.
7. $F_M = \dfrac{Hb\ (Gm/dl)}{D_1 - D_2}$

Determination of F_T

1. Add 2 ml of the unknown (tube No. 1) to 8 ml of distilled water. Mix.
2. Add 2 ml of blank (tube No. 2) to 8 ml of distilled water. Mix.
3. Set the blank at 0 and read the OD of the unknown at 540 mμ. Reading = D_3.
4. $F_T = \dfrac{Hb\ of\ standard\ in\ Gm/dl}{D_3}$

Normal value

0.03 to 0.13 Gm/dl.

Remark

Determination of F_T is not an integral part of the methemoglobin determination, but it is a valuable check for hemoglobinometry.

Note carefully the failure of this method to quantify some abnormal methemoglobins (Chapter 10).

Reference

Hawk et al, 1949

Assay of serum iron concentration
Principle

Iron is dissociated from protein at an acid pH, reduced to the ferrous state, and the proteins precipitated leaving the ferrous iron in the supernate. It is then reacted with a chromogen. The optical density of the developed color is compared with the optical density developed in a standard solution.

Reagents

1. Protein precipitant

Trichloroacetic acid (iron free)	100 Gm
Thioglycollic acid	30 ml
Concentrated HCl	100 ml
Sufficient iron-free water to make 1 liter	

2. Chromogen solution: Ferrozine,* 105 mg/dl of saturated sodium acetate solution. This is stable when stored in a brown bottle at room temperature.
3. Iron standard solution
   a. Stock solution: dissolve 100 mg of dry, polished, certified, electrolytic iron wire in 2 ml of 7M iron-free hydrochloric acid in a boiling water bath. Cool and dilute to 100 ml with iron-free water.
   b. Working solution containing 2 μg/ml of iron: dilute 2.0 ml of stock solution to 1 liter with 0.0005M iron-free HCl.
4. Iron-free water: prepare by passing distilled water through a deionizer containing both charcoal and iron-exchange resin.

Method

1. Use iron-free (acid cleaned) glassware or plastic throughout the procedure.
2. Draw venous blood without trauma and allow to clot. There must be no hemolysis. Centrifuge and transfer serum to clean tube. Recentrifuge to eliminate any contaminating red blood cells.
3. Add 2.0 ml protein precipitant solution to 2.0 ml serum. Mix thoroughly with a vortex mixer and incubate 15 minutes at 56° C.
4. Add 2.0 ml protein precipitant solution to 2.0 ml of working standard. Mix thoroughly and incubate 15 minutes at 56° C.
5. Add 2.0 ml protein precipitant solution to 2.0 ml iron-free water. Mix thoroughly and incubate 15 minutes at 56° C. This is the reagent blank.
6. After incubation, centrifuge the 3 tubes at 3,000 rpm/15 minutes or to an optically clear supernate.
7. Add 0.5 ml chromogen solution to 2.0 ml of serum supernate solution.
8. Add 0.5 ml of chromogen solution to each of 2.0 ml treated standard solution and 2.0 ml treated blank solution supernates.
9. Determine the OD of the three solutions at 562 nm against distilled water.
10. Calculate the serum iron concentration:

$$\text{Serum iron (μg/dl)} = \frac{\text{OD serum specimen} - \text{OD blank}}{\text{OD standard} - \text{OD blank}} \times 200$$

---

*Hach Chemical Co., Ames, Iowa.

Remarks

This is the method proposed by the International Committee for Standardization in Hematology as modified by Rice and Fenner (1974). The modified method is recommended because it gives a clearer serum supernate, and the chromogen is less expensive and more sensitive than the bathophenanthroline salt.

TESTS FOR HEMOLYTIC DISEASE
Osmotic fragility of erythrocytes

The value of osmotic fragility measurements is discussed in Chapter 13. The first method, that of Sanford, is adequate for most clinical purposes. The second method, that of Dacie, is recommended for critical measurements.

Method of Sanford
Reagent

1. Stock 0.5% saline solution
   a. Add exactly 0.5 Gm of chemically pure, freshly dried sodium chloride to about 50 ml of distilled water in a 100-ml volumetric flask.
   b. Dissolve, and make up to volume with distilled water.

Method

1. Set up two rows of 12 small test tubes. One row is for the test on the patient's blood and the other for a normal control. Each set of tubes is handled in the same way.
2. Number the tubes, from left to right, 25, 24, 23, 22, 21, 20, 19, 18, 17, 16, 15, and 14.
3. With a capillary pipet, add to each tube the number of drops of 0.5% saline solution indicated by the number on the tube. With the same pipet, add the number of drops of distilled water required to bring the contents of each tube to a total of 25 drops. Mix by shaking. The salt concentration in each tube is now the number on the tube times 0.02.
4. Obtain blood by venipuncture and, with the needle still attached to the syringe, carefully add 1 drop of blood to each tube. Mix.
5. Let stand at room temperature for 2 hours. Record the salt concentration at which there is first evidence of hemolysis (initial hemolysis). Record the salt concentration at which no sediment of erythrocytes can be seen (complete hemolysis) (Fig. 13-17, p. 583).
6. If the various saline solutions used in the method of Dacie (see following section) are available, these can be used instead of the above method, using 25 drops of each saline dilution plus 1 drop of blood.

Results

See Table 13-11, p. 584.

Method of Dacie
Reagents

1. Stock solution of buffered sodium chloride
   a. Dissolve 90 Gm of NaCl, 13.66 Gm of $Na_2HPO_4 \cdot 2 H_2O$ and 2.43 Gm of $NaH_2PO_4 \cdot 2 H_2O$ in distilled water and make up exactly to 1 liter. This stock solution is osmotically equivalent to 10% NaCl. It is stable for months if kept in a stoppered bottle.
2. Working solutions
   a. First dilute the stock solution 1:10 to make up a solution equivalent to 1% NaCl.
   b. The working solutions can be most conveniently made by delivering the correct amount of 1% solution into 50-ml volumetric flasks and diluting to volume with distilled water as follows:

0.85%; 42.5 ml of 1% solution
0.75%; 37.5 ml of 1% solution
0.65%; 32.5 ml of 1% solution
0.60%; 30.0 ml of 1% solution
0.55%; 27.5 ml of 1% solution
0.50%; 25.0 ml of 1% solution
0.45%; 22.5 ml of 1% solution
0.40%; 20.0 ml of 1% solution
0.35%; 17.5 ml of 1% solution
0.30%; 15.0 ml of 1% solution
0.20%; 10.0 ml of 1% solution
0.10%; 5.0 ml of 1% solution

   c. Label each bottle and store at 4° C. These solutions can be used until they become contaminated with molds.

Method

1. Obtain blood by venipuncture and heparinize.
2. Set up 12 tubes, each containing 5 ml of the various working solutions. Label. Add 0.05 ml of blood to each and mix well.
3. Let stand at room temperature for 30 minutes; then gently resuspend and centrifuge at 2,000 rpm for 5 minutes.
4. Read the supernates in a spectrophotometer, wavelength 545 mμ, using the supernate of the 0.85% tube as the blank and the 0.1% tube as 100%.
5. Plot an osmotic fragility curve, percent hemolysis against salt concentration (see Fig. 13-19, p. 585).

Results

Normal range of osmotic fragility at 20° C, pH 7.4, is as follows:

0.30% salt 97 to 100% hemolysis
0.35% salt 90 to 99% hemolysis
0.40% salt 50 to 90% hemolysis
0.45% salt 5 to 45% hemolysis
0.50% salt 0 to 5% hemolysis
0.55% salt   0% hemolysis

Osmotic fragility after incubation

The method is the same as Dacie's, except that the test is performed with sterile defibrinated blood that has been incubated at 37° C for 24 hours (Chapter 13).

Method

1. Using a sterile technic and equipment, obtain 10 ml of blood by venipuncture and defibrinate by swirling in a bottle containing glass beads.
2. Transfer 2 ml of defibrinated blood to each of two sterile screw-capped tubes. Incubate at 37° C for 24 hours.
3. Mix and pool the two samples.
4. Determine osmotic fragility by the method of Dacie.

Results

Normal range of osmotic fragility after incubation at 37° C for 24 hours is as follows:

0.20% salt 91 to 100% hemolysis
0.30% salt 80 to 100% hemolysis
0.35% salt 72 to 100% hemolysis
0.40% salt 65 to 100% hemolysis
0.45% salt 54 to 96% hemolysis
0.50% salt 36 to 88% hemolysis
0.55% salt 5 to 70% hemolysis
0.60% salt 0 to 40% hemolysis
0.65% salt 0 to 19% hemolysis
0.70% salt 0 to 9% hemolysis
0.85% salt   0% hemolysis

Acid serum test for paroxysmal nocturnal hemoglobinuria

In paraoxysmal nocturnal hemoglobinuria (PNH) the erythrocytes are abnormally susceptible to hemolysis in acidified serum.

Method

1. Obtain blood from the patient, defibrinate it by means of glass beads, and centrifuge to separate the serum from the cells.
2. Obtain, as above, fresh serum from a normal, A-B-O blood group–compatible individual.
3. Wash erythrocytes from both patient and normal control three times with isotonic saline solution and resuspend to make a 50% suspension.
4. Label tubes 1 through 5.
5. Add 0.5 ml of patient's serum to tubes 1 and 2. Add 0.5 ml normal serum to tubes 3, 4, and 5.
6. Add 0.05 ml of 0.2N HCl to tubes 1, 3, and 5.
7. Add 1 drop of patient's erythrocyte suspension to tubes 1, 2, 3, and 4.
8. Add 1 drop of normal erythrocyte suspension to tube 5.
9. Cork and incubate all tubes for 1 hour at 37° C.
10. Centrifuge tubes and observe supernatant for hemolysis.

Results

A positive result shows lysis in the acidified serum samples (tubes 1 and 3), little or no lysis in unacidified serum (tubes 2 and 4), and no lysis of normal erythrocytes in acidified fresh serum (tube 5).

Remarks

The optimum pH for the reaction is 6.5 to 7.

A false-positive test is sometimes seen in congenital spherocytic anemia or if tube 5 shows lysis. If this is suspected, the test should be repeated, using acidified serum previously inactivated at 56° C for 30 minutes. Since PNH erythrocytes require complement for hemolysis, the modified test will be negative in PNH and will remain positive in spherocytosis. Acid hemolysis is also seen in HEMPAS (p. 569), but in this disease the red blood cells are not lysed by the patient's own acidified serum.

Normal red blood cells treated with 2-aminoethylisothiouronium bromide behave like PNH cells and can be used for a positive control.

PNH erythrocytes are unusually susceptible to hemolysis by autoantibodies and isoantibodies and are useful in the detection of hemolytic antibodies.

References

Dacie and Lewis, 1975b
Sirchia and Dacie, 1967

Sugar-water test for paroxysmal nocturnal hemoglobinuria
Principle

PNH erythrocytes lyse when incubated with autologous or isologous compatible normal serum in a sucrose solution of low ionic strength. The reaction is specific for PNH and probably depends on the enhanced fixation of complement to the surface of the erythrocytes when they are incubated with sucrose.

Reagent

1. Isotonic sucrose solution
   a. Dissolve 92.4 Gm of reagent grade sucrose in 910 ml of 0.005M solution of sodium phosphate (monobasic) and 90 ml of solution of 0.005M sodium phosphate (dibasic).
   b. Check pH and adjust to 6.1 if necessary.

Method

1. Obtain clotted venous blood from the patient and a normal donor. Centrifuge and separate serum.
2. From the clots, prepare 50% suspensions of erythrocytes.
3. To separate tubes, add 0.85 ml of sucrose soluton, 0.05 ml of the autologous serum, and 0.1 ml of the corresponding erythrocyte suspension. Mix thoroughly.
4. Incubate at 37° C for 30 minutes, centrifuge, and observe the supernate for hemolysis.

Results

Marked hemolysis is found in PNH but not in control. According to Hartmann and Jenkins (1966) no hemolysis is found in other types of hemolytic anemia (cold agglutinin disease, acquired autoimmune hemolytic anemia, hereditary spherocytosis, pyruvate kinase deficiency, hemoglobinopathies, and acanthocytosis).

Blood collected in EDTA or heparin is not suitable for this test.

Reference

Hartmann et al, 1970

Demonstration of Donath-Landsteiner (D-L) hemolysin

Paroxysmal cold hemoglobinuria is characterized by the presence of a special hemolysin called the D-L hemolysin or D-L antibody (Chapter 13).

Method

1. Obtain venous blood from the patient, divide it into two test tubes, and allow both specimens to clot. Obtain a second set of blood specimens from a normal person and use these two tubes as controls.
2. Place one tube from each person in an ice bath (3° to 4° C) for 20 minutes and then transfer to a 37° C water bath for 1 hour. The second set of tubes is left at room temperature.
3. Observe the supernatant sera for hemolysis.

Results

Hemolysis in the patient's tube that has been chilled and then warmed is presumptive evidence for the presence of D-L antibody. The patient's specimen that was not chilled and both control tubes should be free of hemolysis.

Autohemolysis
Principle

If sterile defibrinated or oxalated normal blood is incubated at 37° C for 24 hours, only minimal hemolysis will take place. In hemolytic anemias, spontaneous hemolysis (autohemolysis) is accelerated (Chapter 13).

Although it is possible to perform the test quantitatively, it is not so specific as to warrant the effort. The simple screening test outlined here is sufficient. See methods for identifying specific types of hemolytic anemia.

Method

1. Obtain sterile oxalated blood from the patient and from a normal control by nontraumatic venipuncture. Avoid hemolysis.
2. Incubate both samples at 37° C for 24 hours.
3. Centrifuge and observe the degree of hemolysis in the plasma.

Results

Autohemolysis is estimated visually by the color of the plasma.

Alkali denaturation test for fetal hemoglobin
Principle

Quantification of fetal hemoglobin is based on the fact that fetal hemoglobin is more resistant to denaturation by a strong alkali than the other hemoglobins.

Reagents

1. Drabkin's soluton

KCN	0.05 Gm
$K_3Fe(CN)_6$	0.20 Gm

   Dissolve in sufficient distilled water to make 1 liter.
2. NaOH, 1.2N
3. NH_4SO_4, saturated solution
4. Hemolysate (p. 888) with hemoglobin concentration of 8 Gm/dl.

Method

1. Add 0.6 ml hemolysate to 10 ml Drabkin's solution.
2. Prepare standards
   a. Mix 1.4 ml cyanmethemoglobin certified standard* solution, 1.6 ml distilled water, and 2.0 ml NH_4SO_4.
   b. Dilute 1:10 with Drabkin's solution.
   c. Filter through a double layer of Whatman No. 6 filter paper.
3. Prepare test
   a. Add 0.2 ml NaOH to 2.8 ml hemolysate solution. Agitate 2 minutes.
   b. Add 2 ml NH_4SO_4, shake, then allow to stand 5 minutes.
   c. Filter through a double layer of Whatman No. 6 filter paper.
4. Read the OD of standard and test solutions at 415 nm.

Interpretation

$$\text{Calculation of } \% \text{ Hb F} = \frac{\text{OD of test}}{\text{OD of standard} \times 20} \times 100$$

Comments

This method (White, 1974) gives more reliable and reproducible results than the original method of Singer. In experienced hands, this technic yields Hb F values of under 2% in normal subjects, whereas with the Singer method, values up to 4% can be found. In a study of 200 normals, 98% had values between 0% and 1%, and 2% had values between 1.0% and 2.5%.

References

Singer et al, 1951a; 1951b
White, 1974

Demonstration of fetal hemoglobin in red blood cells: acid elution technic
Principle

Hemoglobin is precipitated inside the cell by drying and fixing with alcohol. Hemoglobin A and its adult variants are then soluble in citric acid–phosphate buffer. Hemoglobin F remains precipitated inside the cell.

Reagents

1. 80% ethanol
2. Citric acid–phosphate buffer, pH 3.3
   a. Solution A: Dissolve 21 Gm citric acid monohydrate in 1 liter distilled water. Store at 4° C.
   b. Solution B: dissolve 35.6 Gm dibasic sodium phosphate ($Na_2HPO_4 \cdot 2H_2O$) in 1 liter distilled water. Store at 4° C. Combine 73.4 ml solution A with 26.6 ml solution B. Check pH and correct if necessary. This working buffer must be prepared fresh daily.
3. Erythrosin (eosin B) 0.1% in water
4. Ehrlich's acid hematoxylin. Dissolve 4 Gm crystalline hematoxylin in 200 ml 95% ethanol. Add 8 ml 10% sodium iodate. Add 200 ml distilled water and bring to a boil. When cooled, add 200 ml of glycerin, 6.0 Gm aluminum–ammonium sulfate, and 200 ml of glacial acetic acid. Allow solution to stand at least 14 days.

Method

1. Collect blood in EDTA. Obtain a normal adult blood sample and a cord blood sample for controls. Use blood less than 6 hours old.
2. Dilute each blood 1:1 with 0.9% NaCl. For normal control, use the normal adult blood. For the abnormal control, mix 1 drop of normal adult blood with 1 drop of the cord blood cell suspension. (The same A-B-O group should be used.)
3. Prepare thin smears of each diluted blood and allow to air dry, then fix in 80% ethanol for 5 minutes at 20° to 22° C.
4. Rinse with tap water and air dry.
5. Wash smears gently with distilled water.
6. Immerse slides in working buffer at 37° C for 6 minutes. Occasionally lift slides up and down to stir solution.
7. Wash with distilled water and air dry.
8. Stain 3 minutes in hematoxylin stain.
9. Wash with distilled water and air dry.
10. Counterstain with erythrosin for 3 minutes.
11. Wash with distilled water and air dry.
12. Examine under ordinary light microscopy.

Interpretation

Smears from normal blood show little if any stain uptake, and cells appear as ghost cells. The abnormal control shows both densely stained and unstained cells. Most abnormalities will show this "two distinct cell" population. Smears from persons with hereditary persistence of fetal hemoglobin (HPFH) show most all of the cells stained fairly evenly. Reticulocytes that contain a high concentration of Hb F and also some hemoglobin A sometimes resemble intermediate cells and may show some intracellular granulation. Inclusion bodies are visible in eluted cells as compact particles of differing sizes.

Normal values

Normal values for hemoglobin F cells in adults are below 0.01%; in full-term newborns they are above 90%.

Comments

Concentration and temperature (80% ethanol at 20° to 22° C) during fixation are important. Fix smears within 1 hour after making. Make certain pH of wash water is not too acid; pH should be 6.6 to 7.1.

---

*Hycel Inc., Houston, Tex.

References
Kleihauer, 1974
Kleihauer et al, 1957
Schmidt and Brosius, 1975

Susceptibility to Heinz body formation
Principle

When the red blood cells of susceptible individuals are incubated aerobically with certain reducing substances (acetylphenylhydrazine and hydroxylamine), there develops a different pattern of Heinz body formation than occurs in the cells of normal persons. This phenomenon indicates that an individual's erythrocytes are especially liable to hemolyze following administration of a variety of aniline-derived drugs; e.g., primaquine, phenacetin, acetanilid, sulfanilamide, Furadantin, and probenecid.

Reagents

1. Buffer solution
   a. Mix 1.3 parts of 0.067M KH_2PO_4 with 8.7 parts of 0.067M Na_2HPO_4.
   b. Add sufficient glucose to make a final concentration of 200 mg%.
   c. This solution is quite stable if kept refrigerated.
2. Acetylphenylhydrazine solution
   a. Dissolve powdered CP acetylphenylhydrazine* in buffer solution at room temperature to make a 100 mg% solution.
   b. This must be used within 1 hour after preparation.
3. Crystal violet solution
   a. Add 2 Gm crystal violet (CI 681,† certified) to 100 ml of an aqueous 0.73% sodium chloride solution at room temperature.
   b. Shake for 5 minutes; then filter.
   c. Mix filtrate with an equal quantity of 0.73% sodium chloride solution.
   d. This solution is stable for several months at room temperature.

Method

1. Heparinized blood, 3 to 5 ml, from a known normal control and from the patient is transferred into screw-capped vials. Just prior to use, gently agitate blood. Test all samples within 1 hour of collection.
2. Add 0.1 ml of this blood to 2 ml of acetylphenylhydrazine solution in a 12-mm diameter test tube using a 0.1 ml "blowout" pipet. Whiffle mix two or three times, bubbling small amount of air back in suspension (aeration). Leave pipet in tube and incubate at 37° C for 2 hours.
3. At the end of 2 hours, whiffle mix again. Place a small drop on a coverslip and invert onto a microscope slide on which a larger drop (two times as large) of the crystal violet solution has been previously placed. Wait 5 to 10 minutes and then, using oil immersion lens, scan for Heinz bodies in intact undistorted red cells. Count cells containing several Heinz bodies (Fig. 13-24, p. 597) as positive to obtain percentage of positive cells (count 100 to 200 cells). Only a few larger marginal bodies are formed in nonsensitive cells.

Remarks

This is a simple, useful laboratory procedure. It is subject, however, to inherent technical error in the cell counting and to inadequate oxygenation of the blood. Anemia will also alter the results.

---

*Fisher Scientific Co., Pittsburgh, Pa
†National Aniline Div., Allied Chemical Corp., Morristown, N.J.

Reference
Beutler et al, 1955

Tests for unstable hemoglobins
Inclusion bodies (Heinz bodies)
Reagents

1. Brilliant cresyl blue, 1% in 0.9% NaCl
2. Methyl violet 1% in 0.9% NaCl
   Both reagents should be made in small batches and filtered before use.

Method

1. Brilliant cresyl blue stain: Mix one part reagent and 2 parts fresh anticoagulated blood. Incubate one tube at room temperature and one at 37° C. Prepare smears at 20-minute, 1-hour, and 2-hour intervals. Dry, do not counterstain, and observe under oil immersion.
2. Methyl violet stain: Mix equal parts reagent and blood or two parts reagent and one part bone marrow. Incubate at room temperature and prepare slides as in step 1.

Results

Preformed Heinz bodies will be seen with either dye incubated at room temperature. Induced Heinz bodies will be produced by the 37° C incubation.

Hemoglobin H inclusion bodies
Principle

Hemoglobin H is unstable and undergoes denaturation in the presence of brilliant cresyl blue dye. This denatured hemoglobin will show up as stained bodies within the cell.

Reagents

1. Citrate-saline: Mix 1 volume 3% sodium citrate with 4 volumes 0.85% NaCl.
2. 1% brilliant cresyl blue in citrate-saline solution. Store in refrigerator. Filter before use.

Method

1. Add 1 or 2 drops of fresh anticoagulated blood to 2 drops of filtered stain in small tube.
2. Use a normal blood for a control.
3. Label tubes and place in 37° C waterbath.
4. Make smears after 20 minutes, 1 hour, and 2 hours.
5. Dry, do not counterstain, and observe under oil immersion.

Results

Hb H inclusions appear as multiple greenish blue inclusions. Ten percent to 100% of the red cells of a patient with Hb H disease may contain the inclusion bodies. Reticulocytes can be seen, but are distinguished by their dark blue filamentous material. Preformed hemoglobin inclusions (seen in a majority of splenectomized patients) appears as large, spherical, single inclusions.

References
Gouttas et al, 1955
Papayannopoulou and Stamatoyannopoulos, 1974

Heat denaturation test
Principle

Normal hemoglobin is hardly precipitated when heated to 60° C for 30 minutes, while many unstable hemoglobins are completely denatured. Hemoglobin associated with Heinz body formation is partially denatured and will precipitate. If only a small amount of abnormal hemoglobin is present, or if the hemoglobin is relatively insensitive to heat, a negative result may be obtained.

Reagents

Phosphate buffer pH 7.4:
1. *Solution 1:* 0.1M NaH_2PO_4 (13.8 Gm $NaH_2PO_4 \cdot 2H_2O/1$ of distilled water).
2. *Solution 2:* 0.1M Na_2HPO_4 (14.2 Gm anhydrous $Na_2HPO_4/1$ of distilled water).
3. Add 19.2 ml of solution 1 to 80.8 ml solution 2.
4. Mix and let equilibrate 10 minutes. Check pH.

Method

1. Add 1 ml fresh anticoagulated blood to a small test tube.
2. Prepare a control normal blood at the same time as the test specimen.
3. Wash four times in isotonic saline (0.85%) by centrifuging at 3,000 rpm for 5 minutes, removing supernatant, adding saline, and mixing four times.
4. Remove saline from last wash and add 5 ml distilled water to the packed cells. Mix.
5. Transfer hemolysate to a larger tube and add 5 ml phosphate buffer pH 7.4. Mix, then centrifuge for 10 minutes at 3,000 rpm.
6. Transfer upper 2 ml of the clear supernatant to another tube and place in a 50° C water bath for 1 hour or a 60° C bath for 30 minutes.

Results

Normal blood should show little, if any, precipitate. A positive result (denatured hemoglobins present) will show a copious flocculation.

References

Huehns, 1970
Lehmann and Huntsman, 1968
Motulsky and Stamatoyannopoulos, 1968

Isopropanol precipitation test
Principle

Unstable hemoglobins are precipitated by buffered isopropanol, whereas normal hemoglobin is not.

Reagents

1. Buffer pH 7.4. Add 12.11 Gm Tris primary standard (Trizma base) to a 1-liter volumetric flask. Add about 700 ml of distilled water to dissolve the Tris, then add 170 ml of 100% isopropyl alcohol. Mix. Adjust the pH to 7.4 with concentrated HCl. Add enough distilled water to make 1 liter. Keep tightly stoppered at room temperature.
2. Hemolysate. Use only freshly prepared hemolysates in test. Wash test and control cells three times in isotonic saline. Add an equal volume of distilled water to packed cells after last wash and a half volume of CCl_4. Shake for 5 minutes; centrifuge for 10 minutes at 3,000 rpm. To supernate add 2% KCN (1 volume KCN to 5 volumes hemolysate).

Method

1. Add 2 ml buffer to two small stoppered tubes and place in 37° C water bath for 10 minutes.
2. Add 0.2 ml fresh hemolysate from control to one tube and 0.2 ml from the patient in the other tube. Label accordingly.
3. Stopper tubes, mix, and incubate at 37° C for 30 minutes.

Results

After 5 minutes check tubes for formation of a precipitate. The control should remain clear, whereas an unstable hemoglobin will begin to show a precipitate. A flocculent precipitate should form within 20 minutes, while the normal should remain clear.

Reference

Carrell and Kay, 1972

Demonstration of sickle cells

Erythrocytes that contain Hb S sickle when the oxygen tension is lowered (Chapter 14). Oxygen tension can be reduced by various means. The sodium bisulfite method is used for screening purposes. Confirmation is accomplished by electrophoresis and other special studies.

Sodium bisulfite method
Reagent

1. Sodium bisulfite solution
   a. Dissolve one 0.2 Gm tablet of sodium bisulfite* in 10 ml of distilled water.
   b. The solution deteriorates on standing, and a fresh solution should be made every 8 hours and checked for reactivity by use of a known positive Hb S blood sample.

Method

1. Transfer a small drop of capillary or venous blood to a clean slide and add 2 drops of the same size of bisulfite solution.
2. Mix with the corner of a coverslip and then cover with the coverslip. Let stand for 30 minutes.
3. Examine under high dry objective.

Remarks

Sodium bisulfite and sodium metabisulfite can be used interchangeably. The results are reported as negative or positive.

Neither the number nor the morphology of sickle cells can be relied on to differentiate sickle cell trait from sickle cell anemia by this method. Either may show 100% sickling.

Before reporting a preparation as negative, inspect the area just within the edge of the coverslip. We have encountered a few cases of sickle cell trait in which only the erythrocytes around the edge sickled.

Note that there are hemoglobins other than Hb S that sickle (Table 14-10, p. 625).

Solubility test for Hb S
Principle

Sickle cell hemoglobin in the oxygenated form has virtually the same solubility as normal adult hemoglobin. However, in the reduced form, the solubility of sickle cell hemoglobin is markedly less than normal. Itano (1953) described a technic for recognition of a hemolysate of reduced sickle cell hemoglobin by its characteristic insolubility in concentrated phosphate buffer. Later a commercial preparation, Sickledex,† permitted whole blood to be used instead of hemolysate. Since then several tests based on the principle of the Sickledex reaction (i.e., introducing a lysing agent such as saponin into the phosphate buffer) have been published.

---

*Hartman-Leddon Co., Philadelphia, Pa.
†Ortho Pharmaceutical Corp., Raritan, N.J.

Reagents

1. Buffer solution

Potassium dihydrogen phosphate (anhydrous)	33.78 Gm
Dipotassium hydrogen phosphate (anhydrous)	59.33 Gm
White saponin	2.5 Gm

Dissolve in distilled water to a final volume of 250 ml. Store at 4° C.

2. Working solution: Dissolve 0.1 Gm sodium dithionite in 10 ml of buffer prior to testing.

Method

1. Add 2 ml working solution to a small round-bottom test tube (13 × 77 mm).
2. Wash 1 drop of patient's whole blood (0.02 ml) into the working solution and mix.
3. A sample from normal blood and blood with sickle cell hemoglobin should be set up as controls.
4. Assess the turbidity of the solutions after 5 minutes.

Interpretation

Place the tubes in front of a white background containing fine lines. A positive test for sickling hemoglobin is a solution so turbid that small black lines cannot be seen through the solution. Negative controls, or tests with hemoglobins A, F, D, or C, may be *slightly* cloudy, but black lines can be seen through the solution. Hb C Harlem and possibly other hemoglobins give a positive solubility test.

Comments

1. The anhydrous salts for preparing the buffer must be truly anhydrous. In doubt, use a new bottle of reagent.
2. The blood–reagent mixture should be light red to pink in color. A light orange color indicates a deteriorated reagent, most probably the dithionite.
3. Abnormal proteins (dysproteinemias, lupus erythematosus, renal disease) or hyperlipidemia may cause plasma turbidity and false-positive results.
4. Severe anemia may give false-negative results. To overcome this problem when a hemoglobin is below 10 Gm/dl, adjust the packed cell volume of a sedimented sample to approximately 50% by pipetting off excess plasma. Mix and proceed with testing.
5. False-negative results are expected in newborns and in infants within the first few months of life.
6. Transfusions of normal blood to patients with sickle cell hemoglobin, or sickle cell blood transfused to a normal patient will give false-negative and false-positive results, respectively.
7. Other commercial kits are now available besides Sickledex: SCAT, Sickle-Quik, Sik-L-Stat, and Sickle Screne. The test can also be automated with an AutoAnalyzer system.

Centrifugation test to differentiate sickle cell traits from sickle cell anemia

This procedure is carried out on positive samples from the solubility screening procedure.

Reagents

Same as for screening procedure.

Method

1. Add 2 ml of working solution to a 13 × 77 test tube.
2. Wash 4 drops (0.1 ml) patient's whole blood into the working solution and mix thoroughly.
3. Controls of normal and sickle cell hemoglobin are desirable.
4. Centrifuge at 1,500 g for 5 minutes. Do not brake the centrifuge.

Interpretation

1. Hb AA, AC, AD, and AE: a clear or opalescent solution of reduced hemoglobin will be present showing a variable amount of grayish protein on the surface.
2. Hb AS, SC, and Hb S in combination with another variant: the reduced hemoglobin is clear and pink. The sickle hemoglobin separates to the surface as a dark red band, easily distinguished from the gray protein in a normal sample.
3. Hb SS: the solution will be clear and straw colored, all the hemoglobin being found as a dark band at the surface. Usually benign cases of sickle cell anemia associated with splenomegaly and high fetal hemoglobin give a result intermediate between Hb SS and Hb AS.
4. Sickle cell–thalassemia: depending on the level of normal and fetal hemoglobin present, the result will lie anywhere between that seen in sickle cell anemia and sickle cell trait.
5. Dysproteinemia will cause a variable increase in gray surface protein, otherwise no different from normal blood.

Comments

1. Anemic bloods should be handled as in the screening procedure.
2. Solubility testing is particularly valuable in diagnosing sickle cell–Hb D disease. This disease will show a "sickle cell anemia" pattern on cellulose acetate and a "sickle cell trait" on solubility testing. The diagnosis is confirmed by agar gel electrophoresis at acid pH.

References

Huntsman et al, 1970
Schmidt et al, 1974
Serjeant and Serjeant, 1972

Hemoglobin electrophoresis
Preparation of hemolysate

This hemolysate is used for qualitative hemoglobin electrophoresis and for quantification of Hb A_2, Hb F, and serum haptoglobin.

Material and reagents

1. Graduated conical centrifuge tubes
2. Vortex mixer
3. Sodium chloride solution, 0.85%
4. Toluene
5. Whatman No. 1 filter paper

Method

1. Obtain 8 ml of oxalated or EDTA blood (smaller amount may be obtained from babies).
2. Centrifuge sample and remove plasma.
3. Pour cells into one or two graduated, conical centrifuge tubes.
4. Wash cells four times with isotonic saline solution. Centrifuge 5 minutes on each washing.
5. Measure volume of cells in the graduated conical centrifuge tube.

6. Add 1.4 ml of distilled water for each 1 ml of washed, packed cells. Mix on Vortex mixer for 15 seconds.
7. Add 0.4 ml of toluene for each 1 ml of washed packed cells. Mix on Vortex mixer for 15 seconds.
8. Centrifuge for 15 minutes at 3,400 rpm.
9. Remove toluene layer and protein plug by suction.
10. The clear hemolysate is filtered through wet filter paper (Whatman No. 1).
11. The hemolysate, at this point, may be stoppered and stored at 4° C if necessary.

Remarks

Be sure to shake vigorously after addition of distilled water and toluene to packed cells (steps 6 and 7). This aids in obtaining a clear hemolysate. If a very small volume of hemolysate is obtained, the filter paper (step 10) should be cut small.

For preservation of blood during shipping, the cells should be kept cold (0° to 4° C) and sent by airmail. When solution of oxyhemoglobin is sent, fill tube almost completely. Add 1 drop of 1:1,000 Merthiolate or antibiotic. Send washed RBCs in ACD solution. During transport, keep refrigerated at 4° C. It is not recommended to ship whole blood.

Hemoglobin electrophoresis (cellulose acetate: alkaline pH)

Principle

Detection of abnormal hemoglobins with electrophoretic technics is based on differences of their migration within an electric field. These differences in migration velocities are the result of electric charges of each hemoglobin variant brought about by various amino acid substitutions in the polypeptide chains of the molecule. At this alkaline pH, the relative migration is shown in Fig. 14-23, p. 627.

In this procedure, Tris-EDTA-borate buffer (TEB), pH 8.9 to 9.3, and ionic strength of 0.13, is used. Following electrophoresis for 1 hour at 400 volts, the membrane is stained with Ponceau S. Identification of the hemoglobins in the unknown sample is made by comparison of migration velocities of the unknowns with known hemoglobin controls. The controls are Hb A, S, and F.

Apparatus and materials

1. Microzone electrophoresis cell Model R-101* and applicator
2. Regulated power supply
3. Cellulose acetate membranes No. 324330*
4. Flat-tipped forceps for handling membranes
5. Glass plate
6. Blotters
7. Drying oven, temperature 100° to 110° C
8. Staining trays with covers
9. Plastic envelopes to protect completed membranes

Reagents

1. Tris-EDTA-borate buffer, pH 8.9 to 9.3, ionic strength 0.13
   a. Dissolve the following in 700 ml distilled water:
      (1) 32.2 Gm Sigma 7-9 (tris [hydroxymethyl]-aminomethane)†
      (2) 3.12 Gm disodium EDTA
      (3) 1.84 Gm boric acid
   b. Dilute to 2 liters total volume with distilled water and equilibrate overnight at room temperature. Store at refrigerator temperature.

2. Fixative and stain: Ponceau S with trichloroacetic acid and sulfosalicylic acid (same staining solution as used in serum protein electrophoresis, p. 895)
3. Acetic acid solution, 5% (rinsing solution)
4. Alcohol rinse: Denatured ethanol, reagent grade*
5. Cyclohexanone, purified*
6. Clearing solution
   a. Into a 100-ml volumetric flask, pour 30 ml cyclohexanone.
   b. Then add denatured alcohol until contents total 100 ml.
7. Hemoglobin hemolysate of each unknown sample—see Preparation of hemolysate, p. 888
8. Known control samples (Hb A, S, and F)

Method

1. Fill the two electrode compartments of the cell and the pre-buffer tray (tray 1) with refrigerated TEB buffer. Allow the buffer to come to room temperature.
2. Wet the membrane, blot to remove excess surface buffer, and then place on the bridge.
3. Place the bridge in the electrophoresis cell. Avoid splashing of the buffer onto the membrane.
4. Check to see that the ends of the membrane dip into the buffer without touching any surface of the cell. Allow cell and membrane to equilibrate for 2 minutes.
5. Apply sample hemolysates and known Hb A, S, and F controls on each membrane by positioning the applicator in the No. 1 groove (most cathodic position on the cell cover). Allow applicator tip to remain in contact with the membrane for 15 seconds before retracting the top by depressing the red button. (The greater protein content of the hemolysate requires a longer time for absorption then serum samples.)
6. Carefully wash the applicator tip with distilled water, and then blot it gently with soft tissue paper between sample application.
7. Electrophorese for 1 hour at 400 volts, with the output selector switch set on 300 to 500 constant voltage. The starting current should be about 2 mA and the ending current about 4 mA.
8. Turn off current on completion of electrophoresis time.
9. Upon completion of electrophoresis, immerse the membrane immediately in the fixative-dye solution for 10 minutes (tray 2).
10. Remove the membrane from the dye solution and place it in the 5% acetic acid rinse for *1 minute*. Agitate the membrane in this solution (tray 3).
11. Transfer the membrane to the second 5% acetic acid rinse and wash until the background of the membrane is clear (tray 4).
12. Transfer the membrane to a third 5% acetic acid rinse (tray 5).
13. Remove the membrane and place it in alcohol rinse for *1 minute* (tray 6).
14. Transfer the membrane to the tray with the clearing solution and immerse exactly *1 minute*. While the membrane is still in solution, position it over the glass plate. Excess solution is drained from the membrane, leaving even moisture without pools of solution (tray 7).
15. Remove the glass plate with the membrane on it and transfer to a ventilated oven preheated to 100° C for 15 minutes.
16. Remove membrane from glass plate by *carefully* lifting one

---

*Beckman Instruments, Inc., Spinco Div., Palo Alto, Calif.
†Sigma Chemical Co., St. Louis, Mo.

*J. T. Baker Chemical Co., Phillipsburg, N.J.

corner and peel it from the plate. Do this after the glass plate has cooled.

17. Place the dried membrane in a plastic envelope and label.

Remarks

With this technic, two minor cathodal fractions are observed. These are known as CAI and CAII, the latter being the most cathodic fraction. These fractions are nonhemoglobin components and therefore benzidine negative.

The TEB buffer in the electrode compartments is used only four times. After the fourth run, the buffer is discarded.

Quantitative Hb F is determined on all patient samples. Quantitative Hb F should be run the same day the samples are electrophoresed.

As noted by many, hemoglobin solutions deteriorate with time. Aged samples result in distortion and streaking of the fractions. Hemolysates used as controls and prepared by the laboratory should not be used after 3 months of age.

Hemoglobin electrophoretic patterns of young infants should be interpreted with caution. In infants the level of Hb F does not approach adult concentration until the infant approaches the end of the first year.

True hemoglobin patterns can be obscured following blood transfusions. In these cases, it is preferable to wait for a period of at least 3 to 4 months before performing electrophoresis.

Hemoglobin electrophoresis (agar gel, acid pH)

Principle

Electrophoresis on agar at an acid pH differentiates among hemoglobins that have the same migration at an alkaline pH (p. 626 and Fig. 14-23, p. 627).

Apparatus and materials

1. Spinco electrophoresis cell
2. Regulated power supply
3. DuPont Cronar polyester photographic film P-40 B, unperforated, 35 mm, cut in 12.5-cm lengths to make strips
4. Micropipets
5. Chromatography paper, Whatman No. 3 mm
6. Drying oven—temperature 65° C
7. Staining trays
8. 250-ml Erlenmeyer flask

Reagents

1. Phosphate buffer, pH 6.25 to 6.30

Sodium phosphate dibasic anhydrous (Na_2HPO_4)	3.90 Gm
Sodium phosphate monobasic ($NaH_2PO_4 \cdot H_2O$)	15.34 Gm

   Dissolve in distilled water and then adjust the volume to 2 liters.

2. Buffered agar-gel solution: Dissolve 0.50 Gm "Ionagar" No. 2 and 0.50 Gm Noble Agar in 50 ml distilled water mixed with 50 ml phosphate buffer. Use a 250-ml Erlenmeyer flask for this purpose. Bring the agar to a boil, mixing frequently until the agar is completely dissolved. A magnetic stirrer may be used for the mixing. Agar will appear crystal clear when ready.

3. Hemolysate—see Preparation of hemolysate, p. 888

4. Amido black 10B: Dissolve 10 Gm of dye in 100 ml glacial acetic acid. Dilute to 1 liter with distilled water.

5. Clearing solution: 50 volumes methanol, 50 volumes distilled water, and 10 volumes glacial acetic acid.

Method

1. Holding the pipet parallel to the film strip, pour 5 ml of the warm agar onto the strip; spread it evenly. *Be certain that agar is poured on the inside surface of the film strip.*

   Note: These strips may be prepared several days in advance and kept in a moist chamber in the refrigerator (4° to 6° C).

2. After the agar has solidified, aspirate 3 wells in a line perpendicular to, and at the center of, the long axis of the strip.

3. Fill the electrophoresis cell to the fluid line with phosphate buffer.

4. Place the gel strips over the longitudinal divider of the cell so that the sample wells rest on the midlongitudinal divider and the ends of the strips extend directly into the compartments filled with phosphate buffer.

5. Apply 1.0 microliter of the sample hemolysate to the center well. Place the same amount of hemolysate of a known hemoglobin type (A, S, or C) in each of the outside wells.

6. Cover the electrophoresis cell and seal with electric tape.

7. Set the power supply at approximately 10 mA per strip.

8. Electrophoresis time is approximately 1½ hours.

9. The strips are removed from the cell and placed in Amidoschwarz 10B stain for 15 minutes.

10. Remove strips from stain and place *agar side down* on filter paper. Dry in oven set at 65° C.

11. Wash the strips in tap water.

12. Transfer the strips to the clearing solution until cleared.

13. Return the strips to the oven until they are completely dried.

14. Label the strips and apply Krylon spray.

Comments

1. We prefer the use of phosphate buffer over citrate buffer. One difficulty with citrate buffer, which we experienced, was a reversal of pH during electrophoresis.

2. Be certain that only a very small amount of hemolysate is applied. We use only 1 microliter. If larger amounts of sample are applied, the electrophoretic patterns are greatly distorted.

3. The method is sensitive to concentration of the various hemoglobin fractions. Elevations of a single component may influence the migration rate of that particular fraction. For example, if the concentration of Hb C is high, it may migrate the same distance as Hb S of another sample and cause an error in interpretation.

4. The age of the hemolysate influences the results of the separation. The hemolysate should not be over 1 week old.

References

Naiman and Gerald, 1963
Schneider, 1974a

Differential electrophoresis for hemoglobin H

Principle

An electrophoretic technic at pH 7.0 in which only hemoglobin H or Bart's will migrate, serves to differentiate it from other hemoglobins with similar fast anodic mobility at pH 8.0 to 8.6.

Reagents

1. Stock solution 1: 0.2M monobasic sodium phosphate. Dissolve 27.6 Gm $NaH_2PO_4 \cdot H_2O$ in distilled water to make 1 liter. Add 1 drop toluene for storage. Stopper and keep at room temperature.

2. Stock solution 2: 0.2M dibasic sodium phosphate. Dissolve 28.4 Gm anhydrous Na_2HPO_4 in distilled water to make 1 liter. Add 1 drop toluene for storage. Stopper and keep at room temperature.

3. Working buffer pH 6.9 to 7.11. Add 39 ml of stock solution 1 to 61 ml of stock solution 2. Add sufficient distilled water to make 200 ml.

Method

1. Pour working buffer into chamber, soak wicks, and position.
2. Soak mylar-backed cellulose acetate plates ($2\frac{3}{8} \times 3$ in) in working buffer at least 20 minutes before use.
3. Blot plate between two pieces of absorbent paper quickly and evenly to remove excess moisture.
4. Apply samples to cellulose acetate side of plate, 1 inch from the cathode (see Hemoglobin electrophoresis, p. 889). Controls with known Hb A and Hb H should be run on the same strip.
5. Place plate on chamber and glass microscope slide over plate to allow good contact.
6. Apply 50 volts for 60 minutes at room temperature.
7. Remove plates and stain for at least 3 minutes with Ponceau S stain.
8. Remove plates and place in three consecutive 2-minute washes of 5% acetic acid.
9. Stain with benzidene solution, rinse in water, and let air dry.

Interpretation

Only hemoglobin H or Bart's will migrate in this system, thereby allowing differentiation from most fast hemoglobins.

References

Schmidt and Brosius, 1975
Schneider, 1974a

Globin chain separation
At alkaline pH
Principle

Cellulose acetate electrophoresis is used to separate polypeptide chains of hemoglobin that have been dissociated by 6M urea. In the presence of a high concentration of mercaptoethanol, heme is removed from globin, which migrates cathodally while the heme moves to the anode.

Reagents

1. Stock buffer pH 8.6 to 8.7: Add 11.2 Gm acid barbital powder to 1 liter boiling, deionized, distilled water. Stir over heat until dissolved. Turn off heat and add 82.4 Gm sodium barbital powder. Rinse the beakers with deionized, distilled water and add contents to a 4-liter flask. When cool, add sufficient deionized, distilled water to make 4 liters. Refrigerate after solution is completely cool.
2. Working buffer: Dilute stock buffer 1:1 with deionized, distilled water.
3. Urea
4. 2-Mercaptoethanol*
5. Ponceau S

Method

1. On the day of the run, the working buffer is made 6M in respect to urea and 0.05M in respect to 2-mercaptoethanol.

---

*Eastman Kodak Co., Rochester, N.Y.

(The final pH is about 8.9.) To 300 ml of working buffer, add 180 Gm urea. Mix until dissolved.

2. Add 50 microliters of the urea buffer (step 1) and 40 lambda of 2-mercaptoethanol to a small test tube. Add 50 microliters of hemolysate, mix, and refrigerate for 2 to 8 hours.
3. Add 2.5 ml of 2-mercaptoethanol to the remaining urea buffer (step 1). Mix. Soak Titan II* $4\frac{1}{2} \times 2\frac{3}{8}$ inch cellulose acetate strips in this for 2 hours.
4. After the strips have soaked, blot the strips with paper towels. Drape the strip across the supports of a Helena† electrophoresis chamber or any chamber that will accommodate the strips.
5. Apply 2 to 5 microliters of hemolysate to the center of the strip with a Helena applicator, or with a micropipet onto previously pencilled lines on the strip.
6. Electrophorese using buffer from step 3. Surround chamber with cold water with crushed ice in it. Use a cafeteria tray or other suitable large, shallow pan. Electrophorese 1 to $1\frac{1}{2}$ hours at 2 mA/strip.
7. Remove strip from chamber and stain in Ponceau S for 3 minutes. Prepare stain fresh each time.
8. Rinse and preserve strip in 5% acetic acid.

Interpretation

Heme pigmented fractions move rapidly to the anode and disappear in about 20 minutes. All globin chains move to the cathode. See Fig. 14-30, p. 631, for migration patterns using this method.

Comments

Only glass rods should be used to avoid metal contamination when handling urea.

References

Schneider, 1974a
Ueda and Schneider, 1969

At acid pH
Reagents

1. Stock buffer, TEB-citrate, pH 8.4. Dissolve the following in deionized water to make 1 liter:

Tris	10.2 Gm
EDTA	0.6 Gm
Boric acid	3.2 Gm

2. Working buffers: Add 72 Gm urea to 120 ml stock buffer. Adjust pH to 6.0 with 30% citric acid. Add sufficient deionized water to make 200 ml.
   a. Buffer A, to dilute hemolysates and soak plates. Begin with 100 ml of working buffer. To a small test tube add 10 microliters hemolysate (10 Gm%), 10 microliters deionized water, 20 microliters buffer, and 10 microliters 2-mercaptoethanol. (For less concentrated hemolysate, use 20 microliters of hemolysate and no water.) Set aside 15 to 30 minutes. To the remainder of the buffer add 0.5 ml 2-mercaptoethanol, and soak mylar-backed Titan III plates* in this for 15 to 30 minutes.
   b. Buffer B, chamber buffer. To the remaining 100 ml of working buffer, add 0.5 ml 2-mercaptoethanol and put in electrophoresis chambers. Place two wicks (or preferably use sponges) one on top of the other on each side of the chamber.

---

*Helena Laboratories, Beaumont, Tex.

Method

1. Blot the cellulose acetate plate with a paper towel and apply the samples with a Helena applicator about 1 cm from the anodal end of the plate. (Prime the sample applicator several times to ensure thin, even application lines.)
2. Place the plate, mylar side down, on the chamber wicks so that samples run from anode to cathode. Place glass slide on top of plate to ensure good contact.
3. Electrophorese at 2 to 3 mA per plate for 1½ hours. Do *not* use ice. If wicks are used instead of sponges, place two small strips of plain cellulose acetate (presoaked in buffer) on each side of the plate to ensure that the plate does not dry out.
4. Stain with Ponceau S for 3 minutes.
5. Decolorize with 3% acetic acid and air dry.

Interpretation

Migration patterns are similar to those seen using an alkaline buffer (Fig. 14-30, p. 631) with the following exceptions:
1. This buffer differentiates β- and γ-chains.
2. It distinguishes βD Los Angeles from the βG varieties.
3. Hb P separates more anodally than other β variants.
4. Several other mutant hemoglobins, especially those with histidine substitutions, migrate differently under acid compared with alkaline conditions.

Reference

Schneider, 1974a

Quantification of Hb A₂ and Hb S by microchromatography

Principle

This is a simple and accurate chromatographic separation of Hb A₂ from other fractions using the anion exchanger DE-52. This method is superior to the method for quantifying Hb A₂ by cellulose acetate electrophoresis (Huisman, 1974).

Reagents

1. Stock buffer: 1.0M Tris (hydroxymethyl) aminomethane. Dissolve 121.1 Gm Trizma base* in about 500 ml of deionized, distilled water, then add quantity sufficient to make 1 liter.
2. Working buffers: 0.05M Tris/HCl, pH 8.3, pH 8.5, and pH 7.0. Add 100 ml stock buffer and 200 mg KCN to each of three 2-liter flasks. Add deionized water to approximately 1,800 ml, then bring the pH of one flask to 8.3, one to 8.5, and one to 7.0 with concentrated HCl; add sufficient deionized water to each flask to make 2 liters.
3. Anion exchanger DE-52† (diethylaminoethylcellulose): Prepare the DE-52 by washing it several times with large volumes of 0.05M Tris/HCl, pH 8.5. After the material has settled from each wash, pour off the supernatant and "fines." Check the pH of the last wash to ensure that the resin is equilibrated at pH 8.5. Equilibration should be completed within 24 hours. Store the DE-52 as a slurry in a covered container with the supernate volume of buffer about 0.7 that of the settled ion exchanger.
4. Columns: Set up disposable Pasteur pipets (5¾ inch total length) vertically on stands. Position a small cotton plug in the tapered part of the tube. Do not pack cotton too tightly. Moisten the column and plug with pH 8.5 buffer, then fill the column with DE-52, which is in a ratio of 1:1 settled slurry to buffer. One or two fillings should produce a column 6 to 7

cm in height. Cap the tube and store, or use immediately after packing.
5. Hemoglobin solutions
   a. Hemolysate (see p. 888). One drop of hemolysate (3 to 6 mg of hemoglobin, approximately 12 Gm % concentration) is diluted with 6 drops distilled water and 1 drop 2% KCN solution.
   b. Whole blood. The contents of about half of one completely filled heparinized capillary tube is mixed with 8 drops of distilled water and 1 drop 2% KCN solution.
   c. Filter paper, Whatman No. 2 or No. 3, with one drop of falling blood collected on it. The paper is cut into small pieces and submerged for at least 15 minutes in approximately 0.5 ml of an elution reagent containing 0.1% tetrasodium EDTA and 1 mM KCN.

Method

1. Remove all but 5 mm layer of buffer from the top of the column.
2. Apply the hemoglobin solution to the top of the column slowly from another Pasteur pipet.
3. After the hemolysate has settled into the top 5 mm of the column, gently add pH 8.3 buffer to the top of the column and attach rubber tubing with a funnel or reservoir containing approximately 20 ml pH 8.3 buffer.
4. Hb A₂ fraction is eluted as a sharp band in 6 to 8 ml and is collected in a 10-ml volumetric flask.
5. When all the Hb A₂ is eluted (about 15 minutes), change the supernatant buffer on the top of the column and in the reservoir to the pH 7.0 buffer.
6. Catch the effluent in a 25-ml volumetric flask.
7. Adjust the volumes to 10 and 25 ml respectively, mix, and read the optical densities at 415 nm.

Calculation

$$\% \text{ Hb A}_2 = \frac{\text{OD (A}_2) \times 100}{\text{OD (A}_2) + (2.5 \times \text{OD[R]})}$$

where R = Remaining hemoglobin

This procedure is also suitable for quantification of Hb A₂ and Hb S in hemolysates containing Hb S using a 0.5 × 15 cm column, and the following modifications: (1) Hb A₂ zone is eluted with pH 8.35 buffer and is collected into a 10-ml flask, starting when the Hb has reached the lower part of the column; (2) Hb S zone is eluted with pH 8.20 buffer; and (3) the remaining hemoglobin with pH 7.0 buffer. The adjusted volumes of the latter two zones are 25 ml. This modified procedure requires about 5 hours to complete.

Calculation

$$\% \text{ Hb A}_2 = \frac{\text{OD (A}_2) \times 100}{\text{OD (A}_2) + (2.5 \times \text{OD [S]}) + (2.5 \times \text{OD[R]})}$$

where R = Remaining hemoglobin
      S = Hb S
      A₂ = Hb A₂

Results

Normal values: 1.7% to 3.5% (mean, 2.6%)
β-Thalassemia trait: 3.9% to 6.5% (mean, 5.1%)
With 0.5 × 15 cm column:

Hb S heterozygotes	2.8%
Hb S homozygotes	3.05%
Hb S HPFH	2.1%

---

*Sigma Chemical Co., St. Louis, Mo.
†H. Reeve Angel Co., Clifton, N.J.

Comments

1. Because trace amounts of Hb A are eluted with Hb A_2 at pH values of 8.25 and lower, the pH of the first elution buffer must be between 8.3 and 8.35. Because of individual differences in pH meters and standards, it may be that the "correct" pH would be slightly different in another laboratory. If the zone of Hb A_2 should move slower than described or be diffused, the pH or molarity of the buffer may be in error.
2. The amount of hemoglobin in the hemolysate should be fairly accurately determined. Samples with 7 to 8 mg will have contamination with Hb A, and less than 2 mg will give low absorbance readings, tending to decrease the precision.
3. Tests should be run on hemolysates stored for no more than 30 days at 4° C.

References

Efremov et al, 1974

Huisman, 1974

Schmidt and Brosius, 1975

Quantification of serum haptoglobin (cellulose acetate)

Principle

To an aliquot of serum, add a known concentration of hemoglobin in excess of that which binds with the haptoblobin present in the serum. Electrophoretic separation of this mixture is carried out on cellulose acetate, using phosphate buffer with an ionic strength of 0.05 and a pH of 7.0. After electrophoresis, which is completed in 30 minutes, the membranes are stained with o-dianisidine and dried in an oven at 100° to 110° C. The strips are then scanned with the Beckman R-110 Microzone Densitometer and percentages of the separated components determined. The haptoglobin binding capacity of the serum is then calculated from the hemoglobin concentration.

Apparatus and materials

1. Microzone electrophoresis cell, Model R-101*
2. Regulated power supply, Model RD-2 Duostat*
3. Cellulose acetate membranes No. 324330*
4. Flat-tipped forceps for handling membranes
5. Drying oven preheated to 100° to 110° C
6. Plastic staining trays with covers
7. Glass plate
8. Blotters
9. Plastic envelopes to protect completed membranes
10. Beckman R-110 Microzone Densitometer

Reagents

1. 0.05M Phosphate buffer for prebuffering and electrophoresis, pH 7.0
   a. Dissolve 7.1 Gm of sodium phosphate (dibasic) Na_2HPO_4, anhydrous, in 1 liter of distilled water.
   b. Dissolve 3.45 Gm of sodium phosphate (monobasic) $NaH_2PO_4 \cdot H_2O$ in 500 ml of distilled water.
   c. Pool both preparations in a 2-liter Erlenmeyer flask and mix. Store in refrigerator (4° C). Total volume is 1,500 ml.
2. Hemolysate
   a. Prepare as outlined on p. 888. Determine the hemoglobin concentration.
   b. Adjust to approximately 3.5 to 4.0 Gm/dl with distilled water. The adjusted hemolysate is stable at 4° to 6° C for 5 days.
3. Stain
   a. Alcoholic o-dianisidine solution: Dissolve 1 Gm o-dianisidine (3,3'-dimethoxybenzidine)* in 140 ml 95% ethanol.
   b. Acetate buffer, pH 4.7, 20 ml: Mix 53.5 ml sodium acetate (27.22 Gm $Na_2C_2H_3O_2 \cdot 3H_2O$ in 1 liter H_2O) with 46.5 ml acetic acid (11.3 ml of 99% glacial acetic acid in 1 liter).
   c. Distilled water, 35 ml
   d. Hydrogen peroxide, 30%, 5 ml, at room temperature
4. Acetic acid rinse (5% v/v glacial acetic acid in distilled water)
5. Clearing solution
   a. Glacial acetic acid, 25 ml
   b. Ethyl alcohol, 95%, 75 ml

Method

1. Mix well *1 part* hemoglobin solution to *9 parts* serum and allow to stand for 10 minutes at room temperature.
2. Fill the electrophoresis cell to the fluid line with phosphate buffer, pH 7.0, ionic strength 0.05. Wet the membrane with the same buffer, blot, and place on the bridge.
3. With the rider of the sample applicator in the middle groove (No. 2 groove), make a triple application (0.75 microliters total) of each serum-hemoglobin mixture.
4. Set the power supply at 150 volts. Electrophorese for 30 minutes.
5. After electrophoresis is completed, immerse the membrane in o-dianisidine dye for 10 minutes. Cover.
6. Rinse the membrane with distilled water and then immerse in 5% acetic acid for 5 minutes.
7. Remove the membrane and place it in 95% ethyl alcohol for exactly 1 minute.
8. Transfer the membranes to the tray containing freshly prepared clearing solution and immerse exactly *30 seconds*. While it is still in solution, position the membrane over the glass plate. Excess solution is drained from the membrane, leaving even moisture without pools of solution.
9. Remove the glass plate with the membrane on it and transfer to a ventilated oven preheated to 100° C for 10 minutes.
10. After the glass plate has cooled, remove the membrane from the glass plate by *carefully* lifting one corner and peel it from the plate.
11. Place the dried membrane in a plastic envelope.
12. Scan the membrane with the Microzone Densitometer at 450 mμ and a 0.3-mm slit width.

Calculation

Calculate the percent of the haptoglobin band by dividing the total area of the scan into the area of the haptoglobin peak.

Multiply the percent of the haptoglobin by the hemoglobin concentration of the hemolysate.

$$\frac{\% \text{ Haptoglobin} \times \text{Hb conc.}}{10} \times 1,000 = \text{mg\% haptoglobin}$$

Example:

Hemolysate = 3.75 Gm

Area of haptoglobin in % = 45%

Therefore: $0.45 \times 3.75 = 1.68$ Gm%

To covert Gm% to mg%, multiply by 1,000 and divide by dilution factor of 10.

Haptoglobin value = 168 mg%

---

*Beckman Instruments, Inc., Spinco Div., Palo Alto, Calif.

*Eastman Organic Chemicals, Rochester, N.Y.

Remarks

This method is technically simple, reproducible, and requires only 30 minutes of electrophoresis time. Sharp resolution of the various bands is obtained, and there should be no overlapping of the bands.

Under conditions of the test, unbound hemoglobin migrates the slowest from the point of application, while a sharp haptoglobin-hemoglobin band moves toward the anode. Methemalbumin, if present, migrates further than the haptoglobin-hemoglobin complex.

The serum sample to be analyzed should be collected without hemolysis. Prepare hemolysate from normal red blood cells. This standardizes the hemoglobin band in the electrophoretogram. The hemolysate should be fresh.

There is no specific stain for haptoglobin. However, the haptoglobin-hemoglobin complex has peroxidase-like activity, which permits its detection. In addition to *o*-dianisidine, other compounds that can be used to detect haptoglobin-hemoglobin complex are benzidine, *o*-tolidine, and guaiacol. The stain mixture is prepared fresh for each use.

The mixture of hemoglobin with serum should stand at room temperature for 10 minutes. Maximum hemoglobin binding occurs at this time. It is not necessary to allow this binding to take place at 37° C. In our experience, incubation of the hemoglobin-serum leads to increased amounts of methemalbumin in normal serum.

The critical factors in the formation of color caused by peroxidase activity using *o*-dianisidine are similar to those for benzidine.

The staining solution should be prepared in clean glassware; dirty glassware will produce erratic results. The hydrogen peroxide used in the preparation of the stain must be absolutely fresh.

The separated bands including methemalbumin, if present, should stain a deep orange-brown color.

Quantitative hemoglobin in plasma and urine
Reagents

Glassware used for preparing and storing reagents should be acid cleaned. The water and reagents, particularly the hydrogen peroxide, must be free from sulfate. Check by adding $BaCl_2$ solution; if turbidity develops, sulfate ions are present.

1. Benzidine reagent, 1%
   a. Dissolve 1 Gm of benzidine base in 90 ml of glacial acetic acid and dilute to 100 ml with distilled water.
   b. Store in refrigerator.
2. Hydrogen peroxide, 1%
   a. Prepare from reagent grade, sulfate-free stock solution.
   b. Make fresh each time.
3. Standard hemoglobin solution
   a. Pack and wash 2 ml of erythrocytes.
   b. Lyse them by freezing and thawing.
   c. Dilute with saline solution until a solution containing about 10 Gm of hemoglobin/dl is obtained.
   d. Determine the hemoglobin concentration exactly by the cyanmethemoglobin method.
   e. Dilute 0.02 ml of this solution to 10 ml with saline solution; this is that standard hemoglobin solution. It contains 20 mg of hemoglobin per 100 ml if prepared from a concentrated solution of exactly 10 Gm/dl.
4. Diluent
   a. Use 10% acetic acid from glacial acetic acid diluted with distilled water.

Method

1. Label three 15-ml test tubes as "standard," "unknown," and "blank."

2. To each, add 1 ml of benzidine reagent.
3. Add 0.02 ml of plasma (or urine) to the "unknown" tube. Mix.
4. Add 0.02 ml of the standard hemoglobin solution to the "standard" tube. Mix.
5. Add 1 ml of the hydrogen peroxide solution to each of the three tubes. Mix by inversion. Let stand 20 minutes; then add 10 ml of diluent.
6. Let stand for 10 minutes; then read the OD in a spectrophotometer, wavelength 515 mμ, using the "blank" tube as reference.
7. On ordinary graph paper, plot the known concentration of hemoglobin versus OD of the standard solution. Read the hemoglobin concentration of the unknown from the curve.

Remarks

The OD of the unknown should fall between 0.1 and 0.6. If the concentration of hemoglobin in the unknown is higher, the plasma or urine specimen can be diluted until a reading in this range is obtained. If the concentration of hemoglobin is very high, there is no need to use the benzidine method; hemoglobin can then be determined by the cyanmethemoglobin method. If the concentration of hemoglobin in the plasma or urine is too low, the amount of plasma added can be increased to 0.05 ml and the amount of urine to 1 ml. The volume of diluent is reduced accordingly.

The salts present in urine may cause turbidity if present in large amounts. This can be avoided by dialyzing the urine overnight against saline solution. In this case the standard hemoglobin solution should also be dialyzed, and a new curve should be drawn. Measure the volume before and after dialysis and make appropriate correction.

A method that uses orthotolidine instead of benzidine is given by Lewis (1965).

Reference

Crosby and Furth, 1956

PROTEIN ELECTROPHORESIS AND IMMUNOELECTROPHORESIS
Separation of serum proteins using cellulose acetate
Principle

Cellulose acetate as a supporting medium for electrophoresis has several advantages over paper. Some of these advantages are the following:

1. Its application to small samples
2. Short running time
3. Lack of trailing of albumin because adsorption of proteins to the support medium is minimal
4. Sharp separation of fractions

The Microzone electrophoretic system discussed here is a microadaptation of other methods using cellulose acetate.

The Microzone electrophoretic cell is constructed so as to keep evaporation of buffer from the membrane at a minimum by reducing the air space surrounding the membrane. Consistent application of serum sample is ensured by an applicator that picks up a repeatable amount of serum (0.25 microliters) and delivers it in a narrow band perpendicular to the direction of migration. Eight samples of serum are introduced onto each membrane.

After electrophoresis has taken place, the proteins are coagulated and stained in a single solution containing both fixative and dye. The membrane is then rinsed and cleared. Each serum pattern is then scanned with the Beckman R-110 Microzone Densitometer at 520 mμ and a 0.2-mm slit width. The filter holder is set at 1.4.

Apparatus

1. Microzone electrophoresis cell, Model R-101*
2. Regulated power supply, Model RD-2 Duostat*
3. Cellulose acetate membranes No. 324330, prepared with two rows of holes to fit bridge of cell
4. Flat-tipped forceps for handling membranes
5. Plastic trays with covers
6. Glass plate
7. Blotters
8. Ventilated oven preheated to 100° to 110° C
9. Plastic envelopes to protect completed membranes
10. Beckman R-110 microzone Densitometer

Reagents

1. Barbital buffer, pH 8.6, ionic strength 0.075
   a. Beckman buffer B-2 may be used; follow directions on package.
2. Fixative and stain
   a. Dilute the contents of a 30-ml bottle of Beckman fixative-dye solution to 250 ml with distilled water. The relative concentration of the components in this solution are as follows:

   0.2% w/v Ponceau S stain
   3.0% w/v trichloroacetic acid } in distilled water
   3.0% w/v sulfosalicylic acid

3. Acetic acid rinse
   a. Use 5% v/v glacial acetic acid in distilled water. Make 3 to 5 liters at a time.
4. Alcohol rinse
   a. Use specially denatured alcohol No. 3-A,† 95 parts by volume, and isopropanol, 5 parts by volume.
5. Cyclohexanone, purified†
6. Clearing solution
   a. Into a 100-ml volumetric flask, pour 30 ml cyclohexanone. Then add denatured alcohol until contents total 100 ml.
   b. Mix solution under a ventilator hood or in a well-ventilated area.

Method

1. Place the cell with electrode terminal pins facing the operator.
2. Fill the two electrode compartments of the cell with barbital buffer. Check to see that the level of the buffer is within the marked lines on the side of the cell. Fill siphon apparatus and allow fluid level in each compartment to equalize.
3. Place 1 drop of serum on a piece of Parafilm and cover with plastic beaker immediately to prevent evaporation. (Disposable cups used in the AutoAnalyzer may be used for this purpose.)
4. Using tweezers, remove one membrane and gently float it on the surface of some buffer solution previously placed in a plastic tray (tray 1, step 23).
5. Allow the membrane to float until all of the white areas disappear. Now the membrane is completely saturated with buffer.
6. Immerse the entire membrane in buffer.
7. Immediately lift the membrane from the buffer with tweezers.
8. Place the membrane between two blotters. Remove only the excess surface buffer.

9. Mount the membrane on the electrophoretic cell bridge and tension level so that there is no sag in the membrane. Reference hole in membrane must be on the left side and at the bottom.
10. Place the bridge in the electrophoresis cell. Avoid splashing of the buffer onto the membrane.
11. Check to see that the ends of the membrane dip into the buffer without touching any surface of the cell.
12. Check to see that the reference hole on the membrane will line up with the No. 1 strip selection groove.
13. Replace cover on the electrophoresis cell. Allow membrane to equilibrate in the cell for approximately 2 minutes before application of specimens. Do not turn electricity on.
14. Push the white button of the sample applicator so that the two parallel platinum ribbons of the applicator tip run over the top surface of a drop of serum that has already been placed on a piece of Parafilm. Retract the tip by depressing the red button.
15. Position the applicator in the No. 3 groove on the cell cover (most anodal). Depress the white button to lower the applicator tip on the membrane.
16. Wait 10 seconds (actually timed) and then retract the tip by depressing the red button.
17. Carefully wash the applicator tip with distilled water, using a downward jet of water, and then blot it gently with soft tissue paper.
18. Repeat steps 13 to 17 until all seven unknown samples and one control serum are applied.
19. Connect the Duostat to the electrophoresis cell. Set the output selector switch (lower control knob) to *constant voltage* and the range desired (given for each method).
20. Set the meter range switch (upper control knob) to *voltmeter* at the range desired.
    a. Above 150 v, set switch to 0-500 v and read voltage from top scale on the meter; multiply by 10.
    b. Below 150 v, set switch to 0-150 v and read voltage from bottom scale on the meter and multiply by 10.
21. Turn on *output adjust,* wait a few seconds for warm-up (meter pointer begins to move), and then turn output adjust further to the right until meter indicates desired voltage. For protein electrophoresis, apply 250 v and electrophorese for 20 minutes. Check amperage at beginning of run.
22. After completion of the electrophoretic run, turn off current and remove the membrane from the bridge with tweezers.
23. During the electrophoretic run, place seven plastic trays in sequence.

Tray 1	Buffer solution
Tray 2	Fixative-dye solution
Tray 3	5% acetic acid rinse
Tray 4	5% acetic acid rinse
Tray 5	5% acetic acid rinse
Tray 6	Alcohol rinse
Tray 7	Clearing solution with glass plate at bottom of tray

24. Immerse the membrane immediately in the fixative-dye solution for *10 minutes* (tray 2).
25. Remove the membrane from the dye solution and place it in the 5% acetic acid rinse for 1 minute. Agitate the membrane in this solution (tray 3).
26. Transfer the membrane to the second 5% acetic acid rinse and wash until the background of the membrane is clear (tray 4).
27. Transfer the membrane to the third 5% acetic acid rinse (tray 5).

---

*Beckman Instruments, Inc., Spinco Div., Palo Alto, Calif.
†J.T. Baker Chemical Co., Phillipsburg, N.J.

28. Remove the membrane and place it in alcohol rinse for *1 minute* (tray 6).
29. Transfer the membrane to the tray with the clearing solution and immerse exactly *1 minute*. While still in solution, position the membrane over the glass plate. Excess solution is drained carefully from the membrane, leaving even moisture without pools of solution (tray 7).
30. Remove the glass plate with the membrane on it and transfer to a ventilated oven preheated to 100° C for 15 minutes.
31. Remove membrane from glass plate by *carefully* lifting one corner and peel it from the plate. Do this after glass plate has cooled.
32. Place the dried membrane in a plastic envelope.

Calculation

We have found automation of the calculations by means of a Beckman CDS-100 computing densitometer system most useful. This consists of a Model R112 Scanning Densitometer permanently mated to a Model R-115 computer. Scan, computation, and printout of fractional data on chart paper can be obtained from most conventional electrophoretic media.

In the event the automated system is not available, the scans are calculated in the following manner: divide chart into component protein fractions by drawing perpendicular lines between each fraction. Count and record integration teeth marks between verticals. Total number of "blips" divided into number for each band gives percent of protein fraction. To obtain grams percent (Gm%), multiply total serum protein by percent in each band. The total serum protein is determined with the biuret method.

Example:

	Blips	%	Gm%
γ-Globulin =	31	$\frac{31}{186} = 16.66$	$0.1666 \times 5.99 = 1.00$
β-Globulin =	20	$\frac{20}{186} = 10.75$	$0.1075 \times 5.99 = 0.64$
α_2-Globulin =	20	$\frac{20}{186} = 10.75$	$0.1075 \times 5.99 = 0.64$
α_1-Globulin =	9	$\frac{9}{186} = 4.83$	$0.0483 \times 5.99 = 0.29$
Albumin =	106	$\frac{106}{186} = 56.98$	$0.5698 \times 5.99 = 3.41$
TOTALS	186	99.97	5.98

TSP = 5.98

The difference of the total percentage from a hundred ($100 - 99.97 = 0.03$) is not compensated for. Also, after calculations are done, the total protein is rounded off to tenths (5.98 is reported as 6.0).

Remarks

Use membranes from only one manufacturer. It has been reported that cellulose acetate membranes from different manufacturers produce consistently different results in electrophoretic runs on the same serum sample. We have also found some degree of variation in membranes produced by one manufacturer. In checking for this variability among different batches of membranes, a control serum is run eight times on a membrane from each lot number. One sample in every electrophoretic analysis should be a control serum in order to check the other variables affecting the procedure.

When immersing the membrane in buffer, it is important that even penetration of the buffer be achieved. If wetting of the membrane is not properly done, this will prevent even flow of the sample and of the buffer. This leads to irregular separation of protein fractions, giving a distorted electrophoretogram. Blotting of the membrane should remove any uneven pools of excess buffer so as to render the surface of the membrane even and smooth. Failure to achieve this will produce a distorted electrophoretogram.

Avoid any great disparity in amount of sample applied. When washing the tip of the applicator after each sample application, make certain that the tip is adequately dried. A poorly dried tip may introduce a source of error by diluting the serum sample. To avoid this, it is advisable to apply the sample on the applicator tip, completely dry the applicator tip with tissue paper, and then reapply the sample. Keep the serum samples covered except when actually filling the applicator tip. Any change in sample concentration because of evaporation is a source of error. Occasionally the tip of the applicator may become caked with serum sample if the serum is allowed to dry on the tip. The dried serum may be digested off by soaking the tip for several hours in a solution consisting of 9 ml of 0.5% pepsin and 1 ml of HCl. This solution is made fresh whenever needed.

The buffer in the cell is used for four electrophoretic runs. After this, it should be discarded. If the buffer has been stored in the refrigerator (4° C), bring to room temperature before using.

In our laboratory the Ponceau S dye is stored in a closed bottle and used for 6 days only. The alcohol and acetic acid used for rinsing and the clearing solution are replaced daily.

Separation of serum lipoproteins using Agarose gel
Principle

Serum lipoproteins are separated on an Agarose medium supported on Cronar filmstrips. Veronal buffer, pH 8.6 and ionic strength 0.05, is used. Albumin and EDTA are added to the Agarose. Electrophoresis time is 45 minutes at 10 mA per strip. The strips are then dehydrated, stained with Sudan black B, cleared, and dried. In normal fasting serum, three lipoprotein fractions, β, pre-β, and α, are observed. Normally, chylomicrons are absent in a fasting sample. The strips are scanned with the R-110 Densitometer, using a 600 mμ interference filter and a 0.4-mm slit width. Test is done on fresh fasting serum; do not freeze.

Apparatus and materials

1. Spinco electrophoretic cell, Model R, with baffles removed*
2. Regulated power supply
3. Photographic film base (DuPont Cronar P-40B leader film, unperforated 35 mm, cut in 15-cm strips)
4. Drying oven set at 65° C
5. 10-microliter pipets and 5-ml pipet
6. Erlenmeyer flask, 250 ml
7. Capillary tubes (1.5 mm wide, cut 1.5 cm long)
8. Immuno gel board or lipoprotein template board
9. Hot plate
10. Whatman No. 3 MM chromatography paper in rolls 1½ inch wide
11. Staining tank
12. Beckman Microzone Densitometer Model R-110, with 600 mμ interference filter*
13. Blaisdell china marker, white No. 164T
14. Moist chamber

Reagents

1. Barbital buffer, pH 8.6, ionic strength 0.05
   a. Beckman buffer B-1 may be used. This preparation contains:

Diethyl barbituric acid	1.84 Gm
Sodium diethyl barbiturate	10.30 Gm

   b. Prepare according to instructions on package.

---

*Beckman Instruments, Inc., Spinco Div., Palo Alto, Calif.

2. Agarose,* 250 mg
3. Ethylenediamine tetra-acetic acid, disodium salt† (EDTA Na$_2$)
4. Bovine albumin, 30%‡
5. Ethyl alcohol, 55% reagent grade§
6. Sodium hydroxide solution, 25%
7. Sudan black B in 55% alcohol
   a. Dissolve 1 Gm of dye in 1 liter of 55% alcohol.
   b. Filter immediately before use.
   c. Prior to use (after the stain has been filtered as directed above), add 0.1 ml of 25% NaOH for every 50 ml of stain.

Method

1. Wipe the inside surface of the filmstrip with isopropyl alcohol. Allow to air dry.
2. Mix 250 mg Agarose and 150 mg EDTA in an Erlenmeyer flask with 25 ml of barbital buffer and 25 ml of distilled water.
3. Dissolve the Agarose by gentle boiling and stirring over a hot plate at approximately 100° C. A magnetic stirrer may be used. Solution will become crystal clear.
4. Remove flask from the hot plate and let the Agarose cool to approximately 65° C.
5. Add 1.7 ml 30% bovine albumin and mix gently to prevent foaming.
6. Immediately after adding albumin, coat the inside surface of filmstrips with 5 ml of warm gel solution using a pipet. Spread gel evenly using the rounded end of a clean test tube.
7. Using template, place a small capillary tube (1.5 cm long) in the midpoint of the leader film and perpendicular to the major axis of the strips.
8. Place strips in a moist chamber and store in refrigerator for 20 minutes before using.
9. Fill electrophoretic cell with barbital buffer.
10. Remove capillary tube from the strips and place them in the electrophoretic cell so that the sample well of each strip rests in the midlongitudinal divider and the ends of the strips extend directly into the buffer compartments.
11. Apply 10 microliters of serum in the wells.
12. Electrophorese for 45 minutes at 10 mA per strip.
13. Dehydrate strips in 55% ethyl alcohol for 45 minutes (agitate periodically).
14. Place strips in a tray, agar side up, and dry approximately 3 hours in oven at 65° C.
15. Stain the completely dried strips with Sudan black B to which 25% NaOH has been added just prior to staining (use 0.1 ml of NaOH for every 50 ml of stain). Allow strips to remain in dye for 1 hour.
16. Destain and clear the strips in three successive rinses of 55% ethyl alcohol. Allow approximately 5 minutes for each rinse.
17. Dry the strips completely in ventilated oven.
18. Label strips and scan with the Beckman R-110 Densitometer using the 600 mμ interference filter.
19. Calculate the percentage of each lipoprotein fraction from the total area scanned.

Calculation

The lipoprotein fractions are so well separated that they can be easily delimited on the scan by using the deepest part of the valley

---

*Fisher Scientific Co., Pittsburgh, Pa.
†Sigma Chemical Co., St. Louis, Mo.
‡Dade Reagents, Inc., Miami, Fla.
§J.T. Baker Chemical Co., Phillipsburg, N.J.

---

between peaks. In hyperchylomicronemic states and patients with β–pre-β fusion, the fractions can be cut by comparison with a normal lipoprotein pattern if this is necessary. This is done similar to using a control serum in delimiting some serum protein electrophoresis fractions. The percentage each fraction is of the total is calculated in the usual fashion by counting blips, etc. The following four fractions are reported: chylomicrons (nearest to cathode), β-lipoproteins, pre-β-lipoproteins, and α-lipoproteins (nearest to anode).

Remarks

The use of Agarose gel as a supporting medium for the electrophoretic separation of the serum lipoproteins has several advantages over the use of filter paper. Some of these are listed:

1. The separation of the critically important pre-β-lipoprotein band is far superior.
2. The electrophoresis time is shorter.
3. The staining time is shorter.
4. Scanning can be done on the Microzone Densitometer, requiring only a change of the filter.
5. The report and interpretation can be completed on the same day the specimen is received and a permanent and durable record is available.
6. Agarose gel can be easily introduced into a laboratory already using the Microzone system and agar gel without expensive extra equipment.
7. Less background staining occurs.
8. There is better migration and disappearance of the trail artifact.
9. Agarose gel is the nearest to a liquid state of any commonly used medium.
10. The order of migration is the same as on paper; this is not the case with other media such as polyacrylamide gel.

There are some minor disadvantages:

1. Agarose is more expensive than filter paper.
2. In marked hyperchylomicronemic states, not all the chylomicrons stay at the cathodal tip of the application well, but some of the smaller-sized chylomicrons migrate into the gel, resulting in a diffuse blurring of the pattern.

Prestaining of the serum with Sudan black B at various dilutions and with different stain mixtures was unsuccessful because some of the dye precipitated at the cathodal tip of the application well.

When pouring the hot Agarose solution onto the filmstrips, be careful to keep it warm in a 40° C water bath and make all strips at one time. If the Agarose cools too much, it will gel irregularly on the strips.

Electrophoresis should be run at 10 mA per strip. Higher voltage overheats the strips and precipitates the protein. Failure to agitate the strips while dehydrating in 55% ethyl alcohol will cause bubble formation in the gel, thus creating artifacts. Strips in the drying oven must be placed agar side up on filter paper. Irregular drying precipitates some of the Agarose-buffer mixture. The strips must be completely dried or irregular staining results.

The buffer should have an ionic strength of 0.05, because a higher ionic strength causes the buffer salts to precipitate.

With every lipoprotein fractionation, serum cholesterol and triglyceride are determined on the same fasting sample. This permits phenotyping of the hyperlipoproteinemias. Our laboratory report includes a scanned pattern of the strip, percentages of each lipoprotein fraction, and values for serum cholesterol and triglycerides. The most probable hyperlipoprotein phenotype is included with every report.

Immunoelectrophoresis, polyvalent and monovalent
Principle

Immunoelectrophoresis combines the principles of agar gel electrophoresis with that of immunodiffusion. Antigens (proteins) are first separated by electrophoretic methods and then identified with specific antiserum introduced into trenches running parallel to the electrophoretic axis. Precipitin bands are formed where the diffusing antigens and specific antiserum meet.

Apparatus and materials

1. Spinco electrophoretic cell, Model R, with baffles removed*
2. Drying oven, ventilated
3. Photographic film base (DuPont Cronar polyester P-40B leader film, unperforated 35 mm)
4. Whatman No. 3 MM chromatography paper in rolls 1½ inch wide
5. Regulated power supply
6. Hamilton syringe or narrow-tipped microliter pipet
7. 13-gauge needle ground flush to remove bevel
8. Moist incubation chamber or two large serving trays
9. Staining tank
10. Hot plate (optional)
11. Capillary tubes (90 mm long, 1.5 mm wide)
12. Immuno gel board (template)
13. Circulating water bath with activated charcoal

Reagents

1. Stock barbital buffer, pH 8.8, ionic strength 0.24

   | Sodium barbital | 98.9 Gm |
   | Barbituric acid (or barbital–barbituric acid derivative) | 11.1 Gm |

   a. Dissolve and dilute to 2 liters using a volumetric flask.
   b. Add 1 ml of 1:1,000 aqueous solution of Merthiolate to inhibit growth.
   c. Adjust pH with phosphoric acid or NaOH.
2. Working barbital buffer, pH 8.8, ionic strength 0.06
   a. To 1 part stock buffer, add 3 parts distilled water. This can be used about five or six times if polarity is reversed after each run.
   b. Check the pH.
3. Buffered agar gel, 1%, ionic strength 0.03
   a. Dissolve, by gentle boiling and frequent stirring, 1 Gm of ''Ionagar'' No. 2† and 50 ml of working buffer in 50 ml distilled water.
4. Washing solution, 0.85% sodium chloride solution
5. Amido black 10B
   a. Dissolve 10 Gm of dye in 100 ml of glacial acetic acid and dilute to 1,000 ml with distilled water.
6. Acetic acid, 2% (first clearing solution)
7. Methanol, distilled water, glacial acetic acid, 50:50:10 (v/v) (second clearing solution)
8. Isopropyl alcohol, 70%
9. Control serum mixed with minute amount of bromphenol blue dye

Method

1. Cut leader film base into strips 15 cm in length. Clean inside surface of film with 70% isopropyl alcohol. Allow to air dry. Measure and mark from the antigen well toward the end that will be in the anodal side a distance of 4 cm.
2. Attach filmstrips to immuno gel board with cleaned, inside surface up. The template shows the desired trough length and the relationship of antigen wells to both the trough and design as a whole. Strips may be secured by using cellophane tape or masking tape.

---

3. Liquefy the refrigerated agar, using a water bath.
4. Coat film base with 5 ml of warm buffered gel solution, using a 5-ml pipet.
5. Place capillary tube over trough position made on template while agar is still hot. Be sure capillary tube sets well on agar gel.
6. Place strips in moist chamber and transfer to refrigerator for 1 or 2 hours. After agar has solidified, gently extract capillary tubing, leaving a clean cut trough.
7. To make an antigen well, use a 13-gauge needle, with bevel removed. Attach needle to a rubber mouthpiece and aspirate gel. Position wells according to the template. The wells must be cut clean and perfectly round.
8. Place strips in electrophoretic cell that has been filled with working buffer solution. The wells should rest on the plastic divider and ends of strip extended into the buffer. Strips should be placed equidistantly on the plastic divider.
9. Introduce exactly 2 microliters of control serum with added dye into right well and 2 microliters of patient's serum into well on left-hand side of strip. *Do not overload.*
10. Cover and seal electrophoretic cell with masking tape.
11. Electrophoresis is carried out at 150 volts and 80 mA (with eight strips) for *50 minutes* or until stain in control serum reaches the 4-cm mark on the film support.
12. At end of run, disconnect cell and gently transfer strips to plastic support plates or to serving trays lined with moist filter paper. *Be sure that the diffusion chamber is moist.*
13. Aspirate any accumulated moisture in trough with a clean narrow-tipped microliter pipet attached to a rubber mouthpiece.
14. Add 50 microliters of specific antiserum to antibody trough.
15. If moist chamber is used, place support plates in box. If serving trays are used, the second tray is used as a lid to the first and sealed airtight with masking tape.
16. Continue diffusion phase for 18 to 24 hours at room temperature.
17. Following development of the precipitin bands, the strips are washed with 0.85% saline solution in a circulating water bath for a period of 4 to 6 hours. Prior to placing in the water bath, punch a hole at one end of the strip. A single-hole paper punch can be used for this purpose. Then suspend the strips on a glass rod. Alternate each strip on the glass rod with a piece of plastic tubing (spacer) so that strips will not touch each other.
18. After the washing is completed, remove the strips from the water bath and rinse three times by agitating the strips in tap water.
19. Gently lay strips, agar side down, on No. 3 MM chromatography paper and dry at 60° C in ventilated oven.
20. Wash or peel off chromatography paper, and stain strip with Amido black for 5 minutes.
21. Remove excess stain with three successive rinses in 2% acetic acid. Each rinse is for 5 minutes.
22. Then place the strips in clearing solution made of methanol, distilled water, and glacial acetic acid, 50:50:10 (v/v), for approximately 10 minutes.
23. Dry completely in ventilated oven.
24. Label strips.

Sources of error

1. *Inadequate concentration of antibody specific for the protein of interest.* If there is little or no antibody, no precipitin band is formed and no interpretation is possible. Furthermore, if quantitative and qualitative differences exist among the anti-

---

*Beckman Instruments, Inc., Spinco Div., Palo Alto, Calif.
†Consolidated Laboratories, Inc., Chicago Heights, Ill.

sera used, this may make correlation between the results obtained with different antisera impossible.

2. *Excessive concentration of antibody specific for the protein of interest.* This may result in thickening and blurring of precipitin bands, rendering detection of adjacent bands difficult. It is usually possible to dilute the antiserum with isotonic saline solution to obtain sharp precipitin bands.

3. *Solubilization of precipitin bands.* Antibodies produced in certain species such as the horse tend to form soluble complexes in antigen excess. When horse antiserum is diffused against a high concentration of antigen, a precipitin band may form, but subsequently it dissolves as greater quantities of antigen diffuse into the region of the precipitate. Dilution of the test serum with isotonic saline solution to reduce the antigen concentration should eliminate this problem.

4. *Variations in the distance between an antigen well and the antiserum trough.* This may produce false inequalities when precipitin bands are compared. Differences in intensity of the precipitin arcs and in position relative to the antiserum troughs may occur. Too long distances retard the formation of precipitin lines and require larger quantities of reagents.

5. *Differences in solubility of different protein fractions.* The γ-macroglobulins in some macroglobulinemic sera precipitate in the gel because of the low ionic strength buffers that are used frequently in immunoelectrophoresis.

6. *Position of immunoelectrophoretic components influenced by differences in agar preparation.* The cathodal migration of some proteins at high pH is due to flow of water toward the cathode induced by charged groups present on the agar (electroendosmosis). Agar preparations differ in this property, and this is responsible for position of the various serum proteins relative to the point of sample application. Deionized agar, such as Ionagar used in this procedure, has relatively less charge than most types of agar. Because of this, the backward or cathodal migration of γ-globulin is not great.

Remarks

The antiserum prepared against whole normal human serum may produce 20 or more precipitin bands when normal human serum is subjected to immunoelectrophoresis.

In immunoelectrophoresis, it is desirable to produce consistent patterns with sharp bands. This requires a rapid electrophoretic stage, elimination of heat, and prevention of agar and protein interaction. Rapid electrophoresis reduces diffusion of proteins and thereby prevents dilution of antigen. Heat formation is reduced by using a buffer of low ionic strength. This prevents denaturation of proteins that would cause inconsistent precipitin patterns. Interaction of agar and protein is prevented by using a purified agar.

The use of a purified agar that has a diminished charge permits a more rapid separation of proteins. This is because a lower ionic strength buffer may be used with deionized agar. Such a buffer permits higher voltage without increasing the current and generation of heat. The concentration of agar used here contributes also to more rapid separation of proteins and permits rapid diffusion of antiserum into the zone of antigen electrophoresis. Reports in the literature have shown that with high concentrations of agar, poor resolution of proteins may result.

The quantity of precipitate formed during diffusion is influenced by such factors as the pH and electrolytic concentration of the milieu and by the environmental temperature. However, the most important factor is the quantitative ratio of antigen and antibody taking part in the reaction. When optimum antigen-antibody concentration is present, the precipitin lines formed are sharper than those resulting when one of the two reagents is present in excess. Under these circumstances the precipitin arc may get wider, split

up, or even disappear because of the formation of soluble antigen-antibody complexes.

The speed at which the precipitin lines are formed is greater when the temperature is high (37° C), but the quantity of precipitate formed is greater at lower temperatures (4° C). For clinical purposes it is advisable to keep the agar plates during the diffusion stage at a constant temperature of 18° to 20° C and in a slightly moist atmosphere.

The number of precipitin bands developed in immunoelectrophoresis of whole serum can be limited by using monovalent antiserum. For example, monovalent specific antiserum that reacts with only one of the three types of immunoglobulins is available.

The use of a serum control with dye added aids in visualization of proteins during electrophoretic separation. The dye stains the serum albumin fraction so that a bluish front is observed as the proteins progress toward the anode. Visual comparison of the precipitin bands of a test serum with those of a normal serum permits some estimation of the relative concentrations.

In our laboratory, special attention is given to the following:

1. If protein electrophoresis shows a monoclonal peak, or if a suspected peak is apparent on cellulose acetate strip, set up monospecific IgA, IgG, and IgM as well as immunoglobulin chain-specific antisera.

2. With each case, antisera from the same manufacturer are used.

3. The saline solution in the water bath is changed at least once a week.

4. The activated charcoal in the water bath is washed at least once a week.

5. We have found the agar gel IEP system* to be most useful.

Quantification of immunoglobulins
Principle

Immunodiffusion technics are limited to the identification and quantification of those protein fractions for which specific antibodies have been developed. In a single gel or radial gel diffusion method the specific antiserum is incorporated into the gel.

The standards and unknowns are inoculated on the agar strip. The antigen then diffuses actively into the stabilizing medium, meeting the antibody and forming a precipitation ring around the inoculation well. The diameter of the precipitin ring is directly proportional to the initial concentration of the antigen in solution when time, temperature, and antibody concentration remain constant. The greater the concentration of the antigen, the larger the diameter of the precipitin ring.

Apparatus and materials

1. Immuno-Plate* (immunodiffusion plates) containing specific antisera (IgG, IgA, and IgM)
   a. Each plate contains six antigen wells. The plates are labeled according to their antigen specificity.
2. Agar gel incubator–dryer oven (37° to 40° C)* for IgG assay
3. Moist incubation chamber for IgA and IgM assay
4. Hamilton syringe, 10 microliters
5. Reference standards
   a. These are sera with three different concentrations of immunoglobulins.
6. Viewer†

---

*Hyland Laboratories, Los Angeles, Calif.
†Cordis Corp., Miami, Fla.

Method

1. Open the immunodiffusion plate.
2. Fill the wells to the agar surface with unknown serum using the Hamilton syringe. Rinse syringe four times with isotonic saline solution before next application of serum. Three standard dilutions and three unknown serum samples can be applied on each plate. For example, for IgG assay inoculate wells with standards and unknowns as follows:

Well No. 1	Lowest concentration of IgG standard
Well No. 2	Middle concentration of IgG standard
Well No. 3	Highest concentration of IgG standard
Well Nos. 4 to 6	Unknowns

Repeat this for IgA and IgM determinations using the respective standards.
3. Replace plastic cover on plate and allow for diffusion to proceed as follows:
   a. For IgG assay: Incubate 4 hours at 37° C in incubator–dryer oven with a moist sponge.
   b. For IgA and IgM assays: Diffuse for 16 hours in moist chamber at room temperature.
4. After diffusion is completed, remove the cover of the plate. Measure the diameter of the precipitin rings by placing the plate under the viewer. Align one side of the ring with the zero mark on the grid. The diameter of each precipitin ring can be measured to the nearest 0.1 mm.
5. Plot the precipitin ring diameters of the three reference sera on semilogarithmic graph paper using the horizontal or arithmetic scale and the concentration of the corresponding reference serum on the vertical or logarithmic scale. Plotting the squares of the diameters yields a curve that is easier to use.
6. Determine the concentration of the unknown specimens by referring to the standard curve. The quantity of each immunoglobulin is reported in mg/dl of serum.

Remarks

The immunodiffusion plates should be stored at a temperature of between 2° and 8° C. Daily environmental factors such as fluctuations in temperature will produce changes in the diameters of the reference sera and hence the slope and position of the standard curve. Therefore a new standard curve must be prepared with each separate run. In addition, a high and low standard is determined on each separate plate set up during a run. The precipitin ring diameter produced by the standards in the individual plates should be in agreement with the plotted standard curve (0.1 mm).

Underfilling or overfilling of the antigen wells should be avoided. Also avoid introduction of bubbles into the wells. During diffusion, avoid drying of the plates.

Maximum accuracy of the test is obtained when the protein fraction being assayed in the unknown sample is within the range of the three standards used. When levels approach or exceed that of the highest standard, the serum sample should be diluted with isotonic saline solution to reduce the level of the protein fraction to within the range of the standards. The determination should then be repeated on the diluted sample.

Quantification of single immunoglobulins can also be done with the Laurell rocket technique, using monospecific antibody in the gel.

Quantification of ceruloplasmin
Principle

Antigen (patient's serum) placed in a well in antibody-containing agar gel diffuses into the agar and forms a precipitin ring. The diameter of this ring is directly related to the concentration of the testing antigen.

Hereditary deficiency of ceruloplasmin is known to occur and is associated with the disturbed copper metabolism of hepatolenticular degeneration (Wilson's disease). Decreased levels have been noted in tropical and nontropical sprue and scleroderma of the small bowel in which absorption of copper is abnormally low. Elevated levels are seen in a variety of pathologic conditions of both infectious and noninfectious etiology.

Materials and reagents

1. Immuno-Plates and reference standard
2. Hamilton syringe
3. Moist chamber
4. Magnifying comparator (Bausch & Lomb)
5. Viewer (Cordis)

Method

1. Follow technic for quantification of immunoglobulins.
2. Diffuse for 16 hours at room temperature in a moist chamber.

Normal values

Ceruloplasmin is normally present at birth in levels of 1.8 to 13.1 mg/dl; 0.118 to 0.865 μM/1 of serum. After 3 to 6 months of age, *normal adult* levels are attained (20 to 35 mg/dl; 1.32 to 2.31 μM/1).

Fetoglobin (fetuin, α-fetoprotein, α-fetoglobulin)
Principle

This procedure is based on the detection of fetoglobin in human serum by the Ouchterlony immunodiffusion-in-agar technic. This serum α-protein is produced by the liver during fetal life. It reaches a peak serum concentration at about 13 weeks of gestation and then gradually declines, being present in only small amounts at birth and during the first 2 weeks of neonatal life. Thereafter, fetoglobin is not normally detectable in serum.

Fetoglobin reappears in the serum of patients with primary hepatocellular carcinoma. Between 40% and 80% of patients with hepatoma produce fetoglobin detectable with this technic.

Equipment and reagents

1. Feto-Tect Kit,* which contains the following:
   a. Individually packaged plates
   b. Three vials of serum labeled A-positive control, B-antiserum to fetoglobin, and C-negative control
   c. Disposable capillary tubes
2. Viewer (Cordis)

Method

1. Remove plate from plastic bag. Place on a flat, well-lighted table. Label with wax pencil.
2. Using a fresh capillary tube for *each* sample:
   a. Fill well A with A-positive control.
   b. Fill well B with B-antiserum to fetoglobin.
   c. Fill well C with C-negative control.
   d. Fill well X with patient's serum or fluid to be tested.
3. Cover plate and carefully place in refrigerator in a level position.
4. Observe under the viewer at 24, 48, and 72 hours.

Interpretation

Test is either positive or negative. A positive control line should always appear between wells A and B, which runs into the center of well C. If this does not occur, test must be repeated. See com-

---

*Fernwood Laboratories, Inc., Pittsburgh, Pa.

pany insert diagrams for proper visualization of precipitin lines and interpretation of the different ways a positive reaction may look.

Artifacts such as a broad, indistinct halo that partially or completely encircles well X sometimes occur. This is caused by non-specific precipitation of various proteins such as macroglobulins, lipoproteins, and cryoglobulins. These ''rings'' or ''halos'' should be disregarded and attention focused only on the *specific precipitin line*.

Concentration and protein electrophoresis of urine
Principle

The electrophoretic separation of urinary proteins on cellulose acetate medium requires prior concentration if total protein is less than 100 mg/dl. After electrophoresis is completed, the membranes are stained with Ponceau S but not cleared. Membranes are scanned in the R-110 Microzone Densitometer at 520 mμ and a 0.2-mm slit width. For scanning uncleared membranes, the filter holder is set at 2.5 mm.

Apparatus and reagents

1. Glass suction apparatus and collodion bag*
2. Same as for protein electrophoresis

Method

1. Centrifuge urine sample. Measure protein concentration.
2. Fill the collodion bag with 10 ml of the supernatant urine via the glass tube by means of a pipet. If this quantity of urine is not available, follow the requirements listed in Table A-1.
3. Connect suction vessel via side arm to pump and apply vacuum (20 to 22 pounds).
4. Concentrate specimen to 0.5 ml or less. Check the concentration process frequently until the desired degree of concentration is obtained.
5. Remove concentrate from bag with a pipet.
6. Proceed as usual with the Microzone technic for serum proteins using urine rather than serum. Make following applications of the sample:
   a. On one site of the membrane, apply sample one time.
   b. On another site of the membrane, make two applications.
7. After electrophoresis is completed, stain membrane as directed, but delete transfer to clearing solution. After the third acetic acid rinse, transfer membrane to a paper towel and air dry. The membrane is placed stained side up on towel.
8. Place dry membrane in plastic envelope and label.
9. Scan the strip with the R-110 Microzone Densitometer. Select best scan for quantification. Calculate percent of each protein fraction.

Remarks

Electrophoretic patterns of normal and abnormal urine show five zones. From the anode to cathode these are albumin, α_1-globulin, α_2-globulin, β-globulin, and γ-globulin. These fractions correspond to serum protein fractions. However, the quantity of each differs for urine and serum in that the A/G ratio is reversed for urine.

Urine samples having more than 100 mg/dl of protein usually will not require prior concentration.

Urine samples or concentrates may be electrophoresed on the same membrane with CSF samples. Electrophorese a control serum on the same membrane. The use of uncleared membranes increases the sensitivity of the procedure.

*Schleicher & Schuell, Inc., Keene, N.H.

Table A-1. Volume of fluid needed for concentration based on the original protein content

mg/dl of protein	Volume needed	mg/dl of protein	Volume needed
5	16.0 ml	55	1.4 ml
10	8.0 ml	60	1.3 ml
13	6.2 ml	65	1.2 ml
15	5.3 ml	70	1.1 ml
16	5.0 ml	75	1.1 ml
18	4.4 ml	80	1.0 ml
19	4.2 ml	85	1.0 ml
20	4.0 ml	90	0.9 ml
22	3.6 ml	95	0.9 ml
23	3.5 ml	100	0.8 ml
24	3.3 ml	110	0.73 ml
25	3.2 ml	114	0.7 ml
28	2.85 ml	125	0.64 ml
30	2.6 ml	136	0.6 ml
31	2.6 ml	145	0.55 ml
34	2.3 ml	180	0.44 ml
35	2.3 ml	195	0.4 ml
37	2.2 ml	200	0.4 ml
40	2.0 ml	230	0.34 ml
43	1.9 ml	320	0.25 ml
45	1.8 ml	380	0.21 ml
50	1.6 ml	660	0.12 ml

Electrophoresis of urine is useful in the diagnosis of Bence Jones protein. This protein is detected as a single discrete peak, usually in the γ area.

Urine immunoelectrophoresis for κ and λ light chains
Principle

Immunoelectrophoresis can be used to identify specific urine proteins. It is most often used to classify monoclonal spikes observed in urine electrophoretograms. This is usually done with specific antisera for light polypeptide chains (κ and λ) or specific heavy chain.

Apparatus and materials

Same as for immunoelectrophoresis (p. 897).

Method

1. Concentrate urine sample even if negative for protein content. (Follow steps 1 to 5 of procedure for concentration and electrophoresis of urine.) Perform protein electrophoresis on concentrated specimen. If no monoclonal peak is apparent, Bence Jones protein κ and λ light chain typing is not indicated. If pattern shows monoclonal peak in γ area, do routine immunoelectrophoresis. Use 2 microliters of concentrated urine in antigen well. For a control, use known positive Bence Jones κ in one strip and Bence Jones λ in another strip.
2. Cut leader film base into strips 15 cm in length. Wipe inside surface of film with 70% isopropyl alcohol. Allow to air dry.
3. Use a template with one antigen well and two antiserum troughs, with a 2-mm distance between the center well and the troughs. Measure and mark a distance of 4 cm from the antigen well toward the end that will be the anodal end.
4. Proceed as for routine immunoelectrophoresis, using concentrated urine (2 microliters) in the antigen well. For the

diffusion phase, apply 50 microliters of anti-κ serum* in one trough and 50 microliters of anti-λ serum* in the other.

Remarks

Be certain to make the antigen well at the midpoint of the agar gel strip and equidistant between the two troughs. Usually, in patients with a monoclonal gammopathy (multiple myeloma), only one type of light chain is excreted in the urine. In patients with no monoclonal peaks, both light chains may be present. Report as both present and state which one of the light chains appears to be greater.

Cold-precipitable protein study

Principle

In this study the patient's serum and plasma are screened for the presence of proteins precipitating in the cold.

Cryoglobulin is a protein precipitating or gelling when the *serum* is cooled at 4° C for 24 hours. Cryofibrinogen, on the other hand, is precipitated from *plasma* on cooling. This physical characteristic is usually reversible and disappears on warming.

The patient's plasma (blood collected in heparin, preferably) is incubated at 4° C for 24 hours. A fine white precipitate of cryofibrinogen forms but dissolves when the plasma is warmed at 37° C.

Specific identification and classification of each thermoprotein is done by immunoelectrophoresis.

Apparatus and materials

Same as for serum protein electrophoresis and immunoelectrophoresis. In addition, obtain the following:
1. Refrigerated centrifuge (4° C)
2. Wintrobe sedimentation tubes
3. Clotted blood and heparinized blood samples from patient

Reagents

Same as for serum protein electrophoresis and immunoelectrophoresis. Also, 0.85% sodium chloride solutin at 4° and 37° C is needed.

Method

1. Centrifuge blood sample and separate plasma from cells. Handle clotted blood sample in like manner.
2. Fill *two* Wintrobe sedimentation tubes with plasma and *two* Wintrobe tubes with serum. (Label each tube accordingly.)
3. Allow *one set* of tubes (one tube of serum and one of plasma) to stand erect at 4° C for 24 hours.
4. Place second set of tubes at 37° C for 24 hours. (This set is the control.)
5. At the end of this time, observe the tubes at 4° C for fine precipitation or cloudiness. Compare with respective tubes incubated at 37° C.
6. If precipitation or cloudiness is present in any tube incubated at 4° C, centrifuge the tube at 3,000 rpm in a refrigerated centrifuge for 30 minutes.
7. If the plasma shows a precipitate at 4° C, cryofibrinogen is suspected. If serum precipitates at 4° C, cryoglobulin is suspected.
8. At this point in the procedure, follow outline below as indicated.

---

*Meloy Laboratories, Falls Church, Va.

For cryofibrinogen (plasma)

1. Measure amount of precipitate from the sedimentation scale (1 mm of precipitate is equal to 1% of cryofibrinogen). This can be reported as the "cryocrit."
2. Wash precipitate in cold (4° C) isotonic saline solution four times for 5 minutes each.
3. Dissolve precipitate in warm isotonic saline solution in a 37° C water bath.
4. Perform agar gel immunoelectrophoresis with cryofibrinogen-saline suspension. Inoculate four agar gel strips with sample. Fill the antibody troughs with the following specific antisera:

No. 1	Anti-IgG serum
No. 2	Anti-IgA serum
No. 3	Anti-IgM serum
No. 4	Antifibrinogen serum

Control for Nos. 1, 2, and 3 is fresh normal serum, and control for No. 4 is fresh normal plasma.

For cryoglobulin (serum)

1. Measure the amount of precipitate from the Wintrobe scale, 1 mm of precipitate representing 1% of cryoglobulin. *Save the supernatant.*
2. Wash precipitate in cold (4° C) isotonic saline solution four times.
3. Completely dissolve precipitate in saline solution by placing the suspension in a water bath at 37° C. Save the dissolved precipitate suspension for immunoelectrophoretic studies.
4. Do cellulose acetate electrophoresis on the following:
   a. Patient's whole serum
   b. Supernatant (step 1 above)
5. Set up agar gel immunoelectrophoresis using cryoglobulin-saline suspension. Innoculate each strip with one of the corresponding antisera:

No. 1	Anti-IgG
No. 2	Anti-IgA
No. 3	Anti-IgM

The patient's whole serum is used as a control.

Normal values

No cryoglobulin should be present in normal serum. Little (1.5% by volume) to no cryofibrinogen should be detected at the end of 24 hours at 4° C.

Remarks

Most cryoglobulins consist of either IgG (7S) or IgM (19S). Some examples of mixed cryoglobulins, composed of both IgG and IgM fractions, have been reported. In addition, IgA-IgG cryoglobulinemia has been reported.

While some cryoglobulins precipitate at 4° C, others begin to separate just below body temperature as a gel. Therefore the classification of these cold-reacting globulins is as follows: (1) cryoglobulins, (2) cryogelglobulins, (3) macrocryoglobulins, and (4) macrocryogelglobulins.

Cryoglobulins can be associated with multiple myeloma, chronic lymphocytic leukemia, lymphosarcoma, kala-azar, systemic lupus erythematosus, rheumatoid arthritis, periarteritis nodosa, Sjögren's syndrome, subacute bacterial endocarditis, portal cirrhosis, and malignant tumors. The condition may also be primary. Thus cryoglobulins can be associated with monoclonal and polyclonal gammopathies.

Cryofibrinogens are frequently missed because of the practice of searching for cold-precipitable globulins in serum and not in plasma. Cryofibrinogen has been reported in gastric, ovarian, and prostatic carcinoma, fibrosarcoma, multiple myeloma, acute rheumatic fever, ulcerative colitis, and in an "essential" form. The last is the only form associated with cold sensitivity.

SEROLOGY AND IMMUNOLOGY
General laboratory technic
Cell washing
General aspects

When washing red cells, it is important that all plasma proteins be completely removed.

1. After "known" cells are washed, they should be used within 6 hours. A fresh supply should be prepared each morning. Screening cells may be rewashed once or twice for continued use by the evening laboratory shift.
2. For most technics, 3% cell suspensions are used. These may be approximate but should be measured accurately occasionally for controlled performance. Such technics are reverse grouping, antibody titrations, and direct and indirect antiglobulin (Coombs') tests.
3. Three washes in isotonic saline solution (1 vol cells/200 vol saline solution) are adequate for most tests unless hemolysis is present. In this case the cells should be washed until supernatant is clear.
4. Cord cells used for testing should be washed four times in isotonic saline solution. Cells used for absorption and elution technics may require four to eight washings in saline solution.
5. Thorough washing is accomplished only if the proportion of cells to saline solution is proper (1:200).
6. Between washings, complete suspension of red cells is necessary.
   a. After centrifugation the saline solution is decanted as completely as possible by holding the tube mouth down at an angle.
   b. Shake once so the saline solution drops from rim of tube.
   c. Shake the tube (in upright position) to loosen button.
   d. Forcefully add saline solution to tube, holding tip of wash bottle parallel to the tube but not touching the edge.
   e. Repeat as indicated.

Remarks

Do not stir cell suspension with applicator. Do not place finger over tube and invert. After final saline solution wash, decant the same as between washings. Do not blot. Do not attempt to wash too many cells and thus risk "losing cells" during washing procedure.

Reading and grading test tube agglutination

Centrifugation must be performed for the proper length of time with the proper force so that the cells are brought together without being too packed. Every serologic procedure is calibrated, allowing for the variation in centrifuges, viscosity of solutions, amounts, etc.

After proper centrifugation, carefully remove tubes from centrifuge so as not to agitate the cell button. Then tilt the tube so that the cell button is above the liquid. Gently shake the test tube to dislodge the cell button from the bottom of the test tube. Do not strike it against another object. Do not tap or "flick" the test tube. Gently *tilt* the tube several times until all the cells are loosened from the bottom before observing. The tilting motion should loosen the cells.

Observe the way the cells break loose—whether rough or with a smooth, swirling effect. Observe one tube at time.

Grading of agglutination reaction

The degree of agglutination is recorded as follows:

4+	One large clump of cells
3+	Several large clumps of cells
2+	Medium-sized clumps well dispersed
1+	Many small clumps, opaque reddish background
±	Minute clumps, "scratchy" appearance, opaque reddish background
−	No agglutination

Complete or partial hemolysis must be interpreted as a positive reaction if the original serum was free of hemoglobin.

Preparation of red cell suspensions
Cells for A-B-O reverse grouping

Use adult group A_1 and B cells. The following procedure is adhered to in preparation of *fresh* cell suspensions for daily use.

Method

1. Label two test tubes (13 × 100 mm) A_1 and B, respectively.
2. Into respective tubes, put 3 drops of A_1 and B cells (whole blood).
3. Wash cells three times with isotonic saline solution.
4. Aspirate or decant saline solution completely.
5. Make a 3% saline cell suspension (0.3 ml washed cells and 9.7 ml isotonic saline solution).

Remarks

Cells should be fresh, preferably less than 1 week old. These cells may be used when testing eluates in hemolytic disease of the newborn if A-B-O incompatibility is suspected.

Cells for antibody identification

Commercially prepared cells (Selectogen)* are used routinely. These are used according to the manufacturer's directions.

Remarks

The commercially prepared cell suspensions may give better results if washed once before using, 4 to 5 days before their expiration date. Record lot numbers of commercially prepared cells as part of the patient's record. These cells may also be used for testing eluates.

Cells for antibody identification using freshly drawn blood

The use of fresh cells is reserved *only* for special cases. Use cells collected in ACD solution. These cells should be of group O, possessing as many known antigens as possible. It is recommended that the same cells be used regularly.

Method

1. Label test tube (13 × 100 mm) with name of cell donor or in any other designated manner.
2. Into tube, place 2 to 4 drops of whole blood.
3. Wash cells three times with isotonic saline solution.
4. Aspirate or decant saline solution completely.
5. Make a 3% saline cell suspension.

A-B-O blood grouping technics
Principle

It is known that when an antigen is present on the red cells, the corresponding antibody is absent from the serum; conversely,

---

*Ortho Pharmaceutical Corp., Raritan, N.J.

when an antigen is absent, the corresponding antibody is present in the serum.

Blood group	Antigen on cell	Antibodies in serum
O	None	Anti-**A** and Anti-**B**
A	A	Anti-**B**
B	B	Anti-**A**
AB	A and B	None

Therefore, when determining the A-B-O group, the blood is tested two ways:

1. Using known antiserum with the cells to be tested (cell grouping)
2. Using known A_1 and B cells with the serum to be tested (serum grouping)

No cell grouping is complete without results of the serum grouping.

Cell grouping (adults): slide method
Method

1. Place 1 drop of anti-**A** serum on one end of a clean glass slide. Place 1 drop of anti-**B** serum on the other end of the slide.
2. Add ¼ vol of blood next to each drop of antiserum by touching the dropper or applicator stick to the *side of the antiserum*. (The cell suspension must be 40% to 50%.)
3. Place 1 drop of 6% albumin (dilute 3 ml of 22% albumin with 8 ml isotonic saline solution) on slide labeled control. Add ¼ vol of blood as for test.
4. Mix cells and antiserum (also cells and albumin) into a smooth round circle approximately the size of a quarter. Mix each side of the slide with a separate, clean applicator stick held in an almost horizontal position.
5. Both slides should be observed simultaneously for 2 minutes for agglutination while rotating the slide above a light source. *Do not place slide on heated viewbox.*

Interpretation

Agglutination		
Anti-**A** serum	Anti-**B** serum	Interpretation
No	No	Group O
Yes	No	Group A
No	Yes	Group B
Yes	Yes	Group AB

Cell grouping: test tube method
Method

1. Prepare a 3% saline cell suspension of twice-washed red cells to be tested. (Wash cells four times if cord blood is to be tested before making 3% suspension.)
2. Add 1 drop of anti-**A** serum and 1 drop of anti-**B** serum to properly labeled 12 × 75 mm test tubes.
3. Add 1 drop of 6% albumin to a third tube labeled control.
4. Add 1 drop of the above cell suspension to each of the three tubes and mix by shaking.
5. Spin in Sero-Fuge* for 20 seconds.
6. Gently dislodge cells and observe for agglutination.

Interpretation

Same as for slide test.

Serum or reverse grouping: test tube method

Each A-B-O grouping *must be confirmed* by a reverse grouping except in newborn infants.

---

*Clay Adams, Parsippany, N.J.

Method

1. Place 2 drops of serum to be tested into each of two tubes. Label one tube A and the other B.
2. Add 1 drop of 3% saline suspension of washed A_1 cells to tube A and 1 drop of 3% saline suspension of washed B cells to tube B.
3. Mix by shaking.
4. Centrifuge for 20 seconds in Sero-Fuge, 1,000 g.
5. Shake each test tube gently and observe for agglutination.

Interpretation

Reactions with:		
A_1 cells	B cells	Interpretation
Yes	Yes	Group O
Yes	No	Group B
No	Yes	Group A
No	No	Group AB

Remarks

Closely observe reactions with A_1 cells. Anti-A_1 may be found in approximately 2% of A_2 individuals and 25% of A_2B individuals. Group O cells will not be agglutinated by these individuals.

Blood group A_1 individuals may rarely have anti-**H** in their serum. Serum of these individuals will agglutinate group O cells.

If discrepancies are found, repeat tests using group O cells and patient's own cells and serum as a control. Causes of additional discrepancies may be the following:

1. Cold autoagglutinins, with patient's serum agglutinating own cells (a positive control).
2. Cold-reacting isoantibodies such as anti-**P**, anti-**Le**, etc., which react at temperatures below 37° C.
3. Rouleau formation.
4. Absence of expected agglutination with A cells and/or B cells may be caused by agammaglobulinemia or hypogammaglobulinemia.

Cell grouping (cord blood): slide method
Method

1. Place 1 drop of anti-**A** serum on one end of a clean glass slide. Place 1 drop of anti-**B** serum on the other end of the slide.
2. Add ¼ vol of packed cells (washed four times with isotonic saline solution) next to each drop of antiserum by touching the dropper or applicator stick to the *side of the antiserum*. (The cell suspension must be 40% to 50%.)
3. Place 1 drop of 6% albumin on a slide labeled control. Add ¼ vol of packed cells (washed four times with isotonic saline solution) as for test.
4. Mix cells.
5. Observe both slides for agglutination.

Subgroups of A or AB blood
Use of anti-A_1 serum (absorbed anti-A or anti-A lectin)

This serum is specific for A_1 cells. If A cells are not agglutinated by this serum, they are considered a subgroup of A.

Using Ortho antiserum*

1. Place 1 drop of anti-A_1 serum on a clean slide.
2. Add 1 drop of a 10% saline cell suspension.
3. Mix with applicator stick (make a round circle the size of a quarter).

---

*Ortho Pharmaceutical Corp., Raritan, N.J.

4. Rotate slide above light, not on viewbox surface, for *2 minutes only*.
5. If agglutination occurs, record as group A_1.

Using Dade antiserum*

1. Place 1 drop of anti-A_1 serum on a clean slide.
2. Add ¼ vol of fresh blood beside antiserum.
3. Mix with applicator stick.
4. Rotate above light source, not on viewbox surface, for *1 minute only*.
5. If agglutination occurs, record as Group A_1.

Use of group O serum

This serum will *not* agglutinate group O cells. It will agglutinate all other blood groups. It is especially useful in testing for the presence of *weak* A antigens and therefore may be used to verify group O blood.

Method

1. Place 1 drop of anti-**A,B** serum on a clean slide.
2. Put 1 drop of 6% albumin on a slide labeled control.
3. Add ¼ vol whole blood beside antiserum and beside albumin.
4. Mix with applicator stick. (Make a round circle the size of a quarter.)
5. Rotate slide above light source of a viewbox for *1 minute only* (Dade antiserum) or *2 minutes only* (Ortho antiserum).
6. If no agglutination in test or control occurs, record as group 0.

Rh typing

An individual is designated as ''Rh positive'' if the Rh_0 factor is present on the red blood cells, or ''Rh negative'' if this factor is absent. Unlike the A-B-O system, Rh antibody does not occur naturally in the serum of Rh-negative persons. Therefore only direct cell typing is necessary for ascertaining the correct Rh type.

Slide test

Use slide or modified tube test anti-Rh_0 serum. (*Note:* Saline cell suspensions must *not* be used for this test.)

Method

1. Place 1 drop of slide or modified tube test anti-Rh_0 serum on a clean slide.
2. Place 1 drop of 30% albumin on another slide labeled control.
3. To both slides, add 2 drops of unwashed whole blood to be tested (40% to 50% suspension of cells in plasma or serum).
4. Mix well with applicator stick and spread with stick in an almost horizontal position into a smooth oval shape over most of the area of the slide. Stir in both directions. Use a clean applicator stick for each slide.
5. Place both slides on surface of prewarmed viewbox (45° to 50° C).
6. Slowly tilt viewbox back and forth constantly for *2 minutes*.
7. Observe for agglutination at the end of 2 minutes.

Interpretation

Agglutination = Rh_0 positive
No agglutination = Rh_0 negative

---

*Dade Reagents, Inc., Miami, Fla.

Remarks

If no agglutination is observed and the individual is believed to be Rh negative, proceed with D^u procedure. Do D^u testing on all adult individuals who type Rh negative with the slide technic.

Always observe slide reactions for 2 minutes only. Do *not* read after 2 minutes. The control should be negative. If the control is positive, test the cells with saline-agglutinating anti-Rh_0 serum. A positive control may be observed in the presence of rouleaux, strong cold agglutinins, and autoagglutinins.

False-negative reactions in Rh typing occur when hemolyzed blood is used, with weak cells suspensions, and with red cells coated in vivo with antibodies. (This occurs occasionally in acquired hemolytic anemia and hemolytic disease of the newborn.)

In hemolytic disease of the newborn, when the baby's red cells are strongly sensitized with maternal Rh antibody, false-negative results of Rh typing may occur. The correct Rh type of the baby will be indicated best by elution of antibody from the infant's cord blood cells. The eluate then should be tested with Rh_0-positive and Rh_0-negative cells.

False-positive reactions in Rh typing occur when specimens are contaminated, with pseudoagglutination caused by rouleaux, and with autoagglutination caused by autoantibodies.

Modified or rapid tube test
Method

1. Place 1 drop of slide or modified tube anti-Rh_0 serum in a 12 × 75 mm test tube labeled Rh_0.
2. Place 1 drop of 30% albumin into another tube labeled control.
3. Using one applicator stick for each test tube, transfer small amount of blood or 2 drops of 3% saline cell suspension into each of the tubes.
4. Shake the tubes and spin *without incubation* for 30 seconds in Sero-Fuge.
5. Add 1 or 2 drops of saline solution to each tube if stick technic is used.
6. Gently shake the tubes and examine for agglutination over a light source. Interpret as positive or negative as for slide test.

Interpretation

Agglutination in the tube containing the antiserum means that the individual is Rh_0 positive if the control shows no agglutination. If the control is positive (agglutination), then the sample should be tested with saline-agglutinating antiserum.

Tube test

Use saline-agglutinating anti-Rh_0 serum.

Method

1. Place 1 drop of saline-agglutinating antiserum into each of two 12 × 75 mm test tubes. Label one tube Rh_0 and the other *control*.
2. Add 1 drop of patient's 3% saline suspension of twice-washed red cells to test tube Rh_0. Add 1 drop of known group O, Rh_0-positive cells (3% saline suspension) to control tube.
3. Shake tubes and place in 37° C water bath for 30 minutes.
4. Shake tubes gently and then centrifuge for 30 seconds in Sero-Fuge.
5. If results are doubtful, put tubes back in incubator for 30 minutes.
6. Centrifuge tubes for 30 seconds in Sero-Fuge.
7. Gently shake the tubes and examine for agglutination over a light source.

Interpretation

Agglutination in the test tube with the antiserum indicates a positive test if the control test shows agglutination.

Remarks

Rh typing with saline-agglutinating anti-sera is performed in cases having a positive control using slide antiserum. This occurs in the presence of strong rouleaux, strong cold agglutinins, and autoagglutinins. A group O, Rh-positive cell used routinely in the antibody detection test may be used as a control for this test.

Method for Rh$_0$ variant (D^u)

The presence of the D^u variant can be detected by incubating the red cell suspension with 7S anti-**Rh$_0$**. This is then followed with the antiglobulin technic.

Procedure

1. Place 1 drop of anti-**Rh$_0$** slide or rapid tube antiserum into a test tube labeled Rh$_0$.
2. Add 2 drops of 3% saline suspension of red cells to be tested.
3. Mix well and incubate 30 minutes at 37° C.
4. Add 2 drops of 3% saline cell suspension to a test tube labeled control. (This is a direct antiglobulin test.)
5. Wash both tubes three times with tubes full of isotonic saline solution.
6. After the last wash, decant saline solution completely.
7. Add 2 drops of antiglobulin serum (Ortho) to each tube.
8. Mix and then centrifuge for 20 seconds in Sero-Fuge.
9. Gently shake the tubes; observe for agglutination.

Interpretation

If the test and control show no agglutination, the results are negative and the individual is Rh negative. If the test shows agglutination and the control shows no agglutination, the test is positive and the individual is D^u positive. If the control shows agglutination, the test is not valid.

This test should not be performed on cells giving a positive direct antiglobulin test.

Direct antiglobulin (Coombs') test
Principle

The direct antiglobulin (Coombs') test is designed to test for the presence of antierythrocyte antibodies attached to the red cell surface. Antihuman globulin reagent is produced in animals (usually rabbits) by injecting them with human globulin and complement fractions.

Method

1. Put 2 or 3 drops of anticoagulated blood or cells from a clot to be tested in a 12 × 75 mm test tube.
2. Forcefully fill the tube with isotonic saline solution. Centrifuge for 30 seconds in Sero-Fuge. Decant all saline solution and then shake tube to loosen sediment.
3. Repeat for at least three washes, preferably four on cord blood specimens, carefully removing as much saline solution as possible after each wash.
4. After the last wash, add isotonic saline solution to make an approximate 3% saline cell suspension.
5. In a clean test tube, put 2 drops of antiglobulin serum (Ortho).
6. Add 1 drop of the above cell suspension and mix by shaking gently.
7. Spin tube in Sero-Fuge for 20 seconds.
8. Shake tube gently and observe for macroscopic agglutination over a light source.

9. Grade results as negative (−), weak (±), 1+, 2+, 3+, or 4+.
10. If results are *negative*, add 1 drop of Coombs' control cells.
11. Spin tube in Sero-Fuge for 20 seconds. Shake gently and examine macroscopically over light source for agglutination. The reaction now should be positive if the antiglobulin serum is active. If the reaction is negative, the test *must be repeated.*

Remarks

Record on work sheets the degree of agglutination as described in step 9. Report results only as positive (agglutination) or negative (no agglutination). Do not report the degree of agglutination.

Steps 10 and 11 are control procedures to show the reactivity of antiglobulin serum, as a check that the antiglobulin serum was added and that the cells have been thoroughly washed.

Coombs' control cells are presensitized red cells, cells coated with an antibody. These same cells can be used to test the reactivity of the antiglobulin reagent prior to patients' testing.

Screening for irregular antibodies
Principle

It is necessary to use several serologic technics, since no single method detects all irregular antibodies. Always use fresh, *not inactivated,* serum. Red cells for detection tests should be from group O donors and selected to possess as many of the common antigenic determinants as possible.

The technics used in this test are saline solution, immediate spin; high protein, immediate spin; high protein at 37° C; and indirect antiglobulin test.

The indirect antiglobulin is the best technic for the detection of most serum IgG immune antibodies. This part of the test is performed by combining in vitro the antibody in the patient's serum with a specific antigen on the test cells. Following adsorption of antibody to the test cells, antiglobulin serum is added.

We use two cells—Selectogen I and II.* *Working cell suspensions* are prepared daily.

Method

1. Label one tube (12 × 75 mm) S I and another S II.
2. To each tube, add 6 drops of the appropriate cells.
3. To each tube, add 3 drops of isotonic saline solution.
4. Observe outdating date. If within 1 week of expiration, wash cells one time with isotonic saline solution before using.

Screening technic

1. Label three tubes (12 × 75 mm) I, II, and control.
2. Put 2 drops of patient's serum in each tube.
3. Add 1 drop of S I cells to tube I. Add 1 drop of S II cells to tube II. Add 1 drop of patient's 3% saline cell suspension to control tube.
4. Mix and spin 30 seconds in Sero-Fuge.
5. Holding over light source, observe macroscopically for agglutination or hemolysis. Observe one tube at a time, beginning with the control tube. Record as *immediate spin, saline phase.*
6. Add 2 drops of 22% albumin to each tube. Mix and spin 30 seconds in Sero-Fuge.
7. Read as in step 5. Record as *immediate spin, high-protein phase.*
8. Incubate the tubes 30 minutes at 37° C.
9. Spin 30 seconds in Sero-Fuge. Read and record as *37° C, high-protein phase.*

---

*Ortho Pharmaceutical Corp., Raritan, N.J.

10. Proceed with antiglobulin test regardless of results of preceding technics.
11. Wash cells by forcefully filling tubes with isotonic saline solution.
12. Spin 30 seconds in Sero-Fuge. Decant saline solution completely.
13. Repeat cell washing two more times with saline solution as in steps 11 and 12.
14. Add 1 drop of antiglobulin serum (Dade) or 2 drops of antiglobulin serum (Ortho) to each tube.
15. Spin 20 seconds in Sero-Fuge.
16. Read for agglutination as above. Record as *antiglobulin phase*.
17. Add 1 drop of Coombs' control cells if no agglutination is observed in step 16.
18. Spin 20 seconds in Sero-Fuge and then gently shake tubes over light source and observe for agglutination. The reaction now should be positive if the antiglobulin serum is active. If the reaction is negative, the test *must be repeated*.

Interpretation

If no agglutination is observed in any test, "no irregular antibodies demonstrated" should be reported. If the control tube is positive with any test, an autoagglutinin is present in the serum. If it is cold, it may be absorbed out. Antibody identification studies are performed when the screening test is positive with any test. If tests at room temperature are equivocal, it may be helpful to do additional studies at 4° C. This technic helps to detect anti-**P** and anti-**Le** antibodies, since test cells will vary considerably in the strength of these antigens. Always use a control when testing at 4° C.

Remarks

Steps 17 and 18 are control measures to ensure the reactivity of the antiglobulin reagent, as a check that the antiglobulin serum was added and that the cells have been adequately washed.

This test should be done if an indirect antiglobulin test is indicated.

Antibody identification
Principle

It is important to know the blood group and Rh type of the blood containing an antibody to be identified.

If the antibody is discovered with the room temperature tests, additional cells may be added to the commercial panel. If a cold-specific antibody is suspected, group O cord cells may be helpful in identifying anti-**I**.

If the individual is group A or AB, anti-**A** may be ruled out by adding group A_1 and A_2 cells to the panel. For example, if the reactions occur only with A cells and not with O cells or A_2 cells, the antibody probably is anti-**A_1**. However, if the reaction is stronger with group O cells and the A_2 cells and very slight with A_1 or A_1B cells, the cold antibody probably is anti-**H**.

If the pattern does not "fit anti-**A_2** or anti-**H**," the panel may identify such cold antibodies as anti-**P** or anti-**M**.

Antibodies of the Lewis system react at all temperatures. If the antibody appears stronger in the warm phase, such antibodies as Rh, S, or Fy^a may be suspected. If the indirect antiglobulin test demonstrates the antibody best, anti-**Kell**, anti-**Kidd**, or anti-**Duffy** should be considered.

The greater the number of cells in a panel, the more complete the process of elimination and the better the chance of promptly identifying the antibody.

Method

Use Selectogen* and Identogen* as test cells
1. Set up eleven 12 × 75 mm tubes in a rack. Label tubes 1 through 8, S I, S II, and control.
2. Place 2 drops of patient's serum in each tube.
3. Add 1 drop of the appropriate cells to its respective tube. (We repeat the tests with Selectogen I and II in the identification.) Add 1 drop of the patient's 3% cells, washed twice, to the tube labeled control.
4. Use the same procedures as for the screening test, with particular attention paid to the phase in which the antibody was found in the screening procedure.

Remarks

An individual may possess more than one antibody. Record strength of reactions in each phase carefully and consistently. Use clean glassware, fresh saline solutions, and precise amounts of reagents, serum, and cells.

Reagent cells may vary in strength if they are heterozygous or homozygous for a particular antigenic determinant. This may be observed on the antigram chart. Always read the control cell first. This gives a clue to false-positives.

To eliminate possible antigens, select a cell that did not react with the serum. Cross out the antigenic determinants that this cell possesses. Proceed with the next cell that did not react with the serum and cross out antigens not already eliminated. Consider the antigens that you are not able to cross out. See if all the cells reacting possess them. If they all possess one, the antibody is to that antigen. If there are those which cannot be ruled out, more cells may be added to the panel or absorptions made. No single panel can resolve every possible situation.

When the antibody is identified, it is advisable to see if the cells of the patient are lacking the antigen. This is used as confirming evidence.

If the antibody is identified in a pregnant woman, it should be titered. The serum should be labeled, dated, and frozen for further use.

Antibody elution technics
Principle

Elution is the removal by physical or chemical means of antibody that has been adsorbed onto red cells either in vivo or in vitro. Elution technics may be used:
1. To demonstrate and identify antibody causing hemolytic disease of the newborn from the infant's cells if the mother's serum is not available
2. To demonstrate and identify antibody on the red cells of patients with acquired hemolytic anemia
3. To demonstrate and identify antibody on red cells in suspected transfusion reactions
4. To separate and identify a mixture of antibodies
5. To demonstrate and identify weak subgroups or variants within the A-B-O system by the ability of the red cells to adsorb antibody

Heat elution method
Method

1. Obtain approximately 2 ml of cells from an anticoagulated specimen or from clot broken up with applicator stick.
2. Wash the cells four times for 1 minute each time in 15-ml centrifuge tube with large volumes of isotonic saline solution.

---

*Ortho Pharmaceutical Corp., Raritan, N.J.

3. Pack the cells and remove all the supernatant after the last wash. There must be no "free" antibody in the intrinsic solution.
4. To 1 vol of packed cells, add 1 vol of isotonic saline solution or 1 vol of 6% bovine albumin and resuspend.
5. Transfer the cell mixture to a 56° C water bath for 10 minutes, agitating constantly. Preheat centrifuge cup at the same time in the 56° C water bath.
6. *Immediately* centrifuge the cell mixture at high speed for 3 minutes in the heated cup.
7. *Immediately* and *carefully* (so as to avoid cells) aspirate the supernatant fluid (the eluate) and save for testing.
8. The eluate should be tested on the day of preparation or stored frozen.

Remark

The heat elution technic is the method of choice for eluting anti-**A** and anti-**B** antibodies.

Rubin ether method
Method

1. To 1 vol of washed packed red cells, add an equal volume of isotonic saline solution.
2. To this mixture add 2 vol of diethyl ether.
3. Stopper and mix by repeated inversions for 1 minute. *Caution:* Periodically release stopper to prevent "blowing its top." Also, no smoking or flames are permitted while ether is used.
4. Incubate the red cell–ether mixture for 30 minutes at 37° C.
5. Centrifuge for 10 minutes at 3,000 rpm (Sero-Fuge may be used).
6. Three distinct layers result: upper, containing clear ether; middle, containing denatured red cell stroma; and bottom, containing hemoglobin-stained *eluate*.
7. Remove the upper two layers by suction.
8. The remaining layer, which is the eluate, may be used immediately or stored frozen. Before storing, place the eluate in unstoppered tube at 37° C for 15 minutes to evaporate the residual ether.

Remarks

The ether elution method is a satisfactory technic for eluting Rh antibodies. This is not the method of choice for eluting anti-**A** and anti-**B** antibodies.

Testing the heat eluate in A-B-O hemolytic disease
Method

1. Label four test tubes (12 × 75 mm) A, B, I, and II. (I and II refer to group O screening cells—Selectogen.)
2. To each of the four tubes, add 2 drops of the eluate.
3. To the respective tubes, add 1 drop of 3% cell saline suspension of the adult A_1, B, and group O screening cells.
4. Incubate tubes at 37° C for 30 minutes.
5. Forcefully fill tubes with isotonic saline solution. Centrifuge for 30 seconds in Sero-Fuge.
6. Decant all of saline solution and then shake tube to loosen sediment.
7. Repeat steps 5 and 6 for two additional cell washes.
8. Decant all the saline solution and then shake sediment.
9. Add 1 drop of antiglobulin serum (Dade) or 2 drops of antiglobulin serum (Ortho) to each tube.
10. Mix by shaking tubes and then centrifuge in Sero-Fuge for 20 seconds.
11. Shake tubes gently and observe for agglutination over light source.

Remarks

On occasions, an infant with A-B-O incompatibility will give an eluate with an antibody demonstrating both anti-**A** and anti-**B** activity. For example, an eluate from a group A baby may give a reaction with group A and B cells. This is referred to as "cross-reacting antibody" or anti-**C**. (This is not to be confused with rh′ [C].)

If cells I and II are positive, an antibody other than anti-**A** and anti-**B** must be considered.

Testing the eluate for antibody of unknown specificity
Method

1. A cell panel may be used to test the eluate (heat or ether). One should use various technics to demonstrate the behavior of the antibody. However, eluates obtained with the Rubin ether technic should be tested only with the indirect antiglobulin method.
2. The identified antibody in the eluate should be confirmed by testing with four selected red cells, two cells having the suspected antigenic determinant and two cells lacking the antigen.

Absorption of nonspecific cold agglutinins
Collection and preparation of blood sample

1. Draw 20 ml of blood from the patient.
2. Immediately mix blood with standard EDTA anticoagulant in a tube kept at approximately 37° C in a beaker of warm water. Place the remainder of the blood in a plain tube kept in a beaker of ice.
3. Prewarm and store a bottle of isotonic saline solution at 37° C.

Method

1. Wash 3 or 4 drops of the warm anticoagulated blood with the warm isotonic saline solution three times. Prepare a 3% warm saline cell suspension. Keep in 37° C water bath.
2. Do a direct antiglobulin test using 1 drop of the warm washed cell suspension and 2 drops of antiglobulin serum (Ortho).
3. Spin 20 seconds in Sero-Fuge. Observe for agglutination over light source. This will determine the presence or absence of warm autoagglutinins.
4. When the clot has formed in the cold bath (or refrigerator), spin the tube in precooled centrifuge cups. Most of the cold agglutinins will be absorbed onto the patient's red cells.
5. Add 2 drops of the above serum to 1 drop of the cell suspension prepared above.
6. Spin tube immediately and observe for agglutination. If there is none, the nonspecific cold agglutinins have been absorbed. The serum can then be tested for specific agglutinins.
7. If step 6 is positive, further absorption is necessary.
8. Wash the warm anticoagulated blood sample three times with warm isotonic saline solution. Remove as much saline solution as possible.
9. Place the serum from the patient in a clean tube. Add ½ vol of the warm washed packed cells.
10. Mix and place in the cold (4° C) for 30 minutes. Prechill the centrifuge cups.
11. Centrifuge the serum cell mixture and remove the absorbed serum.
12. Test again as in steps 5 and 6 to see if the patient's serum still agglutinates his own cells at room temperature. The absorptions should be repeated using warm freshly washed cells each time until there is no agglutination at room temperature.

13. Test the absorbed serum for specific isoagglutinins with the screening cells that are used routinely.

Investigation of a positive direct antiglobulin test

If the direct antiglobulin test is positive in an individual other than a newborn infant, the following tests are indicated:

1. Prepare a heat eluate using the patient's cells (p. 907).
2. Test the eluate for irregular antibodies using Selectogen I and II (p. 907).
3. Test the patient's serum for irregular antibodies using Selectogen I and II (p. 907).

Note: With each of the previous tests, use patient's serum and patient's washed 3% saline cell suspension as control.

4. These tests are performed with saline solution at refrigerator temperature, with saline solution at room temperature, with albumin at 37° C, and then converting to antiglobulin test.
5. If the "control" is positive at 4° or 18° to 20° C in the serum antibody screening test, a fresh sample must be obtained from the patient and cold agglutinins (usually referred to as "nonspecific") are absorbed out. See p. 911 for absorption of "nonspecific" cold agglutinins.
6. Identification studies are done if the screening tests detect an antibody. Both the serum and eluate can be used for this purpose.

Note: A strongly positive direct antiglobulin test with no antibody present in the eluate should be brought to the attention of the pathologist. This situation may be caused by nonerythrocyte antibodies such as antipenicillin antibodies, and further investigation is required to prove their presence or absence.

Prenatal serologic studies
Patients from labor room

1. If the patient has had prenatal care and is Rh negative, refer to file to determine whether antibody titer is indicated.
2. If antibody titer is not indicated based on previous laboratory studies, perform only antibody screening test.
3. If there is *no record* on file, do the following tests:
   a. A-B-O grouping, direct and reverse.
   b. Rh typing: Perform D^u test if patient is Rh negative.
   c. Antibody screening test: This is done *only* if the patient is Rh negative. If the patient is Rh positive, the cord blood sample that is usually sent to the laboratory will be studied for presence of antibodies. If the studies with cord blood indicate the presence of antibodies, then the maternal blood sample will be studied in detail (i.e., antibody screening test, antibody identification, etc.).

First visit (private outpatient, clinic, etc.)

1. Laboratory studies performed:
   a. A-B-O grouping, direct and reverse.
   b. Rh typing: Perform D^u test if patient is Rh negative.
   c. Antibody screening test: This test is performed *on all* Rh-positive and Rh-negative women.
   d. Antibody identification: This procedure is performed when the antibody detection test indicates the presence of irregular antibodies.
   e. Antibody titration: This is done if antibody is known to cause hemolytic disease of the newborn.

Note: The saline titration is used, together with the albumin-antiglobulin technic, during the initial visit. If the saline test is negative, there is no need to repeat it on the next visit.

2. Laboratory records: Record cards are kept on all Rh-negative. D^u-negative women. Results of all tests, whether positive or negative, are entered on these cards.

Subsequent visit

1. Perform antibody screening test if test has been negative on previous visits.
2. If the screening test was positive previously, and the antibody identified, then only a titer is performed, if indicated.

Titration of irregular antibodies in maternal serum
Principle

The titer or relative amount of antibody in a serum is determined by making serial twofold dilutions of the serum in a suitable medium. A constant volume of cells is added to each tube. The titer is the reciprocal of the highest dilution in which agglutination is observed macroscopically.

Saline titration
Method

1. Place ten 12 × 75 mm test tubes in a rack and label them according to serum dilution: 1, 2, 4, 8, . . . 512, and control.
2. Using a 1-ml pipet, deliver to the bottom of all the tubes except the first, 0.1 ml isotonic saline solution.
3. With a 0.2-ml pipet, add 0.1 ml serum to the bottom of tube No. 1 and 0.1 ml to the bottom of tube No. 2. Blow out.
4. Using a clean 0.2-ml graduated pipet, mix the contents of tube No. 2 four times, keeping the tip of the pipet near the surface of the solution. Blow out gently, carefully avoiding excessive bubbles and coating of the inner surface of the tube. Transfer 0.1 ml of the mixture to tube No. 4.
5. With another clean 0.2-ml pipet, mix four times and transfer 0.1 ml to tube No. 8.
6. Continue mixing and transferring, each time using a clean pipet. Do not transfer diluted serum to the control tube. This contains only diluent and red cell suspension.
7. When the last tube (512) has been mixed, draw up and save 0.1 ml for further dilution if necessary.
8. With a 1-ml pipet, add 0.1 ml of 2% saline suspension of washed cells of appropriate antigenic structure to each tube.
9. Shake rack several times. Incubate tubes at 37° C for 30 minutes.
10. Shake rack again and centrifuge tubes at 2,000 rpm for 1 minute.
11. Gently shake tubes and observe tubes for agglutination one at a time over a light source, starting with control tube, then 512, 256, etc. The tube with the highest dilution that shows macroscopic agglutination is the end point. This is the saline titer.

Albumin-antiglobulin titration
Method

1. Place ten 12 × 75 mm test tubes in a rack and label according to dilution: 1, 2, 4, 8, . . . 512, and control.
2. Using a 1-ml pipet, deliver to the bottom of all the tubes except the first, 0.1 ml of 22% albumin.
3. Follow steps 3 through 7 of method for saline titration.
4. In step 8, use 2% suspension of washed cells suspended in 22% albumin.
5. Shake rack and incubate at 37° C for 30 minutes.
6. Shake rack and then centrifuge tubes at 2,000 rpm for 2 minutes.
7. Gently shake tubes and observe for agglutination over a light source starting with control tube, then 512, etc. The tube with the highest dilution that shows macroscopic agglutination is the end point. This is the albumin titer.

8. All tubes that are negative and the "end point" tube are washed three times with full volumes of isotonic saline solution.
9. After the last wash, decant saline solution completely.
10. Add 2 drops of antiglobulin serum (Ortho) to each of the washed tubes.
11. Spin tubes 20 seconds in Sero-Fuge.
12. Shake tubes gently and observe for agglutination. Begin observations with tube labeled 512 and proceed to 256, etc. The end point is the antiglobulin titer.

Remarks

We use the albumin titration to convert to indirect antiglobulin titer. It is the most sensitive and reliable technic for detection of Rh antibodies. Always use the same titration technic. Use fresh cells (not over 24 hours old) and the same cells that give the strongest reactions possible.

Be certain to dilute cells in saline solution for saline titers and in albumin for albumin titers. Each dilution is made with a separate pipet to eliminate the effect of carry-over.

If the serum is from an obstetric patient, label test tube with patient's name and date when sample was obtained. *Store tube frozen.* This specimen should be tested simultaneously with the next sample obtained on that patient. A difference in the titer of the two specimens done under the same circumstances simultaneously is significant.

Record for the laboratory records the results of both saline and antiglobulin titrations.

Titration of anti-A and anti-B isoagglutinins
Screening for naturally occurring anti-A and anti-B antibodies
Method

1. Add 0.1 ml of serum to be tested to 4.9 ml of isotonic saline solution to make a 1:50 dilution. Mix by inverting.
2. Label two tubes A and B.
3. Add 1 drop of diluted serum to each tube.
4. To tube A, add 1 drop of 2% saline suspension of group A_1 washed red cells.
5. To tube B, add 1 drop of 2% saline suspension of group B washed red cells.
6. Let stand at room temperature for 5 minutes.
7. Shake the tubes and spin in Sero-Fuge for 30 seconds.
8. Gently shake the tubes over light source and observe for agglutination.

Interpretation

Agglutination in either tube indicates presence of corresponding antibody at that dilution, and the titer may be higher.

Even if no agglutination is observed in either tube, further screening must be done for nonneutralizable antibody (immune antibody).

Neutralization of naturally occurring anti-A and anti-B antibodies
Method

1. To 1 ml of serum, add 0.2 ml of NeutrAB.* Mix and let stand at room temperature for 5 minutes.
2. Make a dilution of 1:10 in isotonic saline solution of the neutralized serum.
3. Put 0.9 ml of isotonic saline solution in test tube.
4. Add 0.1 ml neutralized serum to saline solution and mix well.
5. Label two tubes A and B.

---
*Dade Reagents, Inc., Miami, Fla.

6. Add 2 drops of the 1:10 dilution of neutralized serum to both tubes.
7. To tube A, add 2 drops of 2% saline suspension of A_1 cells washed with isotonic saline solution.
8. To tube B, add 2 drops of 2% saline suspension of B cells washed with isotonic saline solution.
9. Centrifuge both tubes for 30 seconds in Sero-Fuge.
10. Gently shake over light source and observe for agglutination. These results should be negative, confirming the neutralization.
11. Incubate the tubes at 37° C for 30 minutes.
12. Remove from incubation.
13. Wash the contents with isotonic saline solution. Forcefully fill the tubes with saline solution so cells will be evenly suspended.
14. Spin 30 seconds in Sero-Fuge.
15. Decant supernatant rapidly and completely and shake the tubes.
16. Repeat steps 13, 14, and 15 for two additional washes.
17. After the last wash, decant completely. Shake the tubes and to each add 2 drops of antiglobulin serum (Ortho).
18. Spin 20 seconds in Sero-Fuge.
19. Gently shake tubes above light source and observe for macroscopic agglutination.

Interpretation

A negative test indicates that no significant titer of nonneutralizable antibodies is present. If a test is positive, a titer should be performed so that the exact amount of antibody can be determined. If a titer of naturally occurring anti-A and anti-B agglutinins is indicated, refer to saline method of titration for irregular antibodies. If a titer of nonneutralizable antibodies is indicated, perform the saline method titration on the neutralized serum and convert it to the antiglobulin test.

Remarks

Titration of these antibodies may be of value when parasitic infections are suspected. Parasitic infections, and sometimes viral and bacterial infections, cause an elevation of anti-A and anti-B titer. In our laboratory, screening of these antibodies is performed mostly for this reason. Low titers may help confirm a diagnosis of hypogammaglobulinemia. Prenatal titers of anti-A and anti-B are not recommended for predicting A-B-O hemolytic disease of the newborn.

Serologic studies on newborn infants

Laboratory studies on infants' cord blood may provide data for the physician even before clinical signs of hemolytic disease can be observed.

The following tests are performed:

1. A-B-O direct grouping: No subgrouping or reverse grouping is performed.
   Note: Use slide test method. If cord blood is submitted, be sure that the cells are washed adequately, four times with isotonic saline, to remove all traces of Wharton's jelly.
2. Rh typing for Rh_0 factor (test tube method)
   Note: If the Rh typing appears negative or questionable, observe the results of the direct antiglobulin test prior to interpretation as Rh positive or Rh negative. Do D^u test on all Rh-negative infants. (Remember that the direct antiglobulin test must be negative for the D^u test to be valid.)
3. Direct antiglobulin test
   Note: If the direct antiglobulin test is strongly positive, the Rh_0 antigen sites of an Rh-positive infant may be blocked with maternal antibody. This results in a false-negative Rh_0 typing. In this case an eluate prepared from the infant's cells

should be used to ascertain the correct Rh type of the infant. If the eluted antibody reacts with Rh-positive cells but not with Rh-negative cells, the infant's blood is recorded as Rh positive. *Caution:* Never report as Rh_0 negative a baby with a positive direct antiglobulin test, especially if the mother is Rh_0 negative.

4. Elution studies

Note: Elution studies are done on all newborn infants with a positive direct antiglobulin test if hemolytic disease of the newborn is suspected to be caused by A-B-O incompatibility. Eluates are tested on newborn infants if direct antiglobulin test is positive and mother's serum is not available for study.

Demonstration of free homologous antibody in cord serum

This test is helpful in confirming hemolytic disease of the newborn caused by A-B-O incompatibility.

Method

1. Label four test tubes (12 × 75 mm) A, B, O, and positive control.
2. Add 2 drops cord serum to each tube.
3. To the respective tubes, add 1 drop of 3% saline suspension of adult A_1, B, O, and patient's cells.
4. Incubate at 37° C for 30 minutes.
5. Wash cells by forcefully adding isotonic saline solution to evenly resuspend cells and fill tube. Spin for 30 seconds in Sero-Fuge.
6. Decant saline solution completely and shake tube to loosen sediment.
7. Repeat steps 5 and 6 for two additional washes.
8. After last wash, add 2 drops antiglobulin serum (Ortho). Mix gently.
9. Centrifuge for 20 seconds in Sero-Fuge.
10. Shake tubes gently over light source and observe for agglutination.

Interpretation

The finding of anti-**A** in an A or AB baby or anti-**B** in a B or AB baby indicates that these antibodies have crossed the placenta. These antibodies are of maternal origin and are potentially hemolytic for the infant's erythrocytes.

Cold agglutinins

Principle

Cold agglutinins are demonstrated by placing a 1% suspension of the patient's washed red blood cells into serial dilutions of the patient's serum. O-negative cells in place of patient's cells may be used, providing there is no incompatibility.

These tubes are refrigerated overnight at 4° C and observed next morning, while still cold, for gross agglutination. After examination, the tubes are warmed at 37° C for 1 hour to demonstrate the reversibility of the agglutination. A 6-hour reading may be taken in emergency cases, but should be left and read again after the overnight refrigeration.

Reagents

1. Sodium chloride, dried, reagent grade
2. Patient's blood, clotted, 5 to 10 ml in a plain tube
3. Distilled water

Preparation of working solution

1. Saline solution, 0.85%
   a. Weigh out 8.5 Gm of sodium chloride.
   b. Dissolve the salt in distilled water.
   c. Make the volume up to 1,000 ml with distilled water.
2. Patient's serum
   a. Separate the serum from the clot on the day the blood is received. If the blood is put in the refrigerator before separation, warm it to 37° C before centrifuging.
   b. Using an applicator stick, rim the clot.
   c. Centrifuge at 1,000 to 1,500 rpm for 5 minutes.
   d. Pour off the serum and save.
3. Patient's washed cells, 1% suspension
   a. Using 0.85% saline solution, wash the patient's cells from the clot remaining after pouring off the serum. Patient's anticoagulated blood or O-negative cells may be used.
   b. Place the cell suspension in a centrifuge tube.
   c. Centrifuge at 1,000 to 1,500 rpm for 5 minutes.
   d. Pour off the supernatant fluid.
   e. Add approximately 10 ml of 0.85% saline solution.
   f. Resuspend the cells by gently inverting the tube, holding the thumb over the opening.
   g. Wash as outlined in *a* three times.
   h. Make a 1% suspension of the cells by adding 10 ml of 0.85% saline solution to 0.1 ml of packed cells and resuspend by gentle inversion.

Method

1. Place nine 13 × 100 mm test tubes in a 20-hole test tube rack.
2. Using a 5-ml serologic pipet, place 0.5 ml of saline solution in each tube.
3. To tube No. 1, add 0.5 ml of serum, using a 1-ml serologic pipet.
4. Mix well by drawing the solution up into the pipet and forcibly expelling it three times.
5. Transfer 0.5 ml of this 1:2 dilution to tube No. 2 and again mix.
6. Continue the twofold serial dilution, as just outlined, through tube No. 8. Tube No. 9 contains only saline solution and is the control.
7. Add 0.5 ml of the 1% patient's cells to all tubes except No. 8, thus giving the following final dilutions:

Tube	Dilution	Tube	Dilution
1	1:4	6	1:128
2	1:8	7	1:256
3	1:16	8	"Hold" tube
4	1:32		*no* cells
5	1:64	9	Control

8. Shake the rack to mix the erythrocytes thoroughly with the diluted serum and place in the refrigerator at 4° C overnight.
9. Examine the tubes immediately after removing them from the refrigerator, holding them in a nearly horizontal position over a well-illuminated white background. Shake each tube gently, but quickly, until all the erythrocytes in the bottom of the tube have been dislodged.
10. Record the titer in terms of the final dilution of serum in the last tube showing grossly detectable agglutination.
11. If titer is above 1:32, place the tubes in a 37° C water bath for 1 hour to determine the reversibility of the agglutination.

Normal values

Titers up to 1:32 may be normal. Titers above 1:32 are suggestive of atypical pneumonia. Titers still positive at 1:256 should be diluted through 12 tubes, starting with tube No. 8.

Remarks

If whole blood was refrigerated before separating the serum, warm the blood to 37° C before centrifuging. Inactivated serum may be used. If the patient's cells are refrigerated with a small amount of serum, there is no loss of reactivity after 24 hours and a minimal loss after 48 hours.

Primary atypical pneumonia is the only respiratory disease in which a high titer or increase in titer can be consistently demonstrated. Reviewing the literature, it would seem that cold agglutinins appear in about half the cases of atypical pneumonia.

Amounts of 0.5 ml are used rather than the smaller amounts used by Young in his investigation, because of the greater ease of pipetting, mixing, and reading the results. Young's recommended procedure, using the final serial dilution of 10, 20, 40, etc., is not used because it is felt the smaller range in the lower dilutions is advantageous.

Patient's cells, rather than group O cells, are used. Young (1946) reports that group O cells from various donors vary in sensitivity. While the wisdom of using the same group O donor for all tests is recognized, the same donor is rarely available to any laboratory for a long period of time. Investigations carried out by Young indicate that absolute values obtained with patient's cells are not often significantly different from those obtained with highly sensitive group O cells. It is therefore concluded that it is more convenient to test each patient's serum with his own cells, which are always obtainable.

Reference

Young, 1946

Demonstration of leukoagglutinins
Principle

Abnormal sera containing antibodies against human leukocytes produced through isoimmunization are tested against normal leukocytes. Negative reactions may result either from antibodies that are occult or from poor sensitivity of this technic. Studies indicate that the leukocyte antigens are inherited. The differences in antigenicity of white cells and red cells have been confirmed by extensive studies on immunologic tolerance. It has been demonstrated that these antigens are located in the nucleus, and antinuclear antibodies have been contrasted with anticytoplasmic antibodies. There is an established relationship between leukocyte antibodies and febrile transfusion reactions.

Method

1. Prepare abnormal sera from defibrinated fasting blood from patients who have received multiple transfusions.
   a. Centrifuge at 3,000 rpm for 30 minutes to remove particulate matter (especially RBCs). This is very important, since particulate matter may produce nonspecific agglutination of leukocytes.
   b. Heat sera for 30 minutes at 56° C (certain sera are inactive unless heated). Store in small aliquots at −20° C.
2. Prepare leukocyte suspension from normal defibrinated blood. One volume of sterile 6% dextran in isotonic saline solution is added to 5 vol of defibrinated blood. The mixture is allowed to sediment for 20 to 30 minutes at room temperature. The leukocyte-rich supernatant is separated, and its WBC count is adjusted to about 5,000/mm^3 (5×10^9/1) by dilution with the donor's own serum. The leukocyte suspension is used as soon as possible, since spontaneous leukocyte clumping often occurs 3 hours after collection, especially if the cells are maintained at temperatures near 37° C.
3. To 0.1 ml of test serum, add 0.05 ml of leukocyte suspension and incubate for 1 hour at 37° C.
4. Resuspend the contents of the test tubes by agitation, pour on a clean slide, and dry at room temperature. Drying is complete within about 1 hour.
5. Fix slides by methyl alcohol, stain in the usual manner with Wright's stain, and examine microscopically for evidence of agglutination (see Fig. 15-7, p. 687).

Results

In the absence of leukoagglutinins, white cells are distributed homogeneously on the slides. Leukoagglutination is considered present when various degrees of white cell clumping are observed; no attempt is made to report the positive reactions quantitatively. Sera tested are specific for leukocyte antibodies when no immune antibodies against erythrocytes can be demonstrated by the indirect Coombs test. Sera from compatible (with respect to red cell antigens and antibodies) donors only should be used. Any equivocal test should be repeated.

Lalezari et al (1960) point out that mixed erythrocyte-leukocyte agglutination is inhibited by 0.1 ml of 10% EDTA to 0.9 ml of cell suspension. This procedure permits the study of leukoagglutinins in incompatible erythrocyte systems. They also noted that in some cases leukoagglutinins are not active in untreated serum but become activated after the serum is heated to 56° C for 30 minutes. Activation was also noted following addition of EDTA.

References

Lalezari and Spaet, 1959
Lalezari et al, 1960

Heterophil antibody: Monospot test
Principle

The diagnosis of infectious mononucleosis requires the demonstration of heterophil antibody not of the Forssman type, i.e., incompletely adsorbed by guinea pig kidney and completely adsorbed by beef cell antigen. The original method for differential adsorption (Davidsohn) has been replaced in our laboratory by the more convenient Monospot* test. In this test, fresh stabilized horse erythrocytes are used. Note discussion on specificity on p. 679.

Reagents

The commercial package consists of adsorbing reagent I (guinea pig kidney antigen), adsorbing reagent II (beef erythrocyte antigen), indicator cells (stabilized horse erythrocytes), and a positive control serum.

Method

The directions given by the manufacturer come with each kit and need not be repeated here. Directions must be followed carefully.

Remarks

While it is possible to use this kit to titrate the antibody present, this is seldom necessary.

Demonstration of LE cells

The LE cell is a neutrophilic leukocyte, monocyte, or eosinophil that has ingested a homogeneous globular mass of altered nuclear material. Formation of the cells depends on the *LE plasma factor*, found in the blood obtained from patients with lupus erythematosus. The factor is a component of the γ-globulin fraction of the serum proteins and is stable in serum stored at refrigerator temperature and in the frozen state and is not destroyed by heat unless the serum is heated to 65° C (Chapter 15).

---

*Ortho Pharmaceutical Corp., Raritan, N.J.

Method

When leukocytes from the patient or from a normal person are incubated in serum containing the LE plasma factor, a depolymerization of DNA in the nucleus of some cells takes place. Depolymerization is accompanied by liberation of nuclear material that appears as free homogeneous globular masses. The typical LE cells are formed when these masses are ingested by neutrophilic leukocytes.

Clotted blood method
Method

1. Obtain blood by venipuncture. Transfer 5 ml to a dry tube and leave at room temperature for 2 to 3 hours after the blood clots.
2. Rim the clot and transfer the serum and clot to a special sieve* and mash through the sieve with the pestle, collecting the strainings in a Petri dish.
3. Fill one or more Wintrobe hematocrit tubes with the material collected.
4. Incubate Wintrobe tube at 37° C for 2 to 2½ hours. Centrifuge tube at approximately 1,000 rpm for 5 to 10 minutes.
5. Discard the supernatant serum, make three or four smears from the buffy coat, and stain with Wright's stain.
6. Examine carefully for the LE cell. Microscopic scanning may be done (with experience) under low power, as the LE cell is characteristically slightly larger than normal cells.

Rotary bead method
Method

1. Place 10 ml of venous blood in a tube containing 5 drops of 1% ammonium heparinate* or balanced ammonium–potassium oxalate and mix. The concentration of heparin is important, and the drops should be delivered through a 25-gauge needle held horizontally.
2. Ten to twenty 4-mm glass beads are added to the tube of blood and mixed on a mechanical tube rotator for 30 minutes.
3. Incubate at room temperature for 1 hour.
4. Two Wintrobe hematocrit tubes are then filled with the blood and incubated at 37° C for not more than 6 nor less than 3 hours (usually 4 hours).
5. The tubes are then centrifuged for 10 minutes at approximately 1,000 rpm.
6. Discard the supernatant plasma, make four smears from the buffy coat, and stain with Wright's stain.

Results

The LE cell is a homogeneous red-purple protein mass engulfed or surrounded by the nucleus of a neutrophil. The inclusion body is *smooth, homogeneous,* and *smoky* in appearance.

The tart cell is a similar cell in which the ingested nucleus retains some characteristic nuclear structure. It is never as "smooth" as the LE cell and usually has a darker-staining rim.

Preparations that contain LE cells may show two other characteristic phenomena:

1. The presence of extracellular globular material having the same homogeneous appearance and staining as the intracellular inclusion.
2. The formation of "rosettes" when neutrophilic leukocytes surround one of these extracellular bodies.

Remarks

In most cases, the finding of LE cells indicates the presence of disseminated lupus erythematosus (see discussion on p. 680). The antinuclear (ANA) technic has been found to be more specific for disseminated lupus erythematosus.

References

Hargraves et al, 1948
Heserick, 1956
Linkham and Conley, 1956
Magath and Winkle, 1952

Fluorescent antinuclear antibody test: qualitative method
Principle

Antinuclear antibody (ANA), which is reported to occur in both the 7S and 19S globulin components of the serum of some patients, will react with various components of the nuclei of tissue cells. Fluorescein-conjugated antihuman γ-globulin will react with the antinuclear antibody within the nuclei of the tissue antigen. When viewed under a microscope equipped with an ultraviolet light source and a dark-field condenser, the nuclei or portions of nuclei will fluoresce.

Equipment

1. Microscope equipped with binocular head, dark-field condenser, Osram HBO 200 high-intensity ultraviolet light source, Schott BG 12 or equivalent primary filter, blue absorbing yellow secondary filter, and tungsten light source. (In our hands, the Leitz system has been most satisfactory.)
2. Alcohol-washed glass slides
3. Alcohol-washed No. 1 or No. 1.5 22-mm square cover glasses
4. Serologic pipets, 0.2- and 1-ml sizes
5. Test tubes, 13 × 100 mm

Reagents

1. FTA hemagglutination buffer, pH 7.3 ± 0.2*
2. Antihuman γ-globulin, fluorescein conjugated†
3. Sodium chloride, kept in a desiccator
4. Fluorescent antibody mounting medium
5. Kidney from healthy young Sprague-Dawley rat
6. Patient's serum
7. Positive control serum of known titer
8. Negative control serum (pooled negative ANA sera)
9. Tween 80

Preparation of working solutions

1. FTA hemagglutination buffer (phosphate-buffered saline, PBS)
   a. Determine the amount of hemagglutination buffer solution necessary to process the test run.
   b. Weigh out hemagglutination buffer powder in the amount recommended by the manufacturer for the volume determined in step *a*.
   c. Dissolve the weighed powder in the correct volume of distilled water and mix well.
2. Rat kidney antigen
   a. To prepare frozen tissue blocks:
      (1) Chloroform and autopsy a young rat, removing the kidneys.

---

(2) Cut the kidneys into cubes approximately 5 mm square.

(3) Place the kidney blocks individually into 13 × 100 mm test tubes and stopper.

(4) Quick-freeze the tissues in a dry ice alcohol bath or in liquid nitrogen.

(5) Store the frozen tissues at dry ice temperature. These tissues will usually last 2 months or until difficulty is encountered with sectioning.

b. On the day of the test run:

(1) Remove a tube containing the frozen tissue from the freezer.

(2) On a cryostat, cut sections of tissue at 4 mμ and mount on alcohol-washed slides.

(3) Prepare sufficient tissue slides for the test run, including the control sera.

(4) Place the slides in a refrigerator until ready to use.

3. Patient's serum

a. Obtain 8 to 10 ml of clotted blood by venipuncture.

b. Rim the clot and centrifuge.

c. Pipet or decant the cell-free serum into a clean 13 × 100 mm test tube, properly labeled.

4. 0.15M saline solution

a. Weight out 8.8 Gm of dry sodium chloride.

b. Place the weighed sodium chloride into a 1,000-ml graduated cylinder.

c. Dissolve in and bring to 1,000 ml volume with distilled water; mix well.

5. Tween 80 solution, 2%, in PBS

a. Warm Tween 80 and an aliquot of PBS in a 56° C water bath.

b. Using a 1-ml serologic pipet, add 0.2 parts of warmed Tween 80 to 9.8 parts of warmed PBS. Mix well with a Vortex mixer until completely dissolved.

c. This solution may be kept refrigerated and used as long as no mold or other particulate matter has formed.

6. Antihuman γ-globulin, fluorescein conjugated

a. Reconstitute the desiccated conjugate according to the manufacturer's directions. Place 0.2-ml aliquots into 13 × 100 mm test tubes and keep frozen.

b. The optimum dilution of conjugate in 2% Tween 80 solution must be determined for each new lot of conjugate before it is put into routine use. The optimum dilution is the highest dilution that will give strong nuclear fluorescence with a minimum of background fluorescence.

(1) Prepare four rat kidney antigen slides.

(2) Prepare twofold serial dilutions, 1:5, 1:10, 1:20, and 1:40, of the untested conjugate in 2% Tween 80.

(3) Run the fluorescent ANA procedure on the antigen slides as described below, using a 1:5 dilution of a known positive ANA serum on all the slides. Label the antigen-antibody complex on each slide with the appropriate conjugate dilution.

(4) Observe the slides under the ultraviolet microscope and determine the best dilution.

c. For the routine test:

(1) Remove an aliquot from the freezer and allow it to warm to room temperature. Shake well.

(2) Make the appropriate dilution of conjugate in 2% Tween 80 in a volume sufficient to allow 0.03 ml of diluted conjugate per slide.

7. Fluorescent antibody mounting medium

a. Add 1 part of buffered saline solution to 9 parts of glycerin, reagent quality.

b. Always check the pH of the mounting medium with 0.04% phenol red solution. A red color denotes a satisfactory pH.

Method

1. Cut the antigen tissues as described in step 2b, allowing one for each serum and the controls.

2. Make a 1:5 dilution of each serum and each control in 0.15M NaCl by adding 0.1 ml of serum to 0.4 ml of saline solution.

3. Apply 1 drop, approximately 0.03 ml of diluted serum, to the antigen slide flooding the tissue.

4. Cover the slides with a tray that contains a moist paper towel.

5. Incubate the covered slides at room temperature for 30 minutes.

6. Drain the slides and place them in a staining dish containing PBS for 10 minutes. Wash two more times for 10 minutes each.

7. Remove the slides from the PBS, drain, and dry as completely as possible by wiping the glass with paper toweling, being careful not to wipe off the tissue.

8. Allow to air dry.

9. Add 1 drop, 0.03 ml, of diluted conjugate to each antigen.

10. Cover the slides with a tray containing a moist paper towel.

11. Incubate for 30 minutes at room temperature.

12. Drain the slides and wash them in PBS three times for 10 minutes each.

13. Remove the slides from the PBS, drain, and dry as completely as possible, being careful not to wipe the tissue off.

14. Add 1 drop of mounting medium, the pH of which has been checked with 0.04% phenol red.

15. Coverslip with alcohol-washed 22-mm square coverslips.

16. Read under the high dry objective of an ultraviolet microscope.

Interpretation

A slide is considered positive if the nuclei or portions of the nuclei fluoresce more brightly than the cytoplasm. The nuclei in negative preparations appear as black holes in the cytoplasm. Read the control slides first to check the reliability of the test run before continuing with the unknown preparations.

Several types of staining may be observed (Fig. 15-6, p. 684):

1. Diffuse: Whole nucleus is evenly stained (most typical of SLE).

2. Peripheral: Periphery of nucleus fluoresces most brilliantly (most frequently seen in acute stages of SLE).

3. Speckled: Discrete spots of the nuclei are stained (not typical of SLE).

4. Nucleolar: The nucleoli of the nuclei stain (not typical of SLE but found in other collagen diseases).

Reporting

Report the test results as negative or positive. If positive, indicate the type of staining pattern. Include in the report, results of positive and negative controls, giving the result of the positive control at its predetermined titer.

Remarks

The frequency with which the test is found to be positive in various diseases is as follows:

Condition	% Positive	Normal	% Positive
SLE	99%	Males 20-60 yr	3%
Lupoid hepatitis	99%	Females 20-60 yr	7%
Scleroderma	73%	Both sexes over 80 yr	49%
Rheumatoid arthritis	60%		
Discoid lupus	47%		
Dermatomyositis	33%		

In some preparations the nuclei on the outer portion of the antigen fluoresce, while those toward the center do not. This is interpreted as a positive test reaction.

References

Barnett and Rothfield, 1969
Rothfield, 1969
Shulman, 1963

Fluorescent antinuclear antibody test: quantitative method

Principle

Twofold serial dilutions of serum are prepared and the fluorescent ANA procedure is run on each dilution.

Method

1. Prepare a 1:5 dilution of serum in 0.15M saline solution as described in the screening procedure.
2. Using 0.5-ml volumes, make twofold serial dilutions of the 1:5 dilution in 0.15M saline solution to give dilutions of 1:10, 1:20, 1:40, etc. In our laboratory the dilutions are not carried beyond 1:40 unless otherwise requested.
3. Process each dilution of serum as described in the screening procedure.
4. Read the slides as described previously.

Reporting

The highest dilution of serum that gives a positive test is reported, i.e., "Positive 1:40 dilution."

Interpretation

Normal	1:1 to 1:20, with the majority 1:5 or below
Rheumatoid arthritis	Range of 1:1 to 1:40,960, with the majority 1:1 to 1:320
Scleroderma	Broad range 1:1 to 1:40,960, with the majority 1:40 to 1:1280
SLE	Broad range 1:20 to 1:40,960, with the majority 1:40 to 1:2,560

Reference

Ritchie, 1967

COAGULATION TESTS
Venous coagulation time: glass technic

The venous coagulation time is the length of time required for a measured amount of blood to form a clot in vitro under standard conditions. The process is dependent on the blood clotting factors necessary for thromboplastinogenesis and on the amount of available fibrinogen.

Equipment

1. Water bath at 37° C or small beaker of water warmed to 37° C
2. Plastic or siliconized syringes; 20-gauge needles
3. Three test tubes, 12 × 75 mm, of unetched glass and chemically clean

Method

1. Mark the test tubes at the 2-ml level and number 1, 2, and 3.
2. Select the patient's best available vein. Using either a plastic or silicone-coated glass syringe and a large-gauge needle, obtain in excess of 6 ml of blood. If the vein is not entered directly, the specimen of blood is unsatisfactory for this test.
3. Start the stopwatch as the blood is dispensed into the first tube (tube No. 3).
4. Remove the needle from the syringe and dispense 2 ml of blood into each tube. Fill tube No. 3 first, then tube No. 2, and tube No. 1 last, allowing the blood to run down the side of the tube (Fig. A-5).
5. Place tubes in water bath at 37° C.
6. Tilt tube No. 1 every 30 seconds until the blood clots; then tilt tube No. 2 in the same manner until the blood in it is clotted, and finally tube No. 3.
7. The venous coagulation time is the length of time required for the blood in tube No. 3 to clot.

Normal values

The average normal coagulation time with this technic is 11.9 minutes, SD 1.77; the minimum and maximum normal time is 8.5 and 15.5 minutes, respectively.

Remarks

A venous coagulation time of less than 7 minutes is usually the result of poor technic.

When blood is drawn into a siliconized syringe and placed in siliconized glass tubes, the coagulation time is normally prolonged to about 30 minutes. A moderate prolongation of the coagulation time in glass is exaggerated when this modification is used.

Clot retraction

About 1 hour after blood is allowed to clot in a clean glass test tube, the clot begins to pull away from the glass surface. In about 24 hours a normal blood clot will show maximum retraction.

Clot retraction is actually a complicated process involving the interaction of at least four effects: (1) the presence of platelets, (2) the concentration of fibrinogen, (3) the activity of a retraction-promoting principle in the serum, and (4) the nature of the surface. The effect of various surfaces is shown in Fig. A-6.

Practically, clot retraction is a useful index of platelet activity. Clot retraction is poor when the platelet concentration is below $100,000/mm^3$ ($0.10 \times 10^{12}/1$) and in thrombasthenia.

Normal clot retraction in a glass tube begins about 1 hour after the blood clots and is complete in 24 hours. When complete clot retraction occurs, about half the total volume consists of clot, and the other half expressed serum. Elaborate technics have been devised to give an accurate measure of clot-to-serum ratio, but they are not necessary for routine purposes. In practice, the test tubes used for determining the venous coagulation time are stoppered, left in the water bath at 37° C, and inspected at 1 and 24 hours. It is sometimes helpful to extract the clot after complete retraction and observe its consistency.

Reference

Budz-Olsen, 1951

Ivy bleeding time using Simplate
Principle

The Simplate is a disposable spring-loaded lancet that makes an incision 5 mm long and 1 mm deep. In our laboratory it has received greater patient acceptance than template devices. The

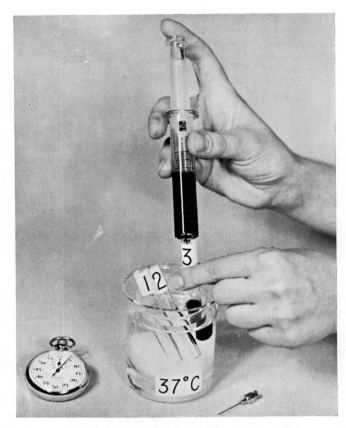

Fig. A-5. Venous coagulation time test at the bedside when a constant temperature water bath is not available. Note that the three tubes are filled in inverse order.

incidence of scar formation is minimized by using a butterfly bandage at the end of the procedure.

Materials

1. Simplate*
2. Sphygmomanometer
3. Stopwatch with sweep-second hand
4. Filter paper discs (Whatman No. 1 or equivalent)
5. Alcohol sponge
6. Butterfly bandage (Johnson & Johnson, medium size)

Method

1. Clean the volar surface of the forearm with the alcohol sponge and allow to dry. Choose an area away from veins or obvious blood vessels.
2. Place sphygmomanometer on upper arm; inflate to 40 mm Hg and maintain this pressure throughout the procedure.
3. Twist off the white tab on the side of the Simplate.
4. Position the Simplate at the chosen site; hold firmly in place; depress the red trigger and simultaneously start the stopwatch.
5. At intervals of 30 seconds, blot the flow of blood with the edge of the filter paper; do not touch the edges of the incision.
6. Note the time when no more blood stains the filter papers. Remove the sphygmomanometer.

---

*General Diagnostics, Div. Warner-Lambert Co., Morris Plains, N.J.

7. Wash arm with a sponge moistened with water, dry, and apply a butterfly bandage. Do not use alcohol at this stage.

Interpretation

Since aspirin may prolong the bleeding time, patients should be instructed not to take aspirin or any aspirin-containing drug for 1 week before the test is performed. Each laboratory should establish its own normal range. Our range of normal values is 2'20" to 7'. Our incision is always made parallel to the fold of the elbow.

Tourniquet test

The methods proposed for measuring capillary fragility fall into two categories: (1) positive pressure methods that depend on increasing the intracapillary pressure and (2) negative pressure methods that depend on applying negative pressure to a small area. Each has disadvantages: (1) the first cannot be repeated more often than every week or two and (2) the second does not take into account the extreme variability in capillary fragility at different sites.

Method

1. Apply a blood pressure cuff on the upper arm, determine a systolic and diastolic pressures, and then deflate to a pressure midway between the two. Usually this falls in the range of 70 to 90 mm Hg.
2. Leave the inflated cuff in place for 5 minutes. Remove the cuff and inspect the arm, wrist, and hand for petechiae.

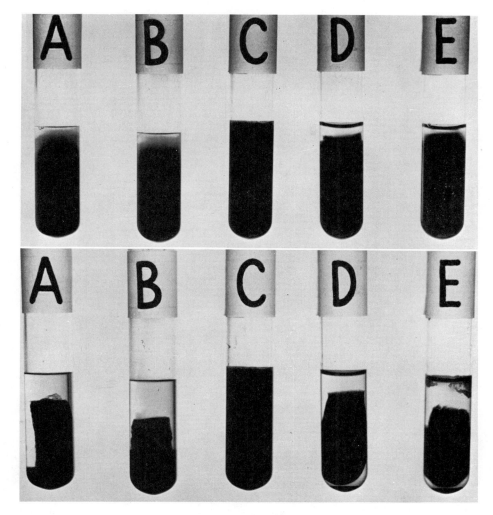

Fig. A-6. Effect of different surfaces on clot retraction. **A,** Silicone. **B,** Paraffin. **C,** Collodion. **D,** Pyrex glass. **E,** Immersion oil. Retraction is shown at 1 hour, top, and 24 hours, bottom.

Remarks

Petechiae commonly appear in the antecubital area, the volar aspect of the wrist, and the dorsum of the hand (Fig. A-7). The distribution of petechiae is usually irregular, and no effort is made to count the number in a given area. The test is graded 1 to 4+, depending on whether there are a few or very many petechiae. Normally only very occasional petechiae are found or none at all.

Petechiae sometimes appear several minutes after the blood pressure cuff is removed.

References

Gothlin, 1933
Hare and Miller, 1951

Platelet adhesiveness: in vivo method
Principle

When a vessel is cut there is almost immediate adhesion of platelets to the site of injury. The in vivo method is based on determining the difference between the platelet count in venous blood and the platelet count from a standard skin incision.

Method

1. Make a standard skin incision as for the bleeding time determination (p. 916).
2. Do not disturb the flow of blood, but let the flow accumulate until the drop is large enough to fill a diluting pipet for a phase platelet count. This usually takes 40 to 50 seconds after the incision is made.
3. At the end of 1 minute fill a platelet count pipet, and each minute thereafter until bleeding has ceased. Take care not to disturb the actual incision, blotting extra blood with filter paper as necessary.
4. Determine the platelet count of a venous blood sample drawn into EDTA anticoagulant.
5. Calculate percent adhesiveness:

Percent adhesiveness =

$$\frac{\substack{\text{Platelet count} \\ \text{in venous blood}} - \substack{\text{Average of counts} \\ \text{in capillary blood}}}{\text{Platelet count in venous blood}} \times 100$$

6. We find it helpful to plot on plain arithmetic graph paper the serial platelet counts against time.

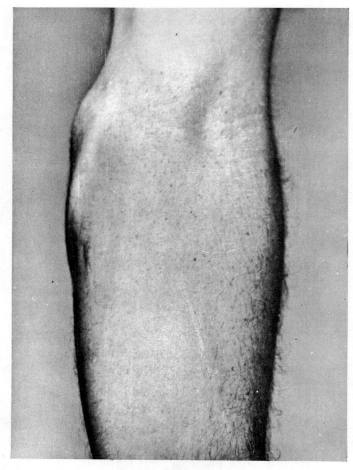

Fig. A-7. Positive tourniquet test.

References

Borchgrevink, 1960a

Didisheim and Bunting, 1966

Platelet aggregation

Principle

Aggregation can be induced by adding aggregating agents to platelet-rich plasma that is being continually stirred. As the platelets aggregate, the plasma becomes progressively clearer. An optical system is used to detect the change in light transmission, and a recorder graphically displays the variations in light transmission from the baseline setting.

Materials

1. Aggregometer and recorder, cuvettes and magnetic stir bars*
2. Plastic graduated centrifuge tubes
3. Pipets
   a. Plastic, 1-ml serologic
   b. Micropipets, 20 and 50 microliters

Reagents

1. Sodium citrate, 3.2% (0.109M)
2. Adenosine 5' diphosphate sodium†

   a. Stock solution: 10.2 mg in 100 ml saline (2×10^{-4}M). Freeze in 1-ml aliquots.

   b. Working solution: Dilute stock 1:10 in saline. When 20 microliters are added to 0.5 ml of PRP, the final concentration is 0.4 µg/ml or 0.8 µM. Other concentrations may be required to obtain a biphasic response.

3. Collagen: Soluble collagen reagent* Reconstitute with 1 ml distilled water. When 50 microliters are used, the final concentration is 0.8 µg/ml.

4. Adrenaline hydrochloride 1:1000 (epinephrine injection, U.S.P.)†

   a. Working solution: Dilute 1:10 with saline. When 20 microliters are added to 0.5 ml of PRP, the final concentration is 4 µg/ml. Further dilutions or higher concentrations may be required.

5. Thrombin (human), Fibrindex‡

   a. Stock solution, 50 units thrombin. Reconstitute vial with 1 ml saline.

   b. Working solution: Dilute 0.1 ml stock with 0.56 ml saline. A further 1:2 dilution may be used. When 20 microliters are used in the test, final concentrations are 0.3 units and 0.15 units/ml, respectively.

---

*Bio Data Corp., Willow Grove, Pa.

†P.L. Biochemicals, Milwaukee, Wis.

---

*General Diagnostics, Div. Warner-Lambert Co., Morris Plains, N.J.

†Parke Davis & Co., Detroit, Mich.

‡Ortho Pharmaceutical Corp., Raritan, N.J.

6. Ristocetin:* Dilute to 10 mg/ml in saline. When 50 microliters are added in the test, the final concentration is 1.0 mg/ml.

Method

1. Draw 9 ml blood with plastic syringe and 20-gauge needle. Add to 1 ml sodium citrate (0.109M) in a plastic centrifuge tube. Spin for 30 minutes at 150 g at *room temperature* to obtain platelet-rich plasma (PRP). Gently withdraw plasma with a plastic pipet. Keep at room temperature and test within 2 hours. Platelet-poor plasma (PPP) is obtained by further centrifugation at 3,000 g for 20 minutes. Dilute the PPP with equal parts of saline for standardizing aggregometer setting. If the plasma is not lipemic, a plain water blank may be used in place of the PPP.
2. Test with aggregating reagent (2, 3, 4, 5, and 6 above).
   a. Dilute 0.025 ml PRP with 0.25 ml saline in cuvette. Add stir bar and place in aggregometer 2 minutes to reach 37° C. Record a baseline for approximately 1 minute.
   b. Add 20 or 50 microliters (as specified in reagent preparation) of aggregating reagent with automatic pipet. Dispense carefully into middle of cuvette.
   c. Record results for approximately 3 to 5 minutes, or until no further change is occurring.
   d. Repeat steps a, b, and c with each aggregating reagent.

Comments

Temperature, pH, and citrate concentration are all very important in aggregation and must be carefully controlled. Plastic or siliconized glassware should be used to handle the platelets.

All plasmas should remain at room temperature for approximately 30 minutes before testing, so shorter or faster centrifugation is of no advantage. Under no circumstances should the platelets be heated or refrigerated.

Results

Epinephrine and ADP should produce biphasic curves. The curve with collagen has a lag phase, then a monophasic curve. Thrombin also has a monophasic curve, frequently forming a clot in the stronger solution, and frequently showing deaggregation in the weaker dilution. Normal ristocetin curves are monophasic, sometimes biphasic. Aspirin and aspirin-containing compounds, antihistamines, etc. may cause reduced aggregation, especially in the secondary wave of the biphasic curves.

References

Day and Holmsen, 1972b
Han and Ardlie, 1974

Platelet factor 3 availability (Celite method)
Principle

Platelets release a phospholipid (platelet factor 3, [PF$_3$]) that has a partial thromboplastin action. To test for the patient's PF$_3$ activity, the patient's platelets can be used as the PF$_3$ reagent in the partial thromboplastin test. Platelet-rich plasma (PRP) (the source of PF$_3$ activity) and platelet-poor plasma (PPP) (low in PF$_3$) are compared with the activated partial thromboplastin reagent for activity.

Reagents

1. Celite 505† 1% suspension in 0.85% NaCl
2. CaCl$_2$, 0.025M
3. Platelin plus Activator‡

---

*Lenau, Copenhagen, Denmark.
†Johns-Manville Products Corp., New York, N.Y.
‡General Diagnostics, Div. Warner-Lambert Pharmaceutical, Morris Plains, N.J.

Method

1. Obtain platelet-rich plasma (PRP) and platelet-poor plasma (PPP) as for platelet aggregation (p. 918). Keep plasmas at room temperature in plastic tubes.
2. Three clotting times are determined.
   a. (Control) Add 0.1 ml Platelin plus Activator to 0.1 ml PPP. Incubate 5 minutes at 37° C, then add 0.1 ml 0.025M CaCl$_2$. Determine clotting time.
   b. Add 0.1 ml 1% Celite suspension to 0.1 ml PRP. Incubate for 5 minutes at 37° C, then add 0.1 ml 0.025M CaCl$_2$. Determine clotting time.
   c. Add 0.1 ml 1% Celite suspension to 0.1 ml PPP. Incubate for 5 minutes at 37° C, then add 0.1 ml 0.025M CaCl$_2$. Determine clotting time.

Results

The PRP and Celite should give a time close to the control with Platelin plus Activator. The PPP will give a prolonged time with the Celite suspension. If the clotting time for the platelet-rich plasma is prolonged, closer to that of the PPP than to the control, there has been a failure to release PF$_3$ from the platelets.

Reference

Hardisty and Ingram, 1965

Plasma recalcification time
Principle

In this test the calcium of *platelet-rich* plasma is replaced, and the clotting time is determined. The test involves the whole blood clotting process, thereby measuring all coagulation factors that are detected by the venous coagulation time. The error of this test is less than that of the venous coagulation time, and we use it instead of the venous coagulation time for the control of heparin therapy (p. 857).

Reagents

1. 0.109M sodium citrate
2. 0.025M CaCl$_2$

Method

1. To 0.5 ml 0.109M sodium citrate, add 4.5 ml venous blood. Mix and centrifuge 5 minutes at 1,700 rpm (500 g).
2. Transfer plasma to a clean, dry test tube, stopper, and refrigerate at 4° C until test can be made.
3. Place a tube containing 0.025M CaCl$_2$ in a 37° C water bath.
4. Pipet 0.2 ml of plasma into a 12 × 75 mm test tube and place in the water bath. Allow to incubate 2 to 3 minutes.
5. Blow 0.2 ml of CaCl$_2$ solution into the tube containing the plasma and simultaneously start a stopwatch.
6. Gently mix and leave undisturbed in the water bath for 45 seconds.
7. Observe the clotting. The end point is the first formation of fibrin threads.

Results

Clotting time is the plasma recalcification time. Normal range is 90 to 120 seconds. A prolonged recalcification time is found in classic hemophilia, Christmas disease (PTC deficiency), factor X deficiency, factor XI deficiency, factor XII deficiency, fibrinogen deficiency, when a circulating anticoagulant is present, and when there are very severe deficiencies of the prothrombin phase.

References

Caldwell, 1957
Owen et al, 1955

Cross-recalcification times for screening circulating anticoagulants

Reagents

Same as for plasma recalcification time.

Method

1. Obtain citrated plasma from a known normal donor in the same manner as previously described for the recalcification test.
2. Make the following mixtures of patient and normal plasmas. Into six 12 × 75 mm test tubes, place the following:
   a. 0.2 ml patient plasma
   b. 0.15 ml patient plasma + 0.5 ml normal plasma
   c. 0.10 ml patient plasma + 0.10 ml normal plasma
   d. 0.05 ml patient plasma + 0.15 ml normal plasma
   e. 0.02 ml patient plasma + 0.18 ml normal plasma
   f. 0.2 ml normal plasma
   Tubes a through e represent 100%, 75%, 50%, 25%, and 10% patient plasma, respectively. Tube f is the control.
3. Incubate at 37° C for at least 60 minutes.
4. To each tube, add 0.2 ml CaCl₂ (0.025M) and determine plasma clotting times in the usual manner.

Results

If the patient's plasma is free of anticoagulant, the long recalcification time will be corrected by the addition of normal plasma. If a circulating anticoagulant is present, the recalcification time of the normal plasma will be greatly prolonged by small amounts of patient plasma.

Antifactor VIII anticoagulant activity is time dependent (p. 828). If the anticoagulant is weak it may be missed if the period of incubation is omitted.

Detection of the lupus anticoagulant

Principle

The lupus anticoagulant is directed against the prothrombin conversion complex (p. 836). When present the plasma shows a moderately prolonged prothrombin time and an even more prolonged activated partial thromboplastin time. The test is based on a marked prolongation of the prothrombin time using a highly diluted thromboplastin.

Equipment

1. Fibrometer*
2. Fibrometer cups and tips*
3. 12 × 75 mm glass test tubes
4. Serologic pipets

Reagents

1. Simplastin†
2. Sodium citrate, 0.109M
3. Calcium chloride, 0.025M
4. Sodium chloride, 0.85%

Specimen

1. Collect blood from the patient and a normal control in 0.109M sodium citrate, 9 parts of blood to 1 part of citrate.
2. Centrifuge bloods at 670 g for 5 minutes to obtain plasma.

Procedure

1. Prepare working solutions of Simplastin, 1:50 and 1:500 in 0.85% saline, as follows:

Tube 1 (1:5)	Tube 2 (1:50)	Tube 3 (1:500)
0.4 ml saline	0.9 ml saline	0.9 ml saline
0.1 ml Simplastin	0.1 ml mixture from tube 1	0.1 ml mixture from tube 2

2. Set up the following in duplicate.
3. In a fibrometer cup, mix 0.1 ml of patient plasma and 0.1 ml of the 1:50 dilution of Simplastin. Final dilution of Simplastin is 1:100.
4. In a second fibrometer cup, mix 0.1 ml patient plasma and 0.1 ml of the 1:500 dilution of Simplastin. Final dilution of Simplastin is 1:1000.
5. Use the two dilutions of Simplastin with normal plasma as in 3 and 4.
6. Incubate the two patient and the two normal plasma mixtures for 5 minutes at 37° C.
7. Add 0.1 ml of the 0.025M CaCl₂ and start timer.
8. Record the clotting time in seconds.

Results

If the patient's plasma contains the lupus anticoagulant, the prothrombin time with 1:100 Simplastin will be prolonged at least 1.5 times the control and at least 1.7 times the control with 1:1000 Simplastin.

Example:

	Simplastin 1:100	Simplastin 1:1000
Control	36.1 sec	73.2 sec
Patient	71.1 sec	175.9 sec
Ratio	1:1.9	1:2.4

Comments

1. The test is normal in patients taking oral anticoagulants and in patients having an inhibitor to VIII:C.
2. The action of the anticoagulant is not time dependent.
3. The test is not valid if the patient is receiving heparin.
4. The test is not valid if the patient is receiving steroids.

Reference

Boxer et al, 1976

One-stage prothrombin time (Quick)

As discussed in Chapter 17, this test measures prothrombin and accessory factors. With tissue thromboplastin, the clotting time depends on the concentration of prothrombin, factor V, factor VII, and factor X (assuming fibrinogen and anticoagulant activity to be normal).

Blood is mixed with a measured amount of citrate, and the plasma is obtained by centrifugation. The test is based on having an optimum concentration of calcium ions and an excess of thromboplastin, the only variable being the concentration of prothrombin and accessory factors in a carefully measured volume of plasma. Technical aspects and quality control are discussed on p. 385.

Reagents

1. Sodium citrate, 0.109M
2. Simplastin.*

---

*BBL, Div. Becton-Dickinson & Co., Cockeysville, Md.
†General Diagnostics, Div. Warner-Lambert Co., Morris Plains, N.J.

*General Diagnostics, Div. Warner-Lambert Co., Morris Plains, N.J.

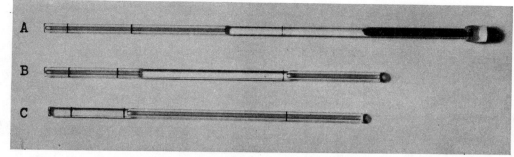

Fig. A-8. Use of disposable micropipet for micro-prothrombin time. **A,** Capped pipet after centrifugation of citrated blood. **B,** The pipet has been scored and snapped and the packed erythrocytes discarded. **C,** Citrated plasma has been run out to the blowout calibration.

Method

1. Into a graduated conical centrifuge tube, measure 0.5 ml of 0.109M sodium citrate (oxalate is not recommended).
2. Obtain venous blood with a carefully performed venipuncture. Add exactly 4.5 ml of blood to the citrate; mix quickly by inversion. We find it useful to use the graduation on the test tube for measuring the citrate and blood.
3. Centrifuge. Aspirate the plasma into a clean tube and place in 37° C water bath or the heating block of the Fibrometer system.
4. Determine the clotting time of a mixture of 0.1 ml of plasma and 0.2 ml of Simplastin.
5. Determine the clotting time of lyophilized normal control plasma.

Normal values

The average normal prothrombin time (471 normals) by this technic and with Simplastin* is 13.1 seconds, SD 0.6 second, 95% range 11.9 to 14.3 seconds, and minimum and maximum value 11.5 and 15.2 seconds, respectively.

Remarks

When a plain thromboplastin is used in place of thromboplastin-CaCl$_2$ reagent, the test is performed by adding 0.1 ml of 0.025M CaCl$_2$ and 0.1 ml of thromboplastin suspension to 0.1 ml of plasma.

One-stage prothrombin time: microtechnic
Materials

1. Disposable, *siliconized*, prothrombin micropipets, (Miale prothrombin pipet†) (Fig. A-8)
2. Thromboplastin-CaCl$_2$ reagent as for standard test‡
3. Sodium citrate solution, 0.109M
4. Sterile No. 11 Bard-Parker blades
5. Plastic microtube closures (disposable plastic caps)
6. Test tubes, 12 × 75 mm, 37° C water bath, stopwatch, and centrifuge

Methods

1. Collect capillary blood as follows:
   a. Draw sodium citrate solution into the micropipet to the 0.015-ml mark, and wipe off the excess.

   b. Cleanse the site chosen for puncture (lateral aspect of finger, toe, or heel) with ether or alcohol and puncture with a sterile Bard-Parker blade. Wipe off the first drop of blood with dry gauze. Then fill the micropipet with blood to the 0.15-ml mark by tilting it slightly below the horizontal and allowing the blood to flow in by gravity. *The puncture should be deep enough to ensure a free flow of blood.*
   c. Keep the pipet in a horizontal position and twirl between the fingers to complete mixing of the blood with the citrate solution.
   d. After mixing is accomplished, cover the collecting end of the micropipet with the fingertip, and seal the other end with a plastic microtube closure.
2. Centrifugation of specimen:
   a. Place the filled and sealed pipet sealed end down into a 13 × 100 mm test tube. Label this tube with the patient's name. Then centrifuge tube and pipet at 1,500 rpm for 10 minutes. The erythrocytes are thus packed at the sealed end of the micropipet, whereas the plasma occupies the graduated end (Fig. A-8, *A*).
   b. After centrifugation, place test tubes and contained pipets in the water bath and leave there for at least 10 minutes. While waiting, add 0.1 ml of thromboplastin-CaCl$_2$ reagent to as many as 12 × 75 mm test tubes as there are tests to be done. These are also placed in the water bath.
3. Obtaining plasma:
   a. Score the micropipet with a file at a point just above the top of the column of packed red blood cells and snap in two. Discard the packed cells (Fig. A-8, *B*).
   b. Run off the plasma contained in the remainder of the pipet to the middle graduation (Fig A-8, *C*). The pipet is now set to deliver, by means of blowing out, 0.05 ml of plasma. Duplicate determinations can be performed on the same specimen by means of running excess plasma into a clean micropipet and adjusting this also to the 0.05-ml mark.
4. Performance of test:
   a. Blow the plasma (0.05 ml) into a test tube that contains 0.1 ml of thromboplastin-CaCl$_2$ mixture at 37° C.
   b. Start a stopwatch simultaneously, and determine the clotting by a visual technic.
5. Evaluation of prolonged prothrombin time:
   a. Correction by fresh normal BaSO$_4$-adsorbed plasma: Fill a micropipet to the 0.015-ml mark with the normal BaSO$_4$-adsorbed plasma and then draw in the abnormal

---

*General Diagnostics, Div. Warner-Lambert Co., Morris Plains, N.J.
†Scientific Products Div., American Hospital Supply Corp., Evanston, Ill.
‡The data presented here were obtained with Simplastin.

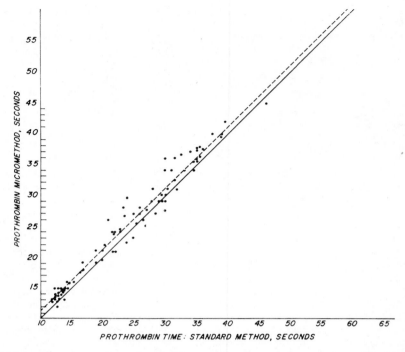

Fig. A-9. Actual versus theoretical regression of micro-prothrombin time results against those obtained by the standard macromethod. Coefficient of correlation is 0.985.

plasma to the 0.15-ml mark. Mix by means of twirling. This makes a mixture of 9 parts of abnormal plasma to 1 part of $BaSO_4$-adsorbed plasma. Run off to the 0.05-ml mark, blow into thromboplastin-$CaCl_2$ mixture, and determine the prothrombin time.

b. Correction by normal stored serum or normal stored oxalated plasma is determined in the same way.

c. Interpretation of results is the same as for the standard macromethod.

Results

In 20 determinations using the microtechnic on the same normal person, the prothrombin time varied between 11 and 12.8 seconds, mean value 11.74 seconds, and SD of the mean ±0.19 second.

In 20 determinations using the standard macrotechnic on the same normal person, the prothrombin time varied between 11.5 and 12 seconds, mean value 11.72 seconds, and SD of the mean ±0.163 second.

Comparison of data for corresponding micro- and macrodeterminations of prothrombin time in 25 normal and 65 abnormal subjects is illustrated graphically in Fig. A-9. The solid line represents the theoretical line of optimal regression (y = ax + b, where a = 1 and b = 0). The dotted line is the best-fit regression line, the slope of which is 0.99. The coefficient of correlation between micro- and macrodeterminations is 0.985. The 95% confidence interval for the population slope is 0.954 to 1.027.

Reference

Miale and Winningham, 1960

Evaluation of a prolonged one-stage prothrombin time

If only the one-stage prothrombin time is prolonged, it is necessary to identify which of the prothrombin factors (prothrombin, factor V, or factor VII) is deficient. Normal stored serum (a source

of factor VII), normal absorbed plasma (a source of factor V), or stored oxalated plasma (a source of prothrombin) is added to aliquots of the abnormal plasma. One-stage prothrombin times are then done to see which of these reagents corrects the defect in the test plasma.

Reagents

The same reagents and equipment are used as in the standard one-stage prothrombin time. The blood specimens are collected in the same manner as for the one-stage prothrombin time. In addition, obtain:

1. Fresh normal adsorbed plasma
   a. Prepare $BaSO_4$-adsorbed plasma as outlined in the evaluation of a prolonged partial thromboplastin time, p. 925, or $Al(OH)_3$-adsorbed plasma as outlined in the thromboplastin generation test, p. 926.
2. Normal stored serum
   a. Normal blood is collected, allowed to clot, and incubated at 37° C for at least 2 hours to ensure maximum prothrombin conversion.
   b. Store serum at 4° C for about 24 hours.
3. Normal aged oxalated plasma.
   a. Store for about 2 weeks at 4° C or for 24 hours at 37° C.
   b. The prothrombin time of the stored plasma should be over 25 seconds.

Method

1. Add 0.8 ml of the abnormal plasma to 0.2 ml of the fresh adsorbed plasma.
2. Add 0.8 ml of the abnormal plasma to 0.2 ml of the stored serum.
3. Add 0.8 ml of the abnormal plasma to 0.2 ml of the stored oxalate plasma.
4. Do one-stage prothrombin times on the above mixtures.

Results

Factor VII is deficient if the stored serum corrects the one-stage prothrombin time. Factor V is deficient if the fresh adsorbed plasma corrects the one-stage prothrombin time. Prothrombin is deficient if the stored oxalate plasma corrects the one-stage prothrombin time.

Factor II assay
Material and reagents

1. Sodium citrate, 0.109M
2. Simplastin*
3. Factor II deficient substrate†
4. Fibrometer with 0.4-ml probe
5. Imidazole-buffered distilled water, pH 7.2 to 7.35
6. Imidazole-buffered saline (0.85% prepared with buffered water)
7. Normal citrate plasma

Method

1. Draw normal blood into 0.109M sodium citrate (1 part sodium citrate plus 9 parts blood).
2. Centrifuge blood for 10 minutes at 1,700 rpm and harvest plasma.
3. Make plasma dilutions by diluting plasma 1:10 with buffered saline, which is equivalent to 100%, and then from that 100% dilution, make a serial dilution of 50%, 25%, 12.5%, 6.25%, 3.13% and 1.56%.
4. Test each of the dilutions as follows:
   a. Prewarm Simplastin for 2 to 5 minutes at 37° C.
   b. Transfer 0.1 ml diluted plasma to a Fibro-cup.
   c. Add 0.1 ml factor II deficient substrate.
   d. Incubate for 60 seconds at 37° C.
   e. Add 0.2 ml Simplastin and activate Fibrometer (use 0.4-ml probe).
5. Plot dilution curve on log-log paper from the seven points.
6. Assay on unknown: Using buffered saline, make 100% and 50% dilutions of unknown plasma, and proceed with method described above for testing dilutions. Plasmas, dilutions, and substrate should always be kept on ice.
7. Read results of unknown in percent from normal dilution curve.

Factor V assay
Materials and reagents

1. Sodium citrate, 0.109M
2. Simplastin*
3. Factor V–deficient substrate*
4. Normal citrate plasma
5. Fibrometer with 0.4-ml probe
6. Imidazole-buffered distilled water, pH 7.2 to 7.35
7. Imidazole-buffered saline (85% in buffered water)

Method

Prepare activity curve as follows:
1. Draw normal blood into 0.109M sodium citrate (1 part sodium citrate plus 9 parts blood).
2. Centrifuge blood for 10 minutes at 1,700 rpm and harvest plasma.
3. Make plasma dilutions by diluting plasma 1:10 with buffered saline, which is equivalent to 100%, and then from that 100% dilution make a serial dilution of 50%, 25%, 12.5%, 6.25%, 3.13% and 1.56%.
4. Test each of the dilute plasmas as follows:
   a. Prewarm Simplastin at 37° C for a minimum of 5 minutes, in aliquots sufficient for four to six tests.
   b. Pipet 0.1 ml factor V substrate into a Fibro-cup and incubate for 2 to 10 minutes at 37° C.
   c. Add 0.1 ml dilute test plasma (which has been held in an ice bath).
   d. Immediately add 0.2 ml prewarmed Simplastin and activate the Fibrometer (use 0.4-ml probe).
5. Plot dilution curve on log-log paper from the seven points.
6. Factor V assay on unknown: Using buffered saline, make 100% and 50% dilutions of the unknown citrate plasma and proceed with the method described above for testing plasma dilutions. Plasmas, dilutions, and substrates should always be kept on ice.
7. Read results of unknown in percent from normal dilution curve.

Factor VII assay
Materials and reagents

1. Sodium citrate, 0.109M
2. Simplastin*
3. Factors VII–and X–free substrate*
4. Factor VII–deficient plasma*
5. Normal citrate plasma
6. Fibrometer with 0.4-ml probe
7. Imidazole-buffered distilled water, pH 7.2 to 7.35
8. Imidazole-buffered saline (0.85% in buffered water)

Method

1. Draw normal blood into 0.109M sodium citrate (1 part sodium citrate plus 9 parts blood).
2. Centrifuge blood for 10 minutes at 1,700 rpm and harvest plasma.
3. Make plasma dilutions by diluting plasma 1:10 with buffered saline, which is equivalent to 100%, and then from that 100% dilution make a serial dilution of 50%, 25%, 12.5%, 6.25%, 3.13%, and 1.56%.
4. Prepare factor VII substrate by mixing 4 parts of Factor VII–and X–free substrate with 1 part of factor VII–deficient plasma.
5. Test each of the saline diluted plasmas as follows:
   a. Prewarm Simplastin for 2 to 5 minutes at 37° C.
   b. Transfer 0.1 ml diluted plasma to a Fibro-cup.
   c. Add 0.1 ml factor VII substrate.
   d. Incubate for 60 seconds at 37° C.
   e. Add 0.2 ml Simplastin and activate Fibrometer (use 0.4-ml probe).
6. Plot dilution curve on log-log paper from the seven points.
7. Factor VII assay on unknown: Using buffered saline, make 100% and 50% dilutions of unknown citrate plasma and proceed with method described above for testing plasma dilutions. Plasmas, dilutions, and substrates should always be kept on ice. Read results of unknown in percent from normal dilution curve.

"Stypven" time

Russell's viper venom (Stypven†) has thromboplastic activity when added to recalcified plasma. The venom is active in high dilutions. Concentrated solutions exhibit inhibitory activity. The thromboplastic action of venom is dependent on platelets, phospholipid, prothrombin, factor V, and factor X. Factor VII does not

---

*General Diagnostics, Div. Warner-Lambert Co., Morris Plains, N.J.
†Dade Reagents, Inc., Miami, Fla.

*General Diagnostics, Div. Warner-Lambert Co., Morris Plains, N.J.
†Burroughs Wellcome Co., Research Triangle Park, N.C.

affect the reaction. This test is a useful measure of prothrombin plus factor V and factor X when it is preformed on platelet-rich nonlipemic plasma.

Reagents

1. Stypven
   a. Dilute 1:10,000 with distilled water according to directions on the package.
2. Other reagents and equipment as for the standard one-stage prothrombin time.

Method

1. Obtain blood from the fasting patient using a plastic syringe. To 0.5 ml of 0.109M sodium citrate in a plastic centrifuge tube, add 4.5 ml of blood. Mix. Centrifuge at 1,500 rpm for 5 minutes. Aspirate the platelet-rich plasma.
2. With all reagents warmed to 37° C, place 0.1 ml of plasma and 0.1 ml of dilute venom in a serologic test tube. Blow in 0.1 ml of 0.02M $CaCl_2$ and simultaneously start a stopwatch. Record the clotting time as for the standard one-stage test.

Remarks

The Stypven time is normally the same as that obtained with tissue thromboplastin.

The Stypven time is prolonged by deficiency of prothrombin, factor V, and factor X.

In factor VII deficiency, the Stypven time is normal.

Prothrombin consumption

When the generation of plasma thromboplastin is normal, prothrombin is normally converted to thrombin, and only small amounts of prothrombin remain in the serum. When thromboplastinogenesis is defective, prothrombin conversion is deficient, and large amounts of prothrombin remain in the serum. The residual prothrombin activity in the serum is measured by the one-stage test, Simplastin-A as the source of thromboplastin, factor V, and fibrinogen.

Reagents

1. Simplastin-A*
2. Patient serum

Method

1. Draw blood from the patient. Place exactly 1 ml of blood in a clean tube and allow it to clot without tilting the tube.
2. Exactly 1 hour after the blood clots, centrifuge the tube of clotted blood for 1 minute at 3,000 rpm. Aspirate the serum and transfer to a clean tube.
3. To a serologic test tube in a 37° C water bath, add 0.2 ml Simplastin-A. Add 0.1 ml of serum and simultaneously start a timer. Record the time required for a clot to form, the end point being the same as for the standard prothrombin time test.

Results

Normally the serum prothrombin time is longer than 21 seconds. Fig. A-10 shows our data obtained from 100 normal persons.

Remarks

Deficient prothrombin consumption, i.e., a high level of serum prothrombin activity, is found in the defects of phases I and II of blood coagulation.

Since normal platelet function is essential for thromboplastino-

*General Diagnostics, Div. Warner-Lambert Co., Morris Plains, N.J.

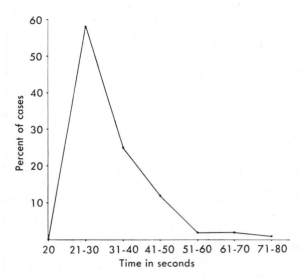

Fig. A-10. Control data for serum prothrombin time (prothrombin consumption test) (100 subjects).

genesis, there is no point in doing a prothrombin consumption test as a screening test for phase II defects when there is thrombocytopenia or a platelet functional abnormality.

In hemophilia the serum prothrombin time is always shorter than the plasma prothrombin time, usually 8 to 9 seconds for the serum prothrombin time as compared with about 13 seconds for the plasma prothrombin time. I believe that this finding has not yet been adequately explained.

For reproducible results, the technic outlined must be followed carefully. The venipuncture must not be traumatic, and a two-syringe technic is recommended. Contamination with tissue thromboplastin accelerates prothrombin consumption. Exactly 1 ml of blood must be allowed to clot without disturbing the tube. Shaking the tube by itself accelerates prothrombin utilization, as does increasing the ratio of glass surface area to blood volume. Centrifugation should be standardized as to time and speed. Hemolysis in the blood specimen enhances prothrombin consumption.

Reference

Quick, 1951

Partial thromboplastin time
Principle

The partial thromboplastin time (PTT) is the clotting time of recalcified citrated plasma on the addition of partial thromboplastin (p. 821). The reagent can be prepared by ether extraction of "complete" thromboplastin, the active material in ether supernate being crude cephalin. Suitably diluted, this will yield a markedly longer clotting time when added to recalcified plasma deficient in factors VIII, IX, X, XI, or XII than is obtained with normal plasma. The PTT is normal with factor VII–deficient plasma and is prolonged with severely factor V–deficient plasma.

Partial thromboplastin reagents using various activating materials are commercially available. Using these reagents the test is called the activated partial thromboplastin time (APTT).

Macromethod, nonactivated
Method

1. Obtain citrated plasma from the patient.
2. Keep plasma on ice or freeze if test is not to be performed immediately.

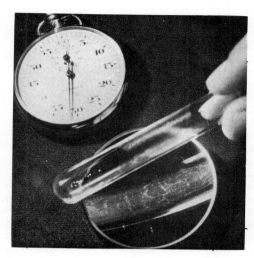

Fig. A-11. End point of the partial thromboplastin time (manual technic). It is important to time the first appearance of fibrin threads.

3. Pipet 0.1 ml patient plasma into Fibrometer cup. Incubate at 37° for 3 to 5 minutes.
4. Incubate a tube containing equal portions of 0.025M $CaCl_2$ and Platelin* for 5 minutes.
5. Add 0.2 ml of Platelin-$CaCl_2$ to plasma and start timer.
6. Record the endpoint.

Normal values

Mean 73.4 seconds, SD 11.4 seconds. The test can be performed manually rather than in a Fibrometer. Using a manual method our normal values are 84.4 seconds, SD 8 seconds.

Macromethod, activated
Method

1. Obtain citrated plasma from the patient.
2. Keep plasma on ice or freeze if test is not to be performed immediately.
3. Pipet 0.1 ml automated APTT reagent* into Fibrometer cup. Add 0.1 ml plasma and incubate for 5 minutes at 37° C.
4. Warm tube of 0.025M $CaCl_2$ to 37° C.
5. After 5 minutes' incubation period add 0.1 ml $CaCl_2$ to the plasma-thromboplastin mixture and start the timer.
6. Record the endpoint.

Normal value

Mean: 35 seconds, SD 4 seconds.

Micromethod, nonactivated or activated
Method

Collect blood as for the microprothrombin time (p. 921).
Perform PTT or APTT using appropriate reagents and technics as for the macromethods. Since the test is performed on half volumes, the Fibrometer system cannot be used, and a manual technic is employed. See endpoint reading in test tube, Fig. A-11.

Normal values

Mean (Platelin): 78.27 seconds, SD 10.2 seconds
Mean (Automated APTT): 35 seconds, SD 4 seconds

---

*General Diagnostics, Div. Warner-Lambert Co, Morris Plains, N.J.

Evaluation of a prolonged partial thromboplastin time
Principle

If the PTT is prolonged, it can be assumed that there is a defect of phase II involving a deficiency of one of the thromboplastic factors: VIII, IX, X, XI, or XII. If the prothrombin time with tissue thromboplastin is normal, this eliminates a deficiency of factor X, since this is characterized by both a prolonged PTT and prolonged prothrombin time. A prolonged PTT and PT will also be found in hypofibrinogenemia (factor I deficiency), severe deficiency of factor V, and when heparin is present.

The specific identification of the factor that is deficient can be made with either the thromboplastin generation test (TGT) (p. 926) or with the PTT system outlined here. The principle of the correction studies is the same as that for the differential studies in the case of a prolonged prothrombin time. The correcting reagents are somewhat different.

Materials and reagents

1. Fibrometer system (desirable but not necessary)
2. Citrated plasma from patient and citrated and oxalated plasma from normal donor.
   a. Use 9 parts venous blood plus 1 part 0.109M sodium citrate, and 9 parts venous blood plus 1 part 0.1M sodium oxalate.
3. Aged normal serum
   a. Allow blood to clot, and incubate at 37° C overnight to ensure maximum prothrombin conversion.
   b. Separate by centrifugation and keep at 4° C for 24 hours.
   c. It then can be frozen in aliquots for later use.
4. $BaSO_4$-adsorbed plasma
   a. Add 100 mg of $BaSO_4$ powder to a dry test tube; then add 1 ml of normal oxalated plasma. Oxalated plasma must be used, as $BaSO_4$ will not adsorb prothrombin etc. from citrated plasma.
   b. Place in a 37° C water bath and stir constantly with a wooden applicator stick or glass rod. Continue mixing for exactly 5 minutes.
   c. Centrifuge immediately for 5 minutes at 3,000 rpm.
   d. Aspirate plasma and check prothrombin time. Properly adsorbed plasma should have a prothrombin time between 1 and 2 minutes. The degree of stirring and shaking will modify the adsorption. Establish a standard technic for your own laboratory and personnel.
5. Celite-adsorbed plasma
   a. Use siliconized glassware or plastic throughout this preparation to avoid activation of the contact factors.
   b. Mix normal platelet-poor citrate plasma with 15 mg Celite/ml of plasma for 10 minutes at room temperature. Celite 545* or Celite Analytical Filter-Aid† may be used.
   c. Centrifuge Celite out for 30 minutes at 3,000 to 4,000 rpm.
   d. Adjust the supernate plasma to pH 7 with 0.1N HCl and incubate at 37° C for 5 hours. It can be frozen in aliquots for later use.
6. Commercial partial thromboplastin reagent
   a. Follow manufacturer's instructions. We use an activated reagent that contains micronized silica that does not settle out on standing (Automated APTT‡). It is important to

---

*Fisher Scientific Co., Pittsburgh, Pa.
†Johns-Manville Products Corp., New York, N.Y.
‡General Diagnostics, Div. Warner-Lambert Co., Morris Plains, N.J.

rinse the probe of the Fibrometer between each test to wash away residual reagent.

7. 0.025M $CaCl_2$

Method

1. Plasmas and correcting reagents should not be incubated until the test is ready to be run.
2. Label five tubes 1 through 5.
3. Prepare mixtures of the unknown and four correcting reagents as follows:
   a. 0.2 ml unknown (baseline)
   b. 0.2 ml unknown plus 0.05 ml normal plasma
   c. 0.2 ml unknown plus 0.05 ml aged normal serum
   d. 0.2 ml unknown plus 0.05 ml $BaSO_4$-adsorbed plasma
   e. 0.2 ml unknown plus 0.05 ml Celite-adsorbed plasma
4. Incubate tube of $CaCl_2$ at 37° C.
5. Incubate 2 cups of partial thromboplastin (0.1 ml each) for 2 minutes at 37° C.
6. Add 0.1 ml unknown (baseline) to 2 cups containing incubated thromboplastin. After 5 minutes of incubation, perform two PTTs.
7. Repeat step on each of the four mixtures prepared from the unknown.
8. Record your results on the following form:

	(sec)	(sec)	(ave)
1. Baseline			
2. 0.2 ml unknown plus 0.05 ml normal plasma			
3. 0.2 ml unknown plus 0.05 ml aged normal serum			
4. 0.2 ml unknown plus 0.05 ml $BaSO_4$-adsorbed plasma			
5. 0.2 ml unknown plus 0.05 ml Celite-adsorbed plasma			

Results

		Corrected by:		
	Normal plasma*	Aged normal serum†	$BaSO_4$ plasma‡	Celite plasma§
VIII deficient	Yes	No	Yes	Yes
IX deficient	Yes	Yes	No	Yes
X deficient‖	Yes	Yes	No	Yes
XI deficient	Yes	Yes	Yes	No
XII deficient	Yes	Yes	Yes	Yes

Thromboplastin generation test

Principle

When a suspension of platelets, deprothrombinized plasma, and serum is allowed to react in the presence of calcium ions, each contributes to the generation of thromboplastic activity in the incubation mixture. The alumina plasma contributes factors V and

---

*Normal plasma contains factors VIII, IX, X, XI, and XII.

†Aged normal serum does not contain factor VIII but contains "activated" IX, X, XI, and XII.

‡$BaSO_4$-adsorbed (oxalated) plasma is deficient in IX and X, but contains VIII, XI, and XII.

§Normal plasma adsorbed with Celite as specified under "materials and reagents" is deficient only in factor XI.

‖Plasma deficient in factor X or factor V will show both a prolonged prothrombin time and a prolonged PTT.

VIII, whereas serum contributes factors VII, IX, X, XI, and XII.

If the three fractions are prepared from normal blood and then allowed to react, powerful thromboplastic activity develops in the mixture, in that aliquots will clot recalcified normal plasma in 8 to 14 seconds. When maximal activity is attained, the reaction can be stopped, and the thromboplastic activity of serial dilutions of the reaction mixture is determined. When these results are plotted (Fig. A-12), a thromboplastin dilution curve is obtained. Abnormal results may then be expressed as *percent of normal activity*.

The localization of a defect in coagulation is achieved by substituting (one at a time) into the normal system the three fractions prepared from an unknown blood; e.g., by substituting an unknown suspension of platelets for the normal, it can be determined whether platelet function (platelet factor 3 release) in the unknown blood is normal or deficient. Likewise, substitution of unknown alumina plasma for normal plasma or unknown serum for normal serum allows a comparison of the activity of these fractions with that obtained with the corresponding normals. Partial thromboplastin reagent may be substituted for the platelet suspension when platelet function is not an issue.

Reagents

1. Aluminum hydroxide gel
   a. Preparation:
      (1) In a 2,000-ml flask, dissolve 76.7 Gm of aluminum ammonium sulfate, $Al(NH_4)(SO_4)_2 \cdot 12H_2O$, in 300 ml of distilled water. Solution is speeded if the flask is put in a water bath at 58° C.
      (2) In a separate 1,000-ml flask, add 22 Gm of ammonium sulfate, $(NH_4)_2SO_4$, to 600 ml of distilled water. Heat gently to approximately 63° C. When dissolved, add 100 ml of 50% NH_4OH solution (sp gr 0.88), stir vigorously, and pour at once into the flask containing the aluminum ammonium sulfate.
      (3) Stir vigorously for approximately 10 minutes. Keep the flask in the water bath at 58° C.
      (4) A gelatinous precipitate forms. Allow to settle; then wash five times:

      First wash: 1,500 ml of distilled water + 0.44 ml of 50% NH_4OH
      Second wash: 1,500 ml of distilled water + 0.88 ml of 50% NH_4OH
      Third through fifth washes: 1,500 ml of distilled water

      Washing may be carried out by allowing the gel to settle after each wash and decanting or aspirating the supernatant fluid. If facilities for centrifuging large volumes are available, the washings may be carried out quite rapidly. After the fifth washing, the pH of the supernatant fluid should be approximately 7 and free of nitrogen (test with Nessler's solution); if not, repeat washings with 1,500 ml of distilled water until these conditions are satisfied.
      (5) After the last washing, resuspend the precipitate in the least amount of water that will yield an easily pipetted suspension. Different preparations of a suspension of $Al(OH)_3$ will vary as to the concentration of the suspended precipitate, and each preparation must be standardized as to its adsorptive activity. However, a single batch is sufficient for hundreds of tests, and it is stable indefinitely. The suspension must be thoroughly shaken before use.
   b. Standardization of $Al(OH)_3$ suspension:
      (1) Obtain fresh citrated plasma from a normal donor (9 ml of blood plus 1 ml of 0.109M sodium citrate solution). Centrifuge at 3,000 rpm for 30 minutes.

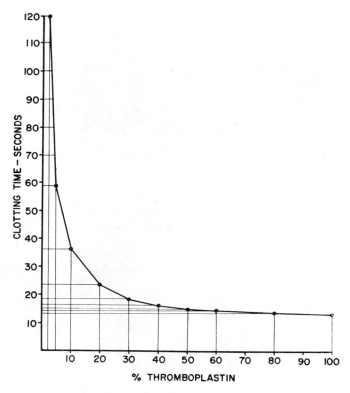

Fig. A-12. Thromboplastin dilution curve for TGT.

(2) To five conical 15-ml centrifuge tubes, add 0.02, 0.03, 0.04, 0.05, and 0.06 ml aliquots of the Al(OH)₃ suspension. Add to each tube 1 ml of citrated plasma.

(3) Stir each tube with a glass rod continuously for 3 minutes at 37° C.

(4) Centrifuge each tube at 4° C at 4,000 rpm (3,500 *g*) for 30 minutes. Decant supernate plasma and centrifuge for another 15 minutes at 3,500 *g* or better. Failure to sediment out very fine particles of Al(OH)₃ will interfere with subsequent steps.

(5) Perform a prothrombin time test on each specimen of supernatant plasma specimen. The amount of Al(OH)₃ to be used for subsequent adsorptions is that which gives a prothrombin time of approximately 2 minutes.

c. An Al(OH)₃ suspension is available commercially as Amphogel.* This should be standardized as for b above.

2. Commercial thromboplastin for standardization of Al(OH)₃ suspension

3. Sodium citrate, 0.109M

4. Sodium chloride, 0.85%

5. 0.025M CaCl₂

Equipment

1. Water bath, thermostatically controlled, 37° C (±1° C), with racks

2. Siliconized glassware†

---

*Wyeth, Philadelphia, Pa.
†General Electric Dri-Film No. SC-87 or Z 4141, Dow-Corning Corp., Midland, Mich., or Siliclad, Clay Adams, Parsippany, N.J.

a. Heavy-duty Pyrex conical centrifuge tubes, 12 ml
b. Syringes, 20 and 50 ml
c. Medicine droppers
d. Glass stirring rods

3. Two automatic pipets to deliver 0.1 ml

4. Six stopwatches and one large timer with sweep-second hand

5. Glass beads

6. Pyrex test tubes (not siliconized), 12 × 75 and 13 × 100 mm

Method

1. Obtain blood from a known normal control and from the patient to be studied by means of nontraumatic and "clean" venipunctures. Use a needle of large gauge and a two-syringe technic. Draw 1 or 2 ml of blood into the first syringe, discard, attach a siliconized syringe, and obtain 15 ml of blood—30 ml of patient's blood will allow a duplicate specimen that can be saved for further studies as well as sufficient blood for complete coagulation studies. Distribute as follows:

a. Centrifuge tube No. 1 (siliconized): 9 ml of *normal* blood + 1 ml of 0.109M sodium citrate. Mix well.

b. Centrifuge tube No. 2 (siliconized): 9 ml of *patient's* blood + ml of 0.109M sodium citrate. Mix well.

c. To a plain glass tube, 13 × 100 mm, containing four glass beads, add 4 ml of *normal* blood. Stopper. Invert repeatedly (do not shake) until clotted. Leave in the water bath at 37° C for at lest 2 hours before using as a source of serum.

d. To a plain glass tube, 13 × 100 mm, containing four glass beads, add 4 ml of *patient's* blood. Stopper. Invert repeatedly (do not shake) until clotted. Leave in the water

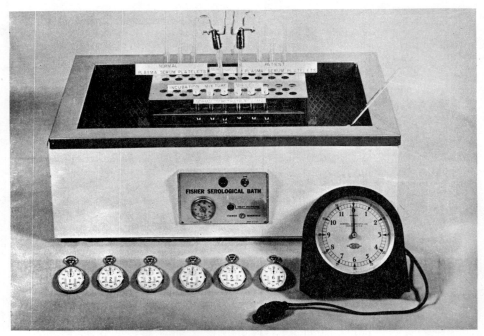

Fig. A-13. Apparatus and reagents for TGT.

bath at 37° C, for at least 2 hours before using as a source of serum.

2. Handle the citrated specimens from the normal person and the patient as follows, using siliconized tubes throughout and labeling carefully at each step.

    a. Centrifuge at 1,500 rpm for 10 minutes. (A refrigerated centrifuge is recommended for all procedures.)

    b. Aspirate the supernatant "platelet-rich" plasma, using siliconized or plastic droppers, into freshly siliconized heavy-duty *conical* centrifuge tubes.

    c. Centrifuge the plasmas at 3,000 rpm for at least 30 minutes. Read the volume of plasma.

    d. Aspirate the "platelet-poor" plasmas into separate siliconized test tubes, label, and store at 4° C. These will be used to prepare Al(OH)$_3$- adsorbed plasma (step f) and as substrate plasmas. Do not disturb the platelet sediments.

    e. Wash the platelet sediments remaining in each tube twice with 2-ml portions of saline solution. After adding the saline solution, thoroughly mix the sediment, using a siliconized stirring rod, and centrifuge it at 3,000 rpm for 10 minutes. After the second wash, resuspend the platelets in an amount of saline solution equal to one third of the amount of plasma as measured in step c. A smooth and even suspension must be prepared.

    f. Handle the platelet-poor plasmas obtained in step d as follows:

        (1) To a conical test tube, add the amount of Al(OH)$_3$ that will give the proper adsorption. Stir constantly for 3 minutes at 37° C. Centrifuge at 4,000 rpm for 30 minutes. Decant plasma and centrifuge a second time (p. 927). Decant the plasma and determine the prothrombin time. It should be about 2 minutes. If it is over 4 minutes, discard the specimen and prepare a fresh specimen adsorbed with less Al(OH)$_3$ suspension. If the prothrombin time is less than 1 minute,

the specimen can be salvaged by repeating the adsorption until the proper prothrombin time is obtained.

        (2) Label the remainder of the plasma as *substrate* plasma, and store it at 4° C until the test is set up. This must have a normal prothrombin time to be suitable for measuring thromboplastic activity. Substrate plasma from the normal control is used in the test.

3. Obtain serum from the tubes of clotted blood that have been in the water bath at 37° C for at least 2 hours. Rim the clot and centrifuge at 2,000 rpm for 10 minutes. Aspirate the sera and label them "normal serum" and "patient serum."

4. Preparation of final reagents:

    a. Prepare normal platelet suspension as outlined in step 2, e.

    b. Prepare patient's platelet suspension as outlined in step 2, e.

    c. Dilute normal alumina plasma (step 2, f, 1) 1:5 with saline solution.

    d. Dilute patient's alumina plasma (step 2, f, 1) 1:5 with saline solution.

    e. Dilute normal serum (step 3) 1:10 with saline solution.

    f. Dilute patient's serum (step 3) 1:10 with saline solution.

Note 1: If the platelet count is below normal, the platelet suspension must be adjusted so that it will contain approximately the same concentration of platelets as the normal suspension (approximately 1 million/mm^3, 1×10^{12}/l).

Note 2: Different plasma and serum dilutions are made as required.

5. Performance of test (Fig. A-13).

    a. Pipet 0.1 ml of normal substrate plasma into each of six plain glass tubes, 12 × 75 mm, in the water bath at 37° C. Use six tubes for testing each incubation mixture.

    b. Prepare, one at a time, the following incubation mixtures and perform the test with each.

(1) 0.3 ml of *normal* 1:5 alumina plasma + 0.3 ml of *normal* 1:10 serum + 0.3 ml of *normal* platelet suspension.

(2) 0.3 ml of *normal* 1:5 alumina plasma + 0.3 ml of *normal* 1:10 serum + 0.3 ml of *patient's* platelets.

(3) 0.3 ml of *normal* 1:5 alumina plasma + 0.3 ml of 1:10 *patient's* serum + 0.3 ml of *normal* platelets.

(4) 0.3 ml of *patient's* 1:5 alumina plasma + 0.3 ml of 1:10 *normal* serum + 0.3 ml of *normal* platelets.

(5) 0.3 ml of *patient's* 1:5 alumina plasma + 0.3 ml of 1:10 *patient's* serum + 0.3 ml of *patient's* platelets.

c. Place two tubes, each containing approximately 5 ml of 0.025M $CaCl_2$ solution, in the water bath at 37° C.

d. Add 0.3 ml of 0.025M $CaCl_2$ to the incubation mixture to be tested and simultaneously start the master timer.

e. Beginning 1 minute after the $CaCl_2$ is added to the incubation mixture, add to tube No. 1 (of substrate plasma) simultaneously (by means of automatic pipets) 0.1 ml of the recalcified incubation mixture plus 0.1 ml of 0.025M $CaCl_2$ solution. Start stopwatch 1 at the same time. At 1-minute intervals repeat with substrate tubes Nos. 2, 3, etc., starting a separate stopwatch for each tube. Time the first appearance of a clot in each tube and record. For this, two persons work together. One adds the $CaCl_2$ to the incubation mixture, starts the master timer, and pipets reagents into the tubes of substrate at 1-minute intervals. The other starts the individual stopwatches and records the time of clotting for each tube. Usually during the second or third minute, a clot forms in the incubation mixture. When this occurs, the first person removes the clot with a wooden applicator stick. Formation of the clot does not interfere with the results, but if it is not removed, it will clog the pipets used for transferring the recalcified incubation mixture.

f. If a serum defect is present that is not caused by deficiency of factor VII or X (as evidenced by a normal prothrombin time in the original blood), it is necessary to determine whether it is a deficiency of factor IX, XI, or XII. This is done by setting up additional incubation mixtures to determine the mutually corrective effects with known substrate plasmas.

g. In testing for anticoagulants the TGT is repeated, adding to a normal incubation mixture serial dilutions of the patient's serum or plasma (1:50, 1:100, 1:250, and 1:500 *final* concentrations in the incubation mixture). To keep the volume and the normal concentration of serum or plasma constant, it is necessary to vary the composition of the mixture. If plasma is being tested for an anticoagulant, the incubation mixture is made up with 0.15 ml of 1:2.5 normal plasma plus 0.15 ml of diluted unknown plasma. If serum is being studied, the incubation mixture is made up with 0.15 ml of 1:5 normal serum plus 0.15 ml of diluted unknown serum. If generation of thromboplastin is good with the high dilutions and poor with the low dilutions, an anticoagulant is present.

Results and interpretation

Fig. A-14 illustrates the range of normal values obtained in 165 normal persons. The average is 11.1 seconds, with an SD of ±2.8 seconds. The variation is not caused by technical factors because repeated tests performed with the same reagents check within a few tenths of a second. We regard a value of 8 to 14 seconds, occurring at any time during the 6 minutes of the test, as evidence of normal

generation of thromboplastin. In most normal tests, maximal activity is reached during the third minute. One run with the three normal reagents is included in all instances in which an unknown blood is studied, as this gives the control value for 100% generation.

The greatest usefulness of the TGT is in the study and differentiation of deficiencies of factors VIII, IX, X XI, and XII, in the demonstration and titration of abnormal circulating anticoagulants, and, when patient's platelets are included in the incubation mixture, as a measure of platelet factor 3 release.

References

Miale and Wilson, 1956a, 1956b

Factor VIII (VIII: C) assay
Materials and reagents

1. Fibrometer with 0.4-ml probe
2. Automated APTT*
3. 0.025M $CaCl_2$
4. Factor VIII–deficient plasma*
5. Sodium citrate, 0.109M
6. Verify Normal* (assayed for factor VIII by manufacturer)
7. Normal saline (0.85%)

Method

1. Preparation of activity curve
   a. Reconstitute Verify Normal as shown on manufacturer's label.
   b. Using serial dilutions, prepare reconstituted Verify Normal with 0.85% saline in the following concentrations: 10%, 5%, 2.5%, 1.25%, 0.625%, 0.313%, and .156% (10% = assayed activity).
   c. Into a 37° C Fibrometer heat block place:
      (1) A test tube containing 0.025M $CaCl_2$
      (2) A Fibro-cup containing:
         0.1 ml automated APTT
         0.1 ml factor VIII–deficient plasma
         0.1 ml diluted Verify plasma
         Incubate for 5 minutes.
      (3) Add 0.1 ml prewarmed $CaCl_2$, activate the Fibrometer, and record time in seconds. Repeat for each plasma dilution. The results of each dilution are plotted on 3 cycles × 60 division semilog graph paper.
2. Testing of patient plasma
   a. Sodium citrate plasma from patient is diluted to 10% with 0.85% saline.
   b. Test a 10% and 5% patient plasma dilution as for Verify Normal dilutions.
   c. The time in seconds is related to percent activity by reading off the normal activity curve.

Remarks

Test plasmas and factor VIII–deficient plasmas must be kept on ice at all times.

Factor VIII–related antigen (VIII: Ag) by electroimmunoassay (EIA)
Principle

Factor VIII: Ag in plasma is electrophoresed through agarose gel containing factor VIII antiserum. The antigen develops a rocket-like immunoprecipitate, the length of which is directly proportional to the concentration of antigen.

---

*General Diagnostics, Div. Warner-Lambert Co., Morris Plains, N.J.

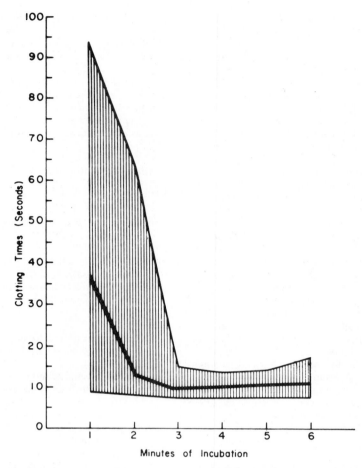

Fig. A-14. Control data for TGT (165 normal subjects). The heavy line is the mean value at each minute; the top and bottom lines represent the upper and lower limits at each minute.

Equipment

1. Behring electrophoresis chamber, water cooled,* and power supply
2. GelBond film, 3½ × 4 inches†
3. Well cutter and template
4. Telfa nonadherent strips
5. Micropipette, 5 microliter

Reagents

1. Tris barbital buffer pH 8.8, ionic strength 0.028‡: Dissolve 17 Gm of high-resolution buffer in deionized water and dilute to 2,000 ml.
2. Agarose, Indubiose A45§ 1%.
3. Coomassie Brilliant Blue R250‖: Dissolve 0.25 gm stain in decolorizing solution and dilute to 1,000 ml.
4. Decolorizing solution: Mix 1,000 ml methyl alcohol, 1,000 ml distilled water, and 200 ml glacial acetic acid.
5. Antiserum to human factor VIII– associated protein.*
6. Frozen normal plasma pool.
7. Fresh patient platelet-poor plasma.

---

*Calbiochem-Behring Corp., La Jolla, Calif.
†Marine Colloids Division, FMC Corp., Rockland, Me.
‡Gelman Instrument Co., Ann Arbor, Mich.
§Fisher Scientific, Philadelphia, Pa.
‖Bio Rad Laboratories, Richmond, Calif.

Method

Preparation of gel

Dissolve 0.15 Gm agarose in 15 ml of tris barbital buffer and heat to boiling on a hot plate with an electric magnet. When all agarose is dissolved and the solution is clear, place in a 50° water bath. When the agarose has reached 50°, add 0.06 ml of factor VIII antiserum. (Amount of antiserum required may vary among batches). Swirl to mix. Place the GelBond film on a level spot. Carefully pour the agarose onto the hydrophilic side of the Gel-Bond film and allow to cool at room temperature for 10 to 15 minutes. Place in a moist chamber and store at 4° overnight to harden. Gels should not be prepared more than 3 days in advance. Just before using, punch 14 holes 3 mm in diameter, approximately 3 mm apart and 2 cm from the edge of the plate.

Electrophoresis

1. Fill the electrophoresis chamber with 2 liters of tris barbital buffer.
2. Thaw normal plasma pool. Prepare the following dilutions with tris barbital buffer: undiluted, 100%; 1:2 dilution, 50%; 1:4 dilution, 25%; and 1:8 dilution, 12.5%.
3. Patient samples are quick thawed or fresh, tested undiluted and 1:2 in buffer.
4. Using a micropipette add 5 microliters of plasma to each well. This should be done as quickly as possible to minimize radial diffusion.
5. Place the gel in the electrophoresis chamber with the wells on the cathode side. Two gels can be electrophoresed at one time.

6. Telfa strips that have been presoaked in buffer are placed on the cathode and anode side of each gel to act as wicks. The wicks should be flat against the agarose with the other end remaining in the buffer.
7. Run the electrophoresis for 16 to 18 hours at approximately 8 or 9 mA per gel. Water-cooled cell temperatures should be approximately 15° C.
8. When electrophoresis is finished, transfer gels to a saline wash to remove excess protein. Wash overnight or for several hours with several changes of saline.

Staining
1. Remove gel from saline. Cover with a layer of wet filter paper, then invert on several dry layers of absorbent paper. Place a plain glass slide on top of the paper directly over the gel and immediately add a weight (approximately 1 pound). Leave weight on 15 minutes to remove excess water from the gel.
2. Carefully remove weight and filter paper. Stand gel up and allow to air dry, or carefully blow warm air from a hand dryer kept at least 2 feet away from gel.
3. Stain dried gel in Coomassie Blue stain for 10 minutes. Longer times may be necessary to obtain darker peaks.
4. Place the gel briefly in several changes of decolorizer solution until background is nearly colorless.

Calculations
1. Measure the length of the rockets from the top of the well to the apex.
2. Construct a reference curve using the four normal plasma dilutions. The height of each dilution peak is plotted on log-log paper against the percent of normal.
3. Plot a best-fit line.
4. Determine the percent of VIII:Ag in each patient sample from the curve.

Results

Normal is 70% to 150%. The level of VIII:Ag is normal or increased in hemophiliacs and carriers, but is decreased or absent in von Willebrand's disease.

Ristocetin cofactor (VIII:vW) assay by aggregometry
Principle

Ristocetin cofactor (VIII:vW) activity is measured in terms of its ability to cause agglutination of normal formalin-fixed platelets in the presence of the antibiotic ristocetin. Platelet-poor plasma and ristocetin are added to a suspension of formalin-fixed platelets, and the agglutination is measured in an aggregometer. The percent agglutination is proportional to the amount of ristocetin cofactor present in the plasma sample.

Reagents and equipment
1. Phosphate buffered saline (PBS) pH 7.2
   a. 13.2 ml 1.0M monobasic sodium phosphate
   b. 53.6 ml 0.5M dibasic sodium phosphate
   c. 34.0 Gm NaCl
   d. QS 4 liters
2. Ristocetin,* 18 mg/ml PBS
3. Bovine serum albumin (BSA),† 100 mg/2.5 ml PBS
4. Formaldehyde 2% in PBS (2 ml of formalin + 98 ml of PBS)
5. Pooled normal platelet-poor plasma, frozen
6. Formaldehyde-fixed platelet suspension, concentration adjusted to about 500,000/mm^3
7. Platelet Aggregation Profiler, Model PAP-3‡

*Lenau, Copenhagen, Denmark.
†Sigma Chemical Co., St. Louis, Mo.
‡Bio Data Corp., Willow Grove, Pa.

Method
Preparation of normal fixed platelets
1. Plastic or siliconized glassware is used throughout the procedure. Fresh whole blood is drawn into 3.2% sodium citrate in a ratio 1:10. Use a normal donor not receiving medication. Centrifuge for 40 minutes at 100 g to obtain PRP. Note yield of plasma and check platelet count.
2. Incubate PRP 1 hour at 37° C.
3. Add an equal volume of 2% formaldehyde to PRP, mix, and incubate 18 to 24 hours at 4° C in round-bottomed 40-ml plastic tubes.
4. Spin 30 minutes at 2,000 g to obtain platelet button. Discard supernate and wash button six times with cold PBS. Each wash is spun 15 minutes at 2,000 g.
5. Resuspend button after final wash in PBS with azide (0.05%). Check count and adjust to about 500,000/mm^3. Store in convenient aliquots at 4° C.
6. Before using, add cold PBS to top of tube, spin 15 minutes at 2,000 g. Resuspend in PBS to original volume to obtain count of about 500,000/mm^3.

Reference plasma
1. Dilute normal pooled platelet-poor plasma 1:2 to 1:16 in BSA. The undiluted plasma is considered to contain 100% VIII:vW.

Test plasma
1. Dilute the test plasma 1:2 and 1:4 in BSA.

Assay
1. In aggregometer cuvette add 0.5 ml fixed-platelet suspension and 0.1 ml plasma. Without incubation, place in aggregometer with stir bar. The blank is prepared by making a 4:3 mixture of the fixed-platelet suspension in BSA (see Comments).
2. Adjust baseline to 0% (± 2 minutes), then add 50 microliters of ristocetin. Readjust to zero after maximum minus deflection has occurred if necessary (see Comments).
3. Record percent OD change. Prepare a reference curve on arithmetic graph paper using the diluted normal plasma pool.
4. Add 0.1 ml of undiluted patient plasma or plasma dilution. Read values from reference curve.

Results

The percent change in OD of the aggregation (agglutination) when undiluted plasma is added to the system is considered 100% ristocetin cofactor (VIII:vW). The percent OD obtained with the patient's plasma is converted to percent VIII:vW from the reference curve.

Normal individuals have 50% to 130% VIII:vW compared with normal pooled plasma. Patients with von Willebrand's disease usually have 0% VIII:vW. Variants range from low to normal.

Comments
1. Assay of VIII:vW by aggregometry requires an instrument that automatically sets the difference between the blank and the test at 0% and also allows for resetting the baseline to 0 when a minus value occurs when ristocetin is added. This occurs frequently with the test as outlined. With a good preparation of fixed platelets the initial minus deflection when ristocetin is added is −40% or less. This is adjusted to 0 when the greatest minus deflection is reached.
2. Within fairly wide limits (400,000 to 600,000 mm^3) the platelet count of the fixed platelets is not critical. However, it may be necessary to vary the platelet concentration in the blank to allow the instrument to record the difference between test and blank. If the platelet count in the blank is not suitable, it will not be possible to zero the baseline. We

find that the blank is usually a 4:3 mixture of fixed platelets and BSA.

3. Because the stability of the stored fixed-platelet preparation is unpredictable, we frequently make only a small batch when an assay is anticipated.

References

Macfarlane and Zucker, 1975
Weiss, 1975
Weiss et al, 1973a, b, c, d

Factor IX assay
Materials and reagents

1. Sodium citrate, 0.109M
2. Automated APTT*
3. Factor IX–deficient plasma*
4. 0.025M calcium chloride
5. Normal citrate plasma
6. Fibrometer with 0.4-ml probe
7. Imidazole-buffered distilled water, pH 7.2 to 7.35
8. Imidazole-buffered saline (0.85% in buffered water)

Method

1. Draw normal blood into 0.109M sodium citrate (1 part sodium citrate plus 9 parts blood).
2. Centrifuge blood for 10 minutes at 1,700 rpm and harvest plasma.
3. Make plasma dilutions by diluting plasma 1:10 with buffered saline, which is equivalent to 100%, and then from that 100% dilution, make a serial dilution of 50%, 25%, 12.5%, 6.25%, 3.13%, and 1.56% with buffered saline.
4. Test each of the saline dilute plasmas as follows:
   a. Prewarm 0.025M CaCl₂ at 37° C.
   b. Transfer 0.1 ml diluted plasma to a Fibro-cup.
   c. Add 0.1 ml factor IX–deficient plasma.
   d. Add 0.1 ml automated APTT.
   e. Mix and incubate for 6 minutes at 37° C.
   f. Add 0.1 ml 0.025M CaCl₂ and activate the Fibrometer (use 0.4-ml probe).
5. Plot dilution curve on log-log paper from the seven points.
6. Factor IX assay on unknown: Using buffered saline, make 100% and 50% dilutions of unknown citrate plasma, and proceed with method described above for testing plasma dilutions. Plasmas, dilutions, and substrates should always be kept on ice.
7. Read result of unknown in percent from normal dilution curve.

Factor X assay
Materials and reagents

1. Sodium citrate, 0.109M
2. Simplastin*
3. Factor X-deficient plasma*
4. Normal citrate plasma
5. Imidazole-buffered distilled water, pH 7.2 to 7.35
6. Imidazole-buffered saline (0.85% in buffered water)
7. Fibrometer with 0.4-ml probe

Method

1. Draw normal blood in 0.109M sodium citrate (1 part sodium citrate plus 9 parts blood).
2. Centrifuge blood for 10 minutes at 1,700 rpm and harvest plasma.
3. Make plasma dilutions by diluting plasma 1:10 with buffered

saline, which is equivalent to 100%, and then from that 100% dilution make a serial dilution of 50%, 25%, 12.5%, 6.25%, 3.13%, and 1.56%.

4. Test each of the dilutions as follows:
   a. Prewarm Simplastin at 37° C for a minimum of 5 minutes in aliquots sufficient for four to six tests.
   b. Pipet 0.1 ml Factor X-deficient substrate into a Fibro-cup.
   c. Add 0.1 ml dilute test plasma (which has been held in an ice bath).
   d. Immediately add 0.2 ml Simplastin and activate the Fibrometer (use 0.4 ml probe).
5. Plot dilution curve on log-log paper from the seven points.
6. Factor X assay on unknown: Using buffered saline, make 100% and 50% dilutions of unknown citrate plasma and proceed with method described above for testing plasma dilutions. Plasmas, dilutions, and substrates should always be kept on ice.
7. Read result of unknown in percent from normal dilution curve.

Factor XI assay
Material and reagents

1. Sodium citrate, 0.109M
2. Automated APTT*
3. Factor XI–deficient plasma*
4. 0.025M calcium chloride
5. Normal citrate plasma
6. Fibrometer with 0.4-ml probe
7. Imidazole-buffered distilled water, pH 7.2 to 7.35
8. Imidazole-buffered saline (0.85% in buffered water)

Method

1. Draw normal blood into 0.109M sodium citrate (1 part sodium citrate plus 9 parts blood).
2. Centrifuge blood for 10 minutes at 1,700 rpm and harvest plasma.
3. Make plasma dilutions of 1:10, 1:100, and 1:1,000 with buffered saline.
4. Test each of the saline-diluted plasmas as follows:
   a. 0.1 ml dilute plasma.
   b. 0.1 ml factor XI–deficient plasma.
   c. 0.1 ml APTT.
   d. Mix and incubate for 6 minutes at 37° C in a Fibro-cup.
   e. Add 0.1 ml 0.025M calcium chloride and activate the Fibrometer (use 0.4-ml probe).
5. Plot dilution curve on log-log paper from three points; 1:10 dilution is equivalent to 100%, 1:100 to 10%, and 1:1,000 to 1%.
6. Factor XI on unknown: Using buffered saline, make a 1:10 dilution of unknown citrate plasma and proceed with method described above for testing plasma dilutions. Plasmas, dilutions, and substrates should always be kept on ice.
7. Read results of unknown in percent from normal dilution curve.

Factor XII assay

Materials, reagents, and method exactly the same as for factor XI assay with one exception, namely, factor XII–deficient plasma is used in place of factor XI–deficient plasma.

---

*General Diagnostics, Div. Warner-Lambert Co., Morris Plains, N.J.

*General Diagnostics, Div. Warner-Lambert Co., Morris Plains, N.J.: or use Celite adsorption method on p. 925.

Table A-2

	Patient—tube no.							Normal control—tube no.						
	1	2	3	4	5	6	7	1	2	3	4	5	6	7
Plasma	—	0.05	0.10	0.20	0.30	0.40	0.50	—	0.05	0.1	0.2	0.3	0.4	0.5
Saline solution	0.7	0.65	0.60	0.50	0.40	0.30	0.20	0.70	0.65	0.6	0.5	0.4	0.3	0.2
Fibrinogen	1.0	1.0	1.0	1.0	1.0	1.0	1.0	1.0	1.0	1.0	1.0	1.0	1.0	1.0
CaCl$_2$-bovine thrombin	1.0	1.0	1.0	1.0	1.0	1.0	1.0	1.0	1.0	1.0	1.0	1.0	1.0	1.0
Monochloroacetic acid*	2.7	2.7	2.7	2.7	2.7	2.7	2.7	2.7	2.7	2.7	2.7	2.7	2.7	2.7

*Add 1 hour after above solutions clot.

Semiquantitative assay of fibrin-stabilizing factor (factor XIII)

The role of factor XIII in the formation of physiologic fibrin clots is discussed in Chapter 17. A fibrin clot forming in normal plasma not deficient in factor XIII is insoluble in 5M urea or 1% monochloracetic acid. A fibrin clot forming in factor XIII–deficient plasma is soluble in urea or monochloroacetic acid. Fibrin clots formed from purified fibrinogen by the addition of thrombin are formed in the absence of factor XIII and are therefore also soluble in urea or monochloroacetic acid. Solubility can be inhibited by normal plasma or serum.

Quantitative methods are available. The method presented here, developed jointly with Dr. Gary Weiss, uses an optimum concentration of mercuric chloride to just inhibit contaminating factor XIII in the crude bovine fibrinogen and in the thrombin. The system is then equivalent to one free of factor XIII. We have adopted this system because (1) we do not find it possible to destroy contaminating factor XIII by heating to 40° C, as reported by others, and (2) we avoid time-consuming procedures for purifying fibrinogen.

Reagents

1. Mercuric chloride solution, 5×10^{-5}M, buffered to pH 7.4 ionic strength 0.15
   a. Mercuric chloride stock

Mercuric chloride	13.575 Gm
Distilled water to	1,000 ml

   b. Tris (hydroxymethylaminomethane) buffer, pH 7.4

Tris base (trizma base*)	18.15 Gm
1N HCl	125.50 ml
Distilled water to	1,000 ml

   Dissolve Tris base in about 500 ml of distilled water, add the HCl, and bring volume to 1,000 ml. Check and adjust pH to 7.4, if necessary.
   c. Bring 1 ml of mercuric chloride stock to 1,000 ml with Tris buffer solution.
2. Fibrinogen solution
   a. Dissolve 0.6 Gm of bovine fibrinogen† in 100 ml of buffered mercuric chloride solution.
   b. Filter through Whatman No. 1 paper.
3. CaCl$_2$-bovine thrombin solution
   a. Dilute lyophilized bovine thrombin‡ to 25 NIH units/ml with 1% CaCl$_2$ solution.
4. Citrated plasma, platelet free, from patient to be studied (9 parts blood plus 1 part 0.109M sodium citrate)

5. Citrated plasma from normal control
6. Monochloroacetic acid, 2%, in distilled water

Method

1. Set up test as shown in Table A-2.
2. One hour after clotting occurs, add 2.7 ml of 2% monochloracetic acid to each tube. Seal with patch of Parafilm; free clot by tapping and inverting the tube.
3. Incubate 2 hours at room temperature and read.
4. Examine each tube for solution of the clot. Grade results as follows:
   a. Tube No. 1 is control tube and should always dissolve.
   b. Normal factor XIII activity: Clots dissolve in tubes Nos. 1 to 3; remain undissolved in tubes Nos. 4 to 7.
   c. Moderate reduction in factor XIII activity: Clots remain in tubes Nos. 5 to 7; are dissolved in tubes Nos. 1 to 4.
   d. Markedly reduced factor XIII activity: No clots remain in any of the tubes.

Remarks

As discussed in Chapter 17, deficiency of factor XIII is accompanied by normal coagulation tests, except for specific assay of factor XIII.

Assay is not valid if patient has received mercurial diuretic within 48 hours of the test.

Seventeen out of twenty normal subjects showed the same pattern, tubes Nos. 1 to 3 dissolved, tubes Nos. 4 to 7 not dissolved. The other three showed only partial solution of the clot in tube No. 3.

References

Lorand, 1964
Lorand and Dickenman, 1955
Nussbaum and Morse, 1964

Detection of Fletcher factor deficiency
Principle

The prolonged APTT of Fletcher factor (prekallikrein)–deficient plasma will be shortened after prolonged incubation with an APTT reagent sensitive to the defect.

Equipment and reagents

See procedure for Activated Partial Thromboplastin Time.

Procedure

1. Perform an activated partial thromboplastin time on the patient's plasma.
2. Repeat the activated partial thromboplastin time on the patient's plasma, increasing the incubation time of the patient's plasma plus activated partial thromboplastin reagent mixture to 10 minutes.

---

*Sigma Chemical Co., St. Louis, Mo.
†Armour Pharmaceutical Co., Chicago, Ill.
‡Parke, Davis & Co., Detroit, Mich.

Results

Correction of the APTT to normal or near normal after the 10-minute incubation period is suggestive of Fletcher factor (prekallikrein) deficiency.

Note: Prolonged incubation with an APTT reagent that uses elagic acid will not correct the APTT in Fletcher factor deficiency. Kaolin, celite, or silica is the activator of choice.

References

Hathaway et al, 1965
Hattersley and Hayse, 1976

Antithrombin III

Antithrombin III is a heparin cofactor that may be decreased in thrombotic disease (p. 820). It can be assayed by a variety of technics, the most frequently used being (1) a clotting test that measures neutralization of thrombin, (2) the Laurell rocket electroimmunoassay, or (3) the Mancini radial immunodiffusion. Our experience with these assays indicates that when performed in parallel they do not always yield comparable results. The reasons for the discrepancies are not obvious, but some of the variables are known.

Antithrombin III makes up about 75% of the total blood antithrombic activity, so that tests based on thrombin neutralization are probably not specific for antithrombin III. Clotting tests can be made somewhat more specific for antithrombin III by using serum harvested after clotted blood stands at room temperature for 2 hours, since antithrombin III activity is said to be "progressive." Some antithrombin is consumed when blood clots, so that thrombin neutralization tests give higher antithrombin III levels when plasma, rather than serum, is used. In addition, antithrombin titers depend on the free procoagulant activity in plasma or serum; this depends in part on platelet breakdown products; e.g., platelet factor 3. Because of these known variables and some unknown variables, a carefully standardized technic should be followed and normal values should be established in each laboratory.

Immunologic technics would appear to be subject to fewer variables, assuming that the antiserum is specific for antithrombin III. Our data indicate that the radial immunodiffusion method is less sensitive than the Laurell technic.

By thrombin neutralization*

Principle

The antithrombin activity is determined by measuring the neutralization of the clotting activity of a standard solution of thrombin.

Equipment

1. Fibrometer
2. 0.1-ml pipets

Reagents

1. Thrombin†
2. Normal human plasma, lyophilized‡
3. Normal saline (0.85% NaCl)

Method

1. Five ml of venous whole blood is allowed to clot in a plain glass tube and allowed to stand at room temperature for exactly 2 hours after it clots.
2. Serum is obtained by centrifugation and maintained at room temperature.

3. Prepare a dilute solution of thrombin in saline that will give a thrombin time of 15 to 16 seconds with normal plasma (0.2 ml of normal plasma + 0.1 ml of thrombin at 37° C). Warm to 37° C.
4. Add 0.2 ml of normal plasma to a Fibro-cup; incubate at 37° C.
5. Add 0.1 ml of serum to 0.9 ml of the standardized thrombin solution. Mix and incubate at 37° C for *exactly* 3 minutes.
6. After the 3-minute incubation add 0.1 ml of the thrombin-serum mixture to the 0.2 ml of normal plasma in the Fibro-cup and activate the Fibrometer.

Normal values

The thrombin time of normals is 32.9 seconds, S.D. 3 seconds. A decreased antithrombin titer results in a shorter than normal (< 26 seconds) thrombin time.

By rocket electroimmunoassay

Principle

Antithrombin III in serum is electrophoresed through agarose gel containing antithrombin III antiserum. The antigen develops a rocket-like immunoprecipitate, the length of which is directly proportional to the concentration of antigen.

Equipment

1. Gelman electrophoresis chamber (Model No. 51170-1) and power supply.
2. Kodak glass slides, 3¼ × 4 inches, precoated with 0.1% agarose.
3. Well cutter and template.
4. Telfa nonadherent strips.*
5. Micropipet to deliver 5 microliters.
6. Template: On a 3¼ × 4 inch rectangle draw a pattern of a single row of 14 holes 3 mm in diameter, approximately 3 mm apart and 2 cm from the edge of the long side of the rectangle.
7. Well cutter: sharp-edged hollow metal tube with OD 3 mm.

Reagents

1. Barbital buffer A, pH 8.6 (for preparing agar)

Diethylbarbituric acid	1.04 Gm
Sodium diethylbarbiturate	6.57 Gm
EDTA, Na$_2$	1.0 Gm

Dissolve barbituric acid in 100 ml of warm distilled water. Add about 850 ml of distilled water and other salts. Adjust pH to 8.6 with 0.1N NaOH and add sufficient distilled water to make 1 liter.

2. Barbital buffer B, pH 8.6 (for electrophoresis chamber)

Diethylbarbituric acid	2.07 Gm
Sodium diethylbarbiturate	13.14 Gm
EDTA, Na$_2$	1.0 Gm

Dissolve and adjust pH as with buffer A. Add sufficient distilled water to make 1 liter.

3. Agarose, Indubiose A45.†
4. Amido black, 2 Gm in 1,000 ml of decolorizing solution.
5. Decolorizing solution: Mix 1,000 ml methyl alcohol, 1,000 ml distilled water, and 200 ml glacial acetic acid.
6. Antiserum to antithrombin III.‡

---

*Modification of the Zuck (1971) method.
†Fibrindex, Ortho Pharmaceutical Corp., Raritan, N.J.
‡General Diagnostics, Div. Warner-Lambert Co., Morris Plains, N.J.

*Kendall Hospital Products Div., Chicago, Ill.
†Fisher Scientific Co., Pittsburgh, Pa.
‡Calbiochem-Behring Corp., La Jolla, Calif.

7. Frozen normal serum pool.
8. Fresh or frozen patient serum (or EDTA-plasma).

Method
Preparation of slides

Carefully clean several glass slides and precoat with a thin layer of 0.1% agarose. Allow to air dry and store in a cool, clean place. Dissolve 0.15 Gm agarose in 15 ml barbital buffer A and heat to boiling on a hot plate with an electric stirring magnet. When all agarose is dissolved and the solution is clear, place in a 55° C water bath. When the agarose has reached 50° to 55° C, add 0.6 ml antithrombin III antiserum. (Amount of antiserum may vary among batches.) Swirl to mix. Warm a precoated slide and place on a level spot. Carefully pour the agarose onto the slide and allow to cool at room temperature for 10 to 15 minutes. Place in a moist chamber and store at 4° C overnight to harden. Slides should not be made more than 3 days in advance. Just before using, place slide over template pattern and punch fourteen 3-mm holes according to the pattern. Aspirate the agar from the gels with a Pasteur pipet attached to suction.

Electrophoresis

1. Fill the electrophoresis chamber with 1 liter of barbital buffer B. Cool in refrigerator.
2. Prepare dilutions of frozen normal serum pool 100% (undiluted) and 50% and 25% (diluted with buffer A).
3. Patient serum is tested 100% (undiluted) and 50% (diluted with buffer A).
4. Using a micropipet add 5 microliters of serum to each well. This should be done as quickly as possible to minimize radial diffusion.
5. Place the slide in the electrophoresis chamber with the wells on the cathode side.
6. Telfa strips that have been presoaked in buffer are placed on the cathode and anode sides of the gel to act as wicks. The wicks should be flat against the agarose with the other end remaining in the buffer.
7. Run at 4° C at 7 to 10 mA for 6 hours.
8. Transfer slide to normal saline; wash for several hours or overnight.

Staining

1. Remove slides from saline. Place on Whatman No. 1 filter paper. Cover with 8 to 10 layers of filter paper. Place a plain glass slide on top of the paper directly over the agarose slide and immediately add a weight (approximately 1 pound). This must be done quickly to prevent the paper from wrinkling and distorting the agarose. Leave weight on for 15 minutes to remove excess water from slide.
2. Carefully remove weight and paper. Stand slide up and allow to air dry completely or carefully blow warm air from a hand dryer held at least 2 feet away from the slide.
3. Stain slide in Amido black for 5 minutes.
4. Place slide in several changes of decolorizing solution until the background is nearly colorless.

Calculations

1. Measure the length of the rockets from the top of the well to apex.
2. Construct a reference curve using the normal serum dilutions. The height of each peak is plotted on log-log paper against the percent of normal.
3. Plot a best-fit line.

4. Determine the percent of antithrombin III antigen in each patient sample from the curve.

Reference
Laurell, 1966; 1972

By radial immunodiffusion
Reagents

1. Phosphate buffer 0.01M, pH 6.5

K$_2$HPO$_4$	0.56 Gm
KH$_2$PO$_4$	0.93 Gm
EDTA, Na$_2$	1.0 Gm

Add sufficient distilled water to make 1 liter.
2. Kodak slides, well cutter, agarose, staining solution, decolorizing solution, control serum, antithrombin III antiserum, and patient serum the same as antithrombin III immunoassay.
3. Template

Method

1. Prepare precoated Kodak slides with 1% agarose in phosphate buffer, pH 6.5. Use technic as outlined for antithrombin III rocket technic, except add 0.25 ml of antiserum to the agar.
2. Prepare a template with 20 equidistant holes 3 mm in diameter. Cut holes in hardened gel using well cutter, and aspirate with suction.
3. Normal or reference serum is prepared 100% (undiluted) and 50% (diluted with phosphate buffer). A 200% value is obtained by using twice as much reference serum (10 microliters) in one well.
4. Patient serum is used as 100% (undiluted) and 50% (diluted with phosphate buffer).
5. Fill wells with 5 microliters of serum (except 10 microliters in 200% reference well).
6. Place plate in moist box at 37° C for 18 hours. Measure diameters of immunoprecipitate circles. After 18 hours the antithrombin III standard well should have reached a diameter of 7.5 to 8 mm. If necessary, reincubate for several hours. If no more migration has occurred, place in a saline wash for 6 to 8 hours. Dry and stain as in the antithrombin III rocket technic.

Calculations

Measure the diameters of the circles in two directions, perpendicular to each other. Construct a standard curve on log-log paper, using the mean diameters of the three control sera. Calculate percent antithrombin III of unknowns from standard curve.

Reference
Mancini et al, 1965

Assays utilizing chromogenic or fluorogenic substrates

Many of the coagulation factors develop proteolytic activity when activated and become serine proteases. One, antithrombin III, is the chief protease inhibitor. Methods have been developed to assay serine proteases or inhibitors that depend on the cleavage of synthetic peptide substrates that yield either a chromogenic or a fluorogenic fragment. The substrates currently available are summarized by Fareed et al (1980).

At this time, assays based on synthetic substrates are used primarily in research laboratories. First, they are expensive, for the synthesis of a given substrate is laborious. Second, there is continuing investigation as to specificity and in the standardization of methodology. Finally, those assays which are acceptably specific (antithrombin III, heparin, Xa) either offer no obvious advantage over other assay technics (antithrombin III, Xa) or have no clinical application (heparin). There is no denying, however, that this is an exciting development in the methodology of quantifying coagulation factors, and it may well happen that in the near future the questions of specificity, methodology, and cost will be answered.

Thrombin time
Principle

The time required for plasma to clot when thrombin is added is a function of the integrity of the fourth phase of coagulation. It is affected by the concentration of fibrinogen, by some dysfibrinogenemias, the concentration of plasmin, the presence of fibrin split products, and the presence of antithrombic agents. It is useful in establishing that a fourth-phase defect is present and in following the progress of therapy. It does not distinguish between DIC and primary fibrinolytic syndromes.

The method as described by Brodsky et al calls for determining the thrombin time serially at intervals of 10 minutes, but the test can be simplified to a single reading, at 20 minutes' incubation, since this allows a sharp distinction between normal and abnormal.

Reagents
1. Fibrindex*
   a. Add 1 ml of saline solution to a vial to make a solution containing some 50 NIH thrombin units/ml.
   b. Dilute this solution with saline solution so that when 0.2 ml is added to 0.2 ml normal plasma, the clotting time will be 15 to 18 seconds.

Method
1. Obtain citrated plasma from the patient and from a normal donor.
2. Add 0.2 ml of each to separate 12 × 75 mm plain glass tubes. Incubate in water bath at 37° C for 20 minutes.
3. Add 0.2 ml of Fibrindex solution to the control tube and measure clotting time with a stopwatch (Fibrometer may be used). Repeat with the tube of patient's plasma.

Results

Normal plasma has a thrombin time of 15 to 18 seconds under the conditions of the test. Abnormal results are usually longer than 30 seconds and, in some instances, no clot will form.

References
Brodsky et al, 1968b
Coleman et al, 1972

Protamine paracoagulation test
Principle

The addition of protamine to citrated plasma containing soluble fibrin monomer complexes and fibrinogen degradation products causes a polymerization of the monomer complexes and visible fibrin formation.

Reagent
1. Protamine (1% solution of protamine sulfate)

Method
1. Obtain citrated plasma from the patient and a normal donor (9 parts venous blood plus 1 part 0.109M sodium citrate).
2. To 1 ml of plasma at 37° C, add 0.1 ml of the protamine sulfate solution.
3. Mix, incubate at 37° C for 15 minutes, and read.

Results
A positive test shows definite fibrin strands. Clear or opalescent tubes are read as negative.

References
Kowalski, 1968
Seaman, 1970

Ethanol gelation test
Principle

Like protamine, ethanol added to plasma that contains soluble fibrin monomers causes them to aggregate, and a visible gel is formed.

Reagent
1. Ethyl alcohol, 50% (v/v)

Method
1. Obtain platelet-poor citrated plasma (9 parts venous blood plus 1 part 0.109M citrate) from the patient and from a normal donor.
2. To 0.5 ml of plasma, add 0.15 ml of 50% ethyl alcohol. Mix and read at intervals of 5 minutes at room temperature.

Results

Visible gel formation, usually within a few minutes, is read as a positive test. The formation of a granular precipitate is read as negative.

References
Breen and Tullis, 1968
Godal and Abilgaard, 1966

Fibrinolysis (screening)

If an excess of fibrinolytic substance is present in blood, the formation of the fibrin clot will be impaired, and the clot will quickly lyse after incubation at 37° C. Lysis of a clot within an hour after the blood is drawn is indicative of a high titer of fibrinolysins. In our laboratory, one or two tubes of blood from the venous coagulation time are kept at 37° C. These are observed periodically for fibrinolytic activity as well as for clot retraction (Fig. A-15).

The following is a more sensitive test for the presence of fibrinolysins. The specimens of plasma to be tested should be fresh.

Reagents and equipment
1. Water bath at 37° ± 1° C
2. Ice bath
3. Sodium citrate, 0.109M
4. 12 × 75 mm glass test tubes
5. Graduated centrifuge tubes
6. Syringes and large-gauge needles
7. Thrombin* 1,000-unit vials dissolved in 10 ml saline solution (100 units/ml)
8. Fibrinogen,† two vials

---

*Ortho Pharmaceutical Corp., Raritan, N.J.

*Parke, Davis & Co., Detroit, Mich.
†General Diagnostics Div. Warner-Lambert Co., Morris Plains, N.J.

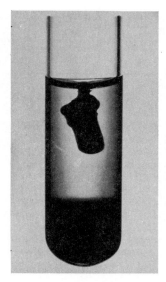

Fig. A-15. Clot retraction in hypofibrinogenemia and excessive fibrinolysin. Note that the small clot reflects the low concentration of fibrinogen, while the "fallout" of red cells that falls to the bottom reflects increased lysis of the clot.

a. Dissolve each vial in 2 ml distilled water and filter before use.
b. This solution contains 300 mg% of fibrinogen.

Method

1. Obtain 9 ml of blood from the patient and mix with 1 ml of 0.109M sodium citrate. Collect just before use and keep the tube of blood chilled in an ice bath.
2. Collect blood from a normal person in the same manner.
3. Separate the plasmas at once by centrifugation for 5 minutes at 2,000 to 2,500 rpm at 4° C. Transfer the plasmas to test tubes in the ice bath.
4. Into 12 × 75 mm test tubes at 37° C place:

   Tube 1: 0.5 ml of normal plasma + 0.5 ml of patient's plasma
   Tube 2: 1.0 ml of normal plasma (control)
   Tube 3: 0.5 ml of fibrinogen solution + 0.5 ml of patient's plasma
   Tube 4: 1 ml of fibrinogen solution (control)

5. To each of the four tubes, add 0.1 ml (10 units) of the thrombin solution.

Results

Fibrin clots should form within a few seconds after the thrombin is added.

Tube Nos. 2 and 4 are control tubes. Lysis in tube No. 2 will be slow compared with lysis in tube No. 1 when the patient's plasma contains increased fibrinolysin. Lysis in tube No. 3 is faster than that in tube No. 1, since fibrinogen contains no antifibrinolysin. There should be no lysis in tube No. 4.

Euglobulin lysis time (fibrinolysin activity)
Principle

This test is based on the fact that the plasma euglobulins contain all the essential factors necessary for clotting and fibrinolysis, but the greatest part of antifibrinolysin is eliminated during the process of plasma preparation. The clotted fraction of human plasma invariably undergoes spontaneous lysis during incubation at 37° C.

When increased fibrinolysin is present in the test plasma, the lysis time will be shortened, the time dependent on the amount present. The test will detect even slight amounts of increased fibrinolysins and is not inhibited by the presence of heparin.

Materials and reagents

1. Sodium citrate, 0.109M
2. Barbital acetate buffer, pH 7.42
   a. 9.714 Gm sodium acetate trihydrate
   b. 14.7 Gm disodium diethyl barbiturate
   c. qs 500 ml H_2O
3. Buffered physiologic saline solution
   a. Mix 1 part sodium barbital acetate buffer and 4 parts 0.85% NaCl.
4. Thrombin*
   a. Dissolve 1,000 NIH units in 5 ml 50% glycerol solution.
   b. Distribute in small amounts and store in deep freeze.
5. Carbon dioxide (pure), obtained by means of a two-stage reduction valve
6. Centrifuge tubes, 12-ml graduated (preferably siliconized) and 40-ml tubes (not siliconized; may or may not be graduated)
7. Water bath, constant temperature at 37° C

Method

1. To 0.5 ml of 0.109M sodium citrate in a 12-ml centrifuge tube, add 4.5 ml venous blood.
2. Mix blood and anticoagulant by gentle inversion and centrifuge immediately at 1,000 g for 4 minutes.
3. Transfer plasma to a clean, dry test tube.
4. To a 50-ml Erlenmeyer flask containing 15 ml distilled water, add 1 ml of the test plasma, mixing carefully with pipet.
5. Allow a stream of CO_2 to flow over the surface of the mixture for 4 minutes, slowly swirling the flask during the entire time. This may be done by hand or with a magnetic stirrer. *Avoid excessive foaming.*
6. Transfer the mixture to a 40-ml centrifuge tube and spin for 3 minutes at 1,000 g.
7. Discard the supernate, invert the tube, and allow to drain for 2 to 4 minutes.
8. Wipe the interior walls of the tube dry without disturbing the euglobulin sediment.
9. To the sediment, add 1 ml of buffered saline solution and stir the mixture, using a siliconized glass rod. After about 1 minute, the euglobulins are dissolved, and an opalescent solution results. *The next steps must be performed quickly to avoid spontaneous clotting of the euglobulin solution.*
10. Transfer 0.3 ml of the mixture into each of two 10 × 75 mm test tubes.
11. To each tube, add 0.01 ml to the thrombin solution by blowing in carefully. Invert tubes once. Clotting occurs within a few seconds.
12. Stopper tubes and place in the water bath. Observe every 15 minutes for lysis of the clots.

Results and interpretation

Normal range for lysis—over 2 hours. Lysis in less than 2 hours indicates increased fibrinolytic activity. The shorter the lysis time, the more powerful the fibrinolytic activity.

The lysis of the euglobulin clot is easily recognized; the end

---

*Parke, Davis & Co., Detroit, Mich.

point is complete dissolution of the clot, with little debris remaining in the bottom of the tube.

The test should be performed immediately after venipuncture because there is a loss of activity if the plasma is stored. The loss of activity is reduced, but not completely checked, when the plasma is frozen.

Reference
von Kaulla and Schultz, 1952

Heparin assay
Principle
The assay of heparin in plasma is based on the neutralization of the anticoagulant activity of heparin by protamine sulfate.

Equipment
1. Fibrometer
2. Pipets, 1.0 ml & 0.1 ml

Reagents
1. Heparin sodium solution (1000 IU/ml)*
2. Protamine sulfate, stock solution (10 mg/ml)†
3. Imidazole-buffered saline (0.85% NaCl), pH 7.4
4. Thrombin‡
5. Normal citrate plasma, lyophilized§

Method
1. Standardization of protamine sulfate versus heparin units
   a. Dilute thrombin with saline so that it clots normal plasma in 18 to 20 seconds (0.1 ml of saline + 0.1 ml of normal citrated plasma + 0.1 ml dilute thrombin at 37° C).
   b. Dilute the stock heparin solution 1:10 in normal citrate plasma, giving a heparin concentration of 100 IU/ml.
   c. Prepare dilutions of protamine sulfate in buffered saline.

	Protamine sulfate (ml)	Buffered saline (ml)	Protamine concentration
Sol. A:	2 ml stock	8.0	2.0 mg/ml
	1.3 ml sol A	0.7	1.3 mg/ml
	1.2 ml sol A	0.8	1.2 mg/ml
	1.1 ml sol A	0.9	1.1 mg/ml
Sol. B:	4 ml sol A	4.0	1.0 mg/ml
	1.8 ml sol B	0.2	0.9 mg/ml
	1.6 ml sol B	0.4	0.8 mg/ml
	1.4 ml sol B	0.6	0.7 mg/ml

   d. Add 0.1 ml of the heparin-plasma mixture to each of eight Fibro-cups. To each cup add 0.1 ml of the protamine sulfate solutions given above. Incubate at 37° C for 1 minute.

*The Upjohn Co., Kalamazoo, Mich.
†Eli Lilly and Co., Indianapolis, Ind.
‡Fibrindex, Ortho Pharmaceutical Corp., Raritan, N.J.
§General Diagnostics, Div. Warner-Lambert Co., Morris Plains, N.J.

Table A-3. Preparation of protamine sulfate solution in buffered saline

Protamine		Buffer	Protamine (mg/ml)	Heparin (U/ml)
Stock 1:	Undiluted	0. ml	10.0	910
Stock 2:	1.0 ml stock No. 1 + 9.0 ml		1.0	91.0
Stock 3:	1.0 ml stock No. 2 + 9.0 ml		0.10	9.1
	1.6 ml stock No. 3 + 0.4 ml		0.08	7.28
	1.2 ml stock No. 3 + 0.8 ml		0.06	5.46
	1.1 ml stock No. 3 + 0.9 ml		0.055	5.05
	1.0 ml stock No. 3 + 1.0 ml		0.05	4.55
	0.9 ml stock No. 3 + 1.1 ml		0.045	4.09
	0.8 ml stock No. 3 + 1.2 ml		0.04	3.6
	0.7 ml stock No. 3 + 1.3 ml		0.035	3.18
	0.6 ml stock No. 3 + 1.4 ml		0.03	2.7
	0.5 ml stock No. 3 + 1.5 ml		0.025	2.27
	0.4 ml stock No. 3 + 1.6 ml		0.020	1.82
Stock 4:	1.0 ml stock No. 3 + 9.0 ml		0.010	0.91
	1.6 ml stock No. 4 + 0.4 ml		0.008	0.73
	1.2 ml stock No. 4 + 0.8 ml		0.006	0.55
	0.8 ml stock No. 4 + 1.2 ml		0.004	0.36
	0.4 ml stock No. 4 + 1.6 ml		0.002	0.18

   e. To each cup add 0.1 ml of the standardized thrombin solution (37° C). Activate the Fibrometer simultaneously and determine the clotting time.
   f. The end point is the lowest concentration of protamine sulfate that gives a clotting time closest to the standardized thrombin time. The specific activity of heparin varies with the preparation, so it is best to calculate the amount of protamine required by titration. In our laboratory, 1 mg of protamine sulfate neutralized 91 IU of heparin.
2. Assay of unknown plasma
   a. Prepare protamine sulfate solutions in buffered saline as shown in Table A-3. The units of heparin neutralized by each concentration of protamine sulfate (based on 91 IU heparin/1 mg protamine) are also shown.
   b. Add 0.1 ml of unknown plasma to 0.1 ml of each protamine sulfate solution in a Fibro-cup and incubate at 37° C for 1 minute.
   c. To each cup add 0.1 ml of standardized thrombin solution (37° C) and activate Fibrometer simultaneously. Determine the end point (the lowest protamine sulfate concentration that corrects clotting time closest to the standardized thrombin time). After this point is reached, the clotting times may become longer because excess protamine has anticoagulant properties.
   d. From Table A-3, calculate the heparin IU/ml in unknown plasma.

References

Abaidoo KJR (1974) Extrarenal lipid inhibitors of human erythropoietin, Acta Haematol **52**:193

Aballi AJ and De Lamerens S (1962) Coagulation changes in the neonatal period and in early infancy, Pediatr Clin North Am **9**:785

Abbott WM et al (1977) The relationship of heparin source to the incidence of delayed hemorrhage, J Surg Res **22**:593

Abbrecht PH and Greene JA Jr (1966) Serum erythropoietin after renal homotransplantation, Ann Intern Med **65**:908

Abdella PM et al (1977) Glycosylation of hemoglobin S by reducing sugars and its effect on gelation, Biochim Biophys Acta **490**:462

Abeles M et al (1979) Eosinophilic fasciitis: a clinicopathologic study, Arch Intern Med **139**:586

Abelson NM (1974) Topics in blood banking, Philadelphia, Lea & Febiger, p 133

Åberg H and Nilsson IM (1972) Recurrent thrombosis in a young woman with a circulating anticoagulant directed against factors XI and XII, Acta Med Scand **192**:419

Abernathy MR (1966) Döhle bodies associated with umcomplicated pregnancy, Blood **27**:380

Abildgaard CF et al (1967) Factor-VIII (antihaemophilic factor) activity in sickle-cell anaemia, Br J Haematol **13**:19

Abildgaard CF and Harrison J (1974) Fletcher factor deficiency: family study and detection, Blood **43**:641

Abildgaard CF et al (1976) Prothrombin complex concentrate (Konyne) in the treatment of hemophilic patients with factor VIII inhibitors, J Pediatr **88**:200

Abilgaard U (1967) Purification of two progressive antithrombins of human plasma, Scand J Clin Lab Invest **19**:190

Ablin RJ et al (1972) Tissue- and species-specific antibodies in antithymocyte globulin, Transplantation **13**:306

Abramov A et al (1980) Hb Shaare Zedek (alpha 56 E5 lys → glu), FEBS Lett **113**:235

Abramson N and Schur PH (1972) The IgG subclasses of red cell antibodies and relationship to monocyte binding, Blood **40**:500

Abramson N et al (1970) The interaction between human monocytes and red cells. Specificity for IgG subclasses and IgG fragments, J Exp Med **132**:1207

Abramson N et al (1974) Post-transfusion purpura: immunologic aspects and therapy, N Engl J Med **291**:1163

Abramson N et al (1976) Immune markers in adult leukemia, Am J Clin Pathol **66**:111

Ackerman BD (1969) Infantile pyknocytosis in Mexican-American infants, Am J Dis Child **117**:417

Ackerman GA and Bellios NC (1955) A study of the morphology of the living cells of blood and bone marrow in vital films with the phase contrast microscope. I. Normal blood and bone marrow. II. Blood and bone marrow from various hematologic dyscrasias, Blood **10**:3, 1183

Ackerman GA and Clark MA (1971) Ultrastructural localization of peroxidase activity in human basophil leukocytes, Acta Haematol **45**:280

Ackroyd JF (1949) Three cases of thrombocytopenic purpura occurring after rubella, with review of purpura associated with infections, Q J Med **18**:299

Ackroyd JF (1953) Allergic purpura, including purpura due to foods, drugs, and infections, Am J Med **14**:605

Adam E et al (1974) Type B hepatitis antigen and antibody among prostitutes and nuns: a study of possible venereal transmission, J Infect Dis **129**:317

Adams JF (1968) The clinical and metabolic consequences of total gastrectomy. II. Anemia. Metabolism of iron, vitamin B_{12}, and folic acid, Scand J Gastroenterol **3**:145

Adams JF and Boddy K (1968) Metabolic equilibrium of tracer and natural vitamin B_{12}, J Lab Clin Med **72**:392

Adams JG et al (1972) Biosynthesis of hemoglobin Ann Arbor: evidence for catabolic and feedback regulation, Science **176**:1427

Adams JG et al (1974) Hemoglobin Rush (beta 101 [G3] glutamine): a new unstable hemoglobin causing mild hemolytic anemia, Blood **43**:261

Adams JG III et al (1975) Hemoglobin J Altgeld Gardens (beta 92 [F8] his → asp): a new hemoglobin variant involving a substitution of the proximal histidine, Proc Am Soc Hematol 18th Meeting, Dallas, Texas

Adams JG et al (1978) Hemoglobin Indianapolis: post-translational degradation of an unstable beta chain variant producing a phenotype of severe heterozygous beta thalassemia, Clin Res **26**:501A

Adams JG and Heller P (1973) Hemoglobin Arlington Park (beta 6 glu → lys 95 lys → glu): electrophoretically "silent" hemoglobin variant with two amino acid substitutions in the same polypeptide chain, Blood **42**:990

Adams JG III and Steinberg MH (1977) Alpha-thalassemia, Am J Hematol **2**:317

Adams KH (1973) A theory for the shape of the red blood cell, Biophys J **13**:1049

Adams RW and Elmore DT (1971) The kinetics of hydrolysis of synthetic substrates by bovine factor Xa, Biochem J **124**:66p

Adamson JW et al (1966) Erythropoietin excretion in normal man, Blood **28**:354

Adamson JW (1968) The kidney and erythropoiesis, Am J Med **44**:725

Adamson JW and Fialkow PJ (1978) The pathogenesis of myeloproliferative syndromes, Br J Haematol **38**:299

Adamson JW and Finch CA (1970) Erythropoietin and the regulation of erythropoiesis in DiGuglielmo's syndrome, Blood **36**:590

Adamson JW et al (1973) Recessive familial erythropoiesis: aspects of marrow regulation in two families, Blood **41**:641

Adamson JW et al (1976) Polycythemia vera: stem-cell and probable clonal origin of the disease, N Engl J Med **295**:913

Adamson JW et al (1978) Analysis of erythropoiesis by erythroid colony formation in culture, Blood Cells **4**:89

Adelson E et al (1961) The platelet as a sponge: a review, Blood **17**:767

Addison GM et al (1972) An immunoradiometric assay for ferritin in the serum of normal subjects and patients with iron deficiency and iron overload, J Clin Pathol **25**:326

Adinolfi M (1970) Levels of two components of complement C'$_4$ and C'$_3$ in human fetal and newborn sera, Dev Med Child Neurol **12**:307

Adinolfi M (1977) Human complement: onset and site of synthesis during fetal life, Am J Dis Child **131**:1015

Adler WH and Smith RT (1969) In vitro stimulation of mouse spleen cell suspensions, Fed Proc **28**:813

Adner MM et al (1969) Used of "compatible" platelet transfusion in treatment of congenital isoimmune thrombocytopenic purpura, N Engl J Med **280**:244

Afifi AM (1974) Spontaneous haemophilia in a genotypically normal female, Acta Haemat **52**:112

Aggeler PM et al (1952) PTC factor deficiency: a previously undescribed hemophilia-like disease due to a deficiency of a heretofore unknown thromboplastin component, Am J Med **13**:90

Aguilar MJ et al (1956) Syndrome of congenital absence of the spleen with associated cardiovascular and gastroenteric anomalies, Circulation **14**:520

Ahern EJ et al (1970) Haemoglobin F Jamaica (alpha 2 gamma 2 61 lys → glu: 136 ala), Br J Haematol **18**:369

Ahern EJ et al (1972) Further characterization of haemoglobin F. Texas I gamma 5 glutamic acid → lysine: gamma 136 alanine, Biochim Biophys Acta **271**:61

Ahern E et al (1975) Haemoglobin F Victoria Jubilee (alpha 2 A gamma 2 80 asp → tyr), Biochim Biophys Acta **393**:188

Ahern E et al (1976a) Haemoglobin Caribbean beta 91 (F7) leu → arg: a mildy unstable haemoglobin with low oxygen affinity, FEBS Lett **69**:99

Ahern E et al (1976b) Haemoglobin Spanish town alpha 27 glu → val (B8), Biochim Biophys Acta **427**:530

Ahlborg B and Ahlborg G (1970) Exercise leukocytosis with and without beta-adrenergic blockade, Acta Med Scand **187**:241

Aiach M et al (1973) Dysfibrinogénémies acquises et affections hépatiques: a propos de 30 observations, Sem Hop Paris **49**:183

Aikawa T et al (1978) Seroconversion from hepatitis Be antigen to anti-HBe in acute hepatitis B virus infection, N Engl J Med **298**:439

Ainley NJ and Lamb DC (1961) Megaloblastic anaemia following operations on the small intestine, Br J Surg **48**:608

Aisen P (1974) The role of transferrin in iron transport, Br J Haematol **26**:159

Aisenberg AC (1972) Updated Hodgkin's disease. Value of immunologic testing, JAMA **222**:1301

Aisenberg AC and Block KJ (1972) Immunoglobulins on the surface of neoplastic lymphocytes, N Engl J Med **287**:272

Aisenberg AC and Long JC (1975) Lymphocyte surface characteristics in malignant lymphoma, Am J Med **58**:300

Aisenberg AC et al (1973a) Cell-surface immunoglobulins in chronic lymphocytic leukemia and allied disorders, Am J Med **55**:184

Aisenberg AC et al (1973b) Reaction of normal human lympho-

cytes and chronic lymphocytic leukemia cells with antithymocyte antiserum, Blood **41**:417

Aiuti F et al (1974) Lymphocyte membrane markers in acute lymphoblastic leukaemia, Br J Haematol **27**:635

Ajlouni K and Doeblin TD (1974) The syndrome of hepatitis and aplastic anaemia, Br J Haematol **27**:345

Aksoy M (1960) The hemoglobin E syndromes. I. Hemoglobin E in Eti-Turks, Blood **15**:606

Aksoy M (1963a) The combination of hereditary elliptocytosis with heterozygous beta-thalassemia. Study of a Turkish Family, Acta Haematol **30**:215

Aksoy M (1963b) The first observation of homozygous hemoglobin S—alpha thalassemia disease and two types of sickle cell—thalassemia disease: (a) sickle cell—alpha thalassemia disease, (b) sickle cell—beta thalassemia disease, Blood **22**:757

Aksoy M and Erdem S (1967) Decrease in the concentration of haemoglobin A$_2$ during erythroleukemia, Nature **213**:522

Aksoy M and Erdem S (1978) Followup study on the mortality and the development of leukemia in 44 pancytopenic patients with chronic exposure to benzene, Blood **52**:285

Aksoy M et al (1972) Hemoglobin Istanbul: substitution of glutamine for histidine in a proximal histidine (F8 [92] beta), J Clin Invest **51**:2380

Aksoy M et al (1974a) Combination of hereditary elliptocytosis and hereditary spherocytosis, Clin Genet **6**:46

Aksoy M et al (1974b) Leukemia in shoe-workers exposed chronically to benzene, Blood **44**:837

Alami SY et al (1969) Lymphosarcoma with two serum IgG M components of different L chain types, Am J Clin Pathol **51**:185

Alarcón-Segovia D (1969) Drug-induced lupus syndromes, Mayo Clin Proc **44**:664

Alarcón-Segovia D et al (1964) Presence of circulating antibodies to gluten and milk fractions in patients with nontropical sprue, Am J Med **36**:485

Alarcón-Segovia D et al (1967) Clinical and experimental studies on the hydralazine syndrome and its relationship to systemic lupus erythematosus, Medicine **46**:1

Albert E et al (1978) Nomenclature for factors of the HLA system, 1977, Bull WHO **56**:461

Alberti R et al (1974) A new haemoglobin variant: J-Rovigo alpha 53 (E-2) alanine → aspartic acid, Biochim Biophys Acta **342**:1

Alberti R et al (1978) Hb A$_2$-Adria (δ 51 Pro → Arg[D2]): a new δ chain variant found in association with beta thalassemia, Hemoglobin **2**:171

Albritton EC (1940) Standard values in blood, ed 3, Philadelphia, WB Saunders Co

Albritton EC (1952) Standard values in blood, Philadelphia, WB Saunders Co

Alder A (1939) Ueber konstitutionell bedingte Granulationsveränderungen der Leukocyten, Dtsch Arch Klin Med **183**:372

Alder A and Schaub F (1952) Gleichzeitiges Vorkommen von Pelgerscher Kernanomalie und von Blutkrankheiten, Dtsch Med Wochenschr **77**:1290

Alexander B et al (1951) Congenital SPCA deficiency: hitherto unrecognized coagulation defect with hemorrhage rectified by serum and serum fractions, J Clin Invest **30**:596

Alexander B et al (1954) Congenital afibrinogenemia: a study of some basic aspects of coagulation, Blood **9**:843

Alexander EL and Wetzel B (1975) Human lymphocytes: similarity of B and T cell surface morphology, Science **188**:732

Alexandre P et al (1975) Maladie de Willebrand et agrégation plaquettaire en présence de ristocétine, Blut **31**:87

Alexanian R (1966) Urinary excretion of erythropoietin in normal men and women, Blood **28**:344

Alexanian R (1969) Erythropoietin and erythropoiesis in anemic man following androgens, Blood **33**:564

Alexanian R and Donohue DM (1965) Neutrophilic granulocyte kinetics in normal man, J Appl Physiol **20**:803

Alexanian R et al (1968) Melphalan therapy for plasma cell myeloma, Blood **31**:1

Alford CA et al (1967) A correlative immunologic, microbiologic, and clinical approach to the diagnosis of acute and chronic infections in newborn infants, N Engl J Med **277**:437

Alfrey CP Jr et al (1967) Characteristics of ferritin isolated from human marrow, spleen, liver and reticulocytes, J Lab Clin Med **70**:419

Ali SY (1967) Purification and properties of tissue activator of plasminogen, Biochem J **104**:1p

Ali MAM et al (1978) Serum ferritin concentration and bone marrow iron stores: a prospective study, Can Med Assoc J **118**:945

Ali NO and Janes WO (1979) Malignant myelosclerosis (acute myelofibrosis): report of two cases following cytotoxic chemotherapy, Cancer **43**:1211

Alkjaersig N et al (1975) Association between oral contraceptive use and thromboembolism: a new approach to its investigation based on plasma fibrinogen chromatography, Am J Obstet Gynecol **122**:199

Allain JP and Krieger GR (1975) Prothrombin-complex concentrate in the treatment of classical haemophilia with factor VIII antibody, Lancet **2**:1203

Allan N et al (1965) Three haemoglobins K: Woolwich, an abnormal, Cameroon and Ibadan, two unusual variants of human haemoglobin A, Nature (London) **208**:658

Allansmith M and Bergstresser P (1968) Sequence of immunoglobulin changes resulting from an attack of infectious mononucleosis, Am J Med **44**:124

Allcock E (1961) Absorption of vitamin B_{12} in man following extensive resection of the jejunum, ileum, and colon, Gastroenterology **40**:81

Allen DM et al (1968) Oxymetholone therapy in aplastic anemia, Blood **32**:83

Allen DW and Jandl JH (1961) Oxidative hemolysis and precipitation of hemoglobin. II. Role of thiols in oxidant drug action, J Clin Invest **40**:454

Allen EL et al (1973) Acute myelomonocytic leukemia with macroglobulinemia, Bence Jones proteinuria, and hypercalcemia, Cancer **32**:121

Allen FH Jr et al (1958) M^g, a new blood group antigen in the MNS system, Vox Sang **3**:81

Allen TD (1964) Sickle cell disease and hematuria: a report of 29 cases, J Urol **91**:177

Allison AC (1954) Protection afforded by sickle-cell trait against subtertian malarial infection, Br Med J **1**:290

Allison AC (1957) The binding of haemoglobin by plasma proteins (haptoglobins): its bearing on the "renal threshold" for haemoglobin and aetiology of haemoglobinuria, Br Med J **2**:1137

Allison AC (1964) Polymorphism and natural selection in human populations, Cold Spring Harbor Symp Quant Biol **29**:137

Ally AI et al (1980) Thromboxane A2 in blood vessel walls and its physiological significance: relevance to thrombosis and hypertension, Prostaglandins Med **4**:431

Almer L-O and Janzon L (1975) Low vascular fibrinolytic activity in obesity, Thromb Res **6**:171

Al-Mondhiry HRB et al (1975) Fibrinogen "New York"—an abnormal fibrinogen associated with thromboembolism: functional evaluation, Blood **45**:607

Alonso K et al (1972) Thymic alymphoplasia and congenital aleukocytosis (reticular dysgenesia), Arch Pathol **94**:179

Alper CA et al (1970) Increased susceptibility to infection associated with abnormalities of complement-mediated functions and of the third component of complement (C3), N Engl J Med **282**:349

Alperin JB (1967) Folic acid deficiency complicating sickle cell anemia. A study on the response to titrating doses of folic acid, Arch Intern Med **120**:298

Al-Rashid RA and Spangler J (1971) Neonatal copper deficiency, N Engl J Med **285**:841

Alsted G (1937) Pernicious anaemia after nitric acid corrosion of the stomach, Lancet **232**:76

Altay C et al (1976) Hemoglobin Hacettepe or alpha 2 beta 2 127 (H5) gln → glu, Biochim Biophys Acta **434**:1

Altay C et al (1978) Hemoglobin S and some other hemoglobinopathies in Eti-Turks, Hum Hered **28**:56

Alter AA et al (1962) Leukocyte alkaline phosphatase in mongolism: a possible chromosome marker, J Clin Invest **41**:1341

Alter BP and Nathan DG (1979) Red cell aplasia in children, Arch Dis Child **54**:263

Alter HJ (1975) Hepatitis B surface antigen and the health care professions. In Greenwalt TJ and Jamieson GA (Eds): Transmissible disease and blood transfusion, New York, Grune & Stratton, Inc, p 115

Alter HJ et al (1975) Clinical and serological analysis of transfusion-associated hepatitis, Lancet **2**:838

Altman LC et al (1973) A human mononuclear leukocyte chemotactic factor: characterization, specificity, and kinetics of production by homologous leukocytes, J Immunol **110**:801

Altman LC et al (1974) Abnormalities of chemotactic lymphokine synthesis and mononuclear leukocyte chemotaxis in Wiskott-Aldrich syndrome, J Clin Invest **54**:486

Altman PL and Dittmer DS (Eds) (1961) Blood and other body fluids, Washington, DC, Federation of American Societies for Experimental Biology

Altman PL and Dittmer DS (1964) Biology data book, Federation of American Societies for Experimental Biology, Washington, DC, pp 267-268

Alving BM et al (1978) Hypotension associated with prekallikrein activator (Hageman-factor fragments) in plasma protein fraction, N Engl J Med **299**:66

Alwall N (1946) On hereditary non-hemolytic bilirubinemia, Acta Med Scand **123**:560

Amare M et al (1978) Aplastic anemia associated with bone marrow suppressor T-cell hyperactivity: successful treatment with antithymocyte globulin, Am J Hematol **5**:25

Amato D et al (1976) Granulopoiesis in severe congenital neutropenia, Blood **47**:531

Amato M (1946) Rilievi anamnestico-clinici, ematologici e biochemici e considerazione pathogenetiche osservate in bambini della prima infanzia, Pediatria **54**:71

Amazon K and Rywlin AM (1980) Ceroid granulomas of the gallbladder, Am J Clin Pathol **73**:123

Ambrus CM and Ambrus JL (1959) Regulation of the leukocyte level, Ann NY Acad Sci **77**:445

American National Red Cross Blood Services Operation Report: Fiscal year 1977-78 (1979), Washington DC, American National Red Cross

Amezcua JL et al (1979) Prolonged paradoxical effect of aspirin on platelet behavior and bleeding time in man, Thromb Res **16**:69

Amman R and Martin H (1961) Blutmastzellen und Heparin, Acta Haematol **25**:209

Ammann AJ et al (1969) Immunoglobulin E deficiency in ataxia-telangiectasia, N Engl J Med **281**:469

Amorosi EL (1965) Hypersplenism, Semin Hematol **2**:249

Amorosi EL and Ultmann JE (1966) Thrombotic thrombocytopenic purpura, Medicine **45**:139

Amos DB (1975) Nomenclature for factors of the HLA system, Bull WHO **52**:261

Amris CJ and Ranek L (1965) A case of fibrin-stabilizing factor (FSF) deficiency, Thromb Diath Haemorrh **14**:322

Amsellem M et al (1978) Dysfibrinogénémie congénitale: deux observations, Nouv Presse Med **7**:3745

Anayo-Galindo R et al (1976) Soluble fibrin complexes in coronary disease, Thromb Res **9**:153

Andersen BR and Terry WD (1968) Gamma G₄-globulin antibody causing inhibition of clotting factor VIII, Nature **217**:174

Andersen J (1960) An inheritable B-like character in persons of blood group A, Blood **16**:1163

Anderson HD et al (1966) The clinical use of dried fibrinogen (human) and the risk of transmitting hepatitis by its administration, Transfusion, **6**:234

Anderson LG and Talal N (1971) The spectrum of benign to malignant lymphoproliferation in Sjögren's syndrome, Clin Exp Immunol **10**:199

Anderson R et al (1960) Hereditary spherocytosis in the deer mouse. Its similarity to the human disease, Blood **15**:491

Anderssen N (1964) The activity of lactic dehydrogenase in megaloblastic anemia, Scand J Haematol **1**:212

Andersson L-O et al (1975) Purification and characterization of human factor IX, Thromb Res **7**:451

Andreasen E and Christensen S (1949) The rate of mitotic activity in the lymphoid organs of the rat, Anat Rec **103**:401

Andresen PH (1948) The blood group system L. A new blood group L₂. A case of epistasy within the blood groups, Acta Pathol Microbiol Scand **25**:728

Andrews EJ (1960) Moon talk: the cyclic periodicity of postoperative hemorrhage, J Fla Med Assoc **46**:1362

Angle RM and Alt HL (1950) Thrombocytopenic purpura complicating infectious mononucleosis. Report of a case and serial platelet counts during infectious mononucleosis, Blood **5**:449

Angles-Cano E et al (1979) Predisposing factors to thrombosis in systemic lupus erythematosus: possible relation to endothelial cell damage, J Lab Clin Med **94**:312

Anner RM and Drewinko B (1977) Frequency and significance of bone marrow involvement by metastatic solid tumors, Cancer **39**:1337

Ansley HR et al (1971) Leucocyte esterase cytochemistry, J Histochem Cytochem **19**:711

Ansell J and Deykin D (1980) Heparin-induced thrombocytopenia and recurrent thromboembolism, Am J Hematol **8**:325

Arakawa ET (1960) Radiation dosimetry in Hiroshima and Nagasaki atomic-bomb survivors, N Engl J Med **263**:488

Arakawa T (1970) Congenital defects in folate utilization, Am J Med **48**:594

Arcasoy A et al (1974) A new haemoglobin J from Turkey—hb Ankara (beta 10 [A7] ala → asp), FEBS Lett **42**:121

Archer GT et al (1965) Studies on rat eosinophil peroxidase, Biochim Biophys Acta **99**:96

Ardeman S et al (1963) The Pelger-Huët anomaly and megaloblastic anemia, Blood **22**:472

Ardeman S et al (1966) Addisonian pernicious anemia and intrinsic factor autoantibodies in thyroid disorders, Q J Med **35**:421

Arends T et al (1977) Haemoglobin North Shore-Caracas beta 134 (H12) valine → glumatic acid, FEBS Lett **80**:261

Argani I and Kipkie GF (1965) The cellular origin of macroglobulins. A study of the protein-secreting cells in Waldenström's disease, Lab Invest **14**:720

Arias IM and London IM (1957) Bilirubin glucuronide formation in vitro: demonstration of a defect in Gilbert's disease, Science **126**:563

Armitage JO et al (1978) Diffuse histiocytic lymphoma complicating chronic lymphocytic leukemia, Cancer **41**:422

Arneson MA et al (1980) A new form of Ehlers-Danlos syndrome: fibronectin corrects defective platelet function, JAMA **244**:144

Arnon DI (1965) Ferrodoxin and photosynthesis: an iron-containing protein is a key factor in energy transfer during photosynthesis, Science **149**:1460

Arnone A (1972) X-ray diffraction study of binding of 2,3-diphosphoglycerate to human deoxyhaemoglobin, Nature **237**:146

Aronow S et al (1962) The medical consequences of thermonuclear war, N Engl J Med **266**:1126

Aronstam A et al (1976) Prophylaxis in haemophilia: a double-blind controlled trial, Br J Haematol **33**:81

Arseneau JC et al (1975) American Burkitt's lymphoma: a clinicopathologic study of 30 cases. I. Clinical factors relating to prolonged survival, Am J Med **58**:314

Arterberry JD et al (1964) Significance of hematoxylin bodies in lupus erythematosus cell preparations, JAMA **187**:389

Ascensao J et al (1976) Aplastic anaemia: evidence for an immunological mechanism, Lancet **1**:669

Aschoff L and Kiyono (1913) Zur Frage der grossen Mononukleären, Folia Haematol (Leipz) **15**:385

Aschoff L (1925) Das reticulo endotheliale System, Ergeb Inn Med Kinderheilkd **26**:1

Ashenhurst JB et al (1976) Hemolytic anemia due to anti-B in antihemophiliac factor concentrates, J Pediatr **88**:257

Ashley DJB (1957) Occurrence of sex chromatin in the cells of the blood and bone marrow in man, Nature **179**:969

Ashworth TR (1869) A case of cancer in which cells similiar to those in the tumours were seen in the blood after death, Aust Med J **14**:146

Aspegren N et al (1963) Basophil leukocytes in lesions of various dermatoses, Acta Derm Venereol (Stockh) **43**:544

Åstedt B (1972) Significance of placenta in depression of fibrinolytic activity during pregnancy, J Obstet Gynaecol Br Common **79**:205

Åstedt B et al (1973) Thrombosis and oral contraceptives: possible predisposition, Br Med J **4**:631

Aster RH (1965) Splenic platelet pooling as a cause of "hypersplenic" thrombocytopenia, Trans Assoc Am Physicians **78**:362

Aster RH (1969) Studies of the fate of platelets in rats and man, Blood **34**:117

Aster RH and Keene WR (1969) Sites of platelet destruction in idiopathic thrombocytopenic purpura, Br J Haematol **16**:61

Aster RH et al (1976) Studies to improve methods of short-term platelet preservation, Transfusion **16**:4

Astrup P and Rørth M (1973) Oxygen affinity of hemoglobin and red cell 2,3-diphosphoglycerate in hepatic cirrhosis, Scand J Clin Lab Invest **31**:311

Astrup P et al (1970) Dependency on acid-base status of oxyhemoglobin dissociation and 2,3-diphosphoglycerate level in human erythrocytes. II. In vivo studies, Scand J Clin Lab Invest **26**:47

Atkins HL et al (1963) Giant hemangioma in infancy with secondary thrombocytopenic purpura, Am J Roentgenol Radium Ther Nucl Med **89**:1062

Atwater J et al (1960) Sickling of erythrocytes in a patient with thalassemia—hemoglobin I disease, N Engl J Med **263**:1215

Auer J (1906) Some hitherto undescribed structures found in large lymphocytes of an acute leukemia, Am J Med Sci **131**:1002

Augener W et al (1971) The reaction of monomeric and aggregated immunoglobulins with C1, Immunochemistry **8**:1011

Austin RF and Desforges JF (1969) Hereditary elliptocytosis: an unusual presentation of hemolysis in the newborn associated with transient morphologic abnormalities, Pediatrics **44**:196

Ayvazian JH (1964) Xanthinuria and hemochromatosis, N Engl J Med **270**:18

Azar HA et al (1957) Malignant lymphoma and lymphatic leukemia associated with myeloma-type serum proteins, Am J Med **23**:239

Aznar J et al (1974) Fibrinogen Valencia. A new case of congenital dysfibrinogenemia, Thromb Diath Haemorrh **32**:564

Baadenhuijsen H et al (1971) Metabolic observations on platelets from patients with familial thrombopathic thrombocytopenia, Br J Haematol **20**:417

Babcock RB et al (1976) Heparin-induced immune thrombocytopenia, N Engl J Med **295**:237

Bach FH et al (1969) Agammaglobulinemic leukocytes—their in vitro reactivity. In Rieke WO (Ed): Proceedings of the fluid leukocyte culture conference, New York, Appleton-Century-Crofts

Bach ML et al (1973) β_2-Microglobulin: association with lymphocyte receptors, Science **182**:1350

Bachman R (1965) Studies on the serum γA-globulin level. III. The frequency of a-γA-globulinemia, Scand J Clin Lab Invest **17**:316

Bacigalupo A et al (1978) Lymphoid antigens on blast cells in the agranular metamorphosis of chronic myelogenous leukaemia, Acta Haematol **60**:280

Bader RA et al (1963) Polycythemia vera and arterial oxygen saturation, Am J Med **34**:435

Badet J et al (1978) α-N-acetyl-D-galactosaminyl and α-D-galactosyltransferase activities in sera of Cis AB blood group individuals, J Immunogenet **5**:221

Badr FM et al (1973) Haemoglobin P-Nilotic: containing a beta-delta chain, Nature New Biol **242**:107

Baehner RL (1975) Microbe ingestion and killing by neutrophils: normal mechanisms and abnormalities, Clin Haematol **4**:609

Baehner RL and Nathan DG (1968) Quantitative nitro-blue tetrazolium test in chronic granulomatous disease, N Engl J Med **278**:971

Baehner RL et al (1970) Correction of metabolic deficiencies in the leukocytes of patients with chronic granulomatous disease, J Clin Invest **49**:865

Baglioni C (1962) The fusion of two peptide chains in hemoglobin Lepore and its interpretation as a genetic deletion, Proc Natl Acad Sci USA **48**:1880

Baglioni C (1962a) The fusion of two peptide chains in hemoglobin Lepore and its interpretation as a genetic deletion, Proc Natl Acad Sci USA **48**:1880

Baglioni C (1962b) A chemical study of hemoglobin Norfolk, J Biol Chem **237**:69

Baglioni C (1962c) Abnormal human haemoglobins. VIII. Chemical studies on haemoglobin D, Biochim Biophys Acta **59**:437

Baglioni C and Ingram VM (1961) Abnormal human hemoglobins. V. Chemical investigation of haemoglobins A,G, C, X from one individual, Biochim Biophys Acta **48**:253

Baglioni C and Lehmann H (1962) Chemical heterogeneity of haemoglobin O, Nature **196**:229

Baglioni C and Weatherall DJ (1963) Abnormal human hemoglobins. IX. Chemistry of hemoglobin J Baltimore, Biochim Biophys Acta **78**:637

Baglioni C et al (1961) Genetic control of foetal and adult haemoglobin, Nature **189**:467

Bain B et al (1964) The development of large immature mononuclear cells in mixed leukocyte cultures, Blood **23**:108

Bainton DF (1975a) Neutrophil granules, Br J Haematol **29**:17

Bainton DF (1975b) Abnormal neutrophils in acute myelogenous leukemia: identification of subpopulations based on analysis of azurophil and specific granules, Blood Cells **1**:191

Bainton DF and Farquhar MG (1970) Segregation and packaging of granule enzymes in eosinophilic leukocytes, J Cell Biol **45**:54

Bainton DF and Finch CA (1964) The diagnosis of iron deficiency, Am J Med **37**:62

Bainton DF et al (1971) The development of neutrophilic polymorphonuclear leukocytes in human bone marrow. Origin and content of azurophilic and specific granules, J Exp Med **134**:907

Bainton DF et al (1977) Abnormalities in granule formation in acute myelogenous leukemia, Blood **49**:693

Baird I et al (1959) The pathogenesis of anaemia after partial gastrectomy. I Development of anaemia in relation to time after operation, blood loss, and diet, Q J Med **28**:21

Baird RN et al (1971) Red-blood-cell survival after splenectomy in congenital spherocytosis, Lancet **2**:1060

Bajaj SP and Mann KG (1973) Simultaneous purification of bovine prothrombin by trypsin-activated factor X, J Biol Chem **248**:7729

Bajoghli M (1961) Generalized lymphadenopathy and hepatosplenomegaly induced by diphenylhydantoin, Pediatrics **28**:943

Bakemeier RF and Leddy JP (1968) Erythrocyte autoantibody associated with alpha-methyldopa: heterogeneity of structure and specificity, Blood **32**:1

Baker H et al (1959) A microbiological method for detecting folic acid deficiency in man, Clin Chem **5**:275

Baker H et al (1964) Mechanisms of folic acid deficiency in nontropical sprue, JAMA **187**:119

Baker SJ (1972) Vitamin B_{12} and tropical sprue, Br J Haematol **23**:135

Baker WG et al (1964) Hypofibrinogenemic hemorrhage in acute myelogenous leukemia treated with heparin: with autopsy findings of widespread intravascular clotting. Ann Intern Med **61**:116

Bakshi SP et al (1967) Sausage cyanosis—acquired methemoglobinemic nitrite poisoning, N Engl J Med **277**:1072

Balcerzak SP et al (1968a) Diabetes mellitus and idiopathic hemodermatosis, Am J Med Sci **255**:53

Balcerzak SP et al (1968b) Discordant occurrence of pernicious anemia in identical twins, Blood **32**:701

Baldini M and Pannacciulli I (1960) The maturation rate of reticulocytes, Blood **15**:614

Baldini MG (1972a) Idiopathic thrombocytopenic purpura and the ITP syndrome, Med Clin North Am **56**:47

Baldini MG (1972b) Nature of the platelet defect in the Wiskott-Aldrich syndrome, Ann NY Acad Sci **201**:437

Baldini MG et al (1976) Permeability changes in the plasma and granular membrane of stored platelets. Their prevention for improved platelet preservation, Transfusion **16**:13

Ball EW et al (1968) Haemoglobin A_2': alpha 2 delta 2 16 glycine $\rightarrow$ arginine, Nature (London) **209**:1217

Ballard HS and Marcus AJ (1970) Hypercalcemia in chronic myelogenous leukemia, N Engl J Med **282**:663

Ballard HS et al (1970) A new variant of heavy-chain disease (μ-chain disease), N Engl J Med **282**:1060

Ballas SK et al (1977) Hemoglobin S-O Arab-thalassemia: globin synthesis and clinical picture, Hemoglobin **1**:651

Baltimore D (1976) Viruses, polymerases, and cancer, Science **192**:632

Bancroft WH et al (1972) Detection of additional antigenic determinants of hepatitis B antigen, J Immunol **109**:842

Banerjee RN and Narang RM (1967) Haematologic changes in malignancy, Br J Haematol **13**:829

Bang HU et al (1972) Plasma protein requirements for human platelet aggregation, Ann NY Acad Sci **201**:280

Bank A (1970) Globin chain synthesis in heterozygotes for beta chain mutations, J Lab Clin Med **76**:616

Bank A and Marks PA (1966) Excess α-chain synthesis relative to β-chain synthesis in thalassemia major and minor, Nature **212**:1198

Bank A et al (1968) Absolute rates of globin chain synthesis in thalassemia, Blood **31**:226

Banks PM et al (1975) American Burkitt's lymphoma: a clinicopathologic study of 30 cases. II. Pathologic correlations, Am J Med **58**:322

Bannerman RM and Renwick JH (1962) The hereditary elliptocytoses: clinical and linkage data, Ann Hum Genet **26**:23

Bannister WH et al (1972) Hemoglobin St Luke's or alpha 2 95 arg (G2) beta 2, Eur J Biochem **29**:301

Barbara JAJ et al (1977) A comparison of different methods of screening blood donations for HBsAg, Vox Sang **32**:4

Barbedo MMR and McCurdy PR (1974) Red cell life span in sickle cell trait, Acta Haematol **51**:339

Barclay GPT et al (1969) Abnormal haemoglobin in Zambia. A new haemoglobin Zambia alpha 60 (E9) lysine → asparagine, Br Med J **4**:595

Bard H (1973) Postnatal fetal and adult hemoglobin synthesis in early preterm newborn infants, J Clin Invest **52**:1789

Barem GH et al (1976) Altered C-terminal salt bridges in haemoglobin York cause high oxygen affinity, Nature **259**:155

Barker BE et al (1965) Mitogenic activity in *Phytolacca americana* (poke weed), Lancet **1**:170

Barker BE et al (1966) Peripheral blood plasmacytosis following accidental systemic exposure to *Phytolacca americana* (poke weed), Pediatrics **38**:490

Barker LF et al (1973) Antibody responses in viral hepatitis, type B, JAMA **223**:1005

Barker LF et al (1975) Viral hepatitis B detection and prophylaxis. In Greenwalt TJ and Jamieson GA (Eds): Transmissible disease and blood transfusion, New York, Grune & Stratton, Inc, p 81

Barker LF and Murray R (1971) Relationship of virus dose to incubation time of clinical hepatitis and time of appearance of hepatitis-associated antigen, Am J Med Sci **263**:27

Barkhan P et al (1964) Haemoglobin Lepore trait: an analysis of the abnormal haemoglobin, Br J Haematol **10**:437

Barkley KL et al (1965) Hemoglobin and packed cell volume in Negro and Caucasian subjects: a comparative study, South Med J **58**:1012

Barnabas J and Muller CJ (1962) Haemoglobin Lepore Hollandia, Nature (London) **194**:931

Barnard DR et al (1979) Coagulation studies in extremely premature infants, Pediatr Res **13**:1330

Barnes DWH and Loutit JF (1967) Haemopoietic cells in the peripheral blood, Lancet **2**:1138

Barnes HD (1958) Porphyria in South Africa: the faecal excretion of porphyrin, S Afr Med J **32**:680

Barnes HD (1963) Porphyria, Int Rev Trop Med **2**:197

Barnes MG et al (1972) A comprehensive screening program for hemoglobinopathies, JAMA **219**:701

Barnett EV and Rothfield NF (1969) The present status of antibody serology, Arthritis Rheum **12**:543

Barnett RN (1966) Interpretation of laboratory data, Israel J Med Sci **2**:519

Barnett RN (1979) Clinical laboratory statistics, Boston, Little, Brown & Co

Barnhart MI and Noonan SM (1973) Cellular control mechanisms for blood clotting proteins, Thromb Diath Haemorrh (supp) **54**:59

Barnhart MI and Riddle JM (1963) Cellular localization of profibrinolysin (plasminogen), Blood **21**:306

Barnhart MI et al (1980) Essential thrombocythemia in a child: platelet ultrastructure and function, Am J Hematol **8**:87

Baron S et al (1962) Antibody production by hypogammaglobulinemic patients, J Immunol **88**:443

Barr ML and Bertram EG (1949) A morphological distinction between neurons of the male and female, and the behavior of the nucleolar satellite during accelerated nucleoprotein synthesis, Nature **163**:676

Barreras L and Diggs LW (1964) Bicarbonates, pH, and percentage of sickled cells in venous blood of patients in sickle cell crisis, Am J Med Sci **247**:710

Barreras L et al (1968) Erythrocyte morphology in patients with sickle cell anemia and pulmonary emboli, JAMA **203**:569

Barrett-Connor E (1971) Bacterial infection and sickle cell anemia, Medicine **50**:97

Barrow ES et al (1979) The separation of Willebrand factor from VIII-related antigen, Br J Haematol **42**:455

Barrowcliffe TW (1980) Studies of heparin binding to antithrombin III by crossed immunoelectrophoresis, Thrombs Haemost **42**:1434

Barrowcliffe TW et al (1977) Anticoagulant activities of lung and mucous heparins, Thromb Res **12**:27

Barrowcliffe TW et al (1979) Anticoagulant activities of high and low molecular weight heparin fractions, Br J Haematol **41**:573

Bar-Shany S and Herbert V (1967) Transplacentally acquired antibody to intrinsic factor with vitamin B_{12} deficiency, Blood **30**:777

Barth WF et al (1965) Antibody deficiency syndrome. Selective immunoglobulin deficiency with reduced synthesis of gamma and alpha immunoglobulin polypeptide chains, Am J Med **39**:319

Bartman J et al (1967) Pigmented lipid histiocytosis and susceptibility to infection: ultrastructure of splenic histiocytes, Pediatrics **40**:1000

Barton EM (1959) Abnormal serum proteins as aids in diagnosis of rheumatoid arthritis and systemic lupus erythematosus, Med Clin North Am **43**:607

Barton JC and Conrad ME (1978) Current status of blastic transformation in chronic myelogenous leukemia, Am J Hematol **4**:281

Bartsch DC et al (1975) Acute non-lymphocytic leukemia. An adult cluster, JAMA **232**:1333

Bass DA and Szejda P (1979) Eosinophils versus neutrophils in host defense: killing of newborn larvae of *Trichinella spiralis* by human granulocytes in vitro, J Clin Invest **64**:1415

Bass DA et al (1980) Eosinopenia of acute infection: production of eosinopenia by chemotactic factors of acute inflammation, J Clin Invest **65**:1265

Bassen FA and Kornzweig AL (1950) Malformation of the erythrocytes in a case of atypical retinitis pigmentosa, Blood **5**:381

Basset P et al (1978) Isoelectric focusing of human hemoglobin: its application to screening, to the characterization of 70 variants, and to the study of modified fractions of normal hemoglobins, Blood **51**:971

Basten A and Beeson PB (1970) Mechanism of eosinophilia. II. Role of the lymphocyte, J Exp Med **131**:1288

Bastiaans MJS et al (1979) A new antigenic determinant on HBsAg; geographic and subtype distribution and association with HBeAg and anti-HBe, Vox Sang **37**:129

Bataille R et al (1980) Myeloma bone marrow acid phosphatase staining: a correlative study of 38 patients, Blood **55**:802

Bateman S et al (1978) Splenic red cell pooling: a diagnostic feature in polycythaemia, Br J Haematol **40**:389

Bateson EM and Lebroy T (1978) Clay eating by aboriginals of the northern territory, Med J Aust (Spec Suppl) **1**:1

Baugh CM and Krumdieck CL (1971) Naturally occurring folates, Ann NY Acad Sci **186**:7

Baugh CM et al (1975) Absorption of folic acid poly-γ-glutamates in dogs, J Nutr **105**:80

Baughan MA et al (1968) An unusual hematological syndrome

with pyruvate-kinase deficiency and thalassemia minor in kindreds, Acta Haematol **39**:345

Bauman AW and Swisher SH (1967) Hyporegenerative processes in hemolytic anemia, Semin Hematol **4**:265

Baumgartner HR et al (1971) Adhesion of blood platelets to subendothelial surface: distinct from adhesion to collagen, Experientia **27**:283

Baumgartner HR (1973) The role of blood flow in platelet adhesion fibrin deposition and formation of mural thrombi, Microvasc Res **5**:167

Baur EW (1968) Hb alpha 2 glu beta 2 (Hb I) in a Caucasian family: independent mutation or common origin? Humangenetik **6**:368

Bayer WL et al (1965) Purpura in congenital and acquired rubella, N Engl J Med **273**:1362

Bayer WL et al (1969) Acquired factor X deficiency in a Negro boy, Pediatrics **44**:1007

Bayer WL and Tegtmeier GE (1976) The blood donor: detection and magnitude of cytomegalovirus carrier states and the prevalence of cytomegalovirus antibody, Yale J Biol Med **49**:5

Bayrakci C et al (1964) A new fast hemoglobin, Proceedings of the Tenth Congress of the International Society of Haematology, Stockholm, Sweden

Bayrd ED et al (1965) Macroglobulinemia. Its recognition and treatment, JAMA **193**:724

Beal RW et al (1967) Neutrophil alkaline phosphatase in pregnancy, J Clin Pathol **20**:749

Beale D and Lehmann H (1965) Abnormal haemoglobins and the genetic code, Nature **207**:259

Beamish MR et al (1974) Transferrin iron, chelatable iron and ferritin in idiopathic haemochromatosis, Br J Haematol **27**:219

Beard ME and Allen DM (1967) Effect of antimicrobial agents on the *Lactobacillus casei* folate assay, Am J Clin Pathol **48**:401

Bearden JD et al (1974) Comparison of the diagnostic value of bone marrow biopsy and bone marrow aspiration in neoplastic disease, J Clin Pathol **27**:738

Bearman RM et al (1978a) Prolymphocytic leukemia: clinical, histopathological, and cytochemical observations, Cancer **42**:2360

Bearman RM et al (1978b) Hodgkin's disease, lymphocyte depletion type: a clinicopathologic study of 39 patients, Cancer **41**:293

Bearman RM et al (1979) Acute ("malignant") myelosclerosis, Cancer **43**:279

Beattie KM et al (1964) Blood group chimerism as a clue to generalized tissue mosaicism, Transfusion **4**:77

Beaumont C et al (1979) Serum ferritin as a possible marker of the hemochromatosis allele, N Engl J Med **301**:169

Beaven GH et al (1960) Studies on human foetal haemoglobin. II. Foetal haemoglobin levels in healthy children and adults in certain haematological disorders, Br J Haematol **6**:201

Beaven GH et al (1963) Occurrence of haemoglobin H in leukaemia, Nature **199**:1297

Beaven GH et al (1964) An abnormal haemoglobin (Lepore/Cyprus) resembling haemoglobin-Lepore and its interaction with thalassemia, Br J Haematol **10**:159

Beaven GH et al (1978) Occurrence of haemoglobin H in leukaemia: a further case of erythroleukaemia, Acta Haematol **59**:37

Beaver PC and Danaraj TJ (1958) Pulmonary ascariasis resembling eosinophilic lung, Am J Trop Med Hyg **7**:100

Beck DW et al (1979) An intrinsic coagulation pathway inhibitor in a 3-year-old child, Am J Clin Pathol **71**:470

Beck EA (1980) Idiopathic thrombocytopenia with giant platelets, Johns Hopkins Med J **146**:281

Beck EA and Lüdin H (1967) Reversible sideroachrestiche Storung bei Behandlung mit Chloramphenicol, Helv Med Acta **34**(supp 147):139

Beck E et al (1961) The influence of fibrin stabilizing factor on the growth of fibroblasts in vitro and wound healing, Thromb Diath Haemorrh **6**:485

Beck EA et al (1971) Functional evaluation of an inherited abnormal fibrinogen: fibrinogen "Baltimore," J Clin Invest **50**:1874

Beck JS (1969) Antinuclear antibodies: methods of detection and significance, Mayo Clin Proc **44**:600

Beck ML et al (1976) Unexpected limitations in the use of commercial antiglobulin reagents, Transfusion **16**:71

Beck WS (1962) The metabolic functions of vitamin B_{12}, N Engl J Med **266**:708, 765, 814

Becker AJ et al (1963) Cytological demonstration of the clonal nature of spleen colonies derived from transplanted mouse marrow cells, Nature **197**:452

Becker EL (1972) The relationship of the chemotactic behaviour of the complement-derived factors, C3a, C5a, and C567, and a bacterial chemotactic factor to their ability to activate the proesterase I of rabbit polymorphonuclear leukocytes, J Exp Med **135**:376

Becker KE et al (1973) Surface IgE on human basophils during histamine release, J Exp Med **138**:394

Bednar B et al (1964) Vascular pseudohemophilia associated with ceroid pigmentophagia in albinos, Am J Pathol **45**:283

Beeken WL (1968) Effect of five salicylate-containing compounds upon loss of ^{51}chromium labelled erythrocytes from the gastrointestinal tract of normal man, Gut **9**:475

Beeson PB and Bass DA (1977) The eosinophil, Philadelphia, WB Saunders Co, p 92

Begemann NH and Campagne A Van L (1952) Homozygous form of Pelger-Huët's nuclear anomaly in man, Acta Haematol **7**:295

Begg TB (1955) Sulfhemoglobinaemia, a report of five cases, Br Med J **1**:701

Behnke O et al (1971) Electron microscopical observations on actinoid and myosinoid filaments in blood platelets, J Ultrastruct Res **37**:351

Behrendt DM et al (1968) Postperfusion nonthrombocytopenic purpura. An uncommon sequel of open heart surgery, Am J Cardiol **22**:631

Beisel WR et al (1959) Absence of leukocyte alkaline phosphatase activity in hypophosphatasia, Blood **14**:975

Beksedic D et al (1975) Hb Serbia (alpha ^{112} [G19] his → arg), a new haemoglobin variant from Yugoslavia, FEBS Lett **58**:226

Belcher RW (1972) Ultrastructure and cytochemistry of lymphocytes in the genetic mucopolysaccharidoses, Arch Pathol **93**:1

Belkin GA (1967) Cocktail purpura. An unusual case of quinine sensitivity, Ann Intern Med **66**:583

Bell TG et al (1976) Decreased nucleotide and serotonin storage associated with defective function in Chediak-Higashi syndrome of cattle and human platelets, Blood **48**:175

Bellevue R et al (1975) Pseudohyperkalemia and extreme leukocytosis, J Lab Clin Med **85**:660

Bellingham AJ (1973) Ninth symposium on abnormal medicine: Proceedings of a conference at the Royal College of Physicians, Turnbridge Wells, Kent, Pitman Medical, p 253

Bellingham AJ (1974) The red cell in adaptation to anaemic hypoxia, Clin Haematol **3**:577

Bellingham AJ et al (1971) The role of hemoglobin affinity for oxygen and red-cell 2,3-diphosphoglycerate in the management of diabetic ketoacidosis, Trans Assoc Am Physicians **83**:113

Belpomme D et al (1974) T and B lymphocyte markers on the neoplastic cell of 20 patients with acute and 10 patients with chronic lymphoid leukemia, Biomedicine **20**:109

Belpomme D et al (1977) An immunological classification of leukemias and non Hodgkin's hematosarcomas based on T and B cell membrane markers with special reference to null "cell" disorders, Eur J Cancer **13**:311

Benedict WF et al (1979) Correlation between prognosis and bone marrow chromosomal patterns in children with acute nonlymphocytic leukemia: similarities and differences compared to adults, Blood **54**:818

Benesch R and Benesch RE (1967) The effect of organic phosphates from the human erythrocyte on the allosteric properties of hemoglobin, Biochem Biophys Res Commun **26**:162

Benesch R and Benesch RE (1969) Intracellular organic phosphates as regulators of oxygen release by haemoglobin, Nature **221**:618

Benesch R et al (1975) Oxygenation properties of hemoglobin variants with substitutions near the polyphosphate binding site, Biochim Biophys Acta **393**:368

Benjamin JT et al (1975) Congenital dyserythropoietic anemia—type IV, J Pediatr **87**:210

Bennett B and Ogston D (1973) Natural and drug-induced inhibition of fibrinolysis, Clin Haematol **2**:135

Bennett E and Bloom AL (1975) Molecular variants of factor VIII. In Brinkhous KM and Hemker HC (Eds): Handbook of hemophilia, New York, American Elsevier Publishing Co, Inc, p 217

Bennett E and Huehns ER (1970) Immunological differentiation of three types of hemophilia and identification of some female carriers, Lancet **2**:956

Bennett JH (1845) Case of hypertrophy of the spleen and liver, in which death took place from suppuration of the blood, Edinburgh Med Surg J **64**:413

Bennett JM et al (1969) Characterization and significance of abnormal leukocyte granules in the beige mouse: a possible homologue for Chediak-Higashi Aleutian trait, J Lab Clin Med **73**:235

Bennett JM and Reed CE (1975) Acute leukemia cytochemical profile: diagnostic and clinical implications, Blood Cells **1**:101

Bennett JM et al (1976) Proposals for the classification of the acute leukemias, Br J Haematol **33**:451

Bennich HH and Johansson SGO (1971) Structure and function of human immunoglobulin E, Adv Immunol **13**:1

Bennich HH et al (1968) Immunoglobulin E, a new class of immunoglobulin, Bull WHO **38**:151

Bensinger TA and Gilette PN (1974) Hemolysis in sickle cell disease, Arch Intern Med **133**:624

Bensinger TA et al (1970) Hemorrhagic thrombocythemia: control of post-splenectomy thrombocytosis with melphalan, Blood **36**:61

Bensusan HB et al (1978) Evidence that fibronectin is the collagen receptor on platelet membranes, Proc Natl Acad Sci USA **75**:5864

Bentley HP Jr and Krivit W (1960) An assay of antihemophilic globulin activity in the carrier female, J Lab Clin Med **56**:613

Bentley HP Jr et al (1961) Eosinophilic leukemia: report of a case, with review and classification, Am J Med **30**:310

Benton JW et al (1962) Systemic lupus erythematosus occurring during anticonvulsive drug therapy, JAMA **180**:115

Benveniste J (1974) Platelet-activating factor, a new mediator of anaphylaxis and immune complex deposition from rabbit and human basophils, Nature **249**:581

Benvenisti DS and Ultman JE (1969) Eosinophilic leukemia. Report of five cases and review of literature, Ann Intern Med **71**:731

Benz EJ Jr and Forget BG (1971) Defect in messenger RNA for human hemoglobin synthesis in beta thalassemia, J Clin Invest **50**:2755

Benz EJ Jr and Forget BG (1974) The biosynthesis of hemoglobin, Semin Hematol **11**:525

Benz EJ Jr et al (1975) Absence of functional messenger RNA activity for beta globulin chain synthesis in β^0-thalassemia, Blood **45**:1

Berard C et al (1969) Histopathologic definition of Burkitt's tumor, Bull WHO **40**:601

Berard CW et al (1978) Immunologic aspects and pathology of the malignant lymphomas, Cancer **42**:911

Berenbaum MC (1956) The use of bovine albumin in the preparation of marrow and blood films, J Clin Pathol **9**:381

Beresford CH et al (1971) Iron absorption and pyrexia, Lancet **1**:568

Beresford CH et al (1972) Haemoglobin Ocho Rios (beta 52 [D3] aspartic acid → alanine); a new beta chain variant of haemoglobin A found in combination with hemoglobin S, J Med Genet **9**:151

Beretta A et al (1968) Haemoglobin Torino—alpha 43 (CD1) phenylalanine → valine, Nature (London) **217**:1016

Berg B and Brandt T (1970) The cytology distribution and function of the neoplastic cells in leukaemic reticuloendotheliosis, Scand J Haematol **7**:428

Bergdahl U et al (1969) Pulmonary hemosiderosis and glomerulonephritis, Acta Med Scand **186**:199

Bergentz SE et al (1963) The viscosity of whole blood in trauma, Acta Chir Scand **126**:289

Berger HC (1921) Eosinophilia occurring in chorea, Am J Dis Child **21**:477

Berglund S (1972) Erythrocytosis associated with haemoglobin Malmö accompanied by pulmonary changes, occurring in the same family, Scand J Haematol **9**:355, 377

Berkson J (1959) The statistical investigation of smoking and cancer of the lung, Mayo Clin Proc **34**:206

Berkson J et al (1940) Error of estimate of blood cell counts as made with the hemocytometer, Am J Physiol **128**:309

Berlin NI and Berk PD (1975) The biological life of the red cell. In Surgenor DM (Ed): The red blood cell, New York, Academic Press, Inc, p 957

Berlin NI et al (1950) Blood volume in polycythemia as determined by P^{32} labeled red blood cells, Am J Med **9**:747

Berlin NI et al (1952) Medical progress: blood volume in various medical and surgical conditions, N Engl J Med **247**:675

Berlin NI et al (1956) Blood volume in chronic leukemia, Acta Med Scand **164**:257

Berman M et al (1979) The chronic sequelae of non-A, non-B hepatitis, Ann Intern Med **91**:1

Bern MM (1975) Variable response of activated partial thromboplastin time to heparin therapy during hemodialysis, Am J Clin Pathol **64**:602

Bernard C et al (1964) Effects of phytohemagglutinin on blood-cultures of chronic lymphocytic leukemia, Lancet **1**:667

Bernard J and Soulier J-P (1948) Sur une nouvelle variéte de dystrophie thrombocytaire hémorragipare congénitale, Sem Hop Paris **24**:3217

Bernard J et al (1963) A cytological and histological study of acute premyelocytic leukaemia, J Clin Pathol **16**:319

Bernard J et al (1965) Anomalie de Pelger homozygote chez l'homme, Sang **27**:819

Bernard JF et al (1975) Hémoglobinurie de marche, Nouv Presse Med **4**:1117

Bernhard W (1966) Ultrastructural aspects of the normal and pathological nucleolus in mammalian cells, Natl Cancer Inst Monogr **23**:13

Bernier GM and Fanger MW (1972) Synthesis of β-2-microglobulin by stimulated lymphocytes, J Immunol **109**:407

Bernier GM and Hines JD (1967) Immunologic heterogeneity of autoantibodies in patients with pernicious anemia, N Engl J Med **277**:1386

Bernstein LH et al (1970) The absorption and malabsorption of folic acid and its polyglutamates, Am J Med **48**:570

Bernstein RE (1955) The correction of mean cell volume and mean cell haemoglobin concentration, J Clin Pathol 8:225

Bernstein RE (1980) Glycosylated hemoglobins: hematologic considerations determine which assay for glycohemoglobin is advisable, Clin Chem 26:174

Berrebi A and Efrati P (1974) Congenital dyserythropoietic anemia in Jews from Morocco, JAMA 229:24

Berrebi A and Levene C (1976) Acanthocytes bearing the i antigen, Vox Sang 30:396

Bessis M and Maigné J (1970) Le diagnostic des varietés de leucémies aiguës par la réactiondes peroxydases au microscope électronique: son intérêt et ses limites, Rev Eur Etud Clin Biol 15:691

Bessis M (1973a) Cytologic diagnosis of leukemias by electron microscopy, Recent Results Cancer Res 43:63

Bessis M (1973b) Living blood cells and their ultrastructure, New York, Springer-Verlag New York Inc

Bessis M (1973c) Red cell shapes: an illustrated classification and its rationale. In Bessis M et al (Eds): Red cell shape. Physiology, pathology, ultrastructure, New York, Springer-Verlag New York Inc

Bessis M (1977) Blood smears reinterpreted, Berlin, Springer International, pp 18, 130

Bessis M and Breton-Gorius J (1960) Aspects de la molécule de ferritine et d'apoferritine au microscope électronique, C R Acad Sci 250:1360

Bessis M and Breton-Gorius J (1961) L'ilot erythroblastique et la rhophéocytose de la ferritine dans l'inflammation, Nouv Rev Fr Hematol 1:569

Bessis M and Bricka M (1952) Aspect dynamique des cellules du sang: son étude par la microcinématographie en contraste de phase, Rev Hematol 7:407

Bessis et al (1973) Red cell shape. Physiology, pathology, ultrastructure, New York, Springer-Verlag New York Inc

Bessman D (1977) Erythropoiesis during recovery from iron deficiency: normocytes and macrocytes, Blood 50:987

Best WR (1967) Chloramphenicol-associated blood dyscrasias, JAMA 201:181

Bethlefalvay NC et al (1975) Hereditary persistence of fetal hemoglobin, thalassemia, and the δ-β locus: further family data and genetic interpretations, J Hum Genet 27:140

Betke K et al (1960) Properties of a further variant of Haemoglobin M, Nature 188:864

Bettigole RE et al (1970) Hypofibrinogenemia due to L-asparaginase: studies of fibrinogen survival using autologous ¹³¹I-fibrinogen, Blood 35:195

Beutler E (1959) The hemolytic effect of primaquine and related compounds: a review, Blood 14:103

Beutler E (1975) Red cell metabolism: a manual of biochemical methods, New York, Grune & Stratton, Inc

Beutler E (1978a) Hemolytic anemia in disorders of red cell metabolism, New York, Plenum Publishing Corp

Beutler E (1978b) Glucose-6-phosphate dehydrogenase deficiency. In Stanbury JB et al (Eds): The metabolic basis of inherited disease, New York, McGraw-Hill Book Co, p 1430

Beutler E (1978c) Why has the autohemolysis test not gone the way of the cephalin flocculation test? Blood 51:109

Beutler E (1979) Red cell enzyme defects as nondiseases and as diseases, Blood 54:1

Beutler E and West C (1979) The storage of hard-packed red blood cells in citrate-phosphate-dextrose (CPD) and CPD-adenine (CPDA-1), Blood 54:280

Beutler E et al (1955) The hemolytic effect of primaquine. VI. An in vitro test for sensitivity of erythrocytes to primaquine, J Lab Clin Med 45:40

Beutler E et al (1960) Iron therapy in chronically fatigued nonanemic women: a double blind study, Ann Intern Med 52:378

Beutler E et al (1962) The normal human female as a mosaic of X-chromosome activity: studies using the gene for G-6-PD deficiency as a marker, Proc Natl Acad Sci USA 48:9

Beutler E et al (1969) Depletion and regeneration of 2,3-diphosphoglyceric acid in stored red blood cells, Transfusion 9:109

Beutler E et al (1974) Hemoglobin Duarte: alpha 2 beta 2 62 (E6) ala → pro: a new unstable hemoglobin with increased oxygen affinity, Blood 43:527

Beuzard Y et al (1972) Structural studies of hemoglobin Saint Etienne beta 92 (F8) his → gln: a new abnormal hemoglobin with loss of beta proximal histidine and absence of heme on the beta chains, FEBS Lett 27:76

Beuzard Y et al (1975) Haemoglobin Saki alpha 2 beta 2 14 leu → pro (A11) structure and function, Biochim Biophys Acta 393:182

Bevelaqua FA et al (1976) Scurvy and hemarthrosis, JAMA 235:1874

Beveridge BR et al (1965) Hypochromic anemia: a retrospective study and followup of 378 inpatients, Q J Med 34:145

Beychok, IA (1978) Precise diagnosis in severe hematochezia, Arch Surg 113:634

Bhende YM et al (1952) A "new" blood group character related to the ABO system, Lancet 1:903

Bianco I et al (1963) Alteration in the alpha chain of haemoglobin L Ferrara, Nature (London) 198:395

Bianco C et al (1970) A population of lymphocytes bearing a membrane receptor for antigen-antibody-complement complexes. I. Separation and characterization, J Exp Med 132:702

Bick RL et al (1976) Bleeding times, platelet adhesion, and aspirin, Am J Clin Pathol 65:69

Bickel YB (1968) Immunofluorescent patterns and specificity of human antinuclear antibodies, Clin Exp Immunol 3:641

Bierman HK and Kelly KH (1956) Multiple marrow aspiration in man from posterior ilium, Blood 11:370

Bierman HR et al (1959) The production and destruction of granulocytes in normal and leukemic man, Ann NY Acad Sci 77:417

Biggs R and Macfarlane RG (1962) Human blood coagulation and its disorders, Oxford, Blackwell Scientific Publications Ltd

Biggs R et al (1952) Christmas disease: a condition previously mistaken for haemophilia, Br Med J 2:1378

Biggs R et al (1968) The coagulant activity of platelets, Br J Haemotol 15:283

Billing BH and Lathe GH (1958) Bilirubin metabolism in jaundice, Am J Med 24:111

Billing BH et al (1957) The excretion of bilirubin as a diglucuronide giving direct van den Bergh reaction, Biochem J 65:774

Billingham RE (1964) Transplantation immunity and the maternal fetal relation, N Engl J Med 270:667

Billo OE and Wolff JA (1960) Thrombocytopenic purpura due to cat-scratch disease, JAMA 174:1824

Bing RJ et al (1948) Physiological studies in congenital heart disease. VI. Adaptation to anoxia in congenital heart disease with cyanosis, Johns Hopkins Med J 83:439

Bingham J (1959) The macrocytosis of hepatic disease. I. Thin macrocytosis, Blood 14:694

Biörck G et al (1964) Leukocytosis during cortico-steroid therapy, Acta Med Scand 176:127

Bird GWG and Wingham J (1976) The action of seed and other reagents on HEMPAS erythrocytes, Acta Haematol 55:174

Bird RM and Jaques WE (1959) Vascular lesions of hereditary hemorrhagic telangiectasia, N Engl J Med 260:597

Bird GWG (1977) Paroxysmal cold haemoglobinuria, Br J Haematol 37:167

Bird GWG et al (1976) Idiopathic non-syphilitic paroxysmal cold haemoglobinuria in children, J Clin Pathol 29:215

Bird T and Proctor SJ (1977) Malignant myelosclerosis: myeloproliferative disorder or leukemia, Am J Clin Pathol **67**:512

Birkhill FR et al (1951) Effect of transfusion polycythemia upon bone marrow activity and erythrocyte survival in man, Blood **6**:1021

Bisno AL (1971) Hyposplenism and overwhelming pneumococcal infection: a reappraisal, Am J Med Sci **262**:101

Bithell TC and Wintrobe MM (1967) Drug-induced aplastic anemia, Semin Hematol **4**:194

Bithell TC et al (1967) Radioactive diisopropyl flourophosphate as a platelet label: an evaluation of in vitro and in vivo technics, Blood **29**:354

Bithell TC et al (1970) Variant of factor IX deficiency in female with 45, X Turner's syndrome, Blood **36**:169

Bithell TC et al (1972) Platelet function studies in the Bernard-Soulier syndrome, Ann NY Acad Sci **201**:145

Bitran JD et al (1977) Chromosomal aneuploidy in a patient with hypereosinophilic syndrome: evidence for a malignant disease, Am J Med **63**:1010

Bjure J et al (1962) Familial neutropenia possibly caused by deficiency of a plasma factor, Acta Pediatr **51**:497

Blackburn EK et al (1962) Christmas disease associated with primary capillary abnormalities, Br Med J **1**:154

Blaese RM et al (1967) The Wiskott-Aldrich (W-A) syndrome, a defect in antigen processing or recognition? Clin Res **15**:465

Blackwell RQ and Liu C-S (1966) The identical structural anomalies of hemoglobins J Meinung and J Korat, Biochem Biophys Res Commun **24**:732

Blackwell RQ and Liu C-S (1968) Hemoglobin G Taiwan-Ami alpha 2 beta 2 25 gly → arg, Biochem Biophys Res Commun **30**:690

Blackwell RQ and Liu C-S (1970) Hemoglobin G Taichung: alpha 74 asp → His, Biochim Biophys Acta **200**:70

Blackwell RQ et al (1968) Hemoglobin variant common to Chinese and North American Indians: alpha 2 beta 2 22 glu → ala, Science **161**:381

Blackwell RQ et al (1969a) Hemoglobin J Taichung: beta 129 ala → asp, Biochim Biophys Acta **194**:1

Blackwell RQ et al (1969b) Hemoglobin G Taipei: alpha 2 beta 2 22 glu → gly, Biochim Biophys Acta **175**:237

Blackwell RQ et al (1969c) Hemoglobin G-Szuhu: beta 80 asn → lys, Biochim Biophys Acta **188**:59

Blackwell RQ et al (1970a) Hemoglobin G Makassar: beta 6 glu → ala, Biochim Biophys Acta **214**:396

Blackwell RQ et al (1970b) Fast hemoglobin variant in Minahassan people of Salawesi, Chinese and Thais: alpha 2 beta 2 56 gly → asp, Am J Phys Anthropol **32**:147

Blackwell RQ et al (1971a) Hemoglobin Ta-li: beta 83 gly → cys, Biochim Biophys Acta **243**:467

Blackwell RQ et al (1971b) Hemoglobin J Kaohsiung: beta 59 lys → thr, Biochim Biophys Acta **229**:343

Blackwell RQ et al (1972a) Hemoglobin J Singapore: alpha 78 asn → asp: alpha 79 ala → gly, Biochim Biophys Acta **278**:482

Blackwell RQ et al (1972b) Hemoglobin C-Hsi-Tsou: beta 79 asp → gly, Biochim Biophys Acta **257**:49

Blackwell RQ et al (1972c) Fast haemoglobin variant found in Hawaiian-Chinese-Caucasian family in Hawaii and a Chinese subject in Taiwan, Vox Sang **22**:469

Blackwell RQ et al (1973) Hemoglobin G Waimanalo: alpha 64 asp → asn, Biochim Biophys Acta **322**:70

Blackwell RQ et al (1974) Hemoglobin J Meerut: alpha 120 ala → glu, Biochim Biophys Acta **351**:7

Blajchman MA et al (1979) Clinical use of blood, blood components and blood products, Can Med Assoc J **121**:33

Blankenship RM et al (1973) Familial sea-blue histiocytes with acid phosphatemia: a syndrome resembling Gaucher disease: the Lewis variant, JAMA **225**:54

Blatt PM et al (1977) Treatment of anti-factor VIII antibodies, Thromb Haemost **38**:514

Blattner WA et al (1976) Familial chronic lymphocytic leukemia: immunologic and cellular characterization, Ann Intern Med **84**:554

Blaud P (1832) Sur les maladies chlorotiques, et sur un mode de traitement, specifique dans ces affections, Rev Med Fr Etrand **45**:341

Blaustein A (1963) The spleen, New York, McGraw-Hill Book Co

Bleyer WA and Skinner AL (1976) Fatal neonatal hemorrhage after maternal anticonvulsant therapy, JAMA **235**:626

Bleyer WA et al (1971) The development of hemostasis in the human fetus and newborn infant, J Pediatr **79**:838

Block MH and Jacobson LO (1950) Splenic puncture, JAMA **142**:641

Block O Jr (1941) Loss of virulence of *Treponema pallidum* in citrate blood at 5° C, Johns Hopkins Med J **68**:412

Bloem TF (1933) The relative value of clinical tests for blood, Biochem J **27**:121

Blondin C and McDuffie FC (1970) Role of IgG and IgM antinuclear antibodies in formation of lupus erythematosus cells and extracellular material, Arthritis Rheum **13**:786

Bloom AL and Hutton RD (1975) Fresh-platelet transfusions in haemophilic patients with factor-VIII antibody, Lancet **2**:369

Bloom BR and Bennett B (1966) Mechanisms of a reaction in vitro associated with delayed-type hypersensitivity, Science **153**:80

Bloom BR and Bennett B (1968) Migration inhibitory factor associated with delayed-type hypersensitivity, Fed Proc **27**:13

Bloom BR and Bennett B (1970) Relation of the migration inhibitory factor (MIF) to delayed-type hypersensitivity reactions, Ann NY Acad Sci **169**:258

Bloom BR and Chase MW (1967) Transfer of delayed-type hypersensitivity. A critical review and experimental study in the guinea pig. Prog Allergy **10**:151

Bloom BR and Jiminez L (1970) Migration inhibitory factor and the cellular basis of delayed-type hypersensitivity reactions, Am J Pathol **60**:453

Bloom GE and Diamond LK (1968) Prognostic value of fetal hemoglobin levels in acquired aplastic anemia, N Engl J Med **278**:304

Bloom GE et al (1966) Chronic myelogenous leukemia in an infant: serial cytogenetic and fetal hemoglobin studies, Pediatrics **38**:295

Bloom W (1960) The embryogenesis of lymphocytic tissue. In Rebuck JW (Ed): The lymphocyte and lymphocytic tissue, New York, Paul B Hoeber, Inc

Bloom W and Bartelmez G (1940) Hematopoiesis in young human embryos, Am J Anat **67**:21

Bloomfield CD et al (1977) The Philadelphia chromosome (Ph[1]) in adults presenting with acute leukaemia: a comparison of Ph[1]+ and Ph[1]− patients, Br J Haematol **36**:347

Bloomfield CD et al (1979) Clinical utility of lymphocyte surface markers combined with the Lukes-Collins histologic classification in adult lymphoma, N Engl J Med **301**:512

Bloomfield FJ and Scott JM (1972) Identification of a new vitamin B_{12} binder (transcobalamin III) in normal human serum, Br J Haematol **22**:33

Blombäck, B et al (1957) Coagulation studies on "Reptilase," an extract of the venom of *Bothrops jararaca*, Thromb Diath Haemorrh **1**:76

Blombäck B and Blombäck M (1972) The molecular structure of fibrinogen, Ann NY Acad Sci **202**:77

Blouquit Y et al (1976) Hb Henri Mondor: beta 26 (B8) glu →

val: a variant with a substitution localized at the same position as that of hb E beta[26] glu → lys, FEBS Lett **72**:5

Blumenfeld TA et al (1979) Recommended site and depth of newborn heel skin punctures based on anatomical measurements and histopathology, Lancet **1**:230

Blumberg BS and Hesser JE (1975) Viral hepatitis, Modes of transmission and the role of the carrier. In Greenwalt TJ and Jamieson GA (Eds): Transmissible disease and blood transfusion, New York, Grune & Stratton Inc. p 67

Blumberg BS et al (1964) Multiple antigenic specificities of serum lipoproteins detected with sera of transfused patients, Vox Sang **9**:128

Blumberg BS et al (1965) A "new" antigen in leukemia sera, JAMA **191**:541

Blumberg BS et al (1968) Hepatitis and leukemia: their relationship to Australia antigen, Bull NY Acad Med **44**:1566

Blume KG et al (1968a) Familienuntersuchungen zum Glutathionreduktasemangel menschlicher Erythrocyten, Humangenetik **6**:163

Blume KG et al (1968b) Beitrag zur Populationsgenetik der Glutathionreduktase menschlicher Erythrocyten, Humangenetik **6**:266

Blume RS et al (1969) The Chediak-Higashi syndrome: continuous suspension cultures derived from peripheral blood, Blood **33**:821

Blundell J (1818) Experiments on the transfusion of blood by the syringe, Med Chir Trans London **9**:56

Blundell J (1828) Observations on transfusion of blood, Lancet **2**:320

Bodansky O (1951) Methemoglobinemia and methemoglobin producing compounds, Pharmacol Rev **3**:144

Boddington MM and Spriggs AI (1969) The epithelial cells in megaloblastic anaemias, J Clin Pathol **12**:228

Boehme WM et al (1978) Acquired hemoglobin H in refractory sideroblastic anemia: a preleukemic marker, Arch Intern Med **138**:603

Boggs DR (1966) Hemostatic regulatory mechanisms of hematopoiesis, Ann Rev Physiol **28**:39

Boggs DR (1974) The frequency of heterozygosity for S and C hemoglobins in western Pennsylvania, Blood **44**:699

Boggs DR (1975) Physiology of neutrophil proliferation, maturation and circulation, Clin Haematol **4**:535

Boggs DR and Boggs SS (1976) The pathogenesis of aplastic anemia: a defective pluripotent hematopoietic stem cell with inappropriate balance of differentiation and self-replication, Blood **48**:71

Boggs DR and Boggs SS (1978) Possible pathogenic mechanisms in aplastic anemia, Transplant Proc **10**:125

Boggs DR et al (1962) The acute leukemias: analysis of 322 cases and review of the literature, Medicine **41**:163

Boggs DR et al (1966) Factors influencing the duration of survival of patients with chronic lymphocytic leukemia, Am J Med **40**:243

Bohn H (1972) Comparative studies on the fibrin-stabilizing factors from human plasma, platelets, and placentas, Ann NY Acad Sci **202**:256

Bohr C (1904) Theoretische Behandlung der quantitativen Verhältnisse bei der Sauerstoff aufnahme der Hamoglobins, Zbl Physiol **17**:682

Boivin P and Eoche-Duval V (1965) Une technique simple de dosage de l'erythropoiétine chez la souris rendue polycythémique par hypoxie, Rev Eur Etud Clin Biol **10**:434

Bolton FG (1956) Thrombocytopenic purpura due to quinidine. II. Serologic mechanism, Blood **11**:547

Bolton FG and Dameshek W (1956) Thrombocytopenic purpura due to quinidine. I. Clinical studies, Blood **11**:547

Bonaventura J and Riggs A (1967) Polymerization of hemoglobins of mouse and man: structural basis, Science **158**:800

Bonaventura J and Riggs A (1968) Hemoglobin Kansas, a human hemoglobin with a neutral amino acid substitution and an abnormal oxygen equilibrium, J Biol Chem **243**:980

Bonaventura J et al (1976) Hemoglobin Providence. Functional consequences of two alterations of the 2,3-diphosphoglycerate binding site at position beta 82, J Biol Chem **251**:7563

Bonaventura J and Riggs A (1967) Polymerization of hemoglobins of mouse and man. Structural basis, Science **158**:800

Bond VP and Cronkite EP (1957) Effects of radiation on mammals, Ann Rev Physiol **19**:299

Bondue H et al (1980) The leucocyte alkaline phosphatase activity in mature neutrophils of different ages, Scand J Haematol **24**:51

Bonnet JD et al (1960) A quantitative method for measuring the gastrointestinal absorption of iron, Blood **15**:36

Bonomo L et al (1965) Characterization of the antibodies producing the homogenous and the speckled flourescence patterns of cell nuclei, J Lab Clin Med **66**:42

Bonsdorff E and Jalavisto E (1948) Humoral mechanism in anoxic erythrocytosis, Acta Physiol Scand **16**:150

Bookchin RM et al (1967) Structure and properties of hemoglobin C-Harlem, a human hemoglobin variant with amino acid substitutions in 2 residues of the β-polypeptide chain, J Biol Chem **242**:248

Bookchin RM et al (1968) Hemoglobin C-Harlem: a sickling variant containing amino acid substitutions in two residues of the β-polypeptide chain, Biochem Biophys Res Commun **23**:122

Booth CC and Mollin DL (1959) The site of adsorption of vitamin B_{12} in man, Lancet **1**:18

Booyse FM and Rafelson ME Jr (1969) Studies on human platelets. III. A contractile protein model for platelet aggregation, Blood **33**:100

Booyse FM and Rafelson ME (1971) Human platelet contractile proteins: location, properties, and function, Ser Haematol **4**:152

Booyse FM et al (1972) Possible thrombosthenin defects in Glanzmann's thrombasthenia, Blood **39**:377

Borchgrevink CF (1959) Myocardial infarction in a haemophilic, Lancet **1**:1229

Borchgrevink CF (1960a) A method for measuring platelet adhesiveness in vivo, Acta Med Scand **168**:157

Borchgrevink CF (1960b) Long-term anticoagulant therapy in angina pectoris and myocardial infarction. A clinical trial of intensive versus moderate treatment, Acta Med Scand **168**:(supp 359):1

Born GV (1970) Observations on the change in shape of blood platelets brought about by adenosine diphosphate, J Physiol **209**:487

Born GV (1972) Current ideas on the mechanism of platelet aggregation, Ann NY Acad Sci **201**:4

Borsook H (1964) A picture of erythropoiesis at the combined morphologic and molecular levels, Blood **24**:202

Bortin MM and Rimm AA (1977) Severe combined immunodeficiency disease: characterization of the disease and results of transplantation, JAMA **238**:591

Botha MC et al (1966) Haemoglobin J Cape Town alpha 2 92 arginine → glutamine beta 2, Nature (London) **212**:792

Bothwell TH et al (1956) The study of erythropoiesis using tracer quantities of radioactive iron, Br J Haematol **2**:1

Bothwell TH et al (1957) Erthrokinetics. IV. The plasma iron turnover as a measure of erythropoiesis, Blood **12**:409

Böttiger LE and Svedberg CA (1967) Normal erythrocyte sedimentation rate and age, Br Med J **1**:85

Böttiger LE and Westerholm B (1973) Acquired haemolytic anaemia. II. Drug-induced haemolytic anaemia, Acta Med Scand **193**:227

Böttner H and Reinecke H (1955) Pelgersche Kernvarietät und diffuses Plasmocytom, Arch Klin Med **202**:510

Bottura C and Ferrari I (1963) Endoreduplication in acute leukemia, Blood **21**:207

Boulton FE et al (1971) Myoglobin variants, Br J Haematol **20**:671

Bouma BN et al (1972) Immunological characterization of purified antihaemophilic factor A (factor VIII) which corrects abnormal platelet retention in von Willebrand's disease, Nature (New Biol) **236**:104

Bouma BN et al (1975) Evaluation of the detection rate of hemophilia carriers, Thromb Res **7**:339

Bouma BN and Griffin JH (1977) Human blood coagulation factor XI. Purification, properties, and mechanism of activation by activated factor XII, J Biol Chem **252**:6432

Bounameaux Y (1957) Dosage des facteurs de coagulation contenus dans l'atmosphere plasmatique des plaquettes humains, Rev Fr Etud Clin Biol **2**:52

Bounameaux Y (1963) Coagulopathies avec temps de saignement prolongé, Throm Diath Haemorrh **9**:417

Bourne HR et al (1974) Modulation of inflammation and immunity by cyclic AMP, Science **184**:19

Bourne MS et al (1965) Familial pyridoxine-responsive anaemia, Br J Haematol **11**:1

Bourne WA (1951) Capillary resistance test: simple negative-pressure method, Br Med J **2**:1322

Bousser J and Neydé R (1947) La neutropénie familiale, Sang **18**:521

Bovell J (1855) On the transfusion of milk, as practiced in cholera, at the cholera sheds, Toronto, 1854, Can J **3**:188

Bowden DH et al (1956) Acute recurrent rhabdomyolysis (paroxysmal myohaemoglobinuria), Medicine **35**:335

Bowdler AJ (1975) The spleen and haemolytic disorders, Clin Haematol **4**:231

Bowen JM et al (1973) Molecular probes in studies of the relationship of viruses to human neoplasia, Am J Clin Pathol **60**:88

Bowers TK et al (1977) Acquired granulocyte abnormality during drug allergic reactions: possible role of complement activation, Blood **49**:3

Bowie EJW and Owen CA Jr (1971) Some factors influencing platelet retention in glass bead columns including the influence of plastics, Am J Clin Pathol **56**:479

Bowie EJW and Owen CA Jr (1973) The value of measuring platelet "adhesiveness" in the diagnosis of bleeding diseases, Am J Clin Pathol **60**:302

Bowie EJW et al (1963) Thrombosis in systemic lupus erythematosus despite circulating anticoagulants, J Lab Clin Med **62**:416

Bowie EJW et al (1964) The stability of antihemophilic globulin and labile factor in human blood, Mayo Clin Proc **39**:144

Bowie EJW et al (1965) Anticoagulant malingerers (the "Dicumarol-eaters"), Am J Med **39**:855

Bowie EJW et al (1969) Platelet adhesiveness in von Willebrand's disease, Am J Clin Pathol **52**:69

Bowie EJW et al (1976) The spectrum of von Willebrands's disease revisited, Mayo Clin Proc **51**:35

Bowles CA et al (1979) Studies of the Pelfer-Huët anomaly in foxhounds, Am J Pathol **96**:237

Bowman JM and Pollock JM (1965) Amniotic fluid spectrophotometry and early delivery in the management of erythroblastosis fetalis, Pediatrics **35**:815

Bowman WD Jr (1961) Abnormal ("ringed") sideroblasts in various hematologic and non-hematologic disorders, Blood **18**:662

Bowman B and Ingram VM (1961) Abnormal human haemoglobins. VII. The comparison of normal human haemoglobin and haemoglobin D Chicago, Biochim Biophys Acta **53**:569

Bowman BH and Barnett DR (1967) Amino-acid substitution in haemoglobin I (Texas variant), Nature **214**:499

Bowan BH et al (1964) Cheical characterization of three hemoglobins G, Blood **23**:193

Bowman BH et al (1966) Chemical characterization of haemoglobin G St-I, Nature **211**:1305

Bowman BH et al (1967) Hemoglobin G Coushatta: a beta variant with a delta-like substitution, Biochem Biophys Res Commun **26**:466

Bowman JM (1978) The management of Rh-isoimmunization, Obstet Gynecol **52**:1

Bowman JM et al (1978) Rh isoimmunization during pregnancy: antenatal prophylaxis, Can Med Assoc J **118**:623

Boxer LA et al (1974) Neutrophil actin dysfunction and abnormal neutrophil behavior, N Engl J Med **291**:1093

Boxer LB et al (1975) Autoimmune neutropenia, N Engl J Med **293**:748

Boxer LA et al (1979) Impaired microtubule assembly and polymorphonuclear leucocyte function in the Chediak-Higashi syndrome correctable by ascorbic acid, Br J Haematol **43**:207

Boxer M et al (1976) The lupus anticoagulant, Arthritis Rheum **19**:1244

Boyden S (1962) The chemotactic effect of mixtures of antibody and antigen on polymorphonuclear leukocytes, J Exp Med **115**:453

Boyer SH and Graham JB (1965) Linkage between the X chromosome loci for glucose-6-phosphate dehydrogenase electrophoretic variation and hemophilia A, Am J Hum Genet **17**:320

Boyer SH et al (1963) Further evidence for linkage between the β and δ loci governing human hemoglobin and the population dynamics of linkage genes, Am J Hum Genet **15**:438

Boyer SH et al (1968) A survey of hemoglobins in the Republic of Chad and characterization of hemoglobin Chad: alpha 2 23 glu → lys beta 2, Am J Hum Genet **20**:570

Boyle TM (1962) Haemorrhagic thrombocythemia, a cause of repeated severe epistaxis, J Laryngol Otol **76**:181

Bozdech MJ et al (1980) Partial peroxidase deficiency in neutrophils and eosinophils associated with neutrologic disease: histochemical, cytochemical and biochemical studies, Am J Clin Pathol **73**:409

Brabec V et al (1970) The A_2 hemoglobin in hematological diseases, Clin Chim Acta **28**:489

Braconnier F et al (1977) Hemoglobin Fort de France (alpha 2 45 [CD3] his → arg beta 2), a new variant with increased oxygen affinity, Biochim Biophys Acta **493**:228

Brachfeld J and Myerson RM (1956) Pyroglobulinemia. Diagnostic clue in multiple myeloma, JAMA **161**:865

Bradley DW et al (1979) Experimental infection of chimpanzees with antihemophilic (factor VIII) materials: recovery of virus-like particles associated with non-A, non-B hepatitis, J Med Virol **3**:253

Bradley TB et al (1967) Hemoglobin Gun Hill: deletion of five amino acid residues and impared heme-globin binding, Science **157**:1581

Bradley TB et al (1972) Properties of hemoglobin Bryn Mawr, beta 85 phe → ser, a new spontaneous mutation producing an unstable hemoglobin with high oxygen affinity, Blood **40**:947

Bradley TR and Metcalf D (1966) The growth of mouse bone marrow cells in vitro, Aust J Exp Biol Med Sci **44**:287

Brady RO (1972) Biochemical and metabolic basic of familial sphingolipidoses, Semin Hematol **9**:273

Brady RO (1975) The lipid storage diseases: new concepts and control, Ann Intern Med **82**:257

Brady RO (1978a) Glucosyl ceramide lipidosis, Gaucher's disease. In Stanbury JB et al (Eds): The metabolic basis of inherited diseases, New York, McGraw-Hill Book Co Inc, p 731

Brady RO (1978b) Sphingomyelin lipidosis: Niemann-Pick disease. In Stanbury JB et al (Eds): The metabolic basis of inherited diseases, New York, McGraw-Hill Book Co Inc, p 718

Brady RO and King FM (1973) Niemann-Pick's disease. In Hers HG and Van Hoof F (Eds): Lysosomes and storage diseases, New York, Academic Press, Inc, p 439

Brahim F and Osmond DG (1970) Migration of bone marrow lymphocytes demonstrated by selective bone marrow labeling with thymidine-H^3, Anat Rec **168**:139

Brain MC (1970) Microangiopathic hemolytic anemia, Ann Rev Med **21**:133

Branda RF et al (1978a) Folate-induced remission in aplastic anemia with familial defect of cellular folate uptake, N Engl J Med **298**:469

Branda RF et al (1978b) Lymphocyte studies in familial chronic lymphatic leukemia, Am J Med **64**:508

Brandt V and Metz J (1961) Serum vitamin B$_{12}$ levels in South African white and Bantu subjects, S Afr J Med Sci **26**:1

Brandtzaeg P and Baklien K (1974) Bowel diseases involving local immunoglobulin systems, Acta Pathol Microbiol Scand (A) (supp) **248**:43

Brante G (1952) Gargoylism—a mucopolysaccharidosis, Scand J Clin Lab Invest **4**:43

Brass EP et al (1976) Fibrin formation: the role of the fibrinogen-fibrin monomer complex, Thromb Haemost **36**:37

Bratu V et al (1971) Haemoglobin Bucuresti beta 42 (CD1) phe → leu, a cause of unstable haemoglobin haemolytic anaemia, Biochim Biophys Acta **251**:1

Braunsteiner H and Pakesch F (1955) Electron microscopy and functional significance of new cellular structure in plasmacytes: a review, Blood **10**:650

Braverman AS et al (1973) Homozygous beta thalassemia in American Blacks: the problem of mild thalassemia, J Lab Clin Med **81**:857

Braylan R et al (1975) The Sézary syndrome lymphoid cell: abnormal surface properties and mitogen responsiveness, Br J Haematol **31**:553

Brayshaw JR et al (1963) The effect of oral iron therapy on the stool guaiac and orthotolidine reactions, Ann Intern Med **59**:172

Brayton RG et al (1970) Effect of alcohol and various diseases on leukocyte mobilization, phagocytosis, and intracellular bacterial kiling, N Engl J Med **282**:123

Brecher G (1949) New methylene blue as a reticulocyte stain, Am J Pathol **19**:895

Brecher G (1973) Nomenclature of red cell shapes. A commentary. In Bessis M et al (Eds): Red cell shape. Physiology, pathology, ultrastructure, New York, Springer-Verlag New York Inc

Brecher G and Bessis M (1973) Present status of spiculated red cells and their relationship to the discocyte-echinocyte transformation. A critical review, Blood **40**:333

Brecher G and Cronkite EP (1950) Morphology and enumeration of human blood platelets, J Appl Physiol **3**:365

Brecher G et al (1953) The reproducibility and constancy of the platelet count, Am J Clin Pathol **23**:15

Brecher G et al (1972) Spiculed erythrocytes after splenectomy: acanthocytes or non-specific poikilocytes? Nouv Rev Fr Hematol **12**:751

Breen FA and Tullis JL (1968) Ethanol gelation: a rapid screening test for intravascular coagulation, Ann Intern Med **69**:1197

Breen FA and Tullis JL (1969) Prothrombin concentrates in treatment of Christmas disease and allied disorders, JAMA **208**:1848

Brennan SO et al (1977a) Haemoglobin F Melbourne G gamma 16 gly → arg and haemoglobin F Carlton G gamma 121 glu → lys, Biochim Biophys Acta **490**:452

Brennan SO et al (1977b) Haemoglobin Port Phillip alpha 91 (FG3) leu → pro. A new unstable haemoglobin, FEBS Lett **81**:115

Brennan SO et al (1977c) A new unstable haemoglobin, beta 134 val → glu, New Zealand Med J **85**:398

Breslow A et al (1968) The effect of surgery on the concentration of circulating megakaryocytes and platelets, Blood **32**:393

Breton-Gorius J et al (1973) Anomalies ultrastructurales des érythroblastes et des érythrocytes dans six cas de dysérythropoiese congenitale, Nouv Rev Fr Hematol **13**:23

Breton-Gorius J et al (1975) Activités peroxydasiques de certaines granulations des neutrophiles dans deux cas de déficit congénital en myéloperoxydase, CR Acad Sci Paris **280**:1753

Breton-Gorius J et al (1978a) Megakaryoblastic acute leukemia: identification by the ultrastructural demonstration of platelet peroxidase, Blood **51**:45

Breton-Gorius J et al (1978b) The blast crisis of chronic granulocytic leukaemia: megakaryoblastic nature of cells as revealed by the presence of platelet-peroxidase: a cytochemical ultrastructural study, Br J Haematol **39**:295

Brewer GJ (1976) A view of the current status of antisickling therapy, Am J Hematol **1**:121

Brewer GJ and Eaton JW (1971) Erythrocyte metabolism: interaction with oxygen transport, Science **171**:1205

Brewer GJ et al (1962) The methemoglobin reduction test for primaquine-type sensitivity of erythrocytes: a simplified procedure for detecting a specific hypersusceptibility to drug hemolysis, JAMA **180**:386

Brewster DC (1973) Splenosis: report of 2 cases and review of the literature, Am J Surg **126**:14

Briggs DW et al (1973) Inactivation of erythropoietin by hepatic lysosomes, Proc Soc Exp Biol Med **144**:394

Briginshaw GF and Shanberge JN (1974) Identification of two distinct heparin cofactors in human plasma. II. Inhibition of thrombin and activated factor X, Thromb Res **4**:463

Brimhall B et al (1969) Structural characterization of hemoglobin Tacoma, Biochemistry **8**:2125

Brimhall B et al (1973) Haemoglobin F Port Royal (alpha 2 G gamma 125 glu → ala), Br J Haematol **27**:313

Brimhall B et al (1974) Structural characterizations of hemoglobins J Buda (alpha 61 [E10] lys → asn) and G Pest (alpha 74 [EF3] asp → asn), Biochim Biophys Acta **336**:344

Brimhall B et al (1975) Two new hemoglobins: hemoglobin Alabama (beta 39 [C5] gln → lys) and hemoglobin Montgomery (alpha 48 [CD6] leu → arg), Biochim Biophys Acta **379**:28

Brines JK et al (1941) Blood volume in normal infants and children, J Pediatr **18**:444

Brink AJ and Weber HW (1963) Fibroplastic parietal endocarditis with eosinophils: Löffler's endocarditis, Am J Med **34**:52

Brinkhous KM (1975) A short history of hemophilia, with some comments on the word "hemophilia." In Brinkhous KM and Hemker HC (Eds): Handbook of hemophilia, New York, American Elsevier Publishing Co, Inc, p 3

Brinkhous KM and Graham JB (1950) Hemophilia in the female dog, Science **111**:723

Brinkhous KM and Hemker HC (1975) Handbook of hemophilia, New York, American Elsevier Publishing Co, Inc

Brinkhous KM et al (1972) Prevalence of inhibitors in haemophilia A and B, Thromb Diath Haemorrh Suppl **51**:315

Brinkhous KM et al (1975) Assay of von Willebrand factor in von Willebrand's disease and hemophilia: use of a macroscopic platelet aggregation test, Thromb Res **6**:267

Brinn L and Glabman S (1962) Gaucher's disease without splenomegaly. Oldest patient on record, with review, New York J Med **62**:2346

Britten A (1966) Hemophilic bleeding on the first day of life. Report of a unique case and review of the relevant literature, Clin Pediatr **5**:123

Brittin GM et al (1968) A primary sideroblastic anemia terminating in bone marrow aplasia, Am J Clin Pathol **50**:467

Brizel HE and Raccuglia G (1965) Giant hemangioma with thrombocytopenia: radioisotopic demonstration of platelet sequestration, Blood **26**:751

Broder S et al (1976) The Sézary syndrome: a malignant proliferation of helper T cells, J Clin Invest **58**:1297

Brodersen R (1977) Prevention of kernicterus, based on recent progress in bilirubin chemistry, Acta Paediatr Scand **66**:625

Brodeur GM et al (1980) Acquired inhibitors of coagulation in nonhemophiliac children, J Pediatr **96**:439

Brodin MB (1978) William Harvey, J Fla Med Assoc **65**:268

Brodsky I et al (1968a) Polycythemia vera: differential diagnosis by ferrokinetic studies and treatment with busulphan (Myleran), Br J Haematol **14**:351

Brodsky I et al (1968b) Laboratory diagnosis of disseminated intravascular coagulation, Am J Clin Pathol **50**:211

Brodsky I (1974) Leukemia and the hypercoagulable state: pathogenic and therapeutic implication, J Med (Basel) **5**:38

Brody JI and Beizer LH (1965) Christmas disease and myocardial infarction, Arch Intern Med **115**:552

Brody JI et al (1962) The Sézary syndrome, Arch Intern Med **110**:205

Brody JI et al (1970) Symptomatic crises of sickle cell anemia treated by limited exchange transfusion, Ann Intern Med **72**:327

Bromberg PA et al (1973) High oxygen affinity variant of hemoglobin Little Rock with unique properties, Nature (New Biol) **243**:177

Bromberg YM et al (1956) Distribution of fetal hemoglobin in layers by centrifugation, Proc Soc Exp Biol Med **92**:214

Bromberg YM et al (1957) Alkali resistant type of hemoglobin in women with molar pregnancy, Blood **12**:1122

Bromberg PA et al (1973) Hemoglobin Little Rock (beta 143 his → gln: [H21]). A high oxygen affinity haemoglobin variant with unique properties, Nature (New Biol) **243**:177

Bronson WR et al (1966) Pseudohyperkalemia due to release of potassium from white blood cells during clotting, N Engl J Med **274**:369

Brouet J-C et al (1973a) Indications of the thymus-derived nature of the proliferating cells in six patients with Sézary's syndrome, N Engl J Med **289**:341

Brouet J-C et al (1973b) Blast cells with monoclonal surface immunoglobulin in two cases of acute blast crisis supervening on chronic lymphocytic leukaemia, Br Med J **4**:23

Brouet J-C et al (1975a) Chronic lymphocytic leukaemia of T-cell origin: immunological and clinical evaluation in eleven patients, Lancet **2**:890

Brouet J-C et al (1975b) Evaluation of T and B lymphocyte membrane markers in human non-Hodgkin malignant lymphomata, Br J Cancer **31**:Suppl II, 121

Brouet J-C et al (1975c) The use of B and T membrane markers in the classification of human leukemias, with special reference with acute lymphoblastic leukemia, Blood Cells **1**:81

Brouet J-C et al (1976) Immunological classification of acute lymphoblastic leukaemias: evaluation of its clinical significance in a hundred patients, Br J Haematol **33**:319

Brouet J-C et al (1979) μ-Chain disease: report of two new cases, Arch Intern Med **139**:672

Brough AJ et al (1967) Dermal erythropoiesis in neonatal infants: a manifestation of intrauterine viral disease, Pediatrics **40**:627

Brown AK and Zuelzer WW (1958) Studies on the neonatal development of the glucuronide conjugating system, J Clin Invest **37**:332

Brown CH (1972) Bone marrow necrosis. A study of seventy cases, Johns Hopkins Med J **131**:189

Brown EE (1955) Evaluation of new capillary resistometer, petechiometer, J Lab Clin Med **34**:1714

Brown NL and Shnitka TK (1956) Constitutional nonhemolytic jaundice with "lipochrome" hepatosis (Dubin-Sprinz disease), Am J Med **21**:292

Brown WMC and Abbatt JD (1955) Effect of a single dose of x-rays on the peripheral blood count of man, Br J Haematol **1**:75

Brown WJ et al (1976) Hemoglobin Athens-Georgia, or alpha 2 beta 2 40 (C6) arg → lys, a hemoglobin variant with an increased oxygen affinity, Biochim Biophys Acta **439**:70

Broxmeyer H et al (1974) Mechanisms of leukocyte production and release. XII. A comparative assay of the leukocytosis-inducing factor (LIF) and the colony-stimulating factor (CSF), Proc Soc Exp Biol Med **145**:1262

Broxmeyer HE et al (1977) Cell-free granulocyte colony inhibiting activity derived from human polymorphonuclear neutrophils, Exp Hematol **5**:87

Brozovic M et al (1975) Plasma heparin levels after low dose subcutaneous heparin in patients undergoing hip replacement, Br J Haematol **31**:461

Brubaker DB and Whiteside TL (1979) Differentiation between benign and malignant human lymph nodes by means of immunologic markers, Cancer **43**:1165

Brubaker DB et al (1979) Correlations of immunologic markers with histologic features of human non-Hodgkin's lymphomas, Am J Clin Pathol **71**:651

Bruce WR and McCulloch EA (1964) The effect of erythropoietic stimulation on the hemopoietic colony-forming cells of mice, Blood **23**:216

Bruninga GL (1971) Complement—a review of the chemistry and reaction mechanisms, Am J Clin Pathol **55**:273

Brunning RD et al (1975) Bilateral trephine bone marrow biopsies in lymphoma and other neoplastic disease, Ann Intern Med **82**:365

Bruton OC (1952) Agammaglobulinemia, Pediatrics **9**:722

Bryant RE et al (1967) Studies on leukocyte motility. II. Effects of bacterial endotoxin on leukocyte migration, adhesiveness, and aggregation, Yale J Biol Med **40**:192

Buchanan GR (1978) Neonatal coagulation: normal physiology and pathophysiology, Clin Haematol **7**:85

Buchanan GR and Kevy SV (1978) Use of prothrombin complex concentrates in hemophiliacs with inhibitors: clinical and laboratory studies, Pediatrics **62**:767

Buchholz DH (1974) Blood transfusion: merits of component therapy. I. The clinical use of red cells, platelets, and granulocytes, J Pediatr **84**:1

Buchholz DH et al (1971) Bacterial proliferation in platelet products stored at room temperature. Transfusion-induced enterobacter sepsis, N Engl J Med **285**:429

Buchholz DH et al (1973) Detection and quantitation of bacteria in platelet products stored at ambient temperature, Transfusion **13**:268

Buckley RH et al (1968) Serum immunoglobulins. I. Levels in normal children and in uncomplicated childhood allergy, Pediatrics **41**:600

Buckley RH et al (1972) Extreme hyperimmunoglobulinemia E and undue susceptibility to infection, Pediatrics **49**:59

Budz-Olsen OE (1951) Clot retraction, Oxford, Blackwell Scientific Publications Ltd

Buffone GJ et al (1979) Limitations of immunochemical measurement of ceruloplasmin, Clin Chem **25**:749

Bujak JS and Root RK (1974) The role of peroxidase in the bactericidal activity of human blood eosinophils, Blood **43**:727

Buka NJ (1965) Eosinophilia associated with uterine leiomyomas, Can Med Assoc J **93**:163

Bull BS (1975) A statistical approach to quality control. In Lewis SM and Roster JF (Eds): Quality control in haematology, New York, Academic Press, Inc, p 111

Bull BS and Brailsford JD (1972) The zeta sedimentation ratio, Blood **40**:550

Bull BS and Kuhn IN (1970) The production of schistocytes by fibrin strands (a scanning electron microscope study), Blood **35**:104

Bull BS et al (1968) Microangiopathic haemolytic anemia: mechanisms of red-cell fragmentation, in vitro studies, Br J Haematol **14**:643

Bull BS et al (1974) A study of various estimators for the derivation of quality control procedures from patient erythrocyte indices, Am J Clin Pathol **61**:473

Bull WT (1884) On the intra-venous injection of saline solutions as a substitute for transfusion of blood, Med Rec **25**:6

Bullock WH et al (1957) Hemophilia in Negro subjects, Arch Intern Med **100**:759

Bunn HF et al (1972) Structural and functional studies on hemoglobin Bethesda ($\alpha 2\beta 2^{145His}$), a variant associated with compensatory erythrocytosis, J Clin Invest **51**:2299

Bunn, HF et al (1975) Hemoglobin Cranston, an unstable variant having an elongated beta chain due to non-homologous crossover between two normal beta chain genes, Proc Natl Acad Sci USA **72**:3609

Bunn HF et al (1976) The biosynthesis of human hemoglobin A_{1c}: slow glycosylation of hemoglobin in vivo, J Clin Invest **57**:1652

Bunn HF et al (1978) The glycosylation of hemoglobin: relevance to diabetes mellitus, Science **200**:21

Bunn HF et al (1979) Structural heterogeneity of human hemoglobin A due to nonenzymatic glycosylation, J Biol Chem **254**:3892

Burch GE and DePasquale NP (1961) Erythrocytosis and ischemic disease, Am Heart J **62**:139

Burch GE and DePasquale NP (1962) Hematocrit, blood viscosity, and myocardial infarction, Am J. Med **32**:161

Bureau Y et al (1959) La réticulose erythrodermique avec réticulémie de Sézary, Presse Med **67**:2276

Burka ER et al (1966) Clinical spectrum of hemolytic anemia associated with glucose-6-phosphate dehydrogenase deficiency, Ann Intern Med **64**:817

Burke JS (1978) The value of the bone-marrow biopsy in the diagnosis of hairy cell leukemia, Am J Clin Pathol **70**:876

Burke JS et al ((1974) Hairy cell leukemia (leukemic reticuloendotheliosis). I. A clinical pathologic study of 21 patients, Cancer **33**:1399

Burkett LB et al (1976) Hemoglobin Mequon beta 41 (C7) phenylalanine → tyrosine, Blood **48**:645

Burkitt D (1958) A sarcoma involving the jaws in African children, Br J Surg **46**:218

Burman JF et al (1979) Inherited lack of transcobalamin II in serum and megaloblastic anaemia: a further patient, Br J Haematol **43**:27

Burne JC (1953) Niemann-Pick disease in a foetus, J Pathol Bacteriol **66**:473

Burnet FM (1959) The clonal selection theory of acquired immunity, Nashville, Vanderbilt University Press

Burnet FM (1969) Cellular immunology, London and New York, Cambridge University Press

Burns CP et al (1973) Biochemical, morphological, and immunological observations of leukemic reticuloendotheliosis, Cancer Res **33**:1615

Burrell JM (1953) A comparative study of the circulating eosinophil level in babies. II. In full term infants, Arch Dis Child **28**:140

Bursaux E et al (1978) Hemoglobin Ty Gard (alpha 2A beta 2 124 [H2] pro → gln): a stable high O_2 affinity variant at the alpha 1 beta 1 contact, FEBS Lett **88**:155

Burwell CS et al (1956) Extreme obesity associated with alveolar hypoventilation—a Pickwickian syndrome, Am J Med **21**:811

Busuttil RW et al (1971) Cytological localization of erythropoietin in the human kidney using the fluorescent antibody technique, Proc Soc Exp Biol Med **137**:327

Butterworth CE Jr et al (1958) Studies on copper metabolism XXVI. Plasma copper in patients with tropical sprue, Proc Soc Exp Biol Med **98**:594

Butterworth CE Jr et al (1963) The pteroylglutamate components of American diets as determined by chromatographic fractionation, J Clin Invest **42**:1929

Butterworth M et al (1967) Influence of sex on immunoglobin levels, Nature **214**:1224

Byrd RB and Cooper T (1961) Hereditary iron-loading anemia with secondary hemochromatosis, Ann Intern Med **55**:103

Byrne GE Jr (1977) Rappaport classification of non-Hodgkin's lymphoma: histologic features and clinical significance, Cancer Treat Rep **61**:935

Cabanel G et al (1973) Myélome hypo-excrétant, Sem Hop Paris **49**:1057

Cabannes R et al (1972) Deux hémoglobines rapides en Cote-D'Ivoire: 1'hb K Woolwich et une nouvelle hémoglobine, 1'hb J Abidjan (alpha 51 gly → asp), Nouv Rev Fr Hematol **12**:289

Cabot EB et al (1978) Splenectomy in myeloid metaplasia, Ann Surg **187**:24

Cabrera HA and Carlson J (1968) Biologic false-positive reactions and infectious mononucleosis, Am J Clin Pathol **50**:643

Caen JP (1972) Glanzmann thrombasthenia, Clin Haematol **1**:383

Caen JP et al (1966) Congenital bleeding disorders with long bleeding time and normal platelet count. I. Glanzmann's thrombasthenia (report of fifteen patients), Am J Med **41**:4

Caen JP et al (1969) Les thrombocytopathies acquises, Nouv Rev Fr Hematol **9**:553

Caen J et al (1973) La dystrophie thrombocytaire hémorragipare (interaction des plaquettes et du facteur Willebrand), Nouv Rev Fr Hematol **13**:595

Caen J and Legrand Y (1972) Abnormalities in the platelet-collagen reaction, Ann NY Acad Sci **201**:194

Cahill RNP et al (1977) Two distinct pools of recirculating T lymphocytes: migratory characteristics of nodal and intestinal T lymphocytes, J Exp Med **145**:420

Cairnie AB et al (Eds) (1976) Stem cells of renewing cell populations, New York, Academic Press, Inc

Calabro JJ et al (1976) Juvenile rheumatoid arthritis: a general review and report on 100 patients observed for 15 years, Semin Arthritis Rheum **5**:257

Caldwell J (1957) Detection of blood coagulation defects in the clinical laboratory, Am J Med Technol **23**:277

Caligaris-Cappio F et al (1979) Idiopathic neutropenia with normocellular bone marrow: an immune-complex disease, Br J Haematol **43**:595

Callender ST and Race RR (1946) A serological and genetical study of multiple antibodies formed in response to blood transfusion by a patient with lupus erythematosus diffusus, Ann Eugen **13**:102

Callender ST and Warner GT (1968) Iron absorption from bread, Am J Clin Nutr **21:**1170

Cameron C et al (1959) Acquisition of a B-like antigen by red blood cells, Br Med J **2:**29

Cameron GL and Staveley JM (1957) Blood group P substance in hydatid cyst fluids, Nature **179:**147

Campbell BC et al (1978) Haem biosynthesis in rheumatoid disease, Br J Haematol **40:**563

Campbell EW et al (1978) Therapy with factor IX concentrate resulting in DIC and thromboembolic phenomena, Transfusion **18:**94

Campbell E et al (1980) Factor VII inhibitor, Am J Med **68:**962

Canali G (1957) Ittero congenito familiare ''epatico,'' Recent Prog Med **23:**69

Canellos GP et al (1976) Chronic granulocytic leukemia without the Philadelphia chromosome, Am J Clin Pathol **65:**467

Cannat A and Seligmann M (1973) Immunological abnormalities in juvenile myelomonocytic leukaemia, Br Med J **1:**71

Cannemeyer W et al (1955) Severe para-aminosalicylic acid hypersensitivity: blood and lymph node studies, Blood **10:**62

Cáp J et al (1968) Kongenitálna atransferinemia u 11-mesačného dietata, Cesk Pediatr **23:**1020

Cape RDT (1954) Iododerma of face and marked eosinophilia, Br Med **1:**255

Capecchi MR and Klein HA (1969) Characterization of three proteins involved in polypeptide chain termination, Cold Spring Harbor Symp Quant Biol **34:**469

Capp GL et al (1970) Evidence of a new haemoglobin chain (ζ-chain), Nature **228:**278

Capra JD et al (1969) An incomplete cold-reactive gamma G antibody with i specificity in infectious mononucleosis, Vox Sang **16:**10

Caramihai E et al (1975) Leukocyte count differences in healthy white and black children 1 to 5 years of age, J Pediatr **86:**252

Carbone JV and Grodsky GM (1957) Constitutional nonhemolytic hyperbilirubinemia in the rat: defect of bilirubin conjugation, Proc Soc Exp Biol Med **94:**461

Carbone PP et al (1967) Plasmacytic myeloma. A study of the relationship of survival to various clinical manifestations and anomalous protein type in 112 patients, Am J Med **42:**937

Carbone PP et al (1971) Report of the committee on Hodgkin's disease staging classification, Cancer Res **31:**1860

Carey RW et al (1976) Carcinocythemia (carcinoma cell leukemia). An acute leukemia-like picture due to metastatic carcinoma cells, Am J Med **60:**273

Carmel R (1972) Vitamin B_{12}-binding protein abnormality in subjects without myeloproliferative disease. II. The presence of a third vitamin B_{12}-binding protein in serum, Br J Haematol **22:**53

Carmel R and Coltman CA (1971) Nonleukemic elevation of serum vitamin B_{12} and B_{12}-binding capacity levels resembling that in chronic myelogenous leukemia, J Lab Clin Med **78:**289

Carmel R and Herbert V (1969) Deficiency of vitamin B_{12}-binding alpha globulin in two brothers, Blood **33:**1

Carmel R and Hollander D (1978) Extreme elevation of transcobalamin II levels in multiple myeloma and other disorders, Blood **51:**1057

Carmel R et al (1977) Circulating antibody to transcobalamin II causing retention of vitamin B_{12} in the blood, Blood **49:**987

Carmena A et al (1967) Urinary erythropoietin in men subjected to acute hypoxia, Proc Soc Exp Biol Med **125:**441

Carnot P and Deflandre (1906) Sur l'activité hémopoiétique du serum au cours de la régenération du sang. C R Acad Sci **143:**384

Carr MC et al (1973) Cellular aspects of the human fetal maternal relationship. II. In vitro response of gravida lynphocytes to phytohemagglutinin, Cell Immunol **8:**448

Carrell RW et al (1966) Haemoglobin Köln (beta 98 valine → methionine): an unstable protein causing inclusion-body anaemia, Nature (London) **210:**915

Carrell RW et al (1967) Haemoglobin Sydney: beta 67 (E ll) valine → alanine: an emerging pattern of unstable haemoglobins, Nature (London) **215:**626

Carrell RW and Owen MC (1971) A new approach to haemoglobin variant identification. Haemoglobin Christchurch beta 71 (E15) phenylalanine → serine, Biochim Biophys Acta **236:**507

Carrell RW et al (1974) Haemoglobin F Auckland G gamma 7 asp → asn—further evidence for multiple genes for the gamma chain, Biochim Biophys Acta **365:**323

Carrell RW (1974) Hemoglobin stability tests. In Schmidt RM et al (Eds): The detection of hemoglobinopathies, Cleveland, CRC Press

Carrell RW and Kay RA (1972) A simple method for the detection of unstable haemoglobins, Br J Haematol **23:**615

Carriere S et al (1966) Intrarenal distribution of blood flow in dogs during hemorrhagic hypotension, Circ Res **19:**167

Carson PE and Frischer H (1966) Glucose-6-phosphate dehydrogenase deficiency and related disorders of the pentose phosphate pathway, Am J Med **41:**744

Carstens PHB (1969) Pulmonary bone marrow embolism following external cardiac massage, Acta Pathol Microbiol Scand **76:**510

Cartei G and Dini E (1975) Coexistence of β-thalassemia trait and Gilbert's syndrome in three families, Acta Haematol **53:**175

Carter NG and Hocking DR (1967) Diverticula of the ileum with megaloblastic anaemia, Med J Aust **1:**444

Carter JW et al (1978) Infectious mononucleosis in the older patient, Mayo Clin Proc **53:**146

Cartwright GE (1949) An unusual case of clonorchiasis with marked eosinophilia and pulmonary infiltration, Am J Med **6:**259

Cartwright GE (1966) The anemia of chronic disorders, Semin Hematol **3:**351

Cartwright GE and Deiss A (1975) Sideroblasts, siderocytes, and sideroblastic anemia, N Engl J Med **292:**185

Cartwright GE and Lee GR (1971) The anemia of chronic disorders, Br J Haematol **21:**147

Cartwright GE and Wintrobe MM (1964) Copper metabolism in normal subjects, Am J Clin Nutr **14:**224

Cartwright GE et al (1960) Studies on copper metabolism. XXIX. A critical analysis of serm copper and ceruloplasmin concentrations in normal subjects, patients with Wilson's disease, and relatives of patients with Wilson's disease, Am J Med **28:**555

Cartwright GE et al (1964) The kinetics of granulopoiesis in normal man, Blood **24:**780

Cartwright GE et al (1979) Hereditary hemochromatosis: phenotypic expression of the disease, N Engl J Med **301:**175

Carvalho AC et al (1974a) Platelet function in hyperlipoproteinemia, N Engl J Med **290:**434

Carvalho AC et al (1974b) Clofibrate reversal of platelet hypersensitivity in hyperbetalipoproteinemia, Circulation **50:**570

Case RAM (1945) Siderocytes in haemolytic diseases: new index of severity and progress, J Pathol **57:**271

Casey R et al (1976) Double heterozygosity for two unstable haemoglobins: hb Sydney (beta 67 E ll) (val → ala) and hb Coventry (beta 141 [H19] leu deleted), Br J Haematol **33:**143

Cass AJ et al (1980) Gastrointestinal bleeding, angiodysplasia of the colon, and acquired von Willebrand disease, Br J Cancer **67:**639

Cassileth PA (1967) Monocytosis in chlorpromazine-associated agranulocytosis, termination in acute leukemia. Am J Med **43:**471

Cassileth PA and Myers AR (1973) Erythroid aplasia in systemic lupus erythematosus, Am J Med 55:706

Cassimos C et al (1960) Aldrich's syndrome (thrombocytopenia, eczema, and recurrent infections): report of a case, Am J Dis Child 100:914

Castaldi PA and Smith IL (1980) The effect of platelets on the in vitro response to prothrombin complex concentrates in f. VIII inhibitor plasma, Pathology 12:111

Castaneda MR and Guerrero G (1946) Studies on the leukocytic picture in brucellosis, J Infect Dis 78:43

Castle WB (1953) Development of the knowledge concerning the gastric intrinsic factor and its relation to pernicious anemia, N Engl J Med 249:603

Castoldi EL et al (1975) Consecutive cytochemical staining for the analysis of the blastic population in the acute phase of chronic myeloid leukaemia, Biomedicine 23:12

Catovsky D (1977) Surface markers in acute lymphoblastic leukaemia and lymphoproliferative disorders. In Hoffbrand AV et al (Eds): Recent advances in haematology, ed 2, London, Churchill Livingstone, p 201

Catovsky D et al (1971a) Sideroblastic anaemia and its association with leukaemia and myelomatosis: report of five cases, Br J Haematol 20:385

Catovsky D et al (1971b) The significance of lysozyme estimations in acute myeloid and chronic monocytic leukaemia, Br J Haematol 21:565

Catovsky D et al (1973) Prolymphocytic leukemia of B and T cell type, Lancet 1:232

Catovsky D et al (1974a) Cytochemical profile of B and T leukaemic lymphocytes with special reference to acute lymphoblastic leukaemia, J Clin Pathol 27:767

Catovsky D et al (1974b) Leukaemic reticuloendotheliosis ("hairy" cell laeukemia): a distinct clinicopathological entity, Br J Haematol 26:9

Cauchi MN et al (1969) Haemoglobin F (Malta): a new foetal haemoglobin variant with a high incidence in Maltese infants, Nature (London) 223:311

Cavill I et al (1976) The measurement of ^{59}Fe clearance from the plasma, Scand J Haematol 17:160

Cavill I et al (1977) Radioiron and erythropoiesis: methods, interpretation and clinical application, Clin Haematol 6:583

Cavins JA et al (1964) The recovery of lethally irradiated dogs given infusions of autologous leukocytes stored at −80° C, Blood 23:38

Cawein MJ et al (1966) Hemoglobin S-D disease, Ann Intern Med 64:62

Cawein M et al (1962) A study of methemoglobinemia due to congenital diaphorase deficiency, J Lab Clin Med 60:866

Cawley JC and Hayhoe GJ (1972) The inclusions of the May-Hegglin anomaly and Döhle bodies of infection: an ultrastructure comparison, Br J Haematol 22:491

Cech P et al (1979) Hereditary myeloperoxidase deficiency, Blood 53:403

Cedarbaum AI et al (1976) Intravascular coagulation with use of human prothrombin complex concentrates, Ann Intern Med 84:683

Ceppellini R and van Rood JJ (1974) The HL-A system: I. Genetics and molecular biology, Semin Heamatol 11:233

Chaganti RSK et al (1979) Cytogenetic evidence of the intrauterine origin of acute leukemia in monozygotic twins, N Engl J Med 300:1032

Chamberlain JK and Lichtman MA (1978) Marrow cell egress: specificity of the site of penetration into the sinus, Blood 52:959

Chamberlain JK et al (1975) Reduction of adventitial cell cover: an early direct effect of erythropoietin on bone marrow ultrastructure, Blood Cells 1:655

Chambers R and Zeveifack WB (1947) Intercellular cement and capillary permeability, Physiol Rev 27:436

Chambers RW et al (1969) Transmission of syphilis by fresh blood components, Transfusion 9:32

Chambers TJ (1978) Multinucleate giant cells, J Pathol 126:125

Chan BS (1972) Ultrastructural changes in guinea-pig bone marrow basophilis during anaphylaxis, Immunology 23:215

Chan TK and Todd D (1972) Characteristics and distribution of glucose-6-phosphate dehydrogenase-deficient variants in South China, Am J Hum Genet 24:475

Chanarin I (1969) The megaloblastic anemias, Philadelphia, FA Davis Co

Chanarin I (1972) Pernicious anaemia as an autoimmune disease, Br J Haematol 23:101

Chanarin I (1976) Investigation and management of megaloblastic anemia, Clin Haematol 5:747

Chanarin I (1979) Alcohol and the blood, Br J Haematol 42:333

Chanarin I and Davey DA (1964) Acute megaloblastic arrest of haemopoises in pregnancy, Br J Haematol 10:314

Chanarin I and James D (1974) Humoral and cell-mediated intrinsic-factor antibody in pernicious anaemia, Lancet 1:1078

Chanarin I et al (1968) Normal dietary folate, iron, and protein intake, with particular reference to pregnancy, Br Med J 2:394

Chandra RK et al (1969) Chronic granulomatous disease. Evidence for an autosomal mode of inheritance, Lancet 2:71

Chandra S and Wickerhauser M (1979) Contact factors responsible for the thrombogenicity of prothrombin complex, Thromb Res 14:189

Chang RS et al (1979) Incidence of infectious mononucleosis at the Universities of California and Hawaii, J Infect Dis 140:479

Chang MY and Campbell WG (1975) Fatal infectious mononucleosis. Association with liver necrosis and herpes-like virus particles, Arch Pathol 99:185

Chanutin A (1967) Effect of storage of blood in ACD-adenine-inorganic phosphate plus nucleosides on metabolic intermediates of human red cells, Transfusion 7:409

Chanutin A and Curnish RR (1967) Effect of organic and inorganic phosphates on the oxygen equilibrium of human erythrocytes, Arch Biochem Biophys 121:96

Chaplin H Jr (1969) Packed red blood cells, N Engl J Med 281:364

Charache S and Conley CL (1964) Rate of sickling of red cells during deoxygenation of blood from persons with various sickling disorders, Blood 24:25

Charache S and Conley CL (1969) Hereditary persistence of fetal hemoglobin, Ann NY Acad Sci 165:37

Charache S and Page DL (1967) Infarction of bone marrow in the sickle cell disorders, Ann Intern Med 67:1195

Charache S and Ostertag W (1970) Hemoglobin Hopkins-2 (alpha 112 asp) 2 beta 2): "low output" protects from potentially harmful effects, Blood 36:852

Charache S et al (1973) Hemoglobin Okaloosa (beta 48 [CD7] leucine → arginine). An unstable hemoglobin with decreased oxygen affinity, J Clin Invest 52:2858

Charache S et al (1975) Polycythemia produced by hemoglobin Osler (beta 145 [HC2] tyr → asp), Johns Hopkins Med J 136:132

Charache S et al (1978) Hb Potomac (beta 101 glu → asp): speculations on placental oxygen transport in carriers of high affinity hemoglobins, Blood 51:331

Charette R and Komp DM (1972) NBT test and incubation temperature, N Engl J Med 287:991

Charm SE et al (1979) Reduced plasma viscosity among joggers compared with non-joggers, Biorheology 16:185

Chase MW (1945) Cellular transfer of cutaneous hypersensitivity to tuberculin, Proc Soc Exp Biol Med 59:134

Chatterjea JB et al (1952) Splenic puncture, Br Med J **1**:987

Chediak M (1952) Nouvelle anomalie leukocytoire de caractère constititionelle et familial, Rev Hematol **7**:362

Chediak JR et al (1977) Platelet function and immunologic parameters in von Willebrand's disease following cryoprecipitate and factor VIII concentrate infusion, AM J Med **62**:369

Chen HP and Walz DV (1958) Leukemoid reaction in the bone marrow, associated with malignant neoplasms, Am J Clin Pathol **29**:345

Chen B and Doolittle RF (1971) γ-γ crosslinking sites in human and bovine fibrin, Biochemistry **10**:4486

Chen-Marotel J et al (1979) Hemoglobin Bougardirey-Mali beta 119 (GH2) gly → val. An electrophoretically silent variant migrating in isoelectrofocusing as hg F, Hemoglobin **3**:253

Chernoff AI (1955) The human hemoglobin in health and disease, N Engl J Med **253**:322

Chernoff AI (1958) The hemoglobin D syndromes, Blood **13**:116

Chernoff AI and Horton BF (1969) Laboratory approach to diagnosis of hemoglobin abnormalities, Clin Obstet Gynecol **12**:76

Chernoff AI and Liu JC (1961) The amino acid composition of hemoglobin. II. Analytic technics, Blood **17**:54

Chernoff AI and Perillie PE (1964) The amino acid composition of HGB New Haven #2 (HGB N New Haven), Biochem Biophys Res Commun **16**:368

Chernoff AI and Pettit N Jr (1965) The amino acid composition of hemoglobin. VI. Separation of the tryptic peptides of hemoglobin Knoxville No 1 on Dowex-1 X-2 and Sephadex, Biochem Biophys Acta **97**:47

Chernoff AI et al (1956) Studies on hemoglobin E. I. The clinical, hematologic, and genetic characteristics of the hemoglobin E syndromes, J Lab Clin Med **47**:455, 490

Cherrick GR et al (1965) Observations on hepatic avidity for folate in Laennec's cirrhosis, J Lab Clin Med **66**:446

Chervenick PA and Boggs DR (1970) Bone marrow colonies: stimulation in vitro by supernatant from incubated human blood cells, Science **169**:691

Chervenick PA and LoBuglio AF (1972) Human blood monocytes: stimulators of granulocyte and mononuclear colony formation in vitro, Science **178**:164

Chesley LC et al (1972) Plasma and red cell volume during pregnancy, Am J Obstet Gynecol **112**:440

Chessels JM et al (1977) Acute lymphoblastic leukaemia in children: classification and prognosis, Lancet **2**:1307

Chien S et al (1968) Centrifugal packing of suspensions of erythrocytes hardened with acetaldehyde, Proc Soc Exp Biol Med **127**:982

Chien S (1976) Clumping (reversible aggregation and irreversible agglutination) of blood cellular elements. Electrochemical interactions between erythrocyte surfaces, Thromb Res **8**(suppl 2):189

Chievitz E and Thiede T (1962) Complications and causes of death in polycythaemia vera, Acta Med Scand **172**:513

Chilcote RR and Baehner RL (1974) Infection in childhood cancer: experiences in management of infection in acute leukemia. Pediatr Ann **3**:71

Chilosi M et al (1979) Eosinophilic acquired Pelger-Huët anomaly in acute myeloblastic leukemia, Acta Haematol **61**:198

Chini V and Valeri CM (1949) Mediterranean hemopathic syndromes, Blood **4**:989

Choi KW and Bloom AD (1970) Biochemically marked lymphocytoid lines: establishment of Lesch-Nyhan cells, Science **170**:89

Choi SI and McClure PD (1967) Idiopathic thrombocytopenic purpura in childhood, Can Med Assoc J **97**:562

Chiorazzi N et al (1974) Recurrent hematuria: occurrence in a white woman with sickle cell trait, JAMA **230**:582

Chisolm JJ Jr (1964) Disturbances in the biosynthesis of heme in lead intoxication, J Pediatr **64**:174

Chojnacki RE et al (1968) Transfusion-introduced falciparum malaria, N Engl J Med **279**:984

Christensen RD and Rothstein G (1979) Pitfalls in the interpretation of leukocyte counts of newborn infants, Am J Clin Pathol **72**:608

Chuang TF et al (1972) The intrinsic activation of factor X in blood coagulation, Biochem Biophys Acta **273**:287

Chung ASM et al (1961) Folic acid, vitamin B$_6$, pantothenic acid, and vitamin B$_{12}$ in human dietaries, Am J Clin Nutr **9**:573

Chung SI et al (1974) Relationships of the catalytic properties of human plasma and platelet transglutaminases (activated blood coagulation factor XIII) to their subunit structures, J Biol Chem **249**:940

Chung KS et al (1980) Factor IX: genetic, chemical, and biophysical characteristics. In Schmidt RM (Section Ed): Handbook Series in Clinical Laboratory Science, Section I: Hematology, vol 3, Boca Raton, CRC Press, Inc, p 85

Chusid MJ et al (1975) The hypereosinophilic syndrome: analysis of 14 cases with review of the literature, Medicine **54**:1

Cimo PL and Aster RH (1972) Post-transfusion purpura. Successful treatment by exchange transfusion, N Engl J Med **287**:290

Cinotti GA et al (1957) Ittero anemolitico familiare a bilirubinemia diretta e splenomegalia, Policlinico (Prat) **64**:1573

Cioli D and Baglioni C (1968) Catabolic origin of a Bence Jones protein fragment, J Exp Med **128**:517

Claman HN (1966) Human thymus cell cultures—evidence for two functional populations, Proc Soc Exp Biol Med **121**:236

Claman HN and Chaperon EA (1969) Immunologic complementation between thymus and marrow cells—a model for the two-cell theory of immunocompetence, Transplant Rev **1**:92

Clark C et al (1973) Frequent association of IgM λ with cystalline inclusions in chronic lymphatic leukemic lymphocytes, N Engl J Med **289**:113

Clark RA and Kimball HR (1971) Defective granulocyte chemotaxis in the Chediak-Higashi syndrome, J Clin Invest **50**:2645

Clark RA et al (1973) Defective neutrophil chemotaxis and cellular immunity in a child with recurrent infections, Ann Intern Med **78**:515

Clark RA et al (1974) Neutrophil chemotaxis in systemic lupus erythematosus, Ann Rheum Dis **33**:167

Clark RAF and Kaplan AP (1975) Eosinophil leucocytes: structure and function, Clin Haematol **4**:635

Clark WF et al (1978) Immunologic findings, thrombocytopenia and disease activity in lupus nephritis, Can Med Assoc J **118**:1391

Clarke BF and Davies SH (1964) Severe thrombocytopenia in infectious mononucleosis, Am J Med Sci **248**:703

Clarkson B et al (1967) Continuous cultures of seven new cell lines (SK-L1 to 7) from patients with acute leukemia, Cancer **20**:926

Clayton EM et al (1973) Fetal cell counting as a guide to prevention of RH sensitization, Transfusion **13**:425

Clegg JB and Charache S (1978) The structure of hemoglobin Hopkins 2, Hemoglobin **2**:85

Clegg JB and Weatherall DJ (1972) Haemoglobin synthesis during erythroid maturation in β-thalassaemia, Nature (New Biol) **240**:190

Clegg JB et al (1965) An improved method for the characterization of human haemoglobin mutants: identification of alpha 2 beta 2 95 glu, haemoglobin N (Baltimore), Nature (London) **207**:945

Clegg JB et al (1966) Abnormal human haemoglobins. Separation and characterization of the alpha and beta chains by chromatography, and the determination of two new variants, hb Chesapeake and hb J (Bangkok), J Mol Biol **19**:91

Clegg JB et al (1969) Two new haemoglobin variants involving proline substitutions, Nature (London) **22**:379

Clegg JB et al (1971) Haemoglobin Constant Spring—a chain termination mutant, Nature **234**:337

Clegg JB et al (1974) Haemoglobin Icaria, a new chain-termination mutant which causes alpha thalassemia, Nature **251**:245

Clem LW et al (1967) Phylogeny of immunoglobulin structure and function. II. Immunoglobulins of the lemon shark, J Immunol **99**:1226

Clement DB et al (1977) 3. Hemoglobin values: comparative survey of the 1976 Canadian olympic team, Can Med Assoc J **117**:614

Clément F (1979) Les hémopathies malignes induites: six nouvelles observations dont l'une avec survie de 45 mois, Schweiz Med Wschr **109**:544

Clendenning WE et al (1964) Mycosis fungoides: relationship to malignant cutaneous reticulosis and the Sézary syndrome, Arch Dermatol **89**:785

Cleton F et al (1963) Synthetic chelating agents in iron metabolism, J Clin Invest **42**:327

Cleveland WW et al (1968) Foetal thymic transplant in a case of Di Georg's syndrome, Lancet **2**:1211

Clift RA et al (1978) Granulocyte transfusions for the prevention of infection in patients receiving bone marrow transplants, N Engl J Med **298**:1052

Cline MJ and Berlin NI (1963) An evaluation of DFP^{32} and Cr^{51} as methods of measuring red cell life span in man, Blood **22**:459

Cline MJ and Lehrer RI (1968) Phagocytosis by human monocytes, Blood **32**:423

Cline MJ and Golde DW (1974) Production of colony-stimulating activity by human lymphocytes, Nature **248**:703

Cline MJ and Golde DW (1978) Immune suppression of hematopoiesis, AM J Med **64**:301

Cline MJ and Golde DW (1979a) Controlling the production of blood cells, Blood **53**:157

Cline MJ and Golde DW (1979b) Cellular interactions in haematopoiesis, Nature **277**:177

Cline MJ et al (1968) Phagocytosis by human eosinophils, Blood **32**:922

Cline MJ et al (1977) Discrete clusters of hematopoietic cells in the marrow cavity of man after bone marrow transplantation, Blood **50**:709

Cline MJ et al (1978) Inhibitors of myelopoiesis, Transplant Proc **10**:99

Cloutier MD and Burgert EO (1966) Congenital nonspherocytic hemolytic disease secondary to glucose-6-phosphate dehydrogenase deficiency. Report of three cases, Mayo Clin Proc **41**:316

Clyne LP et al (1980) In vitro correction of the anticoagulant activity and specific clotting factor assays in SLE, Thromb Res **18**:643

Cochrane CG and Wuepper KD (1971) The first component of the kinin-forming system in human and rabbit plasma. Its relationship to clotting factor XII (Hageman factor), J Exp Med **134**:986

Cohen D et al (1979) Nonfatal graft-versus-host disease occurring after transfusion with leukocytes and platelets obtained from normal donors, Blood **53**:1053

Cohen EJ et al (1944) Characterization of protein fractions of human plasma, J Clin Invest **23**:417

Cohen G and Somerson NL (1967) Mycoplasma pneumoniae: hydrogen peroxide secretion and its possible role in virulence, Ann NY Acad Sci **143**:85

Cohen HJ and Rundles RW (1975) Managing the complications of plasma cell myeloma, Arch Intern Med **135**:177

Cohen HJ et al (1978) New presentation of alpha heavy chain disease: North American polypoid gastrointestinal lymphoma: clinical and cellular studies, Cancer **41**:1161

Cohen HJ et al (1979) Hairy cell leukemia: cellular characteristics including surface immunoglobulin dynamics and biosynthesis, Blood **53**:764

Cohen I et al (1970) Plasma cell myeloma associated with an unusual myeloma protein causing impairment of fibrin aggregation and platelet function in a patient with multiple malignancy, Am J Med **48**:766

Cohen RJ et al (1968) Methemoglobinemia provoked by malarial chemoprophylaxis in Vietnam, N Engl J Med **279**:1127

Cohen S et al (1974) Serum migration-inhibitory activity in patients with lymphoproliferative diseases, N Engl J Med **290**:882

Cohen-Solal M et al (1973) Haemoglobin Saint Louis beta 28 (B10) leucine → glutamine. A new unstable haemoglobin only present in a ferri form, FEBS Lett **33**:37

Cohen-Solal M et al (1974) Haemoglobin Lyon (beta 17-18 [A14-15]) lys → val → 0) determination of sequenator analysis, Biochem Biophys Acta **351**:306

Cohen-Solal M et al (1975) Haemoglobin G Norfolk alpha 85 (F6) asp → asn. Structural characterization by sequenator analysis and functional properties of a new variant with high oxygen affinity, FEBS Lett **50**:163

Coidan RS (1951) The paranucleoli (nucleolar satellite bodies) in neurons of several male and female mammals, including man, Anat Rec **109**:282

Cole WH et al (1958) The dissemination of cancer cells, Bull NY Acad Med **34**:163

Coleman M et al (1972) Inhibition of fibrin monomer polymerization by lambda myeloma globulins, Blood **39**:210

Coleman MS et al (1976) Serial observations on terminal deoxynucleotidyl transferase activity and lymphoblast surface markers in acute lymphoblastic leukemia, Cancer Res **36**:120

Collier RL and Brush BE (1966) Hematologic disorder in Felty's syndrome. Prolonged benefits of splenectomy, Am J Surg **112**:869

Collins RD et al (1974) Abscence of B- and T-cell markers on acute lymphoblastic leukemic cells and persistence of the T-cell marker on mitrogen-transformed T-lymphocytes, Br J Haematol **26**:615

Collins GJ Jr et al (1976) Detection and management of hypercoagulability, Am J Surg **132**:767

Collison HA et al (1968) Determination of carbon monoxide in blood by gas chromatography, Clin Chem **14**:162

Colman RW and Shein HM (1962) Leukemoid reaction, hyperuricemia, and severe hyperpyrexia complicating a fatal case of acute fatty liver of the alcoholic, Ann Intern Med **57**:110

Colman RW and Sturgill BC (1965) Lupus-like syndrome induced by procaine amide: associated with anti-DNA antibody, Arch Intern Med **115**:214

Colman N and Herbert V (1974) Evidence for "granulocyte-related" and "liver-related" folate binder, Clin Res **22**:700A

Colman RW (1978) Platelet function in hyperbetalipoproteinemia, Thromb Haemost **39**:284

Colman RW (1980) Factor V. In Schmidt RM (Section Ed): Handbook Series in Clinical Laboratory Science, Section I: Hematology, vol 3, Boca Raton, CRC Press Inc, p 33

Colman RW and Wong PY (1977) Participation of Hageman factor dependent pathways in human disease states, Thromb Haemost **38**:751

Colombani J et al (1968) Two cases of neo-natal thrombocytopenia due to maternal iso-immunization against leuco-platelet antigens, Vox Sang **14**:137

Colombo B et al (1974) A new haemoglobin J Habana alpha 71 E20) alanine → glutamic acid, Biochim Biophys Acta **351**:1

Colvin RB and Dvorak HF (1975) Fibrinogen/fibrin on the surface of macrophages: detection, distribution, binding requirements, and possible role in macrophage adherence phenomena, J Exp Med **142**:1377

Colwell JA et al (1976) Altered platelet function in diabetes mellitus, Diabetes **25**:826

Comfort MW (1935) Constitutional hepatic dysfunction, Mayo Clin Proc **10**:57

Conard RA (1975) Acute myelogenous leukemia following fallout radiation exposure, JAMA **232**:1356

Conconi F et al (1975) Appearance of β-globin synthesis in erythroid cells of Ferrara β°-thalassaemic patients following blood tranfusion, Nature **254**:256

Condemi JJ et al (1967) Antinuclear antibodies following hydralazine toxicity, N Engl J Med **276**:486

Conley CL and Hartman RC (1952) A hemorrhagic disorder caused by circulating anticoagulant in patients with disseminated lupus erythematosus, J Clin EInvest **31**:621

Conley CL et al (1963) Hereditary persistence of fetal hemoglobin: a study of 79 affected persons in 15 Negro families in Baltimore, Blood **21**:261

Conley CL et al (1964) Hematocrit values in coronary artery disease, Arch Intern Med **113**:170

Conn HO (1954) Sickle-cell trait and splenic infarction associated with high-altitude flying, N Engl J Med **251**:417

Conn RB Jr and Sundberg RD (1961) Amyloid disease of the bone marrow: diagnosis by sternal marrow aspiration, Am J Pathol **38**:61

Connal A (1911) Auto-erythrophagocytosis in protozoal diseases, J Pathol Bacteriol **16**:502

Connell GE and Smithies O (1959) Human haptoglobins: estimation and purification, Biochem J **72**:115

Connell JT (1968) Morphological changes in eosinophils in allergic disease, J Allergy Clin Immunol **41**:1

Conrad FG et al (1965) A clinical evaluation of plasma thromboplastin antecedent (TPA) deficiency, Ann Intern Med **62**:885

Conrad ME (1971) Hematologic manifestations of parasitic infections, Semin Hematol **8**:267

Conrad ME and Crosby WH (1963) Intestinal mucosal mechanisms controlling iron absorption, Blood **22**:406

Conrad ME and Barton JC (1979) The aplastic anemia–paroxysmal nocturnal hemoglobinuria syndrome, Am J Hematol **7**:61

Constantoulakis M et al (1963) Quantitative studies of the effect of red-blood-cell sensitization on in vivo hemolysis, J Clin Invest **42**:1790

Contrera JF et al (1966) Extraction of an erythropoietin-producing factor from a particulate fraction of rat kidney, Blood **28**:330

Cook A and Raper AB (1971) The solubility test for Hb S: a cheap and rapid method, Med Lab Technol **28**:373

Cook JD and Lipschitz DA (1977) Clinical measurements of iron absorption, Clin Haematol **6**:567

Cook JD et al (1974) Serum ferritin as a measure of iron stores in normal subjects, Am J Clin Nutr **27**:681

Cooke JV (1954) The occurrence of leukemia, Blood **9**:340

Cooley TB (1927) Von Jaksch's anemia, Am J Dis Child **33**:786

Cooley TB and Lee P (1925) A series of cases of splenomegaly in children with anemia and peculiar bone changes, Trans Am Pediatr Soc **37**:29

Cooley TB et al (1927) Anemia in children with splenomegaly and peculiar changes in bones: report of cases, Am J Dis Child **34**:347

Coombs RRA et al (1945) New test for detection of weak and "incomplete" Rh agglutinins, Br J Exp Pathol **26**:255

Coombs RRA et al (1946) In vivo iso-sensitization of red cells in babies with haemolytic disease, Lancet **1**:264

Cooper AG et al (1968) Increased agglutinability by anti-i of red cells in sideroblastic and megaloblastic anaemia, Br J Haematol **15**:381

Cooper BA and Lowenstein L (1964) Relative folate deficiency of erythrocytes in pernicious anemia and its correction with cyanocobalamin, Blood **24**:502

Cooper BA and Whitehead VM (1978) Evidence that some patients with pernicious anemia are not recognized by radiodilution assay for cobalamin in serum, N Engl J Med **299**:816

Cooper HA (1980) The factor VIII complex and its associated activities. In Schmidt RM (Section Ed): Handbook Series in Clinical Laboratory Science, Section I: Hematology, vol 3, Boca Raton, CRC Press, Inc, p 61

Cooper HA and Hoagland HC (1972) Fetal hemoglobin, Mayo Clin Proc **47**:402

Cooper M (1957) Pica, Springfield, Illinois, Charles C Thomas, Publisher

Cooper MD et al (1968a) The two-component concept of the lymphoid system. In Bergsman D and Good RA (Eds): Immunologic deficiency disease in man, Birth Defects **4**:7

Cooper MD et al (1968b) Wiskott-Aldrich syndrome. An immunologic deficiency disease involving the afferent limb immunity, Am J Med **44**:499

Cooper MD et al (1973) Classification of primary immunodeficiencies, N Engl J Med **288**:966

Cooper MR and Toole JF (1972) Sickle cell trait: benign or malignant? Ann Intern Med **77**:997

Cooper MR et al (1972) Complete deficiency of leukocyte glucose-6-phosphate dehydrogenase (G6PD) with defective bactericidal activity, J Clin Invest **5**:769

Cooper RA and Jandl JH (1968) Bile salts and cholesterol in the pathogenesis of target cells in obstructive jaundice, J Clin Invest **47**:809

Cooper RA et al (1974) The role of the spleen in membrane conditioning and hemolysis of spur cells in liver disease, N Engl J Med **290**:1279

Cooper RA et al (1975) Modification of red cell membrane structure by cholesterol-rich lipid dispersions, J Clin Invest **55**:115

Cooperband SR et al (1968) Studies on the in vitro behavior of agammaglobuinemic lymphocytes, J Clin Invest **47**:836

Copeland BE (1957) Standard deviation: a practical means for the measurement and control of the precision of clinical laboratory determinations, Am J Clin Pathol **27**:551

Copeland GD et al (1958) Systemic lupus erythematosus: a clinical report of 47 cases with pathologic findings in 18, Am J Med Sci **236**:318

Copley AL (1968) Proceedings of the first International Conference on Hemorheology, New York, Pergamon Press, Inc

Corby DG and Zuck TF (1976) Newborn platelet dysfunction: a storage pool and release defect, Thromb Haemost **36**:200

Corcino JJ et al (1970) Absorption and malabsorption of vitamin B_{12}, Am J Med **48**:562

Cordano A et al (1964) Copper deficiency in infancy, Pediatrics **34**:324

Corder MP et al (1972) Phytohemagglutinin-induced lymphocyte transformation: the relationship to prognosis of Hodgkin's disease, Blood **39**:595

Cordle D et al (1980) The sterility of platelet and granulocyte concentrates collected by discontinuous flow centrifugation, Transfusion **20**:105

Cornelius CE et al (1968) Dubin-Johnson syndrome in immature sheep, Am J Dig Dis **13**:1072

Corrigan GE (1974) An autopsy survey of aplastic anemia, Am J Clin Pathol **62**:488

Corrigan JJ Jr and Earnest DL (1980) Factor II antigen in liver disease and warfarin-induced vitamin K deficiency: correlation with coagulant activity using Echis venom, Am J Hematol **8**:249

Corwin WC and Nettleship A (1959) A solitary erythroblastoma of the liver, J Lab Clin Med **53**:882

Costanzi JJ et al (1965) Cryoglobulinemia associated with a macroglobulin: studies of a 17.5S cryoprecipitating factor, Am J Med **39**:163

Cöster C (1961) Renal polycythemia. Case of primary hyperparathyroidism associated with nephrocalcinosis and erythrocytosis, Acta Med Scand **170**:191

Cotes PM and Bangham DR (1966) The international reference preparation of erythropoietin, Bull WHO **35**:751

Cotran RS (1965) Endothelial phagocytosis: an electronmicrosopic study, Exp Mol Pathol **4**:217

Cotran RS and Litt M (1969) The entry of granule-associated peroxidase into the phagocytic vacuoles of eosinophils, J Exp Med **129**:1291

Cotton HB and Harris JW (1962) Familial pyridoxine responsive anemia, J Clin Invest **41**:1352

Couch WD (1980) Giant lymph node hyperplasia associated with thrombotic thrombocytopenic purpura, Am J Clin Pathol **74**:340

Coughlin C et al (1978) Myelofibrosis associated with multiple myeloma, Arch Intern Med **138**:590

Courouce-Pauty AM et al (1975) Attempt to prevent hepatitis by using specific anti-HBs immunoglobulin, Am J Med Sci **270**:375

Court-Brown WM (1958) Radiation leukaemogenesis in man, Acta Haematol **20**:44

Court-Brown WM and Doll RR (1957) Leukaemia and aplastic anaemia in patients irradiated for ankylosing spondylitis, Medical Research Council Special Report Series No. 295, London, Her Majesty's Stationery Office

Cove H et al (1976) Autologous blood transfusion in coronary artery bypass surgery, Transfusion **16**:245

Coventry WD (1953) Cyclic neutropenia, JAMA **153**:28

Coventry WD and LaBree RH (1960) Heterotopia of bone marrow simulating mediastinal tumor: a manifestation of chronic hemolytic anemia in adults, Ann Intern Med **53**:1042

Covey TJ (1964) Ferrous sulfate poisoning: a review, case summaries, and therapeutic regimen, J Pediatr **64**:218

Cowall DE et al (1979) Paroxysmal nocturnal hemoglobinuria terminating as erythroleukemia, Cancer **43**:1914

Cowdrey SC (1966) Hyperuricemia in infectious mononucleosis, JAMA **196**:107

Cowling DC et al (1978) Lymph node and splenic imprints: their value in diagnosis, Pathology **10**:135

Cox EV and White AM (1962) Methylmalonic acid excretion: an index of vitamin B$_{12}$ deficiency, Lancet **2**:853

Crabbe PA and Heremans JF (1967) Selective IgA deficiency with steatorrhea, Am J Med **42**:319

Craddock CG Jr et al (1956) The dynamics of leukopoiesis and leukocytosis as studied by leukopheresis and isotopic techniques, J Clin Invest **35**:285

Craddock CG Jr et al (1971) Lymphocytes and the immune response, I and II, N Engl J Med **285**:324, 378

Crafts RC (1941) The effects of endocrines on the formed elements of the blood. I. The effects of hypophysectomy, thyroidectomy, and adrenalectomy on the blood of the adult female rat, Endocrinology **29**:596

Crafts RC (1946) Effects of hypophysectomy, castration, and testosterone proprionate on hemopoiesis in the adult male rat, Endocrinology **39**:401

Crafts RC and Meineke HA (1959) The anemia of hypophysectomized animals, Ann NY Acad Sci **77**:501

Craig J et al (1954) Response of lymph nodes of normal and congenital agammaglobulinemic children to antigenic stimulation, Am J Dis Child **88**:626

Craigie D (1845) Case of disease of the spleen, in which death took place in consequence of the presence of purulent matter in the blood, Edinburg Med Surg J **64**:400

Cramer AD et al (1973) The Giemsa stain for tissue sections: an improved method, Am J Clin Pathol **60**:148

Cramer AD et al (1976) von Willebrand disease San Diego, a new variant, Lancet **2**:12

Crane DB et al (1977) Significant hematuria secondary to sickle cell trait in a white family, South Med J **70**:750

Crawford MN et al (1961) The phenotype Lu (a—b—-) together with unconventional Kidd groups in one family, Transfusion **1**:228

Crigler RJ Jr and Najjar VA (1952) Congenital familial nonhemolytic jaundice with kernicterus, Pediatrics **10**:169

Crile GW (1907) Technique of direct transfusion of blood, Ann Surg **46**:329

Crocker AC (1969) Pigmentation in the lipidoses. In Wolman M (Ed): Pigments in pathology, New York, Academic Press, Inc

Crocker AC and Farber S (1958) Niemann-Pick disease: a review of 18 patients, Medicine **37**:1

Croft JD et al (1968) Coombs'-test positivity induced by drugs. Mechanism of immunologic reactions and red cell destruction, Ann Intern Med **68**:176

Crone M et al (1972) The elusive T cell receptor, Transplant Rev **10**:36

Cronkite EP (1967a) Extracorporeal irradiation of the blood and lymph in the treatment of leukemia and for immunosuppression, Ann Intern Med **67**:415

Cronkite EP (1967b) Radiation-induced aplastic anemia, Semin Hematol **4**:273

Cronkite EP and Bond VP (1960) Radiation injury in man, Springfield, Illinois, Charles C Thomas, Publisher

Cronkite EP and Fliedner TM (1964) Granulocytopoiesis, N Engl J Med **270**:1347, 1403

Cronkite EP and Vincent PC (1969) Granulocytopoiesis, Ser Haematol **II**(4):3

Cronkite EP et al (1959) Anatomic and physiologic facts and hypotheses about hemopoietic proliferating systems. In Stohlman F Jr (Ed): Kinetics of cellular proliferation, New York, Grune & Stratton, Inc

Cronkite EP and Feinendegen LE (1976) Notions about human stem cells, Blood Cells **2**:269

Crookston JH et al (1965) A new haemoglobin J Toronto (α5 alanine $\rightarrow$ aspartic acid), Nature (London) **208**:1059

Crookston JH et al (1969) Hemoglobin Etobicoke: alpha 84 (F5) serine replaced by arginine, Can J Biochem **47**:143

Crookston JH et al (1970) Hemoglobin Manitoba: alpha 102 (G9) serine replaced by arginine, Can J Biochem **48**:911

Crosbie A and Scarborough H (1940) Studies on stored blood: leukocytes in stored blood, Edinburgh Med J **47**:553

Crosby WH (1953) Paroxysmal nocturnal hemoglobinuria: relation of the clinical manifestations to underlying mechanisms, Blood **8**:769

Crosby WH (1959) Normal functions of the spleen relative to red cells: a review, Blood **14**:399

Crosby WH and Conrad ME (1960) Hereditary spherocytosis: observations on hemolytic mechanisms and iron metabolism, Blood **15**:662

Crosby WH and Furth FW (1956) A modification of the benzidine method for measurement of hemoglobin in plasma and urine, Blood **11**:380

Crossen PE et al (1969) Chromosomal abnormality, megaloblastosis, and arrested DNA synthesis in erythroleukemia, J Med Genet **6**:95

Crossen PE et al (1972) Chromosome studies in Fanconi's anaemia before and after treatment with oxymetholone, Pathology **4**:27

Crouch SK and Bishop C (1963) The maintenance of ATP in stored blood by adenosine and inosine, Transfusion **3**:349

Croucher BEE et al (1967) Delayed haemolytic transfusion reactions simulating auto-immune haemolytic anaemia, Vox Sang **12**:32

Crowell EB Jr et al (1971) The effect of oral contraceptives on factor VIII levels, J Lab Clin Med **77**:551

Crowley CA et al (1980a) An inherited abnormality of neutrophil adhesion: its genetic transmission and its association with a missing protein, N Engl J Med **302**:1163

Crowley JP et al (1980b) Tests of leukocyte function. In Seligson D (Ed): CRC Handbook Series in Clinical Laboratory Science, Section I: Hematology, vol 2, Boca Raton, Fla, CRC Press Inc, p 247

Crum ED et al (1974) Fibrinogen Cleveland II. An abnormal fibrinogen with defective release of fibrinopeptide Am J Clin Invest **53**:1308

Cuadra M (1958) Selenoid (crescent) bodies, Blood **13**:258

Cucuianu MP et al (1980) Increased ristocetin-cofactor in acute myocardial infarction: a component of the acute phase reaction, Thromb Haemost **1**:43

Cullum C et al (1967) Familial thrombocytopenic thrombocytopathy, Br J Haematol **13**:147

Cumming RL et al (1969) Clinical and laboratory studies on the action of desferrioxamine, Br J Haematol **17**:257

Curry JL and Trentin JJ (1967) Hemopoietic spleen colony studies. I. Growth and differentiation, Dev Biol **15**:395

Curry JL et al (1967) Hemopoietic spleen colony studies. II. Erythropoiesis, J Exp Med **125**:703

Curtis JE et al (1972) Leukapheresis therapy of chronic lymphocytic leukemia, Blood **39**:163

Cushing AH and Smith SJ (1969) Methemoglobinemia with silver nitrate therapy of a burn: report of a case, J Pediatr **74**:613

Cushman P and Maniatis A (1975) Direct antiglobulin tests in narcotic addicted patients, Transfusion **15**:107

Custer RP (1946) Aplastic anemia in soldiers treated with Atabrine (quinacrine), Am J Med Sci **212**:211

Cutler J (1929) The graphic method for the blood-sedimentation test, Am Rev Tuberc **19**:544

Cutting HO and Lang JE (1964) Familial benign chronic neutropenia, Ann Intern Med **61**:876

Czaja, AJ (1979) Serologic markers of hepatitis A and B in acute and chronic liver disease, Mayo Clin Proc **54**:721

Czapek EE et al (1973) Platelet dysfunction in glycogen storage disease type I, Blood **41**:235

Dacie JV (1948) Transfusion of saline-washed red cells in nocturnal haemoglobinuria, Clin Sci **7**:65

Dacie JV (1953) Acquired hemolytic anemia, with special reference to antiglobulin (Coombs') reaction, Blood **8**:813

Dacie JV (1954) The haemolytic anaemias: congenital and acquired, London, J and A Churchill Ltd

Dacie JV (1960) The haemolytic anaemias. Part I. The congenital anaemias, New York, Grune & Stratton, Inc

Dacie JV and Cutbush M (1954) Specificity of auto-antibodies in acquired haemolytic anaemia, J Clin Pathol **7**:18

Dacie JV and Doniach I (1947) The basophilic property of the iron-containing granules in siderocytes, J Pathol **59**:684

Dacie JV and Lewis SM (1972) Paroxysmal nocturnal haemoglobinuria: clinical manifestations, haematology, and nature of the disease, Ser Haematol **5**:3

Dacie JV and Mollin DL (1966) Siderocytes, sideroblasts, and sideroblastic anemia, Act Med Scand (supp) **445**:237

Dacie JV and Worlledge SM (1969) Auto-immune hemolytic anemias, Prog Hematol **6**:82

Dacie JV et al (1964) Hereditary Heinz-body anaemia. A report of studies on five patients with mild anaemia, Br J Haematol **10**:388

Dacie JV and Lewis SM (1975a) Practical haematology, London, Churchill Livingstone, p 13

Dacie JV and Lewis SM (1975b) Practical haematology, London, Churchill Livingstone, p 304-307

Dacie JV et al (1967) Haemoglobin Hammersmith (beta 42 [CD1] phe → ser), Nature (London) **216**:663

Da Costa M and Rothenberg SP (1974) Appearance of a folate binder in leukocytes and serum of women who are pregnant or taking oral contraceptives, J Lab Clin Med **83**:207

Dack S (1957) The present status of the treatment of cor pulmonale, NY State J Med **57**:74

Dagg J et al (1965) The relationship of lead poisoning and acute intermittent porphyria, Q J Med **34**:163

Dagg JH et al (1966) Value of erythrocyte protoporphyrin in the diagnosis of latent iron deficiency (sideropenia), Br J Haematol **12**:326

Dagnini G and Moreschi E (1957) Ittero familiare epatogeno a bilirubina diretta, Recent Prog Med **23**:47

Dainiak N and Hoffman R (1980) Hemoglobin F production in testicular malignancy, Cancer **45**:2177

Dainiak N et al (1979) Erythropoietin-dependent primary pure erythrocytosis, Blood **53**:1076

Daland GA et al (1956) Hematologic observations in bacterial endocarditis, J Lab Clin Med **48**:827

Dale DC et al (1974) Alternate-day prednisone: leukocyte kinetics and susceptibility to infections, N Engl J Med **291**:1154

Dale GL and Beutler E (1976) Enzyme replacement therapy in Gaucher's disease: a rapid, high-yield method for purification of glucocerebrosidase, Proc Natl Acad Sci USA **73**:4672

Dallman PR (1980) Inhibition of iron absorption by certain foods, Am J Dis Child **134**:453

Dallman PR and Siimes MA (1979) Percentile curves for hemoglobin and red cell volume in infancy and childhood, J Pedriatr **94**:26

Dallman PR et al (1978a) Effects of iron deficiency exclusive of anaemia, Br J Haematol **40**:179

Dallman PR et al (1978b) Hemoglobin concentration in white, black, and Oriental children: is there a need for separate criteria in screening for anemia? Am J Clin Nutr **31**:377

Daly PA et al (1980) Platelet transfusion therapy: one-hour post-transfusion increments are valuable in predicting the need for HLA-matched preparations, JAMA **243**:435

Dameshek W (1931) The appearance of histiocytes in the peripheral blood, Arch Intern Med **47**:968

Dameshek W (1951) Some speculations on the myeloproliferative syndromes, Blood **6**:372

Dameshek W (1963) "Immunoblasts" and "immunocytes"—an attempt at a functional nomenclature, Blood **29**:566

Dameshek W (1965) Sideroblastic anaemia: is this a malignancy? Br J Haematol **11**:52

Dameshek W and Baldini M (1958) The Di Guglielmo syndrome, Blood **13**:192

Dameshek W and Singer K (1945) Familial nonhemolytic jaundice: constitutional hepatic dysfunction with indirect van den Bergh reaction, Arch Intern Med **67**:259

Dammacco F et al (1974) A new case of mu heavy chain disease: clinical and immunochemical studies, Blood **43**:713

Dana B et al (1976) Plasma heparin neutralizing activity: its use in evaluation of thrombocytopenia and thrombocytosis, Am J Clin Pathol **65**:964

Dance N and Huehns ER (1962) A haemoglobin containing only delta chains, Biochem Biophys Res Comm **7**:444

Dance N et al (1964) The chemical investigation of haemoglobin G Bristol and G Bristol/C, Biochim Biophys Acta **86**:144

Dancey JT et al (1976) Section preparation of human marrow for light microscopy, J Clin Pathol **29**:704

Daniel MT and Flandrin G (1974) Fine structure of abnormal cells in hairy cell (tricholeukocytic) leukemia, with special reference to their in vitro phagocytic capacity, Lab Invest **30**:1

Daniel WA et al (1971) Obstetric and fetal complications in folate-deficient adolescent girls, Am J Obstet Gynecol **111**:233

Danks DM et al (1972) Menkes' kinky hair syndrome. An inherited defect in copper absorption with widespread effects, Pediatrics **50**:188

Danks DM et al (1973) Menkes' kinky hair disease: further definition of the defect in copper transport, Science **179**:1140

Dao C et al (1977) Anomalies érythrocytaires et immunitaires dans la splénomégalie myéloids, Nouv Rev Fr Hematol **18**:619

Darnborough J et al (1963) A "new" antibody anti-Lu\(^a\)Lu\(^b\) and two further examples of the genotype Lu(a–b–), Nature **198**:796

Darte JM et al (1954) Pelger-like leucocytes in chronic myeloid leukaemia, Acta Haematol **12**:117

Dausset J et al (1970) Genetics of the HL-A system: deduction of 480 haplotypes. In Terasaki PI (Ed): Histocompatibility testing 1970, Baltimore, The Williams & Wilkins, Co. p 53

Davey FR et al (1979) Studies of mixed lymphocyte reactions, surface B cell antigens, and intracytoplasmic immunoglobulins in "null cell" acute lymphocytic leukemia, Cancer **44**:1622

Davey MG and Lander H (1965) Potassium and acid phosphatase levels in serum and plasma of patients with high platelet counts, Med J Aust **1**:272

David JR (1966) Delayed hypersensitivity in vitro: its mediation by cell-free substances formed by lymphoid cell-antigen interaction, Proc Natl Acad Sci USA **56**:72

David JR (1968) Macrophage migration, Fed Proc **27**:6

David JR (1973) Lymphocyte mediators and cellular hypersensitivity, N Engl J Med **288**:143

Davidsohn I and Lee CL (1962) The laboratory in the diagnosis of infectious mononucleosis: with additional notes on epidemiology, etiology, and pathogenesis, Med Clin North Am **46**:225

Davidsohn I and Lee CL (1964) Serologic diagnosis of infectious mononucleosis, Am J Clin Pathol **41**:115

Davidsohn I and Stern K (1955) Diagnosis of hemolytic transfusion reactions, Am J Clin Pathol **25**:381

Davidsohn I et al (1955) The differential test for infectious mononucleosis, J Lab Clin Med **45**:561

Davidson E (1960) The redistribution of the red cells on centrifugation, Acta Haematol **23**:92

Davidson LSP et al (1943) Nutritional iron deficiency anaemia in wartime, Br Med J **2**:95

Davidson RJL (1969) March or exertional haemoglobinuria, Semin Hematol **6**:150

Davidson WA et al (1954) The Pelger-Huët anomaly: investigation of family A, Ann Hum Genet **19**:1

Davidson WM and Smith DR (1954) A morphological sex difference in the polymorphonuclear neutrophil leukocytes, Br Med J **2**:6

Davidson WM et al (1958) Sexing the neutrophil leucocytes in natural and artificial blood chimaeras, Br J Haematol **4**:231

Davidson WM et al (1960) Giant neutrophil leucocytes: an inherited anomaly, Br J Haematol **6**:339

Davie EW and Ratnoff OD (1964) Waterfall sequence for intrinsic blood clotting, Science **145**:1310

Davie EW et al (1975) Properties of bovine factor IX (Christmas factor), Ann NY Acad Sci **240**:34

Davis AT et al (1971) Polymorphonuclear leukocyte myeloperoxidase deficiency in a patient with myelomonocytic leukemia, N Engl J Med **285**:789

Davis JW and Wilson SJ (1966) Platelet survival in the May-Hegglin anomaly, Br J Haematol **12**:61

Davis S (1976) The variable patterns of circulating lymphocyte subpopulations in chronic lymphocytic leukemia, N Engl J Med **294**:1150

Davis SD et al (1966) Job's syndrome. Recurrent "cold" staphylococcal abscesses, Lancet **1**:1013

Davis WC and Douglas SD (1972) Defective granule formation and function in the Chediak-Higashi syndrome in man and animals, Semin Hematol **9**:431

Davis WC et al (1968) A selective neutrophil dysfunction syndrome: impaired killing of staphylococci, Ann Intern Med **69**:1237

Davis WM and Mendez Ross AO (1973) Thrombocytosis and thrombocythemia: the laboratory and clinical significance of an elevated platelet count, Am J Clin Pathol **59**:243

Davis S (1975) Hypothesis: differentiation of the human lymphoid system based on cell surface markers, Blood **45**:871

Davis S et al (1978) Circulating inhibitors of blood coagulation with procainamide-induced lupus erythematosus, Am J Hematol **4**:401

Davison AM et al (1974) Salt-poor human albumin in management of nephrotic syndrome, Br Med J **1**:481

Dawson RB (1977) Hemoglobin function in stored blood. XIX. Inosine maintenance of 2,3-DPG for 35 days in a CPD-adenine preservative, Transfusion **17**:525

Day HJ and Holmsen H (1972a) Platelet adenine nucleotide "storage pool deficiency" in thrombocytopenic absent radii syndrome, JAMA **221**:1053

Day HJ and Holmsen H (1972b) Laboratory tests of platelet function, Ann Clin Lab Sci **2**:63

Day NK et al (1972) Clr deficiency: an inborn error associated with cutaneous and renal disease, J Clin Invest **51**:1102

Dearing WH et al (1958) The effect of oral antibiotics on the intestinal bacteria and the formation of urobilinogen, Mayo Clin Proc **33**:646

Deaton JG et al (1967) Acute hemolytic anemia complicating infectious mononucleosis: the mechanism of hemolysis, Texas Rep Biol Med **25**:309

De Azavedo TFS et al (1974) Factors influencing anhaptoglobinemia in newborns from Salvador, Brazil, Hum Hered **24**:300

DeBartolo HM et al (1973) Torsion of the spleen: a case report, Mayo Clin Proc **48**:783

DeBastos O et al (1964) A study of three cases of familial congenital hypoprothombinaemia (factor II deficiency), Thromb Diath Haemorrh **11**:497

DeBruyn PPH et al (1977) The transmural migration and release of blood cells in acute myelogenous leukemia, Am J Anat **149**:247

Debré R et al (1952) Métabolisme du fer chez les descendants de malades atteints de cirrhose bronzée, Bull Soc Med Hop Paris **68**:665

De Furia FG and Miller DR (1972) Oxygen affinity in hemoglobin Köln disease, Blood **39**:398

De Gabriele G and Penington DG (1967) Regulation of platelet production: "thrombopoietin," Br J Haematol **13**:210

Degenhardt KH and Wiedemann HR (1953) Zum Problem menschlicher Pelger, Klin Wochenschr **31**:26

DeGowin RL et al (1962) A comparison of erythropoietin bioassays, Proc Soc Exp Biol Med **110**:48

deGennes JL et al (1968) Complications vasculaires cérébrales des xanthomatoses tendineuses hypercholesterolémiques familiales, Soc Med Hop Paris **119**:569

DeGoeij AFPM et al (1977) Porphyrin synthesis in blood cells of patients with erythropoietic protoporphyria, Clin Chim Acta **74**:27

Deiss A and Kurth D (1970) Circulating reticulocytes in normal adults as determined by the new methylene blue method, Am J Clin Pathol **53**:481

Deisseroth A et al (1977) Localization of the human α-globin structural gene to chromosome 16 in somatic cell hybrids by molecular hybridization assay, Cell **12**:205

DeJong WWW and Bernini LF (1968) Haemoglobin Babinga (delta 136 glycine → aspartic acid): a new delta chain variant, Nature (London) **219**:1360

DeJong WWW et al (1968) Haemoglobin Leiden: deletion of beta 6 or 7 glutamic acid, Nature (London) **220**:788

DeJong WWW et al (1971) Haemoglobin Rampa: alpha 95 pro → ser, Biochim Biophys Acta **236**:197

DeJong WWW et al (1975) Hemoglobin Koya Dora: high frequency of a chain termination mutant, Am J Hum Genet **27**:81

Delâge JM et al (1977) Hereditary C7 deficiency: diagnosis and HLA studies in a French-Canadian family, J Clin Invest **60**:1061

Delamore IW and Geary CG (1971) Aplastic anaemia, acute myeloblastic leukaemia, and oxymetholone, Br Med J **2**:743

Delamore IW et al (1961) Megaloblastic anaemia in congenital spherocytosis, Br Med J **1**:543

de Leeuw NK et al (1966) Iron deficiency and hydremia in normal pregnancy, Medicine **45**:291

Delivoria-Papadopoulos M et al (1971) Exchange transfusion in the newborn infant with fresh and "old" blood: the role of storage on 2,3-diphosphoglycerate, hemoglobin-oxygen affinity, and oxygen release, J Pediatr **79**:898

Dellipiani AW et al (1968) The uptake of vitamin B₁₂ by *E. coli*: possible significance in relation to the blind loop syndrome, Am J Dig Dis **13**:718

Delsol G et al (1979) Leukoerythroblastosis and cancer frequency, prognosis and physiopathologic significance, Cancer **44**:1009

de Man JCH and Meiners WBH (1962) Crystals of protein nature in the cytoplasm of lymphocytic cells in a case of lymphoreticular malignancy, Blood **20**:492

DeMarsh QB and Alt HL (1948) Post transfusion anemia, Q Bull Northwest Univ Med Sch **22**:99

DeMatteis F (1968) Toxic hepatic porphyrias, Semin Hematol **5**:409

DeMeo AN and Andersen BR (1972) Defective chemotaxis associated with a serum inhibitor in cirrhotic patients, N Engl J Med **286**:735

DeNatale A et al (1955) V, a "new" Rh antigen, common in Negroes, rare in white people, JAMA **159**:247

Denninger M-H et al (1978) Congenital dysfibrinogenemia: fibrinogen Lille, Thromb Res **13**:453

Denson KWE (1975) Methods for the detection of molecular variants of factor VIII. In Brinkhous KM and Hemker HC (Eds): Handbook of hemophilia, New York, American Elsevier Publishing Co, Inc, p 203

Deprez P et al (1978) La maladie de Chédiak-Higashi: a propos d'une nouvelle observation, Ann Dermatol Venereal (Paris) **105**:841

Dern RJ et al (1954a) Hemolytic effect of primaquine. I. The localization of drug-induced hemolytic defect in primaquine-sensitive individuals, J Lab Clin Med **43**:303

Dern RJ et al (1954b) Hemolytic effect of primaquine. II. Natural course of hemolytic anemia and mechanism of its self-limited character, J Lab Clin Med **44**:171

Desforges JF (1976) Genetic implications of G-6-PD deficiency, N Engl J Med **294**:1438

Desforges JF et al (1954) Effects of massive gastrointestinal hemorrhage on hemostasis; blood platelets, J Lab Clin Med **43**:501

de Sousa M et al (1978) Immunological parameters in childhood Hodgkin's disease. II. T and B lymphocytes in the peripheral blood of normal children and in the spleen and peripheral blood of children with Hodgkin's disease, Pediatr Res **12**:143

De Traverse PM et al (1966) Etude d'une hémoglobine J alpha non encore décrite, dans une famille Francaise, CR Soc Biol (Paris) **160**:2270

Deutsch E et al (1955) Differentiation of certain platelet factors related to blood coagulation, Circ Res **3**:110

De Vaal OM and Seynhaeve V (1959) Reticular dysgenesia, Lancet **2**:1123

Devesa SS and Silverman DT (1978) Cancer incidence and mortality trends in the United States: 1935-74, J Natl Cancer Inst **60**:545

DeVries A et al (1963) The first observation of an abnormal haemoglobin in a Jewish family: haemoglobin Beilinson, Br J Haematol **9**:484

de Weinstein BI et al (1973) A new unstable haemoglobin: hb Buenos Aires, beta 85 (F1) phe → ser, Acta Haematol **50**:357

Deykin D et al (1968) Hepatic removal of activated factor X by the perfused rabbit liver, Am J Physiol **214**:414

Deykin D and Hellerstein LJ (1972) The assessment of drug-dependent and isoimmune antiplatelet antibodies by the use of platelet aggregometry, J Clin Invest **51**:3142

Dhumeaux D and Berthelot P (1975) Chronic hyperbilirubinemia associated with hepatic uptake and storage impairment: a new syndrome resembling that of the mutant Southdown sheep, Gastroenterology **69**:988

Diamond I and Schmid R (1966) Experimental bilirubin encephalopathy. The mode of entry of bilirubin-¹⁴C into the central nervous system, J Clin Invest **45**:678

Diamond LK (1974) The Rh problem through a retrospectroscope, Am J Clin Pathol **62**:311

Diamond LK (1978) Congenital hypoplastic anemia; Diamond-Blackfan syndrome: historical and clinical aspects, Blood Cells **4**:209

Diamond LK and Blackfan KD (1938) Hypoplastic anemia, Am J Dis Child **56**:464

Diamond LK et al (1961) Congenital (erythroid) hypoplastic anemia: a 25-year study, Am J Dis Child **102**:403

Diamond LK et al (1976) Congenital hypoplastic anemia, Adv Pediatr **22**:349

DiBella NJ et al (1977) Effect of splenectomy on teardrop-shaped erythrocytes in agnogenic myeloid metaplasia, Arch Intern Med **137**:380

Dick F et al (1974) Incidence, cytology, and histopathology of non-Hodgkin's lymphomas in bone marrow, Cancer **33**:1382

Dicke KA et al (1971) Colony formation in agar: in vitro assay for haemopoietic stem cells, Cell Tissue Kinet **4**:463

Dicke KA et al (1973) Identification of primate cells in bone marrow resembling the hemopoietic stem cell in the mouse, Blood **42**:195

Dickerman JD et al (1973) In vivo aging of transfused erythrocytes and 2,3-diphosphoglycerate levels, Blood **42**:9

Dickerman JD et al (1980) Infectious mononucleosis initially seen as cold-induced acrocyanosis: association with auto-anti-M and anti-I antibodies, Am J Dis Child **134**:159

Dickie A and Hempelmann LH (1947) Morphologic changes in the lymphocytes of persons exposed to ionizing radiation, J Lab Clin Med **32**:1045

Dickler HB and Kunkel HG (1972) Interaction of aggregated γ-globulin with β-lymphocytes, J Exp Med **136**:191

Didisheim P and Bunting D (1966) Abnormal platelet function in myelofibrosis, Am J Clin Pathol **45**:566

Diebold J (1973) Système réticulo-endothélial et système des macrophages mononucléés, Sem Hop Paris **49**:2467

Dietzman DE et al (1977) Hepatitis B surface antigen (HBsAg) and antibody to HBsAg: prevalence in homosexual and heterosexual men, JAMA **238**:2625

DiGeorge AM (1965) Discussion, Society for Pediatric Research, J Pediatr **67**:907

Diggs LW (1965) The crisis in sickle cells anemia: hematologic studies, Am J Clin Pathol **44**:1

Diggs LW (1967) Bone and joint lesions in sickle-cell disease, Clin Orthop **52**:119

Diggs LW and Bell A (1965) Intraerythrocytic hemoglobin crystals in sickle cell–hemoglobin C disease, Blood **25**:218

Diggs LW and Williams DL (1963) Treatment of painful sickle cell crises with papaverine: preliminary report, South Med J **56**:472

Di Guglielmo G (1946) Les maladies érythrémiques, Rev Hematol **1**:355

di Imperato C and Dettori AG (1958) Ipofibrinogenemia congenita con fibrinoastenia, Helv Paediatr Acta **13**:380

Dike GW et al (1972) The preparation and clinical use of a new concentrate containing factor IX, prothrombin, and factor X, and a separate concentrate containing factor VII, Br J Haematol **22**:469

Dinçol K and Aksoy M (1969) On the platelet levels in chronic iron deficiency anemia, Acta Haematol **41**:135

Dinçol G et al (1979) Beta-thalassaemia with increased haemoglobin A_2 in Turkey: a study of 164 thalassaemic heterozygotes, Hum Hered **29**:272

Dintenfass L (1966) A preliminary outline of the blood high viscosity syndromes, Arch Intern Med **118**:427

Dintenfass L (1977a) Theoretical aspects and clinical applications of the blood viscosity equation containing a term for the internal viscosity of the red cell, Blood Cells **3**:367

Dintenfass L (1977b) Viscosity factors in hypertensive and cardiovascular diseases, Cardiovasc Med **2**:337

Dintenfass L and Davis E (1977) Blood viscosity factors and capillary abnormalities in diabetes mellitus, Adv Microcirc **7**:96

DiScipio RG et al (1977) A comparison of human prothrombin, factor IX (Christmas factor), factor X (Stuart factor) and protein S, Biochemistry **16**:698

Ditzel J (1959) Relationship of blood protein composition to intravascular erythrocyte aggregation (sludged blood), clinical and experimental studies, Acta Med Scand **164**(supp 343):11

Dix D et al (1979) Glycohemoglobin and glucose tolerance tests compared as indicators of borderline diabetes, Clin Chem **25**:877

Dixon RH and Ross WF (1975) Platelet antibody in autoimmune thrombocytopenia, Br J Haematol **31**:129

Djaldetti M et al (1975) Paroxysmal cold hemoglobinuria. Transmission and scanning electron microscopy features of erythrocytes, Am J Clin Pathol **63**:804

Djerassi I et al (1972) Continuous flow filtration—leukopheresis, Transfusion **12**:75

Dmochowski L (1960) Viruses and tumors in the light of electron microscope studies: a review, Cancer Res **20**:977

Dmochowski L et al (1976) Viral type A and type B hepatitis: morphology, biology, immunology, and epidemiology—a review, Am J Clin Pathol **65**:741

Dobbs NB et al (1966) Hemoglobin Jenkins or hemoglobin N-Baltimore or alpha 2 beta 2 95 glu, Biochim Biophys Acta **117**:492

Dobyns WB et al (1979) Clinical spectrum of Wilson's disease (hepatolenticular degeneration), Mayo Clin Proc **54**:35

Dock W (1938) Ebb and flow of theories about pernicious anemia, Am J Clin Pathol **8**:620

Dodge JT et al (1967) Peroxidative hemolysis of red blood cells from patients with abetalipoproteinemia (acanthocytosis), J Clin Invest **46**:357

Dods RF and Bolmey C (1979) Glycosylated hemoglobin assay and oral glucose tolerance test compared for detection of diabetes mellitus, Clin Chem **25**:764

D'Oelsnitz M et al (1975) A propos d'un cas de leucémie aiguë lymphoblastique survenue après guérison d'une maladie de Blackfan-Diamond, Arch Fr Pediatr **32**:582

Doebbler GF et al (1966) Cryogenic preservation of whole blood for transfusion. In vitro study of a process using rapid freezing, thawing, and protection by polyvinylpyrrolidone, Transfusion **6**:104

Doery JC et al (1970) Energy metabolism in human platelets: interrelationship between glycolysis and oxidative metabolism, Blood **36**:159

Doig et al (1957) Response of megaloblastic anaemia to prednisolone, Lancet **2**:966

Donaldson RM Jr (1965) Studies on the pathogenesis of steatorrhea in the blind loop syndrome, J Clin Invest **44**:1815

Donaldson VH (1980) Kininogens. In Schmidt RM (Section Ed): Handbook Series in Clinical Laboratory Science, Section I: Hematology, vol 3, Boca Raton, Fla, CRC Press Inc, p 179

Donath J and Landsteiner K (1904) Über paroxysmale Hemoglobinurie, Munch Med Wochenschr **51**:1590

Donné A (1844) Cours de microscopie, Paris, J-B Ballière

Donohue DM et al (1956) Preservation and transfusion of blood, JAMA **161**:784

Donohugh DL (1966) Eosinophils and eosinophilia, Calif Med **104**:421

Doolittle RF (1980) Fibrinogen. In Schmidt RM (Ed): Handbook Series in Clinical Laboratory Science, Section I: Hematology vol 3, Boca Raton, Fla, CRC Press Inc, p 3

Dorado M et al (1974) Molecular weight estimation of human erythropoietin by SDS-polyacrylamide gel electrophoresis, Biochem Med **10**:1

Dorfman A and Lorincz AE (1957) Occurrence of urinary acid mucopolysaccharides in the Hurler syndrome, Proc Natl Acad Sci USA **43**:443

Dorfman RF and Warnke R (1974) Lymphadenopathy simulating the malignant lymphomas, Hum Pathol **5**:519

Dormandy KM et al (1963) Folic acid deficiency in coeliac disease, Lancet **1**:632

Dormandy JA (1980) Haemorheological aspects of thrombosis, Br J Haematol **45**:519

Dorr AD and Moloney WC (1952) Acquired pseudo-Pelger anomaly of granulocytic leukocytes, N Engl J Med **261**:742

Dosch HM et al (1978) Severe combined immunodeficiency disease: a model of T-cell dysfunction, Clin Exp Immunol **34**:260

Dosik H et al (1972) Acquired lipidosis: Gaucher-like cells and "blue cells" in chronic granulocytic leukemia, Semin Hematol **9**:309

Dougherty TF (1959) Adrenal cortical control of lymphatic tissue mass. In Stohlman F Jr (Ed): Kinetics of cellular proliferation, New York, Grune & Stratton, Inc

Dougherty TF (1960) Lymphocytokarryorrhetic effects of adrenocortical steroids. In Rebuck JW (Ed): The lymphocyte and lymphatic tissue, New York, Paul B Hoeber, Inc

Doughtery TF and White A (1944) Influence of hormone on lymphoid tissue structure and function. Role of pituitary adrenotropic hormone in regulation of lymphocytes and other cellular elements of blood, Endocrinology **35**:19

Doughtery TF et al (1964) Hormonal control of lymphatic structure and function, Ann NY Acad Sci **113**:825

Douglas AS and Dacie JV (1953) The incidence and significance of iron-containing granules in human erythrocytes and their precursors, J Clin Pathol **6**:307

Douglas SD and Fudenberg HH (1969) In vitro development of

plasma cells from lymphocytes following poke weed mitogen stimulation: a fine structural study, Exp Cell Res **54**:277

Douglas SD et al (1969) Human lymphocyte response to phytomitogens in vitro: normal agammaglobulinemic and paraproteinemic individuals, J Immunol **103**:1185

Douglas SD et al (1973) Ultrastructural features of phytohemagglutinin and concanavalin A-responsive lymphocytes in chronic lymphocytic leukemia, Acta-Haematol **50**:129

Douglass C and Twomey J (1970) Transient stomatocytosis with hemolysis: a previously unrecognized complication of alcoholism, Ann Intern Med **72**:159

Douwes FR (1972) Clinical value of NBT test, N Engl J Med **287**:822

Dover GJ et al (1979) Production of erythrocytes that contain fetal hemoglobin in anemia: transient in vivo changes, J Clin Invest **63**:173

Dowben RM and Walker JK (1955) Methemoglobinemia induced by X-irradiation, Proc Soc Exp Biol Med **90**:398

Dowdy RP (1969) Copper metabolism, Am J Clin Nutr **22**:887

Downey H (1923) Acute lymphadenosis compared with acute lymphatic leukemia, Arch Intern Med **32**:82

Dreyfus B (1976) Preleukemic states. I. Definition and classification. II. Refactory anemia with an excess of myeloblasts in the bone marrow (smoldering acute leukemia), Nouv Rev Fr Hematol **17**:33

Drummey GD et al (1961) Microscopical examination of the stool for steatorrhea, N Engl J Med **264**:85

D'Souza L et al (1979) An acquired abnormal fibrinogen associated with thromboembolic disease and pseudotumor cerebri, Thromb Haemost **42**:994

Duane GW (1957) Aplastic anemia fourteen years following administration of Thorotrast, Am J Med **23**:499

Dube VE et al (1975) Hemolytic anemia caused by auto anti-N, Am J Clin Pathol **63**:828

Dubin IN and Johnson FB (1954) Chronic idiopathic jaundice with unidentified pigment in liver cells: new clinicopathologic entity with report of 12 cases, Medicine **33**:155

Dubiski S (1972) Genetics and regulation of immunoglobulin allotypes, Med Clin North Am **56**:557

Dubois EL (1975) Serologic abnormalities in spontaneous and drug-induced systemic lupus erythematosus, J Rheumatol **2**:204

DuBois EL (1974) The clinical picture of systemic lupus erythematosus. In DuBois EL (Ed): Lupus erythematosus, ed 2, Los Angeles, University of Southern California Press, p 232

Dubos RJ and Hirsch JG (1965) Bacterial and mycotic infections in man, ed 4, Philadelphia, JB Lippincott Co

DuBose CM et al (1977) Immobilization and kinetic studies of an erythropoietin-generating factor, Biochem Med **17**:310

Duhm J and Gerlach E (1971) On the mechanisms of the hypoxia-induced increase of 2,3-diphosphoglycerate in erythrocytes. Studies on rat erythrocytes in vivo and human erythrocytes in vitro. Pflugers Arch **326**:254

Duhm J and Gerlach E (1974) Metabolism and function of 2,3-diphosphoglycerate in red blood cells. In Greenwalt TJ and Jamieson GA (Eds.): The human red cell in vitro, New York, Grune & Stratton, Inc

Duke M and Abelmann WH (1969) The haemodynamic response to chronic anaemia, Circulation **39**:503

Dukes PP and Goldwasser E (1961) Estrogen inhibition of erythropoiesis, Endocrinology **69**:21

Dukes PP et al (1969) Comparison of erythropoietin preparations yielding different dose-response slopes in the exhypoxic polycythemic mouse assay, J Lab Clin Med **74**:250

Dukes PP et al (1973) Enhancement of erythropoiesis by prostaglandins, J Lab Clin Med **82**:704

Dull HB (1961) Syringe-transmitted hepatitis: a recent epidemic in historical perspective, JAMA **176**:413

Dumonde DC (1970) "Lymphokines": molecular mediators of cellular immune responses in animals and man, Proc R Soc Med **63**:899

Duncalf D and Underwood DS (1970) Transfusion during and after surgical operations. In Laufman H and Erichson RB (Eds): Hematologic problems in surgery, Philadelphia, WB Saunders Co

Duncan SC and Winkelmann RK (1978) Circulating Sézary cells in hospitalized dermatology patients, Br J Dermatol **99**:171

Dunn CDR and Napier JAF (1978) Technical comments on the bioassay of erythropoietin, Exp Hematol **6**:577

Dunn CDR et al (1977) Progenitor cells in canine cyclic hematopoiesis, Blood **50**:1111

Dunn CDR et al (1978) Cell proliferation of canine cyclic hematopoietic marrow in diffusion chambers, Proc Soc Exp Biol Med **158**:50

Dunsford I et al (1956) A rare variety of the human blood group B, Nature **178**:1167

Dunston GM and Gershowitz H (1973) Further studies of Xh, a serum protein antigen in man, Vox Sang **24**:343

Dupuy JM and Preud'homme JL (1968) Exploration de I'hypersensibilité retardée par le dinitrochlorobenzène (DNCB), Press Med **76**:123

Dutcher TF (1971) Erythrocyte indices and corpuscular constants revisited, Lab Med **2**:32

Dutcher TF (1974) Chronic lymphocytic leukemia, leukemic cells containing azurophilic rods indistinguishable from Auer bodies, problem case No. 5 of Problem Cases in Hematology, presented at the annual meeting of the ASCP, October 9, 1974

Dutcher TF et al (1979) A comparative evaluation of automated blood cell differential analyzers: Hematrak, LARC, and Hemalog D. In Koepke JA (Ed): Differential leukocyte counting, Skokie, Ill, College of American Pathologists, p 161

DuVivier A et al (1978) Lymphocyte transformation in patients with staged mycosis fungoides and Sézary syndrome, Cancer **42**:209

Dvorak HF and Dvorak AM (1975) Basophilic leucocytes: structure, function, and role in disease, Clin Haematol **4**:651

Dvorak HF et al (1974) Morphology of delayed type hypersensitivity reactions in man. I. Quantitative description of the inflammatory response, Lab Invest **31**:111

Dvorak AM and Dvorak HF (1979) The basophil: its morphology, biochemistry, motility, release reactions, recovery, and role in the inflammatory responses of IgE-mediated and cell-mediated origin, Arch Pathol Lab Med **103**:551

Dykes G et al (1978) Three-dimensional reconstruction of the fibres of sickle cell haemoglobin, Nature **272**:506

Dyment PG et al (1978) Safety and efficacy of jet anesthesia for bone marrow aspirations, Blood **52**:578

Eales L (1960) Cutaneous porphyria. Observations on 111 cases in three racial groups, S Afr J Lab Clin Med **6**:63

Eastman P et al (1968) Conversion of polycythemia vera to chronic Di Guglielmo's syndrome, JAMA **204**:1141

Eaton JW et al (1969) Role of red cell 2,3-diphosphoglycerate in the adaptation of man to altitude, J Lab Clin Med **73**:603

Eaton JW et al (1979) Membrane abnormalities of irreversibly sickled cells, Semin Hematol **16**:52

Eaves CJ and Eaves AC (1978) Erythropoietin (Ep) dose-response curves for three classes of erythroid progenitors in normal human marrow and in patients with polycythemia vera, Blood **52**:1196

Ebbe S et al (1962) Autoimmune thrombocytopenic purpura ("ITP" type) with chronic lymphocytic leukemia, Blood **19**:23

Eckardt JJ et al (1978) Autologous transfusion and total hip arthroplasty, Clin Orthop **132**:39

Eckel RH et al (1977) Platelet-inhibiting drugs in thrombotic thrombocytopenic purpura, Arch Intern Med **137**:735

Ecker JA et al (1960) Gastrointestinal bleeding in hereditary hemorrhagic telangiectasia, Am J Gastroenterol **33**:411

Eckstein JD et al (1975) Hereditary thrombocytopenia, deafness, and renal disease, Ann Intern Med **82**:639

Eddie-Quartey AC and Gross NJ (1978) Phytohemagglutinin activation of lymphocytes: quantitative comparison of different preparations, Am J Clin Pathol **69**:326

Edelman GM (1971) Antibody structure and molecular immunology, Ann NY Acad Sci **190**:5

Edelman GM and Gally JA (1962) The nature of Bence-Jones proteins. Chemical similarities to polypeptide chains of myeloma globulins and normal γ-globulins, J Exp Med **116**:207

Edelson PJ et al (1973) Disorders of neutrophil function. Defects in the early stages of the phagocytic process. Clin Exper Immunol **13**:441

Edelson RL et al (1974) Morphologic and functional properties of the atypical leukocytes of the Sézary syndrome, Mayo Clin Proc **49**:558

Edenberg, HJ and Huberman JA (1975) Eukaryotic chromosome replication, Annu Rev Genet **9**:245

Ederer F et al (1965) US childhood cancer mortality patterns, 1950-1959: etiologic implications, JAMA **192**:593

Edgin RA et al (1980) Acquired factor X deficiency with associated defects in platelet aggregation: a response to corticosteroid therapy, Am J Med **69**:137

Edwards CL et al (1964) Clinical bone marrow scanning with radioisotopes, Blood **23**:741

Effert S et al (1960) Normoproteinaemic plasmocytoma, Dtsch Med Wochenschr **85**:1

Efrati P and Danon D (1968) Electron-microscopical study of bone marrow cells in a case of Chediak-Higashi-Steinbrinck syndrome, Br J Haematol **15**:173

Efrati P and Jonas P (1958) Chediak's anomaly of leukocytes in malignant lymphoma associated with leukemic manifestations: case report with necropsy, Blood **13**:1063

Efrati P et al (1957) Mast cell leukemia? Malignant mastocytosis with leukemia-like manifestations, Blood **12**:869

Efrati P et al (1979) Myeloproliferative disorders terminating in acute micromegakaryoblastic leukaemia, Br J Haematol **43**:79

Efremov GD et al (1974) Microchromatography of hemoglobins. II. A rapid microchromatographic method for the determination of hemoglobin A$_2$, J Lab Clin Med **83**:657

Efremov GD (1978) Hemoglobins Lepore and anti-Lepore, Hemoglobin **2**:197

Efremov GD et al (1969) Hemoglobin Richmond, a human hemoglobin which forms asymmetric hybrids with other hemoglobins, J Biol Chem **244**:6105

Efremov GD et al (1973) Hemoglobin Beograd or alpha 2 beta 2 121 glu → val (GH4), Biochim Biophys Acta **328**:81

Efremov GD et al (1974) Haemoglobin M Saskatoon and haemoglobin M Hyde Park in two Yugoslavian families, Scand J Haematol **13**:48

Egeberg O (1965) Inherited antithrombin deficiency causing thrombophilia, Thromb Diath Haemorrh **13**:516

Egeberg O (1967) Inherited fibrinogen abnormality causing thrombophilia, Thromb Diath Haemorrh **17**:176

Egeberg JC et al (1969) Ultrastructure of the specific granules of human neutrophil granulocytes. Studies in fatal granulomatous disease and toxic granulation, Scand J Haematol **6**:303

Egeberg O (1965a) On the natural blood coagulation inhibitor system. Investigations of inhibitor factors based on antithrombin deficient blood, Thromb Diath Haemorrh **14**:473

Egeberg O (1965b) Inherited antithrombin deficiency causing thrombophilia, Thromb Diath Haemorrh **13**:516

Eggen RR (1965) Chromosome diagnostics in clinical medicine, Springfield, Ill. Charles C Thomas, Publisher

Ehlenberger AG and Nussenzweig V (1977) The role of membrane receptors for C3b and C3d in phagocytosis, J Exp Med **145**:357

Ehrlich P (1891) Farbenanalytische Untersuchungen zur Histologie und Klinik des Blutes, Berlin, Hirschwald

Eichner ER and Hillman RS (1971) The evolution of anemia in alcoholic patients, Am J Med **50**:218

Eichner ER and Hillman RS (1973) Effect of alcohol on serum folate level, J Clin Invest **52**:584

Ein D and Fahey JL (1967) Two types of lambda polypeptide chains in human immunoglobulins, Science **156**:947

Einarsson R and Andersson L-O (1977) Binding of heparin to human antithrombin III as studied by measurements of tryptophan fluorescence, Biochim Biophys Acta **490**:104

Ekert H and Firkin BG (1975) Recent advances in haemophilia and von Willebrand's disease, Vox Sang **28**:409

Eknoyan G et al (1969) Platelet function in renal failure, N Engl J Med **280**:677

Elias JM (1980) A rapid, sensitive myeloperoxidase stain using 4-Chloro-1-naphthol, Am J Clin Pathol **73**:797

El-Hazmi MAF and Lehmann J (1976) Hemoglobin Riyadh (alpha 2 beta 2 120 [GH3] lys → asn)—a new variant found in association with alpha thalassemia and iron deficiency, Hemoglobin **1**:59

Elion J et al (1973) Two variants of hemoglobin D in the Algerian population: hemoglobin D Ouled Rabah beta 19 (Bl) asn → lys and hemoglobin D Iran beta 22 (B4) gly → gln, Biochim Biophys Acta **310**:360

Elion J et al (1979) Hémoglobine J Amiens B17 (A14) lys → asn. Coïncidence d'une nouvelle hemoglobine anormale sans retentissement fonctionnel et d'une polyglobulie primitive, Nouv Rev Fr Hematol **21**:347

Elliott J et al (1940) Use of plasma as a substitute for whole blood, N Carolina Med J **1**:283

Ellis EF et al (1976) Coronary arterial smooth muscle contraction by a substance released from platelets: evidence that it is thromboxane A$_2$, Science **193**:1135

Ellis FR (1974) Nutritional megaloblastic anaemia, Practitioner **212**:503

Ellis FR and Crawley LP (1957) The third report of agglutinogen A$_0$: occurrence in mother and child, Am J Clin Pathol **27**:438

Ellis LD et al (1964) Needle biopsy of bone and marrow, Arch Intern Med **114**:213

Ellis RE (1961) The distribution of active bone marrow in the adult, Phys Med Biol **5**:255

Ellison ABC (1960) Pernicious anemia masked by multivitamins containing folic acid, JAMA **173**:240

Elmlinger PJ et al (1952) Depression of red cell iron turnover by transfusion, Proc Soc Exp Biol Med **76**:16

Elödi S and Váradi K (1978) Activation of clotting factors in prothrombin complex concentrates as demonstrated by clotting assays for factors IX$_a$ and X$_a$, Thromb Res **12**:797

Elsborg L (1972) Binding of folic acid to human plasma proteins, Acta Haematol **48**:207

Elves MW et al (1966) Pyridoxine-responsive anemia determined by an X-linked gene, J Med Genet **3**:1

Emery AC Jr et al (1974) "Stress" polycythemia and hypertension, JAMA **229**:159

Emery JL and Follett GF (1964) Regression of bone-marrow haemopoiesis from the terminal digits in the foetus and infant, Br J Haematol **10**:485

Emmel VE (1917) A study of erythrocytes in a case of severe

anemia with elongated and sickle-shaped red blood corpuscles, Arch Intern Med 20:586

Emori HW et al (1973) Psuedo-leukocytosis associated with cryoglobulinemia, Am J Clin Pathol 60:202

Enberg RN et al (1974) T- and B-cells in peripheral blood during infectious mononucleosis, J Infect Dis 130:104

Enfield DL et al (1975) Bovine factor X₁ (Stuart factor). Primary structure of the light chain, Proc Natl Acad Sci USA 72:16

Engell HC (1955) Cancer cells in the circulating blood, Acta Chir Scand (supp) 201:1

England JM et al (1972) Re-assessment of the reliability of the hematocrit, Br J Haematol 23:247

England JM et al (1973) Studies on the transcobalamins, Br J Haematol 25:737

Engle RL Jr and Koprowska I (1959) The appearance of histiocytes in the blood of subacute bacterial endocarditis, Am J Med 26:965

Engle RL and Wallis LA (1969) Immunoglobulinopathies, Springfield, Ill. Charles C Thomas, Publisher

Engström K et al (1966) Periodic thrombocytopenia or tidal platelet dysgenesis in a man, Scand J Haematol 3:290

Enno A et al (1979) "Prolymphocytoid" transformation of chronic lymphocytic leukaemia, Br J Haematol 41:9

Enquist RW et al (1972) Type II congenital dyserythropoietic anemia, Ann Intern Med 77:371

Epstein CJ et al (1972) Hereditary macrothrombocytopathia, nephritis, and deafness, Am J Med 52:299

Epstein WL et al (1966) Immunologic studies in ataxia-telangiectasia. I. Delayed hypersensitivity and serum immune globulin levels in probands and first-degree relatives, Int Arch Allergy Appl Immunol 30:15

Erbe RW (1975) Inborn errors of folate metabolism, N Engl J Med 293:753

Erkelens DW and Statius Van Eps LW (1973) Bartter's syndrome and erythrocytosis, Am J Med 55:711

Erlandson ME et al (1958) Studies of congenital hemolytic syndromes. I. Rates of destruction and production of erythrocytes in thalassemia, Pediatrics 22:910

Erlandson ME et al (1964) Comparison of sixty-six patients with thalassemia major and thirteen patients with thalassemia intermedia: including evaluations of growth, development, maturation, and prognosis, Ann NY Acad Sci 119:727

Ernström U (1965) Studies on growth and cytomorphosis in the thymo-lymphatic system. With special reference to the influence of the thymus and the thyroid in guinea-pigs, Acta Pathol Microbiol Scand (supp) 178:5

Ernström U et al (1965) Venous output of lymphocytes from the thymus, Nature 207:540

Erskine AG and Socha WW (1978) The principles and practice of blood grouping, ed 2, St. Louis, The CV Mosby Co

Erslev A (1953) Humoral regulation of red cell production, Blood 8:349

Erslev AJ and Kazal LA (1968) Inactivation of erythropoietin by tissue homogenates, Proc Soc Exp Biol Med 129:845

Erslev AJ (1971a) Feedback circuits in the control of stem cell differentiation, Am J Pathol 65:629

Erslev AJ (1971b) The effect of hemolysates on red cell production and erythropoietin release, J Lab Clin Med 78:1

Erslev AJ et al (1979) Plasma erythropoietin in polycythemia, Am J Med 66:243

Esber E et al (1975) Lymphocyte surface receptors in childhood acute lymphocytic leukemia, Pediatrics 56:788

Eshaghpour E et al (1966) Iron deficiency anemia in a newborn infant, J Pediatr 68:806

Esnouf MP and Williams WJ (1962) The isolation and purification of bovine-plasma protein which is a substrate for the coagulant protein of Russell's viper venom, Biochem J 84:62

Esnouf MP et al (1973) A method for the simultaneous isolation of factor X and prothrombin from bovine plasma, Biochem J 131:781

Espada J et al (1972) Human erythropoietin: studies on purity and partial characterization, Biochim Biophys Acta 285:427

Essen-Möller E (1938) Die Beweiskraft der Ähnlichkeit im Vaterschaftsnachweis; theoretische Grundlagen, Mitt Anthropol Ges (Wien) 68:9

Estes JW (1968) Platelet size and function is the heritable disorders of connective tissue, Ann Intern Med 68:1237

Estevez JM et al (1974) Acute megakaryocytic myelofibrosis: case report of an unusual myeloproliferative syndrome, Am J Clin Pathol 62:52

Estren S and Dameshek W (1947) Familial hypoplastic anemia of childhood: report of eight cases in two families with beneficial effect of splenectomy in one case, Am J Dis Child 73:671

Evans AS (1972) Infectious mononucleosis and other mono-like syndromes, N Engl J Med 286:836

Evans AS (1978) Infectious mononucleosis and related syndromes, Am J Med Sci 276:325

Evans DIK (1975) Acute myelofibrosis in children with Down's syndrome, Arch Dis Child 50:458

Evans DMD et al (1969) Facilitating the laboratory diagnosis of infectious mononucleosis, Am J Clin Pathol 52:702

Evans EP et al (1967) Repopulation of Peyer's patches in mice, Nature 216:36

Evans G et al (1968) The effect of acetylsalicylic acid on platelet function, J Exp Med 128:877

Evans RS et al (1965) Autoimmune hemolytic disease: observations of serological reactions and disease activity, Ann NY Acad Sci 124:422

Evatt BL et al (1976) Relationships between thrombopoiesis and erythropoiesis: with studies of the effects of preparations of thrombopoietin and erythropoietin, Blood 48:547

Everett NB et al (1964) Recirculation of lymphocytes, Ann NY Acad Sci 113:887

Eversole SL Jr (1955) Cases of disseminated lupus erythematosus diagnosed as idiopathic thrombocytopenic purpura, Johns Hopkins Med J 96:210

Ewald O (1923) Die leukämische Reticuloendotheliose, Dtsch Arch Kinderheilkd 142:222

Ewing MC and Mayon-White RM (1951) Cyanosis in infancy from nitrates in drinking water, Lancet 1:931

Exner T et al (1978) A sensitive test demonstrating lupus anticoagulant and its behavioral patterns, Br J Haematol 40:143

Ezdinli EZ et al (1970) Philadelphia-chromosome-positive and -negative chronic myelocytic leukemia, Ann Intern Med 72:175

Facer CA et al (1979) Direct Coombs antiglobulin reactions in Gambian children with Plasmodium falciparum malaria. I. Incidence and class specificity, Clin Exp Immunol 35:119

Fahey JL (1965) Antibodies and immunoglobulins. II. Normal development and changes in disease, JAMA 194:255

Fahey JL and McKelvey EM (1965) Quantitative determination of serum immunoglobulin in antibody-agar plates, J Immunol 94:84

Fahey JL et al (1963) Infection, antibody response, and gamma globulin components in multiple myeloma and macroglobulinemia, Am J Med 35:698

Fairbanks VF (1967) Copper sulfate-induced hemolytic anemia. Inhibition of glucose-6-phosphate dehydrogenase and other possible etiologic mechanisms, Arch Intern Med 120:428

Fairbanks VF (1971) Is the peripheral blood film reliable for the diagnosis of iron deficiency anemia? Am J Clin Pathol 55:447

Fairbanks VF and Fernandez MN (1969) The identification of metabolic errors associated with hemolytic anemia, JAMA **208**:316

Fairbanks VF et al (1971) Clinical disorders of iron metabolism, New York, Grune & Stratton, Inc

Fairbanks VF (1980) Nonequivalance of automated and manual hematocrit and erythrocyte indices, Am J Clin Pathol **73**:55

Fairbanks VF et al (1979) Hemoglobin E trait reexamined: a cause of microcytosis and erythrocytosis, Blood **53**:109

Fairbanks VF et al (1980) Homozygous hemoglobin E mimics β-thalassemia minor without anemia or hemolysis: hematologic, functional, and biosynthetic studies of first North American cases, Am J Hematol **8**:109

Fakhro AM et al (1967) Lupus-like syndromes induced by procainamide, Am J Cardiol **20**:367

Fanger MW and Bernier GM (1973) Subpopulation of human lymphocytes defined by β-2-microglobulin, J Immunol **111**:609

Fantl P and Nance M (1946) Acceleration of thrombin formation by a plasma component, Nature **158**:708

Faramarz Naeim MD et al (1979) Sézary syndrome: tartrate-resistant acid phosphatase in the neoplastic cells, Am J Clin Pathol **71**:528

Farber S et al (1948) Temporary remissions in acute leukemia in children produced by a folic acid antagonist 4-aminopteroylglutamic acid (aminopterin), N Engl J Med **238**:787

Fareed J et al (1980) New perspectives in coagulation testing, Clin Chem **26**:1380

Farr AG and De Bruyn PPH (1975) The mode of lymphocyte migration through postcapillary venule endothelium in lymph node, Am J Anat **143**:59

Farrales FB et al (1977) Causes of disqualification in a volunteer blood donor population, Transfusion **17**:598

Farrant PC (1960) Nuclear changes in squamous cells from buccal mucosa in pernicious anaemia, Br Med J **1**:1694

Faulkner WR et al (1968) Handbook of clinical laboratory data, ed 2, Cleveland, Chemical Rubber Co, p 427

Fay JW et al (1979) Leukopheresis therapy of leukemic reticuloendotheliosis (hairy cell leukemia), Blood **54**:747

Fehr J and Jacob HS (1977) In vitro granulocyte adherence and in vivo margination: two associated complement-dependent functions. Studies based on the acute neutropenia of filtration leukophoresis, J Exp Med **146**:641

Feinberg MR et al (1980) Differential diagnosis of malignant lymphomas by imprint cytology, Acta Cytol **24**:16

Feinstein DI and Rapaport SI (1972) Acquired inhibitors of blood coagulation, Prog Hemost Thromb **1**:75

Feinstone SM et al (1973) Hepatitis A: detection by immune electron microscopy of a viruslike antigen associated with acute illness, Science **182**:1026

Feizi T et al (1973) Lymphocytes forming red cell resettes in the cold in patients with chronic cold agglutinin disease, Blood **42**:753

Feldman F (1974) Myelosclerosis in agnogenic myeloid metaplasia, Semin Roentgenol **9**:195

Feldman JD et al (1966) The vascular pathology of thrombotic thrombocytopenic purpura. An immunochemical and ultrastructural study, Lab Invest **15**:927

Feldman RE and Schiff ER (1975) Hepatitis in dental professionals, JAMA **232**:1228

Felice AE et al (1979) The association of sickle cell anemia with heterozygous and homozygous α thalassemia-2: in vitro HB chain synthesis, Am J Hematol **6**:91

Feremans W et al (1979) A case of γ3 heavy chain disease with vocuolated plasma cells: a clinical, immunological, and ultrastructural study, J Clin Pathol **32**:334

Ferretti JJ et al (1977) Mutagenicity of benzidine and related compounds employed in the detection of hemoglobin, Am J Clin Pathol **67**:526

Fessas P and Stamatoyannopoulos G (1964) Hereditary persistence of fetal hemoglobin in Greece. A study and a comparison, Blood **24**:223

Fessas P et al (1962) Hereditary persistence of foetal haemoglobin and its combination with alpha- and beta-thalassemia. In Proceedings of the Eighth Congress of European Society of Haematology, Basel, S Karger AG

Fessas P et al (1972) Identification of slow-moving haemoglobins in haemoglobin H disease from different racial groups, Lancet **1**:1308

Fessas Ph et al (1969) On the chemical structure of haemoglobin Uppsala, Hum Hered **19**:152

Fessel WJ (1965) Odd men out: individuals with extreme values, Arch Intern Med **115**:736

Fessel WJ (1978) ANA-negative systemic lupus erythematosus, Am J Med **64**:80

Fialkow PJ (1967) "Immunologic" oncogenesis, Blood **30**:388

Fialkow PJ et al (1965) Mental retardation in methemoglobinemia due to diaphorase deficiency, N Engl J Med **273**:840

Fialkow PJ et al (1967) Clonal origin of chronic myelocytic leukemia in man, Proc Natl Acad Sci USA **58**:1468

Fialkow PJ et al (1979) Acute nonlymphocytic leukemia: expression in cells restricted to granulocytic and monocytic differentiation, N Engl J Med **301**:1

Fichtelius KE and Vahlquist B (1955) Incidence of atypical mononuclear cells in the peripheral blood of children, Acta Paediatr Scand **44**:541

Fichter EG (1954) Sulfhemoglobinemia, Am J Dis Child **88**:749

Fiegenberg DS et al (1967) Migratory pneumonia with eosinophilia associated with sulfonamide administration, Arch Intern Med **120**:85

Field EO et al (1968) Marrow-suppressing factors in the blood in pure red-cell aplasia, thymoma, and Hodgkin's disease, Br J Haematol **15**:101

Fillet G et al (1977) Effects of transfusion on serum iron, serum lactate dehydrogenase, and platelets in magaloblastic anemia, Am J Clin Pathol **68**:458

Finch CA (1948) Methemoglobinemia and sulfhemoglobinemia, N Engl J Med **239**:470

Finch CA (1959) Some quantitative aspects of erythropoiesis, Ann NY Acad Sci **77**:410

Finch CA (1972) Pathophysiologic aspects of sickle cell anemia, Am J Med **53**:1

Finch CA et al (1956) Erythrokinetics in pernicious anemia, Blood **11**:807

Finch SC (1969) Clinical symptoms and signs of infectious mononucleosis. In Carter RL and Penman HG (Eds): Infectious mononucleosis, Oxford, Blackwell Scientific Publications, Ltd.

Finch SC (1972) Granulocyte disorders—benign, quantitative abnormalities of granulocytes. In Williams WJ et al (Eds): Hematology, New York, McGraw-Hill Book Co, p 628

Finch SC (1979) The study of atomic bomb survivors in Japan, Am J Med **66**:899

Finch SC et al (1969) Chronic lymphocytic leukemia in Hiroshima and Nagasaki, Japan, Blood **33**:79

Finch SC et al (1974) Immunosuppressive therapy of chronic idiopathic thrombocytopenic purpura, Am J Med **56**:4

Fink DJ et al (1967) Serum haptoglobin—a valuable diagnostic aid in suspected hemolytic transfusion reactions, JAMA **199**:615

Finkler AE et al (1970) Immunological properties of human vitamin B_{12} binders, Biochim Biophys Acta **200**:151

Finlayson DC et al (1964) Diurnal variation in blood volume of man, J Surg Res **4**:286

Finlayson JS (1974) Crosslinking of fibrin, Semin Thromb Hemost **1**:33

Finlayson JS et al (1980) Fibrinopeptide release from fibrinogen Paris I, Thromb Res **17**:577

Finne PH and Halvorsen S (1972) Regulation of erythropoiesis in the fetus and newborn, Arch Dis Child **47**:683

Finney RD et al (1973) Haemolytic disease of the newborn caused by the rare rhesus antibody anti-C^x, Vox Sang **25**:39

Finney R et al (1975) Hb Newcastle: beta 92 (F8) his → pro, FEBS Lett **60**:435

Firkin B et al (1973) Von Willebrand's disease type B: a newly defined bleeding diathesis, Aust NZ J Med **3**:225

Firkin BG and Howard MA (1976) Annotation on von Willebrand's disease (vWd), Br J Haematol **32**:151

Fisch RO et al (1963) Methemoglobinemia in a hospital nursery, JAMA **185**:760

Fisch C et al (1951) Acute thrombophlebitis associated with carcinoma of the stomach, Gastroenterology **18**:290

Fischer CL et al (1967) Red blood cell mass and plasma volume changes in manned space flight, JAMA **200**:579

Fischer DA (1962) The "lupoid hepatitis" syndrome: report of a case followed by serial liver biopsies, Ann Intern Med **57**:988

Fishbach FA et al (1971) On the structure of haemosiderin and its relationship to ferritin, J Ultrastruct Res **37**:495

Fishbein IL (1978) William Harvey remembered, J Fla Med Assoc **65**:265

Fishberg E (1948) Excretion of benzoquinoneacetic acid in hypovitaminosis C, J Biol Chem **172**:155

Fisher B et al (1963) The occurrence of pyroglobulins in unsuspected myeloma, Am J Clin Pathol **40**:291

Fisher ER and Balcerzak SP (1969) Effect of exogenous erythropoietin on juxtaglomerular cells, Proc Soc Exp Biol Med **132**:367

Fisher ER and Fisher B (1972) Local lymphoid response as an index of tumor immunity, Arch Pathol **94**:137

Fisher JW (1972) Erythropoietin: pharmacology, biogenesis, and control of production, Pharmacol Rev **24**:459

Fisher JW and Crook JJ (1962) Influence of several hormones on erythropoiesis and oxygen consumption in the hypophysectomized rat, Blood **19**:557

Fisher JW et al (1965) Localization of erythropoietin in glomeruli of sheep kidney by fluorescent antibody technique, Nature **205**:611

Fisher JW et al (1971) A radioimmunoassay for human urinary erythropoietin, Isr J Med Sci **7**:873

Fisher RA and Race RR (1946) Rh gene frequencies in Britain, Nature **157**:48

Fisher JW (1979) Extrarenal erythropoietin production, J Lab Clin Med **93**:695

Fisher MM et al (1951) Recurrent thrombophlebitis in obscure malignant tumor of the lung: report of 4 cases, JAMA **147**:1213

Fisher WB et al (1973) "Preleukemia": a myelodysplastic syndrome often terminating in acute leukemia, Arch Intern Med **132**:226

Fishkin BG et al (1972) IgE multiple myeloma: a report of the 3rd case, Blood **39**:361

Fitchen JH and Cline MJ (1978) Recent developments in understanding the pathogenesis of aplastic anemia, Am J Hematol **5**:365

Fitchen JH and Lee S (1979) Phagocytic myeloma cells, Am J Clin Pathol **71**:722

Fitchen JH et al (1979) Serum inhibitors of hematopoiesis in a patient with aplastic anemia and systemic lupus erythematosus, Am J Med **66**:537

Fitzgerald PH and Hamer JW (1969) Third case of chronic lymphocytic leukemia in a carrier of the inherited Ch^1 chromosome, Br Med J **3**:752

Fitzgerald PH et al (1971) Clonal origin of the Philadelphia chromosome and chronic myeloid leukaemia: evidence from a sex chromosome mosaic, Br J Haematol **21**:473

Fitzsimmons JM and Morel PA (1979) The effects of red blood cell suspending media on hemagglutination and the antiglobulin test, Transfusion **19**:81

Flanagan CJ (1955) Mechanical fragility of neutrophilic erythrophagocytes, Proc Soc Exp Biol Med **90**:580

Flandrin B and Brouet J-C (1974) The Sézary cell: cytologic, cytochemical, and immunologic studies, Mayo Clin Proc **49**:575

Flandrin G and Daniel MT (1971) Cytochimie des estérases en hématologie, Pathol Biol **19**:547

Flandrin G and Daniel MT (1973) Practical value of cytochemical studies for the classification of acute leukemias, Recent Results Cancer Res **43**:43

Flandrin G et al (1973) Leucémie à "tricholeucocyte" (hairy cell leukemia), étude clinique et cytologique de 55 observations, Nouv Rev Fr Hematol **13**:609

Flatz G (1967) Hemoglobin E: distribution and population dynamics, Humangenetik **3**:189

Flatz G et al (1971) Haemoglobin Tak: a variant with additional residues at the end of the beta chains, Lancet **10**:732

Flaum MA et al (1979) The hemostatic imbalance of plasma-exchange transfusion, Blood **54**:694

Fleischman AI et al (1975) In vivo platelet function in acute myocardial infarction, acute cerebrovascular accidents, and following surgery, Thromb Res **6**:205

Fletcher JW et al (1973) Erythropoiesis and hyperoxia, Proc Soc Exp Biol Med **144**:569

Fletcher AP and Alkjaersig N (1972) Blood screening methods for the diagnosis of venous thrombosis, Millbank Mem Fund Q **50**:172

Fliedner TM et al (1979) Collection, storage and transfusion of blood stem cells for the treatment of hemopoietic failure, Blood Cells **5**:313

Flückiger R and Winterhalter KH (1976) In vitro synthesis of hemoglobin A_{1c}, FEBS Lett **71**:356

Flury W et al (1975) Ein Fall von Thrombozytopenia bei Morbus Waldenström mit spezifischer antithrombozytärer Eigenschaft des IgM-Paraproteins, Schweiz Med Wochenschr **105**:1241

Flynn FV et al (1974) The frequency distribution of commonly determined blood constituents in healthy blood donors, Clin Chim Acta **52**:163

Fogarty WM et al (1974) Absence of haemoglobin A in an individual simultaneously heterozygous in the genes for hereditary persistence of foetal haemoglobin and β-thalassemia⁰, Br J Haematol **26**:527

Folk JE and Chung SI (1973) Molecular and catalytic properties of transglutaminases, Adv Enzymol **38**:109

Fone DJ et al (1961) Co^{58} B_{12} absorption (hepatic surface count) after gastrectomy, ileal resection, and in coeliac disorders, Gut **2**:218

Fong TP et al (1977) Stainable iron in aspirated and needle-biopsy specimens of marrow: a source of error, Am J Hematol **2**:47

Fong TP et al (1979) An evaluation of cellularity in various types of bone marrow specimens, Am J Clin Pathol **72**:812

Fontan G et al (1976) Defective neutrophil chemotaxis and hyperimmunoglobulinemia E—a reversible defect? Acta Paediatr Scand **65**:511

Foon KA et al (1980) Dual band T markers in acute and chronic lymphocytic leukemia, Blood **55**:16

Forbes CD et al (1972) Acute intravascular haemolysis associated with cephalexin therapy, Postgrad Med J **48**:186

Ford DK et al (1962) Familial lipochrome pigmentation of histiocytes with hyperglobulinemia, pulmonary infiltration, splenomegaly, arteritis and susceptibility to infection, Am J Med **33**:478

Forget BG (1977) Nucleotide sequence of human beta globin messenger RNA, Hemoglobin **1**:879

Forman WB et al (1968) An inherited qualitative abnormality in plasma fibrinogen: fibrinogen Cleveland, J Lab Clin Med **72**:455

Forte FA et al (1970) Heavy chain disease of gamma (γM) type: report of the first case, Blood **36**:137

Foster KM and Jack I (1969) A prospective study of the role of cytomegalovirus in post-transfusion mononucleosis, N Engl J Med **280**:1311

Foucar K et al (1979) Therapy-related leukemia: a panmyelosis, Cancer **43**:1285

Fowler WM (1936) Chlorosis—an obituary, Ann Med Hist **8**:168

Fowler WE and Erickson HP (1979) Trinodular structure of fibrinogen, J Mol Biol **134**:241

Frangione B and Franklin EC (1973) Heavy chain disease: clinical features and molecular significance of the disordered immunoglobulin structure, Semin Hematol **10**:53

Franklin EC et al (1964) Heavy chain disease—new disorder of serum γ-globulins, Am J Med **37**:332

Franklin EC et al (1978) Human heavy chain disease protein WIS: implications for the organization of immunoglobulin genes, Proc Natl Acad Sci USA **76**:452

Franzén S et al (1966) Primary polycythaemia associated with multiple myeloma, Acta Med Scand **179**(supp 445):336

Fraumeni JF Jr (1969) Clinical epidemiology of leukemia, Semin Hematol **6**:250

Fraumeni JF Jr and Miller RW (1967) Leukemia mortality: downturn rates in the United States, Science **155**:1126

Frazier PD et al (1965) Identification of L-cystine crystals in bone marrow by x-ray diffraction, J Lab Clin Med **65**:108

Frederici HHR et al (1966) The fine structure of capillaries in experimental scurvy, Lab Invest **15**:1442

Fredrickson DS (1966a) Cerebroside lipidosis: Gaucher's disease. In Stanbury JB et al (Eds): The metabolic basis of inherited disease, New York, McGraw-Hill Book Co

Fredrickson DS (1966b) Sphingomyelin lipidosis: Niemann-Pick disease. In Stanbury JB et al (Eds): The metabolic basis of inherited disease, New York, McGraw-Hill Book Co

Fredrickson DS (1966c) Familial high-density lipoprotein deficiency: Tangier disease. In Stanbury JB et al (Eds): The metabolic basis of inherited disease, New York, McGraw-Hill Book Co

Fredrickson DS et al (1978) Familial lipoprotein deficiency. In Stanbury JB et al (Eds): The metabolic basis of inherited disease, New York, McGraw-Hill Book Co

Freedman AL et al (1956) Hemolytic anemia due to quinidine. Observations on its mechanism, Am J Med **20**:806

Freedman MH et al (1976) Erythroid colony growth in congenital hypoplastic anemia, J Clin Invest **57**:673

Freedman MH et al (1979) Acquired aplastic anemia: antibody-mediated hematopoietic failure, Am J Hematol **6**:135

Freedom RM (1972) The asplenia syndrome: a review of significant extra-cardiac structural abnormalities in 29 necropsied patients, J Pediatr **81**:1130

Freeman HE (1944) Aplastic anemia with acute agranulocytosis, thrombopenic purpura, and complicating mapharsen therapy, Arch Dermatol Syph **50**:320

Freeman JA (1966) Origin of Auer bodies, Blood **27**:499

Freeman T and Smith J (1970) Human serum protein fractionation by gel filtration, Biochem J **118**:869

Fregert S and Rorsman H (1964) Basophil leukocytes in photo contact dermatitis, J Invest Dermatol **42**:405

Freireich EJ et al (1963) Response to repeated platelet transfusions from the same donor, Ann Intern Med **59**:277

Frick PG (1969) Primary thrombocythemia. Clinical, hematological, and chromosomal studies of 13 patients, Helv Med Acta **35**:20

Fried W and Gurney CW (1968) The erythropoietic-stimulating effects of androgens, Ann NY Acad Sci **149**:356

Fried WL et al (1956) Erythropoiesis. II. Assay of erythropoietin in hypophysectomized rates, Proc Soc Exp Biol Med **92**:203

Fried WL et al (1957) Studies on erythropoiesis. III. Factors controlling erythropoietin production, Proc Soc Exp Biol Med **94**:237

Friedenreich V (1936) Eine bisher unbekannte Blutgruppeneigenschaft (A₃), Z Immunitaetsforsch **89**:409

Friedlander RD (1934) Racial factor in pernicious anemia, Am J Med Sci **187**:634

Friedman BI et al (1958) Tissue mast cell leukemia, Blood **13**:70

Friedman S (1935) Eosinophilia in scarlet fever. I. As a diagnostic aid, Am J Dis Child **49**:933

Friman C et al (1970) IgD myeloma associated with multiple extramedullary amyloid-containing tumours and amyloid casts in the renal tubules, Am Clin Res **2**:161

Friou GJ (1967) Antinuclear antibodies: diagnostic significance and methods, Arthritis Rheum **10**:151

Frisancho AR (1975) Functional adaptation to high altitude hypoxia, Science **187**:313

Frisancho AR et al (1973) Influence of developmental adaptation on aerobic capacity at high altitudes, J Appl Physiol **34**:176

Frisch B and Lewis SM (1974) The bone marrow in aplastic anaemia: diagnostic and prognostic features, J Clin Pathol **27**:231

Frisch B et al (1974) The ultrastructure of erythropoiesis in two hemoglobinopathies, Br J Haematol **28**:109

Frisch B et al (1975) The ultrastructure of dyserythropoiesis in aplastic anaemia, Br J Haematol **29**:545

Frishman WH et al (1974) Reversal of abnormal platelet aggregability and change in exercise tolerance in patients with angina pectoris following oral propranolol, Circulation **50**:887

Fritzsche W and Martin H (1957) Properdin und hämalyse. Zur Hemmung der hämalyse der erythrocyten von kranken mit paroxymaler nächtlicher Hämoglobinurie durch Heparin, Klin Wochenschr **35**:1166

Frizzera G et al (1974) Angioimmunoblastic lymphadenopathy with dysproteinemia, Lancet **1**:1070

Frizzera G et al (1979) Predictability of immunologic phenotype of malignant lymphomas by conventional morphology: a study of 60 cases, Cancer **43**:1216

Frolich ED (1958) Pernicious anemia masked by a multivitamin preparation, N Engl J Med **259**:1221

Froment A et al (1965) Hyperkaliémie au cours d'une leucémie lymphoide, cause possible d'une mort subite, Lyon Med **214**:1067

Frota-Pessoa O and Wajntal A (1963) Mutation rates of the abnormal hemoglobin genes, Am J Hum Genet **15**:123

Fuchs G et al (1977) Fibrinogen Marburg, a new genetic variant of fibrinogen, Blut **34**:107

Fudenberg H and Estren S (1958) Non-Addisonian megaloblastic anemia: the intermediate megaloblast in the differential diagnosis of pernicious and related anemia, Am J Med **25**:198

Fudenberg H et al (1971) Primary immunodeficiencies. Report of a World Health Organization Committee, Pediatrics **47**:927

Fujikawa K et al (1974a) A comparison of bovine prothrombin, factor IX (Christmas factor), and factor X (Stuart factor), Proc Natl Acad Sci USA **71**:427

Fujikawa K et al (1974b) The mechanism of activation of bovine factor IX (Christmas factor) by bovine factor XI$_a$ (activated plasma thromboplastin antecedent), Biochemistry **13**:4508

Fujikawa K et al (1974c) The mechanism of activation of bovine factor X (Stuart factor) by intrinsic and extrinsic pathways, Biochemistry **13**:5290

Fujimura T et al (1964) Two kindreds of abnormal hemoglobins: hb Tagawa I and hb Tagawa II, Jpn J Clin Hematol **6**:71

Fujiwara N et al (1971) Hemoglobin Atago (alpha 2 85 Tyr beta 2): a new abnormal human hemoglobin found in Nagasaki, Int J Protein Res **3**:35

Fukagawa N et al (1979) Hereditary spherocytosis with normal osmotic fragility after incubation. Is the autohemolysis test really obsolete? JAMA **242**:63

Fukuda T (1973) Undifferentiated mononuclear cell in human embryonic liver: presumptive hematopoietic stem cell, Virchows Arch (Zellpathol), **14**:31

Fukushi K et al (1972) Electron microscopic study of the Auer body, Acta Pathol Jap **22**:509

Fuleihan FJD et al (1968) Idiopathic pulmonary hemosiderosis. Case report with pulmonary function tests and review of the literature, Am Rev Resp Dis **98**:93

Fulford KWM et al (1973) Australia antigen and antibody among patients attending a clinic for sexually transmitted diseases, Lancet **1**:1470

Fulginiti VA et al (1966) Dissociation of delayed-hypersensitivity and antibody-synthesizing capacity in man. Report of two subships with thymic dysplasia, lymphoid tissue depletion, and normal immunoglobulins, Lancet **2**:5

Fung CHK and Woodson B (1976) Interpretation of plasma protamine paracoagulation test, Am J Clin Pathol **65**:698

Fung RH et al (1969) Screening of pyruvate kinase deficiency and G6PD deficiency in Chinese newborn in Hong Kong, Arch Dis Child **44**:373

Funk C and Straub PW (1970) Hereditary abnormality of fibrin monomer aggregation (Fibrinogen Zürich II), Eur J Clin Invest **1**:131

Furukawa T et al (1975) An association of hepatitis B (Australia) antigen with platelets, Vox Sang **29**:411

Fuster V et al (1973) Assay of platelet factor 4 in plasma, Mayo Clin Proc **48**:103

Gabbay KH et al (1977) Glycosylated hemoglobins and long-term blood glucose control in diabetes mellitus, J Clin Endocrinol Metab **44**:859

Gabuzda TG et al (1963) The turnover of hemoglobins A, F, and A$_2$ in the peripheral blood of three patients with thalassemia, J Clin Invest **42**:1678

Gacon G et al (1975a) Structural and functional study of hb Nancy beta 145 (HC2) try $\rightarrow$ asp: a high oxygen affinity hemoglobin, FEBS Lett **56**:39

Gacon G et al (1975b) A new unstable hemoglobin mutated in beta 98 (FG5) val $\rightarrow$ ala: hb Djelfa, FEBS Lett **58**:238

Gacon G et al (1976) A second case of haemoglobin Belfast (beta 15 [A12] trp $\rightarrow$ arg) observed in a French patient, Acta Haematol **55**:313

Gacon G et al (1977) Structural and functional studies on hb Rothchild beta 37 (C3) trp $\rightarrow$ arg. A new variant of the alpha 1 beta 2 contact, FEBS Lett **82**:243

Gadner H et al (1973) Akute Leukämie nach Chloramphenicol-Exposition? Ein kasuistischer Beitrag mit Literaturübersicht, Monatsschr Kinderheilkd **121**:590

Gaffney GW et al (1957) Vitamin B$_{12}$ serum concentrations in 528 apparently healthy human subjects of ages 12-94, J Gerontol **12**:32

Gagliardo FJ and Curiano RR (1963) A rare form of anti-M antibody associated with pregnancy, Am J Clin Pathol **40**:662

Gagné C et al (1977) Effect of hyperchylomicronemia on the measurement of hemoglobin, Am J Clin Pathol **68**:584

Gajdusek DC et al (1967) Haemoglobin J Tongariki (alpha 115 alanine $\rightarrow$ aspartic acid): the first new haemoglobin variant found in a Pacific (Melanesian) population, J Med Genet **4**:1

Gajl-Peczalska KJ et al (1974) B-cell markers on lymphoblasts in acute lymphoblastic leukemia, Clin Exp Immunol **17**:561

Gajl-Peczalska KJ (1975) B and T cell lymphomas: analysis of blood and lymph nodes in 87 patients, Am J Med **59**:674

Galatius-Jensen F (1958) Rare phenotypes in the Hp system, Acta Genet **8**:248

Gale RP et al (1975) Thymus-dependent lymphocytes in human bone marrow, J Clin Invest **56**:1491

Gall EA (1936) Previously undescribed granule within the lymphocyte, Am J Med Sci **191**:380

Gall EA (1958) The cytological identity and interrelation of mesenchymal cells of lymphoid tissue, Ann NY Acad Sci **73**:120

Gallango ML and Arends T (1965) Inv(a) serum factor in Venezuelan Indians, Transfusion **5**:457

Gallin JI (1975) Abnormal chemotaxis: cellular and humoral components. In Bellanti JA and Dayton DH (Eds): The phagocytic cell in host resistance, New York, Raven Press

Gallin JI and Kaplan AP (1974) Mononuclear cell chemotactic activity of kallikrein and plasminogen activator and its inhibition by C1 inhibitor and alpha 2-macroglobulin, J Immunol **113**(6):1928

Gallin JI and Wolff SM (1975) Leucocyte chemotaxis: physiological considerations and abnormalities, Clin Haematol **4**:567

Gallin JI et al (1975) Defective mononuclear leukocyte hemotaxis in the Chediak-Higashi syndrome in human, mink, and cattle, Blood **45**:863

Gallo RC et al (1970) RNA dependent DNA polymerase of human acute leukaemic cells, Nature **228**:927

Gallop, PM, et al (1980) Carboxylated calcium-binding proteins and vitamin K, N Engl J Med **302**:1460

Gallus AS (1979) Antiplatelet drugs: clinical pharmacology and therapeutic use, Drugs **18**:439

Gallus AS et al (1973a) Relevance of preoperative and postoperative blood tests to postoperative leg-vein thrombosis, Lancet **2**:805

Gallus AS et al (1973b) Small subcutaneous doses of heparin in prevention of venous thrombosis, N Engl J Med **288**:545

Gallus AS et al (1976) Prevention of venous thromboembolism with small subcutaneous doses of heparin, JAMA **235**:1980

Gally JA and Edelman GM (1972) The genetic control of immunoglobulin synthesis, Ann Rev Genet **6**:1

Galton DAG et al (1974) Prolymphocytic leukaemia, Br J Haematol **27**:7

Gambino SR et al (1965) The Westergren sedimentation rate, using K$_3$EDTA, Tech Bull Regist Med Techn **35**:1

Gammelgaard A (1944) Serologische und genetische Untersuchungen über seltene A-Typen bei Menschen. II. Die Bluttypen A$_4$, A$_5$, und A$_x$, Acta Pathol Microbiol Scand **21**:554

Gandalfo GM et al (1977) Circulating anticoagulant against factor XII and platelet antibodies in systemic lupus erythematosus, Acta Haematol **57**:135

Gangarosa EJ et al (1960) Ristocetin-induced thrombocytopenia: site and mechanism of action, AMA Arch Intern Med **105**:83

Ganguly P (1969) Effect of proteolytic activity on the isolation and stability of platelet proteins, Clin Chim Acta **25**:371

Gänsslen M (1941) Konstitutionelle familiäre leukopenie (neutropenie), Klin Wochenschr **20**:922

Garby L (1970) The normal hemoglobin level, Br J Haematol **19**:429

Garby L et al (1969) Iron deficiency in women of fertile age in a

Swedish community. III. Estimation of prevalence based on response to iron supplementation, Acta Med Scand **185**:113

Gardner FH (1965) Idiopathic thrombocytopenic purpura. In Samter M and Alexander HL (Eds): Immunological diseases, Boston, Little, Brown and Co

Gardner FH (1974) Use of platelet transfusions, Br J Haematol **27**:537

Gardner FH and Murphy S (1972) Granulocyte and platelet functions in paroxysmal nocturnal hemoglobinuria, Ser Haematol **5**:78

Gardner FH and Nathan DG (1966) Androgens and erythropoiesis. III. Further evaluation of testosterone treatment of myelofibrosis, N Engl J Med **274**:420

Gardner FH et al (1968) The erythrocythaemic effects of androgen, Br J Haematol **14**:611

Garel MC et al (1975) Hemoglobin Castilla beta 32 (B14) leu → arg: a new unstable variant producing severe hemolytic disease, FEBS Lett **58**:145

Garel MC et al (1976a) Hemoglobin J Cairo: beta 65 (E9) lys → gln, a new hemoglobin variant discovered in an Egyptian family, Biochim Biophys Acta **420**:97

Garel MC et al (1976b) Hb Strasbourg alpha 2 beta 2 20 (B2) val → asp: a variant at the same locus as Hb Olympia beta 20 val → met, FEBS Lett **72**:1

Garel MC et al (1976c) Hemoglobin Dakar–hemoglobin Grady: demonstration by a new approach to the analysis of the tryptic core region of the alpha chain and oxygen equilibrium properties, Biochim Biophys Acta **453**:459

Garfield MD et al (1978) Malaria transmission by platelet concentrate transfusion, JAMA **240**:2285

Garg SK et al (1971) Use of the megathrombocyte as an index of megakaryocyte number, N Engl J Med **284**:11

Garratty G and Petz LD (1975) Drug-induced immune hemolytic anemia, Am J Med **58**:398

Garratty G and Petz LD (1976) The significance of red cell bound complement components in development of standards and quality assurance for the anti-complement components of antiglobulin sera, Transfusion **16**:297

Garrett TJ et al (1976) The role of bone marrow aspiration and biopsy in detecting marrow involvement by nonhematologic malignancies, Cancer **38**:2401

Gaston LW (1966) Studies on a family with an elevated plasma level of factor V (proaccelerin) and a tendency to thrombosis, J Pediatr **68**:367

Gaston LW et al (1971) Spleno renal shunt, cholecystectomy, and appendectomy in a patient with hemophilia A, an abnormal fibrinogen and thrombocytopenia, Ann Surg **173**:234

Geary CG et al (1974) An association between aplastic anaemia and sideroblastic anaemia, Br J Haematol **27**:337

Geary CG et al (1975) Chronic myelomonocytic leukaemia, Br J Haematol **30**:289

Geerdink RA et al (1966) Hereditary elliptocytosis and hyperhaemolysis. A comparative study of 6 families with 145 patients, Acta Med Scand **179**:715

Gehlot GS and Monga JN (1973) Prevalence of Pelger-Huët anomaly of leucocytes in Adivasi population of western Madjya Pradesh, Indian J Med Res **61**:653

Gelin LE (1965) Rheological disturbances following tissue injury. In Copley Al (Ed): Proceedings of the Fourth International Congress on Rheology, New York, Interscience Publishers, Inc, Pt 4, p 299

Gellady AM and Schwartz AD (1973) Hemoglobins S and J coexisting in the same family, J Pediatr **83**:1038

Gelpi AP (1973) Migrant populations and the diffusion of the sickle-cell gene, Ann Intern Med **79**:258

Gelpi AP and Perrine RP (1973) Sickle cell disease and trait in white population, JAMA **224**:605

Gelpi AP (1979) Benign sickle cell disease in Saudi Arabia: survival estimate and population dynamics, Clin Genet **15**:307

Genton E et al (1975) Platelet-inhibiting drugs in the prevention of clinical thrombotic disease, N Engl J Med **293**:1174, 1236, 1296

Gerald PS and Efron ML (1961) Chemical studies of several varieties of hb M, Proc Natl Acad Sci USA **47**:1758

Gerber P and Monroe JH (1968) Studies on leukocytes growing in continuous culture derived from normal human donors, J Natl Cancer Int **40**:855

Gerber P et al (1968) Infectious mononucleosis: complement-fixing antibodies to herpes-like virus associated with Burkitt lymphoma, Science **161**:173

Gerber P et al (1969) Attempts to transmit infectious mononucleosis to Rhesus monkeys and marmosets and to isolate herpes-like virus, Proc Soc Exp Biol Med **130**:14

Gerlach E and Duhm J (1972a) 2,3-DPG metabolism of red cells: regulation and adaptive changes during hypoxia. In Rørth M and Astrup P (Eds): Oxygen affinity of hemoglobin and red cell acid-base status. Alfred Benzon Symposium IV, Copenhagen, Munksgaard, International Book Sellers & Publishers Ltd, p 552

Gerlach E and Duhm J (1972b) Regulation of the concentration of 2,3-diphosphoglycerate in the erythrocyte, Scand J Clin Lab Invest 29 (supp) **126**:5.4

Gerstner HB (1958) Acute radiation syndrome in man: military and civil defense aspects, US Armed Forces Med J **9**:313

Gerstner JB et al (1979) Posttransfusion purpura: therapeutic failure of Pl^{A1}-negative platelet transfusion, Am J Hematol **6**:71

Gery I et al (1972) Stimulation of B-lymphocytes by endotoxin. Reaction of thymus-deprived mice and karyotypic analysis of dividing cells in mice bearing T6 thymus grafts, J Immunol **108**:1088

Getaz EP et al (1980) Cisplatin-induced hemolysis, N Engl J Med **302**:334

Ghadially FN and Skinnider LF (1971) Ropalocytosis—a new abnormality of erythrocytes and their precursors, Experientia **27**:1217

Ghadially FN and Skinnider LF (1972) Ultrastructure of hairy cell leukemia, Cancer **29**:444

Ghosh ML (1972) The sea-blue histiocyte syndrome with hepatic porphyria and infectious mononucleosis, J Clin Pathol **25**:945

Ghosh ML and Harris-Jones JN (1974) Coombs-negative autoimmune hemolytic anemia and immunoglobulin deficiency, Am J Clin Pathol **62**:40

Giardina B et al (1978) Properties of hemoglobin G Ferrara (beta 57 [E1] asn → lys), Biochim Biophys Acta **534**:1

Gibaud A et al (1974) Sur une hemoglobin "S" aquise de l'adulte, Nouv Press Med **3**:2013

Giblett ER (1960) The serum haptoglobins and transferrins. In Eighth International Congress of Blood Transfusion (Tokyo), Basel, S Karger AG

Giblett ER (1969) Genetic markers in human blood, Philadelphia, FA Davis Co

Giblett ER (1977) Blood group alloantibodies: an assessment of some laboratory practices, Transfusion **17**:299

Giblett ER and Brooks LE (1963) Haptoglobin sub-types in three racial groups, Nature **197**:576

Giblett ER and Chase J (1959) Js^a, a "new" red-cell antigen found in Negroes: evidence for an eleventh blood group system, Br J Haematol **5**:319

Giblett ER and Steinberg AG (1960) The inheritance of serum haptoglobin types in American Negroes: evidence of a third allele Hp^{2m}, Am J Hum Genet **12**:160

Giblett ER et al (1956) Damage of the bone marrow due to Rh antibody, Pediatrics **17**:37

Gibson G (1980) Measuring metric, The Sciences **20**:2

Gibson JG Jr and Evans WA Jr (1937) Clinical studies of the blood volume: relation of plasma and total blood volume to venous pressure, blood velocity rate, physical measurement, age, and sex in ninety normal humans, J Clin Invest **16**:317

Gibson KD et al (1961) Biosynthesis of porphyrins and chlorophylls, Nature **192**:204

Gibson QH (1954) Methaemoglobin and sulfhaemoglobin, Biochem J **57**:111

Gibson QH (1970) The reaction of oxygen with hemoglobin and the kinetic basis of the effect of salt on binding of oxygen, J Biol Chem **245**:3285

Giclas PC et al (1979) Immunoglobulin C independent activation of the classical complement pathway by monosodium urate crystals, J Clin Invest **63**:759

Gierer A (1963) Function of aggregated reticulocyte ribosomes in protein synthesis, J Mol Biol **6**:148

Gilbert HS et al (1966) A study of histamine in myeloproliferative disease, Blood **28**:795

Gilbertsen VA (1965) Erythrocyte sedimentation rates in older patients. A study of 4,341 cases, Postgrad Med **38**:A44

Gill JR et al (1976) Bartter's syndrome: a disorder characterized by high urinary prostaglandins and a dependence of hyperreninemia on prostaglandin synthesis, Am J Med **61**:43

Gilles HM et al (1964) Hookworm infection and anemia. An epidemiological, clinical, and laboratory study, Q J Med **33**:1

Gillespie D and Gallo RC (1975) RNA processing and RNA tumor virus origin and evolution, Science **188**:802

Gilliland BC et al (1971) Red cell antibodies in acquired hemolytic anemia with negative antiglobulin serum tests, N Engl J Med **285**:252

Gilman JG and Smithies O (1968) Fetal hemoglobin variants in mice, Science **160**:885

Gilman PA et al (1970) Congenital agranulocytosis: prolonged survival and terminal acute leukemia, Blood **36**:576

Gilmer PR Jr (1979) The Coulter Perkin-Elmer Diff3 automated leukocyte classifier. In Koepke JA, (Ed): Differential leukocyte counting, Skokie, Ill, College of American Pathologists, p 135

Gilmer PR Jr and Koepke JA (1976) The reticulocyte: an approach to definition, Am J Clin Pathol **66**:262

Giloon JR et al (1960) Chediak-Higashi anomaly of the leukocytes: report of a case, Mayo Clin Proc **35**:635

Gimbrone MA Jr et al (1969) Preservation of vascular integrity in organs perfused in vitro with a platelet-rich medium, Nature **221**:33

Gimpert E et al (1975) Vitamin B_{12} transport in blood. I. Congenital deficiency of transcobalamin II, Blood **45**:71

Ginsberg A and Mullinax F (1970) Pernicious anemia and monoclonal gammopathy in a patient with IgA deficiency, Am J Med **48**:787

Girard JP et al (1967) Penicillin hypersensitivity with eosinophilia: a case report with immunologic studies, Am J Med **42**:441

Girolami A (1975) Prothrombin Padua. In Hemker HC and Veltkamp JJ (Eds): Prothrombin and related coagulation factors, Leiden, Leiden University Press, p 213

Girolami A et al (1970) A "new" congenital haemorrhagic condition due to the presence of an abnormal factor X (factor X Friuli): study of a large kindred, Br J Haematol **19**:179

Girolami A et al (1971) Further studies on the abnormal factor X (factor X Friuli) coagulation disorder: a report of another family, Blood **37**:534

Girolami A et al (1975) Factor X Friuli: An immunological study in plasma and in serum using several methods, Blut **30**:203

Girolami A et al (1976) Combined hereditary deficiency of factors VII and VIII: a distinct coagulation disorder due to the "lack" of an autosomal gene controlling factor VII and VIII activation? Acta Haematol **55**:181

Girolami A et al (1977) Normotest—Thrombotest discrepancy in congenital coagulation disorders of the prothrombin complex and in coumarin-treated patients: a nonspecific phenomenon, Am J Clin Pathol **67**:57

Gitel SN et al (1978) The activated factor X-antithrombin III reaction rate: a measure of the increased thrombotic tendency induced by estrogen-containing oral contraceptives in rabbits, Haemostasis **7**:10

Gitlin D and Craig JM (1963) The thymus and other lymphoid tissues in congenital agammaglobulinemia. I. Thymic alymphoplasia and lymphocytic hypoplasia and their relation to infection, Pediatrics **32**:517

Gitlin D et al (1964) Thymic alymphoplasia and congenital aleukocytosis, Pediatrics **33**:184

Gitlin D et al (1973) Multiple immunoglobulin classes among sharks and their evolution, Comp Biochem Physiol **44B**:225

Gittman JE et al (1978) Hypercalcemic crisis associated with the hypereosinophilic syndrome, Am J Med **64**:901

Giuliani ER et al (1961) Anemia of nontropical sprue studied in the radioiron and radiochromium, J Nucl Med **2**:297

Giuliano VJ et al (1974) The nature of the atypical lymphocyte in infectious mononucleosis, Clin Immunol Immunopathol **3**:90

Gjone E et al (1978) Familial lecithin: cholesterol acyltransferase deficiency. In Stanbury, JB et al (Eds): The metabolic basis of inherited disease, ed 4, New York, McGraw-Hill Book Co, Inc, p 589

Gjønnaess H (1972) Cold-promoted activation of factor VII. IV. Relation to the coagulation system, Thromb Diath Haemorrh **28**:194

Gjønnaess H and Fagerhol MK (1974) Studies on plasma coagulation and fibrinolysis during oral contraception of various types with special reference to cold activation of factor VII, Scand J Haematol **12**:232

Glade PR and Chessin LN (1968) Synthesis of B1C-B1a-globulin (C′3) by human lymphoid cells, Int Arch Allergy Appl Immunol **34**:181

Glade PR et al (1969) Lymphoproliferative potential in infectious diseases, Bull NY Acad Med **45**:647

Glader, BE and Nathan DG (1975) Haemolysis due to pyruvate kinase deficiency and other glycolytic enzymopathies, Clin Haematol **4**:123

Gladhaug A and Prydz H (1970) Purification of the coagulation factors VII and X from human serum. Some properties of factor VII, Biochim Biophys Acta **215**:105

Glass R (1971) Factitiously low ESR with chronic lymphocytic leukemia, N Engl J Med **285**:921

Glass D et al (1978) Inherited deficiency of the sixth component of complement: a silent or null gene, J Immunol **120**:538

Glenner GG et al (1973) Amyloidosis: its nature and pathogenesis, Semin Hematol **10**:65

Glick AD (1976) Acute leukemia: electron microscopic diagnosis, Semin Oncol **3**:229

Glick AD et al (1980) Acute leukemia of adults: ultrastructural, cytochemical and histologic observations in 100 cases, Am J Clin Pathol **73**:459

Glick B et al (1956) The bursa of fabricius and antibody production, Poultry Sci **35**:224

Glover SN and Walford RL (1958) A serologic and family study of the rare blood group A_x, Am J Clin Pathol **30**:539

Glueck HI and Herrmann LG (1964) Cold-precipitable fibrinogen, "cryofibrinogen," Arch Intern Med **113**:748

Gobbi F (1966) Heredity of combined deficiency of AHG and proaccelerin, Scand J Haematol **3**:222

Gocke DJ and Kavey NB (1969) Hepatitis antigen: correlation with disease and infectivity of blood-donors, Lancet **1**:1055

Godal HC (1970) An inhibitor to fibrin stabilizing factor (FSF, factor XIII), Scand J Haematol **7**:43

Godal HC and Abilgaard U (1966) Gelation of soluble fibrin in plasma by ethanol, Scand J Haematol **3**:432

Godal HC and Skaga E (1969) Aggravation of congenital spherocytosis during infectious mononucleosis, Scand J Haematol **6**:33

Godal HC and Refsum HE (1979) Haemolysis in athletes due to hereditary spherocytosis, Scand J Haematol **22**:83

Godwin HA and Ginsburg AD (1974) May-Hegglin anomaly: a defect in megakaryocyte fragmentation? Br J Haematol **26**:117

Goebel KM et al (1975) Haemolytic anaemia with hereditary pyruvate kinase instability developing acute leukaemia, Scand R Haematol **14**:249

Goh K and Swisher SN (1965) Identical twins and chronic myelocytic leukemia. Chromosomal studies of a patient with chronic myelocytic leukemia and his normal identical twin, Arch Intern Med **115**:475

Goh K et al (1965) Cytogenetic studies in eosinophilic leukemia: the relationship of eosinophilic leukemia and chronic myelocytic leukemia, Ann Intern Med **62**:80

Gold AP and Michael AF Jr (1959) Congenital adrenal hyperplasia associated with polycythemia, Pediatrics **23**:727

Gold ER and Balding R (1975) Receptor-specific proteins. Plant and animal lectins, New York, American Elsevier Publishing Co, Inc

Goldberg A (1968) Lead poisoning as a disorder of heme synthesis, Semin Hematol **5**:424

Goldberg A et al (1967) Hereditary coproporphyria, Lancet **1**:632

Goldberg AF and Deane HW (1960) A comparative study of some staining properties of crystals in a lymphoplasmacytoid cell, of Russell bodies in plasmocytes, and of amyloids—with special emphasis on their isoelectric points, Blood **16**:1708

Goldberg CAJ (1958) The ferrohemoglobin solubility test: its accuracy and precision together with values found in the presence of some abnormal hemoglobins, Clin Chem **4**:146

Goldberg LS and Barnett EV (1970) Essential Cryoglobulinemia. Immunologic studies before and after penicillamine therapy, Arch Intern Med **125**:145

Goldberg LS and Bluestone R (1970) Hidden gastric autoantibodies to intrinsic factor in pernicious anemia, J Lab Clin Med **75**:449

Goldberg LS and Bluestone R (1973) Studies on serologic abnormalities induced by L-dopa, Vox Sang **24**:171

Golde DW (1975) Disorders of mononuclear phagocyte proliferation, maturation, and function, Clin Haematol **4**:705

Golde DW and Cline MJ (1972) Identification of the colony-stimulating cell in human peripheral blood, J Clin Invest **51**:2981

Golde DW and Cline MJ (1974a) Regulation of granulopoiesis, N Engl J Med **291**:1388

Golde DW and Cline MJ (1974b) Regulation of human bone marrow leucopoiesis, Br J Haematol **26**:235

Golde DW and Cline MJ (1975) Erythropoietin responsiveness in polycythaemia vera, Br J Haematol **29**:567

Golde DW and Cline MJ (1978) Hormonal interactions with hematopoietic cells in vitro, Transplant Proc **10**:95

Golde DW et al (1977a) The Philadelphia chromosome in human macrophages, Blood **49**:367

Golde DW et al (1977b) Growth hormone: species-specific stimulation of erythropoiesis in vitro, Science **196**:1112

Golden HE and McDuffie FC (1967) Role of lupus erythematosus factor and accessory serum factors in production of extracellular nuclear material, Ann Intern Med **67**:780

Goldman AS et al (1967) Thymic alymphoplasia, lymphoma, and dys-gammaglobulinemia, hyper-gamma-A, normo-gamma-M, hypo-gamma-G, a-gamma-D, and gamma-E-globulinemia, plasmacytosis, normal delayed sensitivity, severe allergic reactions, and Coombs' positive anemia, Pediatrics **39**:348

Goldman JM (1974) In vitro colony forming cells and colony stimulating factor in chronic granulocyte leukaemia, Br J Cancer **30**:1

Goldstein AL et al (1966) Preparation, assay, and partial purification of a thymic lymphocytopoietic factor (thymosin), Proc Natl Acad Sci USA **56**:1010

Goldstein BD (1974) Production of paroxysmal nocturnal hemoglobinuria-like red cells by reducing and oxidizing agents, Br J Haematol **26**:49

Goldstein C and Pechet L (1965) Chronic erythrocytic hypoplasia following pernicious anemia, Blood **25**:31

Goldstein E and Porter DY (1969) Fatal thrombocytopenia with cerebral hemorrhage in infectious mononucleosis, Arch Neurol **20**:533

Goldstein IM et al (1971) Leukocyte transfusions: role of leukocyte allo-antibodies in determining transfusion response, Transfusion **11**:19

Goldstein IM et al (1975) Complement and immunoglobulins stimulate superoxide production by human leukocytes independently of phagocytosis, J Clin Invest **56**:1155

Goldwasser E and Kung CKH (1968) Progress in the purification of erythropoietin, Ann NY Acad Sci **149**:49

Goldwasser E et al (1962) Further purification of sheep plasma erythropoietin, Biochim Biophys Acta **64**:487

Goldwasser E et al (1974) On the mechanism of erythropoietin-induced differentiation. XIII. The role of sialic acid in erythropoietin action, J Biol Chem **249**:4202

Golob JK (1960) Normal ranges in clinical work: their uses and methods of determination, Am J Med Technol **26**:167

Golomb HM et al (1975) "Hairy" cell leukaemia (leukaemic reticuloendotheliosis): a scanning electron microscopic study of eight cases, Br J Haematol **29**:455

Golomb HM et al (1978a) Correlation of clinical findings with quinacrine-banded chromosomes in 90 adults with acute non-lymphocytic leukemia: an eight-year study (1970-1977), N Engl J Med **299**:613

Golomb HM et al (1978b) Hairy cell leukemia: a clinical review based on 71 cases, Ann Intern Med **89**:677

Goluboff N (1958) Methemoglobinemia due to Benzocaine, Pediatrics **21**:340

Gomperts ED et al (1972) A red cell membrane abnormality in hereditary spherocytosis, Br J Haematol **23**:363

Gonen B et al (1977) Hemoglobin A_1: an indicator of the metabolic control of diabetic patients, Lancet **2**:734

Good RA (1955) Studies of agammaglobulinemia. II. Failure of plasma cell formation in the bone marrow and lymph nodes of patients with agammaglobulinemia, J Lab Clin Med **46**:167

Good RA and Zak SJ (1956) Disturbances in gamma globulin synthesis as "experiments of nature," Pediatrics **18**:109

Good RA et al (1966) The development of the central and peripheral lymphoid tissue: ontogenetic and phylogenetic considerations. In Wolsenholme GEW and Porter R (Eds): The thymus, Boston, Little, Brown and Co, p 181

Good RA et al (1968) The immunologic deficiency diseases of man. In Bergma D and Good RA (Eds): Immunological deficiency in man, Birth Defects **4**:17

Goodheart CR (1965) Molecular virology and cancer, JAMA **194**:48

Goodman JR and Hall SG (1966) Plasma cells containing iron. An electron microscopic study, Blood **28**:83

Goodman JR and Hall SG (1967) Accumulation of iron in mitochondria of erythroblasts, Br J Haematol 13:335

Goodman JR et al (1957) Electron microscopy of formed elements of normal human blood, Blood 12:428

Goodman RM et al (1962) The Ehlers-Danlos syndrome and multiple neurofibromatosis in a kindred of mixed derivation, with special emphasis on hemostasis in the Ehlers-Danlos syndrome, Am J Med 32:976

Goodman A et al (1978) Gingival biopsy in thrombotic thrombocytopenic purpura, Ann Intern Med 89:501

Goodnight SH et al (1979) Circulating factor IX antigen-inhibitor complexes in a hemophilia B⁻ following infusion of a factor IX concentrate, Blood 53:93

Goossens M et al (1975) Hemoglobin C Ziguinchor alpha 2A beta 26 (A3) glu → val beta 58 (E2) pro → arg: the second sickling variant with amino acid substitutions in 2 residues of the beta polypeptide chain, FEBS Lett 58:149

Gordon SG et al (1975) Cancer procoagulant A: a factor X activating procoagulant from malignant tissue, Thromb Res 6:127

Gordon-Smith EC et al (1973) Haemoglobin Nottingham, beta 98 (FG5) val → gly: a new unstable haemoglobin producing severe haemolysis, Proc Roy Soc Med 66:507

Gordon AS et al (1962) Reticulocyte and leukocyte release from isolated perfused rats legs and femurs. In Gordon AS (Ed): Erythropoiesis, New York, Grune & Stratton, Inc

Gordon AS et al (1964a) Plasma and urinary levels of erythropoietin in Cooley's anemia, Ann NY Acad Sci 119:561

Gordon AS et al (1964b) Plasma factors influencing leukocyte release in rats, Ann NY Acad Sci 113:766

Gordon AS et al (1967) The kidney and erythropoiesis, Semin Hematol 4:337

Gordon-Smith IC et al (1974) Postoperative fibrinolytic activity and deep vein thrombosis, Br J Surg 61:213

Gorshein D et al (1974) Rapid stem cell differentiation induced by 19-nortestosterone decanoate, Br J Haematol 26:215

Gothlin GF (1933) Outline of a method for the determination of the strength of the skin capillaries and the indirect estimation of the individual vitamin C standard, J Lab Clin Med 18:484

Gotoff SP (1968) Lymphocytes in congenital immunological deficiency diseases, Clin Exp Immunol 3:843

Gött E and Pexa H (1964) Über andauernde Ausschwemmung von Gaucher-Zellen ins Blut. Zytologie und Zytochemie, Acta Haematol 31:113

Gottlieb AA et al (1967) Studies on macrophage RNA involved in antibody production, Proc Natl Acad Sci USA 57:1849

Gottlieb AJ et al (1964) Hemoglobin J Medillin: chemical and genetic study, Fed Proc 23:172

Gottlieb AJ et al (1967) Primary structure of Hopkins-I haemoglobin, Nature 214:189

Götze O and Müller-Eberhard HG (1972) Paroxysmal nocturnal hemoglobinuria. Hemolysis initiated by the C3 activator system, N Engl J Med 286:180

Götze O and Müller-Eberhard HJ (1976) The alternative pathway of complement activation, Adv Immunol 24:1

Goudemand M et al (1970) L'anomalie de May-Hegglin a propos de sept cas observés dans deux familles, Lille Med 15:1259

Goudsmit R et al (1972) Congenital dyserythropoietic anaemia, type 3, Br J Haematol 23:97

Gough KR et al (1965) Folic acid deficiency in patients after gastric resection, Q J Med 34:1

Goulian M and Beck WS (1966) Modifications in the *Lactobacillus casei* assay of serum folate activity, Am J Clin Pathol 46:390

Gouttas A et al (1955) Description d'une nouvelle variété d'anémie hémolytique congénitale: étude hématologique, électrophorétique et génétique, Sangre 26:911

Gowans JL (1957) The effect of the continuous re-infusion of lymph and lymphocytes on the output of lymphocytes from the thoracic duct of unanaesthetized rats, Br J Exp Pathol 38:67

Gowans JL (1964) The transfusion of lymphocytes in experimental animals. In Stohlman F Jr (Ed): Kinetics of cellular proliferation, New York, Grune & Stratton, Inc

Gowans JL et al (1962) Initiation of immune response by small lymphocytes, Nature 196:651

Goya N et al (1972) A family of congenital atransferremia, Blood 40:239

Graham GS (1918) Benzidine as a peroxidase reagent for blood smears and tissues, J Med Res 39:15

Graham JB (1975) Mode of inheritance and current research. In Brinkhous KM and Hemker HC (Eds): Handbook of hemophilia, New York, American Elsevier Publishing Co, Inc, p 175

Graham JB et al (1957) Stuart clotting defect. II. Genetic aspects of a "new" hemorrhagic state, J Clin Invest 36:497

Graham JB et al (1975) Dominant inheritance of hemophilia A in three generations of women, Blood 46:175

Graham MA and Barr ML (1952) A sex difference in the morphology of metabolic nuclei in somatic cells of the cat, Anat Rec 112:709

Graham RC Jr and Karnovsky MJ (1966) The early stages of absorption of injected horseradish peroxidase in the proximal tubules of mouse kidney. Ultrastructural cytochemistry by a new technique, J Histochem Cytochem 14:291

Graham RC Jr et al (1965a) Cytochemical demonstration of peroxidase activity with 3-amino-9-ethylcarbazole, J Histochem Cytochem 13:150

Graham RC Jr et al (1965b) Pathogenesis of inflammation. II. In vivo observations of the inflammatory effects of activated Haegeman factor and bradykinin, J Exp Med 121:807

Gralnick HR and Bennett JM (1970) Bone-marrow histology in chronic granulocytic leukemia: observations on myelofibrosis and the accelerated phase. In Clarke WJ et al (Eds) Myeloproliferative disorders of animals and man, Washington, DC, US Atomic Energy Commission, p 583

Gralnick HR and Sultan C (1975) Acute promyelocytic leukaemia: haemorrhagic manifestation and morphologic criteria, Br J Haematol 29:373

Gralnick HR et al (1967) Coombs' positive reactions associated with sodium cephalothin therapy, JAMA 199:725

Gralnick HR et al (1971a) Fibrinogen "Bethesda": a congenital dysfibrinogenemia with delayed fibrinopeptide release, J Clin Invest 50:1819

Gralnick HR et al (1971b) Hemolytic anemia associated with cephalothin, JAMA 217:1193

Gralnick HR et al (1973) A new congenital abnormality of human fibrinogen, Fibrinogen Bethesda II, Thromb Diath Haemorrh 29:562

Gralnick HR et al (1975) Studies of the human factor VIII/von Willebrand factor protein. III. Qualitative defects in von Willebrand's disease, J Clin Invest 56:814

Gralnick HR et al (1976) Carbohydrate deficiency of the factor VIII/von Willebrand factor protein in von Willebrand's disease variants, Science 192:56

Gralnick HR et al (1977) Classification of acute leukemia, Ann Intern Med 87:740

Gralnick HR et al (1978) Dysfibrinogenemia associated with hepatoma: increased carbohydrate content of the fibrinogen molecule, N Engl J Med 299:221

Granger GA and Kolb WP (1968) Lymphocyte in vitro cytotoxicity: mechanisms of immune and non-immune small lymphocyte mediated target L cell destruction, J Immunol 101:111

Granger GA and Williams TW (1968) Lymphocyte cytotoxicity in vitro: activation and release of a cytotoxic factor, Nature 218:1253

Granger GA et al (1970) Production of lymphotoxin and migration inhibitory factor by established human lymphocytic cell lines, J Immunol **104**:1476

Granick S (1946) Ferritin. IX. Increase of the protein apoferritin in the gastrointestinal mucosa as a direct response to iron feeding. The function of ferritin in the regulation of iron absorption, J Biol Chem **164**:737

Granick S (1949) Iron metabolism and hemochromatosis, Bull NY Acad Med **25**:403

Granick S and Kappas A (1968) Steroid induction of porphyrin synthesis in liver cell culture. II. The effects of heme, uridine diphosphate glucuronic acid, and inhibitors of nucleic acid and protein synthesis on the induction process, J Biol Chem **243**:346

Grant WC (1956) The influence of anoxia of lactating rats and mice on blood of their normal offspring, Blood **11**:334

Granville N and Dameshek W (1958) Hemochromatosis with megaloblastic anemia responding to folic acid, N Engl J Med **258**:586

Gräsbeck R et al (1960) Selective vitamin B_{12} malabsorption and proteinuria in young people, Acta Med Scand **167**:289

Graw RG Jr and Appelbaum FR (1977) Granulocyte transfusion therapy—a review of the practical aspects of collection and transfusion techniques, Exp Hematol (Suppl) **5**:39

Graw RG Jr et al (1977) National donor registry and computer transfusion programs for platelet transfusions, Transplant Proc (Suppl 1) **9**:225

Graziano JH et al (1978) Chelation therapy in β-thalassemia major. I. Intravenous and subcutaneous deferoxamine, J Pediatr **92**:648

Greally J et al (1973) Lymphocyte transformation in malignant lymphoma, Isr J Med Sci **142**:255

Greaves MF et al (1972) Lymphocyte activation. 3. Binding sites for phytomitogens on lymphocyte subpopulations, Clin Exp Immunol **10**:537

Greaves MF et al (1975) Antisera to acute lymphoblastic leukemia cells, Clin Immunol Immunopathol **4**:67

Green D and Potter EV (1976) Failure of AHF concentrate to control bleeding in von Willebrand's disease, Am J Med **60**:357

Green D et al (1971) Thrombocytopenia in Gaucher's disease, Ann Intern Med **74**:727

Green D et al (1972) The role of heparin in the management of consumption coagulopathy, Med Clin North Am **56**:193

Green R et al (1968) Body iron excretion in man: a collaborative study, Am J Med **45**:336

Green RL et al (1971) The sickle-cell and altitude, Br Med J **4**:593

Green D and Philip KJ (1980) Variant von Willebrand's disease: a study emphasizing crossed-immunoelectrophoresis, Thromb Haemost **43**:2

Greenberg MS and Grace ND (1970) Folic acid deficiency and iron overload, Arch Intern Med **125**:140

Greendyke RM et al (1965) Studies of the effects of administration of ACTH and adrenal corticosteroids on erythrophagocytosis, J Clin Invest **44**:746

Greene DA (1975) Localized cervical lymphadenopathy induced by diphenylhydantoin sodium, Arch Otolaryngol **10**:446

Greenwalt TJ et al (1954) An allele of the S(s) blood group genes, Proc Natl Acad Sci USA **40**:1126

Greenwalt TJ and Jamieson GA (1975) Transmissible disease and blood transfusion, New York, Grune & Stratton, Inc

Greenwalt TJ et al (Eds) (1977) General principles of blood transfusion, Chicago, American Medical Association

Gregory CH and Watson CJ (1962) Studies of conjugated bilirubin. II. Problems of sulfates of bilirubin in vivo and in vitro, J Lab Clin Med **60**:17

Greipp PR and Gralnick HR (1976) Platelet to leukocyte adherence phenomena associated with thrombocytopenia, Blood **47**:513

Grenet P et al (1967) Thrombopénies neo-natales par isoimmunisation contre des antigènes leucoplaquettaires, Nouv Rev Fr Hematol **7**:663

Greppi E (1928) Ittero emolitico familiare con aumento della resistenza dei globuli, Minerva Med **8**:1

Grey NM et al (1968) Subclass of human γ A globulin (γ A_2) which lacks the disulfide bonds linking heavy and light chains, J Exp Med **128**:1223

Griffin JH and Cochrane CG (1976) Mechanism for the involvement of high molecular weight kininogen in surface dependent reactions of Hageman factor, Proc Natl Acad Sci USA **73**:2554

Griffin JH and Bouma BN (1980) Blood coagulation factor XI. In Schmidt RM (Section Ed): Handbook Series in Clinical Laboratory Science, Section I: Hematology, vol 3, Boca Raton, Fla, CRC Press, Inc p 109

Griffiths KD et al (1977) Haemoglobin Handsworth alpha 18 (A16) glycine → arginine, FEBS Lett **75**:93

Grifoni V et al (1975) A new hb variant: Hb F Sardinia $γ^{75}$ (E19) isoleucine → threonine found in a family with Hb G Philadelphia, β-chain deficiency and a Lepore-like haemoglobin indistinguishable from Hb A_2, Acta Haematol **53**:347

Griggs RC (1964) Lead poisoning: hematologic aspects. In Moore CV and Brown EB (Eds): Progress in hematology, vol 4, New York, Grune & Stratton, Inc

Grignaschi VJ et al (1963) A new cytochemical picture: spontaneous negativity of the peroxidase, oxidase, and lipid reactions in the neutrophil progeny and in the monocytes of 2 siblings, Rev Assoc Med Argent **77**:218

Grimes AJ et al (1968) The autohaemolysis test: appraisal of the method for the diagnosis of pyruvate kinase deficiency and the effect of pH and additives, Br J Haematol **14**:309

Griner PF and Hoyer LW (1970) Amegakaryocytic thrombocytopenia in systemic lupus erythematosus, Arch Intern Med **125**:328

Griner PF and Oranburg PR (1978) Predictive values of erythrocyte indices for tests of iron, folic acid, and vitamin B_{12} deficiency, Am J Clin Pathol **70**:748

Groover RV et al (1972) The genetic mucopolysaccharidoses, Semin Hematol **9**:371

Gross L (1951) "Spontaneous" leukemia developing in C_3H mice following inoculation, in infancy, with AK-leukemic extracts, or AK-embryos, Proc Soc Exp Biol Med **76**:27

Gross M and Goldwasser E (1971) On the mechanism of erythropoietin-induced differentiation. IX. Induced synthesis of 9S ribonucleic acid and of hemoglobin, J Biol Chem **246**:2480

Gross S and Melhorn DK (1971) Exchange transfusion with citrated whole blood for disseminated intravascular coagulation, J Pediatr **78**:415

Gross S et al (1964) The platelets in iron-deficiency anemia. I. The response to oral and parental iron, Pediatrics **34**:315

Gross S et al (1965) Electron microscopy of the red cells in erythropoietic porphyria, Blood **25**:49

Gross DM et al (1976) Effects of prostaglandins A_2, E_2 and $F_{2α}$ on erythropoietin production, J Pharmacol Exp Ther **198**:489

Grossman J et al (1972) Crystal-globulinemia, Ann Intern Med **77**:395

Grossman MI et al (1961) Fecal blood loss produced by oral and intravenous administration of various salicylates, Gastroenterology **40**:383

Grossowicz N et al (1962) Microbiologic determination of folic acid derivatives in blood, Blood **20**:609

Grove-Rasmussen M et al (1952) A new blood subgroup (A_0) identifiable with group O serums, Am J Clin Pathol **22**:1157

Gruber DF et al (1977) Temporal transition in the site of rat erythropoietin production, Exp Hematol **5**:399

Gruenberg JC et al (1975) Inherited antithrombin III deficiency causing mesenteric venous infarction: a new clinical entity, Ann Surg **181**:791

Grumet FC and Yankee RA (1974) Non-red cell reactions. In New approaches to transfusion reactions, Washington DC, American Association of Blood Banks, p 39

Grzesinkowicz H et al (1965) Enzymatic release of folate activity from red cells in megaloblastic anaemia of pregnancy, J Clin Pathol **18**:599

Guasch J (1954) Hérédité des leucémies, Sang **25**:384

Gubler CJ (1956) Copper metabolism in man, JAMA **161**:530

Gubler CJ et al (1957) Studies on copper metabolism. XXIII. Portal (Laennec's) cirrhosis of the liver, J Clin Invest **36**:1208

Guccione MA et al (1971) Reactions of ^{14}C-ADP and ^{14}C-ATP with washed platelets from rabbits, Blood **37**:542

Guerry D et al (1974) Human cyclic neutropenia: urinary colony-stimulating factor and erythropoietin levels, Blood **44**:257

Gugler E and Lüscher EF (1963) Die kongenitale Afibrinogenämie, Ann Pediatr **200**:125

Guibaud P et al (1978) La forme infantile de la maladie de Gaucher étude clinique et biologigue d'une observation, Arch Fr Pédiatr **35**:949

Gulliani GL et al (1976) Blood recalcification time. A simple and reliable test to monitor heparin therapy, Am J Clin Pathol **65**:390

Gunnells JC Jr and Grim CE (1967) Hematuria and A-D hemoglobinopathy, Arch Intern Med **120**:337

Gunson HH and Donohue WL (1957) Multiple examples of the blood genotype (C^WD—/C^WD—) in a Canadian family, Vox Sang **2**:320

Gunz FW (1960) Hemorrhagic thrombocythemia: a critical review, Blood **15**:706

Gunz FW and Baikie AG (1974) Leukemia, New York, Grune & Stratton, Inc.

Gunz FW and Hough RF (1956) Acute leukemia over the age of fifty. A study of its incidence and history, Blood **11**:882

Gunz FW et al (1978) Thirteen cases of leukemia in a family, J Natl Cancer Inst **60**:1243

Gupta S and Good RA (1978) Immunodeficiencies associated with chronic lymphocytic leukemia and non-Hodgkin's lymphoma. In Twomey JJ and Good RA (Eds): The immunopathology of lymphoreticular neoplasms, New York, Plenum Press, pp 565-583

Gupta S and Good RA (1980) Markers of human lymphocyte subpopulations in primary immunodeficiency and lymphoproliferative disorders, Semin Hematol **17**:1

Gurewich V et al (1978) Hemostatic effects of uniform, low-dose subcutaneous heparin in surgical patients, Arch Intern Med **138**:41

Gurney CW et al (1965) Quantitation of the erythropoietic stimulus produced by hypoxia in the plethoric mouse, Acta Haematol **33**:246

Gustafson GT and Pihl E (1967) Histochemical application of ruthenium red in the study of mast cell ultrastructure, Acta Pathol Microbiol Scan **69**:393

Gutniak O et al (1971) Porphyrin biosynthesis in the erythrocytes of patients with sideropenic anaemias, J Clin Pathol **24**:336

Guzzo J et al (1980) Secreted platelet proteins with antiheparin and mitogenic activities in chronic renal failure, J Lab Clin Med **96**:102

Gynn TN et al (1972) Drug-induced thromboctopenia, Med Clin North Am **56**:65

Gyorkey F et al (1967) The fine structure of ceroid in human atheroma, J Histochem Cytochem **15**:732

Haak HL et al (1977a) Acquired aplastic anaemia in adults. I. A retrospective analysis of 40 cases: single factors influencing the prognosis, Acta Haematol **58**:257

Haak HL et al (1977b) Acquired aplastic anaemia in adults. IV. Histological and CFU studies in transplanted and non-transplanted patients, Scand J Haematol **19**:159

Hachiya M (1955) Hiroshima diary, Chapel Hill, University of North Carolina Press

Hadeishi T et al (1975) Type C RNA tumor virus isolated from cultured human acute myelogenous leukemia cells, Science **187**:350

Haden HT (1967) Pyridoxine-responsive sideroblastic anemia due to antituberculous drugs, Arch Intern Med **120**:602

Hadley GG and Weiss SP (1955) Further notes on use of salts of ethylenediamine tetraacetic acid (EDTA) as anticoagulant, Am J Clin Pathol **25**:1090

Haeger B (1958) Urinary δ-aminolaevulinic acid and porphobilinogen in different types of porphyria, Lancet **2**:606

Haeger-Aronsen B (1962) Fecal porphyrins in porphyria acute intermittens, porphyria cutanea tarda and intoxicatio plumbi, Scand J Clin Lab Invest **14**:397

Haegert DG et al (1975) Acute lymphoblastic leukaemia: a heterogenous disease, Br Med J **1**:312

Hahn EV and Gillespie EB (1927) Sickle cell anemia, Arch Intern Med **39**:233

Haim N et al (1977) Spontaneous and stimulated nitroblue tetrazolium tests of leukocytes from patients with solid malignant tumors, Am J Clin Pathol **68**:570

Haim N et al (1978) Comparative study of the endotoxin-stimulated nitroblue tetrazolium test in disease and health, J Clin Pathol (London) **31**:1249

Hajdu SI and Melamed MR (1973) The diagnostic value of aspiration smears, Am J Clin Pathol **59**:350

Hakami N et al (1971) Neonatal megaloblastic anemia due to inherited transcobalamin II deficiency in two siblings, N Engl J Med **285**:1163

Halbrecht I et al (1967) Hemoglobin Hasharon (alpha 47 aspartic acid → histidine), Israel J Med Sci **3**:827

Hall CA (1965) Gaisböck's disease: redefinition of an old syndrome, Arch Intern Med **116**:4

Hall CA (1971) Vitamin B_{12}-binding proteins of man, Ann Intern Med **75**:297

Hall CA (1979) The transport of vitamin B_{12} from food to use within the cells, J Lab Clin Med **94**:811

Hall CA and Begley JA (1977) Congenital deficiency of human R-type binding proteins of cobalamin, Am J Hum Genet **29**:619

Hall CA and Finkler AE (1966) Measurement of the amounts of the individual vitamin B_{12} binding proteins in plasma. II. Abnormalities in leukemia and pernicious anemia, Blood **27**:618

Hall CA and Finkler AE (1969) Vitamin B_{12}-binding protein in polycythemia vera plasma, J Lab Clin Med **73**:60

Hall CA et al (1975) Hereditary factor VII and IX deficiencies in a large kindred, Br J Haematol **29**:319

Hall R and Losowsky MS (1966) The distribution of erythroblast iron in sideroblastic anemias, Br J Haematol **12**:334

Hallberg L et al (1966) Menstrual blood loss and iron deficiency, Acta Med Scand **180**:639

Halliday JW et al (1977) Serum ferritin in haemochromatosis: changes in the isoferritin composition during venesection therapy, Br J Haematol **36**:395

Halsted CH et al (1971) Decreased jejunal uptake of labeled folic acid (^{3}H-PGA) in alcoholic patients: roles of alcohol and nutrition, N Engl J Med **285**:701

Halsted CH et al (1973) Intestinal malabsorption in folate-deficient alcoholics, Gastroenterology **64**:526

Halsted JA (1959) Serum and tissue concentration of vitamin B_{12} in certain pathologic states, N Engl J Med **260**:575

Halsted JA (1968) Geophagia in man: its nature and nutritional effects, Am J Clin Nutr **21**:1384

Halvorsen K (1965) Neonatal leucopenia due to fetomaternal leucocyte incompatibility, Acta Paediatr Scand **54**:86

Halvorsen S (1966) The central nervous system in regulation of erythropoiesis, Acta Haematol **35**:65

Halvorsen S (1974) Inhibitors of erythropoiesis, Scand J Clin Lab Invest **34**:193

Ham TH (1939) Studies on the destruction of red blood cells. I. Chronic hemolytic anemia with paroxysmal nocturnal hemoglobinuria: an investigation of the mechanism of hemolysis, with observations on five cases, Arch Intern Med **64**:1271

Ham TH (1950) A syllabus of laboratory examinations in clinical diagnosis, Cambridge, Harvard University Press

Hamberg M and Samuelsson B (1974) Prostaglandin endoperoxidases. Novel transformations of arachidonic acid in human platelets, Proc Nat Acad Sci USA **71**:3400

Hamilton HE et al (1958) Studies with inagglutinable erythrocyte counts. VII. Further investigation of the hemolytic mechanism in untreated pernicious anemia and the demonstration of a hemolytic property in the plasma, J Lab Clin Med **51**:942

Hamilton HH et al (1969) Hemoglobin Hiroshima (beta 143 histidine → aspartic acid): a newly identified fast moving beta chain variant associated with increased oxygen affinity and compensatory erythremia (Personal communication, P Heller), J Clin Invest **48**:525

Hamilton JB et al (1964) Effect on castration in man upon blood sedimentation rate, hematocrit, and hemoglobin, J Clin Endocrinol **24**:506

Hamilton RW et al (1971) Acquired hemoglobin H disease. N Engl J Med **285**:1217

Hammar JA (1921) The new views as to the morphology of the thymus gland and their bearing on the problem of the function of the thymus, Endocrinology **5**:543, 731

Hammarström S et al (1973) A new surface marker on T lymphocytes of human peripheral blood, J Exp Med **138**:1270

Hammond D et al (1968) Production, utilization, and excretion of erythropoietin. I. Chronic anemia. II. Aplastic crisis. III. Erythropoietic effects of normal plasma, Ann NY Acad Sci **149**:516

Hammond E et al (1969) Ultrastructural characteristics of siderocytes in swine, Lab Invest **21**:292

Hammond KB (1980) Blood specimen collection from infants by skin puncture, Lab Med **11**:9

Hampson JL et al (1955) The syndrome of gonadal agenesis (ovarian agenesis) and male chromosomal patterns in girls and women: psychologic studies, Johns Hopkins Med J **97**:207

Hampson WGJ et al (1974) Failure of low-dose heparin to prevent deep-vein thrombosis after hip-replacement arthroplasty, Lancet **2**:795

Hampton JW (1968) Qualitative fibrinogen defect associated with abnormal fibrin stabilization, J Lab Clin Med **72**:882

Hampton ML (1974) Sickle cell "nondisease," Am J Dis Child **128**:58

Han P and Ardlie NG (1974) The influence of pH, temperature, and calcium on platelet aggregation: maintenance of environmental pH and platelet function for in vitro studies in plasma stored at 37° C, Br J Haematol **26**:373

Han T and Takita H (1972) Immunologic impairment in bronchogenic carcinoma: a study of lymphocyte response to phytohemagglutinin, Cancer **30**:616

Hancock DE et al (1976) Transferrin loss into the urine with hypochromic, microcytic anemia, Am J Clin Pathol **65**:73

Handin RI and Valeri CR (1971) Hemostatic effectiveness of platelets stored at 22° C, N Engl J Med **285**:538

Handin RI et al (1976) Antibody-induced von Willebrand's disease: a newly defined inhibitor syndrome, Blood **48**:393

Handley DA and Lawrence JR (1967) Factor-IX deficiency in the nephrotic syndrome, Lancet **1**:1079

Hanford RB et al (1960) Massive thoracic extramedullary hemopoiesis, N Engl J Med **263**:120

Hanker JS et al (1978) The light microscopic demonstration of hydroperoxidase-positive Phi bodies and rods in leukocytes in acute myeloid leukemia, Histochemistry **58**:241

Hanker JS et al (1979) Facilitated light microscopic cytochemical diagnosis of acute myelogenous leukemia, Cancer Res **39**:1635

Hanks GE et al (1960) Further modification of the benzidine method for measurement of hemoglobin in plasma: definition of a new range of normal values, J Lab Clin Med **56**:486

Hanrahan JB et al (1963) Factitious hypoglycemia in patients with leukemia, Am J Clin Pathol **40**:43

Hansen HA et al (1960) Studies on an abnormal hemoglobin causing hereditary congenital cyanosis, Acta Paediatr **49**:503

Hansen HA and Weinfeld A (1962) Metabolic effects and diagnostic value of small doses of folic acid and B_{12} in megaloblastic anemias, Acta Med Scand **172**:427

Hansen MS et al (1980) Fibrinogen Cophenhagen: an abnormal fibrinogen with defective polymerization and release of fibrinopeptide A, but normal absorption of plasminogen, Scand J Clin Lab Invest **40**:221

Hanzlick RL and Senhauser DA (1979) Subclinical hemolytic disease of the newborn due to anti-e, Am J Clin Pathol **72**:76

Haque AU et al (1980) Postsplenectomy pneumococcemia in adults, Arch Pathol Lab Med **104**:258

Harada K and Zucker MB (1971) Simultaneous development of platelet factor 4 activity and release of ^{14}C-serotonin, Thromb Diath Haemorrh **25**:41

Harber LC et al (1964) Erythropoietic protoporphyria and photohemolysis, JAMA **189**:191

Hardisty RM and Hutton RA (1967) Bleeding tendency associated with "new" abnormality of platelet behaviour, Lancet **1**:983

Hardisty RM and Ingram GC (1965) Bleeding disorders, investigation and management, Oxford, Blackwell Scientific Publications, Ltd

Hardisty RM et al (1964) Granulocytic leukaemia in childhood, Br J Haematol **10**:551

Hardisty RM et al (1972) The platelet defect associated with albinism, Br J Haematol **23**:679

Hardy JB (1971) Cord serum immunoglobulin levels and long-range fetal outcome, Johns Hopkins Med J **128**:297

Hardy WR and Anderson RE (1968) The hypereosinophilic syndromes, Ann Intern Med **68**:1220

Hare FW Jr and Miller AJ (1951) Capillary resistance tests, Arch Dermatol Syph **64**:449

Hargraves MM (1969) The discovery of the L.E. cell and its morphology, Mayo Clin Proc **44**:579

Hargraves MM et al (1948) Presentation of two bone marrow elements: the "Tart" cell and the "L.E." cell, Proc Staff Meet Mayo Clin **23**:25

Harigaya K et al (1977) Multiple bone marrow necrosis and disseminated intravascular coagulation, Arch Pathol Lab Med **101**:652

Harker LA (1970) Thrombokinetics in idiopathic thrombocytopenic purpura, Br J Haematol **19**:95

Harker LA and Finch CA (1969) Thrombokinetics in man, J Clin Invest **48**:983

Harker LA and Slichter SJ (1970) Studies of platelet and fibrinogen kinetics in patients with prosthetic heart valves, N Engl J Med **283**:1302

Harker LA and Slichter SJ (1972a) The bleeding time as a screening test for evaluation of platelet function, N Engl J Med **287**:155

Harker LA and Slichter SJ (1972b) Platelet and fibrinogen consumption in man, N Engl J Med **287**:999

Harker LA and Slichter SJ (1974) Arterial and venous thromboembolism: kinetic characterization and evaluation of therapy, Thromb Diath Haemorrh **31**:188

Harkness DR (1971) The regulation of hemoglobin oxygenation, Adv Intern Med **17**:189

Harm H (1953) Beeinflussung des weissen Blutbildes von Pelger- und Nicht-Pelger-Kaninchen durch Colchicin, Acta Haematol **10**:95

Harm H (1955) Zur Klassifizerung und Vererbung der Neutrophil-in-Kernform bei Mensch und Kaninchen, Blut **1**:3

Harpel PC and Rosenberg RD (1976) α_2-Macroglobulin and antithrombin-heparin cofactor: Modulators of hemostatic and inflammatory reactions, Prog Hemost Thromb **3**:145

Harrington WJ et al (1951) Demonstration of a thrombocytopenic factor in the blood of patients with thrombocytopenic purpura, J Lab Clin Med **38**:1

Harrington WJ et al (1953) Immunologic mechanisms in idiopathic and neonatal thrombocytopenic purpura, Ann Intern Med **38**:433

Harrington WJ et al (1956) The autoimmune thrombocytopenias, Prog Hematol **1**:166

Harris J et al (1971) Immune function in multiple myeloma: impaired responsiveness to keyhole limpet hemocyanin, Can Med Assoc J **104**:389

Harris JW (1963) The red cell: production, metabolism, destruction: normal and abnormal, Cambridge, Harvard University Press

Harris JW (1964) Notes and comments on pyridoxine-responsive anemia and the role of erythrocyte mitochondria in iron metabolism, Medicine **43**:803

Harris PF and Templeton WR (1968) Studies on the extrinsic lymphatic drainage of the guinea-pig thymus, Acta Anat (Basel) **69**:366

Harris TE (1959) A mathematical model for multiplication by fission. In Stohlman F Jr (Ed): Kinetics of cellular proliferation, New York, Grune & Stratton, Inc

Harris TN et al (1957) Paradoxical values of the erythrocyte sedimentation rate in rheumatic fever: a comparison among three acute phase tests, Am J Med Sci **234**:259

Harrison PM (1977) Ferritin: an iron-storage molecule, Semin Hematol **14**:55

Harrison RJ (1966) An unusual cause of leucocytosis, Br J Clin Pract **20**:319

Hart RJ and McCurdy PR (1971) Pernicious anemia in Negroes, Ann Intern Med **74**:448

Hartmann RC and Jenkins DE Jr (1966) The "sugar water" test for paroxysmal nocturnal hemoglobinuria, N Engl J Med **275**:155

Hartmann RC and Kolhouse JF (1972) Viewpoints on the management of paroxysmal nocturnal hemoglobinuria (PHN), Ser Haematol **5**:42

Hartmann RC et al (1958) Studies on thrombocytosis. I. Hyperkalemia due to release of potassium from platelets during coagulation, J Clin Invest **37**:699

Hartmann RC et al (1970) Diagnostic specificity of sucrose hemolysis test for paroxysmal nocturnal hemoglobinuria, Blood **35**:462

Hartmann RC et al (1980) Fulminant hepatic venous thrombosis (Budd-Chiari syndrome) in paroxysmal nocturnal hemoglobinuria: definition of a medical emergency, Johns Hopkins Med J **146**:247

Hartroft WS and Porta EA (1965) Ceroid, Am J Med Sci **250**:324

Hartsock RJ (1968) Postvaccinial lymphadenitis. Hyperplasia of lymphoid tissue that simulates malignant lymphomas, Cancer **21**:632

Hartsock RJ et al (1965) Normal variations with aging of the amount of hematopoietic tissue in bone marrow from the anterior iliac crest, Am J Clin Pathol **43**:326

Hartz JW and Deutsch HF (1969) Preparation and physiochemical properties of human erythrocuprein, J Biol Chem **224**:4565

Hathaway WE and Alsever J (1970) The relation of "Fletcher Factor" to factors XI and XII, Br J Haematol **18**:161

Hathaway WE et al (1965) Evidence for a new plasma thromboplastin factor. I. Case report, coagulation studies, and physiochemical properties, Blood **26**:521

Hathaway WE et al (1973) Paradoxical bleeding in intensively transfused hemophiliacs: alteration of platelet function, Transfusion **13**:6

Hattersley PG (1964) Macrocytosis of the erythrocytes, JAMA **189**:997

Hattersley PG and Hayse D (1970) Fletcher factor disease: a report of three unrelated cases, Br J Haematol **18**:411

Hattersley PG and Hayse D (1976) The effect of increased contact activation time on the activated partial thromboplastin time, Am J Clin Pathol **66**:479

Hattersley PG et al (1971a) Cold agglutinins and the model S, Lab Med **2**:33

Hattersley PG et al (1971b) Erroneous values on the model S Coulter counter due to high titer cold agglutinins, Am J Clin Pathol **55**:442

Haugen RK (1979) Hepatitis after the transfusion of frozen red cells and washed red cells, N Engl J Med **301**:393

Haupt VH (1965) Factor-X-Verwinderung bei Thrombopenien im Kindesalter, Helv Paediatr Acta **20**:40

Haurani FI et al (1965) Iron absorption in hypoferremia, Am J Med Sci **249**:537

Haurani FI et al (1979) Megaloblastic anemia as a result of an abnormal transcobalamin II (Cardeza), J Clin Invest **64**:1253

Haurowitz F (1970) The molecular basis of immunity, Ann NY Acad Sci **169**:11

Hause LL et al (1978) Relations between surface charge and in vitro lysis of red blood cells in paroxysmal nocturnal haemoglobinuria, Scand J Haematol **20**:141

Hawk P et al (1949) Practical physiological chemistry, Philadelphia, The Blakiston Co

Hawkey CM and Jordan P (1967) Sickle-cell erythrocytes in the mongoose, *Herpestes sanguineus,* Trans R Soc Trop Med Hyg **61**:180

Hayashi A et al (1971) Haemoglobin Rainier: β145(HC2) tyrosine → cysteine and haemoglobin Bethesda: β145(HC2) tyrosine → histidine, Nature (New Biol) **230**:264

Hayes DM and Feltz JH (1964) Sulfonamide methemoglobulinemia and hemolytic anemia during renal failure, Am J Med Sci **247**:552

Hayhoe FGJ and Flemans RJ (1970) An atlas of haematological cytology, New York, Wiley-Interscience

Hayhoe FGJ et al (1964) The cytology and cytochemistry of acute leukaemias. A study of 140 cases, London, Her Majesty's Stationery Office

Haynes RH (1960) Physical basis of the dependence of blood viscosity on the tube radius, Am J Physiol **198**:1193

Haynes RH (1962) The viscosity of erythrocyte suspensions: a review of theory, Biophys **2**:95

Haynes RL and Dunn JM (1967) Oral contraceptives, thrombosis, and sickle cell hemoglobinopathies, JAMA **200**:994

Haynes PJ et al (1977) Measurement of menstrual blood loss in patients complaining of menorrhagia, Br J Obstet Gynaecol **84**:763

Hays EF and Craddook CG (1978) Colony-stimulating activity, Arch Pathol Lab Med **102**:165

Heathcote J et al (1974) Hepatitis B antigen in saliva and semen, Lancet **1**:71

Hebbel RP et al (1980) Abnormal adherence of sickle erythrocytes to cultured vascular endothelium: possible mechanism for microvascular occlusion in sickle cell disease, J Clin Invest **65**:154

Hecht HH (1971) A sea level view of altitude problems, Am J Med **50**:703

Hecht HH and Samuels AJ (1952) Observations on oxygen content of sternal bone marrow with reference to polycythemic states, Fed Proc **11**:68

Heckner F (1948) Toxisch-reaktive Kernveranderungen der Leukozyten (Pseudopelger), Dtsch Med Wochenschr **73**:47

Heddle SB et al (1969) Diffuse eosinophilic gastroenteritis, Can Med Assoc J **100**:554

Hedlund S (1953) Studies on erythropoiesis and total red cell volume in congestive heart failure, Acta Med Scand **146**(supp 284):1

Hedner U et al (1975) Factor XIII in a clinical material, Scand J Haematol **14**:114

Hegglin R (1945) Gleichzeitige konstitutionelle Veränderungen an Neutrophilen und Thrombozyten, Helv Med Acta **12**:439

Hegsted DM et al (1949) The influence of diet on iron absorption. II. The interrelation of iron and phosphorus, J Exp Med **90**:147

Hehlmann R et al (1973) Molecular evidence for a viral etiology of human leukemias, lymphomas, and sarcomas, Am J Clin Pathol **60**:65

Heilmeyer L (1942) Handbuch innere Medizin, vol 2, Berlin, Julius Springer-Verlag

Heilmeyer L and Begemann H (1955) Atlas der klinischen Hämatologie und Cytologie, Berlin, Julius Springer-Verlag

Heilmeyer L et al (1961) Kongenitale Atransferrinämie bei einem siebenjähre-alten Kind, Dtsch Med Wochenschr **86**:1745

Heilmeyer L and Clotten R (1964) Die kongenitale erythropoietische Coproporphyrie: eine dritte erythropoetische Porphyrieform, Dtsch Med Wochnschr **89**:649

Heimpel H and Wendt F (1968) Congenital dyserythropoietic anemia with karyorrhexis and multinuclearity of erythroblasts, Helv Med Acta **34**:103

Heinrich HC (1964) Metabolic basis of the diagnosis and therapy of vitamin B_{12} deficiency, Semin Hematol **1**:199

Heinrich HC et al (1973) Absorption of inorganic and food iron in children with heterozygous and homozygous β-thalassemia, z Kinderheilkd **115**:1

Hellem AJ (1968) Platelet adhesiveness, Ser Haematol **1**:99

Heller P and Zimmerman HJ (1956) Nucleophagocytosis: studies on three hundred thirty-six patients: review of incidence of L.E. phenomenon and allied conditions, Arch Intern Med **97**:403

Heller P et al (1960) Enzymes in anemia: a study of abnormalities of several enzymes of carbohydrate metabolism in the plasma and erythrocytes in patients with anemia, with preliminary observations of bone marrow enzymes, Ann Intern Med **53**:898

Heller P et al (1962) Hemoglobin M Kankakee, a new variant of hemoglobin M, Blood **20**:287

Heller P et al (1963) Variation in the amount of hemoglobin S in a patient with sickle-cell trait and megaloblastic anemia, Blood **21**:479

Heller P et al (1966) Hemoglobin M Hyde Park: a new variant of abnormal methemoglobin, J Clin Invest **45**:1021

Heller VG and Paul H (1934) Changes in cell volume produced by varying concentrations of different anticoagulants, J Lab Clin Med **19**:777

Hellström KE et al (1969) Abrogation of cellular immunity to antigenically foreign mouse embryonic cells by a serum factor, Nature **224**:914

Hellum KB and Solberg CO (1977) Human leucocyte migration: studies with an improved skin chamber technique, Acta Pathol Microbiol Scand Sect C **85**:413

Helmly RB et al (1967) Quinine-induced purpura, Arch Intern Med **120**:59

Hemker HC (1975) Interaction of coagulation factors. In Brinkhous KM and Kemker HC (Eds): Handbook of hemophilia, New York, American Elsevier Publishing Co, Inc

Hemker HC and Kahn MJ (1967) Reaction sequence of blood coagulation, Nature **215**:1201

Hemker HC et al (1963) Nature of prothrombin biosynthesis: preprothrombinaemia in vitamin K-deficiency, Nature **200**:589

Hempelmann LH et al (1975) Neoplasms in persons treated with x-rays in infancy: fourth survey in 20 years, J Natl Cancer Inst **55**:519

Hemphill BM (1977) Blood collection and use by AABB institutional members (1975), Transfusion **17**:403

Henderson PH Jr (1955) Multiple migratory thrombophlebitis associated with ovarian carcinoma, Am J Obstet Gynec **70**:452

Henderson AB et al (1961) Sickle cell disease variants and pregnancy: a pathophysiologic report, N Engl J Med **264**:1276

Henderson F et al (1963) Desferrioxamine in the treatment of acute toxic reaction to ferrous gluconate, JAMA **186**:1139

Henle G et al (1968) Relation of Burkitt's tumor-associated herpes-type virus to infectious mononucleosis, Proc Natl Acad Sci **59**:94

Hennessy TG et al (1967) Cerebellar hemangioblastoma: erythropoietic activity by radioiron assay, J Nucl Med **8**:601

Henry P et al (1967) Characteristics of the RNA synthesized in vitro by lymphocytes of chronic lymphocytic leukemia, J Lab Clin Med **69**:47

Henry RJ (1968) Clinical chemistry: principles and techniques, New York, Hoeber Medical Division, Harper & Row, Publishers, p 748

Henry JB and Hubbel RC (1980) Blood policy and strategy: the American Blood Commission and the nation's blood resource, Hum Pathol **11**:1

Henson PM (1969) The adherence of leukocytes and platelets induced by fixed IgG antibody of complement, Immunology **16**:107

Herbert V (1959) Mechanism of intrinsic factor action in everted sacs of rat small intestine, J Clin Invest **38**:102

Herbert V (1962) Minimal daily adult folate requirement, Arch Intern Med **110**:649

Herbert V (1963) A palatable diet for producing experimental folate deficiency in man, Am J Clin Nutr **12**:17

Herbert V (1968) Diagnostic and prognostic values of measurement of serum vitamin B_{12}-binding proteins, Blood **32**:305

Herbert V and Jacob E (1974) Destruction of vitamin B_{12} by ascorbic acid, JAMA **230**:241

Herbert V and Zalusky R (1962) Interrelations of vitamin B_{12} and folic acid metabolism: folic acid clearance studies, J Clin Invest **41**:1263

Herbert V et al (1960) The measurement of folic acid activity in serum: a diagnostic aid in the differentiation of megaloblastic anemias, Blood **15**:228

Herbert V et al (1963) Correlation of folate deficiency with alcoholism and associated macrocytosis, anemia, and liver disease, Ann Intern Med **58**:977

Herbert V et al (1973) The du suppression test using ^{125}I-UdR to define biochemical megaloblastosis, Br J Haematol **24**:713

Herbert PN et al (1978) Familial lipoprotein deficiency. In Stanbury JB et al, (Eds): The metabolic basis of inherited disease, ed 4, New York, McGraw-Hill Book Co, Inc, p 544

Herman SP et al (1978) Neutrophil products that inhibit cell proliferation: relation to granulocytic "chalone", Blood 51:207

Hermans PE et al (1966) Dysgammaglobulinemia associated with nodular lymphoid hyperplasia of the small intestine, Am J Med 40:78

Herrick JB (1910) Peculiar elongated and sickle-shaped red blood corpuscles in a case of severe anemia, Arch Intern Med 6:517

Hers HG and Van Hoof (1973) Lysosomes and storage diseases, New York, Academic Press, Inc

Hershberg PI et al (1972) Hematocrit and prognosis in patients with acute myocardial infarction, JAMA 219:855

Hershgold EJ et al (1966) The potent antihemophilic globulin concentrate derived from a cold insoluble fraction of human plasma: characterization and further data on preparation and clinical trail, J Lab Clin Med 67:23

Hershgold EJ et al (1971) Isolation and some chemical properties of human factor VIII (antihemophilic factor), J Lab Clin Med 77:185

Hershko C et al (1974) Storage iron kinetics. VI. The effect of inflammation on iron exchange in the rat, Br J Haematol 28:67

Hertzog AJ (1938) The phagocytic activity of human leukocytes with special reference to their type and maturity, Am J Pathol 14:595

Herzberg JJ (1968) Purpura télangiectasique arciforme (Touraine): purpura angioscléreux (Gaucher); purpura bei Dermatite lichénoide purpurique et pigmentée (Schamberg, Gougerot-Blum), Thromb Diath Haemorrh (supp) 30:237

Heserick JR (1956) Evaluation of three diagnostic procedures for systemic lupus erythematosus, Ann Intern Med 44:497

Hess CE et al (1976) Mechanism of dilutional anemia in massive splenomegaly, Blood 47:629

Hess M and Hilschmann N (1971) Genetischer polymorphismus im konstanten Teil von humanen Immunoglobulin-L-Ketten vom λ-Typ. II. Hoppe Seylers Z Physiol Chem 352:657

Hewetson JF et al (1973) Neutralizing antibodies to Epstein-Barr virus in healthy populations and patients with infectious mononucleosis, J Infect Dis 128:283

Heyn RM et al (1973) Lymphocyte size distribution. Determination in normal children and adults and in patients with immunodeficiency states, Am J Dis Child 125:789

Heyns A Du P et al (1979) Thrombotic thrombocytopenic purpura: a case investigated with ^{111}In-oxine-labelled platelets, S Afr Med J 56:229

Heyssel RM et al (1966) Vitamin B_{12} turnover in man. The assimilation of vitamin B_{12} from natural foodstuffs by man and estimates of minimal daily dietary requirements, Am J Clin Nutr 18:176

Hibbard BZ Jr et al (1978) Severe methemoglobinemia in an infant with glucose-6-phosphate dehydrogenase deficiency, J Pediatr 93:816

Higashi O (1954) Congenital gigantism of peroxidase granules, Tohoku J Exp Med 59:315

Higby DJ et al (1974) The prophylactic treatment of thrombocytopenic leukemic patients with platelets: a double blind study, Transfusion 14:440

Higginbottom MC et al (1978) A syndrome of methylmalonic aciduria, homocystinuria, megaloblastic anemia and neurologic abnormalities in a vitamin B_{12}–deficient breastfed infant of a strict vegetarian, N Engl J Med 299:317

Higgy KE et at (1977) Discrimination of B, T and null lymphocytes by esterase cytochemistry, Scand J Haematol 18:437

Higgy KE et al (1978) Identification of the hairy cells of leukaemic reticuloendotheliosis by an esterase method, Br J Haematol 38:99

Higuchi M and Bogorad L (1975) The purification and properties of uroporphyrinogen I synthetases and uroporphyrinogen III cosynthetase: interactions between the enzymes, Ann NY Acad Sci 244:401

Hijman van den Bergh AA and Mueller P (1916) Ueber eine direkte und eine indirekte Diazoreaktion auf Bilirubin, Biochem Z 77:90

Hildreth EA et al (1960) Persistence of the "hydralazine syndrome": a follow-up study of eleven cases, JAMA 173:657

Hill AV (1910) The possible effects of the aggregation of the molecules of hemoglobin on its dissociation curve, J Physiol 40:IV-V

Hill HR and Quie PG (1974) Raised serum IgE levels and defective neutrophil chemotaxis in three children with eczema and recurrent bacterial infections, Lancet 1:183

Hill HR et al (1974a) Defect in neutrophil granulocyte chemotaxis in Job's syndrome of recurrent "cold" staphylococcal abscesses, Lancet 2:617

Hill HR et al (1974b) Impaired leukotactic responsiveness in patients with juvenile diabetes mellitus, Clin Immunol Immunopathol 2:395

Hill JM and Duncan CN (1941) Leukemoid reactions, Am J Med Sci 201:847

Hill RL et al (1962) The chemical and genetic relationships between hemoglobins S and G San Jose, Blood 19:573

Hill RL et al (1966) The evolutionary origin of the immunoglobulins, Proc Natl Acad Sci 56:1762

Hill RL et al (1960) Characterization of a chemical abnormality in hemoglobin G, J Biol Chem 235:3182

Hill RS et al (1972) Iron deficiency and dyserythropoiesis, Br J Haematol 23:507

Hill RW and Bayrd ED (1960) Phagocytic reticuloendothelial cells in subacute bacterial endocarditis with negative cultures, Ann Intern Med 52:310

Hilts SV and Shaw CC (1953) Leukemoid blood reactions, N Engl J Med 249:434

Hines JD (1966) Megaloblastic anemia in an adult vegan, Am J Clin Nutr 19:260

Hines JD and Cowan DH (1970) Studies on the pathogenesis of alcohol-induced sideroblastic bone-marrow abnormalities, N Engl J Med 283:441

Hines JD and Grasso JA (1970) The sideroblastic anemias, Semin Hematol 7:86

Hines JD et al (1967) The hematologic complications following partial gastrectomy: a study of 292 patients, Am J Med 43:555

Hines JD et al (1968) Megaloblastic anemia secondary to folate deficiency associated with hypothyroidism, Ann Intern Med 68:792

Hinz CF Jr and Boyer JT (1963) Dysgammaglobulinemia in the adult manifested as autoimmune hemolytic anemia. Serologic and immunochemical characterization of an antibody of unusual specificity, N Engl J Med 269:1329

Hinz CF Jr and Mollner AM (1964) Studies on immune hemolysis. III. Role of 11 S component in initiating the Donath-Landsteiner reaction, J Immunol 91:512

Hinz CF Jr et al (1961) Studies on immune human hemolysis. I. The kinetics of the Donath-Landsteiner reaction and the requirement for complement in the reaction, J Exp Med 113:177

Hirano M et al (1980) Hb Toyoake: beta 142 ala → pro, a new unstable hemoglobin with high oxygen affinity, Proceedings of the Joint Meeting of the 18th Congress of the International Society on Hematology and the 16th Congress of the International Society on Blood Transfusion, Montreal, Abstract no 1057, p 203

Hirschhorn K et al (1969) Pompe's disease: detection of heterozygotes by lymphocyte stimulation, Science 166:1632

Hirsh J and Dacie JV (1966) Persistent post-splenectomy thrombo-cytosis and thrombo-embolism: a consequence of continuing anaemia, Br J Haematol **12**:44

Hirsh J and Doery JCG (1971) Platelet function in health and disease, Prog Hematol **7**:185

Hirsh J et al (1967) Spontaneous bruising associated with a defect in the interaction of platelets with connective tissue, Lancet **2**:18

Hirst E and Robertson TI (1967) The syndrome of thymoma and erythroblastopenic anemia. A review of 56 cases including 3 case reports, Medicine **46**:225

Hitzig WH and Willi H (1961) Hereditäre lymphoplasmocytäre Dysgenesie ("Alymphocytose mit Agammaglobulinamie"), Schweiz Med Wochenschr **52**:1625

Hitzig WH et al (1960) Erythroleukämie mit Hamoglobinopathie und Eisenstoffwechselstörung, Helv Pediatr Acta **15**:203

Hitzig WH et al (1968) Die schweizerische Form der Agammaglo-binämie, Ergeb Inn Med Kinderheilkd **27**:79

Hjort PS et al (1955) Evidence that platelet accelerator (platelet factor I) is adsorbed plasma proaccelerin, Blood **10**:1139

Hlavay E and Svec F (1958) Pseudo-Pelger-Leukocyten bei exper-imenteller Ratten-Leukämie, Acta Haematol **19**:295

Hoagland RJ (1963) Resurgent heterophil-antibody reaction after mononucleosis, N Engl J Med **269**:1307

Hoagland RJ (1967) Infectious mononucleosis, New York, Grune & Stratton, Inc

Hoagland HC and Goldstein NP (1978) Hematologic (cytopenic) manifestations of Wilson's disease (hepatolenticular degenera-tion), Mayo Clin Proc **53**:498

Hoak JC et al (1971) Hemangioma with thrombocytopenia and microangiopathic anemia (Kasabach-Merritt syndrome): an ani-mal model, J Lab Clin Med **77**:941

Hobolth N (1965) Haemoglobin M Arhus. I. Clinical family study, Acta Paediatr Scand **54**:357

Hodapp RV (1962) The case of the red and white Minnesota twins: intrauterine blood transfer between twins, J Lancet **82**:413

Hoffbrand AV and Newcombe BF (1967) Leukocyte folate and vitamin B_{12} and folate deficiency in leukemia, Br J Haematol **13**:954

Hoffbrand AV et al (1967) Incidence and pathogenesis of megalo-blastic erythropoiesis in multiple myeloma, J Clin Pathol **20**:699

Hoffbrand AV et al (1976) Megaloblastic anaemia: initiation of DNA synthesis in excess of DNA chain elongation as the under-lying mechanism, Clin Haematol **5**:727

Hoffman GC (1968) Human erythropoiesis following kidney trans-plantation, Ann NY Acad Sci **149**:504

Hoffman JF (1966) The red cell membrane and the transport of sodium and potassium, Am J Med **41**:666

Hoffman RG (1971) Establishing quality control and normal ranges in the clinical laboratory, New York, Exposition Press

Hoffman R and Zanjani ED (1978) Erythropoietin-dependent erythropoiesis during the erythroblastic phase of juvenile chron-ic granulocytic leukaemia, Br J Haematol **38**:511

Hoffman R et al (1976) Diamond-Blackfan syndrome: lympho-cyte-mediated suppression of erythropoiesis, Science **193**:899

Hoffman R et al (1977) Suppression of erythroid-colony formation by lymphoctyes from patients with aplastic anemia, N Engl J Med **296**:10

Hoffman R et al (1979) Fetal hemoglobin in polycythemia vera: cellular distribution in 50 unselected patients, Blood **53**:1148

Hoffman NR (1970) The relationship between pernicious anemia and cancer of the stomach, Geriatrics **25**:90

Hofmann V et al (1979) Fibrinogen Zurich 1: impaired release of fibrinopeptide A, Thromb Haemost **41**:709

Hogan GR and Jones B (1970) The relationship of koilonychia and iron deficiency in infants, J Pediatr **77**:1054

Hogarth-Scott RS et al (1969) Antibodies to *Toxocara* in the sera of visceral larva migrans patients: the significance of raised lev-els of IgE, Clin Exp Immunol **5**:619

Hollán SR et al (1967) A Boston-type haemoglobin M in Hungary: haemoglobin M Kiskunhales, Haematologia **1**:11

Hollán SR et al (1972) Duplication of haemoglobin genes, Bio-chimie **54**:639

Holland P and Mauer AM (1963) Myeloid leukemoid reactions in children, Am J Dis Child **105**:568

Holland P and Mauer AM (1965) Diphenylhydantoin-induced hypersensitivity reaction, J Pediatr **66**:322

Holland PV and Wallerstein RO (1968) Delayed hemolytic trans-fusion reaction with acute renal failure, JAMA **204**:1007

Hollenberg NK et al (1968) Acute oliguric renal failure in man: evidence for preferential renal cortical ischemia, Medicine **47**:455

Hollender A et al (1969) New unstable haemoglobin Böras: beta 88 (F4) leucine → arginine, Nature (London) **222**:953

Hollingsworth JW and Adams FM (1955) Megaloblastic anemia of pregnancy in two sisters. Case reports and an investigation of the hemolytic mechanism by means of erythrocyte survival studies, Blood **10**:933

Holmberg L and Nilsson IM (1973) Two genetic variants of von Willebrand's disease, N Engl J Med **288**:595

Holmes B and Good RA (1972) Laboratory models of chronic granulomatous disease, J Reticuloendothel Soc **12**:216

Holmes B et al (1970) Chronic granulomatous disease in females, N Engl J Med **283**:217

Holmes EW Jr et al (1967) Hexokinase isoenzymes in human erythrocytes: association of type II with fetal hemoglobin, Sci-ence **156**:646

Holmes AW et al (1975) Differentiation of HAAg and HBAg: Identification of the A virus. In Greenwalt TJ and Jamieson GA (Eds): Transmissible disease and blood, New York, Grune & Stratton, Inc, p 33

Holmquist WA and Schroeder WA (1966) A new N-terminal blocking group involving a Schiff base in hemoglobin A_{1c}, Bio-chemistry **5**:2489

Holmsen H (1972) The platelet: its membrane, physiology, and biochemistry, Clin Haematol **1**:235

Holmsen H and Weiss HJ (1972) Further evidence for a deficient storage pool of adenine nucleotides in platelets from some patients with thrombocytopathia—"storage pool disease," Blood **39**:197

Holmsen H et al (1969a) The blood platelet release reaction, Scand J Haematol (supp) **8**:3

Holmsen H et al (1969b) Adenine nucleotide metabolism of blood platelets. VI. Subcellular localization of nucleotide pools with different functions in the platelet release reaction, Biochim Bio-phys Acta **186**:254

Holmsen H et al (1975) Content and thrombin induced release of acid hydrolases in gel-filtered platelets from patients with stor-age pool disease, Blood **46**:131

Holti G et al (1958) An investigation of "porphyria cutanea tar-da," Q J Med **28**:183

Hom BL (1967) Demonstration of transcobalamin II complex for-mation and binding to Sephadex G-200 at low ionic strength, Clin Chim Acta **18**:315

Honig GR et al (1971) A new familial disorder with abnormal erythrocyte morphology and increased permeability of the eryth-rocytes to sodium and potassium, Pediatr Res **5**:159

Honig GR et al (1973) Hemoglobin Abraham Lincoln, beta 32 (B14) leucine → proline. An unstable variant producing severe hemolytic disease, J Clin Invest **52**:1746

Honig GR et al (1978a) Hemoglobin Lincoln Park: a βδ fusion (anti-Lepore) variant with an amino acid deletion in the δ chain–derived segment, Proc Natl Acad Sci USA **75**:1475

Honig GR et al (1978b) Hemoglobin Nigeria (alpha 81 ser → cys), a new variant having an inhibitory effect on the gelation of sickle hemoglobin, Blood **52** (Supp 1):113

Honig GR et al (1980) Hg Milledgeville (alpha 44 [CD2] pro → leu): a new variant associated with erythrocytosis, Proceedings of the Joint Meeting of the 18th Congress of the International Society on Hematology and the 16th Congress of the International Society on Blood Transfusion, Montreal, Abstract no 1058, p 203

Hood LE (1972) Two genes, one polypeptide chain—fact or fiction? Fed Proc **31**:177

Hoofnagle JH et al (1978) Type B hepatitis after transfusion with blood containing antibody to hepatitis B core antigen, N Engl J Med **298**:1379

Hopkins R and Das PC (1974) Australia antigen (HB-Ag) subtyping by a sensitive tanned cell haemagglutination—inhibition technique, Br J Haematol **27**:501

Hopkins R et al (1980) Improved economics of HBsAg screening with commercial radioimmunoassay reagents, J Clin Pathol **33**:19

Hoppe HH et al (1978) A silent gene (C3⁻) producing partial deficiency of the third component of human complement, Hum Hered **28**:141

Hörlein H and Weber G (1948) Ueber chronische familiäre Methämoglobinämie und eine neue Modifikation des Methämoglobins, Dtsch Med Wochenschr **73**:476

Horn B (1980) Miami Herald, Aug 19, p 1E

Horowitz HI and Fujimoto MM (1965) Association of factors XI and XII with blood platelets, Proc Soc Exp Biol Med **119**:487

Horowitz HI et al (1963) Assay of plasma thromboplastin antecedent (PTA) with artificially depleted normal plasma, Blood **22**:35

Horrigan DL and Harris JW (1964) Pyridoxine-responsive anemia: analysis of 62 cases, Adv Intern Med **12**:103

Horsfall FL and Tamm I (1965) Viral and rickettsial infection of man, ed 4, Philadelphia, JB Lippincott Co

Horster JA (1957) Phagozytose von Blutzellvorstufen im Knochenmark bei Agranulozytose und ähnlichen Erkrankungen, Dtsch Med Wochenschr **82**:1

Horton BF and Huisman THJ (1965) Studies on the heterogeneity of haemoglobin. VII. Minor haemoglobin components in haematological diseases, Br J Haematol **2**:296

Horwitz MS and Moore GT (1968) Acute infectious lymphocytosis: an etiologic and epidemiologic study of an outbreak, N Engl J Med **279**:399

Horwitz CA et al (1977a) Cold agglutinins in infectious mononucleosis and heterophil antibody-negative mononucleosis-like syndromes, Blood **50**:195

Horwitz CA et al (1977b) Heterophil-negative infectious mononucleosis and mononucleosis-like illnesses: laboratory confirmation of 43 cases, Am J Med **63**:947

Horwitz CA et al (1979) Persistant falsely positive rapid tests for infectious mononucleosis: report of five cases with four six-year follow-up data, Am J Clin Pathol **72**:807

Horwitz CA et al (1980) Hepatic function in mononucleosis induced by Epstein-Barr virus and cytomegalovirus, Clin Chem **26**:243

Hougie C and Twomey JJ (1967) Haemophilia B$_M$: a new type of factor-IX deficiency, Lancet **1**:698

Hougie C et al (1957) Stuart clotting defect. I. Segregation of an hereditary hemorrhagic state from the heterogeneous group heretofore called the "stable factor" (SPCA, proconvertin, factor VII) deficiency, J Clin Invest **26**:485

Hougie C et al (1975) Passovoy factor: a hitherto unrecognized factor necessary for haemostasis, Lancet **2**:290

Hougie C et al (1978) The Passovoy defect: further characterization of a hereditary hemorrhagic diathesis, N Engl J Med **298**:1045

Housman D et al (1973) Quantitative deficiency of chain-specific globin messenger ribonucleic acids in the thalassemia syndromes, Proc Natl Acad Sci USA **70**:1809

Hovig T (1963) Release of platelet-aggregation substance (adenosine diphosphate) from rabbit blood platelets induced by saline "extract" of tendons, Thromb Diath Haemorrh **9**:264

Hovig T (1968) The ultrastructure of blood platelets in normal and abnormal states, Ser Haematol **1**:3

Hovig T (1974) The ultrastructural basis of platelet function. In Baldini MG and Ebbe S (Eds): Platelets: production, function, transfusion, and storage, New York, Grune & Stratton, Inc

Hovig T et al (1968) The transformation of hemostatic platelet plugs in normal and Factor IX deficient dogs, Am J Pathol **53**:355

Howard MA and Firkin BG (1971) Ristocetin—a new tool in the investigation of platelet aggregation, Thromb Diath Haemorrh **26**:362

Howard MA et al (1973) Ristocetin: a means of differentiating von Willebrand's disease into two groups, Blood **41**:687

Howarth C et al (1979) Familial erythrocytosis, Scand J Haematol **23**:217

Howell M (1963) Acquired factor X deficiency associated with systematized amyloidosis—a report of a case, Blood **21**:739

Hoyer LW (1972) Immunologic studies of antihemophiliac factor (AHF, factor VIII) IV. Radioimmunoassay of AHF antigen, J Lab Clin Med **80**:822

Hsieh H-S and Jaffé ER (1971) Electrophoretic and functional variants of NADH-methemoglobin reductase in hereditary methemoglobinemia, J Clin Invest **50**:196

Hsu TC (1952) Mammalian chromosomes in vitro. I. The karyotype of man, J Hered **43**:167

Hubbard M et al (1975) Hemoglobin Atlanta or alpha 2 beta 2 75 leu → pro (E19): an unstable variant found in several members of a Caucasian family, Biochim Biophys Acta **386**:538

Huber CH et al (1974) Receptor sites for aggregated gammaglobulin (AGG) on lymphocytes in lymphoproliferative diseases, Br J Haematol **27**:643

Huber J et al (1967) Congenital aplasia of parathyroid glands and thymus, Arch Dis Child **42**:190

Huber W (1939) Gleichzeitiges Vorkommen von Pelgerscher Varietät mit chronischer Myelose, Schweiz Med Wochenschr **69**:556

Hudson G (1964) The marrow reserve of eosinophils. Effect of cortical hormones on the foreign protein response, Br J Haematol **10**:122

Hudson G (1965) Bone-marrow volume in the human foetus and newborn, Br J Haematol **11**:446

Huehns ER (1970) Disease due to abnormalities of hemoglobin structure, Ann Rev Med **21**:157

Huehns ER et al (1964) Human embryonic haemoglobin, Nature **201**:1095

Huehns ER et al (1961) Haemoglobin α^A, Nature **192**:1057

Huennekens FM (1963) The role of dihydrofolic reductase in the metabolism of one-carbon units, Biochemistry **2**:151

Huennekens FM (1968) Folic acid coenzymes in biosynthesis of purines and pyrimidines, Vitam Horm **26**:375

Huennekens FM and Osborn MJ (1959) Folic acid coenzymes and one-carbon metabolism, Adv Enzymol **21**:369

Huestis DW et al (1976) Practical blood transfusion, Boston, Little, Brown & Co

Huff RL and Feller DD (1956) Relation of circulating red cell volume to body density and obesity, J Clin Invest **35**:1

Huggins CE (1963) Prevention of hemolysis of large volumes of red blood cells slowly frozen and thawed in the presence of dimethylsulfoxide, Transfusion **3**:483

Huggins CE (1964) Frozen blood, Ann Surg **160**:643

Huggins CE and Grove-Rasmussen M (1965) Advances in blood preservation, Postgrad Med **37**:557

Hughes NR (1966) Erythrocyte phagocytosis by human lymphocytes, Nature **212**:1575

Huijgens PC et al (1978) Pure red cell aplasia, toxic dermatitis and lymphadenopathy in a patient taking diphenylhydantoin, Acta Haematol **59**:31

Huisman THJ (1972) Normal and abnormal hemoglobins, Adv Clin Chem **15**:150

Huisman THJ (1974) Chromatographic determination of Hb-A$_2$. In Schmidt RM et al (Eds): The detection of hemoglobinopathies, Cleveland, CRC Press, p 27

Huisman THJ (1979) Sickle cell anemia as a syndrome: a review of diagnostic features, Am J Hematol **6**:173

Huisman THJ and Schroeder WA (1970) New aspects of the structure, function, and synthesis of hemoglobins. In King JW and Faulkner WR (Eds): CRC critical reviews in clinical laboratory science, Cleveland, Chemical Rubber Publishing Co

Huisman THJ et al (1963) The oxygen equilibria of some "slow-moving" human hemoglobin types, Biochim Biophys Acta **74**:69

Huisman THJ et al (1969) Hemoglobin C in newborn sheep and goats: a possible explanation for its function and biosynthesis, Pediatr Res **3**:189

Huisman THJ et al (1970) Hemoglobin G Georgia or alpha 2 95 leu (G2) beta 2, Biochim Biophys Acta **200**:578

Huisman THJ et al (1971) Hemoglobin Savannah (B6 [24] beta → glycine → valine): an unstable variant causing anemia with inclusion bodies, J Clin Invest **50**:650

Huisman THJ et al (1972a) Hemoglobin Kenya, the product of fusion of gamma and beta polypeptide chains, Arch Biochem Biophys **153**:850

Huisman THJ et al (1972b) Evidence for four nonallelic structural genes for the γ chain of human fetal hemoglobin, Biochem Genet **7**:131

Huisman THJ et al (1974) Hemoglobin Grady: the first example of a variant with elongated chains due to an insertion of residues, Proc Natl Acad Sci USA **71**:3270

Hultin MB (1979) Activated clotting factors in factor IX concentrates, Blood **54**:1028

Human Chromosome Study Group (1960) A proposed standard of nomenclature of human mitotic chromosomes, Cerb Palsy Bull **2**(supp):1

Hummel K (1961) Die medizinische Vaterschaftsbegutachtung mit biostatistischem Beweis, Stuttgart, Gustav Fisher Verlag

Hummel K et al (1971, 1972) Biostatistical opinion of parentage, based upon the results of blood group tests, vols 1 and 2, Stuttgart, Gustav Fischer Verlag

Humoller FL et al (1960) Enzymatic properties of ceruloplasmin, J Lab Clin Med **56**:222

Humphrey JH and Fahey JL (1961) The metabolism of normal plasma proteins and gamma-myeloma protein in mice bearing plasma-cell tumors, J Clin Invest **40**:1696

Humphrey TJ and Goulston K (1969) Chemical testing of occult blood in faeces: "Haematest," "Occultest," and guaiac testing correlated with [51]chromium estimation of faecal blood loss, Med J Aust **1**:1291

Humphrey JH and Batty I (1974) International reference preparation for human serum IgG, IgA, IgM, Clin Exp Immunol **17**:708

Hungerford DA and Nowell PC (1962) Chromosome studies in human leukemia. III. Acute granulocytic leukemia, J Natl Cancer Inst **29**:545

Hungerford GF and Karson EF (1960) The eosinophilia of magnesium deficiency, Blood **16**:1642

Hunt JA and Lehmann H (1959) Haemoglobin "Bart's": a foetal haemoglobin without α-chains, Nature **184**:872

Hunt JA and Ingram VM (1960) Abnormal human haemoglobins. IV. The chemical difference between normal human haemoglobin and haemoglobin C, Biochim Biophys Acta **42**:409

Hunt JA and Ingram VM (1961) Abnormal human haemoglobins. VI. The chemical difference between haemoglobins A and E, Biochim Biophys Acta **49**:520

Hunter C (1917) A rare disease in two brothers, Proc R Soc Med **10**:104

Huntsman RG (1974) Sickling tests—microscopic and nonmicroscopic. In Schmidt RM et al (Eds): The detection of hemoglobinopathies, Cleveland, CRC Press

Huntsman RG et al (1970) A rapid whole blood solubility test to differentiate the sickle-cell trait from sickle-cell anaemia, J Clin Pathol **23**:781

Hurdle AD et al (1966) Occurrence of lymphopenia in heart failure, J Clin Pathol **19**:60

Hurdle AD et al (1972) Clinical and cytogenetic studies in chronic myelomonocytic leukaemia, Br J Haematol **22**:773

Hurler G (1919) Über einen Typ multipler Abartungen vorwiegend am Skelettsystem, Z Kinderheilkd **24**:220

Hurt GA and Chanutin A (1964) Organic phosphate compounds of erythrocytes from individuals with uremia, J Lab Clin Med **64**:675

Husby G et al (1976) Tissue T and B cell infiltration of primary and metastatic cancer, J Clin Invest **57**:1471

Huser H-J (1966) A Note on Biermer's anemia, Med Clin North Am **50**:1611

Huser H-J et al (1967) Experimental evidence of excess hemolysis in the course of chronic iron deficiency anemia, J Lab Clin Med **69**:405

Hutchinson NE et al (1964) Hereditary Heinz-body anaemia, thrombocytopenia, and haemoglobinopathy (Hb Köln) in a Glasgow family, Br Med J **2**:1099

Hutter JJ Jr et al (1979) Myelogenous leukemia evolving during the course of lymphoid malignancy in children, Am J Hematol **6**:333

Hütteroth TH et al (1972) Cultured lymphoid cell lines from normal subjects: membrane associated immunoglobulins studied by the mixed antiglobulin reaction, Cell Immunol **5**:446

Hutton JJ and Coleman MS (1976) Terminal deoxynucleotidyl transferase measurements in the differential diagnosis of adult leukaemias, Br J Haematol **34**:447

Hyde RD et al (1971) Haemoglobin J Rajappen: alpha 90 (FG2) lys → thr, Biochim Biophys Acta **243**:515

Hyde RD et al (1972) Haemoglobin Southampton, beta 106 (G8) leu → pro: an unstable variant producing severe haemolysis, Lancet **2**:1170

Hyman C and Paldino RL (1960) Possible role of reticuloendothelial system in protein transport, Ann NY Acad Sci **88**:232

Hymes K et al (1979) A solid phase radioimmunoassay for bound anti-platelet antibody: studies on 45 patients with autoimmune platelet disorders, J Lab Clin Med **94**:639

Hymes K et al (1980) Heavy-chain subclass of bound antiplatelet IgG in autoimmune thrombocytopenic purpura, Blood **56**:84

Hynes M and Whitby LEH (1938) Correction of sedimentation rate for anemia, Lancet 2:249

Hyun BH et al (1976) Reactive plasmacytic lesions of the bone marrow, Am J Clin Pathol 65:921

Idelson LI et al (1974) New unstable hemoglobin (hb Moscva, beta 24 [B6] gly → asp) found in the USSR, Nature 249:768

Idelson LI et al (1975) Haemoglobin Volga beta 27 (B9) ala → asp, a new highly unstable haemoglobin with a suppressed charge, FEBS Lett 58:122

Ikkala E et al (1970) Gastric mucosa in iron deficiency anemia. Results of follow-up examinations, Acta Haematol 43:228

Ikkala E et al (1976) Hb Helsinki: a variant with a high oxygen affinity and a substitution at a 2,3-DPG binding site (beta 82 [EF6] lys → met), Acta Haematol 56:257

Illis L (1964) On porphyria and the aetiology of werwolves, Proc R Soc Med 57:23

Imai K and Lehmann H (1975) The oxygen affinity of haemoglobin Tak, a variant with an elongated beta chain, Biochim Biophys Acta 412:288

Imai K et al (1970) Studies on the function of abnormal hemoglobins. II. Oxygen equilibrium of abnormal hemoglobins: Shimonoseki, Ube II, Hikari, Gifu, and Agenogi, Biochim Biophys Acta 200:197

Imamura T (1966) Hemoglobin Kagoshima: an example of hemoglobin Norfolk in a Japanese family, Am J Hum Genet 18:584

Imamura T and Riggs A (1972) Identification of hemoglobin Oak Ridge with hemoglobin D Punjab (Los Angeles), Biochem Genet 7:127

Imamura T et al (1969) Hemoglobin Yoshizuka (G10 [108] beta asparagine → aspartic acid): a new variant with a reduced oxygen affinity from a Japanese family, J Clin Invest 48:2341

Imerslund O (1960) Idiopathic chronic megaloblastic anemia in children, Acta Paediatr (Upps) 49(supp 119):1

Imoto S et al (1971) A case of drug-induced lipidosis with "seablue histiocytes" in the bone marrow, Jpn Arch Intern Med 18:83

Inae S et al (1979) Deficiency of the ninth component of complement in man, J Clin Lab Immunol 2:85

Incefy GS et al (1975) In vitro differentiation of human marrow cells into T lymphocytes by thymic extracts using the rosette technique, Clin Exp Immunol 19:475

Inceman S and Tangun Y (1975) Essential athrombia: study of a new case, Thromb Diath Haemorrh 33:278

Inceman S et al (1962) Essential athrombia, Thromb Diath Haemorrh 8:502

Inceman S et al (1966) Aggregation, adhesion, and viscous metamorphosis of platelets in congenital fibrinogen deficiencies, J Lab Clin Med 68:21

Infante PF et al (1977) Leukaemia in benzene workers, Lancet 2:76

Ingram GIC and Rizza CR (1976) Heterozygous and homozygous factor XI defect in a consanguineous family, Acta Haematol 55:48

Ingram GI et al (1973) Low factor VIII like antigen in acquired von Willebrand's syndrome and response to treatment, Br J Haematol 25:135

Ingram RH Jr and Seki M (1962) Pseudohyperkalemia with thrombocytosis, N Engl J Med 267:895

Ingram VM (1956) A specific difference between the globins of normal human and sickle cell anemia haemoglobins, Nature 178:792

Ingram VM (1958) Abnormal human haemoglobin. I. The comparison of normal human and sickle-cell haemoglobins by "fingerprinting," Biochim Biophys Acta 28:539

Ingram VM (1959) Abnormal human haemoglobins. III. The chemical difference between normal and sickle cell haemoglobins, Biochim Biophys Acta 36:402

Ingram VM (1963) The hemoglobins in genetics and evolution, New York, Columbia University Press

Inkley SR et al (1955) A study of methods for the prediction of plasma volume, J Lab Clin Med 45:841

Inoue (1924) quoted in Aibara: Hokuetsu Igakkai Zasshi 39:256

International Committee for Standardization in Haematology (1978a) Recommendations for measurement of serum iron in human blood, Br J Haematol 38:291

International Committee for Standardization in Haematology (1978b) The measurement of total and unsaturated iron-binding capacity in serum, Br J Haematol 38:281

Ioachim HL (1965) Emperipolesis of lymphoid cells in mixed cultures, Lab Invest 14:1784

Irons GV Jr and Kirsner JB (1965) Routine chemical tests of the stool for occult blood: an evaluation, Am J Med Sci 249:247

Irvine WJ (1965) Immunological aspects of pernicious anemia, N Engl J Med 273:432

Isaacs R and Friedman A (1938) Standards for maximum reticulocyte percentage after intramuscular liver therapy in pernicious anemia, Am J Med Sci 196:718

Isaacson NH and Rapoport P (1946) Eosinophilia in malignant tumors: its significance, Ann Intern Med 25:893

Iscove NN et al (1970) The proliferative states of mouse granulopoietic progenitor cells, Proc Soc Exp Biol Med 134:33

Iscove NN et al (1971) Colony formation by normal and leukemic human marrow cells in culture: effect of conditioned medium from human leukocytes, Blood 37:1

Ishimori T and Hasekura H (1967) A Japanese with no detectable Rh blood group antigens due to silent Rh alleles or deleted chromosomes, Transfusion 7:84

Ishimori T et al (1976) Rare Diego blood group phenotype Di(a + b −). I. Anti-Di^b causing hemolytic disease of the newborn, Vox Sang 31:61

Ishizaka K and Ishizaka T (1969) Immune mechanisms of reversed type reaginic hypersensitivity, J Immunol 103:588

Ishizaka K and Ishizaka T (1970) The significance of immunoglobulin E in reaginic hypersensitivity, Ann Allergy 28:189

Ishizaka K et al (1970) Mechanisms of passive sensitization. I. Presence of IgE and IgG molecules on human leukocytes, J Immunol 105:1459

Ishizaka T and Ishizaka K (1973) Biologic function of immunoglobulin E. In Ishizaka K and Dayton DH (Eds): The biological role of the immunoglobulin E system, Washington, DC, US Government Printing Office

Issitt PD (1974) Auto-immune hemolytic anemia, Am J Med Technol 40:479

Issitt PD and Smith TR (1976) Evaluation of antiglobulin reagents. In A seminar on performance evaluation, Washington, DC, American Association of Blood Banks, p 25

Issitt PD (1977) Autoimmune hemolytic anemia and cold hemagglutinin disease: clinical disease and laboratory findings, Prog Clin Pathol 7:137

Issitt PD (1979) Serology and genetics of the rhesus blood group system, Cincinnati, Montgomery Scientific Publications

Itano HA (1953) Solubilities of naturally occurring mixtures of human hemoglobin, Arch Biochem 47:148

Itano HA and Pauling L (1949) A rapid diagnostic test for sickle cell anemia, Blood 4:66

Ito S et al (1978) Surface immunoglobulin of human lymphocytes, Scand J Haematol 20:399

Itoga T and Laszlo J (1962) Döhle bodies and other granulocytic alterations during chemotherapy with cyclophosphamide, Blood 20:668

Iuchi I et al (1978) Hemoglobin Hoshida (beta 43 [CD-2] glu →

gln), a new hemoglobin variant discovered in Japan, Hemoglobin **2**:235

Iuchi I et al (1980a) Hemoglobin Mizushi (alpha 75 [EF4] asp → gly): a new hemoglobin variant observed in a Japanese family, Hemoglobin **4**:209

Iuchi I et al (1980b) Hemoglobin Takamatsu (β120 [GH3] lys → gln): a new abnormal hemoglobin detected in three unrelated families in the Takamatsu area of Shikoku, Hemoglobin **4**:165

Jackson CM (1980) Factor X. In Schmidt RM (Section Ed) Handbook Series in Clinical Laboratory Science, Section I: Hematology, vol 3, Boca Raton, Fla, CRC Press Inc, p 101

Jackson DP and Beck EA (1970) Inherited abnormal fibrinogens. In Brinkhous KM (Ed): Hemophilia and new hemorrhagic states, Chapel Hill, NC, University of North Carolina Press, p 225

Jackson DP et al (1965) Congenital disorders of fibrinogen, Fed Proc **24**:816

Jackson EW et al (1968) Down's syndrome: variation of leukemia occurrence in institutionalized populations, J Chronic Dis **21**:247

Jackson IM and Clark RM (1965) A case of neutrophilic leukemia, Am J Med Sci **249**:72

Jackson JF (1962) Histochemical identification of megakaryocytes from peripheral blood examined for tumor cells, Cancer **15**:259

Jackson JM and Knight D (1969) Stomatocytosis in migrants of Mediterranean origin, Med J Aust **1**:939

Jackson JM et al (1973) Haemoglobin Perth: beta 32 (B14) leu → pro. An unstable haemoglobin causing haemolysis, Br J Haematol **25**:607

Jackson JR (1979) The histopathology of lymphomas and pseudolymphomas, Baltimore, University Park Press

Jackson WPU et al (1954) Metaphyseal dysplasia, epiphyseal dysplasia, diaphyseal dysplasia, and related conditions. II. Multiple epiphyseal dysplasia: its relation to other disorders of epiphyseal development, Arch Intern Med (Chicago) **94**:886

Jacob F and Monod J (1961) Genetic regulatory mechanisms in the synthesis of proteins, J Mol Biol **3**:318

Jacob HS (1970) Mechanisms of Heinz body formation and attachment to red cell membrane, Semin Hematol **7**:344

Jacob HS (1978) Granulocyte-complement interaction: a beneficial antimicrobial mechanism that can cause disease, Arch Intern Med **138**:461

Jacob HS and Jandl JH (1962) Effects of sulfhydryl inhibition on red blood cells. I. Mechanism of hemolysis, J Clin Invest **41**:779

Jacob HS et al (1964) Extreme eosinophilia with iodide hypersensitivity. Report of a case with observations on the cellular composition of inflammatory exudates, N Engl J Med **271**:1138

Jacob HS et al (1972) The abnormal red-cell membrane in hereditary spherocytosis: evidence for the causal role of mutant microfilaments, Br J Haematol **23**(supp):35

Jacobasch G and Boese C (1969) Regulation des Kohlenhydratstoffwechsels roter Blutzellen bei Pyruvatkinasemangel, Folia Haematol (Leipzig) **91**:70

Jacobi JM et al (1969) Immunochemical quantitation of human transferrin in pregnancy and during the administration of oral contraceptives, Br J Haematol **17**:503

Jacobs A and Cavill I (1968) The oral lesions of iron deficiency anemia: pyridoxine and riboflavin status, Br J Haematol **14**:291

Jacobs A and Kilpatrick GS (1964) The Paterson-Kelly syndrome, Br Med J **2**:79

Jacobs A and Miles PM (1969) Role of gastric secretion in iron absorption, Gut **10**:226

Jacobs A et al (1966) Gastric acid secretion in chronic iron deficiency anemia, Lancet **2**:190

Jacobs A et al (1972) Ferritin in the serum of normal subjects and patients with iron deficiency and iron overload, Br Med J **4**:206

Jacobs F and Monod J (1961) Genetic regulatory mechanisms in the synthesis of proteins, J Mol Biol **3**:318

Jacobs HS (1969) The defective red blood cell in hereditary spherocytosis, Annu Rev Med **20**:41

Jacobs HS (1974) Hypersplenism: mechanisms and management, Br J Haematol **27**:1

Jacobs J et al (1965) Acute iron intoxication, N Engl J Med **273**:1124

Jacobs A and Worwood M (1975) Ferritin in serum: clinical and biochemical implications, N Engl J Med **292**:951

Jacobs A et al (1972) Ferritin in the serum of normal subjects and patients with iron deficiency and iron overload, Br Med J **4**:206

Jacobsen CD and Hoak JC (1973) Fibrinogen Iowa City: an abnormal fibrinogen with clinical symptoms, Thromb Res **2**:261

Jacobsen CD et al (1972) Sea-blue histiocytes in familial lecithin: cholesterol acyltransferase deficiency, Scand J Haematol **9**:106

Jacobson ED et al (1960) An experimental malabsorption syndrome induced by neomycin, Am J Med **28**:524

Jacobson LO et al (1959) Studies of erythropoietin: the hormone regulating red cell production, Ann NY Acad Sci **77**:551

Jacobson RJ et at (1978) Agnogenic myeloid metaplasia: a clonal proliferation of hematopoietic stem cells with secondary myelofibrosis, Blood **51**:189

Jadhav M et al (1962) Vitamin B$_{12}$ deficiency in Indian infants. A clinical syndrome, Lancet **2**:903

Jaffe EA and Nachman RL (1975) Subunit structure of factor VIII antigen synthesized by cultured human endothelial cells, J Clin Invest **56**:698

Jaffé ER (1966) Hereditary methemoglobinemias associated with abnormalities in the metabolism of erythrocytes, Am J Med **41**:786

Jaffe ES et al (1974) Leukemic reticuloendotheliosis: presence of a receptor for cytophilic antibody, Am J Med **57**:108

Jaffe ES et al (1975) Membrane receptor sites for the identification of lymphoreticular cells in benign and malignant conditions, Br J Cancer **31**(suppl II):107

Jaffe ES et al (1977) Functional markers: a new perspective on malignant lymphomas, Cancer Treat Rep **61**:953

Jaffe RM et al (1975) False-negative stool occult blood tests caused by ingestion of ascorbic acid (vitamin C), Ann Intern Med **83**:824

Jager BV (1962) Cryofibrinogenemia, N Engl J Med **266**:579

Jamieson GA (1974) Interaction of platelets and collagen. In Baldini MG and Ebbe S (Eds): Platelets: production, function, transfusion, and storage, New York, Grune & Stratton, Inc

Jamieson WM and Kerr MR (1962) A family with several cases of hypogammaglobulinemia, Arch Dis Child **37**:330

Jamshidi K and Swaim WR (1971) Bone marrow biopsy with unaltered architecture: a new biopsy device, J Lab Clin Med **77**:335

Jandl JH (1968) Hereditary spherocytosis. In Beutler E (Ed) Hereditary disorders of erythrocyte metabolism, New York, Grune & Stratton, Inc

Jandl JH and Aster RH (1967) Increased splenic pooling and the pathogenesis of hypersplenism, Am J Med Sci **253**:383

Jandl JH and Cooper RA (1972) Hereditary spherocytosis. In Stanbury JB et al (Eds): The metabolic basis of inherited disease, New York, McGraw-Hill Book Co, Inc, p 1323

Jandl JH and Cooper RA (1978) Hereditary spherocytosis. In Stanbury JB et al (Eds): The metabolic basis of inherited disease, New York, McGraw-Hill Book Co, Inc, p 1398

Janeway CA et al (1956) Collagen disease in patients with congenital agammaglobulinemia, Trans Assoc Am Physicians **69**:93

Janis M and Bach FH (1970) Potentiation of in vitro lymphocyte reactivity, Nature **225**:238

Janitschke K et al (1974) Untersuchungen über die Möglichkeit der Übertragung von Toxoplasmen durch Bluttransfusionen, Blut **29**:407

Janossy G et al (1976) Target cell in chronic myeloid leukaemia and its relationship to acute lymphoid leukaemia, Lancet **2**:1058

Jansen J et al (1978) Hairy cell leukaemia: clinical features and effect of splenectomy, Scand J Haematol **21**:60

Janssen CL and Vreeken J (1971) Fibrinogen Amsterdam, another hereditary abnormality of fibrinogen, Br J Haematol **20**:287

Jaques LB (1973) Protamine—antagonist to heparin, Can Med Assoc J **108**:1291

Jaques LB (1979) Heparin: an old drug with a new paradigm, Science **206**:528

Jaques LB (1980) Heparins—anionic polyelectrolyte drugs, Pharmacol Rev **31**:99

Jaques LB et al (1973) Variation in commercial heparin and its relation to the problems of heparin standardization for clinical use, Thromb Res **3**:295

Jasin HG et al (1970) Rheumatoid hyperviscosity syndrome, Am J Med **49**:484

Javid J (1965) The effect of haptoglobin polymer size on hemoglobin binding capacity, Vox Sang **10**:320

Javid J (1973) Hemoglobin SO Arabia disease in a Black American, Am J Med Sci **265**:266

Javid J (1978) Human haptoglobins, Curr Top Hematol **1**:151

Jayle MF and Boussier G (1955) Le seromucoids du sang: leur relations avec les mucoproteins de la substance fundamentale de tissu conjonetif, Expos Annu Biochim Med **17**:157

Jeannet M et al (1972) Use of the HL-A antigen system in disputed paternity cases, Vox Sang **23**:197

Jeannet M and Hässig A (1964) Ueber die Beziehungen der Hämagglutination im kolloidalen Milieu zur Geldrollenbildung, Blutkörpershensenkung und Sphärozytose, Blut **10**:297

Jedrzejczak WW et al (1975) Evaluation of the usefulness of nitroblue tetrazolium reduction test (NBT test) for detection of bacterial infection in cancer patients, Neoplasma **22**:323

Jenkins CSP et al (1975) Comparative studies of available ristocetins: proteolytic activity and effect on platelets, Thromb Res **7**:531

Jenkins GC et al (1965) Arsine poisoning: massive haemolysis with minimal impairment of renal function, Br Med J **2**:78

Jenkins GC et al (1967) Haemoglobin F Texas I ($\alpha2\gamma2$ 5 (glu → lys): a variant of haemoglobin F, Br J Haematol **13**:252

Jenkins WJ et al (1960) The I antigen and antibody, Vox Sang **5**:97

Jenkins WJ et al (1965) Infectious mononucleosis: an unsuspected source of anti-i, Br J Haematol **11**:480

Jensen K et al (1962) Multiple passive transfer of the delayed-type hypersensitivity in humans, Am Rev Resp Dis **85**:373

Jensen J et al (1967) Coronary disease in familial hypercholesterolemia, Circulation **36**:77

Jensen M et al (1975) Hemoglobin Syracuse (alpha 2 beta 2 143 [H21] his → pro), a new high affinity variant detected by special electrophoretic methods, J Clin Invest **55**:469

Jensen WN and Klug PP (1973) The cell membrane in sickle cell disease. In Abramson H et al (Eds): Sickle cell disease: diagnosis, management, education, and research, St. Louis, The CV Mosby Co

Jensen WN et al (1965) An electron microscopic description of basophilic stippling in red cells, Blood **25**:933

Jensson O (1958) Observations on the leucocyte blood picture in acute uraemia, Br J Haematol **4**:422

Jepson JH and Lowenstein L (1966) Inhibition of the stem-cell action of erythropoietin by estradiol, Proc Soc Exp Biol Med **123**:457

Jepson JH and Lowenstein L (1967) The effect of testosterone, adrenal steroids, and prolactin on erythropoiesis, Acta Haematol **38**:292

Jepson JH and McGarry EE (1968) Polycythemia and increased erythropoietin production in a patient with hypertrophy of the juxta-glomerular apparatus, Blood **32**:370

Jerry LM et al (1972) Stabilization of dissociable IgA2 proteins by secretory component, J Immunol **109**:275

Jervis GA et al (1962) Cerebral lipidosis of unclear nature. In Aronson SM and Volk BW (Eds): Cerebral sphingolipidoses, New York, Academic Press, Inc

Jesty and Nemerson Y (1974) Purification of factor VII from bovine plasma. Reaction with tissue factor and activation of factor X, J Biol Chem **249**:509

Jesty J (1980) Coagulation factor VII. In Schmidt RM (Section Ed): Handbook Series in Clinical Laboratory Science, Section I: Hematology, vol 3, Boca Raton, Fla CRC Press Inc, p 41

Jeunet F and Good RA (1968) Thymoma, immunologic deficiencies, and hematological abnormalities. In Good RA and Bergsma D (Eds): Immunologic deficiency diseases in man, vol 4, New York, National Foundation Press, p 192

Jobin F and Esnouf MP (1967) Studies on the formation of the prothrombin-converting complex, Biochem J **102**:666

Johansson SGO and Bennich H (1967) Immunological studies of an atypical (myeloma) immunoglobulin, Immunology **13**:381

Johansson SGO et al (1968) A new class of immunoglobulin in human serum, Immunology **14**:265

Johansson SG et al (1970) Some factors influencing the serum IgE levels in atopic diseases, Clin Exp Immunol **6**:43

Johns DG and Bertino JR (1965) Folates and megaloblastic anemia: a review, Clin Pharmacol Ther **6**:372

Johnson CS et al (1980) Hemoglobin Pasadena, $\alpha_2\beta_2$ 75 (E19) leu → arg: identification by high performance liquid chromatography of a new unstable variant with increased oxygen affinity, Biochim Biophys Acta **623**:360

Johnson MH et al (1980) Hemoglobin Tampa: $\beta79$ (EF3) aspartic acid → tyrosine, Biochim Biophys Acta **623**:119

Johnson RL et al (1967) Adult hypogammaglobulinemia with malabsorption and iron deficiency anemia, Am J Med **43**:935

Johnson RR et al (1963) An unusual epidemic of methemoglobinemia, Pediatrics **31**:222

Johnson SA et al (1965) The ultrastructure of platelet participation in hemostasis, Thromb Diath Haemorrh **13**:65

Johnston DWC et al (1980) Tests for hemostasis and their relevance to venous thrombosis, Can J Surg **23**:373

Johnston RB Jr (1978) Oxygen metabolism and the microbicidal activity of macrophages, Fed Proc **37**:2759

Johnston RB Jr et al (1973) An abnormality of the alternate pathway of complement activation in sickle-cell disease, N Engl J Med **288**:803

Joishy SK et al (1976) Sickle β-thalassemia: identical twins differing in severity implicate nongenetic factors influencing course, Am J Hematol **1**:23

Joist JH and Niewiarowski S (1973) Detection of platelet fibrin stabilizing factor during the platelet release reaction and clot retraction, Thromb Diath Haemorrh **29**:679

Joncas JH et al (1974) Limitations of immunofluorescence tests in the diagnosis of infectious mononucleosis, Can Med Assoc J **110**:793

Jones AR and Kaneb L (1960) Some properties of cross reacting antibody of the ABO blood group system, Blood **15**:395

Jones B et al (1970) Sea-blue histiocyte disease in siblings, Lancet **2**:73

Jones CC (1973) Megaloblastic anemia associated with long-term tetracycline therapy, Ann Intern Med **78**:910

Jones G and Roitt IM (1972) Immunoglobulin determinants on lymphoid cells in culture, Cell Immunol **3**:478

Jones JH (1961) Foetal haemoglobin in Fanconi type anaemia, Nature **192**:982

Jones MS and Jones OTG (1969) The structural organization of haem synthesis in rat liver mitochondria, Biochem J **113**:507

Jones P et al (1979) Interpretation of serum and red cell folate results. A comparison of microbiological and radioisotopic methods, Pathology **11**:45

Jones RT and Brimhall B (1967) Structural characterization of two delta chain variants, J Biol Chem **242**:5141

Jones RT and Koler RD et al (1976) Functional studies of seven new abnormal hemoglobins, Proceedings of the 16th International Congress on Hematology, Abstract nos 1-21

Jones RT et al (1959) Gross structure of hemoglobin H, J Am Chem Soc **81**:3161

Jones RT et al (1966a) Hemoglobin Freiburg: abnormal hemoglobin due to deletion of a single amino acid residue, Science **154**:1024

Jones RT et al (1966b) Hemoglobin Sphakia: a delta chain variant of hemoglobin A_2 from Crete, Science **151**:1406

Jones RT et al (1967) Hemoglobin Yakima: I. Clinical and biochemical studies, J Clin Invest **46**:1840

Jones RT et al (1968a) Chemical characterization of hemoglobin Mexico and hemoglobin Chiapas, Biochim Biophys Acta **154**:488

Jones RT et al (1968b) Structural characterization of hemoglobin N Seattle: alpha 2 A beta 2 61 lys → glu, Biochim Biophys Acta **154**:278

Jones RT et al (1976a) Hemoglobin British Columbia (alpha 2 beta 2 101 [G3] glu → lys): a new variant with high oxygen affinity, Hemoglobin **1**:171

Jones RT et al (1976b) Hemoglobin Vancouver (alpha 2 beta 2 73 [E17] asp → tyr): its structure and function, J Mol Evol **9**:37

Jones RT et al (1976c) Hemoglobin Willamette (alpha 2 beta 2 51 pro → arg [D2]): a new abnormal human hemoglobin, Hemoglobin **1**:45

Jones SE (1973) Autoimmune disorders and malignant lymphoma, Cancer **31**:1092

Jones SE et al (1973) Non-Hodgkin's lymphomas. IV. Clinicopathologic correlation in 405 cases, Cancer **31**:806

Jones SR et al (1970) Sudden death in sickle-cell trait, N Eng! J Med **282**:323

Jonxis JHP and Huisman THJ (1968) A laboratory manual of abnormal hemoglobins, ed 2, Oxford, Blackwell Scientific Publishers, Ltd

Jordan GW (1966) Serum calcium and phosphorus abnormalities in leukemia, Am J Med **41**:381

Jordan HE (1942) Extramedullary blood production, Physiol Rev **22**:375

Jordan MC et al (1973) Spontaneous cytomegalovirus mononucleosis: clinical and laboratory observations in nine cases, Ann Intern Med **79**:153

Jordan SW and Larsen WE (1965) Ultrastructural studies of the May-Hegglin anomaly, Blood **25**:921

Jordans GH (1953) The familial occurrence of fat containing vacuoles in the leukocytes diagnosed in two brothers suffering from dystrophia musculorum progressiva, Acta Med Scand **145**:419

Jorpes E (1969) Robin Fåhraeus and the discovery of the erythrocyte sedimentation test, Acta Med Scand **185**:23

Joseph R (1925) Hochgrädige retikulo-endotheliale Monozytosen bei Endocarditis maligna, Dtsch Med Wochenschr **51**:863

Josephs BN et al (1962) Polycythemia secondary to hamartoma of the liver, JAMA **179**:867

Josephson AM et al (1958) Starch block electrophoretic studies of human hemoglobin solutions. II. Results in cord blood, thalassemia, and other hematologic disorders: comparison with Tiselius electrophoresis, Blood **13**:543

Josephson AM et al (1962) A new variant of hemoglobin M disease: hemoglobin M Chicago, J Lab Clin Med **59**:918

Josephson AS et al (1973) H chain fragment and monoclonal IgA in a lymphoproliferative disorder, Am J Med **54**:127

Joshua H et al (1970) The incidence of peroxidase and phospholipid deficiency in eosinophilic granulocytes among various Jewish groups in Israel, Am J Hum Genet **22**:574

Josso F et al (1975) A congenitally abnormal prothrombin: prothrombin Barcelona. In Hemker HC and Veltkamp JJ (Eds): Prothrombin and related coagulation factors, Leiden, Leiden University Press, p 199

Jounela AJ et al (1974) Drug-induced malabsorption of vitamin B_{12}. VI. Malabsorption of vitamin B_{12} during treatment with phenformin, Acta Med Scand **196**:267

Jue DL et al (1979) Hemoglobin Dunn: α6(A4) aspartic acid → asparagine, Hemoglobin **3**:137

Junquiera PC et al (1957) An example of A_x or A_m reactions in group AB, Vox Sang **2**:386

Kabat D (1972) Gene selection in hemoglobin and in antibody synthesizing cells, Science **175**:134

Kacian DL et al (1973) Decreased globin messenger RNA in thalassemia detected by molecular hybridization, Proc Natl Acad Sci **70**:1886

Kadin ME et al (1970) Isolated granulomas in Hodgkin's disease, N Engl J Med **283**:859

Kagan WA et al (1976) Aplastic anemia: Presence in human bone marrow of cells that suppress myelopoiesis, Proc Natl Acad Sci USA **73**:2890

Kagan WA et al (1979) Studies on the pathogenesis of aplastic anemia, Am J Med **66**:444

Kagimoto T et al (1978) A new hemoglobin variant hb Yatsushiro alpha 2A beta 260 val → leu, Biochim Biophys Acta **532**:195

Kahan BD and Reisfeld RA (1969) Transplantation antigens, Science **164**:514

Kahan J and Norén I (1975) Use of a lyophilized reference plasma to compare coagulation test procedures: Normotest, Simplastin-A, and Thrombotest, Thromb Diath Haemorrh **34**:426

Kahn A et al (1975) Gd(−) Abrami: a deficient G-6PD variant with hemizygous expression in blood cells of a woman with primary myelofibrosis, Humangenetik **30**:41

Kahn LB et al (1973) Giant lymph node hyperplasia with haematological abnormalities, S Afr Med J **47**:811

Kahn MJP (1975) Prothrombin Brussels. In Hemker HC and Veltkamp JJ (Eds): Prothrombin and related coagulation factors, Leiden, Leiden University Press, p 223

Kahn RA and Meryman HT (1976) Storage of platelet concentrates, Transfusion **16**:13

Kahn SB et al (1965) Methylmalonic acid excretion, a sensitive indicator of vitamin B_{12} deficiency in man, J Lab Clin Med **66**:75

Kakkar VV (1972) The diagnosis of deep vein thrombosis using the ^{125}I-fibrinogen test, Arch Surg **104**:152

Kakkar VV et al (1972) Efficacy of low doses of heparin in prevention of deep-vein thrombosis after major surgery, Lancet **2**:101

Kalendovsky Z et al (1975) Increased platelet aggregability in young patients with stroke: diagnosis and therapy, Arch Neurol **32**:13

Kalter RD et al (1979) Cardiopulmonary bypass: associated hemostatic abnormalities, J Thorac Cardiovasc Surg **77**:427

Kamel K et al (1970) Ethnological significance of hemoglobin alpha 2 beta 2 121 lys, Am J Phys Anthropol **26**:107

Kamuzora H et al (1974) A new haemoglobin variant hemoglobin J Birmingham alpha 120 (H3) ala → glu, Ann Clin Biochem **11**:53

Kan YW et al (1967) Hydrops fetalis with alpha thalassemia, N Engl J Med **276**:18

Kan YW et al (1972) Gamma-beta thalassemia: a cause of hemolytic disease of the newborn, N Engl J Med **286**:129

Kan YW et al (1974) Haemoglobin Constant Spring synthesis in red cell precursors, Br J Haematol **28**:103

Kan YW et al (1975) Successful application of prenatal diagnosis in a pregnancy at risk for homozygous β-thalassemia, N Engl J Med **292**:1096

Kan YW et al (1975) Demonstration of nonfunctional β-globin mRNA in homozygous β⁰-thalassemia, Proc Natl Acad Sci USA **72**:5140

Kan YW et al (1979) Molecular basis of hemoglobin-H disease in the Mediterranean population, Blood **54**:1434

Kao K-J et al (1980) The bleeding diathesis in human glycogen storage disease type I: in vitro identification of a naturally occurring inhibitor of ristocetin-induced platelet aggregation, Thromb Res **18**:683

Kao YS et al (1978) Anti-M in children with acute bacterial infections, Transfusion **18**:320

Kapadia SB and Kanbour AI (1979) Tumor-simulating retrorectal heterotopia of bone marrow, Am J Clin Pathol **72**:486

Kapadia SB et al (1980) Induced acute non-lymphocytic leukemia following long-term chemotherapy, Cancer **45**:1315

Kaplan E et al (1954) Sideroblasts: a study of stainable nonhemoglobin iron in marrow normoblasts, Blood **9**:203

Kaplan J et al (1974) Childhood lymphoblastic lymphoma, a cancer of thymus-derived lymphocytes, Cancer Res **34**:521

Kaplan KA et al (1977) Autologous blood transfusion during cardiac surgery, J Thorac Cardiovasc Surg **74**:4

Kaplan PM et al (1973) DNA polymerase associated with human hepatitis B antigen, J Virol **12**:995

Kaplow LS (1955) A histochemical procedure for localizing and evaluating leukocytic alkaline phosphatase activity in smears of blood and marrow, Blood **10**:1023

Kaplow LS (1963) Cytochemistry of leukocyte alkaline phosphatase. Use of complex naphthol AS phosphates in azo dye-coupling technics, Am J Clin Pathol **39**:439

Kaplow LS (1965) Simplified myeloperoxidase stain using benzidine dihyrochloride, Blood **26**:215

Kaplow LS (1968) Leukocyte alkaline phosphatase cytochemistry: applications and methods, Ann NY Acad Sci **155**:911

Kaplow LS (1975) Substitute for benzidine in myeloperoxidase stains, Am J Clin Pathol **63**:451

Kappas A and Granick S (1968) Steroid induction of porphyrin synthesis in liver cell culture. II. The effects of heme uridine diphosphate glucuronic acid, and inhibitors of nucleic acid and protein synthesis on the induction process, J Biol Chem **243**:346

Kappas A et al (1968) The regulation of porphyrin and heme synthesis, Semin hematol **5**:323

Karaylacin G et al (1971) Sea blue histiocyte in an octogenarian, Lancet **2**:318

Karayalcin G et al (1972) Pseudoneutropenia in Negroes. A normal phenomenon, NY State J Med **72**:1815

Karayalcin G et al (1973) Quantitative serum immunoglobulins in healthy Negroes, NY State J Med **73**:751

Karcher DS et al (1978) Malignant histiocytosis occurring in patients with acute lymphocytic leukemia, Cancer **41**:1967

Kardinal CG et al (1976) Chronic granulocytic leukemia: review of 536 cases, Arch Intern Med **136**:305

Karp JE et al (1978) Humoral factors in aplastic anemia: relationship of liver dysfunction to lack of serum stimulation of bone marrow growth in vitro, Blood **51**:397

Karpatkin MH and Karpatkin S (1960) In vitro and in vivo binding of factor VIII to human platelets. Thromb Diath Haemorrh **3**:129

Karpatkin S (1967) Studies on human platelet glycolysis. Effect of glycose, cyanide, insulin, citrate, and agglutination and contraction on platelet glycolysis, J Clin Invest **46**:409

Karpatkin S (1972) Human platlet senescence, Ann Rev Med **23**:953

Karpatkin S and Siskind GW (1969) In vitro detection of platelet antibody in patients with idiopathic thrombocytopenic purpura and systemic lupus erythematosus, Blood **33**:795

Karpatkin S et al (1972a) Detection of splenic antiplatlet antibody synthesis in idiopathic autoimmune thrombocytopenic purpura (ATP), Br J Haematol **23**:167

Karpatkin S et al (1972b) Cumulative experience in the detection of antiplatlet antibody in 234 patients with idiopathic thrombocytopenic purpura, systemic lupus erythematosus and other clinical disorders, Am J Med **52**:776

Karpatkin S and Garg SK (1974) The megathrombocyte as an index of platelet production, Br J Haematol **26**:307

Kasakura S and Lowestein LA (1965) A factor stimulating DNA synthesis derived from the medium of leukocyte cultures, Nature **208**:794

Kaslow RA and Masi AT (1978) Age, sex, and race effects on mortality from systemic lupus erythematosus in the United States, Arthritis Rheum **21**:473

Kasper CK and Kipnis SA (1972) Hepatitis and clotting-factor concentrates, JAMA **221**:510

Kasper CK et al (1975) Determinants of factor VIII recovery in cryoprecipitate, Transfusion **15**:312

Kasper CK (1975) Thromboembolic complications, Thromb Diath Haemorrh **33**:640

Kasper CK and Hemophilia Study Group (1979) Effect of prothrombin complex concentrates on factor VIII inhibitor levels, Blood **54**:1358

Kass L (1974a) Pink staining of perniciouis anemia megaloblasts by alizarin red S, Am J Clin Pathol **62**:511

Kass L (1974b) Megakaryocytes in the May-Hegglin anomaly, Arch Pathol **98**:112

Kass L (1975a) Origin and composition of Cabot rings in pernicious anemia, Am J Clin Pathol **64**:53

Kass L (1975b) Cytochemical abnormalities of atypical erythroblasts in acute erythremic myelosis, Acta Haematol **54**:321

Kass L (1977a) Esterase activity in erythroleukemia, Am J Clin Pathol **67**:368

Kass L (1977b) Periodic acid-Schiff-positive megaloblasts in pernicious anemia, Am J Clin Pathol **67**:371

Kass L (1977c) Biochemical abnormalities in chronic erythraemic myelosis, Br J Haematol **35**:169

Kass L (1979) Preleukemic disorders, Springfield, Ill, Charles C Thomas, Publishers

Kass L and Peters CL (1977) Nonspecific-esterase activity in pernicious anemia and chronic erythremic myelosis, Am J Clin Pathol **68**:273

Kass L and Schnitzer B (1975) Refractory anemia, Springfield, Ill, Charles C Thomas, Publishers

Katayama I and Finkel HE (1974) Leukemic reticuloendotheliosis. A clinicopathologic study with review of the literature, Am J Med **57**:115

Katayama I and Yang JPS (1979) Tartrate resistant acid phosphatase reactions not specific for hairy cell leukemia, Am J Clin Pathol **71**:482

Katayama I et al (1980) β-Lineage prolymphocytic leukemia as a distinct clinicopathologic entity, Am J Pathol **99**:399

Kattamis CA et al (1969) Favism: clinical and biochemical data, J Med Genet **6**:34

Kattlove HE et al (1969) Gaucher cells in chronic myelocytic leukemia: an acquired abnormality, Blood **33**:379

Kattlove HE et al (1970) Sea-blue indigestion, N Engl J Med **282**:630

Katz DH and Benacerraf B (1972) The regulatory influence of activated T cells on B cell responses to antigen, Adv Immunol **15**:1

Katz HI et al (1964) Indirect basophil degranulation test in penicillin allergy, JAMA **188**:351

Katz JH (1965) The delivery of iron to the immature red cell: a critical review, Ser Haematol **6**:15

Katz M et al (1972) Vitamin B_{12} malabsorption due to a biologically inert intrinsic factor, N Engl J Med **287**:425

Katz M et al (1974) Isolation and characterization of an abnormal intrinsic factor, J Clin Invest **53**:1274

Kaufman DB and Miller HC (1977) Ataxia telangiectasia: an autoimmune disease associated with a cytotoxic antibody to brain and thymus, Clin Immunol Immunopathol **7**:288

Kaufman RM et al (1965) Origin of pulmonary megakaryocytes, Blood **25**:767

Kaufman S et al (1978) Syndromes myéloprolifératifs familiaux: étude à propos de six familles et revue de la littérature, Nouv Rev Fr Hematol **20**:1

Kaufman RW et al (1969) Paroxysmal nocturnal hemoglobinuria terminating in acute granulocytic leukemia, Blood **33**:287

Kaunitz JD and Lindenbaum J (1977) The bioavailability of folic acid added to wine, Ann Intern Med **87**:542

Kay AB and Austen KF (1971) The IgE-mediated release of an eosinophil leukocyte chemotactic factor from human lung, J Immunol **107**:899

Kay AB and Austen KF (1972) Chemotaxis of human basophil leukocytes, Clin Exp Immunol **11**:557

Kay AB et al (1971) An eosinophil leukocyte chematactic factor of anaphylaxis, J Exp Med **133**:602

Kay HE (1971) Lymphocyte function, Br J Haematol **20**:139

Kaywin P et al (1978) Platelet function in essential thrombocythemia: decreased epinephrine responsiveness associated with a deficiency of platelet α-adrenergic receptors, N Engl J Med **299**:505

Kazazian HG Jr and Woodhead AP (1973) Hemoglobin A synthesis in the developing fetus, N Engl J Med **289**:58

Keeling MM et al (1971) Hemoglobin Louisville (beta 42 [CD1] phe → leu): an unstable variant causing mild hemolytic anemia, J Clin Invest **50**:2395

Keeling M et al (1974) Avascular necrosis and erythrocytosis in sickle-cell trait, N Engl J Med **290**:442

Keitt AS (1966) Pyruvate kinase deficiency and related disorders of red cell glycolysis, Am J Med **41**:762

Keitt AS (1972) Hereditary methemoglobinemia with deficiency of NADH-methemoglobin reductase. In Stanbury JB et al (Eds): The metabolic basis of inherited disease, New York, McGraw-Hill Book Co, Inc, p 1389

Keitt AS et al (1966) Red-cell ''pseudomosaicism'' in congenital methemoglobinemia, N Engl J Med **275**:398

Kelemen E (1973) Granulocyte alkaline phosphatase activity: a measure of the emergence time of mature marrow neutrophils, Acta Haematol **50**:19

Keleman E et al (1977) Chronic idiopathic myelofibrosis. A reversible disease? Acta Haematol **57**:171

Keller AJ et al (1979) Coagulation abnormalities produced by plasma exchange on the cell separator with special reference to fibrinogen and platelet levels, Br J Haematol **42**:593

Keller AR et al (1968) Correlation of histopathology with other prognostic indicators in Hodgkin's disease, Cancer **22**:487

Keller AR et al (1972) Hyaline-vascular and plasma-cell types of giant lymph node hyperplasia of the mediastinum and other locations, Cancer **29**:670

Keller HU et al (1975) Physiology of chemotaxis and random motility, Semin Hematol **12**:47

Kellermeyer RW (1967) Inflammatory process in acute gouty arthritis. III. Vascular permeability enhancing activity in normal human synovial fluid; induction by Hageman Factor activators; and inhibition by Hageman Factor antiserum, J Lab Clin Med **70**:372

Kelly MT and White A (1974) An inhibitor of histamine release from human leukocytes, J Clin Invest **53**:1343

Kelly P and Penner JA (1976) Antihemophilic factor inhibitors: management with prothrombin complex concentrates, JAMA **236**:2061

Kelton JG et al (1980) Sex-related differences in platelet aggregation: influence of the hematocrit, Blood **56**:38

Kendall AG et al (1973a) Haemoglobin J Nyanza: alpha 21 (B2) ala → asp, Biochim Biophys Acta **310**:357

Kendall AG et al (1973b) Hemoglobin Kenya, the product of a γ-b fusion gene; studies of the family, Am J Hum Genet **25**:548

Kendall AG et al (1977) Hb Vaasa or alpha 2 beta 2 (39 [C5] gln → glu), a mildly unstable variant found in a Finnish family, Hemoglobin **1**:292

Kennedy BJ (1962) Stimulation of erythropoiesis by androgenic hormones, Ann Intern Med **57**:917

Kennedy CC et al (1974) Haemoglobin Belfast 15 (A12) tryptophan → arginine: a new unstable haemoglobin variant, Br Med J **4**:324

Kernoff PB et al (1972) Severe allergic pulmonary oedema after plasma transfusion, Br J Haematol **23**:777

Kernoff PB et al (1974) A variant of factor VIII related antigen, Br J Haematol **26**:435

Kerr CB (1965) Genetics of human blood coagulation, J Med Genet **2**:254

Kerr RO et al (1972) Two mechanisms of erythrocyte destruction in penicillin-induced hemolytic anemia, N Engl J Med **287**:1322

Kersey JH and Gajl-Peczalska KJ (1975) T and B lymphocytes in humans, Am J Pathol **81**:446

Kersey J et al (1975) Evidence for origin of certain childhood acute lymphoblastic leukemias and lymphomas in thymus-derived lymphocytes, Cancer **36**:1348

Kevorkian J and Marra JJ (1964) Transfusion of human corpse blood without additives, Transfusion **4**:112

Keyloun VE and Grace WJ (1966) Acute hemolytic anemia complicating infectious mononucleosis, NY State J Med **66**:273

Khaleeli M et al (1973) Sideroblastic anemia in multiple myeloma: a preleukemic change, Blood **41**:17

Khan I et al (1975) Microthrombocytosis and platelet fragmentation associated with idiopathic/autoimmune thrombocytopenic purpura, Br J Haematol **31**:449

Khumbanonda M et al (1969) Coombs' positive hemolytic anemia in myelofibrosis with myeloid metaplasia, Am J Med Sci **258**:89

Kiang S and Choa GH (1949) The blood picture in leprosy, Am J med Sci **217**:269

Kiel FW (1969) Blood substitutes in the Soviet Union: a review, Transfusion **6**:213

Kikushi G et al (1958) The enzymatic synthesis of δ-aminolevulinic acid, J Biol Chem **233**:1214

Killmann S-A et al (1964) Mitotic indices of human bone marrow cells. III. Duration of some phases of erythrocytic and granulocytic proliferation computed from mitotic indices, Blood **24**:267

Kilmartin JV and Rossi-Bernardi L (1973) Interaction of hemoglobin with hydrogen ions, carbon dioxide, and organic phosphates, Physiol Rev **53**:836

Kilpatrick ZM and Katz J (1969) Occult celiac disease as a cause of iron-deficiency anemia, JAMA **208**:999

Kimber CL et al (1965) The mechanism of anemia in chronic liver disease, Q J Med **34**:33

King MAR et al (1972) An unstable haemoglobin with reduced oxygen affinity: haemoglobin Peterborough, beta III (G13) valine → phenylalanine; its interaction with normal haemoglobin and with haemoglobin Lepore, Br J Haematol **22**:125

Kingdon HS et al (1975) Potentially thrombogenic materials in factor IX concentrates, Thromb Diath Haemorrh **33**:617

Kingdon HS and Lundblad RL (1975) Biochemistry of factor IX. In Brinkhous KM and Hemker HC (Eds): Handbook of hemophilia, New York, American Elsevier Publishing Co, Inc

Kingdon HS et al (1975) Potentially thrombogenic materials in factor IX concentrates, Thromb Diath Haemorrh **33**:617

Kinney TR et al (1977) Bone marrow necrosis in children: three instances, Clin Pediatr **16**:565

Kiraly JF III and Wheby MS (1976) Bone marrow necrosis, Am J Med **60**:361

Kirchen ME and Marshall GJ (1976) Marrow storage cells: an ultrastructural study, J Reticuloendothel Soc **19**:109

Kirkpatrick CH and Gallin JI (1975) The chemotactic activity in dialyzable transfer factor. II. Further characterization of the activity in vivo and in vitro. In Bellanti JA and Dayton DH (Eds): The phagocytic cell in host resistance, New York, Raven Press

Kirkpatrick CH et al (1968) Hypogammaglobulinemia with nodular lymphoid hyperplasia of the small bowel, Arch Intern Med **121**:273

Kirov SM et al (1980) Characterization of null cells in chronic lymphocytic leukaemia with B-cell allo- and hetero-antisera, Br J Haematol **44**:235

Kirshbaum BA et al (1967) The basophil degranulation test: a review of the literature, Am J Med Sci **253**:473

Kirtland HH et al (1980) Methyldopa inhibition of suppressor-lymphocyte function. A proposed cause of autoimmune hemolytic anemia, N Engl J Med **302**:825

Kisiel W et al (1977) Activation of Factor VII (Proconvertin) by factor XIIa (activated Hageman factor), Biochemistry **16**:4189

Kissmeyer-Nielsen F et al (1972) The HL-A system in clinical medicine, Johns Hopkins Med J **131**:385

Kistler GS et al (1973) Hepatitis B antigen (HBAg, Australia antigen) in mixed saliva of patients with HB antigenemia, Pathol Microbiol (Basel) **39**:313

Kitahama M et al (1957) On the peculiar group B blood cells, Jpn J Legal Med **11**:952

Kitchen H et al (1964) Hemoglobin polymorphism: its relation to sickling of erythrocytes in white-tailed deer, Science **144**:1237

Kitchen H et al (1968) Structural comparison of polymorphic hemoglobins of deer with those of sheep and other species, J Biol Chem **243**:1204

Kitchens CS (1977) The syndrome of post-splenectomy fulminant sepsis. Case report and review of the literature, Am J Med Sci **274**:303

Kitchens CS (1980) Occult hemophilia, John Hopkins Med J **146**:255

Kjeldsberg CR et al (1974) Spurious thrombocytopenia, JAMA **227**:628

Kjeldsberg CR et al (1980) Prolymphocytic leukemia. An ultrastructural study, Am J Clin Pathol **73**:150

Kjellström T et al (1979) Familial monocytic leukaemia: a report of two families, Scand J Haematol **23**:272

Klebanoff SJ (1970) Myeloperoxidase: contribution of the microbicidal activity of intact leukocytes, Science **169**:1095

Klebanoff SJ and Clark RA (1978) The neutrophil: function and clinical disorders, Amsterdam, North Holland Publishing Co

Kleckner HB et al (1975) Hemoglobin Fort Gordon or alpha 2 beta 2 145 tyr → asp, a new high-oxygen affinity hemoglobin variant, Biochim Biophys Acta **400**:343

Klee GG and O'Sullivan MB (1979) Screening versus diagnostic differential leukocyte counts. In Koepke JA (Ed): Differential leukocyte counting, Skokie, Ill, College of American Pathologists, p 69

Kleihauer EF et al (1968) Hemoglobin Bibba or alpha 2 136 pro beta 2, an unstable alpha chain abnormal hemoglobin, Biochim Biophys Acta **154**:220

Kleihauer E et al (1971) Hb Tübingen, eine neue beta-kettenvariante (beta Tp 10-12) mit erhöhter Spontanoxydation, Klin Wochenschr **49**:651

Kleihauer E (1974) Determination of fetal hemoglobin: elution technique. In Schmidt RM et al (Eds): The detection of hemoglobinopathies, Cleveland, CRC Press

Kleihauer E and Betke K (1963) Elution procedure for the demonstration of methaemoglobin in red cells of human blood smears, Nature **199**:1196

Kleihauer E et al (1957) Demonstration von fetalem Hämoglobin in den Erythrocyten eines Blutausstrichs, Klin Wochenschr **35**:637

Klein E et al (1968) Surface IgM-kappa specificity on a Burkitt lymphoma cell in vivo and in derived culture lines, Cancer Res **28**:1300

Klein PD and Seegers WH (1950) The nature of plasma antithrombin activity, Blood **5**:742

Klein RB et al (1977) Decreased mononuclear and polymorphonuclear chemotaxis in human newborns, infants, and young children, Pediatrics **60**:467

Klemola E et al (1969) Cytomegalovirus mononucleosis in previously healthy individuals. Five new cases and follow-up of 13 previously published cases, Ann intern Med **71**:11

Klipstein FA (1972) Folate in tropical sprue, Br J Haematol **23**:119

Kloeze J (1969) Relationship between chemical structure and platelet-aggregation activity of prostaglandins, Biochim Biophys Acta **187**:285

Knisley MH (1936) Spleen studies. I. Microscopic observations of the circulatory system of living unstimulated mammalian spleens, Anat Rec **65**:23

Knisley MH (1960) Some categories of blood rheology. In Copley AL and Stainsby G (Eds): Flow properties of blood and other biological systems, New York, Pergamon Press, Inc

Knoblich R (1960) Extramedullary hematopoiesis presenting as intrathoracic tumors, Cancer **13**:462

Knodell RG et al (1977) Development of chronic liver disease after acute non-A, non-B post-transfusion hepatitis: role of γ-globulin prophylaxis in its prevention, Gastroenterology **72**:902

Knospe WH and Gregory SA (1971) Smoldering acute leukemia: clinical and cytogenetic studies in six patients, Arch Intern Med **127**:910

Knowles DM II and Holck S (1978) Tissue localization of T-lymphocytes by the histochemical demonstration of acid α-naphthyl acetate esterase, Lab Invest **39**:70

Knudson AG Jr and Kaplan WD (1962) Genetics of the sphingolipidoses. In Aronson SM and Volk BW (Eds): Cerebral sphingolipidoses, New York, Academic Press, Inc

Knuth A et al (1979) Hemoglobin Moabit: alpha 86 (F7) leu → arg. A new unstable abnormal hemoglobin, Acta Haematol **61**:121

Ko HS et al (1976) Amyloid lymphadenopathy, Ann Intern Med **85**:763

Knutti RE and Hawkins WB (1935) *Bartonella* incidence in splenectomized bile fistula dogs, J Exp Med **61**:115

Kocher T (1883) Ueber Kropfexstirpation und ihre Folgen, Arch Klin Chir **29**:254

Koch-Weser J and Sellers EM (1971) Drug interactions with coumarin anticoagulants, N Engl J Med **285**:487

Koenig HM (1976) Classification of microcytic anemia by fluorometric analysis of free erythrocyte porphyrins (FEP), Ann Clin Res **8**(supp 17):151

Koenig RJ et al (1976a) Hemoglobin A_{Ic} as an indicator of the glucose intolerance in diabetes, Diabetes **25**:230

Koenig RJ et al (1976b) The correlation of glucose regulation and hemoglobin A_{Ic} in diabetes mellitus, N Engl J Med **295**:417

Koepke JA et al (1975) A comparison of platelet production methods suitable for a service-oriented blood donor center, Transfusion **15**:39

Koepke JA (Ed) (1979) Differential leukocyte counting, Skokie, Ill, College of American Pathologists

Koerper MA and Dallman PR (1977) Serum iron concentration and transferrin saturation in the diagnosis of iron deficiency in children: normal developmental changes, J Pediatr **91**:870

Kohne E et al (1975) Hb M Erlangen: alpha 2 beta 2 63 (E7) tyr. Eine neue Mutation mit Hämolyse and Diaphorasemangel, Z Kinderheilkd **120**:69

Kohne E et al (1976) Structural and functional characteristics of the hb Tübingen: beta 106 (G8) leu → gln, FEBS Lett **64**:443

Kohne E et al (1977) Hb M Milwaukee in a German family, Hemoglobin **1**:759

Kolb WP and Granger GA (1968) Lymphocyte in vitro cytotoxicity: characterization of human lymphotoxin, Proc Natl Acad Sci USA **61**:1250

Koler RD et al (1973) Hemoglobin Casper: beta 106 (G8) leu → pro, a contemporary mutation, Am J Med **55**:549

Kolhouse JF et al (1978) Cobalamin analogues are present in human plasma and can mask cobalamin deficiency because current radioisotope dilution assays are not specific for true cobalamin, N Engl J Med **299**:785

Kolk-Vegter AJ et al (1975) Some problems concerning the assay of erythropoietin using the haemagglutination inhibition kit, Br J Haematol **30**:371

Koller F (1966) Importance of coagulation besides haemostasis, Acta Haematol **36**:133

Koller M-E et al (1978) The diagnosis of iron deficiency by erythrocyte protoporphyrin and serum ferritin analyses, Acta Paediatr Scand **67**:361

Kolodny EH (1972) Clinical and biochemical genetics of the lipidoses, Semin Hematol **9**:251

Kolodny EH (1976) Lysosomal storage diseases, N Engl J Med **294**:1217

Komiya M et al (1972) Bovine prekallikrein activator with functional activity as Hageman factor, J Biochem **72**:1205

Komninos ZD et al (1965) Folic acid deficiency in hereditary spherocytosis, Arch Intern Med **115**:663

Konotey-Ahulu FID et al (1968) Haemoglobin Korle-Bu (beta 73 aspartic acid → asparagine) showing one of the two amino acid substitutions of haemoglobin C Harlem, J Med Genet **5**:107

Konotey-Ahulu FID et al (1971) Haemoglobin Osu-Christiansborg: a new beta chain variant of haemoglobin A (beta 52 [D3] aspartic acid → asparagine) in combination with haemoblogin S, J Med Genet **8**:302

Konotey-Ahulu FID (1974) The sickle cell disease. Clinical manifestations including the "sickle crisis," Arch Intern Med **133**:611

Kontras SB and Bass JC (1969) Chronic granulomatous disease, Lancet **2**:646

Kopp WL et al (1967) Hyperviscosity syndrome in multiple myeloma, Am J Med **43**:141

Kornfeld S and Kornfeld R (1969) Solubilization and partial characterization of a phytohemagglutinin receptor site from human erythrocytes, Proc Natl Acad Sci USA **63**:1439

Korn D (1960) Demonstration of cystine crystals in peripheral white blood cells in a patient with cystinosis, N Engl J Med **262**:545

Korpman RA and Bull BS (1976) The implementation of a robust estimator of the mean for quality control on a programmable calculator or a laboratory computer, Am J Clin Pathol **65**:252

Korsan-Bengtsen K et al (1962) Acquired factor X deficiency in a patient with amyloidosis, Throm Diath Haemorrh **7**:558

Korst DR et al (1958) Assay of erythropoietic factor using radio-iron uptake in the nitrogen mustard treated rat, J Lab Clin Med **52**:364

Kostmann R (1956) Infantile genetic agranulocytosis (agranulocytosis infantilis hereditaria); new recessive lethal disease in man, Acta Paediatr **45**(supp 105):1

Kough RH and Makary AZ (1978) Chronic lymphocytic leukemia (CLL) terminating in multiple myeloma: report of two cases, Blood **52**:532

Kowalski E (1968) Fibrinogen derivatives and their biologic activity, Sem Hematol **5**:45

Krajny M and Pruzanski W (1976) Waldenström's macroglobulinaemia: review of 45 cases, Can Med Assoc J **114**:899

Kramer JW et al (1977) The Chediak-Higashi syndrome of cats, Lab Invest **36**:555

Krantz SB (1973) Annotation: pure red cell aplasia, Br J Haematol **25**:1

Krantz SB and Jacobson LO (1970) Erythropoietin and the regulation of erythropoiesis, Chicago, University of Chicago Press

Krantz SB and Kao V (1967) Studies on red cell aplasia. I. Demonstration of a plasma inhibitor to heme synthesis and an antibody to erythroblast nuclei, Proc Natl Acad Sci USA **58**:493

Krantz SB and Kao V (1969) Studies on red cell aplasia. II. Report of a second patient with an antibody to erythroblast nuclei and a remission after immunosuppressive therapy, Blood **34**:1

Krantz SB et al (1973) Studies on red cell aplasia V. Presence of erythroblast cytotoxicity in G-globulin fraction of plasma, J Clin Invest **52**:324

Kraus AP and Diggs LW (1956) In vivo crystallization of hemoglobin occurring in citrated blood from patients with hemoglobin C, J Lab Clin Med **47**:700

Kraus AP et al (1965) A new variety of sickle cell anemia with clinically mild symptoms due to an alpha-chain variant of hemoglobin (alpha 23 glu NH2), J Lab Clin Med **66**:886

Kraus AP et al (1967) Hemoglobin Memphis/S. A new variant of sickle cell anemia, Trans Assoc Am Physicians **80**:297

Krause JR (1977) Acquired factor X deficiency and amyloidosis, Am J Clin Pathol **67**:170

Krause JR and Stolc V (1979) Serum ferritin and bone marrow iron stores. I. Correlation with absence of iron in biopsy specimens, Am J Clin Pathol **72**:817

Krause JR et al (1979) Comparison of stainable iron in aspirated and needle-biopsy specimens of bone marrow, Am J Clin Pathol **72**:68

Krause WH et al (1973) Congenital dysfibrinogenemia (fibrinogen Giessen), Thromb Diath Haemorrh **29**:547

Krause WH et al (1975) Hypodysfibrinogenämie: Fibrinogen Giessen III, Klin Wochenschr **53**:781

Krauss S and Sokal JE (1966) Paraproteinemia in the lymphomas, Am J Med **40**:400

Krauss S et al (1964) Comparison of Philadelphia chromosome-positive and -negative patients with chronic myelocytic leukemia, Ann Intern Med **61**:625

Kravitz H et al (1956) Methemoglobin values in premature and mature infants and children, Am J Dis Child **91**:1

Krevans JR and Jackson DP (1955) Hemorrhagic disorder following massive blood transfusions, JAMA **159**:171

Krill CE et al (1964) Chronic idiopathic granulocytopenia, N Engl J Med **270**:973

Krishnan EU et al (1978) Congenital hypoplastic anemia terminating in acute promyelocytic leukemia, Pediatrics **61**:898

Kriss JP et al (1964) Isolation and identification of the long-acting thryoid stimulator and its relation to hyperthyroidism and circumscribed pretibial myxedema, J Clin Endocrinol **24**:1005

Kristensen HP and Gormsen H (1958) Vitamin B_{12} deficiency in uncharacteristic macrocytic anaemia: comparison of bone marrow findings and vitamin B_{12} level in plasma, Acta Med Scand **162**:415

Kristensson K and Sourander P (1966) Occurrence of lipofuscin in inherited metabolic disorders affecting the nervous system, J Neurol Neurosurg Psychiat **29**:113

Krivit W and Good RA (1959) Aldrich's syndrome (thrombocytopenia, eczema, and infection in infants: studies of the defense mechanisms, Am J Dis Child **97**:137

Krivit W et al (1966) Platelet survival studies in Aldrich syndrome, Pediatrics **37**:339

Krizsa F et al (1977) Specific thrombopoietic inhibition by syngeneic platelet homogenates, Biomedicine **27**:145

Kroe D et al (1963) The influence of amino acids on iron absorption, Blood **21**:546

Kropatkin ML and Izak G (1968) Studies on the hypercoagulable state: the regulation of fibrinogen production in experimental hyper- and hypo-fibrinogenemia, Thromb Diath Haemorrh **19**:547

Krugers Dagneaux PGLC et al (1968) Investigations on an immunoassay of erythropoietin, Ann NY Acad Sci **149**:294

Krugman S et al (1967) Infectious hepatitis, JAMA **200**:365

Krugman S et al (1979) viral hepatitis, Type B; studies on natural history and prevention re-examined, N Engl J Med **300**:101

Krumbhaar EB (1936) Pre-Columbian tibia exhibiting syphilitic (?) periostitis with recognizable varieties of bone marrow cells, Ann Med Hist **8**:232

Kryger M et al (1978) Treatment of excessive polycythemia of high altitude with respiratory stimulant drugs, Am Rev Respir Dis **117**:455

Kubasik NP et al (1979) Storage and stability of folate and vitamin B-12 in plasma and blood samples, Clin Chim Acta **95**:147

Kudryk B et al (1976) Fibrinogen Detroit—an abnormal fibrinogen with non-functional NH_2-terminal polymerization domain, Thromb Res **9**:25

Kuis-Reerink JD et al (1976) Hb Volga or alpha 2 beta 2 27 (B9) ala → asp: an unstable hemoglobin variant in three generations of a Dutch family, Biochim Biophys Acta **439**:63

Kumpati JA et al (1978) Interaction between human hemoglobin variants and hemoglobin S, Proc Soc Exp Biol Med **157**:250

Kunkel HG et al (1969) Genetic marker of the gamma-A_2 subgroup of gamma-A immunoglobulins, Nature **223**:1247

Kunkel HG et al (1970) Genetic variants of γG4 globulin. A unique relationship of other classes of γG globulins, J Exp Med **132**:508

Kurachi S et al (1973) Structure of haemoglobin Seattle, Nature (New Biol) **243**:275

Kuramoto A et al (1970) Lack of platelet response to stimulation in the Wiskott-Aldrich syndrome, N Engl J Med **282**:475

Kurczinski EM and Penner JA (1974) Activated prothrombin concentrate for patients with factor VIII inhibitors, N Engl J Med **291**:164

Kurland J and Moore MAS (1977) Modulation of hemopoiesis by prostaglandins, Exp Hematol **5**:357

Kurnick JE et al (1971) In vitro granulocytic colony-forming potential of bone marrow from patients with granulocytopenia and aplastic anemia, Proc Soc Exp Biol Med **137**:917

Kurstjens R et al (1968) Familial thrombopathic thrombocytopenia, Br J Haematol **15**:305

Kurth D et al (1969) Circulating siderocytes in human subjects, Blood **34**:754

Kushner JP et al (1971) Idiopathic refractory sideroblastic anemia: clinical and laboratory investigation of 17 patients and review of the literature, Medicine (Baltimore) **50**:139

Kutti J et al (1980) Plasma beta-thromboglobulin values in thrombocytopenic patients with acute leukemia, Am J Hematol **8**:339

Kwaan HC et al (1972) Increased platelet aggregation in diabetes mellitus, J Lab Clin Med **80**:236

Kyle RA (1975) Multiple myeloma: review of 869 cases, Mayo Clin Proc **50**:29

Kyle RA and Bayrd ED (1965) "Benign" monoclonal gammapathy: a potentialy malignant condition? Am J Med **40**:426

Kyle RA and Bayrd ED (1975) Amyloidosis: review of 236 cases, Medicine **54**:271

Kyle RA and Linman JW (1968) Chronic idiopathic neutropenia: a newly recognized entity? N Engl J Med **279**:1015

Kyle RA and Pease GL (1965) Hematologic aspects of arsenic intoxication, N Engl J Med **273**:18

Laake K and Österud B (1974) Activation of purified plasma factor VII by human plasmin, plasma kallikrein, and activated components of the human intrinsic blood coagulation system, Thromb Res **5**:759

Laan B ter et al (1974) Interaction of human anaphylatoxin C3a with rat mast cells demonstrated by immunofluorescence, Eur J Immunol **4**:393

Labie D et al (1966) The amino acid sequence of the δ-β chains of hemoglobin Lepore$_{Augusta}$ = Lepore$_{Washington}$, Biochim Biophys Acta **127**:428

Labossiere A et al (1971) A new beta Tp V hemoglobin variant: hb Edmonton, Clin Biochem **4**:114

Labossiere A et al (1972) Hemoglobin Deer Lodge: alpha 2 beta 2 2 His → arg, Clin Biochem **5**:46

Lace JK et al (1975) An appraisal of the nitroblue tetrazolium reduction test, Am J Med **58**:685

Lackner H et al (1970) Abnormal fibrin ultrastructure, polymerization, and clot retraction in multiple myeloma, Br J Haematol **18**:625

Lacombe M et al (1973) Fibrinogen Montreal. A new case of congenital dysfibrinogenemia with defective aggregation monomers, Thromb Diath Haemorrh **29**:536

Lagarde M et al (1978) Impairment of platelet thromboxane A_2 generation and of the platelet release reaction in two patients with congenital deficiency of platelet cyclo-oxygenase, Br J Haematol **38**:251

Lajtha LG (1964) Recent studies in erythroid differentiation and proliferation, Medicine (Baltimore) **43**:625

Lajtha LG (1975) Haemopoietic stem cells, Br J Haematol **29**:529

Lake AM et al (1977) Vitamin E deficiency and enhanced platelet function: reversal following E supplementation, J Pediatr **90**:722

Lake-Lewin D et al (1975) Metastatic tumor in bone-marrow biopsy, NY State J Med **75**:1008

Laki K (1968) Fibrinogen, New York, Marcel Dekker, Inc

Laki K (1974) Fibrinogen and metastases, J Med **5**:32

Lala PK and Johnson GR (1978) Monoclonal origin of B lymphocyte colony-forming cells in spleen colonies formed by multipotential hemopoietic stem cells, J Exp Med **148**:1468

Lalezari P and Spaet TH (1959) Studies on the genetics of leukocyte antigens, Blood **14**:748

Lalezari P et al (1960) Neonatal neutropenia due to maternal isoimmunization, Blood **15**:236

Lalezari P et al (1975) Chronic autoimmune neutropenia due to anti-Na$_2$ antibody, N Engl J Med **293**:744

Lam H et al (1977) Hemoglobin Alamo (alpha 2 beta 2 19 [B1] asn $\rightarrow$ asp), Hemoglobin **1**:703

Lamerton LF (1976) Concluding address. In Cairnie AB et al (Eds): Stem cells of renewing cell populations, New York, Academic Press, Inc

Lamon JM et al (1979) Family evaluations in acute intermittent porphyria using red cell uroporphyrinogen I synthetase, J Med Genet **16**:134

Lampasso JA (1968) Changes in hematologic values induced by storage of ethylenediaminetetraacetate human blood for varying periods of time, Am J Clin Pathol **49**:443

Lampert F (1969) Akute lymphoblastische Leukämie bei Geschwistern mit progressiver Kleinhirnataxie (Louis-Bar-Syndrome), Dtsch Med Wochenschr **94**:217

Lampkin BC and Schubert WK (1968) Pernicious anemia in the second decade of life, J Pediatr **72**:387

Lamy J (1973) Hyperhaptoglobinemie des alcooliques chroniques, Clin Chim Acta **46**:257

Lamy M et al (1960) L'absence congénitale de β-lipoproteines, C R Soc Biol (Paris) **154**:1974

Lance EM (1970) The selective action of antilymphocyte serum on recirculating lymphocytes: a review of the evidence and alternatives, Clin Exp Immunol **6**:789

Landau M (1933) Microsedimentation (Linzenmeier-Raunent method), Am J Dis Child **45**:691

Landaw SA et al (1970) Catabolism of heme in vivo: comparison of the simultaneous production of bilirubin and carbon monoxide, J Clin Invest **49**:914

Lander H et al (1965) Reduced platelet survival in patients with Star-Edwards prostheses, Br Med J **1**:688

Landsteiner K (1901) Ueber Agglutinationserscheinungen normalen menschlichen Blutes, Wien Klin Wochenschr **14**:1132

Landsteiner K and Chase MW (1940) Studies on the sensitization of animals with simple chemical compounds. VII. Skin sensitization by intraperitoneal injection, J Exp Med **71**:237

Landsteiner K and Levine P (1927) Further observations on individual differences of human blood, Proc Soc Exp Biol Med **24**:941

Landsteiner K and Wiener As (1940) Agglutinable factor in human blood recognized by immune sera for rhesus blood, Proc Soc Exp Biol Med **43**:223

Lane DA et al (1980) Dysfibrinogenaemia characterized by abnormal fibrin monomer polymerization and normal fibrinopeptide A release, Br J Haematol **44**:483

Lane TA and Windle B (1979) Granulocyte concentrate function during preservation: effect of temperature, Blood **54**:216

Lang A et al (1972) Identification of haemoglobin C Georgetown, Biochim Biophys Acta **278**:57

Langaney A and Pison G (1975) Probability of paternity: useless, Am J Hum Genet **27**:558

Lange RD et al (1954) Leukemia in atomic bomb survivors. I. General observations, Blood **9**:574

Lange RD et al (1955) Refractory anemia occurring in survivors of the atomic bombing in Nagasaki, Japan, Blood **10**:312

Lange RD et al (1968a) Use of silicone rubber membrane enclosures for preparation of erythropoietin assay mice, Ann NY Acad Sci **149**:34

Lange RD et al (1968b) Application of erythropoietin antisera to studies of erythropoiesis, Ann NY Acad Sci **149**:281

Lange RD et al (1969) Antisera to erythropoietin: partial characterization of two different antibodies, J Lab Clin Med **73**:78

Lange RD et al (1971) The hemagglutination-inhibition assay for erythropoietin: its specificity, reproducibility and sensitivity, Israel J Med Sci **7**:861

Langer EE et al (1972) Erythrocyte protoporphyrin, Blood **40**:112

Langevoort HL et al (1970) The nomenclature of mononuclear cells: Proposal for a new classification. In Van Furth R (Ed): Mononuclear phagocytes, Philadelphia, FA Davis Co

Langley GR and Felderhof CH (1968) Atypical autohemolysis in hereditary spherocytosis as a reflection of two cell populations: relationship of cell lipids to conditioning by the spleen, Blood **32**:569

Lanzkowsky P (1961) The influence of maternal iron-deficiency anemia on the haemoglobin of the infant, Arch Dis Child **36**:205

Lanzkowsky P (1970) Congenital malabsorption of folate, Am J Med **48**:580

Lanzkowsky P et al (1965) Pelger-Huët anomaly of the granulocytes in a Cape colored family, J Pediatr **67**:826

Lanzkowsky P et al (1978) Partial exchange transfusion in sickle cell anemia: use in children with serious complications, J Dis Child **132**:1206

Lappat EJ and Cawein MJ (1968) A familial study of procainamide-induced systemic lupus erythematosus: a question of pharmacogenetic polymorphism, Am J Med **45**:846

Larkin ILM et al (1968) Haemoglobin F Texas II (alpha 2 gamma 2 6 glu $\rightarrow$ lys). The second of the haemoglobin F Texas variants, Br J Haematol **14**:233

Larrieu MJ et al (1972) Comparative effects of fibrinogen degradation fragments D and E on coagulation, Br J Haematol **22**:719

Larrimer JH et al (1975) Howell-Jolly bodies. A clue to splenic infarction, Arch Intern Med **135**:857

Larsson SO (1957) Anemia and iron metabolism in hypothyroidism, Acta Med Scand **157**:349

Laszlo J (1975) Myeloproliferative disorders (MPD): myelofibrosis, myelosclerosis, extramedullary hematopoiesis, undifferentiated MPD, and hemorrhagic thrombocythemia, Semin Hematol **12**:409

Laszlo J et al (1969) Effects of hyperbaric oxygenation on sickle syndromes, South Med J **62**:453

Lauer JL et al (1979) Transmission of hepatitis B virus in clinical laboratory areas, J Infect Dis **140**:513

Laurell CB (1966) Quantitative estimation of proteins by electrophoresis in agarose gel containing antibodies, Ann Biochem **15**:45

Laurell CB (1972) Electroimmunoassay, Scand J Clin Lab Invest **29**(supp 124):21

Law IP et al (1976) Acute myelomonocytic leukemia associated with paraproteinemia, Cancer **37**:1359

Lawlor E et al (1979) Acute myeloid leukaemia occurring in untreated chronic lymphatic leukaemia, Br J Haematol **43**:369

Lawrence HS (1969) Transfer factor, Adv Immunol **11**:195

Lawrence HS (1970) Transfer factor and cellular immune deficiency disease, N Engl J Med **283**:411

Lawrence HS (1974) Transfer factor in cellular immunity. In Harvey Lectures, Series 68, New York, Academic Press, Inc

Lawrence HS and Valentine FT (1970) Transfer factor and other mediators of cellular immunity, Am J Pathol **437**:1970

Lawrence HS et al (1960) Transfer of delayed hypersensitivity to skin homografts with leukocyte extracts in man, J Clin Invest **39**:185

Lawrence JH (1955) Polycythemia: physiology, diagnosis, and

treatment based on 303 cases, New York, Grune & Stratton, Inc

Lawrence JH et al (1969) Leukemia in polycythemia vera. Relationship to splenic myeloid metaplasia and therapeutic radiation dose, Ann Intern Med **70**:763

Lawrence JS (1964) Irradiation leukemogenesis, JAMA **190**:1049

Lawrence R Jr et al (1980) Eosinophilia in the hospitalized neonate, Ann Allerg **44**:349

Lawson DH et al (1970) Hypokalemia in megaloblastic anemias, Lancet **2**:588

Lay WH et al (1971) Binding of sheep red blood cells to a large population of human lymphocytes, Nature **230**:531

Layrisse M et al (1973) Iron fortification of food: its measurement by the extrinsic tag method, Blood **41**:333

Leader RW et al (1963) Studies of abnormal leukocyte bodies in the mink, Blood **22**:477

Leavey RA et al (1970) Disseminated intravascular coagulation—a complication of chemotherapy in acute myelomonocytic leukemia, Cancer **26**:142

Leblond PF et al (1978a) Erythrocyte populations in pyruvate kinase deficiency anaemia following splenectomy. I. Cell morphology, Br J Haematol **39**:55

Leblond PF et al (1978b) Erythrocyte populations in pyruvate kinase deficiency anaemia following splenectomy. II. Cell deformability, Br J Haematol **39**:63

Le Bouvier GL (1971) The heterogeneity of Australia antigen, J Infect Dis **123**:671

Lechner K (1974) Acquired inhibitors in nonhemophiliac patients, Haemostasis **3**:65

Lecks HI and Kravis L (1969) The allergist and the eosinophil, pediatr Clin North Am **16**:125

Leder LD (1970) Diagnostic experiences with the naphthol AS-D chloroacetate esterase reaction, Blut **21**:1

Lee CL et al (1968) Horse agglutinins in infectious mononucleosis. II. The spot test, Am J Clin Pathol **49**:12

Lee CL (1980) Numerical expression of paternity test results using predetermined indexes, Am J Clin Pathol **73**:522

Lee DB et al (1970) Haematological complications of chlorate poisoning, Br Med J **2**:31

Lee GR et al (1968a) Iron metabolism in copper-deficient swine, J Clin Invest **47**:2058

Lee GR et al (1968b) Hereditary X-linked sideroachrestic anemia. The isolation of two erythrocyte populations differing in Xg^a blood type and porphyrin content, Blood **32**:59

Lee RE and Ellis LD (1971) The storage cells of chronic myelogenous leukemia, Lab Invest **24**:261

Lee SL et al (1966) Activation of systemic lupus erythematosus by drugs, Arch Intern Med **117**:620

Lee-Potter JP et al (1975) A new cause of haemolytic anemia in the newborn. A description of an unstable fetal haemoglobin: F Poole, alpha 2 G gamma 2 130 tryptophan → glycine, J Clin Pathol **28**:317

Leffler RJ (1957) Aspiration of bone marrow from the anterior superior iliac spine, J Lab Clin Med **50**:482

Legaz ME et al (1973) Isolation and characterization of human factor VIII (antihemophilic factor), J Biol Chem **248**:3946

Legrand YJ et al (1979) Specific and quantitative method for estimation of platelet adhesion to fibrillar collagen, J Lab Clin Med **94**:438

Lehman RAW et al (1977) Neurological complications of infantile osteoporosis, Ann Neurol **2**:378

Lehmann H (1959a) Distribution of variations in human hemoglobin synthesis. In Jonxis JPH and Delafresnaye JF (Eds): Abnormal hemoglobins, Oxford, Blackwell Scientific Publications

Lehmann H (1959b) The maintenance of the haemoglobinopathies

at high frequency. A consideration of the relationship between sickling and malaria and of allied problems. In Jonxis JPH and Delafresnaye JF (Eds): Abnormal haemoglobins, Oxford, Blackwell Scientific Publications

Lehmann H and Carrell RW (1969) Variations in the structure of human haemoglobin with particular reference to the unstable hemoglobins, Br Med Bull **25**:14

Lehmann H and Huntsman RG (1968) Man's hemoglobins, Amsterdam, North-Holland Publishing Co, p 293

Lehmann H and Charlesworth D (1970) Observation on haemoglobin P (Congo type), Biochem J **119**:43

Lehmann H et al (1964) Haemoglobin G$_{Accra}$, Nature **203**:363

Lehmann H et al (1975) Haemoglobin Tak: a beta chain elongation, Br J Haematol **31**:119

Lehmann HP (1976) Metrication of clinical laboratory data in SI units, Am J Clin Pathol **65**:2

Lehrer RI and Cline MJ (1969) Leukocyte myeloperoxidase deficiency and disseminated candidiasis: the role of myeloperoxidase in resistance to *Candida* infection, J Clin Invest **48**:1478

Lehrer RI et al (1972) Refractory megalobastic anemia with myeloperoxidase-deficient neutrophils, Ann Intern Med **76**:447

Leichtman DA and Brewer GJ (1978) Elevated plasma levels of fibrinopeptide A during sickle cell anemia pain crisis—evidence for intravascular coagulation, Am J Hematol **5**:183

Leikin SL (1957) The aplastic crisis of sickle-cell disease. Occurrence in several members of families within a short period of time, J Dis Child **93**:128

Leikola J et al (1973) IgA-induced anaphylactic transfusion reactions: a report of four cases, Blood **42**:111

Leist ER and Banwell JG (1974) Products containing aspirin, N Engl J Med **291**:710

Lejeune F et al (1974) Anomalie de Pelger acquise au cours d'une anémie sidéroblastiques avec myelobastose partielle, Pathol Biol **22**:319

Leland J and Macpherson B (1979) Hematologic findings in cases of mammary cancer metastatic to bone marrow, Am J Clin Pathol **71**:31

Lenfant C et al (1968) Effect of altitude on oxygen binding by hemoglobin and on organic phosphate levels, J Clin Invest **47**:2652

Lenfant C et al (1971) Shift of the O$_2$-Hb-dissociation curve at altitude: mechanism and effect, J Appl Physiol **30**:625

Lepow IH (1965) Serum complement and properdin. In Samter M (Ed): Immunological diseases, Boston, Little, Brown & Co, p 188

Lerner RA et al (1971) Quantitative aspects of plasma membrane-associated immunoglobulin in clones of diploid human lymphocytes, Science **173**:60

Lessin LS and Jensen WN (1972) Structural membrane lesion in the irreversibly sickled cell (ISC), Blood (Abst) **40**:930

Lessin LS and Jensen WN (1974) Sickle cell anemia 1910-1973: an overview, Arch Intern Med **133**:529

Lesuk A et al (1967) Biochemical and biophysical studies of human urokinase, Thromb Diath Haemorrh **18**:293

Lévêque B et al (1966) Les anomalies immunologiques et lymphocytaires dans le syndrome d'ataxie-télangiectasie. Analyse des observations de la littérature. Etude de quatre observations personnelles, Ann Pediatr (Paris) **13**:2710

Levere RD (1966) Stilbestrol-induced porphyria: increase in hepatic δ-aminolevulinic acid synthetase, Blood **28**:569

Levere RD (1967) Porphyrin synthesis in hepatic cirrhosis: increase in δ-aminolevulinic acid synthetase, Biochem Med **1**:92

Levin AS et al (1971) Immunofluorescent evidence for cellular control of synthesis of variable regions of light and heavy chains of immunoglobulins G and M by the same gene, Proc Natl Acad Sci USA **68**:169

Levin WC and Truax WE (1960) The influence of storage on erythrocyte survival in blood obtained from donors with sickle cell trait, J Lab Clin Med **55**:94

Levine B and Redmond A (1967) Immunochemical mechanisms of penicillin induced Coombs positively and hemolytic anemia in man, Int Arch Allergy Appl Immunol **31**:594

Levine BB et al (1966) Benzylpenicilloyl specific serum antibodies to penicillin in man, J Immunol **96**:707

Levine P and Javert C (1941) Cited in Levine, P. (1946) The present status of the Rh factor, Am J Clin Pathol **16**:597

Levine P et al (1941) Isoimmunization in pregnancy: its possible bearing on the etiology of erythroblastosis foetalis, JAMA **116**:825

Levine P et al (1949) The Kell-Cellano (K-k) genetic system of human blood factors, Blood **4**:869

Levine P et al (1951) Isoimmunization by a new blood factor in tumor cells, Proc Soc Exp Biol Med **77**:403

Levine P et al (1956) The Diego blood factor, Nature **177**:40

Levine P et al (1964) A second example of ---/--- blood or Rh$_{null}$, Nature **204**:892

Levine P et al (1973) Hemolytic anemia associated with Rh null but not with Bombay blood. A hypothesis based on differing antigenic structures, Vox Sang **24**:417

Levine PH (1976) The effect of thrombocytopenia on the determination of platelet aggregation, Am J Clin Pathol **65**:79

Levine PH et al (1972) Infectious mononucleosis prior to acute leukemia: a possible role for the Epstein-Barr virus, Cancer **30**:875

Levine S (1959) Chronic familial neutropenia, with marked periodontal lesions. Report of a case, Oral Surg **12**:310

Levine SP and Wohl H (1976) Human platelet factor 4. Purification and characterization by affinity chromatography, J Biol Chem **251**:324

Levinson JP and Kincaid OW (1961) Myxoma of the right atrium associated with polycythemia: report of successful excision, N Engl J Med **264**:1187

Levit EJ et al (1957) Progesterone-induced porphyria, Am J Med **22**:831

Levy HL et al (1970) A derangement in B$_{12}$ metabolism associated with homocystinemia, cystathioninemia, hypomethioninemia, and methylmalonic aciduria, Am J Med **48**:390

Levy R et al (1977) The monoclonality of human B-cell lymphomas, J Exp Med **145**:1014

Lewis CM and Pegrum GD (1978) Immune complexes in myelofibrosis: a possible guide to management, Br J Haematol **39**:233

Lewis GP (1965) Method using ortho-tolidine for the quantitative determination of haemoglobin in serum and urine, J Clin Pathol **64**:519

Lewis JP et al (1975) A comparison of four preparations of erythropoiesis regulatory factors, Biochem Med **14**:399

Lewis LP et al (1970) The inference of antiserum to human erythropoietin on the production of hemoglobin C in goats, Proc Soc Exp Biol Med **134**:990

Lewis ML (1974) Cyclic thrombocytopenia: a thrombopoietin deficiency? J Clin Pathol **27**:242

Lewis SM and Dacie JV (1967) The aplastic anaemia—paroxysmal nocturnal haemoglobinuria syndrome, Br J Haematol **13**:236

Lewis SM and Koster JF (1975) Quality control in haematology: Symposium of the International Committee for Standardization in Haematology, New York, Academic Press, Inc

Lewis SM and Sirchia G (1972) PNH: disease or defect? Br J Haematol **23**:71

Lewis SM et al (1971) Electron microscope study of PNH red cells and AET-treated normal red cells (PNH-like cells), J Clin Pathol **24**:677

Lewis TL et al (1973) A comparison of the frequency of hepatitis-B antigen and antibody in hospital and nonhospital personnel, N Engl J Med **289**:647

Lewisohn R (1915) A new and greatly simplified method of transfusion, Med Rec **87**:141

Lewy RI et al (1979) Leukemia in patients with acquired idiopathic sideroblastic anemia: an evaluation of prognostic indicators, Am J Hematol **6**:323

Li CY et al (1970) Acid phosphatase isoenzyme in human leukocytes in normal and pathologic conditions, J Histochem Cytochem **18**:473

Li CY et al (1973) Esterases in human leukocytes, J Histochem Cytochem **21**:1

Libánská et al (1975) Thrombocytopénie thrombocytopathique hypogranulaire héréditaire. Etude ultrastructurale d'une mégacaryocytopathie, Nouv Rev Fr Hematol **15**:165

Lichtenstein H et al (1961) Vitamin B$_{12}$ microbiological assay methods and distribution in selected foods, Washington DC, Home Economics Research Report No. 13, US Dept of Agriculture

Lichtenstein L (1953) Histiocytosis X: integration of eosinophilic granuloma of bone, "Letterer-Siwe disease," and "Schüller-Christian disease" as related manifestations of a single nosologic entity, Arch Pathol (Chicago) **56**:84

Lichtenstein LM and Henney CS (1974) Adenylate cylase-linked hormone receptors: an important mechanism for the immunoregulation of leukocytes. In Brent L and Holborow EJ (Eds): Progress in immunology, vol 2, Proceedings of the Second International Congress of Immunology, Amsterdam, North-Holland Publishing Co, p 73

Lichtenstein LM et al (1973) Effects of cholera toxin on in vitro models of immediate and delayed hypersensitivity. Further evidence for the role of cyclic adenosine 3',5'-monophosphate, J Clin Invest **52**:691

Lichtman MA (1970) Cellular deformability during maturation of the myeloblast: possible role in marrow egress, N Engl J Med **283**:943

Lichtman MA et al (1976) Detection of mutant hemoglobins with altered affinity for oxygen: a simplified technique, Ann Intern Med **84**:517

Lichtman MA et al (1978) Parasinusoidal location of megakaryocytes in marrow: a determinant of platelet release, Am J Hematol **4**:303

Lichty JA et al (1932) Renal thresholds for hemoglobin in dogs, J Exp Med **55**:603

Liddell J et al (1964) A new haemoglobin J alpha Oxford found during a survey of an English population, Nature (London) **204**:269

Lie JT et al (1968) Anaemias associated with increased foetal haemoglobin content: a study by the acid elution technique, Med J Aust **1**:43

Lieb H and Mladenović M (1929) Cerebrosidspeicherung bei Morbus Gaucher, Z Physiol Chem **181**:208

Lieber CS (1980) Metabolism and metabolic effects of alcohol, Semin Hematol **17**:85

Liebow AA et al (1949) Pathology of atomic bomb casualties, Am J Pathol **25**:853

Lie-Injo LE (1961) Haemoglobin "Bart's" and the sickling phenomenon, Nature **191**:1314

Lie-Injo LE et al (1966) Further cases of hemoglobin Q-H disease (hemoglobin Q-alpha thalassemia), Blood **28**:830

Lie-Injo LE et al (1967) Carbonic anhydrase and fetal hemoglobin in thyrotoxicosis, Blood **30**:442

Lie-Injo LE and Sadono (1958) Haemoglobin O (Buginese X) in Sulawesi, Br Med J **1**:1461

Lie-Injo LE et al (1971) Hemoglobin A$_2$-Indonesia or alpha 2 delta 2 69 (E13) gly → arg, Biochim Biophys Acta **229**:335

Lie-Injo LE et al (1973) Structural identification of haemoglobin F Kuala Lumpur (alpha 2 gamma 2 22 [B4] asp → gly: 136 Ala), Biochim Biophys ACta **322:**224

Lie-Injo LE et al (1974) Haemoglobin F Malaysia: alpha 2 γ2 1 (NA1) glycine → cysteine: 136 glycine, J Med Genet **11:**25

Liem HH et al (1979) Quantitative determination of hemoglobin and cytochemical staining for peroxidase using 3,3′, 5,5′-tetramethylbenzidine dihydrochloride, a safe substitute for benzidine, Anal Biochem **98:**388

Ligumski M et al (1978) Nature and incidence of liver involvement in agnogenic myeloid metaplasia, Scand J Haematol **21:**81

Lille I et al (1973) Thymus-derived proliferating lymphocytes in chronic lymphocytic leukaemia, Lancet **2:**263

Lillibridge CB et al (1967) Childhood pernicious anemia: gastrointestinal secretory, histological, and electron microscopic aspects, Gastroenterology **52:**792

Lillie RD et al (1942) Histogenesis and repair of the hepatic cirrhosis in rats produced on low protein diets and preventable with choline, Public Health Rep **57:**502

Lin KL et al (1973) Blood flow in capillaries, Microvasc Res **5:**7

Lin PS et al (1973) Scanning electron microscopy of human T-cell and B-cell rosettes, N Engl J Med **289:**548

Lindenbaum J (1974) Hemoglobin Munchausen, JAMA **228:**498

Lindenbaum J and Hargrove RL (1968) Thrombocytopenia in alcoholics, Ann Intern Med **68:**526

Lindenbaum J and Lieber CS (1969) Alcohol-induced malabsorption of vitamin B$_{12}$ in man, Nature **224:**806

Lindenbaum J (1980) Folate and vitamin B$_{12}$ deficiencies in alcoholism, Semin Hematol **17:**119

Lindenbaum J and Nath BJ (1980) Megaloblastic anaemia and neutrophil hypersegmentation, Br J Haematol **44:**511

Lindenmann J (1974) Viruses as immunological adjuvants in cancer, Biochim Biophys Acta **355:**49

Lindhout MJ and Kop-Klaassen BMH (1975) Proteins induced by vitamin K antagonists (PIVKAs). In Hemker HC and Veltkamp JJ (Eds): Prothrombin and related coagulation factors, Leiden, Leiden University Press, p 274

Lines JG and McIntosh R (1967) Oxygen binding by haemoglobin J Cape Town (alpha 2 92 arg → gln), Nature **215:**297

Linkham WH and Conley CL (1956) Some factors influencing the formation of L.E. cells, Bull Johns Hopkins Hosp **98:**102

Linman JW and Pierre RV (1962) Thrombocytosis-promoting activity of normal plasma, Proc Soc Exp Biol Med **110:**463

Linman JW and Pierre RV (1963) Studies on thrombopoiesis. III. Thrombocytosis-promoting effects of "thrombocythemic" and "polycythemic" plasmas, J Lab Clin Med **62:**374

Linna TJ (1968) Cell migration from the thymus to other lymphoid organs in hamsters of different ages, Blood **31:**727

Lipinska I et al (1976) Fibrinogen heterogeneity in cancer, in occlusive vascular disease, and after surgical procedures, Am J Clin Pathol **66:**958

Lippert H and Lehmann HP (1978) SI units in medicine, Baltimore, Urban and Schwarzenberg

Lipschitz DA et al (1974) A clinical evaluation of serum ferritin as an index of iron stores, N Engl J Med **290:**1213

Lipson RL et al (1959) The postsplenectomy blood picture, Am J Clin Pathol **32:**526

Lipton A (1969) Chronic idiopathic neutropenia. Treatment with corticosteroids and mercaptopurine, Arch Intern Med **123:**694

Lipton EL (1955) Elliptocytosis with hemolytic anemia: the effects of splenectomy, Pediatrics **15:**67

Lischner HW et al (1967) Lymphocytes in congenital absence of the thymus, Nature **214:**580

Lischner HW et al (1973) Proliferative responsiveness of human B and T lymphocytes to phytohemagglutinin and pokeweed mito-

gen. In Daguillard F (Ed): Proceedings of the Seventh Leukocyte Culture Conference, New York, Academic Press, Inc, p 547

Liso V et al (1974) Leucemia acuta a promielociti cosiddetti basofili, La Recerca Clin Lab **4:**339

Little JB (1968) Cellular effects of ionization radiation, N Engl J Med **278:**308

Litwin SD and Zanjani ED (1977) Lymphocytes suppressing both immunoglobulin production and erythroid differentiation in hypogammaglobulinaemia, Nature **266:**57

Litwins J and Leibowitz S (1951) Abnormal lymphocytes (virocytes) in virus diseases other than infectious mononucleosis, Acta Haematol **5:**223

Livingstone FB (1967) Abnormal hemoglobins in human populations, Chicago, Aldine Publishing Co

Lloyd KO and Kabat EA (1968) Immunochemical studies on blood groups. XII. Proposed structures for the carbohydrate portions of blood group A, B, H, Lewis^a, and Lewis^b substances, Proc Natl Acad Sci **61:**1470

Lock SP et al (1961) Stomatocytosis: a hereditary red cell anomaly associated with haemolytic anaemia, Br J Haematol **7:**303

Lockhard RE and Lingrel JB (1969) The synthesis of mouse hemoglobin β-chains in a rabbit reticulocyte cell-free system programmed with mouse reticulocyte 9S RNA, Biochem Biophys Res Commun **37:**204

Lockhead AC et al (1963) Quantitative measurement of the iron-incorporating enzyme in relation to marrow cells and liver tissue in the rabbit, Br J Haematol **9:**39

Lockman LA et al (1967) The Chediak-Higashi syndrome: electrophysiological and electron microscopic observations on the peripheral neuropathy, J Pediatr **70:**942

Lodish HF (1976) Translational control of protein synthesis, Annu Rev Biochem **45:**39

Loewy AG (1972) Some thoughts on the state in nature, biosynthetic origin, and function of factor XIII, Ann NY Acad Sci **202:**41

Löffler H and Hansen HT (1967) Erythroblasten mit elliptischen Kernen, Blut **15:**7

Loge JP (1948) Spinous process puncture, simple clinical approach for obtaining bone marrow, Blood **3:**198

Logue GL et al (1973) Mechanisms of immune lysis of red blood cells in vitro. I. Paroxysmal nocturnal hemoglobinuria cell, J Clin Invest **52:**1129

Lohrmann H et al (1974) Platelet transfusions from HL-A compatible unrelated donors to alloimmunized patients, Ann Intern Med **80:**9

Lokich JJ et al (1973) Hemoglobin Brigham (alpha 2A beta 2 100 pro → leu). Hemoglobin variant associated with familial erythrocytosis, J Clin Invest **52:**2060

London IM and West R (1950) Formation of bile pigment in pernicious anemia, J Biol Chem **184:**359

London JC and Ellis LB (1969) Leukocyte cultures from chimpanzees. In Rieke WO (Ed): Proceedings of the Third Annual Leucocyte Culture Conference, New York, Appleton-Century-Crofts

London WT et al (1969) An epidemic of hepatitis in a chronic-hemodialysis unit, N Engl J Med **281:**571

Long JC and Aisenberg AC (1975) Richter's syndrome. A terminal complication of chronic lymphocytic leukemia with distinct clinicopathologic features, Am J Clin Pathol **63:**786

Long L et al (1960) Cancer cells in blood, Arch Surg **80:**910

Lopaciuk S et al (1976) Subcellular distribution of fibrinogen and factor XIII in human blood platelets, Thromb Res **8:**453

Lopez A and Lozzio BB (1972) Enhanced hemopoietic regeneration by transplantation of lymphoid cells from donors treated with phytohemagglutinin, J Reticuloendothel Soc **12:**324

Lorand L (1964) Assays for the fibrin stabilizing factor (FSF). In Tocantins LM and Kazol LA (Eds): Blood coagulation, hemorrhage, and thrombosis, New York, Grune & Stratton, Inc

Lorand L (1972) The fibrin-stabilizing factor system of blood plasma, Ann NY Acad Sci **202:**6

Lorand L and Dickenman RC (1955) Assay method for "fibrin-stabilizing factor," Proc Soc Exp Biol Med **89:**45

Lorand L et al (1979) Enzymatic basis of membrane stiffening in human erythrocytes, Semin Hematol **16:**65

Loria A et al (1967) Red cell life span in iron deficiency anaemia, Br J Haematol **13:**294

Lorkin PA et al (1970a) Two new pathological haemoglobins: Olmsted beta 141 (H19) leu → arg and Malmö: beta 97 (FG4) his → gln, Biochem J **119:**68

Lorkin PA et al (1970b) Two haemoglobins Q, alpha 74 (EF3) and alpha 75 (EF4) aspartic acid → histidine, Br J Haematol **19:**117

Lorkin PA et al (1974) Structure of haemoglobin Wien beta 130 (H8) tyrosine → aspartic acid: an unstable haemoglobin variant, Acta Haematol **51:**351

Lorkin PA et al (1975a) Haemoglobin Rahere (beta 82 lys → thr): a new high affinity haemoglobin associated with decreased 2,3-diphosphoglycerate binding and relative polycythaemia, Br Med J **4:**200

Lorkin PA et al (1975b) Haemoglobin G Norfolk: alpha 85 (F6) asp → asn, Biochim Biophys Acta **379:**22

Lorkin PA et al (1970) Two haemoglobins Q, α74 (EF3) and α75 (EF4) aspartic acid → histidine, Br J Haematol **19:**117

Losowsky MS and Hall R (1965) Hereditary sideroblastic anaemia, Br J Haematol **11:**70

Loukopoulos D et al (1969) On the chemical abnormality of hb "Alexandra" a fetal hemoglobin variant, Blood **33:**114

Loutit JF (1968) Versatile haemopoietic stem cells, Br J Haematol **15:**333

Loutit JF and Mollison PL (1943) Advantages of a disodium-citrate-glucose mixture as a blood preservative, Br Med J **2:**744

Low FN and Freeman JA (1958) Electron microscopic atlas of normal and leukemic human blood, New York, McGraw-Hill Book Co, Inc

Lowden JA et al (1970) Wolman's disease: a microscopic and biochemical study showing accumulation of ceroid and esterified cholesterol, Can Med Assoc J **102:**402

Lowenstein LM (1959) The mammalian reticulocyte, Int Rev Cytol **8:**135

Lowey AG (1972) Some thoughts on the state in nature, biosynthetic origin, and function of factor XIII, Ann NY Acad Sci **202:**41

Lubash GD et al (1964) Acute aniline poisoning treated by hemodialysis. Report of a case, Arch Intern Med **114:**530

Lubin J and Rywlin AM (1971) Lymphoma-like lymph node changes in Kaposi's sarcoma. Two additional cases, Arch Pathol **92:**338

Lubin J et al (1976) Malignant myelosclerosis, Arch Intern Med **136:**141

Lucarelli G et al (1967) Effetto della somministrazione di triiodotironina sulla eritropoiesi nel ratto normale a digiuno, policitemico e netroprivo, Boll Soc Ital Biol Sper **43:**139

Lucas PF (1955) Lymph node smears in the diagnosis of lymphadenopathy: a review, Blood **10:**1030

Ludden TE and Harvey M (1962) Pelger-Huët anomaly of leukocytes, Am J Clin Pathol **37:**302

Luddy RE et al (1978) A fatal myeloproliferative syndrome in a family with thrombocytopenia and platelet dysfunction, Cancer **41:**1959

Ludlam CA (1979) Evidence for the platelet specificity of β-thromboglobulin and studies on its plasma concentration in healthy individuals, Br J Hematol **41:**271

Ludlam CA et al (1975) New rapid method for diagnosis of deep vein thrombosis, Lancet **2:**259

Ludman H and Spear PW (1957) Reed-Sternberg cells in the peripheral blood, Blood **12:**189

Lukes RJ (1971) Criteria for involvement of lymph node, bone marrow, spleen, and liver in Hodgkin's disease, Cancer Res **31:**1755

Lukes RJ and Collins RD (1974) Immunologic characterization of human malignant lymphomas, Cancer **34**(suppl):1488

Lukes RJ and Collins RD (1975) New approaches to the classification of lymphomata, Br J Cancer **31**(suppl):1

Lukes RJ and Tindle BH (1975) Immunoblastic lymphadenopathy, N Engl J Med **292:**1

Lukes RJ et al (1966) Natural history of Hodgkin's disease as related to its pathologic picture, Cancer **19:**317

Lukowsky W and Painter RH (1968) Molecular weight of erythropoietin from anemic sheep plasma and human urine, Can J Biochem **46:**731

Lundin P et al (1964) Comparison of hemosiderin estimation in bone marrow sections and bone marrow smears, Acta Med Scand **175:**383

Lüscher EF and Bettex-Galland M (1972) Thrombosthenin, the contractile protein of blood platelets. New facts and problems, Pathol Biol (Paris) (supp):89

Lusher JM et al (1968a) The May-Hegglin anomaly: platelet function, ultrastructure, and chromosome studies, Blood **32:**950

Lusher JM et al (1968b) Antibody nature of an AHG·(factor VIII) inhibitor, J Pediatr **72:**325

Lusher JM et al (1980) Efficacy of prothrombin-complex concentrates in hemophiliacs with antibodies to factor VIII: a multicenter therapeutic trial, N Engl J Med **303:**421

Lutcher CL and Huisman THJ (1975) Hb-Leslie: an unstable variant due to deletion of gln beta 131, occurring in combination with β⁰-thalassemia, hb-S and hb-C, Clin Res **23:**278A

Lutcher CL et al (1976) Hb Leslie, an unstable hemoglobin due to deletion of glutaminyl residue beta 131 (H9) occurring in association with β⁰-thalassemia, hb-C and hb-S, Blood **47:**99

Lutzner MA and Jordan HW (1968) The ultrastructure of an abnormal cell in Sézary's syndrome, Blood **31:**719

Lutzner MA et al (1973) Cytogenetic, cytophotometric, and ultrastructural study of large cerebriform cells of the Sézary syndrome and description of a small-cell variant, J Natl Cancer Inst **50:**1145

Lux SE (1979) Spectrin-actin membrane skeleton of normal and abnormal red blood cells, Semin Hematol **16:**21

Ly B et al (1978) Acute myelogenous leukaemia occurring at the same time in husband and wife, Scand J Haematol **21:**376

Luzzatto L et al (1969) Glucose-6-phosphate dehydrogenase deficient red cells: resistance to infection by malarial parasites, Science **164:**839

Lyon MF (1968) Chromosomal and subchromosomal inactivation, Ann Rev Genet **2:**31

Lyons HA (1976) Centrally acting hormones and respiration, Pharmacol Ther (B) **2:**743

Mabry CC et al (1960) Studies concerning the defect in a patient with acanthrocytosis, Clin Res **8:**371

Macalpine I and Hunter R (1966) The "insanity" of King George III: a classic case of porphyria, Br J Med **1:**1

Macalpine I et al (1968) Porphyria in the Royal Houses of Stuart, Hanover, and Prussia: a follow-up study of George III's illness, Br Med J **1:**17

Macfarlane DE and Zucker MB (1975) A method for assaying von Willebrand factor (ristocetin cofactor), Thromb Diath Haemorr **34:**306

Macfarlane RG (1964) An enzyme cascade in the blood clotting mechanism and its function as a biochemical amplifier, Nature **202**:498

Macfarlane RG (1966) The basis of the cascade hypothesis of blood clotting, Thromb Diath Haemorrh **15**:591

MacGibbon BH and Mollin DL (1965) Sideroblastic anaemia in man: observation on seventy cases, Br J Haematol **11**:59

MacGillivray JB et al (1964) Congenital neutropenia: a report of five cases, Acta Paediatr **53**:188

MacGregor RR et al (1974) Inhibition of granulocyte adherence by ethanol, prednisone, and aspirin, measured with an assay system, N Engl J Med **291**:642

Machin SJ and Miller BR (1980) Congenital combined factor VII and factor VIII deficiency, Acta Haematol **63**:167

Machin SJ et al (1980) Factor X deficiency in the neonatal period, Arch Dis Childhood **55**:406

Machovich R (1975) Mechanism of action of heparin through thrombin on blood coagulation, Biochim Biophys Acta **412**:13

MacIver JE and Back EH (1960) Megaloblastic anaemia of infancy in Jamaica, Arch Dis Child **35**:134

MacIver JE and Parker-Williams EJ (1961) The aplastic crisis in sickle-cell anemia, Lancet **1**:1086

Mackaness GB (1969) The influence of immunologically committed lymphoid cells on macrophage activity in vivo, J Exp Med **129**:973

MacKenzie DH (1959) Reticulin patterns in tumors of lymphoid tissue, Br J Cancer **13**:38

MacKenzie FAF et al (1962) Relapse in hereditary spherocytosis with proven splenunculus, Lancet **1**:1102

MacKenzie IL et al (1972) Ileal mucosa in familial selective vitamin B_{12} malabsorption, N Engl J Med **286**:1021

Mackey JP and Vivarelli F (1954) Sickle-cell anaemia, Br Med J **1**:276

MacLean LD et al (1956) Thymic tumor and acquired agammaglobulinemia: a clinical and experimental study of the immune response, Surgery **40**:1010

MacMahon B (1962) Prenatal x-ray exposure and childhood cancer, J Natl Cancer Inst **28**:1173

MacMillan DC (1966) Secondary clumping effect in human citrated platelet-rich plasma produced by adenosine diphosphate and adrenaline, Nature **211**:140

Maddison SE et al (1975) The relationship of race, sex, and age to concentrations of serum immunoglobulins expressed in international units in healthy adults in the USA, Bull WHO **52**:179

Macpherson BR and Westphal RG (1979) Antileukocyte antibodies in patients refractory to platelet transfusions, Am J Clin Pathol **72**:893

Madden JL and Hume M (1976) Venous thromboembolism: prevention and treatment, New York, Appleton-Century-Crofts

Maddock RK Jr (1965) Incidence of systemic lupus erythematosus by age and sex, JAMA **191**:137

Madison JT (1968) Primary structure of RNA, Ann Rev Biochem **37**:131

Maeda K et al (1973) Multiple myeloma in childhood: report of a case with breast tumors as a presenting manifestation, Am J Clin Pathol **60**:552

Maeda K et al (1980) Type I dyserythropoietic anemia: a 30 year follow-up, Am J Clin Pathol **73**:433

Maekawa M et al (1970) Hemoglobin Nagasaki: alpha A2 beta 2 17 glue. A new abnormal human hemoglobin found in one family in Nagasaki, Int J Prot Res **11**:147

Magath TB and Winkle V (1952) Technic for demonstrating "L.E." (lupus erythematosus) cells in blood, Am J Clin Pathol **22**:586

Maginus LO et al (1975) A new antigen-antibody system. Clinical significance in long-term carriers of hepatitis B surface antigen, JAMA **231**:356

Magnus EM (1967) Folate activity in serum and red cells of patients with cancer, Cancer Res **27**:490

Magnus IA et al (1961) Erythropoietic protoporphyria—new syndrome with solar urticaria due to protoporphyrinaemia, Lancet **2**:448

Magnusson S (1972) On the primary structure of bovine thrombin, Folia Haematol Leipzig **98**:385

Mahmood A (1969) Fibrinolytic activity and sickle-cell crises, Br Med J **1**:52

Mahmood T et al (1979) Macrocytic anemia, thrombocytosis and nonlobulated megakaryocytes: the 5q-syndrome, a distinct entity, Am J Med **66**:946

Mahoney BS and Githens JH (1979) Sickling crises and altitude: occurrence in the Colorado patient populations, Clin Pediatr **18**:431

Main RA et al (1959) Sézary's syndrome, Br J Dermatol **71**:335

Maini RN et al (1969) Lymphocyte mitogenic factor in man, Nature **224**:43

Mainwaring RL and Brueckner GG (1966) Fibrinogen-transmitted hepatitis: a controlled study, JAMA **195**:437

Majeski JA and Upshur JK (1978) Asplenia syndrome: a study of congenital anomalies in 16 cases, JAMA **240**:1508

Majno G and Palade GE (1961) Studies on inflammation. I. The effect of histamine and serotonin on vascular permeability: an electron microscopic study, J Biophys Biochem Cytol **11**:571

Major RH (1945) Classical descriptions of disease, Springfield, Ill, Charles C Thomas, Publishers, p 488

Makler MT et al (1974) A new variant of sickle-cell disease with high levels of fetal hemoglobin homogeneously distributed within red cells, Br J Haematol **26**:519

Malcolm ID et al (1979) Vacuolization of the neutrophil in bacteremia, Arch Intern Med **139**:675

Maldonaldo JE (1976) Platelet granulopathy. A new morphologic feature in preleukemia and myelomonocytic leukemia: light microscopy and ultrastructural morphology and cytochemistry, Mayo Clin Proc **51**:452

Maldonado JE and Hanlon DG (1965) Monocytosis: a current appraisal, Mayo Clin Proc **40**:248

Malenfant AL et al (1968) Spectrophotometric determination of hemoglobin concentration and percent oxyhemoglobin and carboxyhemoglobin saturation, Clin Chem **14**:789

Malloy HT and Lowenstein L (1940) Hereditary jaundice in the rat, Can Med Assoc J **42**:122

Malmgren RA et al (1958) Method or cytologic detection of tumor cells in whole blood, J Natl Cancer Inst **20**:1203

Malmsten C et al (1975) Physiological role of an endoperoxide in human platelets: hemostatic defect due to platelet cyclo-oxygenase deficiency, Proc Natl Acad Sci USA **72**:1446

Mammen EF (1974) Congenital abnormalities of the fibrinogen molecule, Semin Thromb Hemost **1**:184

Mammon Z et al (1976) Philadelphia chromosome with t(6;22)(p25;q12), N Engl J Med **294**:827

Mancini G et al (1965) Immunochemical quantitation of antigens by single radial immunodiffusion, Immunochemistry **2**:235

Mandle RJ et al (1976) Identification of prekallikrein and high-molecular-weight kininogen as a complex in human plasma, Proc Natl Acad Sci USA **73**:4179

Mandle R Jr and Kaplan AP (1980) Human plasma prekallikrein. In Schmidt RM (Section Ed): Handbook Series in Clinical Laboratory Science, Section I: Hematology, vol 3, Boca Raton, Fla. CRC Press Inc. p 171

Maniatis A et al (1979) Hemoglobin Crete (beta 129 ala → pro): a new high affinity variant interacting with β^0- and $\delta\beta^0$-thalassemia, Blood **54**:54

Manley RW (1957) The effect of room temperature on erythrocyte sedimentation rate and its correction, J Clin Pathol **10**:354

Mann FD (1970) Simplification of the concept of coagulation by revival of the inhibitor theory, Thromb Diath Haemorrh **23**:12

Mann JD and Higgins GM (1950) Lymphocytes in thoracic duct, intestinal and hepatic lymph, Blood **5**:177

Mann KG and Elion J (1980) Prothrombin. In Schmidt RM (Section Ed): Handbook Series in Clinical Laboratory Science, Section I: Hematology, Vol 3, Boca Raton, Fla, CRC Press Inc, p 15

Mann RB et al (1976) Non-endemic Burkitt's lymphoma: a β-cell tumor related to germinal centers, N Engl J Med **295**:685

Mann RB et al (1979) Malignant lymphomas—a conceptional understanding of morphologic diversity. A review, Am J Pathol **94**:105

Manoharan A et al (1979) The reticulin content of bone marrow in acute leukaemia in adults, Br J Haematol **43**:185

Manroe BL et al (1979) The neonatal blood count in health and disease. I. Reference values for neutrophilic cells, J Pediatr **95**:89

Mansfield AO (1972) Alteration in fibrinolysis associated with surgery and venous thrombosis, Br J Surg **59**:754

Mant MJ et al (1972) Thrombotic thrombocytopenic purpura: report of a case with possible immune etiology, Blood **40**:416

Mant MJ et al (1973) Von Willebrand's syndrome presenting as an acquired bleeding disorder in association with a monoclonal gammopathy, Blood **42**:429

Mant MJ et al (1976-77) Hb Alberta or alpha 2 beta 2 (101 [G3] glu → gly), a new high oxygen affinity hemoglobin variant causing erythrocytosis, Hemoglobin **1**:183

Marasco WA et al (1980) The ionic basis of chemotaxis: separate cation requirements for neutrophil orientation and locomotion in a gradient of chemotactic peptide, Am J Pathol **98**:749

March HC (1950) Leukemia in radiologists in a 20 year period, Am J Med Sci **220**:282

March HC (1961) Leukemia in radiologists, ten years later. With a review of the pertinent evidence for radiation leukemia, Am J Med Sci **242**:137

Marchalonis J and Edelman GM (1965) Phylogenetic origins of antibody structure. I. Multichain structure of immunoglobulins in the smooth dogfish (Mustelus canis), J Exp Med **112**:601

Marchalonis JJ et al (1978) Evolutionary immunobiology and the problem of the T-cell receptor, Dev Comp Immunol **2**:203

Marchand F (1907) Ueber sog. idiopathische Splenomegalie (Typus Gaucher), München Med Wochenschr **54**:1102

Marchasin S et al (1964) Variation of the platelet count in disease, Calif Med **101**:95

Marchesi VT (1979) Functional proteins of the human red blood cell membrane, Semin Hematol **16**:3

Marchesi VT and Gowans JL (1964) The migration of lymphocytes through the endothelium of venules in lymph nodes: an electron microscope study, Proc R Soc (Biol) **159**:283

Marciniak E et al (1974) Familial thrombosis due to antithrombin 3 deficiency, Blood **43**:219

Marcoullis G et al (1979) Blocking and binding type antibodies against all major vitamin B₁₂-binders in a pernicious anaemia serum, Br J Haematol **43**:15

Marcus AJ et al (1966) Studies on human platelet granules and membranes, J Clin Invest **45**:14

Marcus AJ et al (1971) Studies on human platelet granules and membranes. In Brinkhous KM and Shermer RW (Eds): The platelet, Baltimore, The Williams & Wilkins Co

Markkanen T et al (1972) Transferrin, the third carrier protein of folic acid activity in human serum, Acta Haematol **48**:213

Markowitz H et al (1959) Studies on copper metabolism. XXVII. The isolation and properties of an erythrocyte cuproprotein (erythrocuprein), J Biol Chem **234**:40

Marengo-Rowe AJ et al (1968a) New human haemoglobin variant from southern Arabia: G Audhali (alpha 23 [B4] glutamic acid → valine) and the variability of B4 in human haemoglobin, Nature (London) **219**:1164

Marengo-Rowe AJ et al (1968b) Haemoglobin Dhofar—a new variant from Southern Arabia, Biochim Biophys Acta **168**:58

Marinucci M et al (1977) Hemoglobin Gavello alpha 2 beta 2 47 (CD6) asp → gly, a new hemoglobin variant from Polesine (Italy), Hemoglobin **1**:771

Marinucci M et al (1979) A new abnormal human hemoglobin: Hb Prato (α₂ 31 [B12] Arg → Ser β₂), Biochim Biophys Acta **578**:534

Marinucci M et al (1980) A new human hemoglobin variant: hb Bari (alpha 2 45 [CD3] his → gln beta 2), Biochim Biophys Acta **622**:315

Markkanen T et al (1972) Transferrin, the third carrier protein of folic acid activity in human serum, Acta Haematol **48**:213

Markkanen T et al (1973) Binding of folic acid to serum proteins. II. The effect of diphenylhydantoin treatment and of various diseases, Acta Haematol **50**:284

Markkanen T et al (1974) Binding of folic acid to serum proteins: III. The effect of pernicious anaemia, Acta Haematol **51**:193

Marks SM et al (1978) Multimarker analysis of T-cell chronic lymphocytic leukemia, Blood **51**:435

Marsh WL (1960) The pseudo B antigen. A study of its development, Vox Sang **5**:387

Marshall PN (1979) Romanowsky staining: state of the art and ''ideal'' techniques. In Koepke JA, (Ed): Differential leukocyte counting, Skokie, Ill, College of American Pathologists, p 205

Marston HR et al (1961) Primary metabolic defect supervening on vitamin B₁₂ deficiency in the sheep, Nature **190**:1085

Marti HR et al (1964) Eine neue Hämoglobin I variante: hb I Interlaken, Acta Haematol **32**:9

Marti HR et al (1967) Haemoglobin Koelliker: a new acquired haemoglobin appearing after severe haemolysis: α₂ minus 141 arg β₂, Acta Haematol **37**:174

Marti HR et al (1976) Hb Altdorf alpha 2 beta 2 135 (H13) ala → pro: a new electrophoretically silent unstable haemoglobin variant from Switzerland, FEBS Lett **63**:193

Martin JD et al (1967) Serum folate and vitamin B₁₂ levels in pregnancy with particular reference to uterine bleeding and bacteriuria, J Obstet Gynecol Br Commonw **74**:697

Martinek RG (1965) Spectrophotometric determination of abnormal hemoglobin pigments in blood, Clin Chim Acta **11**:146

Martinez J et al (1974) Fibrinogen Philadelphia: a hereditary hypofibrinogenemia characterized by fibrinogen hypercatabolism, J Clin Invest **53**:600

Martinez G et al (1977) Haemoglobin J Guantanamo (alpha 2 beta 2 128 [H6] ala → asp). A new fast unstable haemoglobin found in a Cuban family, Biochim Biophys Acta **491**:1

Martinez G et al (1978) Hb J Camagüey alpha 2 141 (HC3) arg → gly beta 2. A new abnormal human hemoglobin, Hemoglobin **2**:47

Martland HS (1929) Occupational poisoning in manufacture of luminous watch dials, JAMA **92**:466

Marver HS and Schmid R (1972) The porphyrins. In Stanbury JB et al (Eds): Metabolic basis of inherited diseases, ed 3, New York, McGraw-Hill Book Co, p 1089

Masi AT and Kaslow RA (1978) Sex effects in systemic erythematosus: a clue to pathogenesis, Arthritis Rheum **21**:480

Mason BA et al (1978) Sea-blue histiocytes in a patient with lymphoma, Am J Med **64**:515

Mason P and Rigby BJ (1965) Ehlers-Danlos syndrome: physical and biochemical aspects, Arch Pathol **80**:363

Mason SJ et al (1977) The Duffy blood group determinants: their role in the susceptibility of human and animal erythrocytes to *Plasmodium knowlesi* malaria, Br J Haematol **36**:327

Matchett KM et al (1973) Impaired lymphocyte transformation in Hodgkin's disease. Evidence for depletion of circulating t-lymphocytes, J Clin Invest **52**:1908

Matej H (1962) The use of fluorescent antibodies in the study of blood groups, Arch Immunol Ter Dosw **10**:975

Mathe G et al (1976) Les adénopathies angio-immunoblastiques, Nouv Presse Med **5**:1515

Matson GA et al (1959) A "new" antigen and antibody belonging to the P blood group system, Am J Hum Genet **11**:26

Matsumoto KK and Grossman MI (1959) Quantitative measurement of blood loss during ingestion of aspirin, Proc Soc Exp Biol Med **102**:517

Matter M et al (1960) A study of thrombopoiesis in induced acute thrombocytopenia, Blood **15**:174

Mattern CFT et al (1957) Determination of number and size of particles by electrical gating: blood cells, J Appl Physiol **10**:56

Matthews DM (1962) Observations on the estimation of serum vitamin B_{12} using *Lactobacillus leichmannii*, Clin Sci **22**:101

Matthias FR et al (1977) Dysfibrinogenämie: Zugleich ein neuer Fall: Dysfibrinogenämie Giessen III, Klin Wochenschr **55**:539

Matula G and Paterson PY (1971) Spontaneous in vitro reduction of nitroblue tetrazolium by neutrophils of adult patients with bacterial infection, N Engl J Med **285**:311

Maurer HS et al (1972) Similarities of the erythrocytes in juvenile chronic myelogenous leukemia to fetal erythrocytes, Blood **39**:778

Mauri C and Silingardi V (1964) A cytological and cytochemical study of Chediak's leukocytic anomaly, Acta Haematol **32**:114

Mauzerall O and Granick S (1956) Occurrence and determination of δ-aminolevulinic acid and porphobilinogen in urine, J Biol Chem **219**:435

Mavilio F et al (1978) Hemoglobin Legnano (alpha 2 141 [HC3] arg → leu beta 2): a new abnormal hemoglobin with high oxygen affinity, Hemoglobin **2**:249

Maximow A (1932) The lymphocytes and plasma cells. In Cowdry EV (Ed): Special cytology, vol 2, New York, Paul B Hoeber, Inc, p 601

Maynert EW and Isaac L (1968) Uptake and binding of serotonin by the platelet and its granules, Adv Pharmacol **6**:113

Mayr WR (1971) Die Genetik des HL-A Systems. Populations und Familienuntersuchungen unter besonderer Berücksichtigung der Paternitätsserologie, Humangenetik **12**:195

Mazur A et al (1958) Mechanism of release of ferritin iron in vivo by xanthine oxidase, J Clin Invest **37**:1809

Mazza U et al (1980) γ Chain composition in five Italian newborns heterozygous for Hb F Malta Gγ 117 his → arg, Br J Haematol **44**:93

McBride JA and Jacob HS (1968) Cholesterol loading of acanthocytic red cell membranes causing hemolytic anemia in experimental and genetic abetalipoproteinemia, J Clin Invest **47**:67a

McCann SR et al (1978) Intracellular λ light chanin inclusions in chronic lymphocytic leukaemia, Br J Haematol **38**:367

McCracken GH Jr and Eichenwald HF (1971) Leukocyte function and the development of opsonic and complement activity in the neonate, Am J Dis Child **121**:120

McCulloch EA (1975) Granulopoiesis in cultures of human haemopoietic cells, Clin Haematol **4**:509

McCullough J et al (1974) Effects of anticoagulants and storage on granulocyte function in bank blood, Blood **43**:207

McCullugh J (1978) Leukapheresis and granulocyte transfusion, Arch Pathol Lab Med **102**:53

McCurdy PR (1962) Clinical, genetic, and physiological studies in hereditary elliptocytosis, Proc Cong Int Soc Hematol **1**:53

McCurdy PR et al (1974) Hemoglobin S-G(S-D) syndrome, Am J Med **57**:665

McCurdy PR and Sherman AS (1978) Irreversibly sickled cells and red cell survival in sickle cell anemia: a study with both DF^{32}P and ^{51}Cr, Am J Med **64**:253

McCurdy PR and Rath CE (1980) Vacuolated nucleated bone marrow in alcoholism, Semin Hematol **17**:100

McDevitt DG and Glasgow JF (1967) Lupus-like syndrome induced by procainamide, Br Med J **3**:780

McDevitt NB et al (1972) An acquired inhibitor to factor XIII, Arch Intern Med **130**:770

McDonagh J et al (1974) Factor XIII deficiency: a genetic study of two affected kindreds in Finland, Blood **43**:327

McDonagh J and McDonagh RP (1980) Factor XIII. In Schmidt Rm (Section Ed): Handbook Series in Clinical Laboratory Science, Section I: Hematology, vol 3, Boca Raton, Fla, CRC Press, Inc, p 125

McDonagh RP et al (1971) Crosslinking of human fibrin: evidence for intermolecular crosslinking involving α-chains, FEBS Lett **14**:33

McDonald JM and Davis JE (1979) Glycosylated hemoglobin and diabetes mellitus, Hum Pathol **10**:279

McDonald TP (1973) The hemagglutination inhibition assay for thrombopoietin, Blood **41**:219

McDonald TP (1974a) Immunoassay and bioassay for thrombopoietin. In Baldini G and Ebbe S (Eds): Platelets: production, function, transfusion, and storage, New York, Grune & Stratton, Inc, p 81

McDonald TP (1974b) Immunologic studies of thrombopoietin, Proc Soc Exp Biol Med **147**:513

McDonald TP (1976) Role of the kidneys in thrombopoietin production, Exp Hematol **4**:27

McDonald TP (1978) Neutralizing antiserum to thrombopoietin, Proc Soc Exp Biol Med **158**:557

McDonald TP and Clift R (1979) Effects of thrombopoietin and erythropoietin on platelet production in rebound-thrombocytotic and normal mice, Am J Hematol **6**:219

McDonald TP and Green D (1977) Demonstration of thrombopoietin production after plasma infusion in a patient with congenital thrombopoietin deficiency, Thromb Haemost **37**:577

McFadzean JA et al (1969) The effect of phenothiazines on the sickling phenomenon in vitro, Br J Haematol **16**:173

McFarland W and Dameshek W (1958) Biopsy of bone marrow with Vim-Silverman needle, JAMA **166**:1464

McFarlin DE et al (1972) Ataxia-telangiectasia, Medicine **51**:281

McGarry MP et al (1971) Lymphoid cell dependence of eosinophil response to antigen, J Exp Med **134**:801

McGrath MA and Penny R (1976) Paraproteinemia: blood hyperviscosity and clinical manifestations, J Clin Invest **58**:1155

McIntyre OR (1979) Multiple myeloma, N Engl J Med **301**:193

McIntyre OR and Ebaugh FG Jr (1962) The effect of phytohemagglutinin on leukocyte cultures as measured by P^3 incorporation in the DNA, RNA, and acid soluble fraction, Blood **19**:443

McIntyre OR et al (1965) Permicious anemia in childhood, N Engl J Med **272**:981

McKay DG (1965) Disseminated intravascular coagulation, New York, Harper & Row, Publishers

McKay DG (1972) Participation of components of the blood coagulation system in the inflammatory response, Am J Pathol **67**:181

McKay DG (1973) Intravascular coagulation—acute and chronic—disseminated and local. In Schmer G and Strandjord PE (Eds): Coagulation, New York, Academic Press, Inc, p 45

McKay DG and Corey AE (1964) Cryofibrinogenemia in toxemia of pregnancy, Obstet Gynecol **23**:508

McKee PA et al (1970) Subunit structure of human fibrinogen, soluble fibrin and crosslinked insoluble fibrin, Proc Natl Acad Sci USA **66**:738

McKenna JL and Pisciotta AV (1962) Fluorescence of megakaryocytes in idiopathic thrombocytopenic purpura (ITP) stained with fluorescent antiglobulin serum, Blood **19**:664

McKenna R et al (1977) Thrombo-embolism in patients with abnormally short activated partial thromboplastin time, Thromb Haemost **38**:893

McKusick VA (1962) The earliest record of hemophilia in America? Blood **19**:243

McKusick VA (1969) The nosology of the mucopolysaccharidoses, Am J Med **47**:730

McKusick VA (1978) Mendelian inheritance in man, Baltimore, Johns Hopkins University Press

McKusick VA et al (1965) The genetic mucopolysaccharidoses, Medicine (Baltimore) **44**:445

McKusick VA et al (1978) The mucopolysaccharide storage diseases. In Stanbury JB et al (Eds): The metabolic basis of inherited disease, New York, McGraw-Hill Book Co, Inc

McMillen P and Luftig RB (1973) Preservation of erythrocyte ghost ultrastructure achieved by various fixatives, Proc Natl Acad Sci USA **70**:3060

McNabb PC et al (1979) Transmural eosinophilic gastroenteritis with ascites, Mayo Clin Proc **54**:119

McNicol GP and Davies JA (1973) Fibrinolytic enzyme system, Clin Haematol **2**:23

McPhedran P et al (1972) Multiple myeloma incidence in metropolitan Atlanta, Georgia: racial and seasonal variations, Blood **39**:866

Medawar PB (1968) Biological effects of heterologous antilymphocyte sera. In Rapaport FT and Dausset J (Eds): Human Transplantation, New York, Grune & Stratton, Inc, p 501

Meier HL et al (1976) Enhancement of surface dependent Hageman factor activation by high molecular weight kininogen, Fed Proc **35**:692

Meighan SS (1964) Leukemia in children. Incidence, clinical manifestations, and survival in an unselected series, JAMA **190**:578

Meili EO et al (1968) Myocardial infarction in a haemophiliac. Demonstration of coronary sclerosis by selective angiography, Helv Med Acta **34**:239

Meineke HA and Crafts RC (1968) Further observations on the mechanism by which androgens and growth hormone influence erythropoiesis, Ann NY Acad Sci **149**:298

Mellinger EJ and Duckert F (1971) Major surgery in a subject with factor V deficiency: cholecystectomy in a parahaemophilic woman and review of the literature, Thromb Diath Haemorth **25**:438

Mellins RB et al (1970) Failure of automatic control of ventilation (Ondine's curse). Report of an infant born with this syndrome and review of the literature, Medicine **49**:487

Mellwig KP and Jakobs KH (1980) Inhibition of platelet adenylate cyclase by ADP, Thromb Res **18**:7

Melmon KL and Cline MJ (1967) Kinins, Am J Med **43**:153

Melmon KL et al (1974) Hemolytic plaque formation by leukocytes in vitro. Control by vasoactive hormones, J Clin Invest **53**:13

Meltzer M et al (1966) Cryoglobulinemia—a clinical and laboratory study. II. Cryoglobulins with rheumatoid factor activity, Am J Med **40**:837

Ménaché D and Roberts HR (1975) Summary report and recommendations of the Task Force members and consultants, Thromb Diath Haemorrh **33**:645

Ménaché D and Aronson DL (1978) Heterogeneity of factor IX in therapeutic factor IX concentrates, Thromb Res **13**:821

Mendes NF et al (1973) Technical aspects of the rosette tests used to detect human complement (B) and sheep erythrocyte-binding (T) lymphocytes, J Immunol **111**:860

Menefee MG et al (1978) The Sézary syndrome: a case with fetal-type glycogen and lymphocytic lymphphoma, Arch Dermatol **114**:772

Mengel CE et al (1967) Studies of paroxysmal nocturnal hemoglobinuria erythrocytes: increased lysis and lipid peroxide formation by hydrogen peroxide, J Clin Invest **46**:1715

Mengel CE et al (1972) Biochemistry of PNH cells: nature of the membrane defect, Ser Haematol **5**:88

Menkes JH et al (1962) A sex-linked recessive disorder with retardation of growth, peculiar hair, and focal cerebral and cerebellar degeneration, Pediatrics **29**:764

Mercer DW et al (1977) Acid phosphatase isoenzymes in Gaucher's disease, Clin Chem **23**:631

Merker H and Heilmeyer L (1960) Alkaline phosphatase of neutrophil leukocytes. Cytoenzymatic demonstration and activity in diseases and reactions of the hematopoietic system, Dtsch Med Wochenschr **85**:253

Merrill DA et al (1964) Change in serum haptoglobin type following human liver transplantation, Proc Soc Exp Biol Med **116**:748

Merrill RH and Barrett O Jr (1976) Positive Mono-spot test in histiocytic medullary reticulosis, Am J Clin Pathol **65**:407

Mertelsmann R et al (1978) Improved biochemical assay for terminal deoxynucleotidyl transferase in human blood cells: results in 89 adult patients with lymphoid leukemias and malignant lymphomas in leukemic phase, Leukemia Res **2**:57

Merzbach D and Obedeanu N (1975) Standardisation of the nitro-blue-tetrazolium test, J Med Microbiol **8**:375

Meshaka G et al (1966) Etude des immunoglobulines dans l'ataxie-télangiectasie. In Protides of the biological fluids, XIVᵉ coll., Bruges, Elsevier Press, p 715

Mestecky J et al (1971) Immunoglobulin M and secretory immunoglobulin A: presence of a common polypeptide chain different from light chains, Science **171**:1163

Mestecky J et al (1972) Studies on human secretory immunoglobulin A. III. J chain, Immunochemistry **9**:883

Metcalf D (1967) Lymphocyte kinetics in the thymus. In Yoffey JM (Ed): The lymphocyte in immunology and haemopoiesis, London, Edward Arnold (Publishers) Ltd, p 333

Metcalf D and Wahren B (1968) Bone marrow colony-stimulating activity of sera in infectious mononucleosis, Br Med J **3**:99

Metcalf D (1972) The colony stimulating factor (CSF), Aust J Exp Biol Med Sci **50**:547

Metcalf D (1977) Hemopoietic colonies; in vitro cloning of normal and leukemic cells, Recent Results Cancer Res **61**:1

Metcalf D (1978) Regulation of hemopoiesis, Nouv Rev Fr Hematol **20**:521

Metcalf D and Moore MAS (1971) Haematopoietic cells. In Neuberger A and Tatum EL (Eds): Frontiers in biology, Amsterdam, North Holland, p 489

Metchnikoff E (1887) Sur la lutte des cellules de l'organisme contre l'invasion des microbes, Ann Inst Pasteur **1**:321

Metchnikoff E (1905) Immunity in infective disease (Translated by FG Binnie), Cambridge, Cambridge University Press

Metz J et al (1960) Acetylcholinesterase activity of the erythrocytes in paroxysmal nocturnal hemoglobinuria in relation to the severity of the disease, Br J Haematol **6**:372

Metzger H (1970) The antigen receptor problem, Ann Rev Biochem **39**:889

Metzger H (1978) The IgE-mast cell system as a paradigm for the study of antibody mechanisms, Immunol Rev **41**:186

Meuret G et al (1974) Functional characteristics of chronic monocytic "leukemia," Acta Haematol **52**:95

Meyer CJLM et al (1977) Cerebriform (Sézary-like) mononuclear cells in healthy individuals: a morphologically distinct population of T cells; relationship with mycosis fungoides and Sézary's syndrome, Virchow's Arch (Zellpathol) **25**:95

Meyer D et al (1971) Factor VIII and IX variants. Relationship between haemophilia B$_M$ and haemophilia B$_+$, Eur J Clin Invest **1**:425

Meyer D et al (1975) Problems in the detection of carriers of haemophilia A, J Clin Pathol **28**:690

Meyer LM and Rotter SD (1942) Leukemoid reaction (hyperleukocytosis) in malignancy, Am J Clin Pathol **12**:218

Meyer TC and Angus J (1956) The effect of large doses of "Synkavit" in the newborn, Arch Dis Child **31**:212

Meyer UA and Schmid R (1978) The porphyrias, In Stanbury JB et al (Eds): The metabolic basis of inherited disease, ed 4, New York, McGraw-Hill Book Co, Inc, p 1166

Miale JB (1947) The hematologic response in dogs to the administration of anti-spleen serum, Blood **2**:175

Miale JB (1962) Laboratory control of anticoagulant therapy, JAMA **180**:736

Miale JB (1971) The value of hematology screening. In Advances in automated analysis, vol 1, Technicon International Congress, 1970, Miami, Thurman Associates, p 387

Miale JB (1980) The use of reference plasmas in the control of oral anticoagulant therapy, Scand J Haematol **25** (Supp 37):21

Miale JB and Kent JW (1962) Serum haptoglobin in rabbits after subcutaneous injection of Freund's adjuvant of turpentine, Proc Soc Exp Biol Med **8**:589

Miale JB and Kent JW (1972) Standardization of the theapeutic range for oral anticoagulants based on standard reference plasmas, Am J Clin Pathol **57**:80

Miale JB and Kent JW (1974) The effects of oral contraceptives on the results of laboratory tests. Am J Obstet Gynecol **120**:264

Miale JB and Kent JW (1975) Prothrombin complex proteins as cofactors in platelet aggregation. I. Inhibition of aggregation by antiserum, Blood **45**:97

Miale JB and Kent JW (1979) Standardization of the technique for the prothrombin time test, Lab Medicine **10**:612

Miale JB and LaFond DJ (1969a) Prothrombin time standardization, Am J Clin Pathol **52**:154

Miale JB and LaFond DJ (1969b) Prothrombin time standardization: proposal of the Standards Committee, College of American Pathologists, Thromb Diath Haemorrh (supp) **35**:107

Miale JB and Wilson MP (1956a) Studies on the thromboplastin generation test. I. Method and clinical applications, Am J Clin Pathol **26**:969

Miale JB and Wilson MP (1956b) Studies on the thromboplastin generation test. II. Basic mechanisms and theoretical aspects, Am J Clin Pathol **26**:984

Miale JB and Winningham AR (1960) A true micromethod for prothrombin time, using capillary blood and disposable multipurpose micropipet, Am J Clin Pathol **33**:214

Miale JB et al (1976) Joint AMA-ABA Guildelines: present status of serologic testing in disputed parentage, Fam Law Q **10**:247

Michael AF Jr and Mauer AM (1961) Maternal fetal transfusion as a cause of plethora in the neonatal period, Pediatrics **28**:458

Micheli F et al (1935) Ulteriori ricerche sulla anemia ipocromica splenomegalica con poichilocitosi, Atti Soc Ital di Ematol, Haematol **16**:(supp):10

Michiels JJ et al (1978) Factor VIII inhibitor postpartum, Scand J Haematol **20**:97

Mickenberg ID et al (1972) Bacterial and metabolic properties of human eosinophils, Blood **39**:67

Mielke CH Jr and Rodvien R (1976) Qualitative platelet abnormality due to absent collagen-induced aggregation, Thromb Haemost **36**:283

Mielke CH Jr et al (1969) The standardized normal Ivy bleeding time and its prolongation by aspirin, Blood **34**:204

Miescher PA (1973) Drug-induced thrombocytopenia, Semin Hematol **10**:311

Miescher PA and Miescher A (1978) Immunologic drug-induced blood dyscrasias, Klin Wochenschr **56**:1

Migler R et al (1978) Human eosinophilic peroxidase: role in bactericidal activity, Blood **51**:445

Migliore PJ and Alexanian R (1968) Monoclonal gammopathy in human neoplasia, Cancer **21**:1127

Mihalyi E (1980) Proteolytic fragmentation of fibrinogen. In Schmidt RM (Section Ed); Handbook Series in Clinical Laboratory Science, Section I: Hematology, vol 3, Boca Raton, Fla, CRC Press Inc, p 51

Millar WG (1925) Observation on the haematocrit method of measuring the volume of erythrocyte, Q J Exp Physiol **15**:187

Miller AA (1957) Congenital sulfhemoglobinemia, J Pediatr **51**:233

Miller AM and McGarry MP (1976) A diffusible stimulator of eosinophilopoiesis produced by lymphoid cells as demonstrated with diffusion chambers, Blood **48**:293

Miller AM et al (1978) Modulation of graulopoiesis: opposing roles of prostaglandins F and E, J Lab Clin Med **92**:983

Miller D (1959) Observations on a case of probable bone marrow anthracosis, Blood **14**:1350

Miller DR (1968) Serum folate deficiency in children receiving anticonvulsant therapy, Pediatrics **41**:630

Miller DR (1969) Raised foetal haemoglobin in childhood leukemia, Br J Haematol **17**:103

Miller DR et al (1971) A new variant of hereditary hemolytic anemia with stomatocytosis and erythrocyte cation abnormality, Blood **38**:184

Miller DR et al (1979) Prognostic significance of lymphoblast morphology (FAB classification) in childhood leukemia, Proc Am Soc Clin Oncol **20**:345

Miller EC (1978) Some current perspectives on chemical carcinogenesis in humans and experimental animals (Presidential Address), Cancer Res **38**:1479

Miller G et al (1965) A new congenital hemolytic anemia with deformed erythrocytes (?"stomatocytes") and remarkable susceptibility of erythrocytes to cold hemolysis in vitro. I. Clinical and hematologic studies, Pediatrics **35**:906

Miller LH (1975) Transfusion malaria. In Greenwalt TJ and Jamieson GA (Eds): Transmissible disease and blood transfusion, New York, Grune & Stratton, Inc, p 241

Miller LH et al (1975) Erythrocyte receptors for (*Plasmodium knowlesi*) malaria: Duffy blood group determinants, Science **189**:561

Miller LH et al (1976) The resistance factor to *Plasmodium vivax* in Blacks. The Duffy blood group genotype, *FyFy*, N Engl J Med **295**:302

Miller ME (1967) Thymic dysplasia ("Swiss agammaglobulinemia"). I. Graft versus host reaction following bone-marrow transfusion, J Pediatr **70**:730

Miller ME (1975a) Pathology of chemotaxis and random mobility, Semin Hematol **12**:59

Miller ME (1975b) Developmental maturation of human formability. In Bellanti JA and Dayton DH (Eds): The phagocytic cell in host resistance, New York, Raven Press

Miller ME and Nilsson UR (1970) A familial deficiency of the phagocytosis-enhancing activity of serum related to a dysfunction of the fifth component of complement (C5), N Engl J Med **282**:354

Miller ME et al (1971) Lazy-leukocyte syndrome. A new disorder of neutrophil function, Lancet **1**:665

Miller ME et al (1973) A new familial defect of neutrophil movement, J Lab Clin Med **82**:1

Miller ME et al (1974) Mechanism of erythropoietin production by cobaltous chloride, Blood **44**:339

Miller MJ et al (1956) Distribution of parasites in the red cells of sickle-cell trait carriers infected with *Plasmodium falciparum,* Trans R Soc Trop Med Hyg **50**:294

Millett YL et al (1969) Nodular sclerotic lymphasarcoma: a further review, Br J Cancer **26**:683

Mills DCB and MacFarlane DE (1974) Stimulation of human platelet adenylate cyclase by prostaglandin D_2, Thromb Res **5**:401

Mills DCB and Smith JB (1972) The control of platelet responsiveness by agents that influence cyclic AMP metabolism, Ann NY Acad Sci **201**:391

Mills DC et al (1968) The release of nucleotides, 5-hydroxytryptamine and enzymes from human blood platelets during aggregation, J Physiol **195**:715

Mills H and Lucia SP (1949) Familial hypochromic anemia associated with postsplenectomy erythrocytic inclusion bodies, Blood **4**:891

Milner PF (1974) Oxygen transport in sickle cell anemia, Arch Intern Med **133**:565

Milner PF et al (1970) Hemoglobin O Arab in four Negro families and its interaction with hemoglobin S and hemoglobin C, N Engl J Med **283**:1417

Milner PF et al (1971) Haemoglobin H disease due to a unique haemoglobin variant with an elongated α-chain. Lancet **1**:729

Milner PF et al (1976) Thalassemia intermedia caused by heterozygosity for both beta thalassemia and hemoglobin Saki (beta 14 [All] leu → pro), Am J Hematol **1**:283

Milstein C and Pink JR (1970) Structure and evolution of immunoglobulins, Prog Biophys Mol Biol **21**:209

Min K-W et al (1978) Selective uptake of ^{75}Se-selenomethionine by thymoma with pure red cell aplasia, Cancer **41**:1323

Minden MD et al (1979) Separation of blast cell and T-lymphocyte progenitors in the blood of patients with acute myeloblastic leukemia, Blood **54**:186

Minnefor AB et al (1970) Production of interferon by long-term suspension cultures of leukocytes derived from patients with viral and nonviral diseases, J Infect Dis **121**:442

Minnich V et al (1962) Alpha, beta and gamma hemoglobin polypeptide chains during the neonatal period with description of a fetal form of hemoglobin D St. Louis, Blood **19**:137

Minnich V et al (1965) Hemoglobin Hope: a beta chain variant, Blood **25**:830

Minnich V et al (1968) Pica in Turkey, II. Effect of clay upon iron absorption, Am J Clin Nutr **21**:78

Minot GR and Murphy WB (1926) Treatment of pernicious anemia by special diet, JAMA **87**:470

Mirand EA et al (1968) Extra-renal production of erythropoietin in man, Acta Haematol **39**:359

Mishler JM and Parry ES (1979) Transfusion of hydroxyethylated amylopectin-protected frozen blood in man. I. Plasma clearance and renal excretion of the cryoprotectant, Vox Sang **36**:337

Mishler JM et al (1978) Whole blood storage in citrate and phosphate solutions containing half-strength trisodium citrate: cellular and biochemical studies, J Pathol **124**:125

Mishler JM et al (1979) Viability of red cells stored in diminished concentration of citrate, Br J Haematol **43**:63

Mitchell HK et al (1941) The concentration of "folic acid," J Am Chem Soc **63**:2284

Mitelman F et al (1976) Non-random karyotypic evolution in chronic myeloid leukemia, Int J Cancer **18**:24

Mitrakul C et al (1969) Basophilic leukemia. Report of a case, Clin Pediatr **8**:178

Mittal KK et al (1976) Matching of histocompatibility (HL-A) antigens for platelet transfusion, Blood **47**:31

Mittwoch U (1961) Inclusions of mucopolysaccharides in the lymphocytes of patients with gargoylism, Nature **191**:1315

Mittwoch U (1963) The demonstration of mucopolysaccharide inclusion in the lymphocytes of patients with gargoylism, Acta Haematol **29**:202

Mitus WJ et al (1959) Alkaline phosphatase of mature neutrophils in various "polycythemias," N Engl J Med **260**:1131

Mitus WJ et al (1964) Experimental renal erythrocytosis. I. Effects of pressure and vascular interference, Blood **24**:343

Mitus WJ et al (1968) Erythrocytosis, juxtaglomerular apparatus (JGA), and erythropoietin in the course of experimental unilateral hydronephrosis in rabbits, Ann NY Acad Sci **149**:107

Miyagawa Y et al (1978) Measurement of Donath-Landsteiner antibody-producing cells in idiopathic nonsyphilitic paroxysmal cold hemoglobinuria (PCH) in children, Blood **52**:97

Miyaji T et al (1963a) Hemoglobin Shimonoseki (alpha 2 54 arg beta 2A), a slow moving hemoglobin found in a Japanese family, with special reference to its chemistry, Acta Haematol Jpn **26**:531

Miyaji T et al (1963b) Possible amino acid substitution in the alpha chain (alpha 87 tyr) of hb M Iwate, Acta Haematol Jpn **26**:538

Miyaji T et al (1966) Hemoglobin Agenogi (alpha 2 beta 2 90 lys), a slow-moving hemoglobin of a Japanese family resembling hb-E, Clin Chim Acta **14**:624

Miyaji T et al (1967) Amino acid substitution of hemoglobin Ube 2 (alpha 2 68 asp beta 2): an example of successful application of partial hydrolysis of peptide with 5% acetic acid, Clin Chim Acta **16**:347

Miyaji T et al (1968a) Hemoglobin Hijiyama: a new fast moving hemoglobin in a Japanese family, Science **159**:204

Miyaji T et al (1968B) Japanese haemoglobin variant, Nature (London) **217**:89

Miyaji T et al (1977) Hemoglobin Karatsu: beta 120 (GH3) lysine → asparagine. An example of hb Riyadh in Japan, Hemoglobin **1**:461

Mizoguchi H and Levere RD (1971) Enhancement of heme and glohin synthesis in cultural human marrow by certain 5 β-H steroid metabolites, J Exp Med **134**:1501

Modan B (1965) Polycythemia. A review of epidemiological and clinical aspects, J Chronic Dis **18**:605

Modan B and Lilienfeld AM (1965) Polycythemia vera and leukemia—the role of radiation treatment. A study of 1222 patients, Medicine **44**:305

Moeschlin S (1940) Erythroblastosen, Erythroleukämien, und Erythroblastämien, Folia Haematol **64**:262

Moeschlin S (1951) Spleen puncture, London, William Heinemann Medical Books Ltd

Moeschlin S (1954) Nervous regulation of hematopoiesis. In Proceedings of the Fourth International Society of Hematology, New York, Grune & Stratton, Inc, p 41

Mohler DN et al (1970) Glutathione synthetase deficiency as a cause of hereditary hemolytic disease, N Engl J Med **283**:1253

Mollin DL and Ross GIM (1955) Serum vitamin B_{12} concentrations in leukaemia and in some other haematological conditions, Br J Haematol **1**:155

Mollison PL (1979) Blood transfusion in clinical medicine, ed 6, Oxford, England, Blackwell Scientific Publications

Moloney WC (1955) Leukemia in survivors of atomic bombing, N Engl J Med **253**:88

Moloney WC and Lange RD (1954) Leukemia in atomic survivors. II. Observations on early phases of leukemia, Blood **9**:663

Molthan L et al (1967) Positive direct Coombs tests due to cephalothin, N Engl J Med **277**:123

Moncada S et al (1976) An enzyme isolated from arteries transforms prostaglandin endoperoxidases to an unstable substance that inhibits platelet aggregation, Nature **263**:663

Moncada S et al (1977) Differential formation of prostacyclin (PGX or PGI$_2$) by layers of the arterial wall: an explanation for the anti-thrombotic properties of vascular endothelium, Thromb Res **11**:323

Monn E et al (1968) Hemoglobin Sogn (beta 14 arginine). A new haemoglobin variant, Scand J Haematol **5**:353

Montgomery PO et al (1964) Cellular and subcellular effects of ionizing radiations, Am J Pathol **44**:727

Moo-Penn WF (1978) Hemoglobin Detroit: beta 95 (FG2) lysine → asparagine, Biochim Biophys Acta **536**:283

Moo-Penn WF et al (1975) Hemoglobin Deaconess, a new deletion mutant: beta 131 (H9) glutamine deleted, Biochem Biophys Res Commun **65**:8

Moo-Penn WF et al (1976a) Hemoglobin Providence. A human hemoglobin variant occurring in two forms *in vivo,* J Biol Chem **251**:7557

Moo-Penn WF et al (1976b) Hemoglobin Fannin-Lubbock (alpha 2 beta 2 119 [GH2] gly → asp): a new hemoglobin variant at the alpha 1 beta 1 contact, Biochim Biophys Acta **453**:472

Moo-Penn WF et al (1976c) Hemoglobin Jackson alpha 127 (H10) lys → asn, Am J Clin Pathol **66**:453

Moo-Penn WF et al (1977a) Hemoglobin Raleigh (beta 1 valine- → acetylalanine). Structural and functional characterization, Biochemistry **16**:4872

Moo-Penn WF et al (1977b) Hemoglobin Tarrant: alpha 126 (H9) asp → asn. A new hemoglobin variant in the alpha 1 beta 1 contact region showing high oxygen affinity and reduced cooperativity, Biochim Biophys Acta **490**:443

Moo-Penn WF et al (1977c) Hemoglobin S Travis. A sickling hemoglobin with two amino acid substitutions (beta 6 [A3] glutamic acid → valine and beta 142 [H20] alanine → valine), Eur J Biochem **77**:561

Moo-Penn WF et al (1977d) Hemoglobin Austin and Waco: two hemoglobins with substitutions in the alpha 1 beta 2 contact region, Arch Biochem Biophys **179**:86

Moo-Penn WF et al (1978) Hemoglobin Presbyterian: beta 108 (G10) asparagine → lysine. A hemoglobin variant with low oxygen affinity, FEBS Lett **92**:53

Moo-Penn WF et al (1980a) Structural and functional properties of hemoglobin Brockton, beta 138 ala → pro, Joint Meeting of the 18th Congress of the International Society on Hematology and the 16th Congress of the International Society on Blood Transfusion, Montreal, Abstract no 599, p 128

Moo-Penn WF et al (1980b) Hemoglobin Ohio (β143 ala → asp): a new abnormal hemoglobin with high oxygen affinity and erythrocytosis, Blood **56**:246

Moore BPL et al (1961) A weak example of the blood group antigen A, Vox Sang **6**:151

Moore CV (1961) Iron metabolism and nutrition, Harvey Lect **55**:67

Moore CV et al (1939) Studies in iron transportation and metabolism. IV. Observations on the absorption of iron from the gastrointestinal tract, J Clin Invest **18**:553

Moore EC and Meuwissen JH (1973) Immunologic deficiency disease. Approach to diagnosis, NY State J Med **73**:2437

Moore EW (1964) Iron absorption kinetic studies in the normal dog, J Clin Invest **43**:1282

Moore GE et al (1957) Clinical and experimental observations of the occurrence and fate of tumor cells in the blood stream, Ann Surg **146**:580

Moore HC and Mollison PL (1976) Use of a low-ionic-strength medium in manual tests for antibody detection, Transfusion **16**:291

Moore KL and Barr ML (1954) Nuclear morphology according to sex, in human tissues, Acta Anat **21**:197

Moore KL et al (1955) Sex chromatin in the freemartin, Anat Rec **121**:422

Moor-Jankowski J et al (1964) Blood group antigens and cross reacting antibodies in primates, including man. III. Heterophile-like behavior of the blood factor I, Exp Med Surg **22**:308

Moore MAS et al (1974) Monocyte production of colony stimulating factor in familial cyclic neutropenia, Br J Haematol **27**:47

Moore S and Pepper DS (1976) Identification of a platelet specific release product β-thromboglobulin. In Gordon JL (Ed): Platelet physiology, Amsterdam, Biomedical Press, p 293

Morawitz P (1905) Die Chemie der Blutgerinnung, Erebn Physiol **4**:307. Available in the English translation as: "The chemistry of blood coagulation," translated by: Hartman RC and Guenther PF (1958), Springfield, Ill, Charles C Thomas, Publishers

Morell A et al (1970) Metabolic properties of IgG subclasses in man, J Clin Invest **49**:673

Morgan EH and Appleton TC (1969) Autoradiographic localization of 125-I-labelled transferrin in rabbit reticulocytes, Nature **223**:1371

Morgan WT (1976) The binding and transport of heme by hemopexin, Ann Clin Res **8**:224

Morganti G and Cresseri A (1954) Nouvelles recherches génétiques sur les leucémies, Sang **25**:421

Morita H et al (1971) The occurrence of homozygous hemophilia in the female, Acta Haematol **45**:112

Morley AA (1966) A neutrophil cycle in healthy individuals, Lancet **2**:1220

Morley AA et al (1967) Familial cyclical neutropenia, Br J Haematol **13**:719

Morowitz DA et al (1968) Thrombocytosis in chronic inflammatory bowel disease, Ann Intern Med **68**:1013

Morrell AG et al (1964) Physical and chemical studies on ceruloplasmin, J Biol Chem **239**:1042

Morrison FS and Baldini MG (1969) Antigenic relationship between blood platelets and vascular endothelium, Blood **33**:46

Morrison FS and Mollison PL (1966) Post-transfusion purpura, N Engl J Med **275**:243

Morrison FS et al (1968) Post-transfusion survival of red cells stored in liquid nitrogen, Br J Haematol **14**:215

Morrison JC and Wiser WL (1976) The effect of maternal partial exchange transfusion on the infants of patients with sickle cell anemia, J Pediatr **89**:286

Morrow JJ et al (1968) A controlled trial of iron therapy in sideropenia, Scott Med J **13**:78

Morse BS (1978) Total red cell volume in healthy young males, Ann Clin Lab Sci **8**:413

Morse D et al (1974) Prehistoric multiple myeloma, Bull NY Acad Med **50**:447

Morse EE (1967) Topics in clinical medicine. Posttransfusion thrombocytopenic purpura, Johns Hopkins Med J **121**:365

Morse EE et al (1966a) The transfusion of leukocytes from donors with chronic myelocytic leukemia to patients with leukopenia, Transfusion **6**:183

Morse EE et al (1966b) Thrombocytopenic purpura following rubella infection in children and adults, Arch Intern Med **117**:573

Morse EE (1978) The fibrinogenopathies, Ann Clin Lab Sci **8**:234

Morse EE et al (1966) Repeated leukapheresis of patients with chronic myelocytic leukemia, Transfusion **6**:175

Mortensen E (1976) Determination of erythrocyte folate by competitive protein binding assay preceded by extraction, Clin Chem **22**:982

Morton JH (1969) Surgical transfusion practices, 1967, Surgery **65**:407

Moses HL et al (1968) Infectious mononucleosis: detection of herpes-like virus and reticular aggregates of small cytoplasmic particles in continuous lymphoid cell lines derived from peripheral blood, Proc Natl Acad Sci USA **60**:489

Moses S and Barland P (1979) Laboratory criteria for a diagnosis of systemic lupus erythematosus, JAMA 242:1039

Mosesson MW (1974) Fibrinogen catabolic pathways. Semin Thromb Hemost 1:63

Mosesson MW et al (1976) Studies on the structural abnormality of fibrinogen Paris I, J Clin Invest 57:782

Moss MH (1969) Hypothrombinemic bleeding in a young infant associated with a soy protein formula, Am J Dis Child 117:540

Motulsky AG (1964) Hereditary red cell traits and malaria, Am J Trop Med Hyg 13:147

Motulsky AG (1973a) Frequency of sickling disorders in U.S. blacks, N Engl J Med 288:31

Motulsky AG (1973b) Screening for sickle cell hemoglobinopathy and thalassemia, Isr J Med Sci 9:1341

Motulsky AG (1974) Brave new world? Science 185:653

Motulsky AG and Stamatoyannopoulos G (1968) Drugs, anesthesia, and abnormal hemoglobins, Ann NY Acad Sci 151:807

Mourant AE (1946) A ''new'' human blood group antigen of frequent occurrence, Nature 158:237

Mourant AE (1954) The distribution of the human blood groups. Springfield, Ill, Charles C Thomas, Publishers

Movassaghi N et al (1967) Serum and urinary levels of erythropoietin in iron deficiency anemia, proc Soc Exp Biol Med 126:615

Movat HZ et al (1958) The diffuse intimal thickening of the human aorta with aging, Am J Pathol 34:1023

Movitt ER et al (1963) Idiopathic true bone marrow failure, Am J Med 34:500

Mowat AG and Baum J (1971a) Chemotaxis of polymorphonuclear leukocytes from patients with diabetes mellitus, N Engl J Med 284:621

Mowat AG and Baum J (1971b) Chemotaxis of polymorphonuclear leukocytes from patients with rheumatoid arthritis, J Clin Invest 50:2541

Moynahan EJ (1974) Acrodermatitis enteropathica: a lethal inherited human zinc-deficiency disorder, Lancet 2:399

Muckerheide MM et al (1977) Increased serum folate-binding capacity, a familial trait, Acta Haematol 58:45

Mueh JR et al (1980) Thrombosis in patients with the lupus anticoagulant, Ann Intern Med 92:156

Mueller-Eckhardt C et al (1980) Post-transfusion thrombocytopenia purpura: immunological and clinical studies in two cases and review of the literature, Blut 40:249

Muenzer J et al (1975) Oxygen consumption of human blood platelets. II. Effect of inhibitors on thrombin-induced oxygen burst, Biochem Biophys Acta 376:243

Muggia FM et al (1969) Lysozymuria and renal tubular dysfunction in monocytic and myelomonocytic leukemia, Am J Med 47:351

Muir A and Cossar IA (1959) Aspirin and gastric haemorrhage, Lancet 1:539

Muldowney FP et al (1957) The total red cell mass in thyrotoxicosis and myxedema, Clin Sci 16:309

Muller CJ (1961) A comparative study of the structure of mammalian and avian hemoglobins, Groningen (Holland), Van Gorcum & Co

Muller CJ and Kingma S (1961) Haemloglbin Zürich alpha 2A beta 2 63 arg, Biochim Biophys Acta 50:595

Müler-Eberhard HJ (1975) Complement, Ann Rev Biochem 44:697

Müler-Eberhard HJ (1976) The serum complement system. In Miescher Pa and Müler-Eberhard HJ (Eds): Textbook of immunopathology, New York, Grune & Stratton, Inc

Müler-Eberhard U (1970) Hemopexin, N Engl J Med 283:1090

Mulvihill JJ et al (1977) Multiple childhood osteosarcomas in an American Indian family with erythroid macrocytosis and skeletal anomalies, Cancer 40:3115

Murano G (1974) The molecular structure of fibrinogen, Semin Thromb Hemost 1:1

Murano G and Bick RL (1980) Basic concepts of hemostasis and thrombosis, Boca Raton, Fla, CRC Press Inc, p 45

Muratore R et al (1973) Anomalies morphologiques des polynucléaires neutrophiles au cours des affections prolifératives du tissu myéloïde, Nouv Rev Fr Hematol 13:376

Murawski K et al (1963) A New variant of abnormal methaemoglobin: hb M Radom, Biochim Biophys Acta 69:442

Murayama M (1966) Molecular mechanism of red cell ''sickling,'' Science 153:145

Murayama M (1971) The chemical and the three-dimensional structure of human hemoglobin, Ann Clin Lab Sci 1:1

Murayama M and Nalbadian R (1973) Sickle cell hemoglobin: molecule to man, Boston, Little, Brown & Co

Murphy JR (1965) Erythrocyte metabolism. VI. Cell shape and the location of cholesterol in the erythrocyte membrane, J Lab Clin Med 65:756

Murphy JR (1973) Sickle cell hemoglobin (HB AS) in black football players, JAMA 225:981

Murphy RJC et al (1980) Death following an exchange transfusion with hemoglobin SC blood, J Pediatr 96:110

Murthy MNS and von Haam E (1958) The occurrence of the sex chromatin in white blood cells of young adults, Am J Clin Pathol 30:216

Muss HB and Moloney WC (1973) Chloroma and other myeloblastic tumors, Blood 42:721

Mustard JF and Packham MA (1970) Factors influencing platelet function: adhesion, release, and aggregation, Pharmacol Rev 22:97

Mustard JF et al (1966) Platelet economy (platelet survival and turnover) Br J Haematol 12:1

Myerowitz RL et al (1977) Carcinocythemia (carcinoma cell leukemia) due to metastatic carcinoma of the breast: report of a case, Cancer 40:3107

Myers AJ et al (1953) Quantitative studies of the influence of plasma proteins and hematocrit on the erythrocyte sedimentation rate, Blood 8:893

Myerson RM and Frumin AM (1960) Hyperkalemia associated with the myeloproliferative disorder, Arch Intern Med 106:479

Myhre BA (1974) Quality control in blood banking, London, John Wiley & Sons Ltd

Myhre BA and Nakayama V (1976) Serologic evaluation of the Mono-chek test, Am J Clin Pathol 65:987

Myrhed M et al (1976) Genetic control of serum hemopexin, Ann Clin Res 8:259

Myllylä G et al (1967) Hereditary thrombocytopenia: report of three families, Scand J Haematol 4:441

Nachman RL (1965) Immunologic studies of platelet protein, Blood 25:703

Nachman RL and Jaffe EA (1976) The platelet-endothelial cell-VIII axis, Thromb Haemost 35:120

Nachman RL et al (1967) Platelet thrombasthenia: subcellular localization and function, J clin Invest 46:1380

Nachtscheim H (1950) The Pelger anomaly in man and rabbit, a mendelian character of the nuclei of leukocytes, J Hered 41:131

Nadler HL et al (1969) Enzyme changes and polyribosome profiles in phytohemagglutinin (PHA) stimulated lymphocytes, Blood 34:52

Nadler SB et al (1962) Prediction of blood volume in normal human adults, Surgery 51:224

Naegeli O (1900) Über rothes Knockenmark und Myeloblasten, Dtsch Med Wochenschr 26:287

Naets JP and Wittek M (1968) Presence of erythropoietin in the plasma of one anephric patient, Blood 31:249

Nagaya H (1970) Antilymphocyte serum or antithymus serum, Arch Intern Med **125**:499

Nagel RL and Bookchin RM (1974) Human hemoglobin mutants with abnormal oxygen binding, Semin Hematol **11**:385

Nagel RL and Ranney HM (1964) Haptoglobin binding capacity of certain abnormal hemoglobins, Science **144**:1014

Nagel RL et al (1976) Hemoglobin Beth Israel: a mutant causing clinically apparent cyanosis, N Engl J Med **295**:125

Nagel RL et al (1980) Hb G Manhasset (beta 139 asn → lys): an abnormal hemoglobin with decreased oxygen affinity, Joint Meeting of the 18th Congress of the International Society on Hematology and the 16th Congress of the International Society on Blood Transfusion, Montreal, Abstract no 1059, p 203

Nagel V et al (1972) Unexplained appearance of antibody in an Rh null donor, Vox Sang **22**:519

Naiman JL and Gerald PS (1963) Fetal hemoglobin: improved separation by a modified agar gel electrophoresis, J Lab Clin Med **61**:508

Naiman JL et al (1964) Hereditary eosinophilia: report of a family and review of the literature, Am J Hum Genet **16**:195

Najean Y et al (1966) Le syndrome de May-Hegglin, Presse Méd **74**:1649

Nakao K et al (1968) δ-Aminolevulinic acid dehydratase activity in erythrocytes for the evaluation of lead poisoning, Clin Chim Acta **19**:319

Napoli VM and Wallach H (1976) Pancytopenia associated with a granulosa-cell tumor of the ovary: report of a case, Am J Clin Pathol **65**:344

Naspitz CR and Richter M (1968) The action of phytohemagglutinin in vivo and in vitro, a review, Prog Allergy **12**:1

Natelson EA and Coltman CA Jr (1972) Immunoadsorption of human factor IX, Clin Res **20**:495

Nath BJ and Lindenbaum J (1979) Persistence of neutrophil hypersegmentation during recovery from megaloblastic granulopoiesis, Ann Intern Med **90**:757

Nathan DG and Baehner RL (1971) Disorders of phagocyte function, Prog Hematol **7**:235

Nathan DG et al (1965) Extreme hemolysis and red-cell distortion in erythrocyte pyruvate kinase deficiency. II. Measurements of erythrocyte glucose consumption, potassium flux, and adenosine triphosphate stability, N Engl J Med **272**:118

Nathan DG et al (1966) Studies of erythrocyte spicule formation in haemolytic anaemia, Br J Haematol **12**:385

Nathan DG et al (1968a) Erythroctye production and metabolism in anephric and uremic men, Ann NY Acad Sci **149**:539

Nathan DG et al (1968b) Life span and organ sequestration of the red cells in pyruvate kinase deficiency, N Engl J Med **278**:73

Nathan DG et al (1978a) Human erythroid burst-forming unit: T-cell requirement for proliferation in vitro, J Exp Med **147**:324

Nathan DG et al (1978b) Erythroid precursors in congenital hypoplastic (Diamond-Blackfan) anemia, J Clin Invest **61**:489

Nathwani BN et al (1978) Non-Hodgkin's lymphomas: a clinico-pathologic study comparing two classifications, Cancer **41**:303

National Academy of Sciences, National Research Council (1970) An evaluation of the utilization of human blood resources in the United States, Washington, DC

National Blood Policy (1974) Fed Reg **39**:9329

National Bureau of Standards (1958) Handbook 65: Safe handling of bodies containing radioactive isotopes, Washington, DC, US Department of Commerce

National Center for Health Statistics (1967) Mean blood hematocrit of adults: United States (1960-1962), Series 11, No. 24, Washington, DC, US Government Printing Office

Natvig H (1963) Studies on hemoglobin values in Norway. I. Hemoglobin levels in adults, Acta Med Scand **173**:423

Natvig JB and Kunkel HG (1968) Genetic markers of human immunoglobulins. The Gm and Inv systems, Ser Haematol **1**:66

Natvig JB and Kunkel HG (1973) Human immunoglobulins: classes, subclasses, genetic variants, and idiotypes, Adv Immunol **16**:1

Natvig JB et al (1967) Genetic studies of the heavy chain subgroups of γG globulin. Recombination between the closely linked cistrons. In Kilander J (Ed): Gamma globulins, New York, John Wiley & Sons, Inc.

Naumann HN (1966) A system of testing for Bence Jones protein, South Med J **59**:157

Naumann HN et al (1971) Plasma hemoglobin and hemoglobin fractions in sickle cell crisis, Am J Clin Pathol **56**:137

Necheles TF (1980) Quantitative disorders of leukocytes: differential diagnosis. In Seligson D (Ed): Handbook Series in Clinical Laboratory Science, Section I: Hematology, vol 2, Boca Raton, Fla, CRC Press Inc, p 305

Necheles TF et al (1968) Studies on control of hemoglobin synthesis: nucleic acid synthesis and normoblast proliferation in the presence of erythropoietin, Ann NY Acad Sci **149**:449

Necheles TF et al (1970) Erythrocyte glutathioneperoxidase deficiency, Br J Haematol **19**:605

Needleman P et al (1977) Coronary tone modulation: formation and actions of prostaglandins, endoperoxidases, and thromboxanes, Science **195**:409

Neely CL et al (1969) Lactic acid dehydrogenase activity and plasma hemoglobin elevations in sickle cell disease, Am J Clin Pathol **52**:167

Neiman RS et al (1973) Lymphocyte-depletion Hodgkin's disease. A clinicopathological entity, N Engl J Med **288**:751

Neimann A (1914) Ein unbekanntes Krankheitsbild, Janrb Kinderh **79**:1

Ness PM and Pennington RM (1974) The national blood resource program adenine experience, Transfusion **14**:530

Ness PM et al (1980) An unusual factor-X inhibitor in leprosy, Am J Hematol **8**:397

Nettleship A (1938) Leucocytosis associated with acute inflammation, Am J Clin Pathol **8**:398

Neufeld AH et al (1964) Beta-2 lipoprotein myelomatosis, Can J Biochem **42**:1499

Newcomb T et al (1956) Congenital hemorrhagic diathesis of the prothrombin complex, Am J Med **20**:798

Newman MM et al (1971) Use of banked autologous blood in elective surgery, JAMA **218**:861

Newman MV et al (1979) Hb Vicksburg: a low yield variant which mimics the phenotype of beta thalassemia, Clin Res **27**:745A

Nexø E et al (1975) A rare case of megaloblastic anaemia caused by disturbances in the plasma cobalamin binding proteins in a patient with hepatocellular carcinoma, Scand J Haematol **14**:320

Nezelof C et al (1964) L'hypoplasie Héréditaire du thymus: sa place et sa responsabilité dans une observation d'aplasie lymphocytaire, mormoplasmacytaire et normoglobulinémique du nourrisson, Arch Fr Pediatr **21**:897

Niazi GA et al (1975) Hemoglobin Strumica or alpha 2 112 (G19) his → arg beta 2. (With an addendum: hemoglobin J Paris-I alpha 2 12 [A10] ala → asp beta 2 in the same population), Biochim Biophys Acta **412**:181

Nieburgs HE and Glass GBJ (1963) Gastric-cell maturation disorders in atrophic gastritis, pernicious anemia, and carcinoma, Am J Dig Dis **8**:135

Niederman JC et al (1976) Infectious mononucleosis Epstein-Barr-virus shedding in saliva and the oropharynx, N Engl J Med **294**:1355

Nielsen JO et al (1973) Subtypes of Australia antigen among patients and healthy carriers in Copenhagen. A relation between the subtypes and the degree of liver damage in acute viral hepatitis, N Engl J Med **288**:1257

Nielsen JO et al (1971) Incidence and meaning of persistence of Australia antigen in patients with acute viral hepatitis: development of chronic hepatitis, N Engl J Med **285**:1157

Nielsen JO et al (1974) Incidence and meaning of the "e" determinant among hepatitis-B-antigen positive patients with acute and chronic liver diseases: report from the Copenhagen Hepatitis Acuta Programme, Lancet **2**:913

Nienhuis AW and Anderson WF (1972) Hemoglobin switching in sheep and goats: change in functional globin messenger RNA in reticulocytes and bone marrow cells, Proc Natl Acad Sci **69**:2184

Nienhuis AW and Anderson WF (1974) The molecular defect in thalassemia, Clin Haematol **3**:437

Nienhuis AW and Bunn HF (1974) Hemoglobin switching in sheep and goats: occurrence of hemoglobins A and C in the same red cell, Science **185**:946

Nienhuis AW et al (1971) Translation of rabbit haemoglobin messenger RNA by thalassaemic and nonthalassaemic ribosomes, Nature (New Biol) **231**:205

Nierhaus K and Betke K (1968) Eine vereinfachte Modifikation der sauren Elution für die cytologische Darstellung von fetalem Hämoglobin, Klin Wochenschr **46**:47

Niewiarowski W and Stewart GJ (1978) Interaction of blood cells with fibrinogen and polymerizing fibrin. In de Gaetano G and Garattini S (Eds): Platelets: a multidisciplinary approach, New York, Raven Press

Niléhn J-E and Nilsson IM (1966) Coagulation studies in different types of myeloma, Acta Med Scand **179**(supp 445):194

Nilsson IM et al (1957a) On an inherited autosomal hemorrhagic diathesis with antihemophilic globulin (AHG) deficiency and prolonged bleeding time, Acta Med Scand **159**:35

Nilsson IM et al (1957b) Von Willebrand's disease and its correction with human plasma fraction I-O, Acta Med Scand **159**:179

Nilsson IM et al (1959) Von Willenbrand's disease in Sweden, Acta Med Scand **164**:263

Nilsson LR and Lundholm G (1960) Congenital thrombocytopenia associated with aplasia of the radius, Acta Paediatr **49**:291

Nishi M et al (1979) The migration of lymphocytes across the vascular endothelium in lymph nodes: a scanning electron microscopic study, Lymphology **12**:9

Nishiyama H et al (1973) The incidence of malignant lymphoma and multiple myeloma in Hiroshima and Nagasaki atomic bomb survivors, 1945-1965, Cancer **32**:1301

Nixon RK (1966) The relation of mastocytosis and lymphomatous disease, Ann Intern Med **64**:856

Noble R and Ranney HM (1974) Hemoglobin structure and gas transport. In Greenwalt TJ and Jamieson GA (Eds): The human red cell in vitro, New York, Grune & Stratton, Inc. p 91

Nolf P (1908) Contribution a l'étude de la coagulation du sang: les facteurs primordiaux, leur origine, Arch Int Physiol **6**:1

Norgaard O (1971) Three cases of multiple myeloma in which the preclinical asymptomatic phases persisted throughout 15 to 24 years, Br J Cancer **25**:417

Nøgaard-Pedersen B et al (1972) Hemoglobin pigments. Mixing technique for preparation of known fractions of hemoglobin pigments, Clin Chim Acta **42**:109

Norgard MJ et al (1979) Bone marrow necrosis and degeneration, Arch Intern Med **139**:905

Northam BE et al (1963) Methaemalbumin in the differential diagnosis of acute haemorrhagic and oedematous pancreatitis, Lancet **1**:348

Norum KR et al (1972) Familial lecithin: cholesterol acyl transferase deficiency. In Stanbury JB et al (Eds): The metabolic basis of inherited disease, New York, McGraw-Hill Book Co, Inc, p 531

Nossel HL (1976) Radioimmunoassay of fibrinopeptides in relation to intravascular coagulation and thrombosis, N Engl J Med **295**:428

Nour-Eldin F and Wilkinson JF (1959) Factor VII deficiency with Christmas disease in one family, Lancet **1**:1173

Nowell PC and Finan JB (1977) Isochromosome 17 in atypical myeloproliferative and lymphoproliferative disorders, J Natl Cancer Inst **59**:329

Nowell PC and Hungerford DA (1960) Chromosome studies on normal and leukemic human leukocytes, J Natl Cancer Inst **25**:85

Nowell PC and Wilson DB (1971) Lymphocytes and hemic stem cells, Am J Pathol **65**:641

Nowell PC et al (1970) Evidence for the existence of multipotential lympho-hematopoietic stem cells in adult rat, J Cell Physiol **75**:151

Nowell PC et al (1975) Kinetics of human lymphocyte proliferation: proportion of cells responsive to phytohemagglutinin and correlation with E rosette formation, J Reticuloendothel Soc **17**:47

Nurden AT and Caen JP (1974) An abnormal platelet glycoprotein pattern in three cases of Glanzmann's thrombasthenia, Br J Haematol **28**:253

Nurden AT and Caen JP (1975) Specific roles for platelet surface glycoproteins in platelet function, Nature (London) **255**:720

Nussbaum M and Morse BS (1964) Plasma fibrin stabilizing factor activity in various diseases, Blood **23**:669

Nute PE et al (1974) Hemoglobinopathic erythrocytosis due to a new electrophoretically silent variant, hemoglobin San Diego (beta 109 [G11] val → met), J Clin Invest **53**:320

Nyberg W (1952) Microbiological investigations on antipernicious anemia factors in the fish tapeworm, Acta Med Scand **144**(supp 271):1

Nyberg W and Saarni M (1964) Calculation on the dynamics of vitamin B_{12} in fish tapeworm carriers spontaneously recovering from vitamin B_{12} deficiency. Acta Med Scand (supp) **412**:65

Nyman M et al (1970) Acquired macrocytic anemia and hemoglobinopathy—a paraneoplastic manifestation? Am J Med **48**:792

Ober WB et al (1959) Hemoglobin S-C disease with fat embolism: report of a patient dying in crisis: autopsy findings, Am J Med **27**:647

Oberling Fr et al (1973) Application de certaines colorations à l'histopathologie de routine en coupes semi-fines de la moelle osseuse incluse en "araldite," Nouv Rev Fr Hematol **13**:429

Oberman HA (1969) Early history of blood substitutes: transfusion of milk, Transfusion **9**:74

O'Brien C et al (1964) A survey of cord bloods for abnormal hemoglobin with further observations on hemoglobin I Burlington, Am J Obstet Gynecol **88**:816

O'Brien JR (1966) Changes in platelet membranes possibly associated with platelet stickiness, Nature **212**:1057

O'Brien JR (1967) Platelets: a Portsmouth syndrome? Lancet **2**:258

O'Brien JS (1960) Urinary excretion of folic and folinic acids in normal adults, Proc Soc Exp Biol Med **104**:354

O'Brien JS et al (1971) Ganglioside storage diseases, Fed Proc **30**:956

O'Brien RT (1974) Perspectives in sickle cell disease screening, South Med J **67**:1269

Ochs HD and Igo RP (1973) The NBT slide test: a simple screening method for detecting chronic granulomatous disease and female carriers, J Pediatr **83**:77

O'Conor GT and Davies JNP (1960) Malignant tumors in African children: with special reference to malignant lymphoma, J Pediatr **56**:526

Odada K et al (1976) e antigen and anti-e in the serum of asymptomatic carrier mothers as indicators of positive and negative transmission of hepatitis B virus to their infants, N Engl J Med **294**:746

Odegard OR and Lie M (1978) Simultaneous inactivation of thrombin and factor Xa by AT-III; influence of heparin, Thromb Res **12**:697

Odell GB (1967) "Physiologic" hyperbilirubinemia in the neonatal period, N Engl J Med **277**:193

O'Donnell JF et al (1979) Acute nonlymphocytc leukemia and acute myeloproliferative syndrome following radiation therapy for non-Hodgkin's lymphoma and chronic lymphocytic leukemia: clinical studies, Cancer **44**:1930

Ogawa M et al (1969) Clinical aspects of IgE myeloma, N Engl J Med **281**:1217

Ogle JW et al (1978) The in vitro production of erythropoietin and thrombopoietin, Scand J Haematol **21**:188

O'Grady LF and Lewis JP (1970) Proliferation of erythroid-committed cells in the absence of erythropoietin, J Lab Clin Med **76**:445

Ogston D and Dawson AA (1969) Thrombocytosis following thrombocytopenia in man, Postgrad Med J **45**:754

Ogura T et al (1967) Localization of fibrinogen in the tumor tissue, Gann **58**:403

Ohba Y et al (1973) Identical substitution in hb Ube-1 and Hb Köln, Nature (New Biol) **243**:205

Ohba Y et al (1975a) Hemoglobin Tokuchi: beta 131 glutamine → glutamic acid, an example of hb Camden in Japan, Acta Haematol Jpn **38**:1

Ohba Y et al (1975b) Hemoglobin Chiba: hb Hammersmith in a Japanese girl, Acta haematol Jpn **38**:53

Ohba Y et al (1975c) Hemoglobin Hirosaki (alpha 43 [CE 1] phe- → leu) a new unstable variant, Biochim Biophys Acta **405**:155

Ohba Y et al (1977a) Hemoglobin Mizuho or beta 68 (E12) leucine → proline, a new unstable variant associated with severe hemolytic anemia, Hemoglobin **1**:467

Ohba Y et al (1977b) Hemoglobin Matsue-Oki: alpha 75 (EF4) aspartic acid → asparagine, Hemoglobin **1**:383

Ohba Y et al (1978) Characterization of hb Ube-4: alpha 116 (GH4) glu → ala, Hemoglobin **2**:181

Ohta Y et al (1970) Two unique structural and synthetic variants, Hb Miyada and homozygous δ-thalassemia, discovered in Japanese. Thirteenth International Congress of Hematology, Munich, JF Lehmanns Verlag, Abstracts p 233

Ohta Y et al (1971) Hemoglobin Miyada, a beta-delta fusion peptide (anti-Lepore) type discovered in a Japanese family, Nature (New Biol) **234**:218

Okada K et al (1976) e Antigen and anti-e in the serum of asymptomatic carrier mothers as indicators of positive and negative transmission of hepatitis B virus to their infants, N Engl J Med **294**:746

Okazaki N et al (1979) Hepatocellular carcinoma associated with erythrocytosis. A nine year survival after successful chemotherapy and left lateral hepatectomy, Acta Hepato-Gastroent **26**:248

Oken MM et al (1978) Terminal transferase levels in chronic myelogenous leukemia in blast crisis and in remission, Leukemia Res **2**:173

Okolicsanyi L et al (1978) An evaluation of bilirubin kinetics with respect to the diagnosis of Gilbert's syndrome, Clin Sci Molec Med **54**:539

Okonkwo P et al (1970) Absent plasma second phase platelet aggregation factor in a patient with Hageman trait, Thromb Diath Haemorrh **23**:423

Okuda K (1972) Intestinal mucosa and vitamin B_{12} absorption, Digestion **6**:173

Okun DB et al (1979) Bone marrow granulomas in Q fever, Am J Clin Pathol **71**:117

Okuno T and Crockatt D (1977) Platelet factor 4 activity and thromboembolic episodes, Am J Clin Pathol **67**:351

Olansky S and McCormick GE (1963) Further laboratory studies on the Sézary syndrome, South Med J **56**:824

Old J et al (1977) Molecular basis for acquired haemoglobin H disease, Nature **269**:524

Olesen H and Terp B (1968) Transferrin determination by Laurell electrophoresis in antibody containing agarose gel, Scand J Clin Lab Invest **21**:14

Olinger EJ et al (1973) Intestinal folate absorption. II. Conversion and retention of pteroylmonoglutamate by jejunum, J Clin Invest **52**:2138

Oliva G et al (1968) Sindrome nefrosica atransferrinemica: contributo clinico e valutazioni etio-pathogenetiche, Minerva Med **59**:1297

Oliver JM et al (1975) Concanavalin A cap formation on polymorphonuclear leukocytes of normal and beige (Chediak-Higashi) mice, Nature **253**:471

Oliver JM et al (1977) Mechanisms of microtubule disassembly in vivo: studies in normal and chronic granulomatous disease leucocytes, Br J Haematol **37**:311

Olsen KW (1979) The three-dimensional structure of hemoglobin. In Schmidt RM (Section Ed): Handbook Series in Clinical Laboratory Science, Section I: Hematology, vol 1, Boca Raton, Fla, CRC Press Inc, p 105

Olson JD et al (1975) Evaluation of ristocetin-Willebrand factor assay and ristocetin induced platelet aggregation, Am J Clin Pathol **63**:210

Olson LC et al (1964) Acute infectious lymphocytosis presenting as a pertussis-like illness: its association with adenovirus type 12, Lancet **1**:200

O'Malley BC et al (1975) Platelet abnormalities in diabetic peripheral neuropathy, Lancet **2**:1274

Omura H et al (1975) Hemoglobin F Ube (108 asp → lys), a new abnormal fetal hemoglobin found in a Japanese baby, Chem Abstr **83**:266

Oni SB et al (1970) Paroxysmal nocturnal hemoglobinemia: evidence for monoclonal origin of abnormal red cells, Blood **36**:145

Opelz G et al (1973) Suppression of lymphocyte transportation by aspirin, Lancet **1**:478

Opfell RW et al (1968) Hereditary nonspherocytic haemolytic anaemia with post-splenectomy inclusion bodies and pigmenturia caused by an unstable haemoglobin Santa Ana—beta 88 (F4) leucine → proline, J Med Genet **5**:292

Oppenheimer EH and Andrews EC Jr (1959) Ceroid storage disease in childhood, Pediatrics **23**:1091

Order SE and Hellman S (1972) Pathogenesis of Hodgkin's disease, Lancet **1**:571

O'Reilly RA (1970) The second reported kindred with hereditary resistance to oral anticoagulant drugs, N Engl J Med **282**:1448

O'Reilly RJ et al (1978) Severe combined immunodeficiency: transplantation approaches for patients lacking an HLA genotypically identical sibling, Transplant Proc **10**:187

Orfanakis NG et al (1970) Normal blood leukocyte concentration values, Am J Clin Pathol **53**:647

O'Riordan ML et al (1971) Distinguishing between the chromosomes involved in Down's syndrome (trisomy 21) and chronic myeloid leukemia (Ph[1]) by fluorescence, Nature **230**:161

Orlina AR and Josephson AM (1969) Comparative viability of blood stored in ACD and CPD, Transfusion **9**:62

Orlina AR et al (1978) Post-transfusion alloimmunization in patients with sickle cell disease, Am J Hematol **5**:101

Orringer EP et al (1976) Hemoglobin Chapel Hill or alpha 2 74 asp → gly beta 2, FEBS Lett **65**:297

Orringer EP et al (1976) Hemolysis caused by factor VIII concentrates, Arch Intern Med **136**:1018

Ortega JA et al (1975) Congenital hypoplastic anemia: inhibition of erythropoiesis by sera from patients with congenital hypoplastic anemia, Blood **45**:83

Osgood EE (1954) Number and distribution of human hemic cells, Blood **9**:1141

Osgood EE (1965) Polycythemia vera: age relationships and survival, Blood **26**:243

Oski FA and Delivoria-Papadopoulos M (1970) The red cell, 2,3-diphosphoglycerate, and tissue oxygen release, J Pediatr **77**:941

Oski FA (1972) Fetal hemoglobin, the neonatal red cell and 2,3-diphosphoglycerate, pediatr Clin North Am **19**:907

Oski FA (1979) The nonhematologic manifestations of iron deficiency, Am J Dis Child **133**:315

Oski FA et al (1964) Extreme hemolysis and red-cell distortion in erythrocyte pyruvate kinase deficiency. I. Morphology, erythrokinetics, and family enzyme studies, N Engl J Med **270**:1023

Oski FA et al (1969) Congenital hemolytic anemia with high-sodium, low-potassium red cells. Studies of three generations of a family with a new variant, N Engl J Med **280**:909

Osmond DG (1975) Formation and maturation of bone marrow lymphocytes, J Reticuloendothel Soc **17**:99

Osoba D (1965) The effects of the thymus and other lymphoid organs enclosed in millipore diffusion chambers on neonatally thymectomized mice, J Exp Med **122**:633

Osserman EF (1959) Plasma-cell myeloma. II. Clinical aspects, N Engl J Med **261**:952, 1006

Osserman EF and Takatsuki K (1963) Plasma cell myeloma: gamma globulin synthesis and structure. A review of biochemical and clinical data, with the description of a newly recognized and related syndrome, $H\gamma^2$-chain (Franklin's) disease, Medicine **42**:357

Osserman EF and Takatsuki K (1964) Clinical and immunochemical studies of four cases of heavy ($H\gamma^2$) chain disease, Am J Med **37**:351

Ossias AL et al (1973) Case report: studies on the mechanism of erythrocytosis associated with a uterine fibromyoma, Br J Haematol **25**:179

Ostertag W and Smith EW (1968) Hb Sinai: a new alpha chain mutant alpha 47 His, Humangenetik **6**:377

Ostertag W and Smith EW (1969) Hemoglobin Lepore Baltimore, a third type of a delta beta crossover (delta 50, beta 86), Eur J Biochem **10**:371

Ostertag W et al (1972) Duplicated α-chain genes in Hopkins-2 hemoglobin of man and evidence for unequal crossing over between them, Nature (New Biol) **237**:90

Østerud B and Rapaport SI (1980) Activation of ^{125}I-factor IX and ^{125}I-factor X: effect of tissue factor and factor VII, factor X_A and thrombin, Scand J Haematol **24**:213

Ostrow JD and Schmid R (1963) The protein-binding of C^{14} bilirubin in human and murine serum, J Clin Invest **42**:1286

O'Sullivan MB et al (1970) Some molecular characteristics of human urinary erythropoietin determined by gel filtration and density-gradient ultracentrifugation, J Lab Clin Med **75**:771

Otani S (1957) A discussion on eosinophilic granuloma of bone, Letterer-Siwe disease and Schüller-Christian disease, J Mount Sinai Hosp NY **24**:1079

Ottenberg R (1908) Transfusion and arterial anastomosis, Ann Surg **47**:486

Ottesen J (1954) On age of human white cells in peripheral blood, Acta Physiol Scand **32**:75

Ottolenghi S et al (1976) Delta-beta-thalassemia is due to a gene deletion, Cell **9**:71

Outeirino J et al (1974) Haemoglobin Madrid beta 115 (G17) alanine → proline: an unstable variant associated with haemolytic anaemia, Acta Haematol **52**:53

Over J et al (1980) Heterogeneity of human factor VIII: III. Transitions between forms of factor VIII present in cryoprecipitate and in cryosupernatant plasma, J Lab Clin Med **95**:323

Owen CA and Bowie EJW (1975) Infusion therapy of hemophilia A and B. In Brinkhous KM and Hemker HC (Eds): Handbook of hemophilia, New York, American Elsevier Publishing Co, Inc, p 449

Owen CA et al (1955) Evaluation of disorders of blood coagulation in the clinical laboratory, Am J Clin Pathol **25**:1417

Owen CA et al (1978) Prothrombin Quick: a newly identified dysprothrombinemia, Mayo Clin Proc **53**:29

Owen RD (1945) Immunogenetic consequences of vascular anastomoses between bovine twins, Science **102**:400

Owren PA (1947) Parahaemophilia: haemorrhagic diathesis due to absence of a previously unknown clotting factor, Lancet **1**:446

Owren PA (1948) Congenital hemolytic jaundice: pathogenesis of "hemolytic crisis," Blood **3**:231

Özer L and Mills GC (1964) Elliptocytosis with haemolytic anaemia, Br J Haematol **10**:468

Ozge-Anwar AH et al (1972) The kinin system of human plasma. IV. The interrelationship between the contact phase of blood coagulation and the plasma kinin system in man, Thromb Diath Haemorrh **27**:141

Özsoylu S (1970) Homozygous hemoglobin D Punjab, Acta Haematol **43**:353

Özsoylu S and Balci S (1970) Fetal hemoglobin in various forms of childhood leukemia: relation to relapse and remission, Clin Pediatr **9**:152

Packman CH et al (1979) Complement lysis of human erythrocytes: differing susceptibility of two types of paroxysmal nocturnal hemoglobinuria cells to C5b-9, J Clin Invest **64**:428

Packham MA and Mustard JF (1974) Drug-induced alteration of platelet function. In Baldini MG and Ebbe S (Eds): Platelets: production, function, transfusion, and storage, New York, Grune & Stratton, Inc

Packham MA et al (1969) Effect of adenine compounds on platelet aggregation, Am J Physiol **217**:1009

Padgett GA et al (1964) The familial occurrence of the Chediak-Higashi syndrome in mink and cattle, Genetics **49**:505

Padgett GA et al (1967) Comparative studies of the Chediak-Higashi syndrome, Am J Pathol **51**:553

Padilla F et al (1973) The sickle-unsickle cycle: a cause of cell fragmentation leading to permanently deformed cells, Blood **41**:653

Page AR and Good RA (1957) Studies on cyclic neutropenia, Am J Dis Child **94**:623

Paglia DE et al (1968) An inherited molecular lesion of erythrocyte pyruvate kinase. Identification of a kinetically aberrant isozyme associated with premature hemolysis, J Clin Invest **47**:1929

Pagliardi E et al (1958) Erythrocyte copper in iron deficiency anemia, Acta Haematol **19**:231

Pagnier J et al (1979) Hematological and hemoglobin synthesis in a family with δβ-thalassemia trait, Acta Haematol **61**:27

Painter TS (1923) Studies in mammalian spermatogenesis. II. The spermatogenesis of man, J Exp Zool **37**:291

Palascak JE and Shapiro SR (1977) Anti-factor VIII anamnesis after factor IX complex, N Engl J Med **297**:1403

Palek J et al (1969) 2,3-diphosphoglycerate metabolism in hereditary spherocytosis, Br J Haematol **17**:59

Palek J and Liu S-C (1979) Dependence of spectrin organization in red blood cell membranes on cell metabolism: implications for control of red cell shape, deformability, and surface area, Semin Hematol **16**:75

Pallesen G et al (1979) β-Prolymphocytic leukaemia—a mantle zone lymphoma? Scand J Haematol **22**:407

Palutke M and McDonald JM (1973) Monoclonal gammopathies associated with malignant lymphomas, Am J Clin Pathol **60**:157

Palutke M and Tabaczka P (1979) Functional studies of hairy cell leukemia (leukemic reticuloendotheliosis), Am J Clin Pathol **7**:273

Palutke M et al (1976) Immunologic and electronmicroscopic characteristics of a case of immunoblastic lymphadenopathy, Am J Clin Pathol **65**:929

Panayi GS (1970) Unified concept of cell-mediated immune reaction, Br Med J **2**:656

Pandolfi M et al (1972) Failure of fetal platelets to aggregate in response to adrenaline and collagen, Proc Soc Exp Biol Med **141**:1081

Pangalis GA et al (1978) Cytochemical findings in human nonneoplastic blood and tonsillar B and T lymphocytes, Am J Clin Pathol **69**:314

Paniker NV et al (1978) Haemoglobin Vanderbilt (alpha 2 beta 2 89 ser → arg): a new haemoglobin with high oxygen affinity and compensatory erythrocytosis, Br J Haematol **39**:249

Panlilio AL and Reiss RF (1979) Therapeutic plateletpheresis in thrombocythemia, Transfusion **19**:147

Papac RJ (1970) Lymphocyte transformation in malignant lymphomas, Cancer **26**:279

Papayannis AG and Israëls MC (1970) Glanzmann's disease and trait, Lancet **2**:44

Papayannis EJ et al (1971) Platelet function abnormalities: a report of two familial defects in interaction between collagen and platelets and ADP release, Blood **38**:745

Papayannopoulou T and Stamatoyannopoulos G (1974) Stains for inclusion bodies. In Schmidt R et al (Eds): The detection of hemoglobinopathies, Cleveland, CRC Press

Papayannopoulou T et al (1980) Fetal hb production during acute erythroid expansion. I. Observations in patients with transient erythroblastopenia and post-phlebotomy, Br J Haematol **44**:535

Pappenheimer AM et al (1945) Anaemia associated with unidentified erythrocytic inclusions, after splenectomy, Q J Med **14**:75

Paran M and Sachs L (1968) The continued requirement for inducer for the development of macrophage and granulocyte colonies, J Cell Physiol **72**:247

Paraskevas F et al (1972) The reaction of antilymphocyte serum with lymphocytes. I. The blocking of surface-associated γ-globulin, Transplantation **13**:212

Park BH (1971) The use and limitations of the nitroblue tetrazolium test as a diagnostic aid, J Pediatr **78**:376

Park BH et al (1968) Infection and nitroblue-tetrazolium reduction by neutrophils. A diagnostic aid, Lancet **2**:532

Parker AC (1973) A case of acute myelomonocytic leukaemia associated with myelomatosis, Scand J Haematol **11**:257

Parker JP et al (1972) Androgen-induced increase in red cell 2,3-diphosphoglycerate, N Engl J Med **287**:381

Parkhouse RM (1972) Biosynthesis of J-chains in mouse IgA and IgM, Nature (New Biol) **236**:9

Parmley RT et al (1979) Giant platelet granules in a child with the Chediak-Higashi syndrome, Am J Hematol **6**:51

Parrillo JE et al (1978) Therapy of the hypereosinophilic syndrome, Ann Intern Med **89**:167

Parrot DMV and DeSousa M (1971) Thymus-dependent and thymus-independent populations: origin, migratory patterns, and life span, Clin Exp Immunol **8**:663

Parry DH and Bloom AL (1978) Failure of factor VIII inhibitor bypassing activity (Feiba) to secure haemostasis in haemophilic patients with antibodies, J Clin Pathol **31**:1102

Parsons L Jr and Thompson JE (1959) Symptomatic myelolipoma of the adrenal gland, N Engl J Med **260**:12

Pasmantier MW and Azar HA (1969) Extraskeletal spread in multiple plasma cell myeloma. A review of 57 autopsied cases, Cancer **23**:167

Pasmantier M et al (1977) Value of biopsy in diagnosis of primary lymphosarcoma of marrow, Arch Intern Med **137**:52

Pasternack BS and Heller MB (1968) Genetically significant dose to the population of New York City from diagnostic medical radiology. A dosimetric and statistical study, Radiology **90**:217

Pataryas HA and Stamatoyannopoulos G (1972) Hemoglobins in human fetuses: evidence for adult hemoglobin production after the 11th gestational week, Blood **39**:688

Patek AJ and Taylor FHL (1937) Hemophilia. II. Some properties of a substance detained from normal human plasma effective in accelerating the coagulation of hemophilic blood, J Clin Invest **16**:113

Patel A and Chanarin I (1975) Restoration of normal red cell size after treatment in megaloblastic anaemia, Br J Haematol **30**:57

Patrick AD and Lake BD (1973) Wolman's disease. In Hers HG and Van Hoof F (Eds): Lysosomes and storage disease, New York, Academic Press, Inc

Pattengale PK et al (1974) B-cell characteristics of human peripheral and cord blood lymphocytes transformed by Epstein-Barr virus, J Natl Cancer Inst **52**:1081

Pattison CP et al (1974) Epidemic hepatitis in a clinical laboratory. Possible association with computer card handling, JAMA **230**:854

Patrone F et al (1979) Lazy leukocyte syndrome, Blut **39**:265

Patrono C et al (1980) Low dose aspirin and inhibition of thromboxane B_2 production in healthy subjects, Thromb Res **17**:317

Patt HM et al (1973) Cyclic hematopoiesis in grey collie dogs: a stem-cell problem, Blood **42**:873

Patten E et al (1977) Autoimmune hemolytic anemia with anti-Jk_a specificity in a patient taking Aldomet, Transfusion **17**:517

Paul BB et al (1970) The role of the phagocyte in host-parasite interactions. XXIV. Aldehyde generation by the myeloperoxidase-H_2O_2-chloride antimicrobial system: a possible in vivo mechanism of action, Infect Immunol **2**:414

Paul JR and Bunnell WW (1932) The presence of heterophile antibodies in infectious mononucleosis, Am J Med Sci **183**:90

Pauling L et al (1949) Sickle cell anemia, a molecular disease, Science **110**:543

Paulo LG et al (1973a) Effects of posterior hypothalamic stimulation on reticulocyte release and bone marrow microcirculation, Proc Soc Exp Biol Med **143**:986

Paulo LG et al (1973b) The effects of prostaglandin E_1 on erythropoietin production, Proc Soc Exp Biol Med **142**:771

Paulo LG et al (1974) Effects of several androgens and steroid metabolites on erythropoietin production in the isolated perfused dog kidney, Blood **43**:39

Paulsen EP (1973) Hemoglobin Alc in childhood diabetes, Metabolism **22**:269

Paver WK and Goldman P (1966) The detection of occult blood in faeces, Med J Aust **1**:669

Pavlic GJ and Bouroncle BA (1965) Megaloblastic crisis in paroxysmal nocturnal hemoglobinuria, N Engl J Med **273**:789

Pawlak AL and Kozlowska F (1970) Swiss type hereditary persistence of foetal haemoglobin in a case of acquired haemolytic anaemia, Acta Haematol **43**:184

Payne R (1962) The development and persistence of leukoagglutinins in parous women, Blood **19**:411

Paz RA et al (1969) Fatal simultaneous thrombocytopenic purpura in siblings, Br Med J **4**:727

Pearl R (1941) Introduction to medical biometry and statistics, ed 3, Philadelphia, WB Saunders Co

Pearse AGE (1961) Histochemistry, theoretical and applied, ed 2, Boston, Little, Brown & Co

Pearson HA and Diamond LK (1959) Fetomaternal transfusion, AMA J Dis Child **97**:267

Pearson HA and Lorincz AE (1964) A characteristic bone marrow finding in the Hurler syndrome, Pediatrics **34**:280

Pearson HA et al (1961) "Pseudo-abnormal" hemoglobins, Blood **17**:758

Pearson HA et al (1964) Isoimmune neonatal thrombocytopenic purpura: clinical and therapeutic considerations, Blood **23**:154

Pearson HA et al (1969) Functional asplenia in sickle-cell anemia, N Engl J Med **281**:923

Pearson MA and O'Brien RT (1975) The management of thalassemia major, Semin Hematol **12**:255

Pechet L et al (1966) Previously undescribed hereditary clotting abnormality. In Brinkhous KM et al (Eds): Diffuse intravascular clotting, Stuttgart, FK Schattauer Verlag

Pechet L et al (1967) Further studies on the "Dynia" clotting abnormality, Thromb Diath Haemorrh **17**:365

Pedersen-Bjergaard J et al (1978) Chronic lymphocytic leukaemia with subsequent development of multiple myeloma. Evidence of two B-lymphocyte clones and of myeloma-induced suppression of secretion of an M-component and of normal immunoglobulins, Scand J Haematol **21**:256

Pembrey ME and Weatherall DJ (1971) Maternal synthesis of haemoglobin F in pregnancy, Br J Haematol **21**:355

Peña AS et al (1972) Small intestinal mucosal abnormalities and disaccharidase activity in pernicious anemia, Br J Haematol **23**:313

Penfil RL and Brown ML (1968) Genetically significant dose to the United States population from diagnostic medical roentgenology, 1964, Radiology **90**:209

Penfold JB and Lipscomb JM (1943) Elliptocytosis in man associated with hereditary haemorrhagic telangiectasia, Q J Med **12**:157

Penick GD et al (1966) Predisposition to intravascular coagulation, Thromb Diath Haemorrh **21**(suppl):543

Penn D et al (1979) Comparison of hematocrit determinations by microhematocrit and electronic particle counter, Am J Clin Pathol **72**:71

Penner JA and Kelly PE (1975) Management of patients with factor VIII or IX inhibitors, Semin Thromb Hemost **1**:386

Penny R et al (1966) The splenic platelet pool, Blood **27**:1

Pensky J et al (1968) Properties of highly purified human properdin, J Immunol **100**:142

Pentchev PG et al (1978) Gaucher disease: isolation and comparison of normal and mutant glucocerebrosidase from human spleen tissue, Proc Natl Acad Sci USA **75**:3970

Perillie PE (1967) Studies of the changes in leukocyte alkaline phosphatase following pyrogen stimulation in chronic granulocytic leukemia, Blood **29**:401

Perillie PE and Chernoff AI (1965) Heterozygous beta-thalassemia in association with hereditary elliptocytosis: a family study, Blood **25**:494

Perkins HA et al (1970) Hemostatic defects in dysproteinemias, Blood **35**:695

Perkins HA and Morel PA (1980) Problems in paternity testing: subtypes of AB, Am J Clin Pathol **73**:263

Perkins WD et al (1972) An ultrastructural study of lymphocytes with surface-bound immunoglobulin, J Exp Med **135**:267

Perlman P et al (1969) Cytotoxic effects of lymphocytes triggered by complement bound to target cells, Science **163**:937

Perlroth MG et al (1965) Oral contraceptive agents and the management of acute intermittent porphyria, JAMA **194**:1037

Perman G (1967) Hemochromatosis and red wine, Acta Med Scand **182**:281

Pernis B et al (1970) Immunoglobulin spots on the surface of rabbit lymphocytes, J Exp Med **132**:1001

Perrine RP (1973) Cholelithiasis in sickle cell anemia in a Caucasian population, Am J Med **54**:327

Perry E and Chaudhary RK (1973) Hepatitis B antigen: distribution of ad and ay subtypes in blood donors and hepatitis patients, Can Med Assoc J **109**:857

Perry HM Jr et al (1971) Immunologic findings in patients receiving methyldopa: a prospective study, J Lab Clin Med **78**:905

Perry RP (1966) On ribosome biogenesis, Natl Cancer Inst Monogr No. 3, **23**:527

Persson E and Hansen HA (1963) Interrelations of bone marrow morphology, serum vitamin B_{12}, and the Schilling test in 73 subjects with normal folic acid levels, Scand J Clin Lab Invest **15**:217

Perutz MF (1963) X-ray analysis of hemoglobin, Science **140**:863

Perutz MF (1965) Structure and function of haemoglobin. I. A tentative atomic model of horse oxyhaemoglobin, J Mol Biol **13**:646

Perutz MF (1970a) The Bohr effect and combination with organic phosphates, Nature **228**:734

Perutz MF (1970b) Stereochemistry of cooperative effects in haemoglobin, Nature **228**:726

Perutz MF (1978) Hemoglobin structure and respiratory transport, Sci Am **239**:92

Perutz MF and Lehmann H (1968) Molecular pathology of human haemoglobin, Nature **219**:902

Perutz MF et al (1965) Structure and function of haemoglobin. II. Some relations between polypeptide chain configuration and amino acid sequence, J Mol Biol **13**:669

Perutz MF et al (1968a) Three-dimensional Fourier synthesis of horse oxyhaemoglobin at 2.8 A resolution: (1) x-ray analysis, Nature (London) **219**:29

Perutz MF et al (1968b) Three-dimensional Fourier synthesis of horse oxyhaemoglobin at 2.8 A resolution: the atomic model, Nature (London) **219**:131

Perutz MF et al (1969) Identification of residues responsible for the alkaline Bohr effect in haemoglobin, Nature **222**:1240

Perutz MF et al (1971) Haemoglobin Hiroshima and the mechanisms of the alkaline Bohr effect, Nature (New Biol) **232**:147

Perutz MF et al (1972) Structure and subunit interaction of haemoglobin M Milwaukee, Nature (New Biol) **237**:259

Peskin GW et al (1969) Stroma-free hemoglobin solution: the "ideal" blood substitute, Surgery **66**:185

Peter CR et al (1974) T or B cell origin of some non-Hodgkin's lymphomas, Lancet **2**:686

Peterman ML (1964) The ribosome, New York, American Elsevier Publishing Co, Inc

Peters JC et al (1966) Erythrocyte sodium transport in hereditary elliptocytosis, Can J Physiol Pharmacol **44**:817

Peters JH (1967) Heterophile reactive antigen in infectious mononucleosis, Science **157**:1200

Peters SP et al (1975) A microassay for Gaucher's disease, Clin Chim Acta **60**:391

Peters SP et al (1977) Gaucher's disease, a review, Medicine **56**:425

Peters TJ and Hoffbrand AV (1970) Absorption of vitamin B_{12} by the guinea-pig. I. Subcellular localization of vitamin B_{12} in the ileal enterocyte during absorption, Br J Haematol **19**:369

Petersen WF (1934-1938) The patient and the weather, vol 1 to 5, Ann Arbor, Michigan, Edwards Brothers, Inc

Peterson H deC (1960) Acquired methemoglobinemia in an infant due to benzocaine suppository, N Engl J Med 263:454

Peterson J et al (1979) Splenectomy and antiplatelet agents in thrombotic thrombocytopenic purpura, Am J Med Sci 277:75

Peterson RD et al (1966) Lymphoid tissue abnormalities associated with ataxia-telangiectasia, Am J Med 41:342

Pettit JE et al (1978) Polycythemia vera—transformation by myelofibrosis and subsequent reversal, Scand J Haematol 20:63

Petrucci JV et al (1971) Spurious erythrocyte indices as measured by the Model S Coulter counter due to cold agglutinins, Am J Clin Pathol 56:500

Petz LD and Garratty G (1975) Laboratory correlations in immune hemolytic anemias. In Vyas GN et al (Eds): Laboratory diagnosis of immunologic disorders, New York, Grune & Stratton, Inc, p 139

Petz LD and Garratty G (1978) Antiglobulin sera—past, present and future, Transfusion 18:257

Peytremann R et al (1972) Thrombosis in paroxysmal nocturnal hemoglobinuria (PNH) with particular reference to progressive, diffuse hepatic venous thrombosis, Ser Haematol 5:115

Pfändler U (1946) La maladie de Niemann-Pick dans le cadre des lipoïdoses, Schweiz Med Wochenschr 76:1128

Pick L (1927) Über die lipoidzellige Splenohepatomegalie Typus Niemann-Pick als Stoffwechselerkrankung, Med Klin 23:1483

Pierce LE et al (1963) A new hemoglobin variant with sickling properties, N Engl J Med 268:862

Pierre RV (1974) Preleukemic states, Semin Hematol 11:73

Pierre RV (1979) The technicon Hemalog D automated leukocyte differential system. In Koepke, JA (Ed): Differential leukocyte counting, Skokie, Ill, College of American Pathologists, p 145

Pik C and Tönz O (1966) Nature of haemoglobin M Oldenburg, Nature 210:1182

Pike IM et al (1972) Immunochemical characterization of a monoclonal G_4, lambda human antibody to factor IX, Blood 40:1

Piliero SJ et al (1968) The interrelationships of the endocrine and erythropoietic systems in the rat with special reference to the mechanism of action of estradiol and testosterone, Ann NY Acad Sci 149:336

Pillemer L (1958) The nature of the properdin system and its interactions with polysaccharide complexes, Ann NY Acad Sci 66:233

Pimparker BD et al (1961) Correlation of radioactive and chemical fecal fat determinations in the malabsorption syndrome, Am J Med 30:910

Pineda AA et al (1978a) Hemolytic transfusion reaction: recent experience in a large blood bank, Mayo Clin Proc 53:378

Pineda AA et al (1978b) Delayed hemolytic transfusion reaction: an immunologic hazard of blood tranfusion, Transfusion 18:1

Pineo GF et al (1974) Tumors, mucus production, and hypercoagulability, Ann NY Acad Sci 230:262

Pinkerton PH et al (1970) An assessment of the Coulter Counter Model S, J Clin Pathol 23:68

Pinkerton PH et al (1978) Lazy leucocyte syndrome—disorder of the granulocyte membrane? J Clin Pathol 31:300

Pinkhas J et al (1963) Sulfhemoglobinemia and acute hemolytic anemia with Heinz bodies following contact with a fungicide—zinc ethylene bisdithiocarbamate—in a subject with glucose-6-phosphate dehydrogenase deficiency and hypocatalasemia, Blood 21:484

Pinkus GS and Said JW (1979) Characterization of non-Hodgkin's lymphomas using multiple cell markers, Am J Pathol 94:349

Pirofsky B (1969) Autoimmunization and the hemolytic anemias, Baltimore, The Williams & Wilkins Co

Pirofsky B (1975) Immune haemolytic disease: the autoimmune haemolytic anaemias, Clin Haematol 4:167

Pirofsky B (1976) Clinical aspects of autoimmune hemolytic anemia, Semin Hematol 13:251

Pirofsky B and Mangum M (1959) Use of bromelin to demonstrate erythrocyte antibodies, Proc Soc Exp Biol Med 101:49

Pirofsky B and Vaughn M (1968) Addisonian pernicious anemia with positive antiglobulin tests. A multiple autoimmune disease syndrome, Am J Clin Pathol 50:459

Pirofsky B et al (1961) The present status of the antiglobulin and bromelin tests in demonstrating erythrocyte antibodies, Am J Pathol 36:492

Pirofsky B et al (1962) The nonimmunologic reaction of globulin molecules with the erythrocyte surface, Vox Sang 7:334

Pirofsky B et al (1965) Hemolytic anemia complicating aortic-valve surgery, N Engl J Med 272:235

Pisano JJ et al (1971) Epsilon-(gamma glutamyl) lysine in fibrin: lack of crosslink formation in Factor 13 deficiency, Proc Natl Acad Sci USA 68:770

Pisciotta AV (1973) Immune and toxic mechanism in drug-induced agranulocytosis, Semin Hematol 10:279

Pisciotta AV and Hinz JE (1956) Occurrence of agglutinogens in normoblasts, Proc Soc Exp Biol Med 91:356

Pisciotta AV et al (1959) Clinical and laboratory features of two variants of methemoglobin M disease, J Lab Clin Med 54:73

Pisciotta AV et al (1977) Treatment of thrombotic thrombocytopenic purpura by exchange transfusion, Am J Hematol 3:73

Pitney WR (1971) Disseminated intravascular coagulation, Semin Hematol 8:65

Pittman MA Jr and Graham JB (1964) Glanzmann's thrombopathy: an autosomal recessive trait in one family, Am J Med Sci 247:293

Pittz EP et al (1977) Interaction of polysaccharides with plasma membranes. I. Interaction of human erythrocytes with degraded iota carrageenans and the effect of dextran and DEAE dextran, Biorheology 14:21

Plachetka JR et al (1980) Platelet loss during experimental cardiopulmonary bypass and its prevention with prostacyclin, Ann Thorac Surg 30:58

Plum CM et al (1978) Defective maturation of granulocytes, retinal cysts and multiple skeletal malformations in a mentally retarded girl: a new syndrome, Acta Haematol 59:53

Pluznik DH and Sachs L (1965) The cloning of normal "mast" cells in tissue culture, J Cell Comp Physiol 66:319

Pochedly C (1969) How to perform bone marrow puncture in small children, Clin Pediatr 8:705

Pochedly C et al (1973) "Hypercoagulable state" in children with acute leukemia or disseminated solid tumors, Oncology 28:517

Polesky HF (1979) Parentage testing 1979, Lab Med 10:601

Polesky HF and Krause HD (1977) Blood typing in disputed paternity cases: capabilities of American laboratories, Transfusion 17:521

Polesky HF and Taswell HF (1975) Evaluation of HB_sAg detection methods from AABB-CAP survey data, Am J Clin Pathol 63(supp):1002

Polesky HF et al (1969) Positive antiglobulin tests in cardiac surgery patients, Transfusion 9:43

Pollack S et al (1964) Iron absorption: effects of sugars and reducing agents, Blood 24:577

Pollack W et al (1965) A study of the forces involved in the second stage of hemagglutination, Transfusion 5:158

Pollard TD and Weihing RR (1974) Actin and myosin and cell movement, CRC Crit Rev Biochem 2:1

Poller L (1957) Thrombosis and factor VII activity, J Clin Pathol 10:348

Polley MJ and Nachman R (1978) The human complement system in thrombin-mediated platelet function, J Exp Med **147**:1713

Polliack A (1971) Acute promyelocytic leukemia with disseminated intravascular coagulation, Am J Clin Pathol **56**:155

Polliack A et al (1973) Identification of human B and T lymphocytes by scanning electron microscopy, J Exp Med **138**:607

Polliack A et al (1974a) An electron microscopic study of the nuclear abnormalities in erythroblasts in beta-thalassemia major, Br J Haematol **26**:201

Polliack A et al (1974b) Plasma cell leukemia. Unassembled light and heavy chains in the urine, Arch Intern Med **134**:131

Polliack A et al (1977) Multiple myeloma terminating in lymphocytic leukemia with B-lymphocyte membrane markers, Am J Hematol **3**:153

Pollock A and Cotter KP (1973) Oxygen transport in anaemia, Br J Haematol **25**:631

Pollycove M et al (1966) Classification and evolution of patterns of erythropoiesis in polycythemia vera as studied by iron kinetics, Blood **28**:907

Polmar SH et al (1972) Immunoglobulin E in immunologic deficiency diseases. I. Relation of IgE and IgA to respiratory tract disease in isolated IgE deficiency, IgA deficiency, and ataxia-telangiectasia, J Clin Invest **51**:326

Ponder E (1948) Hemolysis and related phenomena, New York, Grune & Stratton, Inc

Pool JG et al (1964) High-potency antihaemophilic factor concentrate prepared from cryoglobulin precipitate, Nature (London) **203**:312

Pool JG and Shannon AE (1965) Production of high-potency concentrates of antihemophilic globulin in a closed-bag system. Assay in vitro and in vivo, N Engl J Med **273**:1443

Pootrakul S and Dixon GH (1970) Hemoglobin Mahidol: a new hemoglobin alpha chain mutant, Can J Biochem **48**:1066

Pootrakul S et al (1974) Hemoglobin Siam (alpha 2 15 arg beta 2): a new alpha chain variant, Humangenetik **23**:199

Pootrakul S et al (1975) A new haemoglobin variant: haemoglobin Anantharaj alpha 11 (A9) lysine → glutamic acid, Biochim Biophys Acta **405**:161

Pootrakul S et al (1977) Hemoglobin Thailand (alpha 56 [E5] lys → thr): a new abnormal human hemoglobin, Hemoglobin **1**:781

Poplawski A and Niewiarowski S (1965) Method for determining antiheparin activity of platelets and erythrocytes, Thromb Diath Haemorrh **13**:149

Popovic WJ et al (1976) Thyroid hormone (TH)-stimulated erythropoiesis: mediation by a β-adrenergic receptor, Blood **48**(Abst):979

Porter FS Jr (1963) Multiple myeloma in a child, J Pediatr **62**:602

Porter FS Jr and Lowe BA (1963) Congenital erythropoietic protoporphyria. I. Case reports, clinical studies, and porphyrin analyses in two brothers, Blood **22**:521

Porter KA and Cooper EH (1962) Recognition of transformed small lymphocytes by combined chromosomal and isotopic labels, Lancet **2**:317

Porter WG and Lyle CB (1974) Leukemid reaction: an unusual manifestation of autoimmune hemolytic anemia, South Med J **67**:79

Portier A et al (1960) L'hémoglobinose C-thalassémie a propos d'une observation familiale caractéristique, Presse Méd **68**:1760

Porto J (1948) Analyse pathogénique de la cardiopathie noire (maladie d'Ayerza), Schweiz Med Wochenschr **78**:913

Post RM and Desforges JF (1968) Thrombocytopenic effect of ethanol infusion, Blood **31**:344

Povey S et al (1973) Genetic studies on human lymphoblastoid lines: isozyme analysis on cell lines from forty-one different individuals and on mutants produced following exposure to a chemical mutagen, Ann Hum Genet **36**:247

Powars D (1965) Aplastic anemia secondary to glue sniffing, N Engl J Med **273**:700

Powell HC and Wolf PL (1976) Neutrophilic leukocyte inclusions in colchicine intoxication, Arch Pathol **100**:136

Powell LW et al (1967) Idiopathic unconjugated hyperbilirubinemia (Gilbert's syndrome). A study of 42 families, N Engl J Med **277**:1108

Poyart C et al (1976) Structural and functional studies of haemoglobin Suresnes or alpha 2 141 (HC3) arg → His beta 2, a new high oxygen affinity mutant, FEBS Lett **69**:103

Prager D (1972) An analysis of hematologic disorders presenting in the private practice of hematology, Blood **40**:568

Prager D et al (1979) Pennsylvania State-wide Hemophilia Program: summary of immediate reactions with use of factor VIII and factor IX, Blood **53**:1012

Prasad A (1958) The association of hypogammaglobulinemia and chronic lymphatic leukemia, Am J Med Sci **236**:610

Prasad AS et al (1961) Syndrome of iron deficiency anemia, hepatosplenomegaly, hypogonadism, dwarfism, and geophagia, Am J Med **31**:532

Praxedes H and Lehmann H (1972) Haemoglobin Niteroi—a new unstable variant, Proceedings of the 14th International Congress of Hematology, Sao Paulo, Brazil

Prentice CRM (1975) Indications for antifibrinolytic therapy, Thromb Diath Haemorrh **34**:634

Prentice CRM and Davidson JF (1973) Drug-induced activation of fibrinolysis, Clin Haematol **2**:159

Presentey BZ (1968) A new anomaly of eosinophilic granulocytes, Am J Clin Pathol **49**:887

Preston FE et al (1974) Essential thrombocythaemia and peripheral gangrene, Br Med J **3**:548

Pretlow TG II (1969) Chronic monocytic dyscrasia culminating in acute leukemia, Am J Med **46**:130

Preud'homme JL and Seligmann M (1972) Surface bound immunoglobulins as a cell marker in human lymphoproliferative diseases, Blood **40**:777

Price DC et al (1976) The measurement of circulating red cell volume using nonradioactive cesium and fluorescent excitation analysis, J Lab Clin Med **87**:535

Price PM et al (1972) Chromosomal localization of human haemoglobin structural genes, Nature **237**:340

Prieur DJ and Collier LL (1978) Animal model of human disease: Chediak-Higashi syndrome, Am J Pathol **90**:533

Prince AM (1968) An antigen detected in the blood during the incubation period of serum hepatitis, Proc Natl Acad Sci USA **60**:814

Prokop O and Uhlenbruck G (1969) Human blood and serum groups, New York, Interscience Publishers, Inc

Prokop O et al (1965) A "new" human blood group receptor A$_{hel}$ tested with saline extracts from *Helix hortensis* (garden snail), S Afr J Forensic Med **12**:108

Propper RD et al (1976) Reassessment of the use of desferrioxamine B in iron overload, N Engl J Med **294**:1421

Prunieras M (1974) DNA content and cytogenetics of the Sézary cell, Mayo Clin Proc **49**:548

Pruzanski W et al (1969) Leukemic form of immunocytic dyscrasia (plasma cell leukemia), Am J Med **47**:60

Pruzanski W et al (1976) Angioimmunoblastic lymphadenopathy: an immunochemical study, Clin Immunol Immunopathol **6**:62

Prydz H (1965) Some characteristics of purified factor VII preparations, Scand J Clin Lab Invest (suppl)**84**:78

Pryor DS and Pitney WR (1967) Hereditary elliptocytosis: a report of two families from New Guinea, Br J Haematol **13**:126

Puccini C et al (1977) The erythrocyte sedimentation curve: a semiempirical approach, Biorheology **14**:43

Pugh LGCE (1964) Blood volume and haemoglobin concentration at altitudes above 18,000 ft (5500 m), J Physiol **170**:344

Pulvertaft RJV (1959) Cellular associations in normal and abnormal lymphocytes, Proc R Soc Med **52**:315

Purcell RH et al (1975) Recent advances in hepatitis A research. In Greenwalt TJ and Jamieson GA (Eds): Transmissible disease and blood transfusion, New York, Grune & Stratton, Inc, p 11

Putnam SM et al (1968) Infectious lymphocytosis: long-term follow-up of an epidemic, Pediatrics **41**:588

Quaglino D and Hayhoe FGJ (1959) Observations on the periodic acid-Schiff reaction in lymphoproliferative diseases, J Pathol **78**:521

Quan SG et al (1980) Ultrastructure and tartrate-resistant acid phosphatase localization in a T-cell hairy-cell leukemia cell line, J Histochem Cytochem **28**:434

Quastler H (1959) The description of steady-state kinetics. In Stohlman F Jr (Ed): Kinetics of cellular proliferation, New York, Grune & Stratton, Inc

Quattrin N (1973) Leucémies aiguës a basophiles, Nouv Rev Fr Hematol **13**:754

Quattrin N and Ventruto V (1974) Hemoglobin Lepore: its significance for thalassemia and clinical manifestations, Blut **28**:327

Quesenberry PJ et al (1973) Effect of endotoxin on granulopoiesis and the in vitro colony-forming cell, Blood **41**:391

Quick AJ (1943) On the constitution of prothrombin, Am J Physiol **140**:212

Quick AJ (1951) The physiology and pathology of hemostasis, Philadelphia, Lea & Febiger

Quick AJ (1965) Hereditary thrombopathic thrombocytopenia and Minot-von Willebrand syndrome: probable co-existence in a family, Am J Med Sci **250**:1

Quick AJ (1966) Salicylates and bleeding: the aspirin tolerance test, Am J Med Sci **252**:265

Quick AJ and Hickey ME (1960) Influence of erythrocytes on the coagulation of blood, Am J Med Sci **239**:51

Quick AJ and Hussey CV (1963) Hereditary thrombopathic thrombocytopenia, Am J Med Sci **245**:643

Quigley HJ (1967) Peripheral leukocyte thromboplastin in promyelocytic leukemia, Fed Proc **26**:648

Rabiet M-J et al (1978) Abnormal activation of a human prothrombin variant: prothrombin Barcelona, FEBS Lett **87**:132

Rabiner SF and Molinas F (1970) The role of phenol and phenolic acids on the thrombocytopathy and defective platelet aggregation of patients with renal failure, Am J Med **49**:346

Rabinovitz M (1974) Translational repression in the control of globin chain initiation by hemin, Ann NY Acad Sci **241**:322

Rabinowitz Y and Dameshek W (1960) Systemic lupus erythematosus after "idiopathic" thrombocytopenic purpura: a review, Ann Intern Med **52**:1

Rabinowitz Y and Dietz A (1967) Genetic control of lactate dehydrogenase and malate dehydrogenase isozymes in cultures of lymphocytes and granulocytes: effect of addition of phytohemagglutinin, actinomycin D, or puromycin, Biochim Biophys Acta **139**:254

Rabson AR et al (1978) Inhibitory effect of prostaglandin A_1 on neutrophil motility, Br J Exp Pathol **59**:298

Race RR (1942) On the inheritance and linkage relations of acholuric jaundice, Ann Eugenet **11**:365

Race RR (1944) An "incomplete" antibody in human serum, Nature **153**:771

Race RR et al (1950) A probable deletion in a human Rh chromosome, Nature **166**:520

Rachmilewitz B et al (1977) The transcobalamins in polycythemia vera, Scand J Haematol **19**:453

Rachmilewitz EA (1974) Denaturation of the normal and abnormal hemoglobin molecule, Semin Hematol **11**:441

Radmer R and Bogorad L (1972) A tetrapyrrylmethane intermediate in the enzymatic synthesis of uroporphyrinogen, Biochemistry **11**:904

Rado JP and Hammer S (1959) Polycythemia vera turning into myelofibrosis in an individual with Pelger-Huët anomaly of the leukocytes, Blood **14**:1143

Raff MC (1971) Surface antigenic markers for distinguishing T and B lymphocytes in mice, Transplant Rev **6**:52

Raffel S (1965) Delayed (cellular) hypersensitivity. In Samter M (Ed): Immunological diseases, Boston, Little, Brown & Co, p 146

Rahbar S (1968) An abnormal hemoglobin in red cells of diabetics, Clin Chim Acta **22**:296

Rahbar S (1973) Haemoglobin D Iran: beta 22 glutamic acid → glutamine (B4), Br J Haematol **24**:31

Rahbar S et al (1967) Abnormal haemoglobins in Iran. Observation of a new variant: haemoglobin J Iran (alpha 2 beta 2 77 his → arg), Br Med J **1**:674

Rahbar S et al (1969a) Haemoglobin L Persian Gulf: alpha 57 (E6) glycine → arginine, Acta Haematol **42**:169

Rahbar S et al (1969b) Studies of an unusual hemoglobin in patients with diabetes mellitus, Biochem Biophys Res Commun **36**:838

Rahbar S et al (1973) Hemoglobin Daneskgah-Tehran alpha 2 72 (EF1) histidine → arginine beta 2A, Nature (New Biol) **245**:268

Rahbar S et al (1975a) Hemoglobin Arya: alpha 2 47 (CD5) aspartic acid → asparagine, Biochim Biophys Acta **386**:525

Rahbar S et al (1975b) Haemoglobin Hamadan alpha 2A beta 2 56 glycine → arginine (D7), Biochim Biophys Acta **379**:645

Rahbar S et al (1976) Two new haemoglobins: haemoglobin Perspolis (alpha 64 [E13] asp → tyr) and haemoglobin J-Kurosh (alpha 19 [AB] ala → asp), Biochim Biophys Acta **427**:119

Rahbar S et al (1979) Haemoglobin Avicenna (beta 47 [CD6] asp → ala), a new abnormal haemoglobin, Biochim Biophys Acta **576**:466

Rakela J et al (1978) Hepatitis A virus infection in fulminant hepatitis and chronic active hepatitis, Gastroenterology **74**:879

Raker JW et al (1960) Significance of megakaryocytes in the search for tumor cells in the peripheral blood, N Engl J Med **263**:993

Rambach WA et al (1961) Erythropoietic activity of tissue homogenates, Proc Soc Exp Biol Med **108**:793

Rambaud JC and Matuchansky C (1973) Alpha-chain disease. Pathogenesis and relation to Mediterranean lymphoma, Lancet **1**:1430

Ramirez F et al (1976) Abnormal or absent βmRNA in $β^0$ Ferrara and gene deletion in δβ thalassemia, Nature **263**:471

Ramot B et al (1969) Hemoglobin D Punjab in a Bulgarian Jewish family, Israel J Med Sci **5**:1066

Ramot B et al (1972) Cited in WHO Technical Report Series No 509, Annex 1, Geneva

Rampini VS and Adank W (1964) Hämatologische Befunde bei Patienten mit Gargoylismus und heterozygoten Gernträgern, Helv Pediatr Acta **19**:101

Ramsay DHE and Harvey CC (1959) Marking-ink poisoning: an outbreak of methaemoglobin cyanosis in newborn babies, Lancet **1**:910

Rand JH et al (1980) Localization of factor-VIII-related antigen in human vascular subendothelium, Blood **55**:752

Rand JJ et al (1969) Coagulation defects in acute promyelocytic leukemia, Arch Intern Med **123**:39

Randall DL et al (1965) Familial myeloproliferative disease: a new syndrome closely simulating myelogenous leukemia in childhood, Am J Dis Child **110**:479

Ranke EJ (1965) Eosinophilia and hepatocellular carcinoma: report of a case, Am J Dig Dis **10**:548

Rankin GLS et al (1962) Measurement with ^{51}Cr of red cell loss in menorrhagia, Lancet **1**:567

Ranney HM and Jacobs AS (1964) Simultaneous occurrence of haemoglobins C and Lepore in an Afro-American, Nature **204**:163

Ranney HM et al (1967) Haemoglobin New York, Nature **213**:876

Ranney HM et al (1968) Hemoglobin Riverdale-Bronx, an unstable hemoglobin resulting from the substitution of arginine for glycine at helical residue B6 of the beta polypeptide chain, Biochim Biophys Acta **33**:1004

Ranney HM et al (1969) Hemoglobin NYU, a delta chain variant, alpha 2 delta 2 12 lys, J Clin Invest **48**:2057

Rao LM et al (1974) Hereditary splenomegaly with hypersplenism, Clin Genet **5**:379

Rapaport SI et al (1961) A simple, specific one-stage assay for plasma thromboplastin antecedent activity, J Lab Clin Med **57**:771

Rapoport S (1968) The regulation of glycolysis in mammalian erythrocytes, Essays Biochem **4**:69

Rapoport S and Luebering J (1951) Glycerate-2,3-diphosphatase, J Biol Chem **189**:683

Rapoport S and Luebering J (1952) An optical study of diphosphoglycerate mutase, J Biol Chem **196**:583

Rapoport S et al (1972) Control of glycolysis in the erythrocyte on the level of 1,3-DPG. In Rørth M and Astrup P (Eds): Benzon Symposium, Copenhagen, Munksgaard

Rapp F and Buss ER (1974) Are viruses important in carcinogenesis? Am J Pathol **77**:85

Rappaport H (1966) Tumors of the hematopoietic system. Atlas of Tumor Pathology, Section III, Fascicle 8, Washington DC, Armed Forces Institute of Pathology

Rappaport H et al (1956) Follicular lymphoma. A reevaluation of its position in the scheme of malignant lymphoma, based on a survey of 253 cases, Cancer **9**:792

Rappaport H et al (1971) Report of the committee of histopathological criteria contributing to staging of Hodgkin's disease, Cancer Res **31**:1864

Rastrick JM et al (1968) Direct evidence for presence of Ph-1 chromosome in erythroid cells, Br Med J **1**:96

Ratnoff OD (1972) Studies of the product of the reaction between activated Hageman factor (factor XII) and the plasma thromboplastin antecedent (factor XI), J Lab Clin Med **80**:704

Ratnoff OD and Agle D (1968) Psychogenic purpura: a reevaluation of the syndrome of autoerythrocyte sensitization, Medicine **47**:475

Ratnoff OD and Bennett B (1973) The genetics of hereditary disorders of blood coagulation, Science **179**:1291

Ratnoff OD and Crum JD (1964) Activation of Hageman factor by solutions of ellagic acid, J Lab Clin Med **63**:359

Ratnoff OD and Jones PK (1976) The detection of carriers of classic hemophilia, Am J Clin Pathol **65**:129

Ratnoff OD and Miles AA (1964) The induction of permeability-increasing activity in human plasma by activated Hageman factor, Br J Exp Pathol **45**:328

Ratnoff OD and Steinberg AG (1962) Further studies on the inheritance of Hageman trait, J Lab Clin Med **59**:980

Ratnoff OD et al (1968) The demise of John Hageman, N Engl J Med **279**:760

Raven JL et al (1971) Comparison of three methods for measuring vitamin B$_{12}$ in serum: Radioisotopic, *Euglena gracilis*, and *Lactobacillus leichmannii*, Br J Haematol **22**:21

Rawnsley HM and Shelley WB (1968) Cold urticaria with cryoglobulinemia in a patient with chronic lymphocytic leukemia, Arch Dermatol **98**:12

Rawson R et al (1941) Industrial solvents as possible etiology agents in myeloid metaplasia, Science **93**:541

Ray RN et al (1959) In vitro and in vivo observations on stored sickle trait red blood cells, Am J Clin Pathol **32**:430

Rayner S (1952) Juvenile amaurotic idiocy: diagnosis of heterozygotes, Acta Genet **3**:1

Reagan TJ and Okazaki H (1974) The thrombotic syndrome associated with carcinoma: a clinical and neuropathologic study, Arch Neurol **31**:390

Rebuck JW (1978) Basophilic leukemic conversion of chronic granulocytic leukemia, Hematology Check Sample No. H-91, American Society of Clinical Pathologists

Rebuck JW and Crowley JH (1955) A method of studying leukocyte functions in vivo, Ann NY Acad Sci **59**:757

Rebuck JW and LoGrippo GA (1961) Characteristics and interrelationships of the various cells of the RE cell, macrophage, lymphocyte, and plasma cell series in man, Lab Invest **10**:1068

Rebuck JW and Van Slyck EJ (1968) An unsuspected ultrastructural fault in human elliptocytes, Am J Clin Pathol **49**:19

Rebuck JW et al (1958) Potentialities of the lymphocyte, with an additional reference to its dysfunction in Hodgkin's disease, Ann NY Acad Sci **73**:8

Rebuck JW et al (1961) Volumetric ultrastructural studies of abnormal platelets. In Johnson SA (Ed): The blood platelets, Boston, Little, Brown & Co

Rebuck JW et al (1971) Morphologic evaluation of megakaryocytes. In Brinkhous KM et al (Eds): The platelet, Baltimore, The Williams & Wilkins Co

Reece RL and Beckett RS (1966) Epidemiology of single-unit transfusion, JAMA **195**:801

Reed CS et al (1968) Erythrocytosis secondary to increased oxygen affinity of a mutant hemoglobin, hemoglobin Kempsey, Blood **31**:623

Reed RE (1974) False-positive monospot tests in malaria, Am J Clin Pathol **61**:173

Reed RE et al (1974) Haemoglobin Inkster (alpha 2 85 aspartic acid → valine beta 2) coexisting with beta thalassemia in a Caucasian family, Br J Haematol **26**:475

Reeve EB (1980) Steady state relations between factors X, X$_A$, II, II$_A$, antithrombin III and alpha-2 macroglobulin in thrombosis, Thromb Res **18**:19

Reeves JD et al (1979) The hematopoietic effects of prednisone therapy in four infants with osteopetrosis, J Pediatr **94**:210

Rega AR et al (1967) Changes in the properties of human erythrocyte membrane proteins after solubilization by butanol extraction, Biochim Biophys Acta **147**:297

Reichert N et al (1975) Clinical and genetic aspects of Glanzmann's thrombasthenia in Israel: report of 22 cases, Thromb Diath Haemorrh **34**:806

Reidbord HR et al (1972) Splenic lipidoses. Histochemical and ultrastructural differentiation with special reference to the syndrome of the sea-blue histiocyte, Arch Pathol **93**:518

Reilly WA (1941) The granules in the leukocytes in gargoylism, Am J Dis Child **62**:489

Reimann F and Arkun NS (1956) Die Einwirkung der Eisenbehandlung auf das Verhalten der osmotischen Resistenz der Erythrocyten bei den Eisenempfindlichen chronischen Chloranemien (Asiderosen), Z Klin Med **153**:589

Reiss RF et al (1975) An improved method for the quantitation of A$_2$ hemoglobin utilizing cellulose acetate and densitometry, Am J Clin Pathol **63**:841

Reissmann KR (1950) Studies on mechanism of erythropoietic stimulation in parabiotic rats during hypoxia, Blood **5**:372

Remmer H and Merker HJ (1963) Drug-induced changes in the

liver endoplasmic reticulum: association with drug-metabolizing enzymes, Science **142**:1657

Remold HG et al (1970) Studies on migration inhibitory factor (MIF): recovery of MIF activity after purification by gel filtration and disc electrophoresis, Cell Immunol **1**:133

Renteria VG et al (1976) The heart in the Hurler syndrome: gross histologic and ultrastructural observations in five necropsy cases, Am J Cardiol **38**:487

Repine JE et al (1979) An improved nitroblue tetrazolium test using phorbol myristate acetate-coated coverslips, Am J Clin Pathol **71**:582

Report by the International Committee for Standardization in Hematology (ICSH): Panel on diagnostic applications of radio-isotopes in haematology (1973), Standard techniques for the measurement of red-cell and plasma volume, Br J Haematol **25**:801

Retief FP and Huskisson YJ (1969) Serum and urinary folate in liver disease, Br Med J **1**:150

Retief FP et al (1967) Delivery of Co^{57} to erythrocytes from A and B globulin of normal, B_{12}-deficient, and chronic myeloid leukemia serum, Blood **29**:837

Reviron J et al (1968) Un exemple de chromosome "cis A_1B". Étude immunologique et génétique du phénotype induit, Nouv Rev Fr Hematol **8**:323

Rey JJ and Wolf PL (1968) Extreme leucocytosis in accidental electric shock, Lancet **1**:18

Reynafarje C (1968) Humoral regulation of the erythropoietic depression of high altitude polycythemic subjects after return to sea level, Ann NY Acad Sci **149**:472

Reynolds CA and Huisman THJ (1966) Hemoglobin Russ or alpha 2 51 arg beta 2, Biochim Biophys Acta **130**:541

Reynolds EH (1976) Neurological aspects of folate and vitamin B_{12} metabolism, Clin Haematol **5**:661

Reynolds EH et al (1965) Reversible absorption defects in anticonvulsant megaloblastic anaemia, J Clin Pathol **18**:593

Reynolds EH et al (1966) Anticonvulsant therapy, megaloblastic haemopoiesis, and folic acid metabolism, Q J Med **35**:521

Reynolds TB and Ware A (1952) Sulfhemoglobinemia following habitual use of acetanilid, JAMA **149**:1538

Rhodes J et al (1968) Absorption of iron instilled into the stomach, duodenum, and jejunum, Gut **9**:323

Ricco G et al (1974) Hb J Sicilia: beta 65 (E9) lys → asn, a beta homologue of hb Zambia, FEBS Lett **39**:200

Rice WG (1956) Myeloma cryoglobulin: morphologic, electrophoretic, and immunologic studies, Lab Invest **5**:410

Richar WJ and Breakell ES (1959) Evaluation of an electronic particle counter for the counting of white blood cells, Am J Clin Pathol **31**:384

Richmond J and Davidson S (1958) Subacute combined degeneration of the spinal cord in non-Addisonian megaloblastic anaemia, Q J Med **27**:517

Rick ME and Hoyer LW (1975) Molecular weight of human factor VIII procoagulant activity, Thromb Res **7**:909

Rickert RR and Vidone RA (1968) The use of bovine albumin in the examination of bone marrow obtained at autopsy, Blood **31**:74

Rickes EL et al (1948) Crystalline vitamin B_{12}, Science **107**:396

Ricketts C et al (1975) Ferrokinetics and erythropoiesis in man: the measurement of effective erythropoiesis, ineffective erythropoiesis and red cell lifespan using ^{59}Fe, Br J Haematol **31**:65

Rickles FR and O'Leary DS (1974) Role of coagulation system in patho-physiology of sickle cell disease, Arch Intern Med **133**:635

Ricks P Jr (1968) Further experience with exchange transfusion in sickle cell anemia and pregnancy, Am J Obstet Gynecol **100**:1087

Riddle JM et al (1960) Platelet abnormalities in pernicious anemia, Fed Proc **19**:64

Riddle MC (1929) Endogenous uric acid metabolism in pernicious anemia, J Clin Invest **8**:69

Ridway JC and Garrett JV (1974) Demonstration of lymphocyte nucleoli, J Clin Pathol **27**:337

Rieder RF (1972) Translation of β-globin mRNA in β-thalassemia and the S and C hemoglobinopathies, J Clin Invest **51**:364

Rieder RF (1974) Human hemoglobin stability and instability: molecular mechanisms and some clinical correlations, Semin Hematol **11**:423

Rieder RF and James GW III (1974) Imbalance in α and β globin synthesis associated with a hemoglobinopathy, J Clin Invest **54**:948

Rieder RF et al (1969) Hemoglobin Philly (beta 35 tyrosine → phenylalanine): studies in the molecular pathology of hemoglobin, J Clin Invest **48**:1627

Rieder RF et al (1975) Rapid post-synthetic destruction of unstable haemoglobin Bushwick, Nature **254**:725

Rieder RF et al (1976) Hemoglobin A_2-Roosevelt: alpha 2 delta 2 20 val → glu, Biochim Biophys Acta **439**:501

Rietti F (1925) Ittero emolitico primitivo, Atti Accad Scient Med Nat Ferrara **2**:14

Rifkind D et al (1961) Urinary excretion of iron-binding protein in the nephrotic syndrome, N Engl J Med **265**:115

Rigas DA (1959) Dynamics of cell proliferation and isotope incorporation into deoxyribonucleic acid. In Stohlman F Jr (Ed): Kinetics of cellular proliferation, New York, Grune & Stratton, Inc

Rigas DA et al (1956) Hemoglobin H: clinical laboratory, and genetic studies of a family with a previously undescribed hemoglobin, J Lab Clin Med **47**:51

Riisager PM (1959) Eosinophil leukocytes in ulcerative colitis, Lancet **2**:1008

Rindler R et al (1971) Naphthol AS-D chloroacetate esterases in granule extracts from human neutrophil leukocytes, Blut **23**:223

Ringelhann B et al (1977) Homozygotes for the hereditary persistence of fetal hemoglobin: the ratio of $^G\gamma$ to $^A\gamma$ chains and biosynthetic studies, Biochem Genet **15**:1083

Rishpon-Meyerstein N et al (1968) The effect of testosterone on erythropoietin levels in anemic patients, Blood **31**:453

Ritchey AK et al (1979) Antibody-mediated acquired sideroblastic anemia: response to cytotoxic therapy, Blood **54**:734

Ritchie RF (1967) The clinical significance of titered antinuclear antibodies, Arthritis Rheum **10**:544

Ritchie RF (1970) Antinuclear antibodies: their frequency and diagnostic association, N Engl J Med **282**:1174

Ritchie RF (1971) Clinical use of automated precipitin data: a problem of volume and physician acceptance. In Advances in automated analysis, vol 1, Technicon International Congress, 1970, Miami, Thurman Associates, p 123

Ritts RE and Neel HB III (1974) An overview of cancer immunology, Mayo Clin Proc **49**:118

Ritzmann SE et al (1963) Cryoproteinemias. I. The characterization and assay of cryofibrinogen, Texas Rep Biol Med **21**:262

Ritzmann, SE et al (1975) Idiopathic (asymptomatic) monoclonal gammopathies, Arch Intern Med **135**:95

River GL (1966) Erythroid aplasia following thymomectomy. Report of a case with a positive lupus erythematosus cell preparation and elevated plasma erythropoietin level, JAMA **197**:726

River GL et al (1961) SC hemoglobin: a clinical study, Blood **18**:385

Rivero SJ et al (1978) Lymphopenia in systemic lupus erythematosus: clinical diagnostic and prognostic significance, Arthritis Rheum **21**:295

Rivlin RS and Wagner HN Jr (1969) Anemia in hyperthyroidism, Ann Intern Med **70**:507

Rizza CR and Biggs R (1973) The treatment of patients who have factor-VIII antibodies, Br J Haematol **24**:65

Rizza CR and Eipe J (1971) Exercise, factor VIII, and the spleen, Br J Haematol **20**:629

Roberts DF (1971) The genetic basis of variation in factor VIII levels among haemophiliacs. J Med Genet **8**:136

Roberts HR and Cederbaum AI (1975) Molecular variants of factor IX. In Brinkhous KM and Hemker HC (Eds): Handbook of hemophilia, New York, American Elsevier Publishing Co, Inc, p 237

Roberts HR and McMillan CW (1975) Clinical use of high-potency factor VIII concentrate. In Brinkhous KM and Hemker HC (Eds): Handbook of hemophilia, New York, American Elsevier Publishing Co, Inc, p 475

Roberts HR et al (1975) Immunology of acquired inhibition of coagulation factors. In Brinkhous KM and Hemker HC (Eds): Handbook of hemophilia, New York, American Elsevier Publishing Co, Inc, p 647

Roberts JC et al (1957) Antibody-producing lymph node cells and peritoneal exudate cells: morphologic studies of transfers to immunologically inert rabbits, Arch Pathol **64**:324

Roberts S et al (1960) The isolation of cancer cells from the blood stream during uterine curettage, Surg Gynecol Obstet **111**:3

Robertson BR et al (1972) ''Fibrinolytic capacity'' in healthy volunteers at different ages as studies by standardized venous occlusion of arms and legs, Acta Med Scand **191**:199

Robertson JH (1970) Uracil mustard in the treatment of thrombocythemia, Blood **35**:288

Robertson JH and Trueman RG (1964) Combined hemophilia and Christmas disease, Blood **24**:281

Robertson JH et al (1972) Vincristine-induced thrombocytosis studies with ^{75}Se selenomethionine, Acta Haematol **47**:356

Robertson MG (1972) Hematuria and cholelithiasis with β-thalassemia (letter to editor), JAMA **219**:1213

Robinowitz B et al (1975) Sea-blue histiocytes in mycosis fungoides, Arch Dermatol **111**:1165

Robins-Browne RM et al (1977) Thymoma, pure red cell aplasia, pernicious anaemia and candidiasis: a defect in immunohomeostasis, Br J Haematol **36**:5

Robinson DS and Sylwester D (1970) Interaction of commonly prescribed drugs and warfarin, Ann Intern Med **72**:853

Robinson DS et al (1971) Interaction of warfarin and nonsystemic gastrointestinal drugs, Clin Pharmacol Ther **12**:491

Robinson MG and Watson RJ (1963) Megaloblastic anemia complicating thalassemia major, Am J Dis Child **105**:275

Robinson WA and Mangalik A (1975) The kinetics and regulation of granulopoiesis, Semin Hematol **12**:7

Robinson WA and Pike BL (1970) Leukopoietic activity in human urine. The granulocytic leukemias, N Engl J Med **282**:1291

Robinson WS and Lutwick LI (1976) The virus of hepatitis, type B, N Engl J Med **295**:1168

Robitaille GA (1964) Ehlers-Danlos syndrome and recurrent hemoptysis, Ann Intern Med **61**:716

Rockey JH et al (1964) Beta-2A-aglobulinemia in two healthy men, J Lab Clin Med **63**:205

Rocklin RE et al (1970) An in vitro assay for cellular hypersensitivity in man, J Immunol **104**:95

Rockoff AS et al (1978) Myocardial necrosis following general anesthesia in hemoglobin SC disease, Pediatrics **61**:73

Rodey GE et al (1970) Defective bactericidal activity of peripheral blood leukocytes in lipochrome histocytosis, Am J Med **49**:322

Rodgers GM et al (1972) Increased kidney cyclic AMP levels and erythropoietin production following cobalt administration, Proc Soc Exp Biol Med **140**:977

Rodin AE et al (1972) Polysplenia with severe congenital heart disease and Howell-Jolly bodies, Am J Clin Pathol **58**:127

Rodman NF Jr et al (1966) Fibrinogen—its role in platelet agglutination and agglutinate stability: a study of congenital afibrinogenemia, Lab Invest **15**:641

Rodriguez-Erdmann F et al (1971) Kasabach-Merritt syndrome: coagulo-analytical observations, Am J Med Sci **261**:9

Roeser HP et al (1970) The role of ceruloplasmin in iron metabolism, J Clin Invest **49**:2408

Roguin N et al (1978) Polysplenia syndrome: a study of five new cases, Israel J Med Sci **14**:948

Rohner RF et al (1967) Mucinous malignancies, venous thrombosis, and terminal endocarditis with emboli: a syndrome, Cancer **19**:1805

Rohr KL (1952) Reaktive Retikulosen des Knochenmarkes, Acta Haemstol **7**:321

Roland AS (1964) The syndrome of benign thymoma and aregenerative anemia; an analysis of forty-three cases, Am J Med Sci **247**:719

Romain PL et al (1975) Hemoglobin J Chicago (beta 76 [E20] ala → asp): a new hemoglobin variant resulting from a substitution of an external residue, Blood **45**:387

Rominger CJ (1964) Blood volume studies in normal pregnancy, toxemia, and gynecologic patients, Am Surg **30**:357

Root RK et al (1972) Abnormal bactericidal metabolic and lysosomal functions of Chediak-Higashi syndrome leukocytes, J Clin Invest **51**:649

Ropartz C (1971) L'allotypie des immunoglobulines humaines, Bull Inst Pasteur **69**:107

Ropartz C et al (1967) Un troisième locus participant à la synthèse des γG: 1'ISF, Rev Fr Etude Clin Biol **12**:267

Ropartz C et al (1968) Some problems raised by the ISF system of human immunoglobulins, Vox Sang **14**:458

Rørth M (1974) Hypoxia, red cell oxygen affinity, and erythropoietin production, Clin Haematol **3**:595

Rosa J et al (1965) Une nouvelle hémoglobine anormale: l'hémoglobin j alpha Paris 12 ala → asp, Nouv Rev Fr Hématol **6**:423

Rosa J et al (1966) Sur quelques hémoglobines anormales nouvelles recemment isolées en France, International Symposium on Comparative Hemoglobin Structure, Thessaloniki, p 140

Rosa J et al (1969) Haemoglobin I Toulouse: beta 66 (E10) lys → glu: a new abnormal haemoglobin with a mutation localized on the E10 porphyrin surrounding zones, Nature (London) **223**:190

Rosa J et al (1971) Evidence for various types of synthesis of human γ chains of haemoglobin in acquired haematological disorders, Nature (New Biol) **233**:111

Rosai J and Dorfman RF (1969) Sinus histiocytosis with massive lymphadenopathy, Arch Pathol **87**:63

Rose DP (1966) Folic acid deficiency in leukaemia and lymphomas, J Clin Pathol **19**:29

Rose MS and Chanarin I (1969) Dissociation of intrinsic factor from its antibody: application to study of pernicious anemia gastric juice specimens, Br Med J **1**:468

Rose MS and Chanarin I (1971) Intrinsic-factor antibody and absorption of vitamin B_{12} in pernicious anaemia, Br Med J **1**:25

Roseman S (1970) The synthesis of complex carbohydrates by multiglycosyltransferase systems and their potential function in intercellular adhesion, Chem Phys Lipids **5**:270

Rosen FS and Bougas JA (1963) Acquired dysgammaglobuline-mia: Elevation of the 19S gamma globulin and deficiency of the 7S gamma globulin in a woman with chronic progressive bronchiectasis, N Engl J Med **269**:1336

Rosen FS and Janeway CA (1966) The gamma globulins. 3. The antibody deficiency syndromes, N Engl J Med **275**:709

Rosen FS and Merler E (1972) Genetic defects in gammaglobulin synthesis. In Stanbury JB et al (Eds): The metabolic basic of inherited disease, ed 3, New York, McGraw-Hill Book Co, Inc, p 1643

Rosen FS et al (1961) Recurrent bacterial infections and dysgamma-globulinemia: deficiency of 7S gammaglobulins in the presence of elevated 19S gammaglobulins. Report of two cases, Pediatrics **28**:182

Rosen H et al (1969) Spectral properties of hemopexin-heme. The Schumm test, J Lab Clin Med **74**:941

Rosen H and Klebanoff SJ (1979) Bactericidal activity of a superoxide anion-generating system: a model for the polymorpho-nuclear leukocyte, J Exp Med **149**:27

Rosen RB and Kang S-J (1979) Congenital agranulocytosis terminating in acute myelomonocytic leukemia, J Pediatr **94**:406

Rosen RB and Nishiyama H (1968) Leukocyte alkaline phosphatase in chronic granulocytic leukemia of childhood, Ann NY Acad Sci **155**:992

Rosenberg EB et al (1970) Increased circulating IgE in a new parasitic disease—human intestinal capillariasis, N Engl J Med **283**:1148

Rosenberg HS and Taylor FM (1958) The myeloproliferative syndrome in children, J Pediatr **52**:407

Rosenberg IH (1975) Folate absorption and malabsorption, N Engl J Med **293**:1303

Rosenberg JL et al (1973) Viral hepatitis: an occupational hazard to surgeons, JAMA **223**:395

Rosenberg LE et al (1969) Methylmalonic aciduria: an inborn error leading to metabolic acidosis, long-chain ketonuria, and intermittent hyperglycinemia, N Engl J Med **278**:1319

Rosenberg M (1969) Fetal hematopoiesis—case report, Blood **33**:66

Rosenberg RD (1975) Actions and interactions of antithrombin and heparin, N Engl J Med **292**:146

Rosenberg RD and Damus PS (1973) The purification and mechanism of action of human antithrombin-heparin cofactor, J Biol Chem **248**:6490

Rosenberg SA (1971) A critique of the value of laparotomy and splenectomy in the evaluation of patients with Hodgkin's disease, Cancer Res **31**:1737

Rosenberg SA (1975) Bone marrow involvement in the non-Hodgkin's lymphomata, Br J Cancer **31**(suppl II):261

Rosenberg SA et al (1971) Report of the Committee on Hodgkin's Disease Staging Procedures, Cancer Res **31**:1862

Rosenfeld S and Dressler D (1974) Transfer factor: a subcellular component that transmits information for specific immune responses, Proc Natl Acad Sci **71**:2473

Rosenfeld S et al (1961) Syndrome simulating lymphosarcoma induced by diphenylhydantoin sodium, JAMA **176**:941

Rosenfeld SI and Leddy JP (1974) Hereditary deficiency of the fifth component of complement (C5) in man, J Clin Invest **53**:67a

Rosenfeld SI et al (1976) Hereditary deficiency of the fifth component of the complement in man, J Clin Invest **57**:1626

Rosenfield RE (1974) Early twentieth century origins of modern blood transfusion therapy, Mt Sinai J Med NY **41**:626

Rosenfield RE (1975) The past and future of immunohematology, Am J Clin Pathol **64**:569

Rosenfield RE et al (1962) A review of Rh serology and presentation of a new terminology, Transfusion **2**:287

Rosenfield RE et al (1965) Anti-i, a frequent cold agglutinin in infectious mononucleosis, Vox Sang **10**:631

Rosenfield RE et al (1970) A "new" Rh antibody, anti-f, Br Med J **1**:975

Rosenoer VM et al (1970) The thymus and immunocompetence: the target cell of the thymic factor, Proc Soc Exp Biol Med **133**:394

Rosenthal DS and Moloney WC (1977) Occurrence of acute leukaemia in myeloproliferative disorders, Br J Haematol **36**:373

Rosenthal MC (1954) Deficiency in plasma thromboplastin component. II. Its incidence in a hemophilic population. Critique of methods for identification, Am J Clin Pathol **24**:910

Rosenthal MC and Sanders M (1954) Plasma thromboplastin component deficiency. I. Studies on its inheritance and therapy, Am J Med **16**:153

Rosenthal RL and Sloan E (1966) Assay of clotting factors in out-dated blood bank plasma and its potential use for therapy in hemophilia and other hemorrhagic dyscrasias, Transfusion **6**:289

Rosenthal S et al (1977) Blast crisis of chronic granulocytic leukemia: morphologic variants and therapeutic implications, Am J Med **63**:542

Rosenzweig AI et al (1968) Hemoglobin H as an acquired defect of alpha-chain synthesis: report of two cases, Acta Haematol **39**:91

Roskam J (1923) Contribution a l'étude de la physiologie normale et pathologique du globulin, Arch Int Physiol Biochim **20**:241

Roskam J (1954) Arrest of bleeding, Springfield, Ill, Charles C Thomas, Publishers

Rosner F (1969) Hemophilia in the Talmud and rabbinic writings, Ann Intern Med **70**:833

Rosner F et al (1970) Disturbances of hemostasis in acute myeloblastic leukemia, Acta Haematol **43**:65

Ross GD et al (1973) Combined studies of complement receptor and surface immunoglobulin-bearing cells and sheep erythrocyte rosette-forming cells in normal and leukemic human lymphocytes, J Clin Invest **52**:377

Ross GD (1977) Surface markers of B and T cells: recent technical developments reveal a heterogeneity of lymphocyte subpopulations, Arch Pathol Lab Med **101**:337

Ross JF (1945) Hemoglobinemia and the hemoglobinurias, N Engl J Med **233**:732

Rosse C (1971) Lymphocyte production and life-span in the bone marrow of the guinea pig, Blood **38**:372

Rosse C (1972) Migration of long-lived lymphocytes to the bone marrow and to other lymphomyeloid tissues in normal parabiotic guinea pigs, Blood **40**:90

Rosse C et al (1977) Bone marrow cell populations of normal infants; the predominance of lymphocytes, J Lab Clin Med **89**:1225

Rosse WF (1973a) Correlation of in vivo and in vitro measurements of hemolysis in hemolytic anemia due to immune reactions, Prog Hematol **8**:51

Rosse WF (1973b) Variations in the red cells in paroxysmal nocturnal hemoglobinuria, Br J Haematol **24**:327

Rosse WF and Dacie JV (1966) Immune lysis of normal human and paroxysmal nocturnal hemoglobinuria (PNH) red blood cells. II. The role of complement components in the increased sensitivity of PNH cells to immune lysis, J Clin Invest **45**:749

Rosse WF and Gurney CW (1959) The Pelger-Huët anomaly in three families and its use in determining the disappearance of transfused neutrophils from the peripheral blood, Blood **14**:170

Rosse WF and Waldmann TA (1964) A comparison of some physical and chemical properties of erythropoiesis-stimulating factors from different sources, Blood **24**:739

Rosse WF and Waldmann TA (1966) Factors controlling erythropoiesis in birds, Blood **27**:654

Rosse WF et al (1963) Renal cysts, erythropoietin, and polycythemia, Am J Med **34**:76

Rosse WF et al (1974) Mechanisms of immune lysis of the red cells in hereditary erythroblastic multinuclearity with a positive acidified serum test and paroxysmal nocturnal hemoglobinuria, J Clin Invest **53**:31

Rossi EC (1972) Comments on the early history of hemostasis, Med Clin North Am **56**:9

Rossi-Bernardi L and Roughton FJW (1967) The specific effect of carbon dioxide and carbamate compounds on the buffer power and Bohr effects in human hemoglobin selections, J Physiol **189**:1

Roth EF Jr et al (1978) Benign sickle cell anemia in Israeli-Arabs with high red cell 2,3-diphosphoglycerate, Acta Haematol **59**:237

Rothbach C et al (1979) Antibody deficiency with normal immunoglobulins, J Pediatr **94**:250

Rothenberg SP (1973) Application of competitive ligand binding for the radioassay of vitamin B_{12} and folic acid, Metabolism **22**:1075

Rothenberg SP et al (1972a) A radioassay for serum folate: use of a two-phase sequential-incubation, ligand-binding system, N Engl J Med **286**:1335

Rothenberg SP et al (1972b) Evidence for the absorption of immunoreactive intrinsic factor into the intestinal epithelial cell during vitamin B_{12} absorption, J Lab Clin Med **79**:587

Rothenberg SP and DaCosta M (1976) Folate binding proteins and radioassay for folate, Clin Haematol **5**:569

Rothenberg SP and Lawson J (1979) Effect of cyanide on radioassay for serum cobalamin, Clin Chem **25**:639

Rothfield NF (1969) Serologic tests in rheumatic diseases, Postgrad Med **45**:116

Rothfield NF and Pace N (1962) Relation of positive L.E. cell preparations to activity of lupus erythematosus and corticosteroid therapy, N Engl J Med **266**:535

Rothlin E and Undritz E (1946) Zur megakaryozytenbildung durch Polyploidie, Arch Klausstift Verebungsforsch **21**:283

Rothstein G et al (1978) Effect on lithium on neutrophil mass and production, N Engl J Med **298**:178

Rotor AB et al (1948) Familial non-hemolytic jaundice with direct van den Bergh reaction, Acta Med Philipp **5**:37

Rous P and Turner JR (1916) The preservation of living red blood cells in vitro, J Exp Med **23**:219

Rousso C and Cruchaud A (1966) Pernicious anemia. I. Clinical studies of 54 cases, with special reference to associated diseases, Helv Med Acta **33**:175

Rowe DS (1969) Radioactive single radial diffusion: a method for increasing the sensitivity of immunochemical quantitation of proteins in agar gel, Bull WHO **40**:613

Rowe DS et al (1970) A research standard for human serum immunoglobulins IgG, IgA, and IgM, Bull WHO **42**:535

Rowlands DT Jr et al (1974) Characterization of lymphocyte subpopulations in chronic lymphocytic leukemia, Cancer **34**:1962

Rowley JD (1973) A new consistent chromosomal abnormality in chronic myelogenous leukaemia identified by quinacrine fluorescence and Giemsa staining, Nature **243**:290

Rowley MW (1908) A fatal anemia with enormous numbers of circulating phagocytes, J Exp Med **10**:78

Rowley PT (1976) The diagnosis of beta-thalassemia trait: a review. Am J Hematol **1**:129

Rowley PT (1978) Newborn screening for sickle-cell disease: benefits and burdens, NY State J Med **78**:42

Rowley PT and Jacobs M (1972) Hypersplenic thrombocytopenia in sickle cell–beta thalassemia, Am J Med Sci **264**:489

Roy AJ et al (1973) Prophlactic platelet transfusions in children with acute leukemia. A dose response study, Transfusion **13**:283

Roy-Taranger M et al (1965) Lymphocytes binucléés dans le sang d'individus irradiés a faible dose, Rev Fr Etudes Clin Biol **10**:958

Rozenberg MC and Dintenfass L (1964) Thrombus formation in vitro: a rheological and morphological study, Aust J Exp Biol Med Sci **42**:109

Rozenszajn L et al (1963) Acid phosphatase activity in normal human blood and bone marrow cells as demonstrated by the azo dye method, Acta Haematol **30**:310

Rozenszajn L et al (1966) Jordan's anomaly in white blood cells: report of a case, Blood **28**:258

Rubin AL et al (1964) Histocompatibility and immunologic competence in renal homotransplantation, Science **143**:815

Rubin EM and Rowley PT (1979) Sickle cell trait/hereditary persistence of fetal hemoglobin trait: misdiagnosis as sickle cell anemia by newborn screening, Am J Dis Child **133**:1248

Rubin H (1966) Chronic neutrophilic leukemia, Ann Intern Med **65**:93

Rubinow SI and Keller JB (1972) Flow of viscous fluid through an elastic tube with applications to blood flow, J Theor Biol **35**:299

Rubinstein AS and Trobaugh FE Jr (1973) Ultrastructure of presumptive hematopoietic stem cells, Blood **42**:61

Rubinstein E (1962) Blood clotting: the force of retraction, Science **138**:1343

Rucinski B et al (1979) Antiheparin proteins secreted by human platelets. Purification, characterization and radioimmunoassay, Blood **53**:47

Rucknagel DL (1974) The genetics of sickle cell anemia and related syndromes, Arch Intern Med **133**:595

Rucknagel DL et al (1967) Hemoglobin Ypsilanti characterized by increased oxygen affinity, abnormal polymerization and erythremia, Clin Res **15**:270

Rudders RA et al (1973) Double myeloma. Production of both IgG type lambda and IgA type lambda myeloma proteins by a single plasma cell line, Am J Med **55**:215

Ruddy S et al (1972) The complement system of man. Parts I-IV, N Engl J Med **287**:489, 545, 592, 642

Ruhenstroth-Bauer G (1950) Versuche zum Nachweis eines spezifischen erythropoetischen Hormons, Arch Exp Path Pharmakol **211**:32

Ruhrmann G (1963) The history of Schoenlein-Henoch's disease, Ger Med Mon **3**:288

Rümke CL (1976) Nomogrammen voor toetsing van het vershil tussen twee percentages van kansen, Ned T Geneesk **120**:2205

Rümke CL (1979) The statistically expected variability in differential leukocyte counting. In Koepke JA (Ed): Differential leukocyte counting, Skokie, Ill, College of American Pathologists, p 39

Ruscetti FW and Chervenick PA (1974) Release of colony-stimulating factor from monocytes by endotoxin and polyinosinic-polycytidylic acid, J Lab Clin Med **83**:64

Russell D and Snyder SH (1968) Amine synthesis in rapidly growing tissues: ornithine decarboxylase activity in regenerating rat liver, chick embryo and various tumors, Proc Natl Acad Sci USA **60**:1420

Russell FA and Deykin D (1976) The effect of thrombin on the uptake and transformation of arachidonic acid by human platelets, Am J Haematol **1**:59

Russell PS and Monaco AP (1967) Heterologous antilymphocyte sera and some of their effects, Transplantation **5**(supp):1086

Russell PS and Monaco AP (1968) The biology of tissue transplantation, Boston, Little, Brown & Co

Russo G and Mollica F (1962) Sickle cell haemoglobin and two types of thalassaemia in the same family, Acta Haematol **28**:329

Ruthe RC et al (1978) Efficacy of granulocyte transfusions in the control of systemic candidiasis in the leukopenic host, Blood **52**:493

Rutkow IW (1978) Rupture of the spleen in infectious mononucleosis: a critical review, Arch Surg **113**:718

Ryback R and Desforges J (1970) Alcoholic thrombocytopenia in three inpatient drinking alcoholics, Arch Intern Med (Chicago) **125**:475

Ryrie DR et al (1977) Haemoglobin Sherwood Forest beta 104 (G6) arg → thr, FEBS Lett **83**:260

Rywlin AM (1976a) Bone marrow histology, aspiration versus biopsy, Am J Clin Pathol **66**:617

Rywlin AM (1976b) Histopathology of the bone marrow, Boston, Little, Brown & Co

Rywlin AM and Ortega R (1972) Lipid granulomas of the bone marrow, Am J Clin Pathol **57**:457

Rywlin AM et al (1970) A simple technic for the preparation of bone marrow smears and sections, Am J Clin Pathol **53**:389

Rywlin AM et al (1971a) Ceroid histiocytosis of spleen and bone marrow in idiopathic thrombocytopenic purpura (ITP): a contribution of the understanding of the sea-blue histiocytes, Blood **37**:587

Rywlin AM et al (1971b) Ceroid histiocytosis of the spleen in hyperlipemia. Relationship to the syndrome of the sea-blue histiocyte, Am J Clin Pathol **56**:572

Rywlin AM et al (1972) Eosinophilic fibrohistiocytic lesion of bone marrow: a distinctive new morphologic finding, probably related to drug hypersensitivity, Blood **40**:464

Rywlin AM et al (1974) Lymphoid nodules of bone marrow: normal and abnormal, Blood **43**:389

Saab GA et al (1978) Rapid assay for measurement of serum ferritin, Am J Clin Pathol **70**:275

Saarinen UM and Siimes MA (1977) Developmental changes in serum iron, total iron-binding capacity, and transferrin saturation in infancy, J Pediatr **91**:875

Saba TM (1970) Physiology and physiopathology of the reticuloendothelial system, Arch Intern Med **126**:1031

Sabin FR et al (1925) The discrimination of two types of phagocytic cells in connective tissue by the supravital technic, Contrib Embryol **16**:125

Sabo BH et al (1978) The cis AB phenotype in three generations of one family: serological, enzymatic and cytogenetic studies, J Immunogenet **5**:87

Sacker LS et al (1967) Haemoglobin F Hull (gamma 121 glutamic acid → lysine), homologous with haemoglobins O and O Indonesia, Br Med J **3**:531

Sáenz GF et al (1977) Chemical characterization of a new haemoglobin variant haemoglobin J Cubujuqui (alpha 2 141 [HC3] arg → ser beta 2), Biochim Biophys Acta **494**:48

Sagar S et al (1976a) Oral contraceptives, antithrombin III activity and postoperative deep vein thrombosis, Lancet **1**:509

Sagar S et al (1976b) Efficacy of low dose heparin in prevention of extensive deep vein thrombosis in patients undergoing total hip replacement, Lancet **1**:1151

Sagel J et al (1975) Increased platelet aggregation in early diabetes mellitus, Ann Intern Med **82**:733

Sagher F and Even-Paz Z (1967) Mastocytosis and the mast cell, Chicago, Year Book Medical Publishers, Inc

Sagone AL Jr and Balcerzak SP (1973) Absolute erythrocytosis as a result of smoking, Clin Res **21**:566

Sagone AL Jr and Murphy SG (1975) The chronic lymphatic leukemia lymphocyte: correlation of functional, metabolic, and surface immunoglobulin characteristics, Cell Immunol **18**:1

Saidi M et al (1969) Le purpure thrombocytopénique, un nouvel aspect clinique du syndrome de la rubéole congénitale, Can Med Assoc J **101**:340

Saito H and Ratnoff OD (1975) Alteration of factor VII activity by activated Fletcher factor (a plasma kallikrein): a potential link between the intrinsic and extrinsic blood clotting systems, J Lab Clin Med **85**:405

Saito H et al (1964) Whole-body iron loss in normal man measured with a gamma spectrometer, J Nucl Med **5**:571

Saito H et al (1975) Fitzgerald trait: deficiency of a hitherto unrecognized agent, Fitzgerald factor, participating in surface-mediated reactions of clotting, fibrinolysis, generation of kinins, and the property of diluted plasma enhancing vascular permeability (PF/DIL), J Clin Invest **55**:1082

Saldanha PH et al (1969) Distribution and heredity of erythrocyte G-6-PD activity and electrophoretic variants among different racial groups at São Paulo, Brazil, J Med Genet **6**:48

Salen G et al (1966) Malabsorption in intestinal scleroderma: relation to bacterial flora and treatment with antibiotics, Ann Intern Med **64**:834

Salfelder K and Schwarz J (1967) Histoplasmotische Kalkherde in der Milz, Dtsch Med Wochenschr **92**:1468

Salky N and Dugdale M (1973) Platelet abnormalities in ischemic heart disease, Am J Cardiol **32**:612

Salmon C (1971) Immunogénétique des antigénes ABH, Nouv Rev Fr Hematol **11**:850

Salmon SE (1974) "Paraneoplastic" syndromes associated with monoclonal lymphocyte and plasma cell proliferation, Ann NY Acad Sci **230**:228

Salmon SE et al (1970) Myeloperoxidase deficiency. Immunologic study of a genetic leukocyte defect, N Engl J Med **282**:250

Salomon H and Tatarsky I (1969) Preleukemic leukemia: a report of four cases, Israel J Med Sci **5**:1178

Salomon H et al (1965) A new hemoglobin variant found in a Beduin tribe: hemoglobin "Rambam," Israel J Med Sci **1**:836

Salt HB et al (1960) On having no beta-lipoprotein: a syndrome comprising a-beta-lipoproteinaemia, acanthocytosis, and steatorrhoea, Lancet **2**:325

Saltzstein SL and Ackerman LV (1959) Lymphadenopathy induced by anticonvulsant drugs and mimicking clinically and pathologically malignant lymphomas, Cancer **12**:164

Salzman EW (1963) Measurement of platelet adhesiveness. A simple in vitro technique demonstrating an abnormality in von Willebrand's disease, J Lab Clin Med **62**:724

Salzman EW et al (1966) Possible mechanism of aggregation of blood platelets by adenosine diphosphate, Nature **210**:167

Salzman EW et al (1972) Cyclic 3',5'-adenosine monophosphate in human blood platelets. IV. Regulatory role of cyclic AMP in platelet function, Ann NY Acad Sci **201**:61

Salzman EW et al (1975) Management of heparin therapy: controlled prospective trial, N Engl J Med **292**:1046

Samama M et al (1969) Dysfibrinogénémie congénitale et familiale sans tendance hémorragique, Nouv Rev Fr Hematol **9**:817

Samter M (1965) Immunological diseases, Boston, Little, Brown & Co

Sanal SM et al (1979) Pseudoleukemia: when "leukemia" is not leukemia, Postgrad Med **65**:143

Sanchez-Medal L et al (1963) A: Hemolysis and erythropoiesis. I. Influence of intraperitoneal administration of whole hemolysates on the recovery of bled dogs, as measured by changes in the total erythrocytic volume, Blood **21**:586

Sanchez-Medal L et al (1969) Anabolic androgenic steroids in the treatment of acquired aplastic anemia, Blood **34**:283

Sandberg AA and Hossfeld DK (1970) Chromosomal abnormalities in human neoplasia, Ann Rev Med **21**:379

Sandler SG and Zlotnick A (1976) IgA deficiency and autoimmune hemolytic disease, Arch Int Med **136**:93

Sandler SG et al (1973) Post-konyne hepatitis: the ineffectiveness of screening for the hepatitis B antigen (HBAg), Transfusion **13**:221

Sandler SG et al (1978) Blood group phenotypes and the origin of sickle cell hemoglobin in Sicilians, Acta Haemotol **60**:350

Sanger R (1955) An association between the P and Jay systems of blood groups, Nature **176**:1163

Sanguansermsri T et al (1979) Hemoglobin Suan-Dok (alpha 2 109 [G16] leu → arg beta 2): an unstable variant associated with alpha thalassemia, Hemoglobin **3**:161

Sansone G et al (1967) Haemoglobin Genova: beta 28 (B10) leucine → proline, Nature (London) **214**:877

Sansone G et al (1970) Haemoglobin O Indonesia (alpha 116 glu → lys) in an Italian family, Acta Haematol **43**:40

Saphir R (1967) Addison's disease presenting as a lymphocyte dyscrasia, Am J Med **42**:855

Sarin PS and Gallo RC (1974) RNA directed DNA polymerase. In Burton K (Ed): Biochemistry of nucleic acids, (Biochemistry Series one, vol 6, MTP Internation Review of Science), London, Butterworth & Co (Publishers) Ltd, p 219

Sarin PS et al (1976) Terminal deoxynucleotidyl transferase activities in human blood leukocytes and lymphoblast cell lines: high levels in lymphoblast cell lines and in blast cells of some patients with chronic myelogenous leukemia in acute phase, Blood **47**:11

Sas G et al (1974) Abnormal antithrombin III (antithrombin III "Budapest") as a cause of familial thrombophilia, Thromb Diath Haemorrh **32**:105

Sas G et al (1975) Plasma and serum antithrombin III: differentiation by crossed immunoelectrophoresis, Thromb Res **6**:87

Sasakawa S et al (1978) Change of oxygen affinity of hemoglobin in different conditions of blood preservation, Vox Sang **34**:164

Sasaki J et al (1977) Increased oxygen affinity for hemoglobin Sawara: αA4 (6) aspartic acid → alanine, Biochim Biophys Acta **495**:183

Sathiapalan R and Robinson MG (1968) Hereditary haemolytic anaemia due to an abnormal haemoglobin (haemoglobin Kings County), Br J Haematol **15**:579

Sato A (1955) Chediak and Higashi's disease. Probable identity of "a new leucocytal anomaly (Chediak)" and "congenital gigantism of peroxidase granules (Higashi)," Tohoku J Exp Med **61**:201

Sauer H and Wilmanns W (1977) Cobalamin-dependent methionine synthesis and methyl-folate-trap in human vitamin B_{12} deficiency, Br J Haematol **36**:189

Savage RA et al (1978) Diagnostic problems involved in detection of metastiatic neoplasms by bone-marrow aspirate compared with needle biopsy, Am J Clin Pathol **70**:623

Sawitsky A et al (1966) Chromosomal breakage and acute leukemia in congenital telangiectatic erythema and stunted growth, Ann Intern Med **65**:487

Sawitsky A et al (1972) The sea-blue histiocyte syndrome, a review: genetic and biochemical studies, Semin Hematol **9**:285

Sawyer WD (1969) Interaction of influenza virus with leukocytes and its effect on phagocytosis, J Infect Dis **119**:541

Sax SM (1979) SI units in the clinical laboratory, Santa Monica, Clinton Laboratories

Saxon A et al (1978) T-lymphocyte variant of hairy-cell leukemia, Ann Intern Med **88**:323

Schachter M (1980) Kallikreins (kininogenases)—a group of serine proteases with bioregulatory actions, Pharmacol Rev **31**:1

Schade SG et al (1966) Occurrence in gastric juice of antibody to a complex of intrinsic factor and vitamin B_{12}, N Engl J Med **275**:528

Schaefer HE et al (1975) Zytochemischer Polymorphismus der sauren phosphatase bei Haarzell-Leukamie, Blut **31**:365

Schaller J et al (1966) Hypergammaglobulinemia, antibody deficiency, autoimmune hemolytic anemia, and nephritis in an infant with a familial lymphopenia immune defect, Lancet **2**:825

Schechter FR et al (1962) Hemorrhagic thrombocythemia, Am J Gartroenterol **38**:659

Scheinberg IH et al (1954) The concentration of copper and ceruloplasmin in maternal and infant plasma at delivery, J Clin Invest **33**:693

Schiff L et al (1959) Familial nonhemolytic jaundice with conjugated bilirubin in the serum, N Engl J Med **260**:1315

Schiffer CA et al (1978) Some aspects of recent advances in the use of blood cell components, Br J Haematol **39**:289

Schiffer CA et al (1979) Alloimmunization following prophylactic granulocyte transfusion, Blood **54**:766

Schiffman S (1980) Factor XII. In Schmidt RM (Section Ed): Handbook Series in Clinical Laboratory Science, Section I: Hematology, vol 3, Boca Raton, Fla, CRC Press Inc, p 117

Schiffman S and Lee P (1974) Preparation, characterization, and activation of a highly purified factor XI: evidence that a hitherto unrecognized plasma activity participates in the interaction of Factors XI and XII, Br J Haematol **27**:101

Schiffman S et al (1975) Identify of contact activation cofactor and Fitzgerald factor, Thromb Res **6**:451

Schiffman S et al (1977) Factor XI and platelets: evidence that platelets contain only minimal factor XI activity and antigen, Br J Haematol **35**:429

Schilirò G et al (1978) Fetal haemoglobin in early malignant osteopetrosis, Br J Haematol **38**:339

Schleicher EM (1942) Origin and nature of the Cabot ring bodies of erythrocytes, J Lab Clin Med **27**:983

Schleicher EM (1973) Bone marrow morphology and mechanics of biopsy, Springfield, Ill, Charles C Thomas, Publishers

Schleider MA et al (1976) A clinical study of the lupus anticoagulant, Blood **48**:499

Schleip K (1906) Zur Diagnose von Knochenmarkstumoren aus dem Blutbefunde, Z Klin Med **59**:261

Schleupner CJ and Overall JC Jr (1979) Infectious mononucleosis and Epstein-Barr virus. 1. Epidemiology, pathogenesis, immune response, Postgrad Med **65**:83

Schloesser LL et al (1965) Thrombocytosis in iron-deficiency anemia, J Lab Clin Med **66**:107

Schmaier AH et al (1974) Electronically determined red cell indices in a predominantly black urban population of children 4 to 8 years of age, J Pediatr **84**:559

Schmalzl F and Braunsteiner H (1971) The application of cytochemical methods to the study of acute leukemia, Acta Haematol **45**:209

Schmid JR (1963) Acquired pure red cell agenesis: report of 16 cases and review of the literature, Acta Haematol **30**:255

Schmid R (1957) The identification of "direct-reacting" bilirubin as a bilirubin glucuronide, J Biol Chem **229**:881

Schmid R (1960) Urinary total, aqueous, and ether soluble prophyrins, Am J Clin Pathol **39**:531

Schmid R (1972) Hyperbilirubinemia. In Stanbury JB et al (Eds): Metabolic basis of inherited diseases, ed 3, New York, McGraw-Hill Book Co, p 1141

Schmid R (1978) Bilirubin metabolism: state of the art, Gastroenterology **74:**1307

Schmid R and McDonagh AE (1978) Hyperbilirubinemia. In Stanbury JB et al (Eds): The metabolic basis of inherited disease, ed 4, New York, McGraw-Hill Book Co, Inc, p 1221

Schmid R et al (1955) Erythropoietic (congenital) porphyria: a rare abnormality of the normoblasts, Blood **10:**416

Schmid W (1967) Familial constitutional panmyelocytopathy, Fanconi's anemia (F.A.). II. A discussion of the cytogenetic findings in Fanconi's anemia, Semin Hematol **4:**241

Schmidt P et al (1976) Sodium pertechnetate as a red cell label: in vitro and in vivo studies, Br J Haematol **32:**411

Schmidt PJ and Vos GH (1967) Multiple phenotypic abnormalities associated with Rh$_{null}$ (---/---), Vox Sang **13:**18

Schmidt PJ et al (1959) A hemolytic reaction due to the transfusion of A$_x$ blood, J Lab Clin Med **54:**38

Schmidt RM (1973) Laboratory diagnosis of hemoglobinopathies, JAMA **224:**1276

Schmidt RM (1974) Diagnostic products marketed for abnormal hemoglobin detection in the United States. In Schmidt RM et al (Eds): The detection of hemoglobinopathies, Cleveland, CRC Press

Schmidt RM (1975) Abnormal haemoglobins and thalassaemia: diagnostic aspects, New York, Academic Press, Inc

Schmidt RM and Brosius EM (1974) Evaluation of proficiency in the performance of tests for abnormal hemoglobins, Am J Clin Pathol **62:**664

Schmidt RM and Brosius EM (1975) Basic laboratory methods of hemoglobinopathy detection, Atlanta, DHEW Publication No. (CDC) 76-8266

Schmidt RM et al (1974a) The detection of the hemoglobinopathies, Cleveland, CRC Press

Schmidt RM et al (1974b) Quantitation of fetal hemoglobin by densitometry, J Lab Clin Med **84:**740

Schmidt RM et al (1975) Advanced laboratory methods of hemoglobinopathy detection, Atlanta, DHEW Publication No. (CDC) 75-8296

Schmidt RM et al (1977) Hemoglobin Lufkin: beta 29 (Bll) gly → asp: an unstable hemoglobin variant involving an internal amino acid residue, Hemoglobin **1:**799

Schneider RG (1974a) Differentiation of electrophoretically similar hemoglobins—such as S, D, G, and P; or A$_2$, C, E, and O—by electrophoresis of the globin chains, Clin Chem **20:**1111

Schneider RG (1974b) Identification of hemoglobins by electrophoresis. In Schmidt RM et al (Eds): The detection of hemoglobinopathies, Cleveland, CRC Press

Schneider RG and Barwick RC (1978) Measuring relative electrophoretic mobilities of mutant hemoglobins and globin chains, Hemoglobin **2:**417

Schneider RG and Jim RTS (1961) A new haemoglobin variant (the Honolulu type) in a Chinese, Nature **190:**454

Schneider RG et al (1966) Hemoglobin I in an American Negro family: structural and hematologic studies, J Lab Clin Med **68:**940

Schneider RG et al (1968) Hemoglobin Sealy (alpha 2 47 His beta 2): a new variant in a Jewish family, Am J Hum Genet **20:**151

Schneider RG et al (1969a) Hemoglobin Sabine, beta 91 (F7) leu → pro. An unstable variant causing severe anemia with inclusion bodies, N Engl J Med **280:**739

Schneider RG et al (1969b) Hemoglobin P (alpha 2 beta 2 117 arg): structure and properties, J Lab Clin Med **73:**616

Schneider RG et al (1971) Hb Fort Worth: alpha 27 glu → gly (B8) a variant present in unusually low concentration, Biochim Biophys Acta **243:**164

Schneider RG et al (1974) Genetic haemoglobin abnormalities in about 9,000 black and 7,000 white newborns: haemoglobin F Dickinson (A 97 his → arg), a new variant, Br J Haematol **28:**515

Schneider RG et al (1975a) Haemoglobin Titusville: alpha 94 asp → asn, a new haemoglobin with a lowered affinity for oxygen, Biochim Biophys Acta **400:**365

Schneider RG et al (1975b) Hb Mobile (alpha 2 beta 73 [E17] asp → val): a new variant, Biochem Genet **13:**411

Schneider RG et al (1976a) Hemoglobin Baylor (alpha 2 beta 2 81 [EF5] leu → arg)—an unstable mutant with high oxygen affinity, Hemoglobin **1:**85

Schneider RG et al (1976b) Hemoglobin Fannin-Lubbock (alpha 2 beta 119 [GH2] gy → asp): a slightly unstable mutant, Biochim Biophys Acta **453:**478

Schneider WHG (1974) Regulation of energy metabolism in human blood platelets by cyclic AMP. In Baldini MG and Ebbe S (Eds): Platelets: production, function, transfusion, and storage, New York, Grune & Stratton, Inc

Schneiderman LJ et al (1969) Genetic studies of a family with two unusual autosomal dominant conditions: muscular dystrophy and Pelger-Huët anomaly, Am J Med **46:**380

Schnitzer B and Kass L (1973) Leukemic phase of reticulum cell sarcoma (histiocytic lymphoma). A clinicopathologic and ultrastructural study, Cancer **31:**547

Schnitzer B and Kass L (1974) Hairy-cell leukemia. A clinicopathologic and ultrastructural study, Am J clin Pathol **61:**176

Schnitzer B et al (1972) Pitting function of the spleen in malaria: ultrastructural observations, Science **177:**175

Schoefl GI (1972) The migration of lymphocytes across the vascular endothelium in lymphoid tissue: a re-examination, J Exp Med **136:**568

Schoen I and Brooks SH (1970) Judgement based on 95% confidence limits: a statistical dilemma involving multitest screening and proficiency testing of multiple specimens, Am J Clin Pathol **53:**190

Schooley JC and Mahlmann LJ (1971) Stimulation of erythropoiesis in the plethoric mouse by cyclic-AMP and its inhibition by antierythropoietin, Proc Soc Exp Biol Med **137:**1289

Schooley JC and Mahlmann LJ (1972) Evidence for de novo synthesis of erythropoietin in hypoxic rats, Blood **40:**662

Schooley JC and Mahlmann L-J (1975) Hypoxia and the initiation of erythropoietin production, Blood Cells **1:**429

Schooley JC et al (1968) A summary of some studies on erythropoiesis using anti-erythropoietin immune serum, Ann NY Acad Sci **149:**266

Schreiber C and Waxman S (1974) Measurement of red cell folate levels by ^{3}H-pteroylglutamic acid (^{3}H-PteGlu) radioassay, Br J Haematol **27:**551

Schrek R and Donnelly WJ (1966) "Hairy" cells in blood in lymphoreticular neoplastic disease and "flagellated" cells of normal lymph nodes, Blood **27:**199

Schrek R et al (1970) Chromatin and other cytologic indices in chronic lymphocytic leukemia, J Lab Clin Med **75:**217

Schrier SL et al (1974) Erythrocyte membrane vacuole formation in hereditary spherocytosis, Br J Haematol **26:**59

Schröder J (1975) Review article: transplacental passage of blood cells, J Med Genet **12:**230

Schröder J and de la Chapelle A (1972) Fetal lymphocytes in the maternal blood, Blood **39:**153

Schroeder WA and Huisman THJ (1970) Heterogeneity of fetal hemoglobin in beta-thalassemia of the Negro, Am J Hum Genet **22:**505

Schroeder WA and Jones RT (1965) Some aspects of the chemistry and function of human and animal hemoglobins, Fortschr Chem Org Naturst **23:**113

Schroeder WA et al (1968) Evidence for multiple structural genes for the γ-chain of human fetal hemoglobin, Proc Natl Acad Sci USA **60**:537

Schroeder WA et al (1979) Hemoglobin Sunshine Seth - alpha 2 (94 [G1] asp → His) beta 2, Hemoglobin **3**:145

Schubert GE et al (1972) Structure and function of the kidney in multiple myeloma, Virchow's Arch (Pathol Anat) **355**:135

Schubert WK and Lahey ME (1959) Copper and protein depletion complicating hypoferric anemia of infancy, Pediatrics **24**:710

Schulman I (1961) Iron requirements in infancy, JAMA **175**:118

Schulman I and Smith CH (1952) Hemorrhagic disease in an infant due to deficiency of a previously undescribed clotting factor, Blood **7**:794

Schulman I et al (1960) Studies on thrombopoiesis, I. A factor in normal human plasma required for platelet production; chronic thrombocytopenia due to its deficiency, Blood **16**:943

Schulman I et al (1965) Studies on thrombopoiesis. II. Assay of human plasma thrombopoietic activity, J Pediatr **66**:604

Schultz DR and Yunis AA (1975) Immunoblastic lymphadenopathy with mixed cryoglobulinemia: a detailed case study, N Engl J Med **292**:8

Schumacher AE et al (1969) The mononucleosis cell. III. Electron microscopy, Blood **33**:833

Schur PH (1977) Complement testing in the diagnosis of immune and autoimmune diseases, Am J Clin Pathol **68**:647

Schur PH et al (1979) Immunoglobulin subclasses in normal children, Pediatr Res **13**:181

Schwartz AD (1974) A method for demonstrating shortened platelet survival utilizing recovery from aspirin effect, J Pediatr **84**:350

Schwartz E (1969) The silent carrier of beta thalassemia, N Engl J Med **281**:1327

Schwartz IR et al (1957) Sickling of erythrocytes with I-A electrophoretic hemoglobin pattern, Fed Proc **16**:115

Schwartz JM and Jaffé ER (1978) Hereditary methemoglobinemia with deficiency of NADH dehydrogenase. In Stanbury JB et al (Eds): The metabolic basis of inherited disease, ed 4, New York, McGraw-Hill Book Co, Inc, p 1452

Schwartz JP et al (1974) Platelet function studies in patients with glucose-6-phosphate dehydrogenase deficiency, Br J Haematol **27**:273

Schwartz S et al (1944) The quantitative determination of urobilinogen by means of the Evelyn photoelectric colorimeter, Am J Clin Pathol **14**:598

Schwartz S et al (1951) An improved method for the determination of urinary coproporphyrin and analysis of factors influencing the analysis, J Lab Clin Med **37**:843

Schwartz S et al (1960) Determination of porphyrins in biologic materials. In Glick D (Ed): Methods of biochemical analysis, vol 8, New York, Interscience Publishers, Inc, p 221

Scott CR et al (1972) Hereditary transcobalamin II deficiency: the role of transcobalamin II in vitamin B_{12}-mediated reactions, J Pediatr **81**:1106

Scott CS (1978) Cytochemical applications in haematology, with particular reference to acute leukaemias: a review, Med Lab Sci **35**:111

Scott D and Theologides A (1974) Hepatoma, erythrocytosis and increased serum erythropoietin developing in long-standing hemochromatosis, Am J Gastroenterol **61**:206

Scott JM and Weir DG (1976) Folate composition, synthesis and function in natural materials, Clin Haematol **5**:547

Scott RB et al (1964) A clinical study of twenty cases of erythroleukemia (Di Guglielmo's syndrome), Am J Med **37**:162

Scullin DC Jr et al (1979) Pseudo-Gaucher cells in multiple myeloma, Am J Med **67**:347

Seaman AJ (1970) The plasma protamine paracoagulation test, Arch Intern Med **125**:1016

Seaman AJ and Koler RD (1953) Acquired erythrocytic hypoplasia: a recovery during cobalt therapy; report of two cases with review of the literature, Acta Haematol **9**:153

Seaman AJ and Starr A (1962) Febrile postcardiotomy lymphocytic splenomegaly: new entity, Ann Surg **156**:956

Sears DA (1970) Disposal of plasma heme in normal man and patients with intravascular hemolysis, J Clin Invest **49**:5

Sears DA (1978) The morbidity of sickle cell trait: a review of the literature, Am J Med **64**:1021

Sears DA et al (1966) Urinary iron excretion and renal metabolism of hemoglobin in hemolytic diseases, Blood **28**:708

Seeff LB et al (1978) Type B hepatitis after needle-stick exposure: prevention with hepatitis B immune globulin: final report of the Veteran's Administration cooperative study, Ann Intern Med **88**:285

Seegers WH (1965) Basic enzymology of blood coagulation, Thromb Diath Haemorrh **14**:213

Seegers WH and Alkjaersig N (1955) Nature of the blood coagulation mechanisms in SPCA plasma, Cir Res **3**:514

Seegers WH et al (1970) Structural changes in prothrombin during activation: a theory, Thromb Diath Haemorrh **23**:26

Seegmiller JE et al (1964) Xanthine oxidase and iron, N Engl J Med **270**:534

Seeler RA (1972a) Parahemophilia: factor V deficiency, Med Clin North Am **56**:119

Seeler RA (1972b) Congenital "hypoprothrombinemias": deficiency of factors II, VII, and X, Med Clin North Am **56**:127

Segal AW and Loewi G (1976) Neutrophil dysfunction in Crohn's disease, Lancet **2**:219

Segi M and Kurihara M (1964) Cancer mortality for selected sites in 24 countries. No. 3, 1960-1961, Sendai, Japan, June 1964, Department of Public Health, Tohuku University School of Medicine

Seid-Akhaven, M et al (1972) Hemoglobin Wayne: a frameshift variant occurring in two distinct forms, Annual Meeting of the American Society of Hematologists, Miami, Abstract no 9

Seidl S et al (1972) Two siblings with Rh_{null} disease, Vox Sang **23**:182

Sejeny SA et al (1975) Platelet counts during normal pregnancy, J Clin Pathol **28**:812

Seldon M et al (1980) A fatal case of cold autoimmune hemolytic anemia, Am J Clin Pathol **73**:716

Seligmann M (1975) Immunochemical, clinical, and pathological features of α-chain disease, Arch Intern Med **135**:78

Seligmann M and Rambaud JC (1969) IgA abnormalities in abdominal lymphoma (α-chain disease), Isr J Med Sci **5**:151

Seligmann M et al (1968a) A proposed classification of primary immunologic deficiencies, Am J Med **45**:817

Seligmann M et al (1968b) Alpha-chain disease: a new immunoglobulin abnormality, Science **162**:1396

Seligmann M et al (1969) Immunochemical studies in four cases of alpha chain disease, J Clin Invest **48**:2374

Seligmann M et al (1973) Band T cell markers in human proliferative blood diseases and primary immunodeficiencies, with special reference to membrane bound immunoglobulins, Transplant Rev **16**:85

Seligsohn U and Ramot B (1969) Combined factor-V and factor-VIII deficiency: report of four cases, Br J Haematol **16**:475

Seligsohn U et al (1979) Activated factor VII: presence in factor IX concentrates and persistence in the circulation after infusion, Blood **53**:828

Sell S (1969) Antilymphocytic antibody: effects in experimental animals and problems in human use, Ann Intern Med **71**:177

Sell S and Asofsky R (1968) Lymphocytes and immunoglobulins, Prog Allergy **12**:86

Seltser R and Sartwell PE (1965) The influence of occupational exposure to radiation on the mortality of American radiologists and other medical specialists, Am J Epidemiol **81**:2

Selzer G et al (1979) Primary small intestine lymphomas and α-heavy-chain disease. A study of 43 cases from a pathology department in Israel, Israel J Med Sci **15**:111

Sen L and Borella L (1975) Clinical importance of lymphoblasts with T markers in childhood acute leukemia, N Engl J Med **292**:828

Senn HJ and Jungi WJ (1975) Neutrophil migration in health and disease, Semin Hematol **12**:27

Senn JS and Pinkerton PH (1972) Defective in vitro colony formation by human bone marrow preceding overt leukaemia, Br J Haematol **23**:277

Seppänen N and Uusitalo AJ (1977) Carboxyhaemoglobin saturation in relation to smoking and various occupational conditions, Ann Clin Res **9**:261

Serjeant BE and Sergeant GR (1972) A whole blood solubility and centrifugation test for sickle cell hemoglobin: a clinical trial, Am J Clin Pathol **58**:11

Serjeant BE et al (1978) The development of haemoglobin A_2 in normal Negro infants and in sickle cell disease, Br J Haematol **39**:259

Sessarego M et al (1979) A case of chronic myelogenous leukemia with unusual chromosomal abnormality, Leukemia Res **3**:271

Sézary A (1959) Nouvell réticulose cutanée: réticulose maligne leucemique à histio-monocytes monstrueux et à forme d'erythrodermie oedémateuse et pigmentée, Ann Dermatol Syphiligr **9**:5

Shabtai F et al (1978) A new cytogenetic aspect of polycythemia vera, Hum Genet **41**:281

Shadduck RK and Nagabhushanam NG (1971) Granulocyte colony stimulating factor. I. Response to acute granulocytopenia, Blood **38**:559

Shafer RB et al (1973) Hematologic alterations following partial gastrectomy, Am J Med Sci **266**:241

Shah PC et al (1975) Hyperlipemia and spuriously elevated hemoglobin values, Ann Intern Med **82**:382

Shah PC et al (1978) Transient pseudoleukocytosis caused by cryocrystalglobinemia, Arch Pathol Lab Med **102**:172

Shahidi NT (1973) Androgens and erythropoiesis, N Engl J Med **269**:72

Shahidi NT and Hemaidan A (1969) Acetophenacetin-induced methemoglobinemia and its relation to the excretion of diazotizable amines, J Lab Clin Med **74**:581

Shahidi NT et al (1962) Alkali-resistant hemoglobin in aplastic anemia of both acquired and congenital types, N Engl J Med **226**:117

Shahidi NT et al (1964) Iron-deficiency anemia associated with an error of iron metabolism in two siblings, J Clin Invest **43**:510

Shalet M et al (1966) Mechanism of erythropoietic action of thyroid hormone, Proc Soc Exp Biol Med **123**:443

Shalet MF et al (1967) Erythropoietin-producing Wilms' tumor, J Pediatr **70**:615

Shall S (1972) Poly (ADP-ribose). A report on the EMBO workshop held in Hamburg, Germany, March 27-29, 1972, FEBS Lett **24**:1

Shamir H et al (1974) Cryofibrinogen in familial Mediterranean fever, Arch Intern Med **134**:125

Shamov VN (1937) The transfusion of stored cadaver blood, Lancet **2**:306

Shanberge JN et al (1978) Fractionated tritium-labelled heparin studied in vitro and in vivo, Thromb Res **13**:767

Shanbrom E and Tanaka KR (1962) Acquired Pelger-Huët granulocytes in severe myxedema, Acta Haematol **27**:289

Shapira Y et al (1972) Juvenile myeloid leukemia with fetal erythropoiesis, Cancer **30**:353

Shapiro CM and Horowitz H (1959) Infectious mononucleosis in the aged, Ann Intern Med **51**:1092

Shapiro GA et al (1973) The subunit structure of normal and hemophilic factor VIII, J Clin Invest **52**:2198

Shapiro SS (1975) Prothrombin San Juan: a complex new dysprothrombinemia. In Hemker HC and Veltkamp JJ (Eds): Prothrombin and related coagulation factors, Leiden, Leiden University Press, p 205

Shapiro SS and Hultin M (1975) Acquired inhibitors to the blood coagulation factors, Semin Thromb Hemost **1**:336

Shapiro SS et al (1969) Congenital dysprothrombinemia: inherited structural disorder of human prothrombin, J Clin Invest **48**:2251

Sharma RS et al (1974) A new chain variant haemoglobin A_2-Melbourne or alpha 2 delta 2 43 glu → lys (CD2), Biochim Biophys Acta **359**:233

Sharma RS et al (1975) Hemoglobin A_2-Coborg or alpha 2 delta 2 116 arg → his (G18), Biochim Biophys Acta **393**:379

Sharpe LM et al (1950) The effect of phytate and other food factors on iron absorption, J Nutr **41**:433

Shattil SJ et al (1977) Abnormalities of cholesterol-phospholipid composition in platelets and low-density lipoproteins of human hyperbetalipoproteinemia, J Lab Clin Med **89**:341

Shaw MT and Nordquist RE (1975) "Pure" monocytic or histio-monocytic leukemia; a revised concept, Cancer **35**:208

Sheehan RG et al (1978) Evaluation of a packaged kit assay of serum ferritin and application to clinical diagnosis of selected anemias, Am J Clin Pathol **70**:79

Sheldon PJ et al (1973) Thymic origin of atypical lymphoid cells in infectious mononucleosis, Lancet **1**:1153

Shelley WB (1963) Indirect basophil degranulation test for allergy to penicillin and other drugs, JAMA **184**:171

Shelley WB and Parnes HM (1965) The absolute basophil count, technique and significance, JAMA **192**:368

Sheridan BL and Pinkerton PH (1980) von Willebrand's syndrome with abnormal platelet aggregation correctable by cryoprecipitate, Br J Haematol **45**:353

Sheridan BL et al (1976) The pattern of fetal haemoglobin production in leukaemia, Br J Haematol **32**:487

Sherman JD et al (1967) Anemia, positive lupus and rheumatoid factors with methyldopa. A report of three cases, Arch Intern Med **120**:321

Shevach E et al (1974) A human leukemia cell with both B and T cell surface receptors, Proc Natl Acad Sci **71**:863

Shibata F et al (1960) Hemoglobin M: demonstration of a new abnormal hemoglobin and hereditary nigremia, Acta Haematol Jpn **23**:96

Shibata S et al (1961) A comparative study of hemoglobin M Iwate and hemoglobin M Kurume by means of electrophoresis, chromatography and analysis of peptide chains, Acta Haematol Jpn **24**:486

Shibata S et al (1964) Hemoglobin Hikari (alpha 2A beta 2 61 aspNH2): a fast moving hemoglobin found in two unrelated Japanese families, Clin Chim Acta **10**:101

Shibata S et al (1966) Abnormal hemoglobins discovered in Japan, Acta Haematol Jap **29**:115

Shibata S et al (1967) Hemoglobin M's of the Japanese, Bull Yamaguchi Med School **14**:141

Shibata S et al (1969) Hemoglobin M Akita disease, Acta Haematol Jpn **32**:311

Shibata S et al (1970) Hemoglobin Tochigi (beta 56-59 deleted). A new unstable hemoglobin discovered in a Japanese family, Proc Jpn Acad **46**:440

Shibata S et al (1975) Evaluation of precision of procedures for estimating the Hb A_2 and GHb F in hemolysates. In Schmidt

RM (Ed): Abnormal haemoglobins and thalassaemia, diagnostic aspects, New York, Academic Press, Inc

Shih T-B et al (1980) Further studies on the functional properties of hemoglobin M Hyde Park, Hemoglobin 4:125

Shiloh Y et al (1979) Cytogenetic investigation of leukemic and preleukemic disorders, Israel J Med Sci 15:500

Shimizu A et al (1965) The structural study on a new hemoglobin variant, hg M Osaka, Biochim Biophys Acta 97:472

Shimkin MB (1955) Hodgkin's disease. Mortality in the United States, 1921-1951: race, sex, and age distribution: comparison with leukemia, Blood 10:1214

Shimoda SS et al (1968) The Zollinger-Ellison syndrome with steatorrhea. II. The mechanisms of fat and vitamin B_{12} malabsorption, Gastroenterology 55:705

Shirahama T and Cohen AS (1974) Ultrastructural evidence for leakage of lysosomal contents after phagocytosis of monosodium urate crystals: a mechanism of gouty inflammation, Am J Pathol 76:501

Shirakura T (1968) Zur erythropoetischen Wirkung von Testosteron, Acta Haematol 39:366

Shohet SB et al (1973) Hereditary hemolytic anemia associated with abnormal membrane lipid. II. Ion permeability and transport abnormalities, Blood 42:1

Shreffler DC et al (1967) Electrophoretic variation in human serum ceruloplasmin: a new genetic polymorphism, Biochem Genet 1:101

Shreiner DP (1975) Acute lymphoblastic leukemia terminating as histiocytic medullary reticulosis, JAMA 231:838

Shreiner DP and Levin J (1973) Regulation of thrombopoiesis. In Wolstenholme GEW and O'Connor M (Eds): Haemopoietic stem cells, CIBA Foundation Symposium 13 (New Series), New York, Associated Scientific Publishers, p 225

Shulman LE (1963) Serologic abnormalities in systemic lupus erythematosus, J Chronic Dis 16:889

Shulman NR (1964) A mechanism of cell destruction in individuals sensitized to foreign antigens and its implications in autoimmunity, Ann Intern Med 60:506

Shulman NR (1972) Immunologic reactions to drugs, N Engl J Med 287:408

Shulman NR et al (1961) Immunoreactions involving platelets. V. Post-transfusion purpura due to a complement-fixing antibody against a genetically controlled platelet antigen. A proposed mechanism for thrombocytopenia and its relevance in "autoimmunity," J Clin Invest 40:1597

Shulman NR et al (1965) Similarities between known antiplatelet antibodies and the factor responsible for thrombocytopenia in idiopathic purpura. Physiologic, serologic, and isotopic studies, Ann NY Acad Sci 124:499

Shum HY et al (1971) Vitamin B_{12} absorption and the Zollinger-Ellison syndrome, Lancet 1:1303

Shustik C et al (1976) Kappa and lambda light chain disease: survival rates and clinical manifestations, Blood 48:41

Sibley C et al (1973) Comparison of activated partial thromboplastin reagents, Am J Clin Pathol 59:581

Sick K et al (1967) Haemoglobin G Copenhagen and haemoglobin J Cambridge. Two new beta chain variants of haemoglobin A, Biochim Biophys Acta 140:231

Siegel SE et al (1971) Transmission of toxoplasmosis by leukocyte transfusion, Blood 37:388

Siegel W et al (1970) An adult homozygous for persistent fetal hemoglobin, Ann Intern Med 72:533

Siegler M (1975) Pascal's wager and the hanging of crepe, N Engl J Med 293:853

Sienknecht CW et al (1977) Felty's syndrome: clinical and serological analysis of 34 cases, Ann Rheum Dis 36:500

Siggaard-Andersen O et al (1972) Hemoglobin pigments. Spectrophotometric determination of oxy-, carboxy-, met-, and sulfhemoglobin in capillary blood, Clin Chim Acta 42:85

Siimes MA et al (1974) Ferritin in serum: diagnosis of iron deficiency and iron overload in infants and children, Blood 43:581

Silber R (1969) Of acanthocytes, spurs, burrs, and membranes, Blood 34:111

Silber R et al (1966) Spur-shaped erythrocytes in Laennec's cirrhosis, N Engl J Med 275:639

Siltzbach LE et al (1974) Course and progress of sarcoidosis around the world, Am J Med 57:847

Silver H and Frankel S (1971) Normal values for mean corpuscular volume as determined by the Model S Coulter Counter, Am J Clin Pathol 55:438

Silver S (1968) Radioactive nuclides in medicine and biology, New York, Lea & Febiger

Silvergleid AJ (1979) Autologous transfusions: experience in a community blood center, JAMA 241:2724

Silverstein MN and Linman JW (1969) Causes of death in agnogenic myeloid metaplasia, Mayo Clin Proc 44:36

Silverstein MN and Maldonado JE (1970) Asymptomatic splenomegaly, Postgrad Med 48:80

Silverstein MN et al (1970) The syndrome of the sea-blue histiocyte, N Engl J Med 282:1

Silvestroni E et al (1967) Proceedings of the 10th Congress of the European Society of Hematologists, Strasbourg, 1965, New York, Karger, Part II, p 232

Simchowitz L and Spilberg I (1979) Evidence for the role of superoxide radicals in neutrophil-mediated cytotoxicity, Immunology 37:301

Simionescu CI et al (1978) Porphyrins and the evolution of biosystems, Bioelectrochem Bioenerget 5:1

Simmons A and Twaitt J (1975) Another example of a B variant, Transfusion 15:359

Simon G and Varonier HS (1963) Étude au microscope électronique du foie de deux cas d'ictère nonhémolytique congénital de type Gilbert, Schweiz Med Wochenschr 93:459

Simone JV et al (1968) Acquired von Willebrand's syndrome in systemic lupus erythematosus, Blood 31:806

Singer K (1955) Hereditary hemolytic disorders associated with abnormal hemoglobins, Am J Med 18:633

Singer K et al (1951a) Studies on abnormal hemoglobins. I. Their demonstration in sickle-cell anemia and other hematologic disorders by means of alkali denaturation, Blood 6:413

Singer K et al (1951b) Studies on abnormal hemoglobins. II. Their identification by means of method of fractional denaturation, Blood 6:429

Singer K et al (1952) Acanthrocytosis: a genetic erythrocytic malformation, Blood 7:577

Singer SJ and Nicolson GL (1972) The fluid mosaic model of the structure of cell membranes, Science 175:720

Singh G et al (1977) Bone marrow examination for metastatic tumor: aspirate and biopsy, Cancer 40:2317

Singley TL III (1962) Secondary methemoglobinemia due to the adulteration of fish with sodium nitrite, Ann Intern Med 57:800

Sirchia G and Dacie JV (1967) Immune lysis of AET-treated normal red cells (PNH-like cells), Nature 215:747

Sirchia G and Lewis SM (1975) Paroxysmal nocturnal haemoglobinuria, Clin Haematol 4:199

Sixma JJ and Molenaar I (1966) Microtubules and microfibriles in blood platelets, Thromb Diath Haemorrh 16:153

Sixma JJ and Nijessen JG (1970) Characteristics of platelet factor 3 release during ADP-induced aggregation. Comparison with 5 hydroxytryptamine release, Thromb Diath Haemorrh 24:206

Sixma JJ and Wester J (1977) The hemostatic plug, Semin Hematol 14:265

Skalak R and Branemark PI (1969) Deformation of red blood cells in capillaries, Science **164**:717

Skendzel LP and Hoffman GC (1962) The Pelger anomaly of leukocytes: forty-one cases in seven families, Am J Clin Pathol **37**:294

Skjaelaaen P et al (1971) Inhibition of erythropoiesis by plasma from newborn infants, Israel J Med Sci **7**:857

Slack J (1969) Risks of ischaemic heart-disease in familial hyperlipoproteinaemic states, Lancet **2**:1380

Slawsky P and Desforges JF (1972) Erythrocyte 2,3-diphosphoglycerate in iron deficiency, Arch Intern Med **129**:914

Slichter SJ and Harker LA (1976) Preparation and storage of platelet concentrates, Transfusion **16**:8

Sloan HR et al (1969) Deficiency of sphingomyelin-cleaving enzyme activity in tissue cultures derived from patients with Niemann-Pick disease, Biochem Biophys Res Commun **34**:582

Slotta KH (1960) Thromboplastin. I. Phospholipid moiety of thromboplastin, Proc Soc Exp Biol Med **103**:53

Smith ADM (1960) Megaloblastic madness, Br Med J **2**:1840

Smith CH (1936) A method for determining the sedimentation rate and red cell volume in infants and children with the use of capillary blood, Am J Med Sci **192**:73

Smith CH et al (1955) Studies in Mediterranean (Cooley's) anemia. II. The suppression of hematopoiesis by transfusions, Blood **10**:707

Smith CH et al (1957) Hazard of severe infections in splenectomized infants and children, Am J Med **22**:390

Smith CW et al (1972) A serum inhibitor of leukotaxis in a child with recurrent infections, J Lab Clin Med **79**:878

Smith DW and Elliott J (1951) Red blood cell suspension transfusions, JAMA **147**:737

Smith EL (1948) Purification of antipernicious anemia factors from liver, Nature **161**:638

Smith EW and Conley CL (1959) Sickle cell–hemoglobin D disease, Ann Intern Med **50**:94

Smith EW and Krevans JR (1959) Clinical manifestations of hemoglobin C disorders, Johns Hopkins Med J **104**:17

Smith H (1967) Unidentified inclusions in haemopoietic cells, congenital atresia of the bile ducts and livedo reticularis in an infant: a new syndrome? Br J Haematol **13**:695

Smith JA et al (1964) Spur-cell anemia: hemolytic anemia with red cells resembling acanthocytes in alcoholic cirrhosis, N Engl J Med **271**:396

Smith JB et al (1976) Persistence of thromboxane A$_2$-like material and platelet release-inducing activity in plasma, J Clin Invest **58**:1119

Smith JE and Moore K (1980) In vivo and in vitro turnover of spectrin phosphate in erythrocytes, J Lab Clin Med **95**:808

Smith JR and Landaw SA (1978) Smoker's polycythemia, N Engl J Med **298**:6

Smith JW et al (1971) Cyclic adenosine 3',5'-monophosphate in human lymphocytes. Alterations after phytohemagglutinin stimulation, J Clin Invest **50**:432

Smith KL and Johnson W (1974) Classification of chronic myelocytic leukemia in children, Cancer **34**:670

Smith LL et al (1972) Subunit dissociation of the abnormal hemoglobin G Georgia (alpha 2 95 [G2] beta 2) and Rampa (alpha 2 95 ser [G2] beta 2), J Biol Chem **247**:1433

Smith MD and Pannacciulli IM (1958) Absorption of inorganic iron from graded doses: its significance in relation to iron absorption tests and the "mucosal block" theory, Br J Haematol **4**:428

Smith R and Oliver RAM (1967) Sudden onset of psychosis in association with vitamin B$_{12}$-deficiency, Br Med J **3**:34

Smith RJ et al (1974) Liposomal enzyme release: a possible mechanism of action of cobalt as an erythropoietic stimulant, Proc Soc Exp Biol Med **146**:781

Smithies O (1955) Zone electrophoresis in starch gels: group variations in the serum proteins of normal human adults, Biochem J **61**:629

Smithies O (1957) Variations in human serum β$_2$-globulins, Nature **180**:1482

Smithies O and Hiller O (1959) The genetic control of transferrins in humans, Biochem J **72**:121

Smithies O and Walker NF (1956) Notation for serum protein groups and the genes controlling their inheritance, Nature **178**:694

Smithies O et al (1962) Inheritance of haptoglobin subtypes, Am J Hum Genet **14**:14

Smithies O et al (1966) Gene action in the human haptoglobins. 1. Dissociation into constituent polypeptide chains, J Mol Biol **21**:213

Smithson WA et al (1979) Acute lymphoblastic leukemia in children: immunologic, cytochemical, morphologic and cytogenetic studies in relation to pretreatment risk factors, Med Pediatr Oncol **7**:83

Snell EE and Peterson WH (1940) Growth factors for bacteria. X. Additional factors required by certain lactic acid bacteria, J Bacteriol **39**:273

Snyder LM and Reddy WJ (1970) Mechanism of action of thyroid hormones on erythrocyte 2,3-diphosphoglyceric acid synthesis, J Clin Invest **49**:1993

Snyderman R and Stahl C (1975) Defective immune effector function in patients with neoplastic and immune deficiency diseases. In Bellanti JA and Dayton DH (Eds): The phagocytic cell and host resistance, New York, Raven Press

Snyderman R et al (1979) Deficiency of the fifth component of complement in human subjects: clinical genetic and immunologic studies in a large kindred, Am J Med **67**:638

Socha WW and Wiener AS (1973) Problems of blood Factor C of A-B-O system. Critical historical review, NY State J Med **73**:2145

Solomon A (1976) Bence-Jones proteins and light chains of immunoglobulins, N Engl J Med **294**:17, 19

Solomon A (1977) Homogeneous (monoclonal) immunoglobulins in cancer, Am J Med **63**:169

Solomon A and McLaughlin CL (1973) Immunoglobulin structure determined from products of plasma cell neoplasms, Semin Hematol **10**:3

Solomon A et al (1963) Clinical and experimental metabolism of normal 6.6S γ-globulin in normal subjects and in patients with macroglobulinemia and multiple myeloma, J Lab Clin Med **62**:1

Solomon LR and Hillman RS (1979) Vitamin B$_6$ metabolism in idiopathic sideroblastic anaemia and related disorders, Br J Haematol **42**:239

Sonoda T et al (1976) Use of prothrombin complex concentrates in the treatment of a hemophilic patient with an inhibitor of factor VIII, Blood **47**:983

Sørensen PJ et al (1980) Familial functional antithrombin III deficiency, Scand J Haematol **24**:105

Soria J et al (1972a) Fibrinogen Troyes-Fibrinogen Metz. Two new cases of congenital dysfibrinogenemia, Thromb Diath Haemorrh **27**:619

Soria J et al (1972b) Anomalie de structure du fibrinogéne "Metz," localisée sur la chaine (A) de la molécule, Biochimie **54**:415

Soriano RB et al (1973) Defect in neutrophil motility in a child with recurrent bacterial infections and disseminated cytomegalovirus infection, J Pediatr **83**:951

Soulier J-P and Boffa M-C (1980) Avortements à répétition, thromboses et anticoagulant circulant anti-thromboplastine: trois observations, Nouv Presse Med **9**:859

Soulier J-P et al (1964) Fractions "coagulantes" contenant les facteurs de coagulation adsorbables par le phosphate tricalcique, Presse Med **72**:1223

Soulier JP and Steinbuch M (1975) Concentrates of factor IX: preparation and clinical use. In Brinkhous KM and Hemker HC (Eds): Handbook of hemophilia, New York, American Elsevier Publishing Co, Inc, p 531

Soulier JP et al (1974) Paternity research using the HL-A system, Haematologia (Budap) **8**:249

Spaet TH et al (1961) Reticuloendothelial clearance of blood thromboplastin by rats, Blood **17**:196

Spaet TH et al (1969) Defective platelets in essential thrombocythemia, Arch Intern Med **124**:135

Speck B (1968) Diurnal variation of serum iron and the latent iron-binding in normal adults, Helv Med Acta **34**:231

Speck B et al (1978) Immunologic aspects of aplasia, Transplant Proc **10**:131

Spector I and Metz J (1966) Giant myeloid cells in the bone marrow of protein malnourished infants: relationship to folate and vitamin B_{12} nutrition, Br J Haematol **12**:737

Spector JI and Miller S (1978) Acute myelofibrosis with peripheral myeloblastosis, Arch Pathol Lab Med **102**:564

Speiser P (1975) Das HL-A-System in Paternitätsprozess mit Berucksichtigung des Beweiswertes, Wien Klin Wochenschr **87**:321

Sperber A and Tessler AN (1974) Gross hematuria in a white man with a sickling disorder, J Urol **111**:528

Spielmann W et al (1974) Anti-ce (anti-f) in a CDe/cD−mother, as a cause of haemolytic disease of the newborn, Vox Sang **27(5)**:473

Spitler LE and Lawrence HS (1969) Studies on lymphocyte culture: products of sensitive lymphocyte-antigen interactions, J Immunol **103**:1072

Spitznagel JK et al (1974) Character of azurophil and specific granules purified from human polymorphonuclear leukocytes, Lab Invest **30**:774

Spivak JL and Cooke CR (1976) Polycythemia vera in an anephric man, Am J Med Sci **272**:339

Sprague CC and Peterson JCS (1958) Role of the spleen and effect of splenectomy in sickle cell disease, Blood **13**:569

Spray GH and Witts LJ (1958) Results of three years experience with microbiological assay of vitamin B_{12} in serum, Br Med J **1**:295

Springer GF et al (1959) Origin of anti-human blood group B agglutinins in white leghorn chicks, J Exp Med **110**:221

Sprinz H and Nelson RS (1954) Persistant nonhemolytic hyperbilirubinemia associated with lipochrome-like pigments in liver cells: report of 4 cases, Ann Intern Med **41**:952

Sproul EE (1938) Carcinoma and venous thrombosis: frequency of association of carcinoma in body or tail of the pancreas with multiple venous thromboses, Am J Cancer **34**:566

Srikantia SG and Reddy V (1967) Megaloblastic anemis of infancy and vitamin B_{12}, Br J Haematol **13**:949

Stadtman TC (1971) Vitamin B_{12}, Science **171**:859

Stahlberg KG et al (1967) Liver B_{12} in subjects with and without vitamin B_{12} deficiency. A quantitative and qualitative study, Scand J Haematol **4**:312

Stallman PJ and Aalberse RC (1977) Quantitation of basophil-bound IgE in atopic and nonatopic subjects, Int Arch Allergy Appl Immunol **54**:114

Stamatoyannopoulos G and Nute PE (1974) Genetic control of hemoglobins, Clin Haematol **3**:251

Stamatoyannopoulos G et al (1966a) On the familial predisposition to favism, Am J Hum Genet **18**:253

Stamatoyannopoulos G et al (1966b) The distribution of glucose-6-phosphate dehydrogenase deficiency in Greece, Am J Hum Genet **18**:296

Stamatoyannopoulos G et al (1967) Absence of hemoglobin A in a double heterozygote for F-thalassemia and hemoglobin S, Blood **30**:772

Stamatoyannopoulos G et al (1969) F-thalassemia: a study of thirty-one families with simple heterozygotes and combinations of F-thalassemia with A_2-thalassemia, Am J Med **47**:194

Stamatoyannopoulos G et al (1970) Electrophoretic diversity of glucose-6-phosphate dehydrogenase among Greeks, Am J Hum Genet **22**:587

Stamatoyannopoulos G et al (1971) Abnormal hemoglobins with high and low oxygen affinity, Ann Rev Med **22**:221

Stamatoyannopoulos G et al (1973) Hemoglobin Olympia (beta 20 valine → methionine): an electrophoretically silent variant associated with high oxygen affinity and erythrocytosis, J Clin Invest **52**:342

Stamatoyannopoulos G et al (1974) Inclusion-body β-thalassemia trait: a form of β-thalassemia producing clinical manifestations in simple heterozygotes, N Engl J Med **290**:939

Stamatoyannopoulos G et al (1976) Haemoglobin $H_{Hyde Park}$ occurring as a fresh mutation: diagnostic, structural, and genetic considerations, J Med Genet **13**:142

Stamper HB Jr and Woodruff JJ (1976) Lymphocyte homing into lymph nodes: in vitro demonstration of the selective affinity of recirculating lymphocytes for high-endothelial venules, J Exp Med **144**:828

Stanbury JB et al (Eds) (1978) The metabolic basis of inherited disease, New York, McGraw-Hill Book Co, Inc

Standards for blood banks and transfusion services (1976), ed 8, Washington, DC, American Association of Blood Banks, p 5

Stanley ER and Metcalf D (1972) Purification and properties of human urinary colony stimulating factor (CFS). In Harris R and Viza D (Eds): Cell differentiation, Copenhagen, Munksgaard, p 149

Statland BE and Winkel P (1977) Relationship of day-to-day variation of serum iron concentrations to iron-binding capacity in healthy young women, Am J Clin Pathol **67**:84

Statland BE et al (1978) Evaluation of biologic sources of variation of leukocyte counts and other hematologic quantities using very precise automated analyzers, Am J Clin Pathol **69**:48

Steadman JH et al (1970) Idiopathic Heinz body anaemia: hb-Bristol (beta 67 [E11] val → asp), Br J Haematol **18**:435

Stebbins R and Bertino JR (1976) Megaloblastic anaemia produced by drugs, Clin Haematol **5**:619

Steele PP et al (1973) Platelet survival and adhesiveness in recurrent venous thrombosis, N Engl J Med **288**:1148

Steere AC et al (1978) Pyrogen reactions associated with the infusion of normal serum albumin (human), Transfusion **18**:102

Steerman RL et al (1971) Intrinsic defect of the polymorphonuclear leucocyte resulting in impaired chemotaxis and phagocytosis, Clin Exp Immunol **9**:939

Stefanini M and Karaca M (1966) Acquired thrombocytopathy in patients with pernicious anaemia. Revision of biochemical abnormalities after treatment with vitamin B_{12}, Lancet **1**:400

Stefanini M et al (1978) Gaisböck's syndrome: its hematologic, biochemical and hormonal parameters, Angiology **29**:520

Stein H and Kaiserling E (1974) Surface immunoglobulins and lymphocyte-specific surface antigens on leukaemic reticuloendotheliosis cells, Clin Exp Immunol **18**:63

Stein H et al (1972) Malignant lymphomas of B-cell type, Lancet **2**:855

Stein H et al (1976) Lymphoblastic lymphoma of convoluted or acid phosphatase type—a tumor of T precursor cells, Int J Cancer **17**:292

Steinberg AD and Klassen LW (1977) Role of suppressor T cells in lymphopoietic disorders, Clin Haematol **6**:439

Steinberg AG (1969) Globulin polymorphisms in man, Ann Rev Genet **3**:25

Steinberg AG et al (1962) A new human gammaglobulin factor determined by an allele at the Inv locus, Vox Sang **7**:151

Steinberg F (1961) The megaloblastic anemia of regional ileitis: report of a case, N Engl J Med **264**:186

Steinberg MH et al (1975) Alpha thalassemia in adults with sickle cell trait, Br J Haematol **30**:31

Steinberg MH et al (1976) Hemoglobin Hope: studies of oxygen equilibrium in heterozygotes hemoglobin S–Hope disease and isolated hemoglobin Hope, J Lab Clin Med **88**:125

Steinberg MH et al (1979) Diamond-Blackfan syndrome: evidence for T-cell mediated suppression of erythroid development and a serum blocking factor associated with remission, Br J Haematol **41**:57

Steinbrinck W (1948) Uber eine neue Granulationsanomalle der Leukozyten, Dtsch Arch Klin Med **193**:577

Steiner ML and Pearson HA (1966) Bone marrow plasmacyte values in childhood. A morphologic correlation in developmental immunology, J Pediatr **68**:562

Steinglass P et al (1941) Effect of castration and sex hormones on blood of the rat, Proc Soc Exp Biol Med **48**:169

Stemerman MB (1973) Platelet interaction with intimal connective tissue. In Baldini MG and Ebbe S (Eds): Platelets: production, function, transfusion, and storage, New York, Grune & Stratton, Inc, p 157

Stemerman MB and Ross R (1972) Experimental arteriosclerosis. I. Fibrous plaque formation in primates, an electron microscopic study, J Exp Med **136**:769

Stenflo J (1970) Dicumarol-induced prothrombin in bovine plasma, Acta Chem Scand **24**:3762

Stenflo J (1975) Structural comparison of normal and dicoumarol-induced prothrombin. In Hemker HC and Veltkamp JJ (Eds): Prothrombin and related coagulation factors, Leiden, Leiden University Press, p 152

Stenflo J and Ganrot PO (1973) Binding of Ca 2+ to normal and dicoumarol-induced prothrombin, Biochem Biophys Res Commun **50**:98

Stenman U-H (1976) Intrinsic factor and the vitamin B_{12} binding proteins, Clin Haematol **5**:473

Stephens AD (1977) Polycythaemia and high affinity haemoglobins, Br J Haematol **36**:153

Stern C (1960) Principles of human genetics, San Francisco, WH Freeman and Co Publishers

Steward RD et al (1973) Carboxyhemoglobin concentrations in blood donors in Chicago, Milwaukee, New York, and Los Angeles, Science **182**:1362

Stiehm ER and Fudenberg HH (1966a) Serum levels of immune globulins in health and disease: a survey, Pediatrics **37**:715

Stiehm ER and Fudenberg HH (1966b) Clinical and immunologic features of dysgammaglobulinemia type I. Report of a case diagnosed in first year of life, Am J Med **40**:805

Stiehm ER and McIntosh RM (1967) Wiskott-Aldrich syndrome: review and report of a large family, Clin Exp Immunol **2**:179

Stites DP et al (1971) Factor VIII detection by hemagglutination inhibition: hemophilia A and von Willebrand's disease, Science **171**:196

Stobo JD and Tomasi TB Jr (1967) A low molecular weight immunoglobulin antigenically related to 19S IgM, J Clin Invest **46**:1329

Stocker F et al (1968) Selective gamma-A-globulin deficiency, with dominant autosomal inheritance in a Swiss family, Arch Dis Child **43**:585

Stohlman F Jr and Brecher G (1956) Stimulation of erythropoiesis in sublethally irradiated rats by a plasma factor, Proc Soc Exp Biol Med **91**:1

Stohlman F Jr and Quesenberry PJ (1972) Colony-stimulating factor and myelopoiesis, Blood **39**:727

Stohlman F Jr et al (1954) Evidence for humoral regulation of erythropoiesis: studies on patient with polycythemia secondary to regional hypoxia, Blood **9**:721

Stohlman F Jr et al (1973) The regulation of myelopoiesis as approached with in vivo and in vitro techniques, Prog Hematol **8**:259

Stokstad ELR and Koch J (1967) Folic acid metabolism, Phys Rev **47**:83

Stonard MD (1974) Experimental hepatic porphyria induced by hexachlorobenzene as a model for human symptomatic porphyria, Br J Haematol **27**:617

Stone GE and Redmond AJ (1963) Leukopenic infectious mononucleosis: report of a case closely simulating acute monocytic leukemia, Am J Med **34**:541

Storb R et al (1968) Marrow repopulating ability of peripheral blood cells compared to thoracic duct cells, Blood **32**:662

Storb R et al (1978) One hundred ten patients with aplastic anemia (AA) treated by marrow transplantation in Seattle, Transplant Proc **10**:135

Stossel TP (1975) Phagocytosis: recognition and ingestion, Semin Hematol **12**:83

Stossel TP et al (1972) Phagocytosis in chronic granulomatous disease and Chediak-Higashi syndrome, N Engl J Med **286**:120

Stratton F (1975) Recent observations on the antiglobulin test, Wadley Med Bull **5**:182

Streiff F et al (1971) Un nouveau cas d'anomalie constitutionnelle et familiale du fibrinogéne sans diatheses hémorragique, Thromb Diath Haemorrh **26**:565

Strelling MK et al (1966) Megaloblastic anaemia and whole-blood folate levels in premature infants, Lancet **1**:898

Streuli RA et al (1980) Dysmyelopoietic syndrome: sequential clinical and cytogenetic studies, Blood **55**:636

Strouth JC et al (1966) Leukocyte abnormalities in familial amaurotic idiocy, N Engl J Med **274**:36

Strukelj M and Zemva M (1973) Modification of the N.B.T. test, Lancet **1**:149

Strum SB et al (1971) Further observations on the biologic significance of vascular invasion in Hodgkin's disease, Cancer **27**:1

Strumia MM and McGraw JJ Jr (1941) The development of plasma preparations for transfusion, Ann Intern Med **15**:80

Strumia MM and Phillips M (1963) Effect of red cell factors on the relative viscosity of whole blood, Am J Clin Pathol **39**:464

Strumia MM et al (1954) An improved microhematocrit method, Am J Clin Pathol **24**:1016

Strumia MM et al (1970) The preservation of blood for transfusion. VII. Effect of adenine and inosine on the adenine triphosphate and viability of red cells when added to blood stored from zero to seventy days at 1° C, J Lab Clin Med **75**:244

Stryckmans PA (1974) Current concepts in chronic myelogenous leukemia, Semin Hematol **11**:101

Stuart AE and Dewar AE (1979) Properties of anti-hairy cell serum, Br J Haematol **41**:163

Stuart MJ et al (1975) A simple non-radioisotope technic for the determination of platelet life span, N Engl J Med **292**:1310

Stuart MJ et al (1979) The post-aspirin bleeding time: a screening test for evaluating haemostatic disorders, Br J Haematol **43**:649

Studzinski GP (1974) Molecular basis of cell proliferation: the cell cycle, Ann Clin Lab Sci **4**:115

Sturgeon P (1970) Hematological observations on the anemia associated with blood type Rh null, Blood **36**:310

Sturgeon P et al (1964) Notations for two weak A variants: A_{end} and A_{el}, Vox Sang **9**:214

Sugerman HJ et al (1970) The basis of defective oxygen delivery from stored blood, Surg Gynecol Obstet **131**:733

Sugimoto T et al (1978) Plasma levels of carcinoembryonic antigen in patients with ataxia-telangiectasia, J Pediatr **92**:436

Sugino A and Okazaki R (1973) RNA-linked DNA fragments in vitro, Proc Natl Acad Sci USA **70**:88

Sukumaran PK et al (1960) Haemoglobin D–thalassaemia. A report of two families, Acta Haematol **23**:309

Sukumaran PK et al (1972) Haemoglobin Q India (alpha 64 [E13] aspartic acid → histidine) associated with beta thalassemia observed in three Sindhi families, J Med Genet **9**:436

Sullivan AL et al (1971) Electron microscopic localization of immunoglobulin E on the surface membrane of human basophils, J Exp Med **134**:1403

Sullivan LW and Herbert V (1965) Studies on the minimum daily requirement for vitamin B_{12}. Hematopoietic responses to 0.1 microgm. of cyanocobalamin or coenzyme B_{12}, and comparison of their relative potency, N Engl J Med **272**:340

Sullivan JL et al (1978) Immune response after splenectomy, Lancet **1**:178

Sultan C (1977) Pure acute monocytic leukemia, Am J Clin Pathol **68**:752

Sultan Y and Caen JP (1972) Platelet dysfunction in preleukemic states and in various types of leukemia, Ann NY Acad Sci **201**:300

Sultan Y et al (1976) Isolated platelet factor 3 deficiency, N Engl J Med **294**:1121

Sumaya CV (1977) Endogenous reactivation of Epstein-Barr virus infections, J Infect Dis **135**:374

Sumida I (1975) Studies of abnormal hemoglobins in western Japan. Frequency of visible hemoglobin variants and chemical characterization of hemoglobin Sawara (alpha 2 6Ala beta 2) and hemoglobin Mugino (hb L Ferrara alpha 2 47 Gly beta 2), Jpn J Hum Genet **19**:343

Sumida I et al (1973) Hemoglobin Sawara: α6(A4) aspartic acid → alanine, Biochim Biophys Acta **322**:23

Sun NC et al (1974) Blood coagulation studies in patients with cancer, Mayo Clin Proc **49**:636

Sundberg RD and Broman H (1955) The application of the Prussian blue stain to previously stained smears of blood and bone marrow, Blood **10**:160

Sundberg RD et al (1964) Cell debris and blue pigment macrophages in chronic myelogenous leukemia. In Proceedings of the Tenth Congress of the International Society of Hematology, Stockholm, Abstract 837

Sunderman FW and Boerner F (1950) Normal values in clinical medicine, Philadelphia, WB Saunders Co, p 718

Sunderman FW And Sunderman FW Jr (1964) Hemoglobin: its precursors and metabolites, Philadelphia, JB Lippincott Co

Sunderman FW et al (1953) Clinical hemoglobinometry, Baltimore, The Williams & Wilkins Co

Sung JH et al (1969) Neuropathological changes in Chédiak-Higashi disease, J Neuropathol Exp Neurol **28**:86

Surgenor DM (1974) Progress toward a national blood system, N Engl J Med **291**:17

Sussman LN (1978) Paternity blood grouping tests using legally unacceptable testing systems, Am J Clin Pathol **69**:650

Sutherland EW et al (1949) Mechanism of the phosphoglyceric mutase reactions, J Biol Chem **181**:153

Sutow WW and Welsh VC (1958) Acute leukemia and mongolism, J Pediatr **52**:176

Svejgaard A et al (1979) The HLA system: an introductory survey, Basel, S Karger

Swan H and Schecter DC (1962) The transfusion of blood from cadavers: a historical review, Surgery **52**:545

Sweeney L (1965) Case report of Lindau's disease with polycythemia and the relationship of erythropoietin, Am J Roentgenol Radium Ther Nucl Med **95**:880

Swenson RT et al (1962) A chemical abnormality in hemoglobin G from Chinese individuals, J Biol Chem **237**:1517

Szeinberg A et al (1962) Effect of nitrofurantoin in erythrocyte viability, Proc Tel-Hashomer Hosp **1**:49

Szelény JG et al (1980) A new hemoglobin variant in Hungary: Hb Savaria-alpha 49 (CE7) ser → arg, Hemoglobin **4**:27

Tabor E and Gerety RJ (1979) Non-A, non-B hepatitis: new findings and prospects for prevention, Transfusion **19**:669

Taketa F et al (1975) Hemoglobin Wood beta 97 (FG4) his → leu: a new high-oxygen affinity hemoglobin associated with familial erythrocytosis, Biochim Biophys Acta **400**:348

Tan JS et al (1974) Persistent neutrophil dysfunction in an adult. Combined defect in chemotaxis, phagocytosis, and intracellular killing, Am J Med **57**:251

Tanaka KR and Paglia DE (1971) Pyruvate kinase deficiency, Semin Hematol **8**:367

Tanaka KR et al (1960) Diseases or clinical conditions associated with low leukocyte alkaline phosphatase, N Engl J Med **262**:912

Tanaka Y and Brecher G (1971) Effect of surface digestion and metabolic inhibitors on appearance of ferritin in guinea pig erythroblasts in vitro: evidence for the production of apoferritin on the erythroblast cell membrane, Blood **37**:211

Tangheroni W et al (1968) Haemoglobin J Sardegna: alpha 50 (CD8) histidine → aspartic acid, Nature (London) **218**:470

Tanzer J et al (1964) Cytochemical and cytogenetic findings in a case of chronic neutrophilic leukaemia of mature cell type, Lancet **1**:387

Taswell HF and Winkelmann RK (1961) Sézary syndrome—a malignant reticulemic erythroderma, JAMA **177**:465

Tatsis B et al (1976) Hemoglobin Pyrgos alpha 2 beta 2 83 (EF7) gly → asp: a new hemoglobin variant in double heterozygosity with hemoglobin S, Blood **47**:827

Tattersall RB et al (1975) Hemoglobin components in diabetes mellitus: studies in identical twins, N Engl J Med **293**:1171

Tauro GP et al (1976) Dihydrofolate reductase deficiency causing megaloblastic anemia in two families, N Engl J Med **294**:466

Tavassoli M and Weiss L (1973) An electron microscopic study of spleen in myelofibrosis with myeloid metaplasia, Blood **42**:267

Tavassoli M and Shaklai M (1979) Absence of tight junctions in endothelium of marrow sinuses: possible significance for marrow cell egress, Br J Haematol **41**:303

Tavassoli M et al (1979) Cytochemical diagnosis of acute myelomonocytic leukemia, Am J Clin Pathol **72**:59

Taylor KB (1976) Immune aspects of pernicious anemia and atrophic gastritis, Clin Haematol **5**:497

Taylor RF and Farrell RK (1973) Light and electron microscopy of peripheral blood neutrophils in a killer whale affected with Chediak-Higashi syndrome, Fed Proc (Abstr) **32**:822

Taylor RL (1973) Pelger-Huët anomaly and megaloblastic anemia, Am J Clin Pathol **60**:932

Tchernia G et al (1968) Anemie hémolytique avec acanthocytose et dyslysidémie au cours de deux hépatitis néonatales, Arch Fr Pediatr **25**:729

Teien AN and Abildgaard U (1976) On the value of the activated partial thrombo-plastin time (APTT) in monitoring heparin therapy, Thromb Haemost **35**:592

Temin HM (1964) Nature of the protovirus of Rous sarcoma, Natl Cancer Inst Monogr **17**:557

Temin HM (1971) Mechanism of cell transformation by RNA tumor viruses, Ann Rev Microbiol **25**:609

Tenhunen R et al (1970) Reduced nicotinamide-adenine dinucleotide phosphate dependent biliverdin reductase: partial purification and characterization, Biochemistry **9**:298

Tentori L (1974) Three examples of double heterozygosis beta-thalassemia and rare hemoglobin variants, International Symposium on Abnormal Hemoglobin and Thalassemia, Istanbul, Turkey, Abstract 68

Tentori L (1977) Hemoglobin L Ferrara-hemoglobin Hasharon, Hemoglobin **1**:602

Tentori L et al (1972) Hemoglobin Abruzzo: beta 143 (H21) his → arg, Clin Chim Acta **38**:258

Teodorescu M and Mayer EP (1978) Surface imunoglobulin in immunoproliferative diseases, Ann Clin Lab Sci **8**:353

Teodorescu M et al (1976) Simultaneous identification of T and B cells in blood smears using antibody coated bacteria, Cell Immunol **24**:90

Terada H et al (1966) Interaction of influenza virus with blood platelets, Blood **28**:213

te Velde K et al (1964) A family study of pernicious anemia by an immunologic method, J Lab Clin Med **64**:177

Terasaki PI (1978) Resolution by HLA testing of 1,000 paternity cases not excluded by ABO testing, J Fam Law **16**:543

Terasaki PI et al (1978) Twins with two different fathers identified by HLA, N Engl J Med **299**:590

Territo MC (1977) Autologous bone marrow repopulation following high dose cyclophosphamide and allogenic marrow transplantation in aplastic anemia, Br J Haematol **36**:305

Testa JR et al (1979) Evolution of karyotypes in acute nonlymphocytic leukemia, Cancer Res **39**:3619

Therriault DG et al (1957) Influence of thrombin on rate of prothrombin conversion, Proc Soc Exp Biol Med **95**:207

Thiagarajan P et al (1980) Monoclonal immunoglobulin Mλ coagulation inhibitor with phospholipid specificity: mechanism of a lupus anticoagulant, J Clin Invest **66**:397

Thieffry St et al (1961) L'ataxie-télangiectasie (7 observations personnelles), Rev Neurol **105**:390

Thiele H (1953) pelger'sche Kernanomalie und aleukämische Myelose, Folia Haematol **71**:250

Thiéry JP and Bessis M (1956) Mécanisme de la plaquettogénèse: Etude "in vitro" par microcinematographie, Rev Hematol **11**:162

Thillet J et al (1976a) Hemoglobin Creteil beta 89 (F5) ser → asn: high oxygen affinity variant of hemoglobin frozen in quaternary R-structure, J Mol Med **1**:135

Thillet J et al (1976b) Functional and physiochemical studies of hemoglobin St Louis beta 28 (B10) leu → gln, J Clin Invest **58**:1098

Thillet J et al (1977) Hemoglobin Pontoise alpha 63 ala → asp (E12). A new fast moving variant, Biochim Biophys Acta **491**:16

Thomas DP et al (1976) Plasma heparin levels after administration of calcium and sodium salts of heparin, Thromb Res **3**:241

Thomas DB and Yoffey JM (1962) Human foetal haemopoiesis. I. The cellular composition of foetal blood, Br J Haematol **8**:290

Thomas DP et al (1967) Platelet aggregation in patients with Laennec's cirrhosis of the liver, N Engl J Med **276**:1344

Thomas ED et al (1955) Homozygous hemoglobin C disease: report of a case with studies on the pathophysiology and neonatal formation of hemoglobin C, Am J Med **18**:832

Thomas HM III et al (1974) The oxyhemoglobin dissociation curve in health and disease; role of 2,3-diphosphoglycerate, Am J Med **57**:331

Thomas WJ et al (1977) Free erythrocyte porphyrin: hemoglobin ratios, serum ferritin and transferrin saturation levels during treatment of infants with iron deficiency anemia, Blood **49**:455

Thompson AR and Davie EW (1971) Affinity chromatography of thrombin, Biochim Biophys Acta **250**:210

Thompson KW and Eisenhardt L (1943) Further consideration of the Cushing syndrome, J Clin Endocrinol Metab **3**:445

Thompson PR et al (1967) Anti-Di[b]—first and second examples, Vox Sang **13**:314

Thompson RB and Holloway CH (1963) Observations in the sickling phenomenon, Am J Med Technol **29**:379

Thompson RE et al (1977) Interaction of factor XI and kallikrein with high molecular weight kininogen, Thromb Haemost **38**:13

Thomson C et al (1974) Evidence for a qualitative defect in factor-VIII–related antigen in von Willebrand's disease, Lancet **1**:594

Thor DE et al (1968) Cell migration inhibition factor released by antigen from human peripheral lymphocytes, Nature **219**:755

Thurman WG et al (1966) Elevation of erythropoietin levels in association with Wilms' tumor, Arch Intern Med **117**:280

Till JE and McCulloch EA (1961) A direct measurement of the radiation sensitivity of normal mouse bone marrow cells, Radiat Res **14**:213

Till JE et al (1964) A stochastic model of stem cell proliferation, based on the growth of spleen colony-forming cells, Proc Natl Acad Sci USA **51**:29

Tinney WS et al (1943) The liver and spleen in polycythemia vera, Mayo Clin Proc **18**:46

Tio TH et al (1957) Acquired porphyria from liver tumor, Clin Sci **16**:517

Tiselius A (1937) Electrophoresis of serum globulin. II. Electrophoretic analysis of normal and immune sera, Biochem J **31**:1464

Titmuss RM (1971) The gift relationship: from human blood to social policy, New York, Pantheon Books, Inc

Tjio JH (1966) The Philadelphia chromosome and chronic myelogenous leukemia, J Natl Cancer Inst **36**:567

Tjio JH and Levan A (1956) The chromosome number of man, Hereditas **42**:1

Tobler R and Cottier H (1958) Familiäre Lymphopenie mit Agammaglobulinämie und schwerer Moniliasis: die essentielle Lymphocytophthise als besondere Form der fruhkindlichen Agammaglobulinämie, Helv Paediatr Acta **13**:313

Toennies G et al (1956) Blood folic acid activity of normal humans, cancer patients, and noncancer patients, Cancer **9**:1053

Tokuhata GK et al (1968) Chronic myelocytic leukemia in identical twins and a sibling, Blood **31**:216

Tolstoshev P et al (1976) Presence of gene for β-globin in homozygous β⁰ thalaessemia, Nature **259**:95

Tondo CV et al (1974) Functional properties of hemoglobin Porto Alegre (alpha 2A beta 2 9 ser → cys) and the reactivity of its extra cysteinyl residue, Biochim Biophys Acta **342**:15

Tomasi TB (1972) Secretory immunoglobulins, N Engl J Med **287**:500

Tombridge TL (1968) Effect of posture on hematology results, Am J Clin Pathol **49**:491

Tonelli Q and Meints RH (1978) Sialic acid: a specific role in hematopoietic spleen colony formation, J Supramol Struct **8**:67

Tönz O (1968) The congenital methemoglobinemias: physiology and pathophysiology of hemiglobin metabolism, Basel, S Karger

Toolis F et al (1978) Pseudo-Chediak-Higashi anomaly in promyelocytic leukaemia associated with intravascular coagulation, Scand J Haematol **21**:283

Tooney NW and Cohen C (1972) Microcrystals of a modified fibrinogen, Nature **237**:23

Torrance J et al (1970) Intraerythrocytic adaptation to anemia, N Engl J Med **283**:165

Torres J and Bisno AL (1973) Hyposplenism and pneumococcemia: visualization of diplococcus pneumoniae in the peripheral blood smear, Am J Med **55**:851

Toskes PP and Deren JJ (1972) Selective inhibition of vitamin B_{12} absorption by para-aminosalicylic acid, Gastroenterology **62**:1232

Toskes PP and Deren JJ (1973) Vitamin B_{12} absorption and malabsorption, Gastroenterology **65**:662

Tracey R and Smith H (1978) An inherited anomaly of human eosinophils and basophils, Blood Cells **4**:291

Trainin N and Linker-Israeli M (1967) Restoration of immunologic reactivity of thymectomized mice by calf thymus extracts, Cancer Res **27**:309

Tranzer JP and Baumgartner HR (1967) Filling gaps in the vascular endothelium with blood platelets, Nature **216**:1126

Trentin J et al (1967) Antibody production by mice repopulated with limited numbers of clones of lymphoid cell precursors, J Immunol **98**:1326

Trentin JJ and Fahlberg WJ (1963) An experimental model for studies of immunologic competence in irradiated mice repopulated with "clones" of spleen cells. In Conceptual Advances in Immunology and Oncology, New York, Hoeber Medical Division, Harper & Rowe, Publishers, p 66

Trentin JJ (1971) Determination of bone marrow stem cell differentiation by stromal hemopoietic inductive microenvironments (HIM), Am J Pathol **65**:621

Trentin JJ (1978) Hemopoietic microenvironments, Transplant Proc **10**:77

Trentin JJ et al (1967) Antibody production byb mice repopulated with limited numbers of clones of lymphoid cell precursors, J Immunol **98**:1326

Trey C et al (1966) Treatment of hepatic coma by exchange blood transfusion, N Engl J Med **274**:473

Trigg ME (1979) Immune function of the spleen, South Med J **72**:593

Trincao C et al (1968) Haemoglobin J Paris in the south of Portugal (Algarve), Acta Haematol **39**:291

Triplett DA (1979) An objective overview of presently available automated differential counters. In Koepke JA (Ed): Differential leukocyte counting, Skokie, Ill, College of American Pathologists, p 181

Triplett DA et al (1977) Mechanism of acquired factor X deficiency in primary amyloidosis, Blood **50** (suppl l):285

Trobaugh FE Jr and Bacus JW (1979) Design and performance of the LARC automated leukocyte classifier. In Koepke JA (Ed): Differential leukocyte counting, Skokie, Ill, College of American Pathologists, p 119

Trubowitz S and Masek B (1968) A histochemical study of the reticuloendothelial system of human marrow—its possible transport role, Blood **32**:610

Trubowitz S et al (1957) Metal requirements of alkaline phosphatases of human and rabbit leukocytes, Proc Soc Exp Biol Med **95**:35

Trubowitz S et al (1971) Leukemic reticuloendotheliosis, Blood **38**:288

Trucco JI and Brown AK (1967) Neonatal manifestations of hereditary spherocytosis, Am J Dis Child **113**:263

Trujillo JM and Ohno S (1963) Chromosomal alteration of erythropoietic cells in chronic myeloid leukemia, Acta Haematol **29**:311

Trujillo JM et al (1979) Hematologic and cytologic characterization of 8/21 translocation acute granulocytic leukemia, Blood **53**:695

Tsai LC et al (1977) Pseudo-Chediak-Higashi anomaly in chronic myelogenous leukemia with myelofibrosis, Am J Clin Pathol **67**:608

Tsai SY and Levin WC (1957) Chronic erythrocytic hypoplasia in adults, Am J Med **22**:322

Ts'ao C et al (1976) Critical importance of citrate-blood ratio in platelet aggregation studies, Am J Clin Pathol **65**:518

Tschopp TB and Zucker MB (1972) Hereditary defect in platelet function in rats, Blood **40**:217

Tschopp TB et al (1974) Decreased adhesion of platelets to subendothelium in von Willebrand's disease, J Lab Clin Med **83**:296

Tschudy DP et al (1964) Effect of carbohydrate feeding on induction of δ-aminolevulinic acid synthetase, Metabolism **13**:396

Tsukimoto I et al (1976) Surface markers and prognostic factors in acute lymphoblastic leukemia, N Engl J Med **294**:245

Ts'o POP (1962) The ribosomes-ribonucleoprotein particles, Am Rev Plant Physiol **13**:45

Tso SC and Hua ASP (1974) Erythrocytosis in hepatocellular carcinoma: a compensatory phenomenon, Br J Haematol **28**:49

Tubiana M et al (1968) A study of hematological complications occurring in patients with polycythemia vera treated with 32-P (based on a series of 296 patients), Blood **32**:536

Tuchinda S et al (1965) A new haemoglobin in a Thai family. A case of haemoglobin Siriraj-beta-thalassaemia, Br Med J **1**:158

Tuddenham EG et al (1974a) Hyperviscosity syndrome in IgA multiple myeloma, Br J Haematol **27**:65

Tuddenham EG et al (1974b) Tissue localization and synthesis of factor-VIII–related antigen in the human foetus, Br J Haematol **26**:669

Tudhope GR and Wilson GM (1960) Anemia in hypothyroidism. Incidence, pathogenesis, and response to treatment, Q J Med **29**:513

Tuffy P et al (1959) Infantile pyknocytosis: a common erythrocyte abnormality of the first trimester, Am J Dis Child **98**:227

Tulliez M et al (1979) Pseudo-Chediak-Higashi anomaly in a case of acute myeloid leukemia: electron microscope studies, Blood **54**:863

Tullis JL (1947) Effect of experimental hypertonia on circulating leukocytes, J Clin Invest **26**:1098

Türk W (1907) Septische Erkrankungen bei Verkummerung des Granulozytensystems, Wien Klin Wochenschr **20**:157

Tumen J et al (1980) Complement sensitivity of paroxysmal nocturnal hemoglobinuria bone marrow cells, Blood **55**:1040

Turner DR and Wright DJM (1973) Lymphadenopathy in early syphilis, J Pathol **110**:305

Turpin F (1970) Contenu en hémoglobine des érythroblastes humains aux différents stades de maturation. Étude par microspectrophotométrie, Nouv Rev Fr Hematol **10**:747

Turpin F et al (1978) Déficit en peroxydase des granulocytes neutrophiles au cours d'une mastocytose diffuse, Nouv Rev Fr Hematol **20**:77

Tursz T et al (1974) Simultaneous occurrence of acute myeloblastic leukaemia and multiple myeloma without previous chemotherapy, Br Med J **2**:642

Twomey JJ et al (1969) The syndrome of imunoglobulin deficiency and pernicious anemia, Am J Med **47**:340

Tyler et al (1969) Effect of antilymphocytic serum on rat lymphocytes, J Immunol **102**:179

Udall JA (1970) Drug interference with warfarin therapy, Clin Med **77**:20

Ueda S and Schneider RG (1969) Rapid differentiation of polypeptide chains of hemoglobin by cellulose acetate electrophoresis of hemolysates, Blood **34**:230

Ullrich O and Wiedemann HR (1953) Sur Frage der konstitutionellen Granulationsanomalien der Leukozyten in ihrer Beziehung zu enchondralen Dysostosen, Klin Wochenschr **31**:107

Ullyot JL and Bainton DF (1974) Azurophil and specific granules of blood neutrophils in chronic myelogenous leukemia: an ultrastructural and cytochemical analysis, Blood **44**:469

Unanue ER (1976) Secretory function of mononuclear phagocytes, Am J Pathol **83**:396

Unanue ER et al (1973) Antigen receptors on lymphocytes, Fed Proc **32**:44

Undritz E (1937) Die Pelgersche Varietät nebst Mitteilung über eine bisher noch nicht beschriebene besondere Form (Teilträger), Folia Haematol **56**:416

Undritz E (1951) Pathological polyploidy (heteroploidy) of the blood cells and its significance in leukaemia, Proc Soc Int Haematol **3**:284

Undritz E (1954) Les malformations héréditaires des éléments figurés du sang, Sang **25**:296

Undritz E and Schäli H (1964) Eine neue Sippe mit erblichkonstitutioneller Hochsegmentierung der Neutrophilenkerne und das Knochenmarkbild beim homozygoten Träger dieser anomalie, Schweiz Med Wochenschr **94**:1365

Unger LJ and Wiener AS (1959) Observations on blood factors Rh^A, Rhα, Rh^B, Rh^C, Am J Clin Pathol **31**:95

United States Department of Health, Education and Welfare (1972) Summary report: NHLI blood resource studies, Bethesda, DHEW publication No. (NIA) 73-416

Vaes G (1973) Digestive capacity of lysosomes. In Hers HG and Van Hoof F (Eds): Lysosomes and storage diseases, New York, Academic Press, Inc

Vahlquist B et al (1958) Infectious mononucleosis and pseudomononucleosis in childhood, Acta Paediatr **47**:120

Valentine FT and Lawrence HS (1969) Lymphocyte stimulation: Transfer of cellular hypersensitivity to antigen in vitro, Science **165**:1014

Valentine WN and Tanaka KR (1978) Pyruvate kinase and other enzyme deficiency hereditary hemolytic anemias. In Stanbury JB et al (Eds): The metabolic basis of inherited disease, New York, McGraw-Hill Book Co, Inc, p 1410

Valenzuela R et al (1976) Unusual fibrillary inclusions in neutrophils of human renal allografts, N Engl J Med **295**:787

Valeri CR (1975) Blood components in the treatment of acute blood loss: use of freeze-preserved red cells, platelets and plasma proteins, Anesth Analg (Cleve) **54**:1

Valeri CR (1974a) Oxygen transport function of preserved red cells, Semin Hematol **3**:649

Valeri CR (1974b) Hemostatic effectiveness of liquid-preserved and previously frozen human platelets, N Engl J Med **290**:353

Valeri CR and Fortier NL (1969) Red cell mass deficits and erythrocyte 2,3-DPG levels, Försvarsmedicin **5**:212

Valeri CR et al (1965) Quantitation of serum haptoglobin-binding capacity using cellulose acetate membrane electrophoresis, Clin Chem **11**:581

Vallery-Radot P (1957) Introduction. In Benacerraf B and Delafresnaye JF (Eds): Physiopathology of the reticuloendothelial system, Springfield, Ill, Charles C Thomas, Publishers, p 1

van Assendelft OW et al (1979) The differential distribution of leukocytes. In Koepke JA (Ed): Differential leukocyte counting, Skokie, Ill, College of American Pathologists, p 11

Van Den Berghe H et al (1979a) Philadelphia chromosome in human multiple myeloma, J Natl Cancer Inst **63**:11

Van Den Berghe H et al (1979b) Transformation of polycythemia vera to myelofibrosis and late appearance of a 5q− chromosome anomaly, Cancer Genet Cytogenet **1**:157

Van den Bogaert P and Van Hove W (1971) Polycythémia vera suivie d'une érythroleucémie aiguë, Presse Med **79**:1685

van Den Ende J et al (1975) Giant lymph node hyperplasia with haematological abnormality (Letter), S Afr Med J **49**:170

Van Den Engh GJ and Golub ES (1974) Antigenic differences between hemopoietic stem cells and myeloid progenitors, J Exp Med **139**:1621

van der Meer J et al (1973) Antithrombin III deficiency in a Dutch family, J Clin Pathol **26**:532

van Dommelen CK et al (1964a) Cyanocobalamin-dependent depression of the serum alkaline phosphatase level in patients with pernicious anemia, N Engl J Med **271**:541

van Dommelen CK et al (1964b) B$_{12}$ lack ("pernicious anaemia"), possibly caused by "parasitization" (consumption by a neoplasm), in a case of Waldenström's macroglobulinemia, Acta Med Scand **176**:611

van Doornik MC et al (1978) Fatal aplastic anemia complicating infectious mononucleosis, Scand J Haematol **20**:52

Van Dorpe A et al (1973) Gaucher-like cells and congenital dyserythropoietic anaemia, type II (HEMPAS), Br J Haematol **25**:165

Van Dyke DC et al (1966) Erythropoietin in the urine of normal and erythropoietically abnormal human beings, Blood **28**:535

Van Epps DE et al (1974) Characterization of serum inhibitors of neutrophil chemotaxis associated with anergy, J Immunol **113**:189

Van Furth R (1970) Mononuclear phagocytes, Philadelphia, FA Davis Co

Van Furth R (ed) (1975) Mononuclear phagocytes: in immunity, infection, and pathology, Oxford, England, Blackwell Scientific Publications

Van Hoof F and Hers HG (1972) The mucopolysaccharidoses as lysosomal diseases, Adv Exp Med Biol **19**:211

Van Hoof F and Hers HG (1973) Other lysosomal storage disorders. In Hers HG and Van Hoof F (Eds): Lysosomes and storage diseases, New York, Academic Press, Inc

Vanier TM and Tyas JF (1966) Folic acid status in normal infants during the first year of life, Arch Dis Child **41**:658

van Loghem E and Litwin SD (1972) Antigenic determinants on immunoglobulins of nonhuman primates, Transplant Proc **4**:129

Van Mourik JA et al (1975) Biochemistry of factor VIII. In Brinkhous KM and Hemker HC (Eds): Handbook of hemophilia, New York, American Elsevier Publishing Co, Inc, p 77

Van Ros G et al (1968) Haemoglobin Stanleyville-II (alpha 78 asparagine → lysine), Br Med J **4**:92

Van Slyck EJ and Rebuck JW (1974) Psuedo-Chediak-Higashi anomaly in acute leukemia: a significant morphologic corollary? J Clin Pathol **62**:673

Van Slyck EJ and Adamson TC III (1979) Acute hypereosinophilic syndrome: successful treatment with vincristine, cytarabine, and prednisone, JAMA **242**:175

Van Slyck EJ et al (1970) Chromosomal evidence for the secondary role of fibroblastic proliferation in acute myelofibrosis, Blood **36**:729

van Rood JJ (1974) The HL-A system. II. Clinical relevance, Semin Hematol **11**:253

van Vliet G and Huisman THJ (1964) Changes in the hemoglobin types of sheep as a response to anemia, Biochem J **93**:401

Varco RL (1971) Conference on mechanical surface and gas layer effect on moving blood, Fed Proc **30**:1485

Vargas GP (1970) Anomalia de May-Hegglin como etiopatogenia de purpura thrombocitopenica (consideraciones sobre 22 nuevos casos), Bol Asoc Med PR **62**:52

Vatanavicharn S et al (1979) Serum erythrocyte folate levels in thalassemic patients in Thailand, Scand J Haematol **22**:241

Vaughan-Neil EF et al (1975) Post-transfusion purpura associated with unusual platelet antibody (anti-Pl^{B1}), Br Med J **1**:436

Veeger W et al (1962) Effect of sodium bicarbonate and pancreatin on the absorption of vitamin B_{12} and fat in pancreatic insufficiency, N Engl J Med **267**:1341

Veer A et al (1979) Acquired hemoglobin H disease in idiopathic myelofibrosis, Am J Hematol **6**:199

Vella F (1977) Variation in hemoglobin A_2, Hemoglobin **1**:619

Vella F et al (1958) An abnormal haemoglobin in a Chinese: haemoglobin G, Nature **182**:460

Vella F et al (1967a) A new hemoglobin variant resembling hemoglobin E. Hemoglobin E Saskatoon: beta 22 glu → lys, Can J Biochem **45**:1385

Vella F et al (1967b) Hemoglobin G Saskatoon: beta 22 glu → ala, Can J Biochem **45**:351

Vella F et al (1973) Hemoglobin Winnipeg alpha 2 75 asp → tyr beta 2, Clin Biochem **6**:66

Vella F et al (1974a) Haemoglobin Ottawa: alpha 2 15 (A13) gly → arg beta 2, Biochim Biophys Acta **336**:25

Vella F et al (1974b) Hemoglobin St Claude or alpha 2 127 (H10) lys → thr beta 2, Biochim Biophys Acta **365**:318

Vellar OD (1967) Studies on hemoglobin values in Norway. IX. Hemoglobin, hematocrit, and MCHC values in old men and women, Acta Med Scand **182**:681

Veltkamp JJ (1975a) Diagnosis of carriers of hemophilia A. In Brinkhous KM and Hemker HC (Eds): Handbook of hemophilia, New York, American Elsevier Publishing Co, Inc, p 277

Veltkamp JJ (1975b) Clinical features of hemophilia. In Brinkhous KM and Hemker HC (Eds): Handbook of hemophilia, New York, American Elsevier-Publishing Co, Inc, p 371

Veltkamp JJ and van Tilburg NH (1973) Detection of heterozygotes for recessive von Willebrand's disease by the assay of anti-hemophilic factor-like antigen, N Engl J Med **289**:882

Veltkamp JJ et al (1968) Detection of the carrier state in hereditary coagulation disorders. I and II, Thromb Diath Haemorrh **19**:279, 403

Veltkamp JJ et al (1970) Another genetic variant of haemophilia B: haemophila B_{Leyden}, Scand J Haematol **7**:82

Verhaeghe R et al (1974) Fibrinogen "Leuven," another genetic variant, Br J Haematol **26**:421

Verloop MC (1970) Iron depletion without anemia: a controversial subject, Blood **36**:657

Verma RS and Dosik H (1977) The value of reverse banding in detecting bone marrow chromosomal abnormalities: translocation between chromosomes 1,9, and 22 in a case of chronic myelogenous leukemia (CML), Am J Hematol **3**:171

Verstraete M et al (1962) Hemophilia B associated with a decreased factor VII activity, Am J Med Sci **243**:20

Verwilghen R et al (1969) Ineffective erythropoiesis with morphologically abnormal erythroblasts and unconjugated hyperbilirubinemia, Br J Haematol **17**:27

Verwilghen RL et al (1973) HEMPAS: congenital dyserythropoietic anaemia (type II), Q J Med **42**:257

Vettore L et al (1974) A new abnormal hemoglobin O Padova, alpha 30 (B11) glu → lys and a dyserythropoietic anemia with erythroblastic multinuclearity co-existing in the same patient, Blood **44**:869

Veys EM et al (1977) Short term variation of human immunoglobulin levels with an estimation of the day to day physiological variability, Clin Chim Acta **75**:275

Vicic WJ et at (1980) Release of human platelet factor V activity is induced by both collagen and ADP and is inhibited by aspirin, Blood **56**:448

Videbaek A (1947) Heredity in human leukemia, London, HK Lewis & Co Ltd

Videbaek A (1962) Cyclic neutropenia: report on three cases, Acta Med Scand **172**:715

Videbaek AA (1966) On the pathogenesis of human leukaemia, Acta Haematol **36**:183

Vigliani EC and Saita G (1964) Benzene and leukemia, N Engl J Med **271**:872

Vigliano EM and Horowitz HI (1967) Bleeding syndrome in a patient with IgA myeloma: interaction of protein and connective tissue, Blood **29**:823

Vilter RW et al (1960) Refractory anemia with hyperplastic bone marrow, Blood **15**:1

Vinciguerra V and Silver RT (1974) The importance of bone marrow biopsy in the staging of patients with lymphosarcoma, Blood **41**:913

Vinograd JR et al (1959) C^{14}-hybrids of human hemoglobins. II. The identification of the aberrant chain in human hemoglobin S, J Am Chem Soc **81**:3168

Viola MV et al (1976) Reverse transcriptase in leukocytes of leukemic patients in remission, N Engl J Med **294**:75

Virchow R (1845) Weisses Blut, Froriep's Notizen **36**:151

Virchow R (1865) Die Leukämie, in Gesammelte Abhandlungen zer wissenschaftglichen Medizin, Frankfurt, Meidinger

Virmani R et al (1979) Thrombocytosis, coronary thrombosis and acute myocardial infarction, Am J Med **67**:498

Vitale L et al (1969) Congenital and familial iron overload, N Engl J Med **280**:642

Viteri FE et al (1972) Normal haematological values in the Central American population, Br J Haematol **23**:189

Vittal SBV et al (1974) Hepatitis B antigen in saliva, urine, and tears, Am J Gastroenterol **61**:133

Vogel JM and Vogel P (1972) Idiopathic histiocytosis: a discussion of eosinophilic granuloma, the Hand-Schüller-Christian syndrome, and the Letterer-Siwe syndrome, Semin Hematol **9**:349

Vogler LB et al (1978) Pre-B cell leukemia: a new phenotype of childhood lymphoblastic leukemia, N Engl J Med **298**:872

Vogler WR and Winton EF (1977) A controlled study of the efficacy of granulocyte transfusions in patients with neutropenia, Am J Med **63**:548

Vogler WR and Mingioli ES (1968) Porphyrin synthesis and heme synthetase activity in pyridoxine-responsive anemia, Blood **32**:979

Vogler WR and Winton EF (1975) Humoral granulopoietic inhibitors: a review, Exp Hematol **3**:337

Voigt D et al (1967) Uber die Blutkonzentrationen der Leukozyten und Thrombocyten bei Eisenmangel, Blut **14**:267

Voke J and Letsky E (1977) Pregnancy and antibody to factor VIII, J Clin Pathol **30**:928

Volpe E et al (1974) The May-Hegglin anomaly. Further studies in leukocyte inclusions and platelet ultrastructure, Acta Haematol (Basel) **52**:238

von Behrens, WE (1975) Mediterranean macrothrombocytopenia, Blood **46**:199

von Felten A et al (1969a) Studies on fibrin monomer aggregation in congenital dysfibrinogenemia (Fibrinogen "Zürich"): separation of a pathological from a normal fibrin fraction, Br J Haematol **16**:353

von Felten A et al (1969b) Dysfibrinogenemia in a patient with primary hepatoma: first observation of an acquired abnormality of fibrin monomer aggregation, N Engl J Med **280**:405

Von Foerster H (1959) Some remarks on changing populations. In Stohlman F Jr (Ed): Kinetics of cellular proliferation, New York, Grune & Stratton, Inc

von Kaulla KN and Schultz RL (1952) Methods for the evaluation of human fibrinolysins, Am J Clin Pathol **29**:104

Vos GH et al (1961) A sample of blood with no detectable Rh antigens, Lancet **1**:14

Vos GH et al (1973) The incidence of antibodies to leukocytes and gammaglobulin IgG and IgA in a population of multitransfused Southern African Negroes, Transfusion **13**:432

Vossen ME et al (1968) Observations on platelet ultrastructure in familial thrombocytopathic thrombocytopenia, Am J Pathol **53**:1021

Vreeken J and van Aken WG (1971) Spontaneous aggregation of blood platelets as a cause of idiopathic thrombosis and recurrent painful toes and fingers, Lancet **2**:1394

Vullo C and Tunioli AM (1958) Survival studies of thalassemic erythrocytes transfused into donors, into subjects with thalassemia minor, and into normal and splenectomized subjects, Blood **13**:803

Vyas GN and Fudenberg HH (1969) Am(1), the first genetic marker of human immunoglobin A, Proc Natl Acad Sci USA **64**:1211

Vyas GN et al (1968) Anaphylactoid transfusion reactions associated with anti-IgA, Lancet **2**:312

Vyas GN et al (1969) Serologic specificity of human anti-IgA and its significance in transfusion, Blood **34**:573

Waaler BA et al (1959) Contact activation in the intrinsic blood clotting system, Scand J Clin Lab Invest **11**(supp 37):1

Wade PT et al (1967) Haemoglobin variant in a Bushman: haemoglobin D beta Bushman alpha beta 22 16 gly → arg, Nature (London) **216**:688

Wade Cohen PT et al (1973) Amino-acid substitution on the alpha 1 beta 1 intersubunit contact of haemoglobin Camden beta 131 (H9) gln → glu, Nature **243**:467

Wagner PD (1974) The oxyhemoglobin dissociation curve and pulmonary gas exchange, Semin Hematol **11**:405

Wagner RH and Cooper HA (1975) Current approaches to the characterization of factor VIII. In Brinkhous KM and Hemker HC (Eds): Handbook of hemophilia, New York, American Elsevier Publishing Co, Inc, p 61

Wahren B (1969) Diagnosis of infectious mononucleosis by the monospot test, Am J Clin Pathol **52**:303

Waitz R et al (1978) Formes pseudo-tumorales des myéloscléroses, Nouv Rev Fr Hematol **20**:501

Wajcman H et al (1972) Hb Setif: G1 (94) alpha asp → tyr. A new alpha chain hemoglobin variant with substitution of the residue involved in a hydrogen bond between unlike subunits, FEBS Lett **27**:298

Wajcman H et al (1973) Two new hemoglobin variants with deletion. Hemoglobin Tours: thr β87 (F3) deleted and hemoglobin St. Antoine: gly, leu β74-75 (E18-19) deleted. .Consequences for oxygen affinity and protein stability, Biochim Biophys Acta **295**:495

Wajcman H et al (1975) Hemoglobin Cochin-Port Royal—consequences of the replacement of the beta chain C-terminal by an arginine, Biochim Biophys Acta **400**:354

Wajcman H et al (1976) A new hemoglobin variant involving the distal histidine: hb Bicetre (beta 63 [E7] his → pro), J Mol Med **1**:187

Wajcman H et al (1977) Hemoglobin J Lome beta 59 (E3) lys → asn. A new fast moving variant found in a Togolese, FEBS Lett **84**:372

Wajcman H et al (1980) A silent hemoglobin variant: hemoglobin Necker Enfants-Malades alpha 20 (B1) his → tyr, Hemoglobin **4**:177

Wajima T and Kraus AP (1968) Low leukocyte alkaline phosphatase activity in sickle cell anemia, J Lab Clin Med **72**:980

Wald N et al (1978) Carboxyhaemoglobin levels and inhaling habits in cigarette smokers, Thorax **33**:201

Waldenström J (1957) The porphyrias as inborn errors of metabolism, Am J Med **22**:758

Waldenström J (1961) The incidence and cytology of different myeloma types, Lancet **1**:1147

Waldenström J and Haeger-Aronsen B (1967) The porphyrias: a genetic problem, Prog Med Genet **5**:58

Waldenström J and Kjellberg SR (1939) Roentgenological diagnosis of sideropenic dysphagia (Plummer-Vinson's syndrome) Acta Radiol **20**:618

Waldman R et al (1975) Fitzgerald factor: a hitherto unrecognized coagulation factor, Lancet **1**:949

Waldmann TA (1964) Polycythemia and cancer, Proc Natl Cancer Conf **5**:437

Waldmann TA and Blaese RM (1972) Immunodeficiency disease and malignancy, Ann Intern Med **77**:605

Waldmann TA et al (1968) The erythropoiesis-stimulating factors produced by tumors, Ann NY Acad Sci **149**:509

Walker FJ and Esmon CT (1979) Interactions between heparin and factor X_A: inhibition of prothrombin activation, Biochim Biophys Acta **585**:405

Walker ME et al (1977) Biochemical genetics of MN, Vox Sang **32**:111

Walker RH (1978) Probability in the analysis of paternity test results. In Silver H (Ed): Paternity testing, Washington, DC, American Association of Blood Banks, pp 69-135

Walker RH (1975) Bacteria and spirochetes. In Greenwalt TJ and Jamieson GA (Eds): Transmissible disease and blood transfusion, New York, Grune & Stratton, Inc, p 221

Walker RH et al (1963) Js^b of the Sutter blood group system, Transfusion **3**:94

Walker W (1975) Haemolytic anaemia in the newborn infant, Clin Haematol **4**:145

Walker WA and Hong R (1973) Immunology of the gastrointestinal tract: Part I, J Pediatr **88**:517

Walknowska J et al (1969) Practical and theoretical implications of fetal/maternal lymphocyte transfer, Lancet **1**:1119

Waller CW et al (1948) Synthesis of pterolyglutamic acid (liver *L. casei* factor) and pteroic acid. I, J Am Chem Soc **70**:19

Wallner SF et al (1976) The anemia of chronic renal failure and chronic diseases: in vitro studies of erythropoiesis, Blood **47**:561

Wallner SF et al (1978) The effect of serum from patients with chronic renal failure on erythroid colony growth in vitro, J Lab Clin Med **92**:370

Walravens PA (1980) Nutritional importance of copper and zinc in neonates and infants, Clin Chem **26**:185

Walsh PN (1972a) Albumin density gradient separation and washing of platelets and the study of platelet coagulant activities, Br J Haematol **22**:205

Walsh PN (1972b) The role of platelets in the contact phase of blood coagulation, Br J Haematol **22**:237

Walsh PN (1972c) The effects of collagen and kaolin on the intrinsic coagulant activity of platelets. Evidence for an alternative pathway in intrinsic coagulation not requiring factor XII, Br J Haematol **22**:393

Walsh PN (1974) Platelet antiheparin activity: assay based on factor-X_a inactivation by heparin and anti-factor X_a, Br J Haematol **26**:405

Walsh PN et al (1975) Hereditary giant platelet syndrome: absence of collagen-induced coagulant activity and deficiency of factor-XI binding to platelets, Br J Haematol **29**:639

Walters GO et al (1973) Serum ferritin concentration and iron stores in normal subjects, J Clin Pathol **26**:770

Wang TY (1968) Restoration of histone-inhibited DNA-dependent RNA synthesis by acidic chromatin proteins, Exp Cell Res **53**:288

Wangel AG et al (1968) A family study of pernicious anemia. I. Autoantibodies, achlorhydria, serum pepsinogen, and vitamin B_{12}, Br J Haematol **14**:161

Wapnick AA et al (1970) The relationship between serum iron

levels and ascorbic acid stores in siderotic Bantu, Br J Haematol **19**:271

Warburton D and Bluming A (1973) A "Philadelphia-like" chromosome derived from the Y in a patient with refractory dysplastic anemia, Blood **42**:799

Ward HN and Reinhard EH (1971) Chronic idiopathic leukocytosis, Ann Intern Med **75**:193

Ward HP and Block MH (1971) The natural history of agnogenic myeloid metaplasia (AMM) and a critical evaluation of its relationship with the myeloproliferative snydrome, Medicine **50**:357

Ward HP et al (1971) Serum levels of erythropoietin in anemias associated with chronic infection, malignancy, and primary hematopoietic disease, J Clin Invest **50**:332

Ward PA (1969) Chemotaxis of human eosinophils, Am J Pathol **54**:121

Ward PA and Berenberg JL (1974) Defective regulation of inflammatory mediators in Hodgkin's disease. Supernormal levels of chemotactic factor inactivator, N Engl J Med **290**:76

Ward PA and Hill JH (1970) C5 chemotactic fragments produced by an enzyme in lysomal granules of neutrophils, J Immunol **104**:535

Ward PA and Schlegel RJ (1969) Impaired leukotactic responsiveness in a child with recurrent infections, Lancet **2**:344

Ward PA et al (1969) Leukotactic factor produced by sensitized lymphocytes, Science **163**:1079

Ward PA et al (1970) The production by antigen-stimulated lymphocytes of a leukotactic factor distinct from migration inhibitory factor, Cell Immunol **1**:162

Ward PA et al (1971) Chemoattractants of leukocytes, with special reference to lymphocytes, Fed Proc **30**:1721

Ward PA et al (1972) Leukotactic factors elaborated by virus-infected tissues, J Exp Med **135**:1095

Ward PCJ et al (1979) Erythrocyte ecdysis: an unusual morphologic finding in a case of sickle cell anemia with intercurrent cold agglutinin syndrome, Am J Clin Pathol **72**:479

Ward R et al (1972) Hepatitis B antigen in saliva and mouth washings, Lancet **2**:726

Wardrop CAJ et al (1978) Nonphysiological anaemia of prematurity, Arch Dis Child **53**:855

Ware AG and Seegers WH (1948) Plasma accelerator globulin: partial purification, quantitative determination, and properties, J Biol Chem **172**:699

Ware AG and Seegers WH (1949) Two-stage procedure for the quantitative determination of prothrombin concentration, Am J Clin Pathol **19**:471

Warner ED et al (1936) A quantitative study on blood clotting: prothrombin fluctuations under experimental conditions, Am J Physiol **114**:667

Warner HR and Athens JW (1964) An analysis of granulocyte kinetics in blood and bone marrow, Ann NY Acad Sci **113**:523

Warner NL et al (1962) The immunological role of different lymphoid organs in the chicken. I. Dissociation of immunological responsiveness, Aust J Exp Biol Med Sci **40**:373

Warren S (1970) Radiation carcinogenesis, Bull NY Acad Med **46**:131

Wasi P et al (1968) The effect of iron deficiency on the levels of hemoglobins A$_2$ and E, J Lab Clin Med **71**:85

Wasi P et al (1968) Haemoglobin D beta Los Angeles (D Punjab, alpha 2 beta 2 121 glu NH$_2$) in a Thai family, Acta Haematol **39**:151

Wasi P et al (1969) Alpha- and beta-thalassemia in Thailand, Ann NY Acad Sci **165**:60

Wasi P et al (1972) Incidence of haemoglobin Thai: a reexamination of the genetics of alpha-thalassemic diseases, Ann Hum Genet **35**:467

Wasserman K and Mayerson HS (1955) Plasma volume changes compared with hematocrit and plasma protein changes after infusion, Am J Physiol **182**:419

Wasserman LR (1976) The treatment of polycythemia vera, Semin Hematol **13**:57

Watanabe T et al (1979) Disseminated intravascular coagulation in autopsy cases: its incidence and clinicopathologic significance, Path Res Pract **165**:311

Waters WJ and Lacson PS (1957) Mast cell leukemia presenting as urticaria pigmentosa: report of a case, Pediatrics **19**:1033

Watkins WM (1967) The possible enzymic basis of the biosynthesis of blood-group substances. In Proceedings of the Third International Congress of Human Genetics, Baltimore, Johns Hopkins Press

Watson CG and Cooper WM (1971) Thrombotic thrombocytopenic purpura: concomitant occurrence in husband and wife, JAMA **215**:1821

Watson CJ (1950) The erythrocyte coproporphyrin: variation in respect to protoporphyrin and reticulocytes in certain of the anemias, Arch Intern Med **86**:797

Watson CJ (1960) The problem of porphyria: some facts and questions, N Engl J Med **263**:1205

Watson CJ and Hawkinson V (1947) Studies of urobilinogen. VI. Further experience with the simple quantitative Ehrlich reaction. Corrected calibration of the Evelyn colorimeter with a pontacyl dye mixture in terms of urobilinogen, Am J Clin Pathol **17**:108

Watson CJ and Schwartz S (1941) A simple test for urinary porphobilinogen, Proc Soc Exp Biol Med **47**:393

Watson CJ et al (1964) Present status of the Ehrlich aldehyde reaction for urinary porphobilinogen, JAMA **190**:501

Watson J et al (1948) The significance of the paucity of sickle cells in newborn Negro infants, Am J Med Sci **215**:419

Watson J et al (1973) Cyclic nucleotides as intracellular mediators of the expression of antigen-sensitive cells, Nature **246**:405

Watson-Williams EJ et al (1965) A new haemoglobin, D Ibadan (beta 87 threonine → lysine), producing no sickle cell haemoglobin D disease with haemoglobin S, Nature (London) **205**:1273

Wautier JL et al (1976) Acquired von Willebrand's syndrome and thrombopathy in a patient with chronic lymphocytic leukaemia, Scand J Haematol **16**:128

Waxman HS and Rabinovitz M (1966) Control of reticulocyte polyribosome content and hemoglobin synthesis by heme, Biochim Biophys Acta **129**:369

Waxman S (1975) Folate binding proteins, Br J Haematol **29**:23

Waxman S and Gilbert HS (1974) Characteristics of a novel serum vitamin B$_{12}$-binding protein associated with hepatocellular carcinoma, Br J Haematol **27**:229

Waxman S and Schreiber C (1973a) Measurement of serum folate levels and serum folic acid-binding protein by ^{3}H-PGA radioassay, Blood **42**:281

Waxman S and Schreiber C (1973b) Characteristics of folic acid-binding protein in folate-deficient serum, Blood **42**:291

Waxman S et al (1970) Drugs, toxins, and dietary amino acids affecting vitamin B$_{12}$ or folic acid absorption or utilization, Am J Med **48**:599

Weatherall DJ (1960) Enzyme deficiency in haemolytic disease of the newborn, Lancet **2**:835

Weatherall DJ (1964a) Biochemical phenotypes of thalassemia in the American Negro population, Ann NY Acad Sci **119**:450

Weatherall DJ (1964b) Hemoglobin J (Baltimore) coexisting in a family with hemoglobin S, Johns Hopkins Hosp Bull **114**:1

Weatherall DJ (1978) The thalassemias. In Stanbury JB et al (Eds):

The metabolic basis of inherited disease, New York, McGraw-Hill Book Co, Inc, p 1508

Weatherall DJ and Clegg JB (1972) The thalassemia syndromes, Oxford, Blackwell Scientific Publications Ltd

Weatherall DJ et al (1968) Haemoglobin and red cell enzyme changes in juvenile myeloid leukaemia, Br Med J 1:679

Weatherall DJ et al (1977) Haemoglobin Radcliffe (alpha 2 beta 2 99 [G1] ala): a high oxygen affinity variant causing familial polycythaemia, Br J Haematol 35:177

Weatherbee L et al (1974) Coagulation studies after transfusion of hydroxyethyl starch protected frozen blood in primates, Transfusion 14:109

Webb DI et al (1968) Mechanism of vitamin B_{12} malabsorption in patients receiving colchicine, N Engl J Med 279:845

Webster WP et al (1975) Biosynthesis of factors VIII and IX: organ transplantation and perfusion studies. In Brinkhous KM and Hemker HC (Eds): Handbook of hemophilia, New York, American Elsevier Publishing Co, Inc, p 149

Weech AA (1947) The genesis of physiologic hyperbilirubinemia, Adv Pediatr 2:346

Weed RI (1975) Membrane structure and its relation to haemolysis, Clin Haematol 4:3

Weed RI and Bessis M (1973) The discocytes stomatocyte equilibrium of normal and pathologic red cells, Blood 41:471

Weed RI and Chailley B (1972) Calcium-pH interactions in the production of shape change in erythrocytes, Nouv Rev Fr Hematol 12:775

Weeke B and Krasilnikoff PA (1972) The concentration of serum proteins in normal children and adults, Acta Med Scand 192:149

Weick JK et al (1974) Leukoerythroblastosis. Diagnostic and prognostic significance, Mayo Clin Proc 49:110

Weil R (1915) Sodium citrate in the transfusion of blood, JAMA 64:425

Weiner HL and Robinson WA (1971) Leukopoietic activity in human urine following operative procedures, Proc Soc Exp Biol Med 136:29

Weinfeld A et al (1977) Polycythaemia vera terminating in acute leukaemia: a clinical, cytogenetic and morphologic study in 8 patients treated with alkylating agents, Scand J Haematol 19:255

Weinsaft PP and Haltaufderhyde V (1965) Erythrocyte sedimentation rate in the aged, J Am Geriatr Soc 13:738

Weinstein IM and LeRoy GV (1953) Radioactive sodium chromate for the study of survival of red blood cells. II. The rate of hemolysis in certain hematologic disorders, J Lab Clin Med 42:368

Weinstein IM et al (1954) Radioactive sodium chromate for the study of survival of red blood cells. III. The abnormal hemoglobin syndromes, Blood 9:1155

Weinstein L and Taylor ES (1975) Hemolytic disease of the neonate secondary to anti-Fy^a, Am J Obstet Gynecol 121:643

Weinstein MJ and Doolittle RF (1972) Differential specificities of the thrombin, plasmin, and trypsin with regard to synthetic and natural substrates and inhibitors, Biochim Biophys Acta 258:577

Weir DG and Gatenby PBB (1963) Anaemia following gastric operations for peptic ulceration in Dublin. I. Incidence, Ir J Med Sci (6th Series) 447:105

Weir DM and Ögmundsdóttir HM (1977) Non-specific recognition mechanisms by mononuclear phagocytes, Clin Exp Immunol 30:323

Weisenburger DD (1980) Acute myelofibrosis terminating as acute myeloblastic leukemia, Am J Clin Pathol 73:128

Weisenburger DD et al (1976) Thrombotic thrombocytopenic purpura with C′3 vascular deposits, Am J Clin Pathol 67:61

Weiss AE (1975) Circulating inhibitors in hemophilia A and B: epidemiology and methods of detection. In Brinkhous KM and Hemker HC (Eds): Handbook of hemophilia, New York, American Elsevier Publishing Co, Inc, p 629

Weiss AS et al (1974) Fletcher factor deficiency: a diminished rate of Hageman factor activation caused by absence of prekallikrein, with abnormalities of coagulation, fibrinolysis, chemotactic activity, and kinin generation, J Clin Invest 53:622

Weiss HJ (1963) Hereditary elliptocytosis with hemolytic anemia. Report of six cases, Am J Med 35:455

Weiss HJ (1967) Platelet aggregation, adhesion, and adenosine diphosphate release in thrombopathia (platelet factor 3 deficiency). A comparison with Glanzmann's thrombasthenia and von Willebrand's disease, Am J Med 43:570

Weiss HJ (1972) Abnormalities in platelet function due to defects in the release reaction Ann NY Acad Sci 201:161

Weiss HJ (1975a) Platelet physiology and abnormalities of platelet function, N Engl J Med 293:580

Weiss HJ (1975b) Abnormalities of factor VIII and platelet aggregation—use of Ristocetin in diagnosing the von Willebrand syndrome, Blood 45:403

Weiss HJ and Ames RP (1973) Ultrastructural findings in storage pool disease and aspirin-like defects of platelets, Am J Pathol 71:447

Weiss HJ and Eichelberger JW Jr (1963) Secondary thrombocytopathia. Platelet factor 3 in various disease states, Arch Intern Med 112:827

Weiss HJ and Kochwa S (1968) Studies of platelet function and proteins in three patients with Glanzmann's thrombasthenia, J Lab Clin Med 71:153

Weiss HJ and Lages BA (1977) Possible congenital defect in platelet thromboxane synthetase, Lancet 1:760

Weiss HJ and Rogers J (1971) Fibrinogen and platelets in the primary arrest of bleeding—studies in 2 patients with congenital afibrinogenemia, N Engl J Med 285:369

Weiss HJ and Rogers J (1972) Correction of the platelet abnormality in von Willebrand's disease by cryoprecipitate, Am J Med 53:734

Weiss HJ et al (1972) Fatal disseminated intravascular coagulation and hemolytic anemia following stibophen therapy: a study of basic mechanisms, Am J Med Sci 264:375

Weiss HJ et al (1973a) Properties of the platelet retention (von Willebrand) factor and its similarity to the antihemophilic factor (AHF), Blood 41:809

Weiss HJ et al (1973b) Defective ristocetin-induced platelet aggregation in von Willebrand's disease and its correction by factor VIII, J Clin Invest 52:2697

Weiss HJ et al (1973c) Quantitative assay of a plasma factor deficient in von Willebrand's disease that is necessary for platelet aggregation. Relationship to factor VIII procoagulant activity and antigen content, J Clin Invest 52:2708

Weiss HJ et al (1973d) Decreased activity of a platelet cofactor located on the factor VIII molecule in 15 patients with von Willebrands' disease, Abstract, Fourth International Congress on Thrombosis and Hemostasis, Vienna, p 252

Weiss HJ et al (1974) Decreased adhesion of giant (Bernard-Soulier) platelets to subendothelium: further implications on the role of the von Willebrand factor in hemostasis, Am J Med 57:920

Weiss L (1974) A scanning electron microscopic study of the spleen, Blood 43:665

Weissman IL et al (1978) The lymphoid system: its normal architecture and the potential for understanding the system through the study of lymphoproliferative diseases, Hum Pathol 9:25

Wellington MS and Whitcomb JF (1960) Association of cyanocobalamin deficiency with myeloproliferative states: report of three cases, Am J Med Sci 239:750

Wells GM et al (1978) Rocky Mountain spotted fever caused by blood transfusion, JAMA **239**:2763

Wells R and Lau KS (1960) Incidence of leukaemia in Singapore, and rarity of chronic lymphocytic leukaemia in Chinese, Br Med J **1**:759

Wennberg E and Weiss L (1968) Splenic erythroclasia: an electron microscopic study of hemoglobin H disease, Blood **31**:778

Went LN and MacIver JE (1961) Thalassemia in the West Indies, Blood **17**:166

Werre JM et al (1970) Causes of macroplania of erythrocytes in diseases of the liver and biliary tract with special reference to leptocytosis, Br J Haematol **19**:223

Wessler S and Yin ET (1974) On the antithrombotic action of heparin, Thromb Diath Haemorrh **33**:71

West BC et al (1974) Separation and characterization of human neutrophil granules, Am J Pathol **77**:41

Wester J et al (1979) Morphology of the hemostatic plug in human skin wounds, Lab Invest **41**:182

Westergren A (1924) Die Senkungsreaction, Ergeb Inn Med Kinderheilkd **26**:577

Westphal RG (1972) Rational alternatives to the use of whole blood, Ann Intern Med **76**:987

Westlin WF (1966) Deferoxamine in the treatment of acute iron poisoning. Clinical experiences with 172 children, Clin Pediatr **5**:531

Wetli CV et al (1973) A previously unrecognized laboratory hazard. Hepatitis B antigen-positive control and diagnostic sera, Am J Clin Pathol **59**:684

Whang J et al (1963) The distribution of the Philadelphia chromosome in patients with chronic myelogenous leukemia, Blood **22**:664

Whang-Peng J et al (1968) Clinical implications of cytogenetic variants in chronic myelocytic leukemia (CML), Blood **32**:755

Whaun JM et al (1980) Effect of prenatal drug administration on maternal and neonatal platelet aggregation and PF$_4$ release, Haemostasis **9**:226

Wheeler JT and Krevans JR (1961) The homozygous state of persistent fetal hemoglobin and the interaction of persistent fetal hemoglobin with thalassemia, Johns Hopkins Med J **109**:217

Whipple GH and Bradford WL (1936) Mediterranean disease—thalassemia (erythroblastic anemia of Cooley): associated pigment abnormalities simulating hemochromatosis, J Pediatr **9**:279

Whipple GH and Robscheit-Robbins FS (1925) Blood regeneration in severe anemia: favorable influence of liver, heart, and skeletal muscle in diet, Am J Physiol **72**:408

Whitcomb WH and Moore M (1964) Erythropoietic inhibitory effect of plasma from hypertransfused animals, J Lab Clin Med **64**:1017

Whitcomb WH et al (1970) Effect of the South Polar Plateau on plasma and urine erythropoietin levels, Arch Intern Med **125**:638

White GC II et al (1977) Prothrombin complex concentrates: potentially thrombogenic materials and clues to the mechanism of thrombosis in vivo, Blood **49**:159

White JC and Beaven GH (1959) Foetal haemoglobin, Br Med Bull **15**:33

White JG (1966) The Chediak-Higashi syndrome: a possible lysosomal disease, Blood **28**:143

White JG (1968) The dense bodies of human platelets. Origin of serotonin storage particles from platelet granules, Am J Pathol **53**:791

White JG (1969) Observations on the mechanism of erythrocyte sickling, Pediatr Res **3**:220

White JG (1971) Ultrastructural physiology and cytochemistry of blood platelets. In Brinkhous KM and Shermer RW (Eds): The platelet, Baltimore, The Williams & Wilkins Co

White JG (1972a) Ultrastructural defects in congenital disorders of platelet function, Ann NY Acad Sci **201**:205

White JG (1972b) Visualization of the platelet release reaction, Blood **40**:953

White JG (1972c) Interaction of membrane systems in blood platelets, Am J Pathol **66**:295

White JG and Gerrard JM (1976) Ultrastructural features of abnormal blood platelets: a review, Am J Pathol **83**:590

White JG and Witkop CJ (1972) Effects of normal and aspirin platelets on defective secondary aggregation in the Hermansky-Pudlak syndrome: a test for storage pool deficient platelets, Am J Pathol **68**:57

White JG et al (1971) Studies of platelets in a variant of the Hermansky-Pudlak syndrome, Am J Pathol **63**:319

White JG et al (1973) The Hermansky-Pudlak syndrome: ultrastructure of bone marrow macrophages, Am J Pathol **70**:329

White JM (1974) Fetal hemoglobin: whole blood quantitation and intracellular distribution. In Schmidt RM et al (Eds): The detection of hemoglobinopathies, Cleveland, CRC Press, p 23

White JM and Dacie VJ (1971) The unstable hemoglobins—molecular and clinical features, Prog Hematol **7**:69

White JM et al (1970) Mild "unstable haemoglobin haemolytic anaemia" caused by haemoglobin Shepherds Bush (beta 74 [E18] gly → asp), Nature (London) **225**:939

White JM et al (1973) Familial polycythaemia caused by a new haemoglobin variant. Hb Heathrow beta 103 (G5) phenylalanine → leucine, Br Med J **3**:665

White WF et al (1960) Studies on erythropoietin, Recent Prog Horm Res **16**:219

Whitehead VM et al (1972) Intestinal conversion of folinic acid to 5-methyltetrahydrofolate in man, Br J Haematol **22**:63

Whittaker DL et al (1962) Linkage of color blindness to hemophilia A and B, Ann J Hum Genet **14**:149

Whitten CF (1967) Innocuous nature of the sickling (pseudosickling) phenomenon in deer, Br J Haematol **13**:650

Whitten CF et al (1966) Studies in acute iron poisoning. II. Further observations on desferrioxamine in the treatment of acute experimental iron poisoning, Pediatrics **38**:102

Whittingham S et al (1969) The genetic factor in pernicious anemia. A family study in patients with gastritis, Lancet **1**:951

Wick MR et al (1980) Malignant histiocytosis as a terminal condition in chronic lymphocytic leukemia, Mayo Clinic Proc **55**:108

Wickramasinghe SN and Saunders JE (1977) Results of three years' experience with the deoxyuridine suppression test, Acta Haematol **58**:193

Wickramasinghe SN et al (1969) Arrest of cell proliferation and protein synthesis in megaloblasts of pernicious anaemia, Acta Haematol **41**:65

Wide L and Porath J (1966) Radioimmunoassay of proteins with the use of Sephodex-coupled antibodies, Biochim Biophys Acta **130**:257

Widness JA et al (1980) Rapid fluctuations in glycohemoglobin (hemoglobin A$_{Ic}$) related to acute changes in glucose, J Lab Clin Med **95**:386

Wiener AS (1941) Hemolytic reactions following transfusions of the homologous group. II. Further observations on the role of property Rh particularly in cases without demonstrable isoantibodies, Arch Pathol **32**:227

Wiener AS (1944a) The Rh series of allelic genes, Science **100**:595

Wiener AS (1944b) A new test (blocking test) for Rh sensitization, Proc Soc Exp Biol Med **56**:173

Wiener AS (1951) Origin of naturally occurring hemagglutinins and hemolysis: a review, J Immunol **66**:287

Wiener AS (1953) The blood factor C of the A-B-O system, with special reference to the rare blood group C, Ann Eugenet **18**:1

Wiener AS (1961) Principles of blood group serology and nomenclature: a critical review, Transfusion **1**:308

Wiener AS (1963) Blood groups in man and lower primates: a review, Transfusion **3**:173

Wiener AS (1965) Lewis blood types: theoretical implications and practical applications, Am J Clin Pathol **43**:388

Wiener AS (1968a) Serology, genetics, and nomenclature of the P blood group system, Lab Dig **31**:6

Wiener AS (1968b) Problems and pitfalls in blood grouping tests for non-parentage. II. The Rh-Hr blood group system, J Forensic Med **15**:106

Wiener AS (1968c) The Rh-Hr blood types: the anatomy of a controversy, J Forensic Med **15**:22

Wiener AS (1969) Problems and pitfalls in blood grouping tests for nonparentage. 1. Distribution of the blood groups, Am J Clin Pathol **51**:9

Wiener AS and Cioffi AF (1972) A group B analogue of subgroup A_3, Am J Clin Pathol **58**:693

Wiener AS and Gordon EB (1956) A hitherto undescribed human blood group A_m, Br J Haematol **2**:305

Wiener AS and Moor-Jankowski J (1965) The V-A-B blood group system of chimpanzees: a paradox in the application of the 2×2 contingency test, Transfusion **5**:64

Wiener AS and Moor-Jankowski J (1969) Blood groups of apes and monkeys—their practical implications for experimental medicine, Ann NY Acad Sci **162**:37

Wiener AS and Nieberg KC (1963) Exclusion of parentage by Rh-Hr blood tests: revised table including blood factors Rh_0, rh′, rh″, hr′, hr″ and hr, J Forensic Med **10**:6

Wiener AS and Peters HR (1940) Hemolytic reactions following transfusions of blood of the homologous group, with three cases in which the same agglutinogen was responsible, Ann Intern Med **13**:2306

Wiener AS and Silverman IJ (1941) Subdivision of group A and group AB, with special reference to the so-called agglutinogen A_3, Am J Clin Pathol **11**:45

Wiener AS and Socha WW (1976) Methods available for solving medicolegal problems of disputed parentage, J Forensic Sci **21**:42

Wiener AS and Sonn EB (1943) Additional variants of the Rh type demonstrable with a special human anti-Rh serum, J Immunol **47**:461

Wiener AS and Unger LJ (1955) Excess of group O mothers in A-B-O hemolytic disease, with special reference to the blood factor C, Exp Med Surg **13**:204

Wiener AS and Unger LJ (1962) Further observations on the blood factor Rh^A, Rh^B, Rh^C, and Rh^D, Transfusion **2**:230

Wiener AS and Ward FA (1966) The serologic specificity (blood factor) C of the A-B-O blood groups, Am J Clin Pathol **46**:27

Wiener AS and Wexler IB (1958) Heredity of the blood groups, New York, Grune & Stratton, Inc

Wiener AS and Wexler IB (1961) Genetics of blood groups. In Gedda L (Ed): De genetica medica, pars secunda, genetica humana normalis, Rome, Instituto G Mendel

Wiener AS et al (1953) Fatal hemolytic transfusion reaction caused by sensitization to a new blood factor U, JAMA **153**:1444

Wiener AS et al (1956) Type-specific cold autoantibodies as a cause of acquired hemolytic anemia and hemolytic transfusion reactions: biologic test with bovine red cells, Ann Intern Med **44**:221

Wiener AS et al (1957) Observations on the nature of the autoantibodies in a case of acquired hemolytic anemia, Ann Intern Med **47**:1

Wiener AS et al (1963) Blood groups in chimpanzees, Exp Med Surg **21**:159

Wiener AS et al (1964a) Blood groups of apes and monkeys. V. Studies on the human blood group factors A, B, H, and Le in Old and New World monkeys, Am J Phys Anthropol **22**:175

Wiener AS et al (1964b) Problems in the management of erythroblastosis fetalis. III. Further observations on cases with unusual serologic and clinical findings, Exp Med Surg **22**:1

Wiener AS et al (1964c) The Lewis blood groups in man: a review with supporting data on non-human primates, J Forensic Med **11**:67

Wiener AS et al (1965) The blood factors I and i in primates including man, and in lower species, Am J Phys Anthropol **23**:289

Wiley JS and Gill FM (1976) Red cell calcium leak in congenital hemolytic anemia with extreme microcytosis, Blood **47**:197

Wiley JS et al (1979) Hereditary stomatocytosis: association of low 2,3-diphosphoglycerate with increased cation pumping by the red cell, Br J Haematol **41**:133

Wilkinson T et al (1967) Haemoglobin J Baltimore interacting with beta-thalassaemia in an Australian family, Med J Aust **1**:907

Wilkinson T et al (1975) A new haemoglobin variant, haemoglobin Camperdown beta 104 (G6) arginine → serine, Biochim Biophys Acta **393**:195

Wilkinson T et al (1980) Hemoglobin Summer Hill β52 (D3) asp → his: a new variant from Sydney, Australia, Hemoglobin **4**:185

Williams DM et al (1973) Mitochondrial iron metabolism, Fed Proc **32**:924

Williams RC et al (1973) Studies of T- and B-lymphocytes in patients with connective tissue diseases, J Clin Invest **52**:283

Williams TW and Granger GA (1969) Lymphocyte in vitro cytotoxicity: correlation of derepression with release of lymphotoxin from human lymphocytes, J Immunol **103**:170

Williams WJ et al (1972) Hematology, New York, McGraw-Hill Book Co, Inc

Willingham MC et al (1972) Control of DNA synthesis and mitosis in 3T3 cells by cyclic AMP, Biochim Biophys Res Commun **48**:743

Willoughby DA et al (1964) A lymph-node permeability factor in the tuberculin reaction, J Pathol **87**:353

Wilner GD et al (1968) Activation of Hageman factor by collagen, J Clin Invest **47**:2608

Wilson HA et al (1980) Transient pure red-cell aplasia: cell-mediated suppression of erythropoiesis associated with hepatitis, Ann Intern Med **92**:196

Wilson HE and Long MJ (1955) Hereditary ovalocytosis (elliptocytosis) with hypersplenism, Arch Intern Med **95**:438

Wilson HTH and Fielding J (1953) Sézary's reticulosis with exfoliative dermatitis, Br Med J **1**:1087

Wilson JF et al (1961) Loss of proteins in the gastrointestinal tract in iron-deficiency anemia, Am J Dis Child **102**:603

Wilson JF et al (1964) Milk-induced gastrointestinal bleeding in infants with hypochromic microcytic anemia, JAMA **189**:568

Wilson PA et al (1967) Platelet abnormality in human scurvy, Lancet **1**:975

Wilson SJ et al (1958) Blood coagulation in acute iron intoxication, Blood **13**:483

Wiltshire BG et al (1972) Haemoglobin Denmark Hill alpha 95 (G2) pro → ala, a variant with unusual electrophoretic and oxygen binding properties, Biochim Biophys Acta **278**:459

Winckelmann G (1973) Kongenitale Dysfibrinogenämie—Bericht über eine neue Familie, Thromb Diath Haemorrh, Supp **55**:345

Windhorst DB et al (1967) A newly defined X-linked trait in man with demonstration of the Lyon effect in carrier females, Lancet **1**:737

Windhorst DB et al (1968) A human pigmentary dilution based on a heritable subcellular structural defect—the Chediak-Higashi syndrome, J Invest Dermatol **50**:9

Windhorst DB et al (1969) The pattern of genetic transmission of the leukocyte defect in fatal granulomatous disease of childhood, J Clin Invest **47**:1026

Winkelmann RK (1973) T cell erythroderma (Sézary syndrome), Arch Dermatol **108**:205

Winkelmann RK and Hoagland HC (1980) The Sézary cell in the blood of patients with mycosis fungoides, Dermatologica **160**:73

Winkelstein JA and Drachman RH (1968) Deficiency of pneumococcal serum opsonizing activity in sickle-cell disease, N Engl J Med **279**:459

Winn LC et al (1975) ABO discrepancy caused by an auto anti-N, Transfusion **15**:612

Winslow RM and Anderson WF (1978) the hemoglobinopathies. In Stanbury JB et al (Eds): The metabolic basis of inherited disease, New York, McGraw-Hill Book Co, Inc, p 1465

Winslow RM et al (1976) Hemoglobin Mckees Rocks (alpha 2 beta 2 145 tyr → term): a human "nonsense" mutation leading to a shortened beta chain, J Clin Invest **57**:772

Winston RM et al (1970) Enzymatic diagnosis of megaloblastic anaemia, Br J Haematol **19**:587

Winter WP et al (1978) Identification of several rare hemoglobin variants discovered in a population survey including a new variant hb Garden State alpha 82 ala → asp, Clin Res **26**:122A

Winterbourne CC and Carrell RW (1974) Studies of hemoglobin denaturation and Heinz body formation in the unstable hemoglobins, J Clin Invest **54**:678

Winterhalter KH (1964) Hemoglobin synthesis, Path Microbiol (Basel) **27**:508

Wintrobe MM (1934) Anemia: classification and treatment on the basis of differences in the average volume and hemoglobin content of the red corpuscles, Arch Intern Med **54**:256

Wintrobe MM (1939) Diagnostic significance of changes in leukocytes, Bull NY Acad Med **15**:223

Wintrobe MM and Landsberg JW (1935) A standardized technique for blood sedimentation test, Am J Med Sci **189**:102

Wintrobe MM and Shumacker HB (1935) Comparison of hematopoiesis in the fetus and during recovery from pernicious anemia together with a consideration of the relationship of fetal hematopoiesis to macrocytic anemia of pregnancy and anemia in infants, J Clin Invest **14**:837

Wintrobe MM and Shumacker HB (1936) Erythrocyte studies in the mammalian fetus and newborn, Am J Anat **58**:313

Wintrobe MM et al (1940) A familial hemopoietic disorder in Italian adolescents and males, JAMA **114**:1530

Wintrobe MM et al (1974) Clinical hematology, ed 7, Philadelphia, Lea & Febiger

Wiseman BK and Doan CA (1939) A new recognized granulopenic syndrome caused by excessive splenic leukolysis and successfully treated by splenectomy, J Clin Invest **18**:473

Wissler RW et al (1960) The reticuloendothelial system in antibody formation, Ann NY Acad Sci **88**:134

Witts LJ (1969) Hypochromic anaemia, London, William Heinemann Medical Books, Ltd

Woessner S et al (1978) Prolymphocytic leukaemia of T-cell type: immunological, enzymatic and ultrastructural morphometric characteristics, Br J Haematol **39**:9

Wojcik JD et al (1969) Mechanism whereby platelets support the endothelium, Transfusion **9**:324

Wolf P et al (1970) False-positive infectious mononucleosis spot test in lymphoma, Cancer **25**:625

Wolfe MS (1975) Parasites, other than malaria, transmissible by

blood transfusion. In Greenwalt TJ and Jamieson GA (Eds): Transmissible disease and blood transfusion, New York, Grune & Stratton, Inc, p 267

Wong SC et al (1971) Hb J Georgia = Hb J Baltimore = alpha 2 beta 2 16 gly → asp, Clin Chim Acta **35**:521

Wood JK et al (1972) Folic acid and the pill, Scand J Haematol **9**:539

Wood S Jr (1958) Pathogenesis of metastasis formation observed in vivo in the rabbit ear chamber, Arch Pathol **66**:550

Woodard HQ and Higinbotham NL (1962) Development of osteogenic sarcoma in a radium dial painter thirty-seven years after the end of exposure, Am J Med **32**:96

Woodard HQ and Holodny E (1960) A summary of the data of Mechanik on the distribution of human bone marrow, Phys Med Biol **5**:57

Woodrow JC (1970) Rh immunization and its prevention, Ser Haematol **3**:7

Woodruff CW (1977) Iron deficiency in infancy and childhood, Pediatr Clin North Am **24**:85

Woodruff CW et al (1972) The role of fresh cow's milk in iron deficiency. II. Comparison of fresh cow's milk with a prepared formula, Am J Dis Child **124**:26

Woodruff JJ (1974) Role of lymphocyte surface determinants in lymph node homing, Cell Immunol **13**(3):378

Woodruff MFA (1967) Antilymphocyte serum: summary and further observations, Transplantation **5**(supp):1127

Woods WD et al (1960) Vitamin B_{12} Co^{60} readily passes the placenta into fetal organs and nursing provides B_{12} from mother to pup: a record of its distribution, J Exp Med **112**:431

Woodson RD et al (1970) Oxygen transport in hemoglobin San Francisco, Clin Res **18**:134

Workman EF and Lundblad RL (1980) Thrombin. In Schmidt RM (Section Ed): Handbook Series in Clinical Laboratory Science, Section I: Hematology, vol 3, Boca Raton, Fla, CRC Press Inc, p 149

Workman RD et al (1978) Granulocyte transfusions for patients with severe thermal burns, Transfusion **18**:142

World Health Organization (1970) Requirements of ascorbic acid, vitamin D, vitamin B_{12}, folate, and iron, WHO Techn Rep Series 452

Worlledge SM (1969a) Immune drug-induced hemolytic anemias, Semin Hematol **6**:181

Worlledge SM (1969b) Autoantibody formation associated with methyldopa (Aldomet) therapy, Br J Haematol **16**:5

Worlledge SM (1973) Immune drug-induced hemolytic anemias, Semin Hematol **10**:327

Worlledge SM and Dacie JV (1969) Haemolytic and other anaemias in infectious mononucleosis. In Carter RL and Penman HG (Eds): Infectious mononucleosis, Oxford, Blackwell Scientific Publications Ltd, p 82

Worlledge SM and Blajchman MA (1972) The autoimmune haemolytic anaemias, Br J Haematol **23**(Suppl):61

Worlledge SM and Rousso C (1965) Studies on the serology of paroxysmal cold haemoglobinuria (PCH) with special reference to its relationship with the P blood group system, Vox Sang **10**:293

Worton RG et al (1969) Physical separation of hemopoietic stem cells from cells forming colonies in culture, J Cell Physiol **74**:171

Wright AE and Douglas SR (1903) An experimental investigation of the role of the blood fluids in connection with phagocytosis, Proc R Soc (London) **72**:357

Wright DH (1971) Burkitt's lymphoma: a review of the pathology, immunology, and possible etiologic factors, Pathol Immunol **6**:337

Wright IS et al (1954) Myocardial infarction and its treatment with anticoagulants: summary of findings of 1031 cases, Lancet **1**:92

Wright MS and Issitt PD (1979) Anticomplement and the indirect antiglobulin test, Transfusion **19**:688

Wright R et al (1966) Autoantibodies and microscopic appearance of gastric mucosa, Lancet **1**:618

Wruble LD and Kalser MH (1964) Diabetic steatorrhea: a distinct entity, Am J Med **37**:118

Wu AM et al (1968) Cytological evidence for a relationship between normal hematopoietic colony-forming cells and cells of the lymphoid system, J Exp Med **127**:455

Wu KK and Hoak JC (1974) A new method for the quantitative detection of platelet aggregate in patients with arterial insufficiency, Lancet **2**:924

Wu KK and Hoak JC (1975) Increased platelet aggregates in patients with transient ischemic attacks, Stroke **6**:521

Wu KK and Hoak JC (1976) Spontaneous platelet aggregation in arterial insufficiency: mechanisms and implications, Thromb Diath Haemorrh **35**:702

Wu KK et al (1976) Platelet hyperaggregability in idiopathic recurrent deep vein thrombosis, Circulation **53**:687

Wueper KD (1973) Prekallikrein deficiency in man, J Exp Med **138**:1345

Xefteris E et al (1961) Leukocytic alkaline phosphatase in busulfan-induced remissions of chronic granulocytic leukemia, Blood **18**:202

Yachnin S et al (1972) The potentiation of phytohemagglutinin-induced lymphocyte transformation by cell-cell interaction: a matrix hypothesis, Cell Immunol **3**:569

Yam LT et al (1968) Functional cytogenetic and cytochemical study of the leukemic reticulum cells, Blood **32**:90

Yam LT et al (1971) Cytochemical identification of monocytes and granulocytes, Am J Clin Pathol **55**:283

Yamada K and Furusawa S (1976) Preferential involvement of chromosomes No. 8 and No. 21 in acute leukemia and preleukemia, Blood **47**:679

Yamaguchi K et al (1975) Cyclic premenstrual unconjugated hyperbilirubinemia. Report of two cases, Ann Intern Med **83**:514

Yamamoto A et al (1970) Accumulation of acid phospholipids in a case of hyperlipidemia with hepatosplenomegaly, Lipids **5**:566

Yamaoka K (1971) Hemoglobin Hirose: alpha 1 beta 2 37 (C3) tryptophan yielding serine, Blood **38**:730

Yanase T et al (1968) Molecular basis of morbidity—from a series of studies of hemoglobinopathies in western Japan, Jpn J Hum Genet **13**:40

Yang HC and Kuzur M (1977) Procoagulant specificity of factor VIII inhibitor, Br J Haematol **37**:429

Yang SSL et al (1978) Tc-99m human serum albumin: a suitable agent for plasma volume measurements in man, J Nucl Med **19**:804

Yankee RA et al (1973) Selection of unrelated compatible platelet donors by lymphocyte HL-A matching, N Engl J Med **288**:760

Yao AC et al (1969) Distribution of blood between infant and placenta after birth, Lancet **2**:871

Yataganas X et al (1973) Proliferative activity and glycogen accumulation of erythroblasts in β-thalassaemia, Br J Haematol **24**:651

Yeung CY and Hobbs JR (1968) Serum-gamma-G-globulin levels in normal, premature, post-mature, and "small-for-dates" newborn babies, Lancet **1**:1167

Ygge J (1970) Changes in blood coagulation and fibrinolysis during the postoperative period, Am J Surg **119**:225

Yin ET and Gaston LW (1965) Purification and kinetic studies on a circulating anticoagulant in a suspected case of lupus erythematosus, Thromb Diath Haemorrh **14**:88

Yin ET et al (1971a) Rabbit plasma inhibitor of the activated species of blood coagulation factor X. Purification and some properties, J Biol Chem **246**:3694

Yin ET et al (1971b) Identity of plasma-activated factor X inhibitor with antithrombin 3 and heparin cofactor, J Biol Chem **246**:3712

Yoffey JM (1971) The stem cell problem in the fetus, Isr J Med Sci **7**:825

Yoffey JM and Courtice FC (1970) Lymphatics, lymph, and the lymphomyeloid complex, New York, Academic Press, Inc

Yoffey JM et al (1954) A quantitative study of the effects of compound E, compound F, and compound A upon the bone marrow of the guinea pig, J Anat **88**:115

Yoffey JM et al (1964) Further problems of lymphocyte production, Ann NY Acad Sci **113**:867

Yokoyama M and Fudenberg HH (1966) Heterogeneity of immune anti-A antibody in relation to Forssman antigen, J Immunol **96**:304

Yolken RH and Hilgartner MW (1978) Prothrombin complex concentrates: use in treatment of hemophiliacs with factor VIII inhibitors, Am J Dis Child **132**:291

Yon JL et al (1976) Granulomatous hepatitis, increased platelet aggregation, and hypercholesterolemia, Ann Intern Med **84**:148

Yonemitsu H et al (1973) Two cases of familial erythrocytosis with increased erythropoietin activity in plasma and urine, Blood **42**:793

Yoo D et al (1978) Bone-marrow mast cells in lymphoproliferative disorders, Ann Intern Med **88**:753

Yoo D et al (1980) Myeloproliferative syndrome with sideroblastic anemia and acquired hemoglobin H disease, Cancer **45**:78

Yoshida K and Nahmias A (1967) Specific heterophile antibody from infectious mononucleosis serum, Proc Soc Exp Biol Med **124**:515

Yoshida K et al (1961a) Separation of Nishimine factor from fibrinogen and factor VIII (AHF) by the DEAE-cellulose column chromatography, J Nara Med Assoc **12**:1165

Yoshida K et al (1961b) Separation of Tatsumi factor from factor IX PTC, factor X, and factor VII-complex by the DEAE-cellulose column chromatography, J Nara Med Assoc **12**:1173

Yoshida T et al (1973) The production of migration inhibition factor by B and T cells of the guinea pig, J Exp Med **138**:784

Young LE (1946) The clinical significance of cold hemagglutinins, Am J Med Sci **211**:23

Young LE (1955) Hereditary spherocytosis, Am J Med **18**:486

Young LE (1951) Hereditary spherocytosis. I. Clinical, hematologic, and genetic features in 28 cases, with particular reference to the osmotic and mechanical fragility of incubated erythrocytes, Blood **6**:1073

Young LE et al (1956) Studies on spontaneous in vitro autohemolysis in hemolytic disorders, Blood **11**:977

Yount WJ et al (1970) Imbalance of gamma globulin subgroups and gene defects in patients with primary hypogammaglobulinemia, J Clin Invest **49**:1957

Yu JS et al (1971) Osteopetrosis, Arch Dis Child **46**:257

Yü T (1965) Secondary gout associated with myeloproliferative diseases, Arthritis Rheum **8**:765

Yuile CL et al (1949) Hemolytic reactions produced in dogs by transfusion of incompatible dog blood and plasma: renal aspects following whole blood transfusions, Blood **4**:1232

Yunis AA (1973) Chloramphenicol toxicity. In Girdwood RH (Ed): Blood disorders due to drugs and other agents, Amsterdam, Excerpta Medica, p 107

Yunis AA and Bloomberg GR (1964) Chloramphenicol toxicity: clinical features and pathogenesis, Prog Hematol **4**:138

Yunis AA et al (1967) Biochemical lesion in dilantin-induced erythroid aplasia, Blood **30**:587

Zachara B (1977) Synthesis of ITP and ATP and regeneration of 2,3-DPG in human erythrocytes incubated with adenosine pyruvate and inorganic phosphate, Transfusion **17**:628

Zacharski LR and Kyle RA (1967) Significance of extreme elevation of erythrocyte sedimentation rate, JAMA **202**:264

Zacharski LR and Linman JW (1969) Chronic lymphocytic leukemia versus chronic lymphosarcoma cell leukemia. Analysis of 496 cases, Am J Med **47**:75

Zacharski LR and Linman JW (1971) Lymphocytopenia: its causes and significance, Mayo Clin Proc **46**:168

Zadek I (1927) Die Polycythämien, Ergebn D Ges Med **10**:355

Zail SS et al (1964) Studies on the formation of ferritin in red cell precursors, J Clin Invest **43**:670

Zaino EC et al (1971) Gaucher's cells in thalassemia, Blood **38**:457

Zak SJ et al (1974) Hemoglobin Andrew-Minneapolis alpha 2A beta 2 144 lys → asn: a new high-oxygen-affinity mutant human hemoglobin, Blood **44**:543

Zamchek N et al (1955) Occurrence of gastric cancer among patients with pernicious anemia at the Boston City Hospital, N Engl J Med **252**:1103

Zanjani ED et al (1967) The renal erythropoietic factor. III. Enzymatic role in erythropoietin production, Proc Soc Exp Biol Med **125**:505

Zanjani ED et al (1977) Liver as the primary site of erythropoietin formation in the fetus, J Lab Clin Med **89**:640

Zannis-Hadjopoulos M et al (1977) Improved detection of β-thalassaemia carriers by a two-test method, Hum Genet **38**:315

Zarkowsky HS (1979) Heat-induced erythrocyte fragmentation in neonatal elliptocytosis, Br H Haematol **41**:515

Zarkowsky HS et al (1968) Congenital hemolytic anemia with high sodium, low potassium red cells. I. Studies of membrane permeability, N Engl J Med **278**:573

Zarkowsky HS et al (1975) A congenital haemolytic anaemia with thermal sensitivity of the erythrocyte membrane, Br J Haematol **29**:537

Zarrabi MH et al (1979) Immunologic and coagulation disorders in chlorpromazine-treated patients, Ann Intern Med **91**:194

Zawadzki ZA et al (1978) Leukemic myelomatosis (plasma cell leukemia), Am J Clin Pathol **70**:605

Zeidman I (1965) The fate of circulating tumor cells, Acta Cyto **9**:136

Zeimer R et al (1978) A noninvasive method for the evaluation of tissue iron deposition in beta-thalassemia major, J Lab Clin Med **91**:24

Zeman W and Siakotos AN (1973) The neuronal ceroidlipofuscinoses. In Hers HG and Von Hoof F (Eds): Lysosomes and storage diseases, New York, Academic Press, Inc

Zervas J et al (1974) Sideroblastic anemia treated with immunosuppressive therapy, Blood **44**:117

Zeya HI and Spitznagel JK (1969) Cationic protein-bearing granules of polymorphonuclear leukocytes: separation from enzyme rich granules, Science **163**:1069

Ziegler Z et al (1975) Post-transfusion purpura: a heterogeneous syndrome, Blood **45**:529

Zietz BH and Scott JL (1970) An inherited defect in fibrinogen polymerization: fibrinogen Los Angeles, Clin Res **18**:179

Zieve L (1958) Jaundice, hyperlipemia, and hemolytic anemia: a heretofore unrecognized syndrome associated with alcoholic fatty liver and cirrhosis, Ann Intern Med **48**:471

Zieve L and Hill E (1961) Two varieties of hemolytic anemia in cirrhosis, South Med J **54**:1347

Zieve L et al (1953) Normal limits of urinary coproporphyrin excretion determined by an improved method, J Lab Clin Med **41**:663

Zilva JF and Patston VJ (1966) Variations in serum-iron in healthy women, Lancet **1**:459

Zimmerman HJ et al (1953) Production of nucleophagocytosis by rabbit antileukocytic serum, Blood **8**:651

Zimmerman HG et al (1961) Hepatic hemosiderin deposits: incidence in 558 biopsies from patients with and without intrinsic hepatic disease, Arch Intern Med **107**:494

Zimmerman J et al (1974) Sickle crisis precipitated by exercise rhabdomyolysis in a patient with sickle cell trait: case report, Milit Med **139**:313

Zimmerman TS (1976) The coagulation mechanism and the inflammatory response. In Miescher PA and Müller-Eberhard HJ (Eds): Textbook of immunopathology, New York, Grune & Stratton, Inc

Zimmerman TS et al (1971a) Immunologic differentiation of classic hemophilia (factor VIII deficiency) and von Willebrand's disease, J Clin Invest **50**:244

Zimmerman TS et al (1971b) Detection of carriers of classic hemophilia using an immunologic assay for antihemophilic factor (factor VIII), J Clin Invest **50**:255

Zinkham WH (1963) Peripheral blood and bilirubin values in normal full-term primaquine-sensitive Negro infants: effect of vitamin K, Pediatrics **31**:983

Zinkham WH and Diamond LK (1952) In vitro erythrophagocytosis in acquired hemolytic anemia, Blood **7**:592

Zinkham WH et al (1979a) Observations on the rate and mechanism of hemolysis in individuals with hb Zürich (His E7 [63] β → arg). I. Concentrations of haptoglobin and hemopexin in the serum, Johns Hopkins Med J **144**:37

Zinkham WH et al (1979b) Observations on the rate and mechanism of hemolysis in individuals with hb Zürich (his E7 [63] β → arg). II. Thermal denaturation of hemoglobin as a cause of anemia during fever, Johns Hopkins Med J **144**:109

Zittoun R (1976) Subacute and chronic myelomonocytic leukaemia: a distinct haematological entity, Br J Haematol **32**:1

Zittoun R et al (1975) Acute myelomonocytic leukaemia: a terminal complication of paroxysmal nocturnal haemoglobinuria, Acta Haematol **53**:241

Zivkovic M and Baum J (1972) Chemotaxis of polymorphonuclear leukocytes from patients with systemic lupus erythematosus and Felty's syndrome, Immunol Commun **1**:39

Zlotnik A (1967) The plasma cell production pathway of small lymphocytes transferred to a heterologous host. In Yoffey JM (Ed): The lymphocyte in immunology and haemopoiesis, London, Edward Arnold Publishers Ltd, p 317

Zuck TF (1971) Implications of depressed antithrombin III activity associated with oral contraceptives, Surg Gynecol Obstet **133**:609

Zucker MB and Peterson J (1968) Inhibition of adenosine diphosphate-induced secondary aggregation and other platelet functions by acetylsalicylic acid ingestion, Proc Soc Exp Biol Med **127**:547

Zucker MB et al (1966) Platelet function in a patient with thrombasthenia, Blood **28**:524

Zucker S and Mielke CH (1972) Classification of thrombocytosis based on platelet function tests: correlation with hemorrhagic and thrombotic complications, J Lab Clin Med **80**:385

Zucker S et al (1970) Plasma muramidase: a study of methods and clinical applications, J Lab Clin Med **75**:83

Zucker S et al (1972) Bone marrow response to erythropoietin in polycythemia vera and chronic granulocytic leukemia, Blood **39**:341

Zucker S et al (1978) IgM inhibitors of the contact activation phase of coagulation in chlorpromazine-treated patients, Br J Haematol **40:**447

Zucker-Franklin D (1969) The ultrastructure of lymphocytes, Semin Hematol **6:**4

Zucker-Franklin D (1970) The ultrastructure of megakaryocytes and platelets. In Gordon AS (Ed): Regulation of hematopoiesis, New York, Appleton-Century-Crofts, p 1553

Zucker-Franklin D (1974) Properties of the Sézary lymphoid cell. An ultrastructural analysis, Mayo Clin Proc **49:**567

Zucker-Franklin D and Grusky G (1972) The actin and myosin filaments of human and bovine blood platelets, J Clin Invest **51:**419

Zucker-Franklin D et al (1966) The interaction of mycoplasmas with mammalian cells. II. Monocytes and lymphocytes, J Exp Med **124:**533

Zuelzer WW (1978) Childhood leukemia—a perspective, Johns Hopkins Med J **142:**115

Zuelzer WW and Bajoghli M (1964) Chronic granulocytopenia in childhood, Blood **23:**359

Zuelzer WW and Ogden FN (1946) Megaloblastic anemia in infancy: common syndrome responding specifically to folic acid therapy, Am J Dis Child **71:**211

Zuelzer WW et al (1961) Reciprocal relationship of hemoglobins A_2 and F in beta chain thalassemias, a key to genetic control of hemoglobin F, Blood **17:**393

Zuelzer WW et al (1966) Etiology and pathogenesis of acquired hemolytic anemia, Transfusion **6:**438

Zuelzer WW et al (1968) Erythrocyte pyruvate deficiency in nonspherocytic hemolytic anemia: a system of multiple genetic markers? Blood **32:**33

Index

A

A-B-H blood group substances, 496
  and Lewis antigens, 510
A-B-O blood group system, 104, 489, 491-500
  A^b group, 498
  acquired B, 497-498
  agglutinins from snails and other animals, 496
  binary code for, 522
  blood fractions, 499
    A and A_1, 498
    C, 498-499
  Bombay, 498
  cell grouping
    slide method, 904
    test tube method, 904
  chemistry of blood group substances, 496
  "cis-AB," 495
  forms of, 499
  genetics of, 491-492
  genotypes in, 491
    frequency of, 491-492
  and H substance, 498
  in hemolytic disease of newborn, 562
  in hemolytic reactions, 544-555
  inheritance of, 492
  lectins, 495
  missing isoagglutinins in, 495
  origin of isoagglutinins, 494-495
  racial distribution of, 493
  secretion of group-specific substances in saliva, 499-500
  secretors vs nonsecretors in, 499, 500
  serologic characteristics of, 500
  subgroups of A or AB, 496-497
    use of anti-A_1 serum in grouping of, 904-905
    use of group O serum in grouping of, 905
  subgroups of B, 497
  use of, in establishing parentage, 517
Abbott ADC, 500, 667
Abetalipoproteinemia, 479
  clinical aspects of, 595
  hemolysis from, 568
  laboratory findings, 595-596
  lecithin-cholesterol acyltransferase deficiency in, 569
  neutrophilia in, 673
Acanthocyte, 478-481
  in diagnosis of hemolytic disease, 580
  hemolysis of, 479-481
  with pyruvate kinase deficiency in RBC, 567
  vs schizocytes, 483

Acanthocytosis, 478-479
  vs abetalipoproteinemia, 568, 595
  effect of, on rouleau formation of erythrocytes, 352
Acarboxyprothrombin, 834
Accessory spleen, 65, 68
Acenocoumaril, 837
Acetanilid
  as cause of methemoglobinemia, 460
  sulfhemoglobinemia from, 461
Acetophenetidin, 460
Acetylphenylhydrazine, 587
Achlorhydria
  histamine-fast, from iron deficiency, 412
  with pernicious anemia, 429, 434, 443
  in pregnancy, 441
  of tropical sprue, 443
Achylia, 434
Acid-citrate-dextrose solution
  for platelet storage, 536
  for storage of coagulation factors, 536
  for storage of erythrocytes, 532, 535
  transfusion of, toxic effects from, 548
Acid mucopolysaccharide, 53
Acid phosphatase, 209, 210
  vs alkaline phosphatase, 207
  in blastoid transformation of lymphocytes, 82
  in Gaucher's disease, 4
  in leukemic reticuloendotheliosis, 725
  of lymphocytes, 76
  with lysosomal hydrolases, 36
  in Niemann-Pick disease, 41, 44
  in phagocytosis, 664
  release of, from platelet, 794
  in Sezary cells, 165
  stain for, 871-872
Acid-serum test
  in aplastic anemia, 596
  in leukemia, 596
  in myeloproliferative syndromes, 596
  in paroxysmal nocturnal hemoglobinuria, 564, 596
Acidophilic granules, 118
Aconitase, 406
Acrodermatitis enteropathica, 405
ACTH
  and alkaline phosphatase activity, 209
  effect of, on hemopoiesis, 16
  effect of, on leukocyte count, 667
  effect of, on leukocytic response, 673
  effect of, on lymphocytes, 26
  eosinophilia from, 256, 688
  erythrocyte sedimentation rate with, 356

Actinomyces infection, 673
Actomyosin, 789
Addison's disease, 16
Addisonian anemia, 417
Adenosine, 532, 535
Adenyl cyclase, 789, 790
Adjuvants
  action of, 96-98
  aluminum hydroxide, 96
  with antigens, 86
  Freund's, 96
ADP
  in causing platelets to change shape, 792
  in platelet aggregation, 793, 794, 799, 800
  platelet release of, 794
  receptors for, on platelet membrane, 788
  in storage pool disease, 804, 805, 806
ADPase, 788
Adrenal glands
  effect of, on hemopoiesis, 16
  extramedullary hemopoiesis in, 30
  myelolipoma in, 30
Adrenocortical steroid therapy
  abnormal neutrophil adherence with, 662
  effect of, on lymphoid tissue and lymphocytes, 26
Adventitial cells of Marchand, 2
Afibrinogenemia
  acquired, 843
  congenital, 818, 841-842
    platelet aggregation in, 793
  delayed wound healing in, 787
  partial thromboplastin time in, 821
Agammaglobulinemia, 98
  Bruton-type, 100
    phytohemagglutinin response to, 83
  congenital, lymphopenia in, 688
  indicated by missing isoagglutinins, 495
  lymphopenic, 101
  Swiss-type, 101
  with thymoma, 74
  treatment of, in gamma globulin, 538
  X-linked, 100
    lymphoid tissue in, 104
Agglutination, grading of, 903
Agglutinins
  of A-B-O system, 104, 492
  vs agglutinogens, 493
  cold, 911-912
    nonspecific, absorption of, 908-909
  definition of, 492
  irregular, 545
  Rh, 510

Agglutinins—cont'd
from snails and other animals, 495
Agglutinogens, 490
in A-B-O system, 500
in relation to agglutinins, 493
of erythrocytes, 492
in designating blood groups, 492, 493
M-N-S-s, 500, 501
in Rh-Hr blood group, 503
in stimulation of production of isoagglutinins,
494
Agnogenic myeloid metaplasia, 268, 705-708
from benzol or carbon tetrachloride, 696
derivation of, 700
Agranulocytic angina, 685
Agranulocytosis
acute, 685
blood transfusions in treatment of, 531
infantile genetic, 687-688
Ahaptoglobinemia, 464
Albers-Schönberg disease, 708
Albinism, 47, 818
Albumin, 89
administration of, 538
agglutinins of, 510
antifibrinolytic activity of, 841
bilirubin binding to, 469, 472
binding of, to coumarin drugs, 837
binding of, with heme, 469
copper binding to, 403
effect of, on erythrocyte sedimentation rate,
353
in formation of methemalbumin, 571
media with, for agglutination of erythrocytes,
592
for protection of cells from postmortem marrow
tissue, 222
transfusion of, in treatment of hypoproteinemia,
532
Alcoholism
abnormal neutrophil adherence to endothelium
in, 662
decreased neutrophil mobilization with, 660
haptoglobin levels in, 409
in idiopathic hemochromatosis, 397
megaloblastic anemia from folate deficiency
with, 440
stomatocytes in, 478, 568
thrombocytopenia in, 803
Alder's anomaly of leukocytes, 53
Alius-Grignaschi anomaly, 167
Alkaline phosphatase
vs acid phosphatase, 207
in chronic granulocytic leukemia, 727
in cytochemical reactions of blood cells, 207-
209
application of, in study of leukemias, 210
in granulocytes, 125
in leukemoid reaction, 711
measurement of
biochemical, 209
cytochemical, 208-209
in paroxysmal nocturnal hemoglobinuria, 727
in pernicious anemia, 438, 727
in polycythemia vera, 702
in specific granules of phagocytosis, 663
stain for, 871
Allergic reactions, 546
reaginic antibody in, 93
Allografts
neutrophils of, 167
skin, survival of, 88
Alport syndrome, 808

Altitude
effect of, on erythrocyte count, 378-379
hypoxia with increased, 391-392
Aluminum hydroxide, 96
Alymphocytosis, 101
Alymphoplasia, thymic, 688
Amato bodies, 161
ε-Aminocaproic acid, 841, 847
α-Amino-ketoadipic acid, 448
δ-Aminolevulinic acid
in acquired porphyria, 455
in biosynthesis of porphyrins, 448-449
in heme synthesis, 414, 448-449
in intermittent acute porphyria, 454
in lead intoxication, 455
quantitative assay of, 879, 880
calculation, 880
isolation of, 878
method, 879-880
normal values, 880
reagents for, 879-880
in variegate porphyria, 454
δ-Aminolevulinic acid synthetase, 448
effect of heme on, 454
in hepatic porphyria, 454
increase in, with cirrhosis, 455
Aminopterin, 419
Aminopyrine, 252
Ammonia intoxication, 549
Amyloidosis
with factor X deficiency, 831
primary, 226
secondary, 322
Amylophagia, 397
American Blood Commission, 528
Analgesia, local, 212
Anaphylactoid purpura, 852
Anaphylactoid reactions, 548
Anaphylatoxins, 556, 557, 559
Anaphylaxis, 665
Androgens
effect of, on 2,3-DPG, 392
effect of, on erythropoiesis, 16
effect of, on hemopoietic microenvironment,
691
effect of, on reticulocytes, hemoglobin, and
hematocrit, 17
in treatment of aplastic anemia, 697
Anemia
in acute lymphocytic leukemia, 724
in acute monocytic leukemia, 724
addisonian, 417
antiglobulin-positive immunohemolytic, 559
aplastic; see Aplastic anemia
aregenerative, 530
Biermer's, 417
causes of, 1, 392
of chronic disease, 531
in chronic granulocytic leukemia, 727
of chronic renal insufficiency, 21
classification of, 392-394
etiologic, 392-394
morphologic, 392
congenital dyserythropoietic, 569
Cooley's, 68
diagnosis of, 388
laboratory, 392
due to decreased erythrocyte survival, 550-
657
due to deficiency of vitamin B$_{12}$ or folic acid,
426-429
classification, 426-427
concept of megaloblastic dyspoiesis, 427-
429

Anemia—cont'd
due to deficiency of vitamin B$_{12}$ or folic acid—
cont'd
macrocytosis, 427
due to increased plasma volume, 392, 394
effect of, on erythropoietin production, 21
effect of, on stimulation of erythropoietin, 21
erythrocyte sedimentation rate with, 353
familial hypoplastic, of childhood, 698
fetal, 8
in Gaucher's disease, 41
in Hand-Schüller-Christian syndrome, 58
hemolytic; see Hemolytic anemia
hypochromic
with Gaucher's disease, 39, 41
and microcytic
calculation of hematocrit, 360
with chronic hemorrhage, 240
in steatorrheas, 443
in thalassemia, 650
from hypothyroidism, 16
increase of 2,3-DPG in, 532, 535
as an indication for blood transfusion, 530-531
iron-deficiency; see Iron-deficiency anemias
isoantibody immunohemolytic, 559
in Letterer-Siwe disease, 58
macrocytic, 392
from benzol, 696
in infancy, 441
MCH of, 380
morphologic classification of, 426, 427
normoblastic hyperplasia with, 246, 247
pernicious; see Pernicious anemia
in pregnancy, 441
in pregnancy with sickle cell anemia, 274,
275
in steatorrheas, 443
treatment of, 417
tropical, 272
Mediterranean, 68
megaloblastic; see Megaloblastic anemia
microcytic, 392
hypochromic
calculation of hematocrit for, 360
with chronic hemorrhage, 240
in steatorrheas, 443
in thalassemia, 650
in myeloproliferative syndromes, 700
familial, 708
myelofibrosis, 706
osteopetrosis, 708
normocytic, 392
normochromic, 246
in Gaucher's disease, 41
pathogenesis of, 392-394
pernicious; see Pernicious anemia
from pituitary dysfunction, 16
in pregnancy, 274, 275, 394, 441
with red cell aplasia, 698, 699
refractory, 690
with excess blasts, 729
reticulocyte maturation rate in, 23, 24
of the Rietto-Greppi-Micheli type, 603
sickle cell; see Sickle cell anemia
sideroblastic; see Sideroblastic anemia
symptoms of, 392
transferrin deficiency; see Transferrin, deficiency of, anemia in
Anemia infantum pseudoleukemica, 603
Anemia perniciosiforme constituzionale infantile,
698
Angina pectoris, 356
Angioimmunoblastic lymphadenopathy, 102
Angiomatous lymphoid hamartoma, 102

Aniline dyes and derivatives
  as cause of methemoglobinemia, 460
  hemolysis from, 563
Anisindione, 837
Anisocytosis, 379, 476
  effect of, on rouleau formation of erythrocytes, 352
  in hemoglobinopathies, 623
  in hereditary spherocytosis, 593
  in iron-deficiency anemias, 406, 407
  in pernicious anemia, 432
  in sickle cell anemia, 640
  in thalassemia, 650
Anthracosis, 229, 230
Antibiotics
  in bone marrow suppression, 697
  in vitamin K deficiency, 836
Antibodies
  as agglutinins, 492
    complete, 592
  antierythrocyte
    in disseminated intravascular coagulation, 844
    in immunogenetics, 489, 490
  antileukocyte, 547, 548
  antiplatelet, 537, 538
    in diffuse intravascular coagulation, 844
    in idiopathic thrombocytopenic purpura, 531, 801, 802
    reaction of, 547
  in autoimmune diseases, 69
  in autoimmune hemolytic anemia, 559-560, 599
  blocking, 510, 561
  cells producing, 63
  cold-acting, erythrocytic, 560, 561
  D-L, 563
  detection of
    in albumin media, 592
    in direct antiglobulin test, 589-590
    elution technics, 907-908
      heat elution method, 907-908
      Rubin ether method, 908
      testing eluate in ABO hemolytic disease, 908
      testing eluate for unknown antibody, 908
    with enzyme-treated erythrocytes, 592
    in induced antiglobulin test, 591
  in diagnosis of humoral deficiency, 104
  in fixation of complement, 558
  formation and production of
    by B-lymphocytes, 83
    lymph nodes in, 105
    in lymphoid follicles, 79
    in lymphoid nodules, 79
    in spleen, 63
    transfer of antigen from macrophage to lymphocyte in, 83
  Forssman, 678
  free homologous, in cord serum, demonstration of, 911
  in hemolytic anemia, 592
    blood transfusion for, 530
    properties of, 561
    and thrombocytopenic purpura, 577
  to hepatitis antigens, 542
  heterophil, 678-679
    absorption patterns for, 678
    in infectious mononucleosis, 676, 678-679
    Monospot test of, 912
    presumptive test of, 679
  identification of, 907
    cells for, 903
  in immediate hypersensitivity reactions, 88

Antibodies—cont'd
  in immune hemolysis, 556
  incomplete, 510
  inducement of, 74
  against intrinsic factor, 429, 439
    binding, 430
    blocking, 430
  irregular
    screening for, 906-907
    titration of, 909-910
  in lupus erythematosus, 680, 683-684
  in paroxysmal cold hemoglobinuria, 563
  reaginic, in allergic reactions, 93
  Rh, 510
  warm-acting, erythrocytic, 560, 561
Anticoagulants
  bishydroxycoumarin, 837
    effect of, on factor IX, 785
    isolation of, 775
    in treatment of thrombotic disease, 836
  bleeding time with, 797
  in determination of hematocrit, 357
  for disseminated intravascular coagulation, 847
  effect of
    on erythrocyte size and sedimentation rate, 354
    on partial thromboplastin time, 821
  laboratory control of, 856-857
  lupus, 682, 820, 836
    detection of, 920
    in hemophilia, 827
  oral, 836-839
    coumarin derivatives, 837
    derivatives of indandione, 837
    effect of, on vitamin K–dependent coagulation factors, 833
    therapy of
      factors affecting, 837-839
      laboratory control of, 838
  pathologic, against thrombin, factors V and X, 833
  in reducing tumor metastases, 787
  screening, 920
  for storage of coagulation factors, 536
  use of, in obtaining blood specimen, 862
Anticonvulsant drugs
  inducing folate malabsorption, 441
  lupus activity potential of, 683
Antifolate drugs, 418, 419
Antigens
  Australian, 541
  in autoimmune hemolysis, 559, 560
  binding of, to IgE, 665
  in delayed hypersensitivity reactions, 88
    skin tests for, 103
  of erythrocyte membrane, 555
    as agglutinogens, 492
    location of, 489
    reaction of, to antibodies, 490
  Forssman, 678, 679
  hepatitis A, 541, 542
  hepatitis B, 541, 542
  hepatitis Be, 542
  histocompatibility, 89
  HLA, of granulocyte, 531
  in immune hemolysis, 556
  macrophage in phagocytosis of, 86
  nonspecific, in blastoid transformation of lymphocyte, 82
  processing of, 86
  in stimulation of transfer factor release, 85-86
  of transplantation reaction, 89
Antiglobulin test, 589-591

Antiglobulin test—cont'd
  for autoimmune hemolytic anemia, 599
  direct, 589-590, 906
    nature of antiglobulin serum, 589-590
    positive, investigation of, 909
    principle of, 589
    results of, in hemolytic anemia, 590
    values and limitations, 590
  for drug-related hemolysis, 562, 563
  for hemolysis with glucose-6-phosphate dehydrogenase deficiency, 566
  in hereditary elliptocytosis, 595
  indirect, 590-591
  in isoimmune hemolytic disease, 600-601
  for paroxysmal cold hemoglobinuria, 563, 600
  for paroxysmal nocturnal hemoglobinuria, 596
  of patients with cardiac surgery, 569
  for penicillin immunohemolysis, 562
Antihemophilic factor, 784
Antihemophilic globulin, 537
Antilymphocyte globulin, 82
Antilymphocyte serum, 88
  in cellular immunity, 88
  production of, 88
  survival of skin allograft, 88
Antimetabolites, 88
Antinuclear antibody, 680, 683-684
Antinuclear antibody test
  fluorescent, 683, 684
    qualitative method, 913-915
    quantitative method, 915
Antithrombins, 774, 779
Antithrombin I, 820
Antithrombin III, 820
  heparin effect on, 855
  in inhibition of thrombin, 783
  in prethrombotic state, 854, 855
  tests of, 934-935
    by radial immunodiffusion, 935
    by rocket electroimmunodiffusion, 934-935
    by thrombin neutralization, 934
Antithromboplastins, 779
Antitrypsin, 855
Aortic stenosis, 569
Aplasia, red cell; see Red cell aplasia
Aplastic anemia, 690-698
  acquired
    from chemical agents, 695-697
    from ionizing radiation, 692-695
      acute radiation syndrome, 694-695
      chronic exposure to thorium radiation, 694
      chronic exposure to x-radiation, 693-694
      hemopoietic effects of radiation injury, 692
      radiation injury from isotopes, 694
      sensitivity of various tissues, 692
      types of, 692
    laboratory findings, 697-698
  bone marrow with, 213
  bone marrow transplant for cellular recolonization, 6
  classification of, 691
  definition of, 690
  effect of, on erythropoietin production, 21
  familial, 690, 698
  Fanconi type, 690
  from glue sniffing, 696
  from gold salts, 696
  hemoglobin F in, 633
  idiopathic, 698
  lymphocyte-mediated suppression of hemopoiesis in, 25

Aplastic anemia—cont'd
  with paroxysmal nocturnal hemoglobinuria, 596
  pathogenesis of, 690-692
  relationship of, with other blood disorders, 698
  reticulocyte count in, 407, 487
  and viral hepatitis, 698
Apoceruloplasmin, 403
Apoferritin, 396
Appendix, 79, 770
  infection of, 356
Apronalide, 802
APTT; *see* Partial thromboplastin time, activated
Arachidonic acid, 790
Arsenicals, 696
Arsine, 563
Arthritis
  pyogenic, 356
  rheumatoid
    deficient neutrophil chemotaxis in, 663
    erythrocyte sedimentation rate, 356
    haptoglobin levels with, 469
    lupus erythematosus and, 682
    macroglobulinemia secondary to, 748, 751
    splenomegaly with, 69
Aryl sulfatase, 82
Ascorbate test, 587
Ascorbic acid
  effect of, on dietary vitamin B$_{12}$, 425
  effect of, on iron absorption, 397
  in treatment of methemoglobinemia, 458, 460
Aspiration, bone marrow
  as technic for obtaining tissue
    choice of needles, 212, 213
    local analgesia for, 212
    sites for, 212-220
      ileum, 214-216, 218
      rib, 219
      sternum, 213-214
      for study, 219-220
      tibial, 218-219
      vertebral, 216-218
Aspirin
  and abnormal neutrophil adherence to endothelium, 662
  and blood loss with iron deficiency, 401
  effect of, on bleeding time, 797
  effect of, on PHA-induced lymphoblast transformation, 83
  effect of, on platelet function, 538, 790, 792, 818
  effect of, in relation to dose, 790
  sensitivity to, test of, 676
Asplenia, 65
Asthma, bronchial
  in allergic reaction, 546
  eosinophilia in, 256, 674
Ataxia-telangiectasia, 83
  immunodeficiency with, 101
  IgA and IgE in, 94
Atherosclerosis, 790, 791
Athrobia, essential, 804
Athrombin-K; *see* Warfarin sodium
ATP, for platelet activity, 789, 790
ATPase
  of erythrocyte membrane, 555, 556
  of platelet membrane, 788
Atransferremia, 410, 415
Auer bodies, 119, 138, 157, 159, 296-297
  in acute granulocytic leukemia, 724
  in leukemic cells, 192
  with multiple myeloma, 192
  in myelomonoblast, 280, 281

Auer bodies—cont'd
  ultrastructure of, 192, 195
Auer rods, 157, 206
Australian antigen, 541
Autoerythrocyte sensitization, 852
Autohemolysis
  in abetalipoproteinemia, 595
  in diagnosis of hemolytic disease, 586-587
  in hereditary elliptocytosis, 595
  in hereditary spherocytosis, 594
  test of, 884, 885
Autoimmune disease
  immunoglobulin deficiency with, 102
  pernicious anemia with, 429
  spleen in, 69-71
Autoimmune hemolysis, 559-560
Autoimmune hemolytic anemia, 559
  antiglobulin test of, 589, 590
  autohemolysis in, 587
  with chronic lymphocytic leukemia, 726
  cold antibody type, 599
  drug-induced type, 599
  etiology and pathogenesis of, 597-599
  fluctuations in, 575, 579
  with non-Hodgkin's lymphoma, 759
  thrombocytopenia in, 577
  treatment of, 599
  warm antibody type, 599
Autophagy, 37
Autosplenectomy, 65
Azaserine, 419
Azauridine, 419
Azotemia
  in hemolytic reactions, 545, 546
  leukemoid reaction associated with, 254, 255
Azurophilic dust, 137
Azurophilic granules, 119, 182
  and Auer bodies, 157
  esterases associated with, 209
  in lymphocytes, 75, 137
  of megakaryocyte, 148
  of myelocyte, 125
  myeloperoxidase of, 206
  in phagocytosis, 663
  of progranulocyte, 125
  of promegakaryocyte, 148
  of reticulum cell, 125

B

B-lymphocytes
  as bursa-dependent cells, 75
  defect of, in Bruton-type agammaglobulinemia, 100
  dormant, 83
  function of, 86
  identification of, 86
  in immunoblastic lymphadenopathy, 102
  location of, in lymph nodes, 105
  of lymphoid nodules, 79
  rosette formation by, 86
  with severe combined immunodeficiency, 101
  stimulated by nonspecific activator, 83
  stimulated by specific antigens, 83
  stimulation of antibody secretion by, 83
  surface receptors of, 86
  villous surface of, 84
Bacteria
  infection by, with neutrophilic leukocytosis, 673
  killing of, 663
  phagocytosis of, 36
Baker's method in identification of lipids, 207
Barr body, 175
Bartler's syndrome, 21

Bartonella, 582
Basophil, 133
  chemotactic response of, 660, 665
  in chronic granulocytic leukemia, 727
  as diploid cells, 175
  effect of kallikrein on, 660
  granules of, 36, 118, 125, 131, 182, 665, 667
  IgE attachment to, 94, 665
  inclusions in, 167
  in mucopolysaccharidoses, 55, 58
  periodic acid-Schiff reaction, 207
  peroxidase reaction, 206
  in phagocytosis, 665
  in polycythemia vera, 702
  sudanophilic staining of, 207
  ultrastructure of, 185, 191
  Wright-Giemsa stain of, 868
Basophil count, 866
Basophilia
  in cell maturation, 118
  diffuse, 486
  in hemoglobinopathies, 623
  punctate, 486
Bence Jones proteins
  definition of, 91-93
  in immunoblastic lymphadenopathy, 102
  in multiple myeloma, 91, 96, 733, 744, 746
Benzene, 720
Benzol
  chronic red cell hypoplasia from, 699
  as myelotoxic agent, 695-696
Benzoquinone acetic acid, 460
Bernard-Soulier syndrome, 807-808
  platelets in, 797
Biopsy
  obtaining marrow tissue by, 211
  of spleen, 71
    indications and contraindications, 71
    normal and abnormal splenograms, 72
    puncture technic, 71-72
    site of puncture, 71
    trephine, 220-221
Bile, 403
Bile ducts, 471
Bile pigments
  excretion of
    fluctuations in, 572
    related to total hemoglobin, 572
  metabolism of, 570-574
  source of, 572
Bilirubin
  clearance of, in liver, 574
  conjugation of, by newborn, 471-472
  formation of, 469-471, 574
  from hemoglobin breakdown, 572
  in hereditary spherocytosis, 594
  increases in; *see* Hyperbilirubinemia
  in isoimmune hemolytic disease, 600
  metabolism of, 713
  partition of, 574
  regulation of, 574
  serum concentration of, 469, 574
  in thalassemia, 650
  unconjugated, 471
Bilirubin glucuronide, 469
Bilirubinemia, hereditary nonhemolytic, 473
Biliverdin, 469
Biliverdin reductase, 469
Bishydroxycoumarin
  effect of, on factor IX, 785
  isolation of, 775
  in treatment of thrombotic disease, 836, 837
Bismuth, 699
Blastogenic factor, 85, 86

Blastoid cells, 83
Blastoid transformation of lymphocytes, 82-83
  in diagnosis of cellular immunity deficiency, 103-104
Bleeding; *see also* Hemorrhage
  anemia from, 412
  detection of, 411-412
  gastrointestinal, 411, 412
  in Gaucher's disease, 41
  iron loss in, 401
  from Meckel's diverticulum, 411
  menorrhagia, 411
Bleeding time, 791, 797, 856
  in Bernard-Soulier syndrome, 807
  vs coagulation time, 774
  definition of, 794
  effect of aspirin on, 797
  effect of platelet count on, 531
  in evaluation of thromboplastinogenesis, 821
  Ivy, 915-916
  in patients on anticoagulant therapy, 797
  in platelet functional disorders, 797
  prolonged, 779
  in thrombasthenia, 804
  in thrombocytopenic states, 797
  in von Willebrand's disease, 797
Blind loop syndrome, 439
Blister cells, 640
Blood, 350-366
  cadaver, 539
  changes in drawn, 350-351
  composition of, 350
  donation of, 527, 528
    incidence of hepatitis with, 543
  erythrocyte mass of, 362-363
  establishment of, in fetus, 8
  fibrinolytic, 539
  hematocrit; *see* Hematocrit
  plasma volume of, 362-363
  polycythemia vera, 702
  rheology and viscosity of, 351
  sedimentation rate of, 351-357
    clinical correlation, 355-357
    factors affecting, 352-355
      aggregation of erythrocytes, 352
      anticoagulant used, 354
      caliber and length of tube, 354
      changes in plasma composition, 352-353
      delay in performing test, 355
      number of erythrocytes, 353-354
      number of leukocytes, 354
      position of tube, 354
      size of erythrocytes, 354
  stored, in blood banking, 532-537
    chemical changes in, 533
    coagulation factors, 536-537
      factor V and VII, 536
      factor VIII, 537
      factor IX, 537
      factor X, 537
      factor XI, 537
      factor XII, 537
      factor XIII, 537
      fibrinogen, 536-537
      prothrombin, 536
    erythrocytes, 532-535
    leukocytes, 535-536
    platelets, 536
  study of; *see* Hematology
  venous, 357
  viscosity of, 351
    vs hematocrit, 361-362
  whole
    measurement of, 862-867

Blood—cont'd
  whole—cont'd
    measurement of—cont'd
      basophil count, absolute, 866
      eosinophil count, circulating, 866
      erythrocyte count, 863-864
      erythrocyte indices, 867
      hemocytometer, 862-863, 864
      leukocyte count, 863-864
      microhematocrit, 867
      platelet count, 864-865
      reticulocyte count, 865
      sedimentation rate, 867
    transfusion of, 537
      for factor V deficiency, 536
      for hypoprothrombinemia, 536
      for shock, 531, 532
      in treatment of hemorrhage, 530
Blood cells and bone marrow cells, 350
  abnormal forms in, 157-173
  Auer bodies in, 157, 159
  characteristics of, 121
  chromosomal content of, 173-174
  constitutional hypersegmentation of neutrophils, 167
  counts of
    Coulter cell counter, 371-372
    Hemac laser cell counter, 372-373
    hemocytometer, 370-371
    successive, significance of, 373-374
      with electronic cell counts, 374
      with hemocytometer counts, 373-374
  cystine crystals in, 167
  cytochemically abnormal neutrophils and eosinophils, 167
  cytochemistry of, 206-210
    acid phosphatase, 209
    alkaline phosphatase, 207-209
    application of, to study of leukemia, 210
    esterases, 209-210
    glycogen, 207
    lipids, 207
    peroxidase, 206
  derivation of, 2, 3-4
  distribution of, 13
    on centrifugation, 362
  Döhle bodies in, 161-162
  and endothelial cells, 169
  erythroblast, 8
  granulocyte; *see* Granulocytes
  hemocytoblasts, 6
  hemohistioblasts, 6
  homeostasis of, 14
  and Jordans' anomaly in progressive muscular dystrophy, 167
  leukocyte inclusions in, 167
  leukocytes; *see* Leukocytes
  lymphoblast, 131, 134
  lymphocyte; *see* Lymphocytes
  lymphoidocytes, 6
  maturation of, 117-119
    abnormal, 118-119
    cytoplasmic differentiation, 117-118
    hiatus leukemicus in, 119
    multinuclearity in, 119
    nuclear, 119
    size in, 118, 119
  May-Hegglin anomaly in, 161-162
  megakaryoblast; *see* Megakaryoblast
  megakaryocyte; *see* Megakaryocyte
  megaloblast; *see* Megaloblast
  metamyelocyte and juvenile, 125, 129, 131
  monoblast; *see* Monoblast
  monocyte; *see* Monocyte

Blood cells and bone marrow cells—cont'd
  morphology of, observation of, 179-211
    cytochemical methods, 206-210
    electron microscopy, 181-206
      general considerations, 181
      ultrastructure of abnormal cells, 192-205
      ultrastructure of normal cells, 181-192
    phase contrast microscopy, 180-181
      general considerations, 180-181
      time-lapse photography, 181
    supravital methods, 179-180
      advantages of, 180
      general considerations, 179-180
      plus phase contrast, 180
      technical considerations, 180
  myeloblast, 125, 126
  myelocyte, 125, 128
  nomenclature of, 119, 120
  normal values of, 218, 219
  normoblasts; *see* Normoblasts
  Pelger-Huët anomaly in, 157, 160-161
  phagocytic cells in peripheral blood, 170
  with phagocytosis in bone marrow, 170-173
  plasmablast, 148, 154
  plasmacyte, 156, 157
  production and maintenance of, 3
  progranulocyte, 125, 127
  prolymphocyte, 131, 135
  promegakaryocyte, 148, 152
  promegaloblast, 142, 146
  promonoblast, 137, 141, 142
  promonocyte, 137, 139
  proplasmacyte, 148, 155
  release of, 32-34
  reticulum cell, 119-125
  sequestration and destruction of, 64
  sex chromatin of, 179
  in Sezary's syndrome, 162-165
  toxic granulation in, 157, 158
  tumor cells in peripheral blood, 169-170
  ultrastructure of, 181-205
    abnormal, 192-205
    normal, 182-192
  virocytes and, 165-167
Blood chimera, 495
Blood factors, 490
  A, 494, 498
  C, 498-499
  D$_i$, 513
  definition of, 503
  H, 494
  He, 501
  Hu, 501
  Hr, 503
  hr, 503
  I, 494
  Js, 512
  Kell, 512
  Le, 494
  low vs high incidence, 514
  M, 500, 501
  N, 500, 501
  P, 501-502
  Rh, 502, 503, 504, 505, 508
  Tj, 502
  U, 500
  Vw, 501
Blood groups
  A
    agglutinins of, 492
    among American Indians, 490
    inheritance of, 492, 494
    subgroups of, 496-497, 498
    inheritance of, 492, 494

Blood groups—cont'd
A—cont'd
serologic reactions of, 497
A^b, 498
A$_{el}$, 495
A$_{hei}$, 495
AB, 492
A-B-O; see A-B-O blood group system
B
acquired, 497-498
agglutinin of, 492
subgroups of, 492, 497
Bombay, 498
C-D-E, 505-508
cis-AB, 495
medicolegal application of, 494
Diego, 513
distribution of, 490
Duffy, 512-513
in establishing parentage, 520
establishment of, time, 494
in establishment of parentage, 519-520
genes of, notation of, 491
HLA, 521
I-i, 513
Kell, 512
in establishment of parentage, 520
Kidd, 513
in establishment of parentage, 520
Lewis, 510-511
Lutheran, 511-512
M-N-S-s, 500, 501
in establishment of parentage, 519-520
inheritance of, 501
medicolegal application of, 500
variants of, 500-501
O, 490, 498
P, 501, 502
phylogenetic evolution of, 490
Rh, 509
in establishment of parentage, 517-519
Rh-Hr
basic genetics and serology of, 502-505
vs C-D-E nomenclature, 505-508
substances of, chemistry of, 496
Xg, sex-linked, 513-514
Blood islands, 6
Blood Labeling Act, 527
Blood smear, 575
preparation of, 867-868
materials, 867
method, 867-868
Blood specimen, obtaining of, 860-862
capillary, 861-862
use of anticoagulants, 862
EDTA salts, 862
sodium citrate, 862
venous, 860-861
external jugular puncture, 861
femoral puncture, 861
internal jugular puncture, 861
longitudinal sinus puncture, 861
venipuncture, 860-861
Blood tests, 517-519
Blood transfusion; see Transfusion, blood
Blood volume, 362-363
in differential diagnosis of polycythemia, 705
effect of altitude on, 379
effect of, on hematocrit, 360, 361
excessive, in transfusion, 549
increase of, with polycythemia vera, 702
increase of, with pregnancy, 356
loss of, in hemorrhage, 530
loss of, in shock, 532

Blood volume—cont'd
volume of erythrocytes per, 357
Boeck's sarcoid, 256
Bohr effect, 389, 458, 607
Bombay blood group, 498
Bone
destruction of
in eosinophilic granuloma, 58
in Gaucher's disease, 39, 41
in Hand-Schüller-Christian disease, 58
marrow-containing, 222
Bone marrow, 211-349
abnormalities present in, 227
activity of, in compensation for increased RBC
destruction, 552
amegakaryocytosis of, 324-325
aplasia of, 531
aplastic, 248, 249, 250, 251
in aplastic anemia, 690, 697, 698
biopsy of, indications for, 229
blood transfusion into, 540
effect of, 530
bronchogenic carcinoma metastatic to, 338-
339
carcinoma of
mast cells with, 226
normoblastosis associated with, 342-343
cells of; see Blood cells and bone marrow
cells
cellularity of, estimation of, 229
circulation of lymphocytes from, to thymus,
81
in clearance of hemoglobin-haptoglobin complex, 571
in congenital erythropoietic porphyria, 451
depression of, drugs implicated in, 696
destruction of, 4
in diagnosis of Hodgkin's disease, 770
distribution of, by weight, 222
effect of erythropoietin on, 21
effect of thorium radiation on, 694
embolism of, 29
endothelial sinusoidal cells of, 2
in eosinophilic leukemia, 258, 259
in eosinophilic leukocytosis, 262, 263
in erythremic myelosis, 304-305
in erytholeukemia, 306-307
examination of, 218, 219
fatty, 222, 552
following irradiation, 248
in fibroplastic parietal endocarditis, 260, 261
with granuloma, 220
hemopoiesis in, 10, 29, 211
Hodgkin's disease involving, 326-327
hyperplasia of, erythroid
with chronic hemorrhage, 577
in compensation for erythroid destruction,
575
in hereditary spherocytosis, 594
with increased erythropoietic need, 552
normoblasts with, 580
in sickle cell anemia, 639-640
in hyperplasia of eosinophil series associated
with sarcoidosis, 256, 257
in hyperplasia of myeloid series secondary to
infection, 236, 237
hyperplastic with pancytopenia and megaloblastosis, 252, 253
hypoplasia of, 220, 239
anemia with leukopenia in, 576
differential cell count, 238
history and exam, 238
laboratory data, 238

Bone marrow—cont'd
hypoplasia, erythroid, in aplastic type of hemolytic crisis, 576
in infectious mononucleosis, 346-347
in inflammatory reaction, 659
in iron-deficiency anemias, 408
iron storage in, 400
in leukemia
lymphocytic, acute
case study of, 308-311
congenital, 302-303
lymphocytic, chronic, 314-315
with terminal acute exacerbation, 312-
313
monocytic, 278, 279
myelocytic, acute, 292, 293
micromyeloblastic, 296-297
with retrobulbar leukemic tumor, 294-
295
myelocytic, chronic, 290
myelomonocytic, acute, 280, 281, 282, 283,
284, 285
myelomonocytic, chronic, 286, 287, 288,
289
promyelocytic, acute, 300
in leukemoid reactions, 254, 255
eosinophilic, 264, 265, 711
lymphoma of
case study of, 332-335
differential cell count, 332
history and physical examination, 332
laboratory data, 332
non-Hodgkin's, 328-331
in lymphomyeloid complex, 74
in lysosomal storage diseases, 38
in macroglobulinemia, 747
mass of, 222
megaloblastic
in macrocytic anemia of pregnancy with sickle cell disease, 274, 275
in pernicious anemia, 270, 271
in tropical macrocytic anemia, 272, 273
metastatic tumor to, 340-341
miliary tuberculosis involving, 348-349
in multiple myeloma, 316-323, 733
in myeloproliferative syndrome, 220, 268, 269,
700
necrosis of, 229
neuroblastoma metastatic to, 344-345
in neutropenia, 685
normal, 220, 222-226
derivation from, 222-223
differential count of, 234
laboratory data on, 234
smears of, 235
in normoblastic hyperplasia
associated with acute hemolytic crisis of sickle cell anemia, 244, 245
associated with iron-deficiency anemia, 242,
243
associated with macrocytic anemia of liver
disease, 246, 247
due to chronic hemorrhage, 240, 241
obtaining, by aspiration, 212
local analgesia for, 212
sites for, 212-220
ilium, 214-216, 218
rib, 219
sternum, 213-214
for study, 219-220
tibial, 218-219
vertebral, 216-218
obtaining, by biopsy, 211
trephine, 220-221

Bone marrow—cont'd
 obtaining, technics for, 212
 as an organ of reticuloendothelial system, 36
 in pernicious anemia, 434-436
 in phagocytosis of hemoglobin, 469
 in polycythemia vera, 266, 267, 701, 702, 705
 postmortem, 222
 qualitative abnormalities, 226-229
 quantitative abnormalities, 229
 in radium poisoning, 694
 in red cell aplasia, 698
 red vs fatty, 11
 with severe combined immunodeficiency, 101
 in sickle cell anemia, 636, 639-640
 with sideroblastic anemia, 414
 studies on, 212
  preparation of tissue, 217, 219-220
 in thalassemia, 650
 in thrombocytopenia, 803
  idiopathic, 801
  with mesenchymal stomach tumor, 326-327
 in thymoma, 100
 transplantation of, 690, 691, 692
 weight of, 222
 yellow vs red, 222
Bone marrow smear
 nonhemoglobin storage iron in, 874
 Wright-Giemsa stain for, 869
Bone marrow spaces, 222
Brain damage
 in Gaucher's disease, 41
 in Niemann-Pick disease, 43-44
Breast, carcinoma of, 228
Bromelin, 592
Bronchi, lymphoid tissue of, 105
Brucellosis, 124, 544
Bruton-type agammaglobulinemia, 100
 phytohemagglutinin response in, 83
Buhot's cells, 55
Burkitt's lymphoma, 676, 718, 723, 753-759, 770
 lymphocytes of, 82
Burr cells, 483, 595
Bursa of Fabricius, 79
 excision of, 74, 75
Buttock cells, 726

C

Cl, 557, 558, 855
C1a, 556, 557
C1q, 557, 563
C1r, 557
 deficiency of, 661
C1s, 557
C2, 557
 deficiency of, 661
 in lupus erythematosus, 681
C2a, 556, 557
C2b, 557
C3, 559
 in chemotaxis, 665
 deficiency of, 661
  with defective opsonization, 664
 in lupus erythematosus, 681
 as opsonins, 663
 in paroxysmal nocturnal hemoglobinuria, 563, 564
 proactivator, 558-559
C3a, 556, 557, 559
 chemotactic activity of, 660
  basophilic, 660
  eosinophilic, 660
C3d, 589

C4, 557
C4a, 557
C4b, 556, 557
C4,2, 557
C4,2,3, 557, 558
C5, 557, 558, 559
 in chemotaxis, 665
 deficiency of, 661
  with defective opsonization, 664
 as opsonins, 663
C5,6,7, 556
 in chemotaxis, 660, 665
C5a, 556, 557, 559
 in chemotaxis, 660
 inactivation of, 660
C5b, 557
C5b,6,7, 557
C5b,6,7,8,9, 557
C6, 557
C7, 557
C8, 557
C9, 557
C-D-E blood group system, 505-508
Cabot rings, 488
 in erythrocytes with pernicious anemia, 432, 435
Cadaver blood, 539
Calcium
 in activation of factor XIII, 786
 in conversion of prothrombin to thrombin, 782, 833
 effect of, on fibrin, 840
 effect of, on thrombasthenia, 789
 in multiple myeloma, 746
 in platelet adhesion to glass, 792
 in platelet aggregation, 792
 release of, from platelet, 794
 role of, in coagulation, 774
  in classic theory, 778
 transport of, across erythrocyte membrane, 556
Cancer; see also Carcinoma; Neoplasms
 chemotherapy for
  antifolates in, 419
  sideroblastic anemia from, 414
 immunology of, 89
 and tumor cells in peripheral blood, 169, 170
 of uterus, blood loss from, 413
Capillary blood, obtaining, 861-862
Carbon dioxide
 effect of, on affinity of hemoglobin for oxygen, 390
 transport of, 456
Carbon monoxide, 469
Carbonic acid, 456
Carbonic anhydrase, 456
Carboxyhemoglobin
 concentration of, for cyanosis, 456
 with erythrocytosis, 705
 formation of, 456
 hypoxia from, 456
 measurement of, 875
 preparation of, for spectroscopy, 876
 spectroscopic identification of, 456, 461, 462, 464, 876-877
Carcinoma
 blood loss from, 530
 of bone marrow, 226
 of breast, 228
 disseminated intravascular coagulation secondary to, 845
 erythrocyte sedimentation rate with, 357
 of liver, 356
 of lung, 83

Carcinoma—cont'd
 metastatic to bone marrow, 338-339
  case studies of, 342-343
  with monoclonal immunoglobulinopathy, 748
 of prostate, 228
  case study of, 340-341
 of stomach, 429
Catalase, 406, 447, 448
 in peroxisomes, 37
Celiac disease, 443
 effect of, on iron absorption, 397
 hypocupremia, 404
Celite test, 798
Cell, 1, 11
 blood and bone marrow; see Blood cells and bone marrow cells
 cycle of, 11
 death and aging of, 37, 38
Cell stimulatory factor, 85, 86
Cellular immunity, 88-89
 antilymphocytic serum in, 88
 with ataxia-telangiectasia, 101
 in cancer immunology, 89
 delayed hypersensitivity reaction, 88
 lymphocytes in, 74, 85
 in pregnancy, 89
 in severe combined immunodeficiency, 101
 with thymic hypoplasia, 100
 with thymoma, 100
 transplantation reactions, 88-89
Cellular immunity deficiencies
 laboratory diagnosis of, 103-104
  by evaluation of lymphocyte transformation, 103-104
  by hematologic data, 103
  by lymph node exam, 103
  by measurement of complement, 104
  by presence or absence of thymus, 104
  by release of migration inhibition factor, 103-104
  by skin tests for delayed hypersensitivity reaction, 103
Centrifugation
 in determination of hematocrit, 357-359
 distribution of blood cells on, 362
Centrosome, 181
Cephalin, 795
Ceramide, 39
Ceramide glucose, 39
Ceramide glucosyl, 39
Ceramide lactoside, 39
Cerebroside of Gaucher cell, 39, 192
Ceroid, 43, 44, 45
Ceroid lipofuscinosis, 167
Ceroid storage disease, 45
Ceruloplasmin, 403-404
 quantification of, 900
Chalones, 25
Chediak-Higashi syndrome, 36-37, 45-51
 ADP in platelets with, 806
 delayed bacterial killing in, 664
 differential diagnosis of, 45
 granulocytes in, 662
 thrombocytopenia in, 804
Chemotaxis, 660
 defective, 662-663
  and random motility, 660-662
   abnormalities of the kinin-generating system, 661
   decreased cell-derived products, 662
   deficiencies of the complement system, 661
   inhibition of chemotactic factors, 661-662

Chemotaxis—cont'd
  regulation of, 660
Chimera, blood, 495
Chloramphenicol
  aplastic bone marrow following administration of, 250, 251
  effect of, on stem cells and normoblasts, 697
  hemolysis from, 566
  in producing aplastic anemia, 697
Chlorates, 460
Chloride shift, 456
Chloromas, 724
  acute myelocytic leukemia with, 294
Chlorophyll, 447
Chlorosis, 394-395
Chlorpromazine, 562
Cholestasis, 471
Cholesterol
  in abetalipoproteinemia, 595-596
  accumulation of, in histiocytosis, 58
  accumulation of, in Niemann-Pick disease, 43, 44
  biotransformation and excretion of, 3
  of erythrocyte membrane, 555
  in pernicious anemia, 438
Cholinesterase, 438
Chondrodystrophy, 53
Christmas disease, 830
Christmas factor IX, 785
Chromatin, 181
  changes in, with cell maturation, 118
  sex, 173, 175-177
Chromosomal sex, 175
Chromosomes, 491
  abnormalities of, in leukemia, 720-721
  of blood cells, 173-175
  composition of, 15
  effect of ionizing radiation on, 719
  Philadelphia, 175
    in chronic granulocytic leukemia, 700, 711, 720, 727, 728
    in multiple myeloma, 720
    in myelocytic leukemia, 728
    in myelofibrosis, 708
  replication of, 11
  in synthesis of hemoglobin, 622
Chronic granulomatous disease of childhood, 36, 47
Cirrhosis of liver
  acanthocytes in, 479
  coproporphyrin excretion with, 455
  erythrocyte sedimentation rate with, 356
  increase in 2,3-DPG with, 392
  increased fibrinolysis with, 847
  lipoprotein abnormalities with, 568
  megaloblastic anemia from folate deficiency with, 440
  protoporphyrin in, 451
Citrate-phosphate-dextrose solution, 532, 535
Citric acid intoxication, 548
Clasmatocytes of Ranvier, 2, 3
Clavicles, 222
Clot formation, 840
  in disseminated intravascular coagulation, 846
  by drawn blood, 350
Clot retraction, 797-798
  absence of, in purpura, 774
  as coagulation test, 915
  in hyperfibrinogenemia vs hypofibrinogenemia, 798
  with immunoglobulinopathies, 848
  vs platelet count, 797-798
  in thrombasthenia, 789, 804

Clotting factors; see Coagulation factors
Coagulase, staphylococcal, 787
Coagulation, 772-858
  classic theory of, 774, 778
  fibrin formation and fibrinolysis in, 779, 839-848
    hemorrhagic disorders caused by abnormalities in, 841-848
      afibrinogenemia and hypofibrinogenemia, 841-843
      deficiency of factor XIII, 848
      diffuse intravascular coagulation; see Diffuse intravascular coagulation
      dysfibrinogenemia, 841
      immunoglobulinopathies, 848
      increased fibrinolytic activity, 847
    mechanism of, 839-841
  future studies on, 776-777
  and hemostasis, 777-778
  history of, 773-774
  initiation, phase of, 778-779, 787-819
    abnormalities in, laboratory studies of, 779, 797-801
      bleeding time, 797
      clot retraction, 797-798
      deficiency of contact factors, 800-801
      platelet adhesiveness, 798-799
      platelet aggregation, 799-800
      platelet factor 3 release, 798
      platelet factor 4 release, 798
      platelet morphology, 797
      release of serotonin, 798
      tourniquet time, 797
    platelets in, 787-791
      abnormalities of, 804-819
      classification of disorders, 801
      function of, 791-795
      role of factors XI and XII, 795-797
      role of platelet factor 3, 795
      thrombocytopenic states, 801-804
      thrombocytosis and thrombocythemia, 819
  modern theory of, 778
  nonhemostatic functions of, 786-787
  in polycythemia vera, 703-704
  present theories on, 774-776
  prevention of, 351
  role of complement in, 559
  role of kinin system in, 559
  sequence of, 778-781
  thrombinogenesis in, 779, 832-839
    defects of, differential diagnosis of, 834
    hemorrhagic disorders in, 834-839
      acquired deficiencies, 835-839
        hemorrhagic disease of newborn, 836
        lupus coagulant, 836
        oral coagulants, 836-839
        vitamin K in, 835-836
      congenital deficiencies, 834-835
        in factor II, 834-835
        in factors V and VII, 835
    reactions, 832-833
    role of vitamin K in, 833-834
  thromboplastinogenesis in, 779, 819-832
    defects of, differential diagnosis of, 833
    with factor IX deficiencies, 830
    with factor X deficiencies, 830
    with factor XI deficiencies, 831
    with factor XII deficiencies, 831-832
    factors involved, 819-820
    with hemophilia, 823-830
    hemorrhagic disorders in, 820-821
    interaction of factors, 820
    laboratory study of abnormalities in, 821-823

Coagulation—cont'd
  thromboplastinogenesis in—cont'd
    laboratory study of abnormalities in—cont'd
      assays of coagulation factors, 823
      bleeding time, 821
      coagulation time, 821
      factor deficiencies, 823
      partial thromboplastin time, 821
      prothrombin consumption time, 823
      prothrombin time, 821
      recalcification time, 821-823
      thromboplastin generation test, 823
    naturally occurring inhibitors, 820
    therapy for abnormalities, 832
Coagulation factors, 781-786
  I, 781-782
    effect of hyperfibrinolysis on, 847
  II, 538-539, 780, 782; see also Prothrombin
    assay of, 923
    deficiency of, 787, 834-835
    in diffuse intravascular coagulation, 846
    effect of hyperfibrinolysis on, 847
    variant molecules of, 835
    vitamin K dependency of, 781
  V, 783-784
    assay of, 923
    in conversion of prothrombin to thrombin, 782, 783
    deficiency of, 775, 820-821
      congenital, 834, 835
      detection of, 834
      partial thromboplastin time for, 821
      prothrombin consumption test for, 823
      prothrombin time for, 821
      thromboplastin generation test for, 823
    in diffuse intravascular coagulation, 846, 847
    effect of, on factor X, 783
    properties of, 783
    in prothrombin activator complex, 832
    synthesis of, 783
    in thromboplastinogenesis, 820
  VI, 783
  VII, 538, 539, 780, 784
    assay of, 923
    deficiency of, 835
      congenital, 787, 834, 835
    effect of, on factor X, 784
    effect of factor XII on, 784
    effect of Fletcher factor on, 786
    effect of kallikrein on, 784
    effect of tissue thromboplastin on, 784
    inhibition of, 784, 835
    isolation of, 784
    phospholipids complexing with, 778
    source of, 784
    vitamin dependency of, 781, 833, 835
  VIII
    assay of, 929-931
    commercial preparation of, 784
    in correction of abnormal platelet adhesion, 792
    deficiency of, 822, 823, 828
    in disseminated intravascular coagulation, 846
    in evolution of plasma thromboplastin, 785
    history of, 784
    increase in, in sickle cell anemia, 636
    inhibitor of, 826, 828
    isolation and purification of, 784
    in multiple myeloma, 784
    synthesis of, 781, 826
    in thromboplastinogenesis, 820
    in von Willebrand's disease, 808, 809

Coagulation factors—cont'd
  IX, 538-539, 780, 785
    activation of, 778
    assay of, 932
    deficiency of, 821, 822, 830
      thromboplastin generation test for, 823
      treatment of, 832
    dependency of, on vitamin K, 833, 835
    isolation of, 785
    preparation of, 785
    properties of, 785
    in thromboplastinogenesis, 785, 820
    vitamin K dependency of, 781
  X, 538-539, 780, 785
    activation of, 778
    assay of, 932
    in conversion of prothrombin to thrombin, 782, 785
    deficiency of, 785, 787, 821, 822, 823, 830-831, 832
    effect of Russell's viper venom on, 833
    in prothrombin activator complex, 832
    structure of, 785
    in thromboplastinogenesis, 785
    vitamin K dependency of, 781, 833, 835
  XI, 780
    activation of, 785
    assays of, 932
    deficiency of, 787, 821, 822, 823, 831
      treatment for, 832
    in initiating platelet adhesion and aggregation, 779
    role of, 795-797
    in thromboplastinogenesis, 785, 820
  XII
    activation of, 786, 844
    assays of, 932
    deficiency of, 661, 777, 821, 822, 823, 831-832
      treatment for, 832
    effect of, on factor VII, 784
    effect of endotoxin on, 843
    in initiating platelet adhesion and aggregation, 779, 793
    and kinin system, 844
    nonhemostatic functions of, 787
    role of, 795-797
    in thromboplastinogenesis, 785, 820
  XIII, 786, 840
    activation of, 786
    assays of, 933
    deficiency of, 848
      delayed wound healing with, 787
    isolation of, 786
    in stabilization of fibrinogen, 781
    synthesis of, 781, 786
    transfusion of, 543
    as transglutaminase, 786
  assays of, 823
  deficiency of, 833
  effect of coumarin drugs on, 775, 837
  Fitzgerald, 786
  Fletcher, 786
    deficiency of, 933-934
  in prethrombotic state, 854
  standard nomenclature and synonyms, 779
  storage of, 536-537
  survival time of, after transfusion, 539-540
  thrombin; see Thrombin
  thromboplastin; see Thromboplastin
Coagulation tests
  of antithrombin III
    by radial immunodiffusion, 935
    by rocket electroimmunoassay, 934-935

Coagulation tests—cont'd
  of antithrombin III—cont'd
    by thrombin neutralization, 934
    assays using chromogenic or fluorogenic substrates, 935-936
  clot retraction, 915
  cross recalcification of plasma, 920
  detection of lupus anticoagulant, 920
  euglobin lysis time, 937-938
  evaluation of prolonged one-stage prothrombin time, 922-923
  evaluation of prolonged partial thromboplastin time, 925-926
  factor II assay, 923
  factor V assay, 923
  factor VII assay, 923
  factor VIII assay, 929-931
  factor IX assay, 932
  factor X assay, 932
  factor XI assay, 932
  factor XII assay, 932
  factor XIII assay, 933
  fibrinolysis, screening for, 936-937
  Fletcher factor, deficiency of, 933-934
  heparin assay, 938
  Ivy bleeding time, 915-916
  one-stage prothrombin time, microtechnic method, 921-922
  one-stage prothrombin time, Quick's method of, 920-921
  partial thromboplastin time, 924-925
  plasma recalcification time, 919
  platelet adhesiveness, 917-918
  platelet aggregation, 918-919
  platelet factor 3 availability, 919
  protamine paracoagulation test, 936
  prothrombin consumption test, 924
  ristocetin cofactor, 931-932
  semiquantitative assay of fibrin-stabilizing factor, 933
  thromboplastin generation test, 926-929
  tourniquet test, 916-917
  venous coagulation time, 915
Cobalamin, 423
Cobalt, 404
  deficiency of, 404
  effect of, on alkaline phosphatase, 207
  in stimulation of erythropoietin, 19-20
  in vitamin B_{12}, 422, 423
Cobalt unit, 19, 20
Cobaltous chloride, 19
Cobamide coenzymes, 423
Codocytes, 427, 480, 481
  in diagnosis of hemolytic disease, 580
  in Hb C disease, 641
  in Hb D disease, 641
  in Hb E disease, 643
  in hemoglobinopathies, 623
  with lecithin-cholesterol acyltransferase deficiency, 569
  in sickle cell anemia, 640
  in sickle cell–Hb C disease, 644
  in thalassemia, 650
Colchicine, 11
  ingestion of, 167
  in interference with vitamin B_{12} absorption, 440
  intoxication with, 157
  and Pelger-Huët anomaly, 161
Collagen
  in formation of hemostatic plug, 791
  platelet adhesion to, 791, 792
  in platelet aggregation, 793, 794, 799
Collagenase, 663

Colony-stimulating activity, 25
  in differentiation of stem cells, 6
Colony-stimulating factors, 25
  in granulopoiesis, 659
  inhibitors of, 25
Complement system 556-565; see also specific complement component
  activation of, 557
    by activator system, 558-559
    by convertase system, 557-558
  in autoimmune hemolysis, 559-560
  binding of IgG subclasses to, 90
  from blastoid cells, 82
  in chemotaxis, 660
    deficiencies of, 661
  components of, 556
    properties of, 557
  deficiencies of, 564-565
    with defective opsonization, 664
  in diagnosis of cellular immunity deficiencies, 104
  in drug-related hemolysis, 562-563
    with alpha-methyldopa types, 563
    with hapten types, 562
    nonimmunologic, 563
    with positive antiglobulin test, 563
  in hemolytic reactions, 545
  interactions between, 559
  in isoimmune hemolysis, 560-562
  in opsonization, 663
  in paroxysmal cold hemoglobinuria, 563
  in paroxysmal nocturnal hemoglobinuria, 563-564
Concanavalin A, 82
  in action of helper T-cells, 83
  in chronic granulomatous disease, 664
Congenital dyserythropoietic anemia, 569
  abnormal normoblasts in, 624
Congenital erythropoietic prophyria, 451
Congenital erythropoietic protoporphyria, 451-454
Conjugase, 420, 443
Connective tissue disorders, 852
Constitutional hepatic dysfunction, 472-473
Consumption coagulopathy, 843
Contraceptives, oral
  folate deficiency with, 441
  increase in coagulation factor VIII with, 636
  in prethrombotic state, 854, 855
Convertase system of complement activation, 557-558
  components of, 557
  sequence of, 557
  sites of, 557-558
Cooley's anemia, 68, 650
Coombs' test, 589, 906
  in pernicious anemia, 430
Copper, 403-404
  deficiency in, 403
  intoxication by, 404
  metabolism, 403
Copper porphyrin, 447
Coproporphyrin, 447, 454
  in acquired porphyria secondary to griseofulvin, 455
  in acquired porphyria secondary to hepatoma, 455
  in cirrhosis of liver, 455
  in congenital erythropoietic protoporphyria, 451
  in constitutional hepatic dysfunction, 473
  free erythrocyte, 449
  in hepatitis, 455
  in infectious mononucleosis, 455

Coproporphyrin—cont'd
 with ingestion of alcohol, 455
 isolation and measurement of, 877
 in lead intoxication, 455
 in porphyria cutanea tarda, 454
 quantitative assay of, 877-879
 in secondary porphyrinuria, 455
 in variegate porphyria, 454
Coproporphyrin I
 in acquired porphyria secondary to hepatoma,
  455
 changes in, with congenital erythropoietic porphyria, 451
 excretion of, in pernicious anemia, 438
Coproporphyrin III, 449
 in erythropoietic coproporphyria, 454
 in hereditary coproporphyria, 454
Coproporphyrin synthetase, 454
Coproporphyrinogen, 414
Coproporphyrinogen oxidase, 413
Cords of Billroth, 61
Corning LARC, 667
Corticosteroids
 in depletion of lymphocytes, 88
 in treatment of aplastic anemia, 697
 in treatment of pernicious anemia, 430
 in treament of red cell aplasia, 698
Cortisol, 26
Cortisone, 26
 erythrocyte sedimentation rate with, 356
 in inhibition of lymphocytotoxin release, 85
Coulter cell counter, 360
 in erythrocyte counts, 371-372
  Model F, 385
  Model S, 372, 380, 381
 significance of successive cell counts, 374
Coulter diff3, 667
Coulter ZBI, 381
Coumadin; see Warfarin sodium
Coumarin drugs
 absorption of, 837
 administration of, 836-837
 binding of, to albumin, 837
 drug interaction with, 837-839
 effect of, on coagulation factors, 834
 metabolism of, 837
 optimal dose of, 837
 for suicidal purposes, 837
Crigler-Najjar syndrome, 474
Crinophagy, 37
Cristae, 182
Cryofibrinogen, 748
 in disseminated intravascular coagulation, 846
 immunoelectrophoresis of, 902-903
Cryofibrinogenemia, 748
Cryogelglobulins, 902
Cryoglobulinemia, 98, 748-752
 hemorrhagic tendencies in, 848
 in multiple myeloma, 733
Cryoglobulins, 748, 752
 immunoelectrophoresis of, 902
Cryoprotective agents, 532
Crypt-agglutinoids, 510
Cushing's syndrome, 16, 688
Cyanferrihemoglobin, 457
Cyanmethemoglobin, 457
 in measurement of blood hemoglobin concentra-
  tion, 372, 377, 382
  method of, 875
  normal values, 875-876
  principles of, 875
  reagents in, 875
 spectroscopic identification of, 461
Cyanocobalamin, 404, 423

Cyanocobalamin—cont'd
 formula of, 422
Cyanocobamide, 423
Cyanosis, 456
 from acquired methemoglobinemia, 458, 460
 from carboxyhemoglobin, 456
 decreased oxygen affinity with, 649
 in hemoglobinopathy, 624
 in polycythemia vera, 701
 from sulfhemoglobinemia, 411
Cyclic AMP
 in binding antigen to IgE, 665
 in inhibition of immunologic reactions, 87
 in platelet reactions, 789-790
 in stimulation of erythropoietin, 15, 20
Cyclohexamide, 85
Cyclooxygenase
 deficiency of, 818
 inhibition of, 790
 in platelet metabolism, 790
Cyclophosphamide, 161
Cyst, splenic, 61
Cystine crystals, 167
Cystine storage disease, 167
Cystinosis, 167
Cytochrome, 395, 406, 447, 448
Cytochrome-B_5-reductase, 458
Cytofibrinokinase, 841
Cytopenia
 definition of, 4
 in stimulation of proliferation of blood cells,
  14
Cytoside, 39
Cytosine arabinoside, 419
Cytosol, 37
Cytotaxigens, 660, 662
Cytotaxins, 660
Cytotaxin inactivators, 660
Cytotoxins, 652
Cytoxan; see Cyclophosphamide

D

Dacryocyte, 480, 481
Dane particle, 542
Dark-field illumination, 180
Deferrioxamine, 400
Defibrination syndrome, 843
Dehydration, 378
Delayed hypersensitivity reaction
 abolishment of, with thymectomy, 75
 basophils in, 665
 and cellular immunity, 88
 inducement of, 88
 passive transfer of, 88
 skin tests for, 103
 T-lymphocytes in, 83, 85
Deoxyadenosylcobalamin, 424
Deoxyhemoglobin
 in oxygen transport, 389
 vs oxyhemoglobin, 390
 quaternary structure of, 607
Deoxythymidine triphosphate, 419
Deoxyuridine suppression test, 438-439
Deoxyuridylate, 418
Dermatitis, contact, allergic, 665
Diabetes mellitus
 abnormal chemotaxis in, 663
 concentration of Hb A_{1c} in, 608-609
Diabetic steatorrheas, 443
Diaphorase, 460
Diarrhea, 397
Dibothriocephalus infection, 440
DIC; see Diffuse intravascular coagulation
Dicumarol; see Bishydroxycoumarin

Didandin; see Diphenadione
Diego blood group system, 513
Diego factor, 490
Diffuse intravascular coagulation
 aggregation and entrapment of platelets in,
  788
 association of, with hemolytic transfusion reaction, 548
 classification of, 845
 clearance of fibrin in, 3
 definition of, 843
 erythrocytes in, 783
 etiology of, 843
 vs hyperfibrinogenemia, 847-848
 laboratory diagnosis of, 845-847
 pathogenesis of, 843-845
  activation of extrinsic coagulation system,
   844-845
  induction by endotoxin, 843
  role of immune reactions in, 844
  role of inflammation in, 844
 in sickle cell disease, 636
 synonyms of, 843
 thrombocytopenia in, 803
 from thrombogenic phospholipids in blood,
  555
Diffusion methods in measurement of immunoglobulins, 104
Difluorophosphate, 783
DiGeorge's syndrome, 100
 characterization of, 75
Diglucuronide, 469
DiGuglielmo's syndrome, 268, 304, 306, 711-
  714, 725, 729
 megaloblastic anemia in, 444
Dihydrofolate, 418-419
Dihydrofolate reductase, 419
2,4-Dinitrochlorobenzene, 103
Dinitrophenol, 85
Dipaxin; see Diphenadione
Diphenadione, 837
2,3-Diphosphoglycerate
 in cirrhosis of liver, 392
 decrease of, with erythrocyte storage, 535
 effect of, on combination and release of oxygen
  and hemoglobin, 608
 effect of, on oxygen transport, 389
 effect of androgens and thyroid hormone on,
  392
 increases in
  with anemia, 532, 535
  cause of, 392
  at high altitudes, 704
 interaction of, with hemoglobin, 391
 role of, 390-391, 532, 535
 sensitivity of, 392
 in stored erythrocytes, 532
 synthesis and degradation of, 390-391
 in uremia, 392
Diphosphoglycerate mutase, 390, 391
2,3-Diphosphoglycerate phosphatase, 390
Diplococcus pneumoniae, 673
Diploid cells, 175
Dipyridamole, 790
Discocyte, 476
 transformation of, to echinocyte, 477, 478
 transformation of, to spherocyte, 483
 transformation of, to stomatocyte, 478
Disseminated fibrin thromboembolism, 843
Diverticulosis, 439
DNA
 of chromosomes in blood cells, 15
 deoxyribonuclease digestion of, 873
 Feulgen reaction for staining, 873, 874

DNA—cont'd
impaired synthesis of, 418, 419, 429
in protein synthesis, 15
replication of, 11
Döhle bodies, 119, 161-162, 192, 674
Donath-Landsteiner hemolysin, 563
Down's syndrome, 209
Downey cells, 78
2,3-DPG; *see* 2,3-Diphosphoglycerate
Drepano-discocyte, 481
Drepano-echinocyte, 481
Drepano-stomatocytes, 481
Drepanocytes, 480, 481, 623, 624
in diagnosis of hemolytic disease, 579, 580
effect of oxygenation on, 638
in sickle cell anemia, 640
Drepanoechinocyte, 477-478
Drumstick of leukocytes, 173
as sex characteristic, 177-179
Dubin-Johnson syndrome, 473-474
Duffy blood group system, 512-513
and resistance to infection, 641
use of, in establishing parentage, 520
Dynia defect, 786
Dyserythropoietic anemia, congenital, 569
Dysfibrinogenemia, 841
Dysgammaglobulinemia, 98
Dysmyelopoietic syndrome, 729
preceding acute leukemia, 695
Dysotosis multiplex, 53

E

Ecchymosis, 779
ECF-A, 660
Echino-acanthocyte, 477
Echinocytes, 477-478
vs schizocyte, 483
Ectopic hemopoiesis
bone marrow embolism vs, 29
extramedullary hemopoiesis vs, 28-29
sites of, 32
Ectopic lymphopoiesis, 29
Eczema, 101
EDTA
effect of, on erythrocyte, 354-355
effect of, on platelet, 792
for obtaining blood specimens, 862
Ehlers-Danlos syndrome, 852
platelet dysfunction, 818
Ehrlich's aldehyde reaction, 469, 471, 572, 573
specificity of, 574
Electron microscopy, 181-205
in classification of acute leukemias, 723
general considerations, 181
ultrastructure of blood cells
abnormal, 192-205
Gaucher cells, 192
leukemic cells, 192
May-Hegglin anomaly, 192
Pelger-Huët anomaly, 192
phagocytic histiocytes, 192
plasma cells in myeloma, 192
normal, 182-192
granulocytes, 182, 192
lymphocytes, 192
megakaryocytes and platelets, 192
monocytes, 192
normoblasts, 192
plasma cells, 192
Electrophoresis
acrylamide gel, 631
cellulose acetate, 630
in identification of Hb S, 640, 641
in quantification of Hb A_2, 626

Electrophoresis—cont'd
hemoglobin; *see* Hemoglobin electrophoresis
precautions in use of, 633
protein; *see* Protein electrophoresis
starch block, 631
zone, 626-631
Elliptocytes, 481-483, 594
in diagnosis of hemolytic disease, 580
Elliptocytosis, 481, 483
cells in, 580
hereditary
clinical aspects of, 594
hemolysis from, 568
laboratory findings in, 594-595
treatment of, 595
Embden-Meyerhof pathway, 458, 459, 565
Embolism, 787
Embryo, hemopoiesis in, 6-11
control of, 8-9
hepatic, 9-10
medullary, 10-11
mesoblastic period, 6-7
primitive erythroblasts vs definitive normoblasts, 8
Emperipolesis, 32, 76
Endocarditis, fibroplastic parietal, 258, 260, 261
Endocarditis lenta cells, 170
Endocrines in hemopoiesis, 15-16
Endocytic vacuole, 36
Endocytosis, 36
Endoplasmic reticulum
in autophagy, 37
of blood cell, ultrastructure of, 182, 183
of leukemic cell, 192
of lymphocyte, 76
lysosomes from, 36, 37
of myeloblast, 182
of myelocyte, 182
of plasma cell, 192
in myeloma, 192, 200
Endothelial cells
in connecting blood islands, 6
in peripheral blood, 169
of reticuloendothelial cells, 2, 3
Endothelium
as inhibitor of coagulation, 779, 787
as nonthrombogenic surface, 791
Endotoxin
in activation of complement, 558
clearance and detoxification of, 3
in diffuse intravascular coagulation, 843, 844
staphylococcal, 82
in stimulation of colony-stimulating factor, 25, 659
Enzymes
erythrocytic, deficiency of, with hemolysis, 565-567
iron-containing, 395
lysosomal, 37, 38
in blastoid transformation, 82
deficiency of, 38, 39
respiratory, 447
Eosinopenia, 688
from ACTH, 256
definition of, 685
in Good's syndrome, 100
from radiation, 692
Eosinophil, 126, 127, 133, 138, 156
band, 130
in Chediak-Higashi syndrome, 47
chemotactic responses of, 660, 665
in chronic granulocytic leukemia, 727
cytochemically abnormal, 167
cytoplasmic granules of, 36, 118, 125, 131, 182

Eosinophil—cont'd
drumsticks found in, 179
effect of ACTH on, 16, 667
in erythrocytosis, 570
inclusion in, 167
in killing of bacteria, 665
in mucopolysaccharidoses, 55, 58
periodic acid–Schiff reaction of, 207
peroxidase reaction of, 206
in phagocytosis, 663, 665
segmented, 130
sudanophilic staining of, 207
ultrastructure of, 184, 190
Wright-Giemsa stain of, 868
Eosinophil chemotactic factor of anaphylaxis, 665
Eosinophil count, circulating, 866
Eosinophilia, 86
associated with sarcoidosis, 256, 257
conditions manifesting, 256
with fibroplastic parietal endocarditis, 258, 260, 261
in leukemoid reaction, 264, 265
and leukocytosis, 261, 262
from radiation, 692
Eosinophilic granuloma of bone, 58-61
Eosinophilic leukemia, 258, 259
Eosinophilic leukocytosis, 675
Eosinophilotropic factor, 85, 86
Epinephrine
effect of, on erythropoietin, 15
in mobilization of leukocytes, 659
in platelet aggregation, 793, 794, 799, 800
receptors for, on platelet membrane, 788-789
Epstein-Barr virus, 676
Erythremia, 701
vs erythrocytosis, 379
Erythremic myelosis, 711, 712, 713
chronic, 726, 729
with terminal acute myelocytic leukemia, 304-305
Erythroblast, 8
Erythroblastoma, solitary, 30
Erythroblastosis fetalis, 600
Rh factor in, 502
Erythrocuprein, 404
Erythrocyte; *see also* Red blood cell
abnormal forms of, 476-489
in shape, 476-486, 567
acanthocyte, 478-481
codocyte, 481
dacryocyte, 481
discocyte, 476
drepanocyte, 481
echinocyte, 477-478
elliptocyte, 481, 483
keratocyte and schizocyte, 483
knizocyte, 486
leptocyte, 483
megalocyte, 483
spherocyte, 483
stomatocyte, 478
in size, 476
anisocytosis, 476
macrocytosis, 476
microcytosis, 476
agglutination of, 352
cause of, 352
effect of, on sedimentation velocity, 352
with lectins, 495
with phytohemagglutinins, 82
in aplastic anemia, 697
autoerythrocyte sensitization, 852
centrifugation of, 362

Erythrocyte—cont'd
 cholinesterase levels in, with pernicious anemia, 438
 in congenital erythropoietic porphyria, 451
 in congenital erythropoietic protoporphyria,
   451
 copper in, 404
 deficiency of, in anemia
   aregenerative, 530
   blood transfusion for, 530
 deformability of, 555, 556
 disruption of, by mechanical trauma, 569-570
   from cardiac valves, 569
   in exertional hemoglobinuria, 570
   in microangiopathic hemolytic anemia, 569-
     570
 in diffuse intravascular coagulation, 844, 846
 effect of adrenocortical hormones in, 16
 end point of elimination of, 552
 enzyme deficiencies of, with hemolysis, 565-
   567
 enzyme-treated, agglutination with, 592
 equilibrium between production and destruction
   of, 552
 fetal, 11
 fluorescent, 409
   with lead poisoning, 455, 456
 folate of, assay of, 420-421
 fragments of, lymphocytic phagocytosis of, 78
 free protoporphyrin of, 449
 function of, 389
 globoside of, 39
 half-life of, 552-553
 hematocrit; see Hematocrit
 hematoside of, 39
 hemoglobin of; see Hemoglobin
 immunology of; see Immunology of erythrocyte
 inclusions in
   Cabot rings, 488
   with diffuse basophilia and basophilic stip-
     pling, 486-487
   Heinz bodies, 460, 488
   Howell-Jolly bodies, 488
   with polychromatophilia, 486-487
   reticulocytes, 486
   siderotic granules, 488-489
 increases in; see Erythrocytosis
 interior of, ions in, 556
 life span of, 551, 552
 mass of
   in body hematocrit, 357
   clinical correlation, 362-363
   during pregnancy, 356
   effect of altitude on, 379
   method of measurement, 363
   normal values, 363-366
   vs relative blood viscosity, 351
   response of 2,3-DPG to, 392
 mean cell life, 552
 mean corpuscular hemoglobin of, 379-380
 mean corpuscular hemoglobin concentration of,
   379, 380
 mean corpuscular volume of, 360, 379
 membrane of, 181
   biochemical composition of, 553-555
   charges on, 352
     effect of centrifugation on, 353
   permeability changes in, 558
   structure of, 553-555
   ultrastructural appearance of, 553
 metabolism within, glucose
   aerobic and anaerobic, 459
   Embden-Meyerhof pathway in, 458

Erythrocyte—cont'd
 metabolism within—cont'd
   hexose monophosphate shunt, 458
   methemoglobin in, distribution of, 460
 mitotic index of, 11
 morphology of, 577-582
 number of
   and distribution of, 12
   effect of, on erythrocyte sedimentation rate,
     353-354
   vs reticulocyte count, 23
 osmotic fragility of, 584
   in abetalipoproteinemia, 595
   in diagnosis of hemolytic anemia, 503-506
     after incubation, 586
     interpretation of results, 583
     significance of measurements, 583
   with hereditary spherocytosis, 567, 594
   in sickle cell anemia, 640
   tests for, 883
   in thalassemia, 650
 packing of, 357, 359
 of pernicious anemia, 429, 432, 438
 phagocytosis of, 64, 570
   time-lapse photography in study of, 181
 poikilocytosis of, 242
 in polycythemia vera, 702
 porphyrin of; see Porphyrin
 production of; see Erythropoiesis
 protoporphyrin of, 411
 release of, from marrow, 32
 removal of granular inclusions from, 64
 rouleau formation of, 352
   in acanthocytosis and anisocytosis, 352
   effect of plasma protein composition on,
     352
   effect of, on sedimentation velocity, 352
   in hemolytic anemia, 352
   increased, with decreased zeta potential,
     352
   in sickle cell disease, 352
 sedimentation rate of, 351-357
   clinical correlations of, 355-357
   factors affecting, 352-355
     aggregation of erythrocytes, 352
     anticoagulant used, 354-355
     caliber and length of tube, 354
     changes in plasma composition, 352-353
     delay in performing test, 355
     number of erythrocytes, 354
     number of leukocytes, 354
     position of tube, 354
     size of erythrocytes, 354
     temperature, 355
 senescence of, 552
   disposal of, 570
 sequestration and destruction of, 64
 shape of, 556
   sequence of, 577
 sickling of, 68
   tests for, 624-625
 size of, 354
   effect of, on relative blood viscosity, 351
   measurement of, 379
   spheroid, 66, 68
 stored, 532-535
   deterioration of, 532
   2,3-DPG in, 535
   effect of temperature on, 532
   solution for, 532
   survival of, effect of adenosine on, 534
   survival of, after transfusions, 532, 533,
     534
 sulfhemoglobin in, 461

Erythrocyte—cont'd
 survival of, 552
   decreased, anemia due to, 602-657
   susceptibility of, to radiation injury, 692
 teardrop
   in myelofibrosis, 706, 708
   in myeloproliferative disorders, 700, 701
 transfusion of, 537
   for hereditary spherocytosis, 567
   in transport of oxygen and carbon dioxide,
     456
 volume of, per volume of blood; see Hematocrit
 Wright-Giemsa stain of, 868
 zeta potential of, 352
Erythrocyte count, 360, 530
 Coulter cell counter, 371-372
 in diagnosis of anemia, 392
 in diagnosis of hemolytic disease, 575-576
 diluting fluid for, 864
 effect of age on, 378
 effect of altitude on, 378-379
 effect of dehydration on, 378
 effect of exercise or excitement on, 378
 effect of sex on, 378
 error of, 370-373
 Hemac laser cell counter, 372-373
 hemocytometer method, 370-371
   calculation of SD from control data
     duplicate analysis, 371
     standard method, 371
   inherent errors, 370
   technical and human errors, 370
 at high altitudes, 704
 method, 863-864
 normal values, 864
   determination of, 376-377
   physiologic variations, 377-379
 in pernicious anemia, 431, 432
 in polycythemia vera, 700-701
 successive, significance of, 373-374, 375
   with electronic cell counts, 374
   with hemocytometer counts, 373-374
Erythrocyte indices, 379-380
 calculated by electronic counters, 380
 in diagnosis of hemolytic disease, 577
 in iron-deficiency anemias, 407
 mean corpuscular hemoglobin, 379-380, 867
 mean corpuscular hemoglobin concentration,
   367, 379, 380
 mean corpuscular volume, 379, 867
 normal values of, 867
 use of, 380
Erythrocytin, 783, 820
Erythrocytosis
 from abnormal hemoglobin pigments, 705
 benign familial, 705
 in chronic hemolytic anemia, 576
 vs erythremia or polycythemia vera, 379
 erythrocyte mass in, 363
 from heart disease, 705
 in hemoglobinopathies, 624
 at high altitudes, 704
 from high doses of testosterone, 16
 from hypoventilation, 705
 increased oxygen affinity with, 646-649
 in newborn, 705
 plasma volume in, 363
 from pulmonary disease, 704-705
 relative, 701, 705
 with tumors, 705
Erythrocytosis megalosplenica, 701
Erythrodermia
 basophilic leukocytosis, 675

Erythrodermia—cont'd
in Sezary's syndrome, 162, 163
Erythrodontia, 451
Erythrogenin, 21
Erythroleukemia, 268, 596, 712
case study of, 306-307
Hb A$_2$ in, 633
Hb H in, 633
megaloblastic anemia in, 444
Erythromatosis, 711
Erythron, 22
Erythrophagocytes, 580
Erythrophagocytosis, 570, 571
C4b, 2a in, 556
in paroxysmal cold hemoglobinuria, 600
Erythropoiesis, 17-24
vs degree of reticulocytosis, 487, 552
effect of, on iron absorption, 396
effect of blood transfusion on, 530
effect of estrogen on, 378
effect of hormones on, 16
effect of hypoxia on, 379
effect of iron on, 402
effective vs total, 22-24
and erythron, 22
erythropoietin in, 17-22
assay and normal values of, 18-20
chemistry of, 20
formation and metabolism of, 20-21
immunology of, 20
physiologic and pathologic significance of,
21-22
evaluation of, with radioactive iron, 395
megaloblastic, 418
metabolic inhibition of, 699
normal, 22
quantitative aspects of, 22-24
in red cell aplasia, 698
in sickle cell anemia, 636-638
site of, 11
splenomegaly with, 69
unconjugated hyperbilirubinemia in, ineffective, 472
Erythropoietic coproporphyria, 454
Erythropoietic factor, renal, 21
Erythropoietic porphyria, congenital, 451
Erythropoietin, 17-22
in aplastic anemia, 697
assay and normal values of, 18-20
chemistry of, 20
in differential diagnosis of polycythemia, 705
discovery of, 17-18
effects of, 24
effect of cobalt on, 404
effect of hormones on, 15, 16
fetal, 8
in liver vs kidney, 8
formation and metabolism of, 20-21
immunology of, 20
increase of, 704, 705
International Reference Preparation for, 20
physiologic and pathologic significance of, 21-
22
in polycythemia vera, 701
in red cell aplasia, 698
associated with thymoma, 699
in secondary polychythemia, 704
in stimulation of differentiation of stem cells, 4,
14
urinary excretion of, 20
Erythropoietin-responsive cell, 21
Erythropoietin Standard A, 20
Erythropoietin Standard B, 20
Erythropoietinogen, 21

Escherichia coli
in assay of vitamin B$_{12}$, 437
as sickling agent, 624
Esterases, 209, 210
application of, to study of leukemias, 210
Estrogen
effect of, on erythropoiesis, 16, 378
effect of, on hemopoiesis, 15
effect of, in intermittent acute porphyria, 454
Ethanol gelation test, 846, 854
Ethyl alcohol, 440
Ethyl biscoumacetate, 837
Euglena gracilis, 422, 437
Euglobin lysis test, 847, 855, 937-938
Evans' syndrome, 577, 598, 599, 802
Exchange transfusion, 540-541
Excitement, effect of, on erythrocytes, 378
Exercise
effect of, on erythrocytes, 378
in mobilization of leukocytes, 659
Exocytosis, 37
Extramedullary hemopoiesis; see Hemopoiesis,
extramedullary
Extramedullary lymphopoiesis, 29
Extramedullary megakaryocytosis, 268
Extrinsic factor, 417

F
Fabricius, bursa of, 74, 75
Fairley's pigment, 461, 571
Farber's disease, 39
Fat, subepicardial, extramedullary hemopoiesis
in, 30, 33
Fat cells, 223, 224
Fava bean, 566
Favism, 566, 575
Felty's syndrome, 663, 803
Ferrata reticulum cell, 124, 125
Ferric hydroxide, 396
Ferrihemoglobin, 456
Ferritin
concentration of, in evaluation of iron metabolism, 409
effect of xanthine oxidase on, 397
electron microscopic appearance of, 400
ferric hydroxyphosphate molecules of, 400
formation of, 396
as storage iron, 395, 400
transfer of, to normoblasts, 402
Ferrochelatase, 449
in acquired porphyria secondary to griseofulvin,
455
in congenital erythropoietic protoporphyria,
451, 454
Ferrodoxin, 395
Ferrohemoglobin, 626
Ferroxidase, 403
Fetal hemoglobin, 608, 609, 610
acid elution technic in demonstration of, 886
interpretation, 855
method, 855
normal values, 855
principle, 855
reagents, 855
in acute erythroleukemia, 725
vs adult, 8-9
alkali denaturation test of
calculation of, 885
method, 885
principle of, 885
reagents, 885
binding of, to 2,3-DPG, 390
in centrifugation of blood, 362
in chronic granulocytic leukemia, 727

Fetal hemoglobin—cont'd
conversion of, to adult hemoglobin, 8
conversion of, to methemoglobin, 460
distribution of, 626
effect of, on sickling reaction, 624-625
effect of alkali on, 608
electrophoretic identification of, 626
elevation of, in disease, 633
hereditary persistence of, 608, 622, 626, 885
Greek type, 655
heterozygous with another hemoglobinopathy, 656
Negro type, 655
Swiss type, 655-656
history of, 603
increase of, in aplastic anemia, 697
in polycythemia vera, 702
properties of, 608
with sickle cell anemia, 636, 640
structure of, 604, 606
switch from, to Hb A, 622-623
synthesis of, 622
in thalassemias, 460, 650, 653
testing for, 625-626
Fetal hemopoiesis, 29
Fetoglobulin
in ataxia-telangiectasia, 101
electrophoresis of, 900-901
Fetus
erythropoiesis of, 6, 7
control of, 8-9
hepatic period of, 9-10
erythropoietin of, 8
production, conjugation, and excretion of bilirubin by, 471
Feulgen reaction
method, 873-874
reaction, 873
results, 874
Fibrin
clearance of, 3
in clotting mechanism, 350
conversion of, from fibrinogen, 779
products of, in prethrombotic state, 554-555
deposition of, 570
in bacterial infection, 787
discovery of, 773
effect of, on thrombin, 783
formation of, 818, 839-840
in implantation of metastatic tumor cells, 787
physiologic, 840
split products of, 846
in wound healing, 787
Fibrin-stabilizing factor, 786, 840; see also Coagulation factors, XIII
Fibrin thromboembolism, disseminated, 843
Fibrinogen
abnormal, 781-782
administration of, 537, 538
in afibrinogenemia; see Afibrinogenemia
in classic theory of coagulation, 778
in clotting mechanism, 350, 781
cold form of, 748
concentration of, 781
conversion of, to fibrin, 779
products of, in prethrombotic state, 854-855
in diffuse intravascular coagulation, 846
in dysfibrinogenemia, 841
effect of, on zeta potential of erythrocytes,
352
history of, 773
in hyperfibrinolysis, 847
in hypofibrinogenemia; see Hypofibrinogenemia

Fibrinogen—cont'd
 increases in, effect of, on ESR, 352, 353
 macrophage binding of, 36
 molecular variants of, 841, 843
 in plasma vs serum, 350
 in platelet aggregation, 793
 properties of, 781
 storage of, 536-537
 structure of, 781
 transfusion of, 543
Fibrinoligase, 840
Fibrinolysin, 840
 in hypofibrinogenemia, 842
Fibrinolysis, 778, 780
 activation of, 840
  by bacterial filtrates, 841
  by tissue activation, 841
  by urokinase, 841
 increased, 847
  vs diffuse intravascular coagulation, 847-848
 inhibition of, 841, 847
 in prethrombotic state, 854-855
 screening for, 936-937
Fibrinolytic agents, 787
Fibrinolytic blood, 539
Fibrinolytic thromboembolism, 843
Fibroblasts, 3
 effect of lymphocytotoxin on, 85
 in elaboration of corrective factors for mucopolysaccharidoses, 53
Ficin, 592
Fick's equation, 390
Fingerprint technic, 631
Fitzgerald factor, 786, 797
Flaujeac factor, 786
Fletcher factor, 661, 786, 795, 797
 deficiency of, detection of, 933-934
Fluorescytes, 449, 455, 486
Fluoride ions
 effect of, on acid and alkaline phosphatase, 207
 inhibition of esterase reaction by, 209
5-Fluorouracil, 419
Foam cells, 45, 58, 69
Folic acid
 absorption of, 419, 420
 assays of, 419-420, 437
 chemistry of, 417-418
 deficiency of, 142
  abnormal blood cell sizes with, 119
  anemia due to, 426-429
   caused by cellular proliferation, 441
   classification of, 426-427
   concept of megaloblastic dyspoiesis in, 427-429
   defective folate interconversion, 443
   dietary, 440
   due to malabsorption, 441-443
   macrocytosis, 427
   megaloblastic, of infancy, 441
   megaloblastic, of pregnancy, 440-441
  impaired DNA synthesis with, 418, 419
  with leukemia, 724
  macrocytosis with, 476
  Schilling test of, 436, 437
  vitamin B₁₂ levels with, 437
 excretion of formiminoglutamic acid, 421
 in foods, 419-420
 historical background, 416-417
 interrelation of, and vitamin B₁₂, 426
 malabsorption of, 441-443
  congenital, 441
  drug-induced, 441

Folic acid—cont'd
 malabsorption of—cont'd
  in steatorrheas, 441-443
 metabolism of, 418-419
  disturbance of, 419
  drugs that interfere with, 418, 419
 requirements of, 441
 reticulocyte response to, 437, 438
 in treatment of vitamin B₁₂ deficiency, 427, 429
Follicular artery, 61
Formiminoglutamic acid
 excretion of, 421
 transformation of, to glutamic acid, 421, 422
N-Formyl-methionyl-leucyl-phenylalanine, 660
Forssman antigen, 678, 679
Free erythrocyte coproporphyrin, 449, 455
Free erythrocyte protoporphyrin, 449
Freemartin, 175
Freund's adjuvant, 96
Fructose, 397

G

G0 phase of cell cycle, 11
G1 phase of cell cycle, 11
G2 phase of cell cycle, 11
Gaisbock's disease, 705
Gallstones, 451-454
Gamma-Gandy bodies, 65, 66
Gamma globulin neutralization test, 591-592
Gamma heavy chain disease, 102, 103
Gammopathy, 98
Ganglioside, 39
 vs acid mucopolysaccharide, 53
 turnover of, in Gaucher's disease, 41
Gargoylism, 53, 54
 hematologic findings in, 55, 56, 57, 58
Gasser cells, 55
Gastrectomy, 439
 defective iron absorption with, 412
Gastric juice, 397
Gastric ulcer, 530
Gastrointestinal bleeding, 411-412
Gaucher cell, 43
 cells similar to, 45, 47
 histologic description of, 41-42
 location of, 41
 staining of, 42
 ultrastructure of, 192, 204
Gaucher's disease
 classification of, 39, 41
 clinical features of, 39-41
 diagnosis of, 41-43
 inheritance pattern of, 39
 metabolic defect of, 39
 sphingolipids of, 39
 splenomegaly of, 61
 thrombocytopenia in, 803
Gene, 490
 allelomorphic, 491
 blood group, notation of, 491
 concept of, 491
 Hb C, 635, 636
 Hb D, 636
 Hb E, 635, 636
 in inheritance of blood group, 492
 sickle cell, 634
 in switching from fetal to adult hemoglobin, 623
 in synthesis of polypeptide chains of globin, 620, 621, 622
 in thalassemia, 635, 636, 649, 650
Genetic dysequilibrium, 521
Genotype, 491

Genotype—cont'd
 in ABO blood group system, 491, 492
  frequency of, 491-492
Geometric Data Hemotrak, 667
Geophagia, 397
Germ cells, 175
Giant lymph node hyperplasia, 102
Giemsa stain, 869
Gilbert's syndrome, 472-473, 650
Glanzmann and Riniker's lymphocytophthisis, 101
Glanzmann's thrombasthenia, 804
Globoside, 39
Globulin
 antihemolytic, storage of, 537
 secretion of, by plasma cell, 181
α-Globulin, 89
β-Globulin, 89, 397
γ-Globulin, 74, 89
 affinity of Cia for, 556
 B-lymphocyte receptors for, 86
 in Coombs' test, 589
 LE plasma factor, 680
 long-acting thyroid stimulator, 82
 use of, in therapy, 538
Glomerulonephritis, 683
Glucocerebrosidase, 41, 42, 43
 deficiency of, 39
  in Gaucher's disease, 39, 41-42
Glucose-6-phosphate dehydrogenase, 565, 566
 deficiency of, 565-566, 575
  ascorbate test in, 587
  clinical aspects of, 596-597
  differences in, among racial and geographic groups, 566
  fluorescent test for, 588
  glutathione stabilizer, 587
  Heinz bodies in, 580, 587, 632
  inheritance of, 566
  laboratory findings, 597
  methemoglobin reduction test for, 588
  treatment, 597
 effect of, on glutathione system, 565-566
 variants of, 566
α-Glucosidase, 82
Glucosyl ceramide lipidosis, 38
Glucosyl transferase, 788, 792
Glucuronic acid, 469, 470
β-Glucuronidase
 in Sezary cells, 165
 of T-lymphocytes, 85
Glucuronyl transferase, 469
 deficiency of
  hyperbilirubinemia with, 471
  in newborn, 472
Glue sniffing, 696
Glutamic acid, 421, 422
Glutathione, 556
Glutathione peroxidase, 565
 deficiency of, 587
  Heinz body formation with, 587
 in exertional hemoglobinuria, 570
Glutathione reductase, 565
 deficiency of, 587
  fluorescence test for, 588
  Heinz body formation with, 587
 in exertional hemoglobinuria, 570
Glutathione stability test, 587
Glutathione synthetase, 565
Glutathione system
 deficiency of, 565
 effect of glucose-6-phosphate dehydrogenase on, 565-566
Gluten, 397

Gluten-sensitive enteropathies, 443
Glycine, 418
Glycogen
 of platelets, 789
 in Sezary cell, 165
 staining of, 207
Glycogen storage disease, 818
Glycohemoglobin, 608-610
Glycolipids, 555
Glycophorin A, 555
Glycoproteins
 of erythrocyte membrane, 553, 555
 in proliferation and differentiation of stem cells,
  4, 6
Glycosaminoglycuronoglycan, 53
Gold salts, 696
Golgi apparatus, 36, 37, 76
Good's syndrome, 100
Goodpasture's syndrome, 401
Gout, 37, 559
Graft reaction, 83, 85
Granulation, toxic, 157, 158
Granules, cytoplasmic, 118
 acidophilic, 118
 azurophilic, 125, 182
 basophilic, 118, 125, 131, 182, 665, 676
 eosinophilic, 118, 125, 131, 182
 of leukocytes, 182
  staining of, 207
 of lymphocytes, 192
 of monocytes, 192
 neutrophilic, 118, 131, 182
 nonspecific, 157, 182
  in phagocytosis, 663
 siderotic, 402, 488-489
 specific, 157, 182, 663
α-Granules
 of platelets, 789
 in storage pool disease, 805
Granules of Palade, 182
Granulocytes, 699-700
 abnormal cytoplasmic maturation of, 118
 in activation of C5, 558
 azurophilic granules in, 36
 band, 130
  cytoplasm of, 131
  granules of, 131
  nucleus of, 131
  size of, 131
 basophilic; see Basophil
 breakdown products of, 660
 in Chediak-Higashi syndrome, 47
 in chronic granulomatous disease, 664
 circulating and marginating pool of, 24, 659
 eosinophilic; see Eosinophil
 HLA antigens of, 531
 of marrow, 659
 migration of, through endothelium and basement membrane, 660
 mitotic index of, 11
 in mucopolysaccharidoses, 55
 neonatal, rigidity of, 662
 neutrophilic; see Neutrophil
 Pelger-Huët anomaly in, 157
 release of, 659-660
 role of, in inflammation, 659
 segmented, 132
  cytoplasm of, 131
  granules of, 131
  in leukopoiesis, 24
  nucleus of, 131
  size of, 131
 sensitivity of, to radiation injury, 692
 spreading phenomenon of, 181

Granulocytes—cont'd
 stab, 131
 ultrastructure of, 182, 192
Granulocytic sarcomas, 724
Granulocytopenia
 from chronic exposure to radiation, 694
 chronic idiopathic, 688
Granulocytopoiesis
 inhibitors of, 25
 kinetics of, 24-25
  metamyelocyte, band, and segmented compartments, 24-25
  myelocyte compartment, 24
  progranulocyte compartment, 24
  stem cell compartment, 24
 and leukocytosis, 25
 splenomegaly with, 69
Granuloma, 220, 229
Granulomatous disease, chronic, 36, 47, 664
Granulopoiesis, 6
 in inflammation, 659
 site of, 11
Granulopoietin, 659
Griseofulvin, 455
Guanosine, 532, 535
Guillain-Barré, 677
Gumprecht ghosts, 726
Günther's disease, 451

H

H blood group substances, 498
H chain disease, 93, 98, 102-103
Hageman factor; see also Coagulation factors,
  XII
 deficiency of, 537, 777
Hageman trait, 831-832
"Hairy cell" leukemia, 725
Ham test, 596
Hamartoma, angiomatous lymphoid, 102
Hand-Schüller-Christian syndrome, 58, 61
Haploid cells, 175
Haptens
 in autoimmune hemolysis, 560
 in drug-related hemolysis, 562
Haptoglobin
 in abetalipoproteinemia, 595
 alleles, 464, 491
 binding of, to hemoglobin, 468, 469, 571
 concentration of, measurement of, 468
 electrophoresis of, 464, 465, 466, 468
 in hereditary elliptocytosis, 594-595
 as index of hemolysis, 546
 in lupus erythematosus, 681
 in paroxysmal nocturnal hemoglobinuria, 596
 quantification of, 893-894
 in sequestration hemolysis, 570
 types of, 464, 465, 466
  frequency of, 467
  predicted inheritance of, 467
Haptoglobin-hemoglobin complex, 546
Hassall's corpuscle, 101
 in thymus, 81
Heart disease, 705
Heat stability test of hemoglobin, 631
Heavy chain disease, 748
Hedulin; see Phenindione
Heinz bodies, 488
 with deficiency of glucose-6-phosphate dehydrogenase, 566, 632
 in diagnosis of hemolytic disease, 580, 587
 in erythrocytes from toxic dyes, 460
 formation of, 587
 in sickle cells, 638
 tests for, 886

Heinz bodies—cont'd
 in thalassemias, 632
 with unstable hemoglobin, 632, 644
Helmet cells, 483, 580
Hemac laser cell counter, 360
 in calculation of erythrocyte indices, 380
 in erythrocyte counts, 372-373
  significance of successive cell counts, 374
Hemangiomas, 803
Hematin, 461
 conversion of, to biliverdin, 469
Hematobium infection, 412
Hematocrit, 357-362
 amount of trapped plasma, 359
 body, 357, 360, 394
 calculation, 360
 clinical correlation of, 361-362
 conditions of centrifugation, 357-359
 definition of, 357
 measurement of, 372
  by Coulter S model, 381
  effect of posture on, 378
  manually, by microhematocrit technic, 381,
   383-384
 microhematocrit methods, 360, 383-384
 normal values, 360-361
 in polycythemia vera, 702
 in prethrombotic states, 853, 855
 vs relative blood viscosity, 351, 361-362
 response of 2,3-DPG to, 392
 use of data from, 359-360
 venous, 357, 360, 394
Hematology
 adoption of SI units, 386, 387
 application of statistics in, 367-380
  erythrocyte counts, 370-372
   Coulter cell counter, 371-372
   hemocytometer method, 371-372
   Hemac cell counter, 372-373
  erythrocyte indices, 379-380
   calculated by electronic counters, 380
   mean corpuscular hemoglobin, 379-380
   mean corpuscular hemoglobin concentra-
    tion, 380
   mean corpuscular volume, 379
   use of, 380
  interpretation of quantitative data, 367-373
  normal values
   determination of, 376-377
   effect of age on, 378
   effect of altitude on, 378-379
   effect of dehydration on, 378
   effect of exercise or excitement on, 378
   effect of posture on, 378
   effect of sex on, 378
   physiologic variations on, 377-379
  significance of successive cell counts, 373-
   374
   with electronic cell counter, 374
   with hemocytometer counts, 373-374
 quality assurance in, 381-387
  blood hemoglobin, 382-383
  Coulter Model S, 381-382
  leukocyte differential counts, 384
  microhematocrit, 383-384
  partial thromboplastin time, 387
  platelet counts, 384-385
  prothrombin time, 385-387
Hematopoietic hypoplasia, 101-102
Hematoporphyria, 447
Hematoside, 39
Heme
 binding of, by serum protein, 469
 binding of, to globin, 644

Heme—cont'd
  biosynthesis of, 448-449
  from dissociation of methemoglobin, 571
  effect of, on δ-aminolevulinic acid, 454
  in formation of hemoglobin, 447
  from hemoglobin catabolism, 469
  as iron-containing porphyrin, 447
  location of, in structure of hemoglobin, 606,
    607
  oxygenation of, 607
  spectroscopic identification of, 461
  structure of, 448
  synthesis of
    disruption of, with lead intoxication, 414
    effect of lead on, 455
    from protoporphyrin and iron, 402
  in synthesis of hemoglobin, 395
Heme oxygenase, 469
Heme synthetase, 449
Hemichromes, 461
Hemiglobin, 457
Hemin, 461
Hemochromatosis
  with excessive absorption of iron, 397
  iron overload in, 409
  megaloblastic anemia in, 444
  secondary, 355
  transferrin saturation in, 410
Hemochromes, 447, 448
Hemocyanin, 403, 447
Hemocytoblast, 6, 78
Hemocytometer, 862-863, 864
Hemocytometer method
  for blood cell counts, 370-371
    calculation of standard deviation, 370-371
    inherent errors, 370
    in successive cell counts, significance of,
      373-374, 375
    technical and human errors, 370
  for calibration of Coulter Model S, 381
Hemoglobin, 447
  affinity of, for oxygen, 389, 390
  allosteric model of, 607
  bile pigment excretion related to total, 572
  breakdown of, 38, 64
    bile pigments from, 572
    bilirubin from, 572, 574
    porphyrins from, 352, 447
    urobilinogen from, 572, 573, 574
  carboxyhemoglobin, 456
  catabolism of, 469-474
    formation of bilirubin, 469-471
    hyperbilirubinemia, 471-474
      chronic idiopathic jaundice, 473-474
      congenital nonhemolytic jaundice, 474
      constitutional hepatic dysfunction, 472-
        473
      familial nonhemolytic jaundice, 474
      hemolytic disease, 472
      hereditary, in rats and sheep, 472
      neonatal, 471-472
      unconjugated, 472
  changes in, with oxygenation and deoxygen-
    ation, 535
  combination and release of oxygen with, 607-
    608
  concentration of, in blood, 530
    determination of, 372, 377
  conversion of, to cyanmethemoglobin, 382
  decrease in, from increased plasma volume,
    394
  denatured, in Heinz bodies, 488
  in diagnosis of anemia, 392
  in diagnosis of hemolytic disease, 575-576

Hemoglobin—cont'd
  dissociation and recombination of, 632
  effect of, on erythropoietic cells, 22
  effect of altitude on, 378-379, 704
  effect of benzoquinone acetic acid on, 460
  effect of erythrocytic deficiency on, 565
  elaboration of, in cell maturation, 118
  electrophoresis of, 888-892
    agar gel, acid pH, 890
    cellulose acetate, alkaline pH, 889-890
    differential, for hemoglobin H, 890-891
    and globin chain separation, 891-892
    preparation of hemolysate, 888-889
  estimation of erythrocyte content of, 360
  exposure of, to carbon monoxide, 456
  fetal; see Fetal hemoglobin
  geographic distribution of, 633
  haptoglobin, 464-469
  in hemolytic reaction, 545
    presence in blood, 546
    presence in urine, 546
  interaction of 2,3-DPG with, 391, 392, 535
  iron content of, 401, 409
  in isoimmune hemolytic disease, 600
  location of, within erythrocytes, 553
  massing of, in elliptocytes, 481
  measurement of, 378, 875-882
    abnormal compounds, 876-883
      and assay of serum iron concentration,
        882-883
      identification of, 876-877
      methemoglobin, 881-882
      porphobilinogen, 877, 880-881
      porphyrins, 877-880
      by spectroscopy, 876
    in measurement of mean corpuscular hemoglo-
      bin, 379-380
    in measurement of mean corpuscular hemoglo-
      bin concentration, 380
  metabolism of, 570-574
  methemalbumin, 461
  methemoglobin, 456-460
    in acquired methemoglobinemia, 460
    in hereditary methemoglobinemia
      deficient reducing systems, 458-460
      excessive oxidative activity, 460
      Hb M variants, 457-458
    minimal renal threshold of, 468
    from normoblasts, 192
  permeability of, to erythrocyte membrane,
    555
  in pernicious anemia, 432
  of polychromatophilic normoblast, 142
  in polycythemia vera, 702
  from primitive erythroblasts, 8
  quantification of, 894
  relaxed vs tense state of, 607
  in sickle cell disease, 68
  in sickling reactions, 625
  spectroscopic identification of, 461, 464
  structure of, 391, 423, 603-608
    primary, 604
    quaternary, 607-608
    secondary, 604
    tertiary, 606-607
  sulfhemoglobin, 461
  synthesis of
    effect of blood transfusions on, 530
    failure of, in iron-deficiency anemias, 395
    genetic control of, 610-623
      inheritance patterns, 610, 620
      polypeptide chains, 620-622
      in switch from fetal to adult, 622-623
    iron in, 395

Hemoglobin—cont'd
  in thalassemia, 68
  unstable, 600, 644-646
    associated with hemolytic anemia, 644
    glutathione stability test with, 587
    Heinz bodies with, 580, 587
    tests for, 587, 631-632
      heat denaturation test, 886-887
      inclusion bodies, 886
      isopropanol precipitation test, 887
  variants of, 610-620
    α chain, 611-613
    β chain, 614-618
    δ chain, 618
    γ chain, 619
    classification of, 610
    with deleted residues, 619
    with extended chains, 620
    with more than one point mutation, 620
    nomenclature of, 610
Hemoglobin A, 460, 603
  erythrocyte with, sickling of, 624
  switch from fetal hemoglobin to, 622-623
Hemoglobin A_1, 608-610
  denaturation of, 625
  electrophoretic identification of, 626, 629
  with sickle cell anemia, 636
  in sickle cell trait, 640
  structure of, 604, 605, 606
  in thalassemia, 633, 650
Hemoglobin A_2, 608, 609
  electrophoretic identification of, 629, 630,
    631
  elevation of, 633
  quantification of, 626
    by microchromatography, 892-893
  with sickle cell anemia, 636
  structure of, 604, 605
  in thalassemia, 650, 653
Hemoglobin A_3, 604, 608
Hemoglobin Agenogi, 649
Hemoglobin Bart, 625, 655
Hemoglobin Beth Israel, 649
Hemoglobin Bibba, 646
Hemoglobin C, 626
Hemoglobin C disease, 641
  codocytes in, 481
  with sickle cell anemia, 643-644
Hemoglobin C Harlem, 626
Hemoglobin C trait, 641
  elliptocytosis with, 483
  and resistance to malaria, 641
Hemoglobin C-β-thalassemia, 653
Hemoglobin Constant Spring, 655
Hemoglobin Coventry, 656
Hemoglobin D, 626
  electrophoretic identification of, 626, 628,
    641
Hemoglobin D disease and trait, 641
  with sickle cell anemia, 644
Hemoglobin D Ibadan, 644
Hemoglobin D Punjab, 644
Hemoglobin D-thalassemia, 653
Hemoglobin E, 626
Hemoglobin E disease and trait, 641-643
Hemoglobin E-β-thalassemia, 653
Hemoglobin Freiburg, 646, 649
Hemoglobin G-thalassemia, 653
Hemoglobin Genova, 646
Hemoglobin Gower, 604
Hemoglobin Gun Hill, 646
Hemoglobin H, 632, 633
  electrophoresis of, 890-891
Hemoglobin Hope, 649

Hemoglobin I, 632
Hemoglobin I-α-thalassemia, 655
Hemoglobin J, 625
Hemoglobin J-thalassemia, 653
Hemoglobin Kansas, 649
Hemoglobin King's County, 626
Hemoglobin Leiden, 644, 645, 646
Hemoglobin Lepore syndromes, 656, 657
Hemoglobin Lincoln Park, 656
Hemoglobin Little Rock, 648
  electrophoretic identification of, 626
Hemoglobin M
  abnormal function of, 458
  abnormal pigments of, 456
  variants of, 457, 458
Hemoglobin Miyada, 656
Hemoglobin Munchausen syndrome, 636
Hemoglobin P Congo, 656
Hemoglobin P Nilotic, 656
Hemoglobin Peterborough, 649
Hemoglobin Philly, 646
Hemoglobin Portland 1, 604
Hemoglobin Q-α-thalassemia, 655
Hemoglobin Rainier, 625
Hemoglobin S
  centrifugation test of, 888
  in drepanocyte, 481
  electrophoretic identification of, 624, 626
  hereditary persistence of fetal hemoglobin with, 644
  identification of, 640
  molecular rearrangement of for sickling reaction, 625
  peptide pattern of, 632
  quantification of, 892-893
  screening for, 641
  in sickle cell anemia, 603
  in sickle cell trait, 640
  solubility test for, 626, 887-888
  structural formula of, 636
  tests for, 624
Hemoglobin S–Hemoglobin E hemoglobinopathy, 644
Hemoglobin S–Hemoglobin G Philadelphia hemoglobinopathy, 644
Hemoglobin S–Hemoglobin J Baltimore hemoglobinopathy, 644
Hemoglobin S–Hemoglobin K hemoglobinopathy, 644
Hemoglobin S–Hemoglobin O Arab hemoglobinopathy, 644
Hemoglobin Sabine, 646
Hemoglobin Santa Ana, 646
Hemoglobin Seattle, 649
Hemoglobin Stanleyville II, 626
Hemoglobin Tacoma, 646
Hemoglobin Titusville, 649
Hemoglobin Tübingen, 649
Hemoglobin Yoshizuka, 649
Hemoglobin-haptoglobin complex, 464, 468, 469
  clearance of, 571
Hemoglobinemia
  in glucose-6-phosphate dehydrogenase, 597
  in hemolytic disease, 571
  in paroxysmal cold hemoglobinuria, 600
  in paroxysmal nocturnal hemoglobinuria, 596
Hemoglobinometry, 875
  cyanmethemoglobin method, 875-876
  oxyhemoglobin method, 875
Hemoglobinopathies, 575
  alteration of hemoglobin molecule in, 608
  ascorbate test for, 587

Hemoglobinopathies—cont'd
  associated with abnormal oxygen transport, 646
    congenital methemoglobinemia, 649
    with cyanosis, 649
    with erythrocytes, 646-649
  classification of, 603, 623
  erythrocyte survival time in, 553
  geographic distribution, 633-636
  Hb C disease and trait, 641
  Hb D disease and trait, 641
  Hb E disease and trait, 641-643
  history of, 603
  interaction between two structurally abnormal hemoglobins, 643-644
    sickle cell–Hb C disease, 643-644
    sickle cell–Hb D disease, 644
  laboratory diagosis of, 623-633
    ferrohemoglobin solubility, 626
    fingerprint technic, 631
    alkali denaturation test for Hb F, 625-626
    erythrocyte distribution by acid elution for Hb F, 626
    hybridization technic, 632
    ion-exchange chromatography, 631
    precautions in, 632-633
    quantification of Hb A_2, 626
    tests for erythrocyte sickling, 624-625
    tests for unstable hemoglobin, 631-632
    zone electrophoresis, 626-631
  red cell morphology in, 407
  screening for Hb S, 641
  sickle cell anemia, 636-640
    clinical features, 638-640
    hemoglobin synthesis, 636
    laboratory diagnosis and findings, 640
    pathogenesis, 636-638
  sickle cell trait, 640-641
  with sickling of erythrocytes, 625
  thalassemia; *see* Thalassemia
  unstable hemoglobin disease, 644-646
Hemoglobinuria, 468, 575
  exertional or march, 570
  in hemolytic disease, 571
  paroxysmal cold, 563
  paroxysmal nocturnal, 552, 558, 563-564
Hemohistioblast, 6
Hemolysin
  Donath-Landsteiner, 884
Hemolysis
  caused by deficiency of erythrocytic enzymes, 565-567
  caused by hereditary abnormality of red cell membrane, 567-569
    abetalipoproteinemia, 568
    congenital dyserythropoietic anemia, 569
    hereditary elliptocytosis, 568
    hereditary spherocytosis, 567-568
    hereditary stomatocytosis, 568-569
    high phosphatidylcholine hemolytic anemia, 569
    lecithin-cholesterol acyltransferase deficiency, 569
    Zieve's syndrome, 569
  colloid osmotic, 555-556
    antibodies in, 558
    with hereditary spherocytosis, 567
  complement-dependent, 563-564
    paroxysmal cold hemoglobinuria, 563
    paroxysmal nocturnal hemoglobinuria, 563-564
  drug-related, 562-563
    of alpha-methyldopa type, 563

Hemolysis—cont'd
  drug-related—cont'd
    with glucose-6-phosphate dehydrogenase, 566
    of hapten type, 562
    of innocent bystander type, 562-563
    nonimmunologic, 556, 563
    positive antiglobulin test with, 563
  isoimmune, 560-562
  sequestration, liver and spleen in, 570
Hemolytic anemia, 551-601
  acanthocytes in, 479
  acquired, idiopathic
    increased osmotic fragility of erythrocytes in, 583
    survival curves of RBC in, 552
  associated with lymphoma, 552
  with atrophy of spleen, 65
  autoimmune; see Autoimmune hemolytic anemia
  blood transfusion for, 530
  characteristics of, 593-601
    abetalipoproteinemia, 595-596
      clinical aspects of, 595
      etiology and pathogenesis of, 595
      laboratory findings, 595-596
      treatment of, 596
    autoimmune, 597-600
      cold antibody type, 599
      drug-induced type, 599
      etiology and pathogenesis, 597-599
      warm antibody type, 599
    elliptocytic, 594-595
      clinical aspects, 594
      etiology and pathogenesis, 594
      laboratory findings, 594-595
      treatment, 595
    enzymatic defects, 597
    glucose-6-phosphate dehydrogenase, 596-597
      clinical aspects, 596-597
      etiology and pathogenesis, 596
      laboratory findings, 597
    isoimmune, 600-601
      clinical aspects, 600
      etiology and pathogenesis of, 600
      laboratory findings, 600-601
      prevention, 601
    hereditary spherocytosis, 593
      clinical aspects, 593
      etiology and pathogenesis of, 593
      laboratory findings, 593-594
      treatment, 594
    paroxysmal cold hemoglobinuria, 600
    paroxysmal nocturnal hemoglobinuria, 596
  of Chaauffard-Minkowski syndrome, 567
  classification of, 553
    etiologic, 554
  compensated, 552
  congenital, 567
  with congenital erythropoietic porphyria, 451
  with congenital spherocytic, 66
  decompensated, 552
  drug-induced, 565
  dyserythropoietic, 552
  effect of, on marrow space, 222
  elliptocytosis, 483
  erythrocyte sedimentation rate in, 352
  erythrocytes in, 103
  erythroid hyperplasia in, 699
  and extramedullary hemopoiesis, 30, 32, 33
  folate deficiency from, 441
  free erythrocyte protoporphyrin, 449
  haptoglobins in, 468

Hemolytic anemia—cont'd
Heinz bodies in, 488
hemoglobin catabolism in, 469
Howell-Jolly bodies in, 488
in immunoblastic lymphadenopathy, 102
in infectious mononucleosis, 677, 678
isoimmune; see Isoimmune hemolytic anemia
knizocytes of, 486
laboratory diagnosis of, 574-593
  clinical-pathologic approach to, 574-575
  erythrocyte count and hemoglobin concentration, 575-576
  erythrocyte indices, 577
  erythrocyte morphology in, 577-582
    acanthocytes, 580
    codocytes, 580
    distorted and disrupted, 578-580
    drepanocytes, 580
    erythrophagocytes, 580
    giant platelets, 580
    Heinz bodies, 580
    normoblasts, 580
    parasites, 582
    polychromatophilia, 578
    siderocytes, 580-582
    spherocytes, 577-578
    stomatocytes, 580
  importance of peripheral blood smear, 575
  leukocyte count, 576
  metabolic abnormalities, 586-588
    ascorbate test for, 587
    autohemolysis, 586-587
    fluorescence test for glucose-6-phosphate dehydrogenase, 588
    fluorescence test for glutathione reductase, 588
    fluorescence test for pyruvate kinase, 588
    fluorescence test for triosephosphate isomerase, 588
    glutathione stability test, 587
    Heinz body formaton, 587
    methemoglobin reduction test, 588
    orthocresol reduction test, 588
    unstable hemoglobin test, 587
  osmotic fragility, 582-586
    after incubation, 586
    interpretation of results, 583-586
    significance of measurements, 583
  platelet count, 577
  reticulocyte count, 577
  serologic investigations, 588-593
    agglutination in albumin and serum-albumin media, 592
    agglutination of enzyme-treated erythrocytes, 592
    complete agglutinating antibodies, 592
    direct antiglobulin test, 589-590
    γ-globulin neutralization test, 591-592
    hemolytic antibodies, 592
    indirect antiglobulin test, 590-591
    in isoimmune hemolytic disease, 592-593
    use of low-ionic strength suspending media, 592
in lupus erythematosus, 681, 682
metabolism of hemoglobin and bile pigments in, 570-574
  hemoglobinemia, 571
  hemoglobinuria, 571
  hemosiderinuria, 571
  methemalbumin, 571
  quantitative relationships, 571-574
    bilirubin urobilinogen, 573-574
    corrected fecal urobilinogen excretion, 572

Hemolytic anemia—cont'd
metabolism of hemoglobin and bile pigments in—cont'd
  quantitative relationships—cont'd
    fecal urobilinogen, 572-573
    fluctuations in pigment excretion, 572
    hemolytic index, 572
    pigment excretion related to total hemoglobin, 572
    source of bile pigments, 572
    specificity to Ehrlich's aldehyde reaction, 574
    urinary urobilinogen, 573-574
microangiopathic, 569-570, 843
with neoplasms, 30
normoblastic hyperplasia with, 246, 247
in paroxysmal nocturnal hemoglobinuria, 552
pathogenesis of, 553-570
  colloid osmotic hemolysis, 555-556
  complement, 556-565
    activator system, 558-559
    in autoimmune hemolysis, 559-560
    convertase system, 557-558
    definition of, 564-565
    in drug-related hemolysis, 562-563
    interactions of, 559
    in isoimmune hemolysis, 560-562
    special types of complement-dependent hemolysis, 563-564
  erythrophagocytosis, 570
  due to deficiency of erythrocytic enzymes, 565-567
    glucose-6-phosphate dehydrogenase, 565-566
    glutathione-dependent systems, 565
    pyruvate kinase, 566-567
  due to hereditary abnormalities of red cell membrane, 567-570
    abetalipoproteinemia, 568
    congenital dyserythropoietic anemia, 569
    hereditary elliptocytosis, 568
    hereditary spherocytosis, 567-568
    hereditary stomatocytosis, 568-569
    high phosphatidylcholine, 569
    lecithin-cholesterol acyltransferase deficiency, 569
    Zieve's syndrome, 569
  immune hemolysin, 556
  mechanical fragmentation, 569-570
    from cardiac valves, 569
    exertional hemoglobinuria, 570
    microangiopathic hemolytic anemia, 569-570
  spleen and liver sequestration, 570
  due to structure of erythrocyte membrane, 553-555
  transport of sodium and potassium, 555
reticulocyte count in, 407, 487
reticulum cell in, 124
with Rh_null type blood, 508
rouleau formation in, 352
spherocytes of, 483
spleen in, 66-69
stomatocyte in, 478
from toxic dyes, 460
treatment of, 540-541
with unstable hemoglobin, 644
Hemolytic disease
  with abetalipoproteinemia, 479
  definition of, 551
  hyperbilirubinemia in, 471, 472
  normoblasts of, staining of, 207
  of sickle cell disease, 636
  tests for
    acid serum test, 884

Hemolytic disease—cont'd
tests for—cont'd
  alkali denaturation test, 885
  autohemolysis, 884-885
  demonstration of Donath-Landsteiner hemolysin, 884
  demonstration of fetal hemoglobin by acid elution technic, 885-886
  demonstration of sickle cells, 887
  hemoglobin electrophoresis, 888-892
    in agar gel, 890
    in cellulose acetate, 889-890
    differential, 890-891
    globin chain separation, 891-892
    preparation of hemolysate, 888-889
  osmotic fragility of erythrocytes, 883
    after incubation, 883
    method of Dacie, 883
    method of Sanford, 883
  quantification of Hb A_2 and Hb S by microchromatology, 892-893
  quantification of serum haptoglobin, 893-894
  quantitative hemoglobin in plasma and urine, 894
  solubility test for Hb S, 887-888
  sugar water test, 884
  susceptibility to Heinz body formation, 886
  unstable hemoglobins, 886-887
    Hb H inclusion bodies, 886
    heat denaturation test, 886-887
    inclusion bodies, 886
    isopropanol precipitation test, 887
Hemolytic crisis, 575
  aplastic type of, 575, 576
  in hereditary spherocytosis, 593
Hemolytic disease of newborn, 8, 500-501, 600
  A-B-O in, 562
  antiglobulin test of, 589
  Diego blood group system in, 513
  from Duffy blood group, 512
  from Kell factor, 512
  from Kidd blood group system, 513
  from Lutheran blood group, 511 512
  increased osmotic fragility of erythrocyte in, 583
  from isoantibodies, 589
  Rh in, 559, 561
Hemolytic index, 572
Hemolytic reactions, 544-546
  clinicopathologic correlation, 545-546
  delayed, 545
  etiology of, 544-545
  investigation of, 546
Hemolytic-uremic syndrome, 570
Hemopexin, 469, 571
Hemophilia, 779, 823-830
  clinical findings, 827-828
  genetics, 825-826
  incidence, 826
  laboratory diagnosis, 828-830
  multiple factor deficiencies, 828
  severity, 826-827
  sex-linked inheritance of, 774
  therapy for, 832
  treatment of, 538
    prior to surgery, 540
Hemophilia B, 830
Hemophilia B Chapel Hill, 830
Hemophilia B Leyden, 830
Hemophilia Bm, 830
Hemopoiesis, 1-34
  abnormal, synchronism in cell maturation in, 117

Hemopoiesis—cont'd
  in adult, 9-10
  canine cycle, 6
  definition, 3
  derivation of blood cells, 3-4
  ectopic, 28-29
    bone marrow embolism distinguished from, 29
    vs extramedullary, 29
  in embryo, 6-11
    control of erythropoiesis in fetus and new-born, 8-9
    hepatic, 9-10
    medullary, 10-11
    mesoblastic period, 6-8
    primitive erythroblasts vs definitive normo-blasts, 8
  erythropoiesis, 17-24
    effective vs total, 22-24
    and erythron, 22
    erythropoietin in, 17-22
      assay of, and normal values, 18-20
      chemistry of, 20
      formation and metabolism of, 20-21
      immunology of, 20
      physiologic and pathologic significance of, 21-22
    normal, 22
    quantitative aspects of, 22-24
  extramedullary, 10, 28-32
    ectopic vs, 28-29
    and hemopoietic potential of mesenchymal cells, 30
    in liver and spleen, 30
    in lymph nodes, 31
    lymph node imprint of, 106
    in myeloproliferative syndrome, 268
    in normal infants, 29
    possible mechanisms of, 29-30
    relation between fetal and, 29
    relation of medullary to, 30-32
    simulating tumor, 30
    sites of, 32
    study of, 211
    with thalassemia, 69
  endocrines in, 15-16
    adrenal, 16
    pituitary, 15-16
    sex hormones, 16
    thyroid, 16
  hepatic, 9-10
  kinetics of, 11-14
    feedback rate-regulating systems, 14
    quantitative aspects, 11-14
  leukopoiesis, 24-27
    granulocytopoiesis and leukocytosis, 25
    inhibitors, 25
    kinetics of granulocytopoiesis, 24-25
      metamyelocyte, band, and segmented compartments, 24-25
      myelocyte compartment, 24
      progranulocyte compartments, 24
      stem cell compartments, 24
    lymphocytes, 25-27
      adrenocortical influence on, 26-27
      definition, 25
      fate of, 26
      life span of, 25
      origin of, 25
  through lymphomyeloid complex, 74
  medullary, 9, 10-11
    qualitative and quantitative data on, 211
  neurogenic control of, 17
  nucleic acids in, 15

Hemopoiesis—cont'd
  pathologic, with abnormal cell maturation, 118
  and release of blood cells, 32-34
  stem cell for, 4-6
  thrombocytopoiesis, 27-28
Hemopoietic inducive microenvironment, 6
Hemopoietin, 17-18
  in stimulation of differentiation of stem cells, 4
Hemorheology, 351
Hemorrhage; see also Bleeding
  acute, increased fibrinolysis in, 847
  anemia due to
    blood transfusion for, 530
    reticulocytosis in, 577
  cerebral, associated with leukemoid reaction, 254, 255
  in hemophilia, 827-828
  normoblastic hyperplasia with, 240
  in polycythemia vera, 703
  reticulocytosis with, 487
  thrombocytopenia from, 802
  vitamin B$_{12}$ levels with, 437
Hemorrhagic diseases, 774
  caused by vascular defects, 848-855
    allergic purpura, 852
    autoerythrocyte sensitization, 852
    connective tissue disorders, 852
    hereditary hemorrhagic telangiectasia, 848-852
    prethrombotic state, 852-855
      coagulation factors in, 854
      platelets in, 853-854
      products of fibrinogen to fibrin conversion, 854-855
      products of fibrinolysis, 854-855
      reduced fibrinolytic acitivity, 855
      serum lipoproteins, 855
    scurvy, 848
    thrombotic thrombocytopenic purpura, 852
  investigation of, 857-858
  laboratory diagnosis of
    preoperative tests, 855-856
    through anticoagulant therapy, 856
      heparin, 856-857
      oral, 856
  of newborn, 836
  recurrent patterns in, 858
Hemorrhoids, 411
Hemosiderin, 64, 409
  appearance of, 400
  from breakdown of hemoglobin, 571
  in histologic sections, 410
  identification of, 400
  location of, 400
  with sickle cell disease, 68
  as storage iron, 395, 400
Hemosiderinuria, 571
Hemosiderosis, 401
  pulmonary, idiopathic, 401
Hemostasis, 777-778
  mechanism of, 778
  in newborn, 787
  platelets in, 787
Henoch-Schönlein purpura, 852
Heparin
  administration of, lowered PT with, 833
  assay for, 938
  control of therapy of, 856-857
  for diffuse intravascular coagulation, 847
  effect of, 856
  effect of, on sedimentation rate, 354
  thrombocytopenic purpura from, 802

Heparin—cont'd
  in treatment of hypofibrinogenemia, 536
Hepatic dysfunction, constitutional, 472-473
Hepatic hemopoiesis, 9-10
Hepatic porphyria, 454
Hepatitis, 541-543
  with aplastic anemia, 698
  as complication of infectious mononucleosis, 677, 678
  coproporphyrin excretion in, 455
  incidence of, with administration of fibrinogen, 537
  viral, 541-543
  infectious, 541
    transmission of, 541
  non-A, non-B, 541, 542
  with red cell aplasia, 699
  serum
    and Australian antigen, 541
    transmission of, 541, 543
  transfusion, 527, 528
Hepatitis A, 541, 542
  antigen, 541
Hepatitis B, 541, 542
  antigen, 541, 542
Hepatitis Be antigen, 542
Hepatocytes, 85
Hepatoma, 455
Hepatomegaly, 36
  in acute myelocytic leukemia, 724
  in Chediak-Higashi syndrome, 47
  with Gaucher's disease, 39, 41
  in hemolytic anemia, 575
  in Hunter-Hurler syndrome, 53
  in idiopathic jaundice, 473
  with immunoblastic lymphadenopathy, 102
  in infectious mononucleosis, 677
  in isoimmune hemolytic disease, 600
  in Letterer-Siwe disease, 58
  in myeloproliferative syndrome, 700
    familial, 708
    myelofibrosis, 706
    polycythemia vera, 701
  in Niemann-Pick disease, 43, 44
  in sea-blue histiocyte syndrome, 45
Hereditary coproporphyria, 454
Hereditary erythroblastic multinuclearity with pos-itive acidified serum test, 569
Hermansky-Pudlak syndrome, 806
Herpes zoster, 673
Heterochromatin mass, 173
Hexachlorobenzene, 454-455
Hexokinase deficiency, 587
Hexose monophosphate shunt, 458
  in glucose metabolism in RBC, 565
  increased activity of, in neutrophil with phago-cytosis, 663
Hiatus leukemicus, 119
Hill equation, 389
Histamine
  in basophils, 665
  effect of, in immune reaction, 87
  in eosinophil chemotaxis, 660, 665
  release of
    from basophil, 94
    from mast cell, 94
    mediated by complement system, 359
Histidine, 421
Histiocyte, 3
  blue-staining, 45
  in chronic granulomatous disease, 664
  in eosinophilic granuloma, 61
  in Hand-Schüller-Christian disease, 58
  in Letterer-Siwe disease, 58

Histiocyte—cont'd
  in immunoblastic lymphadenopathy, 102
  in iron storage, 64
  of lymph nodes, 105
  phagocytic, 36
    ultrastructure of, 192, 197, 203
Histiocytes of Maximow, 2
Histiocyte syndrome, sea-blue, 45
Histiocytosis
  idiopathic, 58-61
  sea-blue, 45, 46
  sinus, with lymphadenopathy, 102
Histiocytosis X, 58
Histoplasma, 229, 231
HLA system, 89, 521
  use of, in establishing parentage, 514, 516, 521
Hodgkin's disease, 759-771
  blastoid transformation of lymphocytes in, 83
  case study of, 109, 336-337
    differential cell count, 326
    history and physical exam, 326
    laboratory data, 326
  classification of, 759
  clinical correlations, 771
  clinical presentation and staging, 770
  criteria for diagnosis, 770-771
  eosinophilia in, 256
  ferritin levels in, 409
  histologic types of, 763
  lymph node aspiration with, 109
  lymph node imprints, 108, 109
  lymphocyte depletion type, 688, 763, 770
  lymphocytic predominance type, 763
  MIF activity in, 85
  mixed cellularity type, 763
  nodular sclerosis type, 763
  Reed-Sternberg cells in, 175
  reticulum cell in, 124
  staging laparotomy, 770
  survival rate, 771
  T-lymphocyte in, 85
Homeostasis of blood cells, 14
Homocysteine, 423
Homograft rejection, 75
Hookworm infection, 412
Hormones
  effect of, on ESR, 355-356
  in hemopoiesis, 15-16
Howell-Jolly bodies, 64, 65, 488
  in Evans' syndrome, 598
  in iron-deficiency anemias, 407
  in pernicious anemia, 432, 435
  in sickle cell anemia, 640
Humoral immunity, 89-98
  with ataxia-telangiectasia, 101
  B-lymphocyte in, 74, 86
  bursa of Fabricius in, 74
  deficiencies in, 104
  immunoglobulins in, 89-98
    allotypes, 95-96
    catabolism of, 98
    definition of, 89
    function of, 93-94
    normal serum concentrations in, 98
    structure of, 89-93
    synthesis of, 96-98
      genetics of, 94-95
  with severe combined immunodeficiency, 101
  with thymoma, 100
  with X-linked agammaglobulinemia, 100
Hunter-Hurler syndrome, 53, 54, 55
Hurler's syndrome, 53, 54, 55
Hyaluronidase, 848

Hydralazine, 682, 683
Hydroa aestivale, 451
Hydrogen peroxide
  in chronic granulomatous disease, 664
  in phagocytosis, 664
Hydrolases, lysosomal, 36
Hydrops fetalis, 600
Hydroxyethyl starch, 532
Hydroxyethylated amylopectin, 532
Hydroxyurea, 419
Hyperbilirubinemia, 471-474, 574
  in chronic idiopathic jaundice, 473-474
  classification of, 472
  in congenital nonhemolytic jaundice, 474
  in constitutional hepatic dysfunction, 472-473
  in familial nonhemolytic jaundice, 474
  in glucose-6-phosphate dehydrogenase deficiency, 597
  in hemolytic anemia, 575
  in hemolytic disease of newborn, 562
  in hemolytic reactions, 545, 546
  hereditary, in rats and sheep, 472
  with increased erythrocyte destruction, 552
  in isoimmune hereditary disease, 600
  neonatal, 471-472
  in paroxysmal nocturnal hemoglobinuria, 596
  in pernicious anemia, 429
  physiologic, 8
  treatment of, 540
  unconjugated, 472
Hypereosinophilic syndrome, 675
Hyperglycemia, 804
Hyperimmunoglobulinemia, 100, 101, 102-103, 320
  chronic lymphocytic leukemia, 103
  drug-induced lymphadenopathy, 103
  infectious mononucleosis, 103
  gamma heavy chain diseases, 102-103
  giant lymph node hyperplasia, 102
  immunoblastic lymphadenopathy, 102
  lymphadenopathy with sinus histiocytosis, 102
Hyperpituitarism, 16
Hyperproteinemia, 98
Hypersensitivity reactions, 546-548
  acute pulmonary edema, 548
  allergies, 546
  anaphylactoid reactions, 548
  delayed; *see* Delayed hypersensitivity reaction
  febrile reaction, 547
  immediate reactions, 87, 88, 546-547
  serum sickness, 547-548
Hypersplenism, 65
Hypertension, portal, 61
Hyperthyroidism, 16
Hyperviscosity syndrome, 351
Hypoalbuminemia, 538
Hypofibrinogenemia, 841
  acquired, 842-843
  in acute promyelocytic leukemia, 300
  congenital, 777
Hypogammaglobulinemia, 98, 538, 663
Hypoimmunoglobulinemia, 98-100
Hypophysectomy, 16
Hypophysis, 2, 3
Hypopituitarism, 16
Hypoproteinemia, 538
  blood transfusion in treatment of, 532
  hypocupremia in, 404
  plasma transfusion for, 537
Hypothyroidism, 16
Hypoxia
  adaptations to, 392
  cause of, 388-389
  in causing secondary polycythemia, 704, 705

Hypoxia—cont'd
  due to high altitudes, 391-392
  effect of, on 2,3-DPG, 391
  effect of, on erythropoiesis, 379
  with formation of carboxyhemoglobin, 456
  vs hemoglobin concentration, 456
  in regulation of erythropoietin, 21
  in sickle cell anemia, 636
  symptoms of, 704

I

I-i blood group system, 513
Icterus, 567
Idiogram, 173
IgA, 74, 89, 92
  with absence of plasma cells, 104
  with ataxia-telangiectasia, 94, 101
  concentration of, in serum, 98
  as cryoglobins, 748
  deficiency of, 102
    with pernicious anemia, 430
  evolution of, 95
  in giant lymph node hyperplasia, 102
  half-life of, 98
  in hyperviscosity syndrome, 351
  lupus erythematosus, 683
  in lymphadenopathy with sinus histiocytosis, 102
  molecular weight of, 91
  in monoclonal immunoglobulinopathy, 748
  in penicillin sensitivity reaction, 562
  polypeptide chain of, 90
    secretory, 90, 91
    transplacental passage of, 91
IgA heavy chain disease, 443
IgD, 74, 86, 89
  polypeptide chains of, 90, 91
IgE, 74, 86, 89, 93-94
  action of, 94
  with ataxia-telangiectasia, 94, 101
  binding of, 665
  deficiency of, 102
  elevated levels of, in Job's syndrome, 663
  polypeptide chains of, 90, 91
  reaginic activity of, 93
  in secretion of histamine from basophils, 665
IgG, 74, 86, 89, 510
  catabolism of, 98
  in commercial gamma globulin, 538
  in complement fixation, 557
  concentration of, in serum, 98
  in Coombs' test, 589
  as cryoglobin, 748, 902
  D-L antibody, 563
  deficiency of, 102
    in pernicious anemia, 430
  evolution of, 95
  in giant lymph node hyperplasia, 102
  half-life of, 98
  in hyperviscosity syndrome, 351
  in immunoblastic lymphadenopathy, 102
  in immunohemolysis from stibophen, 562
  with infectious mononucleosis, 103, 510
  in lupus erythematosus, 683, 836
  in lymphadenopathy with sinus histiocytosis, 102
  in monoclonal immunoglobulinopathy, 748
  as opsonins, 663
  in penicillin sensitivity reaction, 562
  polypeptide chains of, 90, 91
  production of, 63
  transplacental passage of, 91, 98
IgM, 74, 86, 92
  in ataxia-telangiectasia, 101

IgM—cont'd
as cold-acting erythrocytic antibody, 561
in complement fixation, 557
concentration of, serum, 98
as cryoglobin, 748, 902
deficiency of, 102
of elasmobranchs, 95
half-life of, 98
in immunoblastic lymphadenopathy, 102
in immunohemolysis from stibophen, 562
in infectious mononucleosis, 678
in lupus, 683, 836
in lymphadenopathy with sinus histiocytosis, 102, 510
in monoclonal immunoglobulinopathy, 748
as opsonin, 663
in penicillin-sensitivity reactions, 562
polypeptide chains of, 90
in primary macroglobulinemia, 747
production of, 63
in Waldenstrom's macroglobulinemia, 91
IgND, 94
Ileitis, 439
Iliac crest, aspiration of marrow tissue from, 214-216
anterior, 215
in infants vs adults, 214
posterior, 218, 220, 221
Ilium
absorption of vitamin B_{12} in, 439
aspiration of marrow tissue from, 214-216, 218
crest of; see Iliac crest, aspiration of marrow tissue from
in infants vs young children, 214
posterior, 218
spine of, 216
technic, 214-216
Imerslund-Gräsbeck syndrome, 439, 440
I mucoids, 496
Immunity
cellular; see Cellular immunity
humoral; see Humoral immunity
Immunization, 104
Immunoblasts, 74
in immunoblastic lymphadenopathy, 102
Immunoblastic sarcoma, 102
Immunocyte, 74
synthesis of immunoglobulins in, 96
Immunodeficiencies
with ataxia-telangiectasia, 101
with hemopoietic hypoplasia, 101-102
laboratory diagnosis of, 103-104
with normal immunoglobulins or hyperglobulinemia, 101
primary, 100, 102
selective immunoglobulin deficiencies, 102
severe combined, 100-101
with thrombocytopenia and eczema, 101
thymic hypoplasia, 100
with thymoma, 100
X-linked agammaglobulinemia, 100
Immunoelectrodiffusion, 104
Immunoelectrophoresis, 89, 894-903
fetoglobin, 900-901
polyvalent and monovalent, 897-899
quantification of immunoglobulins, 899-900
urine, for κ and λ light chains, 901-902
Immunogenetics, 490
Immunoglobinopathies, 848
classification of, 98-100
monoclonal, associated with neoplasm, 748
case study of, 332-335

Immunoglobinopathies—cont'd
monoclonal, with non-Hodgkin's lymphoma, 759
Immunoglobulins
in activation of complement, 558
as allotypes, 95-96
as antigens, 95
from blastoid cells, 82
catabolism of, 98
characteristics of, 94
deficiencies of; see Immunodeficiencies
definition of, 74, 89
effect of, on zeta potential of erythrocytes, 352
Fc component of, 36
function of, 93-94
in hemolytic reactions, 545
hypersensitivity to, 547
as idiotypes, 95
increase of, 352, 353, 730
as isotypes, 95
measurement and quantification of, 104
apparatus and materials, 899
in diagnosis of humoral deficiencies, 104
immunoelectrodiffusion methods, 104
isotopically tagged antisera in, 104
method of, 900
principles of, 899
radioimmunoassay methods, 104
single radial diffusion method, 104
in multiple myeloma, 91, 730, 731, 733-746
of newborn, 98
in opsonization, 663
from preimmunoglobulins, 94-95
proteolytic digestion of, 91, 92
structure of, 92
antigen combining sites on, 90
constant regions, 89, 91
heavy chains of, 89, 91
light chains of, 89, 90, 91
variable regions, 89, 90, 91
synthesis of, 96-98
genetics of, 94-95
Immunohematology, 494
Immunohemolysis, 562-563
Immunology of erythrocyte, 489-514
A-B-O blood group system; see A-B-O blood group system
Diego blood group system, 513
Duffy blood group system, 512-513
I-i blood group system, 513
immunogenetics, fundamentals of, 491
Kell blood group system, 512
Kidd blood group system, 513
Lewis blood group system, 510-511
Lutheran blood group system, 511-512
M-N-S-s blood group system, 500-501
P blood group system, 501-502
paleoimmunohematology, 491
private and public blood factors, 574
Rh-Hr blood group system, 502-510
Xg, sex-linked blood group system, 513-514
Immunology of erythropoietin, 20
Immunology and serology; see Serology and immunology
Inclusion, cellular, 37
erythrocytic; see Erythrocyte, inclusion of
in Jordan's anomaly, 167
leukocytic, 167
within lymphocytes, 75, 76
in plasmacyte, 156
in tests for unstable hemoglobins, 886
Indandione, 837
Indomethacin, 790

Indon; see Phenindione
Infants and children
aspiration of marrow tissue from, 212, 214, 218
ceruloplasmin concentration in, 403
erythrocyte count of, 378
erythrocyte sedimentation rate of, 355
hematocrit of, 360
hemorrhagic disease of, 836
hyperbilirubinemia of, 471
iron-deficiency anemia in, 242, 406
iron requirement of, 401, 412
lymphocytes of, 137
marrow spaces of, 222
MCH in, 380
MCHC in, 380
MCV, 379
megaloblastic anemia of, 441
pernicious anemia of, 439
schizocytes in, 883
serologic studies of, 910-911
Infantile X-linked agammaglobulinemia, 100
Infection
anemia of, 449
by bacteria, neutrophilic leukocytosis due to, 673
diminished iron absorption with, 412
effect of, on antianemic therapy, 487
eosinophilia with, 674
erythrocyte sedimentation rate with, 356
hyperfibrinogenemia with, 353
hyperplasia of myeloid series secondary to, 236, 237
leukocyte transfusions for, 535
normoblastic hyperplasia with, 240
in precipitation of sickle cell crisis, 636
susceptibility to, in Chediak-Higashi syndrome, 47
susceptibility to, in chronic granulomatous disease, 664
susceptibility to, in multiple myeloma, 731
susceptibility to, after splenectomy, 63-64
Infectious mononucleosis; see Mononucleosis, infectious
Inflammation
C3a and C5a in, 556
granulocytes in, 659
interaction between endothelial cells and lymphocytes in, 76
leukocytic response to, 659
mobilization in, 659
role of, in diffuse intravascular coagulation, 844
Inosine, 532, 535
Insulin, 562
Interferon, 82
Intestinal tract, lymphoid tissue of, 105
Intestine, nodular lymphoid hyperplasia of, 102
Intrinsic factor
absence of, in pernicious anemia, 439
antibody against, 429-430
binding, 430
blocking, 430
congenital deficiency of, 439
historical background of, 417
lack of, in pernicious anemia, 429, 430
in Schilling test, 436
secretion of, 425
in vitamin B_{12} absorption, 425
Iron
absorption of, 396-397
defects in, 412
enhancement of, factors in, 397
excessive, 397

Iron—cont'd
absorption of—cont'd
regulation of, 396
retardation of, factors in, 397
assay of, 882
binding capacity of, 409-410
latent vs total, 400
in sideroblastic anemia, 398, 400, 413
deficiency of, 403
dietary, 395-396
distribution of, 395
ferric form, 396
ferrous form, 396, 397
general considerations of, 394-403
intoxication with, 398, 400
loss and excretion of, 401
metabolism of, 395-403
evaluation of, in diagnosis of iron-deficiency
anemias, 409-411
estimation of iron stores, 410
free erythrocyte protoporphyrin in, 410-411
serum ferritin concentration, 409
serum iron-binding capacity, 409-410
serum iron concentration, 409
in pernicious anemia, 438
in polycythemia vera, 702
overload, congenital and familial, 401
phagocytic elimination of, 35
radioactive, 395
in studies of iron, 411
requirements of, 401-402
increased, during pregnancy, 394
physiologically increased, 412
in serum, 400
in sideroblastic anemia, 413
sources of, 395-396
storage of, 400-401
ceruloplasmin in release of, 403
estimation of, 410
in histiocytes, 64
nonhemoglobin, staining for, 874
transport of, 397-400
in treatment of anemia, 394
turnover rate of, 398
utilization of, 402-403
Iron-containing pigments, 38
Iron-deficiency anemias, 388-415
abnormal normoblasts in, 624
associated with an error in iron metabolism,
401
cause of, 395
classification of, 405
clinical picture of, 405-406
codocytes in, 481
copper concentration in, 404
effect of, on erythropoietin production, 21
free erythrocyte protoporphyrin in, 449
Hb A₂ in, 633
laboratory diagnosis of, 406
bone marrow exam, 408
degree of anemia, 406
detection of blood loss, 411-412
estimation of iron stores, 410
free erythrocyte protoporphyrin, 410-411
leukocytes, 407
osmotic fragility of red cells, 409
platelets, 407-408
red cell indices, 407
red cell morphology, 406-407
reticulocytes, 407
serum ferritin concentration, 409
serum iron-binding capacity, 409-410
serum iron concentration, 409

Iron-deficiency anemias—cont'd
leptocyte in, 483
MCH in, 380
microcytosis in, 476
normoblasts of, staining of, 207
normoblastic hyperplasia with, 240, 242, 243
response of 2,3-DPG to, 392
reticulocyte count in, 487
sideroachrestic anemia, 405, 413
anemia of chronic disorders, 413
hereditary iron-loading anemia, 414
sideroblastic anemias, 413-414
sideropenic, 405, 412-413
anemia due to blood loss, 412-413
anemia due to physiologically increased iron
requirements, 412
anemia due to poor iron absorption, 412
nutritional iron deficiency, 412
transferrin deficiency, 405, 415
Irradiation; see Radiation
Isoagglutinins of A-B-O system, 492
age of detection of, 494
missing, 495
origin of, 494-495
titration of, 910
Isoantibodies; see also Isoagglutinins of A-B-O
system
in hemolytic disease, 560-561, 588, 589
Isoimmune hemolytic anemia, 91, 699
antiglobulin test of, 589, 590, 593
clinical aspects, 600
laboratory findings, 600-601
prevention and treatment, 601
serologic studies in, 592-593
Isoniazid, 562
Isopropanol precipitation test, 631
Isotopes, 694
Ivy bleeding time, 915-916

J

Jaundice, 575
acholuric, 567
chronic idiopathic, 473-474
in constitutional hepatic dysfunction, 473
hemolytic, 546, 552, 574
blood transfusion for, 530
in hereditary elliptocytosis, 594
in hereditary spherocytosis, 593
with Niemann-Pick disease, 43
nonhemolytic
congenital, 474
familial, 472, 473, 474
obstructuve, 472
in rats, 472
regurgitation, 471
of sickle cell anemia, 639
Job's syndrome, 662
Jordan's anomaly, 167
Jugular puncture, 861
Juvenile cells, 125, 131

K

Kallikrein
chemotactic activity of, 660
effect of, on coagulation factor VII, 784
from prekallikrein, 786, 795
Karyotype, 173
Kell blood group system, 512
use of, in establishing parentage, 520
Keratocyte, 482, 483
in abetalipoproteinemia, 595
in hemolytic anemia, 578
in sickle cell anemia, 640
Kernicterus, 471, 472

Kernicterus—cont'd
exchange transfusion in treatment of, 541
in hemolytic disease of newborn, 562
Kidd blood group system, 513
use of, in establishing parentage, 520
Kidney
breakdown of hemoglobin in, 571
effect of hemolysis on, 545
extramedullary hemopoiesis in, 30
in production of erythropoietin, 20-21
in synthesis of erythropoietin, 8
Kinins
from kininogens, 795
in diffuse intravascular coagulation, 844
role of, in coagulation, 559
Kininogens
conversion of, to kinins, 795
deficiency of, 785
function of, 785, 786, 797
Kinky hair syndrome, 403
Knizocyte, 486
Kuf's disease, 167
Kupffer cells, 2
in erythropoietin production, 20
Kwashiorkor, 404
megaloblastic anemia secondary to, 441

L

L chain disease, 98
Lactation
increased iron requirements with, 412
iron loss in, 401
Lactic dehydrogenase
activity of, in pernicious anemia, 438
in sickle cell anemia, 640
Lactobacillus lactis, 422, 437
Lactobacillus leichmannii, 422, 436, 437
Lactoferrin
in phagocytosis, 664
in specific granules, 663
Laparotomy, staging, 770
Lazy leukocyte syndrome, 662
Lead, 563
Lead intoxication and poisoning, 411
anemia of, 409
basophilic stippling of RBC with, 486
Cabot rings in, 488
free erythrocyte protoporphyrin in, 449
heme synthesis with, disturbance in, 455-456
sideroblastic anemia from, 414
Lecithin-cholesterol acyltransferase, deficiency
of
codocytes with, 481
hemolysis from, 569
Lectins, 495
Leishmaniasis, 544
Lepore syndromes, 656-657
Leptocyte, 427, 483, 485
formation of, 568
Leptospira icterohaemorrhagiae, 673
Letterer-Siwe disease, 58, 60
case study of, 114
lymph node imprint of, 114
Leukemia, 721
abnormal nuclear maturation in, 119
acute
cells of, 721
from chloramphenicol toxicity, 697
chromosomal abnormalities of, 720
cytochemical reactions of, 723
electron microscopy, 723
French-American-British classification of,
721-723
hypofibrinogenemia in, 300

Leukemia—cont'd
  acute—cont'd
    immunologic cell markers in, 723
    incidence of, 717
    life expectancy with, 721
    pseudo-Chediak-Higashi anomaly, 47
    from red cell aplasia, 698
    stem cell, 723-724
  age and sex distribution of, 716, 717
  from aplastic anemia, 698
  basophilic, 727
  bone pain as symptom of, 330
  chromosomal abnormalities of, 175
  chronic, 726
    blood transfusion for, 531
    cells of, 721
    incidence of, 717
    life expectancy with, 721
  classification of, 721
  cytochemistry of blood cells in study of, 206,
    210
  definition of, 715-717
  diagnosis of, 576
  eosinophilic, 133, 727
    case study of, 258, 259
      differential cell count, 258
      history and physical exam, 258
      laboratory data, 258
  epidemiology of, 717
  erythremic myelosis, chronic, 729
  erythroleukemia, acute, 725
  etiology of, 717-721
    chemicals, 720
    chromosomal abnormalities, 720-721
    ionizing radiation, 719
    role of viruses, 719-720
  extramedullary hemopoiesis in, 30
  familial, 718
  from familial myeloproliferative disease, 708
  ferritin levels in, 409
  folate deficiency with, 441
  granulocytic
    abnormal cytoplasmic maturation in, 119
    acute, 724
      from myelofibrosis, 706
    chronic, 714-715
      alkaline phosphatase in, 208
      blood and bone marrow in, 727-729
      chromosomal characteristics of, 700
      incidence of, 717
      pseudo-Chediak-Higashi anomaly, 47
      thrombocytosis in, 708
    vs leukemoid reaction, 206
  hairy cell, 725
    cells in, stain for, 871-872
  Hb H in, 633
  hematologic disorders with high risk of develop-
    ing into, 729
  historical background, 714-715
  immunoglobulin deficiency with, 102
  incidence of, 717
  from ionizing radiation, 692-693
    and acute radiation syndrome, 695
  vs leukemoid reaction, 711
  leukosarcoma, 726
  lymphoblastic, acute, 721
  lymphocytic
    following infectious mononucleosis, 676
    lymphoblast in, 131
    lymphocytes in, 25, 165
  lymphocytic, acute
    B-cell, 723
    case study of, 284, 308-310
      differential cell counts, 308, 310

Leukemia—cont'd
  lymphocytic, acute—cont'd
    case study of—cont'd
      history and physical exam, 308, 310
      laboratory data, 308, 310
    congenital, 302-303
    FAB classification of, 722
    lymphoblast in, 134
    null, 723
    prolymphocyte in, 135
    response to chemotherapy in, 722, 724
    symptoms of, 724
  lymphocytic, chronic, 137, 715, 726-727
    blastoid transformation of lymphocyte with,
      83
    blood and bone marrow, 220, 726
    case study, 314
    chromosomal abnormalities in, 720
    with hypergammaglobulinemia, 103
    hyperkalemia with, 673
    incidence of, 717, 718
    increased mast cells with, 226
    leukophoresis, 536
    with lymphadenopathy, 103
    lymphocytes in
      small, 75, 78
      ultrastructure of, 198
    MIF activity with, 85
    Rieder cells in, 298
    with terminal acute exacerbation, case study
      of, 312-313
      differential cell count, 312
      history and physical exam, 312
      laboratory data, 312
    with thrombocytopenic purpura, 802
  lymphosarcoma cell in, chronic, 726
  marrow tissue with, 222
    aspiration of, 212
  mast cell, 725
  megakaryoblastic, acute, 725
  monocytic
    Auer bodies of, 157, 192
    monocytosis in, 680
    peroxidase reaction of cells in, 206
    Schilling type, 278, 280
    supravital methods in study of, 180
  monocytic, acute, 724-725
    case study of
      differential cell count, 278
      history and physical exam, 278
      laboratory data, 278
    lysozyme concentration in, 723
    monoblast from, 138, 192
    promonocyte in, 139
  myeloblastic, acute, 721, 724
    FAB classification of, 722
  myelocytic
    abnormal cell sizes in, 119
    Auer bodies in, 157, 192
    eosinophilia with, 256, 258
    vs myelocytic leukemoid reaction, 254
    Pelger-Huët anomaly with, 160
    vitamin B_{12} levels in, 437
  myelocytic, acute, 126, 724
    abnormal nuclear maturation with, 119
    case study of
      differential cell count, 292
      history and physical exam, 292
      laboratory data, 292
    with erythremic myelosis, case study of
      differential cell count, 304
      history and physical exam, 304
      laboratory data, 304

Leukemia—cont'd
  myelocytic, acute—cont'd
    with hypergammaglobulinemia, case study
      of
      differential cell count, 298
      history and physical exam, 298
      laboratory data, 298
    micromyeloblastic, 119
      case study of, 296
    myeloperoxidase deficiency in neutrophils,
      664
    with retrobulbar leukemic tumor, case study
      of, 294-295
      differential cell count, 294
      history and physical exam, 294
      laboratory data, 294
    Rieder cells in, 298
  myelocytic, chronic, 126, 127
    alkaline phosphatase activity in, 209
    basophils in, 133, 675
    case study of, 290, 291
      differential cell count, 290
      history and physical exam, 290
      laboratory data, 290
    chromosomal content of blood cells, 175
    Döhle bodies with, 161
    eosinophils in, 133
    fetal hemoglobin in, 633
    Gaucher-like foamy cells in, 39
    high granulocytic count in, 24-25
    increased production of colony-stimulating
      factor in, 659
    leukopheresis for, 536
    with pseudo-Pelger-Huët anomaly, 160
    spherocytes in, 578
  myelogenous, 185
  myelomonocytic, 278
  myelomonocytic, acute, 725
    case study of
      differential cell count, 280, 282, 284
      history and physical exam, 280, 282, 284
      laboratory data, 280, 282, 284
    lysozyme concentration in, 723
    monoblast in, 138
    myeloperoxidase deficiency in neutrophils
      with, 664
    Naegeli type, 280, 282
    promonocyte in, 138
  myelomonocytic, chronic, 197, 725, 726
    case study of
      differential cell count, 286
      history and physical exam, 286
      laboratory data, 286
    with dysmyelopoietic syndrome, 729
    incidence of, 717
    lysozyme concentration in, 723
    terminal acute relapse of, 288, 289
  from myeloproliferative syndromes, 700
  neutrophilic, chronic, 726
  null cells with, 86
  plasma cell, 732
    blood and bone marrow, 725
  from polycythemia vera, 702
  progranulocytic, hypergranular, 724
  in pseudo-Chediak-Higashi anomaly, 47
  promyelocytic, acute, 843
    blood transfusion in treatment of, 531
    case study of, 300-301
      course of, 300
      history and physical exam, 300
      laboratory data, 300
  reticuloendotheliosis, 725
  splenic aspiration in study of, 72
  stem cell, 723-724

Leukemia—cont'd
 subacute, 721
  cells of, 721
  life expectancy with, 721
Leukemic reticuloendotheliosis, 725
 acid phosphatase in, 209
 lymphocyte of, 206
 stain for cells in, 871-872
 tartrate resistance with, 76
Leukemoid reactions, 236, 709-711
 basis for diagnosis of, 254
 conditions causing, 711
 eosinophilic, 264, 265
  differential cell count, 264
  history and physical exam, 264
  laboratory data, 264
 in glucose-6-phosphate dehydrogenase deficiency, 597
 lymphocytic, 254
 monocytic, 254
 of myelocytic type, 254, 255
  differential cell count, 254
  history and physical exam, 254
  laboratory data, 254
 in polycythemia vera, 702
 from radiation exposure, 694
Leukoagglutinins, 912
Leukocytes, 350, 658-688
 Alder's anomaly of, 53
 alkaline phosphatase activity in, 208
 anomaly of, with mucopolysaccharide storage diseases, 53
 basophilic; see Basophil
 centrifugation of, 362
 in Chediak-Higashi syndrome, 45
 chemotaxis of, 556, 557
 in diagnosis of hemolytic disease, 576
 drumstick of, 173
 eosinophilic; see Eosinophil
 vs erythrocytes, 658-659
 in erythrophagocytosis, 570
 esterases of, 209
 granules of, 182
 ingestive and digestive functions of, 36
 in iron-deficiency anemias, 407
 life cycle of, 24
 mobilization of, 659
 monocytic; see Monocyte
 in mucopolysaccharidoses, 55
 neutrophilic; see Neutrophil
 number of, effect of, on erythrocyte sedimentation rate, 354
 with Pelger-Huët anomaly, 160, 161
 in pernicious anemia, 435
 sequestration and destruction of, 65
 sex chromatin of, 175-177
 sex patterns in, 177
 sexual dimorphism of, 173-179
 storage of, 535-536
 transfusion of
  for agranulocytosis, 531
  indications for, 535-536
 as virocytes, 165
 zinc content of, 208
Leukocyte count, 24, 667
 in acute lymphocytic leukemia, 724
 in chronic granulocytic leukemia, 727
 in chronic lymphocytic leukemia, 726
 in classification of leukemia, 721
 in deviations from basal conditions, 667
 differential
  in aplastic anemia, 697
  method, 869
  normal values, 667-671, 869

Leukocyte count—cont'd
 differential—cont'd
  quality assurance of, 384
  relative vs absolute values, 670-671
 diluting fluid, 864
 effect of age on, 667
 method, 864
 in polycythemia vera, 702
 principles of, 864
 significance of successive counts, 375
Leukocytosis, 24, 25, 665-688
 in acute monocytic leukemia, 724
 balanced, 671
 basophilic, 675-676
 cause of, 17
 definition of, 671
 digestive, 667
 in electric shock, 667
 from emotional stress, 667
 eosinophilic, 671-675
  fibroplastic parietal endocarditis with, 260, 261
  of unknown etiology, 262, 263
 after exercise, 667
 following anesthesia, 667
 following paroxysmal tachycardia, 667
 following seizures, 667
 in glucose-6-phosphate dehydrogenase deficiency, 597
 in hemoglobinopathies, 623
 with hyperactivity of marrow, 266
 in immunoblastic lymphadenopathy, 102
 in isoimmune hemolytic disease, 600
 lymphocytosis, 676-680
  in infectious lymphocytosis, 679-680
  in infectious mononucleosis, 676-679
   clinical picture, 676-677
   differential absorption test, 679
   heterophil antibody, 678-679
   laboratory findings, 677-678
   monospot test, 678
   presumptive test, 678
 monocytosis, 680
 in myeloproliferative syndrome, 700
  familial, 708
  polycythemia vera, 702, 705
 neutrophilic, 673-674
 pathologic, 671
 physiologic, 671
 from radiation exposure, 694
 releasing factors in, 659
 in sickle cell anemia, 640
 significance of, 671-673
 vitamin B_{12} levels in, 437
Leukoerythroblastosis, 708
Leukopenia, 665-688
 balanced, 685
 from benzol, 696
 in Chediak-Higashi syndrome, 47
 definition of, 684-685
 eosinopenia, 688
 etiology, 685
 with Gaucher's disease, 39, 41
 in hemolytic disease, 576
 in Letterer-Siwe disease, 58
 lymphopenia, 688
 malignant, 685
 in mononucleosis, 677
 neutropenia, 685-688
  chronic, in children, 685
  cyclic, 687
  familial, 687
  neonatal, 685-687
 in paroxysmal cold hemoglobinuria, 600

Leukopenia—cont'd
 in pernicious anemia, 432
 in refractory anemia with excess blasts, 729
 in sickle cell anemia, 640
 with splenomegaly, 65
 in thalassemia, 650
 from X-irradiation, 692, 694
Leukopheresis, 535, 536
Leukopoiesis, 24-27
 effect of leukocyte transfusion on, 531
 feedback rate regulation of, 14
 granulocytopoiesis and leukocytosis, 25
 inhibitors, 25
 kinetics of, 24-25
  metamyelocyte, band, and segmented compartments, 24-25
  myelocyte compartment, 24
  progranulocyte compartment, 24
  stem cell compartments, 24
 lymphocytes, 25-27
  adrenocortical influences in lymphoid tissue, 26-27
  definition, 25
  fate, 26
  life span, 25
  origin, 25
 stimulated by leukopoietin, 17
Leukopoietins, 24
 in stimulation of differentiation of stem cells, 4
 in stimulation of leukopoiesis, 17
Leukosarcoma cells, 328
Lewis blood group system, 510-511
Lewis substance, 510-511
 chemistry of, 496
Lidocaine, 212
Lignac-Fanconi disease, 167
Lindau's disease, 705
Lipases, 663
Lipidosis
 glucosyl ceramide; see Gaucher's disease
 sphingomyelin; see Niemann-Pick disease
Lipids
 abnormalities of, 479, 481
 in cytochemical reactions of blood cells, 207
 identification of, 207
Lipochondrodystrophy, 53
Lipofuscin pigment, 38
Lipomucopolysaccharides, 53-58
Lipopolysaccharidosis, 53
Lipoprotein
 in abetalipoproteinemia, 568, 595
 of erythrocyte membrane, 553, 555
 inhibitors of granulopoiesis, 25
 plasma, 568
 in prethrombotic state, 855
 separation of serum, 896-897
  approaches and materials, 896
  calculations, 897
  method, 897
  reagents, 896-897
Lithium carbonate, 660
Littoral cells, 105
Liver
 in bilirubin clearance, 574
 carcinoma of, 356 ✗
 as chief fetal hemopoietic organ, 6
 cirrhosis of; see Cirrhosis of liver
 in clearance of hemoglobin-haptoglobin complex, 571
 in conjugation of bilirubin, 471
 in diagnosis of Hodgkin's disease, 770 ✗
 effect of thorium radiation on, 694
 endothelial cells of capillaries of, 3

Liver—cont'd
 enlargement of; see Hepatomegaly
 extramedullary hemopoiesis in, 30, 32, 33
 fetal, in hemopoiesis, 8, 9-10, 29
 folate storage in, 420
 in hereditary spherocytosis, 594
 Kupffer cells of, 2, 20
 in lysosomal storage diseases, 38
 in phagocytosis of hemoglobin, 469
 protoporphyria of, 451
 in sequestration hemolysis, 570
 in sickle cell anemia, 636
 siderosis of, 401
 as site of abnormal porphyrin synthesis, 454
 as site of erythropoietin production and inactivation, 20-21
 storage of iron in, 400, 401
 storage of vitamin B$_{12}$ in, 426
 synthesis of coagulation factors in, 781
 synthesis of haptoglobin in, 464, 468
 in thalassemia, 650
 urobilinogen of, 573
Löffler's syndrome, 256
Lungs, hemosiderin in, 401
Lupus anticoagulant, 820, 836
 detection of, 920
 in hemophilia, 827
Lupus erythematosus, 680-684
 clinical picture, 680
 demonstration of cell in, 912-913
  clotted blood method, 913
  rotary bead method, 913
 diffuse intravascular coagulation in, 847
 identification of, through blood preparations,
  229
 lymphopenia in, 688
 macroglobulinemia secondary to, 748, 750
 red cell aplasia with, 699
 spleen in, 69
 thrombocytopenia with, 577, 802
Lupus erythematosus cell phenomenon, 680-684
 antinuclear antibodies, 683-684
 formation of cells, 680-681
 laboratory findings in, 681-682
 morphology of cells, 681
 significance of, 682
 specificity of, 682-683
 tart cells, 681
Lupus erythematosus plasma factor, 680
Lutheran blood group system, 511-512
Lymph, 74
 filtration of, 105
 T-lymphocytes of, 84
 thoracic duct, 88
Lymph nodes
 aspiration and imprint preparations of, 105-
  115
 biopsy of, 103
 capsule of, 105
 circulation of lymphocytes from thymus to, 81
 development of, 25
 effect of cortisol on, 26
 endothelial cells of, 2, 3
 exam of, 103
 excision of, 105
 in fetal erythropoiesis, 9
 in filtration of lymph, 105
 in formation of lymphocytes, 105
 function of, 104
 giant, hyperplasia, 102
 in immunoblastic lymphadenopathy, 102
 imprints of, 108
  differential counts from, 105
  in drug-induced lymphadenopathy, 112

Lymph nodes—cont'd
 imprints of—cont'd
  in extramedullary hemopoiesis, 106
  in Hodgkin's disease, 108, 109
  in infectious mononucleosis, 106
  in Letterer-Siwe disease, 114
  in lymphoblastic lymphoma, 110
  in lymphocytic lymphoma, 107, 111
  preparation of, 115
  supravital methods in study of, 180
 in lymphocytopoiesis, 25
 lymphoid nodules of, 105
 in lymphomyeloid complex, 74
 in lymphopoiesis, at birth, 10
 medullary area of, 105
 paracortical areas of, 105
  with thymic hypoplasia, 100
  in Wiskott-Aldrich syndrome, 101
 in production of antibodies, 105
 reticulum and lymphoid cells of, 3
 in staging of Hodgkin's disease, 770
 structure of
  cytologic, 105
  histologic, 104-105
 T-lymphocyte localization in, 84
 trabeculae of, 105
Lymph node permeability factor, 85, 86
Lymphadenopathy
 angioimmunoblastic,   with   dysproteinemia,
  102
 drug-induced, 103
  case study of, 113
  lymph node imprint with, 112
 with gamma heavy chain disease, 102-103
 with hyperimmunoglobulinemia, 100
 immunoblastic, 102
 with sinus histiocytosis, 102
Lymphangiectasia, intestinal, 102
Lymphatic vessels, 105
 circulation of lymphocytes through, 81
Lymphoblasts, 134
 in acute lymphocytic leukemia, 724
 cytoplasm of, 131
 form of, 181
 nucleoli of, 131
 nucleus of, 131
 periodic acid–Schiff reaction of, 207
 size of, 131
Lymphocyte(s), 124, 129, 133, 135, 136, 143,
  144
 in antibody production, 63
 in aplastic anemia, 697
 atypical, 165, 167
 B; see B-lymphocyte
 blastoid transformation of, 103-104
 Buhot's cells, 55
 Burkitt's lymphoma, 82
 in cellular immunity, 88-89
 in Chediak-Higashi syndrome, 47
 chemotactic responses of, 660
 in chronic lymphocytic leukemia, 198, 298
 culture of, 83
 cytoplasm of, 137
 definition of, 25
 in delayed hypersensitivity reaction, 88
 as diploid cells, 175
 effect of adrenocortical hormones on, 16, 26-
  27, 667
 factors released by
  blastogenic, 82
  leukotactic, 82
  macrophage migration inhibition, 82
  transfer, 82
 fate of, 26

Lymphocyte(s)—cont'd
 fetal, during pregnancy, 89
 formation of, 105, 181
  site of, 79
 in formation of antibodies, 74
 function of, 83-87
 Gasser cells, 58
 granules of, 137
 histamine-releasing factor of, 665
 in immunologic reactions, 87-98
 in infectious mononucleosis, 677-678
 in inflammatory response, 76, 78
 large, 105, 137
  in chronic lymphosarcoma cell leukemia,
   726
  cytoplasm of, 75
  dimensions of, 75
  nucleus of, 75
  proliferation of, in immunoblastic lymphadenopathy, 102
  vs small, 75
 life span of, 25, 78-79
 localization of, 81
 long-lived vs short-lived, 78, 79
  migrations of, 81
 of lymph nodes, 105
 medium, 105, 137
 migrations of, 76
  tropisms in, 81
 Mittwoch cells, 54
 morphology of, 75-78
  with lymphopenia, 103
 in mucopolysaccharidoses, 55, 58
 nucleoli of, 137
 nucleus of, 137
 number and distribution of, 13
 origin of, 25
 Pelger-Huët anomaly of, 157
 periarteriolar sheath of, 81
 periodic acid–Schiff reaction of, 207
 peripheralization of, 81
 peroxidase reaction of, 206
 plasmacytoid, 102
 in production of colony-stimulating factor, 25
 reactive, 83, 165-167
 resistance of, to lymphocytotoxin, 85
 sensitivity of, to radiation injury, 692
 sensitized, in antibody formation, 83
 sex chromatin of, 179
 in Sézary's syndrome, 162, 163, 164
 size of, 137
 small, 137
  in chronic lymphocytic leukemia, 726
  of corona of lymphoid nodule, 105
  in cortex of thymus, 80
  cytoplasm of, 75
  dimensions of, 75
  in Hodgkin's disease, 763
  vs large, 75
  life span of, 78
  nucleus of, 75
  of paracortical area of lymph node, 105
  recirculation of, through blood and lymph,
   79
  as stem cells, 82
 in spleen, 61
 in splenograms, 72
 sudanophilic staining of, 207
 supravital methods in study of, 180
 surface receptors of, 82
 in synthesis of immunoglobulins, 96
 T; see T-lymphocytes
 thoracic duct, 79
 entering thymus, 81

Lymphocyte(s)—cont'd
    from thymus, 81
    thymus-derived, 81
    transformation of, to macrophage, 83
    transformation of, to plasma cells, 83
    transformation of, in vitro, to blastoid cells,
        82
    transformation of, in vivo, 83
    transplacental passage of, 89
    ultrastructure of, 184, 185, 192
    vacuolated, 54-55
    Wright-Giemsa stains of, 868
Lymphocyte count, 666
Lymphocyte stimulating factor, 81
Lymphocyte transforming factor, 85, 86
Lymphocytic system, 74-75, 79
Lymphocytopoiesis, 25, 78
    bone marrow in, 79
    defective, with thymectomy, 75
    fetal, 9
        and at birth, 10
    in thymus, 81
        vs peripheral lymphoid tissue, 81
Lymphocytosis
    in acute lymphocytic leukemia, 724
    from chronic exposure to radiation, 694
    in Gaucher's disease, 41
    from hyperthyroidism, 16
    infectious, 679-680
    in infectious mononucleosis, 346
    in pernicious anemia, 432
Lymphocytotoxin, 85
Lymphoid follicles
    corona of, 81, 84
    in formation of lymphocytes, 79
    hyperplasia of, 102
    in X-linked agammaglobulinemia, 100
Lymphoid hamartoma, angiomatous, 102
Lymphoid hyperplasia, 102, 113
Lymphoid nodule
    in bone marrow, 223, 226
    corona of, 105
    germinal centers of, 105
    in intestine, 74
    of lymph nodes, 105
    lymphocytes of, 105
    in lymphocytopoiesis, 25
    structure of, 79, 80
Lymphoid tissue
    at birth, 81
    in diagnosis of humoral deficiencies, 104
    effect of adrenocortical hormones on, 26
    in gastrointestinal tract, 25
    gut-associated, 79
    location of, 104-105
    in Nezelof's syndrome, 101
    with thymoma, 100
    in Wiskott-Aldrich syndrome, 101
    in X-linked agammaglobulinemia, 100
Lymphoidocytes, 6
Lymphokines, 83, 85
    abnormal production of, 662
    in basophilic chemotaxis, 660
Lymphoma
    blastoid transformation of lymphocytes with,
        83
    of bone marrow, 332-335
    Burkitt, 676, 753-759
    classification of, 752-753
    diagnosis of, 229
    erythrocyte sedimentation rate, 357
    ferritin levels in, 409
    folate deficiency with, 441
    hemolytic anemia with, 552

Lymphoma—cont'd
    histiocytic, diffuse, 726
    Hodgkin's disease; see Hodgkin's disease
    immunoglobulin deficiencies with, 102
    lymphoblastic
        lymph node imprint with, 110
    lymphocytic
        case study of, 110
        lymph node imprint of, 107, 111
    Mediterranean abdominal, 748
    with monoclonal immunoglobulinopathy, 748
    non-Hodgkin's, 753-759
        Burkitt's, 753-759
        case study of, 328-331
        clinical correlations, 759
        diffuse, 753
        MIF activity with, 85
        nodular, 753
        null cells with, 86
    with thrombocytopenic purpura, 802
Lymphomyeloid complex, 74
Lymphopenia, 26, 688
    with ataxia-telangiectasia, 101
    definition of, 685
    in Good's syndrome, 100
    from irradiation, 692
    in lupus erythematosus, 681
    T-lymphocyte deficiency with, 103
Lymphopenia agammaglobulinemia, 101
Lymphoplasmacytoid cells, 747-748
Lymphoproliferative disorders, 83, 730, 752
    staining of cells with, 207
    types of lymphocytes found in, 87
Lymphoreticular cells, 747-748
Lymphosarcoma, 723
    cells of, 328
        glycogen staining of, 207
    lymphocytes of, 165
    lymphopenia in, 688
    thrombocytopenia in, 803
        and amegakaryocytosis of bone marrow, 324-
            325
Lymphosarcoma cell leukemia, chronic, 726
Lysosomes
    azurophilic granules as, 36
    basophilic granules as, 36
    definition of, 36
    derivation of, 36, 37
    digestive capacity of, 37-38
    enzymes of
        action of, 38
        in blastoid transformation, 82
        deficiency of, 38, 39
        glucocerebrosidase, 39
        hydrolases, 36
        peroxisomes, 37
        source of, 37
    mechanism of overloading of, 38
    in phagocytosis of antigens, 86
    primary, 36, 37
        as nonspecific granules, 125
        staining of, 157
    secondary, 36, 37
        in storage of mucopolysaccharidoses, 53
    self-digestion of, 37
Lysosomal storage diseases, 38-61
    cause of, 36
    Chediak-Higashi syndrome, 45-52
    Gaucher's disease, 38-43
        clinical features, 39-41
        metabolic defect, 39
        sphingolipids, 39
    idiopathic histiocytosis, 58-61
    of lipomucopolysaccharides, 53-58

Lysosomal storage diseases—cont'd
    Niemann-Pick disease, 43-45
        clinical features, 43-44
        diagnosis, 44-45
        metabolic defect, 43
    sea-blue histiocyte syndrome, 45
Lysozyme
    increased activity of
        in Chediak-Higashi syndrome, 47
        in chronic myelomonocytic leukemia, 729
    levels of, in leukemia, 723
    in phagocytosis, 664
    in specific granules of phagocytosis, 663

M

M phase of cell cycle, 11
M-N-S-s blood group substances, 496
    use of, in establishing parentage, 519-520
    variants of, 500-501
Macrocryogelglobulins, 902
Macrocryoglobulins, 902
Macrocytes
    appearance of, 427
    in hemoglobinopathy, 623
    in hemolytic anemia, 578
    in myeloproliferative syndrome, 700
    in paroxysmal nocturnal hemoglobinuria, 596
Macrocytosis, 476
    in cirrhosis of liver, 440
    measurement of, 379
    in pernicious anemia, 432
    pseudomacrocytosis, 427
    true, 427
Macroglobulins, 89
    effect of, on clot formation, 840
    in inhibition of chemotaxis, 662
    in inhibition of plasmin, 855
    vitamin B_{12} bound to, 426
    Waldenström's, 747-748, 749
Macroglobulinemia, 83
    hemorrhagic tendencies in, 848
    increased mast cells with, 226
    in multiple myeloma, 733
    primary, 747-748
    secondary to lupus erythematosus, 748, 750
    secondary to rheumatoid arthritis, 748, 751
    treatment of, 539
Macrophages, 2
    aggregation of blastoid cells around, 83
    breakdown products of, 660
    in Chediak-Higashi syndrome, 47
    in delayed hypersensitivity reaction, 88
    derived from monocytes, 83
    in erythrophagocytosis, 570
    fixed, 3
    in formation of antibodies, 74
    ingestive and digestive functions of, 36
        pinocytosis, 36
    migration of, inhibition of, 85
    in phagocytosis, 96, 663
    in presenting antigen to lymphocyte, 86
    in production of colony-stimulating activity, 6,
        25, 659
    receptors at surface of, 36
    synthesis of complement components in, 556
    transformation of lymphocytes to, 83
    transformation of monocytes to, 3
Macrophage chemotactic factor, 85
Macrophage migration inhibition factor, 82
Macropolycytes, 432
Macrothrombocytopathia, hereditary, 797, 808
Magnesium ions, 207, 208
Malabsorption syndromes, 412

Malaria
  antiglobin test of, 589
  erythrocyte sedimentation rate with, 356
  as hazard of blood transfusions, 543-544
  and Hb C trait, 641
  relationship of, to sickle cell trait, 641
Mammary gland, 30
Marchand, adventitial cells of, 2
Marrow; *see* Bone marrow
Mast cells, 223, 224
  IgE binding to, 94, 665
  increases in, conditions with, 226
  receptors of, for C3a, 559
Mast cell disease, systemic, 676
Mast cell leukemia, 725
Mastocytosis, systemic, 725
Maxinow, fixed histiocytes of, 2
May-Grünwald-Giemsa stain, 869
May-Hegglin anomaly, 161-162
  cells of, ultrastructure of, 192
  defective thrombocytopoiesis in, 804
  platelets in, 797
  platelet dysfunction in, 818
MCH; *see* Mean corpuscular hemoglobin
MCHC; *see* Mean corpuscular hemoglobin concentration
MCV; *see* Mean corpuscular volume
Mean, 369
Mean corpuscular hemoglobin, 379-380
  in hereditary spherocytosis, 593
  in iron-deficiency anemias, 407
  measurement of, 372
  in pernicious anemia, 432
  in polycythemia vera, 702
  in thalassemia, 650
Mean corpuscular hemoglobin concentration, 379, 380
  in diagnosis of hemolytic disease, 577
  in hereditary spherocytosis, 577, 593
  in iron-deficiency anemias, 407
  measurement of, 372
  in pernicious anemia, 432
  in polycythemia vera, 702
  in thalassemia, 650
Mean corpuscular volume
  with anisocytosis, 476
  in diagnosis of hemolytic disease, 577
  in Hb E trait, 643
  in hereditary spherocytosis, 577, 593
  in iron-deficiency anemia, 407
  with macrocytosis, 476
  measurement of, 372
  with microcytosis, 476
  in pernicious anemia, 432
  with polycythemia vera, 702
  in thalassemia, 650
Median, 369
Mediterranean anemia, 68
Mediterranean giant platelet syndrome, 808
Medullary hemopoiesis, 9
  fetal, 10-11
  qualitative and quantitative data on, 211
  relation of, to extramedullary hemopoiesis, 30-32
Megakaryoblast, 27, 151
  cytoplasm of, 148
  nucleoli, 148
  nucleus of, 148
  periodic acid–Schiff reaction of, 207
  size of, 148
Megakaryocytes, 151, 153
  basophilic, 148
  in chronic granulocytic leukemia, 727

Megakaryocytes—cont'd
  cytoplasm of, 148
  in formation of platelets, 787
  granular, 148
  in idiopathic thrombocytopenic purpura, 801
  maturation of, 27
  multinucleated, 175
  nucleoli of, 148
  nucleus of, 148
  vs osteoclasts, 223
  periodic acid–Schiff reaction of, 207
  in pernicious anemia, 435, 436
  platelet-forming, 148
  in polycythemia vera, 266, 702
  sensitivity of, to radiation injury, 692
  size of, 148
  sudanophilic staining of, 207
  synthesis of platelet factor XIII in, 781
  in thrombocytopenic purpura, 326
  ultrastructure of, 192
Megakaryocytic myelosis, 706, 707
Megakaryocytosis, extramedullary, 268
Megaloblast(s), 417
  basophilic, 142, 146, 147, 150
    cytoplasm of, 148
    nucleoli of, 142
    nucleus of, 142
    size of, 142
  in DiGuglielmo's syndrome, 713, 714
  as diploid cells, 175
  identification of, 226
  orthochromic, 146, 149, 150
    cytoplasm of, 148
    nucleus of, 148
    in pernicious anemia, 432, 434
    size of, 148
  periodic acid–Schiff reaction of, 207
  in pernicious anemia, 270, 434-435, 715
  polychromatophilic, 147, 149, 150
    cytoplasm of, 148
    nucleus of, 148
    size of, 148
  resemblance of, to primitive erythroblasts, 8
  size of, 119
Megaloblastic anemia, 160
  blood transfusions for, 530-531
  due to deficiency of folate, 420, 440-443
    caused by increased cellular proliferation, 441
    in defective interconversion, 443
    dietary, 440
    in infancy, 441
    in malabsorption, 441-443
      congenital, 441
      drug-induced, 441
      in steatorrheas, 441-443
    in pregnancy, 440-441
  due to deficiency of vitamin B_{12}, 429-440
    with biologically inert intrinsic factor, 439
    deficiency of transcobalamin II, 440
    in disease of small intestine, 439-440
    drug-induced malabsorption, 440
    familial selective malabsorption, 440
    after gastrectomy, 439
    inadequate intake, 429
    increased requirements of vitamin B_{12}, 440
    pernicious anemia in adults, 429-439
    pernicious anemia in infants and children, 439
    in Zollinger-Ellison syndrome, 440
  Hb A_2 in, 633
  macrocytosis in, 476
  megalocyte in, 483
  in Pelger-Huët anomaly, 160

Megaloblastic anemia—cont'd
  reticulocyte count in, 487
  of uncertain etiology, 444
    in DiGuglielmo's syndrome, 444
    in hemochromatosis, 444
    OSLAM syndrome, 444
    in sideroblastic anemias, 444
Megaloblastic dyspoiesis, 427-429
  biochemical basis of, 419
  hypersegmented macropolycyte in, 167
Megaloblastic erythropoiesis, 418
Megaloblastosis
  of DiGuglielmo's syndrome, 306
  pancytopenia with hyperplastic bone marrow and, 252, 253
  case study of
    differential cell count, 252
    history and physical exam, 252
    laboratory data in, 252
Megalocyte, 483, 485
Menorrhagia, 411
Menstruation
  blood loss from, 411, 412
  effect of, in intermittent acute porphyria, 454
  erythrocyte sedimentation rate during, 356
  iron loss in, 401
Mephenytoin, 697
6-Mercaptopurine, 419
Mesenchymal cells, hemopoietic potential of, 30
Mesobilene-B, 574
Mesobilirubinogen, 469, 574
Metamyelocyte, 141, 147, 149, 150
  basophilic, 131
  in chronic granulocytic leukemia, 727
  cytoplasm of, 131
  drumsticks found in, 179
  eosinophilic, 131, 133
  giant, 119
  granules of, 125
  juveniles, 125
  in leukopoiesis, 24-25
  in megaloblastic bone marrow, 270
  neutrophilic, 132, 133, 143, 146, 188
    granules of, 157
  nucleoli of, 125
  nucleus of, 125, 131
  in pernicious anemia, 435
  peroxidase reaction in, 206
  proliferation of, with severe infection, 236
  with severe neutrophilia, 673
  size of, 131
  ultrastructure of, 182, 188
Methemalbumin, 461, 469
  in hemolytic disease, 546, 571
  identification of, 877
  preparation of, for spectroscopy, 876
Methemalbuminemia, 596
Methemoglobin
  accumulation of, with formation of Heinz bodies, 488
  acquired, 457, 460
  as cause of hypoxia, 456
  concentration of, for cyanosis, 456
  concentration of, in normal blood, 456-457
  conversion of Hb F and Hb A to, 460
  dissociation of, 571
  formation of, 456
  identification of, 571
  measurement of, quantitative method of
    method, 882
    normal values, 882
    reagents, 881-882
    remarks, 882
  in paroxysmal cold hemoglobinuria, 600

Methemoglobin—cont'd
preparation of, for spectroscopy, 876
Methemoglobinemia
classification of, 457
congenital, 649
hereditary
deficient reducing systems, 458-460
excessive oxidative activity, 460
Hb variants, 457-458
secondary polycythemia with, 705
spectroscopic identification of, 461, 463
with sulfhemoglobinemia, 461
Methionine, 423
Methionine methyl, 423-425
Methotrexate, 419
Methylcobalamin, 419
Methyldopa, 683
Methylene blue, 458, 460
Methylfolate transferase, 419
Methylmalonic acid, 437
Methylmalonic aciduria, congenital, 437
Methylmalonyl CoA, 423, 424
Methylmalonyl CoA isomerase, 423, 424
Microangiopathic hemolytic anemia, 569-570
Microcytosis, 476
in hemoglobinopathies, 623
measurement of, 379
Microfilaments
of neutrophils exhibiting abnormal migration, 662
of platelet membrane, 789
of pseudopodia in phagocytosis, 663
Microglobulin, 82
as marker on T-lymphocyte, 84
Microhematocrit, 383-384
method, 360, 867
normal values, 867
principle, 867
quality assurance of, 383-384
Micromyeloblasts, 119, 126
in acute myelocytic leukemia, 296
Microperoxisomes, 37
Microphages, 2
Microscope
electron, 181
phase, 180-181
use of, in supravital methods of blood cell study, 180
Microscopy
electron, 181-205
in classification of acute leukemias, 723
general considerations, 181
ultrastructure of blood cells
abnormal, 192-205
normal, 182-192
phase contrast
general considerations, 180-181
time-lapse photography, 181
Microspherocyte, 484, 485, 578
in Hb C disease, 641
Microtubules
of neutrophils in Chediak-Higashi syndrome, 47
of platelet membrane, 789
in shape change, 792
Migration inhibitory factor, 85
in diagnosis of cellular immunity deficiency, 104
Miradon; *see* Anisindione
Mitochondria
of blood cells, ultrastructure of, 182
intrinsic factor and vitamin B_{12} in, 425
iron utilization by, 402
of leukemic cells, 192

Mitochondria—cont'd
of lymphocytes, 76, 192
of metamyelocyte, 182
of monocytes, 192
of myeloblast, 182
of myelocyte, 182
of plasma cell, 192
of platelets, 789
staining of, 207
Mitogen, 85, 86
concanavalin A, 82
as nonspecific antigen, 82
phytohemagglutinin, 82
Mittwoch cells, 54
Mode, 369
Monge's disease, 704
Monoblasts, 138
in acute monocytic leukemia, 192, 724
cytoplasm of, 137
nucleoli of, 137
nucleus of, 137
size of, 137
ultrastructure of, 195, 196
Mono-chek test, 679
Monocyte, 136, 140, 144
azurophilic granules of, 36
in Chediak-Higashi syndrome, 47
in chronic granulomatous disease, 664
cystine crystals in, 167
cytoplasm, 137
as diploid cells, 175
effect of kallikrein on, 660
effect of lymphokine production on, 662
effect of plasminogen activator on, 660
in erythrophagocytosis, 570
esterases of, 209
form of, 181
granules of, 36
location of, 3
macrophages derived from, 83
migration of, 660
in mucopolysaccharidoses, 55, 58
nucleoli of, 137
nucleus of, 137
periodic acid–Schiff reaction of, 207
peroxidase reaction of, 206
in phagocytosis, 663
in production of colony-stimulating factor, 6, 25
random motility and chemotaxis of, 660
reduction in numbers of, 685
sex chromatin of, 179
in sideroblastic anemia, 413
size of, 137
as source of colony-stimulating factor in granulopoiesis, 659
spreading phenomenon of, 181
sudanophilic staining of, 207
supravital methods in study of, 180
transformation of, 3
ultrastructure of, 184, 192
Wright-Giemsa stain of, 868
Monocyte counts, 666
Monocytosis, 680
causes of, 680
in Gaucher's disease, 41
Mononuclear phagocyte system, 3
Mononucleosis, infectious, 83
aplastic anemia from, 697, 698
case study of, 346-347
bone marrow differential cell count, 346
history and physical exam of, 346
laboratory data, 346
clinical picture of, 678

Mononucleosis, infectious—cont'd
coproporphyrin excretion in, 455
differential absorption test, 679
Downey cells of, 78
glandular type, 677
heterophil antibodies in, 678-679
immunoglobulin levels in, 93
increases of IgG with, 103
in increasing colony-stimulating activity of granulopoiesis, 659
laboratory findings in, 677-678
lymph node imprint of, 106
lymphocytes with, vs virocytes, 165
lymphocytosis in, 676-679
monospot test of, 679
pharyngeal type, 676
posttransfusion, 544
presumptive test for, 679
spleen in, 66
with thrombocytopenic purpura, 802
typhoidal type, 676
typical serologic findings in, 679
Monospot test, 912
in infectious mononucleosis, 679
Moschkovitz syndrome, 852
Mountain sickness, acute, 704
Mucolipids, 53
Mucopolysaccharide, acid, 53
Mucopolysaccharidosis I, 53
Multiple myeloma, 83, 730-747
Auer bodies with, 192
Bence Jones proteins in, 91, 733, 746
blood, 732-733
bone marrow, 733
case study of, 316-323
bone marrow differential cell count, 316, 318, 320, 322
history and physical exam, 316, 318, 320, 322
laboratory data, 316, 318, 320, 322
cells of, identification of, 226
coagulation in, 747
cryofibrinogenemia in, 748
definition of, 730-732
electrophoretic patterns in, 733-745
erythrocyte sedimentation rate in, 353, 357
excess formation of immunoglobulins in, 91
folate deficiency with, 441
hemorrhagic tendencies of, 848
hypercalcemia in, 746
immunoglobulins in, 733-746
deficiency of, 731
incidence of, 731
increased coagulation factor VIII in, 784-785
Philadelphia chromosome in, 720
plasma cells in, 157
ultrastructure of, 192, 199, 200, 201, 202
and plasma cell leukemia, 725
plasmablast in, 154
proplasmacyte in, 155
protein abnormalities of, 733-746
pyroglobulins in, 752
splenic aspiration in study of, 72
symptoms of, 731
vitamin B_{12} levels in, 437
Mumps antigen, 103
Munchausen syndrome, hemoglobin, 636
Muramidase
in monocytic and myelomonocytic leukemia, 724-725
in pernicious anemia, 438
Murayama test, 624
Muscular dystrophy, progressive, 167
Mustard gas, 696-697

Mycobacteria, 38
  case history of infection from, 49
  histiocytes engorged with, 45, 48
Mycobacterium tuberculosis
  bone marrow smears of, 232
  identification of, 219
  in miliary tuberculosis of bone marrow, 348
  neutrophilia from, 673
Mycosis fungoides, 770
  blastoid transformation of lymphocytes with, 83
  eosinophilia with, 256
  and Sézary's syndrome, 162
Myeloblast, 126, 715
  in acute granulocytic leukemia, 724
  in acute myelocytic leukemia with hypergammaglobulinemia, 298
  alterations in size of, 119
  cytoplasm of, 125
  giant, 119
  in leukopoiesis, 24
  movement of, 181
  nucleoli of, 125
  nucleus of, 125
  peroxidase reaction of, 206
  size of, 125
  in splenograms, 72
  sudanophilic staining of, 207
  ultrastructure of, 182, 186
Myeloblastomas, 724
Myelocyte, 128, 143
  in acute monocytic leukemia, 724
  in chronic granulocytic leukemia, 727
  in classification of granulocytes, 131
  cytoplasm of, 125
  eosinophilic, 129, 133
  granules of, 125
  in leukopoiesis, 24
  neutrophilic, 187
  nucleoli of, 125
  nucleus of, 125
  in pernicious anemia, 435
  peroxidase reactions in, 206
  vs progranulocyte, 125
  size of, 125
  ultrastructure of, 182, 187
Myelocytes A, 125
Myelocytes B, 125
Myelofibrosis, 705-708
  acute, 706
  megakaryocytic, 706
  primary, derivation of, 700
  symptoms of, 706
Myelolipoma, 30
Myeloma
  ferritin levels, 409
  multiple; see Multiple myeloma
  plasma cell, 175
  solitary, 730
Myeloperoxidase, 36, 206, 406
  in phagocytosis, 664
Myelopoiesis, fetal, 9
Myeloproliferative syndromes, 699-714
  case study of, 268, 269
    bone marrow differential cell count, 268
    history and physical exam, 268
    laboratory data, 268
  clinical and laboratory features, 700
  dacrocyte in, 481
  derivation of, 700
  DiGuglielmo's syndrome, 711-714
  Döhle bodies with, 161
  erythrocytes in, teardrop, 700, 701
  familial, 708

Myeloproliferative syndromes—cont'd
  increase in basophils with, 675
  leukemoid reactions, 709-711
  leukoerythroblastosis, 708
  megakaryoblast in, 151
  with myelofibrosis
    and agnogenic myeloid metaplasia, 705-708
    bone marrow from, 220
  osteopetrosis, 708
  platelets in, 797
  polycythemia; see Polycythemia
  spherocytes in, 578
  splenic aspiration in study of, 72
  splenomegaly from, 61
  stimulation of blood cells in, 14
  thrombocytopenia in, 803
  thrombocytosis and thrombocythemia, 708
  vitamin B_{12} depletion in, 440
  vitamin B_{12} levels in, 437
Myelosclerosis, 727
  acute, 706
  malignant, 708
Myocardial infarction, 356
Myoglobin, 409, 447
  identification of, 877
  iron in synthesis of, 395
Myositis, 256

N

Naphthol ASD acetate, stain for
  interpretation of, 873
  method, 872-873
  principle of, 872
  reagents, 872
National Blood Policy, 527-529
Needles for aspiration of marrow tissue, 212, 213
  Jamshidi-Swain needle, 221
  Klima-Rosseger needle, 214
  Vim-Silverman needle, 218, 220, 221
Neoarsphenamine, 699
Neomycin, 440
Neonatal neutropenia, 687
Neoplasm; see also Cancer; Carcinoma
  with ataxia-telangiectasia, 101
  cells of, multinucleated, 173, 175
  and cellular immunity, 89
  monoclonal immunoglobulinopathy associated with, 332-335
  of stomach, thrombocytopenia associated with, 326-327
Nervous system
  effect of Niemann-Pick disease on, 43
  involvement of, in Gaucher's disease, 41
Neuroblastoma
  cells of, 344, 345
  metastatic to bone marrow
    case study of
      bone marrow differential cell count, 344-345
      history and physical exam of, 344
      laboratory data, 344
Neutrons, 692
Neutropenia
  cause of, 686
  chronic, in childhood, 685
  chronic hypoplastic, 687
  congenital, 688
  cyclic, 687
  definition of, 685
  from excessive margination of neutrophils, 662
  familial, 687
  leukocyte transfusions for, 535

Neutropenia—cont'd
  neonatal, 685-687
  in pernicious anemia, 432
  primary splenic, 687
  from radiation, 692
  in relation to colony-stimulating factor, 659
Neutrophils
  in activation of C5, 558
  adherence of, to vascular endothelium, 662
  alkaline phosphatase activity in, 208, 209
  in aplastic anemia, 697
  band, 127, 128, 143
    increase in, with moderate neutrophilia, 673
    in pernicious anemia, 432
    ultrastructure of, 182, 192
  changes in, with toxic conditions, 161
  with Chediak-Higashi syndrome, 47
  chemotaxis of, 559, 660-663
  in chronic granulocytic leukemia, 727
  circulation of, 24
  constitutional hypersegmentation, 167
  cyclic variation in numbers of, 667
  cystine crystals in, 167
  cytochemically abnormal, 167
  cytoplasmic granule of, 118
  in diagnosis of hemolytic disease, 576
  drumsticks found in, 179
  effect of adrenocortical hormones on, 16, 667
  effect of kallikrein on, 660
  effect of plasminogen activator on, 660
  esterases of, 209
  function of, 658-665
  in generalized hyperplasia of bone marrow, 238
  glucocerebroside in, 39
  granules of, 119, 125, 131, 157, 182
  granulopoiesis in inflammation, 659
  histamine releasing factor of, 665
  hypersegmentation of, 417
    in pernicious anemia, 432, 433, 436
  increased production of, 660
  ingestive function of, 36
  in iron-deficiency anemias, 406
  lupus erythematosus cell, 681
  as microphages, 2
  in mucopolysaccharidoses, 55
  myeloperoxidase of, 36
  number and distribution of, 12
  with Pelger-Huët anomaly, 160
  in phagocytosis, 663-665
  in polycythemia vera, 702
  production of, 25
  random migration of, 660
    abnormal, 662
  random motility and chemotaxis of, 659-660
  release of, 25
  segmented, 127, 129, 130, 131, 132, 133, 144, 157, 206
    drumsticks in, 179
    with oxalate crystals, 168
    in pernicious anemia, 674
    ultrastructure of, 182, 189, 192
  sex chromatin of, 179
  sexual dimorphism of, 179
  in splenograms, 72
  stab, 124, 126, 129, 132, 133, 144, 146, 156, 157, 206
    drumsticks in, 179
  sudanophilic staining of, 207
  time-lapse photography in study of, 181
  ultrastructure of, 184, 185
  Wright-Giemsa stain of, 868
Neutrophil counts, 666
Neutrophil immobilizing factor, 660

Neutrophilic leukocytosis, 673-674
  in myelofibrosis, 796
  from radiation, 692
Nezelof's syndrome, 101
Niemann-Pick disease, 72
  acid phosphatase in, 41
  cholesterol storage in, 58
  clinical features of, 43-44
  diagnosis of, 44-45
  histology of, 44-45
  location of, 44
  metabolic defect of, 43
  staining of, 45
Nigremia, hereditary, 457
Nishimini factor, 786
Nitrates and nitrites, 460
Nitrobenzene derivatives, 563
Nitroblue tetrazolium test, 874-875
  for chronic granulomatous disease, 664
  materials and reagents, 874
  method, 874
  normal values of, 875
  in phagocytosis, 663
  principle of, 874
  remarks, 875
Nitrogen mustard, 697
Normoblasts, 138
  in alcoholism, 440
  antigens of, 489
  basophilic, 143, 144
    cytoplasm of, 142
    nucleoli of, 142
    nucleus of, 142
    size of, 142
  in biosynthesis of porphyrins and heme, 449
  in chronic granulocytic leukemia, 727
  in congenital erythropoietic porphyria, 451
  in congenital erythropoietic protoporphyria, 454
  in diagnosis of hemolytic disease, 580
  as diploid cells, 175
  effect of chloramphenicol toxicity on, 697
  elliptical, 483
  hemoglobin elaboration by, 118
  in hemoglobinopathies, 623
  in hereditary spherocytosis, 593-594
  hyperplasia of
    associated with acute hemolytic crisis of sickle cell anemia, 244, 245
      case study of, 244
    due to chronic hemorrhage, 240, 241
      case study of, 240
    associated with iron-deficiency anemia, 242, 243
      case study of, 242
    associated with macrocytic anemia of liver disease and hemolytic anemia, 246, 247
      case study of, 246
  in myeloproliferative syndromes, 268
  iron utilization of, 402
    ceruloplasmin in, 403
  in leukoerythroblastosis, 708
  megaloblastoid, 427
  orthochromic, 124, 129, 133, 141, 143, 144, 154, 194
    cytoplasm of, 142
    loss of nucleus of, 32, 486
      with formation of Howell-Jolly bodies, 488
    nucleus of, 142
    size of, 142
  passage of, through endothelial cells, 32
  Pelger-Huët anomaly in, 157

Normoblasts—cont'd
  periodic acid–Schiff reaction of, 207
  in pernicious anemia, 434
  polychromatophilic, 124, 127, 128, 135, 141, 142, 143, 144
    cytoplasm of, 142
    nucleus of, 142
    size of, 142
  in polycythemia vera, 702
  in porphyria erythropoietica, 229, 230
  in red cell aplasia, 698
  sensitivity of, to radiation injury, 692
  in sickle cell anemia, 640
  as sideroblasts, 408
  as siderotic granules, 488
  in splenograms, 72
  in thalassemia, 650
  ultrastructure of, 192, 193, 194
Normoblastosis associated with carcinoma metastatic to bone marrow, case study of, 342-343
  history and physical exam, 342
  laboratory data, 342
Novobiocin, 541
Nuclear membrane, 182
Nucleic acids, 15
Nucleolar satellite, 173
Nucleolus
  of blood cell, 182
  changes in, with cell maturation, 118
  chromatin of, 175
  of lymphoblast, 131
  of lymphocyte, 137
  of megakaryoblast, 148
  of megakaryocyte, 157
  of megaloblast, 142
  of monoblast, 137
  of monocyte, 137
  of multinucleated cells, 175
  of myeloblast, 125, 182
  of myelocyte, 125
  of normoblast, 142
  of osteoblast, 223
  of plasma cells in myeloma, 192
  of plasmablast, 148
  of plasmacyte, 157
  of progranulocyte, 125
  of prolymphocyte, 131
  of promegakaryocyte, 148
  of promegaloblast, 142
  of promonocyte, 137
  of proplasmacyte, 148
  of reticulum cell, 125
Nucleoside diphosphokinase, 788
Nucleus
  of cells with Pelger-Huët anomaly, 192
  chromosomal content of, 173
  of granulocyte, 131
    band, 131
  of lymphoblast, 131
  of lymphocytes, 75, 131, 192
  maturation of
    abnormal, 119
    in blood and bone marrow cells, 118
      changes in shape, 118
      structure and cytochemistry, 118
  of megakaryoblast, 148
  of megakaryocyte, 148
  of megaloblast
    basophilic, 142
    orthochromic, 148
    polychromatophilic, 148
  of metamyelocyte, 131, 182
  of monoblast, 137

Nucleus—cont'd
  of monocyte, 137, 192
  of multinucleated cells, 175
  myeloblast, 125
  of myelocyte, 125, 182
  of normoblasts, 192
    basophilic, 142
    orthochromic, 142
    polychromatophilic, 142
  of osteoblast, 223
  of Pelger-Huët cells, 192
  of phagocytic histiocytes, 192
  of plasmablast, 148
  of plasmacyte, 157
  polyploidy of, 119
  of progranulocytes, 125, 182
  of prolymphocyte, 137
  of promegakaryocyte, 148
  of promegaloblast, 142
  of promonocyte, 137
  of proplasmacyte, 148
  of reticulum cell, 125
  of Sézary cell, 164
  ultrastructure of, 181-182
  of virocytes, 165
Null cells, 83, 86
  vs Sézary cells, 165

O

Ochromonas malhamensis, 437
Ondine's curse, 705
Oral contraceptives
  folate deficiency with, 441
  increase in coagulation factor VIII with, 636
  in prethrombotic state, 854, 855
Opsonins, 36, 663
OSLAM syndrome, 444
Osler's disease, 701
Osteoarthritis, 356
Osteoclasts, 224
  vs megakaryocytes, 223
  as multinucleated cells, 175
  vs plasma cells, 223, 224
  as polykaryon, 119
Osteopetrosis, 708
Ova, 175
Oxalate crystals, 167, 168
Oxygen
  affinity of hemoglobin for, 389, 390
  dissociation curves of, 177-178, 389, 390, 607, 608, 647
  effect of, on hemoglobin, 456
  hypoxia; *see* Hypoxia
  partial pressure of
    effect of, on combination with hemoglobin, 389
    at varying altitudes, 391
  role of, in control of respiration, 175
  role of, in radiation injury, 692
  transport of
    abnormal, hemoglobinopathy associated with, 646-649
      congenital methemoglobinemias, 649
      decreased oxygen affinity with cyanosis, 649
      increased oxygen affinity with erythrocytosis, 646-649
    and delivery of, to tissues, 388-392, 532
      role of 2,3-DPG in, 390-391
Oxyhemoglobin
  conversion of, 389, 456
  denaturation of, 625, 626
  vs deoxyhemoglobin, 390
  effect of alkali on, 608

Oxyhemoglobin—cont'd
  identification of, 876
    spectroscopic, 461, 462, 464
  measurement of, 875
  preparation of, for spectroscopy, 876

P

P blood group system, 501-502
Pagophagia, 397
Palade, granules of, 182, 183
Paleoimmunohematology, 490
Pancytopenia
  following administration of chloramphenicol, 250, 251
    bone marrow differential count, 250, 251
    history and physical exam, 250
    laboratory data, 250
  with hyperplastic bone marrow and megaloblastosis, 253
    bone marrow differential count, 252
    history and physical exam, 252
    laboratory data, 252
  following therapeutic irradiation, 248, 249
    bone marrow differential count, 248
    history and physical exam, 248
    laboratory data, 248
Panwarfin; *see* Warfarin sodium
Papain, 592
Papaverine
  in platelet inhibition, 790
  in treatment of sickle cell anemia, 638
Pappenheimer bodies, 488, 582
Para-aminosalicylic acid
  in drug-related hemolysis, 562
  in interference with vitamin B_{12} absorption, 440
Parahemophilia, 834, 835
Paraimmunoglobulinopathy, 100
Paraproteinemia, 98
Parasites
  in diagnosis of hemolytic disease, 582
  identification of, in blood preparation, 229
  eosinophilia with infestation of, 256
Parathyroid glands, 100
Parentage, serologic tests in disputed; *see* Serologic tests in disputed parentage
Paroxysmal cold hemoglobinuria
  autohemolysis in, 587
  clinical aspects of, 600
  laboratory findings on, 600
  treatment, 600
Paroxysmal nocturnal hemoglobinuria
  acid serum test for, 884
  from aplastic anemia, 698
  clinical aspects of, 596
  fetal hemoglobin in, 633
  hemolytic antibodies in, 592
  laboratory findings in, 596
  leukopenia with, 576
  osmotic fragility of erythrocyte in, 583
  sugar-water test, 884
  thrombocytopenia in, 577
  treatment of, 596
Partial thromboplastin time
  activated, 786
    in control of heparin therapy, 857
    in factor IX deficiency, 831
    in factor X deficiency, 831
    in factor XI deficiency, 831
    in factor XII deficiency, 832
    in identification of factor deficiencies, 823
    in lupus coagulant, 836
    in prethrombotic state, 854, 855
  in diffuse intravascular coagulation, 846

Partial thromboplastin time—cont'd
  in evaluation of thromboplastinogenesis, 821
  in factor VIII and IX deficiency, 828
  Fletcher factor deficiency, 797
  in hemophilia, 828
  in increased fibrinolysis, 847
  in lupus erythematosus, 682
  methods of measurement, 924-925
  in newborn, 787
  in premature infant, 787
  prolonged, 779, 786
    evaluation of, 925-926
  quality assurance in measurement of, 385
  technic, 855, 856
Passovoy factor, 786
Paterson-Kelly syndrome, 406
Paul-Bunnell test, 678
Pelger-Huët anomaly
  cells of, 160, 161
    ultrastructure of, 192, 205
  with chronic granulocytic leukemia, 727
  incidence of, 157, 160
  inheritance of, 157, 160
  morphology of cells with, 160
Pelvic inflammatory disease, 356
Pelvis
  extramedullary hemopoiesis in, 30
  as marrow-containing bone, 222
Pemphigus leprosus, 447
Penicillar arterioles, 61
Penicillin
  in autoimmune hemolytic anemia, 599
  erythrocyte sedimentation rate with, 356
  immunohemolysis from, 562
  reaction of, LE cell phenomenon with, 683
  sensitivity to, test of, 676
Peptic ulcer, 530
Periarteritis nodosa tumors, 256
Periodic acid–Schiff reaction, 207
  method, 872
  principle of, 872
  reagents in, 872
  results of, 872
  in study of leukemia, 210
Peripolesis, 83
Pernicious anemia, 142, 146, 147, 149
  in adult, 429-439
  anisocytosis with, 477
  atrophy of gastric mucosa with, 430
  Cabot rings in, 488
  carcinoma of stomach with, 429
  case study of, 270, 271
    bone marrow differential count, 270
    history and physical exam, 270
    laboratory data, 270
  in chlorosis, 394
  clinical features, 430
  Döhle bodies with, 161
  effect of blood transfusion on, 531
  eosinophilia with, 256
  formiminoglutamic acid excretion in, 421
  glossitis of, 406
  haptoglobin levels in, 468
  Hb F in, 633
  historical background in, 417
  Howell-Jolly bodies in, 488
  increased methylmalonic acid excretion in, 423, 424
  in infants and children, 439
  laboratory diagnosis of, 432-439
    assay of vitamin B_{12}, 437
    biochemical findings, 438
    bone marrow, 434-436
    deoxyuridine suppression test, 438-439

Pernicious anemia—cont'd
  laboratory diagnosis of—cont'd
    erythrocyte survival, 438
    excretion of labeled vitamin B_{12}, 436-437
    excretion of methylmalonic acid in urine, 437
    gastric analysis, 434
    iron metabolism, 438
    peripheral blood, 432-434
    pigment excretion, 438
    reticulocyte response after therapeutic trial, 437-438
    urine and renal function, 438
  macrocytosis with, 477
  as malignant disease, 715
  marrow with, 222
  MCV and MCH of, 380
  megaloblasts in
    orthochromic, 150
    polychromatophilic, 148
    staining of, 207
  vs megaloblastic anemia of pregnancy, 440, 441
  megaloblastic dyspoiesis in, 427
  pathogenesis of, 429-430
  with Pelger-Huët anomaly, 161
  reticulocyte count in, 487
  reticulocyte maturation rate of, 23-24
  segmented neutrophils with, 674
  spinal cord in, 431, 432
Peroxidase, 406, 447, 448, 869-870
  in cells of acute myelomonocytic leukemia, 282
  in cells with chronic myelomonocytic leukemia, 286
  in cytochemical reactions, 206-207
  of hemoglobin and haptoglobin, 464, 468
  method for staining, 870
  in nonspecific vs specific granules, 125
  reagents for staining, 870
Peroxide, 565
Peroxisomes, 37
Petechiae, 791
Peyer's patches, 79, 770
  in lymphomyeloid complex, 74
Phagocytes
  in Chediak-Higashi syndrome, 47
  in lymph sinus, 105
  sea-blue staining, conditions with, 45, 47
Phagocytic cells
  fixed, 3
  in peripheral blood, 170, 171
Phagocytic vacuole, 36
Phagocytosis, 3, 36, 663-665
  of erythrocytes, 64, 570
  as function of spleen, 64
  relationship of, to immunity, 2
  by small lymphocytes, 78
Phagosome, 36, 663
Phase contrast microscopy
  general considerations, 180-181
  time-lapse photography, 181
Phenacetin
  direct hemolysis from, 563
  in drug-related hemolysis, 562
Phenformin, 440
Phenindione, 837
Phenothiazines, 624
Phenotypes, 490, 491
  in A-B-O system, 492
  coding of, 523
Phenprocoumon, 837
Phenylhydrazine, 563
Phenytoin, 697

Philadelphia chromosome, 175
  in chronic granulocytic leukemia, 727, 728
  in granulocytic leukemia, 711
  in leukemia, 720
  in multiple myeloma, 720
  in myelocytic leukemia, 728
  in myelofibrosis, 708
Phosphatases, 207
  acid; *see* Acid phosphatase
  alkaline; *see* Alkaline phosphatase
Phosphates
  effect of, on iron absorption, 397
  of red blood cell, 390
Phosphatidylcholine, 555
Phosphatidylcholine hemolytic anemia, 569
Phosphatidylserine, 555
Phosphatidylthanolamine, 555
Phosphodiesterase, 789, 790
Phosphofructokinase, 390, 391
Phospholipids
  in abetalipoproteinemia, 596
  from damaged cell membranes, 778
  effect of, on recalcification time of plasma, 796
  of erythrocyte membrane, 555
Phosphomonoesterases, 207
Photosensitivity
  in congenital erythrocytic porphyria, 451
  in variegate porphyria, 454
Photosynthesis, 395
Phytates, 397
Phytohemagglutinin
  in activation of T-lymphocytes, 83
  in blastoid transformation of lymphocyte, 82
  as nonspecific antigen, 82
  in study of lymphocyte competence and immune response, 83
Pica, 397
  defective iron absorption with, 412
Pickwickian syndrome, 705
Pigments
  iron-containing, 38
  lipofuscin, 38
Pingueculae
  definition of, 39
  in Gaucher's disease, 39
Pinocytic vacuole, 36
Pinocytosis, 36
Pituitary gland, 15-16
Plasma, 350-351
  extenders of, and substitutes for, 539
  protein composition of
    effect of, on erythrocyte sedimentation rate, 352-353
    effect of, on rouleau formation of erythrocytes, 352
    vs relative blood viscosity, 351
  recalcification of, 821-823, 919
    in hemophiliac, 828
  stored, 537
    transfusion of, indications for, 537
  transfusion of
    for factor V deficiency, 536
    for factor VII deficiency, 536
    for hypoprothrombinemia, 536
    in shock, 531
    transmission of hepatitis with, 543
    in treatment of hypoproteinemia, 532
Plasma cell, 83, 124, 128, 147
  absence of, 104
    with lymphoid hyperplasia of intestine, 102
  in antibody production, 63
  Auer bodies in, 157
  binucleated or multinucleated, 119

Plasma cell—cont'd
  in diagnosis of humoral deficiency, 104
  as diploid cells, 175
  esterase of, 209
  in formation of antibodies, 74
  glycogen staining of, 207
  in hematologic exam, 103
  in immunoblastic lymphadenopathy, 102
  lamellar structures within, 181
  lymphocytoid, 102
  of lymphoid nodules, 105
  in multiple myeloma, 316, 318, 730, 731, 732
  in myeloma, multinucleated, 175
  in myeloma, ultrastructure of, 192, 199, 200, 201, 202
  vs osteoblasts, 223
  in synthesis of immunoglobulins, 96
  transformation of lymphocyte to, 83
  ultrastructure of, 183, 192, 196
Plasma cell leukemia, 725
Plasma cell myeloma, 748
Plasma contact factor, 820
Plasma fractions, 538-539
  albumin, 538
  factor II, VII, IX, and X concentrates, 538-539
  factor VIII concentrate, 538
  fibrinogen, 538
  gamma globulin, 538
Plasma thromboplastin component, 785
Plasma thromboplastin component deficiency, 830
Plasma volume, 362-366
  clinical correlation of, 362-363
  in differential diagnosis of polycythemia, 705
  decrease in
    with relative erythrocytosis, 705
    relative polycythemia from, 701
  increase in
    as cause of anemia, 392, 394
    with pregnancy, 356, 363
  methods of measurement, 363
  normal values, 363-366
  in polycythemia vera, 702
Plasmablasts, 154, 733
  cytoplasm of, 148
  in multiple myeloma, 316
  nucleoli of, 148
  nucleus of, 148
  size of, 148
Plasmacytes, 154, 156
  cytoplasm of, 157
  nucleoli of, 157
  nucleus of, 157
  size of, 157
Plasmacytomas, 148
Plasmacytosis
  in cirrhosis, 226
  in immunologic reactions, 226
  in infectious diseases, 226
  vs multiple myeloma, 733
Plasmapheresis, 539
  in treatment of aplastic anemia, 692
Plasmin
  in fibrinolysis, 840, 841
  inhibitors of, 855
Plasminogen
  in fibrinolysis, 840, 841
  chemotactic activity of, 660
Plasmodium, 582
Plasmodium falciparum, 543, 589
Plasmodium knowlesi, 641

Plasmodium malariae, 543
Plasmodium vivax, 543, 544
Platelets, 350
  adhesion of, 778, 788
    abnormal, 799
      in von Willebrand's disease, 792
    to basement membrane, 791, 792
    to collagen, 791, 792
    to damaged blood vessels, 787
    determination of, 798, 799
    inhibitor of, 792
    measurement of, 853-854, 917-918
  aggregation of, 778
    abnormal, in thrombasthenia, 804
    agents in, 799
    enhancement of, by complement, 559
    inhibitor of, 792
    measurement of, 853, 918-919
    role of cAMP in, 790
    thromboxane A$_2$ in, 790
  antibodies against, 537, 538
    in immunologic thrombocytopenic purpura, 531
  autoaggregation of, 853
  centrifugation of, 362
  in chronic myelocytic leukemia, 290
  circulation of, 788
  concentration of, vs thrombin formation, 795
  destruction of, 788, 802, 803
  in diffuse intravascular coagulation, 788
  effect of adrenocortical hormones on, 16
  effect of spleen on, 65
  energy metabolism of, 789-791
  formation of, 27
  function of, 791-794
    adhesion, 792, 798-799
    aggregation, 792-794, 799-800
    release reactions, 794-795
    shape change, 792
  functional abnormalities of, 804-819
    absent collagen-induced aggregation, 818
    Bernard-Soulier syndrome, 807-808
    congenital afibrinogenemia, 818
    congenital enzymatic deficiency, 818
    storage pool disease, 804-807
    thrombasthenia, 804
    thrombocytopathy, acquired, secondary to other diseases, 818
    thrombocytopathy with congenital syndromes, 818
    thrombocytopenia, acquired, caused by drugs, 818
    thrombopathic thrombocytopenia, 808
    von Willebrand's disease, 808-818
    in Wiskott-Aldrich syndrome, 101
  giant, in diagnosis of hemolytic disease, 580
  historical background on, 774
  interaction of, with endothelium and subendothelial tissues, 778, 791
  in iron-deficiency anemia, 407-408
  life span of, 788
  with May-Hegglin anomaly, 161, 162
  from megakaryoblast, 148
  membrane of, 788-789
  morphology of, 787-788
    abnormalities of, 797
  of newborn, 787
  organelles of, 789
  periodic acid–Schiff reaction, 207
  in pernicious anemia, 432-434
  in polycythemia vera, 266
  in prethrombotic state, 853-854
  in refractory anemia with excess blasts, 729
  regulation of, 28

Platelets—cont'd
release of, 34
from marrow, 32
in storage pool disease, 804
in release of components in hypercoagulation state, 778, 854
sequestration of, in spleen, 788
storage of, 536
study of, with phase contrast microscopy, 180
sudanophilic staining of, 207
survival and turnover in hypercoagulation state, 854
in thrombocytopenic purpura, 326
transfusion of
indications for, 531, 538
in treatment of leukemia, 531
in treatment of thrombocytopenia, 531
ultrastructure of, 184, 185, 192
"wash-out" effect on, in hemorrhagic transfusion reactions, 548
Wright-Giemsa stain of, 868
Platelet basic protein, 794
Platelet count, 801
in chronic granulocytic leukemia, 727
in diagnosis of hemolytic disease, 577
in diffuse intravascular coagulation, 846
equipment and reagents, 864
in infectious mononucleosis, 678
method, 864-865
normal values, 865
phase contrast microscopy method, 384
in polycythemia vera, 702
in prethrombotic state, 853, 855
semiautomated, 384-385
successive, significance between, 375
in thrombocytosis, 708
Platelet disorders
classification of, 810
Platelet factor 3, 778, 789, 832
availability of, 919
in Bernard-Soulier syndrome, 807
measurement of, 798
release of, 798
role of, 395, 795
abnormal, 798
in thromboembolic disease, 854
in thrombopathic thrombocytopenia, 808
in thromboplastinogenesis, 819, 820
Platelet factor 4, 789
release of, 394, 798
abnormal, 798
Platelet factor 5, 794
Platelet factor 10, 794
Platelet factor XIII, 786
synthesis of, 781
Platelet-like aggregating factor, 665
Platelet shock, 793
Platelet tidal dysgenesis, 819
Plateletpheresis, 536
Plumbism, 455
basophilic stippling of erythrocyte in, 456
Plummer-Vinson syndrome, 406
Pneumoconiosis, 37
Poikilocytosis
definition of, 476
in hemoglobinopathy, 623
with iron-deficiency anemias, 406, 407
in pernicious anemia, 432
in sickle cell anemia, 640
in thalassemia, 650
Pokeweed mitogen, 82
Poliomyelitis, 673
Polychromatophilia
definition of, 486

Polychromatophilia—cont'd
in hemoglobinopathies, 623
in hemolytic anemia, 575, 578
in thalassemia, 650
Polycythemia
cryptogenia, 701
differential diagnosis of, 705
myelopathic, 701
in myeloproliferative syndrome, 700
primary, 701
from radiation exposure, 694
relative, 701
diagnosis of, 705
secondary, 701
at birth, diagnosis of, 705
erythropoietin in, 21, 22
etiology of, 704-705
abnormal hemoglobin pigments, 705
benign familial erythrocytosis, 705
chronic acquired heart disease, 705
congenital heart disease, 705
erythrocytosis in newborn, 705
hemoglobinopathies, 705
high altitude, 17, 704
from high dosages of testosterone, 16
hypoventilation hypoxia, 17, 705
pulmonary disease, 704-705
relative erythrocytosis, 705
tumors, 705
sickling reactions with, 625
Polycythemia rubra, 701
Polycythemia vera
blood volume, 363
case study of, 266, 267
bone marrow differential count, 266
history and physical exam, 266
laboratory data, 266
clinical picture of, 701-702
definition of, 700-701
derivation of, 700
diagnosis of, 705
erythrocyte mass in, 363
vs erythrocytosis, 379
erythropoietin levels in, 22
with gastric ulcers, 530
increase in basophils with, 675
laboratory findings in, 702-704
blood coagulation and hemostasis, 702-704
blood as a whole, 702
bone marrow, 702
erythrocyte count, 702
hemoglobin concentration, 702
iron metabolism and erythrocyte survival, 702
leukocyte count, 702
peripheral blood smear, 702
platelet count, 702
plasma volume in, 363
and thrombosis, 853
vitamin B_{12} binder in, 426
Polyglutamates, 419, 420
Polykaryons, 119
Polyploidy, 173, 175
Polysomes, 15
Polysplenia, 65
Porphobilinogen, 414, 448-449
in acquired porphyria secondary to griseofulvin, 455
in Ehrlich's aldehyde reaction, 574
in intermittent acute porphyria, 454
qualitative measurement of, 877
method, 877
reagents, 877
results, 877

Porphobilinogen—cont'd
quantitative assay of, 879, 880
calculation of, 880
method, 880
normal values, 880
reagents, 879-880
semiquantitative method, 880-881
calculation, 881
method, 881
principle, 880
reagents, 880-881
in variegate porphyria, 454
Porphyrias
acquired, 454-456, 460
classification of, 449-451
congenital, 447
classification and characteristics of, 450
isomers of, 447
congenital erythropoietic, 447, 451
congenital erythropoietic protoporphyria, 451-454
erythropoietic coproporphyria, 454
hepatic, 447, 454
hereditary coproporphyria, 454
history of, 445-447
intermittent acute, 454
secondary to griseofulvin, 455
secondary to hepatoma, 455
secondary to hexachlorobenzene, 454-455
variegate, 454
Porphyria cutanea tarda, 454
Porphyria erythropoietica
normoblasts in, 229, 230
Porphyrin
biosynthesis of, 448-449
catabolism of, carbon monoxide from, 456
chemical structure of, 447-448
excretion of, normal values for, 450
identification of, 877
metabolism of, 445-456
preparation of, for spectroscopy, 876
qualitative measurement of
method, 877
reagents, 877
remarks, 877
quantitative assay of, 877-880
collection of urine, 878
principle, 877-878
Porphyrinuria, secondary, 455
Potassium, 354
increases in
in chronic granulocytic leukemia, 728
with high WBC count, 673
in thrombocytosis, 708
in pernicious anemia, 438
in polycythemia vera, 702
release of, from platelet, 794
transport of, across erythrocyte membrane, 555, 556
Prausnitz-Küstner test, 94
Pregnancy
and alkaline phosphatase activity, 209
anemia during, 394
and cellular immunity, 89
copper concentration in, 404
effect of, in intermittent acute porphyria, 454
erythrocyte sedimentation rate in, 356
fibrin split products in, 846
Hb F levels in, 633
hematocrit in, 360
hyperfibrinogenemia with, 353
iron loss in, 401
macrocytic anemia of, with sickle cell disease, 274, 275

Pregnancy—cont'd
  macrocytic anemia of, with sickle cell disease—
    cont'd
    case study of
      bone marrow differential count, 274
      history and physical exam, 274
      laboratory data, 274
    megaloblastic anemia of, 440-441
  and obstetric complications, diffuse intravascu-
    lar coagulation secondary to, 845
  physiologically increased iron requirements
    with, 412
  plasma volume in, 363
  with sickle cell–Hb C disease, 644
  thrombocytopenic levels in, 801
  toxemia of, 748
  vitamin B_{12} levels in, 437
Preimmunoglobulin, 94-95
Prekallikrein, 661
  in activation of factor VII, 785
  conversion of, to kallikrein, 786, 795
  and Fletcher factor, 786
Primaquine, 587
Proaccelerin, 783
Procainamide hydrochloride, 683
Procaine hydrochloride, 212
Progranulocyte, 126, 127
  in acute granulocytic leukemia, 724
  in acute monocytic leukemia, 724
  in acute promyelocytic leukemia, 300-301
  in chronic granulocytic leukemia, 726
  crescentic zone of, 192
  cytoplasm of, 125
  in hypergranular progranulocytic leukemia, 724
  in leukopoiesis, 24
  nucleoli of, 125
  nucleus of, 125
  peroxidase reaction of, 206
  size of, 125
  ultrastructure of, 182
Prolymphocyte, 135
  cytoplasm of, 131
  nucleoli of, 131
  nucleus of, 131
  size of, 131
Promegakaryocyte, 151, 152
  cytoplasm of, 148
  nucleoli of, 148
  nucleus of, 148
  periodic acid–Schiff reaction of, 207
  size of, 148
Promegaloblast, 146
  cytoplasm of, 142
  nucleoli of, 142
  nucleus of, 142
  size of, 142
Promonocyte, 137, 139
  cytoplasm of, 137
  in monocytic leukemia, 139
  in myelomonocytic leukemia, 138, 286
  nucleoli of, 137
  nucleus of, 137
  size of, 137
Pronormoblast, 137, 141
  cytoplasm of, 137, 142
  nucleoli of, 137, 142
  nucleus of, 137, 142
  size of, 142
Properdin, 558-559
Propionibacterium, 422
Propionic acid, 423
Proplasmacyte, 155, 733
  cytoplasm of, 148
  nucleoli of, 148

Proplasmacyte—cont'd
  nucleus of, 148
  size of, 148
Prostaglandins
  in activation of platelet function, 790
  in differentiation of stem cells, 6
  effect of, in immune reaction, 87
  in inhibition of granulopoiesis, 25
  in inhibition of platelet function, 790
  in stimulation of erythropoiesis, 20, 21
Prostaglandin A_1, 660
Prostaglandin endoperoxidases, 790
Prostate, carcinoma of
  case study of
    bone marrow differential count, 340
    history and physical exam, 340
    laboratory data, 340
  tumor cells of, 228
Protamine sulfate, 857
Protamine sulfate paracoagulation test, 846, 854,
  936
Protectins, 495
Protein
  electrophoresis, 894-903
    cold-precipitable study, 902-903
    quantification of ceruloplasmin, 900
    in separation of lipoproteins, 896-897
    in serum, separation of, using cellulose ace-
      tate, 894-896
    of urine, 901
  synthesis of, 15
Prothrombin
  in classic theory of coagulation, 778
  concentration of, 782
  conversion of, to thrombin, 782, 832-833
    effect of platelet factor 3 on, 795
  deficiency of, detection of, 834
  dependency of, on vitamin K, 833, 835
  derivatives of, 776
  history of, 774
  measurement of, 782
  storage of, 536
  synthesis of, 782
Prothrombin activator complex, 782, 832, 833
  effect of lupus anticoagulant on, 836
Prothrombin Barcelona, 835
Prothrombin Brussels, 835
Prothrombin Cardeza, 835
Prothrombin consumption test
  in Bernard-Soulier syndrome, 807
  in evaluation of thromboplastinogenesis, 823
  for hemophilia, 828
  in measurement of platelet factor 3, 798
  method of measurement, 924
Prothrombin Padua, 835
Prothrombin Quick, 835
Prothrombin San Juan, 835
Prothrombin time
  in congenital deficiency of factor II, 835
  in control of anticoagulant therapy, 833, 837
  in diffuse intravascular coagulation, 846
  in evaluation of thrombinogenesis, 833
  in evaluation of thromboplastinogenesis, 821
  in hemorrhagic disease of newborn, 836
  in increased fibrinolysis, 847
  with lupus anticoagulant, 836
  in lupus erythematosus, 682
  microtechnic, 921-922
  in newborn, 787
  in premature infant, 187
  prolonged, 779
    causes for, 833
    evaluation of, 922-923
  quality assurance in measurement of, 385

Prothrombin time—cont'd
  Quick's method, 920-921
  standardization of, 839
  with tissue extract and Russell's viper venom,
    533
Protoporphyrin
  accumulation of, in RBC with lead intoxication,
    414
  in acquired prophyria secondary to griseofulvin,
    455
  in acquired porphyria secondary to hepatoma,
    455
  in cytoplasm of orthochromic normoblast, 486
  in erythropoietic coproporphyria, 454
  in evaluation of iron metabolism, 410-411
  free erythrocyte, 449
  in lead intoxication, 455
  metabolism of, 445-456
  in pernicious anemia, 438
  in porphyria cutanea tarda, 454
  in variegate porphyria, 454
Protoporphyrin III, 447, 448, 449
Protoporphyrin IX, 451
Protoporphyrinogen, 414
Protoporphyrinogen oxidase, 454
Pseudo-Pelger-Huët anomaly, 160-161
Pseudohermaphroditism, 175
Pseudoleukemia, 709
Pseudolymphoma, 771
Pseudomononucleosis, 165
Pseudosickling, 624
PT; *see* Prothrombin time
Pteroylmonoglutamic acid, 417, 418
PTT; *see* Partial thromboplastin time
Pulmonary disease, 704-705
Purpura, 779, 791
  allergic, 852
  anaphylactoid, 852
  associated with scurvy, 848, 850
  associated with thrombocytopenia, 774
  cause of, 848
  Henoch-Schönlein, 852
  relationship of, to blood abnormalities, 774
  relationship of, to platelets, 774
Pyelonephritis, chronic, 254, 255
Pyknocytosis, infantile, 483
Pyrimethamine, 419
Pyrogens, 549
Pyroglobulins, 752
Pyroglobulinemia, 98, 748-752
  in multiple myeloma, 733
Pyruvate kinase
  action of, 566
  deficiency of, 597
    ascorbate test of, 587
    fluorescence test for, 588
    glutathione stability test, 587
    hemolysis from, 566-567
    inheritance of, 566
    orthocresol red test for, 588

Q

Quinacrine hydrochloride, 697
Quinidine
  hemolysis with, 566
  hypersensitivity to, 562, 802
Quinine
  hemolysis with, 566
  hypersensitivity to, 562, 802

R

Rad, 692
Radiation
  absorbed dose of, 692

Radiation—cont'd
  aplastic bone marrow and pancytopenia from
      therapeutic, 248, 249
  case study of
    bone marrow differential count, 248
    history and physical exam, 248
    laboratory data, 248
  ionizing
    in acute radiation syndrome, 694-695
    in aplastic anemia, 692-695
    biologic effects of, 693
    cellular effects of, 692
    effect of, on hemopoietic tissues, 692
    injury from
      in chronic exposure to thorium radiation,
          694
      in chronic exposure to x-radiation, 693-
          694
      hemopoietic effects, 692-693
      from isotopes, 694
    leukemia from, 719
    sensitivity of various cells and tissues to, 692,
        693
    types of, 692
  leukopenia from, 685
  measurement of, 692
  methemoglobinemia from, 460
  neutrons, 692
  α-rays, 692
  β-rays, 692
  γ-rays, 692
  X-rays, 692
Radiation syndrome, acute, 694-695
  gastrointestinal effects, 695
  hemopoietic effects, 695
Radioimmunoassay methods, 104
Radium, hemopoietic effects of exposure to, 694
Ranvier, clasmatocytes of, 2, 3
Rapoport-Luebering cycle, 390
Rapoport-Luebering shunt, 392
Rebuck technic, 660
Red blood cells; see also Erythrocytes
  abnormality of, hereditary
    with hemolysis, 567-569
      in abetalipoproteinemia, 568
      in congenital dyserythropoietic anemia,
          569
      in elliptocytosis, 568
      in high phosphatidylcholine hemolytic ane-
          mia, 569
      in lecithin-cholesterol acyltransferase defi-
          ciency, 569
      in spherocytosis, 567-568
      in stomatocytosis, 568-569
      in Zieve's syndrome, 569
  in erythron, 22
  folate of, assay of, 420-421
  glucose metabolism in, 565
    major pathways of, 564
  life span of, 551
  morphology of, with iron deficiency anemia,
      406-407
  morphology of, with sideroblastic anemia,
      413
  normal values of, 374-380
    mean corpuscular hemoglobin, 379-380
    mean corpuscular hemoglobin concentration,
        379, 380
    mean corpuscular volume, 379
    physiologic variations, 377-379
      age, 378
      altitude, 378-379
      dehydration, 378
      exercise or excitement, 378

Red blood cells—cont'd
  normal values of—cont'd
    physiologic variations—cont'd
      posture, 378
      sex, 378
    statistical determination of, 376-377
  osmotic fragility of, 409
  packed
    transfusion of, 537
      in treatment of aregenerative anemia, 530
      in treatment of hemorrhage, 530
  shapes of, nomenclature of, 477
  size of, 117
  survival of, 552-553
  transfusion of, transmission of hepatitis with,
      543
Red blood cell count, 372
Red cell aplasia, 698-699
  association with thymoma, 699
  chronic hypoplasia in adults, 698-699
    erythroid hypoplasia in hemolytic anemia,
        699
    idiopathic, 698-699
    metabolic inhibition of erythropoietin, 699
  Diamond-Blackfan type, 698
  effect of, on erythropoietin production, 21
  fetal hemoglobin in, 633
  lymphocyte-mediated suppression of hemopoie-
      sis in, 25
Reductases, 458
Reed-Sternberg cells, 72, 109, 169, 175
  in Burkitt's lymphoma, 759
  in Hodgkin's disease, 326, 327, 759, 763,
      770
Reid factors, 786
Reilly cells in gargoylism, 53
Rem unit, 692
Renal erythropoietic factor, 21
Renal tubular cells, 85
Rendu-Osler-Weber disease, 848
Replicons, 11
Reptilase, 781
Reticular dysgenesia, 101, 688
Reticular dysgenesia, 101, 688
Reticular system, 3
Reticulin, 229
  collagenous, 229
  increased, in pathologic tissue, 229
  true, 229
Reticulocyte count
  in diagnosis of hemolytic disease, 577
  vs erythrocyte number, 23
  in hemolytic crisis, aplastic type, 575
  in hereditary elliptocytosis, 594
  method, 865
  reagents, 865
  statistical error of, 487
Reticulocytes
  in aplastic anemia, 697
  basophilia of, 486
  in centrifugation of blood, 362
  classification of, by age, 486
  concentration of, among erythrocytes, 487
  effect of hypothalamic stimulation on, 17
  in erythron, 22
    of marrow, 22
    peripheral, 22, 23
  in hereditary spherocytosis, 593
  identification of, 487
  increase in, with iron administration, 402
  in iron-deficiency anemias, 407
  vs leptocytes, 427
  vs macrocytes, 476
  maturation rate of, 23

Reticulocytes—cont'd
  in measurement of MCV, 379
  in pernicious anemia, 429, 432
  protoporphyrin in, 449
  response of, to folic acid or vitamin B_{12}, 425,
      437-438
  vs reticulated siderocytes, 408
  siderotic granules in, 488
Reticulocytosis
  in abetalipoproteinemia, 595
  vs erythropoiesis, 487
  in glucose-6-phosphate dehydrogenase deficien-
      cy, 597
  in hemoglobinopathy, 625
  in hemolytic anemia, 487, 575, 777
  in hemolytic crisis, 576
  with hemorrhage, 487
  at high altitudes, 379, 704
  with increased erythropoiesis, 552
  in iron-deficiency anemia, 487
  in isoimmune hemolytic disease, 600
  in megaloblastic anemia, 487
  in paroxysmal nocturnal hemoglobinuria, 596
  in pernicious anemia, 487
  with pyruvate kinase deficiency, 567
  with Rh$_{null}$ type blood, 508
  in sickle cell anemia, 640
  in thalassemia major, 487
Reticuloendothelial cells
  cystine crystals in, 167
  erythrocytes sticking to, 570
  ferritin in, 409
  formation of bilirubin in, 574
  function of, 3, 35
  in Gaucher's disease, 42
  hemosiderin in, 400
  of lymph nodes, 105
  in removal of erythrocytes, 469
Reticuloendothelial system
  cellular composition of, 3
  in Chediak-Higashi syndrome, 45-52
  definition of, 2
  derivation of blood cells from, 2
  function and reactions of, 3
  in Gaucher's disease, 38-43
  in hemopoiesis, 1-34
    derivation of blood cells, 3-4
    in embryo, 6-11
    endocrines, 15-16
    erythropoiesis, 17-24
    extramedullary hemopoiesis, 28-32
    kinetics of hemopoietic proliferation, 11-15
    leukopoiesis, 24-27
    neurogenic control, 17
    nucleic acids, 15
    release of blood cells, 32-34
    stem cells, 4-6
    thrombocytopoiesis, 27-28
  in histiocytosis, 58-61
  ingestive and digestive functions, 36-38
    digestive capacity of liposomes, 37-38
    endoplasmic reticulum and lysosomes, 36-
        37
  and lipomucopolysaccharides, 53-58
  lymphocytes and immunocyte complex, 73-115
    duality of lymphocyte system, 79
    hyperimmunoglobulinemia, 102-103
    immunodeficiencies, primary, 100-102
    immunoglobulinopathies, 98-100
    in immunologic reactions, 87-98
    laboratory diagnosis of immunodeficiency,
        103-104
    lymphocyte function, 83-87
    lymphocytic migration streams, 81

Reticuloendothelial system—cont'd
lymphocytes and immunocyte complex—cont'd
role of bone marrow, 79-80
transformation of lymphocytes, 81-83
lysosomal storage diseases, 38-61
Gaucher's disease, 38-43
Niemann-Pick disease, 43-45
pathophysiology of, 3
phagocytosis and pinocytosis in, 36-38
proliferation of, in idiopathic histiocytosis, 58-61
in sea-blue histiocyte syndrome, 45
spleen as organ of, 61-72
atrophy of, 65
biopsy of, 71-72
indications and contraindications, 71
normal and abnormal splenograms, 72
puncture technic, 71-72
site of puncture, 71
congenital anomalies of, 65
in diseases of blood and blood-forming organs, 69
functions of, 63-65
hemopoietic and immunologic, 63-64
phagocytosis of foreign particles and microorganisms, 64
sequestration and destruction of blood cells, 64-65
storage of iron and other metabolites, 64
in hemolytic anemia, 66-69
structure of, 61-63
in systemic infections, 65-66
Reticuloendotheliosis, leukemic, 725
acid phosphatase in, 209
lymphocyte in, 206
leukopheresis for, 536
tartrate resistance with, 76
Reticulum cells, 2, 3, 119
cytoplasm of, 125
in iron utilization, 402
of lymphoid nodules, 105
nucleoli of, 125
nucleus of, 125
in pernicious anemia, 436
size of, 125
staining of, 486
Retina
in Chediak-Higashi syndrome, 47
effect of Niemann-Pick disease on, 43
Reverse transcriptase, 719-720
Rh antibodies, 510
Rh blood group systems, 509
in establishing parentage, 517-519
in hemolytic disease of newborn, 561-562
in hemolytic reactions, 545
incompatibility, 32
Rh typing, 905-906
method for Rh_0 variant, 905
modified or rapid tube test, 905
slide test, 905
tube test, 905
Rh_{null} disease, 508
stomatocytosis in, 478, 568, 580
Rh_0
negativity, 490
positivity, 490
Rh-Hr blood group system
binary code for, 523
vs C-D-E nomenclature, 505-508
genetics and serology of, 502-505
Rheology, 351
Rheumatoid arthritis
deficient neutrophil chemotaxis in, 663

Rheumatoid arthritis—cont'd
erythrocyte sedimentation rate, 356
haptoglobin levels with, 469
lupus erythematosus cell phenomenon in, 682
macroglobulinemia secondary to, 748, 751
splenomegaly with, 69
Ribosomes
in lymphocytes, 76
in protein synthesis, 15
in synthesis of hemoglobin, 620
Ribs
aspiration of marrow tissue from, 219
as marrow-containing bones, 222
in multiple myeloma, 731
Richter's syndrome, 726
Rieder cells, 119
in chronic lymphocytic leukemia, 298
in myelocytic leukemia, 298
Ristocetin, 794, 804, 807
assay of, 931-932
in platelet aggregation, 799
in von Willebrand's disease, 808, 809, 810, 811
RNA
in cytoplasm of orthochromic normoblast, 486
vs degree of basophilia, 118
of nucleolar chromatin, 175
in protein synthesis, 15
ribonuclease reaction for identification of, 873
in synthesis of erythropoietin, 21-22
types of, in blood cells, 15
Rocky Mountain spotted fever, 544
Roentgen, 692
Ropalocytosis, 600
Ropheocytosis, 402
Rotor's syndrome, 474
Rouleau formation; see Erythrocyte, rouleau formation of
Russell bodies, 207
plasma cells from myeloma with, 192, 202
Russell's viper venom, 833

S

S phase of cell cycle, 11
Salicylate therapy, 356
Saliva, secretion of group-specific substances in, 499-500
Salmonella typhosa, 673
Sanfilippo's syndrome, 55
Sarcoid, Boeck's, 256
Sarcoidosis
hyperplasia of eosinophilic series associated with, 256, 257
bone marrow differential count, 256
history and physical exam, 256
laboratory data, 256
thrombocytopenia in, 803
Sarcoma, immunoblastic, 102
Scapulae, 222
Schilling test, 436-437
Schistocytes, 483
Schizocyte, 482, 483, 484
in abetalipoproteinemia, 595
in diffuse intravascular coagulation, 846
in hemolytic anemia, 578, 579, 580
in microangiopathic hemolytic anemia, 570
in paroxysmal nocturnal hemoglobinuria, 596
in sickle cell anemia, 640
Schumm's test, 571
Schwartzman reaction, 843, 844
Scleroderma, 683, 684
of small intestine in vitamin B_{12} deficiency, 439

Scurvy, 848
Sea-blue histiocytosis, 45, 46
Sedimentation rate, erythrocyte
clinical correlations of, 355-357
factors affecting, 352-355
aggregation of erythrocytes, 352
anticoagulant used, 354-355
caliber and length of tube, 354
changes in plasma composition, 352-353
delay in performing test, 355
number of erythrocytes, 354
number of leukocytes, 354
position of tube, 354
size of erythrocytes, 354
temperature, 355
measurement of
Laudau-Adams method, 867
Westergren method, 867
Selenoid bodies, 483
Septic splenitis, 65
Septicemia, thrombocytopenia in, 803
Serine, 418
Serologic tests in disputed parentage
exclusion of paternity or maternity, 514-516
types of, 516
likelihood of paternity, 516-517
procedures and forms in introduction of evidence, 522-523
guidelines for experts, 522-523
identification of parties, 522
identification of specimens, 522
initial request, 522
report of expert, 523
use of individual systems, 517-521
A-B-O blood group system, 517
Duffy blood group system, 520
HLA system, 521
Kell blood group system, 520
Kidd blood group system, 520
M-N-S-s blood group system, 518-520
Rh blood group system, 517-519
Serology and immunology, 903-915
A-B-O blood grouping technics, 903-905
cell grouping, 904
slide method, 904
tube method, 904
serum or reverse grouping, 904
subgroups of A or AB blood, 904
absorption of nonspecific cold agglutinins, 908-909
antibody elution technics, 907-908
antibody identification, 907
cold agglutinins, 909, 911-912
demonstration of free homologous antibodies in cord serum, 911
demonstration of leukoagglutinins, 912
demonstration of lupus erythematosus cells, 912-913
clotted blood method, 913
rotary bead method, 913
direct antiglobulin test, 906-907
fluorescent antinuclear antibody test, 913-915
qualitative method, 913-915
quantitative method, 915
general laboratory technics, 903
cell washing, 903
preparation of red cell suspensions, 903
reading and grading test tube agglutinations, 903
heterophil antibody: Monospot test, 910
investigation of positive direct antiglobulin test, 909
prenatal serologic studies, 909
Rh typing, 905-906

Serology and immunology—cont'd
Rh typing—cont'd
modified or rapid tube test, 905
slide test, 905
tube test, 905-906
screening for irregular antibodies, 906
serologic studies on newborn infants, 910
titration of anti-**A** and anti-**B** isoagglutinins
neutralization of, 910
screening for, 910
titration of irregular antibodies in maternal
serum, 909
albumin-antiglobulin, 909-910
saline, 909
Serotonin
receptors for, on platelet membrane, 788
release of, from platelets, 798
vasoconstriction caused by, 778
Serum
in neutralizing chemotaxis, 660
vs plasma, 350-351
total iron-binding capacity of, 398
Serum sickness, 547-548
heterophil antibody in, 679
lupus erythematosus in, 683
Sex, effect of, on erythrocyte count, 378
Sex chromatin, 173, 175-177
of blood cell, 179
Sex chromatin body, 175-177
in blood cells, 179
Sexual dimorphism in leukocytes, 173-179
drumstick, 177-179
genetic, 177
nuclear, 175-177
Sézary cell, 162, 163, 164
cytochemistry of, 165
periodic acid–Schiff reaction, 210
ultrastructure of, 164
Sézary's syndrome, 86, 162-165
T-lymphocytes of, 662
Shock
administration of albumin for, 538
in anaphylactoid reaction, 548
blood transfusion for, 531-532, 537
increased fibrinolysis in, 867
platelet, 793
SI units, 386, 387
Sickle cell anemia
acute hemolytic crisis, normoblastic hyperplasia
of, 244-245
atrophy of spleen in, 67
clinical features of, 638-640
codocytes in, 481
crisis in, 636
drepanocyte of, 481, 580
effect of, on erythropoietin production, 21
erythrocyte sedimentation rate of, 357
folate deficiency in, 441
hemoglobin S in
genetic control of, 636, 637
sythesis of, 636
hematocrit in, 379
history of, 603
laboratory findings, 640
MCV in, 379
osmotic fragility of erythrocyte in, 583
pathogenesis of, 636-638
reticulocytosis in, 577
sickling of RBC in, 624
with β-thalassemia, 653
Sickle cell disease
erythrocytes in
sedimentation rate of, 352
shape of, and rouleau formation, 352

Sickle cell disease—cont'd
macrocytic anemia of pregnancy with, 274,
275
case study of
bone marrow differential count, 274
history and physical exam, 274
laboratory data on, 274
spleen in, 67, 68
Sickle cell–Hb C disease, 643-644
codocytes in, 481
crisis in, 636
Sickle cell–Hb D disease, 644
Sickle cell–β-thalassemia
codocytes in, 481
crisis in, 636
Sickle cell trait, 640-641
contraindications or oral contraceptives with,
636
diagnosis of, 641
elliptocytosis in, 483
genetic control of hemoglobins in, 637
hemoglobins in, 640
relationship of, to malaria, 641
vs sickle cell anemia, 624
centrifugal test to differentiate, 888
Sickle cells, 480, 481, 887
Sickledex test, 641
Sickling of erythrocytes, 624
mechanism of, 624
methods demonstrating, 624
Sideroachrestic anemias, 405
from chronic disorders, 413
ferritin concentration in, 409
from hereditary iron-loading anemia, 415
sideroblastic anemias, 413-414
Sideroblastic anemia, 206, 209, 210
anisocytosis in, 476
from aplastic anemia, 698
classification of, 413
dimorphism of RBC in, 413
drug-induced, 408
as dysmyelopoietic syndrome, 729
folate deficiency with, 441
free erythrocyte protoporphyrin in, 449
Hb F in, 633
idiopathic, 408
iron-containing cells in, 408
megaloblastic anemia with, 444
monocytosis with, 413
primary vs secondary, 413-414
red cell morphology with, 407
transferrin saturation in, 410
Sideroblasts, 210, 402, 408
ringed, 408, 413, 414
in sideroblastic anemias, 206
Siderocytes, 408, 488
demonstration of, 874
in diagnosis of hemolytic disease, 580-582
reticulated, 408
Sideropenic dysphagia, 406
Sideropenic iron-deficiency anemia, 405
due to blood loss, 412-413
ferritin concentration in, 409
vs free erythrocyte protoporphyrin, 411
iron-binding capacity in, 409
iron concentration in, 409
morphology of erythroid cells in, 408
nutritional, 412
due to physiologically increased iron requirements, 412
due to poor iron absorption, 412
transferrin saturation in, 410
Siderosis, 401
with hereditary spherocytosis, 594

Siderosis—cont'd
iron overload in, 409
in paroxysmal nocturnal hemoglobinuria, 596
pulmonary, idiopathic, 410
of spleen, 64
Siderotic granules, 402, 408, 488-489
incidence of, with hemolytic anemia, 582
Silica particles, 37
Sintron; see Acenocoumarol
Sinus histiocytosis, 102
Sinus of lymph node, 105
Sinusoids of spleen, 61, 63
Sjögren's syndrome, 684
Skin, allografts of, 88
Skin tests for delayed hypersensitivity reaction,
103
Skull
as marrow-containing bone, 222
in multiple myeloma, 731
Small intestine, 439
Snake venom, 781
Sodium, transport of, in erythrocyte, 555, 556
imbalance in
with elliptocytosis, 568
with spherocytosis, 567
with stomatocytosis, 568
Sodium bisulfite, 887
Sodium chlorate, 563
Sodium citrate, 355
administration of, effects of, 548
in obtaining blood specimens, 862
in treatment of sickle cell crisis, 638
Sodium dithionite, 624
Sodium lactate, 638
Sodium metabisulfite, 887
sickling of erythrocytes with, 624
Sodium oxalate, 354
Spectrin, 555, 556
Spectroscope, 876
Spectroscopy in identification of hemoglobin compounds, 461-464, 876
Spermatozoa, 175
Spherocyte, 483, 567, 577
acquired, 577
congenital, 577
in hereditary spherocytosis, 593, 594
true, 578
production and destruction of, 66
Spherocytosis
congenital
autohemolysis in, 587
increased osmotic fragility of erythrocytes in,
583
spherocytes in, 483
in diagnosis of hemolytic disease, 577-578
familial, 567
hereditary, 66, 68
ascorbate test of, 587
autohemolysis in, 587
clinical aspects of, 593
folate deficiency of, 441
glutathione stability test for, 587
hemoglobin concentration in, 380
hemolysis from, 567-568
laboratory findings, 593-594
MCHC and MCV, 577
microspherocyte in, 483
knizocyte in, 486
response of 2,3-DPG to, 392
reticulocytosis in, 577
sodium influx with, 583
treatment of, 594
true spherocytes in, 578
isoimmune hemolytic disease in, 600

Spherocytosis—cont'd
with Rh$_{null}$ type blood, 508
Sphingolipids, 39
Sphingomyelin, 39
of erythrocyte membrane, 555
in Niemann-Pick disease, 43, 44
Sphingomyelinase, 43, 44
Sphingosine, 39
Spinous process puncture, 216-218
Spleen
accessory, 65, 68
agenesis of, 65
atrophy of, 36, 61-62, 65
in autoimmune disease, 69-71
biopsy of, 71-72
indications and contraindications, 71
normal and abnormal splenograms, 72
puncture technic, 71-72
site of puncture, 71
in changing siderocyte to erythrocyte, 582
circulation of lymphocytes from thymus to, 81
congenital anomalies of, 65
in diseases of blood and blood-forming organs, 69
effect of thorium radiation on, 694
endothelial sinusoidal cells of, 2, 3
enlargement of; see Splenomegaly
erythroid colonies of, 6
extramedullary hemopoiesis in, 30, 32, 33
in fetal erythropoiesis, 9
in fetal hemopoiesis, 29
functions of, 63-65
in hemopoiesis and immunology, 63-64
in phagocytosis of foreign particles and microorganisms, 64
in sequestration and destruction of blood cells, 64-65
in storage of iron and other normal metabolites, 64
fusion of, with gonads, 65
in hemolytic anemia, 66-69
in hereditary elliptocytosis, 568
in hereditary spherocytosis, 567, 594
hyperplasia of, acute reactive, 65, 66
iron storage in, 400
irradiation of, 692
lymphoid tissue of, 105
in lymphomyeloid complex, 74
in lymphopoiesis at birth, 10
in lysosomal storage diseases, 38
in phagocytosis of hemoglobin, 469
in production of lymphocytes, 25
red pulp of, 61, 63
reticulum and lymphoid cells of, 3
in sequestration hemolysis, 570
in sequestration of platelets, 788, 802-803
in sickle cell anemia, 636
in sickle cell disease, 68
in sickle cell trait, 640
siderosis of, 64, 401
in staging of Hodgkin's disease, 770
structure of, 61-63
in systemic infections, 65-66
T-lymphocyte localization in, 84
in β-thalassemia, 65-69, 650
in thrombocytopenia, 28
vascular system of, 61, 62
white pulp of, 61, 81
Splenic artery, 61
Splenic aspiration, 71, 72
Splenic puncture, 70, 71-72
Splenic tumor, 65
Splenitis, septic, 65
Splenomegaly, 36

Splenomegaly—cont'd
acute inflammatory, 65
in acute myelocytic leukemia, 724
with acute systemic infections, 65
with autoimmune diseases, 69
body to venous hematocrit in, 394
causes of, classification of, 61, 62
in Chediak-Higashi syndrome, 47
in congenital erythropoietic porphyria, 451
effect of, on antibody production, 63, 64
effect of, on platelet count, 65
with Gaucher's disease, 39, 41
in Hand-Schüller-Christian disease, 58
with hematologic disorders, 69
hemoglobin breakdown in, 64
in hemoglobin C disease, 641
in hemoglobinopathy, 624
in hemolytic anemia, 68, 575
in hereditary elliptocytosis, 594
in hereditary spherocytosis, 593
in Hunter-Hurler syndrome, 53
in immunoblastic lymphadenopathy, 102
increased plasma volume with, 394
in infectious mononucleosis, 677
in isoimmune hemolytic disease, 600
in Letterer-Siwe disease, 58
in leukemic reticuloendotheliosis, 725
lipoid cell, 43
in myeloproliferative syndrome, 700
familial, 708
myelofibrosis, 706
polycythemia vera, 701, 702, 705
with neutropenic syndromes, 687
in Niemann-Pick disease, 43, 44
in sea-blue histiocyte syndrome, 45
in sickle cell anemia, 639
spherocytosis with, 578
in thrombocytopenia, 802-803
Splenosis, 65
Sprue, 102
effect of, on iron absorption, 397
hypocupremia in, 404
tropical, 441
malabsorption of vitamin B$_{12}$ with, 443
Spur cells, 483, 595
Stabkernige cells, 131
Stains
acid phosphatase with tartrate resistance, 871, 872
alkaline phosphatase, 871
for deoxyribonuclease digestion, 873
Feulgen reaction, 873-874
Giemsa, 869
May-Grünwald-Giemsa, 869
naphthol ASD acetate, 872-873
nitro blue tetrazolium test, 874-875
periodic acid–Schiff reaction, 872
peroxidase, 870
for ribonuclease reaction, 873
Sudan black B for lipids, 870
Wright-Giemsa, 868-869
Staphylococcal endotoxin, 82
Staphylococcus aureus
in fibrin deposition, 787
neutrophilia from, 673
Staphylococcus clumping test, 846, 854
Staphylokinase, 841
Status thymicolymphaticus, 74
Steatorrheas, 102, 441-443
celiac disease, 443
diabetic, 443
in folate malabsorption, 441-443
gluten-sensitive enteropathies, 443
idiopathic, 443

Steatorrheas—cont'd
pathogenesis of, 443
tropical sprue, 443
with vitamin K deficiency, 836
Stem cell
of blood cells, 3-6
differentiation of, stimulation of, 4, 6
evidence of, 4
location of, 4
multipotentiality of, 4
committed vs uncommitted, 24
defect of, in aplastic anemia, 690, 691
effect of androgens on, 15
effect of chloramphenicol toxicity on, 697
of lymph nodes, 25
role of, in rate-regulation of hemopoiesis, 14
Stem cell leukemia, 723-724
Stercobilin, 469
Stercobilinogen, 469
oxidation of, 469
Sternum
aspiration of marrow tissue from, 213-214
contraindications
in apprehensive adult, 213
congenital anomalies, 213
in infants, 212
technics, 213-214
as marrow-containing bones, 222
in multiple myeloma, 731
Steroids, 3
Stibophen, 562, 599
Stokes equation, 352
Stomatocytes, 478, 479
in alcoholism, 568
in diagnosis of hemolytic disease, 580
in Rh$_{null}$ disease, 568
Stomatocytosis, hereditary, 478
hemolysis from, 568-569
with Rh$_{null}$ type blood, 508
Stomatospherocytes, 483
Storage pool disease, 804-807
Streptococcal antigens, 103
Streptococci, 78
Streptococcus hemolyticus, 673
Streptodornase, 841
Streptokinase, 787, 841
Streptolysin S, 82
Streptomyces aureofaciens, 422
Streptomyces griseus, 422
Streptomycin, 697
Stuart factor, 785
Stypven time
in factor X deficiency, 831
measurement of, 923-924
Succinate, 397
Succinic dehydrogenase, 406
Succinyl CoA
in biosynthesis of porphyrins and heme, 448
conversion of methylmalonyl CoA to, 423, 424
Sudan black B stain for lipids, 870-871
Sudanophilic inclusions, 167
in Jordan's anomaly, 167
in lymphocytes, 76
Sugar-water test, 564
in paroxysmal nocturnal hemoglobinuria, 596
Sulfhemoglobin, 461
concentration of, for cyanosis, 456
identification of, 877
preparation of, for spectroscopy, 876
spectroscopic, 463
Sulfhemoglobinemia, 461
with secondary polycythemia, 705
Sulfonamides, 697

Sulfonamides—cont'd
chronic red cell hypoplasia from, 699
in drug-related hemolysis, 562
Supravital methods of studying blood cells, 179-180
advantages of, 180
general characteristics of, 179-180
plus phase contrast, 180
technical considerations, 180
Sweat glands, 30
Sweet clover disease of cattle, 774, 775
Swiss type of agammaglobulinemia, 101
Syndrome of sea-blue histiocytosis, 45, 46
Syphilis, 600
transmission of, through blood transfusion, 544

T

T-lymphocyte
in antigen response, 85
in aplastic anemia, 691
in cancer, 89
defect of, with thymic dysplasia, 100
deficiency of, with lymphopenia, 103
in diagnosis of cellular immunity deficiency, 104
effector, 83
efferent, from thymus, 81
esterase activity of, 85
factors produced by
cytotoxic and growth-inhibiting, 85
eosinophilotropic, 86
lymph node permeability, 86
lymphocyte transforming, 86
migration inhibition, 85
transfer, 85-86
glucuronidase activity of, 85
helper, 83, 86
surface receptors of, 84
identification of, 85
in immunoblastic lymphadenopathy, 102
immunoglobulin receptors in, 84
localization of
in blood and lymph, 84
in lymph nodes, 84, 105
in spleen, 84
lymphocytotoxin elaboration by, 85
of lymphoid nodule, 79
membrane features of, 81
in production of colony-stimulating activity, 6
in production of lymphokines, 83
responsiveness of, to phytohemagglutinin, 82
rosette formation by, 85
with severe combined immunodeficiency, 101
vs Sézary cells, 165
of Sézary's syndrome, 662
smooth surface of, 84
in stimulation of B-lymphocyte antibody secretion, 83
suppressor, 83, 86
surface receptors of, 83-84
surface markers on, 84
thymus-dependent, 75
transformation of, 498
Tangier disease, 58
Tar baby syndrome, 806
Target cells, 580
Tart cell, 681
Tatsumi factor, 786
Technicon Autocounter, 384
Technicon Hemalog-D, 667, 669
Telangiectasia
congenital, hemorrhagic, 412
hereditary hemorrhagic, 848-852

Telangiectasia—cont'd
hereditary hemorrhagic—cont'd
elliptocytosis in, 483
Temperature
effect of, on affinity of hemoglobin for oxygen, 389
effect of, on erythrocyte metabolism, 532
effect of, on erythrocyte sedimentation rate, 355
Testosterone proprionate
for anemia of hypopituitarism, 16
effect of, on erythropoiesis, 16
Tetracycline, 441
Tetrahydrofolate, 418-419
deficiency of, 421, 422
Thalassemia, 575, 649-657
α-, 654-655
geographic distribution of, 649
heterozygous with another hemoglobin, 655
homozygous, 654-655
β-, 650-653
geographic distribution, 649
heterozygous, 652-653
with Hb C disease, 653
with Hb E disease, 653
with sickle cell anemia, 653
δ-, 655
δβ-, 653-654
classification of, 649
codocytes of, 481
effect of, on erythropoietin production, 21
elliptocytosis in, 483
folate deficiency with, 441
genetics of, 649-650
geographic distribution, 649
Heinz bodies in, 580, 632
hemoglobin Lepore syndromes, 656
hereditary persistence of fetal hemoglobin, 655-656
with another hemoglobinopathy, 656
history of, 603
leptocyte in, 483
microcytosis in, 476
normoblasts of, staining of, 207
osmotic fragility of RBC in, 409
reticulocyte count in, 487
reticulocyte maturation rate in, 23'
with sickle cell trait, 640
spleen in, 68-69
transferrin saturation in, 410
Thalassemia intermedia, 649, 650
Thalassemia major, 69, 649, 650
Thalassemia minima, 649
Thalassemia minor, 30, 640, 650
Theophylline, 15
Thomsen phenomenon, 498
Thoracic duct, 79
Thorium radiation, 694
Thrombasthenia, 531, 789, 804
abnormal platelet aggregation in, 805, 806
clot retraction in, 797
Thrombin
in activation of factor XIII, 786
catalytic action of, 779, 780
in classic theory of coagulation, 778
in clotting of fibrinogen, 781, 783
in conversion of fibrinogen to fibrin, 839-840
formation of, 779, 832-839
defects of, differential diagnosis of, 834
hemorrhagic disorders of, 834
acquired deficiencies, 835-839
congenital deficiencies, 834-835
reactions, 832-833

Thrombin—cont'd
formation of—cont'd
role of vitamin K in, 833-834
history of, 774
inhibition of, 783
in platelet aggregation, 799-800
preparation of, 783
properties of, 783
from prothrombin, 795
as prothrombin accelerator, 783
receptors for, on platelet membrane, 788-789
structure of, 783
Thrombin time, 936
Thrombocytes, 558
Thrombocythemia, 708, 819
treatment of, 536
Thrombocytopathy, 531
abnormal platelet factor 3 release in, 798
acquired
caused by drugs, 818
secondary to other diseases, 819
association with congenital diseases, 818
platelet aggregation in, 807
storage pool disease, 804
Thrombocytopenia, 103
in acute lymphocytic leukemia, 724
in acute monocytic leukemia, 724
following administration of chloramphenicol, 250
in autoimmune hemolytic anemia, 577
from benzol, 696
bleeding time in, 797
blood transfusions in treatment of, 531
cause of, 28, 558
by deficient production, 803-804
due to bone marrow suppression, 803
congenital, neonatal, familial syndromes, 803-804
deficient thrombocytopoiesis, 803
by excessive destruction or sequestration, 801-803
due to immunologic mechanism, 801-802
due to mechanical destruction, 803
due to sequestration not in spleen, 803
due to splenomegaly and sequestration in spleen, 802-803
in Chediak-Higashi syndrome, 47
classification of, 800
in diffuse intravascular coagulation, 846
with Gaucher's disease, 39, 41
giant platelets in, 580
hereditary, 804
in immunoblastic lymphadenopathy, 102
with immunodeficiency, 101
in iron-deficiency anemia, 407-408
in isoimmune hemolytic disease, 600
in Letterer-Siwe disease, 58
in lupus erythematosus, 577, 681
with May-Hegglin anomaly, 161-162
in myeloproliferative syndrome, 700
familial, 708
osteopetrosis, 708
in paroxysmal nocturnal hemoglobinuria, 577
in pernicious anemia, 432
platelet suspensions in treatment of, 537, 538
from quinidine and quinine sensitization, 562
from radiation, 692
recalcification time of plasma with, 823
in refractory anemia with excess blasts, 729
in sea-blue histiocyte syndrome, 45
in sickle cell anemia, 640
with splenomegaly, 65
in β-thalassemia, 650
thrombopathic, 808

Thrombocytopenia—cont'd
  thrombopathic—cont'd
    platelets in, 797
    from transfusion of platelet-deficient stored blood, 548
Thrombocytopenic purpura, 27, 28
  with acute hemolytic anemia, 577
  associated with mesenchymal stomach tumor
    case study of, 326-327
      bone marrow differential count, 326
      history and physical exam, 326
      laboratory data, 326
  in Gaucher's disease, 41
  idiopathic, 69, 71, 801-802
    clinical correlation, 801
    with non-Hodgkin's lymphoma, 759
    symptoms of, 801
  immunologic, 69, 71
    platelet transfusion for, 531
  with lymphosarcoma and amegakaryocytosis of bone marrow
    case study of, 324-325
      bone marrow differential count, 324
      history and physical exam, 324
      laboratory data, 324
  neonatal, 802
  posttransfusion, 548
  spleen in, 69-71
  symptomatic, 801, 802
  thrombotic, 71, 843, 852
    as microangiopathic hemolytic anemia, 510
Thrombocytopoiesis, 27-28
  deficient, 803
  site of, 11
Thrombocytosis, 708, 819
  giant platelets in, 580
  in glucose-6-phosphate dehydrogenase, 597
  with hyperactivity of marrow, 266
  in iron-deficiency anemia, 408
  in myeloproliferative syndromes, 700
    polycythemia vera, 702, 703, 704, 705, 708
  stimulation of, 27
  associated with thrombosis, 853
Thromboembolism
  disseminated fibrin, 843
  fibrinolytic, 843
  pathologic hemostasis, 778
Thrombogen, 783
β-Thromboglobulin, 794
  in thromboembolic disease, 854
Thrombokinase, 774
Thromboplastin
  in classic theory of coagulation, 778
  commercial preparation of, 783
    therapeutic levels for, 839
  in conversion of prothrombin to thrombin, 782
  intrinsic, 783
  partial, 782
  plasma, 782, 783
    effect of platelet factor 3 on, 795
    factor VIII in evolution of, 785
  tissue
    activation of, in DIC, 845
    effect of, on factor VII, 836
    effect of lupus anticoagulant on, 836
    release of, in sickle cell anemia, 630
Thromboplastin generation test, 783
  equipment for, 928
  in evaluation of thromboplastinogenesis, 823
  in measurement of platelet factor 3, 798
  method, 927-929
  principle of, 927

Thromboplastin generation test—cont'd
  reagents, 927-928
  results and interpretation of, 929
Thromboplastinogen, 785
Thromboplastinogenesis, 779, 819-832
  defects of, differential diagnosis of, 833
  with factor IX deficiency, 830
  with factor X deficiency, 830
  with factor XI deficiency, 831
  with factor XII deficiency, 831-832
  factors involved, 819-820
  with hemophilia, 823-830
  hemorrhagic disorders in, 820-821
  interaction of factors, 820
  laboratory study of abnormalities in, 821-823
    assays of coagulation factors, 823
    bleeding time, 821
    coagulation time, 821
    factor deficiencies, 823
    partial thromboplastin time, 821
    prothrombin consumption time, 823
    prothrombin time, 821
    recalcification time, 821-823
    thromboplastin generation test, 823
  naturally occurring inhibitors, 820
  therapy for abnormalities, 832
Thromboplastin time, partial; *see* Partial thromboplastin time
Thrombopoietic stimulating factor, 27, 28
Thrombopoietin, 27, 28
  congenital deficiency of, 804
  in stimulation of differentiation of stem cells, 4
Thrombosis, 777, 787
  bishydroxycoumarin in treatment of, 836
  as complication of postoperative state, 853
  in hemophiliacs, 828
  with lupus anticoagulant, 836
  prethrombotic state, 852-855
    coagulation factors in, 854
    platelets in, 853-854
    products of fibrinogen to fibrin conversion, 854-855
    products of fibrinolysis, 854-855
    reduced fibrinolysis, 855
    serum lipoproteins, 855
  situations predisposing to, 853
Thrombosis-fibrinolysis-thrombocytopenia syndrome, 843
Thromboxane A$_2$, 806
  effect of, on smooth muscle, 790
  in platelet aggregation, 790
Thromboxane synthetase, 806
  deficiency of, 818
Thymic alymphoplasia, 101, 688
Thymic hypoplasia, 688
Thymidylate, 418
Thymidylate synthetase, 419
Thymocytes, 80
Thymoma, 74
  immunodeficiency with, 100
  red cell aplasia with, 699
Thymosin, 81
Thymus
  absence of, 104
  in cellular immunity deficiency, 103-104
  cortex and medulla of, 80-81
  development of, 80
  dysplasia of, 83, 100-101
  effect of cortisol on, 26
  excision of, 74-75
  in fetal erythropoiesis, 9
  hypoplasia of, 100
    in Nezelof's syndrome, 101

Thymus—cont'd
  in lymphocyte system, 79, 80-81
  lymphocytopoiesis in, 10, 81
  lymphoid tissue of, 105
  phytohemagglutinin response to, 83
  reticulum and lymphoid cells of, 3
  in staging of Hodgkin's disease, 770
  in status thymicolymphaticus, 74
  tumor of, 74
Thyroid gland, 16
Thyroid hormones, 16
Thyrotoxicosis, 633
Tibia, 218-219
Time-lapse photography, 181
Tonsils, 74, 79
Tonsillectomies, 74
Tourniquet test, 797, 916-917
  theory of, 797
  in thrombocytopenia, 797
  in von Willebrand's disease, 797
Toxoplasmosis, 544
Transcobalamin I, 425, 426, 728
  deficiency of, 440
Transcobalamin II, 425
  congenital absence of, 439
  deficiency of, 440
  in multiple myeloma, 747
Transcobalamin III, 425, 426
  in polycythemia, 701
Transcobalamin 0, 426
Transcobalamin Cardeza, 440
Transfer factor, 85-86, 662
Transferrin
  absence of, congenital, 415
  in binding of iron, 395
  concentration of, serum, 409
  deficiency of, 405
    anemia in, 415
  identification of, 397-398, 399
  in iron transport, 397-398
  in measurement of iron-binding capacity, 409
  saturation of, 409, 410
    in sideroblastic anemias, 413
  types of, 398, 399
  utilization of, by normoblasts, 402
Transfusion, blood
  autologous, 539
  exchange, 540-541
  fetal-to-fetal, 413, 705
  fetal-maternal, 413, 705
  frequency of, 539-540
    for coagulation disorders, 539-540
    single-unit, 540
  hazards of, 541-549
    transmission of disease, 541
      malaria, 543-544
      posttransfusion mononucleosis, 544
      syphilis, 544
      viral hepatitis, 541-543
  hemolytic, from factor U, 501
  hemolytic disease from, 589
  history of, 524-529, 575
    National Blood Policy, 527-529
  indications and contraindications, 529-532
    agranulocytosis, 531
    anemia, 530-531
      acute hemolytic, 530
      aregenerative, 530
      of chronic disease, 531
      chronic hemolytic, 530
      due to hemorrhage, 530
      megaloblastic, 530-531
    general supportive therapy, 532
    hemorrhagic disorders, 531

Transfusion, blood—cont'd
  indications and contraindications—cont'd
    leukemia, 531
    shock, 531-532
    thrombocytopenia, 531
  intra-arterial, 540
  intravenous, 540
  material for, 532-539
    autologous blood, 539
    cadaver blood, 539
    fresh whole blood, 537
      packed red cell, 537
      plasma, 537
      plasma fractions, 538-539
      platelet suspension, 537-538
    plasma extenders and substitutes, 539
    plasmapheresis, 539
    stored blood, 532-537
      coagulation factors, 536-537
      erythrocytes, 532-535
      leukocytes, 535-536
      platelets, 536
  routes of administration, 540
  for β-thalassemia, 650
  thrombocytopenic purpura following, 802
  in treatment of aplastic anemia, 697
  in treatment of autoimmune hemolytic anemia, 599
  in treatment of hemophilia, 774
  in treatment of red cell aplasia, 698
Transfusion reactions, 544-549
  ammonia intoxication, 549
  circulatory overload, 549
  citric acid intoxication, 548
  from Duffy factor, 512
  due to HLA antigen of granulocyte, 531
  hemolytic, 579
    clinicopathologic correlation, 545-546
    etiology of, 544-545
    haptoglobin levels in, 468
    investigation of, 546
    isoantibodies in, 561
  hemorrhagic, 548
    diffuse intravascular coagulation, 548
    posttransfusion thrombocytopenia, 548
    "wash-out" effect on platelets, 548
  hypersensitivity, 546-548
    acute pulmonary edema, 548
    allergic reaction, 546
    anaphylactoid reactions, 548
    febrile reactions, 547
    immediate dermal reactions, 546-547
    serum sickness, 547-548
  from Kell factor, 512
  from Kidd blood group antibodies, 513
  from Lewis sensitization, 511
  from Lutheran blood group, 511
  Rh factor in, 502
Transplantation reactions, 88-89
Trephine biopsy, 212, 220-221
Treponema pallidum, 544
Triamterane, 419
Trichinosis, 256
Trichophyton, 103
Trichuris infection, 412
Triglycerides, 596
Trimethadione, 697
Trimethoprim, 419
Trinitrotoluene, 461
Triosephosphate isomerase deficiency, 587
  fluorescence test for, 588
Trypanosomiasis, 544
Trypsin
  in activation of factor XI, 785

Trypsin—cont'd
  in activation of fibrinolysis, 841
  in agglutination of erythrocytes, 592
  in conversion of factor X, 785
  in digestion of hemoglobin, 631
Tryptophan pyrrolone, 406
Tuberculin reaction, 85
Tuberculosis
  of bone marrow, 229, 232
  drugs for, 414
  miliary
    increased mast cells with, 226
    involving bone marrow, case study of, 348-349
  pulmonary, 685
  sedimentation rate as index of, 356
  of spleen, 803
Tumor cells, 226, 228
  in peripheral blood, 169-170
Tumors, 30
Turk cell, 165
Tyrosinosis, 804

U

Ulcer
  duodenal, 828
  gastric, 530
  in hereditary elliptocytosis, 594
  in hereditary spherocytosis, 593
  peptic, 530
  in sickle cell anemia, 640
Ulcerative colitis, 675
Uremia
  anemia of, 23
  increase in 2,3-DPG in, 392
Uric acid
  effect of, on lysosomal membranes, 37
  levels of, in pernicious anemia, 438
  in polycythemia vera, 702
Urobilin, 469, 574
  in pernicious anemia, 438
Urobilinogen, 574
  excretion of
    with hemolytic reaction, 546
    in pernicious anemia, 429, 438
  fecal, 572-573
    excretion of, 572
    in hereditary spherocytosis, 574
    limitations, 573
    normal values, 572-573
  as indication of hemoglobin breakdown, 572
  from mesobilirubinogen, 469
  oxidation of, 469
  urinary, 572, 573, 574
    collection of urine specimen, 573
    determination by dilution of random sample, 573
    from twenty-four hour sample, 574
    from a two-hour sample, 574
Urobilinogen equivalents, 574
Urohematin, 447
Urokinase, 841
Uropodasis, 83
Uroporphyrin, 447
  in acquired porphyria secondary to hepatoma, 455
  in erythrocyte coproporphyria, 454
  isolation and identification of, 877
  quantitative assay of, 877-879
Uroporphyrin I
  biosynthesis of, 449
  in congenital erythropoietic porphyria, 451
  in porphyria cutanea tarda, 454

Uroporphyrin III
  in acquired porphyria secondary to hepatoma, 455
  biosynthesis of, 449
  in porphyria cutanea tarda, 454
Uroporphyrinogen decarboxylase
  in acquired porphyria, 454-455
  in porphyria cutanea tarda, 454
Uroporphyrinogen I synthetase, 449
  in congenital erythropoietic porphyria, 451
  in intermittent acute porphyria, 454
Uroporphyrinogen III cosynthetase, 449
  in hepatic porphyria, 454
Urorubrohematin, 447
Urticaria
  in allergic reactions, 546
  in dermal reactions, immediate, 547
  eosinophilia with, 256
  and basophilic leukocytosis, 675
Urticaria pigmentosa, 675
Uterus, 413

V

Vacuole
  endocytic, 36
  phagocytic, 36
  pinocytic, 36
Valves, cardiac, 569
Vaquez' disease, 701
Variegate porphyria, 454
Venipuncture, 860-861
Venous blood, obtaining, 860-861
Venous coagulation time, 915
Vertebrae, 222
Vertebral spinous process, aspiration of marrow tissue from, 241
  in infants and young children, 214
  technic, 216-218
Vim-Silverman needle, 218, 220, 221
Vincristine, 819
Viral infection, erythrocyte sedimentation rate for, 356
Virocytes, 165-167
  in spleen, 66
  transformation of small lymphocyte to, 83
Viruses
  adsorbed by megakaryocytes, 802
  in leukemia, 719-720
Viscosity of blood, 351
Vitamin A, 596
Vitamin B_{12}
  absorption of, 425
  administration of, in pernicious anemia, 577
  assay of, 437
  chemical structure of, 422-423
    corrin ring of, 422, 423
    vs structure of hemoglobin, 423
  cobalt in, 404
  in chronic granulocytic leukemia, 728
  coenzyme form of, 423
  deficiency of
    abnormal blood cell size with, 119
    anemia due to, 426-429
      due to biologically inert intrinsic factor, 439
      classification, 426-427
      due to deficiency of transcobalamin II, 440
      due to disease of small intestine, 439-440
      due to drug-induced malabsorption, 440
      due to familial selective malabsorption, 440
      after gastrectomy, 439
      due to inadequate intake, 429

Vitamin B₁₂—cont'd
  deficiency of—cont'd
    anemia due to—cont'd
      due to increased requirement for vitamin, 440
      macrocytosis with, 427, 476
      megaloblastic dyspoiesis, 418, 427-429
      pernicious anemia, 429-430
      in Zollinger-Ellison syndrome, 440
    impaired DNA synthesis from, 418, 419
    with leukemia, 724
    methylmalonic acid excretion with, 423, 424, 437
    serum and red cell folate levels in, 421
  dietary, 425
  in DiGuglielmo's syndrome, 713
  history of, 416-417
  interrelation of, and folate, 426
  intrinsic factor, 425
  malabsorption of
    congenital, 439
    familial selective, 440
    in steatorrheas, 443
  metabolic role, 423
    cobamide coenzymes, 423
    DNA synthesis, 425
    methylmalonyl CoA isomerase, 423
    synthesis of methionine methyl, 423-425
  in pernicious anemia, 436-437
  requirements of, 440
  reticulocyte response to, 437
  in Schilling test, 436
  source, 422
  storage, 426
  transport, 425
Vitamin C, 848
  effect of, on dietary vitamin B₁₂, 425
Vitamin E, 596
Vitamin K, 775
  action of, 835

Vitamin K—cont'd
  in conversion of prothrombin to thrombin, 782
  deficiency of
    acquired, 835-836
      effect of, on synthesis of coagulation factors, 834
  effect of, on oral coagulation therapy, 839
  factors dependent on, 833, 835
  hemolytic properties of, 541, 563
  role of, in thrombinogenesis, 833-834
  sources of, 835
  in treatment of factor VII deficiency, 536
  in treatment of hypoprothrombinemia, 536
von Willebrand's disease and variants, 776, 808-818
  bleeding time in, 797
  features of, 810
  PTT in, 821
  treatment of, 538, 818
von Willebrand factor, 808, 809
  for platelet aggregation, 793
  receptors for, on platelet membrane, 788-789

W

Waldenström's macroglobulinemia, 747, 749
  IgM in, 91
  periodic acid–Schiff reaction in, 210
  vitamin B₁₂ depletion in, 440
Waldeyer's ring, 770
Warfarin sodium, 837
Wilson's disease, 404
Wiskott-Aldrich syndrome, 101
  ADP in platelets in, 806
  lymphokine production in, 662
  phytohemagglutinin response with, 83
  platelets in, 797, 803, 818
Whipple's disease, 229
White blood cells; see Leukocytes

White blood cell count
  derivation of, from basal conditions, 667
  effect of age on, 667
  influences on, 667
  normal, 372, 665-667
Wolman's disease, 58
Wound healing, 787
Wright-Giemsa stain, 868-869
  method, 868
  reagents, 868
  remarks on, 868-869

X

X-linked agammaglobulinemia, 100
  lymphoid tissue in, 104
X-radiation
  chronic exposure to, 693-694
  leukopenia from, 692
  in roentgenology, 692
  for therapeutic purposes, 719
Xanthine oxidase, 406
  in regulation of iron release from ferritin, 397
Xanthopterin, 417
Xenografts, 88
Xg blood group system, sex-linked, 513-514

Z

Zeta potential of erythrocytes, 352
Zeta sedimentation ratio, 353
Zieve's syndrome, hemolysis from, 569
Zinc, 405
  in activation of alkaline phosphatase, 207, 208
  deficiency of, 405
Zinc ethylene bisdithiocarbamate, sulfhemoglobinemia from, 461
Zollinger-Ellison syndrome, 440
  with interference of vitamin B₁₂ absorption, 440